NURSING MANAGEMENT PLANS—*cont'd*

CRITICAL CARE NURSING

DIAGNOSIS AND MANAGEMENT

CRITICAL CARE NURSING

DIAGNOSIS AND MANAGEMENT

LYNNE A. THELAN, MN, RN

Critical Care Consultant and Lecturer
San Diego, California

JOSEPH K. DAVIE, MSN, RN

Dean, School of Nursing
The Long Island College Hospital
Brooklyn, New York

LINDA D. URDEN, DNSc, RN, CNA

Administrative Director, Nursing Services
Quality, Education, and Research
Butterworth Hospital
Grand Rapids, Michigan

MARY E. LOUGH, MS, RN, CCRN

Critical Care Cardiovascular Clinical Nurse Specialist
Sequoia Hospital
Redwood City, California

Assistant Clinical Professor
University of California, San Francisco

SECOND EDITION

with 476 illustrations

Mosby

St. Louis Baltimore Boston Chicago London Madrid Philadelphia Sydney Toronto

Mosby

Editors: Terry Van Schaik, Timothy M. Griswold
Project Manager: Patricia Tannian
Senior Production Editor: Betty Hazelwood
Senior Book Designer: Gail Morey Hudson
Manufacturing Supervisor: John Babrick

SECOND EDITION

Printed in the United States of America
Composition by Graphic World, Inc.
Printing/binding by Von Hoffmann Press, Inc.

Mosby-Year Book, Inc.
11830 Westline Industrial Drive
St. Louis, Missouri 63146

Library of Congress Cataloging in Publication Data

Critical care nursing : diagnosis and management / Lynne A. Thelan . . .
[et al.]. – [2nd ed.]
p. cm.
Rev. ed. of.: Textbook of critical care nursing / Lynne Ann Thelan, Joseph Kevin Davie, Linda Diann Urden. c1990.
Includes bibliographical references and index.
ISBN 0-8016-7167-1
1. Intensive care nursing. 2. Emergency nursing. I. Thelan, Lynne A. Textbook of critical care nursing.
[DNLM: 1. Critical Care—nurses' instruction. WY 154 C93296 1993]
RT120.I5T48 1993
610.73'61—dc20
DNLM/DLC
for Library of Congress 93-14177
CIP

93 94 95 96 97 / 9 8 7 6 5 4 3 2 1

Contributors

JENNIFER BLOOMQUIST, RN, MN

Cardiothoracic Surgery Clinical Nurse Specialist
Department of Veterans Affairs Medical Center
San Diego, California

Chapter 14; Case Study (physical assessment) in Chapter 18

WENDY BODWELL, RN, MSN, CCRN

Director of Clinical Education
Presbyterian Heathcare Services
Albuquerque, New Mexico

Chapters 37, 38, 39, 40; section on Nutrient Metabolism in Chapter 50

KAREN BRASFIELD, RN, MSN

Nephrology Nurse Consultant
Seattle, Washington

Chapters 31, 32, 33, 34, 35, 36

DOROTHY J. BRUNDAGE, RN, PhD, FAAN

Associate Professor
Duke University School of Nursing
Durham, North Carolina

Chapter 7

REBECCA WILLS BUTLER, RN, MN

Liver Transplant Coordinator
Emory University Hospital
Atlanta, Georgia

Section on Liver Transplantation in Chapter 49; Case Study (liver transplantation) in Chapter 49

JoANN M. CLARK, RN, MSN

Professor of Nursing
Grossmont College
El Cajon, California

Chapters 41, 42, 43, 44

JOSEPH K. DAVIE, RN, MSN

Dean, School of Nursing
The Long Island College Hospital
Brooklyn, New York

Chapter 1

JONI L. DIRKS, RN, MS, CCRN

Clinical Nurse Specialist, SICU
Department of Veterans Affairs Medical Center
Palo Alto, California

Chapter 17

MARILYN KUHEL DOUGLAS, RN, DNSc, CCRN

Clinical Nurse Specialist, MICU/CCU
Department of Veterans Affairs Medical Center
Palo Alto, California

Chapter 4

LORRAINE FITZSIMMONS, RN, DNS

Chair, Critical Care Nurse Specialist Concentration
San Diego State University School of Nursing
San Diego, California

Chapter 47

JEANNINE M. FORREST, RN, MS

University of Illinois at Chicago
Chicago, Illinois

Chapter 51

KATHERINE M. FORTINASH, RNCS, MSN

Professor and Certified Clinical Specialist
Adult Psychiatric-Mental Health Nursing
Grossmont College
El Cajon, California

Chapter 9; Nursing Management Plans in Chapter 45

SUSAN FRYE, RN, MSN, JD

Bartley Law Offices
Health Care Consultant
Attorney at Law
Iowa City, Iowa

Chapter 3; All Legal Reviews

SHEANA WHELAN FUNKHOUSER, RN, DNSc

Research and Education Consultant
Palo Alto, California

Chapter 13

BONNIE MOWINSKI JENNINGS, AN, RN, COL, DNSc, FAAN

Nurse Consultant to the Army Surgeon General
US Army Nurse Corps
Office of the Surgeon General
Falls Church, Virginia

Chapter 6

KAREN L. JOHNSON, RN, MSN, CCRN

Critical Care Clinical Nurse Specialist/Instructor
University of Kentucky Hospital
University of Kentucky College of Nursing
Lexington, Kentucky

Chapter 45

JACQUELINE L. KARTMAN, RN, MS, CCRN, CS

Clinical Nurse Specialist—Critical Care
Lutheran Hospital—LaCrosse
LaCrosse, Wisconsin

Chapters 10, 11, 12

MARY E. LOUGH, RN, MS, CCRN

Critical Care Cardiovascular Clinical Nurse Specialist
Sequoia Hospital
Redwood City, California

Chapters 15, 18

MARTHA J. LOVE, RN, MN, CCRN

Cardiovascular Clinical Nurse Specialist
Department of Veterans Affairs Medical Center
San Diego, California

Chapter 15

HELEN LUIKART, RN, MSN, CCRN

Nurse Educator/Transplant Coordinator
Department of Cardiothoracic Surgery
Stanford University
Stanford, California

Sections on Heart, Heart and Lung, and Single-Lung Transplantation in Chapter 49

MARY COURTNEY MOORE, RN, PhD, RD

Research Associate
Vanderbilt University
Nashville, Tennessee

Chapter 50

COLLEEN O'DONNELL, RN, MS, CCRN

Cardiovascular Clinical Nurse Specialist
Swedish Medical Center
Englewood, Colorado

Chapter 5

MADELINE M. O'DONNELL, RN, MS, CCRN

Cardiovascular Clinical Nurse Specialist
Massachusetts General Hospital
Boston, Massachusetts

Chapter 16

ANGELA S. PALOMA, RN, MN

Cardiothoracic Surgery Clinical Nurse Specialist
University Hospital
Denver, Colorado

Chapter 17

JEANNE RAIMOND, RN, MSN, CCRN

Nursing Instructor, Grossmont College
El Cajon, California

Sections on Hypothalamic Tumors, Unilateral Neglect, Impaired Communication, Acute Pain in Chapter 28; Chapter 30

MARIANN REBENSON-PIANO, RN, PhD

Assistant Professor, University of Illinois at Chicago
Chicago, Illinois

Chapter 51

KATE RELLING-GARSKOF, RN, MSN, CS

Head Nurse, Psychiatry
New York University Medical Center
New York, New York

Chapter 8

JULIE A. SHINN, RN, MA, CCRN, FAAN

Cardiovascular Clinical Nurse Specialist
Stanford University
Stanford, California

Section on Immunology of Transplant Rejection in Chapter 49; Case Study (heart transplantation) in Chapter 49

KATHLEEN M. STACY, RN, MS, CCRN

Critical Care Clinical Nurse Specialist
Tri-City Medical Center
Oceanside, California

Chapters 19, 20, 21, 22, 23, 24, 46

LINDA D. URDEN, RN, DNSc, CNA

Administrative Director, Nursing Services
Quality, Education, and Research, Butterworth Hospital
Grand Rapids, Michigan

Chapters 2, 34, 35; All Research Abstracts

LINDA M. VALENTINO, RN, BSN

Nurse Manager, The Burn Center at New York Hospital
Cornell Medical Center
New York, New York

Chapter 48

HELEN VOS, RN, MS

Quality Services Leader
Thornton Hospital, University of California–San Diego
Medical Center
San Diego, California

Chapters 25, 26, 27, 28, 29; Portions of sections on head injuries and spinal cord injuries in Chapter 45

SUSAN WINDHAM, RN, MN

Staff Nurse, Emory University Hospital
Atlanta, Georgia

Sections on Kidney and Pancreas Transplantation in Chapter 49; Case Study (kidney-pancreas transplantation) in Chapter 49

Acknowledgments for Previous Contributions

Carol Archibald, RN, MPH
Joy Boarini, RN, MSN, CETN
Ruth Bryant, RN, MS, CETN
Kathleen S. Crocker, RN, MSN, CNSN
Jane Frein, RN, MN
Judith R. Heggie, RN, MS, CCRN
Christine Kennedy-Caldwell, RNc, MSN, CNSN
Gere Harris Lane, RN, MSN, MEd, GNP
Gail B. Lewis, RN, MSN, CCRN
Cynthia E. Northrop, RN, MS, JD
Thomas W. Oertel, RN, MSN
Judith Hartman Ruekberg, RN, MSN
Penny Schoenmehl, RN, MN, CS
Sondra Thiederman, PhD
Laura Toledo, RN, MS
David Unkle, RN, MSN, CCRN, CEN
Evelyn Wassli, RN, DNSc

Reviewers

SHARON AUGUSTINE, RN, MS
The Johns Hopkins Hospital
Baltimore, Maryland

TALLY BELL, RN, MN
Wesley Medical Center
Wichita, Kansas

KATHY BIZEK, RN, CCRN, CS
Detroit Receiving Hospital
Detroit, Michigan

ELAINE BOND, RN, MSN, CCRN
Brigham Young University
Provo, Utah

SHAREN BROSCIUS, RN, MSN, CCRN
Old Dominion University
Norfolk, Virginia

TERESA HALLORAN, RN, MSN
St. John's Mercy Medical Center
St. Louis, Missouri

MARGO HALM, RN, MA, CCRN
University of Iowa Hospital
Iowa City, Iowa

PAMELA HARRISON, RN, BSN
Indiana Wesleyan University
Marion, Indiana

MARGARET M. HEITKEMPER, RN, PhD, FAAN
University of Washington
Seattle, Washington

LINDA HOLLINGER, RN, PhD
Rush University
Chicago, Illinois

PEGGY JENKINS, RN, MS, BS
Hartwick College
Oreonta, New York

ROSEMARY LUQUIRE, RN, MSN
St. Luke's Episcopal Hospital
Houston, Texas

GAIL TOMBLIN MURPHY, RN, MSN
Dalhousie University
Halifax, Nova Scotia, Canada

JOHN PARKER, RN, MN, CNS
Foothills Hospital School of Nursing
Calgary, Alberta, Canada

MARY QUINLAN, RN, MA
University of Kansas
Kansas City, Missouri

TERRY RUDD, RN, MSN, CCRN
Mt. San Antonio College
Walnut, California

VIRGINIA H. SECOR, RN, MSN
Vanderbilt University
Nashville, Tennessee

KATHLEEN SOLOTKIN, RN, BSN
Wishard Regional Trauma Center
Indianapolis, Indiana

DEBORAH WRIGHT SPRITZ, RN, MS
University of Maryland
Baltimore, Maryland

JANYCE STREETER, RN, MS, CNS
Brigham Young University
Provo, Utah

NANCY THORKILDSEN, RN, MS
Ellis Hospital School of Nursing
Schenectady, New York

GERALDINE VARASSI, RN, EdD
Columbia-Presbyterian Medical Center
New York, New York

SHEILA ZIELINSKI, RN, MN
Methodist Hospital
Indianapolis, Indiana

To
Christopher *and* Nicole
with love

L.A.T.

To
Nancy Mahoney *and* Mary Davie
womenfolk who bring refreshment, light,
and peace to my life and work

J.K.D.

To
***my* Mother**
for her patience and understanding

L.D.U.

To
***my* Father *and* Mother**
Michael *and* Agnes Lough
the two nurses who first inspired me

M.E.L.

Preface

We are most grateful to the many students and nurses who made the first edition of this book successful. The success validated our commitment in the first edition to proclaim the outstanding contibutions of critical care nurses and to promote research-based nursing in the complex critical care environment. We actively solicited feedback from users of the first edition and eagerly incorporated their comments and suggestions regarding format, content, and organization. And so, with this second edition, we again present to you a book that is thorough in all that is most pertinent to critical care nurses in a format that is organized for clarity and comprehension.

Nurses and students familiar with the first edition of *Textbook of Critical Care Nursing: Diagnosis and Management* will notice that the title of the book has been changed to *Critical Care Nursing: Diagnosis and Management.* We have modified the title because, although nursing students use the book as a textbook in critical care and advanced medical-surgical nursing courses, practicing nurses also use it as a reference. The new title more accurately reflects the comprehensive use of the book.

ORGANIZATION

The book's ten units are again organized around alterations in dimensions of human functioning that span biopsychosocial realms.

The content of Unit 1, ***Foundations of Critical Care Nursing,*** forms the basis of practice regardless of the physiologic alterations of the critically ill patient. Although chapters in the book may be studied in any sequence, we recommend that Chapter 1, ***The Nursing Process: Critical Thinking in Critical Care,*** be studied first because it clarifies the major assumptions on which the entirety of the book is based. Chapter 2, ***Ethical Issues,*** delineates ethical theories and strategies for dealing with the ethical dilemmas that arise on a daily basis in critical care. Chapter 3, ***Legal Issues,*** provides a basis of information to help the critical care nurse be cognizant of practice issues that may have legal implications. Chapter 4, ***Cultural Issues,*** provides information and strategies to deal with multicultural influences on patients in critical care. Teaching and learning theory, strategies to best meet the learning needs of critical care patients, and sample teaching plans are delineated in Chapter 5, ***Patient Education.*** Chapter 6, ***Stressors of Critical Care Nursing,*** addresses the impact the critical care environment has on the nurse and presents excellent strategies for management of this stress.

The interrelationship of human biopsychosocial dimensions is explored and applied to practice in this book to a genuine degree. Unit II, ***Psychosocial Alterations,*** consists of three chapters that examine the theoretic basis and nursing process for alterations in self-concept, coping, and sexuality as consequences of critical illness and care. Unit III, ***Sleep Alterations,*** examines a perennial problem in critical care and is divided into three chapters: ***Sleep Physiology and Assessment, Sleep Disorders,*** and ***Sleep Nursing Diagnosis and Management.***

Unit IV, ***Cardiovascular Alterations;*** Unit V, ***Pulmonary Alterations;*** Unit VI, ***Neurologic Alterations;*** and Unit VII, ***Renal Alterations,*** are each structured with the following chapters:

- Anatomy and Physiology
- Clinical Assessment
- Diagnostic Procedures
- Disorders
- Therapeutic Management
- Nursing Diagnosis and Management

This organization permits easy retrieval of information for students and clinicians and provides for flexibility for the instructor to individualize teaching methods by assigning chapters that best suit student needs. Unit VIII, ***Gastrointestinal Alterations,*** and Unit IX, ***Endocrine Alterations,*** are organized similarly. However, in these units the assessment parameters, such as clinical and diagnostic procedures, are discussed in one chapter. In addition, disorders and therapeutic management are combined into one chapter.

Unit X, ***Multisystem Alterations,*** covers disorders that affect multiple body systems and necessitate discussion as a separate category. Unit X consists of seven chapters:

Trauma
Shock
Systemic Inflammatory Response Syndrome and Multiple Organ Dysfunction Syndrome
Burns
Transplantation
Nutritional Alterations and Management
Gerontologic Alterations and Management

Finally, three appendixes are included, which contain useful information for all students and practitioners of critical care. Appendix A, **North American Nursing**

Diagnosis Association's (NANDA) Taxonomy I Revised, contains all diagnostic categories approved up through the Tenth Conference on the Classification of Nursing Diagnoses in 1992. Appendix B, **Advanced Cardiac Life Support (ACLS) Guidelines**, presents the American Heart Association's decision trees for use in treating life-threatening dysrhythmias, administering emergency drugs, and defibrillation during cardiopulmonary resuscitation. Appendix C, **Physiologic Formulas for Critical Care,** features commonly encountered hemodynamic, oxygenation, and other calculations and are presented in easily understood formulas. Recommendations for nutritional supplement are also included.

NURSING DIAGNOSIS AND MANAGEMENT

A dominant theme of the book continues to be nursing diagnosis and management, reflecting the strength of critical care nursing practice. The power of research-based critical care practice is incorporated into nursing interventions. To foster critical thinking and decision making, a boxed "menu" of nursing diagnoses complete with specific etiologic or related factors accompanies each medical disorder and major medical treatment discussion and directs the learner to the section in the book where appropriate nursing management is detailed. To facilitate student learning, the nursing management plans incorporate nursing diagnosis definition, etiologic or related factors, clinical manifestations, and intervention with rationale. The nursing management plans are liberally cross-referenced throughout the book for easy retrieval by the reader.

NURSING RESEARCH ABSTRACTS AND LEGAL REVIEWS

Research abstracts are integrated throughout the book to encourage incorporation of research findings into clinical practice. The abstracts are derived from published research in research, critical care, and specialty journals of 1991 and 1992 and are distinguished by having at least one nurse author.

Reviews of medical malpractice case law pertinent to critical care are highlighted throughout the book to focus on the importance of safe delivery of patient care and to illustrate actions for which the nurse may be liable.

NEW TO EDITION

New to this second edition are the following chapters:
Shock
Transplantation
Gerontologic Alterations and Management
Systemic Inflammatory Response Syndrome and Multiple Organ Dysfunction Syndrome

Also new to this edition is the inclusion of case studies, along with the nursing management plans in the last chapter of each body system alteration unit and in the following chapters: Shock, Transplantation, Burns, Trauma, and Multiple Organ Dysfunction Syndrome and Systemic Inflammatory Response Syndrome. The case studies enhance student learning and promote critical thinking by illustrating the clinical course of a patient experiencing the history, clinical manifestations, treatment, and outcomes discussed in the related unit or chapter. Case studies are organized in the following manner: clinical history, current problems, medical and nursing diagnoses, plan of care, medical and nursing management and patient outcome, and revised plan of care.

Finally, the teaching and learning package accompanying this book has been greatly expanded for this edition. The *Instructor's Resource Manual* provides a variety of aids to help enhance the course instruction. Provided for each chapter in the text is an overview, objectives, concepts, content outline, and detailed teaching strategies paralleling the chapter content. Student review sheets for each chapter focus on analysis and critical thinking. A separate section includes work sheets and exercises that enhance and complement the use of multimedia within the course. A comprehensive NCLEX coded test bank presenting approximately 650 multiple-choice questions has been added. Guidelines for integrating multimedia components with text and classroom instruction help to enhance the content presentation. Adapted course outlines provide content recommendations for varying course lengths and settings. In addition to the *Manual*, an IBM *Computerized Testbank* is available for exam generation. A *Multimedia Learning Guide* includes the critical thinking activities relating to the text and multimedia components. Fifty two-color *Transparency Acetates* complete the comprehensive teaching and learning package.

MULTIMEDIA CURRICULUM

With this edition of *Critical Care Nursing,* we are proud to introduce Mosby's Critical Care Nursing Teaching and Learning System. Instructors can augment the book through the use of *Mosby's Critical Care Nursing Video Series* and *Critical Care Nursing—Critical Thinking: An Interactive Video Series.*

The *Video Series* consists of eight tapes that are correlated in content in *Critical Care Nursing.* The tapes are as follows:

- Introduction to Critical Care Nursing
- Concepts of Mechanical Ventilation
- Nursing Management of the Patient on Mechanical Ventilation
- Clinical Assessment and Evaluation of Oxygenation Status
- Concepts of Hemodynamic Pressure Monitoring
- Nursing Management of the Patient Undergoing Hemodynamic Pressure Monitoring
- Intracranial Pressure Monitoring: Concepts and Nursing Management
- Ethical Issues in Critical Care Nursing

Critical Care Nursing—Critical Thinking: An Interactive Video Series, developed by Fuld Institute for Technology in Nursing Education (FITNE) in cooperation with Mosby, correlates to content in *Critical Care Nursing.* The program consists of four one-sided discs. Disc 1, "Orientation to Critical Care Nursing," contains an orientation to the program and a critical thinking segment that reviews use of the nursing process in critical care nursing. With the other three discs, "Cardiovascular Care," "Pulmonary Care," and "Neurologic Care," the student can study via a tutorial component that reviews and provides exercises on related critical care concepts, techniques, equipment, and nursing diagnoses. Students can also learn via a case study format that allows them to make a variety of critical thinking decisions about patients as they progress through their stay in the critical care unit.

Critical Care Nursing: Diagnosis and Management represents our continued commitment to bringing you the best and brightest in all things a textbook can offer: the best and brightest in contributing and consulting authors from around the United States; the latest in scientific research befitting the current state of health care and nursing; an organizational format that exercises diagnostic reasoning skills and is logical and consistent; and outstanding artwork and illustrations that enhance student learning. We are honored that the first edition received a Book of the Year Award from the *American Journal of Nursing* in 1990, and we pledge our continued commitment to excellence in critical care education.

Lynne A. Thelan
Joseph K. Davie
Linda D. Urden
Mary E. Lough

Acknowledgments

A project of this book's magnitude is never merely the work of its authors. The concerted talent, hard work, and inspiration of a multitude of people have produced *Critical Care Nursing: Diagnosis and Management,* second edition, and helped to make it the state-of-the-science text we affirm it to be. A "tradition of publishing excellence" has been evident throughout our partnership with Mosby–Year Book. We deeply appreciate the assistance of our acquisition editor, Terry Van Schaik, and developmental editors, Jeanne Rowland, Jane Petrash, and Louann Morrow, who have helped us document and refine our ideas and transform our book into a reality. Their creativity, expertise, availability, and generosity of time and resources have been invaluable to us throughout this endeavor. We are also grateful to Betty Hazelwood, senior production editor, for her scrupulous attention to detail. We remain indebted to artists George J. Wassilchenko and Donald O'Connor for their extraordinary talent. Their detailed work appears throughout the text, and its beauty is in itself an inspiration to learning. Finally we wish to thank those authors who contributed work to the first edition of this book. Without the foundation they provided, a second edition would not have been born.

Contents

APPENDIX

Detailed Contents

I

FOUNDATIONS OF CRITICAL CARE NURSING

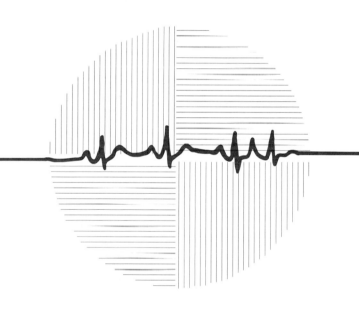

1

The Nursing Process
CRITICAL THINKING IN CRITICAL CARE

CHAPTER OBJECTIVES

- Discuss the role of critical thinking, intuition, and clinical expertise in the critical care decision-making process.
- Define taxonomy.
- Differentiate the methods of stating actual, high-risk, and wellness nursing diagnoses.
- Formulate nursing diagnosis statements from the North American Nursing Diagnosis Association's (NANDA) taxonomy of approved diagnoses, their etiologic/related factors, and defining characteristics.
- Designate nursing actions capable of resolving actual and high-risk nursing diagnoses in critically ill adults.
- Identify the two tasks associated with the evaluation phase of the nursing process.
- Propose a relationship among the phases of the nursing process and such professional practice issues as reimbursement for nursing services, allocation of nursing manpower, and professional autonomy.

Very early in your critical care education and practice you will no doubt be impressed, perhaps even intimidated, by the magnitude and complexity of clinical decisions made by critical care nurses. This reaction is reasonable because, in actuality, *critical* care is critical *nursing* care—of highly unstable, highly at-risk patients whose health conditions change not day by day, but minute by minute.

To the casual observer, critical care in the 1990s might appear to be characterized solely by the application of highly sophisticated technology, but as you shall soon see, in itself, technology is abysmally ignorant. Its application in health care is adjunct to nursing and medical critical thinking and decision making. The core of critical care nursing practice—clinical decision making—is the focus of this chapter and of most of this book.

THE NURSING PROCESS

The nursing process is a method for making clinical decisions. It is a way of thinking and acting in relation to the clinical phenomena of concern to nurses. Classically, the nursing process comprises five phases or dimensions: data collection, nursing diagnosis, planning, implementation, and evaluation. The nursing process is a systematic decision-making model that is cyclic, not linear (Fig. 1-1). By virtue of its evaluation phase, the nursing process incorporates a feedback loop that maintains quality control of its decision-making outputs.

The nursing process is indeed a method for solving clinical problems, but it is not merely a problem-solving method. Similar to a problem-solving method, the nursing process offers an organized, systematic approach to clinical problems. Unlike a problem-solving method, the nursing process is continuous, not episodic. The five phases constitute a continuous cycle throughout the nurse's moment-to-moment data interpretation and management of patient care. Kritek[1] describes the phases of the nursing process as being not only continuous, but "interactive"; in other words, all phases operate and influence each other and the patient simultaneously. Fig. 1-2 illustrates this interactive nature of the nursing process, wherein each phase is represented by a line that intersects with the others and converges at a point in time to which the nurse attends.[1]

Why a nursing process? Why a systematic method for approaching, analyzing, and managing clinical problems? Because it yields sound decisions. And it grooms the novice critical care practitioner for expert practice by necessitating organized thinking and maximizing the nurse's analytic skills.

The nursing process, then, serves as a template for clinical practice reasoning: data collection and analysis; the nursing conclusion about the data's collective meaning; the approach to planning and implementation of treatment; and evaluation. Two important elements strongly influence the nursing process: (1) intuition and (2) breadth of clinical practice experience.

Intuition, or intuitive reasoning, may be defined as a person's insight into a situation without his or her conscious analysis. An intuitive insight can be likened to a "strong hunch." Intuition has been described as an individual's capacity to solve problems with relatively few data.[2]

The status of intuitive problem solving in nursing has an interesting history. At one time, long before clinical decision making formally became an object of interest to the profession, it was acknowledged and accepted that nurses relied heavily on intuitive hunches or "gut

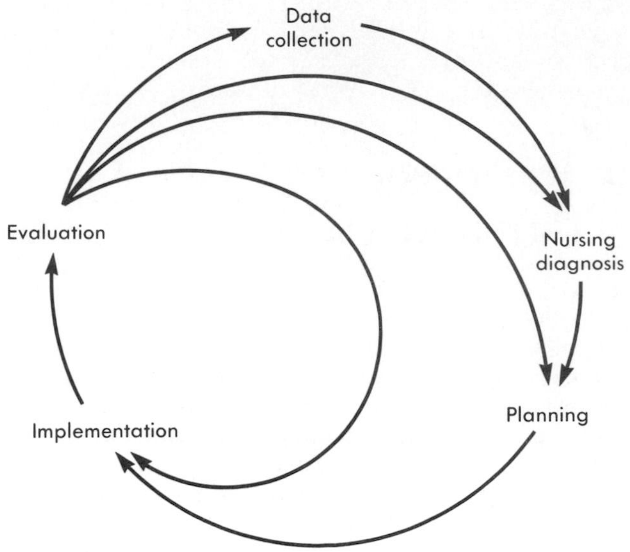

Fig. 1-1 The cyclic nature of the nursing process.

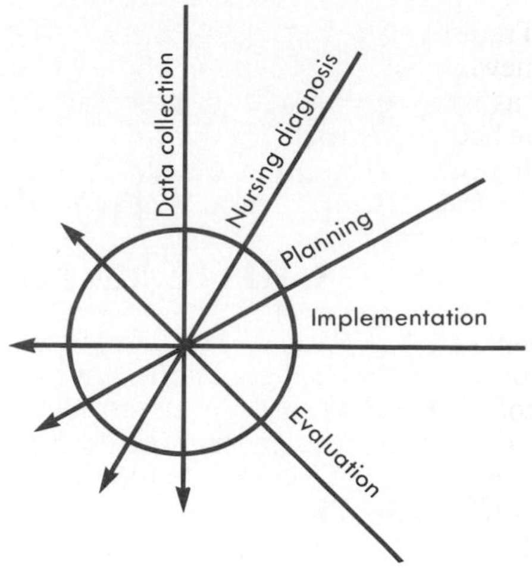

Fig. 1-2 The interactive nature of the nursing process.

feelings" to guide their clinical assessments and direct their nursing actions. Then, with the development of nursing as a science, came a scrutiny of nurses' clinical processes and methods of "knowing." Intuition as a method or ingredient of clinical problem solving was seen as "embarrassing" to the profession because of its historical association with gender and things unscientific.[3] Consequently, nursing endeavored to divest itself of intuitive processes and any lingering associations thereof. What emerged in its place, as if by reaction formation, were some very narrow, stark paradigms of clinical reasoning, which eradicated all elements of subjectivity and intuition from the process. The vast complexity of nurses' decision making was reduced to what amounted to a linear equation: $a + b + c = d$.

In recent years, the nature of intuition and the complexity of clinical reasoning have begun to surface in the scientific literature. The usefulness, indeed the advantage, of intuitive reasoning as an influence on the assessment and management of clinical health states is now given considerable attention in the literature.[4-8]

Patricia Benner's landmark work *From Novice to Expert: Excellence and Power in Clinical Nursing Practice*[4] analyzes the reasoning processes used by expert nurse clinicians. It was found that many of these nurses were not consciously aware of the mental processes that they employed in the assessment and management of patient care problems, but that the sense on which they operated yielded remarkably superior insights.

Smith analyzed the phenomenon of deterioration in critically ill adults. It was found that critical care nurses consistently sensed or felt a patient's impending crisis before any discernible physiologic changes had actually taken place.[8]

Intuition can influence the nursing process in any of its five phases. It has been reported, however, as being more commonly associated with data collection and implementation of nursing interventions.[7] The usefulness of intuition and the process of intuitive reasoning will likely occupy a priority position on nursing's research agenda well into the twenty-first century.

Expertise, which is developed through clinical experience, is a second important element influencing the nursing process and has much to do with the first, intuition. In fact, the empiric limitation of intuitive problem solving is that it cannot be taught and, other than through clinical experience, cannot be learned. Clinical practice experience, beyond all other variables, is what consistently characterizes the nurse expert.[4]

Expertise in the specialty practice of clinical care nursing might seem to the beginning specialist to be dishearteningly far off, and intuition, a domain of the expert, even farther. This is an understandable perception, but one that will gradually be replaced with a more realistic perception that, given time and experience, these qualities are attainable.

Data Collection: Assessment Frameworks

By virtue of nursing's unique orientation and commitment to holism, nurses collect an enormous amount of data about a patient's biopsychosocial health status. And by virtue of an array of technophysiologic monitoring devices, critical care nurses process an additional layer of data in the form of physiologic parameter measurements. Consequently, in the process of assembling this data base, the critical care nurse needs some place to file the information as it is collected. Ideally, this storage system would contain compartments, which could keep the data separated and organized. Such a system is called an *assessment* or *organizational framework.* Organizational frameworks can also serve as guides for assessment, and their compartments consist of headings corresponding to the attributes the nurse accepts as constituting the nature of humans, health, illness, and nursing. In this way, the framework helps guide the identification of diagnoses that are within the domain of nursing.

Assessment frameworks are neither new nor unique to nursing. Traditionally, nursing used medicine's assessment framework for the collection and organization of data, but as nursing's knowledge base and conceptual orientation became increasingly differentiated and complex, the biologic, mechanistic scheme of medicine was found to be insufficiently comprehensive for its use by nurses as a tool for holistic assessment. The assessment framework for generalist medical practice and two frameworks for nursing practice are shown in Table 1-1.

◆ **Functional health pattern typology.** Developed by Marjory Gordon, functional health patterns are categories of human biologic, psychologic, developmental, cultural, social, and spiritual assessments. Health patterns, or sequences of health behavior across time, are identified and interpreted by the nurse and determined to be either functional or dysfunctional. Functional health patterns are the patient's strengths; dysfunctional health patterns form the basis for the patient's nursing diagnoses.[9] The functional health pattern typology has gained wide acceptance in nursing service and education systems as an assessment/organizational framework.

◆ **Unitary person assessment tool.** In 1986 at the Seventh Conference of the North American Nursing Diagnosis Association (NANDA), a classification system for nursing diagnoses was endorsed. Named Taxonomy I, now "Revised," this classification system is based on unitary person framework (NANDA's conceptual framework) and replaces the alphabetized listing of diagnoses used previously.[10] A taxonomy is a system of classification that organizes known phenomena into a hierarchic structure and helps direct the discovery of new phenomena. An example of a taxonomic system from zoology is the familiar categorization: kingdom, phylum, class, order, family, genus, and species. Strictly speaking, the alphabetized list of approved nursing diagnoses (discussed later in this chapter) constitutes a nomenclature, or system of names. The specification of a nomenclature and its successor, a taxonomy, is an important preliminary step in building nursing theory and science.

Developed by Guzzetta and associates,[11] the Unitary Person Assessment Tool is an assessment framework for use in cardiovascular critical care, though adaptable to other critical care specialties. The major categories of the tool are those of Taxonomy I Revised, the nine human response patterns (Table 1-2).

Assessment frameworks are necessary to process the volume of information nurses accrue in the assessment of a patient. Frameworks facilitate diagnostic reasoning (discussed later in this chapter) by guiding data collection and organizing it into manageable parts. Organizing incoming information in this way increases its availability for retrieval and facilitates subsequent identification of relationships among the data.

The selection of any one framework over another, as long as it is designed to organize nursing data, is an individual choice.

Nursing Diagnosis

The concept of nursing diagnosis, a process whereby nurses interpret assessment data and apply standardized labels to health problems they identify and anticipate treating, is rapidly evolving in clinical and educational settings. Not coincidentally, this evolution is taking place parallel to the overall process of professionalization of nursing. Critical attention is being focused on aspects of nursing practice and education that either foster or inhibit the establishment of the discipline of nursing as a profession.

Table 1-1 Comparison of selected organizational frameworks

Medicine	Nursing	
BODY SYSTEMS	**NANDA TAXONOMY I REVISED[10]**	**FUNCTIONAL HEALTH PATTERNS[9]**
Cardiovascular	Exchanging	Health perception Health management
Respiratory	Communicating	Nutritional-Metabolic
Neurologic	Relating	Elimination
Endocrine	Valuing	Activity-Exercise
Metabolic	Choosing	Sleep-Rest
Hematopoietic	Moving	Cognitive-Perceptual
Integumentary	Perceiving	Self-perception—Self-concept
Gastrointestinal	Feeling	Role-Relationship
Genitourinary	Knowing	Sexuality-Reproductive
Reproductive		Coping-Stress tolerance
Psychiatric		Value-Belief

Table 1-2 Nine human response patterns of Taxonomy I Revised[10]

1. Exchanging	A human response pattern involving mutual giving and receiving
2. Communicating	A human response pattern involving sending messages
3. Relating	A human response pattern involving establishing bonds
4. Valuing	A human response pattern involving the assigning of relative worth
5. Choosing	A human response pattern involving the selection of alternatives
6. Moving	A human response pattern involving activity
7. Perceiving	A human response pattern involving the reception of information
8. Knowing	A human response pattern involving the meaning associated with information
9. Feeling	A human response pattern involving the subjective awareness of information

LEGAL REVIEW: Nursing diagnosis and advanced nursing practice legislation

It is well accepted that application of the nursing process to patient problems, with associated statements of nursing diagnosis, is a standard of professional nursing practice for all patients regardless of medical diagnosis.

The nursing diagnosis is now part of the definition of nursing in a typical state nurse practice act and is integral to the nursing regulatory framework as well. The nursing diagnosis has also been the subject of judicial commentary and analysis, as the following case illustrates.

In the case of *Sermchief v. Gonzales,* two nurse practitioners were sued by the Missouri State Board of Registration For the Healing Arts for the unauthorized practice of medicine. Both nurses had postgraduate training in obstetrics and gynecology. Their functions, among others, under standing orders and protocols included performing breast and pelvic examinations, obtaining Papanicolaou smears, dispensing certain medications and contraceptive devices, treating vaginitis and other conditions, inserting intrauterine devices, and providing counseling and education to patients.

The court held in favor of the nurses, stating their conduct constituted professional nursing as defined by the state's nurse practice act and did not constitute the unauthorized practice of medicine. The court noted that the language of the statute reflected legislative intent to expand the scope of authorized nursing practices and avoid statutory constraints on the evolution of new nursing functions. The court further concluded that the nurses' functions were the types of acts the legislature contemplated when it gave nurses the legal right to make assessments and nursing diagnoses. Of particular interest was the court's statement that the nurse undertakes only a nursing diagnosis, as opposed to a medical diagnosis, when he or she finds or fails to find clinical manifestations described by physicians in protocols and standing orders for the purpose of administering care and treatment prescribed by physicians in such protocols and orders.

Kim MF, McFarland GK, McFarlane AM: *Pocket guide to nursing diagnosis,* ed 4, St. Louis, 1991, Mosby–Year Book.
Lounsbury P, Frye SJ: *Cardiac rhythm disorders: a nursing process approach,* ed 2, St. Louis, 1992, Mosby–Year Book.
North American Nursing Diagnosis Association: *Classification of nursing diagnoses: proceedings of the eighth conference, North American Nursing Diagnosis Association,* Philadelphia, 1989, JB Lippincott.
North American Nursing Diagnosis Association: *Taxonomy I Revised 1990 with official nursing diagnoses,* St. Louis, 1990, The Association.
Sermchief v Gonzales, 660 S.W.2d 683 (Mo. 1983).
Tucker SM and others: *Patient care standards: nursing process, diagnosis, and outcome,* ed 5, St. Louis, 1992, Mosby–Year Book.

A traditional reliance on the language and therapeutics of other sciences is inhibiting the establishment of nursing as a free-standing profession. Efforts to identify and name the conditions that nurses study and treat, on the other hand, foster nursing's professional identity by clarifying its distinct services to society and providing a vehicle for the building of its science.

◆ Historical development of nursing diagnosis

Pre–North American Nursing Diagnosis Association (NANDA) era. The term *nursing diagnosis* first appeared in the literature in the 1950s. Gordon points out that along with the genesis of this term, a fundamental change in the process whereby nurses moved from data collection to care planning began to occur: a pause in which the data collected are analyzed and grouped, the signs and symptoms of a suspected health problem identified, a possible cause uncovered, and the diagnostic conclusion stated. Only *then* is care planning begun.[9]

Historically, nursing interventions tended to be disjointed and episodic. The nurse often considered each piece of assessment data as a separate, discrete entity, neither seeking nor perceiving relationships among groups of symptoms. Intervention strategies were planned and carried out in relation to what were considered to be series of independent findings. For example, if soft tissue swelling, frequent infections, and delayed healing were observed in a patient, it was likely these would be interpreted and managed separately, that is, interventions slated to reduce swelling, some to avoid or control infection, and others to promote healing. Consider the gains if the nurse instead takes into account the possibility of a relationship among these symptoms, uncovers a cause, and organizes a treatment plan corresponding to the diagnosis, Altered Nutrition: Less Than Body Protein Requirements.

With nursing diagnosis as a component of our decision-making methods, we necessarily become more systematic in the collection and interpretation of data and accomplish a change in the substance of our clinical operations, from symptom management to problem solving.

NANDA era. In 1973, motivated initially by a need to clarify the nurse's role and to distinguish it from that of other health professionals in their own practice setting, two faculty members at St. Louis University, Kristine Gebbie and Mary Ann Lavin, convened the First National Conference on the Classification of Nursing Diagnoses.[12] The group organized around the task of identifying, standardizing, and classifying health problems treated by nurses. This conference has heralded a now-international professional movement. The organization, now known as the *North American Nursing Diagnosis Association (NANDA),* consists of nurse theorists, nurse researchers, nurse educators, and advanced and grass roots clinicians.

The impetus for the work of NANDA and its scientific sessions derives from the necessity of establishing a vocabulary that specifically reflects the treatment domain of nursing practice. In addition to it being requisite to nursing's status as a profession, such a vocabulary coordinates communication among nurses in relation to the health problems they are observing and treating and is as much for purposes of social policy as it is, says Carpenito, for "clarifying nursing for nurses."[13]

Approved nursing diagnoses are listed on the inside front cover of this book. Though not included in the table, accompanying each diagnosis are possible causative factors (etiologic/related factors) and the signs and symptoms of the health state (defining characteristics). These are used by the nurse to help formulate the diagnostic statement and tailor it to the individual patient characteristics and circumstance.

An "approved" nursing diagnosis is one accepted by NANDA as having been refined to the point of clinical usefulness and approved for clinical validation through formal research methods. Practitioners using approved nursing diagnoses, their etiologies, and defining characteristics are in fact participating in the preliminary testing of the diagnoses as they relate to the health states described by the diagnostic labels. NANDA actively seeks input from practicing nurses regarding the development and refinement of nursing diagnoses. The Association publishes guidelines for submitting new diagnoses to its Diagnosis Review Committee, and direct input into the proceedings of the biennial conferences is possible through membership and participation in NANDA and any of its regional associations.

The immediate goals of NANDA include (1) further validation and refinement of existing diagnoses, their etiologies, risk factors, and defining characteristics, (2) the generation of new diagnoses, (3) the development of *Taxonomy II,* and (4) the incorporation of approved diagnoses into the tenth revision of the World Health Organization's *International Classification of Diseases,*[12] which will feature an axial diagnostic model incorporating unit of analysis (individual, family, community) age-group, wellness, illness, and possibly others.[14,15]

◆ **Definition of nursing diagnosis.** At its Ninth Conference in 1990, the NANDA assembly endorsed the following working definition of nursing diagnosis[16]:

> A nursing diagnosis is a clinical judgment about individual, family or community responses to actual or potential health problems/life processes. Nursing diagnoses provide the basis for selection of nursing interventions to achieve outcomes for which the nurse is accountable.

The term *inference* also is useful in defining nursing diagnosis because it emphasizes the tentative and assumptive nature of diagnoses. Webster's Collegiate Dictionary defines inference as the "process of arriving at a conclusion by reasoning from evidence" and warns that "if the evidence is slight the term comes close to *surmise.*"[17] In recognizing that elements of both judgment and inference are part of nursing diagnosis, one can appreciate the need to limit or control the influence of bias on the part of the diagnostician and in the act of diagnosing so that the diagnostic conclusion reached is as logical and factually based as possible. Inference in the context of diagnostic reasoning is discussed in greater detail later in this chapter.

The human response to health and illness situations constitutes the focus, or phenomenon, of concern to nurses, and it is the object of nurses' diagnostic activities. In 1980 the American Nurses Association (ANA) issued *Nursing: A Social Policy Statement,* which defined the nature and scope of the profession as follows: "Nursing is the diagnosis and treatment of human responses to actual or potential health problems."[18] Actual or potential health problems to which nurses direct their diagnosis and treatment, then, are human responses—human responses to the health challenges encountered in birth, illness, wellness, growth and development, and death.

The most essential and distinguishing feature of any nursing diagnosis is that it describe a health condition *primarily resolved by nursing interventions or therapies.* There is, however, some difficulty in applying this criterion to the broad spectrum of health states that nurses have historically, do currently, and will in the future identify and treat. The boundaries of nursing and particularly those that it shares with other health professions are dynamic and not at once easily delineated.[18]

To assist in clarifying the boundaries of nursing and provide a framework for the development and classification of nursing diagnoses, the ANA outlines the following categories of health problems, the treatment of which lies within the profession's domain[18]:

1. Self-care limitations
2. Impaired functioning in such areas as rest, sleep, ventilation, circulation, activity, nutrition, elimination, skin, and sexuality
3. Pain and discomfort
4. Emotional problems related to illness and treatment; life-threatening events; or daily life experiences, such as anxiety, loss, loneliness, and grief
5. Distortion of symbolic functions, reflected in interpersonal and intellectual processes, such as hallucinations
6. Deficiencies in decision making and ability to make personal choices
7. Self-image changes required by health status
8. Dysfunctional perceptual orientations to health
9. Strains related to processes that occur during life, such as birth, growth and development, and death
10. Problematic affiliative relationships

Although the above categories are not in themselves nursing diagnoses, standardization of diagnostic labels developed from within this framework helps to ensure a discipline-specific perspective for the intervention activities of professional nurses.

◆ **Nursing diagnosis in critical care.** Controversy exists regarding the application of nursing diagnosis in critical care.[19-24] The appropriateness of critical care nurses contending that they diagnose and treat such phenomena as decreased cardiac output, impaired pulmonary gas exchange, and altered tissue perfusion is disputed, although some of the strongest reservations appear to have come from nurses who are outside the critical care specialty.

In addition to the scientific and general assembly sessions of the biennial NANDA Conference, the American Association of Critical-Care Nurses (AACN) and Marquette University have cosponsored national conferences addressing nursing diagnosis in critical care and the professional issues from which it is inseparable. The basic elements of the controversy follow.

The physiologic diagnosis controversy. Since the inception of an organized nursing diagnosis movement, controversy surrounds the question of what is and is not the domain of nursing diagnosis. On one side of this issue, it is held that the term *nursing diagnosis* should refer only to health states that professional nurses manage independent of other health care professionals. Health problems for which nurses do not assume exclusive responsibility, it is argued, do not meet the criteria for a nursing diagnosis. Out of this argument has come a persistent focus on "the physiologic diagnoses" (e.g., Decreased Cardiac Output and Dysreflexia) as being the outliers from mainstream nursing diagnoses.

However, it is not the physiologic diagnoses alone that necessitate or profit from interdisciplinary collaboration. Body Image Disturbance, Rape-Trauma Syndrome, Impaired Verbal Communication, Dysfunctional Grieving, and others are diagnoses not uniformly managed independently by nurses—independent, that is, of the perspective of such allied disciplines as psychiatry, psychology, speech pathology, social work, and thanatology. So, the argument goes, what is the actual distinction between the domain of "physiologic" and "nonphysiologic" diagnoses?

Moreover, Roberts[23] points out that since the original formulations on the application of nursing diagnosis, "times have changed and critical care nursing has become a highly technical and advanced area of practice in which most nursing diagnoses are primarily physiologic." Critical care nurses work intimately with physiologic phenomena and, through a research-based practice, may independently and successfully manipulate such variables as left ventricular afterload, ventilation-perfusion ratios, and intracranial pressure. The deliberate, substantive, and research-based contribution of any health discipline to a therapeutic regimen constitutes the practice domain of that discipline.[20] That which nurses treat should be described with nursing diagnoses.

For clarity, the position taken in this book is one of inclusion rather than exclusion: all phenomena—physiologic, psychologic, and social—of concern to critical care nurses and the object of their treatment are represented by nursing diagnoses throughout this text. The factors contributing to their development (their etiologic factors) are modifiable by nursing intervention.

Kritek[1] asserts that the categorization of nursing diagnoses as *independent* or *collaborative* constitutes a political distinction, not a conceptual one. If this designation is desired, however, it can be easily superimposed by the practitioner.

◆ Formulating nursing diagnosis statements

Guidelines for use of the taxonomy of approved nursing diagnoses. It is important to recognize that classification of the phenomena to which a profession addresses itself is a sizable and ongoing task. The development and refinement of nursing's nomenclature of health states are in their earliest stages and subject to much revision based on the research and clinical reports presented and reviewed at each of NANDA's conferences and by the Diagnosis Review Committee. Work on existing diagnoses also is incomplete. Several have etiologies and defining characteristics yet to be developed, making clinical use difficult and frustrating. Other diagnoses may be deleted from the approved list from conference to conference. Such changes are both necessary and usual in the process of taxonomy development. One has only to look at the system of names describing health problems treated by physicians not many years ago (for example, chilblains, consumption, dropsy) to appreciate nursing's progress to date.

Guidelines for diagnostic labels

DEFINITIONS OF HEALTH PROBLEMS. Nearly all approved diagnoses have accompanying definitions to better explain the health state they represent. These definitions are important for the student of nursing diagnosis to consider, because they clarify more about the health state than is apparent from the label alone. For example, the definitions accompanying the diagnoses Fear and Anxiety draw a particularly useful distinction between the two problems: Fear is an emotion that has an identifiable source or object that the patient validates, whereas Anxiety is an emotion whose source is nonspecific or unknown to the patient.[25] Other good examples of such definitions accompany the diagnoses Social Isolation, Powerlessness, Altered Parenting, and Caregiver Role Strain.

Until definitions accompany all approved diagnoses, it is important for nurses collaborating in care to establish consensus about the meaning and scope of the health problems stated.

MAKING DIAGNOSTIC LABELS SPECIFIC. Some nursing diagnoses need accompanying qualifiers or specifiers based on the characteristics of the health problem as it manifests itself in a particular patient. For example, the diagnosis Fear needs specification as to the object of the patient's particular fear, such as death, pain, disfigurement, or malignancy. Similarly, the diagnosis Knowledge Deficit needs specification about the content of the deficit, such as use of incentive spirometer, counting the pulse rate, or respiratory muscle strengthening exercise. Following is a list of nursing diagnoses needing specification, each with an example of a particular patient circumstance so specified:

Fear: *Postoperative Pain*
Knowledge Deficit: *Self-Monitoring of Oral Anticoagulation Therapy*

Altered *Peripheral* Tissue Perfusion
Altered Nutrition: Less than Body *Potassium* Requirements
Altered Nutrition: More Than Body *Kilocalorie* Requirements
Self-Care Deficit: *Bathing and Feeding*
Noncompliance: *Prescribed Activity Restrictions*

Guidelines for ETIOLOGIC/RELATED FACTORS

MAKING ETIOLOGIES SPECIFIC. In many instances, NANDA's etiologies are broad categories or examples needing to be made specific based on characteristics of the health state and the patient being treated. For example, one of several possible etiologies for the diagnosis Fluid Volume Excess is *compromised regulatory mechanism.* Considering this the cause of the fluid excess in a particular patient, the nurse needs to specify which regulatory mechanism and in what way compromised (for example, inappropriate ADH secretion by the neurohypophysis) before the diagnosis can be formally stated (disregarding the question of whether this problem is treatable by nurses or needs referral).

Several etiologies needing to be made specific follow, along with examples of such specification in parentheses:

- Situational crisis (recent diagnosis of terminal illness)
- Psychologic injuring agent (hurtful relationship, verbal abuse)
- Developmental factors (developmental arrest, extremes of age)

NURSING DIAGNOSES AS ETIOLOGIES. Nursing diagnostic labels may rightfully serve as etiologies for other diagnoses. Examples are Anxiety R/T* knowledge deficit, and Activity Intolerance R/T decreased cardiac output.

ETIOLOGIES AS THE FOCUS OF TREATMENT. The treatment plan formulated for a given diagnosis must include interventions aimed at resolution or management of the etiologic factors, as well as the health state. In fact, in some instances nursing treatment is directed exclusively at the etiology of a diagnosis, with the logical expectation that, if the causative factors are reduced in influence, the problem should begin to resolve. This is true especially in instances where a nursing diagnosis has as its etiology another nursing diagnosis. Consider treatment approaches to the diagnosis Ineffective Breathing Pattern R/T high abdominal incision pain. Predictably, little effectiveness is shown if the interventions are focused solely on reviewing the rationale for slow, deep, symmetrical breathing; demonstrating the technique; and encouraging the patient in its performance without some plan for manipulation of the pain variable.

MEDICAL DIAGNOSES AS ETIOLOGIES. Because, as mentioned, the etiology of a nursing diagnosis becomes a focus of intervention in the management of the overall health state, citing a medical condition or diagnosis as the etiology is conceptually inadvisable if the diagnostic statement is to retain its identity as a health problem primarily resolved by nursing therapies. And yet many health states of concern to critical care nurses and amenable to their treatment *are* consequent to medical conditions. Examples are the Ineffective Airway Clearance that results from chronic obstructive pulmonary disease (COPD), and Sensory-Perceptual Alterations that result from coronary artery bypass graft surgery. In these instances, the nurse should isolate those aspects of the contributing pathologic state that are modifiable by nursing intervention and cite these factors as etiologic, for instance, Ineffective Airway Clearance R/T thick tracheobronchial secretions, respiratory muscle weakness, and knowledge deficit: effective cough and hydration techniques; and Sensory-Perceptual Alterations R/T sensory overload, sensory deprivation, and sleep pattern disturbance. These diagnostic statements are more clearly worded and provide a much sharper focus for nursing intervention.

Guidelines for DEFINING CHARACTERISTICS

MAKING DEFINING CHARACTERISTICS SPECIFIC. As with diagnostic labels and statements of etiology, defining characteristics cited for diagnoses are in nonspecific form and often need to be modified to reflect the particular situation presented by the patient being diagnosed. For example, the diagnosis Impaired Gas Exchange has as one of its possible defining characteristics *abnormal blood gases.* In the nurse's formulation of this diagnostic statement for clinical use, the specific blood gas value used to diagnose the problem should be cited in the statement (e.g., Po_2: 54 mm Hg and/or Pco_2: 50 mm Hg) versus the nonspecific sign category, abnormal blood gases.

Several defining characteristics are cited as follows in nonspecific form, with accompanying examples of proper specification:

- Respiratory depth changes (hypoventilation)
- Blood pressure changes (hypotension)
- Autonomic responses (dilated pupils, tachycardia)
- Altered electrolytes (hypokalemia)
- Change in mental state (confusion, obtundation, apprehension)

MAJOR OR CRITICAL DEFINING CHARACTERISTICS. Major or critical defining characteristics are designated signs and/or symptoms that *must be present for the health problem to be considered present.* Major defining characteristics, when applicable, must be present in the nurse's assessment profile to diagnose the corresponding health state with any degree of certainty. For example, the diagnosis Unilateral Neglect has as its major defining characteristic *consistent inattention to stimuli on affected side.* It is essential, then, that this characteristic be present in the patient's situation (in addition, perhaps, to several other noncritical signs) for the diagnosis of this problem. The assignment of major or critical status to a defining characteristic is based on research or extensive clinical experience in which the signs and symptoms of a health problem are tested for their ability to most reliably predict the presence of the diagnosis and can therefore be used with confidence by the nurse diagnostician.

---

* Related to.

Guidelines for diagnosing high-risk states

DETERMINING A RISK STATE FOR DIAGNOSIS. Predicting a potential health problem in a given patient involves an estimation of probability. The potential for an event, or pattern of response, to occur can truly be said to exist in almost any situation. Consider the high-risk health problems facing the postoperative patient. This risk state includes High Risk for Noncompliance with the rehabilitative regimen, High Risk for Body Image Disturbance, High Risk for Sleep Pattern Disturbance, High Risk for Ineffective Airway Clearance, High Risk for Constipation, and High Risk for Aspiration, to name only a few. To state each of these diagnoses on a treatment plan without regard for probabilities and develop desired patient outcomes and interventions for each is pointless.

What should occur is an appraisal of the patient's health status and the identification of risk factors that place him or her at higher risk for the health problem than the general population. For example, all persons recovering from abdominal surgery have High Risk for Constipation because of the effects of general anesthesia and narcotic analgesics, manipulation of abdominal viscera, and postoperative immobility. All nurses have a tacit understanding of this risk, and monitoring and intervention are carried out as part of routine nursing care to avert the problem; hence there is no need to state the problem.* A patient is at higher risk than the general population of postoperative patients if there is, for example, a history of dependence on laxatives, fluid volume deficit, prolonged immobility, or noncompliance with nursing prescriptions for ambulation. The diagnosis indicating this potential and its risk factors would be stated so that additional and/or more intensified interventions, over those that are routine, can be planned.

STATING HIGH-RISK DIAGNOSES. Several of the approved diagnoses address potential dysfunctional states and cite risk factors. Examples of such diagnoses are the following:

- Altered Nutrition: High Risk for More Than Body Requirements
- High Risk for Aspiration
- High Risk for Disuse Syndrome
- High Risk for Impaired Skin Integrity
- High Risk for Infection
- High Risk for Injury
- High Risk for Poisoning
- High Risk for Suffocation
- High Risk for Trauma
- High Risk for Violence

In addition to those diagnoses formally listed as high risk, any diagnosis from the approved list can be stated as an at-risk problem by simply adding the modifier *high risk* to the label. For example, Self-Esteem Disturbance can be written High Risk for Self-Esteem Disturbance by virtue of the presence of factors but not yet the actual health problem.

High-risk nursing diagnoses have only two parts to the statement: the *health problem at risk* and the *risk factors*[9] (e.g., High Risk for Ineffective Individual Coping, risk factors: malignant biopsy results, absence of interpersonal support system, and history of alcohol abuse).

Guidelines for stating wellness diagnoses. Wellness nursing diagnoses represent clinical judgments regarding an individual, family, or community in transition from a specific level of wellness and functioning to a higher level of wellness and functioning. The term *Potential for Enhanced (specify)* is the designated diagnostic label. Wellness diagnoses are one-part statements, for example, Potential for Enhanced Parenting; Potential for Enhanced Coping.[10]

◆ **Diagnostic reasoning.** Diagnostic reasoning is the critical thinking process through which the nurse moves to arrive at a nursing diagnosis. Like any process, it is often orderly and systematic. However, unlike a process, not all of its factors and operations exist in one's conscious awareness. The challenge of refining one's diagnostic reasoning is to bring into awareness the factors and operations that influence the process and are necessary in arriving at an accurate "answer," or diagnosis. Four key components of diagnostic reasoning are collecting and organizing the data base, identifying cues, making inferences, and validating inferences.

Components

COLLECTING AND ORGANIZING THE DATA BASE. Collecting and organizing a data base was discussed earlier in this chapter, under Data Collection.

IDENTIFYING CUES. A *cue* is a piece of information, a raw fact. Nurses notice and seek cues regarding patients' health status and functioning. Sweaty palms, restlessness, and a heart rate of 102 beats/min are cues. In the process of diagnostic reasoning, cues are the units of information that are collected and recorded for later analysis.

MAKING INFERENCES. An *inference* is the assignment of meaning to cues. A nursing diagnosis is an example of an inference. When individual cues are clustered and interpreted collectively, they begin to assume an identity different from what each represented individually. Sweaty palms, restlessness, and a heart rate of 102 beats/min, when interpreted as a cluster, could now represent anxiety, shock, fear, or pain.

Inferences are created, whereas cues exist. The process of creating inferences from cues, therefore, carries with it the risk of error in logic. If the cues sweaty palms, restlessness, and a heart rate of 102 beats/min were grouped and interpreted in a patient who also manifested gurgling respiratory sounds and a rapid, shallow breathing pattern—and these additional cues were overlooked or ignored by the person assigning meaning to the cluster—the inference might be erroneous, the more probable inference now being ineffective airway clearance. Nursing diagnoses are inferences, and defining characteristics and risk factors are the cues that lead to these inferences.

VALIDATING INFERENCES. Once a diagnostic inference is formulated, the nurse will develop and implement a

---

* No need to state the problem on an individualized nursing care plan; however, this high-risk diagnosis should be on record in a standards-of-care manual or standardized care plan.

treatment plan designed to resolve or reduce the problem represented by that inference. Erroneous inferences carry an obvious implication in terms of potential patient harm resulting from treatment of a nonexistent health problem or from treatment withheld for a missed diagnosis: nursing malpractice. Consequently, it is essential to seek validation of diagnostic inferences before implementing treatment.

Four approaches to the validation of inferences are recommended. First, consult with an authoritative source. This may be a clinical nurse specialist, nurse educator, textbook, or published research, for example. Seek confirmation of the logical and scientific integrity of your diagnostic statement. Second, reexamine the cues: could the ones in this diagnostic statement support any other diagnosis or only the one chosen? Could the cues from the data base believed *not* to be a part of the cluster supporting this diagnosis belong to some other cluster, or could several of them, together with cues supporting this diagnosis, suggest an altogether different diagnosis? Third, validate inferences with the patient. Nurses may share with the patient the cluster of cues identified and what is represented. Patients often have remarkable insight into what underlies their patterns of response and can be a great resource in validating the nurse's conclusions. Additionally, people benefit significantly from having their situations reflected back to them. Indeed, collaborating with the patient in this way may be all the intervention that is necessary. Fourth, seek evidence of the reliability of the diagnostic inference from within the appropriate reference group. Do most professional peers conclude the same explanation for the available cues?

These approaches are workable strategies for seeking validation of diagnostic inferences before the institution of treatment; however, the only way to achieve or confirm validation of a diagnosis is to treat the problem and evaluate the outcome. If favorable and predicted outcomes result, strong evidence exists that the problem and its etiology or risk factors and defining characteristics were accurately inferred.

Sources of diagnostic error. Much scientific curiosity exists within the nursing profession regarding the diagnostic reasoning process, strategies effective in increasing diagnostic accuracy, and sources of diagnostic error. Many of the principles identified through research thus far have come from studying differences in the diagnostic strategies employed by experts and those used by novices.[4,26,27,28] The following discussion focuses only on the most common type of diagnostic error, *the inferential leap,* and several of its sources. For more in-depth examinations of the skills of clinical problem solving and decision making, the reader is referred to Gordon, Carnevali, Tanner, and Benner.

INFERENTIAL LEAP. As the term implies, the inferential leap involves a jump to a conclusion based on premature termination of the data gathering/data analysis phase of the nursing process. Numerous studies show that this jump to an erroneous conclusion is most frequently made because not all of the variables are known or examined at the time the inference is formulated.[4,27,29,28] Of interest, the novice often closes the *search* for cues prematurely, whereas the expert will more often prematurely terminate the *analysis* of cues.

The novice may close the search for cues prematurely because of a lack of understanding of the scope of the problem to be diagnosed. Diagnoses such as Disturbance in Self-Concept and Ineffective Individual Coping are reported to be at the highest level of abstraction among nursing diagnoses and are therefore more difficult to fully grasp, let alone discriminate from other diagnostic possibilities.[30] The expert has an advantage in this regard by virtue of a greater breadth of experience, both with the label and the clinical presentation of patients demonstrating the diagnosis.

◆ Professional advantages of nursing diagnosis. Baer assembled from the literature the following statements in advocacy of nursing diagnosis. They are presented here to highlight the advantages nursing diagnosis brings to the profession. Nursing diagnosis does the following[31]:

- Assists in organizing, defining, and developing nursing knowledge
- Aids in identifying and describing the domain and scope of nursing practice
- Focuses nursing care on the patient's response to problems
- Prescribes diagnosis-specific nursing interventions that should increase the effectiveness of nursing care
- Facilitates the evaluation of nursing practice
- Provides a framework for testing the validity of nursing interventions
- Provides a standardized vocabulary to enhance intraprofessional and interprofessional communication
- Prescribes the content of nursing curricula
- Provides a framework for developing a system to direct third-party reimbursements for nursing services
- Indicates specific rationales for patient care based on nursing assessment
- Leads to more comprehensive and individualized patient care

In summary, nursing diagnoses are standardized labels that represent clinical judgments made by professional nurses and describe health states resolved primarily by nursing therapies. Nursing diagnosis focuses nursing assessment and intervention on the human response to altered health states, thus constituting a unique, distinct, and imperative component to critical health care. Nursing diagnosis is mandated as part of competent registered nurse performance criteria by most state nurse practice acts, as well as constituting the core of the ANA's formal definition of nursing.

Planning

Two things are accomplished in the planning phase of the nursing process: (1) patient *outcome criteria* are established and (2) *nursing interventions* are selected.

◆ Outcome criteria. Outcome statements consist of highly specific indicators that will be used by the nurse in the evaluation phase as criteria that either (1) the

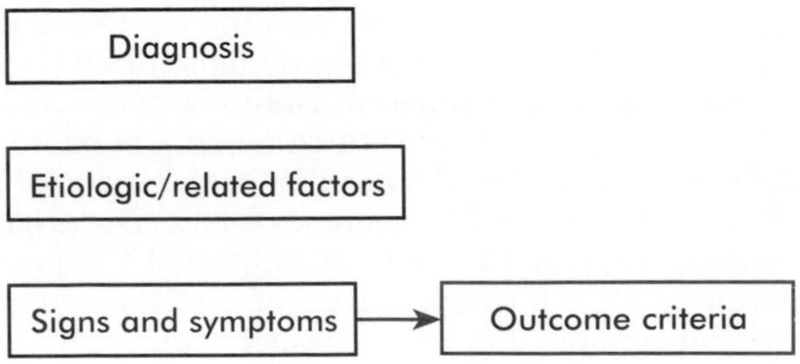

Fig. 1-3 Developing outcome criteria for an actual diagnosis.

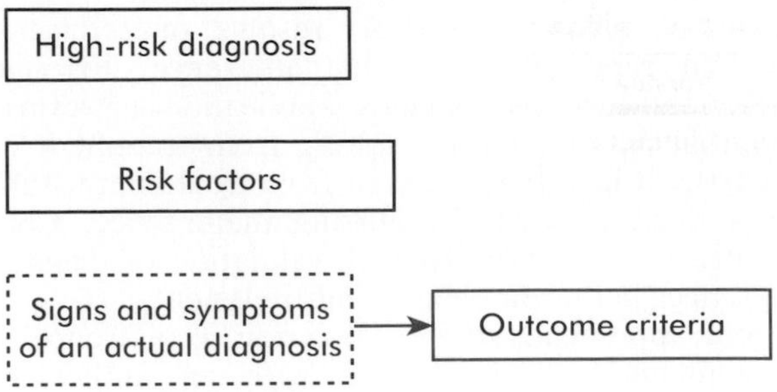

Fig. 1-4 Developing outcome criteria for a high-risk diagnosis.

actual diagnosis has been resolved or reduced or (2) the high-risk diagnosis has not occurred. An outcome statement is a projection of the expected influence that the nursing intervention will have on the patient in relation to the identified diagnosis. Though often confused, statements of expected patient outcome are *not* patient goals or nursing goals, nor should they describe nursing interventions.

As shown in Fig. 1-3, outcome criteria for an *actual* diagnosis are developed from the signs and symptoms of the nursing diagnosis. In other words, the assessment findings that were used to certify the existence of a diagnosis should also be used to establish its resolution or improvement. For example:

Nursing diagnosis	*Outcome criteria*
Ineffective Breathing Pattern R/T respiratory muscle fatigue AEB*: P_{CO_2} = 52 RR = 28	P_{CO_2} ≤45 RR ≤20 at rest

Outcome criteria for a *high-risk* diagnosis differ only in that, being a two-part statement, clinical manifestations will be absent from the diagnostic statement. Fig. 1-4 illustrates how the outcome criteria are developed from what would be the signs and symptoms of the high-risk problem *were it to become actual.* For example:

Nursing diagnosis	*Outcome criteria*
High Risk for Aspiration RISK FACTORS: Endotracheal tube Continuous intraenteral feedings Decreased level of consciousness	Lungs clear to auscultation Absence of blue tinge to tracheal aspirate Afebrile Sv_{O_2} ≥94%

Outcome criteria should be measurable, desirable, and, given full consideration to the resources of the patient and those of the nurse, attainable.

Measurable outcome criteria consist of patient behaviors, statements, and/or physiologic parameters that are recognizable on their occurrence. Many of the phenomena critical care nurses diagnose and treat are readily measurable, such as adequacy of spontaneous ventilation, cardiac output, and tissue perfusion. Many, however, are not readily measurable and thus present a challenging task to care planning in general and outcome criteria development specifically. Phenomena such as anxiety, powerlessness, disturbed body image, and ineffective coping involve the patient's subjective perception and, as such, resist the nurse's quantification. Outcome statements such as "less anxiety," "perceives personal power," or "copes effectively" represent favorable goals for nursing interventions but offer little in the way of criteria against which successful patient attainment can be measured. Again, here it is helpful to consider the signs and symptoms of the problem being treated and to modify them to reflect a situation in which the problem is absent or reduced. Several examples follow:

Clinical manifestations	*Outcome criteria*
"Why is it I have no say in any of this?"	Patient makes five decisions regarding his or her care
Distracted, preoccupied	Maintains eye contact throughout interactions
Looks away during stoma care	Visually regards stoma

Outcome statements are made further measurable by indicating the date and time of anticipated attainment. Projecting outcome attainment seems in some situations to be an arbitrary exercise, such as predicting the date or hour for the return of clear lung fields. However, the importance of this aspect of outcome criteria development lies in the fact that a specific deadline for evaluation of outcome attainment has been designated. Evaluating attainment of the outcome at designated intervals ensures that certain problems do not persist beyond acceptable time periods (such as Altered Peripheral Tissue Perfusion, Urinary Retention, Pain, and Dysfunctional Ventilatory Weaning Response) and that modification of the treatment approach occurs regularly. The outcome criteria applied throughout this text purposefully do not include date and time projection for attainment because this should be a reflection of actual, not hypothetical, patient characteristics.

The desirability and attainability of patient outcome criteria are other important aspects of planning nursing management. Individual patient baseline, patterns, and nurse and patient resources are the dominant considerations given to a projection of desired outcome, versus normative values. An example of an *undesirable* outcome

* As evidenced by.

Table 1-3 Correct and incorrect outcome criteria statements

Nursing diagnosis	Incorrect outcome	Correct outcome
Fluid volume deficit	Improved hydration Patient will be offered 100 ml fluid q 2 hr	Systolic blood pressure ≥100 mm Hg 24 hr fluid intake ≥body surface area fluid requirements Skin turgor ≤3 seconds
Decreased cardiac output	Hemodynamic stability	Cardiac index 2.5-4.0
High risk for disuse syndrome	Patient will be taught active leg exercises Patient will perform active leg exercises 10 times q 1 hr	No calf tenderness No ankle swelling
Pain	Patient will have a reduction in pain	Pain ≤"4/10" 10 minutes after IV narcotic
Powerlessness	Patient will perceive greater control over situation	Patient will make five decisions regarding his or her care

is "RR <16 at rest" for a patient with an unmodifiable chest wall restriction. "Absence of pain" in a patient with a sternotomy incision is also an undesirable target for early postoperative intervention. Examples of outcome criteria that are *unattainable* (and therefore undesirable) are "P_{CO_2} <40" in a patient who chronically retains carbon dioxide and "no anxiety" preoperatively for open heart surgery (see Table 1-3 for examples of correct and incorrect outcome criteria statements for assorted nursing diagnoses).

Developing outcome criteria statements has particular relevance to critical care nursing, because the statements describe in measurable terms the effects or results of critical care nursing. Also, they communicate the influence nursing intervention has in preventing, resolving, or improving various health states and provide a basis for justifying the allocation and reimbursement of professional nursing resources.

Critical pathways. One prominent nursing care delivery system, *case management,* uses expected patient outcomes to measure the effectiveness of nursing management and patient progress against a timeline of essential therapeutic events and responses, called a *critical pathway.* The critical pathway is a trajectory of the patient's hospital stay detailing intervention and outcome each day of the hospitalization from admission through day of discharge. The critical pathways of case management help ensure timely lengths of stay, prevention of complications, and overall coordinated management of each patient's care and progress by the RN case manager. Table 1-4 is an example of a critical pathway for the patient with congestive heart failure. The expected outcomes are under each nursing diagnosis and are stated in broad terms. The specific, measurable criteria used to evaluate daily patient progress along the pathway follow the horizontal headings *Key Pt./S.O. (patient/significant other) Activities/Outcomes.*

Nursing intervention

THE POWER OF NURSING INTERVENTION. Interventions are the power of nursing and a distinct strength of this text. Also known as *nursing orders* or *nursing prescriptions,* interventions constitute the treatment approach to an identified health alteration. Interventions are selected to satisfy the outcome criteria and prevent or resolve the nursing diagnosis.

A common shortcoming of nursing interventions, as much in the literature as in individual practice, is the prescription of vague, weak, nonsubstantive nursing actions. By definition, a nursing diagnosis is a health problem that nurses treat. *Treatment* implies producing a change in a situation, not merely maintaining equilibrium. And *prescribe* connotes recommending a course of action, not simply supporting an existing regimen. Intervention strategies that consist solely of monitoring, measuring, checking, obtaining physician orders, documenting, reporting, and notifying do not fulfill criteria for the treatment of a problem. Nursing intervention for nursing diagnoses should designate therapeutic activity that assists the patient in moving from one state of health to another. The growing body of research-based independent nursing therapies should be liberally applied to treatment plans for nursing diagnoses in critical care. Exciting advances in nurse management of such phenomena as ventilation-perfusion inequalities, excessive preload and afterload, increased intracranial pressure, and sensory-perceptual alterations associated with critical illness afford the critical care nurse the opportunity to incorporate potency into treatment plans.

FOCUS FOR INTERVENTIONS. As discussed earlier in this chapter, interventions have the greatest impact when they are directed at the etiologic/related factors of the diagnosis (Fig. 1-5) or, in the case of a high-risk diagnosis, the risk factors (Fig. 1-6). This stipulates that the etiologic factors of a problem be modifiable by nursing. To achieve the most favorable patient outcome, the multiple etiologic factors of a problem should be studied carefully and interventions selected to modify each.

SPECIFICITY OF INTERVENTIONS. Planned interventions should provide clarity, specificity, and direction to the spectrum of nurses implementing care for a patient. Statements such as "check vital signs" and "measure I&O" provide no real direction to nursing care and are therefore quite useless. Instead, "monitor for heart rate elevations 30 beats/min over baseline" and "look for 24-hr positive fluid balances" are preferable.

Table 1-4 A critical pathway for the patient with congestive heart failure

Nursing diagnosis/ patient problem	Date	ER/Day 1	Day 2	Day 3	Day 4
		/ /	/ /	/ /	/ /
Altered fluid volume R/T excessive accumulation of body fluid Expected outcome: Pt. will achieve and maintain an adequate fluid balance.	Key nsg. activities/ teaching	1. Observe & document excess fluid accum. & wt. gain: –edema –ascites – abdominal girth as ordered –neck vein distention 2. Wts. on admiss. & as ordered. 3. Maintain adequate I&O. 4. Maintain fluid restriction as ordered, help Pt. plan distribution of fluids. 5. Assess/observe adventitious breath sounds.	Continue to assess 1-5 q shift.		
	Key Pt./S.O. activities/outcomes	Understands signs and symptoms of altered fluid volume and need for fluid restriction as ordered	Begins monitoring, I&O, daily weights, edema		
Impaired gas exchange R/T pulmonary congestion Expected outcome: Pt. will experience decreased: –dyspnea –orthopnea –tachypnea –cough –diaphoresis	Key nsg. activities/ teaching	1. Assess/observe for SOB, cough, diaphoresis. 2. Maintain in semi-Fowler or high-Fowler position PRN. 3. Administer O_2 as ordered.	Continue to implement 1-3 q shift.		
	Key Pt./S.O. activities/outcomes	Verbalizes discomfort appropriately to nurse.			

High risk for activity intolerance Expected outcome: Pt. will balance energy demands and experience decreased fatigue.	Key nsg. activities/ teaching	1. Assess/observe activity tolerance. 2. Schedule frequent rest periods. 3. Instruct regarding rationale for conserving energy.	Continue to implement 1-2. Increase activity gradually as per MD & as tol. by Pt.		
	Key Pt./S.O. activities/outcomes	Tolerates ADLs with minimal c/o fatigue.	Understands energy conservation techniques.		
Pt. education and discharge planning	Key nsg. activities/teaching	1. Orient to room, routine, nsg. care delivery model. 2. Assess/observe knowledge deficit. 3. Document response to teaching.	Continue to implement 2-3. Anatomy and physiology of heart, signs and symptoms of CHF, importance of recording weight and edema daily. Introduce stress management/ relaxation techniques. Explain rationale for Na^- restricted diet.	Reinforce stress management/ relaxation techniques.	Review diet, activity progression, and energy conservation techniques, work simplification.
Expected outcome: Pt./S.O. will verbalize knowledge of following: –symptoms of early heart failure –importance of maintaining prescribed diet and fluid restrictions –medications, including name, dose, action, frequency, and side effects –fatigue avoidance –MD follow-up	Key Pt./S.O. activities/outcomes	Can state why admitted. Demonstrates a readiness to learn.	Understands heart failure and reason for Na^+ restricted diet.	States what CHF is. Identifies risk factors.	Demonstrates understanding diet. Makes appropriate menu choices. Verbalizes significance of activity progression balanced with rest.

From the Division of Nursing, The Long Island College Hospital, Brooklyn, N.Y.

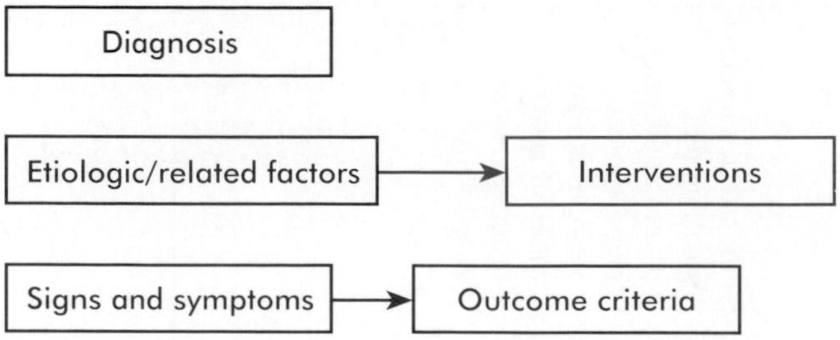

Fig. 1-5 Developing interventions for an actual diagnosis.

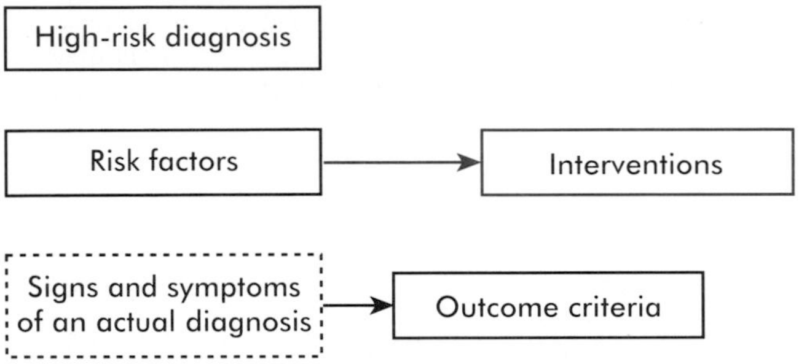

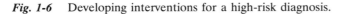

Fig. 1-6 Developing interventions for a high-risk diagnosis.

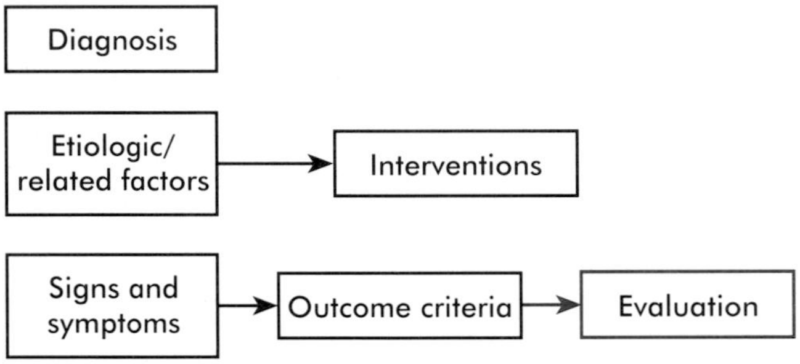

Fig. 1-7 Evaluating an actual diagnosis.

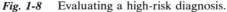

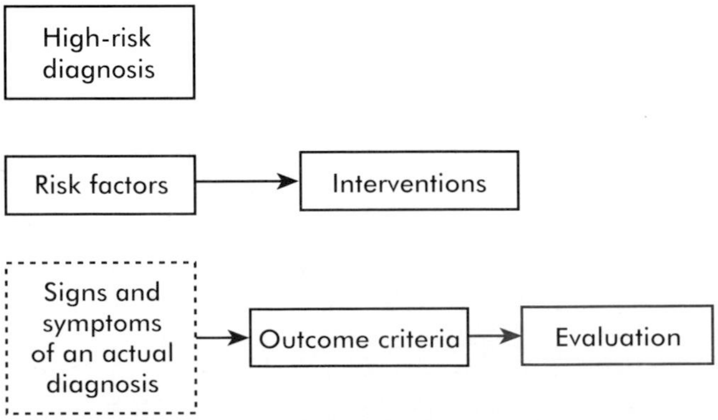

Fig. 1-8 Evaluating a high-risk diagnosis.

Include a brief rationale as part of intervention statement where this would enhance understanding of the treatment maneuver. For example, "change position dynamically q 2 hr, *to best match ventilation with perfusion.*" Rationales are *italicized* throughout the nursing management sections of this book.

Medically delegated actions, such as administering medications and initiating ventilator setting changes, should be included in the interventions but with the emphasis placed squarely on the assessments and judgments the nurse makes in evaluating their effectiveness, patient tolerance, safety, dosage, titration, and discontinuance. In critical care there is no such thing, for example, as "administer nitroprusside as ordered." Adequate specificity of nursing orders has been achieved when one is reasonably certain that a nurse unfamiliar with the patient can review the management plan and implement the kind of care intended by the primary nurse or case manager.

Implementation

Implementation is the action component of planning. It is the phase of the nursing process in which the nursing treatment plan is carried out. Data collection and evaluation are continuous throughout this phase.

Evaluation

Evaluation of attainment of the expected patient outcomes occurs formally at intervals designated in the outcome criteria. Informal evaluation occurs continuously. Fig. 1-7 and Fig. 1-8 illustrate how evaluation is conducted in relation to the outcome criteria for actual and high-risk diagnoses, respectively. There are two components to the evaluation phase of the nursing process. First, the nurse should compare the patient's current state with that described by the outcome criteria: Are breath sounds clear and equal bilaterally? Is the tidal volume of spontaneous respirations >500 ml, as were projected to be by this point in time? An evaluation of nursing effectiveness is done by commenting on the extent to which a predicted outcome has been attained.

Second, the nurse should query: If not, why not? Is it too soon to evaluate? Should implementation of the plan be continued for 24 hours longer and then reevaluated? Should the interventions be intensified; perhaps increase the frequency of respiratory muscle strengthening exercises? Are the outcome criteria impractical for this patient? Is the validity of the nursing diagnosis questionable? Are more data needed? Specific recommendations are then proposed that include either continuing implementation as outlined or returning to the data collection, nursing diagnosis, planning, or implementation phase of the process.

The evaluation phase and the activities that take place within it are perhaps the most important dimensions of the nursing process (see Fig. 1-1). Evaluation of patient progress against a standard of nursing care incorporates accountability into the process—accountability to the standard of care. Lack of progress in outcome attainment or lack of progress in problem solving is readily identified and kept in check, and alternate solutions can then be proposed.

REFERENCES

1. Kritek PB: Generation and classification of nursing diagnoses: toward a theory of nursing, *Image J Nurs Sch* 10:33, 1978.
2. Wescott MR: *Antecedents and consequences of intuitive thinking.* Final report to US Department of Health, Education & Welfare, Poughkeepsie, NY, 1968, Vassar College.
3. Munhall PL, Oiler CJ: *Nursing research,* Norwalk, Conn, 1986, Appleton-Century-Crofts.
4. Benner P: *From novice to expert: excellence and power in clinical nursing practice,* Menlo Park, Calif, 1984, Addison-Wesley.
5. Cosier RA, Alpin JC: Intuition and decision-making: some empirical evidence, *Psychol Rep* 51:275, 1982.
6. Dreyfus H, Dreyfus S: *Mind over machine: the power of human intuition and expertise in the era of the computer,* New York, 1985, Free Press.
7. Rew L: Intuition in decision-making, *Image J Nurs Sch* 20:150, 1988.
8. Smith SK: An analysis of the phenomenon of deterioration in the critically ill, *Image J Nurs Sch* 20:12, 1988.
9. Gordon M: *Nursing diagnosis: process and application,* New York, 1987, McGraw-Hill.
10. North American Nursing Diagnosis Association: *Taxonomy I revised-1990 with official diagnostic categories,* St. Louis, 1990, The Association.
11. Guzzetta CE and others: *Clinical assessment tools for use with nursing diagnoses,* St. Louis, 1989, Mosby–Year Book.
12. Gebbie KM, Lavin MA: *Classification of nursing diagnoses: proceedings of the First National Conference,* St. Louis, 1975, Mosby–Year Book.
13. Carpenito LJ: *Nursing diagnosis: application to clinical practice,* Philadelphia, 1992, JB Lippincott.
14. Hoskins LM and others: Axes: focus of taxonomy II, *Nursing Diagnosis* 3(3), 1992.
15. Warren JJ: Implications of introducing axes into a classification system. In Carroll-Johnson RM, editor: *Classification of nursing diagnoses: proceedings of the Ninth Conference,* Philadelphia, 1991, JB Lippincott.
16. Carroll-Johnson RM: *Classification of nursing diagnoses: proceedings of the Ninth Conference,* Philadelphia, 1991, JB Lippincott.
17. *Webster's New Collegiate Dictionary,* ed 9, Springfield, Mass, 1986, Merriam-Webster.
18. American Nurses Association: *Nursing: a social policy statement,* Kansas City, Mo, 1980, The Association.
19. Briody ME and others: Toward further understanding of nursing diagnosis: an interpretation, *Nursing Diagnosis* 3(3), 1992.
20. Davie JK: Independent and interdependent/collaborative nursing practice, *Newsletter of the Southern California Nursing Diagnosis Association* 5:3, 1988.
21. Kern L, Omery A: Decreased cardiac output in the critical care setting, *Nursing Diagnosis* 3(3), 1992.
22. Kim M: The dilemma of physiological problems: Without collaboration, what's left? *Am J Nurs* 85:281, 1985.
23. Roberts SL: Physiologic nursing diagnoses are necessary and appropriate for critical care, *Focus Crit Care* 15:42, 1988.
24. Tanner C: Overview: symposium on nursing diagnosis in critical care, *Heart Lung* 14:423, 1985.
25. Whitley GG: Concept analysis of anxiety, *Nursing Diagnosis* 3(3), 1992.
26. Benner P, Tanner C: How expert nurses use intuition, *Am J Nurs* 87:23, 1987.
27. Carnevali DL and others: *Diagnostic reasoning in nursing,* Philadelphia, 1984, JB Lippincott.
28. Tanner C and others: Diagnostic reasoning strategies of nurses and nursing students, *Nurs Res* 36:358, 1987.
29. Elstein A and others: Medical problem solving: a ten-year retrospective, *Evaluation and the Health Professions* 7:13, 1990.
30. Kritek PB: *Advantages and limitations of using nursing diagnostic categories as a framework for nursing practice research.* Audiotape transcription: Debate at the National Teaching Institute of American Association of Critical-Care Nurses, Anaheim, Calif. May 1986.
31. Baer CL: Nursing diagnosis, *Top Clin Nurs* 5:89, 1984.

SUGGESTED READINGS

1. American Association of Critical-Care Nurses: *Demonstration project,* Newport Beach, Calif, 1988, The Association.
2. Aspinall NJ: Nursing diagnosis: the weak link, *Nurs Outlook* 24:433, 1976.
3. Carnevali DL: Nursing care planning: diagnosis and management, Philadelphia, 1983, JB Lippincott.
4. Gebbie KM, Lavin MA: Classification of nursing diagnoses: proceedings of the First National Conference, St Louis, 1975, Mosby–Year Book.
5. Guzzetta CE and others: Unitary person assessment tool: easing problems with nursing diagnoses, *Focus Crit Care* 15:12, 1988.
6. Kritek PB: Nursing diagnosis in perspective: response to a critique, *Image J Nurs Sch* 17:3, 1985.
7. Kritek PB: Development of a taxonomic structure for nursing diagnoses: a review and an update. In Hurley ME, editor: *Classification of nursing diagnoses: proceedings of the Sixth Conference,* St Louis, 1986, Mosby–Year Book.
8. Prescott PA, Dennis KE, Jacox AK: Clinical decision making of staff nurses, *Image J Nurs Sch* 19:56, 1987.
9. White JE and others: Content and process in clinical decision making by nurse practitioners, *Image J Nurs Sch* 24:2, 1992.

2

Ethical Issues

CHAPTER OBJECTIVES

- Differentiate between morals and ethics.
- Relate the ethical theories of consequentialism and formalism to decision making in critical care.
- Discuss ethical principles as they relate to the critical care patient.
- Delineate ways in which resources are allocated in critical care.
- Discuss the concept of medical futility.
- Describe what constitutes an ethical dilemma.
- List steps for making ethical decisions.
- Delineate strategies for ethical decision making in critical care.

A revolution has occurred in health care in the past 50 years as the result of new technologies and treatments that were used during World War II. Issues that require ethical decisions about treatments, therapies, and life support are found in all health care settings and are most evident in technologically advanced critical care units. As more treatment modalities are introduced, ethical dilemmas will become harder to resolve.[1] A number of factors surround ethical decisions and have an impact on both the health care recipient and the health care provider: autonomy, philosophic views of health and life, moral and ethical beliefs, societal trends, cultural background, legal directives, health care costs, and bureaucratic constraints.

Almost 18% of the U.S. population under the age of 65 do not have health insurance. Inadequate health care access, along with escalating health care costs, will ultimately force hard decisions regarding rationing of resources.[2] Likewise, the most common ethical issues that occur in critical care units are those of foregoing treatment and allocating the scarce critical care unit resource. Historically, the critical care professionals believed that life had to be maintained at all costs and that death signified the failure of medicine and technology. More recently, long-term prognosis in terms of quality of life has replaced the earlier emphasis on sanctity of life as a major factor in ethical decision making.

Critical care units emerged in the 1950s as areas in which patients who required close observation could be placed together in a central setting.[1,3] Fairman[3] described nurses as historic protectors of patients in two ways: by providing "watchful vigilance" or close observation and by a triage manner in which they grouped patients according to their physiologic status and care needs.

The contemporary critical care nurse is confronted with moral and ethical conflicts on a frequent, sometimes daily, basis and is the health care professional who is most involved with all persons affected by the decision.[4] It is essential that the critical care nurse have an understanding of professional nursing ethics and ethical theories and principles and that she or he is able to use a decision-making model to guide nursing actions. The purpose of this chapter is to provide an overview of ethical theories and principles and professional nursing ethics. An ethical decision-making model will be described and illustrated. In addition, recommendations will be given about methods to discuss ethical issues in the critical care setting.

MORALS AND ETHICS

Morals Defined

The word *moral* is derived from the Latin *moralis,* which is defined as "good or right in conduct or character . . . making the distinction between right and wrong . . . principles of right and wrong based on custom."[5] Morals are the "shoulds," "should nots," "oughts," and "ought nots" of actions and behaviors and have been related closely to sexual mores and behaviors in Western society. Religious and cultural values and beliefs largely mold one's moral thoughts and actions. Morals form the basis for action and provide a framework for evaluation of behavior.

Ethics Defined

The word *ethics* is derived from the Greek *ethos,* which is defined as "the system or code of morals of a particular person, religion, group, or profession . . . the study of standards of conduct and moral judgment."[5] The term *ethics* is sometimes used interchangeably with the word *morals*. However, ethics is more concerned with the "why" of the action rather than with whether the action is right or wrong, good or bad.[6] Ethics implies that an evaluation is being made that is theoretically based on or derived from a set of standards. *Normative ethics* is the division of ethics that focuses on "norms or standards of behavior and value and their ultimate application to daily life"[7] with an emphasis on evaluation for purposes of guiding moral action. *Bioethics* incorporates all aspects of life but most frequently refers to health care ethics and the application of ethical principles to individual cases.

ETHICAL THEORIES

Philosophers have described ethical theories to be the combination of thinking processes, related principles, and rationales. The approach is normative, because it attempts to provide a basis for action. There are two traditional ethical theories that will be briefly discussed in this chapter: teleologic and deontologic.

Teleologic Theory (Consequentialism)

The focus of this theoretic approach is on the consequence of an action. Individuals are obligated to provide the greatest amount of happiness for the greatest number or the least amount of harm to the greatest number. The underlying assumption is that harm and benefit can be weighed and measured and that the outcome will demonstrate a good over evil for most people.[8] According to Fowler, utilitarian ethics is the most important teleologic theory for use in health care today.[7] Two common aphorisms summarize the utilitarian approach: "the greatest good for the greatest number" and "the end justifies the means."[6]

Philosophers Jeremy Bentham and John Stuart Mill professed the utilitarian theory and presented arguments for the approach with what has been described as "calculus morality." The outcomes of all alternative actions on the welfare of present and future generations are calculated. Based on these possibilities, a decision is made as to which alternative best benefits the greatest number.[8] Rather than determining utility of an action on a single situation or act (act utilitarianism), rule utilitarians judge actions on moral rules, which leads to the greatest good for the greatest number.[7]

The effect of consequences on present and future conditions of persons and groups takes precedence in utilitarianism.[9,10] Given the scarce resources of health care dollars, this approach for ethical decision making may be increasingly important. Future productivity of patients may serve to determine the types and amount of treatment or health care services that they receive.[9,10] Emergency situations may require a standard to be violated, such as omitting a sterile procedure to save a life or safely triage patients. According to utilitarian theory, truth telling may not be upheld if it is determined not to be in the best interest of the patient.[9,11]

Deontologic Theory (Formalism)

The focus of the deontologic approach to ethical problems is on the rules that determine the rightness or wrongness of the action.[7,10] Immanuel Kant, a German philosopher, has been credited with the formulation of this approach. Democratic principles or laws are stressed and universality is the basis for decisions.[10] Past moral or ethical judgments are considered, and value is assigned to significant relationships, commitments, and promises. Actions are independently assessed for their own value, and the consequences are not part of the decision.[9]

Kant espoused the belief that moral actions would supercede all other reasons for action and issued a "categorical imperative" that only actions that should become universal law be demonstrated.[11] Categorical imperatives are unconditional commands that are morally necessary and required under any circumstances. One has a duty to obey categorical imperatives with no exceptions and under all circumstances. The aphorism inherent in formalism is "the end does not justify the means." Decisions based on formalism are normally congruent with one's moral convictions and serve to validate one's strong sense of duty when acting out of principle regardless of consequences.[9,12] Strict adherence to rules, policies, and standards may stifle creativity and examination of alternatives in the fast-paced health care environment of today.

ETHICAL PRINCIPLES

There are certain ethical principles that were derived from classic ethical theories that are used in health care decision making.[9] Principles are general guidelines that govern conduct, provide a basis for reasoning, and direct actions.[8] The six ethical principles that are discussed in this chapter are autonomy, beneficence, nonmaleficence, veracity, fidelity, and justice.

Autonomy

The concept of autonomy appears in all ancient writings and early Greek philosophy. Immanuel Kant described an ethical person as one who is guided and motivated in response to one's own inward obedience, free from coercion, desire, or fear of future consequences.[11] Persons are not to be treated as a means to an end but rather as an end themselves.[13] In health care, autonomy can be viewed as the freedom to make decisions about one's own body without the coercion or interference of others. Autonomy is a freedom of choice or a self-determination that is a basic human right. It can be experienced in all human life events.

The obligation for health care professionals is to respect the values, thoughts, and actions of patients and not to let their own values or morals influence treatment decisions.[14] Fry described this as a respect for the "unconditional worth of the individual."[13] Often there is a conflict between the values of the patient and the health care professionals when dealing with life-sustaining matters in critical care. For patient autonomy to be maintained, patient decisions regarding treatments—such as resuscitation—must be supported.[15]

The critical care nurse is often "caught in the middle" in ethical situations, and promoting autonomous decision making is one of those situations. As the nurse works closely with patients and families to promote autonomous decision making, another crucial element becomes clear. Patients and families must have all of the information about a certain situation to make a decision that is best for them. Not only should they be given all of the information and facts, but they must also have a clear understanding of what was presented. This is where the nurse is a most important member of the health care team—that is, as patient advocate, providing more information, clarifying points, reinforcing information, and providing support during the process.[16] The legal implications of informed consent are discussed in Chapter 3. The Patient Self-Determination Act (PSDA) legislates that patients are informed of their right to designate health care treatments (see Chapter 3).[17]

Beneficence

The concept of doing good and preventing harm to patients is a *sine qua non* for the nursing profession. However, the ethical principle of beneficence—which requires that one promote the well-being of patients—points to the importance of this duty for the health care professional. According to Davis and Aroskar,[8] the principle of beneficence presupposes that harms and benefits are balanced, leading to positive or beneficial outcomes.

Murphy described the ethical mandate of the nurse as being different from that of the physician in some aspects of care. Because nurses diagnose and treat human responses to health problems, it is they who deal most closely with quality of life issues.[17] In these situations, the nurse is obligated to act different from the physician, whose duty is to preserve life at all means.

In approaching issues related to beneficence, there is frequently conflict with another principle, that of autonomy. *Paternalism* exists when the nurse or physician makes a decision for the patient without consulting or including the patient in the decision process. *Paternalism* is "making people do what is good for them" and "preventing people from doing what is bad for them."[11] Jameton[11] described two types of paternalists: strong paternalists who make decisions for obviously competent persons and weak paternalists who make decisions for persons who are mentally or physically unable to make their own decision.

Traditional health care has been based on a paternalistic approach to patients. Many patients are still more comfortable in deferring all decisions about care and treatment to their health care provider. Active involvement by various organizations and agencies regarding health care has demonstrated a trend toward the public's need and desire for more information about health care and alternative treatments and providers. Paternalism, or maternalism in the case of female providers, may always be a possibility in the health care setting, but enlightened consumers are changing this practice of health care professionals.

In the critical care setting, there are many instances and possibilities for paternalistic actions by the nurse. Postoperative care, which is designed to assist the patient with a quick recovery, is a good example of paternalistic action by the nurse. Encouraging the patient to turn, cough, and deep breathe and increasing activity in the form of dangling, sitting in a chair, and ambulating are all paternalistic when the patient is in pain, sleep deprived, and wanting to be left alone. However, there are times when the priorities of benefits and harms must be balanced. In this instance, the duty to do no harm—which is the next principle to be discussed—takes precedence over paternalistic actions. When there are conflicts in ethical principles, one must weigh all of the benefits and choose the best one.[8]

Nonmaleficence

The ethical principle of nonmaleficence, which dictates that one prevent harm and remove harmful situations, is a *prima facie* duty for the nurse.[8] Thoughtfulness and care is necessary, as is balancing risks and benefits, which was discussed earlier with beneficence. Beneficence and nonmaleficence are on two ends of a continuum and are often carried out differently, depending on the views of the practitioner. A practitioner using a utilitarian approach will consider long-term consequences and the good to society as a whole. The practitioner operating from a deontologic basis will consider the principle and its effect on the single individual in the situation.

Such complex situations as quality of life versus sanctity of life are always difficult to analyze in the critical care setting as well as in non–critical care settings. Flynn described such decisions as withholding and withdrawing treatments as being based on not one ethical principle alone, but rather on a balance of all ethical principles so that the most appropriate moral decision can be made.[18] Nonmaleficence should serve as the guide for practice of health care professionals.[9]

Veracity

Veracity, or truth-telling, is an important ethical principle that underlies the nurse-patient relationship. In 1860 Florence Nightingale described veracity with patients: "Far more now than formerly does the medical attendant tell the truth to the sick who are really desirous to hear it about their own state."[19] Nightingale's philosophy was not agreed on by other health care providers of the time (i.e., physicians), but she was sensitive to the needs of patients who sought information about their own conditions.

Veracity is important in soliciting informed consent, so that the patient is aware of all potential risks and benefits from specific treatments or their alternatives. Once again, the critical care nurse can be in the middle of a situation where all of the facts and information about a particular treatment option are not disclosed. Sometimes information has been given accurately but has been delivered with bias or in a way that is misleading. In this case and other instances with veracity, the ethical principle of autonomy has been violated.[20]

Are there ever any situations in which nurses should lie to patients? This subject was discussed in depth by Schmelzer and Anema,[21] who posed that nurses make many value judgments in their daily practice, some of which are made after careful consideration and some of which are made quickly with minimal thought. Veracity is also related closely to the principle of beneficence in which the nurse must consider whether the lie will benefit the patient and if so, how. They stressed the importance of designating lies as negative benefits when comparing them with the positive benefits of the truth.

When faced with a veracity dilemma, one should analyze the personal abilities, values, and beliefs of the patient. All possible options and truthful alternatives should be examined. The long-term effects of a lie may

LEGAL REVIEW: Confidentiality and disclosure of human immunodeficiency virus and acquired immunodeficiency syndrome patient information

Physicians, nurses, and other pertinent hospital employees have a duty to maintain the confidentiality of medical records and patient communications. This duty is derived broadly from the privilege doctrine. There is ethical privilege for both physicians and nurses. In every state there is statutory privilege (duty of confidentiality) between physicians and patients; a minority of states have codified the nurse-patient privilege. Every institution has policies and procedures regarding nurse-patient confidentiality, and the nurse must be familiar with them. Finally, the common law theories of invasion of privacy, breach of confidential relationship, professional malpractice, breach of contract, and defamation have been advanced to impose liability on health care professionals who disclose medical information.

Exceptions to the privilege include implicit or explicit waiver by the patient of the right to confidentiality, legal discovery procedures, court order and subpoena, and government agency requests for vital statistics, communicable disease data, abuse data, and wounds of violence. The scope of the privilege duty involves the balancing of the patient's right to privacy and confidentiality with other public or private interests, including the right to know.

In the following cases, the Washington Supreme Court ordered the blood bank to disclose the identity of the HIV-infected donor of transfused blood. However, the Maryland Appeals Court held that a patient with AIDS was entitled to anonymity in his lawsuit against a hospital for violation of the confidentiality of his medical record and invasion of privacy. Several states have enacted statutes specifically addressing confidentiality and AIDS or HIV patient data.

See *The AIDS epidemic: private rights and the public interest,* Boston, 1989, Beacon Press; *AIDS and ethics,* New York, 1991, Columbia University Press; Bureau of National Affairs: *AIDS in the workplace: resource material,* ed 3, Washington, DC, 1989, Bureau of National Affairs; *Doe v Puget Sound Blood Center,* No 56236-9 (Wash Sup Ct, Nov 14, 1991); *Doe v Shady Grove Adventist Hosp,* No. 1058 (Md Ct Spec App, Nov 27, 1991); *HIV/AIDS: a guide to nursing care,* ed 2, Philadelphia, 1992, WB Saunders; Jarvis AM: *AIDS law in a nutshell,* St Paul, 1991, West Publishing; Lambda Legal Defense and Education Fund, Inc.: *AIDS legal guide: a professional resource on AIDS-related legal issues and discrimination,* ed 2, New York, 1990, The Fund; Pratt RJ: *AIDS: a strategy for nursing care,* ed 3, London, 1991, Edward Arnold.

be the loss of credibility of the nurse with the patient, the need for additional "cover-up" lies, and stress to the nurse who told the lie. Schmelzer and Anema concluded that "nurses should be committed to telling the truth and, when faced with situations where they are tempted to lie, should instead seek alternative actions based on honesty."[21] This principle should guide all areas of practice for the nurse, that is, colleague relationships and employee relationships, as well as the nurse-patient relationship.

Fidelity

Another ethical principle that is closely related to autonomy and veracity is fidelity. Fidelity, or faithfulness and promise-keeping to patients, is also a *sine qua non* for nursing. It forms a bond between individuals and is the basis of all relationships, both professional and personal. Regardless of the amount of autonomy that patients have in the critical care areas, they still depend on the nurse for a multitude of types of physical care and emotional support. A trusting relationship that establishes and maintains an open atmosphere is one that is positive for all involved.[22]

Aroskar[20] pointed out that making a promise to a patient is voluntary for the nurse, whereas respect for a patient's making decisions is a moral obligation. She described the critical care nurse as experiencing a great deal of moral conflict. "Fidelity to patients in "high-tech" care units may require that nurses question the use of specific technologies for a specific patient or even the admission of a hopelessly ill patient . . . to such a unit."[20]

As do all the other principles, fidelity extends to the family of the critical care patient. When a promise is made to the family that they will be called if an emergency arises or that they will be informed of other special events, the nurse should make every effort to follow through on the promise. Not only will fidelity be upheld for the nurse-family relationship, but there will also be a positive reflection on the nursing profession as a whole and on the institution in which the nurse is employed.

Confidentiality is one element of fidelity that is based on traditional health care professional ethics. According to Veatch and Fry,[23] the nursing and medical professions have established ethical codes that allow no patient-centered reasons for breaking the principle of confidentiality. Confidentiality is described as a right whereby patient information can only be shared with those involved in the care of the patient. An exception to this guideline might be when the welfare of others is at risk by keeping patient information confidential. Again in this situation, the nurse must balance ethical principles and weigh risks with benefits. Special circumstances, such as mandatory reporting laws, will guide the nurse in certain situations.

Privacy has also been described as inherent in the principle of fidelity. It may be closely aligned with confidentiality of patient information and a patient's right to privacy of his or her person, such as maintaining privacy for the patient by pulling the curtains around the bed or making sure that he or she is adequately covered.

Justice/Allocation of Resources

The principle of justice is often used synonymously with the concept of allocation of scarce resources. Contrary to the belief of many people, health care is not a right guaranteed by the Constitution of the United States. Rather, *access* to health care should be provided to all people. With escalating health care costs, expanded technologies, an aging population with its own special health care needs, and (in some instances) a scarcity of health care personnel, the question of health care allocation becomes even more complex.

The application of the justice principle in health care is concerned primarily with divided or portioned allocation of goods and services, which is termed *distributive justice.*[24] According to Jameton, distributive justice appears at three levels of health care: national policies and budget, state or local distribution of resources, and distribution in the individual health care settings.[11] Traditionally, six criteria for making decisions about allocation of resources have been used.[11,25] Distribution has been based on the following:

- Equality for all persons
- Individual merit
- Societal contributions
- Availability in an open market
- Individual need
- Similar treatment for similar cases

◆ **Equality for all persons.** Equality for all persons has been a traditional stance of health care and has been evidenced in ethical codes and in the practices of professionals. With equality, all persons are given equal treatments and resources, such as access to health care, technologies, specialists, personnel to perform necessary care and treatment, and support for physical and emotional needs during the process. This clearly is not the case in current health care. Is a rural or small community health care agency equal to larger urban centers or medical centers in the ability to provide such comprehensive services described? Is there equality in care across the health care continuum, that is, access to treatment and home, community, or follow-up care for all persons? The answer to both questions is "no" for myriad reasons and circumstances.

Escalating health care costs and technologic advances of expensive treatments have resulted in the inability to provide equality in health care services to all. Elderly retired persons on Medicare, unemployed persons with no insurance, and the middle-class working family with moderate insurance coverage receive differing types and amounts of services. Most persons do not receive health care along the entire continuum, that is, from health care *promotion* to health care *illness.* The quality of care provided has traditionally been the same. But might this also be changing in the future, or has it already changed to varying degrees in some instances?

Veatch[26] delineated three objections to the egalitarian interpretation of justice. First, he raised the question of whether equality should be applied to health status—that is, specific illness or condition—or to equality of health welfare in general—that is, overall health care services across the continuum. Second, he posited that the egalitarian approach does not allow for any consideration of other ethical principles. And third, he raised concern that there might be infinite patient demands for services and that the individual patient-centered principle of autonomy would take precedence over societal needs.

◆ **Individual merit.** Distribution of services based on individual merit has not been a traditional practice of health care professionals and is an area that may be subtle to observe. Individual merit might be based on that which has already been achieved or that which is expected to occur in the future, such as in the case of an infant or child or a person who may have potential for success in some endeavor. Basically, the issue at hand is whether this type of person deserves a particular treatment. The decision is based on values that are subjective and not driven by a set of rules or principles.

Greater merit may be given to those who are rich and famous, have a particular profession or type of work, or lead a certain life-style. Thus a person who smokes, drinks excessively, or uses recreational drugs may have a lower priority for treatments, surgery, and care. Health care professionals may judge that persons have abused themselves, such as in the case of the alcoholic or drug abuser, or have neglected themselves, such as in the case of one who has not sought necessary health care. Such persons may receive varying levels of care or might be denied care altogether.

◆ **Societal contribution.** Decisions based on the societal contribution of the individual examine the worth of that individual in society and are subjective and value-based. Using this as a framework for making decisions causes elderly persons, young persons, those who have conditions that are socially undesirable such as alcoholism or mental diseases, and those who are handicapped to a degree that makes them dependent to be considered to not have worth to society.

Societal worth has not been a factor traditionally espoused by health care professionals as a basis for decisions. However, in the early days of renal transplantation, criteria such as age and personal demographics were considered in the decision to transplant, which resulted in public discomfort with the decision method.[25,27]

◆ **Free market acquisition.** Justice determined by free market acquisition is guided by money and what individuals can acquire with their money. Persons both in the past and in the present who have unlimited money are able to receive the ultimate in services and are able to quickly search for and find services to meet their needs and desires. They are usually limited only by the

RESEARCH ABSTRACT

Severity of illness and resource allocation in DNR patients in ICU.

Tittle MB, Moody L, Becker MP: *Nurs Econ* 10(3):210, 1992.

PURPOSE

The purpose of this study was to examine the differences in severity of illness and resource allocation between DNR patients in ICU and non-DNR patients in ICU.

DESIGN

Comparative descriptive design

SAMPLE

The convenience sample consisted of 124 patients with equal representation of DNR and non-DNR subjects. The mean age of the DNR patients was 74 years, with a mean of 67.7 years for the non-DNR group; males and females were equally represented in the groups. Subjects were from three community hospitals: less than 200-bed, investor-owned, for-profit hospital; 500-bed, not-for-profit, teaching hospital; and 700-bed, not-for-profit hospital. All patients designated as DNR were included in the study, and all subjects were in the CCU a minimum of 24 hours. Excluded from the study were patients in CCU for overnight monitoring, those in CCU to rule out myocardial infarction, and those undergoing CABG or open heart surgery.

INSTRUMENTS

The APACHE II Severity of Disease Classification System (Acute Physiology and Chronic Health Evaluation) measured severity of illness of 12 routine physiologic measurements, patient's age, and chronic health status. The Therapeutic Intervention Scoring System (TISS) measured resource allocation by quantifying the therapeutic interventions used by patients. Construct validity of the instruments in this study was established with a correlation coefficient of 0.72.

PROCEDURE

Data were collected daily using information from the medical record and individual patient observations. Subjects were followed until transferred from the ICU or until death.

RESULTS

Of the non-DNR patients, 92% were transferred from ICU and 74% of DNR patients died either in ICU or a general nursing unit. Of the DNR patients, 47% were transferred from ICU and 26% of the total DNR sample were discharged from the hospital. The mean daily APACHE II score of the DNR subjects was 22.51, with 12.07 for the non-DNR group (significant difference with $p < .001$). There was a linear relationship between resources consumed and severity of illness for the DNR patients (i.e., the amount of resources consumed increased as severity of illness increased). The relationship of resources to severity was nonlinear for the non-DNR patients. There were minimal differences in the consumption of resources between the two groups when the severity score approximated 16. Patients with DNR orders received significantly more resources after the DNR order than before the order ($p < .001$).

DISCUSSION AND IMPLICATIONS

An interesting finding of this study was that patients consumed more resources after the DNR order was given than before. This finding appears to indicate that aggressive therapy continued even after the DNR order was given and that the DNR status did not indicate a withdrawal of treatment modalities. The 26% survival rate of the DNR patients may indicate a response to continued or initiated therapies after the DNR order. It may also indicate that the terminal condition or fatal prognosis was incorrect. In addition, the physical status and quality of life of those DNR patients who survived is not known. This study has implications for ICUs and hospitals regarding the importance of establishing policies for placement of DNR patients from both a human resource and material resource basis. Future studies can use the findings of this study to examine the following issues: What are the fiscal implications of DNR versus non-DNR patients in the ICU? What physical indicators best predict positive patient outcomes? What are the specific care requirements for non-DNR patients? What is the best care environment for the non-DNR patient?

technologies and services available. However, when time is not crucial, money will pay for technologies or services that can be developed if money is available to support such efforts.

Differences can be noted through private rooms; many nurses or attendants; the best, world-renowned specialist brought to the patient; or the patient taken anywhere in the world to obtain treatment. Money and the free market open lines of communication that do not exist for others. Through free market, those with money and necessary resources may be the first in line for a treatment and take priority over others.

◆ **Individual need.** Jameton described individual need as most applicable to health care in deciding allocation of resources.[11] The dilemma arises when one considers one individual's need for heart transplantation or other technologies versus the possibility of using those resource dollars for early education on preventing heart disease for many people. In delineating problematic areas in the determination of individual needs, Levine-Ariff asserted that level and type of need should be identified.[25] If harm would come to the individual were the need not met, the need takes precedence and should be met.

◆ **Similar treatment for similar cases.** The concept of similar treatment for similar cases expands on the concept of equality and applies the same basic principle at the societal level. However, consideration of contribution to society is also inherent in this method of decision. For instance, criteria may be established that designate that all who have a certain condition and who are under a certain age will be given the treatment, surgery, or service. This allows equal access of all who meet those criteria but disallows others who do not meet the criteria. Decisions based on this standard cover groups of people, whereas decisions based on individual need hold only for that one person.

ALLOCATION OF SCARCE RESOURCES IN CRITICAL CARE

Englelhardt and Rie[27] described critical care units as providing optimal care to all who require it. Yet those responsible for the costs of critical care can no longer afford to pay for the advanced treatments and technologies that have been developed and refined and made available.

There have been reductions in federally funded health care programs and a leveling off of monies for health care research funds from previous years. Resources available for health needs are no longer unlimited, as they previously appeared to be. It has become evident that both resource allocation and allocation decisions will become inevitable and may appear in forms of public policies and guidelines.[28,29] Allocation will be discussed in two areas: allocation of technologies and treatments and allocation of health care energy.

Allocation of Technologies and Treatments

Limitations of resources force society and the critical care health professionals to reexamine the goals of critical care for patients. Once considered experimental, coronary artery bypass surgery, magnetic resonance imaging, kidney dialysis, and heart transplantation are now widely accepted and funded by payers.[30] Because the possibilities and number of organ transplants are increasing, there are not enough available organs. To increase the availability of donated organs, most states have enacted "required request" laws, which mandate that families must be approached about donation of organs on the death of their loved ones.[31,32,33] Procurement of organs has posed new ethical dilemmas for health care professionals, who must now act in accordance with state laws (see Legal Review on organ transplantation, Chapter 49, p. 848).

Other technologies found in critical care that were considered experimental only a few years ago are the intraaortic balloon pump (IABP),[34] the left ventricular assist device (LVAD), and the artificial heart.[35] Essential in the use of all technologies and critical care treatments are veracity, autonomy, and informed consent,[34] which have been discussed earlier in this chapter. Legal implications about informed consent are discussed in Chapter 3. In cases in which research protocols are used with patients in the critical care units, all ethical principles apply.[36]

According to Danis and Churchill,[37] the ethical principles of autonomy and justice sometimes need to be carefully separated. An example of this is when a patient requests a costly treatment of debatable utility. Health care rationing is a current subject of great debate and discussion and will continue to be placed at the forefront of health care decisions.[37-40] The state of Oregon has passed legislation dealing with rationing of health care costs for the inhabitants of the state.[41] Regardless of the methodology to allocate health care dollars, it is hoped that compassionate care is delivered along with reduced interventions and costs.[42]

Quality of life is an issue that should be considered when examining the use of technologies. It is an area that is personal and value-laden and one that will be different for all involved and dependent on the content.[43,44] Quality of life has dual dimensions of both objectivity and subjectivity. Objectivity examines the person's functionability, whereas subjectivity analyzes his or her psychosocial state. An evaluation of quality of life issues can take place only after one has received the technology and "lived" that "new" life.[45]

Allocation of Health Care Energy

Knaus stated that "access to an expensive and complex resource like intensive care can never be absolute."[46] Critical care nurses are faced with rationing of critical care beds and nursing staff on a daily basis. Strengths and weaknesses of the staff must be balanced with the needs of the patient. Orientation and other special circumstances—such as designation for charge nurse, trauma nurse, and code nurse—must be considered when scheduling staff and making assignments. Any inexperienced staff, float staff, or registry staff must be given appropriate orientation and backup during the shift.

There is frequently a triage system for critical care units that is called on when there are more admissions than available beds. The critical care nurse is instrumental in assisting the medical director to determine patient selection for transfer, if appropriate. Some hospitals use a set of standards, criteria, or guidelines for determining patient admission and transfer to and from critical care areas. The *Guidelines for Admission/Discharge Criteria in Critical Care* developed by the American Association of Critical-Care Nurses are provided in the box on p. 25. These guidelines can serve as the basis for development of criteria specific to the critical care nurse's institution.

Theory-Based Allocation of Resources

Pinch described allocation of scarce resources in terms of three theories: goal-based theory, duty-based theory, and rights-based theory.[47] Use of the *goal-based theory*

AACN POSITION STATEMENT
Guidelines for admission/discharge criteria in critical care

THE CHALLENGE FOR TODAY'S health care providers is to deliver quality patient care in a changing health care environment. Health care agencies have become increasingly competitive in response to the prospective reimbursement system, with a focus on cost containment, enhanced efficiency, and marketing efforts directed towards consumer satisfaction. Additionally, the expansion of new technology and complex treatment therapies have contributed to the escalating costs of health care. Acute care facilities now must attempt to attract the consumer and deliver quality patient care within the confines of restricted financial and health care resources. These current changes and trends in the health care system are exerting impact on critical care which intensifies the need to appropriately select patients to be cared for in the critical care setting.

Since the inception of critical care, health care personnel have had to decide which patients require admission to critical care units. This selection process has always been a multifaceted one and today, critical care admission/discharge decisions are even more complex. More pronounced ethical dilemmas have resulted from the combination of increasing patient acuity, advanced available technology, and limited resources. Consequently, the critical care admission/discharge process significantly affects the nature of care rendered and the use of limited resources to deliver that care.

WHEREAS, to promote quality care by matching patient requirements for treatment and nursing care with available human and financial resources,

THEREFORE, BE IT RESOLVED THAT, objective admission and discharge criteria must be written, implemented and evaluated for each critical care setting by a multidisciplinary health care team which includes representation from medicine, critical care nursing, and hospital administration.

AND THAT, the development of admission/discharge criteria be based on the following data and resources:

- ◆ Standards of nursing care for the critically ill
- ◆ Current unit admission and discharge patterns
- ◆ Available resources within the critical care unit: level and quantity of nursing care, expertise and qualifications of personnel, and equipment and technology
- ◆ Number and distribution of critical care beds within the institution
- ◆ Institutional occupancy trends
- ◆ Data provided by existing measurement tools in the institution (e.g., patient classification tools, severity of illness indexes)
- ◆ Alternative institutional and community resources available for discharged or triaged patients

AND THAT, the admission/discharge criteria contain or address the following elements:

- ◆ Physiological parameters which define the need for critical care
- ◆ Physiological parameters which define readiness for discharge
- ◆ Definition of unit–specific patient population
- ◆ Frequency and type of medical evaluation and/or treatment required by the patient's condition
- ◆ Frequency and type of critical care nursing assessments and interventions needed by the patient
- ◆ Technological monitoring and intervention only available in the critical care setting
- ◆ Requirements by external regulatory bodies
- ◆ Institutional policies which mandate or preclude critical care for specific patient populations
- ◆ Designation of the health team member(s) accountable for admission/discharge decisions
- ◆ A plan for triage when the need exceeds available physical and human resources
- ◆ A plan for conflict resolution between health care team members utilizing the admission/discharge criteria

AND THAT, the admission/discharge criteria will be approved through appropriate institutional channels and disseminated to all health team members involved in the process,

BE IT FURTHER RESOLVED THAT, compliance to the admission/discharge process will be regularly monitored and evaluated annually by the multidisciplinary team.

Adopted by AACN Board of Directors, May 1987.

From American Association of Critical-Care Nurses.

results in the most happiness or good for the majority. Utilitarian theory is applied, which seeks the best solution to benefit the most. Weighing benefits and establishing criteria for patient selection into critical care areas is an example of this theoretic application.

By analyzing the dilemma with a *duty-based theory,* one acts according to obligations. The basic principle of nonmaleficence governs actions, and all individuals are treated alike. No priority is assigned to any one individual, and all are cared for equally. In the event that no beds are available for admission, the nurse's first and prime consideration is the patients already in the unit under his or her care. Other alternatives are explored, such as admitting the patient elsewhere in the hospital with a critical care nurse in attendance or transporting the patient to another institution that has adequate resources.

The last theory to be discussed is that of the

rights-based theory. The focus here is on the benefits that the individual deserves or is entitled to receive from that individual's point of view and value system. Individual autonomy is the major ethical principle in this theory. In the critical care setting, all patients appear to be voluntary patients in need of critical care. If there are any cases in which individual patients question treatments or do not want certain procedures done, they may self-select a transfer out of the unit. In other cases in which all patients are medically competitive for the critical care bed, random selection is the recommended method of decision making.

The final decision in any of the three theoretically based decision models involves examining several ethical principles and many factors related to each case. No easy answers can be given, and no set rules or standards exist for these difficult issues. Pinch suggested the application of sound management principles and the adherence to legal guidelines as essential to decision situations.[47]

WITHHOLDING AND WITHDRAWING TREATMENT

The technologic support of life at all costs has recently come to be questioned by both health care professionals and health care consumers. Physicians and nurses who are closest to the issues have debated the moral and ethical implications and have looked to ethicists for guidance and legal opinion. Both medical and nursing associations have developed guidelines for their practitioners about withholding and withdrawing treatments. The American Association of Critical-Care Nurses position statement *Withholding and/or Withdrawing Life-Sustaining Treatment* is presented in the box on p. 27.

The decision not to employ aggressive measures or to discontinue treatments that have been in place is always difficult and stressful for all involved in the decision, particularly those who continue to care for the patient on a daily basis.[48,49] Legal implications for withholding or withdrawing treatments and orders not to resuscitate the patient are delineated in Chapter 3.

There appears to be more reluctance to withdraw treatments, which is reflective of ethical and moral conflicts within each of the practitioners. Withholding usually means that there is no hope for success from the onset, whereas withdrawing means surrendering hope. Also, difficult discussions must take place between the health care professionals and the family. The nurse must be sure to examine the treatment with regard for the patient's best interests and wishes and to act accordingly.[14,17,35,50]

MEDICAL FUTILITY

The concept of medical futility has been discussed recently in terms of definition and ethical implications.[51] Medical futility has both a qualitative and a quantitative basis and can be defined as "any effort to achieve a result that is possible but that reasoning or experience suggests is highly improbable and that cannot be systematically reproduced."[51]

Therapy or treatment that achieves its predictable outcome and desired effect is, by definition, effective. But effect must be distinguished from benefit. If that predictable and desired effect is of no benefit to the patient, it is nonetheless futile. It is suggested that when physicians conclude from either personal or colleague experiences or from empiric data that a particular treatment in the most recent 100 cases in which it has been used has been useless, the treatment should be considered futile.[51] It is incumbent on physicians to make optimal use of health-related resources in a technically appropriate and effective manner. Therefore in this era of escalating health care costs and limited resources, the physician has a particular responsibility to avoid futile treatment.[51]

ETHICS AS A FOUNDATION FOR NURSING PRACTICE

Traditional theories of professions include a code of ethics as the basis for the practice of professionals. The moral foundation of nursing is discussed in the literature by various authors who describe the unique relationship of the professional nurse with the patient, which establishes a caring, trusting approach.[52-54] It is by adherence to a code of ethics that the professional fulfills an obligation for quality practice to society.

According to Curtin,[55] nursing ethics is concerned with duties that are assumed by nurses and with the consequences of decisions that affect patients, colleagues, society, and the nursing profession. A professional ethic is based on three elements: the professional code of ethics, the purpose of the profession, and the standards of practice of the profession. The need for the profession and its inherent promise to provide certain duties form a contract between nursing and society. The code of ethics developed by the professionals is the delineation of its values and relationships with and among members of the profession and society. The professional standards describe specifics of practice in a variety of settings and subspecialties. Each element is dynamic, and ongoing evaluations are necessary as societal expectations change, technologies increase, and the profession evolves.

Nursing Code of Ethics

The American Nurses Association (ANA) provides the major source of ethical guidance for the nursing profession.[56,57] According to the preamble of the *Code for Nurses,* "When individuals become nurses, they make a moral commitment to uphold the values and special moral obligations expressed in their code."[58] The 11 statements of the Code are found in the box on p. 28. They are based on the underlying assumption that nursing is concerned with protection, promotion, and restoration of health; prevention of illness; and the alleviation of suffering of patients.[58]

The *Code for Nurses* was adopted by the ANA in 1950 and has undergone revisions over the years. It provides a framework for the nurse in ethical decision making and provides society with a set of expectations of the profession. The Code is "not open to negotiation in employment settings, nor is it permissible for individuals or groups of nurses to adapt or change the language of

AACN POSITION STATEMENT

Withholding and/or withdrawing life-sustaining treatment

ADVANCES IN HEALTHCARE technology have dramatically increased the ability to prolong life. Because of these advances, ethical and legal dilemmas arise when complex therapy is instituted to sustain vital functions, even when there is no hope of reversing the disease processes.

The American Association of Critical-Care Nurses recognizes that critical care nurses have a significant role in supporting a patient's preferences and beliefs about ending treatments of this type.

THEREFORE, AACN resolves that when choices about withholding and/or withdrawing life-sustaining treatments are being considered, critical care nurses should collaborate with individual patients or their surrogates, physicians and other healthcare providers. This should happen in an atmosphere that promotes reasoned deliberation and communication of a patient's preferences and best interests.

To support this resolution, AACN believes that the following elements are essential for nursing practice:

- ◆ Critical care nurses will participate in ongoing assessment of a patient's ability to make decisions about their own health care.
- ◆ Critical care nurses will participate in discussions exploring the patient's beliefs about end of life care at the earliest appropriate time. The best time for discussions and decision-making about withholding and/or withdrawal of life-sustaining treatment is before entry into the health care system.
- ◆ When patients cannot make decisions for themselves, their preferences may be determined from advanced directives (such as living wills or durable power of attorney for health care), previous spoken or written information, and personal lifestyle.
- ◆ Critical care nurses, as patient advocates, will initiate and promote the decision-making process and assure that nursing care goals are consistent with patient preferences or best interests.
- ◆ In the event that life-sustaining treatment is withheld or withdrawn, critical care nurses will participate in planning, implementing, and evaluating supportive care. Supportive care includes providing comfort, hygiene, safe surroundings and emotional support for patients and the family.

Thus AACN believes that health care institutions must have policies that direct a process to withhold and/or withdraw life-sustaining treatment. These policies should include:

- ◆ A process for ongoing review of treatment goals and interventions. The scope of the care the patient will receive should be specified in writing.
- ◆ A process for designating a surrogate when the patient does not have decision-making capacity.
- ◆ A process for dispute resolution among patients, surrogates, and health care team members when there is disagreement about the decision-making process.
- ◆ A process for transferring care of a patient to another qualified critical care nurse, when a decision to withhold and/or withdraw life-sustaining treatment conflicts with the nurse's personal beliefs and values.

This position on withholding and/or withdrawing life-sustaining treatment is based on these beliefs and ethical principles:

1. Individuals have a moral and legal right and responsibility to make decisions about their health care and the use of life-sustaining treatment.
2. There is no moral or legal difference between withholding and withdrawing treatment. Considerations that justify not initiating treatment also justify withdrawing treatment.
3. A person's capacity to make decisions is shown by their ability to understand relevant information, reason, and deliberate about choices, reflect on information according to their individual values and preferences, and communicate their decision to health care providers.
4. The process for decision-making on behalf of incapacitated patients should be directed by the established standards of substituted judgment or best interests.

DEFINITIONS

Advance directives

A document in which a person gives advance directions about medical care or designates who should make medical decisions on their behalf if they should lose decision-making capacity. There are two types of advance directives: treatment directives, such as living wills, and proxy directives, such as durable power of attorney for health care.

Best interest standard

This standard gives priority to the protection of the patient's welfare. In these cases the designated surrogate tries to make a choice on the patient's behalf that seeks to implement what is in the patient's best interests by reference to more objective, societally shared criteria.

Substituted judgment

The doctrine of substituted judgment requires that the surrogate attempt to reach the decision that the incapacitated person would make if he/she were able to choose. This standard preserves the patient's interest in self-determination.

BIBLIOGRAPHY

American Association of Critical-Care Nurses (1989). *Role of the critical care nurse as a patient advocate.* Newport Beach, Ca: Author.

American Nurses' Association (1985). *Code for nurses with interpretive statements.* Kansas City, Mo: Author.

President's Commission for the Study of Ethical Problems in Medicine and Biomedical and Behavioral Research (March 1983). Washington, DC: Government Printing Office.

The Hastings Center (1987). *Guidelines on the termination of life-sustaining treatment and the care of the dying.* Briarcliff Manor, NY: Author.

Adopted by AACN Board of Directors, February 1990.

From American Association of Critical-Care Nurses.

CODE OF ETHICS FOR NURSES

1. The nurse provides services with respect for human dignity and the uniqueness of the client, unrestricted by considerations of social or economic status, personal attributes, or the nature of health problems.
2. The nurse safeguards the client's right to privacy by judiciously protecting information of a confidential nature.
3. The nurse acts to safeguard the client and the public when health care and safety are affected by the incompetent, unethical, or illegal practice of any person.
4. The nurse assumes responsibility and accountability for individual nursing judgments and actions.
5. The nurse maintains competence in nursing.
6. The nurse exercises informed judgment and uses individual competence and qualifications as criteria in seeking consultation, accepting responsibilities, and delegating nursing activities to others.
7. The nurse participates in activities that contribute to the ongoing development of the profession's body of knowledge.
8. The nurse participates in the profession's efforts to implement and improve standards of nursing.
9. The nurse participates in the profession's efforts to establish and maintain conditions of employment conducive to high quality nursing care.
10. The nurse participates in the profession's effort to protect the public from misinformation and misrepresentation and to maintain the integrity of nursing.
11. The nurse collaborates with members of the health professions and other citizens in promoting community and national efforts to meet the health needs of the public.

From American Nurses Association: *Code for nurses with interpretive statements,* Kansas City, Mo, 1985, The Association.

this code."[58] The ANA also suggests that the requirements of the Code may not be in concert with the law and that it is the nurse's obligation to uphold the Code because of the societal commitment inherent in nursing.

The Nurse as Patient Advocate

Winslow[59] described the evolution of nursing ethics from traditional loyalty to physicians to contemporary advocacy of patient rights. The loyalty ethic was based on a military model; advocacy is based on a legal model. He further discussed areas of concern for the nurse when serving in an advocacy role. Patients and their families are sometimes not ready or willing to accept the nurse as an advocate. Advocacy is frequently associated with controversy, and the nurse may experience conflict between interests and loyalties.[59,60] Advocacy "involves an act of free will and a studied choice to view ourselves in a particular way in our relationship to others."[60] Active advocacy reflects the nurse's responsibility and obligation to the patient and incorporates both personal and professional values and standards.[7,61,62]

Curtin[63] delineated four major conditions that cause patients and families to be more vulnerable: loss of independence, loss of freedom of action, interference with the ability to make choices, and the power of health care professionals. If these issues are not addressed, "patients' values are ignored, or replaced with others' values, [and] patients cease to exist as unique human beings."[63]

◆ **Rights protection model.** The legal model of nursing advocacy espoused by Winslow is reflective of the nurse as the protector of patient rights.[13,59] The underlying assumption is that one's rights are violated in the patient role and that assistance is needed in the form of an advocate.

◆ **Values-based decision model.** Inherent in this model is the nurse's respect for the individual's own values and beliefs. It is the responsibility of the nurse to provide information and to clarify it as necessary so that the patient can make informed decisions. Personal values and decisions of the nurse are not imposed on the patient and family.[13] Supporting the patient and family during this process does not necessarily mean agreement with the decision, but rather support of the patient and family to make their own decision.

◆ **Respect-for-persons model.** Respect for the individual as an autonomous decision maker whose human dignity and privacy are to be protected forms the basis for this model. In cases in which patients are unable to determine their own choices, the nurse defers to a surrogate decision maker or advocates in these patients' best interests.[13]

The Risks of Advocacy

As discussed previously, there are occasions in which conflicts exist between professional loyalties. Becker[63a] asserted that assessing risks in an advocate situation will serve to minimize risks to both nurse and patient. There are five important conditions for advocacy. First, the members of the profession must communicate to clarify obligations and responsibilities. Second, open lines of communication among professionals about patient rights must be maintained. Third, it is essential for trust to be established and maintained between the nurse and the patient. Fourth, the nurse must be aware of all conditions and situations related to the health care decision. The fifth condition is that the nurse must remain educated about current legal and ethical trends.

The American Association of Critical-Care Nurses adopted a position statement regarding patient advocacy. The position statement is found in the box on p. 29 and can be used as a guideline for the critical care nurse in any setting.

The Nurse's Obligation to Self

According to Christensen,[64] ethical autonomy forms the basis for professional nursing practice. In this sense,

AACN POSITION STATEMENT
Role of the critical care nurse as patient advocate

THE AMERICAN ASSOCIATION of Critical-Care Nurses believes that patient advocacy is an integral component of critical care nursing practice. Therefore, definitions of advocacy and the behaviors that typify advocacy are essential.

WHEREAS, the *Code for Nurses* (American Nurses Association, 1985) requires that nurses safeguard the patient and the public when health care and safety are affected by the incompetent, unethical, or illegal practice of any person, and

WHEREAS, many definitions of advocacy exist, and

WHEREAS, critical care nurses are confronted with situations that require them to act immediately on the patient's behalf, and

WHEREAS, personal and professional risks are associated with being a patient advocate, and

WHEREAS, state nurse practice acts may require the nurse to be a patient advocate, and

WHEREAS, the process of informed consent mandates that the patient or the patient's surrogate be informed fully and give consent freely, and

WHEREAS, the continuum of advocacy is not limited to the individual but may extend to societal concerns,

THEREFORE, BE IT RESOLVED THAT the American Association of Critical-Care Nurses believes the critical care nurse is a patient advocate,

AND THAT the American Association of Critical-Care Nurses defines advocacy as respecting and supporting the basic values, rights, and beliefs of the critically ill patient.

BE IT FURTHER RESOLVED THAT the American Association of Critical-Care Nurses believes that as a patient advocate, the critical care nurse shall do the following:

1. Respect and support the right of the patient or the patient's designated surrogate to autonomous informed decision making.
2. Intervene when the best interest of the patient is in question.
3. Help the patient obtain necessary care.
4. Respect the values, beliefs, and rights of the patient.
5. Provide education and support to help the patient or the patient's designated surrogate make decisions.
6. Represent the patient in accordance with the patient's choices.
7. Support the decisions of the patient or the patient's designated surrogate or transfer care to an equally qualified critical care nurse.
8. Intercede for patients who cannot speak for themselves in situations that require immediate action.
9. Monitor and safeguard the quality of care the patient receives.
10. Act as liaison between the patient, the patient's family, and health care professionals.

BE IT RESOLVED THAT the American Association of Critical-Care Nurses recognizes that health care institutions are instrumental in providing an environment in which patient advocacy is expected and supported.

ALSO, BE IT FURTHER RESOLVED THAT as patient advocate, critical care nurses initiate and promote actions to improve the health care of the critically ill through social change.

REFERENCE

American Nurses' Association (1985). *Code for nurses with interpretive statements.* Kansas City, Mo: Author.

Adopted by AACN Board of Directors, August 1989.

From American Association of Critical-Care Nurses.

autonomy denotes thinking for oneself, not unlimited freedom of choice. Both clinical practice and ethical elements are inherent in professional nursing competence, and the nurse must incorporate both elements into practice.

Ethical dilemmas surround the critical care nurse on a daily basis. Exposure to frequent moral and ethical conflicts may affect the nurse in the form of burnout or resignation.[9] Dallery[52] posited that there is a moral dilemma of mixed loyalties for the professional. Scientific and theoretic knowledge learned outside the practice setting are difficult to fully incorporate in a different social context, such as the critical care setting. Nursing is based both on caring and on a contract with society to perform nursing. Thus a conflict in professional loyalties occurs.

Results from a survey of more than 1100 critical care nurses revealed that ethical issues encountered in daily critical care practice revolve around many areas[65] (see box, p. 30). Other issues dealt with on a daily basis include "floating,"[66] "covering-up" for colleagues,[67] confidentiality and computerization,[68] and inadequate staffing patterns.[69]

Jameton[70] described one's integrity as being compromised when professional and personal conflicts arise. This most frequently occurs when the nurse is highly dedicated, which leads to a conflict between professional care and self-care. The emotional strains of caring for critically ill patients must balance with personal rewards for the nurse. Personal values and principles may conflict with those of the profession or institution. This conflict with personal identity must be resolved. The duty to self in this situation is to express one's own moral convictions to others. Jameton purported, however, that integration of one's own personal identity with professional identity is possible.[70]

IMPORTANT ETHICAL ISSUES FOR CRITICAL CARE NURSES

ISSUE	% RESPONSE
Conflicts with physicians related to ethical issues	29%
Long-term patients in critical care	20%
Withholding and withdrawing of treatment	8%
Withholding and withdrawing of food and fluids	8%
Conflict with families or designated patient surrogate	7%
DNR policy	6%
Whistleblowing	4%
Ethics management	4%
Advance directives (durable power of attorney for health care/living wills)	3%
Conflict with nursing staff related to ethical issues	3%
Informed consent	2%

STEPS IN ETHICAL DECISION MAKING

1. Identify the health problem.
2. Define the ethical issue.
3. Gather additional information.
4. Delineate the decision maker.
5. Examine ethical and moral principles.
6. Explore alternative options.
7. Implement decisions.
8. Evaluate and modify actions.

ETHICAL DECISION MAKING IN CRITICAL CARE

The Nurse's Role

As discussed earlier in this chapter, the critical care nurse encounters ethical issues on a daily basis. Although the nurse may feel powerless regarding the ability to influence ethical decisions,[71] this need not be the case. Because the nurse is on the "front line" with such issues as DNR, response to treatments, and application of new technologies and new protocols, she or he may be the one who best knows the patient's and/or family's wishes about treatment prolongation or cessation. Therefore it is important that the nurse be included as part of the health care team that determines ethical dilemma resolution.

What is an Ethical Dilemma?

In general, ethical cases are not always clear-cut or black and white, but rather arise in settings and circumstances that involve innumerable side issues and distractions.[72,73] The most common ethical dilemmas encountered in critical care are foregoing treatment and allocating the scarce resource of critical care. But how does one know that a true ethical dilemma exists?

Before the application of any decision model, a decision must be made about the existence of a true ethical dilemma. Thompson and Thompson[6] delineated the following criteria for defining moral and ethical dilemmas in clinical practice:

1. Awareness of different options
2. An issue with different options
3. Two or more options with true or "good" aspects and the choice of one over the other compromises the option not chosen

Krekeler asserted that ethical situations arise when "the moral decision of one person conflicts with the moral decision of another. Both decisions may be good for each individual in question and undoubtedly are made according to their traditional values."[9] What complicates this process is when there is a third person involved, as is the case in most treatment care decisions in the critical care areas.

Steps in Ethical Decision Making

To facilitate the ethical decision process, a model or framework must be used so that all involved will consistently and clearly examine the multiple ethical issues that arise in critical care. Steps in ethical decision making are listed in the box above.

◆ **Step one.** First, the major aspects of the medical and health problem must be identified. In other words, the scientific basis of the problem, potential sequelae, prognosis, and all data relevant to the health status must be examined.

◆ **Step two.** The ethical problem must be clearly delineated from other types of problems. Systems problems—that is, those resulting from failures and inadequacies in the organization and operation of the health care facility and the health care system as a whole—are often misinterpreted as being ethical issues. Occasionally, a social problem that stems from conditions existing in the community, state, or country as a whole is also confused with ethical issues. Social problems can lead to a systemic problem, which can constrain responses to ethical problems.

◆ **Step three.** Although categories of necessary additional information will vary, whatever is missing in the initial problem presentation should be obtained. If not already known, the health prognosis and potential sequelae should be clarified. Usual demographic data—such as age, ethnicity, religious preferences, and educational and economic status—may be considered in the decision process. The role of the family or extended family and other support systems needs to be examined. Any desires that the patient may have expressed either in writing or in conversation about treatment decisions are essential to obtain.

◆ **Step four.** The patient is the primary decision maker and autonomously makes these decisions after receiving information about the alternatives and sequelae of

LEGAL REVIEW: Understaffing and nursing liability

Application of the professional malpractice standard to critical care nursing and increased recognition afforded to nurses by state and federal legislation and the judiciary have extended nursing liability into new areas. These include overwork, understaffing, and "floating" nurses into unfamiliar care settings, all of which potentially compromise patient care. The resulting legal dilemma is that, although hospitals and nurse supervisors can be derelict in their staffing decisions, it is the staff nurse who may be liable in tort or subject to sanctions by the state for the results of those decisions.

As a general rule, nurses do not have statutory protection against understaffing or excessive consecutive number of hours worked. However, many states have regulations that address the minimal competency and training requirements for nurses who "float" or are assigned to unfamiliar areas.

The ANA *Code for Nurses* addresses nursing accountability for individual judgment and actions and criteria for accepting responsibilities, delegating activities to others, and seeking consultation. Nurse supervisors have legal duties (1) to supervise, (2) to properly assign tasks, and (3) to allocate and assign sufficient numbers of trained staff.

In the case of *Leavitt v. St. Tammany Parish Hospital,* the plaintiff-patient fell after the staff failed to respond to her call for help. The defendant-hospital was found liable for failure to have on duty a sufficient number of staff members to respond to the patients' needs. In this particular case, nurses were not named as defendants. However, the court stated in its opinion that the nurses knew of the patient's debilitated condition, yet despite this knowledge failed to take measures to prevent a foreseeable injury. The court concluded that the nurses breached their duty of reasonable care owed to the plaintiff.

It is inadvisable to document inadequate staffing in the medical record. However, nurses subject to understaffing and assignments in unfamiliar units should be thoroughly familiar with their state board of nursing position statement on the issue and their hospital's policies and procedures. Nurses should also keep notes of all efforts taken to remedy the problem, consistently communicate the problem to their superiors, and refuse to acquiesce to a pattern of understaffing or assignments to patient care areas with which they are unfamiliar.

The 1974 amendments to the National Labor Relations Act (NLRA) extended the jurisdiction of the National Labor Relations Board (NLRB) to voluntary and nonprofit hospitals. In *Misericordia Hosp. Medical Center v. NLRB,* the NLRB ordered the reinstatement of a nurse terminated for submitting data that described nursing staff shortages in a JCAH report. The court upheld the jurisdiction extended to the NLRB and the protections the agency gave nurses from dismissal and termination as a result of efforts to improve their working conditions.

See Hoffman NA: Nursing and the future of health care: the independent practice imperative, *Specialty L Dig.: Health Care* 160:7, 1992; *Leavitt v St. Tammany Parish Hosp.,* 396 So.2d 406 (La App 1981); *Misericordia Hosp Medical Center v NLRB,* 623 F2d 808 (2d Cir 1980); and Politis EK: Nurses' legal dilemma: when hospital staffing compromises professional standards, *USFL Rev* 18(1):109, 1983.

treatments or lack of treatments. However, in many ethical dilemmas, the patient is not competent to make a decision, as occurs when he or she is comatose or otherwise physically or mentally unable to make a decision. It is in these situations that surrogates are designated or court appointed, because the urgency of the situation requires a quick decision. Although the decision process and ultimate decision are more important than who makes the decision, delineating the decision maker is an important step in the process.[6]

Others who are involved in the decision should also be identified at this time, such as family, nurse, physician, social worker, clergy, and any other members of disciplines having close contact with the patient. The role of the nurse should be examined. There may not be a need for a nurse decision; rather the nurse may provide additional information and support to the decision maker.

◆ **Step five.** Personal values, beliefs, and moral convictions of all involved in the decision process should be known. Whether actually achieved through a group meeting or through personal introspection, values clarification facilitates the decision process. Professional ethical codes of the nurse and physician will serve as a foundation for future decisions. At this time, legal constraints or previous legal decisions for circumstances at hand will need to be assessed and acknowledged.

General ethical principles need to be examined in relation to the case at hand. For instance, are veracity, informed consent, and autonomy promoted? Beneficence and nonmaleficence will be analyzed as they relate to the patient's condition and desires. Close examination of these principles will reveal any compromise of ethical or moral principles for either the patient or the health care provider and assist in decision making.

◆ **Step six.** After the identification of alternative options, the outcome of each action must be predicted. This analysis helps one to select the option with the best "fit" for the specific situation or problem. Both short-range and long-range consequences of each action must be examined, and new or creative actions should be encouraged. Consideration should also be given to the "no action" option, which is also a choice.[6]

◆ **Step seven.** When a decision has been reached, it is usually after much thought and consideration, and rarely does complete agreement occur among all interested persons.[6] Krekeler described following the action until the actual results of the decision can be seen.[9] Fowler stated that the decision may need to be modified to meet legal or policy requirements.[74]

◆ **Step eight.** Evaluation of an ethical decision serves to both assess the decision at hand and use it as a basis for future ethical decisions. If outcomes are not as predicted, it may be possible to modify the plan or to use an alternative that was not originally chosen.

STRATEGIES FOR PROMOTION OF ETHICAL DECISION MAKING

The complexity of health care and frequent ethical dilemmas encountered in clinical practice demand the establishment of mechanisms to address ethical issues found in hospitals and health care facilities. Four types of mechanisms are discussed briefly: institutional ethics committees, inservice and education, nursing ethics committees, and ethics rounds and conferences.

Institutional Ethics Committees (IECs)

Although not required by law, many health care facilities have developed IECs as a way to review ethical cases that are problematic for the practitioner.[75,76] The three major functions of IECs are education, consultation, and recommendation to policy-making bodies. Kemp[77] identified three models of IECs. In the *optional-optional model,* committees serve as consultants and make recommendations that are not binding. The *optional-mandatory model* requires that health care providers consult with the committees when there is an ethical problem, but recommendations are again not binding. The *mandatory-mandatory model* requires that ethical dilemmas be presented to the committee and recommendations must be followed.

IECs are very often committees comprising executive medical staff. Membership may include staff physicians, administrators, legal counsel, nurses, social workers, clergy, and community public volunteers. To fulfill its requirement for consultation, the committee must include members that not only have expertise, but also are representative of various groups. Regardless of the type of committee model, consultation and support become available to the practitioners.

Inservice and Education

Basic education about ethical principles and decision making is an important first step in facilitating ethical decision making among nursing staff in the critical care area. It is important for nurses to examine their own values, beliefs, and moral convictions. The ANA *Code for Nurses* should be known and used by nurses in their daily clinical practice. Treatment choices for patients and ethical issues involving patients, nurses, and medical colleagues should be explored and discussed in the classroom setting where no time constraints or extraneous distractions exist to interrupt the decision process.

Nursing Ethics Committees

Nursing ethics committees provide a forum in which nurses can discuss ethical issues that are pertinent to nurses at the individual, unit, or department level.[78] Unlike the IEC, which involves treatment choices of patients, the nursing committee may or may not involve a patient situation. Depending on the specific goals of the committee, it can also serve as a resource to nursing staff, make recommendations to a policy-making body about a variety of professional issues, or actually formulate policies. It may also serve to educate the department on ethical and professional issues. Membership usually comprises representatives from all major clinical areas or divisions, educators, clinical nurse specialists, administrators, and other specialty staff. Some departments such as critical care may have their own unit or division committee.

Ethics Rounds and Conferences

Ethics rounds at the unit level on patients in the unit can be done by nurses on a weekly or otherwise established basis. Rounds educate the staff to problems and serve to be "preventive" when facilitated appropriately.[74] During the discussions, potential problems may be identified early and actions taken to decrease or prevent a future problem. An individual patient ethics conference can be scheduled to include only the nursing staff or to include a multidisciplinary group to discuss unit issues. A patient ethics conference may function either as a liaison with the IEC or as an end in itself.

SUMMARY

The emergence of critical care as a specialty and the introduction of sophisticated technologic innovations into critical care units have had a great impact on health care professional practices. Ethical dilemmas are encountered daily in the practice of critical care. The criticality of the situation and speed that is required to make decisions often prevent practitioners from gaining insight into the desires, values, and feelings of patients. The practitioner is often left with no clear ethical or legal guidelines, particularly in the fast-paced modern critical care unit. By assuming a solely technologic approach, practitioners will violate the rights of patients and their professional codes of ethics.

By using an ethical decision-making process, the rights of the patient will be protected and logical analysis of the case will lead to a decision that is made in the best interests of the patient. It is through moral reasoning and examining, weighing, justifying, and choosing ethical principles that patient rights and individuality will be upheld. The practice of nursing is built on a foundation of moral and ethical caring, and the critical care nurse is pivotal in identifying ethical patient situations and can participate in the decision-making process.

REFERENCES

1. Rudy E, Grenvik A: Future of critical care, *Am J Crit Care* 1(1):33, 1992.
2. Scott JL: Ethical issues: a Washington perspective, *Nurs Manage* 23(1):52, 1992.
3. Fairman J: Watchful vigilance: nursing care, technology, and the development of intensive care units, *Nurs Res* 41(1):56, 1992.
4. Wlody G, Smith S: Ethical dilemmas in critical care, *Focus Crit Care* 12:41, 1985.
5. Guralnik D, editor: *Webster's new world dictionary of the American language,* New York, 1981, Simon & Shuster.
6. Thompson J, Thompson H: *Bioethical decision-making for nurses,* Norwalk, Conn, 1985, Appleton-Century-Crofts.
7. Fowler M: Introduction to ethics and ethical theory: a road map to the discipline. In Fowler M, Levine-Ariff J, editors: *Ethics at the bedside,* Philadelphia, 1987, JB Lippincott.
8. Davis A, Aroskar M: *Ethical dilemmas and nursing practice,* Norwalk, Conn, 1983, Appleton-Century-Crofts.
9. Krekeler K: Critical care nursing and moral development, *Crit Care Nurs* 10(2):1, 1987.
10. Young S: The nurse manager: clarifying issues in professional role responsibility, *Pediatr Nurs* 13(6):430, 1987.
11. Jameton A: Duties to self: professional nursing in the critical care unit. In Fowler M, Levine-Ariff J, editors: *Ethics at the bedside,* Philadelphia, 1987, JB Lippincott.
12. Luckenbill-Brett J, Stuhler-Schlag M: Mandatory reporting: legal and ethical issues, *J Nurs Adm* 17(12):32, 1987.
13. Fry S: Autonomy, advocacy, and accountability: ethics at the bedside. In Fowler M, Levine-Ariff J, editors: *Ethics at the bedside,* Philadelphia, 1987, JB Lippincott.
14. Miller B: Autonomy and the refusal of lifesaving treatment, *Hasting's Cent Rep* 11:22, 1981.
15. Ott B, Nieswiadomy RM: Support of patient autonomy in the do not resusitate decision, *Heart Lung* 20(1):66, 1991.
16. Singleton KA, Dever R: The challenge of autonomy: respecting the patient's wishes, *DCCN* 10(3):160, 1991.
17. Omery A: The new patient self-determination act: increasing emphasis on patient autonomy, *DCCN* 10(3):123, 1991.
18. Flynn P: Questions of risk, duty, and paternalism: problems in beneficence. In Fowler M, Levine-Ariff, editors: *Ethics at the bedside,* Philadelphia, 1987, JB Lippincott.
19. Nightingale F: *Notes on nursing,* Toronto, 1969, Dover Publications.
20. Aroskar M: Fidelity and veracity: questions of promise keeping, truth telling and loyalty. In Fowler M, Levine-Ariff J, editors: *Ethics at the bedside,* Philadelphia, 1987, JB Lippincott.
21. Schmeltzer M, Anema M: Should nurses ever lie to patients? *Image J Nurs Sch* 20:110, 1988.
22. Washington G: Trust: a critical element in critical care nursing, *Focus Crit Care* 17(5):418, 1990.
23. Veatch R, Fry S: *Case studies in nursing ethics,* Philadelphia, 1987, JB Lippincott.
24. Omery A: A healthy death, *Heart Lung* 20(3):310, 1991.
25. Levine-Ariff J: Justice and the allocation of scarce nursing resources in critical care nursing. In Fowler M, Levine-Ariff J, editors: *Ethics at the bedside,* Philadelphia, 1987, JB Lippincott.
26. Veatch R: DRGs and the ethical reallocation of resources, *Hastings Cent Rep* 16:32, 1986.
27. Englehardt T, Rie M: Intensive care units, scarce resources, and conflicting principles of justice, *JAMA* 255:1159, 1986.
28. Evans R: Health care technology and the inevitability of resource allocation and rationing decisions. Part I, *JAMA* 249:2047, 1983.
29. Callahan D: Terminating treatment: age as a standard, *Hastings Cent Rep* 17:21, 1987.
30. White J: Rationing health care resources, *Nurs Connect* 4(1):22, 1991.
31. Norris MK: Required request: why it has not significantly improved the donor shortage, *Heart Lung* 19(6):685, 1990.
32. Vernale C, Packard S: Organ donation as gift exchange, *Image J Nurs Sch* 22(4):239, 1990.
33. Vernale C: Critical care nurses' interactions with families of potential organ donors, *Focus Crit Care* 18(4):335, 1991.
34. Birkholz G: IABP: legal and ethical issues, *DCCN* 4:285, 1985.
35. Nolan K: In death's shadow: the meaning of withholding resuscitation, *Hastings Cent Rep* 17:8, 1987.
36. Davison R, Davison L: Medical experimentation: ethics in high technology, *Crit Care Nurs* 10:27, 1987.
37. Danis M, Churchill LR: Autonomy and the common weal, *Hastings Cent Rep* 21:25, 1991.
38. O'Malley NC: Age-based rationing of health care: a descriptive study of professional attitudes, *Health Care Manage Rev* 16(1):83, 1991.
39. Koska M: Can outcomes data help patients make end-of-life decisions? *Hospitals* June 5, 1991, p. 42.
40. Levine M: Ration or rescue: the elderly patient in critical care, *Crit Care Nurse Q* 12(1):82, 1989.
41. Wood C: Health care rationing: the Oregon experiment, *Nurs Econ* 9(4):239, 1991.
42. Campbell M, Field B: Management of the patient with do not resusitate status: compassion and cost containment, *Heart Lung* 20(4):345, 1991.
43. Oleson M: Subjectively perceived quality of life, *Image J Nurs Sch* 22(3):187, 1990.
44. Kleinpell RM: Concept analysis of quality of life, *DCCN* 10(4):223, 1991.
45. O'Mara R: Dilemmas in cardiac surgery: artificial heart and left ventricular assist device, *Crit Care Nurs* 10:48, 1987.
46. Knaus W: Rationing, justice, and the American physician, *JAMA* 255:1176, 1986.
47. Pinch W: Allocation of scarce resources: critical care nursing dilemma, *DCCN* 4:164, 1985.
48. Quigley FM: Withdrawing treatment, *Focus Crit Care* 17(6):464, 1990.
49. Wurzbach ME: The dilemma of withholding or withdrawing nutrition, *Image J Nurs Sch* 22(4):226, 1990.
50. Cranford R: The persistent vegetative state: the medical reality (getting the facts straight), *Hastings Cent Rep* 18:27, 1988.
51. Schneiderman LJ, Jecker NS, Jonsen AR: Medical futility: its meaning and ethical implications, *Ann Int Med* 112(12):949, 1990.
52. Dallery A: Professional loyalties, *Holistic Nurs Prac* 1:64, 1986.
53. Packard J, Ferrara M: In search of the moral foundation of nursing, *ANS* 10:60, 1988.
54. Yarling R, McElmurry B: The moral foundation of nursing, *ANS* 8:63, 1986.
55. Curtin L: Ethics in nursing practice, *Nurs Manage* 19:7, 1988.
56. Cianci M: The code of ethics and the role of nurses: an historical perspective, *Nurs Connect* 5(1):37, 1992.
57. Miller BK, Beck L, Adams D: Nurses' knowledge of the code for nurses, *J Contin Educ Nurs* 22(5):198, 1991.
58. American Nurses Association: *Code for nurses with interpretive statements,* Kansas City, Mo, 1985.
59. Winslow G: From loyalty to advocacy: a new metaphor for nursing, *Hastings Cent Rep* 14:32, 1984.
60. Nelson M: Advocacy in nursing, *Nurs Outlook* 36:136, 1988.
61. Evans SA: Critical care nursing: the ordinary is extraordinary, *Heart Lung* 20(3):21A, 1991.
62. Johanson WL: A scarce and available resource, *Heart Lung* 20(5):19A, 1991.
63. Curtin L: The nurse as advocate: a philosophic foundation for nursing, *ANS* 1:1, 1979.

63a. Becker PH: Advocacy in nursing: perils and possibilities, *Holistic Nurs Pract* 1(1):54, 1986.

64. Christensen P: An ethical framework for nursing service administration, *ANS* 10:46, 1988.
65. Hartwell JL, Lavandero R: What's important to critical care nurses? *Focus Crit Care* 18(5):364, 1991.
66. Yocke JM: Floating out of ICU: the ethical dilemmas. I. The ethical case, *DCCN,* 11(2):104, 1992.
67. Pinch WJ: Nursing ethics: is "cover-up" ever "harmless"? *Nurs Manage* 21(9):60, 1990.
68. Faaoso N: Automated patient systems: the ethical impact, *Nurs Manage* 23(7):46, 1992.
69. Berger MC, Seversen A, Chvatal R: Ethical issues in nursing, *West J Nurs Res* 13(4):514, 1991.
70. Jameton A: Duties to self: professional nursing ethics in the critical care unit. In Fowler M, Levine-Ariff J, editors: *Ethics at the bedside,* Philadelphia, 1987, JB Lippincott.
71. Erlen JA, Frost B: Nurses' perceptions of powerlessness in influencing ethical decisions, *West J Nurs Res* 13(3):397, 1991.
72. Broom C: Conflict resolution strategies: when ethical dilemmas evolve into conflict, *DCCN* 10(6):354, 1991.
73. Wicclair MR: Differentiating ethical decisions from clinical standards, *DCCN* 10(5):280, 1991.
74. Fowler M: Piecing together the ethical puzzle: operationalizing nursing's ethics in critical care. In Fowler M, Levine-Ariff J, editors: *Ethics at the bedside,* 1987, Philadelphia, JB Lippincott.
75. Bushy A, Raub JR: Implementing and ethics committee in rural institutions, *JONA* 21(12):18, 1991.
76. Feutz-Harter SA: Ethics committees: a resource for patient care decision-making, *JONA* 21(4):11, 1991.
77. Kemp V: The role of critical care nurses in the ethical decision-making process, *DCCN* 4:354, 1985.
78. Buchanan S, Cook L: Nursing ethics committees: the time is now, *Nurs Manage* 23(8):40, 1992.

3

Legal Issues

CHAPTER OBJECTIVES

- Identify legal and professional obligations of critical care nurses.
- Define sources of law and types of enforcement.
- Identify classifications of tort law.
- Describe the elements of certain torts that may result from critical care nursing practice.
- Describe theories of liability.
- Identify sources of critical care nursing standards of practice.
- Relate critical care practices and risk management strategies.
- Define the state's role in regulating critical care nursing practice.
- Identify and discuss specific legal issues in critical care nursing practice in the text and in legal abstracts.

CRITICAL CARE NURSING PRACTICE: LEGAL OBLIGATIONS OVERVIEW

The efforts of nurses to be recognized as independent health care practitioners have recently begun to reach fruition in the legal system.[1] The American Nurses Association (ANA) Code for Nurses offers, among others, the following guidelines[2]:

1. Nurses assume accountability and responsibility for individual nursing judgments and actions.
2. Nurses exercise informed judgments and use individual competence and qualifications as criteria for seeking consultation, accepting responsibility, and delegating nursing activities to others.
3. Nurses collaborate with others to meet the health needs of their patients.
4. Nurses maintain the professional image and integrity of the nursing profession.
5. Nurses maintain employment conditions conducive to high quality nursing care and strive to implement and improve nursing standards.
6. Nurses engage in ongoing professional development.
7. Nurses respect their patients' right to privacy and provide patients with protection and safeguards.

The scope of critical care nursing practice has been defined by the American Association of Critical-Care Nurses (AACN) as follows[3]:

Critical care nursing practice is a dynamic process, the scope of which is defined in terms of the critically ill patient, the critical care nurse and the environment in which critical care nursing is delivered; all three components are essential elements for the practice of critical care nursing. The critically ill patient is characterized by the presence of real or potential life-threatening health problems and by the requirement for continuous observation and intervention to prevent complications and restore health. The concept of the critically ill patient includes the patient's family and/or significant others. The critical care nurse is a registered professional nurse committed to ensuring that all critically ill patients receive optimal care.

In *Nursing: A Social Policy Statement,* the ANA defines nursing as the diagnosis and treatment of human problems.[4] Critical care nursing is that specialty within nursing that deals specifically with human responses to life-threatening problems.[5] The AACN has developed standards of practice specifically for the care of critically ill persons.[6]

These standards and definitions raise important legal and professional issues[7]:

- The critical care nurse has legal obligations to the patient, the critical care setting, and the environment.
- The above-referenced ANA and AACN definitions speak to the fact that the nurse deals with life-threatening health problems. In this context, nursing errors are quite likely to cause substantial injuries, if not death, to a patient. Risk of liability is significant.
- The nurse has an obligation to provide continuous observation and intervention.
- The patient includes more than the individual for whom care is being provided; the family or significant other must also receive attention.
- The nurse is licensed by the state and has legal obligations to the public to perform her or his duties in a safe and competent manner.
- The critical care nurse's legal duties are those of a specialist, one with specialized knowledge and skill. These duties involve a higher standard of care, and the courts are applying with increasing frequency the professional malpractice standard in claims alleging nursing negligence.

Legal Relationships

When a nurse commences employment in a critical care facility and assumes the care of a patient, a relationship is created between patient and nurse and between employer and nurse. Every state has a law mandating entry level educational requirements to become licensed to practice nursing. Thus the act of licensing creates a legal relationship between the nurse and the state.

These relationships impose legal obligations. For example, the nurse owes a patient the duty of reasonable and prudent care under the circumstances. The nurse owes the employer the duty of competency and the ability to follow policies and procedures; other contractual duties may exist as well. The nurse owes the state and public the duty of safe, competent practice as legally defined by practice standards.

The critical care nurse's legal duties are enforceable, and the nurse can be held legally accountable for breach or violation through a variety of laws and legal processes. The boxes below list sources of law and systems of enforcement. Nurses, hospitals, patients, and other health care providers are involved in a variety of legal disputes, including negligence and professional malpractice, incompetence, unauthorized practice, unprofessional or illegal conduct, and workers' compensation, contract, and labor disputes.[8]

Membership in professional associations obliges the nurse to subscribe and adhere to standards defined by the associations. For example, in addition to its own standards for nursing care, the AACN advises the critical care nurse to adhere to the Code of Ethics of the American Nurses Association.

Nurses' professional duties are further delineated and clarified by the practice standards of professional associations to which a nurse belongs and by the policies and procedures of the employing institution. For example, state nurses' associations are required to enforce the ANA's Code for Nurses and have established standards of nursing practice. Likewise, the AACN, Association of Operating Room Nurses (AORN), Emergency Department Nurses' Association (EDNA), American Association of Pediatric Nurse Practitioners (AAPNP), and myriad other professional organizations have identified standards of practice and guidelines in a variety of areas. Many of these organizations offer certification after completion of a specialized course of study and an examination. Certification is renewed periodically on satisfaction of academic and/or clinical practice requirements. The box on p. 37 offers a comprehensive list of sources of critical care nursing standards.

The scope of legal issues in nursing is broad. For example, in the past 2 decades health law as a specialty has evolved, embracing more than 60 subspecialty areas of practice.[9] Because of this, this chapter's discussion is necessarily limited to the objectives delineated at the beginning of the chapter. Nurses should seek their own legal advice and counsel for any questions and concerns and not rely on the overview of material provided in this chapter.

TORT LIABILITY

The area of civil law is divided into many categories, two of which are *contracts* and *torts*. The law of contracts contains a set of rules governing the creation and enforcement of an agreement between two or more parties (entities or individuals). A tort is a type of civil wrong, meaning that a dispute resulted from an occurrence between the parties.

Tort law is generally divided into intentional and unintentional torts, strict liability, and specific torts. The box below classifies torts and lists examples within each category.

SOURCES OF LAW

- Federal and state statutes/legislation (Statutory law)
- Federal and state rules and regulations (Administrative law)
- Federal and state constitutions (Constitutional law)
- Federal and state judicial opinions (Case law or common law)

DIFFERENT SYSTEMS THROUGH WHICH LAW IS ENFORCED

- Civil
- Criminal
- Administrative (Regulatory administration)

CLASSIFICATION OF TORTS

INTENTIONAL TORTS

Assault
Battery
False imprisonment
Trespass
Infliction of emotional distress

SPECIFIC TORTS

Defamation
  Slander
  Libel
Invasion of privacy

UNINTENTIONAL TORTS

Negligence
Medical/nursing treatment torts
  Professional malpractice
Abandonment

STRICT LIABILITY

Products liability

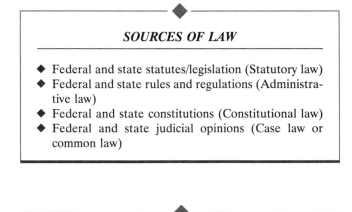

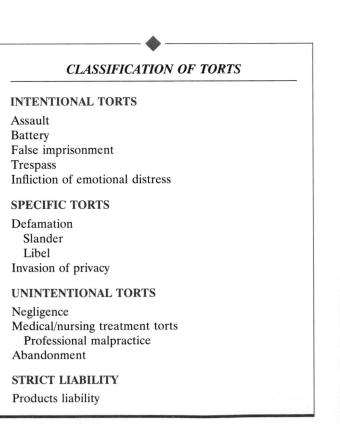

SOURCES OF CRITICAL CARE NURSING STANDARDS AND GUIDELINES

Federal and state statutes
- Americans with Disabilities Act (ADA)
- Basic Health Care for All Americans Act
- Consolidated Omnibus Reconciliations Act of 1985 (COBRA)
- Employee Retirement Income Security Act (ERISA)
- Federal Food, Drug, and Cosmetic Act of 1938
- Federal Privacy Act of 1974
- Federal and state public health statutes
- Federal Rehabilitation Act
- Health Care Quality Improvement Act
- Individuals with Disabilities Act (IDA)
- Medical Devices Amendments of 1976 of the Federal Food, Drug, and Cosmetic Act
- National Organ Transplant Act of 1984
- National Research Act of 1974
  - National Commission for Protection of Human Subjects of Biomedical and Behavioral Research of 1974
  - President's Commission for the Study of Ethical Problems in Medicine and Biomedical and Behavioral Research of 1978
- Omnibus Budget Reconciliations Act (OBRA) of 1986 and 1987
- Patient Self-Determination Act (OBRA of 1990)
- Social Security Act
- State nurse practice acts
- Uniform Anatomical Gift Act of 1968
- Uniform Determination of Death Act of 1980

Federal and state regulations and recommendations
- Centers for Disease Control (CDC) Recommendations
  - Guidelines for Protecting the Safety and Health of Health Care Workers (1988)
  - Prevention of HIV Transmission in Health Care Settings
- Department of Health and Human Services (DHHS)
- Food and Drug Administration
- Medicare and Medicaid regulations of the Federal Social Security Act
- Occupational Safety and Health Administration (OSHA)
  - Regulations enforcing CDC recommendations
  - Regulations enforcing the worker's right to a safe workplace
- State Board of Nursing Rules and Regulations
  - Declaratory Rulings
  - Position Statements
- State Health Department Regulations and Guidelines

Accrediting organizations
- Joint Commission on Accreditation of Healthcare Organizations (JCAHO)
  - Accreditation Manual for Hospitals (1991)
  - Education Medical Device Users (1989)
  - Standards of Nursing Practice (1991)

Hospital policy and procedure manuals

Professional association statements and standards
- American Association of Critical-Care Nurses
  - Certification Standards
  - Position Statements
    - Certification in Cardiopulmonary Resuscitation for all Health Professionals (1981)
    - Collaborative Practice Model: The Organization of Human Resources in Critical Care Units (1982)
    - Definition of Critical Care Nursing (1984)
    - Ethics in Critical Care Research (1984)
    - Principles of Critical Care Nursing Practice (1981)
    - Scope of Critical Care Nursing Practice (1986)
    - Use of Technical Personnel in Critical Care Settings (1983)
  - Standards for Nursing Care of the Critical Ill (1989)
  - Ethics at the Bedside: A Source Book for the Critical Care Nurse (1987)
- American Heart Association
  - Cardiovascular Nursing (serial)
  - Textbook of Advanced Cardiac Life Support (1987)
- American Hospital Association
  - Nurse Staffing Based on Patient Classification (1983)
  - American Hospital Association Society for Healthcare Planning and Marketing: Planning for AIDS Care (1990)
  - American Hospital Association Special Committee on Biomedical Ethics: Values in Conflict Resolving Ethical Issues (1985)
- American Nurses Association
  - Standards of Clinical Nursing Practice (1991)
  - Classification System for Describing Nursing (1989)
  - Code for Nurses with Interpretive Statements (1985)
  - Nursing: A Social Policy Statement (1981)
  - Statutory Requirements for Licensure of Nurses (1985)
  - Scope of Nursing Practice (1987)
  - Position Statements:
    - Guidelines on Withholding/Withdrawing Feedings
    - HIV Testing in Health Care Workers

Testimony by nurse expert witnesses

Literature: Textbooks and journals

Professional education programs and continuing nursing education programs

Intentional torts involve (1) intent and (2) an act. Intent exists when the actor intends to achieve a particular outcome and consequence. Assault, battery, false imprisonment, trespass, and infliction of emotional distress are all examples of intentional torts. In each of these torts, a specific act is required and there is intentional interference with the person or property.

In *assault,* the act is behavior that places the plaintiff (the one being wronged who later sues) in fear or apprehension of offensive physical contact. The person being sued for wronging another in civil law is referred to as the *defendant. Battery* is the unlawful or offensive touching of, or contact with, the plaintiff or something attached to the plaintiff. *False imprisonment* is detaining, confining, or restraining another against his or her will.

There are two types of *trespass:* one type involves a person's land, and the other involves his or her personal property. These acts are defined as unauthorized entry onto land of another or unauthorized handling of another's personal property. In addition, the law protects a person's interest in peace of mind through the tort claim of *infliction of mental or emotional distress.* The act here, however, must be one of extreme misconduct or outrageous behavior.

Nurses can avoid allegations of such torts by the following:

- Reasonably assuring patients that the nursing care is part of an acceptable treatment plan.
- Asking patients for their consent before giving care. (In addition, many hospital policies require that the nurse validate that the patient's physician has also obtained informed consent for medical treatment.)
- Determining whether and when the patient needs self-protection or needs to be restrained to protect others from harm, and taking steps to protect the patient or others by following established protocols, hospital policies, and state regulations governing the use of restraints. (It is important to note that an erroneous decision regarding the use of physical restraints may lead to allegations of malpractice, failure to obtain informed consent, false imprisonment, or battery. It is the nurse's responsibility to exercise independent judgment in making a nursing diagnosis where restraints may be clinically indicated. In some jurisdictions a physician order may also be required. The nurse must also assess whether the patient has the capacity to give or withhold informed consent. One should determine whether the patient has been legally declared incompetent or whether the patient has a guardian or surrogate decision maker. Most jurisdictions apply the "least restrictive alternative" standard. The nurse should know the institutional policy and procedure for the use of restraints and request the patient who refuses restraints to sign a release of liability.[10])
- Handling the patient's personal effects in a safe, secure manner and following hospital policies regarding patient valuables.
- Avoiding extreme, outrageous behavior by delivering care according to generally accepted standards of care.

Unintentional torts involve failures or breach of nursing duties that lead to harm, including negligence, malpractice, and abandonment. *Negligence* is the failure to meet an ordinary standard of care, resulting in injury to the patient or plaintiff. *Malpractice* is a type of professional liability based on negligence and includes professional misconduct, breach of a duty or standard of care, illegal or immoral conduct, or failure to exercise reasonable skill, all of which lead to harm. A more complete outline of the elements of these torts will follow.

Abandonment is a type of negligence in which a duty to give care exists, is ignored, and results in harm to a patient. It is the absence of care and the failure to respond to a patient that may give rise to an allegation of abandonment.

Nurses can avoid allegations of unintentional torts by the following:

- Identifying the duty owed, knowing what the duty consists of, and providing nursing care that meets that duty or standard of care.
- Applying the nursing process to patient care problems: consistent and timely assessment, diagnosis, plan and implementation, and evaluation.
- Documenting the care that was delivered and participating in activities that minimize the opportunity for patient harm and exposure to liability. (These are commonly known as risk management strategies, several of which will be discussed.)

Specific torts involve privacy interests and interests one has in his or her reputation. Invasion of privacy and defamation are both examples of such torts. *Defamation* is composed of two torts, *slander* (oral defamation) and *libel* (written defamation). Defamation is not the mere statement or writing of words that injures one's reputation or good name. The words must be communicated to another, and if the words are true, this may provide a defense against a defamation claim. *Invasion of privacy* involves the violation of a person's right to privacy. Nurses can invade another's privacy by revealing confidential information without authorization or by failing to follow the patient's health care decisions.

Nurses can avoid allegations of these specific claims by (1) making statements about another's reputation only when necessary and substantiated by fact and (2) respecting another's privacy and autonomy and maintaining a confidential relationship with the patient.

ADMINISTRATIVE LAW AND LICENSING STATUTES

A second type of law and legal process in which nurses are involved is administrative law and the regulatory process. This area of law governs the nurse's relationship with the government, either state or federal. *Administrative law* involves the rules of the government's activities in regulating health care delivery and practice. Several government health care agencies are involved in such regulation.

A state has the power to regulate nursing because the state is responsible for the health, safety, and welfare of its citizens. Therefore establishing minimal entry level requirements, standards of nursing practice, and educational requirements is an acceptable state action. The state legislatures create laws (generally termed *nurse practice acts*) governing nursing practice, and a unit of the state government within the executive branch of government is responsible for the enforcement of nursing laws. This unit is often called the State Board of Nursing or Board of Nurse Examiners. However, states do vary. This is another important reason that nurses must seek advice from counsel licensed to practice law within their own state.

In administrative law, the rules of investigation, procedure, and evidence differ from the civil and criminal law.

NEGLIGENCE AND MALPRACTICE

As defined earlier, negligence is an unintentional tort involving a breach of duty or failure (through an act or an omission) to meet a standard of care, causing patient harm. Malpractice is a type of professional liability based on negligence in which the defendant is held accountable for breach of a duty of care involving special knowledge and skill. These torts have several elements, all of which the plaintiff has the burden of proving.

Definition of Elements

The law recognizes the following four elements of negligence and malpractice:

- ◆ Duty and standard of care
- ◆ Breach of duty
- ◆ Causation
- ◆ Injury or damages

A *duty,* or legal obligation, must be one recognized by law requiring the actor to conform to a certain standard of conduct for the protection of others against unreasonable risks.[11] The critical care nurse's legal duty is to act in a reasonable and prudent manner, as any other critical care nurse would act under similar circumstances. The standard is that of a critical care nurse, one with special knowledge and skill in critical care. The standard is one that is owed at the time the incident or injury occurred, not at the time of litigation. In most jurisdictions the standard of care is a national standard, as opposed to a local, community standard. The box (upper right) lists general critical care nursing duties as implied by statute, administrative rules and regulations, and as stated explicitly in judicial decisions.

Breach of duty involves a failure on the actor's part to conform to the standard required. *Causation,* the third element, involves proving that the actor's breach was reasonably close or causally connected to the resulting injury. This is also referred to as *proximate cause.*

The fourth element, *injury,* must involve an actual loss or damage to the plaintiff or his or her interest. A plaintiff may claim different types of damages, such as compensatory or punitive. Patient injury can range in value, depending on what happened to the patient. The plaintiff must produce evidence of the damages and their value. If the nurse breaches a standard of care that leads to injury, the plaintiff must show what amount of money will compensate for his or her injuries. The goal of the compensation is to provide the amount of money that will place the plaintiff back in the position he or she was in before the injury occurred.

Res ipsa loquitur is a rule of evidence used by plaintiffs in negligence or malpractice litigation. It literally means "the thing speaks for itself." It is a rebuttable presumption or inference of negligence by the defendant, which arises on plaintiff's proof that (1) the injury is one that ordinarily does not happen in the absence of negligence and (2) the instrumentality causing the injury was in the defendant's exclusive management and control. The burden then shifts to the defendant to prove absence of negligence. For example, negligence can be inferred when muscle ischemia and necrosis occur as a result of improper body positioning and the application of splints or restraints. Negligence can also be inferred from a foreign object left in a patient's body cavity after surgery.

Because critical care nurses deal with life-threatening situations, patient injury is potentially severe or may result in death. Should this occur as a result of negligence, the nurse may be held liable for the patient's death and also for the resulting loss to surviving family members. All states have wrongful death acts, and a number of states have both death acts and survival acts, which are prosecuted concurrently. With the two causes of action, the expenses, pain and suffering, and loss of earnings of the decedent up to the time of death are allocated to the survival action and the loss of benefits of the survivors is allocated to the wrongful death action.

The first box on p. 40 illustrates specific examples of critical care nurse actions that have resulted in litigation. In cases such as these, the nurse's action is central to the lawsuit. However, nurses are named as sole or codefendants in a comparatively small percentage of cases. Although this pattern is changing, physicians and hospitals are generally named as defendants.

Typically, nursing negligence cases involve breach or failure in six general categories listed in the second box on p. 40. The first category includes the use of defective equipment or the failure to perform safety and maintenance assessments. Nurses commonly make errors in

---

LEGAL DUTIES

Critical care nurses have a legal duty to do the following:

- ◆ Observe
- ◆ Assess
- ◆ Conduct ongoing observations and assessments
- ◆ Recognize significance of information
- ◆ Report
- ◆ Plan, implement, and evaluate care
- ◆ Respond to changes
- ◆ Interpret and carry out orders
- ◆ Take reasonable measures to ensure patient safety
- ◆ Exercise professional judgment
- ◆ Properly perform procedures
- ◆ Follow hospital policies and procedures
- ◆ Record and document

EXAMPLES OF CRITICAL CARE NURSING ACTIONS INVOLVED IN NEGLIGENCE SUITS

GENERAL

- Failure to advise physician and/or supervisor of change in patient's health status
- Failure to monitor patients at requisite intervals
- Failure to adhere to established institutional protocols
- Failure to adequately assess clinical status
- Failure to respond to alarms
- Failure to maintain accurate, timely, and complete medical records
- Failure to properly carry out treatment and evaluate results of treatment
- Failure to use safe, functional equipment

SPECIFIC

- Failure to provide supplemental oxygen when the ventilator cannot be promptly reattached
- Failure to properly use intravenous infusion equipment, causing extensive extravasation of fluid
- Failure to monitor intravenous infusions, recognize infiltration, and discontinue intravenous therapy
- Failure to recognize signs of intracranial bleeding
- Failure to investigate patient's complaint of pain and discover hematoma under blood pressure cuff

COMMON AREAS OF NURSING NEGLIGENCE

- Improper administration of treatments
- Improper administration of medications
- Inadequate or false written and verbal communication
- Insufficient supervision of patients
- Improper postoperative treatment and wound care
- Incorrect perioperative instrument and sponge counts

drug identification, administration, and dosages. Nurses have failed to timely report to physicians changes in patient status and have also failed to communicate to supervisors a physician's failure to respond to the nurse's communication. Failure to supervise and assist patients who subsequently fall is also a source of nursing negligence. Improper wound care with resulting infection, and incorrect instrument and sponge counts in the surgical setting are areas of practice that have led to patient injury and lawsuits.

Legal Doctrines and Theories of Liability

In tort law there are several theories of liability under which the nurse's action may be examined and legal duties defined:

1. Personal
2. Vicarious: *respondeat superior*
3. Corporate
4. Other doctrines, such as temporary or borrowed servant, and captain of the ship

Under the theory of *personal liability,* each individual is responsible for his or her own actions. This includes the critical care nurse, the supervisor, the physician, the hospital, and the patient. Each has responsibilities that are uniquely his or her own. In contrast to personal liability, one may be afforded the protection of *personal immunity.* In certain health care situations, Congress or state legislatures have determined that nurses do not have personal liability and are therefore immune from liability. Again, it is wise to seek advice to review what employment settings and laws apply to a particular situation.

As a general rule in most jurisdictions, mandatory reporting statutes include personal immunity provisions. For example, child abuse and dependent adult abuse statutes provide that a nurse who makes a good faith report will not be liable for making that report or the consequences of the report. Similarly, physicians, nurses, and hospitals that are mandated to report communicable and infectious diseases to state or federal authorities are immune from liability for good faith reporting in a confidential manner. Also, nurses who in good faith render voluntary emergency care in the field to a stranger are immune from liability for negligence under state good samaritan laws. Finally, federally employed nurses are protected by immunity provisions under the Federal Tort Claims Act.[12] However, many states have greatly restricted immunity at state and local levels. Certain personal immunities are not a guarantee against lawsuits; rather, they are potential defenses.

Vicarious liability is indirect responsibility—for example, the liability of an employer for the acts of the employee. Under the doctrine of *respondeat superior,* a master is liable for certain wrongful acts of a servant, as is a principal for those of an agent. An employer may be liable for an employee's acts that are performed within the legitimate scope of employment. In critical care, the nurse typically is an employee of a hospital. However, nurses may be independent contractors with the hospital through critical care nursing agencies or businesses. If the latter is the case, the nurse is not an employee of the hospital and the hospital is not vicariously liable for the nurse's action.

Critical care nurses who are hospital employees are given work assignments and provided equipment and supplies to perform those assignments by the employer's agent, a supervisor. As a general rule, the hospital is responsible for the patient census and staffing on the critical care unit and for clinical orientation of the staff as well. Because of these responsibilities, the hospital-employer generally is responsible for the employee's performance within parameters determined by the employer. Thus it would appear unjust to hold the individual nurse solely responsible for errors as a result of patient care assignments and staffing patterns controlled primarily by the hospital. However, that is sometimes the case.

Corporate liability is the liability that attaches to the corporate entity (e.g., the hospital) for its own corporate activities and decisions.

Other doctrines, such as *temporary or borrowed servant* and *captain of the ship,* may apply to the critical care nurse and the critical care unit. These doctrines are used when the plaintiff argues that the physician is responsible for the nurse's actions, even though the nurse is an employee of the hospital and not the physician. If it can be shown that the nurse acted under the direction and control of the physician, it is possible that the physician may be accountable for the nurse's actions. However, these doctrines are becoming increasingly uncommon. What viability remains is typically found in cases involving nurse anesthetists and operating room nurses.

Risk Management and Reduction

Critical care nurses can minimize patient harm and subsequent claims of malpractice in a variety of ways. The hallmark of risk reduction is knowledge of the professional standards of care, delivery and documentation of that care, and a consistent showing that the standards are met.

In addition to the sources previously listed, the boxes on pp. 42 and 43 summarize the critical care nursing standards of the AACN. Many of these sources are admissible as evidence in negligence and malpractice litigation. The question for which these sources serve as measuring sticks of nursing action or inaction is "Did the nurse breach the professional standard of care and the duty owed?"

Another important component is the individual institution's risk management (RM) program. Nurses should be acutely aware of potential harms to patients and take affirmative steps to avoid and correct deficiencies identified through the RM program. For example, many hospital RM programs require that reports or other documentation be completed for unusual incidents. Institutional policy defines which incidents are to be reported.

It behooves nurses to consider obtaining their own professional liability insurance as an RM strategy. Insurance is a mechanism whereby one can shift to another the potentially devastating economic burden of a lawsuit in which one is found to have been negligent or to have committed malpractice.

Insurance is a contract between the insured (the nurse) and the insurer (the insurance company). Therefore the written agreement between these parties should be examined carefully. It spells out the premium, the coverage, the terms, and the requirements the nurse must fulfill if he or she is sued. For example, most policies state that the insurance company will pay the nurse's legal fees, expenses related to litigation, and the final award. However, the nurse is obligated to notify the insurance company within a reasonable time of knowledge of a possible or pending lawsuit and to cooperate in the defense. The nurse should also know what type of policy he or she has: "occurrence" coverage or "claims made" coverage.

On the other hand, self-insurance has serious drawbacks if it encourages plaintiffs to name nurses as defendants instead of or in addition to hospitals. Traditionally, nurses have not insured themselves, but instead have relied on their employers' (usually the hospitals') liability insurance. However, the judicial trend toward rendering a nurse's liability as nursing malpractice has made this reliance uncertain and hazardous. Today many hospital liability policies have exclusionary clauses by which the insurer disclaims liability for malpractice claims brought against the insured hospital.[1] This means the insurer may have no contractual duty to defend nurse malpractice actions or pay awards for plaintiff verdicts.

Peer review and quality assurance programs are also important processes that can minimize patient harm and nursing liability. Peer review involves self-review, self-evaluation, and the audit of others' actions and records. Similarly, an accurate, timely, and complete medical record is imperative. Patient medical records are legal documents admissible in court as evidence of negligence or malpractice. As a general rule, peer review records and incident reports remain confidential and are inadmissible as evidence.

Other risk management techniques include strengthening communication skills and improving public relations. Risk management experts emphasize prompt reporting of an accident or injury and direct communication to the patient involved. The underlying rationale is that straightforward communication about the incident and what is being done to correct or alleviate the injury often decreases the patient's likelihood of suing. Maintaining the patient's trust is critical to reducing exposure to liability and managing risk.

NURSE PRACTICE ACTS

The practice of nursing is regulated by the state. As a general rule, the state's police power to regulate prevails, so long as the state's actions are not arbitrary or capricious. All nurses must be licensed to practice under their individual state's licensure statutes. Licensure authorizes (1) the right to practice and (2) access to employment. Therefore licensure is a property right that is constitutionally protected.[13] Every state has legislation that defines the legal scope of nursing practice and defines unprofessional and illegal conduct that may lead to investigation and disciplinary action by the state and sanctions on the right to practice. The state nurse practice act establishes entry requirements, definitions of practice, and criteria for discipline. Although licensure is mandatory for registered nurses, statutory content varies among the states.

Generally, state law contains two definitions of nursing: one for the registered (or professional) nurse and one for the licensed practical (or vocational or technical) nurse. These definitions determine titles that may be used by nurses, the scope of nursing practice, and requirements for entering the nursing profession. In some states, advanced registered nursing practice, prescriptive authority for certain nurses, and third-party reimbursement are also defined by statute.[1] Mandatory continuing education requirements are also defined by statute in most states. The state authorizes the board of

STANDARDS FOR NURSING CARE OF THE CRITICALLY ILL

STRUCTURE

I. The critical care unit shall be designed to ensure a safe and supportive environment for critically ill patients and for the personnel who care for them.
II. The critical care unit shall be constructed, equipped, and operated in a manner that protects patients, visitors, and personnel from electrical hazards.
III. The critical care unit shall be constructed, equipped, and operated in a manner that protects patients, visitors, and personnel from fire hazards.
IV. The critical care unit shall have essential equipment and supplies immediately available at all times.
V. The critical care unit shall have a comprehensive infection control program.
VI. The critical care unit shall be managed in a manner that ensures the delivery of safe and effective care to the critically ill.
VII. The critical care unit shall have appropriately qualified staff to provide care on a 24-hour basis.
VIII. The critical care nurse shall be competent and have current knowledge in critical care nursing.
IX. The critical care nurse's performance appraisal shall be based on the roles and responsibilities identified in the job description.
X. The critical care unit shall have a well-defined, organized written program to evaluate care of the critically ill.
XI. Critical care nursing practice shall include both conducting and using clinical research.
XII. The critical care nurse shall ensure the delivery of safe nursing care to patients, being cognizant of the various "causes of action" for which she or he may be liable.

PROCESS

I. Data shall be collected continuously on all critically ill patients wherever they may be located.
II. The identification of patient problems or needs and their priority shall be based on collected data.
III. An appropriate plan of nursing care shall be formulated.
IV. The plan of nursing care shall be implemented according to the priority of identified problems or needs.
V. The results of nursing care shall be continuously evaluated.

OUTCOME

Value statement: The critical care nurse shall be cognizant of the intended results of care provided to the critically ill. For example, critical care delivery is consistent with policies and procedures specific to the patient population.

From American Association of Critical-Care Nurses: *Standards for nursing care of the critically ill,* Newport Beach, Calif, 1989, The Association.

nursing to monitor practice, implement standards of care, enforce rules and regulations, and issue sanctions. Sanctions include additional education, restricted practice, supervised practice, license suspension, and license revocation. Some form of disciplinary action generally occurs as a result of unauthorized practice, negligence or malpractice, incompetence, chemical or other impairment, criminal acts, or violations of specific nurse practice act provisions.

The scope of medical practice is also statutorily defined, and in most states a physician is given broad discretion to delegate tasks to others. Physicians may delegate to critical care nurses through written protocols or standing orders, which must be written, dated, and signed by the physician; standing orders and protocols must be updated regularly. The nurse must be adequately prepared to follow the protocol and perform with a reasonable degree of skill, care, and diligence as performed by similar nurses under similar circumstances. Protocol and standing orders should identify unambiguously the corresponding roles of hospital administrators, nurses, and doctors. However, one must keep in mind that, within a state's jurisdiction, the scope of medical practice and nursing practice frequently overlap because each practice may authorize the same functions. Such overlapping creates problems at the regulatory level and will surely extend as the role of nursing continues to evolve.

Because it is afforded constitutional protection, the right to practice cannot be violated without due process of the law. The amount of due process in administrative law differs from other legal processes. Due process involves notice to the nurse that a complaint has been filed (voluntarily or by mandate); the notice is written and contains the charges against the nurse. Nurses in this situation should seek independent legal counsel immediately; the state will not provide it. The nurse must be given an opportunity to be heard, often in more than one forum, and be given the right to present her or his own evidence.

Chemical impairment is a common reason for disciplinary action. In some states, the impaired nurse may avoid serious sanctions by voluntarily suspending practice and entering a rehabilitation program. This should be done with the advice of counsel (the nurse's own lawyer). Generally, this option is available so long as no patient has been harmed because of the nurse's impairment.

SUPPORTING STANDARDS OF STANDARD XII

The critical care nurse shall ensure the delivery of safe nursing care to patients as defined by professional standards of care and legal duties. The critical care practitioner shall perform with the degree of skill, care, and diligence as performed by similar practitioners under similar circumstances. The nurse shall likewise be cognizant of the various causes of action for which the nurse may be liable if the duty of care owed the patient is breached and patient injury occurs as a result of that breach.

1. Patients shall be fully advised in advance of all nursing and/or medical procedures to which they are subjected, signing a written informed consent when required. (Causes of action may include abandonment, battery, failure to obtain informed consent, malpractice, negligence, and negligent nondisclosure.)
2. Patients shall be allowed freedom of movement within their hospital rooms and are allowed to discharge themselves from the hospital. (Causes of action may include battery, failure to obtain informed consent, false imprisonment, infliction of emotional distress, negligence, and malpractice.)
3. Patients shall receive nursing care in accordance with competent nursing practice and those policies specifically established by the hospital. (Causes of action may include negligence and malpractice.)
4. Patients shall be assured that any medical information will be shared only with health professionals treating the patient, and any other communication is restricted or occurs only with the consent of the patient. (Causes of action may include defamation, infliction of emotional distress, and invasion of privacy.)
5. The patient's family members or significant others shall not be subjected to incorrect information concerning the patient or careless treatment of the patient. (Causes of action may include infliction of emotional distress, negligence, and malpractice.)
6. Patients shall be treated in a dignified manner; only those professionals directly involved in their care have access to their medical information, and this information will not be released or disclosed to others without the approval of the patients. (Causes of action may include infliction of emotional distress and invasion of privacy.)

From American Association of Critical-Care Nurses: *Standards for nursing care of the critically ill,* Newport Beach, Calif, 1989, The Association.

SPECIFIC PATIENT CARE ISSUES

Myriad legal issues and controversies exist in the field of critical care. Concerns frequently arise in the areas of (1) informed consent and authorization for treatment and (2) the patient's right to accept or refuse medical treatment.

Informed Consent and Authorization for Treatment

The common law right not to be touched without giving consent has existed since the early eighteenth century. In the 1914 case of *Schloendorff v. Society of New York Hospital,* a court held that every adult of sound mind has a right to determine what shall be done with his or her own body, including the right to give consent and the right to refuse consent to treatment.[14] Most states now have informed consent statutes, and the body of case law on this subject has developed impressively since the early days of *Schloendorff.*

Intrinsic to the doctrine of informed consent is the physician's legal duty to disclose certain information to the patient and the patient's legal right to *informed* consent and to subsequently refuse or accept medical treatment. Central to critical care nursing is the issue of the extent to which the nurse is involved in obtaining consent. As a general rule, the physician cannot delegate this function entirely to a registered nurse and the nurse's exposure to liability increases if the nurse accepts full responsibility for obtaining the patient's consent. It is common nursing practice to witness and document the procedure and to obtain the patient's signature after the physician has disclosed the required information. However, the nurse should be thoroughly familiar with the state's informed consent statute and the individual institution's policy and procedure for obtaining informed consent. General exceptions to this common practice are the higher standards to which nurse anesthetists, nurse midwives, and nurse researchers are held.[15]

There are two types of consent: express and implied. *Express consent* may be written or verbal and is the consent given specifically for nonroutine procedures. *Implied consent* may be implied in fact, an assumption based on patient behavior (e.g., the patient extending an arm for venipuncture or nodding approval), or it may be implied in law (e.g., an unconscious, hemorrhaging patient in the emergency department).

The following discussion summarizes the elements of valid informed consent, the adequacy of consent and negligent nondisclosure, and exceptions to consent requirements and the duty to disclose.

Valid consent must be (1) voluntary, (2) obtained, and (3) informed. Although consent can be either verbal or written, most hospital policies require that informed, voluntary consent to nonroutine procedures be obtained and confirmed in writing: signed and dated by the patient, physician, and witness (if required). Most informed consent statutes provide that a consent, in writing, to a medical or surgical procedure that meets the consent and disclosure requirements of the statute creates a legal presumption that informed consent was given.

In the vast majority of jurisdictions the decision maker (the one giving the consent) must be a legally competent adult (i.e., having reached majority or, in most states, the age of 18 years). Competence is a legal judgment, and, as a general rule, there is a legal presumption of patient competence.[16] One is mentally incompetent (thereby rendering a consent invalid) if adjudicated incompetent. One must likewise have the capacity (a medical and nursing judgment) to give consent: the patient must be oriented and understand what he or she has been told; medications the patient is taking must be documented. In those adults legally adjudicated incompetent, the guardian may give consent if the guardian has been given this authority.

Minors are legally incompetent, and consent is obtained from the parent or guardian. However, in many jurisdictions there are two important exceptions to this rule: (1) mature minors may consent to treatment for substance abuse, sexually transmitted disease, and matters involving contraception and reproduction; and (2) emancipated minors may consent to treatment in general: minors are considered emancipated if married or divorced before the age of majority, in the military service, or living independently with parental consent.

Consent must also be informed and timely. The physician has a duty to disclose the following: diagnosis, condition, prognosis, material risks and benefits associated with the treatment or procedure, explanation of the treatment, providers of the treatment (who is performing, supervising, and/or assisting in the procedure), material risks and benefits of alternative therapy, and the probable outcome (including material risks and benefits) if the patient refuses the treatment or procedure. Failure to disclose such information or inadequate disclosure with resultant injury may constitute negligence and give rise to tort claims of malpractice, battery, negligent nondisclosure, and abandonment. Consent is generally valid for 7 to 30 days. However, the time at which consent expires must be explicitly stated in the institutional policy and procedure manual.

There are many exceptions to consent requirements and the duty to disclose, and clearly the exceptions vary according to jurisdiction. Emergencies constitute one exception, unless the patient refuses treatment or has previously made a competent and informed refusal. States vary significantly in the following treatment situations: endangered fetal viability, alcohol or other drug detoxification, emergency blood transfusions, caesarean sections, and substance abuse during pregnancy. Jurisdictions also vary on the issue of sources of consent . (informal directives) for the incompetent patient or the patient in an emergency who has no legal guardian. Alternatives include consensus from as many next of kin as possible, with evidence that (1) the treatment is reasonable and necessary and (2) the family's decision would not be contrary to the patient's wishes (this is known as *substituted judgment* made by a surrogate decision maker). Another alternative is court order for treatment. In the absence of substituted judgment, many courts use what is known as the *best interests standard.*

Lawsuits involving informed consent and the duty to disclose generally require three elements: (1) proof that the health care provider failed to disclose an existing material risk unknown to the patient or alternatives to the proposed treatment, (2) proof that the patient would not have consented if the risk had been disclosed (in other words, that disclosure of the risk would have led a reasonable patient in the plaintiff's position to refuse the procedure or choose a different course of treatment, and (3) proof of injury occurring as a result of the failure to disclose.[15,17]

The Right to Accept or Refuse Medical Treatment and the Law of Advance Directives

◆ **The competent patient's right to refuse treatment.** The right to consent and informed consent includes the right to refuse treatment. In most cases a competent adult's decision to refuse even life-sustaining treatment is honored.[18-22] The underlying rationale is that the patient's right to withdraw or withhold treatment is not outweighed by the state's interest in preserving life.

There are some situations in which the right to refuse treatment is not honored. These include, but are not limited to, the following situations:

- The treatment relates to a contagious illness that threatens the health of the public (e.g., immunizations are required, even over religious objections, if there is substantial danger to the community).
- Innocent third parties will suffer (e.g., a parent's wish to refuse a blood transfusion most likely would be overruled to save the life of a child; these cases are often decided on a case-by-case basis, and legal counsel should always be sought).
- The refusal violates ethical standards (e.g., a Massachusetts court held that a hospital was not required to compromise its ethical principles by following a patient's decision, but must cooperate in the transfer of the patient to a hospital that is willing to cooperate.[23] However, a New Jersey court ruled to the contrary. A patient indicated that she did not want to be fed if she became incapacitated; the hospital opposed this. The court upheld the patient's right and refused to order her transfer.[24] Again, obtaining legal counsel in these instances is highly advisable.).
- Treatment must be instituted to prevent suicide and to preserve life (courts have clearly indicated, however, that terminally ill and/or comatose patients with no hope of recovery do not intend suicide when treatment has been refused).

When patients refuse treatment, complex ethical, legal, and practical problems arise. Hospitals should have specific policies to guide nurses in these areas, and nurses' participation in hospital ethics committees or institutional ethics committees is strongly advisable.

◆ **Withholding and withdrawing treatment.** As indicated earlier, an adult has the right to refuse treatment, even treatment that sustains life. This right means that the

LEGAL REVIEW: New or investigational drugs, devices, procedures, and treatments

The federal Food and Drug Administration (FDA) regulates through licensing the prescription, administration, and use of investigational or experimental drugs and devices. This regulation is governed primarily by the 1938 Federal Food, Drug, and Cosmetic Act and the Medical Device Amendments of 1976. The Food, Drug, and Cosmetic Act is a valid exercise of Congressional power to control interstate commerce. The broad purpose of the statute and its amendments is to protect public health and safety by prohibiting in interstate commerce the sale or transport of misbranded, adulterated, defective, or unsafe products intended for human use or consumption.

The Medical Device Amendments of 1976 preempt state law regarding certain standards for warning of risks or labeling of a product. The amendments also govern certain areas of product design and design defect. In the case of *Slater v. Optical Radiation Corporation,* the plaintiff filed a products liability action alleging injury from a product rendered unsafe as a result of a design defect. The plaintiff had undergone cataract removal with subsequent implantation of an intraocular lens. The lens had not been approved by the FDA as safe and effective, but it had received an exemption under the experimental device exception of the Amendments to permit clinical trials of the lens. The plaintiff signed a consent form stating he had been advised that the lens was an experimental device. After pain and diminished vision in the affected eye resulted, the lens was removed but the plaintiff suffered permanent damage that had not been caused by the cataract.

The U.S. Court of Appeals, Seventh Circuit, ruled that the plaintiff's claim was preempted by the investigational device exemption, and the lawsuit was dismissed. The court reasoned that the investigational device exception is intended to encourage the study and development of medical devices by permitting controlled clinical trials of a product for which effectiveness and safety have not yet been established. The court stated that the Medical Device Amendments prohibit states from imposing by regulation, statute, or judicial ruling requirements for the safety and effectiveness of medical devices that differ from those established by the FDA. The court further noted that imposing liability for defective design on the manufacturer of a device (which had received investigational status by the FDA) would undermine the purpose and intent of the investigational device exception.

However, the Court stated that preemption by the Medical Device Amendments is limited to the issue of safety and effectiveness and does not preclude lawsuits alleging negligent implantation, removal, or contamination of a device, or failure to obtain informed consent to the use of an investigational device.

If the institution is funded in whole or in part by the federal government, human research involving investigational procedures, tests, or treatments is regulated generally under the authority of the Department of Health and Human Services (DHHS). Federal regulations were first established in 1975 and revised in 1981. Institutions sponsoring the research are required by regulation to establish institutional review boards (IRBs). The purpose of the IRB is to evaluate research proposals before implementation to determine whether human research subjects may be at risk, assess the risks involved, identify ways to protect human subjects, and approve or disapprove the proposal. Because IRBs' structure and role are defined by federal regulation, they operate similarly throughout the country.

The DHHS policy for protection of human research subjects contains the following salient provisions: (1) a description of the types of research governed by the regulations, (2) pertinent definitions, including definitions of research, human subject, and risk, (3) requirements for IRB membership, (4) duties and functions of the IRB, (5) review procedures for minimal risk research, (6) criteria for IRB approval of research proposals, (7) requirements for informed consent, and (8) procedures for documentation of informed consent.

It behooves the critical care nurse who participates in any form of clinical research, including the administration of FDA-unapproved or investigational drugs, to be familiar with these regulations and the sponsoring institution's IRB findings and recommendations on the research proposal.

See Federal Food, Drug, and Cosmetic Act, 21 U.S.C.A. Section 301 *et seq.* and Medical Device Amendments of 1976; Lynn JSR: Implantable medical devices: a survey of products liability case law, *Med Trial Tech Q* 38:44, 1991; Protection of Human Research Subjects, 45 C.F.R. Section 46.101 *et seq.* (1985); Shimm DS, Spece RG: Conflict of interest and informed consent in industry-sponsored clinical trials, *J Legal Med* 12:477, 1991; *Slater v. Optical Radiation Corp.,* No. 91-1544 (7th Cir. Apr. 22, 1992).

critical care nurse may participate in the withholding or withdrawing of treatment. Historically, the distinction between withholding and withdrawing treatments was considered the issue of importance, but that is no longer the case. Health care decisions become most complex when patients lose competency and capacity to personally make their own decisions.

◆ **Orders not to resuscitate and other orders.** Hospital policies that address orders to withhold or withdraw treatment should exist in all critical care units. For example, orders not to resuscitate—commonly referred to as do-not-resuscitate (DNR) orders—should be governed by written policies, including, but not limited to, the following:

1. DNR orders should be entered in the patient's record with full documentation by the responsible physician about the patient's prognosis, the patient's agreement (if he or she is capable), or alternatively the family's consensus.
2. DNR orders should have the concurrence of another physician, designated in the policy.
3. Policies should specify that orders are reviewed periodically (some policies require daily review).
4. Patients with capacity must give their informed consent.
5. For patients without capacity, that incapacity must be thoroughly documented, along with the diagnosis, prognosis, and family consensus.
6. Judicial intervention before writing a DNR order is usually indicated when the patient's family does not agree or there is uncertainty or disagreement about the patient's prognosis or mental status. As a general rule, however, in the absence of conflict or disagreement, DNR orders are legal in a majority of jurisdictions if executed clearly and properly.
7. Policies should specify who is to be contacted and notified within the hospital administration.

Other orders to withhold or withdraw treatment may involve mechanical ventilation, dialysis, nutritional support, hydration, and medications, such as antibiotics. The legal and ethical implications of these orders for each patient must be carefully considered. Hospitals should have written policies on all orders to withhold and withdraw treatment. Policies must cover how decisions will be made: who will decide and what the roles of patient, family, health care providers, and the institution will be. Policies must be developed that consider state laws and judicial opinions.

◆ **Advance directives and the Patient Self-Determination Act (OBRA 1990).** Rarely has a case so galvanized public opinion as the case of Nancy Cruzan.[25-32] The tragic experience and hardships of Nancy Cruzan and her family left an indelible mark in American jurisprudence, legislation, and health care.

In *Cruzan* the issue before the U.S. Supreme Court was to consider whether Cruzan had a federal constitutional right that would require the hospital to withdraw life-sustaining treatment from her under the circumstances. The court rejected the request for authority to withdraw artificial nutrition and hydration and held that the U.S. Constitution did not prohibit the state of Missouri from requiring clear and convincing evidence of Cruzan's wishes before treatment withdrawal.

The court stated that where a person is incompetent and unable to exercise the right to refuse treatment and a surrogate must act on his or her behalf, the state may institute procedural safeguards to ensure that the surrogate honors the wishes expressed by the person while competent. The court also held that the U.S. Constitution does not require a state to accept the substituted judgment of the family; the state may recognize only a personal right to make such health care

LEGAL REVIEW: The durable power of attorney for health care

The durable power of attorney for health care is the second and most recently developed advance directive. Approximately 30 states have statutes or pending legislation on this document.

As a general rule, the durable power of attorney for health care is more flexible than is the living will and has broader application: it is not restricted to traditional life-sustaining procedures, nor is it restricted to terminally ill patients.

The document authorizes the agent (attorney in fact) to make health care decisions for the principal when the principal is unable to make those decisions. The principal is the competent adult who executes the power of attorney document and designates the agent to make decisions on his or her behalf.

Similar to the living will, the durable power of attorney for health care is written, signed, dated, witnessed, and notarized. It is part of the medical record. As a general rule, it may be revoked at any time and in any manner. If the nurse's state has a statute governing this document, the nurse should also be familiar with (1) witness disqualifier provisions, (2) agent disqualifier provisions, (3) guardian preemption provisions, (4) revocation conditions, (5) effect on life insurance policies, if any, (6) the effect of out-of-state documents, and (7) immunity provisions.

See *In Re Estate of Greenspan,* 558 N.E.2d 1194 (Ill. 1990); *The durable power of attorney for health care law: a Catholic perspective,* Iowa Catholic Conference, 818 Insurance Exchange Building, Des Moines, Ia, 50309, 515-243-6256; Pozgar GD: *Legal aspects of health care administration,* ed 4, Rockville, Md, 1990, Aspen Systems.

decisions. A state may choose to defer only to the person's express wishes, rather than relying on the family's decision.

Perhaps more important, the court also held that a competent adult has a federal constitutional right to refuse medical treatment, including life-sustaining hydration and nutrition. This right falls under the Fourteenth Amendment due process clause and is not a fundamental privacy right under the First Amendment.

The Cruzan decision quickly mobilized Congress to pass landmark legislation known as the Patient Self-Determination Act/Omnibus Budget Reconciliation Act of 1990.[33-42] The statute requires that all adults must be provided written information on an individual's rights under state law to make medical decisions, including the right to refuse treatment and the right to formulate advance directives.

The Act mandates that providers of health care services under Medicare and Medicaid must comply with requirements relating to patient advance directives, written instructions recognized under state law for provisions of care when persons are incapacitated. Providers may not be reimbursed for the care they provide unless the requirements of this provision are met.

Providers must have written policies and procedures to (1) inform all adult patients at the time treatment is initiated of their right to execute an advance directive and of the provider's policies on the implementation of that right, (2) document in medical records whether an individual has executed an advance directive, (3) not condition care and treatment or otherwise discriminate on the basis of whether a patient has executed an advance directive, (4) comply with state laws on advance directives, and (5) provide information and education to staff and the community on advance directives. The provisions became effective in December 1991.

Patients themselves can provide clear direction by preparing in advance written documents that specify their wishes. These documents are termed *advance directives* and include the living will and durable power of attorney for health care. To be effective in a jurisdiction, both of these directives must be statutorily or judicially recognized. The living will specifies that if certain circumstances occur, such as terminal illness, the patient will decline specific treatment, such as cardiopulmonary resuscitation and mechanical ventilation. The living will does not cover all treatment. For example, in some states nutritional support may not be declined through a living will. The durable power of attorney for health care is a directive through which a patient designates an agent, someone who will make decisions for the patient if the patient becomes unable to do so. Critical care nurses whose patients have executed advance directives must follow state law provisions and the hospital's policies.

Some states have also passed laws providing that a county, municipality, region, or medical center may establish a substitute medical decision-making board composed of health care professionals and lay persons. The board acts as a substitute decision maker if the patient does not have his or her own surrogate. It is of utmost importance that the critical care staff consult with hospital legal counsel in the event the patient has a designated surrogate or has executed one or more advance directives and also has had a court-appointed guardian in the past. Various statutory provisions in the context of guardianship are incongruous with many of the new laws relating to surrogate or substitute decision making and the laws of advance directives. The staff must know without question who has primary legal authority for the patient, and this information must be documented unambiguously.

LEGAL REVIEW: The living will

One type of advance directive is the living will, which typically is a signed, written, witnessed statement that explains the patient's preferences about withholding or withdrawing life-sustaining treatment at the time of terminal illness. This document is part of the medical record. The patient should be advised to periodically review his or her living will. In some states this is required by law, or the effect of the will is void. Living wills may be revoked at any time.

The vast majority of states have living will statutes; all states have pending legislation. The limitations to life-sustaining treatment and terminal illness are being revised in many state statutes to make the living will more compatible with the durable power of attorney for health care.

In the absence of state statute, the will should clearly define life-sustaining treatment and address whether nutrition and hydration are among the measures to be withheld or withdrawn and under what conditions.

See Choice in Dying: *A living will,* New York, Choice in Dying, 200 Varick Street, New York, 10014; Choice in Dying: *Questions and answers about the living will,* New York, Choice in Dying, 200 Varick Street, New York, 10014; Collins E, Weber D: *The complete guide to living wills,* 1991, Bantam Books; Crisham P: Living wills—controversy and certainty, *J Prof Nurs* 6(6):321, 1990; Emanuel L: Beyond the living will, *Harv Med Sch Health Letter* 15(8):4, 1990; *In Re Estate of Greenspan,* 558 N.E.2d 1194 (Ill. 1990); *In Re Peter,* 529 A.2d 419 (N.J. 1987); Killian WH: Knowledge of living will laws essential, *Am Nurse* 22(7):33, 1990; Ney CA: Living wills: the ethical dilemmas, *Crit Care Nurse* 9(8):20, 1989.

REFERENCES

1. Hoffman NA: Nursing and the future of health care: the independent practice imperative. *Specialty L Dig: Health Care* 160:7, 1992.
2. American Nurses Association Committee on Ethics: *Code for nurses with interpretative statements,* Kansas City, Mo, 1985, American Nurses Association.
3. American Association of Critical-Care Nurses Board of Directors: *AACN position statement: scope of critical care nursing practice,* Newport Beach, Calif, 1986, American Association of Critical Care Nurses.
4. American Nurses Association: *Nursing: a social policy statement,* Kansas City, Mo, 1980, American Nurses Association.
5. American Association of Critical-Care Nurses: *Position statement: definition of critical care nursing,* Newport Beach, Calif, 1984, American Association of Critical-Care Nurses.
6. American Association of Critical-Care Nurses: *Standards for nursing care of the critically ill,* ed 2, Norwalk, Conn, 1989, Appleton & Lange.
7. *Fraijo v. Hartland Hosp.,* 99 Cal. App. 3d 331; 160 Cal. Rptr. 246 (1979).
8. Northrop CE, Kelly ME: *Legal issues in nursing,* St Louis, 1987, Mosby–Year Book.
9. Christoffel T: *Health and the law: a handbook for health professionals,* New York: Free Press; London: Collier Macmillan, 1982.
10. Feutz-Harter SA: Legal implications of restraints, *J Nurs Adm* 20(10):8, 1990.
11. Prosser WL, Keeton WP, Dobbs DB, and others: *The law of torts,* ed 5, St Paul, Minn, 1988, West.
12. 28 U.S.C. Secs. 2671-80 (1986).
13. Walker DJ: Nursing 1980: new responsibility, new liability, *Trial* 16(12):43, 1980.
14. *Schloendorff v. Soc'y of N.Y. Hosp.,* 105 N.E. 92 (1914), *overruled on other grounds.*
15. Murphy EK: Informed consent doctrine: little danger of liability for nurses, *Nurs Outlook* 39(1):48, 1991.
16. Northrop CE: Nursing practice and the legal presumption of competency, *Nurs Outlook* 36(2):112, 1988.
17. *Pauscher v. Iowa Methodist Med. Center,* 408 N.W.2d 355 (Iowa 1987).
18. *Bouvia v. Superior Court,* 225 Cal. Rptr. 297; 179 C.A.3d 1127, *review denied* (Cal. App. 1986).
19. *In Re Farrell,* 529 A.2d 404 (N.J. 1987).
20. *McKay v. Bergstedt,* 801 P.2d 617 (Nev. 1990).
21. *State v. McAfee,* 385 S.E.2d 651 (Ga. 1989).
22. Wilson-Clayton ML, Clayton MA: Two steps forward, one step back: *McKay v. Bergstedt, Whittier L Rev* 12:439, 1991.
23. *Brophy v. New England Sinai Hosp.,* 497 N.E.2d 626 (Mass. 1986).
24. *In Re Requena,* 517 A.2d 869 (N.J. App. Div. 1986).
25. *Cruzan v. Director, Missouri Dept. of Health,* 110 S. Ct. 2841 (U.S. S. Ct. 1990).
26. *Cruzan v. Director, Missouri Dept. of Health* and the right to die: a symposium, *Ga L Rev* 25:1139, 1991.
27. *Cruzan v. Missouri, USLW* 58:4916, 1990.
28. Guarino KS, Antoine MP: The case of Nancy Cruzan: the Supreme Court's decision, *Crit Care Nurse* 11(1):32, 1991.
29. Kyba F: Decisions at the end of life: implications following Cruzan, *Tex Nurse* 65(2):13, 1991.
30. Morgan RC: How to decide: decisions on life-prolonging procedures, *Stetson L Rev* 20:77, 1990.
31. Quill T: Death and dignity, *N Engl J Med* 324(10):691, 1991.
32. Right to die symposium, *Issues L & Med* 7:169, 1991.
33. *Advance directives for health care: deciding today about your care in the future,* Iowa Hospital Association, Iowa Medical Society, Iowa State Bar Association, 1991.
34. American Hospital Association: *Put it in writing: a guide to promoting advance directives,* American Hospital Association, 840 North Lake Shore Drive, Chicago, Ill, 60611, 800-242-2626.
35. Cate FH, Gill BA: The Patient Self-Determination Act: implementation issues and opportunities, Washington, DC, 1991, The Annenberg Washington Program.
36. Choice in Dying: *Advance directive protocols and the Patient Self-Determination Act: a resource manual for the development of institutional protocols,* Choice in Dying, 200 Varick Street, New York, NY, 10014, 212-366-5540, 1991 (formerly Society for the Right to Die/Concern for Dying, 250 West 57th Street, New York, NY, 10107, 212-246-6962).
37. Emanuel L, Emanuel E: The medical directive: a new comprehensive advance care document, *JAMA* 261(22):3, 288, 1989.
38. Iowa Hospital Association: *The Patient Self-Determination Act of 1990: implementation in Iowa hospitals,* Iowa Hospital Association, 100 East Grand, Suite 100, Des Moines, Ia, 50309, 515-288-1955, 1991.
39. National Hospice Organization: *Advance medical directives,* National Hospice Organization, 1901 North Moore Street, Suite 901, Arlington, Va, 22209, 703-243-5900, 1991.
40. National Health Lawyers Association: *The patient self-determination directory and resources guide,* National Health Lawyers Association, 1620 Eye Street NW, Suite 900, Washington, DC, 20006, 202-833-1100, 1991.
41. Patient Self-Determination Act/Omnibus Budget Reconciliation Act of 1990, Pub L No 101-508, Sec. 4206; 42 U.S.C. Sec. 1395cc(a)(1) (1990).
42. Unisys Corp: *Advance directives,* informational release general no 122, Unisys Corp, PO Box 10394, Des Moines, Ia 50306, 800-776-6045, 1991.

4

Cultural Issues

CHAPTER OBJECTIVES

- Define the term *stereotyping* and explain how this practice can interfere with the accurate perception of the critical care patient.
- List five questions to ask oneself to become aware of one's own cultural values.
- List two ways in which patients' feelings of powerlessness can interfere with the delivery of care.
- Explain how the doctrine of fatalism can affect the attitude of the critically ill patient.
- List three ethnic groups to whom visits from the extended family are very important in the healing process.
- Explain possible reasons for a patient to cry out in pain or to conceal his or her pain.
- Propose seven techniques for improving communication despite the presence of language barriers.

Two female patients are admitted to the coronary care unit within 30 minutes of each other with the diagnosis of "rule out acute anterior myocardial infarction." The first patient is Mrs. Giovanni, a 71-year-old woman who has lived in "little Italy" since arriving in this country many years ago. The second patient is Mrs. Yamaguchi, a 74-year-old woman who moved from Japan 5 years ago to live with her son and daughter-in-law in California. Both patients are limited in their ability to communicate in English.

Electrocardiograms (ECGs) show ST-segment elevation and T-wave inversion in Leads V_2 through V_4 in both patients. Morphine sulfate (4 mg) had been administered intravenously to both patients just before their transfer from the emergency department. Upon admission to the coronary care unit, Mrs. Giovanni is crying, moaning, very restless, and clutching her chest. Her vital signs show an elevated systolic blood pressure, heart rate, and respiratory rate. The laboratory report indicates that her initial serum creatine phosphokinase (CPK) level is 927 mU/ml.

On the other hand, in the next bed, Mrs. Yamaguchi is lying very still, with her eyes closed and arms held rigidly at her side. The admitting nurse observes that her vital signs are also elevated. The laboratory reports that Mrs. Yamaguchi's CPK level is 879 mU/ml, while her ECG is showing an increasing number of extrasystoles. Further questioning by the nurse reveals that both patients are still experiencing chest pain and require further medication.

Physiologically, these cases are very similar. In the early stages of acute myocardial infarction, both patients are showing the classic physiologic signs of pain, yet their behaviors in the presence of this pain are vastly different. Several reasons are possible for this variation in response to pain, such as individual personality or psychologic status. But another possible explanation for this difference is the culture of each patient.

The impact of cultural and ethnic diversity on both American society and the nursing profession has intensified as the number of immigrants and refugees has steadily increased throughout recent decades. While enriching the lives of us all, diversity has generated numerous challenges for health care professionals who are attempting to deliver effective, compassionate care to patients whose values, beliefs, and language can be very different from their own. Although much remains to be done, in recent years there has developed a substantial body of theoretic and applied literature designed to help overcome the challenges of what has become known as "transcultural nursing."

This chapter covers the most commonly encountered challenges in this new and growing field. After discussing some of the general principles behind successful cross-cultural communication (e.g., the importance of overcoming ethnocentrism and the danger of making unwarranted generalities), the perspectives and values of the patient will be discussed. Emphasis is placed on patients' attitudes toward the health care professional, family roles, and responses to pain and grief and, finally, techniques for overcoming accent and language barriers.

THE CHALLENGE OF DIVERSITY

Culture consists of socially transmitted beliefs about the proper ways of behaving, the nature of the world, and the structure and purpose of the universe. On a more practical level, culture supplies a design for living that delineates how to interpret and react to the world.

Before discussing the challenges presented to the critical care nurse by cultural diversity, an even more fundamental difficulty must be addressed—the resistance that many individuals feel to admitting that cultural diversity does indeed exist. To see diversity may seem like an easy matter, but some who come into regular contact with people from other cultures are reluctant to recognize that cultural differences are interfering with communication and mutual understanding. The tendency is to feel that if language differences could be eliminated, so would communication difficulties.

For many reasons, people deny the impact that cultural diversity can have on effective human and professional relationships. Perhaps the most common cause is the fear that to admit that people's values, etiquette, and even world views might be different is to appear guilty of stereotyping the population in question. Quite the contrary is true. To deny a person his or her cultural distinctiveness is to deny an important part of the individual's being and to limit dramatically one's accurate perception of that person.

Another reason that people tend to deny the importance of cultural diversity is that to do so necessitates confronting and dealing with a complex set of behavioral variables that otherwise could be ignored. The information that follows focuses on those culturally generated behavioral variables that most often arise in critical care settings. Cultural assessment guidelines are described for use in planning care. Particular emphasis is placed on the importance of understanding one's own culture, the perspectives of the immigrant patient and family, cultural variations in the pain response, and techniques for minimizing the difficulties created by language barriers.

THE NURSE'S PERSPECTIVE

Culture is a phenomenon common to all human beings. The critical care nurse has personal beliefs, attitudes, perspectives, and behaviors that depend on ancestral and geographic background. For example, the nurse of Italian ancestry who was brought up in New York but currently lives in southern California is a representative of the cultural styles of Italy, New York, and California. In addition to these layers of culture, the hospital in which the nurse works also has a culture of its own that can be quite distinct from those of other facilities. The hospital culture consists of goals, priorities, heroes, traditional ways of doing things, and even terminology that becomes a part of each health professional's cultural "baggage."

Culture, in short, is not just something that belongs to the ethnic or immigrant patient and family, but it affects—often in very subtle ways—the manner in which each nurse responds to colleagues, patients, and families. Within these culturally conditioned responses lie a great many of the pitfalls to cross-cultural communication. The primary reasons for these pitfalls are (1) the tendency to be ethnocentric and (2) the temptation to stereotype others as a means of eliminating ambiguity from the environment.[1]

Ethnocentrism

Ethnocentrism is the view that one's own culture does things in the best way possible and that cultures that appear different are merely lesser versions of one's own. The dangerous corollary of this belief—that all cultures are striving to be similar to his or her own—leads to the assumption that the behavior of culturally diverse patients can be accurately interpreted in light of traditional American values and priorities. In short, it is easy to forget that the patient's behavior, developed in the context of a certain culture, is based on a different perspective of the world, and behaviors might have very different meanings from those ordinarily expected.

One simple example can clarify how this type of misunderstanding can arise. Although it is always dangerous to generalize about the behavior of any group, it is nonetheless not unusual for critical care nurses to encounter Hispanic men who do not initially express much grief at the loss of a wife. According to mainstream American notions of appropriate grief responses, this lack of response may indicate that the husband cared little for his wife and was feeling little grief. This interpretation would probably be inaccurate; the ethnocentric view that all cultures teach the same responses to grief causes the nurse to project personal values onto the Hispanic man and therefore arrive at the wrong conclusion.

The correct conclusion can be reached only when the Hispanic man's lack of response is interpreted in the context of Hispanic cultural mores. In Hispanic culture, although grieving is generally done quite openly, it is not uncommon to find the male head of the household exhibiting little emotion on the death of a loved one, because he keenly feels his duty as head of the household and postpones his expression of grief until the rest of the family has recovered enough to cope with the duties of everyday life.[2] The cultural value is that someone (the man) must stay in charge and in control until calm has been restored.

Once the Hispanic culture is examined and the behavior evaluated in light of this newfound knowledge, it becomes clear that the initial conclusion that the husband cared little for his wife is probably quite incorrect. Instead, the Hispanic husband was probably feeling a great deal of love, not only for the deceased wife, but for his entire family to whom he owed a most difficult duty. This case clearly illustrates the danger of projecting one's own cultural values onto another.

It is not an easy task to avoid this trap. Indeed, culture is so much a part of us that it is almost impossible to be aware of it; it is like the air we breathe—we experience it but are not conscious of its existence. The key to avoiding the pitfalls of ethnocentrism is to become as aware as possible of how one's own culture stands on the situation being considered. The box below contains a list of questions designed to help facilitate this process of

PROMOTING CULTURAL SELF-AWARENESS

Before arriving at any conclusions about the behavior of someone from a different culture, become aware of your own culturally conditioned perspective by asking yourself the following:

- If I observed my parents behaving in this way, what would the behavior have meant for them?
- How was I raised to behave in a similar situation?
- How would I behave now if I were in the patient's position?
- If I were to behave just as the patient has, what would my motivation be?
- What is my idea of "proper" behavior in a situation such as this?

cultural self-awareness and is to be used anytime a situation arises in which the nurse suspects that cultural differences may be involved. Becoming aware of how one's own culture feels about a given behavior enables the nurse to separate his or her own views from those of the patient. Thus the automatic process of projection and ethnocentrism is short-circuited.

Working Generalities Versus Stereotypes

The second primary pitfall to effective cross-cultural communication involves the human tendency to place people and events into neat, unambiguous categories. Stereotyping involves the assumption that all members of a given group will behave in the same way and for the same reasons. Generally, these stereotypes are created out of the values and fears of one's own culture.

For practical purposes, it is important to distinguish between working generalities and stereotypes. A *working generality* is a guideline—a starting point—formed from intelligently considered experiences and study. These generalities help sort out the universe and help predict, with some reasonable accuracy, what to expect from others. Without them, it would be impossible for human beings to carry out even the simplest interaction.

The main feature of a working generality is that it is abandoned immediately when one suspects that the assumptions on which the generality was based are incorrect. For example, nothing is intrinsically wrong in assuming that newly arrived Vietnamese families prefer a more formal approach from a health professional; this guideline helps us know what tone to strike when approaching people with whom we are not familiar.[3] If it is discovered, however, once the nurse meets the family, that the individuals are casual and spontaneous and prefer to be addressed by first names, the culturally aware nurse will quickly abandon the initial guideline and relate less formally to that particular family.

A *stereotype* differs from a working generality in that it is rarely abandoned in the face of contradictory evidence. One reason stereotypes are adhered to so tenaciously is they make the believer feel more secure by providing a systematic, static way of sorting the world and its inhabitants. Stereotypes also differ from working, flexible generalities in that they tend to limit one's definition of the individual toward whom they are directed. It does not matter whether the stereotypical statement is negative or positive—it still draws limits on who and what the observer believes that person can be. There is, for example, nothing negative in saying that Asians prefer a holistic approach to medicine, Hispanics tend to value the present moment over the future, and Moslems believe in the will of Allah when it comes to matters of illness and death. The problem arises when such statements are used to limit a definition of the person and to distort an accurate perception of who and what that individual really is. Because there is a wide range of behaviors *within* each ethnic group, the patient must be assessed as an individual first, then as a part of a family, and finally as part of a culture. The result of an inflexible stereotype is that it causes one to see what is expected—that is, the stereotype, not the real individual.

Similar to ethnocentrism, which distorts the accurate perception of the individual because of the cultural screen it erects, stereotypical thinking distorts reality by causing us to see what we are predisposed to see, not what is actually there. Nurses who can avoid the temptation to categorize people and behaviors into inflexible boxes will function most effectively in a multicultural hospital setting.

THE PATIENT'S PERSPECTIVE

Some of the greatest challenges ethnic and cultural diversity present to the critical care nurse arise out of differing attitudes toward health care and toward the health care professional. These variations in attitude include differing views on the position and responsibility of the health care professional and differing beliefs about the patient's ability to control health and destiny.

The Nurse as Authority Figure

It is impossible to generalize about patient attitudes toward health care professionals. However, two perspectives vary so dramatically from those found among mainstream, native-born Americans that they must be mentioned. They are the patient's perception of the health professional as an authority figure and as the individual who is ultimately responsible for the success or failure of treatment.

One manifestation of this attitude is the tendency, when given the opportunity, for some patients—and their families—to resist making choices about their treatment, such as whether to intubate a terminally ill patient or initiate renal dialysis in such a patient. During recent years in the United States, there has been a growing trend toward patient involvement and patient responsibility in the treatment process.[4] Indeed, the provision of choice, whenever possible, has become one of the basic tenets of sound, effective nursing care.

In many nations of the world, the movement toward patient involvement and decision making has yet to manifest itself. The patient, instead, looks to the health professional to make decisions and accept full responsibility for these decisions. In short, it cannot be assumed that the patient and family are uncooperative, lazy, or unintelligent when its members do not wish to participate in the decision-making process. This behavior quite simply reflects a different health care hierarchy.

Powerlessness and Fatalism

Related to the desire to give the responsibility for treatment to health professionals is a psychologic phenomenon known as powerlessness. *Powerlessness* is an acquired belief that the individual has little or no control over his or her life. Although this belief is usually not based on reality, its emotional roots lie in historical situations that have left individuals and entire populations with a sense of being out of control.

Decades of discrimination, for example, can leave a people with the belief that it cannot succeed no matter what efforts are forthcoming. In addition, living for generations at the poverty level can result in the overwhelming and paralyzing belief that no effort will allow the individual to break out of this pattern.[5] Short-term historical events can have an equally devastating impact on individual and group feelings of control. Southeast Asian immigrants, for example, who have spent as long as 5 years in refugee camps where every effort at planning for the future was thwarted, experience the same feelings of powerlessness that have taken decades to develop in other peoples.

The ramifications of powerlessness for effective critical care nursing can be dramatic. Foremost is the fact that feelings of powerlessness interfere with a patient's willingness to participate in ongoing treatment. When a patient or family member believes that he or she has no control over the future, lengthy and sometimes uncomfortable treatment seems pointless and fruitless, particularly when attempting to develop therapies for a terminally ill patient.

The problems created by this perspective for patient compliance and morale are obvious; the solutions can be more obscure. Ordinarily, the best way to restore power to the "powerless" patient is to supply him or her with decision-making power and with information. Although these techniques sometimes apply, there is often a disinterest in choice and information among these population groups. Supplying the patient and family with the opportunity to exhibit personal power in a way that is meaningful to them is one of the most effective ways of overcoming this difficulty and, in turn, improving compliance. The nurse must be careful to first assess what the "perceived needs" of the patient and family member really are.

To accurately ascertain the ways in which the patient or family would most like to exhibit power, the nurse must first learn as much as possible about the culture in question. The importance, for example, of allowing the extended family to gather around the patient cannot be overemphasized. Likewise, appointing one individual as the hospital spokesperson so that the family always knows whom to approach for information can have a dramatic effect on how powerful, and therefore cooperative, the family feels. A hospital ombudsman or patient representative could serve this function. The patient and family must be allowed to exhibit power in a way that is meaningful to them, in the context of their culture, not in a way that would be important to persons born and raised in mainstream American culture.

Fatalism—that is, the view that the course of life is dictated by a higher power—is a positive version of powerlessness. The difference between the two is that feelings of powerlessness arise out of discrimination, poverty, and historical adversity, and fatalism is generated out of faith in a higher power and in the preordained perfection of the universe. Although the impact of fatalism on health care can sometimes be adverse (e.g., resistance to invoking heroic measures during critical illness), the effect is a positive one because it leaves the patient and family in a more peaceful, accepting state of mind.

The impact of fatalism is seen most dramatically in those who are critically ill. The notion of calling on the individual's "will to live" is an important feature of American health care attitudes. The fatalistic attitudes found among Hispanic and Middle Eastern immigrants, on the other hand, hold that the will of God dictates the fate of the critically ill.[6] The Arabic phrase *in shallah* (if God wills it) sums up this perspective and illustrates the importance of critical care nurses recognizing and honoring this distinction.

For example, to speak to the Hispanic patient of his or her "will to live" will, in all probability, be fruitless and misunderstood. On the other hand, to speak of the importance of relying on and having faith in God's will may prove both comforting and productive. However, this reliance on God's will among terminally ill patients can create problems for the nursing staff. Because in many cultures it is considered God's will whether a person lives or dies, many family members will not want the patient told that he or she is terminally ill, because in their eyes, this would be second-guessing God and therefore defying His will.[6] There is little that the critical care nurse can or should do about this preference. However, awareness is necessary so that misunderstandings that could result in family alienation can be avoided.

THE FAMILY'S PERSPECTIVE

The ability to communicate effectively with the family of the critical care patient is a most important psychosocial element for the critical care nurse. To succeed at this task, the nurse must understand the structure of the family, who its leaders are, and who its members are.

In contrast to traditional Anglo-American families that consist of comparatively few important members, immigrant families are generally *extended units* in which aunts, uncles, cousins, and grandparents are closely bound and have a central importance in each other's eyes. Many families extend even beyond blood relatives to include *fictive kin*—individuals who are loved and regarded as family members but who are not related by biology or marriage—especially within the African-American culture, as well as within the *compadres* and *comadres* (godparents) tradition of the Hispanic culture.

The implication for critical care of the extended and fictive family lies primarily in the importance of respecting the wishes of the patient concerning visiting rights. Hospital rules must also be respected, but the nurse should make no rash judgments about who really matters to the patient, who is capable of rendering valuable support, and who is not. In addition, the nurse must not believe that he or she has been lied to if a patient refers to a nonblood "relative" as "brother," "sister," "aunt," or "uncle." These designations are merely affectionate and are not meant to manipulate the nurse into allowing a nonfamily member to visit the patient.

With respect to visitation, the importance of family support to the critically ill immigrant patient cannot be overemphasized. In Gypsy culture, to cite an extreme, the presence of the family is believed to bring healing energy to the patient. Among those from the Middle East, the family brings very tangible hope to the critically ill patient.[6] In short, the family functions not just as a support system but as a central component in the healing process.[7]

Because of the central role played by the extended family in the care of the immigrant patient, the nurse must know how to address the family to ensure mutual respect and cooperation.[8] Above all else, the nurse must use last names, proceed slowly, and generally respect the more formal social rules of immigrant cultures. The nurse must also be able to establish who the spokesperson and decision maker is for the family. Only in this way will the professional be able to establish rapport, maintain respect, and ensure good communication.

Within Middle Eastern families, for example, the spokesperson is likely to be the father or eldest brother, although the eldest female is likely to hold a great deal of power within the home. This distinction between public power and private control is an important one and must be honored by the health worker. In Hispanic culture, the public head of the household is very likely the father, but within the home, it is the woman who controls many of the decisions. A similar situation occurs within the Italian household.[9] Despite this covert power of the woman, the nurse must respect the male in public and address him with respect and formality.

The issue of whom to address becomes even more complicated when considering the existence of tribal systems within certain immigrant cultures. The Samoans, Laotians, and Gypsies, for example, each practice a form of tribal culture that has as one of its components a tribal leader who functions as the spokesperson and decision maker for the community. By showing respect for the family and the tribal structure of the group, the nurse can dramatically improve patient and family cooperation.

CULTURAL VARIATIONS IN THE PAIN RESPONSE

One of the most bewildering aspects of cultural diversity is the cultural variations that critical care nurses observe in the response to pain. First, a careful distinction must be drawn between the pain threshold and pain tolerance. The *pain threshold* is that point at which a given sensation is first physically perceived as painful—in other words, when the patient first begins to feel pain. *Pain tolerance* is the level of stimulus at which the patient requests cessation or spontaneously withdraws from the painful stimulus—that is, the maximal level the patient is willing to endure. Because of the lack of well-controlled studies, conclusive evidence has yet to be shown whether either or both of these differ cross-culturally; however, pain tolerance seems to be a more useful cross-cultural measure than is pain threshold.[10]

The pain response reflects the patient's attitude toward the pain and is a learned behavior in response to the pain. Pain response is a behavior that reflects the values and priorities of the culture in which the patient was reared. The response is learned both through observation of how parents and other members of the immediate society responded to pain and through the experience of how parents reacted to children in pain.

Responses to pain have been described as either expressive or stoic.[11,12] But this simple dichotomy is too restrictive to encompass the wide range of responses seen. It may be more helpful to imagine a continuum, with emotive (expressive) behaviors at one end and stoic behaviors at the other. As a working generality, pain responses of immigrants from the Latin countries, southern Europe, and the Middle East tend to lie closer to the emotive end of the scale.[13] Those from northern Europe and Asia and the Native American (American Indian) tend to be more stoic in responding to discomfort.[14] There are, of course, numerous exceptions to these guidelines. Factors such as gender, degree of assimilation into mainstream American culture, socioeconomic status, age, and individual personality create considerable diversity within any one cultural group. Nevertheless, these guidelines can be a good starting point in evaluating the behavior of a given patient.

Before examining some of the reasons for an emotive or stoic response to pain and some possible interventions, it must be noted that there is no intrinsic right or wrong in either of these responses—the patient is behaving in a fashion that, because of cultural background, functions under the circumstances. The danger of the nurse projecting personal cultural beliefs onto the patient again comes into play. It is not uncommon for the Anglo-American nurse who has been taught to restrain the expression of pain and "act like a big girl or boy" to assume that those who express pain are being childlike or self-indulgent.[15] This conclusion merely reflects the nurse's culture and has little to do with the motivation or motives of the patient. The behavior must be evaluated in the context of the patient's culture—not by comparison with American values and norms.

The first box on p. 54 lists some of the possible reasons that a patient might emote when in pain and the appropriate nursing interventions for emotive patients. The item "grief over loss of role" deserves special attention, because it addresses one of the most important values of many immigrant cultures: the desire to properly fulfill one's role as a man or a woman.[16] It is not unusual to see a male patient whose critical illness has deprived him of potency or of the ability to support his family display a great deal of apparent pain even in the absence of actual physical discomfort, in which case, he is probably grieving over loss of manhood and not, as it may appear on the surface, crying out in physical pain. The obvious intervention, as indicated in the second part of the box mentioned above, is to reassure the patient about the severity of his illness. If the perceived loss has indeed taken place, suggestions about alternative ways of performing the desired role might be provided.[17]

The intervention listed in the box as "Provide attention promptly" cannot be overemphasized. When the patient is feeling frightened and lonely, is needing attention, and is afraid of not getting it, nothing is more distressing than having to wait for the desired help. The more the patient must wait, the more his or her fear that the help will not be forthcoming increases. The realities of a busy unit should not be denied, but neither should the realities of punctuality when it comes to relieving patient anxiety.

At the opposite end of the continuum is the stoic patient—the individual who will not push the button to ask for help and will not admit to discomfort when asked (see second box, p. 54). On the surface, this sort of

THE EMOTIVE PATIENT

REASONS FOR EMOTING

Fear of the situation
Desire for help and fear of not receiving it
Loneliness and need for attention
Grief over loss of role, dignity, life
Anger
Desire to pay a price
Exorcism of pain through the act of crying out
Appropriateness of emotive behavior
Self-absorption
Great pain

APPROPRIATE INTERVENTIONS

Ask what is needed.
Listen carefully to the reply.
Provide information about medications, procedures, pain.
Provide attention promptly.
Be prompt with medications and treatments.
Provide distractions.
Provide the chance to give to others.
Reassure patient about role fulfillment.
Speak softly.
Touch (if culturally appropriate).
Use relaxation techniques.
Contact consultant, spiritual leader, family member.
Provide appropriate pain medications.

THE STOIC PATIENT

REASONS FOR STOICISM

To facilitate denial
To perform as the "perfect patient"
To gain self-worth and power
To avoid loss of control
Fear of addiction
Fear of overdose and side effects
Fear of intravenous treatment
To avoid calling attention to oneself
To avoid worrying family
To pay a price for past sins and future joys
Low self-esteem
Desire to experience the process
Desire for meditation
Acceptance of condition
No pain

APPROPRIATE INTERVENTIONS

Careful observation

Check the patient frequently for symptoms of pain.
Observe for objective symptoms of distress.

Elicitation of patient cooperation

Explain that pain retards healing.
Explain that medication is more effective if given at onset of pain.
Explain that medications are safe.
Describe what to expect from pain medication.
Give praise when appropriate.

patient may seem the ideal, but in reality, the concealment of pain can be detrimental to the patient. For one thing, pain inhibits healing. If the nurse does not know that the patient is in pain, the proper medications will not be administered and, in turn, the proper rest and its healing effects will not be experienced by the patient. In the case of acute myocardial infarction (AMI), pain can have more serious effects. The sympathetic response to pain, such as increased heart rate and systolic pressure, increased afterload as reflected in higher peripheral vascular resistance, and increased tendency to ventricular ectopy places the patient at greater risk of lethal dysrhythmias, as well as increases the myocardial oxygen demand. Effective pain management aimed at decreasing the sympathetic input on the cardiovascular system results in a decrease in myocardial oxygen demand and restores a more optimal supply/demand ratio.

Providing explanations to the patient who is afraid to take analgesics can help to improve communication. Many immigrant patients are fearful that medications will become addictive and that too much will be given. For example, an Asian patient with small body stature may fear that the effects of a drug will render him or her out of control, or he or she may believe that pain is an essential part of the healing process.[18,19]

Intervention in these cases obviously involves providing correct information about these concerns. It is particularly helpful for nurses to ask the patient to help them do their job by revealing the amount of pain, explaining that only in this way can the nurse—as the person responsible for the patient's well-being—do a good job. This approach, particularly in view of the Asian emphasis on avoiding failure or embarrassment for all concerned, can have remarkable results.

Observing objective symptoms and noting recent procedures that might cause extreme pain are two of the best ways to assess the amount of pain present. Clenched fists, raised blood pressure, flush, pallor, lack of movement, grimace, rapid pulse, and perspiration are a few of the ways in which the presence of pain can be determined. Even the patient who smiles perpetually should be suspected as one who is trying to maintain dignity and stoicism at all costs.

CULTURAL VARIATIONS IN THE GRIEF RESPONSE

Just as it is necessary for the critical care nurse to understand cultural variations in the response to physical pain, it is equally important to be aware of culturally specific ways of expressing grief and emotional loss, especially if the nurse is to avoid the danger of misinterpreting the meaning of a family's reaction—or

Table 4-1 Death-related behaviors in six cultural groups

Culture	Religious attitudes	Grief expressions	Death rituals	Resources for support
Japanese/Chinese	Very protective of people's feelings Believe in afterlife Decedents return to Nirvana	Not publicly expressive	Chanting ceremony at bedside after death Accepting clothes of deceased may not be appropriate Japanese prepare gift food packs for mourners	Families
Indo-Chinese	After death, soul lives in land of Tian	May weep/wail aloud	Mourning attire consists of white outfit worn by women mourners and black arm-band worn by men	Families
African-Americans	Commonly recognized Western concept of heaven/hell Deceased do not watch over earthlings	Very expressive	Funeral rite is an informal gathering, including prayers, scripture reading, songs, crying/screaming	Minister, family, friends Strong family kinship
Mexican-Americans	Illness/death are God's will	Very expressive	Dependent on religious beliefs	Families
Native Americans	No life after death—return to ancestors Navajos are fearful of death; will burn decedent's possessions Belief in spirits and need to be in harmony with nature	May or may not be publicly expressive	May take form of beasts, chanting, monotonous singing over the dead to frighten away evil spirits	Families, shaman, tribal group
Arabs	Anticipatory grief work not acceptable Children are integral part of family activities	Express grief openly Much touching of decedent's body	Remain with body until transported to funeral home Do life review at decedent's bedside	Family

Modified from York C, Stichler J: *Dimens Crit Care Nurs* 4(2):122, 1985.

lack of reaction—to a loved one's critical condition or death. As in the case of the Hispanic husband mentioned previously, if an individual does not react as expected, it is easy to label the behavior as callousness, denial, or overreaction. In short, the norms for proper grief behavior in one culture may appear strange or even repugnant in the context of another culture. Table 4-1 delineates death-related behaviors associated with six cultural groups.

East Indian culture, for example, allows and indeed calls for a public display of grief. The "stiff upper lip" and brave face that is often called for in British and Anglo-American culture is considered by East Indians as neither appropriate nor necessary.[20]

Although it is impossible to generalize about grief behavior, a good "working generality" with respect to the Jewish family is that in its culture, too, open grieving is encouraged. This grieving is generally confined to a prescribed period, which begins with 7 days of intense mourning and terminates after 1 year when the official season of mourning has ended. During the initial period of mourning, Jewish culture dictates that those who are present to comfort the bereaved would do well to simply listen rather than attempt to mouth empty words of consolation. For this reason, it is important that the family be allowed to congregate at the time of death to provide this necessary support.[21]

Because of the great diversity of Asian cultures within the United States today, it is difficult to predict the grieving pattern of any given Asian family. Japanese people, for example, are likely to be stoic when grieving, whereas certain Chinese persons will feel comfortable venting their feelings even when in public.[21,22] The critical care nurse should bear in mind that the stoicism that is often seen among Asian patients when they have physical pain is likely to be missing when that pain is emotional.

Dr. Lois Davitz and colleagues[23] raised an interesting question during their research into nurses' responses to patient pain. She pointed out that Anglo-American nurses tend to be less tolerant of patients who emote when in physical and psychologic pain than they are of those who are more stoic. This attitude can raise serious problems for the nurse who comes in contact with large numbers of Hispanic families, whose culture dictates an open expression of grief.[22] It must be remembered that each individual learns to react to emotional pain in a way that provides the most effective relief and elicits the most desired support. Hispanic, African-American, and emotive Asian families must be allowed the time and the physical room in which to express their pain.[24,25]

THE LANGUAGE BARRIER

Although language differences form the most obvious barrier to effective cross-cultural communication, they are, paradoxically, among the easiest to overcome, because actual verbiage is only one relatively small element in the communication process. Researchers indicate that nonverbal communication accounts for 70% to 90% of the communication. Gestures, facial expression, body stance and space, eye contact, touch, and tone of voice can go far to soothe the foreign-language–speaking patient's fears and to establish rapport.[26]

An awareness of the meaning of nonverbal communication can also help the critical care nurse overcome one of the most serious barriers to patient compliance and family cooperation – the tendency for newly arrived immigrants to pretend to understand an instruction when in fact they do not.[27] Although this behavior can be very frustrating to the attending nurse, understanding the reasons behind the behavior and some techniques for dealing with it can diffuse this frustration.

Immigrants will pretend to understand for a number of reasons.[28] First, they do not wish to appear inadequate by admitting that their English comprehension is incomplete. Second, they do not wish to have the nurse repeat the material because it is likely that they will still not understand and will therefore feel even more inadequate. Finally, they will pretend comprehension because to not do so would be insulting to the nurse, who – it might be said – failed to explain the material adequately.

Once the motivation of the foreign-born patient is understood, it becomes much easier both to be compassionate and to devise effective interventions. Before interventions can be devised, it is necessary to assess whether the learner does in fact understand what the nurse is saying. To simply ask "Do you understand?" is not an effective means of assessment, because the immigrant will possibly say "yes" to please the nurse and avoid embarrassment for all concerned.

Nonverbal communication is one of the most valuable tools available in dealing with this problem. By observing body language closely, the nurse can readily perceive that the patient or relative does not understand. Such signs as a blank expression, constant nodding of the head and smiling, and a quizzical expression can indicate that true understanding is not taking place. Contrary to popular belief, the avoidance of eye contact (particularly if the family is Asian) does not always mean that the listener is not comprehending.[29] Such behavior is often merely a way of showing respect and deference to the speaker. Another means of assessing the degree of understanding is by the number of questions asked. Paradoxically, if few questions are asked, it can often indicate a lack of understanding, not the opposite. In this case, the patient has not understood enough material to formulate a worthwhile question.

The box (upper right) contains a number of suggestions for facilitating mutual understanding in situations in which it appears that the patient or relative has indeed not understood the information. The final item ("Learn a few words of the language") is a particularly valuable suggestion. By learning just a few words of the languages most often encountered, the nurse can improve rapport with the foreign speaker, make the patient feel emotionally and physically more comfortable, and, perhaps most important, communicate a respect for the patient's own culture.

CROSSING LANGUAGE BARRIERS

Face the patient or relative.
Observe and use nonverbal cues.
Speak simply.
Avoid slang.
Speak slowly.
Speak in short units.
Learn a few words of the language (e.g., "I'm here to help you"; "Do not be afraid"; "You will be all right").

It is not always necessary to use an interpreter to communicate effectively. On the occasions, however, when an interpreter is necessary, a few guidelines are indicated. If possible, do not use family members as interpreters, because relatives frequently will keep information from each other in an attempt to spare feelings or avoid conflict.[30] Further, be certain that the interpreter speaks the correct dialect. This may seem obvious, but numerous errors in this regard are being reported. It is not unknown, for example, for hospitals to have called in an Arabic interpreter when dealing with an Iranian Farsi-speaking family. Finally, if at all possible, arrange for the interpreter and patient to be of the same class, because differences in class can result in severe discomfort and reticence for both parties.

The key to overcoming cultural barriers to effective critical care nursing lies in the nurse's willingness to examine with an open mind the perspective of the immigrant patient and family. The ability to understand another's way of looking at the world arises, not only out of experience and repeated interaction, but also from careful study of the literature in the field.

REFERENCES

1. Baxter C: Culture shock, *Nurs Times* 84:36, 1988.
2. Herrera J: The effectiveness of a cultural milieu on hospitalized Hispanic patients, *Int J Psychosom* 34:6, 1987.
3. Sheikh A, Sheikh K: *Eastern and Western approaches to healing: ancient wisdom and modern healing,* New York, 1989, John Wiley & Sons.
4. Balsmeyer B: Locus of control and the use of strategies to promote self-care, *J Community Health Nurs* 1(3):171, 1984.
5. Mays V: Identity developing of black Americans: the role of history and the importance of ethnicity, *Am J Psychother* 40(4):582, 1986.
6. Lipson J, Meleis A: Issues in health care of Middle-Eastern patients, *West J Med* 139(6):854, 1983.

7. Leininger M: *Culture care diversity and universality: a theory of nursing,* New York, 1991, National League for Nursing Pub. No. 15-2402.
8. Beinfield H, Korngold E: *Between heaven and earth: a guide to Chinese medicine,* New York, 1991, Ballantine Books.
9. Quadagno J: The Italian-American family. In Mindel C, Habenstein R, editors: *Ethnic families in America,* ed 2, New York, 1981, Elsevier Science Publishing.
10. Zatzick D, Dimsdale J: Cultural variations in response to painful stimuli, *Psychosom Med* 52(5):544, 1990.
11. Greenwald H: Interethnic differences in pain perception, *Pain* 44(2):157, 1991.
12. Thomas V, Rose F: Ethnic differences in the pain experience, *Soc Sci Med* 32(9):1063, 1991.
13. Gaston-Johansson F and others: Similarities in pain descriptions of four different ethnic-culture groups, *J Pain Symptom Management* 5(2):94, 1990.
14. Vogel V: *American Indian medicine,* Norman, Okla, 1990, University of Oklahoma Press.
15. Vavasseur J: Psychosocial aspects of chronic disease: cultural and ethnic implications, *Birth Defects* 23:144, 1987.
16. Calvillo E, Flaskerud J: Review of literature on culture and pain of adults with focus on Mexican-Americans, *J Transcult Nurs* 2(2):16, 1991.
17. Strogatz D: Use of medical care for chest pain: differences between blacks and whites, *Am J Public Health* 80(3):290, 1990.
18. Shapiro D: A sense of control, health and illness: exploring the mind-body relationship and the socio-cultural and spiritual context: reflections on Bali, *Int J Psychosom* 37(1-4):40, 1990.
19. Harrell S: Pluralism, performance and meaning in Taiwanese healing: a case study, *Cult Med Psychiatry* 15(1):45, 1991.
20. Mayor V: The family, bereavement and dietary beliefs, *Nurs Times* 80:40, 1984.
21. Johnson T and others: Providing culturally sensitive care: intervention by a consultation-liaison team, *Hosp Community Psychiatry* 39(2):200, 1988.
22. York C, Stichler J: Cultural grief expressions following infant death, *Dimens Crit Care Nurs* 4(2):120, 1985.
23. Davitz J, Davitz L: Inferences of patients' pain and psychological distress: studies of nursing behaviors, New York, 1981, Springer Publishing.
24. Katz P, Kirkland F: Traditional thought and modern western surgery, *Soc Sci Med* 26(12):1175, 1988.
25. Pang K: Hwabyung: The construction of a Korean popular illness among Korean elderly immigrant women in the United States, *Cult Med Psychiatry* 14(1):495, 1990.
26. Erzinger S: Communication between Spanish-speaking patients and their doctors in medical encounters, *Cult Med Psychiatry* 15(1):91, 1991.
27. Muecke M: In search of healers—South East Asian refugees in the American health care system, *West J Med* 139(6):835, 1983.
28. Thompson W, Thompson T: Taking care of culturally different and non–English speaking patients, *Int J Psychiatry Med* 20(3):235, 1990.
29. Ots T: The angry liver, the anxious heart and the melancholy spleen. The phenomenology of perceptions in chinese culture, *Cult Med Psychiatry* 14(1):21, 1990.
30. Reinert B: The health care beliefs and values of Mexican-Americans, *Home Health Care Update* 4:23, 1986.

5

Patient Education

CHAPTER OBJECTIVES

- Describe the educational role of the critical care nurse in health promotion activities.
- List three factors that influence an individual's health maintenance practices.
- Adapt and apply teaching-learning theory to the critical care setting.
- Describe the stages of adaptation to illness and the implications of each for the patient teaching plan.
- Perform a learning needs assessment.
- Construct a teaching plan for a patient in the critical care unit.
- Describe an optimal learning environment.
- Discuss four methods of instruction and the appropriateness of each to the critical care setting.

Persons entering the health care system bring with them unique medical, social, and educational histories that affect their interactions with health care providers. These experiences also form the basis of the philosophies and perceptions of health and illness and of behaviors related to health maintenance and promotion. When a patient is admitted to the hospital with an acute or critical problem, the problem is often the result of a failure to manage and maintain his or her own health. Frequently the illness creates new requirements in the areas of health maintenance and promotion that must be practiced by the patient during recovery and sometimes for a lifetime. Learning needs arise out of the new requirements. Hence the nurse in the critical and telemetry care units often needs to incorporate educational techniques into the plan of care.

This chapter is intended to assist the nurse in identifying factors related to health management and promotion that affect the educational plan of care and the patient's response to that care in the critical care and telemetry units. An exploration of educational theory and techniques is presented to assist the nurse in meeting identified learning needs. The dynamics of compliance and noncompliance with the health care plan as they relate to patient education are also discussed.

HEALTH MAINTENANCE AS A NURSING RESPONSIBILITY

Nursing has played a major role in health promotion since the mid-nineteenth century.[1] In 1980 the American Nurses Association published its *Social Policy Statement* for nursing, which outlines the social context of nursing and the nature and scope of nursing practice. This document highlights the importance of health promotion and maintenance as a responsibility of the nursing profession. Health promotion refers to activities directed toward developing the patient resources that maintain or enhance well-being. In the past several years the focus has shifted from a disease-oriented system of care to one that values wellness and optimal health, including the prevention or control of disease. The focus is on gaining, attaining, and maintaining health. At the same time, both health professionals and the public recognize an increasing responsibility on the part of the individual and family for health maintenance.

Nurses continue to make major contributions to the evolution of the health-oriented system of care and are uniquely qualified to assist patients in planning for short-term and long-term health management and maintenance needs while treating the condition for which the patient was admitted.[2] Nursing management plans for care of the patient with Altered Health Maintenance are included at the end of this chapter.

HEALTH PROMOTION IN THE CRITICAL CARE SETTING

Critical care nurses usually focus on the life-threatening physiologic problems of their patients. Constraints of time and the necessity to set priorities of care have limited health promotion activities of the critical care nurse. However, in the current climate of health care, hospitalized patients are more acutely ill and generally have shorter lengths of stay. This shorter length of stay and other changes in the process of health care mandate efficiency in health care management.[3] Hence the role of health promotion in the critical care unit must be examined. It is important to consider that hospitalization may be the patient's first encounter with health care professionals and health promotion information. The nurse with whom the patient interacts has the potential to influence perceptions about future health care practices.[4] Critical care nurses must recognize that their attitudes directly affect patients' decisions about future health behaviors. In addition, educational activities in the hospital setting have been found to increase patient satisfaction with the care received.[5]

Priorities set by the critical care nurse must place maintenance of immediate physical and psychologic safety above long-term health promotion needs. However, when the patient's clinical condition allows, the therapeutic relationship between the patient and nurse provides an excellent learning environment for discussion of health promotion issues. If patient education, role modeling, effective communication, and skilled nursing care are combined in the experience of the critically ill patient, the patient may begin to identify his or her continuing role in health maintenance and promotion as recovery continues and discharge nears. The educational plan of care begun in the critical care unit forms the basis for successful outcomes in the telemetry setting.

Families also can benefit from health promotion activities during hospitalization, and valuable information concerning the family environment to which the patient will return can be gained during health promotion assessment and teaching.[6] Creative nursing strategies that combine the holistic, long-term goals of health promotion with the critical, short-term goals and behaviors in the critical care setting can add an important and satisfying aspect to the care of acutely ill patients.

NURSING HISTORY OF HEALTH PERCEPTION AND MANAGEMENT

How has the patient's general health been?

Has the patient had any other illnesses in the past year, including colds and minor illnesses?

What are the most important things the patient does to keep healthy? Do these things make a difference? Include folk remedies if appropriate.

Does the patient use cigarettes, alcohol, or drugs? Are appropriate self-screening examinations performed (e.g., regular breast self-examinations for women)?

In the past, has the patient found it easy to follow the advice of health professionals?

Are there financial, social, cultural, or geographic barriers to access to proper health care?

What caused this illness? What actions were taken when the symptoms were noticed? What were the results of those actions?

What things are most important to the patient while in the hospital? How can the staff be most helpful?

Factors Influencing Health Practices

The patient's health practices and perceptions provide some guidance in the planning of care in the critical care and telemetry units. Patient education should be based on a careful assessment, correct diagnosis, and individualization of the plan of care.[7] The educational plan of care in the critical care unit, continued on the telemetry unit, should reflect consideration of individual differences in the patient's health care beliefs. Assessment of factors influencing an individual's health practices provides insight into the patient's perceived health status, the importance he or she places on health, and the level of his or her commitment to health maintenance. Careful assessment in this area also identifies actual or potential health problems or risks that are unrelated to the reason for admission but may adversely affect recovery and the success of educational interventions. The nursing assessment in the critical care unit should include information related to these primarily nonacute health patterns.

The box (upper right) gives general information about health perception and management that should be obtained during the nursing history gathered for the assessment.[8] This assessment should be carried out as soon after admission as the patient's condition allows.

◆ **Health belief model.** All human behavior is motivated by one or more factors. The Health Belief Model is one framework to explain predictable sources of motivation for specific health behaviors. The Health Belief Model was developed in its original form in the 1950s. It was designed to predict those individuals who would or would not use the growing resources in disease prevention. In the 1970s, Becker revised the model to the form that is used today. It identifies the individual perceptions, modifying factors, and variables that affect the likelihood of taking preventive action.

◆ **Individual perceptions.** Individual perceptions refers to the degree to which individuals perceive that they are susceptible to a particular disease and how serious it is believed to be. Research has shown that the more individuals perceive they are susceptible, the greater the likelihood of their engaging in preventive behaviors.[9] This concept also extends to continued or renewed susceptibility to an illness experienced in the past. Although less strongly supported as a motivator of preventive behavior, the degree to which the disease is perceived as serious can affect the health care–seeking actions.[9]

Studies have shown that the greater the perceived threat of an illness, the more likely are preventive behaviors.[9] However, a very high level of perceived severity can produce overwhelming threats and subsequent avoidance of preventive behavior, because of the immobilizing effects of severe anxiety.[10] The perception of threat should be considered when planning the educational care of the patient.

◆ **Modifying factors.** Modifying factors are those demographic, sociopsychologic, and structural variables that may affect an individual's likelihood of practicing behaviors. These factors may include gender, socioeconomic status, race, ethnicity, or level of education. Pressure to conform to social norms appears to play a role in promoting use of preventive measures, as does the expectation of significant others. Structural variables, such as knowledge about the disease and prior contact with it, are motivating factors.

Also considered modifying factors are various cues to action that may trigger preventive action. These may be internal cues, such as uncomfortable symptoms or unpleasant memories of a family member's illness. External cues include reminder cards from health professionals or exposure to media campaigns, news articles, or advice from others.

◆ **Likelihood of action.** The likelihood of practicing the recommended preventive health action also depends on the perceived benefits and barriers. The belief that the action taken will be effective in preventing illness is an important determining factor of the preventive behavior. In addition, barriers such as cost, inconvenience, fear of pain, or significant changes in life-style are negative motivators for health promotion.

COMPLIANCE

One successful outcome of the patient's educational plan is compliance with the treatment regimen. Indeed, what patients view as most important to learn in the hospital is related to what they plan to comply with after discharge.[11] Although not all education will lead to compliance, it is the desired phenomenon. Compliance is defined as "the extent to which a person's behavior coincides with medical or health advice."[12] Compliance can be improved by affecting attitudes, beliefs, and understanding.[13] The concepts of compliance and noncompliance are generally discussed in reference to the chronically ill patient whose care and treatment regimen continues past hospitalization and requires commitment and energy by the patient and family. The use of the nursing diagnosis of Noncompliance, however, refers to the individual who wants to comply but the presence of certain factors prevents him or her from doing so.[14] Using this definition, noncompliance issues concerning the hospitalized patient and the short-term problems of compliance with the medical and nursing treatments in the critical care unit can be considered. The nurse can concentrate on identifying, reducing, or eliminating the factors that affect the patient's ability to comply with treatment. These factors focus on alterations in cognition and perception, inadequacies in the social system, and deficits in the health care system and will be discussed separately. Nursing management plans are included at the end of this chapter related to the nursing diagnosis of Noncompliance.

Factors Influencing Compliance

◆ **Alteration in cognition.** Patients may be noncompliant because they do not know the reason for or the importance of the recommended behaviors. This group of patients includes those who, for whatever reason, do not want information that would lead to compliance. In addition, patients may have false or inaccurate information on which they are basing their behaviors. Some hold to folk beliefs that interfere with their motivation to follow the prescribed medical treatments. Any disturbance in thought processes, such as memory loss, inability to concentrate, and inability to solve problems or to follow directions, can affect compliance. This often occurs in the critical care areas because of side effects of pain medications, sleep deprivation, sensory overload, anxiety, or neurologic deficits. Nurses must also consider the patient's ability to read, write, and understand the language and any real or potential visual or hearing deficits.

◆ **Alteration in perception.** Beliefs, feelings, and values may affect compliance. The Health Belief Model, one theory explaining motivation for compliance, has been discussed in this chapter. Psychologic and emotional responses to illness are often seen in the critical care areas and can adversely affect the patient's ability to comply. For example, the defense mechanism of denial, although serving a useful purpose in protecting the patient from unmanageable levels of anxiety, allows him or her to discount the illness or its severity or the need for cooperating with health care personnel or for making life-style changes. Denial is frequently encountered in the critical care setting, because the reality of the hospitalization can be overwhelming in this period. As the patient progresses to the telemetry unit, nurses can be instrumental in promoting his or her realistic appraisal of the clinical condition.

Depression, anger, or fear can also establish barriers to compliant behavior, as can a conflict in values. In this case, the patient agrees with the desirability of a behavior, but the necessary time, money, or energy resources are not available or the goals are low priority. Finally, some patients agree with the need to comply but feel unable to make the required changes. This is often seen as a return to habitual behaviors despite the attempt to change. In the case of the dependent individual, including children and many disabled and elderly persons, the health beliefs and attitudes of the responsible party determine the extent to which the treatment regimen is followed.[15]

◆ **Inadequacies in the social system.** Factors related to the patient's environment—including significant others, job, community, religious beliefs, and material resources—may affect the ability to comply with treatment. The support of significant others may be the important determinant in the patient's compliance, especially in long-term compliance.[12] Inadequate financial resources may be a barrier to compliance (e.g., an individual on a fixed income who has been prescribed an expensive medication). Adequate financial resources, however, do not ensure compliance. Geographic and transportation difficulties may also affect the ability to comply.

◆ **Deficits in the health care system.** Health care system deficits that may affect compliance include a treatment regimen that is perceived by the patient as too complex or unmanageable, the failure of the system to provide specific and complete instructions, and a patient–health provider relationship that is not supportive and mutually respectful. It is necessary to examine the system and the caregivers as possible factors in patient compliance. Efforts should be made to keep the patient and family involved in the planning of care, including educational efforts, so as to promote meeting individual needs successfully.

Discontinuation of Treatment

A discussion of noncompliance in the critical care setting must include cases in which patients choose to refuse or discontinue treatment. More patients are becoming involved in making life-and-death decisions proactively through the process of living wills, advance directives, and designations for durable powers of attorney for medical care. Both patients with chronic diseases and those who have never been hospitalized are seeking to confirm their wishes in the event of significant or hopeless disease states. Patients, families, and health professionals face difficult decisions when the patient in the critical care unit has advanced disease. Although a thoughtful decision by a person with advanced disease to terminate treatment is not universally viewed as noncompliance,[16] it does represent a rejection of medical advice and can be frustrating to the nurse whose goals are the restoration of optimal health and functional status. Nurses should be aware of their own personal feelings about these dynamics so as to maintain objective viewpoints to assist the patient in determining health care and educational needs. The educational care plan should reflect consideration of the patient's right to determination with realistic goals based on these decisions.

PATIENT EDUCATION

The education of the patient and family is now universally accepted as an important nursing function in all settings of practice. The critical care unit offers additional challenges in that it is often a foreign and threatening environment to the patient and family. Nursing has a legal and ethical responsibility to meet standards of care related to patient education. These standards include identifying the patient's and family's learning needs, assessing their readiness to learn, teaching the appropriate content, documenting the teaching plan, and evaluating and documenting the results of the patient teaching.[17] The American Association of Critical-Care Nurses highlights the importance of patient education in critical care by stating in their "Standards of Care": "The critical care nurse shall identify areas of education of the patient and significant others."[18] Subsequently, authors have explored the questions of whether critically ill patients can be taught[19] and how best to approach patient and family education in the critical care areas.[6,20-23]

The basis for all educational activities for patients and families is the belief that they have the right to information about diagnosis, treatment, and prognosis in terms that are understandable to them.[24] Part of this belief is that rational individuals can, on some level, understand all but the most technical aspects of their care.[23] It also involves the knowledge that each patient is unique, learns in a unique way, and has motivation and skill in applying new knowledge that differs from that of other patients. These individual differences are the reasons for varied responses to the same teaching strategies.

Along with a belief in the patient's right to know, the patient's right not to know must also be recognized in some cases. This is correlated to the dynamics of compliance discussed previously. The patient's right not to know must be respected in those cases in which patients prefer not to learn about their illnesses. Simple basic information about monitors and unit policy, for example, usually suffices in these cases. Indeed, more information than can be processed and integrated can greatly increase anxiety and may result in slower recovery.[3,23] Individuals have the right to accept, adopt, or reject the information provided in educational encounters, however frustrating this may be to the nurse.[3]

Adult Learning Theory

Central to successful implementation of an educational plan in the critical care and telemetry environment is the incorporation of the principles of adult learning theory. An educational plan that does consider the uniqueness of the adult population can potentially fail. It is beneficial for the nurse to have an understanding of this theory before planning or implementing the educational plan of care. Unfortunately, it has been noted that more is known about how animals and children learn than adults.[25] Nonetheless, Knowles described several assumptions on adult learning theory that differ from those of children.[25] Adults must be ready to learn, having moved from one developmental or educational task to the next. They need to know why it is important to learn something before they can actually learn it. Inherent in their attitudes is a responsibility for their own decisions. Consequently, they may resent when others try to force different beliefs on them. Adults bring a wealth of experience to the learning environment that should be recognized and promoted in educational techniques. Their orientation to learning is life-centered, so that tasks being taught should focus on current problem resolution. Finally, motivation for the adult learner arises out of such internal pressures as self-esteem and quality of life.

Teaching-Learning Process

The teaching-learning process used in the health care setting incorporates the dynamics of adult learning theory. This process can be defined as a set of activities organized and structured to maximize the results for the patient and to minimize the amount of time and effort on the part of the health care practitioner.[26] It can be divided into the five steps summarized in the box below. These steps can be closely related to the nursing process. Table 5-1 shows the application of the nursing process to the teaching-learning process in the care of the critically ill patient.

◆ **Assessment.** The assessment step in patient teaching involves gathering a data base to assist the nurse in meeting the patient's and family's learning needs.[26] It is a vital part of any successful educational plan. Among the components of this assessment in the critical care unit are identification of the various physiologic, psychologic, environmental, and sociocultural stressors present; the patient's response to these stressors; adaptation to illness; and an examination of motivation and readiness to learn. In reality, these issues are often

THE TEACHING-LEARNING PROCESS

1. Assessment of the need to learn
2. Assessment of readiness to learn
3. Setting of objectives
4. Teaching-learning activities
5. Evaluation and reteaching if necessary

Table 5-1 Application of the nursing process to the teaching-learning process

Nursing process	Teaching-learning process
Assessment	Physiologic Psychologic Environmental Sociocultural Assessment of physiologic and psychologic stress response Physiologic Heart rate Blood pressure Peristalsis Mental acuity Blood glucose Dilated pupils Psychologic Anxiety Depression Panic Withdrawal Denial Hostility Regression Frustration Assessment of readiness to learn
Nursing diagnosis and plan	Identification of specific knowledge deficit Identification of causes and associated factors Identification of expected outcomes and behavioral objectives Development of teaching plan
Nursing intervention	Teaching-learning activities and experience
Evaluation	Evaluation and documentation of effectiveness of teaching-learning process Measurement of knowledge gain Measurement of behavior changes

related to one another and cannot be assessed as separate entities. For ease of illustration, however, they are discussed separately.

Stressors

PHYSIOLOGIC STRESSORS. One main physiologic stressor for the critically ill patient is the illness, often life-threatening, for which the patient was admitted. In addition, usually other physiologic changes in critically ill patients act as further stressors. These may include pain, hypoxia, cardiac arrhythmias, hypotension, fluid and electrolyte imbalances, infection, fever, or neurologic deficits. The presence of the illness and other stressors may completely consume the patient's available energy and leave none for any type of orientation to stimuli or education.

A physical assessment will yield information about physiologic reactions to stress. The following factors should be considered:

- Is the patient in pain or some other type of distress?
- What is the patient's level of consciousness and orientation?
- Has the patient been sedated?
- Is the patient hypoxic or hypercapnic?
- Are the heart rate, blood pressure, cardiac output, and perfusion adequate?
- Can the patient see and hear?

These questions add to the data base for formulation of an effective educational plan.

PSYCHOLOGIC STRESSORS. Serious illness affects a patient not only physically, but also psychologically. Intense emotions can alter a person's normal way of coping and ability to learn and retain information. Psychologic stressors often present in the critically ill person include helplessness, powerlessness, loneliness, changes in role in the family and at work, changes in body image, fear of future life-style changes, and fear of death. These and other psychologic stressors not only can result in physiologic changes, but also can trigger behavior consistent with anxiety, denial, and depression.

The psychologic assessment is also important in determining the patient's ability to respond to the teaching-learning experience. An important factor is the patient's stage in adaptation to illness during the time teaching is undertaken. The general characteristics of the *stages of adaptation to illness* are outlined in Table 5-2 with corresponding applications for the teaching-learning process. Salient points are reviewed here. It should be noted that each individual moves at his or her own pace through the stages and it is not uncommon to skip or move back and forth through the stages. Because of individual variations, the stages can be encountered in both the critical care and telemetry units. The nurse should also consider that the family goes through stages of adaptation to their loved one's illness as well. Family members may or may not progress at the same rate as the patient, so teaching strategies may need modification to ensure meeting the individual needs of both the patient and the significant others.

The first response to acute illness is generally *disbelief and denial.* Although this response has some psychologic benefit for the patient, it acts as a barrier to learning. During this stage it is acceptable for the nurse to allow denial if it does not put the patient in danger. Teaching should be focused on the present, and comments referring to the future should be avoided.

After a few days the denial mechanism usually breaks down and the patient moves into the stage of *developing awareness.* The patient must accept that he or she is ill. This stage generally coincides with the assumption of the sick role. At this time a patient may respond with anger or guilt. If these emotions are turned inward, he or she may experience depression. If emotions are expressed outwardly, behavior may be hostile toward persons and

Table 5-2 Teaching-learning process in adaptation to illness

Stage of adaptation	Characteristic patient response	Implications for teaching-learning process
Disbelief	Denial	Orient teaching to present. Teach during other nursing activities. Reassure patient about safety. Explain all procedures and activities clearly and concisely.
Developing awareness	Anger	Continue to orient teaching to present. Avoid long lists of facts. Continue to foster development of trust and rapport through good physical care.
Reorganization	Acceptance of sick role	Orient teaching to meet patient needs. Teach whatever patient wants to learn. Provide necessary self-care information. Reinforce with written material.
Resolution	Identification with others with same problem; recognition of loss	Use group instruction. Use patient support groups and visits by recovered patients with same problem.
Identifying change	Definition of self as one who has undergone change and is now different	Answer patient's questions as they arise. Recognize that as basic needs are met more mature needs will arise.

things in the environment, including the nurse. It is important at this time to listen to the expressions of anger but not to argue with the patient. The nurse should remember that the patient is reacting to factors other than the nurse. Teaching during this time should continue to be oriented to the present but may relate more to the disease process, which is now recognized by the patient. The patient is still too anxious to learn and assimilate lists of facts but may be interested in the meaning of symptoms and treatments as they relate to his or her experience at the moment.

The third stage of adaptation to illness is *reorganization.* At this time the patient has begun to work through the anger and guilt and to reorganize his or her self-concept and relationships with others consistent with the acceptance of the sick role. During this time the nurse should teach whatever the patient wants to learn, thus helping the patient to achieve the reorganization necessary to move on to adaptation.

The final stages of adaptation are *resolution* and *identity change.* They occur late in recovery, even as late as the sixth week in the case of a patient with a myocardial infarction.[27] During these times the patient is more receptive to teaching based on objectives and to learning about long-term needs. Group instruction that includes the spouse and significant others can be an effective method at this time.

Also included in the psychologic assessment of the patient is an assessment of the patient's coping style. Coping can affect learning.[28] Weinberger et al.[29] identified two types of coping styles: repression and sensitization. A sensitizer is information-seeking and will respond positively to nursing educational interventions, often keeping the nurse in the room with numerous questions. On the other hand, a repressor is information-escaping and therefore wants minimal information and may dismiss the nurse quickly from educational efforts. It is important for the nurse to recognize the patient's coping style and respect it during educational efforts.[30]

ENVIRONMENTAL STRESSORS. The physical surroundings in a critical care unit contribute to the stress of the experience for a patient. Such factors as sleep deprivation, observation of other patients, loss of privacy, bright lights, unfamiliar noises, unpleasant odors, and loss of contact with loved ones contribute to stress. Management and control of these factors have become important nursing functions, especially in the creation of a learning environment.

SOCIOCULTURAL STRESSORS. Such variables as age, gender, ethnic origin, economic status, religious beliefs, level of education, and occupation may add to the stress of illness and alter learning ability. The nurse-patient interaction should be structured to recognize the effects of these variables on the process and outcome of the teaching-learning experience.

Motivation and readiness to learn. Assessment of motivation and readiness to learn are important parts of the teaching-learning process. This assessment incorporates an analysis of multiple factors that have previously been discussed. These include an appreciation of multiple stressors and their response and the patient's stage of adaptation to illness. In addition, an examination of motivation theory is helpful. One well-known and important theory describing human behavior motivation is Maslow's hierarchy of needs, which provides background for the discussion of motivation to learn.

Maslow described a number of needs that were postulated as motivating all behavior. According to this theory, human beings have a number of needs that are interrelated and hierarchic. In other words, the lower-level needs must be met before higher-level needs can emerge and be satisfied. The basic needs are physiologic, safety, belongingness, love, esteem, and self-actualization.[31] The need to know and understand are among the highest-level needs. During a time of critical illness, a patient's energy is often consumed by the lower-level physiologic and safety needs and it would be impossible for the patient to attend to learning interactions. Attempting to teach a patient who fears for his or her life and safety is of little use unless the patient is being taught that he or she is safe and in no immediate danger of dying. Once the lower-level needs are met and the patient feels out of danger, he or she will be more ready to learn and higher-level needs can be addressed. Therefore if the assessment discloses significant needs in lower areas, the nurse should address those needs before attempting any teaching. Once met, these needs cease to be the primary motivators of behavior and the patient can attend to his or her learning and other higher-level needs.

◆ **Nursing diagnosis and plan.** The assessment of the multitude of factors that have been discussed assists the critical care nurse in the establishment of an adequate data base from which to formulate nursing diagnoses and devise an educational plan of care. In this plan of care, expected outcomes and behavioral objectives are identified. A plan of care for Knowledge Deficit is included at the end of this chapter. Also, various teaching content areas frequently identified in the critical care unit are presented here for review.

Teaching content. Determination of the content presented in the critical care unit depends on the patient's clinical and emotional status and varies with each patient. The nurse sets learning needs priorities based on the assessment as soon as possible. However, at times an acute event precludes full assessment at the time of admission. In this case, behavior crucial to the patient's treatment and his or her participation in care can be taught as soon as appropriate. The teaching should be guided by the patient and family—that is, teach what they want to know when they want to know it. If the patient's questions and concerns are left unanswered during this time of high anxiety, the unmet needs will serve as a block to further communication and prevent the patient from focusing his or her energy appropriately.

Although the specific content taught varies, depending on the condition for which the patient is admitted, certain areas should be covered with any patient who is conscious. *Environmental factors* in a critical care unit can be frightening to patients and should be explained as soon as possible. Cardiac monitors, oxygen equipment, indwelling lines and catheters, frequent laboratory tests, and vital signs checks may cause the patient undue anxiety unless their purpose or function is understood. The reason for procedures, as well as their associated sensations or discomfort, should be briefly explained. This information may not be retained and may require several repetitions, but it will assist in decreasing anxiety and providing a sense of control for the moment.

Most of the time it is appropriate to give *information about the illness or diagnosis* in the critical phase of care. The nurse must often interpret and explain information provided by physicians. Despite the denial often present, some patients want to know about their illness, prognosis, complications, and reason for admission to the critical care unit. A patient may ask if he or she is going to die. This is a traumatic question for both the patient and the nurse. Nurses may reluctantly talk about death with colleagues or a family but are often very uncomfortable in discussing it with patients. It is important for the nurse to remember that the entire experience of the critical care unit, although routine for the staff, is frightening for the patient who may be confronting mortality for the first time. Questions should be answered as honestly, compassionately, and sensitively as possible and should be followed by supportive care as necessary.

Patients in critical care units experience many stressful *medical and nursing procedures* during the course of their care, including radiologic procedures, placement of vascular access or monitoring devices, intubation, suctioning, spinal taps, and many others. Educational and psychologic preparation for these procedures can decrease anxiety and increase patient cooperation with care. Two types of information can be offered to patients in preparation for these procedures. *Procedural information* refers to what will be done, when and where it will happen, and who will provide the service. *Sensory information* refers to what the patient should expect to feel during and after the procedure.[32] When time permits, allowing the patient to ask questions, see equipment that will be used, and practice movements or body positions that will be required can be very helpful in reducing anxiety. In addition, teaching the patient basic relaxation techniques, such as deep breathing or guided imagery, can be effective in helping patients relax during a stressful or uncomfortable procedure.[32,33] When these procedures must occur on an emergent basis without time for patient preparation, the nurse should explain what happened and why as soon as the patient stabilizes and is able to understand the information.

Another important educational consideration in the critical care environment is that the patient learns not only by what is said directly, but also by inadvertent comments or nonverbal cues. Nurses should be especially attuned to staff or physician discussions at the patient's bedside, where information heard by the patient can be misinterpreted and possibly lead to increased anxiety and misinformation. In addition, if nonverbal cues from the nurse do not coincide with the reality of the situation or the severity of the patient condition, mistrust can ensue and alter the nurse-patient therapeutic relationship. These dynamics can also affect educational effort with the family.

Objectives. Inherent in any educational plan of care is careful consideration of desired objectives. Objectives state the desired behaviors expected from the implementation of the plan.[24] They are based on the patient's learning needs and serve as a guide for the teaching-learning process. Objectives are written in behavioral terms that are measurable and are stated in terms of what the patient is to learn, rather than what the nurse is to teach. Terms such as "to know," "understand," "be familiar with," "realize," and "appreciate" are open to many interpretations and are difficult to measure. Rather, active verbs such as to *"identify," "state," "list," "describe,"* or *"demonstrate"* should be used, because they are readily understood by all and easily lend themselves to evaluation.

Both long-term and short-term objectives are appropriate, although in many cases it takes days, weeks, or even months of repetition and practice for a new skill to be mastered. Indeed, constraints of time in both the critical care and telemetry units may indicate considering only those needs identified as important and realistic to the patient with follow-up education after discharge.[34] However, a nurse in the critical care setting should not hesitate to identify goals that surpass the critical care phase, because the educational plan of care continues as the patient improves and is transferred to the telemetry unit. Generalized objectives have been developed for teaching programs used for large numbers of patients, such as cardiac teaching plans for patients recovering from myocardial infarctions. Standardized plans can be useful resource materials in developing a teaching plan but must not take the place of individualized, specific objectives designed for each patient.

◆ Nursing intervention

The teaching-learning experience. Patients in the critical care environment are educated in many informal interactions with the nurse, and knowledge gained fosters patient understanding and well-being. Educational opportunities can be present during various nursing care activities, such as bathing and administration of medication. Each encounter with the patient and family should be viewed as a teaching opportunity. There are times, however, during the hospitalization when more formal or structured educational experiences are in order. Structured educational approaches have been found to be beneficial for immediate knowledge gain.[28] Included in this discussion are techniques in creating a learning environment and various teaching activities or methods that can be used to accomplish the desired outcomes based on the patient's individual learning objectives.

Creating a learning environment. Patient barriers to learning related to physiologic, emotional, and motivational factors have been discussed. To structure a successful teaching-learning experience in a critical care area, the nurse must also carefully assess the environmental and iatrogenic barriers that affect the interaction. Bright lights, unpleasant odors, unfamiliar noises, and untidy surroundings can distract patients and add to cognitive impairment. Control of these factors can facilitate the learning process. Factors that cannot be controlled should be explained to the patient to alleviate anxiety and facilitate a trusting relationship between patient and nurse.

The nurse should examine possible barriers to learning that he or she brings to the interaction. Nurses have been found to set up barriers both consciously and unconsciously to the patient's learning and understanding.[27] The use of medical terms that are not understood by the patient and the use of language inappropriate to the patient's educational level are examples of ways in which nurses may adversely affect the teaching-learning process.[35] There may also be a failure to set aside time just for teaching, resulting in hurried and fragmented sessions. Nonverbal cues on the part of the nurse, such as glancing at the clock or breaking eye contact, may interrupt patient interactions. The manner in which the teaching sessions are planned and executed can have as important an effect on patient learning as the material presented.

Teaching methods. The three basic methods of teaching are lecture, discussion, and demonstration.[3] The choice of method depends on the material to be taught.

LECTURE. Lecture is the presentation of information in a highly structured format to a group. In this method the teacher provides a great deal of material but may not provide ample opportunities for teacher-learner interaction. This style of teaching is inappropriate for acutely ill individuals in the critical care unit. However, it may be useful in the telemetry unit. Optimally, the group size should be arranged to enable the learners to ask questions and get appropriate feedback on content presented.

DISCUSSION. Discussion is less structured than is lecturing and allows an exchange and feedback between the teacher and learner. The teacher can adapt the material to meet the needs of the individual or group. The discussion approach is probably most useful when learning should result in behavior change or in development of an attitude.[3] Discussion groups can be effective with hospitalized patients when a group with similar problems and at similar stages of adaptation can be gathered. Individual discussion with patients and families is appropriate and valuable during the acute phase of illness, because it allows them to express their feelings and interpretations. This approach is the ideal way to teach about sensitive issues, such as resuming sexual activity after myocardial infarction.[3]

DEMONSTRATION. Demonstration involves acting out a procedure while giving appropriate explanations to provide the learner with a clear idea of how to perform a task. The patient can then practice the skill and be given feedback about his or her performance. This method is often used in the acute care setting, such as when coughing and deep breathing, or taking one's own pulse is taught.

OTHER METHODS OF INSTRUCTION. In addition to the three basic methods just presented, several other approaches to delivering or augmenting information in a patient teaching program are available. They include commercially prepared or custom-designed printed materials, bedside videotape programs, and computer-assisted patient education programs. Computer programs, relatively new to health education, have been used in community-based education programs, hospital waiting rooms, designated teaching rooms, and, in some cases, at the bedside with microcomputers on transportable carts.[36] These programs allow the learner to set the program pace and are generally presented in an attractive, colorful format.[37]

Written materials can be very useful tools in patient and family education. They allow repetition and reinforcement of content and provide basic information in printed form for reference at a later time. To be useful, however, the content must be accurate and current and the patient and family must be able to read and understand it. The varied comprehensibility of instructions has been associated with compliance with medical regimens.[38]

It is estimated that the median literacy level of the U.S. population is at the tenth grade level, with about 20% of the population having reading skills at the fifth grade level or lower.[24] Other research indicates that approximately 50% of health care clients have serious difficulty reading instructional materials written at the fifth grade level.[39] The vast majority of patient education materials are written at or above the eighth grade level.[40] To ensure that the reading level of the educational material and the learner are well matched, the patients should be questioned about the last grade level completed in school. Because this level may not equal the grade level in reading ability, written material two to four grade levels below that should be selected.[41] The box below depicts examples of an instruction written at various reading levels.

In recent years the use of educational videotapes at the bedside or in group settings has gained increasing popularity. A recent review of the literature on the use of videotapes verifies that the medium can be used to address the basic and repetitive aspects of patient education and that it is effective for short-term knowledge gain.[42] The use of videotapes, however, should not be considered a substitute for individualized patient teaching, and it is most effective when it is promoted by staff as reinforcing other educational activities.[42,43] Staff members should preview the tapes before showing them to patients to ensure the accuracy and appropriateness of the content and to assess the best way to introduce and reinforce the material. In addition, it is essential that the nurse realize that audiovisual accessories are an adjunct to teaching but do not replace the central role of the nurse in objective accomplishment. Indeed, the credibility of the nurse or educational care plan can be seriously affected when discrepancy exists between the videotapes and information that is reinforced.

Teaching the critically ill patient may require modification of traditional teaching methods and strategies. In critical care units, patient goals are generally short-term and objectives are concrete. Teaching should be kept brief and concise and should be in terms the patient can understand. The many stressors of illness and critical care and the effects of sedation and other drugs may cause the patient to require frequent repetitions and reinforcement of information. This is to be expected with the critically ill person and is not considered failure of the teaching experience. Each educational interaction between patient and nurse is of value, despite the fact it often will not result in long-term behavior change. Nurses should remember that family members are also stressed and may forget pertinent information that has been provided about visiting hours, unit policies, and how to contact a staff member for information about the patient. It is helpful to provide them with written information to supplement and reinforce verbal instructions.[20,44]

◆ **Evaluation.** Evaluation of the educational plan of care focuses on the ability of the plan to accomplish the objectives and outcomes developed in the planning phase. This includes the documentation of the effectiveness of the teaching-learning process with measurement of the knowledge gain and behavior changes identified.

In addition to the traditional evaluation of the educational plan based on objectives, other subtle effects of patient education can be identified. If the nurse in the critical care setting limits measurement of teaching effectiveness to long-term behavior changes, many critical educational activities necessary for the well-being of the patient will be judged failures. If the teaching meets a momentary need, the effect is no less valuable and successful. Less concrete but equally valuable outcomes, such as signs of relaxation when the

SAMPLES OF DIFFERENT READING LEVELS

COLLEGE READING LEVEL

Consult your physician immediately with the onset of chest discomfort, shortness of breath, or increased perspiration.

TWELFTH GRADE READING LEVEL

Call your physician immediately if you experience chest discomfort, shortness of breath, or increased sweatiness.

EIGHTH GRADE READING LEVEL

Call your doctor immediately if you start having chest pain or shortness of breath or feel sweaty.

FOURTH GRADE READING LEVEL

Call your doctor right away if you start having chest pain, can't breathe, or feel sweaty.

information provided decreases anxiety or greater participation in self-care, also document beneficial effects of the educational plan. This does not negate the fact that in many situations written, measurable objectives are necessary and useful, but it does mean that they should not be the sole measures of educational success.[45] A good example of this is the interaction that occurs when a patient is taught about the cardiac monitor on admission to the critical care unit. In teaching the reason for and function of this equipment, the nurse not only increases the patient's knowledge about cardiac monitoring, but may also decrease the patient's anxiety about the critical care setting, thereby promoting rest and healing.

TRANSFER FROM THE CRITICAL CARE UNIT

Transfer from the critical care unit to a telemetry or another acute care area can be an anxiety-producing time for patients. During the stay in the critical care unit, constant interaction with the nurse, monitoring devices, and controlled environment has offered security to the patient. Transfer from that environment can destroy the sense of security and create acute anxiety.[23] To avoid this anxiety, nurses should prepare patients for imminent or eventual transfer—that is, teach toward transfer. To do this, the nurse should point out early in the stay that the patient will be there only temporarily until his or her condition improves and stabilizes, and these improvements should be made known to the patient on an ongoing basis. As the time for transfer approaches, careful explanations can reassure patients and families that close observation and monitoring are no longer necessary. When possible, tubes, machines, and equipment used in the critical care unit—which the patient may see as important to survival—should be removed gradually rather than discontinued all at once. This will alleviate feelings of dependence on equipment.

At the time of transfer, patients can be told how care will change and what changes in activity, self-care, and visiting hours to expect. It is helpful to emphasize that the transfer represents an improvement in patient condition and, contrary to common references to a "step-down" unit, telemetry units are, in fact, a "step-up." The critical care unit nurse should accompany the patient to the new floor and introduce the new staff members to the patient. The patient can be told that a complete report on his or her condition will be given and that nursing care needs at this stage of recovery will be met in the new setting. Family members should be contacted and informed of the transfer. The management plan and educational plan developed in the critical care area should accompany the patient to the floor, and the new nurses should be informed about current short-term and long-term goals and the patient's progress.

Although careful preparation and planning for transfer are always desirable, a patient may be transferred unexpectedly to make room for a more critically ill patient. When this situation occurs, the patient to be moved from the unit must be notified and prepared for the possibility of a quick transfer. Tangible evidence of improvement, such as more favorable vital signs or need for fewer medications or tubes, can be helpful in pointing out advances in condition before unplanned transfers.

SAMPLE EDUCATIONAL PLANS AND NURSING MANAGEMENT PLANS

The boxes on p. 68 include a format for the construction of medication cards and a sample medication card, which can be useful in preparing a patient for discharge. The box on p. 69, which shows a sample plan for the patient undergoing coronary artery bypass surgery, is an example of one way to devise a holistic approach that addresses all phases of hospitalization. Examples of nursing management plans related to patient education begin on p. 70.

MEDICATION CARD FORMAT

GENERAL CONSIDERATIONS

1. Use simple, layman's language.
2. Keep information clear and concise.
3. Give medication information to patient in advance of discharge so that material can be absorbed and questions asked.

PERTINENT POINTS TO INCLUDE ON CARD

1. Basic physiology of how the medication works
2. Action of medication (i.e., why the patient is taking the medication)
3. Importance of taking medication exactly as described
   Include information on timing (i.e., before or after meals, before bedtime, before other medications taken)
4. Aids to medication administration
   Calendar
   Wallet ID
   Medic-alert band
   Small plastic boxes to organize the day's medications
5. Possible side effects
   Most common side effects
   Side effects or symptoms that require notification of physician
6. Prevention of complications
   Activities that should be avoided while on the medication
   Drug interactions
   Food interactions
   Special monitoring, such as blood work

SAMPLE MEDICATION CARD

DIGOXIN

Digoxin is a medication ordered by your doctor to improve and strengthen the pumping action of your heart. It also is used to control heart rate and to promote regular heart rhythm. Overall, the effect is to help blood circulation.

Digoxin can be toxic if not taken properly and as prescribed by your doctor. Take it at the same time each day, even if you feel well. If a dose is forgotten and not remembered within 12 hours, do not double the dose the next time. However, if you remember within 12 hours, take the dose as soon as you remember.

Possible side effects

Because digoxin is a potent drug, it is important to recognize the possible signs of overdosage:

Extreme fatigue
Muscle weakness
Loss of appetite
Nausea or vomiting
Lower stomach pain
Diarrhea
Slow or irregular heartbeat
Blurred vision
Seeing green, yellow, or white halos around objects
Confusion

If you notice these side effects, call your doctor immediately.

Prevention of complications

Do not stop taking this medication without asking your doctor.

Do not take other medications (including nonprescription drugs) unless ordered by your doctor, because they can interfere with this medication.

If you are also taking a diuretic ("water pill"), ask your doctor about the need to eat foods high in the electrolyte potassium. Potassium is lost frequently when taking a water pill, and sometimes a low potassium level can cause digoxin overdosage.

Talk with your doctor about the need to weigh yourself daily. Also, ask whether you should check your pulse daily before taking digoxin, since this drug can affect your heart rate.

TEACHING PLAN FOR THE PATIENT UNDERGOING CORONARY ARTERY BYPASS SURGERY

PREOPERATIVE PHASE

During the preoperative educational interactions, the nurse should assess the patient's and family's levels of anxiety and their effect on the ability or desire to learn. The preoperative education should be individualized to prepare the patient appropriately for the surgery, to educate him or her about postoperative care, and to minimize anxiety. Before the teaching-learning experience, the nurse:

- ◆ Assesses the patient's level of anxiety and desire to learn about the upcoming surgery
- ◆ Individualizes the preoperative teaching plan, based on assessment findings

The following content may be included in the preoperative teaching session:

- ◆ Review of the coronary artery bypass graft (CABG) procedure
- ◆ Time leaving room for surgery, length of surgery
- ◆ Location of family waiting area
- ◆ Surgical preparation and shave
- ◆ Nothing by mouth after midnight
- ◆ What to expect when awakening from anesthesia
- ◆ Sights and sounds of the recovery room and/or critical care unit
- ◆ Tubes and drains: chest tubes, hemodynamic monitoring lines, Foley catheter, intravenous lines, pacemaker wires (if appropriate), endotracheal tube
- ◆ Inability to speak with endotracheal tube in place
- ◆ Discomfort to expect from incisions, availability of pain medication
- ◆ Coughing and deep breathing practice
- ◆ Use of incentive spirometer
- ◆ When family can visit, how long, how often
- ◆ Usual length of critical care unit stay

In addition to this content, the nurse:

- ◆ Reassures patient that many staff members and much activity around bedside is normal and does not indicate complications
- ◆ Elicits and answers any specific questions patient and family have at that time
- ◆ Determines specific needs and desires for day of surgery (e.g., patient needs hearing aid or glasses as soon as possible)
- ◆ Meets with the family alone to offer support and address concerns they may not wish to voice to the patient

CRITICAL CARE UNIT PHASE

During the critical care unit phase, patient and family education is designed to meet immediate needs and reduce anxiety. The following are examples of content appropriate for this time:

- ◆ Basic explanation of bedside equipment
- ◆ Review of tubes and drains
- ◆ Turning, coughing, deep breathing
- ◆ Use of incentive spirometer
- ◆ Use of oxygen equipment
- ◆ Orientation to time, place, situation
- ◆ Explanation of procedures
- ◆ Basic purpose of medications
- ◆ Explanation of normal progression in early postoperative period
- ◆ Basic range-of-motion exercises (e.g., ankle circles, point and flex)

During this phase, the nurse also:

- ◆ Reassures patient and family of normal progression
- ◆ Repeats and reinforces information as necessary
- ◆ Answers questions as they arise
- ◆ Begins early to prepare patient for transfer to prevent transfer anxiety
- ◆ Determines family learning needs and addresses them together with patient or in separate teaching sessions as appropriate

STEP-DOWN UNIT PHASE

After transfer from the critical care unit, the patient's and family's educational needs increase. Short daily educational sessions should be planned to cover the following content:

- ◆ Basic pathophysiology of coronary artery disease
- ◆ Review of surgical procedure
- ◆ Risk factors for coronary artery disease
- ◆ Upper-extremity range-of-motion exercises
- ◆ Dietary recommendations (salt- and fat/cholesterol-modified diet)
- ◆ Taking of own pulse
- ◆ Recognition and treatment of angina (use of nitroglycerin)

During this phase, the nurse also:

- ◆ Uses audiovisual materials in teaching sessions or as reinforcement of content
- ◆ Provides printed take-home materials outlining important content
- ◆ Answers questions as they arise

DISCHARGE TEACHING

Before discharge, the following content should be covered with the patient and family:

- ◆ Activity guidelines
- ◆ Lifting restrictions
- ◆ Incision care
- ◆ Possibility of patient being extremely fatigued or depressed after discharge
- ◆ Guidelines for return to work, driving, sexual activity
- ◆ Medication safety and administration

Before discharge, the nurse also:

- ◆ Reassures patient that ups and downs are normal
- ◆ If necessary, reassures patient and family that likelihood of cardiac emergencies at home is small
- ◆ Provides printed material for further study by patient and family
- ◆ Answers questions as they arise
- ◆ Provides phone number for patient or family to call when further questions arise

ALTERED HEALTH MAINTENANCE RELATED TO LACK OF RESOURCES (financial, interpersonal support systems, health care access)

DEFINING CHARACTERISTICS

- ◆ Lack of participation in primary and/or secondary preventive activities such as obtaining appropriate screenings, proper nutrition, routine medical and dental care
- ◆ Finances inadequate to support medical care
- ◆ Health maintenance behaviors of low priority to family or significant others
- ◆ Access to health care limited because of geographic, transportation, or social barriers
- ◆ Frequent or chronic health problems such as chronic cough, loss of teeth at an early age, frequent infections, chronic fatigue, or anemia
- ◆ Physical signs such as poor hygiene or lesions associated with lack of oral care

OUTCOME CRITERIA

- ◆ Patient gains access to necessary health care.
- ◆ Patient can state self-care and health maintenance behaviors appropriate to his or her age and developmental level.

NURSING INTERVENTIONS AND *RATIONALE*

1. Continue to monitor the assessment parameters listed under "Defining Characteristics."
2. Assist patient and family in identifying social, financial, and environmental factors that limit ability to practice appropriate health maintenance measures.
3. Assist patient and family in identifying appropriate self-care and health maintenance behaviors (e.g., dental hygiene every 6 to 12 months, monthly breast self-examination for women, or complete physical examinations every 2 years for adults age 60 years or older).
4. Include family and/or other support systems in the planning for immediate and long-term health needs.
5. Provide early referral to social services if indicated ***so that appropriate resources and assistance can be obtained.***

ALTERED HEALTH MAINTENANCE RELATED TO LACK OF PERCEIVED THREAT TO HEALTH

DEFINING CHARACTERISTICS

- ◆ Lack of participation in primary and/or secondary preventive activities such as obtaining appropriate screenings, proper nutrition, routine medical and dental care
- ◆ Denial of susceptibility to a particular disease or problem
- ◆ Denial of the seriousness of a health problem or its consequences
- ◆ Absence of cues for action such as uncomfortable symptoms
- ◆ Failure to assume appropriate sick role behaviors

OUTCOME CRITERIA

- ◆ Patient is able to state the health consequences of specific behaviors (e.g., smoking is directly related to the onset of heart and lung disease).
- ◆ Patient assumes appropriate sick role behaviors.
- ◆ Patient states plans for appropriate primary and secondary preventive activities after discharge.

NURSING INTERVENTIONS AND *RATIONALE*

1. Continue to monitor the assessment parameters listed under "Defining Characteristics."
2. Assist patient to see the connection between specific behaviors and the short-term onset of symptoms or long-term progression of disease.
3. Assist patient to set short-term and long-term health management goals related to self-care and life-style.
4. Assist patient to prioritize goals and to make plans to pursue them in a manageable and realistic fashion.
5. Initiate health education ***to give the patient skills necessary to meet the immediate goals.*** (See nursing management plans for Knowledge Deficit.)
6. Initiate referrals for long-term follow-up after discharge (e.g., health educators, counselors, home health personnel, primary care practitioners, or rehabilitation programs).

NONCOMPLIANCE _______ (SPECIFY) RELATED TO KNOWLEDGE DEFICIT

DEFINING CHARACTERISTICS

- ◆ Lack of participation in necessary therapeutic measures
- ◆ Lack of prior experience with the recommended treatment or action
- ◆ Verbalization of inadequate knowledge or skills
- ◆ Questioning the need for the treatment or action

OUTCOME CRITERIA

- ◆ Patient verbalizes adequate knowledge or demonstrates adequate skills necessary for participation in treatment.
- ◆ Patient demonstrates compliance with treatment.

NURSING INTERVENTIONS AND *RATIONALE*

1. Continue to monitor the assessment parameters listed under "Defining Characteristics."
2. Determine specific knowledge or skills necessary ***for adherence to therapeutic plan.***

For other interventions, see nursing management plans for Knowledge Deficit, pp. 72 and 73.

NONCOMPLIANCE _______ (SPECIFY) RELATED TO LACK OF RESOURCES
(see Altered Health Maintenance)

DEFINING CHARACTERISTICS

- ◆ Lack of participation in necessary therapeutic measures
- ◆ Interpersonal or financial resources inadequate to support patient's appropriate participation in treatment
- ◆ Expression of concern about the cost of hospitalization and treatments
- ◆ Reinforcement of patient's behaviors and lack of proper participation in therapy by family/significant others

OUTCOME CRITERIA

- ◆ Patient demonstrates compliance with treatment.
- ◆ Family/significant others appropriately support and encourage patient in health-related and treatment-related behaviors.

NURSING INTERVENTIONS AND *RATIONALE*

1. Continue to monitor the assessment parameters listed under "Defining Characteristics."
2. Educate family and significant others about the prescribed treatments, their importance, and patient's need to participate ***so that support and assistance can be given to the patient.***
3. Assist family/significant others to identify specific ways in which they can assist patient ***so that he or she can comply with plan.***

For other interventions, see nursing management plan for Altered Health Maintenance related to lack of resources, p. 70.

KNOWLEDGE DEFICIT _______ (SPECIFY) RELATED TO LACK OF PREVIOUS EXPOSURE TO INFORMATION

DEFINING CHARACTERISTICS

- ◆ Verbalized statement of inadequate knowledge or skills
- ◆ New diagnosis or health problem requiring self-management or care
- ◆ Lack of prior formal or informal education about the specific health problem
- ◆ Demonstration of inappropriate behaviors related to management of health problem

OUTCOME CRITERIA

- ◆ Patient verbalizes adequate knowledge about or performs skills related to disease process, its causes, factors related to onset of symptoms, and self-management of disease or health problem.
- ◆ Patient actively participates in health behaviors required for performance of a procedure or in those behaviors enhancing recovery from illness and preventing recurrence or complications.

NURSING INTERVENTIONS AND *RATIONALE*

1. Continue to monitor the assessment parameters listed under "Defining Characteristics."
2. Determine existing level of knowledge or skill.
3. Assess factors affecting the knowledge deficit:
   - Learning needs, including patient's priorities and the necessary knowledge and skills for safety
   - Learning ability of client, including language skills, level of education, ability to read, preferred learning style
   - Physical ability to perform prescribed skills or procedures; consider effect of limitations imposed by treatment such as bedrest, restriction of movement by intravenous or other equipment, or effect of sedatives or analgesics
   - Psychologic effect of stage of adaptation to disease
   - Activity tolerance and ability to concentrate
   - Motivation to learn new skills or gain new knowledge
4. Reduce or limit barriers to learning:
   - Provide consistent nurse-patient contact ***to encourage development of trusting and therapeutic relationship.***
   - Structure environment ***to enhance learning;*** control unnecessary noise, interruptions.
   - Individualize teaching plan ***to fit patient's current physical and psychologic status.***
   - Delay teaching until patient is ready to learn.
   - Conduct teaching sessions during period of day when patient is most alert and receptive.
   - Meet patient's immediate learning needs as they arise, e.g., give brief explanation of procedures when they are performed.
5. Promote active participation in the teaching plan by the patient and family:
   - Solicit input during development of plan.
   - Develop mutually acceptable goals and outcomes.
   - Solicit expression of feelings and emotions related to new responsibilities.
   - Encourage questions.
6. Conduct teaching sessions, using the most appropriate teaching methods:
   - Discussion
   - Lecture
   - Demonstration/return demonstration
   - Use of audiovisual or printed educational materials
7. Repeat key principles and provide them in printed form ***for reference at a later time.***
8. Give frequent feedback to patient when practicing new skills.
9. Use several teaching sessions when appropriate. ***New information and skills should be reinforced several times after initial learning.***
10. Initiate referrals for follow-up if necessary:
    - Health educators
    - Home health care
    - Rehabilitation programs
    - Social services
11. Evaluate effectiveness of teaching plan, based on patient's ability to meet preset goals and objectives, and determine need for further teaching.

KNOWLEDGE DEFICIT ______________ (SPECIFY) RELATED TO COGNITIVE/PERCEPTUAL LEARNING LIMITATIONS

(e.g., sensory overload, sleep deprivation, medications, anxiety, sensory deficits, language barrier)

DEFINING CHARACTERISTICS

- ◆ Verbalized statement of inadequate knowledge of skills
- ◆ Verbalization of inadequate recall of information
- ◆ Verbalization of inadequate understanding of information
- ◆ Evidence of inaccurate follow-through of instructions
- ◆ Inadequate demonstration of a skill
- ◆ Lack of compliance with prescribed behavior

OUTCOME CRITERIA

- ◆ Patient participates actively in necessary and prescribed health behaviors.
- ◆ Patient verbalizes adequate knowledge or demonstrates adequate skills.

NURSING INTERVENTIONS AND *RATIONALE*

1. Continue to monitor the assessment parameters listed under "Defining Characteristics."
2. Determine specific cause of patient's cognitive or perceptual limitation. (See also table of contents for Impaired Verbal Communication, Anxiety, Sleep Pattern Disturbances, Sensory/Perceptual Alterations.)
3. Provide uninterrupted rest period before teaching session ***to decrease fatigue and encourage optimal state for learning and retention.***
4. Manipulate environment as much as possible ***to provide quiet and uninterrupted learning sessions:***
   Ensure lights are bright enough to see teaching aids but not too bright.
   Close door if necessary ***to provide quiet environment.***
   Schedule care and medications ***to allow uninterrupted teaching periods.***
   Move patient to quiet, private room for teaching *if possible.*
5. Adapt teaching sessions and materials to patient's and family's levels of education and ability to understand:
   Provide printed material appropriate to reading level.
   Use terminology understood by the patient.
   Provide printed materials in patient's primary language *if possible.*
   Use interpreters during teaching sessions *when necessary.*
6. Teach only present-tense focus during periods of sensory overload.
7. Determine potential effects of medications on ability to retain or recall information. Avoid teaching critical content while patient is taking sedatives, analgesics, or other medications affecting memory.
8. Reinforce new skills and information in several teaching sessions. Use several senses when possible in teaching session (e.g., see a film, hear a discussion, read printed information, and demonstrate skills related to self-injection of insulin).
9. Reduce patient's anxiety:
   Listen attentively and encourage verbalization of feelings.
   Answer questions as they arise in a clear and succinct manner.
   Elicit patient's concerns and address those issues first.
   Give only correct and relevant information.
   Continually assess response to teaching session and discontinue if anxiety increases or physical condition becomes unstable.
   Provide nonthreatening information before more anxiety-producing information is presented.
   Plan for several teaching sessions so information can be divided into small manageable packages.

REFERENCES

1. Novak J: The social mandate and historical basis for nursing's role in health promotion, *J Prof Nurs* 4(2):80, 1988.
2. American Nurses' Association: *A social policy statement,* Kansas City, Mo, 1980, The Association.
3. Burke LE, Scalzi CC: Education of the patient and family. In Underhill S and others, editors: *Cardiac nursing,* Philadelphia, 1982, JB Lippincott.
4. Flynn JB, Griffin PA: Health promotion in acute care settings, *Nurs Clin North Am* 19(2):239, 1984.
5. Thompson D and others: In-hospital counselling for first time myocardial infarction patients and spouses: effect on satisfaction, *J Adv Nurs* 15(9):1064, 1990.
6. Keeling AW: Health promotion in coronary care and step down units: focus on the family—linking research to practice, *Heart Lung* 17(1):28, 1988.
7. Hill M: Strategies for patient education, *Clin Exp Hypertens [A]* 11(5-6):1107, 1989.
8. Gordon M: *Nursing diagnosis: process and application,* New York, 1991, McGraw-Hill.
9. Pender NJ: *Health promotion in nursing practice,* Norwalk, Conn, 1987, Appleton-Century-Crofts.
10. Becker MH and others: Some influences on program participation in a genetic screening program, *Community Health* 1:3, 1975.
11. Surgeon General: *Healthy people: the Surgeon General's report on health promotion and disease prevention,* Washington, DC, 1980, Department of Public Health and Human Service.
12. Gerber KE: Compliance in the chronically ill: an introduction to the problem. In Gerber KE, Nehemkis A: *Compliance—the dilemma of the chronically ill,* New York, 1986, Springer-Verlag.
13. Roccella EJ: Measures for developing education of the hypertensive patient, *J Hum Hypertens* 4(suppl 1):9, 1990.
14. Carpenito L: *Nursing diagnosis: application to clinical practice,* Philadelphia, 1992, JB Lippincott.
15. Bertakis KD: An application of the health belief model to patient education and compliance: acute otitis media, *Fam Med* 18(6):347, 1986.
16. Nehemkis AM, Gerber KE: Compliance and the quality of life. In Gerber KE, Nehemkis AM, editors: *Compliance—the dilemma of the chronically ill,* New York, 1986, Springer-Verlag.
17. Smith E: Patient teaching—it's the law, *Nursing '87,* 17(7):67, 1987.
18. Theirer J and others: *Standards for nursing care of the critically ill,* Englewood Cliffs, NJ, 1981, Reston Publishing.
19. Guzzetta CE: Can critically ill patients be taught? In Billie DA, editor: *Practical approaches to patient teaching,* Boston, 1981, Little, Brown.
20. Burke LE: Learning and retention in the acute care setting, *Crit Care Q* 4:3, 1981.
21. Informational needs of families of intensive care unit patients, *Quality Rev Bull* 12:1, 1986.
22. Provine R: The challenge of patient education in critical care, *Crit Care Nurs* 6(2):22, 1986.
23. Storlie F: *Patient teaching in critical care,* New York, 1975, Appleton-Century-Crofts.
24. Redman BK: *The process of patient teaching in nursing,* ed 7, St Louis, 1993, Mosby–Year Book.
25. Knowles M: *The adult learner: a neglected species,* ed 3, Houston, 1990, Gulf Publishing.
26. Billie DA: The teaching-learning process. In Billie DA: *Practical approaches of patient teaching,* Boston, 1981, Little, Brown & Co.
27. Nite G, Willis F: *The coronary patient: hospital care and rehabilitation,* New York, 1979, Macmillan.
28. Murphy MC and others: Education of patients undergoing coronary angioplasty: factors affecting learning during a structured educational program, *Heart Lung* 18(1):36, 1989.
29. Weinberger DA and others: Low-anxious, high-anxious and depressive coping styles: psychometric patterns and behavioral physiological responses to stress, *J Abnorm Psychol* 88:369, 1979.
30. Creamer-Bauer C, Webber M: Patient teaching strategies for peripheral laser procedures, *Progress Cardiovasc Nurs* 5(2):50, 1990.
31. Narrow B: *Patient teaching in nursing practice,* Salt Lake City, 1978, John Wiley & Sons.
32. Williams CL, Kendall PC: Psychological aspects of education for stressful medical procedures, *Health Educ Q* 12(3):135, 1985.
33. Frenn M, Fehring R, Kartes S: Reducing the stress of cardiac catheterization by teaching relaxation, *Dimens Crit Care Nurs* 5(2):108, 1986.
34. Chan V: Content cardiac teaching: patient's perceptions of the importance of teaching content after myocardial infarction, *J Adv Nurs* 15(10):1139, 1990.
35. Eaton S, Davis G, Brenner P: Discussion stoppers in teaching, *Nurs Outlook* 25(9):578, 1977.
36. Bell JA: The role of microcomputers in patient education, *Comput Nurs* 4(6):255, 1986.
37. Dobberstein K: Computer-assisted patient education, *Am J Nurs* 87(5):697, 1987.
38. Ley P and others: Improving doctor-patient communication in general practice, *J Royal Coll Gen Practitioners* 25:558, 1975.
39. Doak L, Doak C: Patient comprehension profiles: recent findings and strategies, *Patient Coun Health Educ* 3:101, 1980.
40. Streiff LD: Can clients understand our instructions? *Image J Nurs Sch* 18(2):48, 1986.
41. Boyd MD: A guide to writing effective patient education materials, *Nurs Manage* 18(7):56, 1987.
42. Neilsen E, Sheppard MA: Television as a patient education tool: a review of its effectiveness, *Patient Educ Couns* 11:3, 1988.
43. Durand RP, Counts CS: Developing audio-visual programs for patient education, *Am Neph Nurs Assoc* 13(3):158, 1986.
44. Foster DS: Written reinforcement for teaching, *MCN* 11(5):347, 1986.
45. Billie DA: Process oriented patient education, *Dimens Crit Care Nurs* 2:2, 1983.

6

Stressors of Critical Care Nursing

CHAPTER OBJECTIVES

- Define stress.
- Discuss at least three attributes of stress that contribute to its being a complex construct.
- Compare the historic perspective of stress in critical care with the more contemporary view that became evident in the early 1980s.
- Identify at least three major sources that give rise to stress in critical care, and provide two examples of each.
- List at least two signs of stress for each of three categories—physical, psychologic, and behavioral.
- Describe the individual and organizational effects of stress.
- Discuss three individual and three organizational strategies that might reduce the effects of stress.

Vital signs, pulmonary pressures, cardiac rhythms, blood gas values, cardiac outputs, and other physiologic parameters; anger, depression, anxiety, ethical dilemmas, communication, and additional psychosocial indicators; infusion pumps, central lines, ventilators, chest tubes, mouth care, turning, feeding, and bathing—these all are but a glimmer of the myriad features constituting the work environment of a critical care nurse. What response is generated by thoughts of this critical care world? Do they evoke energy, opportunity, and a sense of challenge, or do they elicit exhaustion, danger, and a feeling of threat? In either case, the term *stress* describes the reaction.

Cannon pioneered the study of stress in the early 1900s.[1,2] Since then, various individuals have continued to examine stress from various perspectives: Selye followed a physiologic orientation, Pearlin pursued a sociologic view, and Lazarus considered a psychologic perspective. Stress as a workplace concern first received attention in the mid-1950s.[3] Occupational stress continues to be a pressing concern because of its potentially negative relationship with health.[4-7]

Nursing is an occupation in which stress has been scrutinized. Menzies[8] was one of the first individuals to address the stress experienced by nurses, and a multitude of additional reports have followed.[9-11] As Marshall[11] commented, "The nurse's role is . . . implicitly and chiefly one of handling stress." The physical labor, the human suffering, the work hours, the staffing, and the interpersonal relationships have all been mentioned repeatedly as sources of stress in nursing.

Not only are there stressors inherent in nursing, but stress is exacerbated when traditional beliefs, norms, and structures are realigned. Therefore the prevalence of high technology, high patient acuity, high census, prospective payment, and ongoing concern about the spiraling cost of health care are creating additional turbulence in the health care environment. These issues have the potential to escalate the stress experienced by nurses.

The concept of stress is therefore important to nurses. The purpose of this chapter is to consider the issue of stress in nursing—particularly critical care nursing. The chapter covers six topics: (1) a brief overview of stress, (2) special challenges of critical care nursing, (3) potential sources of stress in critical care, (4) signs of stress, (5) effects of stress, and (6) stress management.

AN OVERVIEW OF STRESS

Definition

Stress is commonly discussed and commonly experienced, but what is stress? Although it has a negative connotation, stress is not inherently deleterious. Stress has the potential for positive outcomes. In fact, Selye[12] emphasized that the complete freedom from stress is death. Nevertheless, despite its pervasive, persistent, and popular use, a precise definition of stress remains elusive. The term has generated much confusion and controversy. Some individuals have even suggested that the usefulness of stress as a concept is doubtful.[13,14]

Pearlin[15] concurs that stress is complicated but suggests that the usefulness of the complex stress concept outweighs the problems inherent in it. However, ambiguity and the lack of consensus about the meaning of stress complicate using the term. Fortunately, models such as the person-environment (P-E) fit framework, presented below, afford a way to discuss work stress more meaningfully.

◆ **The person-environment (P-E) fit model.** The P-E fit model is a framework that considers relationships between job stress and health. According to the P-E fit model, occupational stress is experienced when discrepancies exist between perceived environmental demands and individual abilities.[16,17] This definition is congruent with that proposed by Lazarus and Folkman,[18] who state that stress is "a particular relationship between the person and the environment that is appraised by the person as taxing or exceeding his or her resources and endangering his or her well-being." Stress can therefore be minimized by balancing the abilities and needs of the person with the supplies and demands of the environment.

It is apparent that demands and abilities are influenced, in part, by a subjective evaluation that affects an individual's interpretation of situations and events. It is not so much what happens to people, but the way they interpret it. This subjective interpretation is known as *perception.* Through their perception of events, individuals determine whether the event is viewed as a challenging, positive force or a negative threat. The person ponders, "am I in trouble or being benefited . . . and in what way."[18]

However, because perception and interpretation give meaning to events, it is not possible to specify which circumstances will engender stress. What might be distressing and bothersome for one individual could be satisfying and challenging for another. In addition, perception contributes to the ever-changing nature of stress, establishing stress as a process, not an event.[13,18,19]

◆ **Coping.** Another aspect of stress involves coping, or how the individual evaluates what can be done about the event. Stress and coping are clearly interrelated; both are dynamic processes. The purpose of coping is to help an individual manage demands that are perceived as stressful.[18] This may be accomplished by modifying the situation itself, modifying the perception of the situation, or managing symptoms provoked by the situation.[20] The way a person copes is partially determined by the individual's personal and environmental resources. Therefore coping evolves from such personal characteristics as health, energy, and positive beliefs or from such constituents of the environment as social support.

Coping differs between the genders. For example, Johnson and Johnson[21] found that men used more denial than did women in coping with the stress of parenthood. It is therefore possible that stress experienced by working women from occurrences external to the work milieu might transfer into the work setting. These gender differences were corroborated by Pearlin and Schooler,[22] who found that men were more likely than were women to use such coping modes as maintaining optimism and a positive outlook and possessing a sense of mastery over events. In addition, they found that coping for both genders was more useful in attenuating problems related to marriage and children and less effective in thwarting stress engendered by work. These issues are extremely cogent to a female-dominant profession such as nursing. If socialization constrains women's repertoire of coping skills and nonwork stress is carried into the work setting, the stresses in the workplace might be perceived more harshly.

Related Concepts

Additional confusion in the stress nomenclature arises from the lack of precision in using various terms that are similar to, but different from, stress. Strain and burnout represent the problem. In the occupational literature, stress and strain are typically separated, with stress preceding strain. For example, role-related stress could contribute to strain, which might be manifested as job dissatisfaction.[4,6,16]

Burnout, similar to strain, is a consequence of stress. It is a more extreme state, however, because burnout is the final stage of coping with negative conditions. Burnout is a psychologic response to the chronic stress experienced by professionals employed in human service occupations, and it is characterized by emotional exhaustion, depersonalization, and loss of personal motivation.[23-26]

This overview is only a sketchy beginning of the complex concept of stress. Nevertheless, it does help to convey that stress is indeed complicated. Making definitive statements about stress is both dangerous and difficult because, as French and Caplan[27] conveyed more than 20 years ago, what may be psychologic poison for some people may be less toxic for others, and vice versa. With these cautions in mind, it is possible to turn more specifically to stress in critical care units.

SPECIAL CHALLENGES OF CRITICAL CARE

Historical Perspective

The advent of recovery rooms in the 1940s marked the actual origin of critical care.[28,29] However, coronary care units, which are more prototypical of contemporary critical care settings, did not evolve until 1962.[30] From the 1960s through the 1980s, an ongoing interest in critical care stress led to a number of studies that indicated the critical care environment is filled with stress.

In addition to noting the valuable knowledge gained from early studies of stress in critical care, it is equally important to address their limitation. The most evident limitation is the emphasis on critical care irrespective of other patient care areas. As early as 1960, Menzies[8] stated, "Nurses experience a great deal of stress in their work. This may seem so obvious as hardly to merit comment. For nurses confront suffering and death as few other people do." Nevertheless, the implicit message in many early studies was that critical care was more stressful than were other hospital-based nursing settings.[31-38] Perhaps this belief evolved from a study in which critical care and non–critical care nurses were compared.[39] The findings suggested that critical care nurses were more inclined to experience negative affective states, thereby perpetuating the belief that critical care nursing was more stressful. However, a disproportionately small number of non–critical care nurses in the sample may have skewed the comparison. The caution appropriate to such a limitation was not transmitted along with the results.

Contemporary Perspective

Despite a lapse of 10 years, the idea of comparing critical care nurses with those in other patient areas surfaced again in the 1980s. Perhaps there never really was a difference in the stress experienced by critical care and non–critical care nurses. Perhaps the current health care environment, typified by escalating patient acuity and accelerating technologic advances, has obliterated whatever differences there were at one time. In either case, studies indicate that stress is an occupational problem in the nursing profession regardless of specialty.[40-42] During the late 1980s and early 1990s, however, few studies examined stress in critical care.

As patient care becomes more complicated in all health care areas, the critical care population truly represents the sickest of the sick. Advances in health care enable people to live longer despite aging and chronic illness. It is also possible to treat patients with problems that were previously untreatable. All of these changes have an impact on nursing and nurses. Critical care nurses, therefore, are exposed to the most acutely ill patients and the most sophisticated, state-of-the-art technology. Consequently, even though stress is common in all facets of nursing, it has become important to consider stress as it relates to critical care nurses.

POTENTIAL SOURCES OF STRESS IN CRITICAL CARE

Major Origins of Critical Care Stress

Despite the passing of time, the sources of stress in critical care have not changed. The major sources of stress in the critical care setting, which are summarized in two review articles,[42a, 42b] can be organized into five general categories: (1) the environment, (2) the workload, (3) patient acuity, (4) interpersonal relationships, and (5) responsibility for life and death decisions. Examples of conditions representing each of these categories are in Table 6-1.

The complexity of stress, however, makes it impossible to predict with certainty whether potential sources of stress will in fact generate stress. The following discussion briefly addresses how perception, personality, life's spheres, and chronic versus acute stress complicate identifying origins of stress in critical care.

Complexity of Stress in Critical Care

◆ **Perception.** The importance of perception in the stress process is underscored by reemphasizing that the same situation can evoke different responses among individuals. In the critical care setting this means the same activities labeled as threatening by some staff members are stimulating for others.[32,33,43,44] The positive aspects of stress, however, are often overlooked because of its predominantly negative connotation. Furthermore, the positive side of stress highlights the difficulty that can arise when trying to moderate stress—it would be unwise to remove or reduce sources of satisfaction. As expressed by one critical care nurse, "Cardiac arrest and the amount of rapid decisions that must be made are what I would call positive stressors—without these, my job wouldn't be exciting, challenging, and interesting."[45]

The dynamics of perception are further exemplified in a series of remarks originating from one of the early accounts of stress experienced by coronary care nurses.[35] A well-known cardiologist responded to the article by commenting in part, "It seems to me that coronary care is one of the less stressful and more restful atmospheres in which a nurse can work."[46] However, a registered nurse took issue with the cardiologist's remarks and stated, "Every coronary-care unit is different in terms of its demands" and "Awaiting the unexpected can be more anxiety provoking than active physical engagement."[47]

Table 6-1 Sources of stress in critical care

Category	Examples

Environment	Equipment
	  Complexity
	  Malfunction
	  Nonavailability
	Physical features
	  Inadequate storage
	  Inadequate work space
	  Inaccessible supplies
	  Too much noise
	  Too few windows

Workload	Patient
	  Patient : staff ratio
	  Patient acuity
	  Frequent, repetitive routine
	Nonpatient
	  Documentation
	  Family interactions
	  Staff competence and mix

Severity of illness	Emergencies Death and dying Requisite knowledge: physiologic, psychosocial, pharmacologic, technologic Requisite repertoire of skills

Interpersonal relations and communication	Interactions with the following:
	  Unit staff
	  Other nursing units
	  Hospital departments
	  Other health care professionals
	  Nurse managers
	  Hospital administrators
	  Families
	  Patients

Decision making	Responsibility for decisions Conflicting opinions Adequacy of knowledge and information Accountability for effects of decisions Ethical dilemmas Fear of making mistakes

This situation is not a case of who is right and who is wrong. Rather, it clearly portrays how perception affects one's interpretation of stress. Nevertheless, sufficient sources of stress are perceived only in a negative sense. These stressors are those that warrant modification.

◆ **Personality traits.** The influence of personality further complicates understanding critical care stress. Why are some people seemingly tolerant of stress, whereas others are more vulnerable to its effects? Many personality variables have been identified as relevant to the stress process, including hardiness, locus of control, and type A and type B behaviors. The effect of personality on the stress experienced by the critical care nurse has only recently been explored.

Hardiness—a three-faceted trait comprising challenge, commitment, and control—is purported to enhance tolerance for stress. Characteristics of the hardy personality have been found among both critical care and non–critical care nurses,[48,49] with less burnout experienced by nurses with high hardiness scores. Nurses with higher internal locus of control—a belief that the individual can influence life events to some degree—had fewer deleterious responses to stress.[44,50,51] Nurses with both type A and type B personalities experienced stress, although the sources of stress differed.[10]

These studies demonstrate the existing relationship between personality and stress. That is, studies have not yet been published to demonstrate the effects of programs that try to alter personality to enhance one's ability to work in a stress-filled environment. This is typical of stress research in general, however. It is somewhat easier to conduct descriptive investigations that document existing conditions than it is to design and test interventions that might alter the stress response.

◆ **Life's spheres.** A third complexity in determining sources of stress arises because it is not possible to compartmentalize the many components of one's work and nonwork life. As a result, stress may be experienced in the work environment because of the work itself or stress may actually be provoked by occurrences external to the work environment.[7,52,53]

The interrelatedness of life's spheres is particularly salient for nursing, a profession that is predominantly composed of women. The movement of women out of the home and into the work world has been cited as a chief source of female role strain, or the dissonance experienced when expectations and demands of different roles conflict with one another.[53,54] However, the stress imposed by combining work, marriage, and family, for example, cannot be attributed solely to work.[55-58]

Consequently, it may be very difficult to isolate work stress. Although staffing constraints may be an obvious source of stress, for example, it could be that dealing with a sick child, unpredictable child care, or an unsupportive spouse is the real genesis of stress, the effects of which may be experienced at work. For example, it was determined that the most stressful situation for a group of 79 critical care nurses was dealing with a personal crisis while working.[59] Similarly, in a study of head nurses from a variety of clinical settings, stress from both work and nonwork sources was positively related to psychologic symptoms.[60]

◆ **Chronic versus acute stress.** A final consideration demonstrating the complex process of stress is the influence of two different sources of stress. At one end of the continuum are the sudden, recent, acute events. It is possible to state rather precisely when these events occur. Examples include motor vehicle accidents, death, divorce, policy changes, the arrival of new physicians, and starting a new job. Acute stressors are bothersome, not simply because they generally provoke change, but because they are often viewed as undesirable or uncontrollable.[18,19,52,53]

On the other end of the continuum are the less apparent, daily occurrences that are chronic sources of stress. Lazarus and Folkman[18] refer to them as daily hassles. These ongoing, enduring, wearing conditions are often taken for granted. Although they do not leave the same immediate impression as do many acute stressors, the chronic stressors are nonetheless stressful.[18,19,52,53] Chronic stressors can arise from all segments of life, such as family discord, conflict among one's roles, life-cycle changes, the medical hierarchy, inadequate staffing, and shift work. It is also possible that enduring features of acute stressors move them into the chronic end of the continuum. Feelings engendered by loss encountered because of death or divorce, for example, may linger for a considerable time. These intricacies of the stress process compound the complexity of occupational stress in general and critical care stress in particular.

SIGNS OF STRESS

Despite its complexities, stress does occur. When it does, stress evokes many clinical manifestations. However, the indicators of stress are somewhat nonspecific because they are not unique to stress. Selye[12] referred to stress as a nonspecific response of the person to demands that are either pleasant or noxious. Regardless of the demand or response, the body makes compensatory adjustments to maintain a harmonic balance.

Probably all people have experienced the pounding heart, sweaty palms, and knotted stomach that frequently accompany stressful events. Many of these responses arise from the neuroendocrine effects of preparing to deal with stress and attempting to sustain one's equilibrium. The box on p. 79 represents a composite of physical, psychologic, and behavioral manifestations of stress. Although these indicators might be associated with a variety of conditions, they could be signs of stress. The nonspecificity of these manifestations also further conveys the vagueness that is inherent to the entity known as stress.[62,63]

EFFECTS OF STRESS

Although stressors in the critical care setting have been identified, a reasonable next question might be, "So what?" Remember, the presence of stress may not be detrimental. What are the sequelae of stress? To reiterate a point made at the beginning of this chapter, occupational stress—specifically stress in nursing—is a concern because of the serious health problems it can generate.[4-7] Both individual and organizational health suffers from the deleterious effects of stress. Employers have been held legally accountable for stress-related mental injuries.[64,65] Lowered work quality, increased absenteeism, and increased turnover are additional sequelae of work stress.[65a]

Physical problems induced by work stress must be considered too. This issue is often overlooked by those who have underscored that the demands of stress may be viewed as either a challenge or a threat. Regardless of whether a nurse views events in the critical care setting as positive or negative stressors, the biologic sequelae are the same. Neuroendocrine responses evoke the same physiologic reactions, which, over time, may give rise to disease.[66] It is not surprising that Pelletier[7] warns, "Caution: Work May Be Hazardous To Your Health."

INDICATORS OF STRESS

PHYSICAL MANIFESTATIONS

Cardiovascular

- Tachycardia
- Increased blood pressure
- Chest pain
- Palpitations
- Cold hands and feet

Neurologic

- Headache
- Hyperreflexia
- Trembling; excessive energy
- Insomnia
- Lethargy

Pulmonary

- Tachypnea
- Cough

Endocrine

- Increased metabolic rate
- Increased appetite
- Anorexia

Gastrointestinal

- Decreased peristalsis
- Intestinal cramping
- Indigestion
- Diarrhea
- Nausea

Genitourinary

- Urinary urgency
- Sensation of full bladder
- Urinary frequency

Integumentary

- Cool, pale skin
- Blushing
- Increased perspiration
- Rashes

Musculoskeletal

- Back pain
- Joint pain

Other

- Dry mouth, eyes
- Dysphagia

PSYCHOLOGIC MANIFESTATIONS

- Anger
- Frustration
- Depression
- Apathy
- Fear
- Hostility
- Denial
- Other defensive responses

BEHAVIORAL MANIFESTATIONS

- Complaining
- Crying
- Panicking
- Quarreling
- Withdrawing
- Disorientation
- Indecisiveness
- Helplessness
- Irritability
- Reduced productivity
- Reduced quality of performance
- Forgetfulness
- Inattention to detail
- Preoccupation with other things
- Inability to concentrate
- Reduced creativity
- Increased use of drugs, alcohol, tobacco
- Increased absenteeism and illness
- Lethargy
- Accident proneness
- Disinterest
- Blaming others
- Increased errors
- Inefficiency
- Speech changes

Another relevant issue involves a curious paradox: although the goal of health care providers is to enhance the health of others, their own health may be at risk.[67] Although the preceding statements have an intuitive appeal, some of the effects of critical care stress are more speculative than factual at present. It is therefore helpful to examine the research-based evidence regarding the effects of stress on critical care nurses.

Individual Effects

Cleland's early investigations of stress in nursing are unique in that they considered stress in relation to select effects. In one report the expected curvilinear relationship between nurses' performance and stress was demonstrated,[68] and in another an inverse relationship was found between the quality of nurses' thinking and stress.[69] Most research concerning stress in nursing, however, has been limited to identifying stressors.[43] Only recently has critical care stress been considered in relation to outcome variables. Some of the information is conflictive, and all of it is preliminary, but the findings are nonetheless compelling. For example, most of the stressors identified by a large group of critical care nurses were *not* related to two outcome measures—job satisfaction and psychologic distress.[45]

No pathology was found in two small groups of critical care nurses whose psychologic health was examined.[50,70] However, in a group comprising 180 critical care nurses, 87% of the participants' psychologic symptom scores exceeded normal, with 10% of them reaching levels comparable with psychiatric outpatients.[45] The findings from this latter study suggest that stress does have an undesirable effect. Although additional evidence is needed to elucidate clearly the effect of stress on mental health, it is important to pursue this problem.

Another important outcome to individuals is job satisfaction. Job satisfaction also affects organizations because it relates to retention. Although it is often suggested that stress contributes to job *dis*satisfaction, the empiric evidence is weak. In the previously mentioned study of 180 critical care nurses, only 3 of 16 stressful situations were related to job dissatisfaction.[45] Further, personality traits—characteristics that vary greatly among individuals—have been noted to alter job satisfaction.[51]

Burnout is also a possible outcome of stress. Here, too, the relationship is complicated, but an association between job stress and burnout has been found among critical care nurses.[48,71] A preliminary profile of the burnout-prone critical care nurse is beginning to emerge. Symptoms of burnout are often found in male nurses, younger nurses, and nurses educated at the baccalaureate level and higher.[48,72] Nurses who are inclined to burnout were also found to be less experienced in nursing and to have less effective coping skills.[20] This profile emphasizes that predicting the sequelae of stress is complicated by many factors. Although it is probable that a similar profile could be developed for organizational features that enhance and reduce the development of burnout, no such studies have yet been published.

The physiologic effects of stress and physical illnesses have not been studied. Nevertheless, stress has been related to many disorders, such as headache, hypertension, coronary artery disease, asthma, gastric and duodenal ulcers, diabetes, arthritis, allergies, cancer, and mental disorders.[73-76] Knowing how or whether the stress of nursing contributes to the development of any of these maladies would be valuable.

Organizational Effects

An index of organizational health might be determined by considering such stress-related issues as absenteeism, turnover, or the quality of work. Although these factors are reflections of individual responses to stress, they may also affect the productivity and financial status of the organization. For example, stress-induced illnesses contribute to the escalating costs of medical benefits. Similarly, the cost of turnover is also higher simply because of inflation.

Despite the importance of these organizational effects of stress, they have been studied only limitedly in critical care nursing. Furthermore, the studies that have been done are more than a decade old.[31,77,78]

To date, no published work has examined the rela-

RESEARCH ABSTRACT

ICU nurses' coping measures: response to work-related stressors.

Lewis DJ, Robinson JA: *Crit Care Nurse* 12(2):18, 1992.

PURPOSE

The purpose of this study was to determine the relationship of adaptive coping measures with the perception of stress in critical care nurses.

DESIGN

Descriptive correlational design

SAMPLE

The sample consisted of 577 nurses who worked in a variety of critical care units in 23 Veteran's Administration facilities nationwide, each with a total bed capacity of greater than 400. The majority of respondents were women, between the ages of 30 and 44, and educated at the baccalaureate level in nursing and had fewer than 10 years of critical care unit experience. The subjects worked primarily full time, rotated shifts, and worked in one of three specialty units: SICU, MICU, or CCU. Less than one third had participated in a stress management program.

INSTRUMENTS

The Work-Related Stressor Questionnaire (WRSQ) measured the individual's perceived severity of work-related stressors. The Response to Stressor Questionnaire (RSQ) measured reaction to stressors. The Coping Measures Questionnaire (CMQ) identified the frequency of adaptive/maladaptive strategies used to manage the stress response. Validity and reliability of the instruments had been established in a pilot study by the investigators.

RESULTS

A significant positive relationship ($r = 0.61$, $p < .001$) was found between the perceived severity of stressors and the stress response (i.e., the greater the perceived severity of stressors, the greater the stress response). A significant negative relationship ($r = -0.26, p < .001$) was noted between the perceived severity of the stressors and overall coping measures, as well as between the responses of stressors and the overall coping effectiveness ($r = -0.36, p < .001$). Use of maladaptive coping measures significantly increased as either the severity of perceived stress ($r = -0.36$, $p < .001$) or responses ($r = -0.50, p < .001$) increased. Based on factor analysis of the instruments, five subscales were identified for the WRSQ: interpersonal relationships, environment, patient care, professionalism, and knowledge. For the RSQ, six subscales were identified: overt behavior, physical ailment, kinetics, covert behavior, tedium, and productivity. There were seven subscales for the CMQ: mind control, activity, communication, escape mechanisms, burnout indicator, nutrition, and chemical stimulants.

DISCUSSION/IMPLICATIONS

This study was important in quantifying perceived severity of work-related stressors, reaction to stressors, and adaptive and maladaptive behaviors. In addition, it validated earlier studies in which there was an increased stress response as perception of work-related stressors increased. Stress, inherent in all aspects of nursing, is a condition that must be monitored and controlled in critical care unit staff. Both the staff nurse and key clinical management staff (i.e., manager, clinical nurse specialist, educator) must be aware of factors that produce stress and strategies that can minimize these stressful situations. Orientation and ongoing educational offerings can be designed to assist the staff to deal with the stressors of critical care units and nursing in general. Support groups, effective communication mechanisms, and stress-management programs easily available to the staff are essential. Future research efforts can be directed toward evaluation of such programs to determine which are the most effective from both a personal and a cost perspective. In addition, impact of nurse stressors can be examined regarding their effect on patient outcomes.

tionship between the stress nurses experience and patient outcomes. This important linkage begs to be explored! To expect a connection between nurses' stress, the quality of care delivered, and acceptable patient outcomes is reasonable. In a classic study conducted in the critical care units of 13 hospitals, it was demonstrated that interaction and coordination among physicians and nurses working in critical care units had more effect on patient outcomes than did other variables.[79] In another multisite study currently in progress, various professional nursing practice models and their relationship to nurse satisfaction, quality of care, and fiscal outcomes are being evaluated.[80] More specific to critical care is work being done to restructure the patient care delivery system in the critical care units of a large hospital in the northeast United States.[81] Stress, however, is not a variable in any of these models.

Perhaps the three reports just mentioned reflect a shift in emphasis for the 1990s. The emphasis on stress experienced by nurses has given way to interest in the cost and quality of care, work redesign, and other issues that are of paramount importance to all health care providers. This is not to suggest that stress is no longer an issue. Quite the contrary. Stress is probably higher than ever before, as patient acuity increases and length of stay decreases. However, reports of stress have been replaced by reports concerning other health care issues. This shift in emphasis must be considered with some degree of concern. Although additional reports are not needed to substantiate the existence of stress among nurses, the impact of stress for individuals and organizations cannot be overlooked in a labor-intensive occupation such as nursing. Some work has been done to test approaches to help individuals and organizations better manage stress. Thus far, effects of these approaches are modest at best.

STRATEGIES TO MANAGE WORK STRESS

INDIVIDUAL STRATEGIES

Recognize the presence of stress or feelings of disequilibrium.
Enhance clinical knowledge and skills.
Manage time and set priorities.
Improve all facets of communication.
Assess one's assets and abilities.
Evaluate one's attitudes, values, beliefs, and expectations.
Reconsider expectations of self and work.
Reframe the meaning of situations.
Assert one's needs.
Break out of the "stressed-out" mold.
Adopt self-care measures:
- Exercise
- Proper diet
- Imagery, meditation, relaxation
- Recreation
- Vacation

ORGANIZATIONAL STRATEGIES

Recognize stress and its undesirable effects.
Support educational endeavors.
Develop leadership styles that reduce stress.
Offer group-based experiences:
- Facilitated staff meetings
- Support groups
- Liaison psychiatric involvement

Create a stress-resistant environment:
- Promote high social support.
- Structure or restructure the physical features.
- Assess effects of shift changes and scheduling.
- Introduce a shared-governance model.

STRESS MANAGEMENT

The most obvious way to manage stress is to intervene in the process. That is not as simple as it seems. After considering the innumerable sources of stress and the influence of perception, it is unclear which interventions are truly effective. Furthermore, there are not ready answers to such questions as what is adequate staffing, where can both space and money be obtained to renovate the environment, and exactly how can interpersonal relationships be made more satisfactory?

House[5] offers a valuable insight by noting that work organizations may believe their responsibility is only to help individuals learn how to deal with stress. This approach is necessary but not sufficient. First, it is not clear how effective the use of individual stress remedies are. Second, attending only to the individual detracts from examining the organization. Although restructuring work environments to reduce stress is a difficult task, it may ultimately be the only tenable approach to dealing with work stress.

To date the dominant methods of stress reduction in nursing are those that focus on helping the individual cope. Coping, to reiterate, is an individual response used to reduce internal tension; it protects against stress and represents individual attempts to reestablish a harmonic balance. One of the first steps in coping with stress is to trace its origin. Because of the interrelationship among life's spheres, sources of stress originating from the nonwork setting must be contemplated along with work factors. By pinpointing the problem (e.g., is it child care or critical care), it is possible to mobilize coping resources that are best suited to manage the particular difficulty. This discussion, however, focuses on those individual and organizational coping strategies, as summarized in the box above, relevant to stressors intrinsic to the work setting.

Individual Strategies

Individual coping strategies are those techniques arising from self-awareness and a sense of responsibility for self. Several reports have suggested that the most crucial step in the coping process is recognizing that stress is present and that either one's equilibrium is endangered or that the imbalance has already occurred.[52,59,82] Only after stress is recognized can decisions be made about which specific tactics might enhance coping. There is an extensive array of individual coping strategies, and the approaches may be used either separately or in various combinations (see box, p. 81). However, it is important to emphasize that although approaches to stress management are eagerly sought, the efficacy of most approaches remains unclear.

Clinical knowledge and skills can be expanded to enhance one's sense of competence in the critical care setting. Techniques for time management and priority setting may enhance one's sense of control and accomplishment. Stress might also be reduced by learning better communication skills, such as expressing one's needs and concerns, truly listening to and hearing what is being said, and recognizing the divisiveness and destructiveness of ineffective communication tactics.

Another vital clinical skill is learning to adapt to the ever-changing demands of the critical care environment. Plans must be sufficiently fluid so that they can be altered to meet the patient needs; staff must realize that real-time plan alteration is inherent to critical care. Stress will increase if staff members do not realign their plans of care to meet changing circumstances.

A large collection of self-care measures, such as exercise and proper diet, might also be tried.[52,83] Taking a personal asset inventory may also help to improve personal coping skills.[83a] Although perceived individual limitations are often sources of frustration, identifying one's strengths helps to accentuate the positive. This process enables the individual to cultivate strengths and potentials rather than succumb to a false sense of inadequacy.

Another coping technique involves recognizing how individual attitudes, values, beliefs, and expectations affect the stress experience. It is possible that job stress is largely the product of unfulfilled expectations. In the past, work was primarily viewed as a source of income. At present, work is also expected to contribute to personal fulfillment. These are cogent issues for nurses, because nursing is a female-dominated profession. The doors of opportunity have been opened to new sources of gratification and satisfaction for women. These doors also open to a spectrum of new demands as women juggle a variety of potentially conflicting responsibilities not encountered by previous generations.[84]

Expectations may also affect the sense that the "grass is greener" elsewhere. Things may seem better at another institution. Conversely, this may be merely an illusion created by wishful thinking. By reframing situations, reconsidering expectations, and reevaluating the real significance of events, some of the self-induced stress dynamics can be diminished. Harris[62] phrases it well by stating, "Is . . . dropping a bedpan really a major life threat?" Whether an event is viewed as a major catastrophe or as a somewhat humorous, human error will alter the stressfulness of the occurrence.[83a]

Finally, individual coping has to do with the contemporary reputation surrounding stress. Being "stressed out" is almost an expectation of current life. Perhaps part of coping with stress is to realize that life is busy and demanding but that it is truly a part of living; it is okay to feel exhilarated by all life offers. Furthermore, it is acceptable *not* to be stressed; it is okay to feel relaxed and contented. Perhaps one of the best ways to break the cycle of stress is to express more vocally the good sensations, the happy thoughts, and the pleasantries that are not as stylish to discuss as is stress.

Organizational Strategies

Along with individual coping efforts, a variety of organization-based approaches are available to attenuate stress (see box, p. 81). For example, not only is education an important individual intervention, it is also a viable organizational strategy. Education includes programs to enhance a staff member's knowledge about both critical care and stress. This education might be offered as in-service workshops, university courses with tuition assistance from the health care agency, or continuing education seminars.[85-87]

Group activities aimed at facilitating stress management might also be offered by the health care organization. Well-managed staff meetings, support groups, and consultation with liaison psychiatric personnel have the potential to diminish stress.[50,88] To maximize the effectiveness of group approaches to stress reduction, at least one facilitator must be skilled in the dynamics of group interactions. In addition, group approaches to stress management also require commitment from participants to keep the group viable over a sufficient period to allow the group process to reach its full potential.

Another organizational tool for managing stress is to establish a climate that fosters social support. Social support is typified by interactions that have the potential to both diminish stress and enhance health. There are many definitions of social support, but the essence of it is based in positive relationships that leave the participants feeling cared for, esteemed, and respected.[5] Supportive relationships are not always pleasant or free from conflict. However, even when disagreement prevails, the persons continue to feel valued.[67] Such dynamics require maturity and insight from both the recipient and the giver of support.[83] In the work environment, supervisors and co-workers are obvious sources of social support. For nurses, social support has demonstrated efficacy in reducing burnout[71,89] and lowering symptoms of psychologic distress.[3,90]

Leadership characteristics are also relevant organizational features that may reduce stress. Leadership has two components: (1) consideration or concern for group members and (2) structure or emphasis on task completion. A study of neonatal critical care nurses demonstrated that staff members experienced less burnout and more job satisfaction when they perceived their head nurses as considerate leaders.[91] Other authorities have also cited the importance of the head nurse as an influence on stress.[92,93] The responsibilities and possibilities for administrators to modify the effects of stress are apparent from the investigations of both social support and leadership.

Restructuring the critical care environment is a costly alternative to managing stress, but it may be a necessary consideration. For example, Norbeck[45] found that, more than any other stressors, such features of the physical environment as inaccessible supplies and inoperable equipment contributed to psychologic distress and job dissatisfaction. Gorny[94] also underscored that critical care nurses are predisposed to sensory disequilibrium because of the excessive sensory stimuli present in the critical care environment. Such information must be heeded by those responsible for planning and constructing new critical care settings, as well as those responsible for remodeling existing units. It is imperative that environmental stressors be acknowledged as more than insignificant disgruntlement or idle complaining.

An important point must be considered in regard to managing stress with the aforementioned individual and organizational techniques. With a few exceptions, intervention strategies have been neither extensively nor rigorously evaluated. Although many of the suggestions are extremely appealing, their effectiveness in reducing work stress is not really known. Consequently, it is important to be cautious in regard to which interventions are implemented.

Potentially stressful aspects of the interventions themselves must be considered. For example, at what point does an exercise program become a source of stress rather than a way to cope? The cost of the fitness club membership, dislike for the activities, or time conflicts in using the facilities could all serve to negate the intended benefits of exercise. None of the strategies for managing stress is a panacea nor are the strategies substitutes for directly modifying the actual sources of stress.

SUMMARY

Stress is a complex entity that evokes responses and problems that are equally complicated. It is therefore not surprising that managing stress is also intricate and elusive. *Stress is a common aspect of life, nursing, and critical care.* Developing an understanding of stress is one way to begin to deal with this pervasive process. Nursing represents a very stressful profession. The stresses originate not only from the work and the work environment, but also from nonwork problems, such as how to manage career, home, and family. Those presently in critical care settings have the responsibility to use the information that does exist about critical care stress to establish a more harmonious equilibrium for critical care nurses.

REFERENCES

1. Mason JW: A historical view of the stress field, part I, *J Hum Stress* 1(1):6, 1975.
2. Mason JW: A historical view of the stress field, part II, *J Hum Stress* 1(2):22, 1975.
3. Hirsch BJ, Rapkin BD: Social networks and adult social identities: profiles and correlates of support and rejection, *Am J Community Psychol* 14:395, 1986.
4. Caplan RD and others: *Job demands and worker health. Main effects and occupational differences*, Washington, DC, 1975, NIOSH Government Printing Office.
5. House JS: *Work stress and social support,* Reading, Mass, 1981, Addison-Wesley.
6. Margolis BL, Kroes WH, Quinn RP: Job stress: an unlisted occupational hazard, *J Occup Med* 16:659, 1974.
7. Pelletier K: *Healthy people in unhealthy places,* New York, 1984, Delacorte Press.
8. Menzies IEP: Nurses under stress, *Int Nurs Rev* 7:9, 1960.
9. Holsclaw PA: Nursing in high emotional risk areas, *Nurs Forum* 4(4):36, 1965.
10. Ivancevich JM, Matteson MT: Nurses and stress: time to examine the potential problem, *Superv Nurs* 11(6):17, 1980.
11. Marshall J: Stress amongst nurses. In Cooper CL, Marshall J, editors: *White collar and professional stress,* New York, 1980, John Wiley & Sons.
12. Selye H: *The stress of life,* ed 2, New York, 1976, McGraw-Hill.
13. Karamus W: Working conditions and health: social epidemiology, patterns of stress and change, *Soc Sci Med* 19:359, 1984.
14. Sharit J, Salvendy G: Occupational stress: review and reappraisal, *Hum Factors* 24(2):129, 1982.
15. Pearlin LI: The social contexts of stress. In Goldberger L, Breznitz S, editors: *Handbook of stress: theoretical and clinical aspects,* New York, 1982, The Free Press.
16. French JRP, Rodgers W, Cobb S: Adjustment as person-environment fit. In Coelho GV, Hamburg DA, Adams JE, editors: *Coping and adaptation,* New York, 1974, Basic Books.
17. Harrison RV: Person-environment fit and job stress. In Cooper CL, Payne R, editors: *Stress at work,* New York, 1978, John Wiley & Sons.
18. Lazarus RS, Folkman S: *Stress, appraisal, and coping,* New York, 1984, Springer Publishing.
19. Pearlin LI and others: The stress process, *J Health Soc Behav* 22:337, 1981.
20. Stone GL and others: Identification of stress and coping skills within a critical care setting, *West J Nurs Res* 6:201, 1984.
21. Johnson CL, Johnson FA: Attitudes toward parenting in dual-career families, *Am J Psychiatry* 134: 391, 1977.
22. Pearlin LI, Schooler C: The structure of coping, *J Health Soc Behav* 19:2, 1978.
23. Cherniss C: *Staff burnout: job stress in the human services,* Beverly Hills, Calif, 1980, Sage Publications.
24. Farber BA: Introduction: a critical perspective on burnout. In Farber BA, editor: *Stress and burnout in the human service professions,* New York, 1983, Pergamon Press.
25. Maslach C: Understanding burnout: definitional issues in analyzing a complex phenomenon. In Paine WS, editor: *Job stress and burnout,* Beverly Hills, Calif, 1982, Sage Publications.
26. Seuntjens AD: Burnout in nursing—what it is and how to prevent it, *Nurs Adm Q* 7(1):12, 1982.
27. French JRP, Caplan RD: Organizational stress and individual strain. In Marrow AJ, editor: *The failure of success,* New York, 1972, AMACOM.
28. Conboy CF: A recovery room, *Am J Nurs* 47:686, 1947.
29. Dunn FE, Shupp MG: The recovery room: a wartime economy, *Am J Nurs* 43:279, 1943.
30. Hilberman M: The evolution of intensive care units, *Crit Care Med* 3(4):159, 1975.
31. Anderson CA, Basteyns M: Stress and the critical care nurse reaffirmed, *J Nurs Adm* 11(1):31, 1981.
32. Bailey JT, Steffen SM, Grout JW: The stress audit: identifying the stressors of ICU nursing, *J Nurs Educ* 19(6):15, 1980.
33. Bilodeau CB: The nurse and her reactions to critical-care nursing, *Heart Lung* 2:358, 1973.
34. Cassem NH, Hackett TP: Sources of tension for the CCU nurse, *Am J Nurs* 72:1426, 1972.
35. Cassem NH, Hackett TP: Stress on the nurse and therapist in the intensive-care unit and the coronary-care unit, *Heart Lung* 4:252, 1975.
36. Hay D, Oken D: The psychological stresses of intensive care unit nursing, *Psychosom Med* 34:109, 1972.
37. Huckabay LMD, Jagla B: Nurses' stress factors in the intensive care unit, *J Nurs Adm* 9(2):21, 1979.
38. Vreeland R, Ellis GL: Stresses on the nurse in the intensive-care unit, *JAMA* 208:332, 1969.
39. Gentry WD, Foster SB, Froehling S: Psychologic response to situational stress in intensive and nonintensive nursing, *Heart Lung* 1:793, 1972.
40. Kelly JG, Cross DG: Stress, coping behaviors, and recommendations for intensive care and medical surgical ward registered nurses, *Res Nurs Health* 8:321, 1985.

41. Maloney JP: Job stress and its consequences on a group of intensive care and nonintensive care nurses, *Adv Nurs Sci* 4(2):31, 1982.
42. Vincent P, Coleman WF: Comparison of major stressors perceived by ICU and non-ICU nurses, *Crit Care Nurse* 6(1):64, 1986.
42a. Caldwell T, Weiner MF: Stresses and coping in ICU Nursing. *Gen Hosp Psychiatry* 3:119, 1981.
42b. Stehle JL: Critical care nursing stress: the findings revisited, *Nurs Res* 30:182, 1981.
43. Norbeck JS: Coping with stress in critical care nursing: research findings, *Focus Crit Care* 12(5):36, 1985.
44. Numerof RE, Abrams MN: Sources of stress among nurses: an empirical investigation, *J Hum Stress* 10(2):88, 1984.
45. Norbeck JS: Perceived job stress, job satisfaction, and psychological symptoms in critical care nursing, *Res Nurs Health* 8:253, 1985.
46. Marriott HJL: Letter to the editors regarding Cassem and Hackett: Stress on the nurse and therapist in the intensive-care unit and the coronary-care unit, *Heart Lung* 4:802, 1975.
47. Babbini LJ: Letter to the editors regarding Cassem and Hackett: Stress on the nurse and therapist in the intensive-care unit and the coronary-care unit, *Heart Lung* 5:328, 1976.
48. Keane A, DuCette J, Adler DC: Stress in ICU and non-ICU nurses, *Nurs Res* 34:231, 1985.
49. Maloney JP, Bartz C: Stress-tolerant people: intensive care nurses compared with non-intensive care nurses, *Heart Lung* 12:389, 1983.
50. Fawzy FI and others: Preventing nursing burnout: a challenge for liaison psychiatry, *Gen Hosp Psychiatry* 5:141, 1983.
51. Kosmoski KA, Calkin JD: Critical care nurses' intent to stay in their positions, *Res Nurs Health* 9:3, 1986.
52. Hartl DE: Stress management and the nurse, *Adv Nurs Sci* 1(4):91, 1979.
53. Pearlin LI: Role strains and personal stress. In Kaplan HB, editor: *Psychological stress: trends in theory and research,* New York, 1983, Academic Press.
54. Perun PJ, Bielby DD: Towards a model of female occupational behavior: a human development approach, *Psychol Women Q* 6:234, 1981.
55. Haw MA: Women, work and stress: a review and agenda for the future, *J Health Soc Behav* 23:132, 1982.
56. Kandel DB, Davies M, Raveis VH: The stressfulness of daily social roles for women: marital, occupational and household roles, *J Health Soc Behav* 26:64, 1985.
57. Long J, Porter KL: Multiple roles of midlife women. A case for new directions in theory, research, and policy. In Baruch G, Brooks-Gunn J, editors: *Women in midlife,* New York, 1984, Plenum Press.
58. Verbrugge LM: Role burdens and physical health of women and men, *Women Health* 11(1):47, 1986.
59. Oskins SL: Identification of situational stressors and coping methods by intensive care nurses, *Heart Lung* 8:953, 1979.
60. Jennings BM: Stress, locus of control, social support, and psychological symptoms among head nurses, *Res Nurs Health* 13:393, 1990.
61. Deleted in proofs.
62. Harris JS: Stressors and stress in critical care, *Crit Care Nurse* 4(1):84, 1984.
63. Lindsey AM, Carrieri V: Stress response. In Carrieri V, Lindsey AM, West C, editors: *Pathophysiological phenomena in nursing: human responses to illness,* Philadelphia, 1986, WB Saunders.
64. Brodsky CM: Long-term work stress, *Psychosomatics* 25:361, 1984.
65. Minnehan RF, Paine WS: Bottom lines. Assessing the economic and legal consequences of burnout. In Paine WS, editor: *Job stress and burnout,* Beverly Hills, Calif, 1982, Sage Publications.
65a. Lawler EE: Can the quality of work life be legislated? *The Personnel Administrator* 21:17, 1986.
66. Grout JW, Steffen SM, Bailey JT: The stresses and the satisfiers of the intensive care unit: a survey, *Crit Care Q* 3(4):35, 1981.
67. Jennings BM: Social support: a way to a climate of caring, *Nurs Adm Q* 11(4):63, 1987.
68. Cleland VS: The effect of stress on performance, *Nurs Res* 14:292, 1965.
69. Cleland VS: Effects of stress on thinking, *Am J Nurs* 67:108, 1967.
70. Esteban A, Ballesteros P, Caballero J: Psychological evaluation of intensive care nurses, *Crit Care Med* 11:616, 1983.
71. Cronin-Stubbs D, Rooks CA: The stress, social support, and burnout of critical care nurses: the results of research, *Heart Lung* 14:31, 1985.
72. Bartz C, Maloney JP: Burnout among intensive care nurses, *Res Nurs Health* 9:147, 1986.
73. Dembrowski TM and others: Moving beyond Type A, *Advances* 1(1):16, 1984.
74. Dimsdale JE, Herd JA: Variability of plasma lipids in response to emotional arousal, *Psychosom Med* 44:413, 1982.
75. Holroyd KA, Appel MA, Andrasik F: A cognitive-behavioral approach to psychophysiological disorders. In Meichenbaum D, Jaremko JE, editors: *Stress reduction and prevention,* New York, 1983, Plenum Press.
76. Selye H: Stress and a holistic view of health for the nursing profession. In Claus KE, Bailey JT, editors: *Living with stress and promoting well-being: a handbook for nurses,* St Louis, 1980, Mosby–Year Book.
77. Wandelt MA, Pierce PM, Widdowson RR: Why nurses leave nursing and what can be done about it, *Am J Nurs* 81:72, 1981.
78. Wolf GA: Nursing turnover: some causes and solutions, *Nurs Outlook* 29:233, 1981.
79. Knaus WA and others: An evaluation of outcome from intensive care in major medical centers, *Ann Intern Med* 104:410, 1986.
80. Milton D and others: Differentiated group professional practice in nursing: a demonstration model, *Nurs Clin North Am* 27:23, 1992.
81. Ritter J, Tonges MC: Work redesign in high-intensity environments. ProACT for critical care, *J Nurs Adm* 21(12):26, 1991.
82. Stillman SM, Strasser BL: Helping critical care nurses with work-related stress, *J Nurs Adm* 10(1):28, 1980.
83. Noroian EL, Yasko J: Care for the critical care-giver: strategies for the prevention of burnout, *Dimens Crit Care Nurs* 1:97, 1982.
83a. Scully R: Stress: in the nurse, *Am J Nurs* 80:912, 1980.
84. Jennings BM: *Stress, social support, and locus of control: effects on head nurses' mental health,* doctoral dissertation, San Francisco, 1987, University of California.
85. Newlin B: Stress reduction for the critical care nurse: a stress education program, *Occup Health Nurs* 32:315, 1984.
86. Randolph GL, Price JL, Collins JR: The effects of burnout prevention training on burnout symptoms in nurses, *J Contin Educ Nurs* 17(2):43, 1986.
87. Warren JJ: Developing a stress-management program, *Dimens Crit Care Nurs* 1:307, 1982.
88. Bohannan-Reed K, Dugan D, Huck B: Staying human under stress: stress reduction and emotional support in the critical care setting, *Crit Care Nurse* 3(3):26, 1983.
89. Constable JF, Russell DW: The effect of social support and the work environment upon burnout among nurses, *J Hum Stress* 12(1):20, 1986.
90. Norbeck JS: Types and sources of social support for managing job stress in critical care nursing, *Nurs Res* 34:225, 1985.
91. Duxbury ML and others: Head nurse leadership style with staff nurse burnout and job satisfaction in neonatal intensive care units, *Nurs Res* 33:97, 1984.
92. Gil R, Sumner M: Establishing a leadership style that shows you do care, *Nurs Success Today* 2(4):32, 1985.
93. Guy ML: Leadership style and approaches in critical care nursing, *Crit Care Q* 5(1):17, 1982.
94. Gorny DA: Maintenance of sensory equilibrium for the critical care nurse, *Top Clin Nurs* 6(4):44, 1985.

II

PSYCHOSOCIAL ALTERATIONS

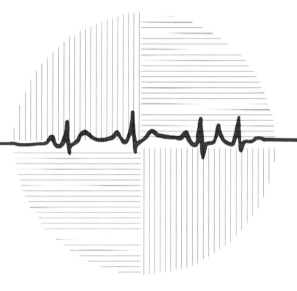

7

Self-Concept Alterations

CHAPTER OBJECTIVES

- Describe the theoretic bases of self-concept and related nursing diagnoses: Body Image Disturbance, Self-Esteem Disturbance, Altered Role Performance, Powerlessness, and Hopelessness.
- Identify defining characteristics and causes of these nursing diagnoses.
- Identify situations that increase the risk of disturbances of self-concept.
- Point out assessment strategies of use with patients experiencing a disturbance in self-concept.
- Given a situation in which a patient experiences a self-concept alteration, match relevant interventions with expected outcomes.

The human self-concept comprises attitudes about oneself; perceptions of personal abilities, body image, and identity; and a general sense of worth. Included in this chapter are discussions of the nursing diagnoses of disturbances in self-concept—that is, Body Image Disturbance, Self-Esteem Disturbance, Altered Role Performance, Powerlessness, and Hopelessness. The nursing diagnosis Personal Identity Disturbance, included as a subcomponent of the human self-concept by the North American Nursing Diagnosis Association (NANDA), is omitted because it is not yet sufficiently developed for useful application to clinical practice. The four subcomponents of the human self-concept appear in Fig. 7-1.

This chapter focuses on the theoretic basis for each diagnosis. Each nursing diagnosis is defined and then discussed in terms of defining characteristics, expected outcomes, and interventions. The problems common to critical care nursing are the major concerns.

SELF-CONCEPT

Over the years many writers in the behavioral sciences have been interested in the self-concept, its development, and its importance to the individual.[1-4] In Rogers' writings on patient-centered psychotherapy,[2] he focused on the patient's self-concept as currently organized and functioning. He believed that there were elements of the self that the person could not face or clearly perceive; therefore he defined self-concept as an organized body of perceptions that were admissible to awareness. Included were perceptions of one's characteristics, abilities, relationships with others and the environment, values, goals, and ideals.

Sullivan[3,4] first used the concepts of *significant others* and *reflected appraisals* in his interpersonal theory of psychiatry. He believed that the self is developed from social interaction, particularly in dynamic patterns of interaction with significant people, especially the mother. Based on interactions that provide reward and punishment, the individual develops a self-concept that reflects the appraisals of others.

Perception is the focus of the theory of self-concept of Combs and Snygg.[1] The part that one regards as *I* or *me* (the beliefs about oneself and one's abilities) determines what one thinks and how one behaves. Although self-concept controls perceptions and eventual behavior, these perceptions and behaviors also affect the self-concept in a cyclic process. Some of the perceptions of self are basic or central and are highly resistant to change. Others are less important and more readily subject to change. Self-perceptions become more clear as the individual matures. These perceptions exist in a framework that is the individual's own private conception of himself or herself. Combs and Snygg named this construction the *phenomenal self,* which encompasses the central, vital concepts of the person. The phenomenal self is set in a *perceptual field,* which includes all the perceptions about the person plus the things outside the person.

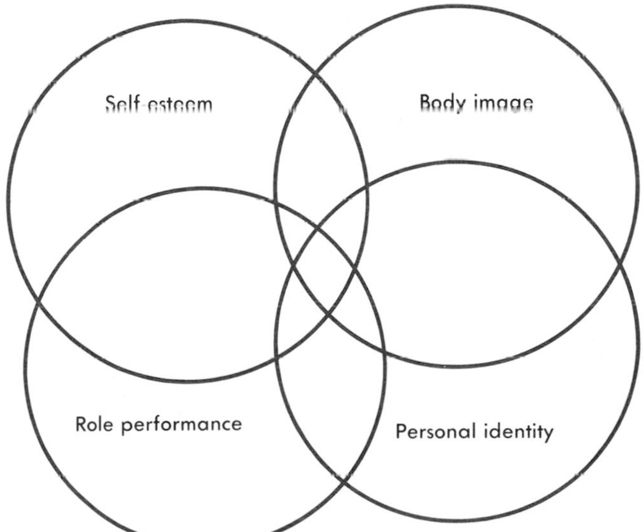

Fig. 7-1 Four subcomponents of the human self-concept (NANDA).

Self-concept is a construct that is useful for understanding individuals and their behavior. Although it is relatively stable, it can be modified. It influences how one reacts to and manages problems in daily life. Self-concept is a major concern for nurses who care for patients, because nursing interventions that do not consider the individual in his or her wholeness—including the self-concept—will probably be ineffective.

DISTURBANCES IN SELF-CONCEPT

Three major subcomponents of the self-concept are discussed in this chapter: body image, self-esteem, and role performance. Alterations may involve any or all of these interrelated components. Pertinent to all these diagnoses are the following key factors that affect an individual's self-concept[5]:

1. Previous perception of appraisals about self from significant others
2. Experience with developmental and situational crises and how they were managed
3. Experiences with success and failure and current expectations of self
4. Positive and negative feelings of self-worth from interpersonal experiences
5. Level of physiologic functioning

Causes of Disturbances of Self-Concept

Causative factors related to self-concept disruptions may be categorized as biophysical, cognitive-perceptual, psychosocial, cultural, or spiritual. Major causative factors include the following[6]:

1. Cognitive-perceptual difficulties—that is, knowing deficit, altered thought processes, and sensory-perceptual alterations
2. Biochemical changes in the body
3. Inability to adjust to and integrate body changes
4. Repeated negative interpersonal experiences
5. Absence of significant role models
6. Inability to learn new behaviors in response to transitional states
7. Poor identity development
8. Loss of control related to health care environment and illness-related regimen
9. Prolonged activity restriction
10. Deteriorating physical health

Assessment of the Self-Concept

The self-concept is what one believes about oneself; the self-report is what one is willing to share about oneself. When assessing the self-concept of the critically ill patient, Lee's phases of response to illness or injury[9] are useful. She identified four phases: impact, retreat, acknowledgment, and reconstruction. Patients in critical care units are primarily in the first two phases. During phase one—impact—signs of despair, discouragement, passive acceptance, anger, and hostility may be present. Shock, anxiety, numbness, strangeness, and unreality may be the immediate responses. During the retreat phase the patient may try to avoid reality; denial is common. Patients are not ready to look at the meaning or implications of the situation. They may repress or suppress reality and then, when this is no longer possible, become intensely angry. The patient is usually transferred to an intermediate unit before the acknowledgment phase occurs. This phase is marked by the conflicting emotions associated with recognition of the changes or losses that have occurred or will occur. In the final phase, there is an attempt at a new approach to life.

When Mr. A. awoke in the surgical critical care unit after amputation of his right arm and left leg, he asked repeatedly what had happened. His nurse and his wife explained that he had touched a "live" wire while atop an electric company pole checking the lines. A jolt of electricity had entered his right arm and exited through his left leg. His coworkers helped him down and revived him. At first he said how lucky he was to be alive. As the impact of the event became clear to him, he focused only on his losses, which resulted in major alterations in self-concept—body image, self-esteem, and role performance.

The disturbances of self-concept are examined individually in this chapter. It must be remembered, however, that although each subcomponent has unique characteristics, some characteristics are shared with several or all the other subcomponents.

BODY IMAGE DISTURBANCE

Body image is the mental picture an individual has of his or her body and its physical functioning at any given time. It is based on past and present perceptions and includes one's attitudes and feelings about one's body. The body image develops over time from internal-sensation postural changes, contact with people and objects in the environment, emotional experiences, and fantasies.[10] Although the body image is a stable part of the self-concept, it changes over time; it is influenced by cognitive growth and physical changes in the body. Fisher[11] suggested that body experiences can be dampened or minimized or they can be magnified to the point where they are the center of attention. He also described the *body boundary,* the demarcation between the self and the environment and the pattern of body awareness. The latter refers to the variation in attention given to different parts of the body; more attention is given to the parts that have symbolic significance or that are currently being threatened.

A change in the body's appearance, structure, and/or function necessitates a change in the body image. Such changes may be caused by disease, trauma, or surgery. The cause of body image disturbance may be biophysical, cognitive-perceptual, psychosocial, cultural, or spiritual. Body image disturbances arise when there is disruption in the way one perceives one's body. The person fails to perceive or adapt to the changed body (Table 7-1). Such disturbances are manifested by verbal or nonverbal response to the actual or perceived change in appearance, structure, or function.[12] Some patients must extend their body image to incorporate environmental objects.[13] The patient temporarily requiring assisted respirations must extend his or her body image to include the ventilator and its accessories. Explanations to patient and family are helpful in this situation. A patient admitted to a surgical critical care unit after a traumatic amputation may awake to find his or her leg missing with

Table 7-1 Body image problems

Structure	Altered by	Treatment	Alteration
Skin	Burns Lacerations	Grafts Sutures	Scars Contractures Change in skin color, texture
Teeth	Automobile accident	Dentures	Altered speech, eating habits
Leg	Traumatic amputation	Artificial limb	Altered gait
Heart	Myocardial infarction, with abnormal rhythms	Automatic implantable cardiodefibrillators	Dependence on equipment
Spinal cord	Diving accident	Rehabilitation	Altered mobility
Kidney	Renal failure	Hemodialysis Peritoneal dialysis Renal transplant	Dependence on equipment Acceptance of a donated organ

no prior knowledge of the loss. Reliving the accident and receiving explanations about the need for the amputation are priorities for such a patient. The critical care nurse must begin the process of helping the patient live with this permanent alteration. Interventions by the nurse and others on the health team focus on helping the person manage the physical changes and the changes in the psychosocial areas affected. Helping the person recognize, accept, and live with the resultant change requires recognition that self-esteem and role performance may also be affected.

Body image has received considerable attention in the nursing literature.[6,13–21] This body of knowledge forms the basis for interventions with patients experiencing the losses associated with altered body image. Body image may also be altered by the need to incorporate a prosthetic device or a donated body part.[22]

The meaning of the alteration (appearance, structure, or function) varies with the individual. What is lost? What value is placed on it? What did the body part or function enable the person to enjoy or accomplish? What disability results? The values of the culture are important; wholeness, independence, and attractiveness are important in society today. The person's ability to cope, the responses from others significant to him or her, and the help available to him or her and the family are important factors in the outcome of body image disturbances.

SELF-ESTEEM DISTURBANCE

Self-esteem develops as a part of self-concept through the reflected appraisals of significant others. The way in which such information is interpreted is probably more important than is the content. Self-esteem is only partly related to material, economic, or social conditions. The need for self-esteem is a part of the hierarchy of human needs postulated by Maslow.[23] Having high self-esteem helps one deal with the environment and face more easily the maturational and situational crises of life. A low self-regard impairs one's ability to adapt. Overall, the goal is to maintain a high positive regard for oneself in the midst of ever-changing views of oneself. This goal, when met, contributes to the quality of life of the individual. Persons with a well-developed self-esteem are at less risk for disturbances of self-esteem than those with poorly developed self-esteem.

Disturbances in self-esteem arise when a person experiences a decrease in self-worth, self-respect, self-approval, or self-confidence. Causative factors of the decrease include repeated negative interactions with significant others, as well as cognitive-perceptual difficulties. Low self-esteem may be manifested by the following[17]:

1. Inability to accept positive reinforcement
2. Expressions of shame/guilt
3. Nonparticipation in therapy
4. Not taking responsibility for self-care (self-neglect)
5. Self-destructive behavior
6. Hesitancy to try new things
7. Denial of problems obvious to others
8. Projection of blame/responsibility for problems
9. Hypersensitivity to criticism

Self-esteem is an important concept for nurses and other health professionals. It has been studied frequently in a variety of contexts.[24-33] Nurses have a significant impact on patients who are ill. When the illness is critical, a patient's self-esteem level may be imperiled. Perhaps the patient caused the accident that injured him or her and others, including family members. Perhaps he or she was under the influence of alcohol or drugs. Perhaps he or she will be subject to arrest if he or she survives. Perhaps he or she will lose his or her job or be unable to return to his or her previous occupation. Topics that make the nurse uncomfortable are frequently avoided. Patients and families can easily get the message not to discuss them. The nurse who expresses negative reactions to a patient, either openly or covertly, will reinforce a patient's low self-esteem. An aloof, insensitive, or superficial relationship with a patient who has acquired immunodeficiency syndrome (AIDS), for example, can cause the patient to feel rejected, humiliated, and stigmatized.[34,35]

Antonucci and Jackson[24] point out that, although a link between self-esteem and mental illness has been confirmed, the link with physical health is not clear. Self-esteem level may be an outcome, a predisposing factor, or an insulating factor in situations involving physical health. In their study of self-esteem and physical health, self-esteem was lower as the severity of the health problem increased, as the perception of ill health increased, and as the degree of disability increased. The study stresses the need for awareness that patients with health problems probably have a lowered self-esteem that may negatively affect behavior during illness.

The antecedents of self-esteem were the focus of Coopersmith's book.[25] He identified four major factors that contribute to the development of self-esteem:

1. The amount of acceptance and concern from significant persons in one's life
2. The successes in one's past and one's status and position in the world
3. The values and aspirations to which one commits oneself
4. The manner in which one responds to devaluing experiences

Of special importance to the development of high self-esteem are three conditions: (1) total or near-total acceptance of the child by the family, (2) clearly defined limits that are reasonable, rational, and enforced, and (3) respect and allowance for individual actions within the defined limits.

Basic self-esteem as described by Crouch and Straub[36] is that which is established early in life and, once firmly established, is relatively unchanging. They also described a functional level of self-esteem that varies from day to day according to ongoing evaluations of interactions. Such self-esteem may be more or less than the basic self-esteem. The functional level can be changed in response to interventions of the person himself or herself, the family, coworkers, or health professionals. Functional or situational self-esteem may be increased through individually oriented, short-term approaches that attempt to improve the person's view of his or her worth.

Self-esteem throughout the life span was discussed by Stanwyck.[33] He found that overall self-esteem was relatively stable and was based on critical elements of experience, including significant others, social role expectations, psychosocial developmental crises, and the communication and coping patterns of the family. In adulthood, self-esteem is affected by intimate relationships, progress in social relationships, and career development. One's self-esteem thrives on the esteem of others. Experiences may confirm or modify self-esteem. Both failures and successful experiences are important. Such information may be ignored or disqualified as useful evidence. Hence the focus on perception of reflected appraisals is important.

In old age, a person faces loss of autonomy that may lower self-esteem. Changes in the expectations of others for one's behavior and capacity may occur. Losses related to health alterations and sensory impairment related to aging, dependency, retirement, and deaths of friends and family may affect self-esteem. If nurses are impatient with performance deficits, the patient may feel inadequate and guilty. If patients are treated as children, they may believe themselves burdens and react with resentment. Failure to include them in decision making may cause them to feel useless and rejected. On the other hand, people with a strong sense of self-worth are likely to be adjusted, happy, and competent.

Defensive self-esteem is used to defend against the person's perception of a gap between his or her real self and ideal self. High self-esteem is associated with a low need for social approval, comfort with intimacy and self-disclosure, and the ability to acknowledge personal failures. Rubin[32] discussed the loss of self-esteem that accompanies the loss of control of functioning in relation to time and place. This loss is associated with a decrease in self-esteem. A sense of shame accompanies this private judgment of failure.

A person's level of self-esteem is an important factor in the response to a critical illness, and behavior during illness may be negatively affected by lowered self-esteem. The patient with severe burns may interpret the avoidance behavior of nurses and family who are appalled by the appearance of the patient and the odor in his or her room as a devaluation of himself or herself. The patient may refuse to cooperate with the treatment regimen and may judge himself or herself a failure and be unable to see a future in which he or she will return to a productive life. Anticipatory interventions that assist the staff and family members in their care of the patient would help to avoid such a situation. Nurses should communicate acceptance, genuine interest, and concern and avoid being judgmental.

ALTERED ROLE PERFORMANCE

Interactions with others that create and modify roles are an important part of the self-concept. The roles one chooses reflect one's beliefs and feelings. Persons have primary, secondary, and tertiary roles. Primary roles are those associated with gender, age, and developmental stage. Secondary roles are those of daughter, sister, and so forth. Tertiary roles are those assumed by choice, such as scout leader or churchgoer. Illness, when it occurs, disrupts secondary and tertiary roles.

Role performance alterations are those problems that arise when a person experiences difficulties in making life transitions. Causative factors include lack of significant role models, inability to learn new roles because of life transitions, and cognitive-perceptual difficulties. Altered role performance may be manifested by the following[12]:

1. Change in self-perception of role
2. Denial of role
3. Change in others' perception of role
4. Conflict in roles
5. Change in physical capacity to resume role
6. Lack of knowledge of role
7. Change in usual patterns of responsibility

Meleis[37,38] examined role theory from a nursing perspective and pointed out that nursing deals with people who are experiencing transitions—that is, a change in role status. They may be completing a transition or about to begin one. Such transitions involve loss and addition to role relationships and may involve developmental, situational, or health status–related events. Each of the types of transition can have implications for nursing. Examples include the teen-aged girl who becomes pregnant (developmental), a young adult whose father dies (situational), and an older adult who experiences an acute onset of illness (health-illness event). All these transitions require changes in roles of the persons and families involved. The individuals concerned must incorporate new knowledge, alter behaviors, and change their self-concepts.

Role transitions occur in patients with critical illness. Role change in the transition from wellness or chronic illness to acute illness is a concern for the critical care nurse because role transitions mean changes in role relationships, expectations, or abilities and can be major concerns for the critically ill patient.

Mrs. B. is a 23-year-old woman (para 1, gravida 1) who is admitted to the medical critical care unit on her second postpartum day. She has pregnancy-induced hypertension complicated by hemolysis, elevated liver enzymes, and a low platelet count—the so-called "HELLP syndrome." Her baby boy, who was almost full-term, is doing well. The need for this admission means separation during the crucial first days of a new role. Her assumption of the mothering role is delayed. Photographs of the baby, brief visits so she can see him, and assurance that he is being well cared for are important interventions to help her bridge this important transition.

The rapid and potentially drastic changes that accompany critical illness may seriously interfere with role performance. The male patient after a myocardial infarction wonders about his role as husband, breadwinner, and worker. If the patient is unable to resume previous roles, he may refuse to accept the new roles associated with the chronic cardiac condition. The psychosocial needs of the patient in such a situation depend on age, gender, occupation, family roles, previous experience with illness, suddenness of onset, extent of illness, and prognosis. Nurses are frequently involved with situations that include alterations in role performance in individuals and families.[39]

The patient may be unable to meet the demands of such changes and thus experience role insufficiency.[37] The use of role supplementation is an approach nurses can use in such a situation. As described by Meleis,[37] this intervention involves both preventive and therapeutic efforts. By communicating and interacting with the patient and family, nurses may convey information or experiences that increase the awareness of the new roles and interrelationships necessary because of the role transition. For example, role insufficiency may be displayed in behaviors that reflect fear of moving from the critical care unit to the intermediate care unit. A variety of nursing activities can anticipate and facilitate this transition.

POWERLESSNESS

The concept of powerlessness may be defined as the perceived inability to influence or control an outcome. Powerlessness as a nursing diagnosis is defined as the perception of the individual that one's own action will not significantly affect an outcome.[12] Powerlessness is a perceived lack of control over a current situation or immediate happening. Unrelieved powerlessness may result in hopelessness, which is discussed in the next section.

The causes of powerlessness include factors in the health care environment, interpersonal interactions, illness-related regimen, and a life-style of helplessness. A severe level of powerlessness may be manifested by the following:

1. Verbal expressions of having no control or influence over the situation
2. Verbal expressions of having no control or influence over the outcome
3. Verbal expressions of having no control over self-care
4. Depression over physical deterioration that occurs despite the patient's compliance with regimens
5. Apathy

Moderate levels of powerlessness may be reflected by nonparticipation in care or decision making when opportunities are provided; expressions of dissatisfaction and frustration over inability to perform previous tasks and/or activities; not monitoring progress; expression of doubt about role performance; reluctance to express true feelings, fearing alienation from caregivers; passivity; inability to seek information about care; dependence on others that may result in irritability, resentment, anger, and guilt; and no defense of self-care practices when challenged. A low level of powerlessness may be reflected in passivity.

Both actual and perceived control over present or impending events are important.

An alert patient with widely spread metastatic carcinoma of the breast is admitted to the medical critical care unit for treatment of septic shock. She is Japanese and has been married for many years to a U.S. serviceman. After a conference with the physician, the husband gives permission for a "do not resuscitate" order. The nurses caring for her soon find that the patient is expecting to get better and to go home. A conference involving the patient, her husband, and the staff clarify the situation. Treatments for her cancer continue, but heroic measures will not be used. Every effort to get her ready to go home again will be made.

In this situation, there are cultural expectations that the husband will make all decisions. However, every effort should be made to allow the patient to exercise her right to make decisions about care to the extent she desires.

Most people expect to have the power to participate in making decisions that affect them. Feelings of powerlessness are avoided if possible. When patients feel their choices are limited, they may act against their own best interests.[40] Given enough frustration, any exercise of control—even one with negative outcomes, such as signing out of the hospital against medical advice (AMA)—can become attractive.

Individuals vary in the amount of control they prefer.[41] A patient may feel power but may or may not desire it. Important variables in this regard are the illness; values, traits, attitudes, and experiences; the hospital setting; and social displacement. Personality, age, religion, occupation, income, residence, and race may all be pertinent factors. Apparently there is an increase in variability in the amount of control preferred as people age. Rodin[41] pointed out that giving a person more control than desired may result in negative outcomes: stress, worry, and self-blame. The critical care unit routines may oppose or preclude any control by the patient. The person to whom control is important should be helped to continue to control as many areas of life as possible. On the other hand, a patient must be given the opportunity to choose not to control.[42]

One explanation of this variable interest in control is the concept of *locus of control.* This idea of expectancy of control developed by Rotter[43] has been particularly helpful in explaining the variability of responses of people to similar situations. The locus of control is a personality characteristic, a relatively stable tendency to perceive events and outcomes as within or outside one's control regardless of the situation.

The Internal-External Locus of Control Scale developed by Rotter is useful in assessing this personality trait. A person with an internal locus of control tends to believe that events are under one's personal control. A person with an external locus of control, however, tends to believe that events are related to chance, fate, or powerful others. Situations exist in which the person with an internal locus of control has made serial life-style changes based on medical advice and then has experienced a major illness, typically a myocardial infarction. This experience forces him or her to believe that his or her own actions will not (because they have not) significantly affect the outcome. Repeated or significant experiences with illness may reinforce belief in an external locus of control for people who originally possessed an internal locus of control. Nursing interventions that support the power or influence the individual does wield help prevent an all-encompassing sense of powerlessness.

Another aspect of powerlessness is *learned helplessness.* Seligman[44] suggested that repeated experiences with uncontrollable events result in diminished motivation, lessened ability to perceive success, and increased emotionality. Interventions suggested to prevent or reverse learned helplessness include opportunities to exert control.

In the critical care unit, threats to a patient's control include the unusual signs and symptoms of his or her illness and inadequate knowledge about the situation.[45] The disease process and the personal, psychologic, and social situation interact to affect the patient's perception of control or lack of control. If control is defined as the ability to determine the use of time, space, and resources, admission to a critical care unit strips away control to varying extents. Patients no longer can decide about physical care, socializing, or privacy. They are under the close scrutiny of the nurses and physicians and have decreased physical strength.

On admission, persons lose their independent status. They become patients. Use of clothes and other personal belongings is usually restricted in a critical care unit. Patients cannot decide who enters the room, provides personal care, or intrudes with painful treatments. Hospital rules usually are not open to modification. Patients may feel anxious because they are separated from a familiar environment, have restrictions on visitors, and must depend on others for their care. They may fear death or permanent loss of function and may feel guilty if they have contributed to the cause of their illness or injury. They may resent the invasion of their privacy.

By virtue of their experiences of critical illness and care, people may lose sight of areas of influence they retain over themselves because so much control is taken from them. Nursing emphasizes this intact influence and control and thus helps to preserve it.

The extent of powerlessness is determined by the situation. Critically ill patients generally have experienced a rapid onset of illness without time to acquire the illness role. A sense of powerlessness in such situations is not unexpected. Poor interactions with the health care providers may make the situation worse. Patients may react aggressively, may try bargaining, or may refuse to comply with diagnostic and treatment regimens.

To assist further in understanding powerlessness, a brief examination of the bases of power is useful. French and Raven[46] identified five bases: *reward, coercive, legitimate, referent, and expert.* The perceived ability to reward or punish, an acknowledged right to influence, possession of personal characteristics with which another person identifies, and possession of special knowledge may be attributed to a person and thus enable this person to control or influence others. In the critical care unit, legitimate and expert power are usually most important. On admission the patient agrees to the rules and regulations of the setting (legitimate) and accepts the directives of the nurses and physicians (expert). In reality, patients may not be in the hospital voluntarily and may believe they are being coerced. They may fear retaliation if they refuse to agree to tests or to follow treatment regimens.

Miller[47,48] wrote extensively about powerlessness in the chronically ill patient. Her ideas are useful in thinking about the acutely ill patient. Many patients in the critical care unit are chronically ill or will become so as a result of the event that precipitated the admission to the unit. Miller developed a powerlessness assessment tool to be used with chronically ill patients.[48] Control factors that increase or decrease a patient's control are categorized as (1) behavioral—responses available to influence or modify the situation, (2) cognitive—the interpretation of the situation, and (3) decisional—the choice of alternative.

Powerlessness in acutely ill persons is related to (1) the uncertainty of the outcome, (2) the strange, threatening, overwhelming experience in the critical care unit, including diagnostic and treatment events, and (3) the lack of knowledge about the situation. The need to relinquish some control and then work to regain it during recovery should be supported.[49] The nurse has a primary role in preventing and alleviating the perception of personal powerlessness in the patient and family.

HOPELESSNESS

Hopelessness is a subjective state in which an individual sees limited or no alternatives or personal choices available and is unable to mobilize energy on his or her own behalf. To help clarify this nursing diagnosis, a definition of hope is included—a feeling that what is wanted will happen, a desire that is accompanied by anticipation or expectation. Most people agree that an element of hope must be maintained no matter how hopeless things appear. Hope is a force that helps one survive. It is an attitude toward the future, and it occupies a key position between the present and future. The absence of hope is a serious situation.

Causative factors related to hopelessness include (1) prolonged activity restriction, creating isolation, (2) a failing or deteriorating physiologic condition, (3) long-term stress, (4) abandonment, and (5) a lost belief in transcendent values or God.[12]

Hopelessness is defined in terms of negative expectations concerning oneself and one's future life.[51] Motivation is lost; a decision is made not to want anything, to give up, and not to try to get something. The future seems dark, vague, and uncertain. Hope often arises in the presence of crisis. The idea of giving up is vigorously resisted. The help of others in the situation supports the patient's belief. Caregivers who label hope-reflecting behavior in the critically or terminally ill patient as denial are less than helpful.[52] Hope wards off despair, mental anguish, disorganization, helplessness, and hopelessness.

A female patient with cancer who is receiving chemotherapy develops pneumonia and is placed on neutropenia precautions in the medical critical care unit. She may believe she has no chance of recovery, since she feels isolated from staff and family and believes that her body will not fight the infection successfully because the drugs for the cancer have lowered her ability to combat infection. She may despair and become desperate and despondent. What causes these feelings in critically ill patients? Why do they feel helpless? Their bodies have lost control. No longer do their physiologic mechanisms adapt to changes. They need external help.

Hopelessness can take control and immobilize the patient. The sense of impossibility can block attempts to change the situation. A system of negative expectancies about oneself and the future may result in a sense of overwhelming defeat. The hopeful person can imagine a future and that the storm will pass. The hopeless one gives up.

Jones[53] points out that one tends to find what one expects in interactions with others. Processing information is selective. Expectancies cause an individual to act in ways that elicit behaviors that can be interpreted as confirming those expectancies, even when such expectancies are mistaken. This response is the behavioral confirmation of an expectancy, the self-fulfilling prophecy. This idea is important in instances of hopelessness. Staff members may feel helpless when patients do not respond to their care; they may label patients as hopeless. Patients recognize this attitude and react to confirm this expectancy by giving up. Engel[54] identified the "giving up–given up" syndrome and included hopelessness as one component. Other components were a depreciated self-image; lack of gratification from roles and role relationships; interference with continuity of the past, present, and future; and reawakened painful memories. Acutely ill persons are highly susceptible to such situations. Persons may give up hope, believing that they have been given up on by others—a self-fulfilling prophecy.

Illness influences hopelessness by threatening internal resources (one's ability to cope) and external resources (one's perceptions of who can help). A patient's autonomy, self-esteem, independence, strength, and integrity may be at risk.

The critically ill patient is a multiproblem patient. Nurses and physicians are tempted to focus on the crisis and overlook the patient in his or her totality. The critical care unit is noisy and frightening; it increases the patient's sense of vulnerability and the fear of death.

Families also need hope. To have hope has been identified in a number of studies as the most important need of families of critically ill patients.[55] Miller[56] proposes a model of nursing strategies to inspire hope in families, believing that if family hope is developed and maintained, patient hope will be developed and maintained. Hope-inspiring strategies for families include activities that accomplish the following:

1. Maintain caring relationships
2. Clarify distorted thinking
3. Provide opportunities to be with the patient
4. Decrease uncertainty
5. Increase patient comfort and well-being
6. Project feelings of hope
7. Avoid unrealistic expectations
8. Consider spiritual needs
9. Decrease environmental hazards
10. Explore the meaning of the crisis
11. Use social support
12. Consider the use of humor
13. Support unique modes of personal comfort
14. Expand the coping repetoire of the family

The patient's degree of hopelessness is related to the perception and duration of his or her powerlessness. Thus feelings of hopelessness are not uncommon in critical care units. It is therefore important to foster a realistic sense of hope.[57] Science has progressed and can accomplish many things. Even if long-term survival is not likely, patients can be helped to plan to live the remaining life to the fullest. The critical care nurse must try to feel hopeful and identify some aspect of the situation in which hope is warranted, no matter how grave the situation, and must try to channel feelings toward some positive outcome.

When the situation moves from hopeful to hopeless in the critical care unit, careful consideration must be given to the process of deciding to write a "do not resuscitate" order.[58] Of special importance is the need to recognize that the nurse, physician, and family may reach this decision at varying times. Careful medical and nursing assessments and the use of family conferences to foster communication can make these situations less frustrating for all concerned.

BODY IMAGE DISTURBANCE RELATED TO ACTUAL CHANGE IN BODY STRUCTURE, FUNCTION, OR APPEARANCE

DEFINING CHARACTERISTICS

- Actual change in appearance, structure, or function
- Avoidance of looking at body part
- Avoidance of touching body part
- Hiding or overexposing body part (intentional or unintentional)
- Trauma to nonfunctioning part
- Change in ability to estimate spatial relationship of body to environment
- Verbalization of the following:
  - Fear of rejection or reaction by others
  - Negative feelings about body
  - Preoccupation with change or loss
  - Refusal to participate in or accept responsibility for self-care of altered body part
- Personalization of part or loss with a name
- Depersonalization of part or loss by use of impersonal pronouns
- Refusal to verify actual change

OUTCOME CRITERIA

- Patient verbalizes the specific meaning of the change to him or her.
- Patient requests appropriate information about self-care.
- Patient completes personal hygiene and grooming daily with or without help.
- Patient interacts freely with family or other visitors.
- Patient participates in the discussions and conferences related to planning his or her medical and nursing care in the critical care unit and transfer from the unit.
- Patient talks with trained visitors (support group representatives) about his or her loss at least twice.

NURSING INTERVENTIONS AND *RATIONALE*

1. Continue to monitor the assessment parameters listed under "Defining Characteristics." In addition, assess patient's mental, physical, and emotional state; recognize assets, strengths, response to illness, position in Lee's phases (see p. 88), coping mechanisms, past experience with stress, support systems, and coping mechanisms.
2. Appraise the response of family and significant others. ***Body image is derived from the "reflected appraisals" of family and significant others.***
3. Determine the patient's goals and readiness for learning.
4. Provide the necessary information to help the patient and family adapt to the change. Clarify misconceptions about future limitations.
5. Permit and encourage the patient to express the significance of the loss or change; note nonverbal behavioral responses.
6. Allow and encourage the patient's expression of anxiety. ***Anxiety is the most predominant emotional response to a body image disturbance.***
7. Recognize and accept the use of denial as an adaptive defense mechanism when used early and temporarily.
8. Recognize maladaptive denial as that which interferes with the patient's progress and/or alienates support systems. Use confrontation.
9. Provide an opportunity for the patient to discuss sexual concerns (see Chapter 9).
10. Touch the affected body part ***to provide patient with sensory information about altered body structure and/or function.***
11. Encourage and provide movement of altered body part ***to establish kinesthetic feedback. This enables the person to know his or her body as it now exists.***
12. Prepare the patient to look at the body part. Call the body part by its anatomical name (e.g., stump, stoma, limb) as opposed to "it" or "she." ***The use of impersonal pronouns increases a sense of fantasy and depersonalization of the body part.***
13. Allow the patient to experience excellence in some aspect of physical functioning—walking, turning, deep breathing, healing, self-care—and point out progress and accomplishment. ***This helps to balance the patient's sense of dysfunction with function.***
14. Avoid false reassurance. Acknowledge the difficulty of incorporating the altered body part or function into one's body image. ***This evidences the nurse's sensitivity and promotes trust.***
15. Talk with the patient about his or her life, generativity, and accomplishments. ***Patients with disturbances in body image frequently see themselves in a distortedly "narrow" sense. Encouraging a wider focus of themselves and their life reduces this distortion.***
16. Help the patient explore realistic alternatives.
17. Recognize that incorporating a body change into one's body image takes time. Avoid setting unrealistic expectations and ***thereby inadvertently reinforcing a low self-esteem.***
18. Suggest the use of additional resources such as trained visitors who have mastered situations similar to those of the patient. Refer patient to a psychiatric liaison nurse or psychiatrist if needed.

BODY IMAGE DISTURBANCE RELATED TO FUNCTIONAL DEPENDENCE ON LIFE-SUSTAINING TECHNOLOGY
(ventilator, dialysis, IABP, halo traction)

DEFINING CHARACTERISTICS

- Actual change in function requiring permanent or temporary replacement
- Refusal to verify actual loss
- Verbalization of the following: feelings of helplessness, hopelessness, powerlessness, fear of failure to wean from technology

OUTCOME CRITERIA

- Patient verifies actual change in function.
- Patient does not refuse or fight technologic intervention.
- Patient verbalizes acceptance of expected change in life-style.

NURSING INTERVENTIONS AND *RATIONALE*

1. Continue to monitor the assessment parameters listed under "Defining Characteristics." In addition, assess patient's response to the technologic intervention.
2. Assess responses of family and significant others. ***Body image is derived from the "reflected appraisals" of family and significant others.***
3. Provide information needed by patient and family.
4. Promote trust, security, comfort, and privacy.
5. Recognize anxiety. Allow and encourage its expression. ***Anxiety is the most predominant emotion accompanying body image alterations.***
6. Assist patient to recognize his or her own functioning and performance in the face of technology. For example, assist the patient to distinguish spontaneous breaths from mechanically delivered breaths. ***This activity will assist in weaning the patient from the ventilator when feasible. To establish realistic, accurate body boundaries, a patient needs help to separate himself or herself from the technology that is supporting his or her functioning. Any participation or function on the part of the patient during periods of dependency is helpful in preventing and/or resolving an alteration in body image.***
7. Plan for discontinuation of the treatment, e.g., weaning from ventilator. Explain procedure that will be followed, and be present during its initiation.
8. Plan for transfer from the critical care environment.
9. Document care, ensuring an up-to-date care plan is available for all involved caregivers.

SELF-ESTEEM DISTURBANCE RELATED TO FEELINGS OF GUILT ABOUT PHYSICAL DETERIORATION

DEFINING CHARACTERISTICS

- Inability to accept positive reinforcement
- Lack of follow-through
- Nonparticipation in therapy
- Not taking responsibility for self-care (self-neglect)
- Self-destructive behavior
- Lack of eye contact

OUTCOME CRITERIA

- Patient verbalizes feelings of self-worth.
- Patient maintains positive relationships with significant others.
- Patient manifests active interest in appearance by completing personal grooming daily.

NURSING INTERVENTIONS AND *RATIONALE*

1. Continue to monitor the assessment parameters listed under "Defining Characteristics." In addition, assess the meaning of health-related situation. How does the patient feel about himself or herself, the diagnosis, and the treatment? How does the present fit into the larger context of his or her life?
2. Assess the patient's emotional level, interpersonal relationships, and feelings about himself or herself. Recognize the patient's uniqueness (how the hair is worn, preference for name used).
3. Help the patient discover and verbalize feelings and understand the crisis by listening and providing information.
4. Assist the patient to identify strengths and positive qualities that increase the sense of self-worth. Focus on past experiences of accomplishment and competency. Help patient with positive self-reinforcement. Reinforce the obvious love and affection of family and significant others.
5. Assess coping techniques that have been helpful in the past. Help the patient decide how to handle negative or incongruent feedback about the situation.
6. Encourage visits from family and significant others. Facilitate interactions and ensure privacy. Help family members entering critical care unit by explaining what they will see. Increase visitors' comfort with equipment; offer chairs and other courtesies.
7. Encourage the patient to pursue interest in individual or social activities, even though difficult in the critical care unit.
8. Reflect caring, concern, empathy, respect, and unconditional acceptance in nurse-patient relationships.
9. Remember that for the patient the nurse is a significant other who provides important appraisals of the patient and who can facilitate the change process.
10. Help the family support the patient's self-esteem.
11. Provide for continuity of nurse assignment to ensure consistent contacts that can ***facilitate support of the patient's self-esteem.***

ALTERED ROLE PERFORMANCE RELATED TO PHYSICAL INCAPACITY TO RESUME USUAL OR VALUED ROLE

DEFINING CHARACTERISTICS

- Lack of acknowledgement of role change
- Change in usual patterns of responsibility
- Change in self-perception of role
- Denial of role
- Change in other's perception of role
- Conflict in roles

OUTCOME CRITERIA

- Patient verbalizes a beginning plan to alter life-style to meet restrictions imposed by physical incapacity.
- Patient verbalizes plans to adjust personal and family goals rather than to abandon them.
- Patient expresses willingness to interact with significant others.

NURSING INTERVENTIONS AND *RATIONALE*

1. Continue to monitor the assessment parameters listed under "Defining Characteristics." In addition, identify the primary, secondary, and tertiary roles of the patient. Assess the patient's developmental stage and whether there are maturational and situational crises in addition to the health-related event. ***Illness disrupts role performance and makes life transitions difficult.***
2. Assess past experiences with role change, the degree of attachment to the role, and the ability or capacity to modify the role.
3. Assess the patient's perception of the role change or role loss, the responses of others, and the likelihood of a new role performance consistent with role expectations.
4. Explore with the patient the expected role change; permit patient to express his or her fears and concerns. Recognize role(s) that will continue.
5. Help the patient establish realistic goals and expectations.
6. Reinforce and support positive behaviors with verbal praise. Help the patient face any conflicts.
7. Teach the new skill(s) needed. Convey information and experience necessary to the patient and family. Provide environmental supports that permit mastery of new skills (equipment and time for practice). Be sure expectations are clear. Reward mastery behavior.
8. Use role supplementation strategies (role clarifying, role taking, role modeling, role rehearsal, and reference group interaction).

POWERLESSNESS RELATED TO HEALTH CARE ENVIRONMENT OR ILLNESS-RELATED REGIMEN

DEFINING CHARACTERISTICS

Severe

- Verbal expressions of having no control or influence over situation
- Verbal expressions of having no control or influence over outcome
- Verbal expressions of having no control over self-care
- Depression over physical deterioration that occurs despite patient's compliance with regimens
- Apathy

Moderate

- Nonparticipation in care or decision making when opportunities are provided
- Expressions of dissatisfaction and frustration about inability to perform previous tasks and/or activities
- Lack of progress monitoring
- Expressions of doubt about role performance
- Reluctance to express true feelings, fearing alienation from caregivers
- Passivity
- Inability to seek information about care
- Dependence on others that may result in irritability, resentment, anger, and guilt
- No defense of self-care practices when challenged

Low

- Passivity

OUTCOME CRITERIA

- Patient verbalizes increased control over situation by wanting to do things his or her way.
- Patient actively participates in planning care.
- Patient requests needed information.
- Patient chooses to participate in self-care activities.
- Patient monitors progress.

NURSING INTERVENTIONS AND *RATIONALE*

1. Continue to monitor the assessment parameters listed under "Defining Characteristics." In addition, assess the patient's feelings and perception of the reasons for lack of power and sense of helplessness.
2. Determine as far as possible the patient's usual response to limited control situations. Determine through ongoing assessment the patient's usual locus of control, i.e., believes influence over his or her life is exerted by luck, fate, powerful persons (external locus of control) or influence is exerted through personal choices, self-effort, self-determination (internal locus of control).
3. Support patient's physical control of the environment by involving him or her in care activities; knock before entering room if appropriate; ask permission before moving personal belongings. Inform the patient that, although an activity may not be to his or her liking, it is necessary. ***This gives the patient permission to express dissatisfaction with the environment and regimen.***
4. Personalize the patient's care using his or her preferred name. ***This supports the patient's psychologic control.***
5. Provide the therapeutic rationale for all the patient is asked to do for himself or herself and for all that is being done for and with him or her. Reinforce the physician's explanations; clarify misconceptions about the illness situation and treatment plans. ***This supports the patient's cognitive control.***
6. Include patient in care planning by encouraging participation and allowing choices wherever possible, e.g., timing of personal care activities and deciding when pain medicines are needed. Point out situations in which no choices exist.
7. Provide opportunities for the patient to exert influence over himself or herself and his or her body, thereby affecting an outcome. For example, share with the patient the nurse's assessment of his or her breath sounds and explain that they can be improved by self-initiated deep breathing exercises. ***Feedback that the patient has been successful in helping clear his or her lungs reinforces the influence he or she does retain.***
8. Encourage family to permit patient to do as much independently as possible ***to foster perceptions of personal power.***
9. Assist the patient to establish realistic short-term and long-term goals. ***Setting unrealistic or unattainable goals inadvertently reinforces the patient's perception of powerlessness.***
10. Document care to provide for continuity ***so the patient can maintain appropriate control over the environment.***
11. Assist the patient to regain strength and activity tolerance as appropriate, ***thus increasing a sense of control and self-reliance.***
12. Increase the sensitivity of the health team members and significant others to the patient's sense of powerlessness. Use power over the patient carefully. Use the words "must," "should," and "have to" with caution, ***because they communicate coercive power and imply that the objects of "musts" and "shoulds" are of benefit to the nurse versus the patient.***
13. Plan with the patient for transfer from the critical care unit to the intermediate unit and eventually to home.

POWERLESSNESS RELATED TO PHYSICAL DETERIORATION DESPITE COMPLIANCE

DEFINING CHARACTERISTICS

- Verbal expressions of having no control over the situation
- Verbal expressions of having no control or influence over outcome
- Despondency over physical deterioration
- Nonparticipation in care or decision making when opportunities are provided
- Dependence on others that may result in irritability, resentment, and anger
- Apathy

OUTCOME CRITERIA

- Patient verbalizes a sense of control.
- Patient verbalizes an increased ability to cope with the stress of illness.
- Patient demonstrates commitment to option(s) selected.
- Patient recognizes that efforts to delay the progression of the disease are worth his or her effort.

NURSING INTERVENTIONS AND *RATIONALE*

1. Continue to monitor the assessment parameters listed under "Defining Characteristics." In addition, assess the patient's feelings and perceptions of the reasons for lack of power and a sense of hopelessness.
2. Determine through ongoing assessment the patient's usual locus of control, i.e., believes influence over his or her life is exerted by luck, fate, powerful persons (external locus of control) or influence is exerted through personal choices, self-effort, self-determination (internal locus of control).
3. Redefine the situation to change the patient's thought process about hospitalization to modify inappropriate beliefs and expectations.
4. Actively involve the patient in care and decision making.
5. Provide choices; make clear the realistic options available.
6. Assist the patient to exercise physical control when possible. Provide information that patient's efforts have had desired effects. For example, suggest that the patient can reduce his or her heart rate and even dysrhythmias by performing relaxation techniques. Then provide feedback that heart rate and ectopy have decreased when true.
7. Communicate desirable, positive behaviors by subtly providing examples.
8. Focus on attainable goals ***so as to not inadvertently reinforce perceptions of person's powerlessness.***
9. Make explicit the positive appraisal of patient's personal resources and expectations for a successful outcome.

HOPELESSNESS RELATED TO FAILING OR DETERIORATING PHYSICAL CONDITION

DEFINING CHARACTERISTICS

Major

- Passivity
- Decreased verbalization
- Decreased affect
- Verbal cues (despondent content, "I can't," sighing)

Minor

- Lack of initiative
- Decreased response to stimuli
- Decreased affect
- Verbal cues (hopeless content, "I can't," sighing)
- Turning away from speaker
- Closing eyes
- Shrugging in response to speaker
- Decreased appetite
- Increased sleep
- Lack of involvement in care or passive allowance of care

OUTCOME CRITERIA

- Patient looks at speaker.
- Patient verbalizes, "I will try" (hopeful content).
- Patient initiates conversation with staff, family.
- Patient requests involvement in self-care activities.
- Patient's conversation reflects affect (hope, anger, disagreement, anticipation).

NURSING INTERVENTIONS AND *RATIONALE*

1. Continue to monitor the assessment parameters listed under "Defining Characteristics." In addition, assess the patient's total health situation realistically. Do not offer false reassurance. What is the patient's perception of treatment and the environment?
2. Assist the patient to look for alternatives. Help patient establish realistic short-term and long-term goals.
3. Offer help and assist the patient as needed, ***thus conserving the patient's energy for things the patient wants to do.***
4. Encourage and help the patient to have something for which to plan. Help him or her imagine a future, even a short-term one. Support the possibilities.
5. Offer information before events occur. Facilitate control and predictability of events when possible.
6. Be careful not to create a hopeless environment. Convey hopefulness despite being helpless to alter the outcome.
7. Support the patient's sense of security and inner strengths. Enhance his or her feelings of being understood. Support what the patient finds in the situation as grounds for hope. Do not renounce hope prematurely.
8. Facilitate close personal contacts between patient and nurse, as well as between patient and family and significant others. Help them to feel involved.
9. Inspire hope. Consider the patient's religious and cultural background. ***Faith and hope in God are strengthening for some patients and families.***
10. Recognize the influences of others such as family, clergy, and friends.
11. Communicate an attitude of quiet confidence, genuine interest, and mutual trust. ***This does much to support the patient's hope.***
12. Help the family members not to "give up." ***Their struggle, as well as that of the nurse, is important. The family can regain and sustain hope from the nurse's example.***

REFERENCES

1. Combs AW, Snygg D: *Individual behavior: a perceptual approach to behavior,* New York, 1959, Harper & Row.
2. Rogers CR: *Client-centered therapy: its current practice, implications, and theory,* Boston, 1951, Houghton-Mifflin.
3. Sullivan HS: *Conceptions of modern psychiatry,* Washington, DC, 1946, William A White Psychiatric Foundation.
4. Sullivan HS: *The interpersonal theory of psychiatry,* New York, 1953, WW Norton & Co.
5. Driever MJ: Theory of self-concept. In Roy C, Sr, editor: *Introduction to nursing: an adaptation model,* Englewood Cliffs, NJ, 1976, Prentice Hall.
6. McFarland GK, McCann J: Self-perception–self-concept. In Thompson JM and others, editors: *Mosby's manual of clinical nursing,* ed 3, St Louis, 1993, Mosby–Year Book.
7. Deleted in proofs.
8. Deleted in proofs.
9. Lee JM: Emotional reactions to trauma, *Nurs Clin North Am* 5(4):577, 1970.
10. Salkin J: *Body ego technique,* Springfield, Ill, 1973, Charles C Thomas.
11. Fisher S: *Body experience in fantasy and behavior,* New York, 1970, Appleton-Century-Crofts.
12. Kim M and others: *Pocket guide to nursing diagnosis,* ed 5, St Louis, 1993, Mosby–Year Book.
13. Smith S: Extended body image in the ventilated patient, *Intensive Care Nurs* 5(1):31, 1989.
14. Baxley KO and others: Alopecia: effect on cancer patient's body image, *Cancer Nurs* 7(6):499, 1984.
15. Brown MS: *Distortions in body image in illness and disease,* New York, 1977, John Wiley & Sons.
16. Brown MS: *Normal development of body image,* New York, 1977, John Wiley & Sons.
17. Brundage DJ, Broadwell DC: Altered body image. In Phipps WJ, Long BC, Woods NF, editors: *Medical-surgical nursing: clinical concepts and practice,* ed 4, St Louis, 1991, Mosby–Year Book.
18. Champion VL, Austin JK, Tzeng O: Assessment of relationships between self-concept and body image using multivariate techniques, *Issues Ment Health Nurs* 4(4):299, 1982.
19. Murray RLE: Symposium on the concept of body image, *Nurs Clin North Am* 7(4):593, 1972.
20. Norris CM: The professional nurse and body image. In Carlson C, Blackwell B, editors: *Behavioral concepts and nursing intervention,* ed 2, Philadelphia, 1978, JB Lippincott.
21. Price B: A model for body-image care, *J Adv Nurs* 15:585, 1990.
22. Muslin HL: On acquiring a kidney, *Am J Psychiatry* 127:1185, 1971.
23. Maslow AH: *Motivation and personality,* New York, 1954, Harper & Row.
24. Antonucci TC, Jackson JS: Physical health and self-esteem, *Fam Community Health* 6(4):1, 1983.
25. Coopersmith S: *The antecedents of self-esteem,* San Francisco, 1967, WH Freeman & Co.
26. Cormack D: *Geriatric nursing: a conceptual approach,* Oxford, 1985, Blackwell Scientific Publications.
27. Driever MJ: Problems of low self-esteem. In Roy C, Sr, editor: *Introduction to nursing: an adaptation model,* Englewood Cliffs, NJ, 1976, Prentice-Hall.
28. Hirst SP, Metcalf BJ: Promoting self-esteem, *J Gerontol Nurs* 10(2):72, 1984.
29. Meisenhelder JB: Self-esteem: a closer look at clinical interventions, *Int J Nurs Stud* 22(2):127, 1985.
30. Meisenhelder JB: Self-esteem in women: the influence of employment and perception of husband's appraisals, *Image J Nurs Sch* 18(1):8, 1986.
31. Norris J, Kunes-Connell M: Self-esteem disturbance, *Nurs Clin North Am* 20(4):745, 1985.
32. Rubin R: Body image and self-esteem, *Nurs Outlook* 16:20, 1968.
33. Stanwyck DJ: Self-esteem through the life span, *Fam Community Health* 6(4):11, 1983.
34. Wolff PH, Colletti MA: AIDS: getting past the diagnosis and on to discharge planning, *Crit Care Nurs* 6(4):76, 1986.
35. Bennett MJ: Stigmatization: experiences of persons with acquired immune deficiency syndrome, *Issues Ment Health Nurs* 11:141, 1990.
36. Crouch MA, Straub V: Enhancement of self-esteem in adults, *Fam Community Health* 6(4):65, 1983.
37. Meleis AI: Role insufficiency and role supplementation: a conceptual framework, *Nurs Res* 24(4):264, 1975.
38. Meleis AI: The evolving nursing scholarliness. In Chinn PL, editor: *Advances in nursing theory development,* Rockville, Md, 1983, Aspen Systems.
39. Gortner SR, Jenkins LS: Self efficacy and activity level following cardiac surgery, *J Adv Nurs* 15:1132, 1990.
40. Janis IL, Rodin J: Attribution, control, and decision-making: social psychology and health care. In Stone GC, Adler NC, editors: *Health psychology—a handbook,* San Francisco, 1979, Jossey-Bass.
41. Rodin J: Aging and health: effects of the sense of control, *Science* 233:1271, 1986.
42. Roberts SL, White BS: Powerlessness and personal control model applied to the myocardial infarction patient, *Progress Cardiovasc Nurs* 5(3):84, 1990.
43. Rotter JB: Generalized expectancies for internal versus external control of reinforcement, *Psychol Monogr 80* (609):1, 1966.
44. Seligman ME: *Helplessness: on depression, development and death,* San Francisco, 1975, WH Freeman & Co.
45. Roberts SL: *Behavioral concepts and the critically ill patient,* ed 2, Norwalk, Conn, 1986, Appleton-Century-Crofts.
46. French JRP, Jr, Raven BH: Bases of social power. In Cartwright D, editor: *Studies in social power,* Ann Arbor, Mich, 1959, University of Michigan Press.
47. Miller JF: *Coping with chronic illness: overcoming powerlessness,* ed 2, Philadelphia, 1992, FA Davis.
48. Miller JF: Development and validation of a diagnostic label: powerlessness. In Kim MJ, McFarland GK, McLane AM, editors: *Classification of nursing diagnoses: proceedings of the fifth national conference,* St Louis, 1984, Mosby–Year Book.
49. Johnson JL, Morse JM: Regaining control: the process of adjustment after myocardial infarction, *Heart Lung* 19:126, 1990.
50. Deleted in proofs.
51. Beck AT and others: The measurement of pessimism: the hopelessness scale, *J Couns Clin Psychol* 42(6):861, 1974.
52. Hall BA: The struggle of the diagnosed terminally ill person to maintain hope, *Nurs Sci Quart* 3(4):177, 1990.
53. Jones EE: Interpreting interpersonal behavior: the effects of expectancies, *Science* 234:41, 1986.
54. Engel GL: A life setting conducive to illness: the giving up–given up syndrome, *Ann Intern Med* 69:293, 1968.
55. Leske JS: Needs of relatives of critically ill patients: a follow-up, *Heart-Lung* 15(2):189, 1986.
56. Miller JF: Developing and maintaining hope in families of the critically ill, *AACN Clin Issues in Critical Care Nursing* 2(2):307, 1991.
57. Herth K: Fostering hope in terminally-ill people, *J Adv Nurs* 15:1250, 1990.
58. Slater AL and others: From hopeful to hopeless . . . when do we write "Do not resuscitate"? *Focus Crit Care* 18:476, 1991.

8

Coping Alterations

CHAPTER OBJECTIVES

- Explain the following coping strategies as they relate to the critically ill patient: regression, suppression, denial, trust, religious beliefs, and family support.
- List and discuss aspects of care that enhance coping.
- Describe the components of the mental status examination.
- Describe mental status changes that require further medical evaluation.
- Describe the needs and coping mechanisms of families of critically ill patients.
- Explain interventions and nursing management for patients with coping alterations.

Patients requiring critical care must cope with a variety of stressors (see box on right). A patient's response to these stressors depends on individual differences, such as age, gender, social supports, medical diagnosis, cultural background (see Chapter 4), current hospital course, and prognosis. The nurse's knowledge of assessment, diagnosis, and intervention in effective coping will also affect how well the patient copes.

STRESSORS IN THE CRITICAL CARE SETTING

Patients' experience of critical illness and care will vary. However, each patient must cope with at least some of the following stressors:

- Threat of death
- Threat of survival, with significant residual problems related to the illness/injury
- Pain or discomfort
- Lack of sleep
- Loss of autonomy over most aspects of life and daily functioning
- Loss of control over environment, including loss of privacy and exposure to light, noise, and general activity of the critical care unit, including the care of other patients
- Loss of usual role and with that, the arena in which usual coping mechanisms serve the patient
- Separation from family and friends
- Loss of dignity
- Boredom broken only by brief visits, threatening stimuli, and frightening thoughts
- Loss of ability to express self verbally when intubated

THE CONCEPT OF COPING

According to White,[1] coping is an adaption strategy. People use coping when faced with serious problems that they cannot master with familiar behaviors. Uncomfortable affects such as anxiety or grief accompany coping.

Lazarus and Folkman[2] define coping as "constantly changing cognitive and behavioral efforts to manage specific external and/or internal demands that are appraised as taxing or exceeding the resources of the person." Coping is a process that serves to manage a problem and modulate the emotional response to that problem.

Aquilera[3] states that coping activities encompass all the diverse behaviors that people use to meet actual or potential demands. The available coping mechanisms are those behaviors that a person typically uses to problem solve and relieve anxiety associated with the problem. The individual draws on what he or she has found to be effective in the past.

Weissman sees coping as a problem-solving process that draws on cognition, judgment, memory, and defense mechanisms.[4] He describes a variety of coping skills that people tend to use, including the steps for problem solving, the defense mechanisms, interpersonal strategies such as sharing concerns, and conscious coping mechanisms such as distracting oneself or laughing off a problem. Weissman emphasizes that no one strategy is superior. The key to effective coping is using the best strategy or mix of strategies in a given situation.[5]

NANDA[6] defines Ineffective Individual Coping as "the impairment of adaptive behaviors and problem solving abilities of a person meeting life's demands and roles." The defining characteristics of Ineffective Individual Coping usually associated with critical illness include the following:

- Verbalization of inability to cope or inability to ask for help
- Inability to meet basic needs
- Inability to problem solve
- Alteration in societal participation
- Inappropriate use of defense mechanisms
- Change in usual communication patterns

COPING MECHANISMS

When a patient copes effectively, what he or she is doing to cope often goes unnoticed. Emotionally the patient seems relatively comfortable, is a cooperative recipient of care, and exhibits nonproblematic behavior. Such a patient is using appropriate coping mechanisms and to the degree that is effective without interfering with care. The patient may be using multiple coping mechanisms.

Regression

Regression is an unconscious defense mechanism that involves a retreat, in the face of stress, to behavior characteristic of an earlier developmental level.[7] Regression allows the patient to give up his or her usual role, autonomy, and privacy to become the passive recipient of medical and nursing care. In fact, the patient who does not regress jeopardizes his or her own care. For example, a patient may insist on conducting business from the bedside or demand bathroom privileges when getting out of bed would be unsafe. Conversely, the patient who becomes too regressed presents another problem. The patient may become childlike in interactions with staff, whine, cling to staff, and attempt to keep the nurse at the bedside constantly.

In both cases, the patient needs limits set on behavior to receive essential care. The patient is best served when limits are set in a supportive manner. For example, the nurse may respond to the patient who shows inappropriate regression by saying, "I understand how frightened you are, but I cannot be at your bedside constantly. I will be checking on you every 15 minutes whether you call or not." To the patient who has not regressed and is jeopardizing his or her safety, the nurse might say, "I realize how difficult it is for you, but we cannot jeopardize your safety by allowing you to get out of bed. Maybe there is something we can do to make the restriction more tolerable for you."

Although the behavior of these patients can be very provocative, avoiding confrontations or reprimands is advisable. Such responses from staff may only worsen a situation in which a patient is already struggling with issues of dependence and autonomy.

Suppression

Suppression is a conscious, intentional process in which patients push ideas, problems, or desires out of their conscious thoughts.[7] Patients often use suppression when their problems are overwhelming and they are in no position to resolve them. Weissman describes strategic suppression as a conscious attempt to focus only on the problems patients can solve in the present.[5] For example, a patient who has lost a job before emergency coronary artery bypass surgery uses suppression appropriately by postponing worry about employment until after recovery from surgery.

Denial

Denial is an unconscious defense mechanism that reduces anxiety by eliminating or reducing the seriousness of the perceived threat. According to NANDA, denial includes both conscious and unconscious attempts to disavow knowledge or the meaning of an event.[6] In this text, the psychoanalytic definition is used rather than the nursing diagnosis to allow for the distinction between denial and suppression. When used by a critically ill patient, denial reduces the anxiety and the threat of the illness.[8] The degree to which denial is used varies among patients and may vary in the same patient at different times.

Patients may also deny different aspects of the illness. Some deny the probable medical significance of symptoms, as in the case of the 55-year-old cardiologist who interprets severe substernal chest pain as indigestion or the quadriplegic who cheerfully insists he will be back on his feet in no time. Other patients are unable to recognize signs of illness that are obvious to others, as in the case of the patient who cannot "see" the gangrenous foot requiring amputation.[9]

Other people cannot readily influence the beliefs of a patient using denial. For example, the patient who is denying a myocardial infarction (MI) is not convinced of its occurrence by being shown the cardiogram interpretation or laboratory reports. The patient is best served by the nurse who recognizes the need to deny at the present time but who observes for cues that indicate readiness to accept the reality of the medical diagnosis.

Research does not support the belief that denial protects the patient with acute MI from the stress reactions associated with complications and/or death.[10] This finding suggests that anxiolytic medications and the nursing interventions that reduce anxiety should not be withheld from patients with acute MI who are in denial.

Trust

Trust manifests itself in the critical care patient as the belief that the staff will get him or her through the illness, managing any untoward event that might occur. Trust is an unconscious process in which the patient transfers the trust learned in early significant relationships onto caregivers in the present.[11] This coping mechanism not only reduces fear of death, but also allows the patient to put himself or herself "in your hands" in every sense, thereby fostering compliance with all aspects of care.

Hope

Although hope has long been recognized as a significant factor in patient recovery and survival, the phenomenon receives little attention until the patient becomes hopeless. Hope is the expectation that a desire will be fulfilled. It can exist even in the face of a realistic appraisal of a grim situation.[12] Hope supports the patient and helps him or her endure the physical and psychologic insults that are a part of the daily experience.

Religious Beliefs and Practices

Religious beliefs and practices may provide the patient with some measure of acceptance of an illness, a sense of mastery and control, a source of hope and trust beyond the limits the staff can provide, and the strength to endure the current stress. A patient may discuss religious beliefs and concerns openly or view the subject as a private and personal matter. Patients who rely on religious beliefs benefit from the nurse who is accepting and respectful of those beliefs and who remains sensitive to the patient's willingness or reluctance to discuss these beliefs.[13]

Use of Family Support

The patient can use the presence of a supportive family to cope with critical illness. The patient with a supportive family knows that family members share a past and hope for a future with the patient. They love the patient as a person and member of the family. The patient also realizes that family members know him or her in ways the staff cannot. With them, the patient may know that his or her experience is truly understood, even when little is said. Family members can also attend to the practical problems the patient cannot, such as managing finances.

Sharing Concerns

Sharing concerns with a caring and understanding listener can relieve some of the patient's emotional distress. The patient is consoled knowing that he or she is not alone and that someone knows and cares about what is being experienced.[5] The patient may share concerns with family members. However, the patient may be reluctant to upset loved ones further or may have a family in which such communication is not the norm. A patient who relies on this coping mechanism will benefit from a nurse who recognizes when a patient needs to talk and who knows how to listen.

ENHANCING COPING

Although the delivery of physical care is essential for patient survival and recovery, several aspects of nursing care enhance the patient's capacity to cope. (See the nursing management plans for Ineffective Coping and Anxiety on pp. 762 and 763 for detailed interventions.)

Display of Competence

The critical care nurse who executes physical and technical aspects of care competently and conscientiously enhances patient trust.

Display of Caring

Many of the stressors in the critical care unit are distinct insults to the patient's emotional and biologic integrity. The technical environment may appear cold and impersonal. A gentle touch, an understanding look, and careful attention to the patient's physical comfort instill hope and promote comfort, assurance, and relaxation.[14]

Display of Quiet Optimism

Patients are keen observers of their caregivers, and they read them well. The nurse who displays a positive outlook enhances the patient's sense of hope as long as the optimism is appropriate to the patient's prognosis and also is sensitive to the patient's fears and concerns.

Empathic Understanding

For those patients who cope by sharing their concerns with others, the empathic nurse can facilitate effective coping. Through empathic understanding the nurse learns what the patient is experiencing and conveys that understanding back to the patient.[15] The process is based on information that the patient validates, rather than on assumptions the nurse makes about how the patient must be feeling or how the nurse would be feeling in similar circumstances. Such understanding involves an awareness, an appreciation, and an acceptance of the patient's feelings.[7]

Although empathic understanding may be one of the most important aspects of nursing care for enhancing the patient's ability to cope, delivering it in the critical care setting is difficult. First, it requires a nurse who has the emotional energy and the willingness to be exposed to painful emotions in others. To look into the face of despair or terror can be extremely difficult. Empathic understanding also requires communication skills that encourage patients to disclose their feelings. Effective communication takes time that the nurse may feel unable to give. Finally, it requires understanding that the nurse need not have any special responses to alleviate the patient's distress. Rather, the process of empathic understanding itself enhances the patient's ability to cope.

Empathic understanding is a therapeutic tool and a skill the nurse can develop.[15] By following a few guidelines, the critical care nurse can use it effectively to enhance patient coping.

- Allow the patient to choose the agenda. Try asking, "How has this been for you?" Although the question may seem awkward, it leaves the topic of concern open for the patient.
- Listen carefully and ask the patient to clarify statements if necessary.
- Communicate understanding and acceptance of the patient's feelings with both verbal and nonverbal communication.
- Maintain the focus on the patient. Avoid relating similar experiences in an effort to convey understanding.
- Evaluate your own emotional resources before delving into the patient's. Because empathic listening can be emotionally demanding, postpone difficult interactions until the attentive listening is possible.
- After the interaction has occurred, consider saying something to bring it to closure. For example, ask, "Is there anything I can do for you right now?" When asked in this context, the question conveys a sense of caring and brings patient and nurse back to the concrete world of the critical care unit.

Supporting Family Members

The nurse's support of family members at the bedside can enhance the value of the visits for the patient. Patients often look to the family for love, understanding, support, and care of matters to which they cannot attend themselves. Although the nurse cannot perform full

RESEARCH ABSTRACT

Critical care patients' perceptions of visits.

Simpson T: *Heart Lung* 20(6):681, 1991.

PURPOSE

The purpose of this study was to examine the relationships among coronary care unit (CCU) and surgical intensive care unit (SICU) patients' preferences for visits, select personal and illness-related characteristics, and patients' evaluations of the impact of visits they received while in critical care.

DESIGN

Comparative descriptive design

SAMPLE

The sample consisted of 50 subjects in CCU (29 men, 21 women) and 50 subjects in SICU (35 men and 15 women) in a 550-bed, acute care teaching hospital in the Northeast. The mean age of the CCU sample was 64.9 years, with an average of 60.9 years for the SICU sample. One third of the CCU sample had documented MIs, and the majority of SICU subjects had cardiovascular-related surgeries.

INSTRUMENTS

A modified version of the Eysenck Personality Inventory measured patients' usual preferences for being with others. The Acute Physiologic and Chronic Health Evaluation (APACHE II) classification system measured the severity of illness. A questionnaire developed by the investigator for this study measured patients' preferences for visit policies, the impact of visitors on patients, and patients' perceptions of illness severity while in critical care.

PROCEDURE

The investigator determined eligible patients daily from a list of patients to be transferred from each critical care unit. A brief letter describing the study was placed in the chart for physician review. One to three days after transfer, the investigator approached the patient during nonvisiting hours to solicit participation and administer the instruments. The instruments were administered in the following order: perceptions of visits in critical care (30 minutes to complete) and Eysenck Personality Inventory (5 minutes to complete). Each questionnaire was verbally administered by the researcher, and subject responses were written verbatim at the time of the interview.

RESULTS

The SICU sample had significantly higher ($p < .0005$) physiologic illness severity scores compared with the CCU sample. A significantly greater number of the SICU patients were unable to remember the visiting policy for critical care when compared with the CCU patients ($p < .003$). Patients from CCU preferred longer visits with more visitors than did SICU patients. Age was positively correlated ($p < .007$) with the preferred length of visits, particularly in the CCU group (i.e., older patients preferred longer visits and younger patients preferred shorter visits). Patients' perceptions of their illness severity were positively related ($p < .001$) to the preferred number of visitors, particularly for the SICU patients; that is, the greater the perceived severity of illness, the greater the number of visitors that was desired. Both groups preferred three or four visits per day. The majority of both groups preferred not to have family assistance with personal care. Although not statistically significant, there was a trend toward a greater proportion of SICU patients compared with CCU patients indicating some level of fatigue after receiving visitors. Both groups evaluated the visits as helpful to them.

DISCUSSION/IMPLICATIONS

This study adds to the existing body of knowledge regarding critical care unit patient needs. Findings illustrate that multiple individual physiologic and personality characteristics have an impact on the patients' perception toward visitors in the critical care unit. Although results will vary among units, hospitals, and patient populations, the results from this study can be used to establish visitor guidelines for the critical care areas. Nurses and other critical care staff should be aware of the importance of visiting practices on the patients. This information can be incorporated into orientation and in-service presentations for open discussion and integration into daily practice. Future research studies could incorporate visitor policies with patient outcomes, such as length of stay, impact on physiologic variables, and relationship with adaptation to illness.

family assessment and give ongoing support to all family members, the critical care nurse can observe the quality of the patient-family interaction and formulate interventions that will aid the family in supporting the patient. The following are some examples:

- ◆ If the family member is at a loss for what to say or do, the nurse might find some words to put the family member at ease and offer a suggestion for what to say to his or her loved one. For example, the nurse who observes a family member staring helplessly at an intubated, confused patient might say, "You can take his hand and tell him you are here."
- ◆ If the family member is so upset that he or she completely loses composure, a brief attempt at supporting this family member away from the bedside may be adequate. In doing so, the nurse may determine that the member needs a consistent outside source of support and may make a referral according to department guidelines.
- ◆ If the family member becomes more focused on the technical aspects of care than on the patient, the nurse can gently redirect him or her to the patient with the assurance that the staff will attend to the technical care.
- ◆ If the family member is angry, hostile, cold, or aloof during visits, the nurse may reflect those observations back to the family member. For example, "I've been noticing an angry tone in your voice during visits with your wife." If this approach does not result in some resolution or explanation of the problem, a referral for family evaluation may be indicated.
- ◆ If the family member seems unattuned to the patient's experience, the nurse could try to convey what the patient is experiencing and how to best provide support.

ASSESSMENT OF INEFFECTIVE COPING

Ineffective coping may be suggested in patient behaviors. Overt hostility, severe regression, or noncompliance with treatment may suggest ineffective coping. The patient may also report such problems as severe anxiety or despondence. The nurse who suspects that coping is ineffective should consider a number of factors before questioning the patient directly.

Witnessing problematic behavior can be very uncomfortable, especially when that behavior is directed at the nurse. The nurse can examine his or her own feelings by asking, Have I taken the behavior personally? Do I find the behavior particularly distasteful? Can I proceed with objectivity to serve the patient's needs, or should I consult with others?

It is not always clear whether coping is truly ineffective and whether intervention is indicated. The nurse might ask, Is the patient's ineffective coping going to jeopardize his or her care or the care of others? Does the staff have anything to offer the patient that will help him or her cope more effectively?

Because coping involves unconscious defenses, the nurse may feel that addressing the behaviors will do more harm than good or that the patient will feel exposed rather than supported or understood. The following guidelines are useful for preventing psychologic harm:

- ◆ Approach the patient with an earnest expression of concern. The patient will sense insincerity.
- ◆ Be direct and supportive. The goal is to learn something more about the patient, so ask questions that allow for full, honest expression from the patient. For example, "I noticed that you were tearful (angry, restless) during your wife's visit. How was that visit for you?" or "You haven't closed your eyes once since the death of the woman in the next bed. How has that been for you?" When questioned in this way, the patient may convey that he or she is not in touch with his or her feelings if incongruence exists between the subjective emotional state and the behavior. For example, a patient who is restless and hypervigilant may deny feeling anxious.

CLINICAL EXAMPLES

One aspect of critical care nursing is knowing what emotional and behavioral responses should be expected in a given patient care situation and recognizing atypical responses. When such responses are observed, careful assessment and appropriate intervention are essential.

When the patient is restless or agitated and the nurse has ruled out physical causes such as hypoxia, other evidence of anxiety should be sought. Is the patient hypervigilant? Does he or she report fear or anxiety? If nursing measures do not reduce the patient's anxiety, the nurse might then recommend evaluation for an anxiolytic medication or consider consultation with a psychiatric clinical nurse specialist.

When the patient appears downcast and disinterested in his or her care, the nurse may suspect despondence or even depression. After assessing the patient's mood (see section on assessment of mental status, p. 107), the nurse may determine the needs for a psychiatric evaluation for a mood disorder or suicidality.

When the patient overtly expresses distress about issues of autonomy and control, such as evidenced by unreasonable demands for attention or privileges in the critical care unit, a unified, consistent plan is essential. All staff members should agree to the plan, which is then written in the patient's record and presented to the patient in a caring and supportive manner. The plan should consider the patient's feeling of powerlessness and make the limits on unreasonable behavior clear to the patient. Whenever possible, the staff should attempt to give the patient any control, autonomy, or privilege that is reasonable in the critical care setting.

When the patient is so mistrustful of staff that his or her questions seem like interrogation, the nurse should recognize that mistrust has a number of possible sources. The nurse may learn from family members that the patient has a lifelong history of being mistrustful or that the mistrust stems from experience with medical or nursing care that did not meet expectations or resulted in a negative outcome. In either case, the staff can only continue to work conscientiously and competently with the patient. However, if direct questioning reveals paranoid ideation or delusional thinking, the nurse should recommend a psychiatric evaluation.

MENTAL STATUS CHANGES REQUIRING MEDICAL EVALUATION

Two medical diagnoses are associated with mental status changes that should be distinguished from ineffective coping. These clinical states call for a medical and/or nurse specialist psychiatric evaluation and medical intervention.

Delirium

Delirium is an organic mental syndrome characterized by disorganized thinking, reduced ability to attend to external stimuli, and at least two of the following signs and symptoms: reduced level of consciousness, perceptual disturbances such as hallucinations, disruption of usual sleep-wake cycle, change in psychomotor activity, disorientation, or memory impairment. The clinical manifestations of delirium develop over a short period and tend to wax and wane in the course of a day.[16]

The clinical presentation of delirium may be the same as Sensory/Perceptual Alteration related to sensory overload, sensory deprivation, or sleep pattern disturbances. However, delirium—by definition—has an organic cause such as medication or electrolyte imbalance. Appropriate changes in the medical regimen are needed to correct the underlying cause.

The nursing care of the patient with delirium will depend on the presenting symptoms. For nursing management strategies for the various symptoms of delirium, refer to the nursing management plan for Sensory/Perceptual Alterations on p. 573.

Major Depressive Episode

A major depressive episode is a mood disorder of at least 2 weeks' duration, characterized by depressed mood, diminished interest or pleasure in usual activities, insomnia, poor appetite, psychomotor retardation or agitation, and loss of energy. Patients will also report feelings of hopelessness, worthlessness, and guilt. Recurrent thoughts of death (not just fear of dying) and recurrent suicidal ideation may be present.[16]

A major depressive episode is not a natural consequence of major medical illness. It is a psychiatric disorder that may complicate the patient's course with such clinical manifestations as psychosis, suicidality, or psychomotor agitation. Apathy and hopelessness may lead the patient to refuse essential medical and nursing care.[17]

Major depression may also complicate the underlying medical illness. Depressed patients have been shown to have a significantly higher mortality from cardiovascular disease than the nondepressed population,[18,19] and adequate pharmacologic treatment of depression is associated with a lower mortality from myocardial infarction than is untreated or undertreated depression.[20]

The nurse who suspects that the patient is depressed can ask about the patient's thought content (see section on assessment of mental status). If expressions of hopelessness, worthlessness, guilt, or suicidal ideation accompany a depressed mood, a psychiatric evaluation is indicated.

A major depressive episode is generally treated with antidepressant medication. Unfortunately, a therapeutic effect is not seen until several weeks after therapeutic blood levels are reached. Stimulants such as methylphenidate (Ritalin) may also be used for their antidepressant effect in the medically ill patient. Benzodiazepines are occasionally prescribed to treat the associated anxiety, if present. Antipsychotic medication is prescribed if the patient's depression has psychotic features.

The nurse can listen empathically and convey that recovery from the depression is expected while respecting that the patient's depression cannot be overcome by cheerfulness or reassurance. If the patient is on suicide precautions, the nurse safeguards the patient according to department policy and procedure. The nurse also communicates to the patient that precautions are being taken to safeguard the patient until his or her mood improves.

ASSESSMENT OF MENTAL STATUS

The Mental Status Examination is a full, formal assessment of the patient's cognitive function and thought processes. Although the examination is rarely conducted in its entirety in the critical care setting, knowledge of its main components will enhance the nurse's effectiveness by providing the proper formal labels for mental status data that the nurse collects informally. Knowing the content of the examination will also enable the nurse to perform further assessment when indicated and to communicate those findings using accepted terminology.

Patients often find formal questioning stressful. A fully competent adult may be uncomfortable being asked repeatedly, "Do you know the date?" or "Who is the President of the United States?" The patient may wonder, "Do they think I'm crazy? Maybe they have good reason!" For the patient who has to struggle with the answers, the questioning is even more difficult. The nurse can minimize the patient's distress by following a few simple guidelines:

- Introduce yourself.
- State the reason for questioning the patient. For example, "Mr. Jones, it is often difficult for patients to keep track of time in this setting, so I would like to ask you some questions to see how you are doing in that regard."
- Give the patient feedback. If the patient answers correctly, acknowledge the correct answer and tell the patient that he or she is doing very well under difficult circumstances. If the patient answers incorrectly, reorient him or her and assure the patient that the confusion is temporary and is caused by the illness and environmental factors.
- Do not question the patient formally when information can be obtained indirectly. The nurse who encourages dialogue during direct care activities can obtain abundant information.

THE MENTAL STATUS EXAMINATION

GENERAL OBSERVATIONS

- Appearance
- Reaction to interviewer
- Behavior and psychomotor activity

SENSORIUM AND INTELLIGENCE

- Level of consciousness
- Orientation
- Memory
- Intellectual function
- Judgment
- Comprehension

THOUGHT PROCESSES

- Form of thought
- Content of thought
- Mood
- Affect
- Insight

The Components of the Mental Status Examination (see box above)

◆ General observations

Appearance. Described in terms of its consistency with age and station in life. Include general health and nutritional status. EXAMPLE: Patient is a normally developed, but emaciated, 37-year-old man, looking older than his stated age. Patient is lying in bed, well groomed, and wearing hospital gown.

Reaction to interviewer. Provides some indication about the reliability of the patient's answers. Is the patient friendly, cooperative, seductive, guarded, hostile, or evasive? EXAMPLE: Patient is cooperative, but appears suspicious and answers questions evasively.

Behavior and psychomotor activity. Include a description of nonverbal communication, such as hand wringing or picking at the sheets. Describe motor activity in terms of agitation or psychomotor retardation. Include speech characteristics. Is speech fast or slow, high pitched or monotone? EXAMPLE: Patient is slightly agitated, frequently shifting his position in bed. Speech is normal in volume, but somewhat rapid and pressured.

◆ Sensorium and intelligence

Level of consciousness. Described as alert, somnolent, stuporous, or unresponsive.

Orientation. Note orientation to person, place, and time. Note disorientation, keeping the overall status in mind. For instance, a patient who is constantly disoriented to place and time differs from the patient who has temporarily forgotten the date. While assessing orientation, take the opportunity to reorient the patient and then record what the patient does know. EXAMPLE: Patient is alert. He is oriented to person. He knows he is in a hospital, but cannot name it. He knows the month and year, but not the day or date.

Memory. Assess the three components. *Immediate recall* involves material in the present. Retaining new information requires that the patient's attention and concentration are intact. To test immediate recall, ask the patient about something that was discussed a few minutes earlier. *Recent memory* includes events in the past 24 hours. EXAMPLE: "Did you have any visitors last evening?" *Remote memory* includes important life events and personal data such as home address or phone number.

Intellectual function. Note vocabulary, fund of general knowledge, ability to abstract, and ability to calculate. Test fund of general knowledge by asking the patient to name the past four presidents, the name of the mayor, or the state capitol. To test ability to abstract, ask the patient to interpret proverbs. To test ability to calculate, ask the patient how many nickels are in $1.35.

Judgment. The nurse has two alternatives for assessing judgment. Give the patient a hypothetical situation and ask what he or she would do in that situation. Or observe the patient's attitude about the illness and hospitalization. The patient who refuses routine, essential treatment may be showing poor judgment.

Comprehension of new information. During the interview process, observe the patient's response when asked to demonstrate understanding of information provided earlier in the interview.

◆ Thought processes

Form of thought. Form of thought is observed in the patient's speech. Normally speech is logical, coherent, and goal directed. Describe any exceptions.

Content of thought. Record any disturbances, three of which are commonly seen in the critical care setting:

- *Hallucinations* are sensory perceptions without environmental stimuli. Although these manifest in any of the senses, visual and auditory hallucinations are the most common. Visual hallucinations tend to be associated with delirium. Auditory hallucinations are more typical of other psychiatric disorders that have psychotic features. When hallucination is suspected, question the patient directly. For example, "Do you see something on the sheets?" or "Are you hearing any voices or sounds that are disturbing you?" The patient may admit to or deny hallucinations and may or may not be distressed by them. Note all observations, as well as the patient's report. For example, "Patient appears to be responding to auditory hallucinations, but he denies having them," or "Patient reports hearing voices and states that they are frightening him."
- *Delusions* are fixed false beliefs that do not change in the face of evidence to the contrary. They can range from somewhat realistic to extremely bizarre. For example, a patient may express the belief he is

the subject of medical experiments to determine how much a person can take before he breaks down. Another patient may believe that monitoring equipment is connected to a computer in Washington that will eventually control his mind. Generally, the more bizarre delusions are associated with serious psychiatric disorders that have psychotic features. The nurse can assess the patient for delusional thoughts by asking, "Being here can be very stressful. Does it ever cause you any troubling or frightening thoughts?"

◆ *Paranoid ideation* is a suspiciousness about being persecuted or harassed. It does not involve fixed and false beliefs, so the patient will accept an explanation of reality. However, suspiciousness is often recurrent and/or pervasive.

Mood. Note the patient's description of his or her relatively enduring, prevalent emotional state. For example, the mood may be described as depressed, anxious, irritable, angry, or euphoric. If the patient reports feeling depressed or discouraged, evaluate for suicidal ideation. The nurse might ask, "Do you ever feel so discouraged that you feel your life is not worth living?" If the patient expresses the wish to die, the nurse could ask, "Do you think about taking your own life?" "How might you accomplish it?" "Do you really think you would do it?" Do not hesitate to question the patient because of fear of giving the patient the idea of committing suicide. *Suicidal ideation stems from hopelessness and not from suggestion.* Most patients find the thoughts distressing. Some are ashamed to admit them. Questioning will relieve most patients with suicidal ideation, because it tells the patient that the staff senses how bad the patient is feeling.

All patients who express a wish to die require psychiatric evaluation. The patient who expresses both suicidal ideation and a serious plan to commit suicide also needs protection from self-harm with one-to-one constant observation until a full psychiatric evaluation can be conducted.

Affect. Note whether the patient's facial expression is appropriate to the patient's mood, whether the patient shows a full or constricted range of expression, or whether the affect is lacking expression.

Insight. Note the patient's ability to understand the meaning of the current situation. For example, a patient who has been told of a confirmed and serious diagnosis but states he or she is in the hospital "for tests" demonstrates poor insight.

Mental Status Examination for the Intubated Patient

When a patient is intubated, both patient and nurse lose the ease of verbal communication. Communication from the patient to the nurse tends to decrease to a bare minimum, and the patient may lose the motivation needed to express himself or herself at all. Consequently, considerable information about the patient's thought content and subjective experience is lost.

The nurse can use the following segments of the Mental Status Examination to evaluate the intubated patient. The patient's clinical status and ability to communicate will determine the wording of questions. The nurse should avoid multiple choice and open-ended questions. To increase the reliability of the assessment of the intubated patient, yes or no questions should be used whenever possible.

◆ **General observations**

Appearance

Note *reaction* to the interview, including eye contact. This reaction provides cues about the reliability of the patient's answers, e.g., "Patient appeared indifferent. Eye contact poor."

Note *psychomotor activity.* Limit description of behavior to nonverbal communication.

◆ **Sensorium**

Describe *level of consciousness.*

Test *orientation.*

Test *recent memory* by asking about events from the past 24 hours.

◆ **Thought processes**

Determine the *presence of hallucinations, delusions, or paranoid ideation* by using the direct questioning described in the Mental Status Examination. Complete descriptions of the symptoms may be difficult to discern; however, they are not essential, e.g., "Patient indicates he is hearing voices" or "Patient acknowledges that he is having frightening thoughts, but because of intubation, cannot describe them."

Assess *mood* with direct questioning. If the patient is depressed, do not omit questions about suicidality.

Describe *affect.*

REFERENCES

1. White RW: Strategies of adaption: an attempt at systematic description. In Monat A, Lazarus RS, editors: *Stress and coping: an anthology,* ed 2, New York, 1985, Columbia University Press.
2. Lazarus RS, Folkman S: *Stress, appraisal and coping,* New York, 1984, Springer Publishing.
3. Aguilera DC: *Crisis intervention: theory and methodology,* ed 6, St Louis, 1990, Mosby–Year Book.
4. Weissman AD: Coping with illness. In Hackett TP, Cassem NH, editors: *Massachusetts General Hospital Psychiatry,* ed 2, Littleton, Mass, 1987, PSG Publishing.
5. Weissman AD: *The coping capacity,* New York, 1984, Human Sciences Press.
6. North American Nursing Diagnosis Association: *Taxonomy I Revised,* St Louis, 1990, The Association.
7. Stuart GW, Sundeen SJ, editors: *Principles and practice of psychiatric nursing,* ed 4, St Louis, 1991, Mosby–Year Book.
8. Hackett TP, Weissman AD: Reactions to the imminence of death. In Monat A, Lazarus RS, editors: *Stress and coping: an anthology,* ed 2, New York, 1985, Columbia University Press.
9. Shelp EE, Perl M: Denial in clinical medicine: a re-examination of the concept and its significance, *Arch Intern Med* 145:697, 1985.
10. Lowery BJ: Psychological stress, denial, and myocardial infarction outcomes, *Image J Nurs Sch* 23:51, 1991.

11. Relling-Garskof K: Transferring the past to the present, *Am J Nurs* 87:476, 1987.
12. *Webster's ninth new collegiate dictionary,* Springfield, Mass, 1991, G&C Merriam.
13. Shaffer JL: Spiritual distress and critical illness, *Crit Care Nurse* 2:42, 1991.
14. Drew N: Exclusion and confirmation: a phenomenology of patients, experience with caregivers, *Image J Nurs Sch* 18:39, 1986.
15. Wheeler K: A nursing science approach to understanding empathy, *Arch Psych Nurs* 2:95, 1988.
16. American Psychiatric Association: *Diagnostic and statistical manual of mental disorders,* ed 3 revised, Washington, DC, 1987, The Association.
17. Roose SP: Diagnosis and treatment of depression in the medical setting, *J Clin Psychiatry* 51(suppl):3, 1990.
18. Malzberg B: Mortality among patients with involutional melancholia, *Am J Psychiatry* 93:1231, 1937.
19. Rabins PV, Harvis K, Koven S: High fatality rates of late life depression associated with cardiovascular disease, *J Affective Disord* 9:165, 1985.
20. Avery D, Winokur G: Mortality in depressed patients treated with electroconvulsive therapy and antidepressants, *Arch Gen Psychiatry* 33:1029, 1976.

9

Sexuality Alterations

CHAPTER OBJECTIVES

- Formulate nursing diagnoses for a patient whose sexual activity is compromised because of cardiovascular or chronic lung disease.
- Conduct a nursing interview that assesses the sexual concerns of patients with cardiovascular or chronic lung disease.
- Provide an environment that eases transmittal of sexual information to postcoronary and COPD patients and their partners.[1]
- Contrast the symptoms and causes of anginal pain, the pain of myocardial infarction, and chest wall pain.
- List appropriate patient responses and treatment strategies for the three types of chest pains that may occur during sexual activity.
- Describe nursing management of cardiac patients who demonstrate adaptive and maladaptive denial related to sexual concerns.
- Assist patients in correlating expended sexual energy with comparable MET equivalents.
- Inform patients with cardiovascular or chronic lung disease and partners about alternate positions recommended for safe sexual activity.
- Facilitate opportunities for patients and partners to experience physical contact as a precursor to healthy sexual expression.
- Develop education programs that assist other health care disciplines to effectively counsel postcoronary patients and their partners about sexual concerns, myths, and realities.

Sexuality is a unique, highly individual expression and experience of the self as a sexual, erotic being. It is a holistic experience in that it encompasses both the mind and the body and a part of the character of a person also termed the *personality.*

To express oneself in a sexual way means to define who one is and what one feels in the most basic sense on one hand and yet in the most deep, profound sense on the other. Sexuality does not solely reflect the technique and mastery of sexual intercourse but is part of a being's relationship to and with all other beings throughout one's lifetime.

Sexuality may therefore be expressed in the most simple ways, such as in the solitary activities of studying or walking in the park, and also in the more physical demonstrations, such as kissing, embracing, and sexual intercourse. Whichever way sexuality is expressed, most authorities agree that rapport and communication are two vital aspects of the sexual experience.

SEXUAL EXPRESSION

Sexual expression at its best is more than just attainment of coitus and orgasm. It also encompasses love, warmth, sharing, and touching between people and an emotional union of hearts and minds, all of which transcend purely physical pleasure. It is the culmination and coming together within the individual of biologic, psychologic, and cultural influences that result in sex-role behavior or sexual expression of self (Fig. 9-1).[2]

Sensuality, although a necessary component of sexual fulfillment, does not in itself reflect sexual activity. It refers to the pleasure one derives through the senses, such as touch, smell, sight, and sound, which enhance the total sexual experience.

Sexual health is defined as "the integration of the somatic, emotional, intellectual and social aspects of a sexual being, in ways that are positively enriching and that enhance personality, communication and love."[3]

Sexual function is limited by very few inevitable, physiologic truths—men normally impregnate women, and women are normally able to ovulate, menstruate, lactate, and gestate. All other differences, including aggressive behavior and even sex roles, have not been found specifically related to either man or woman.[4]

Most authorities concur that in today's society there is a wide range of accepted behaviors leading to sexual gratification. Sex without love or marriage has long been practiced, and although double standards exist, small vociferous groups claiming moral and religious propriety have failed to quell the sexual revolution.

A larger portion of society may frown on extramarital sex, or what is loosely defined as promiscuity, but unless one is engaged in illegal sexual practices such as prostitution or incest, sexual behavior is considered an individual decision. Legalized abortion and inexpensive, accessible birth control methods have enhanced freedom of sexual expression.

All sexual practices are currently being more closely scrutinized as the result of information about the life-threatening sexually transmitted disease acquired immunodeficiency syndrome (AIDS) and HIV-related illnesses.

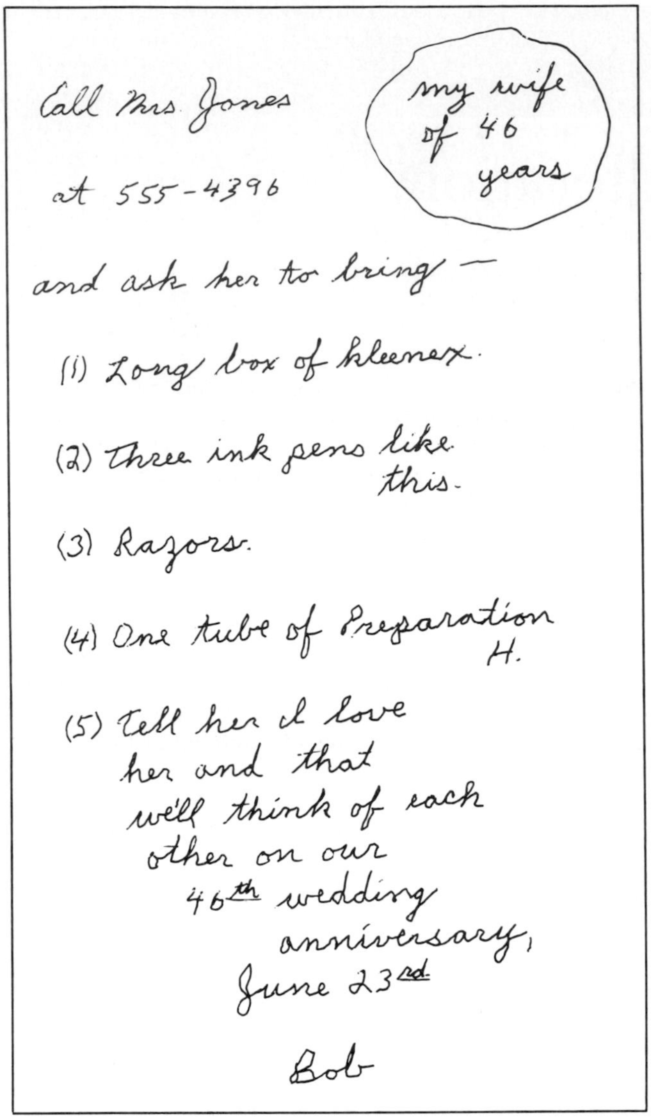
Call Mrs Jones
at 555-4396
(my wife of 46 years)
and ask her to bring —
(1) Long box of kleenex.
(2) Three ink pens like this.
(3) Razors.
(4) One tube of Preparation H.
(5) Tell her I love her and that we'll think of each other on our 46th wedding anniversary, June 23rd.
Bob

Fig. 9-1 Handwritten note from patient.

SEXUAL DYSFUNCTION

Masters and Johnson[5] originally introduced the term *sexual dysfunction* in 1970. It was originally interpreted to mean "sexual problem" or "sexual disorder." Later (1979), Masters and Johnson, along with their associates,[6] first discussed sexual apathy and sexual aversion, calling these conditions "nondysfunction," or problems stemming from a "lack of desire or arousal," differentiating them from organic dysfunctions related to the sex organs themselves. It was thus clarified that sexual dysfunctions, according to Masters and Johnson,[6] are "those sex problems that appear as difficulties on the physical level, such as problems with orgasms, erections or penetration." These physical symptoms are absent from or play only a small part in the bulk of sex problems.[7,8]

It is beyond the scope of this chapter to do justice to the works of leading authorities in the field of human sexuality. The literature is vast, interesting, and in some areas contradictory. For further information about things such as sexual anatomy and physiology, the phases of the human sexual response cycle, organic and nonorganic impotence, and intensive counseling related to sexual expression, refer to the works of experts such as Masters and Johnson, Robert Kolodny, Helen Singer Kaplan, and Bernard Apfelbaum.

This chapter uses the term *sexual dysfunction* as defined by the North American Nursing Diagnosis Association (NANDA) – the state in which an individual experiences or is at risk of experiencing a change in sexual health or sexual function that is viewed as unrewarding or inadequate.[9]

This chapter emphasizes common problems related to physiologic and psychologic stressors that threaten the sexual function of the male and female patient with cardiac disease, with some attention given to the patient with chronic lung disease. The role of sexual partners is included throughout the discussion. Patients with sexual dysfunction related to neurologic deficits are not discussed in this chapter, since the major portion of sexual assessment and intervention for that group of patients is better addressed during the rehabilitation phase versus critical care.

ASSESSMENT OF SEXUAL ACTIVITY INTOLERANCE

Most sources agree that critical care nurses should teach patients and their partners as early as possible about myocardial infarction and how to recognize and manage the different types of chest pain and control the symptoms of fatigue, dyspnea, and rapid heart rate during times such as sexual activity. Because chest pain is the most frightening symptom, the nurse needs to begin by teaching patients the specific language that describes the characteristics of the various types of chest pain. In this way he or she can help patients differentiate chest wall pain from anginal pain and anginal pain from the pain of myocardial infarction. The nurse can then assist patients and partners in connecting each type of pain with its probable cause, symptoms, duration, and mode of prevention and treatment. The nurse can instruct patients how to monitor changes in breathing and heart rates and to determine whether they are within normal parameters in relation to the amount of energy expended. The nurse can alert patients to be aware of thoughts that may invoke anxious feelings that can contribute to the physical symptoms and then demonstrate strategies to reduce anxiety. "Thoughts that attempt to fight chest pain are more likely to increase anxiety than are those that go beyond the immediate pain experience and focus on the idea that the pain will quickly pass."[10]

The nurse needs to inform patients and partners that some or all of these symptoms may occur during sex, partly because the work-load of the damaged cardiac muscle increases to provide the oxygen needed to satisfy the body's demands for energy. Also, anxiety could arouse the nervous system into provoking or sustaining the physical symptoms.[10,11]

Angina pectoris is the chest pain associated with myocardial ischemia. Patients with ischemia have an imbalance of regional myocardial perfusion in relation to the demand for myocardial oxygenation. This transient imbalance is precipitated by conditions that increase the heart rate, such as exercise, anger, anxiety, or postural changes. The location of the pain may be substernal or extrathoracic (neck, jaw, shoulder, arm) and may include variable degrees of discomfort. Patients who experience anginal pain during sexual activity may benefit from the prophylactic use of nitroglycerin, the use of long-acting nitrate preparations, or the use of beta-blocking agents such as propranolol. Some types of anginal pain may be experienced as indigestion or a toothache. Because anginal pain is precipitated by activities and exercise, it is relieved within minutes by rest or the use of nitroglycerin.[11,11a]

Myocardial infarction (MI) involves cellular damage and death of a portion of the cardiac muscle as a result of prolonged ischemia of more than 30 to 45 minutes. Permanent cessation of contractile function occurs in the necrotic or infarcted area. The degree of ventricular dysfunction depends on the size, location, collateral circulation, compensatory mechanisms, and function of the uninvolved myocardium. The patient suffering from MI typically experiences severe, prolonged chest pain, frequently associated with sweating, nausea, vomiting, and a feeling of impending doom. If symptoms of chest pain, chest tightness, or severe shortness of breath persist, sexual activities must cease and the physician must be notified immediately. Hospitalized patients should be instructed that this type of pain can always be treated with narcotic analgesics.[11,11a]

Chest wall pain is caused by a "tightening" of the chest wall muscles, which generally results from poor posture and is exacerbated by anxiety. "Hunching" of the back during sexual intercourse can strain the chest wall muscles and produce dyspnea. Patients should be taught to decrease anxiety by focusing on the idea that the pain will pass versus attempting to fight the pain. Dyspnea can be controlled by straightening the back and performing slow, deep-breathing exercises. Patients can learn to associate anxiety-producing thoughts such as fear of recurrent MI and/or death with the occurrence of chest wall pain and recognize that such thoughts exacerbate otherwise normal symptoms of activity intolerance. Once patients successfully master relaxing the chest wall muscles, the cessation of pain will afford them confidence and control during sexual activity and will help them better distinguish among the three types of chest pain.[10]

PSYCHOLOGIC FACTORS AFFECTING SEXUAL FUNCTION

Many authorities agree with the substantial evidence that recovery from MI can be viewed from a psychologic as well as biologic perspective.

> The meaning one ascribes to one's heart in human terms encompasses a multitude of emotions and feelings such as love, courage, sympathy, affection and survival itself. The heart and its attributes are romanticized throughout literature, music and the art world, to the extent that the very thought of it failing is to reduce it to the mere organ that it is and to bring one face to face with mortality.[10]

According to several outcome studies researched by Mayou, Foster, and Williamson,[12] and Wishnie, Hackett, and Cassem,[3] approximately 50% of post–myocardial infarct patients continue to suffer from fear, anxiety, and depression, as well as low energy and fatigue, for as long as 1 year after the heart attack. Between 20% and 30% of individuals suffer from a morbid fear of returning to normal functions and activities, including sexual activity. Adverse effects from severe anxiety and heightened somatic concern during the early phase of recovery have been associated with dysrhythmias, chest pain, and death. Patients who experience sexual problems as a result of drug therapy and who complain of chest pain, even with mild exertion, are in the minority.[7,10]

During interviews with spouses and partners of myocardial infarct patients, varying degrees of anxiety, depression, and sexual dissatisfaction were expressed. Both British and American studies[10,13] revealed that wives coped by overprotecting their husbands (e.g., attempting to restrict husband's activities in general). Some resentment was also identified and was attributed to the wives' perceived loss of emotional support from their ill husbands. It probably contributed to the ensuing marital discord, although clear causality was not established.

Several authorities document the following psychologic fears[7]:

1. Sudden death will occur from exertion.
2. Sexual activity will impose physical difficulties in sexual function.
3. Heart attack is a "warning" that the aging process reflects a deterioration of sexual capacity.
4. Excitement and orgasm will cause another heart attack.

A study[14] was designed to demonstrate the influence of a brief marriage enrichment relationship skills training program (ME-RSTP) on marital satisfaction and quality of life in couples in the recovery phase of cardiovascular disease. It was established that adequate adaptation to life-threatening and life-style-threatening illness required that couples draw on previous relationship skills and coping styles honed from many years of marriage and experience with stressful situations. It was concluded that only couples whose relationship skills and coping styles were inadequate to meet the demands of adapting to physical illness would truly benefit from such a program. Sexual counseling, no matter how well-intentioned, is not for everyone.

Couples who find in each other "a confidant—one with whom a person can have a close intimate relationship—. . . will be better able to sustain intimacy and satisfy the emotional needs of the relationship in illness as they did in health."[15]

Assessment of Sexual Concerns

Patients with myocardial infarct who are at high risk for sexual dysfunction because of psychologic concerns may be identified early in the critical care unit. For the critical care nurse, eliciting the patient's adaptive or maladaptive responses to MI points the way to distinct interventions that may help him or her vent feelings and overcome loss of sexual function and fear of death.

Remember, any discussion about sex should be done tactfully and gradually, according to the patient's pace and preference[1] (see box below).

One study by Sulman and Verhaeghe[17] revealed two distinct groups of patients in need of sexual counseling.

Group I patients demonstrate grieving behaviors, such as poor appetites, saddened affects, and passive resistance to treatment and exercise regimen. These patients can develop growing anxiety or depression as a result of exaggerated concern about the effect of the illness on their sexual integrity and self-esteem and may require psychiatric consultation.

Group II patients demonstrate angry, "bullying" behaviors, such as being uncooperative and noncompliant to treatment in a belligerent manner. These patients may deny the extent of their illness by continuing to smoke and work while in the hospital and threatening to resume sexual relations at a dangerous pace on discharge. They generally exhibit difficulty in absorbing important information about their illness and frequently verbalize their eagerness for discharge with impatience and frustration.

The researchers identified a third group of patients who comply with treatment in spite of their anxiety and depression. Unlike the patients who clearly display their need for intervention, these patients demonstrate more subtle symptoms, which may be deceptive. They are generally perceived as "good patients," since they make benign requests for encouragement and readily acknowledge apprehension and sadness. Often their compliance is credited to their expressed feelings, so staff members fail to recognize their growing anxiety and depression. This group of patients requires preventive intervention, such as positively acknowledging their participation in treatment regimens. Their consequent sense of mastery reinforces ego strength and promotes adaptive denial.

This same study stipulates that, occasionally, male patients with myocardial infarct will verbalize sexually explicit comments interspersed with humor, jokes, and "adolescent"-type behaviors directed at the staff or visitors. This is considered a "normal" means by which some patients cope with the fear of sexual dysfunction and threat of death. The denial is considered adaptive as long as they *comply* with the treatment and exercise program. In dealing with this personality type, the nurse is advised to ignore the content of the conversation and "go along with the intent" in a light exchange of banter, as long as it allows the patient to cope in a healthful manner.

INTERACTIVE STRATEGIES

1. Provide privacy for the patient and partner. This illustrates respect and consideration, and puts the patient and partner at ease.
2. Demonstrate how the patient and partner can comfort, touch, and hold each other. Explain the equipment so that they are not intimidated by it. A sample statement might be, "Do you wonder how you can touch each other with all these wires and I.V. lines?"[1] If they demonstrate interest in your query, tell them they can touch each other despite wires and lines. If they are not interested or appear anxious, postpone the topic and move on to steps 3 and 4. If they are comfortable with the topic, proceed further in your interactions, up to step 7.
3. Begin slowly, with less personal topics, to build trust and rapport. Discuss topics such as diet, medications, and breathing treatments.
4. Bring in topics such as activities and discuss restrictions that this illness may impose on them (e.g., housework, gardening, playing golf).
5. Ask the patient whether he or she has any concerns about how these restrictions may affect sexual relations as well. If it is expressed that sex has not played a big part in the lives of the patient and partner for years but that they are still close in many ways, there is no need to pursue the subject. Simply move on to other areas. If a sexually active life-style is revealed, proceed to step 6.
6. Determine whether the patient feels that the disease has affected, or may affect, his or her sexual activity and to what extent.
7. Ask whether he or she would like to continue sexual relations but is concerned or anxious about the shortness of breath that accompanies the sex act.

Modified from Cohelo A and others: Treadmill testing in patients with sustained ventricular tachycardia, *Circulation* 64:IV, 1981.

EXERCISE PHYSIOLOGY AND PATIENT EDUCATION

The public has become increasingly aware that exercise throughout the life span can positively influence health. Most authorities agree that a well-planned physical activity program can increase aerobic capacity by 20% to 30%, improve cardiorespiratory endurance, promote muscle strength, and improve flexibility.[18] Individuals with cardiovascular or cardiorespiratory problems will find it easier to adjust to an exercise program if they had previously incorporated some type of aerobic activity into their daily routine.

Experts suggest that during the acute phase of hospitalization (first 3 to 4 days), the critical care nurse should inform the patient and partner that walking, running, sex, and other activities will be possible and can be regained gradually through participation in a progressive cardiac rehabilitation program. Of postcoronary patients, 80% can resume sexual relations 2 to 4 weeks after discharge (4 to 8 weeks after MI), as long as there is no history of complications (50% are uncomplicated) and if exercise can be tolerated to the extent of raising the heart rate to approximately 110 to 120 beats per minute (bpm) without precipitating angina or severe shortness of breath. Exercise tolerance can be ascertained by formal testing, such as the use of a calibrated bicycle ergometer or a submaximal treadmill test.[14,19]

Although sexual intercourse is one of the most physically demanding exercises, conjugal sexual activity in middle-aged men (and women) with uncomplicated cardiac pathology invokes only modest physiologic exertion with maximal cardiac stress lasting only 10 to 15 seconds. In general, the energy needed for intercourse equals that of a brisk walk on level ground, or up and down two flights of stairs for 4 to 6 minutes.[20] Sexual activity, including coitus and orgasm, can be compared in terms of oxygen consumption and workload of the heart with activities equal in energy expenditure. Activity progression is based on METs, a term used to describe the energy expenditure for many activities. An MET is a metabolic equivalent that can be assigned to activities regardless of a person's weight. One MET represents the energy expenditure of a person at rest and equals approximately 3.5 ml of oxygen per kilogram of body weight per minute.[21]

Most patients will need to perform three to four MET-level activities when they return home, and hospitals gear exercise programs toward that goal. Some of the activities that are considered comparable in oxygen consumption and energy expenditure to sexual activity, including coitus and orgasm, are as follows[21]:

1. Climbing two flights of stairs (20 steps in 10 seconds) without difficulty (this task is considered by experts to be the most standard test)
2. Taking a brisk walk (3 to 4 METs equal 4.8 km or 2½ mph)
3. Performing ordinary tasks in many occupations and recreations, such as pushing a light power mower or pulling a light golf bag cart (Table 9-1)

The nurse can also teach the patient to assess his or her own readiness to return to sexual intercourse by checking the pulse rate during comparable activities. When it rises to 110 to 120 bpm without causing shortness of breath, chest pain, or fatigue, sexual activity can be resumed. This generally occurs 4 to 6 weeks after discharge when the patient is still under the care and scrutiny of the physician.[22] One author[23] says 6 to 8 weeks but defers to the physician's final assessment for decision.

Authorities[22-24] cite four danger signals that may indicate that sexual intercourse is causing physiologic problems because of increased workload of the heart beyond the patient's endurance and should be ceased and a physician notified immediately: (1) dyspnea or increased heart rate that lasts longer than 5 minutes after intercourse, (2) extreme fatigue the day after intercourse, (3) insomnia after intercourse, and (4) chest pain during intercourse that is unrelieved by vasodilators, cessation, rest, and/or use of relaxation and breathing techniques.

Sexual activities such as hugging, kissing, and embracing should begin gradually in the critical care unit to prepare for the more strenuous activity of sexual intercourse and to provide a more natural transition to sex for the patient and partner. Continuation of intimacy in illness also maintains healthy sensual relations between couples, which promotes overall wellness. Some patients may find it reassuring to attempt masturbation (3 to 4 METs) before intercourse for these same reasons.[25]

Patients also need information about the medications that act to decrease cardiac workload, because they may be prescribed by the physician for use before intercourse to prevent chest pain.[24,26]

It is also important for nurses to inform patients about medications that can alter or interfere with sexual function and performance. Sometimes simply adjusting the dose of some drugs or using different combinations can ameliorate the problem. For example, propanolol (Inderal) and methyldopa (Aldomet), as well as many antihypertensive medications, can affect sexual function, such as causing diminished libido or erectile problems. Drugs used to treat depression—such as amitriptyline (Elavil), desipramine (Norpramine), and other tricyclic antidepressants—can either heighten or diminish libido.[20]

A commonly shared perception has been that during the sex act the partner with the heart disease should assume the dependent or "patient-on-bottom" position. However, experts[14] have reported no significant difference in either heart rate or blood pressure when healthy men were studied while they engaged in sexual intercourse in either position. Peak heart rates were 114 bpm for the "male-on-top" position, with a peak, mean blood pressure of 163/81 mm Hg. Findings during the "male-on-bottom" position were a peak heart rate of 117 bpm and a blood pressure of 161/77 mm Hg.[14,32]

Experts agree that patients with coronary artery disease who can perform a comparable level of activity without symptoms can safely resume sexual activity as long as they *avoid* sex in the following situations:

- After a heavy meal—food and/or drink disrupts circulatory efficiency and diverts blood flow from the heart and great vessels to the gut.[27]
- For at least 3 hours after alcohol ingestion—alcohol, even in small amounts, decreases cardiac index and stroke index in patients with heart disease;[12] avoid heavy drinking.[27]
- Positions requiring isometric exertion—they are more apt to increase the heart rate or precipitate dysrhythmias.[24,28]
- Anal intercourse—this could cause vagal stimulation and bradycardia.
- Extreme room temperatures—extreme hot or cold can add stress on the heart.
- When fatigued or during an emotional outburst—rest is beneficial before intercourse; and workload on the heart is increased during extreme tiredness, and there is increased stress on the heart during a highly emotional state.[12]

Most authorities agree that patients should avoid sex with unfamiliar partners because it is assumed that a greater level of excitement occurs, which may act as a stressor on the heart. However, no current scientific information supports this belief.[7]

Sex and Sudden Death

In a frequently cited study done in Japan,[29] 34 of 5559 cases of sudden endogenous death (0.6%) occurred during coitus. Of the 34 deaths, 18 were thought of cardiac origin, and 27 of them occurred during or after extramarital sex.

It may be, however, that alcohol use or other unknown variables affected the outcome of this study, since there are no reliable data to indicate the actual magnitude of the risk involved.[6]

Table 9-1 Approximate metabolic cost of activities

	Occupational	**Recreational**
1½-2 METs* 4-7 ml O_2/min/kg 2-2½ kcal/min (70-kg person)	Desk work Auto driving† Typing Electric calculating machine operation	Standing Walking (strolling 1.6 km or 1 mile/hr) Flying,† motorcycling† Playing cards† Sewing, knitting
2-3 METs 7-11 ml O_2/min/kg 2½-4 kcal/min (70-kg person)	Auto repair Radio, television repair Janitorial work Typing, manual Bartending	Level walking (3.2 km or 2 miles/hr) Level bicycling (8.0 km or 5 miles/hr) Riding lawn mower Billiards, bowling Skiing,† shuffleboard Woodworking (light) Powerboat driving† Golf (power cart) Canoeing (4 km or 2½ miles/hr) Horseback riding (walk) Playing piano and many musical instruments
3-4 METs 11-14 ml O_2/min/kg 4-5 kcal/min (70-kg person)	Brick laying, plastering Wheelbarrow (45.4 kg or 100-lb load) Machine assembly Trailer-truck in traffic Welding (moderate load) Cleaning windows	Walking (4.8 km or 3 miles/hr) Cycling (9.7 km or 6 miles/hr) Horseshoe pitching Volleyball (6-person, noncompetitive) Golf (pulling bag cart) Archery Sailing (handling small boat) Fly-fishing (standing with waders) Horseback riding (sitting to trot) Badminton (social doubles) Pushing light power mower Energetic musician
4-5 METs 14-18 ml O_2/min/kg 5-6 kcal/min (70-kg person)	Painting, masonry Paperhanging Light carpentry	Walking (5.6 km or 3½ miles/hr) Cycling (12.9 km or 8 miles/hr) Table tennis Golf (carrying clubs) Dancing (foxtrot) Badminton (singles) Tennis (doubles) Raking leaves Hoeing Many calisthenics
5-6 METs 18-21 ml O_2/min/kg 6-7 kcal/min (70-kg person)	Digging garden Shoveling light earth	Walking (6.4 km or 4 miles/hr) Cycling (16.1 km or 10 miles/hr) Canoeing (6.4 km or 4 miles/hr) Horseback riding ("posting" to trot) Stream fishing (walking in light current in waders) Ice or roller skating (14.5 km or 9 miles/hr)

From Fox SM, Naughton JP, Gorman PA: *Mod Concs Cardiovas Dis* 41:6, 1972.
NOTE: Includes resting metabolic needs.
*MET is the energy expenditure at rest, equivalent to approximately 3.5 ml O_2/kg body weight/minute.
†A major excessive metabolic increase may occur because of excitement, anxiety, or impatience during some of these activities, and a physician must assess his or her patient's psychologic reactivity.

PATIENT WITH SEVERE HEART DISEASE

Physical activity in general does not tend to induce ventricular tachycardia in patients whose conditions are well-controlled; but for the patients with severe heart disease, possible heart failure is a problem, and symptoms of angina, fatigue, and dyspnea must be considered warning signals. For these patients it is difficult to allay the fear of an impending episode of ventricular tachycardia and possible death.[16]

Experts suggest more investigation into the effect of sexual intercourse in provoking episodes of ventricular tachycardia. Because reliable data do not exist for this

Table 9-1 Approximate metabolic cost of activities—cont'd

	Occupational	Recreational
6-7 METs 21-25 ml O_2/min/kg 7-8 kcal/min (70-kg person)	Shoveling for 10 min (4.5 kg or 10 lb)	Walking (8.0 km or 5 miles/hr) Cycling (17.7 km or 11 miles/hr) Badminton (competitive) Tennis (singles) Splitting wood Snow shoveling Hand lawn mowing Folk (square) dancing Light downhill skiing Ski touring (4.0 km or 2½ miles/hr) (loose snow) Water skiing
7-8 METs 25-28 ml O_2/min/kg 8-10 kcal/min (70-kg person)	Digging ditches Carrying 36.3 kg or 80 lb Sawing hardwood	Jogging (8.0 km or 5 miles/hr) Cycling (19.3 km or 12 miles/hr) Horseback riding (gallop) Vigorous downhill skiing Basketball Mountain climbing Ice hockey Canoeing (8.0 km or 5 miles/hr) Touch football Paddleball
8-9 METs 28-32 ml O_2/min/kg 10-11 kcal/min (70-kg person)	Shoveling for 10 min (6.4 kg or 14 lb)	Running (8.9 km or 5½ miles/hr) Cycling (20.9 km or 13 miles/hr) Ski touring (6.4 km or 4 miles/hr) (loose snow) Squash (social) Handball (social) Fencing Basketball (vigorous)
10+ METs 32+ ml O_2/min/kg 11+ kcal/min (70-kg person)	Shoveling for 10 min (7.3 kg or 16 lb)	Running: 6 mph = 10 METs 7 mph = 11½ METs 8 mph = 13½ METs 9 mph = 15 METs 10 mph = 17 METs Ski touring (8+ km or 5+ miles/hr) (loose snow) Handball (competitive) Squash (competitive)

category of patients, a guarantee of safe sexual experience cannot be made.[12]

The importance of the nurse's role as a caring, concerned communicator cannot be stressed enough. For patients who express difficulty in maintaining satisfying love relationships because of the realistic possibility of future abstinence, the nurse should remind them that intimate relationships can be sustained by less vigorous demonstrations, such as hand holding, caressing each other, and possibly conjugal masturbation; the latter activity requires the physician's approval and depends on the patient's cultural beliefs, preferences, and activity tolerance.[10]

Loss of physical capacity is frequently perceived as a severe threat to self-esteem and concepts of masculinity or femininity (body image). Without appropriate counseling, the patient may well transfer these negative feelings to other areas of life, such as work, recreation, and the parenting role. The nurse should be aware of the possibility of the patient's developing overwhelming anxiety or depression and should seek psychiatric consultation if necessary.[23]

PATIENT WITH CHRONIC LUNG DISEASE

Another commonly seen group of patients who may have sexual dysfunction as a result of activity intolerance and shortness of breath are patients with chronic lung disease, for example, chronic obstructive pulmonary disease (COPD), cancer of the lung, or bronchiectasis. Since chronic illness such as COPD tends to progress slowly over a long period, alterations in sexual dysfunction develop insidiously.[20] Because of the advanced age of some of these patients, the nurse should review the medical history carefully for other possible causes of sexual dysfunction unrelated to the respiratory problem, such as excessive alcohol intake, renal disease, hypertension, diabetes mellitus, or use of medications. Also, individuals with such chronic diseases tend to have inaccurate or incomplete information as to the impact of their illness on sexual expression. They often know little about available treatments.[20] The history may uncover long-standing sexual problems that existed before the chronic respiratory illness. Such variables would alter the focus of the approach to sexual counseling.[16]

Anxiety caused by the shortness of breath related to exertional dyspnea and frequent coughing spells[31] is the most common complaint of patients with respiratory disease. The fear is so great that all physical activity, including sex, is avoided, often resulting in a decreased desire for sex and subsequent feelings of worthlessness and isolation. The desire for intimacy and close contact is also diminished because of the coughing, sputum production, and foul mouth odor that accompany respiratory disease.[30] Fear of suffocation takes precedence over desire for sexual expression.[20]

Nurses can reduce their own anxiety by increasing their knowledge about respiratory disease and sexuality and by recognizing the importance of sexual expression regardless of age, illness, disability, and course of treatment.

SUMMARY

Knowledge based on the long-term findings of experts in the field of cardiac pathology and exercise physiology and their effects on the workload of the heart during sexual activity, including intercourse and orgasm, can provide the critical care nurse with two major tools: (1) the scientific data base that affords accurate and inclusive information to the patient and his or her partner about sexual function and activity tolerance of the heart and (2) the impetus to promote nursing research in the critical areas of cardiopulmonary physiology and human sexuality.

Clearly . . . nursing programs must integrate sexuality into their curriculum to adhere to the concept of man and woman as "holistic" beings.[8,33]

SEXUAL DYSFUNCTION RELATED TO ACTIVITY INTOLERANCE SECONDARY TO MYOCARDIAL INFARCTION

DEFINING CHARACTERISTICS

- Verbalized reluctance to resume preillness levels of sexual activity because of decrease in energy and increase in fatigue (EXAMPLE STATEMENT: "I won't be the same in bed after this setback. I just don't have the stamina.")
- Chest pain, dyspnea, and increased heart rate during routine hospital activities, which patient assumes will occur during sexual activity (EXAMPLE STATEMENTS: "I get chest pain and out of breath just by moving around in my room, and my heart speeds up when I exert myself. How is this going to affect my sex life?" "How will I know when I'm in danger of having another heart attack during sexual activity?")

OUTCOME CRITERIA

- Patient lists activities that are comparable in METs to energy expenditure and oxygen consumption during sexual activity, including orgasm (see Table 9-1).
- Patient states with accuracy the specific vocabulary that describes and contrasts the three types of chest pain (chest wall, anginal, and infarct), their individual symptoms, conditions that provoke them, and actions taken for relief.
- Patient demonstrates correct monitoring of pulse rate while performing activities comparable, according to METs, in energy expenditure to sexual intercourse.
- Patient states which medications may alter or decrease sexual desire or performance.
- Patient verbalizes understanding of activities and situations to avoid before and during sexual intercourse.
- Patient describes symptoms related to sexual activity and orgasm that are considered life-threatening and must be reported immediately to a physician.
- Patient participates in progressive cardiac rehabilitation program.
- Patient and partner express they have achieved a mutually gratifying preillness level of sexual function as measured by patient's increased energy and decreased fatigue, dyspnea, heart rate, and chest pain 6 weeks after myocardial infarction.

NURSING INTERVENTIONS AND *RATIONALE*

1. Continue to monitor the assessment parameters listed under "Defining Characteristics." (See box entitled "Sample Interview Guidelines.")
2. Review METs (see Table 9-1) with the patient and partner and explain which activities are comparable to sexual activity in energy expenditure and oxygen consumption (3-4 METs), such as climbing twoflights of stairs in 10 seconds, walking briskly (2½ miles in 1 hour), pushing light power mower, or pulling light golf bag cart.
3. Demonstrate monitoring of heart rate to be practiced by patient during activities that are equivalent to energy expenditure during intercourse and explain that coitus can be performed safely when heart rate is maintained within 110 to 120 bpm without precipitating angina or severe shortness of breath.

SEXUAL DYSFUNCTION RELATED TO ACTIVITY INTOLERANCE SECONDARY TO MYOCARDIAL INFARCTION—cont'd

4. Teach the patient the specific vocabulary that describes each type of chest pain, and ask him or her to associate each type of pain with its symptoms, provocation, and actions for relief such as the following:
   - ◆ *Chest wall pain. Symptoms:* tightness in chest muscles, sore to touch, shortness of breath. *Caused by:* "hunching" of back, which strains chest muscles and/or anxiety. *Actions:* straighten back; relax chest muscles; take slow, deep breaths; and focus on idea that pain will go away. If not relieved within 5 minutes, notify physician.
   - ◆ *Anginal pain. Symptoms:* jaw pain or substernal pain that may radiate to left arm and/or shoulder; may be felt as indigestion or toothache. *Caused by:* increased stress (exercise, anger, extremes of hot or cold temperatures). *Actions:* prevent by taking vasodilator before sex; should be relieved in minutes by use of vasodilator (nitroglycerin), cessation of sex, and rest. If pain persists or worsens, notify physician immediately.
   - ◆ *Infarct pain. Symptoms:* severe, persistent, "crushing" chest pain may be accompanied by sweating, severe shortness of breath, and feeling of impending doom. *Caused by:* inability of narrowed coronary arteries to meet oxygen needs of heart muscle. *Actions:* notify physician and alert emergency facility immediately to obtain relief with narcotic-analgesics and oxygen.
5. Inform the couple that studies indicate the "patient-on-bottom" position during sex uses nearly as much energy as "patient-on-top" position but that isometric exercises (tightening of muscles, including heart) may increase heart rate more than do safe parameters and should be avoided.
6. Construct a list of the patient's medications that may alter or decrease libido, performance, and/or sexual activity, and explain that the physician's adjusting the dose of some drugs may correct the problem.
7. Reassure the couple that safe sexual activity is possible, provided that situations that dangerously increase the workload of the heart are avoided before sexual activity. Such activities include ingesting a large meal, consuming alcohol either excessively or 3 hours before sexual activity, fatigue, and emotional outburst.
8. Instruct the couple to avoid the following situations during sexual activity, and state the reasons that they should be avoided: anal intercourse, isometrics or "tightening" of muscles, extreme hot or cold temperatures, and sexual intercourse with a new partner.
9. Inform couple that if the following symptoms occur as a result of sexual activity, the physician should be notified immediately, ***since it is a signal that the heart's workload is greater than its capacity to meet the body's energy demands:*** shortness of breath that persists more than 5 minutes after orgasm, increased heart rate or palpitations that persist more than 5 minutes after orgasm, extreme fatigue the day after intercourse, insomnia the day after intercourse and chest pain during or after intercourse that is unrelieved by measures listed in interventions for chest wall pain and anginal pain (may indicate infarct pain).
10. Teach patient that, while in the hospital, his or her exercise tolerance during sex will be ascertained by formal testing such as monitoring heart rate during treadmill tests, the use of calibrated bicycle ergometer, and before and after walking briskly down the hospital corridor.
11. Reassure patient and partner that compliance with treatment regimen and participation in rehabilitation program will reduce workload of the heart and promote mutually satisfying sexual activity, with increased energy and decreased fatigue, chest pain, and shortness of breath, within 4 to 6 weeks after myocardial infarction.

SAMPLE INTERVIEW GUIDELINES

LESS PERSONAL (TO BUILD TRUST AND RAPPORT)

Reflect observed behaviors: "Mr. Jones, you've been very quiet for the last 2 days and not eating very much. You hardly spoke to your wife today."

Voice concerns: "The staff and I are concerned that you don't seem interested in your treatment program. How can we help you?"

Sit in silence: "I'd like to sit here with you for a few moments." (Patient may choose to vent feelings or cry, in which case gently touching the patient's hand or arm is appropriate.)

Elicit feelings (open-ended approach): "Tell me, what is it about your illness that troubles you the most?"

Offer information: "I have some information about your heart condition that will help you understand that there are some activities you will still be able to do, but they must begin now while you're in the hospital."

Praise accomplishments: "Mr. Jones, you are doing very well with your exercise program. If you continue, you'll be able to play golf again in about 6 weeks."

PERSONAL

Refocusing (open-ended approach): "Mr. Jones, you said that you've been married for 25 years. Tell me about your relationship. What kind of activities do you enjoy together?"

Open (direct approach): "Has this illness been associated with any problems in sexual relations?"

Offering reassurance (effective in connecting patient with others and alleviating fear and embarrassment and isolation): "Other patients have expressed some concerns about their sexual relations after an illness such as yours. Do you have any such concerns?"

Confrontive: "I'd like to clear up some concerns you have about your ability to experience healthy sexual relations in the future."

Positive closure: "It sounds as though you and your partner enjoy a close, intimate relationship. Hugging and kissing while in the hospital are healthy expressions of love. With your continued work toward recovery, you should enjoy healthy, satisfying sexual relations in 6 to 8 weeks."

ALTERED SEXUALITY PATTERNS RELATED TO FEAR OF DEATH DURING COITUS SECONDARY TO MYOCARDIAL INFARCTION

DEFINING CHARACTERISTICS

- Patient and partner demonstrate behaviors indicating sexual intercourse is a threat to patient's cardiac integrity and life function (EXAMPLE STATEMENTS *[patient]:* "I guess I'll have to take life easy from now on." "My [sexual partner] and I will have to be satisfied with holding hands" [affect anxious, voice tremulous].)
- Partner demonstrates overprotective attitude toward patient, which invokes a shared sense of anxiety (sense of impending doom); partner verbalizes that patient "won't have to lift a finger from now on" (facial expression strained).
- Patient demonstrates grieving behaviors, indicating diminished sense of self-worth related to threat to sexual performance and perceived body image change, including the following:
  - Saddened affect (stares into space with blank facial expression)
  - Lack of interest in food, treatment, and exercise program
  - Apathy toward sexual information offered by nurses
  - Resistance to sexual partner's intimate attempts such as kissing and hugging
- Patient exhibits behaviors indicative of maladaptive denial (unconscious defense mechanism used to decrease anxiety and protect the ego against a painful, unacceptable reality—in this case, fear of death and threat to sexual integrity) such as the following:
  - Lack of cooperation with staff (uses loud, "bullying" tones)
  - Nonparticipation in treatment and exercise program
  - Refusal to pace activities (states intentions to ". . . work, drink, smoke, and have sex as usual")
  - Strong rejection of information about sexuality

OUTCOME CRITERIA

- Patient demonstrates positive attitude with decreased anxiety (steady voice tone, calm body movement, eye contact when discussing illness, recovery, and sexual potential).
- Patient rejects overprotective behaviors of partner (feeds and grooms self). This defuses partner's anxiety and builds mutual confidence in future sex roles.
- Patient does the following:
  - Exhibits brightened affect (animated facial expression and expressive voice tone) and indicates interest in life and a positive self-esteem

ALTERED SEXUALITY PATTERNS RELATED TO FEAR OF DEATH DURING COITUS SECONDARY TO MYOCARDIAL INFARCTION—cont'd

Actively participates in treatment and exercise program and reflects acceptance of body image change and potential for sexual participation

Accepts sexual information offered by nurses about METs and repeats it accurately in a calm manner

Responds to intimate advances of sexual partner and indicates decreased fear of resuming sexual activity on discharge

◆ Patient does the following:

Refrains from using "bullying" behaviors (angry, demanding voice tone), and displays calm, cooperative attitude toward staff and sexual partner

Requests information about how safely to pace activities such as work, drink, cigarette smoking, and sex and repeats information accurately

Long-term outcome (after discharge)

◆ Patient and partner will verbalize transition to mutually satisfying preillness sexual function within 4-6 weeks without fear of recurrent myocardial infarction or fear of death (measured by increase in desire and frequency of the sex act and absence of feeling of impending doom during sex).

NURSING INTERVENTIONS AND *RATIONALE*

1. Continue to monitor the assessment parameters listed under "Defining Characteristics."
2. Clarify any misconceptions about myocardial infarction, contrasting realistic concerns with irrational fears about future sexual function and performance (Refer to "Sexual Dysfunction related to activity intolerance secondary to myocardial infarction" for specific information about cardiac workload during sexual activity.)
3. Inform the patient and partner early in the rehabilitation program that activity and independence are crucial to the patient's emotional and physical recovery in which sexual function plays a role. The ability to feed oneself is one indication of such progress.
4. Do the following:

◆ Use therapeutic communication skills to elicit feelings of fear and anxiety about the effect of sexual intercourse on the function of the heart muscle and the life of the patient.

◆ Encourage and provide privacy for intimate behaviors between patient and partner and for masturbation if feasible.

◆ Provide clear, concise information about rationale for medical protocol and provide role-modeling of calm, controlled, adult behavior. ***Knowledge provides power, which builds self-esteem and decreases anxiety. Use of adult behavior influences patient to respond in like manner.***

◆ Praise the patient generously for participation in cardiac rehabilitation program, for pacing activities of daily living, for displays of intimacy, and for calm, controlled, adult behavior.

◆ Discuss resumption of sexual activity in nonthreatening, matter-of-fact manner, beginning with discussion of the least personal activities such as gardening to the most personal areas. See box entitled "Sample Interview Guidelines." (EXAMPLE STATEMENT: "I'd like to discuss how you can safely incorporate activities, including sexual activity, back into your life.")

Interventions for long-term outcome

1. Refer patient to cardiac rehabilitation support group on discharge for help with continued sexual participation and enrichment.
2. Consult psychiatrist or sex therapist if patient demonstrates progressively depressed mood and affect related to sexual fear and anxiety that are unrelieved by nursing interventions.

SEXUAL DYSFUNCTION RELATED TO ACTIVITY INTOLERANCE SECONDARY TO CHRONIC LUNG DISEASE

DEFINING CHARACTERISTICS

- ◆ Patient and partner express the need to avoid or experience decreased frequency in sexual activities because of patient's dyspnea on exertion during all activities. (EXAMPLE STATEMENT: "It's too hard to breathe during any kind of exertion, so sex is probably out of the question.")
- ◆ Patient verbalizes anxiety or fear about life-threatening respiratory distress and increased heart rate during sexual activity. (EXAMPLE STATEMENT: "Sex is just not worth the risk to my life. I need to conserve my energy to survive.")
- ◆ Patient expresses feelings that increased mucus production, which is exacerbated by activities, including sex, may be repulsive to partner. (EXAMPLE STATEMENT: "My breath smells horrible with all this sputum, and it's worse during activities. How can anyone come close to me?")
- ◆ Patient avoids or rejects efforts by partner to kiss or embrace in the critical care unit.

OUTCOME CRITERIA

- ◆ Patient demonstrates intimate behaviors with partner and masturbates, if feasible, while in critical care unit (affords patient the opportunity to monitor return of pulse and respiratory rate to normal after orgasm).
- ◆ Patient expresses willingness to engage in sexual intercourse after taking appropriate rest periods to conserve energy, decrease mucus production, and reduce dyspnea.
- ◆ Patient verbalizes desire to try alternative, energy-saving positions during sexual intercourse.
- ◆ Patient lists appropriate medications or treatments for use before sexual activity.
- ◆ Patient states knowledge of effects of drug therapy, alcohol consumption, and heavy meals on sexual activity.

Long-term outcomes (after discharge)

- ◆ Patient monitors pulse and respiratory rates before, during, and after sexual activity to note return of rates to normal after coitus.
- ◆ Patient and partner expresses they have mutually gratifying sexual activity and patient has increased energy, decreased mucus production, and minimal episodes of dyspnea.
- ◆ Patient and partner enroll in pulmonary rehabilitation program.

NURSING INTERVENTIONS AND *RATIONALE*

1. Continue to monitor the assessment parameters listed under "Defining Characteristics."
2. The nurse will inform the patient about the following:
   - ◆ Sexual intercourse will increase the pulse and respiratory rates, but they will normally return to baseline very quickly. (Demonstrate how to monitor pulse rate.)
   - ◆ Sexual intercourse with orgasm uses approximately the same amount of energy as climbing two flights of stairs in 10 seconds, walking briskly (2½ miles in 1 hour), pushing light mower, or pulling light golf bag cart (see Table 9-1).
   - ◆ The "patient-on-top" position, although shown in most studies to require nearly the same amount of energy expenditure as the "patient-on-bottom" position, should be avoided by the respiratory patient ***because it may tend to produce more dyspnea. On the other hand, the "patient-on-bottom" position could lead to compression of the chest, which may also lead to shortness of breath.*** Thus the following alternative positions should be tried:

     Side-to-side, rear, or front entry (by man) except for the hypoxemic individual ***who may not be able to tolerate having head and upper chest in a flat position.*** In this situation, ***upright position augments ventilation and perfusion and improves oxygenation status.***[31]

     Patient in chair with feet on floor and partner (woman) astride.

     Masturbation and oral-genital sex (if feasible). Remember that age, religion, cultural beliefs, and desire should be considered before suggesting these alternatives. Although oral-genital sex may be difficult because of the dyspnea, cough, and sputum production, it is up to the patient to determine how bothersome this is compared with the pleasure of sexual fulfillment. Some authorities believe that masturbation can begin in the critical care unit, depending on the couple's inclination and the condition of the patient. They believe that ***patients who masturbate while in the critical care unit set the stage for a smoother transition toward resumption of "normal" or "near-normal" sexual function after discharge as their conditions allow.***
   - ◆ Holding, touching, and caressing are acceptable behaviors in the critical care unit. Also, whenever couples express anxiety about having sex when at home, they should be advised to relax, "cuddle up," and enjoy a glass of wine together at home.
   - ◆ Diaphragmatic or purse-lipped breathing ***will increase energy level and improve tolerance for sexual activity.***[20]
   - ◆ Inhaled bronchodilators can be used by patients with asthma before, during, and after sex ***to decrease anxiety and shortness of breath.***

SEXUAL DYSFUNCTION RELATED TO ACTIVITY INTOLERANCE SECONDARY TO CHRONIC LUNG DISEASE—cont'd

- ◆ Taking medications 30 to 60 minutes before sexual activity ***may decrease dyspnea.***
- ◆ Use of steroids and theophylline have no effect on sexual functioning. (In some instances, adjusting the dose with physician's advice may increase libido and potency.)
- ◆ If oxygen is used at home, increase the liter flow by 1 L/min during intercourse with the recommendation of the physician.
- ◆ Intercourse should be avoided after a heavy meal. ***A full stomach can restrict ventilatory movement because of the raised diaphragm.***
- ◆ Excessive alcohol consumption decreases sexual function.
- ◆ Sexual intercourse is best initiated after a rest period such as in the morning hours, but if there is excessive sputum production at that time, it may be better to plan sexual activities for the afternoon after a nap.
- ◆ Sexual activities should be planned at nontraditional times such as late morning and mid-afternoon, ***since breathing and energy levels are greater during those times.***[20]
- ◆ The use of a waterbed is recommended by some[2] who believe that ***there is decreased demand for energy during sexual intercourse because of the rhythm of the bed.***
- ◆ Attending a pulmonary rehabilitation program to learn about the techniques that aid breathing and conserve energy and about exercises that can increase activity tolerance during sex is crucial after discharge.[16]

REFERENCES

1. Boykoff SL: Strategies for sexual counseling of patients following a myocardial infarction, *Dimens Crit Care Nurs* 8(6):368, 1989.
2. Cooper D: Sexual counseling of the patient with chronic lung disease, *Focus Crit Care* 13(3):18, 1986.
3. Wishnie MA, Hackett TP, Cassem N: Psychological hazards of convalescence following myocardial infarction, *JAMA* 215:1291, 1971.
4. Hellerstein HK, Friedman EH: Sexual activity and the postcoronary patient, *Arch Intern Med* 125:987, 1970.
5. Masters WH, Johnson VE: *Human sexual inadequacy,* Boston, 1970, Little, Brown.
6. Kolodny RC and others: *Textbook of human sexuality for nurses,* Boston, 1979, Little, Brown.
7. Johnson BS: *Psychiatric mental health nursing, adaptation and growth,* Philadelphia, 1986, JB Lippincott.
8. Masters WM, Johnson VE: *Human sexual response,* Boston, 1966, Little, Brown & Co.
9. Carpenito LJ: *Nursing diagnosis: application to clinical practice,* ed 4, Philadelphia, 1992, JB Lippincott.
10. Puksta NS: All about sex . . . after a coronary, *Am J Nurs* 77:602, 1977.
11. Phipps WJ, Long BC, Woods ND: *Medical-surgical nursing,* ed 4, St Louis, 1991, Mosby–Year Book.

11a. Price SA, Wilson LM: *Pathophysiology,* ed 3, New York, 1986, McGraw-Hill.

12. Mayou R, Foster A, Williamson B: Psychosocial adjustment in patients 1 year after myocardial infarction, *J Psychosom Res* 22:447, 1978.
13. Watts RJ: Dimensions of sexual health, *Am J Nurs* 79:1572, 1979.
14. Moore K, Folk-Lightly M, Nolen MJ: The joy of sex after a heart attack, *Nurs '77* 7(6):52, 1977.
15. Cassels C, Eckstein A, Fortinash K: Retirement: aspects, response, and nursing implications, *J Gerontol Nurs* 7(6):335, 1981.
16. Cohelo A and others: Treadmill testing in patients with recurrent sustained ventricular tachycardia, *Circulation* 64:IV, 1981.
17. Sulman JY, Verhaeghe N: Myocardial infarction patients in the acute care hospital: a conceptual framework for social work intervention, *Soc Work Health Care* 11:1, 1986.
18. Volden C and others: The relationship of age, gender, and exercise practices to measures of health, life-style, and self-esteem, *Appl Nurs Res* 3(1):20, 1990.
19. Gould L and others: Cardiac effects of a cocktail, *JAMA* 218:1799, 1971.
20. Katzin L: Chronic illness and sexuality, *Am J Nurs* 90(1):54, 1990.
21. American College of Sports Medicine: *Guidelines for graded exercise testing and exercise prescription,* ed 2, Philadelphia, 1980, Lea & Febiger.
22. O'Shea MD: *An evaluation of a marriage enrichment and relationship skills training program (ME-RSTP) for couples coping with heart disease,* doctoral dissertation, Atlanta, 1984, Georgia State University.
23. Runions J: A program for psychological and social enhancement during rehabilitation after myocardial infarction, *Heart Lung* 14(2):117, 1985.
24. McCauley K and others: Learning to live with controlled ventricular tachycardia: utilizing the Johnson Model, *Heart Lung* 13(6):633, 1984.
25. Kravetz H: Sexual counseling for the patient with chronic lung disease, *Sex Med Today* 17(3):377, 1981.
26. Baggs J: Nursing diagnosis: potential sexual dysfunction after myocardial infarction, *Dimens Crit Care Nurs* 5(3):178, 1986.
27. Ebersole P, Hess P: *Toward healthy aging, human needs, and nursing response,* ed 3, St Louis, 1989, Mosby–Year Book.
28. Stein RA: The effect of exercise training on heart rate during coitus in the post-myocardial infarction patient, *Circulation* 55:738, 1977.
29. Ueno M: The so-called coition death, *Jpn J Legal Med* 17:333, 1952.
30. Krajicek MJ: Developmental disability and human sexuality, *Nurs Clin North Am* 17:173, 1982.
31. Campbell ML: Sexual dysfunction in the COPD patient, *Dimens Crit Care Nurs* 6(2):70, 1987.
32. Nemec ED, Mansfield L, Kenneley J: Heart rate and blood pressure responses during sexual activity in normal males, *Am Heart J* 92:274, 1976.
33. Whipple B: Sexuality education in a nursing curriculum: the whys and hows, *Imprint* 36(4):54, 1989.

III

SLEEP ALTERATIONS

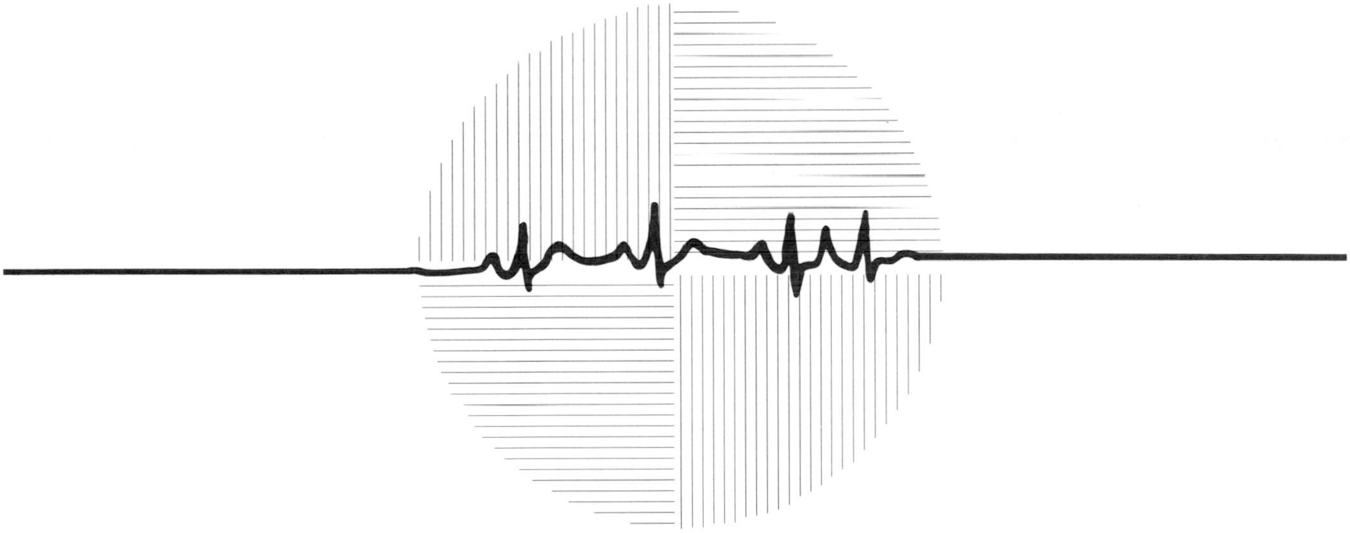

10

Sleep Physiology and Assessment

CHAPTER OBJECTIVES

- State the stages of sleep.
- Explain three physiologic effects that occur during rapid eye movement (REM) sleep.
- State two major physiologic effects of slow wave sleep.
- Define REM rebound.
- Describe circadian desynchronization and its primary effects.
- Describe the changes in sleep resulting from the aging process.
- Define dysfunctional sleep.
- Name three commonly prescribed critical care medications that decrease REM sleep.
- Describe common symptoms of sleep deprivation.

William Shakespeare early recognized the therapeutic value of sleep: "O sleep, o gentle sleep, nature's soft nurse!" Because critical illness requires frequent treatments and 24-hour intensive monitoring, patients admitted to critical care units often suffer an altered sleep pattern. The inability to rest and sleep is one of the causes as well as one of the outcomes accompanying illness. Bahr[1] stated, "The phenomenon of sleep has the potential for relieving an individual of stress and responsibility when a break is needed to recharge the person's spirit, mind and body; or, it can remain maddeningly aloof when it is needed most." A lack of sleep can have disastrous results for the critically ill patient. The critical care nurse can promote recovery and healing through facilitating sleep for patients. To do this, the nurse must understand the physiology of normal sleep and recognize events that can potentially disrupt sleep in the critical care environment. The purpose of this chapter is to familiarize the reader with the phenomenon of sleep and the types of sleep pattern disturbances that may occur in critical care and to describe the assessment of sleep pattern disturbances in critically ill patients.

PHYSIOLOGY OF SLEEP

Sleep has been defined as "a state of unconsciousness from which a person can be aroused by appropriate sensory or other stimuli."[2] Adults normally spend approximately one third of their lives asleep. Research involving the simultaneous monitoring of the electroencephalogram (EEG), electrooculogram (EOG), and electromyogram (EMG) has shown that there are two distinct stages of sleep: *rapid eye movement (REM)* and *non–rapid eye movement (NREM)*.

NREM Sleep

NREM sleep is divided into four stages (NREM 1 through 4), which are associated with progressive relaxation. NREM stage 1 is a transitional state, with the EEG being similar to that seen in the awake stage. See Fig. 10-1 for a comparison of EEG patterns of subjects that were either awake or asleep. Stage 1 is the lightest level of sleep, lasting only 1 to 2 minutes (Fig. 10-2). This stage is characterized by aimless thoughts, a feeling of drifting, and frequently, myoclonic jerks of the face, hands, and feet. The individual is easily awakened during this stage.

NREM stage 2 differs from stage 1 in that the background wave frequency on the EEG is slower with *sleep spindles* (characteristic waveforms) superimposed and high voltage spikes known as *K-complexes* (Fig. 10-3).[3] This stage lasts from 5 to 15 minutes, during which time the individual becomes more relaxed but is still easily awakened. Stages 1 and 2 in the average young adult constitute 50% to 60% of the total sleep time.

Stages 3 and 4 are characterized by large, slow-frequency delta waves on the EEG and are primarily

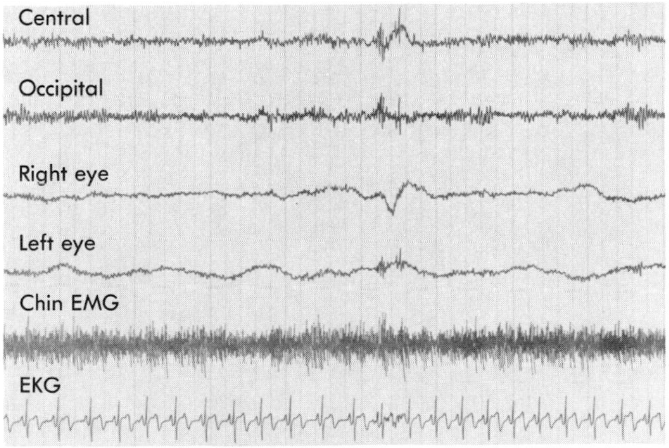

Fig. 10-1 Awake.

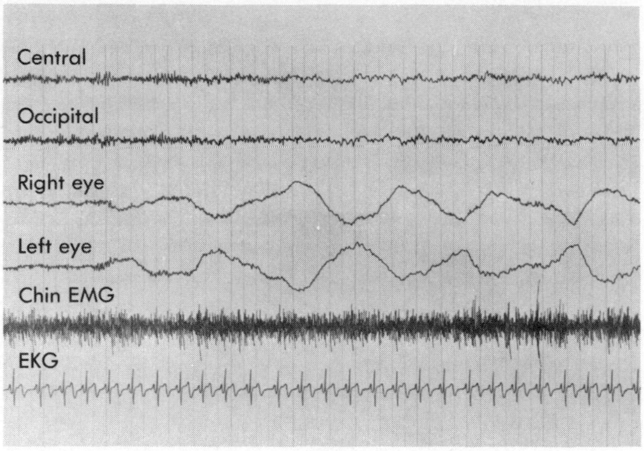

Fig. 10-2 NREM stage 1 sleep.

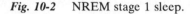

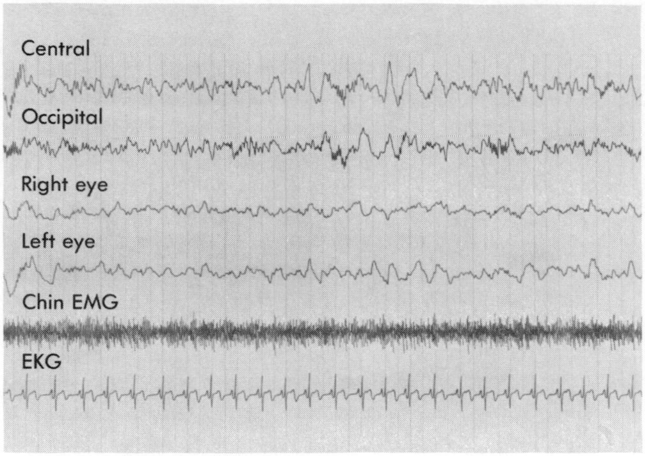

Fig. 10-4 Delta sleep NREM stage 3.

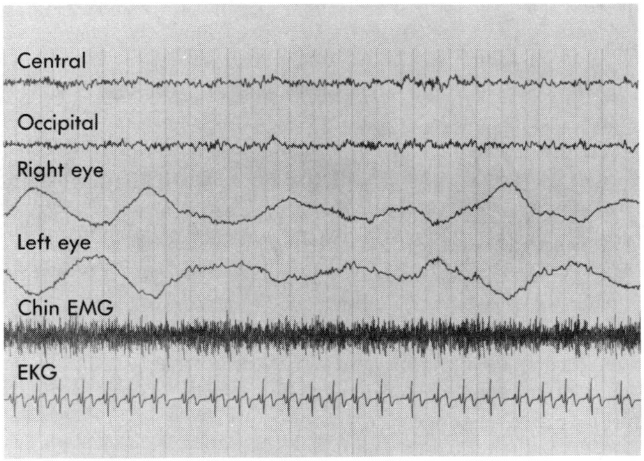

Fig. 10-3 NREM stage 2 sleep.

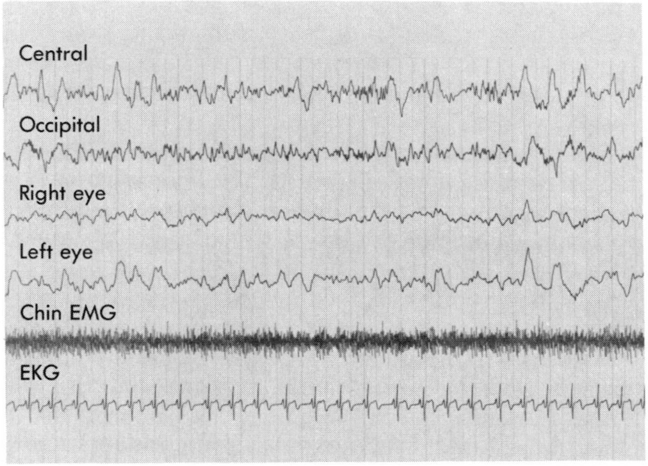

Fig. 10-5 Delta sleep NREM stage 4.

differentiated by the relative percentage of these waves (Figs. 10-4 and 10-5). Random stimuli do not arouse the individual from these deepest levels of sleep. The time spent in stages 3 and 4 varies from 15 to 30 minutes and constitutes approximately 20% of the total sleep time. During NREM sleep, the EOG gradually slows and eye movements cease. The EMG also declines, indicating profound muscle relaxation; however, it does not reach the low levels that it does in REM sleep. The parasympathetic nervous system predominates during NREM sleep. The cardiac and respiratory rates, the metabolic rate, and the blood pressure decrease to basal levels. Thus the supply/demand ratio of coronary blood flow is likely to improve.[4] NREM sleep may in fact have antidysrhythmic properties.

In addition, during slow wave sleep, growth hormone (GH) is secreted by the anterior pituitary gland and functions to promote protein synthesis while sparing catabolic breakdown. Elevated GH and other anabolic hormones, such as prolactin and testosterone, imply that anabolism is taking place during NREM stage 4, particularly in tissues with a high protein content. Thus activities associated with NREM stage 4 include protein synthesis and tissue repair, such as the repair of epithelial and specialized cells of the brain, skin, bone marrow, and gastric mucosa.[5] NREM dreams are often realistic and thoughtlike, rarely in color, and often similar to a recent activity. These dreams are generally more difficult to remember than are REM dreams. NREM sleep, then, is a time of energy conservation and renewal.

REM Sleep

REM, or *paradoxical,* sleep constitutes 20% to 25% of the total sleep time in the young adult. This type of sleep is paradoxical in that some areas of the brain are quite active during REM sleep, while other areas are suppressed. During REM sleep, bursts of eye movements are seen on the EOG that are often associated with periods of dreaming. The EMG becomes essentially flat, indicating immobility and functional paralysis of the skeletal muscles. The cerebral cortical activity increases during REM so that the EEG resembles one taken during the waking state (Fig. 10-6). During REM sleep, the individual is more difficult to awaken than in any

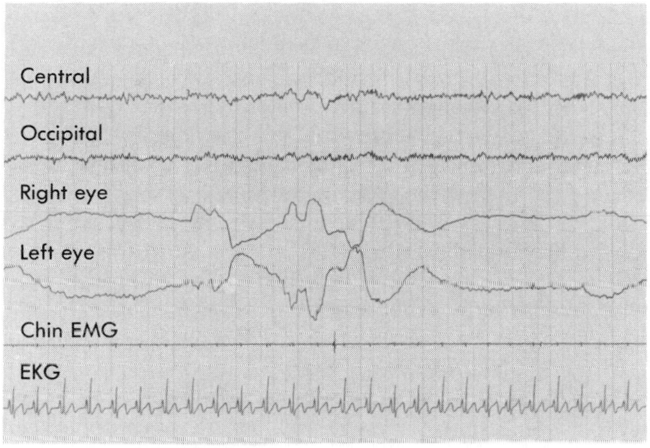

Fig. 10-6 REM sleep.

other stage of sleep.[3] In this regard, REM sleep can be thought of as a "dissociative state."

The sympathetic nervous system predominates during REM sleep. Oxygen consumption increases, and cardiac output, blood pressure, heart rate, and respiratory rate may become erratic. An increase in premature ventricular contractions (PVCs) and tachydysrhythmias associated with respiratory pauses may occur during REM sleep.[4] Evidence suggests that the adrenalin surge that more than doubles during REM sleep may be responsible for episodes of ischemia, sudden cardiac death, and strokes in the early morning hours.[4a] Serum cholesterol and antidiuretic hormone levels increase, and perfusion to the gray matter in the brain doubles. The dreams of REM sleep tend to be colorful, vivid, and implausible, often containing an element of paralysis. REM sleep filters information stored from the day's activities, sifting the important from the trivial, helping to psychologically integrate activities such as problem solving. REM sleep seems to facilitate emotional adaptation to the physical and psychologic environment and is needed in large quantities after periods of stress or learning. The adequacy of sleep is judged by the relative periods spent in each of the stages of sleep.[6]

REM sleep, like the other stages of sleep, is essential to physiologic and psychologic well-being. REM sleep is of great importance to nurses because as the patient is entering this stage of sleep, the nurse may notice a change in vital signs and become concerned that the patient's condition is worsening. If the nurse increases the monitoring of the patient, adjusts drips, and measures vital signs in response to this perceived change in condition, she or he may awaken the patient. Thus the patient may not get the sleep he or she needs. Further research must address the ways in which the nurse can assess sleep and all of its stages without unnecessarily disrupting the patient from the much-needed sleep. An accurate knowledge of sleep will assist nurses in monitoring patients safely while ensuring that they achieve optimal quality of sleep.

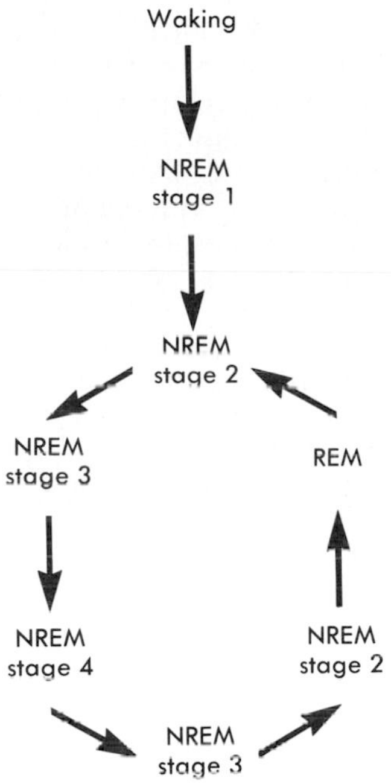

Fig. 10-7 The cyclic nature of sleep.

Cyclic Aspects

At the onset of sleep, the individual normally progresses through repetitive cycles beginning with NREM stages 1 through 4 and then back again to stage 2. From stage 2, the individual enters REM. Stage 2 is then reentered, and the cycle repeats (Fig. 10-7). These cycles occur at approximately 90-minute intervals, so that four or five cycles are normally completed in the sleep period. Early in the sleep period, NREM predominates. During the end of the sleep period, REM periods tend to be longer than those of NREM sleep.

The rhythmic nature of sleep is not unique. The body experiences rhythms in temperature, blood pressure, heart rate, respiratory rate, and hormone secretion. This cyclic 24-hour rhythm has been termed *the circadian rhythm*. Within the central nervous system, the bilaterally paired suprachiasmatic nuclei are the major endogenous pacemaker for the circadian rhythms.[7] Sleep normally occupies the low phase of the circadian rhythm, whereas wakefulness and activity normally occupy the higher phase. Although regular nighttime sleep is synchronized with other circadian rhythms, such as hormone levels, temperature, and metabolic rate, the major determinants of human sleeping are external time cues, light/dark changes, and particular social events, such as meal times.[8]

The cyclic nature of sleep and wakefulness is thought to be regulated by complex neurochemical reactions arising in the tissues of the brain stem known as the *reticular formation*. The sleep-wakefulness cycles, as well as the REM/nonREM cycle, are thought to be mediated by the neurotransmitters *serotonin, dopamine, norepinephrine,* and *epinephrine*. According to Fordham, "simple explanations or single controls of sleep do not fit with the evidence." Current research suggests that the control of sleep is a very complex process not confined to one localized part of the brain.[9]

It is interesting to note that the neurotransmitters dopamine and serotonin are major determinants of mood and affect. The changes in mood and affect in persons with sleep deprivation and desynchronization may partially be explained by the functioning of these transmitters. It is also interesting to note in light of the major role of neurotransmitters in sleep that sleep disorders are frequently seen in psychiatric illness; that is, early morning awakenings are classically found with major depressive disorders that are thought to be biochemically induced.

The sleep-wake cycle follows the circadian rhythm in a 24-hour cycle synchronized with other biologic rhythms. Nighttime sleep is the normal pattern for most adults. Serotonin, for example, is usually released around 8 PM to prepare the body for sleep. Conversely, adrenocorticotropic hormone (ACTH), corticotropin-releasing hormone (CRH), and cortisol all normally peak in the early morning hours to prepare the individual for the day's stresses. If a person is deprived of sleep, especially the deeper stages, these hormones will still be released, but at times that may or may not coordinate appropriately with the stresses he or she is about to face. Thus an abnormal sleep pattern will compromise the patient's ability to cope with the stress of critical illness, thereby complicating his or her recovery. When sleep occurs during the low phase of the circadian rhythm, circadian synchronization is present. Sleep that occurs during normal waking hours is out of phase or desynchronized (Fig. 10-8). Desynchronized sleep is rated as poor-quality sleep and causes a decreased arousal threshold; therefore frequent awakenings are more likely. Irritability, restlessness, depression, anxiety, and decreased accuracy in task performance are characteristic effects of desynchronized sleep. Resynchronization with the circadian rhythm must occur whenever sleep has become desynchronized for the individual to establish a normal sleep-activity pattern. Although variable among individuals, the resynchronization process is thought to require a minimum of 3 days with a consistent sleep-wake schedule. During resynchronization, the individual often feels fatigued and unable to perform all of his or her activities of daily living.

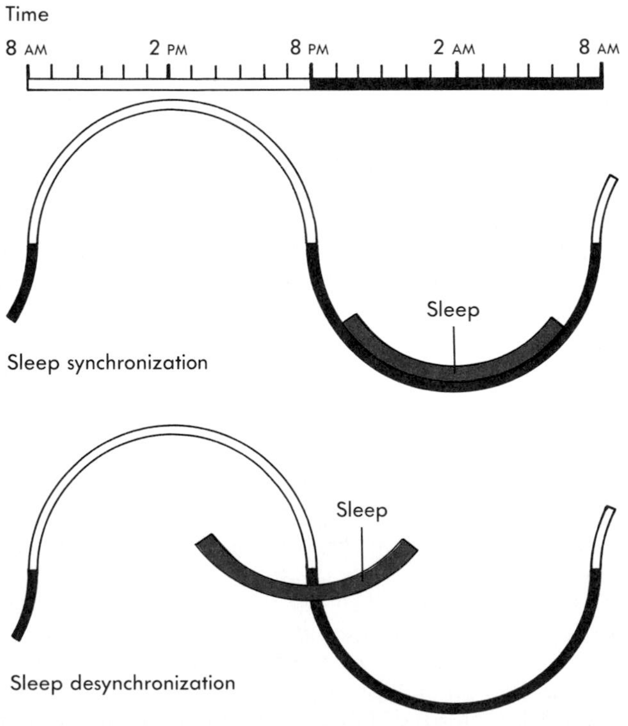

Fig. 10-8 Sleep synchronization and desynchronization with circadian rhythm.

SLEEP CHANGES WITH AGE

Of the factors that influence the quality of sleep, age is one of the most prominent. The sleep of a normal infant is divided into two types. The first is characterized by no eye or body movements and regular respirations. The second type is associated with eye and body movements and a predominant suck reflex. The first type of sleep develops into NREM sleep and the latter into REM sleep. The infant, unlike the adult, goes from wakefulness directly into REM sleep. By approximately 3 months of age, the full-term infant develops the normal adult pattern of falling from wakefulness into NREM sleep.[10] Infants spend a relatively large proportion of their sleep time in REM sleep. For the full-term newborn this percentage is approximately 40% to 50% of total sleep time. By the age of 3 years, REM sleep is approximately one third of the total sleep time, and by late childhood, REM is one fourth of total sleep.[11]

As the biologic systems change during the normal aging process, stress is placed on the human system and the delicate mechanism of sleep is altered.[12] Hayter,[6] in a study of 212 healthy, noninstitutionalized older adults ages 65 to 93, found extreme variability in the sleep behaviors of different subjects within age-groups. Sleep behaviors between men and women had few differences, although women did report more difficulty getting to sleep and more frequent use of sleep aids than did men. The number of daytime naps and nighttime awakenings and variability in sleep behaviors increased with age. By age 75, the number of naps and length of naptime increased, resulting in a gradual increase in the total sleep time. Therefore both the time needed to fall asleep and the amount of time spent in bed increased with age.

The number of awakenings increases significantly, from one or two to as many as six per night; thus elderly persons experience an increase in the total duration of NREM stage 1 sleep and an increase in the number of shifts into stage 1. The duration of NREM stage 2 sleep changes very little; however, awakenings from NREM stage 2 sleep become more frequent. NREM stage 3 tends to be normal. The duration of NREM stage 4, however, declines rapidly so that by age 50 it is reduced by 50%. Little or no stage 4 sleep may be found in 25% of the population in the sixth decade of life. Stage 4 sleep is virtually absent in old age, with REM sleep remaining stable, although more equally distributed through the night. These changes—along with more fragmentation, increased sleep-onset problems, and frequent long periods of wakefulness at night—cause elderly persons to perceive an impairment in their quality of sleep. In caring for older persons, it is important to remember that individuals differ widely in terms of both the age of onset of these changes and individual adaptations.

Advanced age involves losses of functional capabilities, health, friends, spouse, and material belongings. Because these losses can lead to depression, a state that is relatively common in the older population, the relationship between depression and sleep disturbance is important for the nurse to consider when working with elderly persons. By disrupting the psychologic state of the elderly patient, these losses may compound existing sleep difficulties.

SLEEP CHANGES WITH CHRONIC ILLNESS

Chronic illnesses, common in elderly persons, tend to increase the frequency and severity of sleep disorders. Illnesses that commonly affect sleep are arthritis, angina pectoris, chronic obstructive pulmonary disease (COPD), congestive heart failure, diabetes mellitus, peptic ulcers, alcoholism, parkinsonism, thyroid disorders, chronic pain, and depression. Both situational stress and long-term anxiety are causes of disrupted and restless sleep. As anxiety and depression increase, so does lack of sleep, and as sleep decreases, anxiety and depression increase—a vicious cycle resulting in disrupted sleep and not feeling rested on awakening.[8]

DYSFUNCTIONAL SLEEP

In the acutely ill patient, the amount, quality, and consistency of sleep may all decrease. Total sleep deprivation rarely occurs outside the experimental setting; however, in the critical care unit sleep is often interrupted or fragmented, which alters the normal stages and cycles and produces dysfunctional sleep. With frequent interruptions in sleep, the patient spends a larger proportion of time in the transitional stages (i.e., NREM stages 1 and 2) and less time in the deeper stages of sleep (NREM stages 3 and 4 and REM). Thus patients may suffer a decrease in total sleep time (TST) if they do not receive their usual amount of sleep, and they may also experience selective deprivation of the deeper stages of sleep.[13]

CIRCADIAN DESYNCHRONIZATION

Circadian disruption, or desynchronization, is another form of sleep pattern disturbance that may affect critically ill patients. The loss of rhythmicity may result from external stressors, which then alters the timing relationships of neural, hormonal, and cellular systems. Animals and humans respond to stressors, such as surgery, immobilization, and pain, with increased levels and altered timing of adrenal and other hormones. Farr and others[14] reported that circadian levels; the timing of temperature, blood pressure, and heart rate; and urinary excretion of catecholamines, sodium, and potassium were altered after surgery in hospitalized patients. Nurses should closely observe patients for clinical manifestations of such alterations and anticipate such problems as poor responses to physiologic challenges, disruption of sleep, gastrointestinal disturbances, decreased vigilance and attention span, and malaise. Nursing interventions that maintain normal rhythmicity of the day-night cycle—such as opening window blinds, placing clocks and calendars within the patient's view, allowing the patient to retire and rise at familiar times, and following individual sleep-related rituals—should be encouraged. Attention should be given to minimizing disruption during rest periods.[14]

PHARMACOLOGY AND SLEEP

Patients hospitalized in critical care units often receive pharmacologic therapy, which may affect their quality of sleep and compound sleep disturbances. The critical care nurse should be aware of the effects that commonly used drugs have on sleep. In fact, hypnotic drugs have been found to promote the lighter stages of sleep (i.e., NREM stage 2) and may, paradoxically, be the cause of night terrors, hallucinations, and agitation in the elderly.[15] This area has great potential for nursing research.

Barbiturates and sedative-hypnotic and analgesic medications may compound sleep disorders by further decreasing NREM stages 3 and 4 and REM sleep. Amobarbital, secobarbital, and pentobarbital reduce REM and increase NREM stage 2 sleep. Phenobarbital decreases REM sleep in doses greater than 200 mg. REM *rebound* (discussed later in this chapter) has been documented after the patient is withdrawn from phenobarbital therapy.[13]

Diazepam increases NREM stage 1 and reduces both NREM stages 3 and 4 and REM. REM suppression depends on the dose, with the larger doses leading to greater suppression. Flurazepam hydrochloride may be an effective hypnotic if administered in dosages equaling less than 60 mg/day. However, the long half-life of flurazepam may lead to morning drowsiness and may increase sleep apneic episodes in susceptible persons. Chloral hydrate has been shown to be an effective sedative that does not simultaneously disrupt sleep. Chlordiazepoxide and methaqualone also minimally disrupt sleep. Triazolam is effective for short-term use in increasing the total sleep time and decreasing the number of nocturnal awakenings, although it decreases REM sleep during the first 6 hours of sleep. These REM changes have been predominantly noted in young adults. An early morning "hangover" may occur with triazolam, and rebound insomnia may occur in the first 2 nights after discontinuation of the drug.[16] Morphine increases spontaneous arousals during sleep and shortens the sleep time by reducing both REM and NREM stages 3 and 4, resulting in overall lighter sleep.[17]

The prolonged half-life of medications, coupled with altered metabolism or decreased excretion of the drug resulting from renal or liver disease that may occur in

Table 10-1 Common drugs that affect sleep

Drug	Effect on sleep	Comments
BARBITURATES		
Amobarbital Pentobarbital Secobarbital	Increases NREM 2 Suppresses REM	Not considered drugs of choice because of toxicity and long-lasting effects. Often patients experience rebound insomnia, restless sleep, and frequent dreaming and nightmares when drugs are discontinued.
Phenobarbital	Decreases REM in doses greater than 200 mg	REM rebound (increased REM in subsequent sleep) after withdrawal of phenobarbital.
BENZODIAZEPINES		
Diazepam	Increases NREM 1 Decreases NREM 3 and 4 Decreases REM	NREM suppression is not dose related. REM suppression is dose related. May increase sleep apneic episodes.
Flurazepam	Increases total sleep time Decreases NREM 2, 3, and 4 Decreases REM	Conflicting reports about effects on sleep. Long half-life may produce daytime drowsiness.
Midazolam hydrochloride	No reports available as of yet	
Triazolam	Decreases sleep latency (time it takes to get to sleep) Decreases awakenings Increases total sleep time	Drug has a short half-life. Should not be used for a prolonged time because of decreased effectiveness. Use decreased doses with elderly patients.
MISCELLANEOUS		
Chloral hydrate	Thought to be an effective sedative that does not disrupt sleep	Drug has a short half-life, and some reports of nightmares. Increased daytime drowsiness.
Chlordiazepoxide Methaqualone	Minimally disrupts sleep	
Morphine sulfate	Decreases NREM 3 and 4 Decreases REM	Results in increased spontaneous arousals and overall lighter sleep.

elderly persons, can cause the effects of sedatives to continue into the daytime, leading to confusion and sluggishness. Sedative and analgesic medications should not be withheld, but rather, drugs that minimally disrupt sleep should be used to complement comfort measures, with dosages reduced gradually as the medication is no longer necessary. It is the responsibility of the critical care nurse to assess the need for sedative and analgesic medications, to administer them in the most effective manner to promote sleep, and to monitor their effectiveness (Table 10-1).

SLEEP DEPRIVATION

Much of what is known about the function of sleep has been learned from observations made when people are deprived of sleep in the laboratory setting. Both physiologic and psychologic symptoms of sleep deprivation have been reported[16] (see box on right). These symptoms may be, but are not always, associated with the length of sleep deprivation. The symptoms vary among individuals

EFFECTS OF SELECTIVE SLEEP DEPRIVATION

SYMPTOMS OF NREM SLEEP DEPRIVATION

Fatigue
Anxiety
Increased illness

SYMPTOMS OF REM SLEEP DEPRIVATION

Restlessness
Disorientation
Combativeness
Delusions
Hallucinations

with such factors as age, premorbid personality, motivation, and environmental factors.[10]

Selective *REM deprivation* leads to irritability, apathy, decreased alertness, and increased sensitivity to pain. Continued loss of REM sleep may lead to perceptual distortion and significant disturbance in mental-emotional function, often within 72 hours of REM deprivation. Manifestations of sleep deprivation range from disorientation and restlessness to frank auditory and visual hallucinations, with personality changes including withdrawal and paranoia.[10]

Selective *NREM deprivation* is less well studied, but it appears that fatigue is the primary result of NREM deprivation.[17] Because of the renewal, repair, and conservation functions of NREM sleep, deprivation may impair the immune system and depresses the body's defenses, rendering the individual vulnerable to disease.

The critical care environment affects both the quantity and quality of sleep the critically ill patient receives. The patient admitted to the critical care unit is bombarded with combined sensory overload and deprivation and unfamiliar sights, sounds, people, and perceptions. Little time for sleep is available in the critical care unit; noise, lights, and patient care activities interfere with sleep patterns.[18] Such environmental conditions have been shown to be of primary importance in sleep deprivation in the critical care unit. Dlin and others[19] showed that the chief deterrents to sleep in the critical care unit in order of importance were (1) activity and noise, (2) pain and physical condition, (3) nursing procedures, (4) lights, (5) vapor tents, and (6) hypothermia. Woods and Falk[20] found that 10% to 17% of noises in the critical care unit were of a level capable of arousing patients from sleep (greater than 70 decibels).

Using EEGs, Hilton[21] documented quantity and quality of sleep of nine patients in a respiratory critical care unit. Total sleep time ranged from 6 minutes to 13.3 hours. Only 50% to 60% of the sleep occurred at night, and no patients had complete sleep cycles. NREM stage 1 sleep predominated, to the deprivation of all other stages. Significant deprivation of restorative sleep (NREM stages 3 and 4) was demonstrated with only 4.7% to 10.5% of sleep time being spent in these stages (normally 30% to 35%). Sleep-disturbing events validated by EEG were mainly staff and environmental noise, which occurred on the average of every 20 minutes. Quality and quantity of sleep were reported as poor in all subjects. Nightmares, hallucinations, restlessness, or other behavioral changes were observed in 60% of the patients in the sample.

Psychologic stresses and fear associated with the critical care environment and the critical illness make it difficult for patients to relax and fall asleep. Fear and stress precipitate sympathetic nervous system stimulation, which decreases the arousal threshold and results in frequent awakenings and sleep stage transitions.[13]

The relationship between sleep deprivation and delirium in the critical care unit has been shown to be significant.[22] In a study of 62 patients in critical care units and surgical critical care units who ranged in age from 16 to 70 years, Helton and others[22] correlated mental status alterations (disorientation, combativeness, hallucinations, paranoia, and delusions) and sleep deprivation. A 33% increase in mental status alterations was found in severely sleep-deprived patients, defined as those who received less than 50% of their normal sleep time. Shaver, in a review of sleep research, notes that sleep deprivation is considered to be a contributing factor in postoperative psychosis.[22a]

Mortality is higher in critical care patients who exhibit symptoms of psychosis or delirium.[23] Perhaps persons experiencing hallucinations and paranoia (the most severe consequences of sleep deprivation and critical care unit psychosis) are in fact dreaming in the awake state. This hypothesis remains to be verified by research; however, caution needs to be taken in diagnosing a previously nonconfused elderly patient as having organic mental disorder (OMD) until the possibility of sleep deprivation has been ruled out.

"There is substantial evidence to support the fact that 4 days of sleep deprivation results in a decreased production of ATP, the critical energy substance. Sleep returns this balance to normal."[24] An understanding of the stages of sleep and the effects of sleep deprivation assists the nurse in evaluating the quantity and quality of sleep her or his patients receive.

RECOVERY SLEEP

When an individual has sleep deprivation, the changes in physiologic and psychologic performance can be reversed through recovery sleep. Rosa and others[25] found that recall returned to baseline with 4 to 8 hours of recovery sleep after 40 to 64 hours of total sleep deprivation (Fig. 10-9).

Deprivation of REM and NREM stage 4 results in rebounds in an attempt to compensate for "debts." The phenomenon of *REM rebound* occurs after selective REM deprivation. In an attempt to make up for lost REM and NREM stage 4 sleep, REM and NREM stage 4 periods quantitatively increase in the sleep periods after the deprivation. NREM stage 4 sleep is preferentially restored first, presumably because of its anabolic function. Because REM sleep is replenished last, it is more likely that REM debts will occur. REM rebound can exacerbate angina, dysrhythmias, duodenal ulcer pain, or sleep apneic episodes.[13] When a patient is exhibiting any of these symptoms and has had a period of sleep deprivation, REM rebound should be considered when determining the cause. Although the symptoms of angina, dysrhythmias, duodenal ulcer pain, and sleep apnea are treated as usual, further REM deprivation should be avoided.

ASSESSMENT OF SLEEP PATTERN DISTURBANCE

Assessment of the patient on admission to the critical care unit should include a description of the normal sleep pattern, including awakenings, naps, normal bedtime and waking time, and customary habits that enhance sleep (e.g., number of pillows, extra blankets,

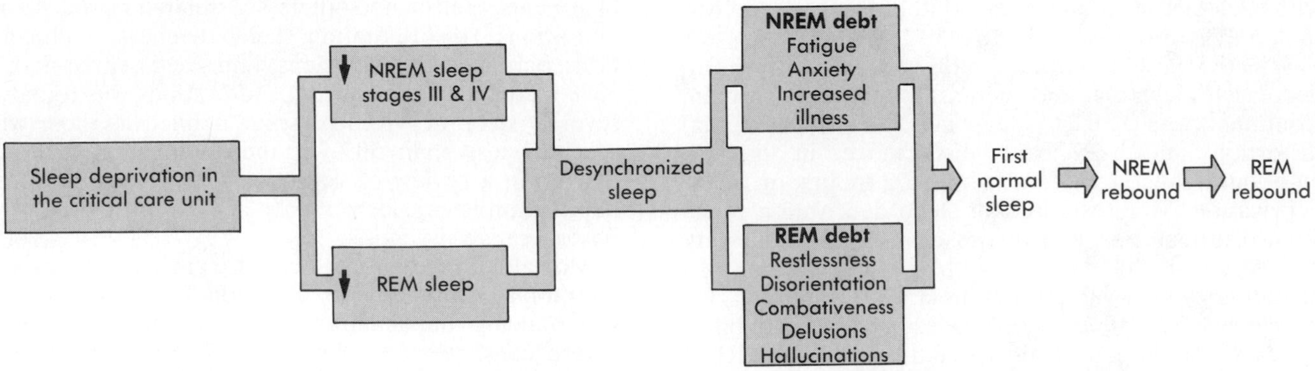

Fig. 10-9 The effects of sleep deprivation on sleep cycling, debt, and rebound. (Modified from Slota M: *Focus Crit Care* 15(3):41, 1988.)

nighttime clothing, bedtime rituals, and medications); any recent changes in the patient's normal pattern resulting from the acute illness; recent and more distant history of sleep disturbances; the severity, duration, and frequency of the problem; and history of chronic illnesses and physical conditions that may disturb sleep, such as COPD, bronchial asthma, bronchitis, arthritis, nocturnal angina, hyperthyroidism, hypertension, duodenal ulcer, or reflux esophagitis and nocturia. The patient's response to the critical care environment should be assessed, along with the noise level in the patient's immediate environment. The critical care nurse should elicit history of snoring because of its relationship to sleep apnea and sleep disturbances. One effective way to assess the quality of the patient's sleep is for the nurse to ask the patient how his or her sleep in the hospital compares with sleep at home. Because of the extreme variations in sleep behaviors, individual differences must be recognized and a flexible, individualized plan of care formulated to promote rest and sleep. Sleep, like pain, is a multidimensional process with considerable individual variations making the assessment of sleep a difficult process. For this reason, both qualitative and physiologic indices are needed to measure sleep.[26] The scientific standard for the measurement of sleep is the polysomnogram (PSG). While the PSG is considered a medical diagnostic and research tool, the nurse can employ it to validate the results of observational and perceptual tools used to measure sleep. In normal, healthy individuals, a high correlation exists between the person's subjective assessment of sleep recorded on a sleep log or questionnaire and PSG data. However, in hospitalized persons this correlation does not always exist.[5,27]

Another problem in the measurement of sleep is that nurses' observations of patients' sleep have demonstrated both overestimation and underestimation of sleep when compared with PSG recordings. When a tool with specific sleep criteria was used, however, the amount of time a patient actually spent awake during the night (a measure of sleep efficiency) was valid when compared with PSG data.[26]

Sleep efficiency is an important sleep variable—it is defined as the proportion of actual sleep time in the total sleep period. Usual adult sleep efficiency is 95% of actual sleep time, whereas in multisystem trauma patients in the critical care area, it may be as low as 65%.[26]

For patients most at risk for a sleep pattern disturbance (e.g., patients with invasive monitoring, those requiring hourly or more frequent assessments and interventions, patients whose illness will require an extended stay in critical care, patients in pain, or patients exhibiting initial signs of sleep deprivation), the nurse's keeping a sleep chart for 48 to 72 hours may assist in assessing actual quantity of sleep in addition to assessing necessary and unnecessary wakenings. The sleep chart should include the date and time, whether the patient was awake or asleep, and any procedures for which it was necessary to awaken the patient. A 24-hour flow sheet such as is common in critical care units could include an area for documentation of sleep. Just as nurses document other data relevant to the patient's recovery, sleep periods of more than 90 minutes in duration, number and length of awakenings, and total possible sleep time should be recorded and evaluated.

REFERENCES

1. Bahr R: Sleep-wake patterns in the aged, *J Gerontol Nurs* 9(10):534, 1983.
2. Guyton AC: *Medical physiology,* ed 8, Philadelphia, 1991, WB Saunders.
3. Rechtschaffen A, Kales A: *A manual of standardized terminology, techniques and scoring systems for sleep stages of human subjects,* 1968, US Department of Health, Education and Welfare.
4. Verrier RL, Kirby DA: Sleep and cardiac arrhythmias, *Ann N Y Acad Sci* 533:238, 1988.

4a. Somers VL and others: Sympathetic/nerve activity during sleep in normal subjects, *N Engl J Med 328*(5):303, 1993.

5. Closs SJ: Assessment of sleep in hospitalized patients: a review of methods, *J Adv Nurs* 13:501, 1988.
6. Hayter J: Sleep behaviors of older persons, *Nurs Res* 32(4):242, 1983.
7. Brock MA: Chronobiology and aging, *J Am Geriatr Soc* 39(1):74, 1991.
8. Hodgson L: Why do we need sleep: Relating theory to nursing practice, *J Advanced Nurs 16*:1503, 1991.

9. Fordham M: In Wilson Bennett J, Butemp L, editors: *Patient problems: a research base for nursing care*, p. 148, London, 1988, Scutain Press.
10. Freemon F: *Sleep research,* Springfield, Ill, 1972, Charles C Thomas.
11. Slota MC: Implications of sleep deprivation in the pediatric critical care unit, *Focus Crit Care* 15(3):35, 1988.
12. Wilse WB: Age related changes in sleep, *Clin Geriatr Med* 5(2):275, 1989.
13. Sanford S: Sleep and the cardiac patient, *Cardiovasc Nurs* 19(5):19, 1983.
14. Farr LA, Campbell-Grossman C, Mack JM: Circadian disruption and surgical recovery, *Nurs Res* 37(3):170, 1988.
15. Deleted in proofs.
16. Brewer MJ: To sleep or not to sleep: the consequences of sleep deprivation, *Crit Care Nurse* 5(6):35, 1985.
17. Wotring K: Using research in practice, *Focus Crit Care* 9(5):34, 1982.
18. Kido L: Sleep deprivation and intensive care unit psychosis, *Emphasis: Nursing 4*(1):23, 1991.
19. Dlin B, Rosen H, Dickstein K: The problems of sleep and rest in the intensive care unit, *Psychosomatics* 12:155, 1971.
20. Woods N, Falk S: Noise stimuli in the acute care area, *Nurs Res* 23:144, 1974.
21. Hilton B: Quantity and quality of patient's sleep and sleep disturbing factors in a respiratory intensive care unit, *Adv Nurs* 1:453, 1976.
22. Helton M, Gordon S, Nunnery S: The correlation between sleep deprivation and ICU syndrome, *Heart Lung* 9(3):464, 1980.
23a. Shaver JL, Giblin EC: Sleep, *Annual Review of Nursing Research*, Chapter 4:71-93. 1989.
23. Noble M: Communication in the ICU: therapeutic or disturbing, *Nurs Outlook* 27:195, 1979.
24. Fabijan M, Gosselin M: How to recognize sleep deprivation in your ICU patient and what to do about it, *Can Nurse* 4:20, 1982.
25. Rosa R, Bonnet M, Warm J: Recovery of performance during sleep following sleep deprivation, *Psychophysiology* 20:152, 1983.
26. Fontaine DK: Measurement of nocturnal sleep patterns in trauma patients, *Heart Lung* 18(4):402, 1989.
27. Richards KC, Bairnsfather L: A description of night sleep patterns in the critical care unit, *Heart Lung* 17(1):35, 1988.

11

Sleep Disorders

CHAPTER OBJECTIVES

- State the four major categories for classifying sleep disorders.
- Define obstructive sleep apnea syndrome.
- Discuss the major complications of obstructive sleep apnea and the implications for critical care nursing practice.
- Describe the treatment of sleep apnea syndrome and state the implications for critical care nursing practice.
- Define central sleep apnea.
- Describe how the medical treatment for central sleep apnea differs from that of obstructive sleep apnea.

CLASSIFICATION OF SLEEP DISORDERS

Sleep disorders have been classified by the Association of Sleep Disorders Centers.[1] In this classification, sleep disorders are divided into four major groups (see box on right). The first is "disorders of initiating and maintaining sleep" (DIMS). The second major category is "disorders of excessive somnolence" (DOES). The third and fourth categories are "disorders of sleep-wake schedule" and "dysfunctions associated with sleep, sleep stages, or partial arousals." This chapter focuses exclusively on sleep apnea syndrome and its management.

SLEEP APNEA SYNDROME

Sleep apnea syndrome (SAS) can be further differentiated as periodic cessation of breathing that results from upper airway obstruction (obstructive sleep apnea), a lack of respiratory muscle activity (central sleep apnea), or a combination of both (mixed apnea). Guilleminault and others[2] have suggested that in all populations except the elderly more than 30 episodes of apnea per 7 hours of sleep or an *apnea index* (the number of apneas per hour) of 5 or greater is diagnostic of SAS. Because a relationship exists between advanced age and sleep apnea episodes, further research must be done to determine diagnostic criteria for every age-group. It has been shown that an apnea index exceeding 20 results in greater mortality. Treatment is recommended for patients with an apnea index of 5 to 20 if additional risk factors, such as smoking, hypercholesterolemia, or high blood pressure, are present. An apnea index less than 20 complicated by daytime sleepiness also requires treatment.[3] SAS results in daytime somnolence, systemic or pulmonary hypertension, arterial blood gas abnormali-

CLASSIFICATION OF SLEEP DISORDERS

I. Disorders of initiating and maintaining sleep (DIMS)
   A. Psychophysiologic DIMS
   B. DIMS with affective disorders
   C. DIMS with tolerance to or withdrawal from central nervous system (CNS) depressants
   D. DIMS with sustained use of CNS stimulants
   E. DIMS with chronic alcoholism
   F. Sleep apnea DIMS syndrome
   G. Alveolar hypoventilation DIMS syndrome
   H. Sleep-related (nocturnal) myoclonus DIMS syndrome
   I. "Restless legs" DIMS syndrome
   J. Etc.

II. Disorders of excessive somnolence (DOES)
   A. Psychophysiologic DOES
   B. DOES with affective disorders
   C. DOES with sustained use of CNS depressants
   D. Sleep apnea DOES syndrome
   E. Alveolar hypoventilation DOES syndrome
   F. Sleep-related (nocturnal) myoclonus DOES syndrome
   G. "Restless legs" DOES syndrome
   H. Narcolepsy
   I. Idiopathic CNS hypersomnolence
   J. Etc.

III. Disorders of the sleep-wake pattern
   A. Rapid time-zone change ("jet lag") syndrome
   B. "Work shift" change in conventional sleep-wake schedule
   C. Frequently changing sleep-wake schedule
   D. Non–24-hour sleep-wake schedule
   E. Irregular sleep-wake pattern
   F. Etc.

IV. Dysfunctions associated with sleep, sleep stages, or partial arousals (parasomnias)
   A. Sleepwalking (somnambulism)
   B. Sleep-related enuresis
   C. Dream anxiety attacks (nightmares)
   D. Sleep-related epileptic seizures
   E. Familial sleep paralysis
   F. Sleep-related painful erections
   G. Sleep-related cluster headaches
   H. Sleep-related asthma
   I. Sleep-related cardiovascular symptoms
   J. Sleep-related hemolysis
   K. Etc.

From Williams RL and others: *Heart Lung* II(3):263, 1982.

ties, life-threatening dysrhythmias, chronic respiratory failure, sexual dysfunction, and mental insufficiency. Hence it is clearly a life-threatening disorder that requires proper diagnosis and treatment.[4]

Obstructive Sleep Apnea

◆ **Definition.** Obstructive sleep apnea (OSA) is the most common form of sleep apnea. OSA is characterized by cessation of air flow resulting from upper airway obstruction, although respiratory effort is exerted. Manifestations can range from a few mild symptoms to very severe symptoms that often constitute Pickwickian syndrome. The syndrome most commonly affects men over age 50 and postmenopausal women, with predominant symptoms being snoring and excessive daytime sleepiness. Patients often have associated obesity, large jowls, and thick necks.[5] Other symptoms include systemic and pulmonary hypertension, arterial blood gas abnormalities, life-threatening cardiac dysrhythmias, chronic respiratory failure, sexual dysfunction, and mental insufficiency. An understanding of OSA is helpful to the critical care nurse, because the physiologic effects of the syndrome can be life threatening.

◆ **Etiologic factors.** The cause of obstructive sleep apnea is not entirely understood; however, upper airway structure, hormonal balance, and neural control are implicated. Factors that contribute to OSA are (1) anatomic narrowing of the upper airway, (2) increased compliance of the upper airway tissue, (3) reflexes affecting upper airway caliber, and (4) pharyngeal inspiratory muscle function.[6] Computerized tomographies of awake subjects have shown that patients with SAS have narrower airways than do normal subjects. The narrower the airway, the more easily it becomes obstructed.

Upper airway patency is also affected by upper airway function, which is under the control of the respiratory motor neurons. During sleep, this control varies and causes decreased neural activity, thereby narrowing the airway. This effect is especially prevalent during REM sleep when the motor neurons are hypotonic. Unstable control of the respiratory nerves of the diaphragm, intercostal, and upper airway muscles can cause sleep apneas.[7] Hypothyroidism can alter respiratory controls and therefore contribute to sleep apnea. Other contributing disorders are exogenous obesity, kyphoscoliosis, and autonomic dysfunction.

◆ **Pathophysiology.** Although the pathophysiology of OSA is unclear, hypotheses suggest that the various types of sleep apnea are all actually part of a disease continuum. Failure of the central respiratory rhythm control center to generate a stable rhythm is thought to be the basic defect responsible for sleep apnea syndrome. Cyclic oscillations occur with greater frequency at night and are further exacerbated by mouth breathing.[8]

The patient with obstructive sleep apnea develops cycles of hypoxemia, hypercapnia, and acidosis with each episode of apnea until he or she is aroused and resumes breathing. Alveolar hypoventilation accompanies each episode of apnea and results in hypercapnia. Between episodes, alveolar ventilation improves so that overall there is not retention of CO_2. Morning headaches may result from lingering hypercapnia.

All types of sleep apnea are accompanied by arterial desaturation and hypoxemia, which may cause pulmonary vasoconstriction and an increased systemic vascular resistance. However, desaturation and hypoxemia are most severe in the obstructive type. With obstruction, inspiratory subatmospheric intrathoracic pressures are abnormally elevated. This leads to a tendency for airways to collapse, resulting in both hemodynamic and electrocardiographic changes.

The extremely elevated pressures that occur in individuals with obstructive sleep apnea who have apneic spells in both REM and NREM stages cause systemic and pulmonary hypertension. Systemic pressures of 200/120 mm Hg (awake control: 130/80 mm Hg) and pulmonary artery pressures of 80/54 mm Hg (awake control: 30/20 mm Hg) have been reported.[7] Cardiac dysrhythmias associated with obstructive apnea include bradycardias, sinus arrest, and occasionally, second-degree heart blocks. After resumption of air flow, tachycardias commonly occur. Thus bradycardia-tachycardia syndrome is associated with obstructive sleep apnea. Careful monitoring can help the nurse identify this syndrome and assist in its diagnosis and treatment.

◆ **Assessment and diagnosis.** The classic features of sleep apnea syndrome are daytime sleepiness and nocturnal snoring. Often the patient's sleep partner originally reports the disrupted sleep, because of episodes of apnea and loud, abrupt sounds as breathing resumes. Patients become excessively sleepy during the day because of sleep fragmentation. Daytime napping and dozing at inappropriate times may be reported. Morning headaches are a complaint of many patients with OSA. The headache is frontal and diffuse, disappearing in several hours. Patients with OSA have increased motor activity during sleep. One significant difference between OSA and narcolepsy is that with the former, patients are able to keep themselves awake, whereas patients with narcolepsy cannot. Memory loss, poor judgment, decreased attention span, irritability, personality changes, exercise intolerance, and impotence often lead to employment difficulties and marital problems for sleep apnea patients.[7] Examination of the throat typically reveals enlarged tonsils, uvula, or tongue or excessive pharyngeal tissue.

Diagnosis of sleep apnea syndrome is made by polysomnogram, a sleep study. The polysomnogram is used to determine the number and length of apnea episodes and sleep stages, number of arousals, air flow, respiratory effort, oxygen desaturation, and vital signs. This monitoring is done using the electroencephalogram, electrooculogram, electromyogram, and electrocardiogram. Respiratory air flow and effort are measured with nasal and oral thermistors and thoracic and abdominal strain gauges, respectively. Gas exchange is monitored with an ear oximeter or a transcutaneous Sao_2 (oxygen saturation) electrode.

After OSA is diagnosed, the patient's hematocrit (Hct) levels are checked for signs of hypoxia-induced polycythemia. Arterial blood gases are checked to assess for daytime hypoxia or hypercapnia. Thyroid function and the pharynx are evaluated for causes of sleep apnea that can possibly be surgically corrected.

◆ **Medical management.** Medical management includes mechanical and surgical approaches, as well as the use of medication. Treatment is varied depending on the type and extent of the patient's illness. Weight loss for those who are overweight is extremely important in the treatment of obstructive sleep apnea. Alcohol should be avoided, particularly before bedtime.

Nasal continuous positive airway pressure (CPAP) has been the most exciting development in recent years in the treatment of obstructive sleep apnea and is currently the treatment of choice.[3] Positive pressure is delivered via a mask placed over the nose splinting the airway open. This improves oxygenation and stimulates afferent impulses from the upper airways, resulting in reflex dilation of the upper airways and stimulation of ventilation. Obstructive sleep apnea is improved by nasal CPAP, which in turn improves the sleep pattern and decreases daytime hypersomnolence.

Uvulopalatopharyngoplasty (UPPP) is a surgical approach to the treatment of obstructive sleep apnea. This procedure is used when anatomic abnormalities are the cause of the obstruction and a surgical approach is indicated. Essentially, a large tonsillectomy is performed and redundant tissue is removed. After this procedure most patients no longer snore; however, only 50% experience sleep apnea improvement.[9] Because of the extensive resection of the posterior pharynx, regurgitation may be a problem for as many as 33% of patients. Patient selection by means of cephalometry of pharyngoscopy to identify the specific site of airway obstruction is important to the success of UPPP and other pharyngeal reconstructive surgeries.

Tracheostomy is rarely used in the treatment of obstructive sleep apnea since the devleopment of nasal CPAP. Fewer than 5% of patients currently require tracheostomy.[3] It is indicated for severe apnea with life-threatening dysrhythmias, cor pulmonale, hypersomnolence, and failure of conservative treatment. The complications of tracheostomy are significant, including infection, bleeding, bronchitis, and granulation tissue, as well as the psychosocial complications of an altered body image.

Because obstructive sleep apnea is so well treated by nasal CPAP, drug therapy is used only if CPAP is ineffective or unavailable. In selected cases medroxyprogesterone acetate (Provera), a central respiratory stimulant, is used and has been shown to improve waking CO_2 retention. Protriptyline HCL (Vivactil), a nonsedating tricyclic antidepressant that suppresses REM sleep, has been shown to decrease the number of apnea episodes and reduce daytime hypersomnolence. Oxygen may be used to relieve hypoxemia and nocturnal desaturations. In general, drug therapy has been disappointing in the treatment of obstructive sleep apnea.

◆ **Nursing management.** Nursing management for patients diagnosed with OSA includes educating the patient, monitoring the effects of drug therapy, providing preoperative teaching, and monitoring for and preventing postoperative complications of UPPP or tracheostomy. Medroxyprogesterone acetate stimulates alveolar hypoventilation but in the dosages required for sleep apnea may be too expensive for some patients, and it may have feminizing effects in men. For these reasons, patient compliance with therapy may be jeopardized. Protryptyline reduces daytime hypersomnolence and nocturnal apneas. In addition to these effects, however, it has the anticholinergic effects of urinary retention and tolerance with prolonged use. Oxygen, as with other drugs, needs careful monitoring to verify its effectiveness and proper dosage.

Nasal CPAP is most effective when patients are properly fitted with the nasal mask and have adequate instruction in the application of the mask and blower. Allowing patients to develop comfort with the equipment facilitates the success of the therapy.

UPPP reduces the number of apneas. Complications of UPPP include hemorrhage, infection, swallowing difficulty, impaired speech, nasal reflux, dry mouth, increased gag reflex, and recurrence of snoring.[9] Patients need close postoperative observation of their airways because of airway edema (refer to Chapter 24, Ineffective Airway Clearance). Postoperative pain is common but manageable with analgesics. Precautions to avoid respiratory depression in this group of patients are imperative. Patients should be observed for regurgitation phenomena and signs of infection.

In the event that a tracheostomy is indicated, patients need to be evaluated for their ability to care for the tracheostomy at home. Careful preoperative instruction should include airway management techniques, such as suctioning and routine tracheostomy changes; information about communication techniques with the tracheostomy; explanation of comfort measures, such as pain relief; and close nursing observation. Emphasis should be placed on the relief of the apnea symptoms accom-

NURSING DIAGNOSIS AND MANAGEMENT
Status post-uvulopalatopharyngoplasty (UPPP)

- ◆ High Risk for Aspiration risk factors: impaired laryngeal sensation or reflex; impaired laryngeal closure or elevation; decreased lower esophageal sphincter pressure, p. 472
- ◆ Acute Pain related to transmission and perception of cutaneous, visceral, muscular, or ischemic impulses secondary to UPPP, p. 566
- ◆ Sleep Pattern Disturbance related to fragmented sleep, p. 142
- ◆ Anxiety related to threat to biologic, psychologic, and/or social integrity secondary to uncertain outcome of UPPP, p. 763
- ◆ Knowledge Deficit: Reportable Symptoms related to lack of previous exposure to information, p. 72

plished by the tracheostomy. Patients with UPPP may temporarily require a tracheostomy for airway management after the UPPP procedure. The critical care nurse must support the patient and family during the critical phase after the operation and be especially sensitive to long-term adjustments to changes in body image. In this case, the nurse can assist the patient to deal with possible disenchantment during convalescence.

Central Sleep Apnea

◆ **Definition, etiology, pathophysiology, assessment, and diagnosis.** Central sleep apnea (CSA) is not a single disease, but rather a heterogenous group of disorders in which breathing ceases momentarily during sleep because of transient withdrawal of central nervous system (CNS) drive to the muscles of respiration.[10] Central sleep apnea is characterized by decreased respiratory output along with the absence of thoracic and abdominal muscle movements. Patients complain of disrupted sleep and waking with a choking feeling. Snoring may be present. Central sleep apnea is a relatively rare disorder, occurring at perhaps 10% the rate of OSA. Patients tend to be older and have less pronounced oxygen desaturation and hemodynamic effects. The mechanisms involved in central sleep apnea include defects in the respiratory control mechanism or muscles, transient instabilities in respiratory drive, and reflex inhibition of central respiratory drive. Central sleep apnea can be viewed clinically by hypercapnic and nonhypercapnic responses. Hypercapnic CSA arises in the situation of central alveolar hypoventilation or respiratory neuromuscular disease. This type of CSA is associated with encephalitis, brain stem neoplasm or infarction, spinal cord injury, muscular dystrophy, myasthenia gravis, bulbar poliomyelitis, and postpolio syndrome. Nonhypercapnic CSA occurs most frequently in patients with Cheyne-Stokes respiration secondary to other medical disorders or as an idiopathic disorder.[10]

Because the underlying mechanisms are heterogenous, the presenting symptoms are variable as well. Patients presenting with hypercapnic CSA characteristically present with symptoms of chronic respiratory failure. Patients presenting with nonhypercapnic CSA present with a pattern of breathing characterized by a waxing and waning of tidal volume. This type of CSA can occur in patients with congestive heart failure and in patients with renal/metabolic disturbances.

◆ **Medical management.** Central sleep apnea associated with central alveolar hypoventilation is managed generally by noninvasive measures—such as advice not to use sedative medications—and supplemental O_2 at nighttime after an assessment has been made of gas exchange during both sleep and wakefulness. Respiratory stimulants such as medroxyprogesterone can improve ventilation during sleep in selected patients. If noninvasive and pharmacologic measures fail, consideration is given to a phrenic nerve pacemaker for nocturnal diaphragmatic stimulation or some form of assisted ventilation. Assisted ventilation may be intermittent positive pressure ventilation via a snug-fitting nasal mask or may require a tracheostomy to assist ventilations. When there is associated neuromuscular weakness, supplemental O_2 and assisted ventilation with a nasal mask is generally very effective.[10]

◆ **Nursing management.** The nursing management of the patient with central sleep apnea involves careful nighttime observation and assessment of breathing pattern. Anxiety about or fear of sleep because of apneic episodes is common and should be confronted. Patient reassurance of continuous nursing observation and monitoring is helpful.

For the patient with a chest cuirass, observation for upper airway collapse as a result of this treatment is essential. Supplemental oxygen may help some patients.[7]

REFERENCES

1. Association of Sleep Disorders Centers, prepared by the Sleep Disorders Classification Committee, Roffwarg HP, chairman: Diagnostic classification of sleep and arousal disorders, *Sleep* 2:1, 1979.
2. Guilleminault C, van den Hoed J, Milter M: Clinical overview of sleep apnea syndrome. In Guilleminault C, Dement WC, editors: *Sleep apnea syndromes,* New York, 1978, Alan R Liss.
3. Kryger MH: Management of obstructive sleep apnea, *Clin Chest Med* 13(3):481, 1992.
4. Mishoe S: The diagnosis and treatment of sleep apnea syndrome, *Respir Care* 32(3):183, 1987.
5. Katz I, Stradling J, Slutsky AS, and others: Do patients with obstructive sleep apnea have thick necks? *Am Rev Resp Disorders* 141:1228, 1990.
6. Hudgel DW: Mechanisms of obstructive sleep apnea, *Chest* 101:541 1992.
7. Weaver T, Millman R: Broken sleep, *Am J Nurs* 86(2):146, 1986.
8. Bjurstrom R, Schoene R, Pierson D: The control of ventilatory drives: physiology and clinical applications, *Respir Care* 31(11):1128, 1986.
9. Sanders M and others: The acute effects of uvulopalatopharyngoplasty on breathing during sleep in sleep apnea patients, *Sleep* 11(1):75, 1988.
10. Bradley TD, Phillipson EA: Central sleep apnea, *Clin Chest Med* 13(3):493, 1992.

12

Sleep Nursing Diagnosis and Management

This chapter is designed to supplement the preceding chapters in the *Sleep Alterations* unit by integrating theoretic content into clinically applicable case studies and nursing management plans.

The case study is designed to illustrate clinical problem solving and patient care management occurring in actual patients. The case, reviewed retrospectively, demonstrates how medical and nursing diagnoses may be effectively used in critical care. The case study also demonstrates revisions to the plan of care and the nursing and medical management outcomes that are apt to occur during the course of a complicated hospitalization as the patient responds physiologically to treatment. Often in a short case anecdote, such as presented in this chapter, the clinical answer may appear to be obvious from the day of admission. In practice, however, critical care patient management is sometimes investigative and the "correct" diagnosis for an individual patient may not become apparent until midway in the hospitalization. Or a patient with an apparently straightforward diagnosis may develop an unexpected complication, and the plan of care and potential outcomes will then require revision. Many of the case studies demonstrate this principle.

The nursing management plans, which—unlike the case study—are not patient-specific, provide a basis nurses can use to individualize care for their patients. In the previous *Sleep Alterations* chapters, each medical diagnosis is assigned a Nursing Diagnosis and Management box. Using this box as a page guide, the reader can access relevant nursing management plans for each medical diagnosis. For example, nursing management of *status post-uvulopalatopharyngoplasty* (UPPP), described on p. 138, may involve several nursing diagnoses and management plans outlined in this chapter and in other Nursing Diagnosis and Management chapters. Specific examples are (1) *Sleep Pattern Disturbance related to fragmented sleep,* on p. 142 and (2) *Anxiety related to threat to biologic, psychologic, and/or social integrity secondary to uncertain outcome of UPPP*, on p. 763. These examples highlight the interrelationship of the various physiologic systems in the body and the fact that pathology often has a multisystem impact in the critically ill.

Use of the case study and management plans can enhance the understanding and application of the *Sleep* content in clinical practice.

SLEEP CASE STUDY

CLINICAL HISTORY

Mr. T is a 73-year-old, muscular, well-nourished, retired construction worker. He has a history of moderate restrictive lung disease. Also, he has had several cerebral vascular accidents, which affected Broca's speech area, but he is now without residual effects. He has a permanent VVI pacemaker for sick sinus syndrome.

CURRENT PROBLEMS

Mr. T arrived at the clinic with chest discomfort that did not radiate and shortness of breath with exertion. Echocardiogram evaluation showed a large aneurysm of the ascending aorta and aortic dilation, stenosis, and insufficiency.

EMERGENCY MEDICAL MANAGEMENT

Surgical intervention was recommended. Mr. T had an unstable intraoperative course that involved a 4-hour run on heart-lung bypass, including circulatory arrest with profound hypothermia (to 16° C) and retrograde cerebral perfusion for 63 minutes. He was admitted to the surgical intensive care unit. His postoperative course was complicated by excessive bleeding secondary to coagulopathy; this required massive blood product replacement. He also experienced pulmonary shunting, which required an FIO_2 of .80 with positive end-expiratory pressure (PEEP) of 15 cm H_2O to maintain adequate oxygenation. Three days postoperatively Mr. T was responsive to commands, although he required Versed at 1 mg/hr. Mr. T received Lasix per IV drip and as a result diuresed some of the 25-pound weight gain. He made slow but definite progress, with decreasing oxygen needs.

SLEEP CASE STUDY—cont'd

MEDICAL DIAGNOSIS

Elective resection and grafting of ascending aortic aneurysm complicated by coagulopathy and adult respiratory distress syndrome (ARDS)

NURSING DIAGNOSES

◆ Impaired Gas Exchange related to ventilation/perfusion mismatch secondary to non-cardiac pulmonary edema associated with ARDS
◆ High Risk for Altered Nutrition: Less than Protein-Calorie Requirements risk factor: inability to ingest nutrients secondary to endotracheal intubation
◆ High Risk for Sleep Pattern Disturbance risk factors: fragmented sleep and/or circadian desynchronization

◆ PLAN OF CARE

1. Continue to monitor for impaired gas exchange.
2. Monitor for altered tissue perfusion.
3. Monitor for altered nutrition including effects on healing, infection, and skin integrity.
4. Monitor for sleep pattern disturbance by initiating a sleep record to document actual sleep cycles.

MEDICAL AND NURSING MANAGEMENT AND PATIENT OUTCOME

Mr. T's cardiopulmonary status stabilized such that he could be weaned successfully from epinephrine, Levophed, and amrinone drips, requiring only a dobutamine drip. He started total parenteral nutrition on the 5th postoperative day. Mr. T continued to require mechanical ventilation; however, the FIO_2 he required could be decreased to .40 with PEEP of 5 cm H_2O. Mr. T continued to require sedation; every time it was decreased, he became so restless that there was danger of dislodging the endotracheal tube. A neurologist was consulted, and a CT scan documented a recent cerebral infarct. Mr. T was following commands with both sides of his body although the left side was weaker than the right. The sleep record indicated that for the past week Mr. T had potentially accomplished only two sleep cycles in any 24-hour period. Eleven days postoperatively, Mr. T began to show signs of extreme agitation. Haldol was ordered and scheduled to be administered q 4 hours.

MEDICAL DIAGNOSIS

Resolving ARDS and inability to wean from mechanical ventilation

NURSING DIAGNOSES

◆ Sleep Pattern Disturbance related to circadian desynchronization and fragmented sleep secondary to sensory overload secondary to critical illness and care
◆ Activity Intolerance related to postural hypotension secondary to prolonged immobility

◆ REVISED PLAN OF CARE

1. Modify environmental factors to promote sleep.
2. Assess patient's sleep history as reported by spouse. Assess bedtime rituals, daily routines, factors that contribute to comfort and relaxation.
3. Balance patient's activity with rest periods. Schedule activity to decrease 2 hours before bedtime.
4. Help patient maintain a consistent sleep/wake cycle.
5. Continue to document sleep pattern with periods of time awake.
6. Encourage patient to assist in his personal care. Begin with low energy ADLs, such as face washing and oral care.

MEDICAL AND NURSING MANAGEMENT AND PATIENT OUTCOME

Mr. T was moved to a private room. Designated times for rest were initiated, with one rest period in the morning and one in the afternoon. At home, Mr. T customarily had fallen asleep watching TV at 10:30 PM. His family brought in pictures of family members for his room and an afghan Mr. T used when he slept on the couch at home. Mr. T's agitation decreased. His sleep pattern was now four or five sleep cycles at night, with one consistent nap per day. He was gaining energy and was able to sit in a chair for 2 hours without tiring. He was able to wash his face and perform oral care with assistance. A tracheostomy was performed on the fourteenth postoperative day.

Continued.

SLEEP CASE STUDY—cont'd

MEDICAL DIAGNOSIS

Same

NURSING DIAGNOSIS

- Sleep Pattern Disturbance related to fragmented sleep and circadian desynchronization

◆ REVISED PLAN OF CARE

1. Continue with measures to promote sleep.
2. Continue to encourage small increments of self-care. Teach strengthening exercises that patient can perform in bed.
3. Encourage participation in decision making related to care through use of a communication board.
4. Begin oral feedings with patient assisting as tolerated.

MEDICAL AND NURSING MANAGEMENT AND PATIENT OUTCOME

Mr. T continued to gain strength and maintained 4 or 5 sleep cycles per night. He was able to be weaned from the ventilator to a tracheostomy cradle at 40% oxygen. Tube feedings were continued at night to supplement a full liquid diet. Mr. T was transferred to the intermediate care area in good spirits and was able to communicate his wishes. He was making steady progress in his ability to ambulate to and from the chair in his room.

SLEEP PATTERN DISTURBANCE RELATED TO FRAGMENTED SLEEP

DEFINING CHARACTERISTICS

- Decreased sleep during one block of sleep time
- Daytime sleepiness
- Sleep deprivation
  - Less than one half of normal total sleep time
  - Decreased slow wave, or REM, sleep
- Anxiety
- Fatigue
- Restlessness
- Disorientation and hallucinations
- Combativeness
- Frequent wakenings
- Decreased arousal threshold

OUTCOME CRITERIA

- Patient's total sleep time approximates patient's normal.
- Patient can complete sleep cycles of 90 minutes without interruption.
- Patient has no delusions, hallucinations, illusions.
- Patient has reality-based thought content.
- Patient is oriented to four spheres.

NURSING INTERVENTIONS AND *RATIONALE*

1. Continue to monitor the assessment parameters listed under "Defining Characteristics."
2. Assess normal sleep pattern on admission and any history of sleep disturbance or chronic illness that may affect sleep or sedative/hypnotic use. Promote normal sleep activity while patient is in critical care unit. Assess sleep effectiveness by asking patient how his or her sleep in the hospital compares with sleep at home. (Refer to Chapter 30, *Sensory/Perceptual Alterations,* for the management of acutely psychotic/suspicious patient.)
3. Minimize awakenings ***to allow for at least 90-minute sleep cycles.*** Continually assess the need to awaken the patient, particularly at night. Distinguish between essential and nonessential nursing tasks. Organize nursing care to allow for maximum amount of uninterrupted sleep while ensuring close monitoring of the patient's condition. Whenever possible, monitor physiologic parameters without waking the patient. Coordinate awakenings with other departments, such as respiratory therapy, laboratory, and x-ray, ***to minimize sleep interruptions.***

SLEEP PATTERN DISTURBANCE RELATED TO FRAGMENTED SLEEP–cont'd

4. Minimize noise, particularly that of the staff and noisy equipment. Reduce the level of environmental stimuli.
5. Plan nap times to assist in equilibrating the normal total sleep time. Discourage or prevent catnaps (sleep lasting longer than 90 minutes at a time) ***because these physically refresh the individual and thereby decrease the stimulus for longer sleep cycles in which REM sleep is obtained.*** Early morning naps, however, may be beneficial in promoting REM sleep ***because a greater proportion of early morning sleep is allocated to REM activity.***
6. Promote comfort, relaxation, and a sense of well-being. Treat pain. Eliminate stressful situations before bedtime. Use of relaxation techniques, imagery, backrubs, or warm blankets may be helpful. Other interventions may include increased privacy or a private room and providing the patient with his or her own garments or coverings. Individual patients may prefer quiet or may prefer the background noise of the television ***to best promote sleep.***
7. Be aware of the effects of commonly used medications on sleep. ***Many sedative andhypnotic medications decrease REM sleep.*** Sedative and analgesic medications should not be withheld, but rather, drugs that minimally disrupt sleep should be used to complement comfort measures, with dosages reduced gradually as the medication is no longer necessary. Do not abruptly withdraw REM-suppressing medications, ***because this can result in "REM rebound."***
8. Foods containing tryptophan (e.g., milk or turkey) may be appropriate ***because these promote sleep.***
9. Be aware that the best treatment for sleep deprivation is prevention.
10. Facilitate staff awareness that sleep is essential and health promoting. Assess the critical care unit for sleep-reducing stimuli and work to minimize them.
11. Document amount of uninterrupted sleep per shift, especially sleep episodes lasting longer than 2 hours. This can be effectively documented as part of the 24-hour flow sheet and reported routinely, shift to shift. ***Sleep pattern disturbance is diagnosed, treated, and resolved more efficiently when formally documented in this manner.***

SLEEP PATTERN DISTURBANCE RELATED TO CIRCADIAN DESYNCHRONIZATION

DEFINING CHARACTERISTICS

- ◆ Sleep is out of synchronization with biologic rhythms, resulting in sleeping during the day and awakening at night
- ◆ Anxiety and restlessness
- ◆ Decreased arousal threshold

OUTCOME CRITERIA

- ◆ Majority of patient's sleep time will fall during low cycle of the circadian rhythm (normally at night).

NURSING INTERVENTIONS AND *RATIONALE*

1. Continue to monitor the assessment parameters listed under "Defining Characteristics."
2. Assist patient to maintain normal day-night cycles by decreasing lighting, noise, and sensory stimulation at night and critically evaluating the need to awaken the patient at night. Maintain a regular schedule for external time cues, such as mealtimes and favorite telvision shows.
3. Activity during the daytime should be increased to stimulate wakefulness. Increased physical activity until 2 hours before bedtime is useful in ***promoting naturally induced sleep.*** Limiting caffeine intake after early afternoon will promote sleep in the evening.
4. Do not schedule routine procedures at night.
5. Be aware that cardiac dysrhythmias can be precipitated by the decreased arousal threshold secondary to desynchronization.
6. If desynchronization occurs, plan for resynchronization by maintaining constancy in day-night pattern for at least 3 days (may require 5 to 12 days to reacclimatize). Plan for activities during the day ***to stimulate wakefulness*** and use comfort measures (comfortable body position, warm blankets, backrub, etc.) ***to promote sleep*** at night. Resynchronization is characteristically associated with chronic fatigue, malaise, and a decreased ability to perform life tasks.

IV

CARDIOVASCULAR ALTERATIONS

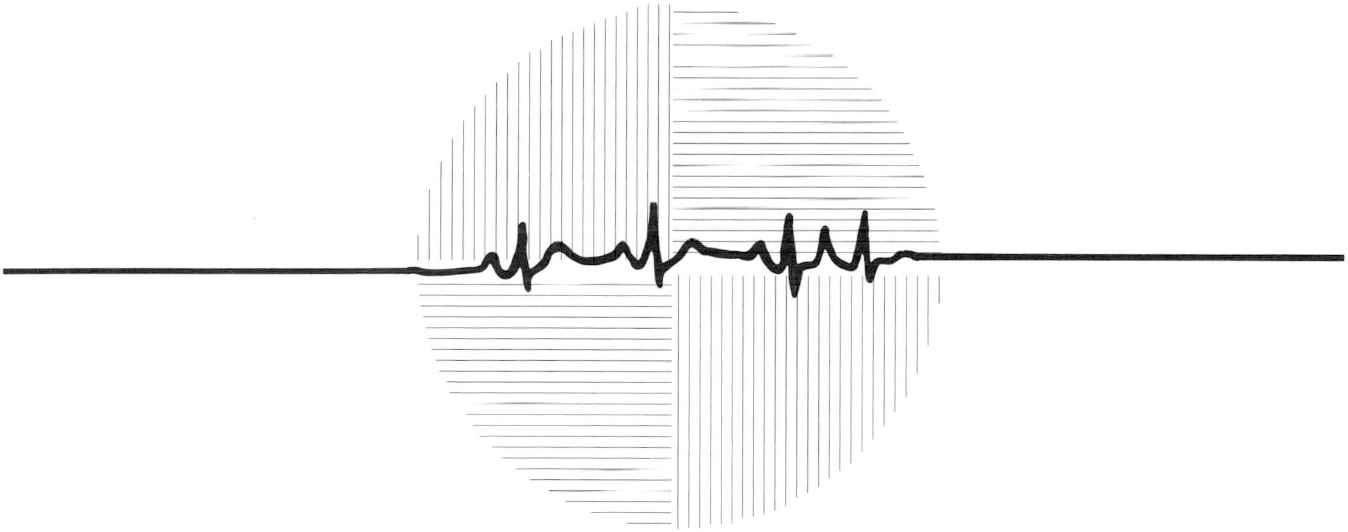

13

Cardiovascular Anatomy and Physiology

CHAPTER OBJECTIVES

- Identify and briefly describe the physiology of the normal anatomic structures of the heart and blood vessels.
- Discuss the ionic and electrical basis of the resting membrane potential and the phases of the action potential.
- Discuss the role of calcium and the contractile proteins in excitation-contraction coupling.
- Trace the normal sequence of depolarization through the cardiac conduction system.
- Identify the determinants of cardiac output.
- Describe the nervous system control of the heart and blood vessels.

The study of the structure and function of the heart and circulatory system will enhance the working knowledge in any area of critical care. This chapter provides the critical care nurse with concepts that will enable the delivery of more thorough and comprehensive nursing care. It is hoped that the information presented here will not only enlighten, but also inspire further study and thought.

ANATOMY

Discussion of the structure of the heart and blood vessels will begin on a macroscopic level and progress to the cellular and molecular level.

Macroscopic Structure

◆ **Structures of the heart.** The heart is situated in the anterior thoracic cavity, just behind the sternum (Fig. 13-1). Posterior to the heart are several structures, including the esophagus, aorta, vena cava, and vertebral column. The position of the heart is such that the right ventricle constitutes the majority of the inferior (or diaphragmatic) and anterior surfaces, and the left ventricle makes up the anterolateral and posterior surfaces. The broader side (base) of the heart is superior, and the tip (apex) is inferior. The base of the heart includes not only the superior portion of the heart itself, but also the roots of the aorta, vena cava, and pulmonary vessels.

Size and weight of the heart. The average human heart is about the size of the clenched fist of that individual. In the adult, this averages 12 cm in length and 8 to 9 cm in breadth at the broadest part. In adult men, the weight of

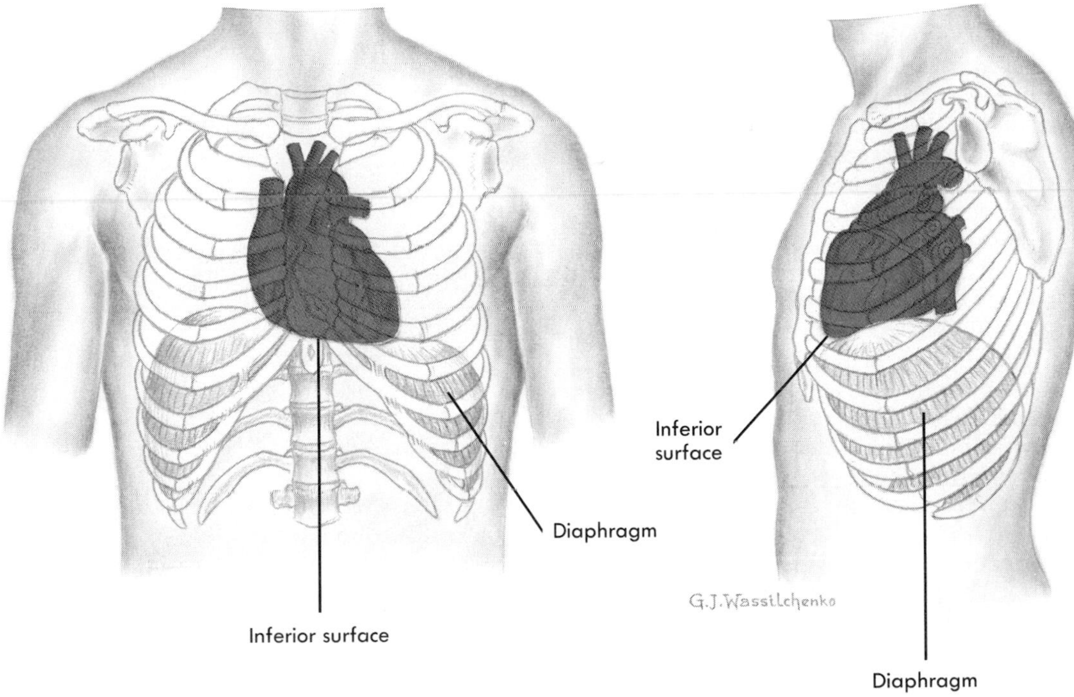

Fig. 13-1 Anatomic location of the heart within the thoracic cavity.

the heart averages 310 g, and that of women averages 255 g. Although there are no significant differences in ventricular wall thickness between men and women, mean values of heart weights increase in women between the third and tenth decades of life. In general, body weight appears to be a better predictor of normal heart weight than is body surface area or height.[1]

Layers of the heart. There are four distinct layers of the heart. The heart and roots of the great vessels are surrounded by a fibrous sac called the *pericardium,* also known as the *parietal pericardium.* The pericardium functions to hold the heart in a fixed position, as well as to provide a physical barrier to infection. The *epicardium* is tightly adhered to the heart and base of the great vessels and is sometimes referred to as the *visceral pericardium.* Together, the pericardium and epicardium form a sac around the heart. This sac normally contains a very small amount of pericardial fluid (approximately 10 ml) that serves as a lubricant between the pericardium and the epicardium. The pericardium is noncompliant to rapid increases in cardiac size or amount of fluid in the sac. For example, blood or serum can abnormally collect in this sac, as occurs in cardiac tamponade or pericardial effusion. If the fluid collection in the sac impinges on ventricular filling, ventricular ejection, or coronary artery perfusion, a clinical emergency may exist that would necessitate removal of the excess pericardial fluid to restore cardiac function.

Next is the thick muscular layer – the *myocardium,* or mid-wall. This layer includes all of the atrial and ventricular muscle fibers necessary for contraction. The fibers of the myocardium are not organized along a single plane throughout the thickness of the ventricular wall, but they have a distinct arrangement such that the force of contraction is most efficient in ejecting blood toward the outflow tracts in a wringing motion (Fig. 13-2).

The innermost layer is the *endocardium,* which is a thin layer of endothelium and connective tissue lining the heart. The endothelial lining is continuous with the blood vessels and includes intracardiac structures such as the papillary muscles and valves. Disruption in the endothelium as a result of surgery, trauma, or congenital abnormality can predispose the area to infection. This infective endocarditis is a devastating disease that, if left untreated, can lead to massive valve damage or sepsis and death.

Cardiac chambers. The human heart has four chambers – the left and right atria and the left and right ventricles. The atria, or auricles, are thin-walled and normally low-pressure chambers. They function to receive blood from the vena cava and pulmonary arteries and to pump blood into their respective ventricles. Atrial contraction (also called *atrial kick*) contributes approximately 30% to ventricular filling, whereas the other 70% occurs passively during diastole. The ventricles are the main pumping forces of the heart. The right ventricle is approximately 3 mm thick, whereas the left ventricle is 10 to 13 mm thick (Fig. 13-3). The right ventricle pumps blood into the low-pressured pulmonary circulation, which has a normal mean pressure of approximately 15

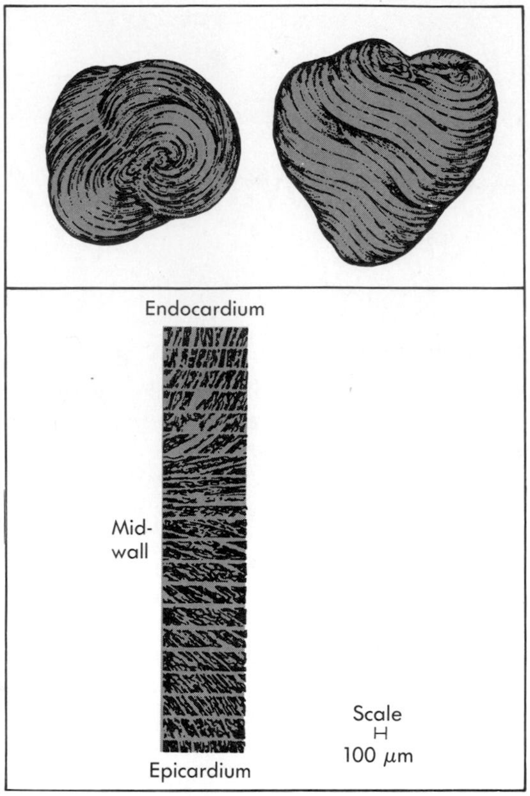

Fig. 13-2 Macroscopic and microscopic structure of the ventricular musculature. **A,** Spiral musculature of the ventricular walls. **B,** Sequence of photomicrographs showing fiber angles in successive sections taken from the middle of the free wall of the left ventricle from a heart in systole. The fiber angle changes at various depths in the heart wall. Compare with **A** to obtain a concept of nonparallel forces generated during ventricular systole. (**B** from Streeter DD, Jr and others: *Circ Res* 24:339, 1969. Reprinted with permission of the American Heart Association.)

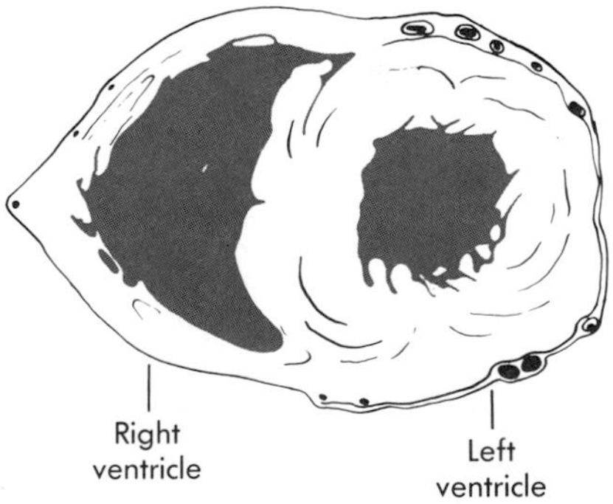

Fig. 13-3 A transverse section of the ventricles of the adult heart. The right ventricle forms the greater part of the anterior surface of the heart, and the wall of the left ventricle is 3 times as thick as the wall of the right ventricle. (From Quaal S: *Comprehensive intraaortic balloon pumping,* St Louis, 1984, Mosby–Year Book.)

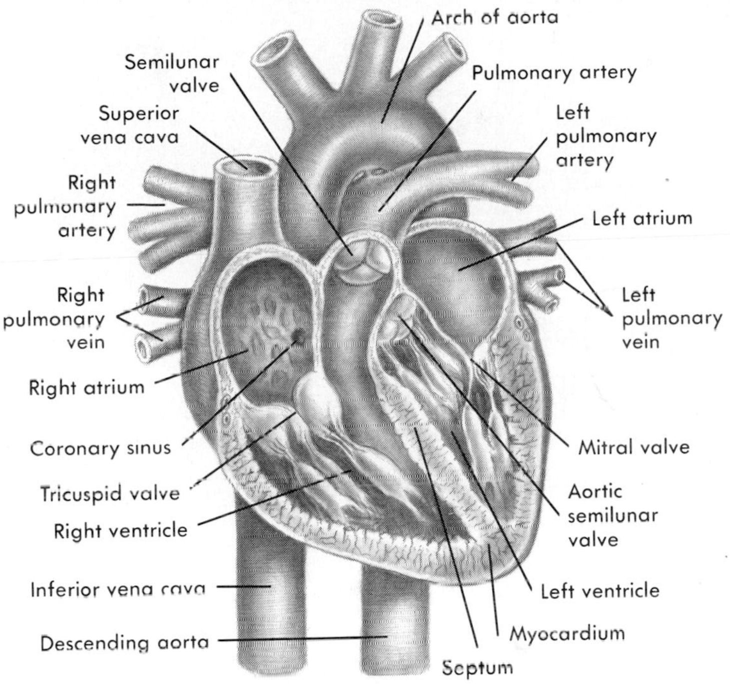

Fig. 13-4 Cross-sectional view of the heart. Note the position of the four cardiac valves. (From Thompson JM and others: *Mosby's clinical nursing,* ed 3, St Louis, 1993, Mosby-Year Book.)

mm Hg. The left ventricle must generate tremendous force to eject blood into the aorta (normal mean pressure of approximately 100 mm Hg). Because of left ventricular thickness and the great force it must generate, the left ventricle is considered the major pump of the heart. When the left ventricular muscle thins out as the result of dilation or disease, the effective pumping pressure may be diminished, leading to left atrial congestion, pulmonary vasculature congestion, and ultimately systemic venous congestion.

Cardiac valves. Cardiac valves are composed of flexible, fibrous tissue that is thinly covered by endocardium. The structure of the valves allows blood to flow in only one direction. The opening and closing of the valves is essentially passive and depends on pressure gradients on both sides of the valve.

There are four cardiac valves, all of which are essential to proper cardiovascular function (Fig. 13-4). The two atrioventricular (AV) valves, so named for their location, are the *tricuspid* (three cusps) valve and the *mitral* (two cusps) valve. The AV valves prevent backflow of blood into the atria during ventricular contraction. The *chordae tendineae* and *papillary muscles,* which attach to the tricuspid and mitral valves, give the valves stability and prevent valve leaflet eversion during systole (Fig. 13-5). Papillary muscles, located in the apical area of the endocardium, derive their blood supply from the coronary arteries. Each papillary muscle gives rise to approximately four to ten main chordae that divide into finer and finer cords as they approach the valve leaflets. The chordae tendineae are basically avascular structures covered by a thin layer of endocardium. A dysfunction of the chordae tendineae or of a papillary muscle can cause incomplete closure of an AV valve, which can result in a murmur. For example, after an acute myocardial infarction (AMI), the papillary muscles may be at risk for rupture as a result of inadequate blood supply from the coronary circulation. When a papillary muscle in the left ventricle ruptures, the mitral valve leaflets do not close completely. Clinically, this situation can cause a mitral regurgitation murmur that can potentially worsen the pulmonary congestion and lower cardiac output.

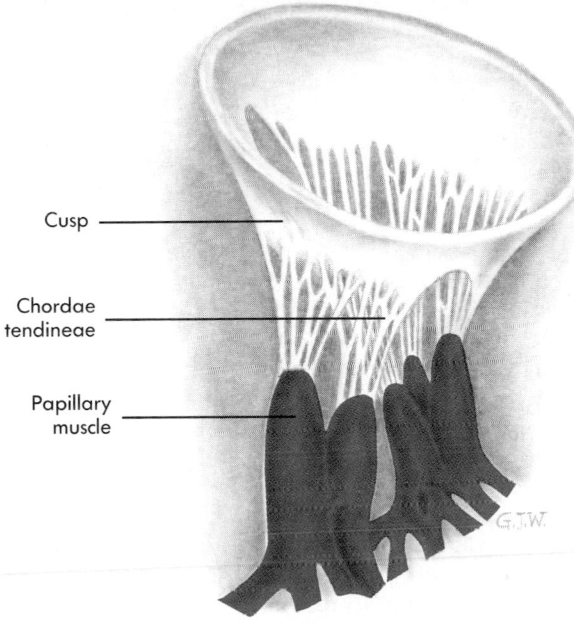

Fig. 13-5 Diagram of the mitral valve and the relationships of the cusps, chordae tendineae, and the papillary muscles.

The semilunar valves, the *pulmonic* and *aortic* valves, each has three main cuplike cusps (Fig. 13-6). These valves separate the ventricles from their respective

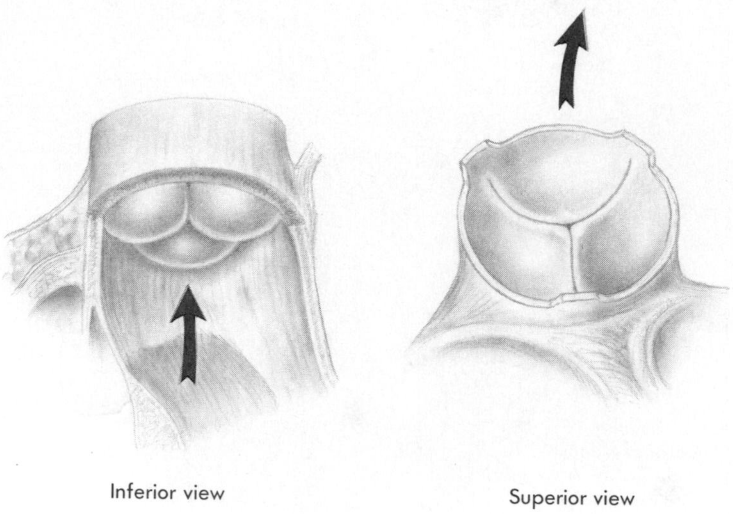

Fig. 13-6 Diagram of the aortic valve and the cuplike cusps.

Table 13-1 Summary of the cardiac valves and their locations

Valve	Type	Situated between
Tricuspid	AV	Right atrium, right ventricle
Pulmonic	SL	Right ventricle, pulmonary artery
Mitral	AV	Left atrium, left ventricle
Aortic	SL	Left ventricle, aorta

AV, atrioventricular; *SL*, semilunar.

Table 13-2 Intrinsic pacemaker rates of cardiac conduction tissue

Location	Rate (beats/min)
SA node	60-100
AV node	40-60
Purkinje fibers	15-40

outflow arteries (Table 13-1). During ventricular systole, the semilunar valves open, allowing blood to flow out of the ventricles. As systole ends and the pressure in the outflow arteries exceeds that of the ventricles, the semilunar valves close, thus preventing blood regurgitation back into the ventricles.

◆ **The conduction system.** The history of the discovery of the conduction system dates back to 1845, when Purkinje wrote a classic paper describing ventricular conductive cells. Recently, breakthroughs in electrophysiology have advanced not only clinical cardiology, but also the cardiac surgery arena.[2,3] Despite these advances and the well-characterized nature of the cardiac conduction system, there are still many concepts in the area of impulse propagation that require further research.[4,5] This section discusses the three main areas of impulse propagation and conduction—the SA node, the AV node, and the His/Purkinje fibers.

The sinoatrial node. The sinoatrial (SA) node is considered the natural pacemaker of the heart, because it has the highest degree of automaticity or intrinsic heart rate (Table 13-2). The node is usually a spindle-shaped structure located near the mouth of the superior vena cava, on the posterior aspect of the right atrium. There is some normal variability in the position and shape of the node. The SA node contains basically two types of cells, the specialized pacemaker cells found in the node center and the border zone cells. Both the pacemaker cells and the border zone cells have inherent depolarization capabilities (they automatically depolarize 60 to 100 times per minute). The cells in the nodal center are responsible for the ac ual pacemaking of the heart. The fibers in the border zone cells also have intrinsic pacemaker properties, but depolarization is depressed by the surrounding atrial tissue.[6]

Once the center nodal cells depolarize, the impulse is conducted through the nodal border zone toward the atrium. Atrial depolarization occurs both cell to cell and also through four specialized conduction pathways that exit the SA node (Fig. 13-7, *A*). These conduction pathways are Bachman's bundle, which is directed to the left atrium, and three internodal pathways that are directed to the AV node.

The atrioventricular node. The atrioventricular (AV) node is located posteriorly on the right side of the interatrial septum. Because the atria and ventricles are separated by nonconductive tissue, all electrical impulses initiated in the atria will be conducted to the ventricles solely via the AV node. Although the AV node also possesses pacemaker cells, the intrinsic rhythmicity is less than that of the SA node (Table 13-2). So, as an impulse from the SA node arrives at the AV node, the AV node will be depolarized (Fig. 13-7, *B*), resetting its own pacemaker potential. This prevents the AV node from initiating its own pacemaker impulse that would compete with the SA node.

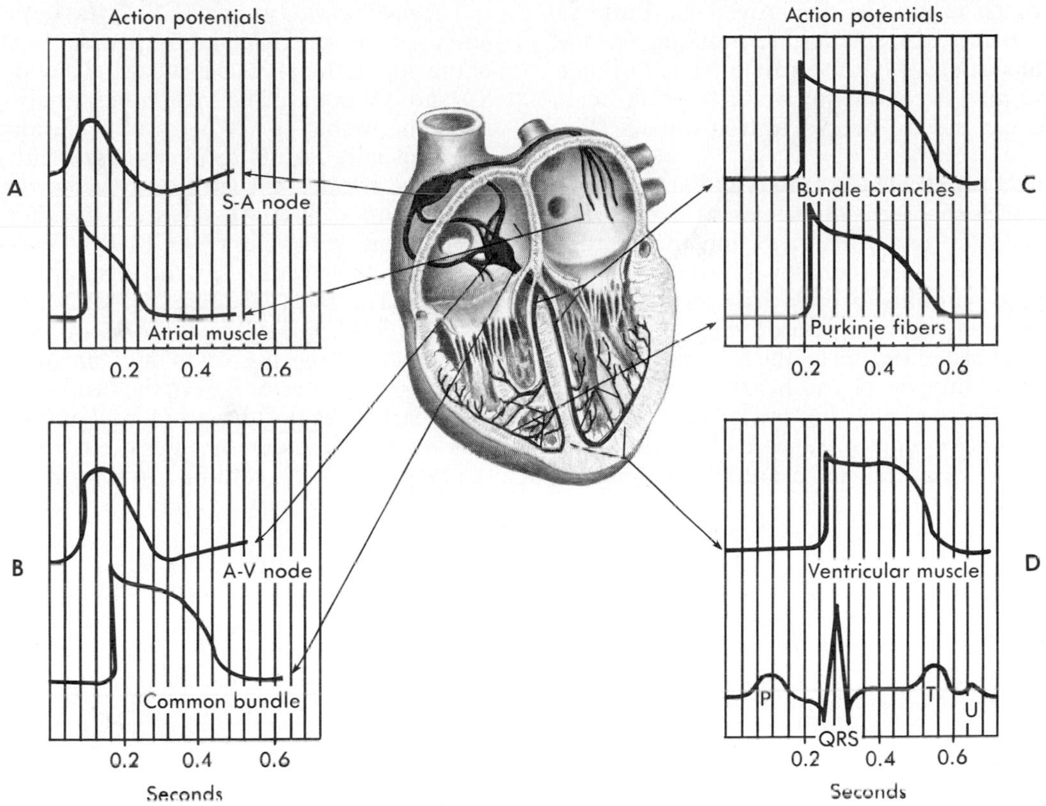

Fig. 13-7 Heart with normal conduction pathways and transmembrane action potentials of **A,** SA node and atrial muscle; **B,** AV node; **C,** bundle branches; and **D,** ventricular muscle. (From Thompson JM and others: *Mosby's clinical nursing,* ed 3, St Louis, 1993, Mosby–Year Book.)

As the depolarization impulse from the SA node arrives at the AV node, a slight conduction delay occurs through the AV node. This delay is a result of the inherent properties of the nodal structures that cause a slowing of conduction velocity. The purpose of this delay is to allow adequate time for optimal ventricular filling from atrial contraction. If no electrical delay occurred, the mechanical event of atrial contraction would not have sufficient time to add to ventricular filling. This would lower end-diastolic ventricular volume and potentially lead to lowered cardiac output. The AV nodal delay also functions as a protection mechanism for the ventricles. As a result of the slowed conduction velocity through the AV node, conduction is thus time dependent and hence limits the contraction frequency of the ventricles. For example, when an abnormal number of electrical impulses bombard the AV node during atrial flutter or atrial fibrillation, the AV nodal delay limits the number of impulses that move through to the ventricles. Without this delay, the ventricles would receive each atrial impulse and the heart would quickly decompensate.

Another property in the AV node is that of retrograde (backward) conduction. This means that an electrical impulse that is initiated in or below the AV node can be conducted in a backward fashion. When this happens, the propagation time is generally longer than that of antegrade (forward) conduction. This may manifest itself in a variety of heart and conduction disease conditions, as well as in the postoperative recovery period after certain cardiac surgical procedures. In this instance, the coordinated efforts of atria and ventricles are diminished or lost, resulting in lack of atrial kick to ventricular filling. Detection of this condition is made by the electrocardiogram (ECG).

Bundle of His and Purkinje fibers. Electrical impulses are conducted in the ventricles through the bundle of His and the Purkinje fibers (Fig. 13-7, *C*). The bundle of His fibers runs through the subendocardium down the right side of the interventricular septum. About 12 mm from the AV node, the bundle of His divides into the right and left bundle branches. The right bundle branch continues down the right side of the interventricular septum toward the right apex. The left bundle branch is thicker than the right and takes off from the bundle of His at almost a right angle. It then traverses the septum to the subendocardial surface of the left interventricular wall, where it divides into a thin anterior and a thick posterior branch. Functionally, when one of the left branches is blocked, it is referred to as a *hemiblock.* All of the bundle branches are subject to conduction defects (bundle branch blocks) and give rise to characteristic changes in the ECG.

The right bundle branch and the two divisions of the

left bundle branch eventually divide into the Purkinje fibers. These divide many times, terminating in the subendocardial surface of both ventricles. The Purkinje fibers have the fastest conduction velocity of all heart tissue. Ventricular muscle depolarization follows (Fig. 13-7, *D*).

◆ **Coronary blood supply.** The coronary circulation consists of those vessels that supply the heart structures with oxygenated blood (coronary arteries) and then return the blood to the general circulation (coronary veins). The right and left coronary arteries arise at the base of the aorta immediately above the aortic valve (Fig. 13-8). After leaving the base of the aorta, the coronary arteries traverse along the outside of the heart in the natural grooves (sulci). To perfuse the thick heart muscle, branches from these main arteries arise at acute angles, penetrating the muscular wall and eventually feeding the endocardium (Fig. 13-9).

The *right coronary artery* (RCA) serves the right atrium and the right ventricle in most people. In more than half of the population, it also is the usual blood supply for the SA and AV nodes. The *left coronary artery* (also referred to as the *widow maker* because occlusion of this main vessel usually results in immediate death) divides into two large arteries, the *left anterior descending* (LAD) and the *circumflex.* These vessels serve the left atria and most of the left ventricle (Fig. 13-10). There is a huge spectrum of variation in the disposition of coronary arteries. The term *dominant* coronary artery was introduced in 1940. The *dominant coronary artery* is the artery that traverses the posterior interventricular sulcus and supplies the posterior part of the ventricular septum and often part of the posterolateral wall of the left ventricle.[7]

After blood passes through the coronary capillaries, the majority of it is returned to the right atrium via the coronary veins, exiting via the coronary sinus. In

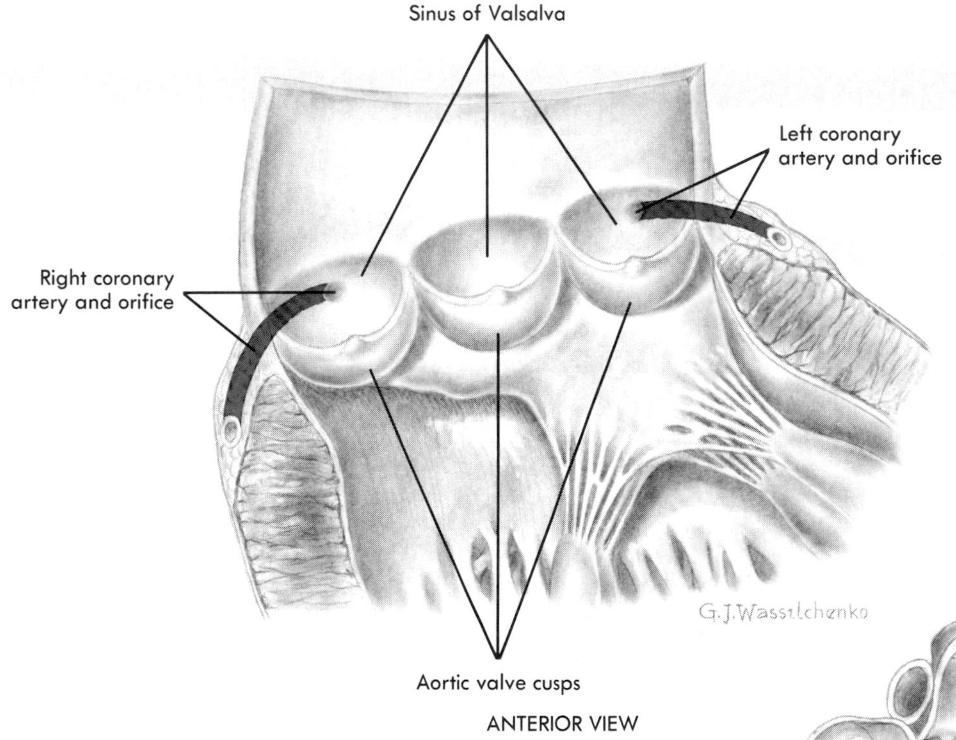

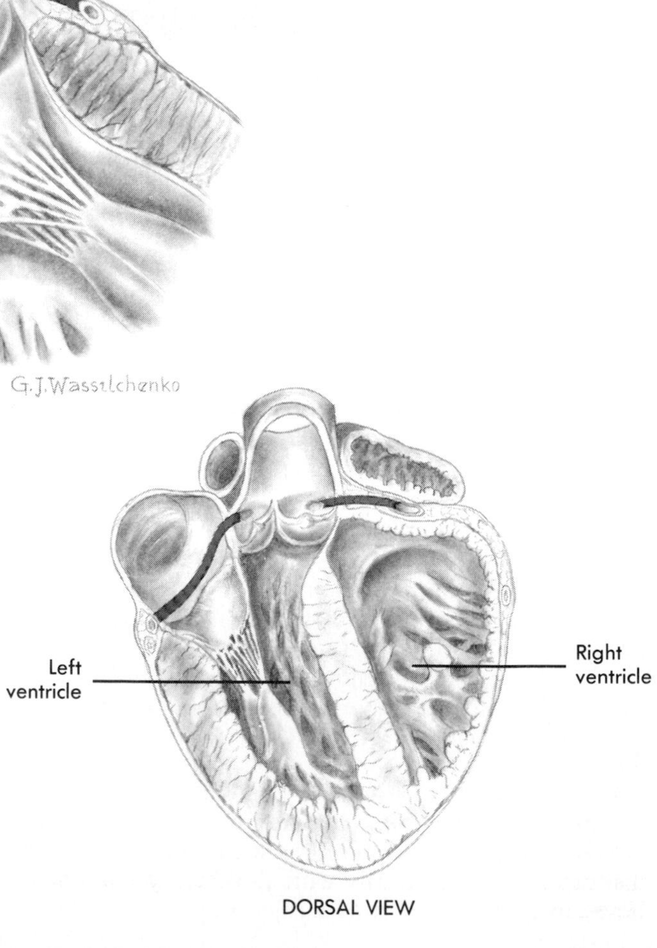

Fig. 13-8 Proximity of the right and left coronary arteries to the aortic valve and the sinus of Valsalva.

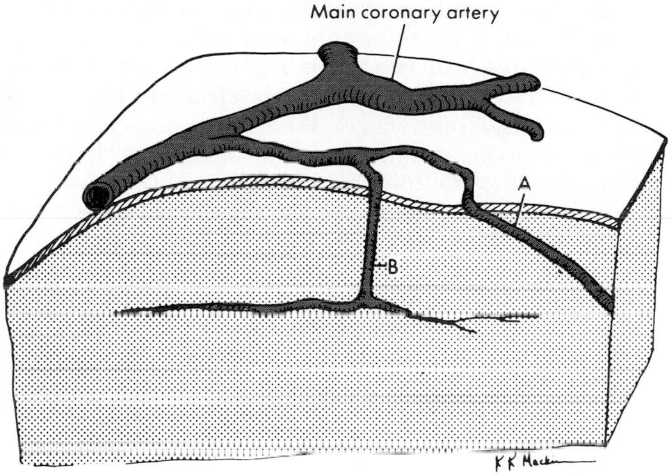

Fig. 13-9 Intramyocardial distribution of coronary arteries. *A*, Epicardial arteries rise at acute angles from main coronary vessels to supply epicardial surface of the heart. *B*, Smaller vessels branch at oblique angles from main coronary vessels that penetrate deeper into the myocardium and endocardium (intramural arteries). (From Quaal S: *Comprehensive intraaortic balloon pumping,* St Louis, 1984, Mosby–Year Book.)

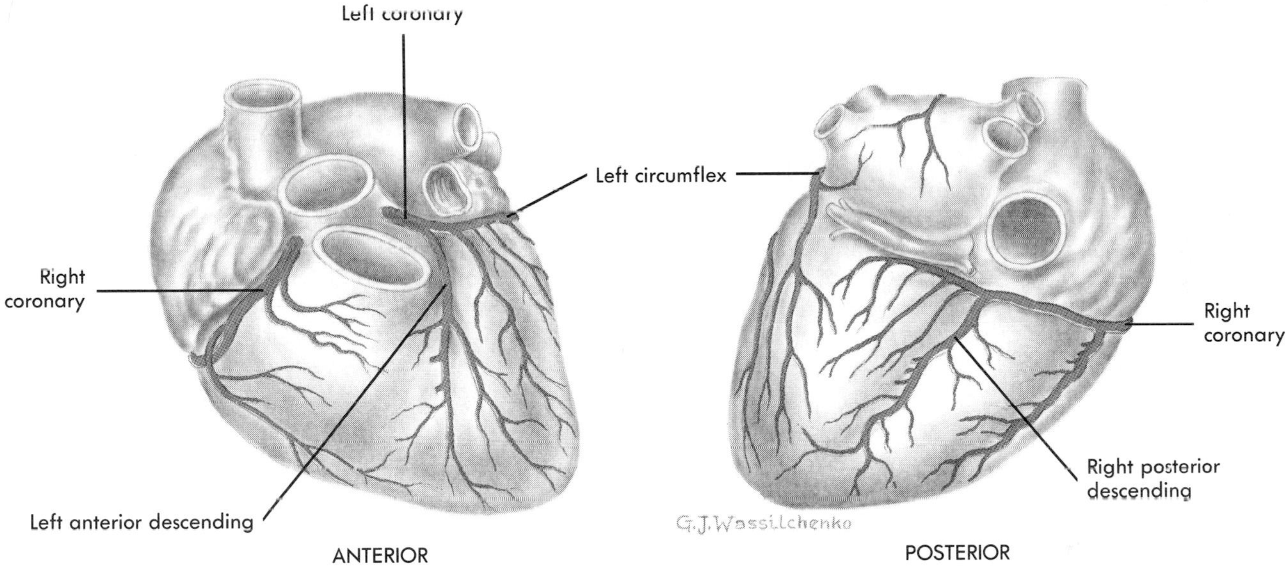

Fig. 13-10 Anterior and posterior views of the coronary artery circulation.

addition, the *Thebesian vessels* are small veins that connect capillary beds directly with the cardiac chambers and also communicate with cardiac veins and other Thebesian veins. However, some of the blood returns directly to the chambers via vascular communications of irregular endothelium-lined sinuses within the muscular structure. These veins that drain into the left ventricle would therefore add unoxygenated blood to the freshly oxygenated blood. When unoxygenated blood mixes with freshly oxygenated blood in the left ventricle, it is called a *physiologic shunt.* An example of a normal shunt is the previously mentioned situation in which unoxygenated blood from the myocardium drains into the left ventricle. An example of an abnormal shunt is an opening in the ventricular septum, called a *ventricular septal defect (VSD),* which allows large amounts of venous blood from the right ventricle to mix with the freshly oxygenated blood in the left ventricle.

Several clinical situations merit a brief discussion here. During ventricular contraction, no blood flows to the cardiac tissue because of the contracted state of the cardiac muscle and resulting occlusion of arteries within the musculature. Coronary artery circulation is highest during early diastole, after the aortic valve has closed. During an episode of tachycardia, diastolic time is greatly diminished; hence coronary perfusion time is diminished. This offers a possible explanation for compromised coronary blood flow during times of rapid heart rate. Conversely, during bradycardia, diastole is prolonged. However, coronary inflow may also be compromised as a result of the lack of adequate pressure and aortic recoil in late diastole to perfuse the myocardium.[8]

◆ **The systemic circulation.** If the purpose of the heart is to generate enough pressure to pump the blood, it is the function of the vascular structures to act as conduits to carry vital oxygen and nutrients to each cell and also to carry away waste products. Also of primary importance is the ability to exchange those nutrients and waste products at the cellular level. The vascular system acts not only as a conducting system for the blood, but as a control mechanism for the pressure in the heart and vessels. So, it is actually the complex interplay between the heart and the blood vessels that maintains adequate pressure and velocity within this system for optimal functioning.

The arterial system. Arteries are constructed of three layers (Fig. 13-11). The innermost layer, or the *intima,* is a thin lining of endothelium and a small amount of elastic tissue. This smooth lining decreases resistance to blood flow and minimizes the chance for platelet aggregation. The *media,* or middle layer, is made up of smooth muscle and elastic tissue. This muscular layer changes the lumen diameter when necessary. The *adventitia,* which is the outermost layer, is largely a connective tissue coat that helps strengthen and shape the vessels.

The intima and the adventitia layers remain relatively constant in the vascular system, whereas the elastin and smooth muscle in the media change proportions, depending on the type of vessel. The aorta contains the greatest amount of elastic tissue, necessary because of the sudden shifts in pressure created by the left ventricle. The arterioles, or smaller arteries, and precapillary sphincters have more smooth muscle than do the larger arteries and aorta, because they function to change the luminal diameter when regulating blood pressure and blood flow to the tissues (Fig. 13-12).

Blood flow and blood pressure. The pulsatile nature of arterial flow is caused by intermittent cardiac ejection and the stretch of the ascending aorta.[9] The pressure wave initiated by left ventricular ejection (Fig. 13-13) travels considerably faster than does the blood itself. Thus when an examiner palpates a pulse, it is this propagation of the pressure wave that is perceived.

In the normal arterial system, the blood flow is called *laminar,* or *streamlined,* because the fluid moves in one direction. However, there are small differences in the linear velocities within a blood vessel.[10] The layer of blood immediately adjacent to the vessel wall moves relatively slowly, because of the friction caused as it comes in contact with the motionless blood vessel wall. In contrast, the fluid more central in the lumen travels more rapidly. The most central blood travels at the highest velocity (Fig. 13-14). Clinical implications include conditions in which the vessel wall has an abnormality, such as a small clot or plaque deposit. This disruption in the streamlined flow can set up eddy currents that may predispose the area to platelet aggregation and thus enlargement of the abnormality.

Blood pressure (BP) measurement has several components. The systolic blood pressure (SBP) represents the ventricular volume ejection and the response of the arterial system to that ejection. The diastolic value (DBP) indicates the ventricular resting state of the arterial system. The pulse pressure is the difference between the SBP and DBP. The mean arterial pressure (MAP) is the mean value of the area under the BP curve (Fig. 13-15). BP may be measured several ways.[11] Direct measurement is accomplished by means of a catheter

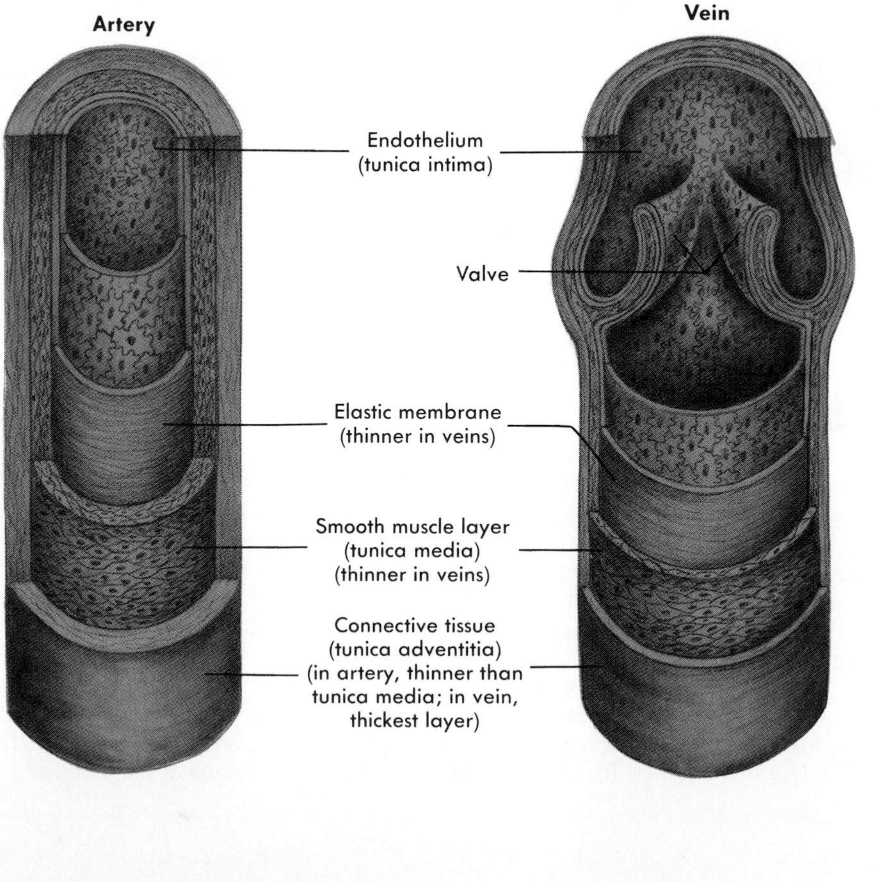

Fig. 13-11 Cross-section of an artery and vein showing the three layers: tunica intima, tunica media, and tunica adventitia. Note the difference in wall thickness between the artery and the vein and the lack of valves within the artery. (From Thompson JM and others: *Mosby's clinical nursing,* ed 3, St Louis, 1993, Mosby–Year Book.)

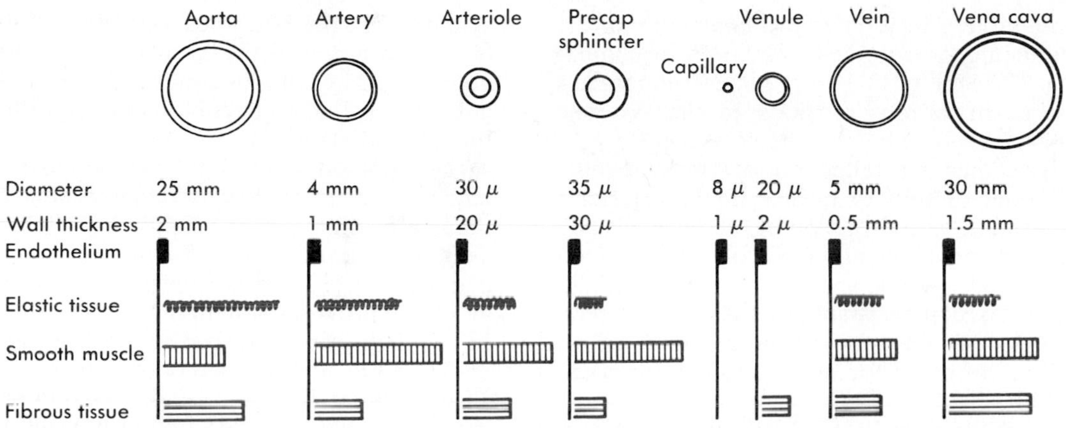

Fig. 13-12 Internal diameter, wall thickness, and relative amounts of the principal components of the vessel circulatory system. Cross-sections of the vessels are not drawn to scale because of the huge range from aorta to vena cava to capillaries. (From Berne RM, Levy MN: *Cardiovascular physiology,* ed 6, St Louis, 1991, Mosby–Year Book.)

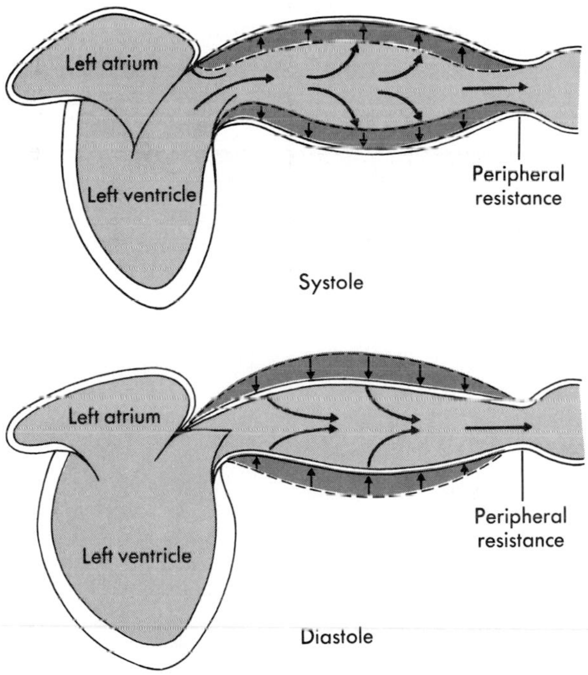

Fig. 13-13 Elastic and recoil properties of the aorta. (From Berne RM, Levy MN: *Cardiovascular physiology,* ed 6, St Louis, 1991, Mosby–Year Book.)

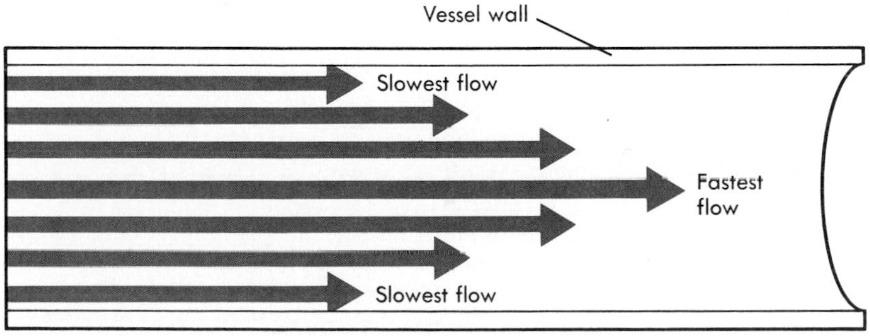

Fig. 13-14 Laminar flow in an artery.

inserted into a large artery. The most common indirect method is by means of a stethoscope and sphygmomanometer (Fig. 13-16). Fig. 13-17 graphically summarizes blood pressures in various portions of the systemic circulatory system.

Vascular resistance is a reflection of arteriolar tone. The large amount of smooth muscle in the arterioles allows for relaxation or contraction of these vessels and causes changes in resistance and redistribution of blood flow. The values of systemic vascular resistance (SVR) and pulmonary vascular resistance (PVR) are based on calculations from other hemodynamic parameters (see Appendix C for formulas for normal values for SVR, PVR, and MAP).

Precapillary sphincters and the microcirculation. Where present, the precapillary sphincters are small cuffs of smooth muscle that control blood flow at the junction of the arterioles and the capillaries. The precapillary sphincters allow selective blood flow into capillary beds, depending on their contractile state. The precapillary sphincters are not innervated by the autonomic nervous system as are the arterioles; rather, they respond to local or circulating vasoactive agents. This means that they do not have direct nervous connection to sympathetic input but will respond to circulating epinephrine released by the adrenal gland.

As the blood reaches the capillary level, the pulsatile nature of arterial flow is damped (Fig. 13-17). Even though the diameter of a capillary is less than that of the arteriole, the pressure and flow velocity in the capillary bed is relatively low as a result of the branching nature and large cross-sectional area of the capillary bed (Fig. 13-18). The capillary consists of a single cell layer of endothelium and is devoid of muscle or elastin (Fig. 13-12). Hence diffusion of solutes into and out of the capillary is not impeded by mechanical barriers. Thus the capillaries normally retain large structures, such as red blood cells, but are permeable to smaller solutes, such as electrolytes. Although true capillaries do not contain smooth muscle, there is evidence that the endothelium can change its shape and may even secrete substances that influence smooth muscle in other vessels.

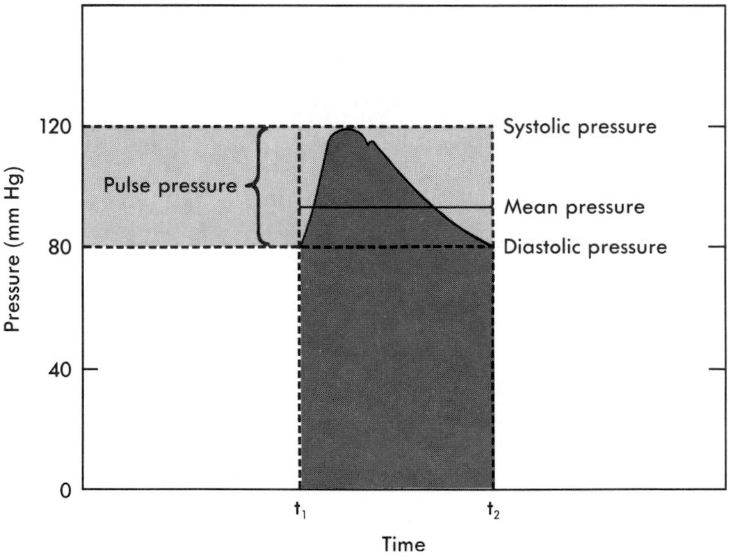

Fig. 13-15 Arterial systolic, diastolic, pulse, and mean pressures. (From Berne RM, Levy MN: *Cardiovascular physiology,* ed 6, St Louis, 1991, Mosby–Year Book.)

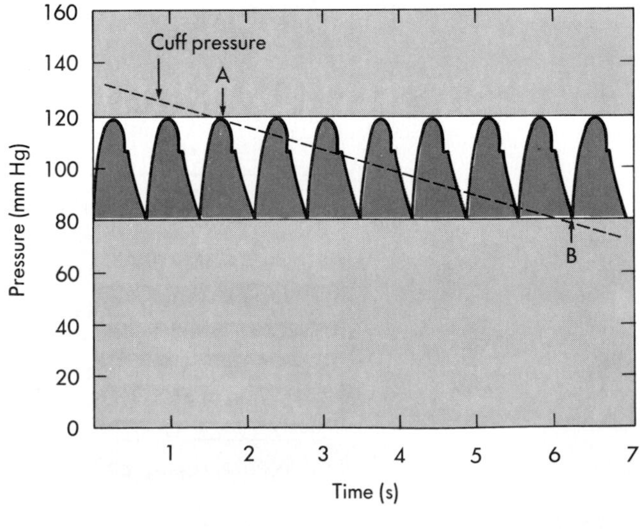

Fig. 13-16 Principles of blood pressure measurements with a sphygmomanometer. The oblique line represents pressure in the inflatable bag in the cuff. At cuff pressures greater than the systolic pressure (*to the left of* **A**), no blood progresses beyond the cuff and no sounds can be detected below the cuff with the stethoscope. At cuff pressures between the systolic and diastolic levels (*between* **A** *and* **B**), spurts of blood traverse the arteries under the cuff and produce Korotkoff's sounds. At cuff pressures below the diastolic pressure (*to the right of* **B**), arterial flow past the region of the cuff is continuous and no sounds are audible. (From Berne RM, Levy MN: *Cardiovascular physiology,* ed 6, St Louis, 1991, Mosby–Year Book.)

Also, different capillary beds have greater permeability than do others (e.g., liver), and some sites along the same capillary have greater permeability (venous versus arterial end).

The venous system. As the blood leaves the capillary system, it passes through the venules and into the veins. Both venules and veins contain elastic tissue, smooth muscle, and fibrous tissue (Fig. 13-12). The veins, however, contain a greater percentage of smooth muscle and fibrous tissue to accommodate the large venous volume and demands for reserve capacity. The majority of circulating blood is contained in the veins that are referred to as *capacitance vessels* (Fig. 13-19). Approximately 60% of the total blood volume is found in the veins and is hemodynamically "inactive," meaning that this blood volume does not directly contribute to blood pressure and other hemodynamic parameters. This enables the body to tap into a ready reserve during times of need. For example, when a person changes from a supine to a sitting position, approximately 7 to 10 ml blood/kg of body weight is pooled in the legs. Cardiac output decreases by approximately 25%, but arterial BP is maintained by reflex vasoconstriction. Thus the primary function of capacitance vessels under reflex control is to redistribute the blood to or from the heart

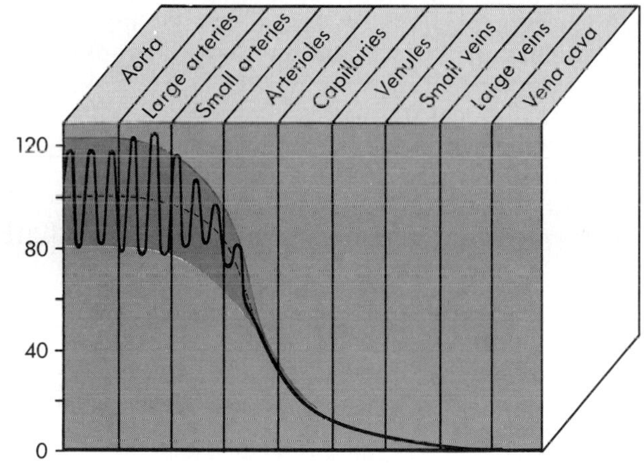

Fig. 13-17 Blood pressures in the different portions of the systemic circulatory system.

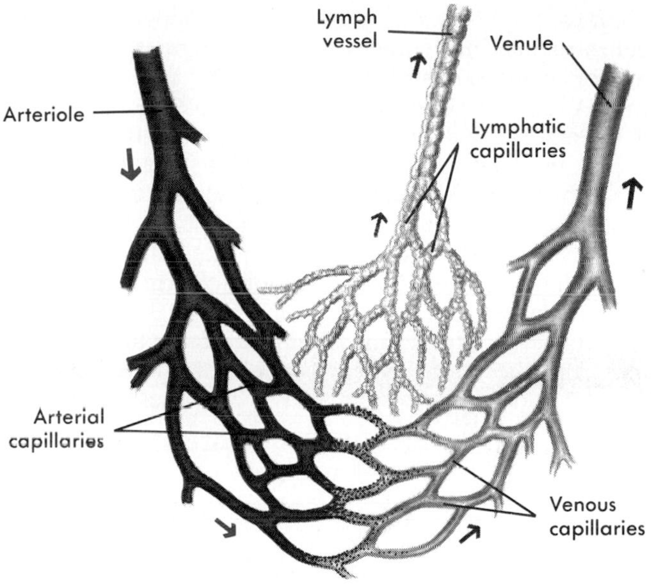

Fig. 13-18 Microcirculation. Note the branching nature and large cross-sectional area of the capillary bed. (From Thompson JM and others: *Mosby's clinical nursing,* ed 3, St Louis, 1993, Mosby–Year Book.)

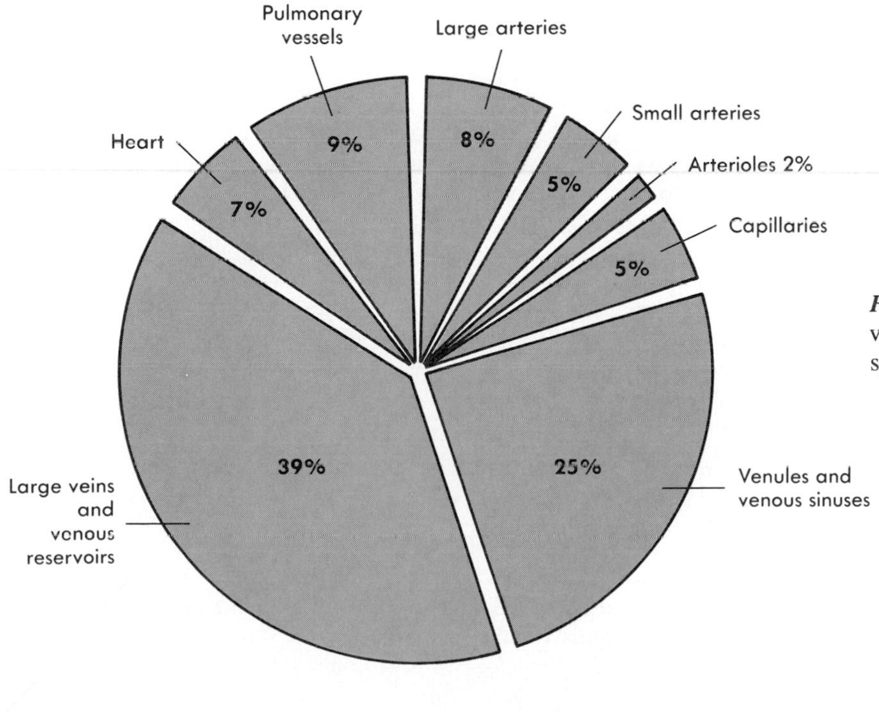

Fig. 13-19 Percentage of the total blood volume in each portion of the circulation system.

to maintain optimal cardiac filling pressures. In human beings, these reservoirs are greatest in the splanchnic bed (liver and intestines). Thus patients with decreased blood reserves, such as occurs in a dehydrated or hypovolemic individual, require special caution during position changes, especially from supine to standing. Before helping such a patient to stand, one should allow him or her to "dangle" (sit on the side of the bed) to check for adequate venous reserves.

Microscopic Structure

To understand and appreciate the unique pumping ability of the heart, one must have knowledge of cardiac cell structure and function. This section reviews the anatomic mechanisms responsible for the contractile process in cardiac muscle cells.

◆ **Cardiac fibers.** Cardiac muscle fibers are typically found in a latticework arrangement. The fiber cells (myofibrils) divide, rejoin, and then separate again, but they retain distinct cellular walls and possess a single nucleus. This differs greatly from skeletal muscle, in which the cells have fused together to form a fiber and have many nuclei.

In general, cardiac myofibrils run on a longitudinal axis, and the fibers appear striped, or striated. When viewed under an electron microscope, these striations are actually the contractile proteins (Fig. 13-20). The areas separating each myocardial cell from its neighbor are called *intercalated disks,* which are continuous with the *sarcolemma,* or cell membrane. The point where a longitudinal branch of the cell meets another cell branch is the tight junction (or *gap junction*), which offers much less of an impedance to electrical flow than does the sarcolemma. Because of this, depolarization will occur from one cell to another with relative ease.[12] Also, the cardiac muscle is a *functional syncytium,* in which depolarization started in any cardiac cell will quickly be spread to all of the heart.

◆ **Cardiac cells.** Each cardiac cell contains two types of intracellular contractile proteins, *actin* and *myosin.* These proteins abound in the cell in organized longitudinal arrangements. When visualized by electronmicroscopy, the myosin filaments appear thick, whereas the almost double amounts of actin filaments appear thin. The actin filaments are connected to the Z bands on one end, leaving the other end free to interact with the myosin crossbridges. In the resting muscle cell, the actin and myosin partially overlap. The ends of the myosin filament that overlap with the actin have tiny projections (Fig. 13-21). For contraction to occur, these projections interact with the actin to form crossbridges (Fig. 13-21). The portion of the muscle fiber between two Z bands is

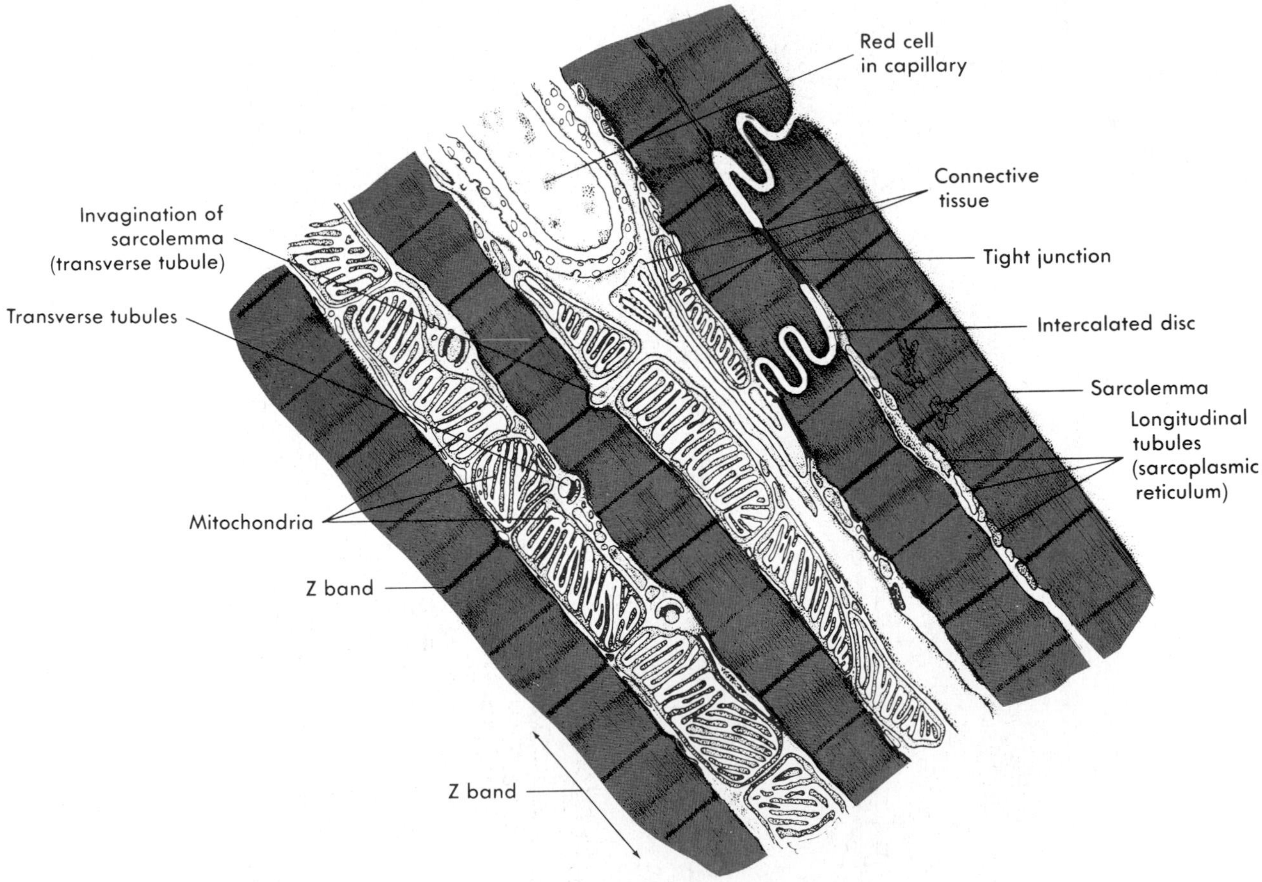

Fig. 13-20 Diagram of an electron micrograph of cardiac muscle showing the large numbers of mitochondria, the intercalated disks with tight junctions, the transverse tubules, and the longitudinal tubules (also known as the sarcoplasmic reticulum) (approximately × 30,000). (From Berne RM, Levy MN: *Cardiovascular physiology,* ed 6, St Louis, 1991, Mosby–Year Book.)

called a *sarcomere.* In a normal resting state, the sarcomere is about 2.0 to 2.2 μm. Another extremely important intracellular structure necessary for successful contraction is the *sarcoplasmic reticulum* (SR). Calcium ions are stored in the SR and released for use after depolarization (Fig. 13-22). Deep invaginations into the sarcomere are called *transverse tubules,* or T tubules. The T tubules are essentially an extension of the cell membrane and thus function to conduct depolarization to structures deep within the cytoplasm, such as the SR. The cardiac cells abound with *mitochondria,* which contain respiratory enzymes necessary for oxidative phosphorylation. This enables the cell to keep up with the tremendous energy requirements of the repetitive contraction.

The importance of these precise and complex anatomic structures is evidenced in several clinical conditions. For example, chronic cardiomyopathy is a disease of the myocardium that most frequently results from viral, alcoholic, or idiopathic causes. The ventricular dilation commonly associated with this condition leads to poor approximation of the actin and myosin filaments. This results in decreased contraction at the microscopic level that is manifested by impaired myocardial contractility, low cardiac output, and increased diastolic volume. Eventually, biventricular heart failure may result.

PHYSIOLOGY

The study of the electrical and mechanical properties of cardiac tissue has fascinated scientists for more than 100 years. These properties include excitability, conductivity, automaticity, rhythmicity, contractility, and refractoriness. The following section relates these concepts specifically to cardiac cells (Table 13-3).

Electrical Activity

◆ **Transmembrane potentials.** Electrical potentials across cell membranes are present in essentially all cells of the body. Some cells, such as nerve and muscle cells, are specialized for conduction of electrical impulses along their membranes. This electrical potential, or transmembrane potential, refers to the relative electrical difference between the interior of a cell and that of the fluid surrounding the cell. Ionic channels are pores in cell membranes that allow for passage of specific ions at specific times or signals. Transmembrane potentials and ionic channels are extremely important in myocardial cells because they form the basis for electrical impulse conduction and muscular contraction.[13]

Resting membrane potential. In a myocardial cell, the normal resting membrane potential (RMP) is approximately −80 to −90 millivolts (mV). This means that the interior of the cell is relatively negative compared with the exterior medium when the cell is at rest. The relative negativity of the cell interior is created by an uneven distribution of positively charged ions and negatively charged ions. Hence there are relatively more of the positively charged ions outside of the cell than there are inside.

When the cell is at rest, the intracellular potassium (K^+) is very high, and sodium (Na^+) is low. Conversely, the extracellular K^+ is relatively low, compared with a high concentration of Na^+ (Table 13-4). Similar to Na^+, calcium (Ca^{++}) also has a much higher concentration outside the cell. These large differences in individual ion concentrations are responsible for the *chemical gradients,* that is, the tendency of a ion to move from the area of higher concentration to the area of lower concentration. However, there is also an *electrical gradient,* in which the positively charged ions will move to the area of relative negativity. For example, the chemical gradient of K^+ is to move out of the cell, because the intracellular concentration is so much higher than the outside medium. But, as a result of the relative negativity inside the cell, the electrical gradient works to retain the positively charged K^+ ion. An important factor influencing both gradients is *membrane permeability,* or the selectivity of the membrane to ionic movements. Even at rest, there is some slight movement of ions across the cell membrane. For example, the cell membrane is approximately 50 times more permeable to K^+ than it is to Na^+. Because K^+ movement out of the cell creates more negativity inside the cell, K^+ is therefore the most important ion for maintaining the negative RMP.[14]

Phases of the action potential. In a myocardial cell, when a sudden increase in the permeability of the membrane to Na^+ occurs, a rapid sequence of events follows that lasts a fraction of a second. This sequence of events is

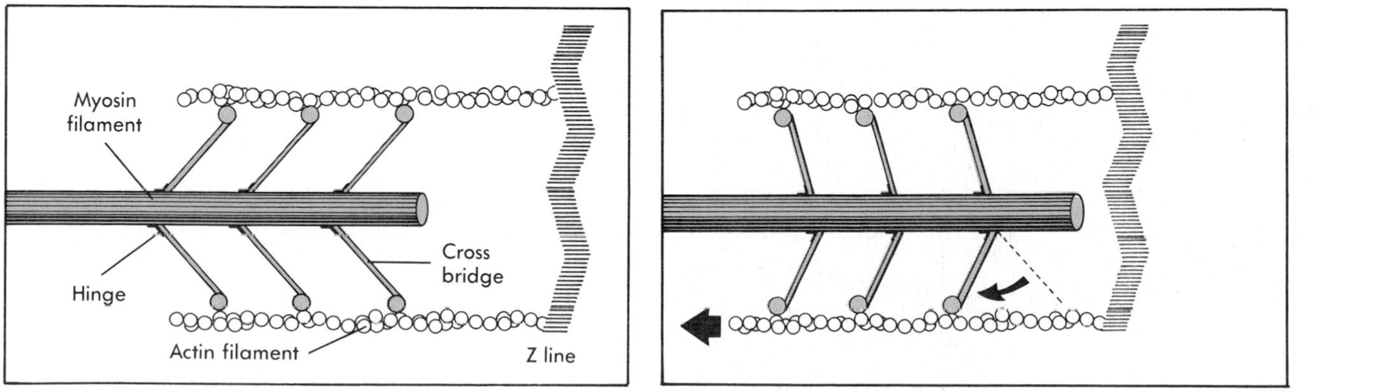

Fig. 13-21 Actin and myosin filaments and cross-bridges responsible for cell contraction.

termed *depolarization.* The graphic representation of depolarization is the *action potential* (AP) (Fig. 13-23). As the membrane is depolarized, Na^+ begins to enter the cell, thus causing the interior of the cell to become more positive. At approximately −65 mV, the membrane reaches *threshold,* the point at which the inward Na^+ current overcomes the efflux of K^+. This is accomplished by means of the fast Na^+ channels. With the fast Na^+ channels open, the inward rush of Na^+ is extremely rapid and briefly causes the inside of the cell to become slightly more positive than the outside of the cell. This is known as *phase 0 of the AP* and is reflected in the overshoot of the AP where the charge is +20 to +30 mV.

When the rapid influx of Na^+ is terminated, a brief period of partial repolarization occurs (phase 1 of the

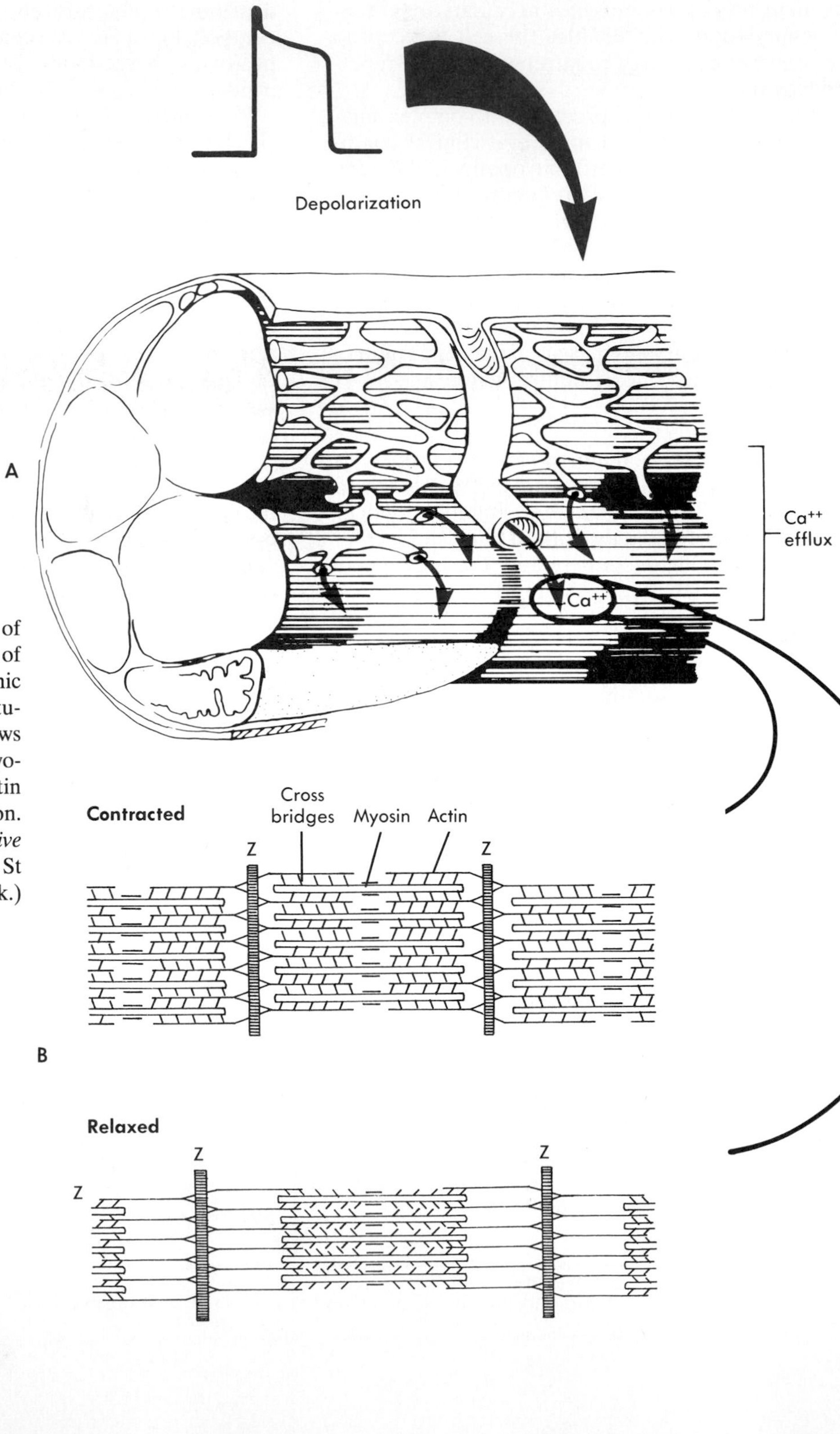

Fig. 13-22 **A,** Depolarization of a myocardial cell causes release of calcium from the sarcoplasmic reticulum and the transverse tubules. **B,** Calcium release allows for the cross-bridges on the myosin filaments to attach to the actin filaments to effect cell contraction. (From Quaal S: *Comprehensive intraaortic balloon pumping,* St Louis, 1984, Mosby–Year Book.)

Table 13-3 Definitions of terms related to cardiac tissue function

Term	Definition
Excitability	The ability of a cell or tissue to depolarize in response to a given stimulus
Conductivity	The ability of cardiac cells to transmit a stimulus from cell to cell
Automaticity	The ability of certain cells to spontaneously depolarize ("pacemaker potential")
Rhythmicity	Automaticity generated at a regular rate
Contractility	The ability of the cardiac myofibrils to shorten in length in response to an electrical stimulus (depolarization)
Refractoriness	The state of a cell or tissue during repolarization when the cell or tissue either cannot depolarize regardless of the intensity of the stimulus or requires a much greater stimulus than is normally required

Table 13-4 The approximate extracellular and intracellular concentrations of K^+, Na^+, and Ca^{++} in a resting myocardial cell

Ion	Extracellular concentration (mM/L)	Intracellular concentration (mM/L)
K^+	4	135
Na^+	145	10
Ca^{++}	2	0.0001

From Berne RM, Levy MN: *Cardiovascular physiology*, ed 6, St Louis, 1991, Mosby–Year Book.

AP). This is followed by phase 2, or the plateau. During this phase, another set of channels—the slow Na^+ and Ca^{++} channels—open and allow the influx of Ca^{++} and Na^+. Also during phase 2, K^+ tends to diffuse out of the cell, balancing the slow inward flux of Na^+ and Ca^{++}, thereby maintaining the plateau of the AP. The Ca^{++} entering the cell at this phase causes cardiac contraction, which is described later in this chapter. The inward flux of Ca^{++} during this phase can be influenced by many factors.[15,16] For example, agents such as verapamil, nifedipine, and diltiazem inhibit the inward Ca^{++} current and thus are known as *calcium channel blockers.*[17]

Phase 3 of the AP is the final repolarization phase and depends on two processes. The first is the inactivation of the slow channels, thereby preventing further influx of Ca^{++} and Na^+. The other is the continued efflux of K^+ out of the cell. Both of these processes cause the intracellular environment to become more negative, thereby reestablishing the RMP. Phase 4 of the AP is the return to RMP. The excess Na^+ that entered the cell during depolarization is now removed from the cell in exchange for K^+ by means of the Na^+ and K^+ pump. This mechanism returns the intracellular concentrations of Na^+ and K^+ to the levels before depolarization and is essential for normal ionic balance[18] (Table 13-5).

◆ **Fiber conduction and excitability.** Propagation of an AP along a cardiac fiber occurs as a result of ionic shifts discussed previously. As a local section of the cell becomes depolarized, reaches threshold, and completely depolarizes, it affects the adjacent area of the cell and begins depolarization in that area. Thus the AP propagates down the fiber in a wavelike fashion (Fig. 13-24). This is somewhat analogous to a trail of gunpowder. When the gunpowder is lit at one end, a small area ignites, burns, and then ignites the area of gunpowder immediately adjacent, and so on.

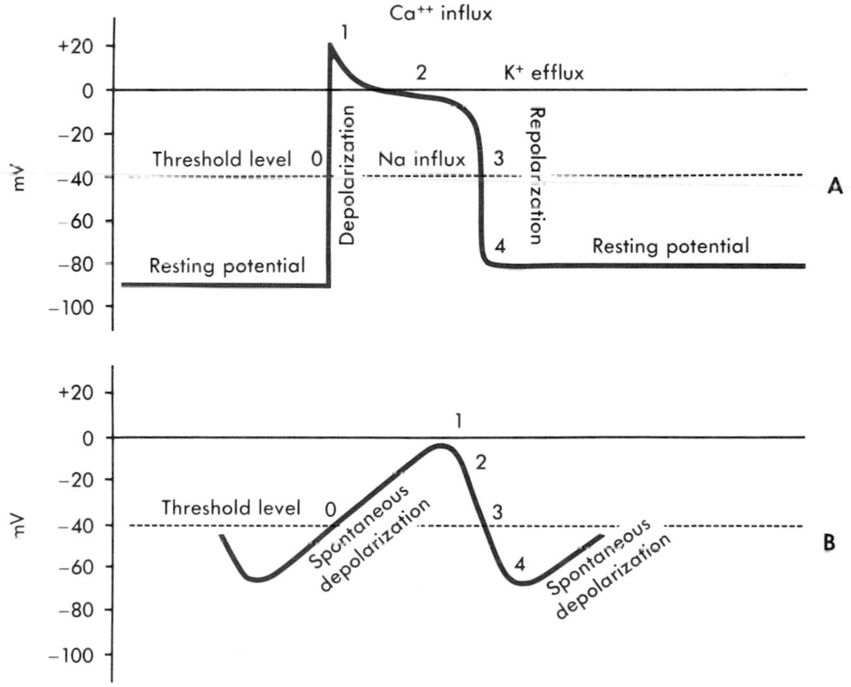

Fig. 13-23 Cardiac action potentials. **A,** Action potential phases 0 to 4 of a nonpacemaker cell. **B,** Action potential of a pacemaker cell. (From Thompson JM and others: *Mosby's clinical nursing,* ed 3, St Louis, 1993, Mosby–Year Book.)

Table 13-5 Summary of phases 0 through 4 of a cardiac cell action potential (AP)

Phase	Description	Ionic movement	Mechanisms
0	Upstroke	Na^+ into cell	Fast channels open
1	Overshoot		Fast channels close
2	Plateau	Na^+, Ca^{++} into cell, K^+ out	Slow channels open
3	Repolarization	K^+ out of cell	Slow channels close
4	RMP	Na^+ out, K^+ in	Na^+/K^+ pump

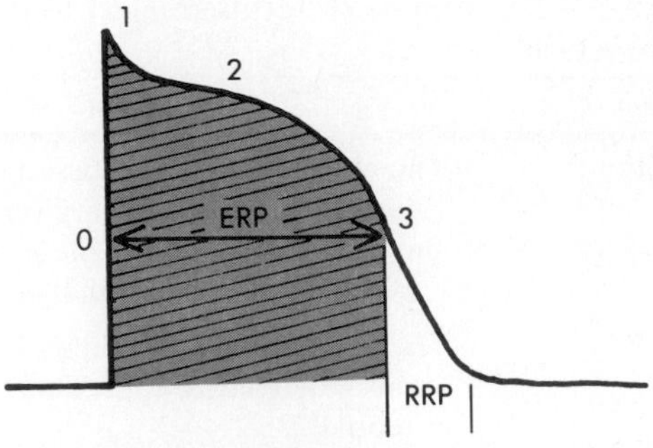

Fig. 13-25 The two parts of the refractory period. The effective (absolute) refractory period (ERP) extends from phase 0 to approximately −50 mV in phase 3. The remainder of the action potential is the relative refractory period (RRP). (From Conover MB: *Understanding electrocardiography,* ed 6, St Louis, 1992, Mosby–Year Book.)

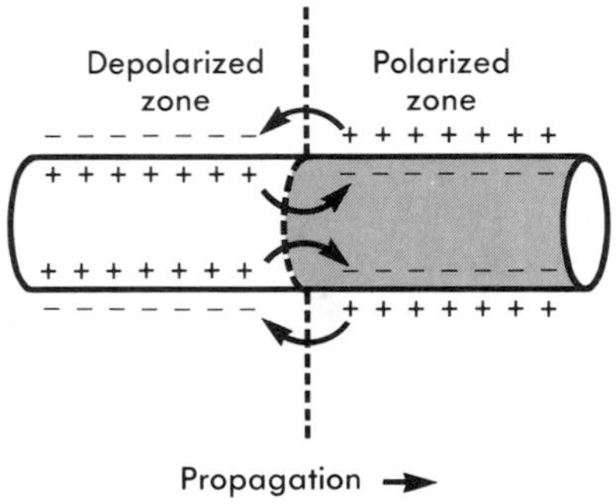

Fig. 13-24 Schematic representation of the propagation of an action potential along a cell membrane.

The time from the beginning of the AP until the time when the fiber can accept another AP is called the *effective* or *absolute refractory period.* During this period, the cell cannot be depolarized regardless of the amount or intensity of the stimulus. This period lasts from the beginning of depolarization to approximately −50 mV during phase 3. Immediately after the absolute refractory period is the *relative refractory period.* At this time, the cell is not fully repolarized, but could depolarize with a strong enough stimulus (Fig. 13-25). This period lasts from approximately −50 mV during phase 3 to when the cell returns to RMP. At phase 4, the cell is fully repolarized and is again at RMP, ready to respond to the next stimulus.

◆ **Pacemaker versus nonpacemaker action potentials.** The action potential as just discussed is representative of the depolarization of nonpacemaker myocardial cells. The AP generated by a Purkinje fiber is similar to that of a ventricular myocardial cell, except that phase 2 is usually more prolonged in the Purkinje fiber. Atrial myocardial cells exhibit a shortened plateau (phase 2) as compared with ventricular cells.

The pacemaker cells of the SA node have an AP that is very different from that of a myocardial or Purkinje cell. In the SA node, the RMP is approximately −65 mV. And, rather than an RMP that remains constant, the cells slowly depolarize at a steady rate until threshold is reached (Fig. 13-23, *B*). Because there are no fast Na^+ channels in the pacemaker cells, the SA node AP has a different configuration from that of a myocardial cell and is referred to as the *slow response.* The lack of a true RMP is largely the result of a steady Na^+ influx through the slow channels. This mechanism explains how the cells can spontaneously depolarize (automaticity). It also provides the basis for understanding alterations in the pacemaker cells. The frequency of the pacemaker cell discharge may be altered by a change in the rate of depolarization (changing the slope of phase 4), changing the level of the threshold, or raising or lowering the RMP.

Mechanical Activity

◆ **Excitation-contraction coupling.** The electrical activity discussed in the previous section is the basis for mechanical contraction. As the myocardial cell is depolarized, specifically during phase 2 of the AP, some Ca^{++} enters the cytoplasm through the cell membrane via special Ca^{++} channels. The majority of Ca^{++} enters the cytoplasm from stores in the sarcoplasmic reticulum (SR).[19] The cytoplasmic Ca^{++} then binds with troponin and tropomyosin, molecules that are present on the actin filaments, resulting in contraction. Occurring throughout the myocardium, the result is myocardial contraction. Once contraction has occurred, Ca^{++} is taken back up into the SR and the cytoplasmic concentration of Ca^{++} falls, leading to muscular relaxation. Both contraction and relaxation are active processes, because they require adenosine triphosphate (ATP) and because the Ca^{++} is removed from the cell by way of a Na^+/Ca^{++} pump. The role of this pump is not fully established, but it clearly contributes to intracellular Ca^{++} regulation during diastole.[20] The question of increased contractility is also not completely elucidated. Variations in strength of contraction may involve recruitment of more or fewer crossbridges, or a change in the Ca^{++}-binding properties of the contractile proteins. There is also probably an increase in Ca^{++} sensitivity as the muscle fiber is stretched. However, the role of Ca^{++} is much more complex than is presented here, because it involves not only the mechanical events in the cell, but also several metabolic and regulatory processes.[21]

The Cardiac Cycle

The cardiac cycle refers to one complete mechanical cycle of the heartbeat, beginning with ventricular contraction and ending with ventricular relaxation.

◆ **Ventricular systole.** As the ventricles are depolarized, the septum and papillary muscles tense first. This provides a stable outflow tract and competent AV valves. The ventricles begin to tense (endocardium to epicardium), causing a rise in pressure. When the intraventricular pressure exceeds that of the intraatrial pressure, the mitral and tricuspid valves close. This stage is known as *isovolumic contraction* because, even though the ventricular muscle is tensing, the ventricular volume does not change. As the ventricular tension increases, the intraventricular pressures exceed those of the aorta and pulmonary arteries, causing the aortic and pulmonic valves to open. The blood ejected from the ventricles is called the *stroke volume.* Usually more than half of the total ventricular blood volume is ejected; the blood that remains in the ventricles is the *residual* or *end-systolic volume.* The *ejection fraction* is the ratio of the stroke volume ejected from the left ventricle per beat to the volume of blood in the left ventricle at the end of diastole (left ventricular end-diastolic volume, or LVEDV). It is expressed as a percent, normal being at least greater than 50%. An ejection fraction of 30% could indicate either poor ventricular function (as in cardiomyopathy), poor ventricular filling, obstruction to outflow (as in some valve stenosis conditions), or a combination of these. Both ejection fraction and LVEDV are widely used clinically as indexes of contractility and cardiac function.

◆ **Ventricular diastole.** After ventricular systole is ventricular diastole. The first phase is *isovolumic relaxation,* which occurs between closure of the semilunar (aortic and pulmonic) valves and the opening of the AV (mitral and tricuspid) valves. Immediately after is the rapid filling phase, in which the AV valves open and the majority of the ventricular filling occurs. The next phase is ventricular diastasis or a reduced ventricular filling period. This is passive flow of blood from the periphery and pulmonary vasculature into the ventricles. The last part of ventricular diastole, known as *atrial kick,* provides approximately 30% of total ventricular filling. With this, the cycle is complete and begins once again with systole (Fig. 13-26).

Interplay of the Heart and Vessels: Cardiac Output

Cardiac output (CO) is defined as the volume of blood ejected from the heart over 1 minute. Therefore the determinants of CO are heart rate (HR) in beats per minute and stroke volume (SV) in milliliters per beat. The equation is as follows:

$$\text{CO} = \text{HR} \times \text{SV}$$

CO is normally expressed in liters per minute (L/min). The normal CO in the human adult is approximately 4 to 6 L/min. Cardiac index (CI) is the CO divided by the individual's estimated body surface area, expressed in square meters (m^2). The normal range for CI is 2.5 to 4.5 L/min/m^2. Changes in either the SV or HR can change the CO. However, all three parameters must be individually assessed. For example, for a person with an HR of 72 and SV of 70 ml,

$$\text{CO} = 72\ (\text{beats/min}) \times 70\ (\text{ml/beat}) = 5.04\ \text{L/min}$$

If, however, the parameters change to an HR of 140 and SV of 40 ml,

$$\text{CO} = 140\ (\text{beats/min}) \times 40\ (\text{ml/beat}) = 5.6\ \text{L/min}$$

Clearly, although the latter CO is greater, it does not reflect improved cardiac status. Rather, it could mean that cardiac decompensation is imminent. Although HR is influenced by many neurochemical factors, as discussed in the next section, this section focuses on the components of the SV (Fig. 13-27). These are preload, afterload, and contractility.

◆ **Preload.** The concept of preload was introduced in the early 1900s when Ernest Starling described his findings in an isolated dog heart preparation. Starling found that as he increased the volume infused into a denervated heart, the cardiac output increased. And as the volume increased, so did the CO, until it reached a point at which further infusion actually caused the CO to decrease. This is now known as *Starling's law of the heart,* and it is graphically described as the Starling curve (Fig. 13-28). It can best be described on a molecular basis, using as a foundation the discussion of the actin and myosin crossbridges in the myofibril. As the diastolic volume increases, it stretches the actin and myosin molecules in their resting state. As contraction occurs, the contractility increases as a result of the increased stretch. However, if the stretch is excessive and causes the actin and myosin to be stretched beyond their crossbridging limits (i.e., greater than 2.2 μm), contractility will decrease. This is the basis for Starling's curve. With the advent of critical care units and sophisticated monitoring, this principle has grown to great significance in clinical practice. For example, after a myocardial infarction (MI), the ability of the left ventricle to pump may be impaired. It is desirable to optimize the contractility of the remaining viable heart muscle by "stretching" it with added volume. But if the intravascular volume exceeds the stretch limit, CO will diminish.

Preload, then, is a function of the volume of blood presented to the left ventricle and also the compliance (the ability of the ventricle to stretch) of the ventricles at the end of diastole.[22] It has been described as left ventricular end-diastolic pressure (LVEDP). Factors affecting the volume aspect include venous return, total blood volume, and atrial kick. Factors affecting the compliance of the ventricles are the stiffness and thickness of the muscular wall. For example, the hypovolemic patient will have too little preload, whereas the patient with heart failure will have too much preload. One way to measure preload is through the pulmonary artery wedge pressure (see the section on hemodynamic monitoring in Chapter 15).

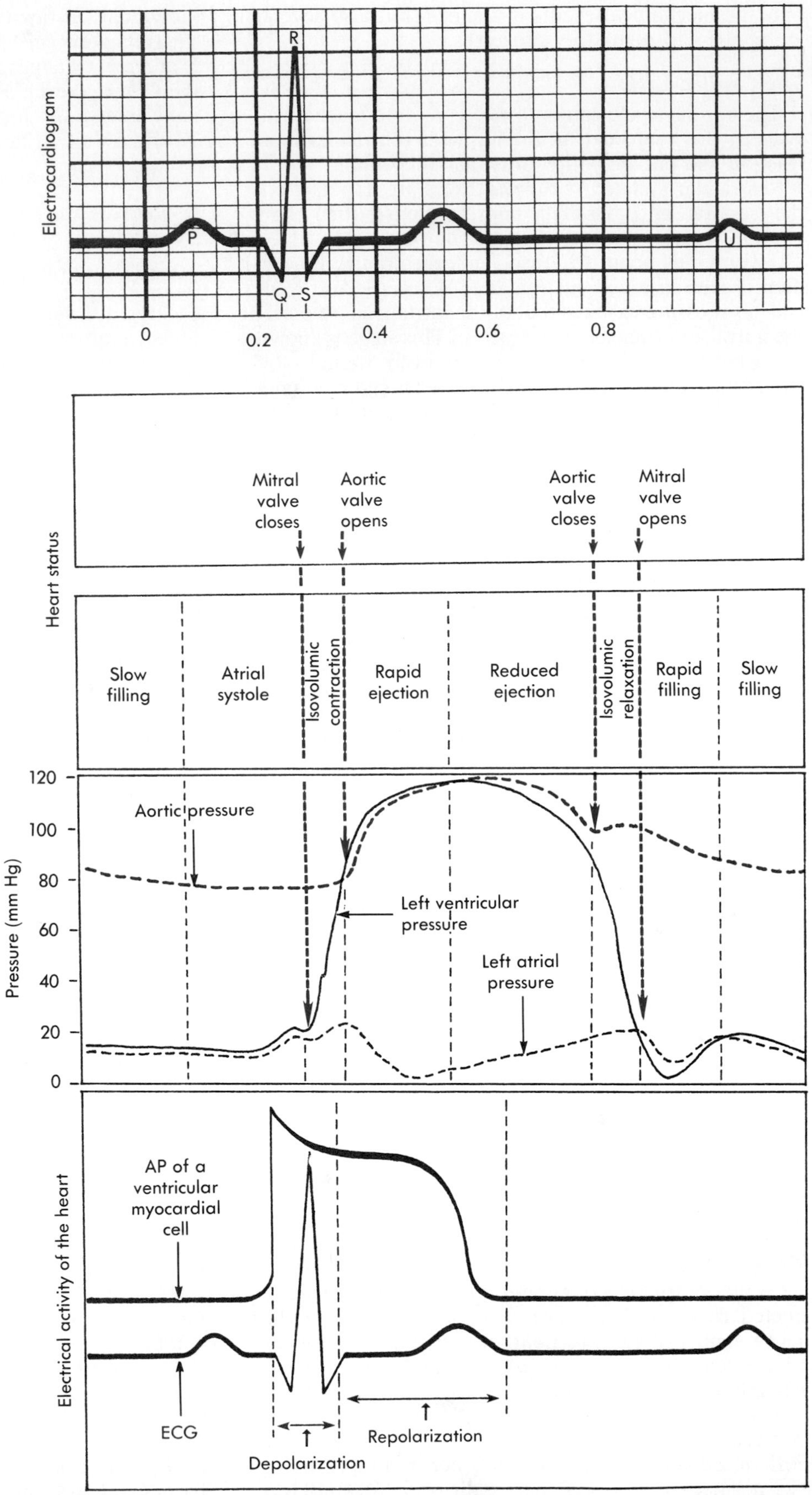

Fig. 13-26 The cardiac cycle.

Fig. 13-27 Determinants of cardiac output.

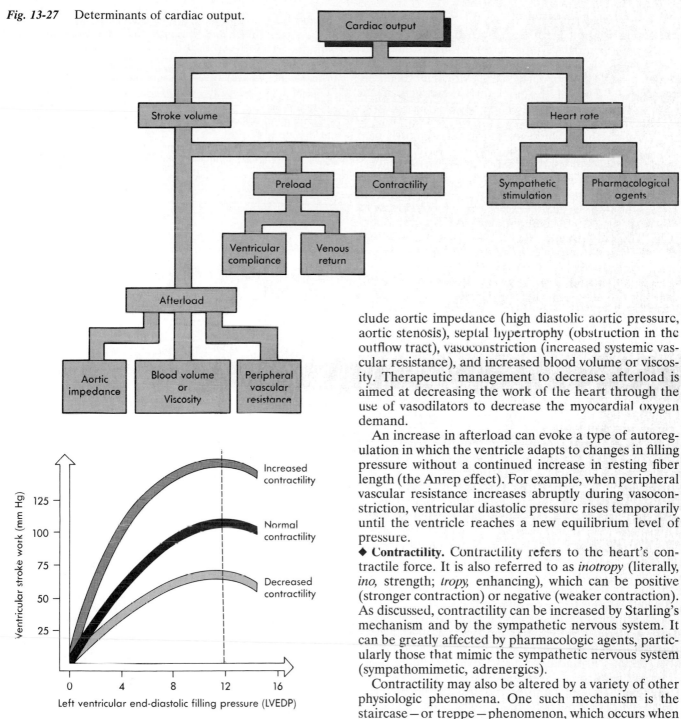

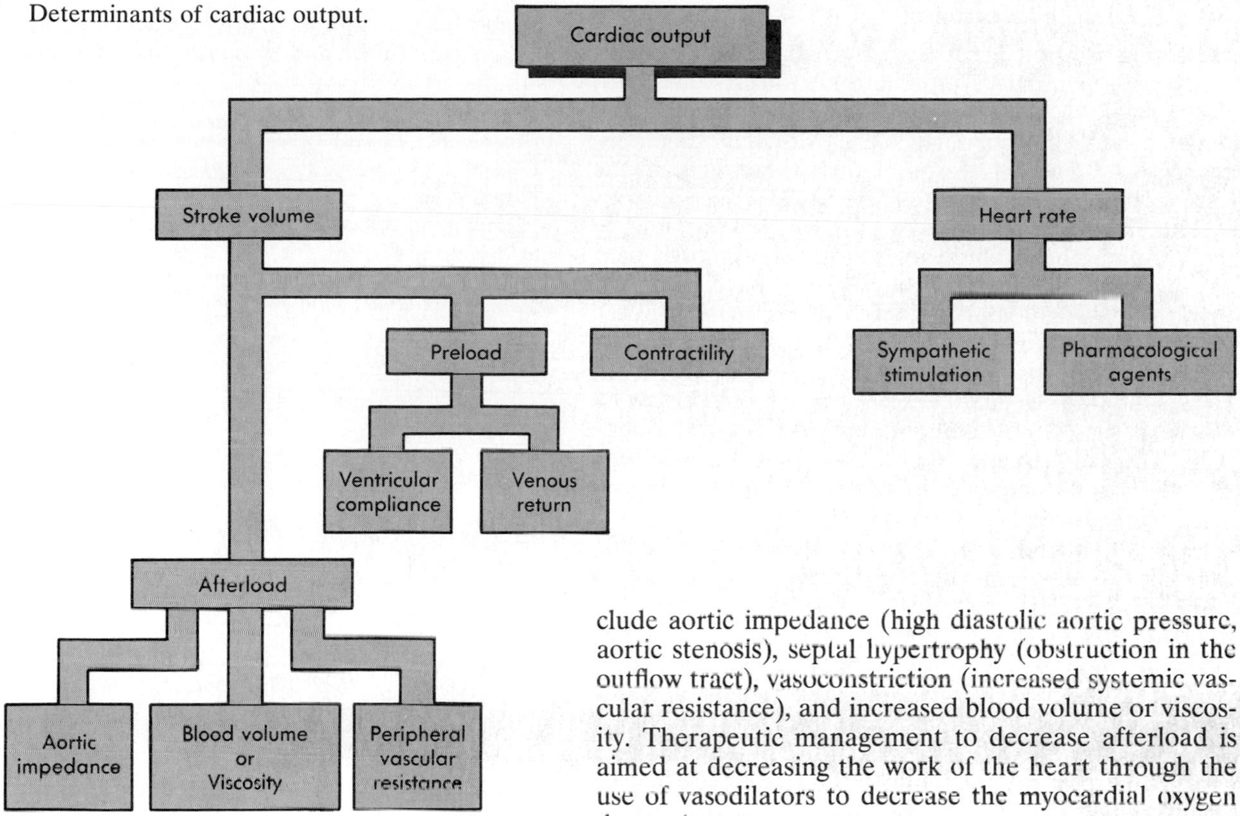

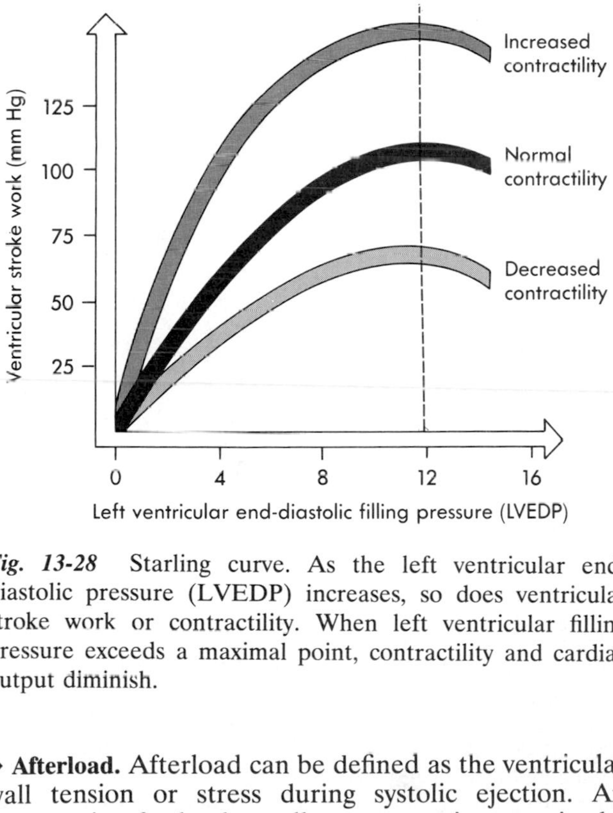

Fig. 13-28 Starling curve. As the left ventricular end-diastolic pressure (LVEDP) increases, so does ventricular stroke work or contractility. When left ventricular filling pressure exceeds a maximal point, contractility and cardiac output diminish.

◆ **Afterload.** Afterload can be defined as the ventricular wall tension or stress during systolic ejection. An increase in afterload usually means an increase in the work of the heart. Afterload is increased by factors that oppose ejection. Examples of increased afterload include aortic impedance (high diastolic aortic pressure, aortic stenosis), septal hypertrophy (obstruction in the outflow tract), vasoconstriction (increased systemic vascular resistance), and increased blood volume or viscosity. Therapeutic management to decrease afterload is aimed at decreasing the work of the heart through the use of vasodilators to decrease the myocardial oxygen demand.

An increase in afterload can evoke a type of autoregulation in which the ventricle adapts to changes in filling pressure without a continued increase in resting fiber length (the Anrep effect). For example, when peripheral vascular resistance increases abruptly during vasoconstriction, ventricular diastolic pressure rises temporarily until the ventricle reaches a new equilibrium level of pressure.

◆ **Contractility.** Contractility refers to the heart's contractile force. It is also referred to as *inotropy* (literally, *ino,* strength; *tropy,* enhancing), which can be positive (stronger contraction) or negative (weaker contraction). As discussed, contractility can be increased by Starling's mechanism and by the sympathetic nervous system. It can be greatly affected by pharmacologic agents, particularly those that mimic the sympathetic nervous system (sympathomimetic, adrenergics).

Contractility may also be altered by a variety of other physiologic phenomena. One such mechanism is the staircase—or treppe—phenomenon, which occurs when cardiac muscle contracts rapidly after a period of normal rate. During this tachycardia, the force of contraction progressively increases until a new steady state is reached. In addition, situations that cause an increase in the cytoplasmic Ca^{++} may result in positive inotropy. An example of this is the drug *digoxin.* Digoxin inhibits the Na^+/K^+ pump, which causes a slight rise in the intracellular Na^+. This rise in turn slows the Na^+/Ca^{++} pump that is responsible for removing the cytoplasmic Ca^{++} during diastole. The impaired Na^+/Ca^{++} pump causes a slight increase in cytoplasmic Ca^{++}, which is the basis for the increased inotropic properties of digoxin.

Regulation of the Heartbeat

◆ **Nervous control.** Both the parasympathetic nervous system (PNS) and the sympathetic nervous system (SNS) are normally active to create a balance between maintenance and fight-or-flight cardiovascular functions, respectively. Table 13-6 summarizes the effects on the heart of these divisions of the autonomic nervous system.[23]

Parasympathetic fibers are concentrated mostly near the SA and AV conduction tissue. Specifically, this involves the right and left vagus nerves (Fig. 13-29). Stimulation of the vagus nerve produces bradycardia as a result of hyperpolarization of phase 4 of the AP, which causes the slope to take a longer time to reach threshold. There is also a concomitant decrease in sympathetic tone. Thus adjustments can be made by changes in both the PNS and the SNS or, under certain conditions, selective changes in one.

Sympathetic nerve fibers parallel the coronary circulation to some degree before the fibers penetrate the myocardium. The right and left sympathetic chains probably have slightly different effects on the myocardium. It appears that the right chain has more effect on acceleration properties, whereas the left chain has a greater influence on contractility.

◆ **Intrinsic regulation.** Supplementing the nervous control are several reflexes that serve as feedback mechanisms to the brain. These reflexes work to maintain even blood flow and perfusion.

The *baroreceptors,* or pressure sensors, are located in the aortic arch and the carotid sinuses. They are more sensitive to wall changes (wall strain) in these areas than to the absolute pressure. As the receptors sense a change in wall conformation, usually as a result of a decrease or increase in pressure, the autonomic nervous system is activated to either raise or lower the heart rate, respectively. For example, a drop in blood pressure alters the baroreceptor input to the vasomotor center in the medulla, causing a reflex tachycardia. Evidence also suggests that the baroreflex initiates changes in vascular capacity to alter CO according to need. Clinically, this is evidenced not only by a reflex tachycardia in response to a decreased BP, but also by venoconstriction to increase blood return to the heart and augment stroke volume. In the opposite situation, an elevated arterial pressure causes the baroreceptors to reset their sensitivity in a way that increases the threshold pressure necessary for baroreceptor activation. This helps to explain why hypertension is not controlled by the baroreceptor response.[24]

The arterial *chemoreceptors,* or aortic bodies, are located in the bifurcation of the aortic arch. They possess a rich capillary blood supply and extensive innervation of the PNS. Their main function is to signal changes in oxygen tension (usually less than 80 mm Hg), a drop in the pH level below 7.40, or a carbon dioxide tension (P_{CO_2}) of greater than 40 mm Hg. Stimulation of the chemoreceptors normally causes an increase in respiratory rate and depth.

The *Bainbridge reflex* is attributed to receptors in the

Table 13-6 Summary of the effects of the parasympathetic and sympathetic nervous systems on the heart

Function	Parasympathetic	Sympathetic
Automaticity	Decrease	Increase
Contractility	Decrease	Increase
Conduction velocity	Decrease	Increase
Chronotropy (rate)	Decrease	Increase

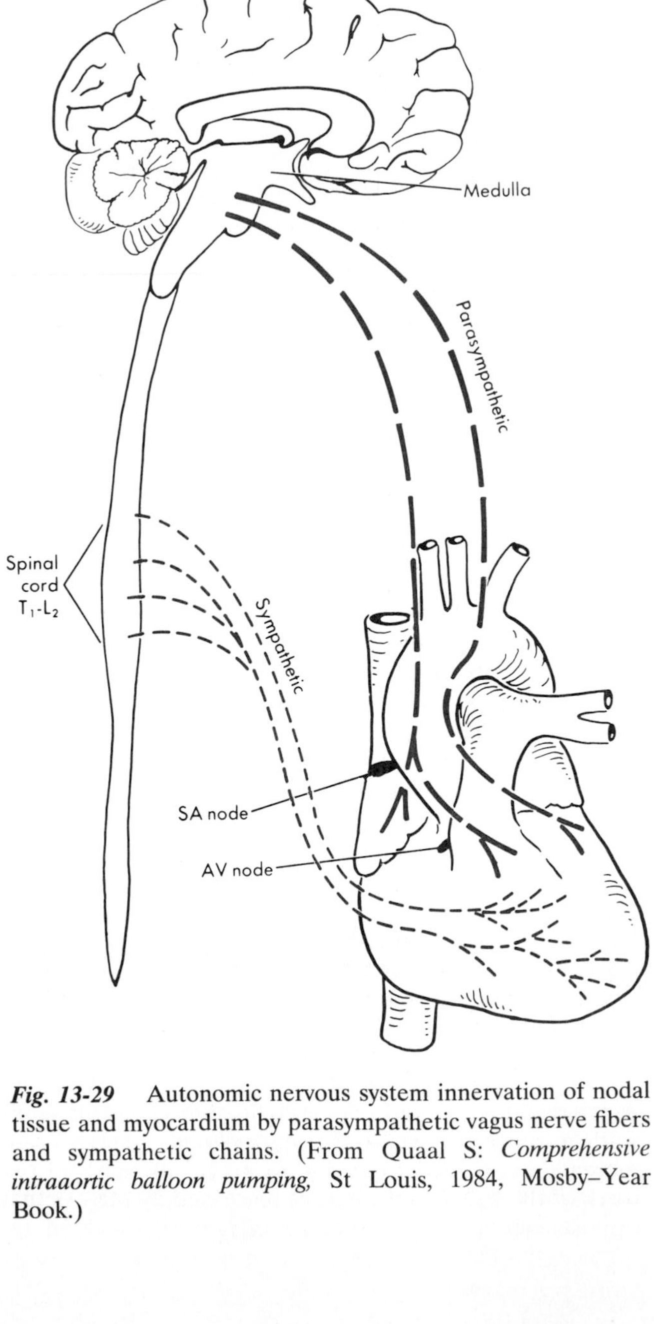

Fig. 13-29 Autonomic nervous system innervation of nodal tissue and myocardium by parasympathetic vagus nerve fibers and sympathetic chains. (From Quaal S: *Comprehensive intraaortic balloon pumping,* St Louis, 1984, Mosby–Year Book.)

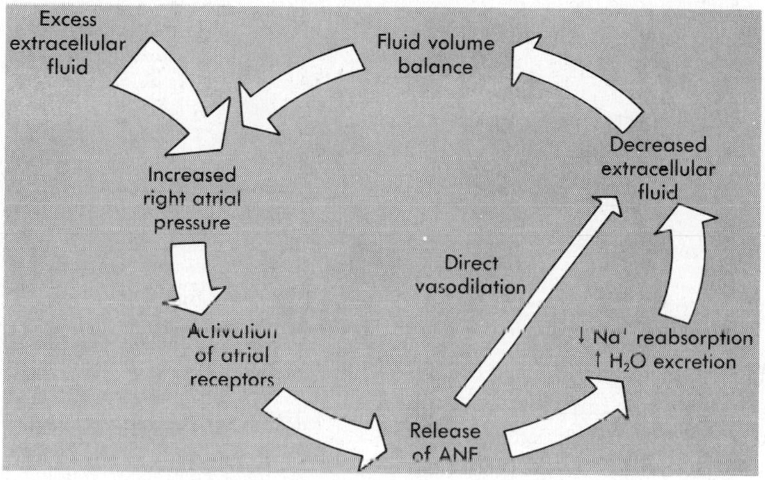

Fig. 13-30 The atrial natriuretic factor system.

right atrium. When the pressure in the right atrium rises sufficiently to stimulate these receptors, it causes a reflex tachycardia. The purpose of this reflex is probably to protect the right side of the heart from an overload state and to quickly equalize filling pressures of the right and left sides of the heart.

A recently described control mechanism involves the *atrial natriuretic factor* (ANF). It was described in rats in 1981[25] and is now known to be present in all mammalian atria. It is a hormone secreted by the atria in response to increases in atrial pressure. This hormone causes Na^+ and water to be excreted by the kidneys and is also a potent vasodilator. Thus the body rids itself of excess extracellular volume and increases the capacity of the veins to restore total body blood volume. It is possible that ANF is the opposite regulatory mechanism countering the renin-angiotensin system, because the renin-angiotensin system works to conserve Na^+ and water and raise blood pressure[26-28] (Fig. 13-30).

Other reflexes involve the respiratory cycle and its effect on heart rate and stroke volume. Normally the heart rate varies slightly with the respiratory cycle. The heart usually accelerates on inspiration and decelerates with exhalation. Also, left ventricular stroke volume decreases during normal inspiration. There may be so many contributing factors to these phenomena that a single explanation would be inadequate. Possible contributors may include normal fluctuations in sympathetic and vagal tone during respiration, changes in intrathoracic pressure involving increased venous return and the Bainbridge reflex, stretch receptors in the lungs, interactions between the respiratory and cardiac centers in the medulla, increased capacity of the pulmonary vessels during lung inflation, decreased left ventricular compliance resulting from increased right ventricular return, increased impedance to left ventricular outflow related to the pleural pressure changes, or neural reflex mechanisms that are independent of mechanical influences.[29] Thus many complex hemodynamic changes occur throughout the respiratory cycle. Consideration must also be given to underlying lung and cardiac disease, intravascular volume status, respiratory rate, and added effects of mechanical ventilation.[30]

Control of Peripheral Circulation

◆ **Intrinsic control.** Intrinsic or local control of the peripheral circulation is most influential at the arteriolar level. The arterioles are the major *resistance vessels* because of the amount of smooth muscle in the vessel walls (Fig. 13-12). Although the vascular smooth muscle differs in arrangement and amount in different organ beds, it is still subject to many influences. Because the smooth muscle is normally under dual influence between the vasodilator and vasoconstrictor mechanisms, the arteriole has the potential for either increasing or decreasing its lumen substantially. Several local factors influence this balance. One is pharmacologic stimuli, such as locally released catecholamines, histamine, acetylcholine, serotonin, angiotensin, adenosine, and prostaglandins. These can be initiated by a variety of mechanisms, such as tissue injury, hypoxemia, or hormones. Other factors that influence circulation locally are temperature and carbon dioxide.

◆ **Extrinsic control.** Extrinsic control is mediated by several mechanisms of the central nervous system. The first is that of the autonomic nervous system and the second that of the vascular reflexes, as discussed.

The autonomic nervous system exerts dual antagonistic control over most organ systems via the sympathetic and parasympathetic fibers.[31,32] The vasoconstrictor region in the medulla is normally tonically active. Experimentally, the neuronal activity of this region is essential for maintenance of arterial BP and heart rate. Stimulation causes increases in mean arterial pressure and heart rate by enhancing sympathetic outflow and possibly inhibiting PNS outflow. The sympathetic outflow targets the resistance vessels, causing vasoconstriction. Inhibition of these areas causes the opposite effect—vasodilation. Sympathetic fibers causing vasoconstriction supply the arteries, arterioles, and veins. However,

Table 13-7 Regions in the medulla affecting cardiovascular activity

Region	Activity
Dorsal lateral medulla (pressor region)	Vasoconstriction Cardiac acceleration Enhanced contractility
Ventromedial medulla (depressor region)	Direct spinal inhibition Inhibition of the pressor region

the capacitance vessels (veins) are probably more responsive to sympathetic stimulation, but the effects are not as readily observed as are those on the arterial side. Table 13-7 summarizes the sympathetic receptors, including location and effects of stimulation.

Control of peripheral circulation is a combination of intrinsic and extrinsic mechanisms.[33] Additional influences include emotions, temperature, and humoral substances.[34]

REFERENCES

1. Kitzman DW: Age-related changes in normal human hearts during the first 10 decades of life. II (Maturity). A quantitative anatomic study of 765 specimens from subjects 20 to 99 years old, *Mayo Clin Proc* 63:137, 1988.
2. Rosen M: The links between basic and clinical cardiac electrophysiology, *Circulation* 77(2):251, 1988.
3. Sealy W: Morphology of the conduction system and arrhythmia surgery, *PACE* 11:362, 1988.
4. Cranefield P: The conduction of the cardiac impulse 1951-1986, *Experientia* 43:1040, 1987.
5. Weidmann S: Cardiac cellular electrophysiology: past and present, *Experientia* 43:133, 1987.
6. Bonke F and others: Impulse propagation from the SA-node to the ventricles, *Experientia* 43:1044, 1987.
7. Allwork S: The applied anatomy of the arterial blood supply to the heart in man, *J Anat* 153:1, 1987.
8. Hoffman JI, Spaan JA: Pressure-flow relations in coronary circulation, *Physiol Rev* 70(2):331, 1990.
9. Silver FH, Christiansen DL, Buntin CM: Mechanical properties of the aorta: a review, *Crit Rev Biomed Eng* 17(4):323, 1989.
10. Xu XY, Collins MW: A review of the numerical analysis of blood flow in arterial bifurcations, *J Eng Med* 204(4):205, 1990.
11. Kajiya F: Progress and recent topics in blood flow measurements, *Front Med Biol Eng* 1(4):271, 1989.
12. Deleze J: Cell-to-cell communication in the heart: structure-function correlations, *Experientia* 43:1068, 1987.
13. Pelzer D, Trautwein W: Currents through ionic channels in multicellular cardiac tissue and single heart cells, *Experientia* 43:1153, 1987.
14. Carmeliet E and others: Potassium currents in cardiac cells, *Experientia* 43:1175, 1987.
15. Reuter J: Calcium channel modulation by beta-adrenergic neurotransmitters in the heart, *Experientia* 43:1173, 1987.
16. Tsien R, Hess P, Nilius B: Cardiac calcium currents at the level of single channels, *Experientia* 43:1169, 1987.
17. McCall D: Excitation-contraction coupling in cardiac and vascular smooth muscle: modification by calcium-entry blockade, *Circulation* 75:V3, 1987.
18. Vassalle M: Contribution of the Na^+/K^+-pump to the membrane potential, *Experientia* 43:1135, 1987.
19. Langer G: The role of calcium at the sarcolemma in the control of myocardial contractility, *Can J Physiol Pharmacol* 65:627, 1987.
20. Noble D: Experimental and theoretical work on excitation and excitation-contraction coupling in the heart, *Experientia* 43:1146, 1987.
21. Lucchesi BR: Role of calcium on excitation-contraction coupling in cardiac and vascular smooth muscle, *Circulation* 80:IV1, 1989.
22. Lorell BH: Significance of diastolic dysfunction of the heart, *Annu Rev Med* 42:411, 1991.
23. Venables PH: Autonomic activity, *Ann N Y Acad Sci* 620:191, 1991.
24. Chapleau M, Hajduczok G, Abboud F: Mechanisms of resetting of arterial baroreceptors: an overview, *Am J Med Sci* 295(4):327, 1988.
25. deBold AJ and others: A rapid and potent natriuretic response to intravenous injection of atrial myocardial extract in rats, *Life Sci* 28:89, 1981.
26. Blaine E: Emergence of a new cardiovascular control system: atrial natriuretic factor, *Clin Exp Hypertens* 7(5-6):835, 1985.
27. Blaine E: Role of atriopeptin in blood pressure regulation, *Am J Med Sci* 295(4):293, 1988.
28. Richards AM: Is atrial natriuretic factor a physiological regulator of sodium excretion? A review of the evidence. *J Cardiovasc Pharmacol* 7:S39, 1990.
29. Biondi J, Schulman D, Matthay R: Effects of mechanical ventilation on right and left ventricular function, *Clin Chest Med* 9(1):55, 1988.
30. Grassi G and others: Cardiogenic reflexes and left ventricular hypertrophy, *Eur Heart J* G:95, 1990.
31. Julius S: The blood pressure seeking properties of the central nervous system, *J Hypertens* 6(3):177, 1988.
32. Cohn JN: Sympathetic nervous system activity and the heart, *Am J Hypertens* 2:353S, 1989.
33. Jacob J and others: Studies on neural and humoral contributions to arterial pressure lability, *Am J Med Sci* 295(4):341, 1988.
34. Reis D, Ledoux J: Some central neural mechanisms governing resting and behaviorally coupled control of blood pressure, *Circulation* 76(suppl I):2, 1987.

14

Cardiovascular Clinical Assessment

CHAPTER OBJECTIVES

- Describe the appearance of a patient in cardiac failure using the technique of inspection.
- Describe jugular venous distention (JVD) and its importance as a clinical sign.
- Use the technique of palpation to thoroughly assess the vascular system.
- Locate the apical impulse on the precordium and describe how its characteristics indicate cardiac size.
- Locate the cardiac auscultation areas on the precordium.
- Verbalize the difference between the first and second heart sounds according to anatomic cause and the auscultation areas where each sound is best heard.
- Define and explain the significance of physiologic and paradoxical splitting of the second heart sound, ventricular and atrial gallops, and systolic and diastolic murmurs.
- Describe the murmurs that may occur after a myocardial infarction.

Nothing is more valuable to a patient in the critical care unit than a nurse who is proficient in physical assessment, a nurse who knows "normal" from "abnormal" appearances or behavior, a nurse who recognizes subtle physical or behavioral changes. The cardiovascular abnormal signs can quickly develop, accelerate, and prove fatal without skilled nursing observation and intervention.

The purpose of this chapter is to demonstrate how the techniques of inspection, palpation, percussion, and auscultation are implemented in the monitoring of cardiovascular patients. Noninvasive assessment of the cardiovascular system provides easily attainable and valuable data on cardiac and vascular status and on any immediate localized or systemic response to treatment. This information, combined with the cardiovascular history and the data from any hemodynamic monitoring equipment, will guide patient treatment and preserve the "excellence of care" reputation that critical care units have established.

What this chapter cannot so readily convey is the professional challenge offered by—and commensurate personal satisfaction derived from—becoming proficient with these techniques. The reward will be the patient who does not succumb to acute cardiac failure, because JVD was detected early in his or her course; or the patient whose thrombophlebitis was discovered on a routine midshift vascular examination and treated appropriately, reducing his or her risk for pulmonary embolism.

HISTORY

The patient history (see box, p. 170) is important for providing data that contribute to the cardiovascular diagnosis and the treatment plan.

The patient's presenting symptoms or complaints should direct the history-taking part of the assessment. Each symptom should be further explored with the questions detailed in Table 14-1. For example, the vague complaint of *chest pain* can become "classic angina" when the patient is more specific (e.g., ". . . a midchest pressure that radiates into my jaw and makes me short of breath when I walk more than a block—if I sit down, it goes away in about 5 minutes"). Other symptoms that may be indicative of cardiovascular problems are listed in the box (on p. 170) under "common cardiovascular symptoms" and should be inquired about even if the patient does not complain of them.

Table 14-1 Clarification of symptoms by asking specific questions

Determine	Typical question
Location, radiation	Where is it? Does it move or stay in one place?
Quality	What's it like?
Quantity	How severe is it? How frequent? How long does it last?
Chronology	When did it begin? How has it progressed?
Aggravating and alleviating factors	What are you doing when it occurs? What do you do to get rid of it?
Associated findings	Are there any other symptoms you feel at the same time?
Treatment sought and effect	Have you seen a doctor in the past for this same problem? What was the treatment?

DATA COLLECTION FOR CARDIOVASCULAR HISTORY

COMMON CARDIOVASCULAR SYMPTOMS

Chest pains
Palpitations
Dyspnea
Cough
Nocturia
Edema
Dizziness/syncope
Claudication

PATIENT PROFILE

Personal habits
- Use of tea, coffee, alcohol, recreational drugs, over-the-counter drug use, smoking, exercise, and dietary habits

Life-style pattern
- Working, relaxing, coping

Recent life changes
- Within the past 6 months

Emotional state
- Evidence of psychologic stress, worry, anxiety

Perception of illness and its meaning for the future

RISK FACTORS

Gender/age
Family history
Hypertension
Diabetes mellitus
Obesity
Smoking history
High serum cholesterol
Sedentary lifestyle

FAMILY HISTORY

Coronary artery disease
Myocardial infarction
Hypertension
Stroke
Diabetes mellitus
Lipid disorders

CARDIAC STUDIES IN PAST

Cardiac catheterization
Cardiac ultrasound
ECG
Exercise tolerance test
Myocardial imaging with radiographic isotopes
Percutaneous transluminal coronary angioplasty
Atherectomy
Valvuloplasty

MEDICAL HISTORY

Childhood
- Murmurs, cyanosis, streptococcal infections, rheumatic fever

Adult
- Heart failure, coronary artery disease, heart valve disease, mitral valve prolapse, myocardial infarction, peripheral vascular disease, diabetes mellitus, hypertension, hyperlipidemia, dysrhythmias, murmurs, endocarditis, psychiatric illnesses

Allergies
- Especially to radiographic contrast agents or iodine

Surgical history
- Coronary artery bypass grafting, valve replacement, peripheral vascular bypasses or repairs

CURRENT MEDICATION USAGE

Digitalis
Diuretics
Potassium
Antidysrhythmics
Beta blockers
Calcium channel blockers
Nitrates
Antihypertensives
Anticoagulants

The box above also lists the other parts of the patient history with specific cardiovascular information that should be solicited in each category. Obtaining information about the medical history, current medication usage, and cardiac studies that may have been performed in the past is useful in determining health/illness patterns and treatment of the current medical problem. Taking the time to obtain this information may prevent repetitive tests or ineffective therapy. Cardiac rehabilitation should be focused on the risk factor variables and personal life-style choices (patient profile) that place the patient at continued risk for cardiovascular disease.

PHYSICAL EXAMINATION

Inspection

The degree to which the body proclaims its condition is surprisingly explicit. To the educated observer, skin color, body posture, and facial expression speak volumes in the absence of a single word from the patient. Inspection of the cardiovascular system focuses on the patient's general appearance—face, extremities, neck, thorax, and abdomen. Although experience will eventually allow one to inspect the patient in a more spontaneous, less compartmentalized fashion, attending to each area suggested ensures the comprehensiveness of the inspection.

◆ **General appearance and face.** The weight in proportion to the height is assessed to determine whether the patient is obese (a cardiac risk factor) or cachectic (which can indicate chronic heart failure). The face is observed for the color of the skin (cyanotic, pale, or jaundiced) and expressions of apprehension or pain. Body posture can indicate the amount of effort it takes to breathe or the position of comfort the patient chooses (e.g., needing to sit upright can result from acute heart failure, and leaning forward may be the least painful position for the patient with pericarditis).[1] The patient should be observed for diaphoresis, confusion, or lethargy, each of which could indicate hypotension or low cardiac output. It is important to systematically inspect the skin, lips, mucous membranes, and conjunctiva for pallor or cyanosis and for signs indicating an alteration in fluid or nutritional status. The first box on the right summarizes the necessary information to obtain from the initial inspection of the patient.

◆ **Extremities.** The nailbeds should be inspected for cyanosis and clubbing. Central cyanosis is a bluish discoloration of the skin, lips, circumoral area, mucous membranes, and nailbeds. It indicates a decreased oxygen saturation of the circulating hemoglobin molecule and may occur as a result of right-to-left intracardiac shunting, impaired pulmonary function, or hypoxia from any cause.[1] Peripheral cyanosis indicates reduction of peripheral blood flow as a result of vascular disease or decreased cardiac output and is usually seen in the nailbeds or the tip of the nose.[1]

Clubbing of the nailbeds is associated with central cyanosis as a sign of chronic oxygen deficiency. Clubbing is evaluated by assessing the angle between the nail and the nail base, which is normally less than 180 degrees. A flattened angle (180 degrees) with a springy or spongy nail base is "early" clubbing, and an angle greater than 180 degrees with a swollen nail base is "late" clubbing (see Fig. 20-2).

The extremities yield multiple signs of vascular disease. The parameters to be assessed are hair distribution (sparse or lacking), skin condition (dry, scaly, cracked, or shiny), temperature (cool or warm), color (pale, dusky, or hyperpigmented), and the presence of edema. With arterial insufficiency pallor is present when the legs are elevated and rubor when the legs are dependent. With venous thrombosis the color of the extremity may be dusky and the circumference of the affected calf or thigh may be slightly larger compared with the other extremity. The lower extremities should be inspected for varicosities that may predispose a patient to develop thrombophlebitis and/or require special venous radiographic studies if the patient were to need coronary artery bypass grafting. The second box on the right lists the specific information to be obtained by inspecting the extremities.

◆ **External jugular vein.** Normally, in the upright position (patient sitting erect), the jugular veins are nondistended. Jugular venous distention (JVD) occurs when central venous pressure is elevated as it is with right heart failure. The procedure for assessing JVD is as follows. With the patient reclined at a 30- to 45-degree angle, the examiner stands on the patient's right side and turns the patient's head slightly toward the left. If the jugular vein is not visible, light finger pressure is applied across the sternocleidomastoid muscle, just above and parallel to the clavicle. This will fill the external jugular vein by obstructing flow (Fig. 14-1). Once the location of the vein has been identified, the pressure is released and the presence of JVD is assessed. Because inhalation decreases venous pressure, JVD should be assessed at the end of exhalation. Any fullness in the vein extending more than 3 cm above the sternal angle is evidence of increased venous pressure.[2] Generally, the higher the sitting angle of the patient when JVD is discovered, the higher the central venous pressure. This finding is reported by including the angle of the head of the bed at the time JVD was evaluated (e.g., "presence of JVD with head of bed elevated to 45 degrees"). The JVD is a clinical sign of high right atrial pressure[3] and may appear without an appreciable change in clinical status. Prompt

INSPECTION OF THE CARDIOVASCULAR SYSTEM
General appearance and face

GENERAL APPEARANCE

Weight
Nutritional status
Position of comfort
Color of skin

FACE

Expression
Emotional state
Presence of diaphoresis
Color of lips
Color of mucous membranes
Color of conjunctiva

INSPECTION OF THE CARDIOVASCULAR SYSTEM
Extremities

Nail bed color
Nail bed clubbing
Skin color
Skin condition
Hair distribution
Presence of edema
Presence of varicosities
Comparison of circumferences

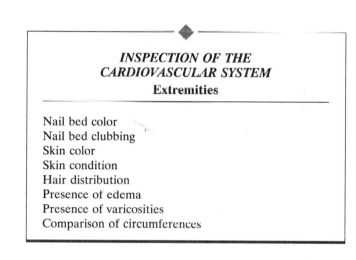

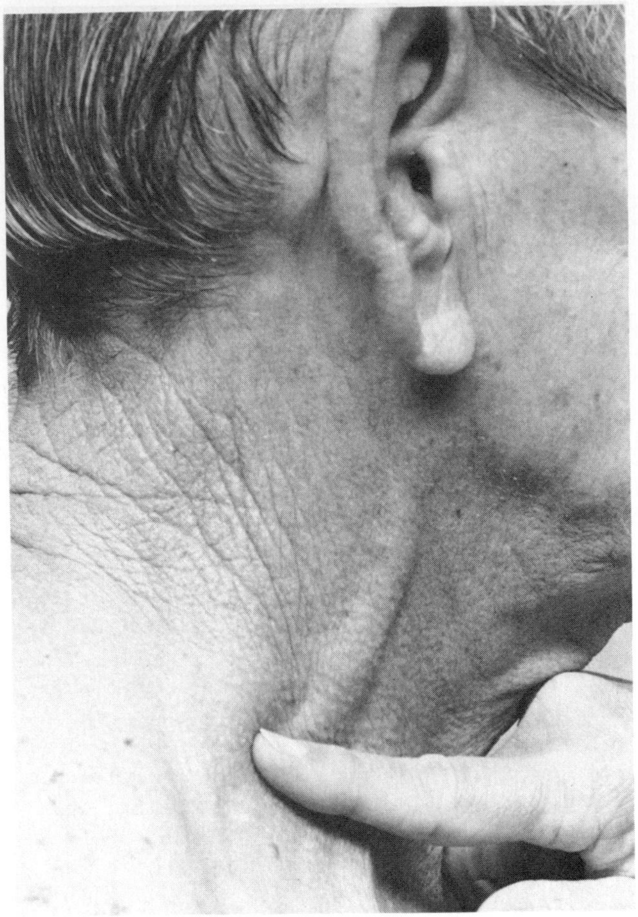

Fig. 14-1 Assessment of jugular vein distention (JVD). Applying light finger pressure over the sternocleidomastoid muscle, parallel to the clavicle, helps identifiy the external jugular vein by occluding flow and distending it. Release the finger pressure and observe for true distention, >3 cm, above sternal angle, indicating JVD.

treatment may prevent sudden deterioration into acute heart failure.[4]

◆ **Internal jugular vein.** The fluid column of the internal jugular vein is also used to estimate the amount of central venous pressure (in centimeters). This vein lies anterior to the external jugular at the level of the clavicle (Fig. 14-2) and follows a parallel path with the carotid artery and the trachea. The highest point of pulsation in this vein is observed during exhalation. The vertical distance between this pulsation, which is at the top of the fluid level, and the sternal angle is estimated in centimeters. This number is then added to 5 cm for an estimation of central venous pressure. The 5 cm is the approximate distance of the sternal angle above the level of the right atrium. The degree of elevation of the patient is included in reporting this finding (e.g., "central venous pressure estimated at 13 cm, using the internal jugular vein pulsation, with the head of the bed elevated 45 degrees").[2]

◆ **Hepatojugular reflex.** Right-sided cardiac failure is one cause of elevated central venous pressure. To further assess for right-sided heart failure, the right ventricle's ability to accomodate volume can be assessed by testing for a hepatojugular reflex.[3] This is accomplished by observing the pulsation of the internal jugular vein as pressure is firmly applied over the right upper quadrant of the patient's abdomen for 30 seconds. The normal response is a slight rise in the fluid level of the internal jugular vein, followed by a prompt return to normal. If there is a sustained rise in the fluid level in the vein that is greater than 1 cm, the test is considered positive. This test is accurate because pressure on the abdomen causes increased venous return to the right atrium, which—if failing—cannot pump away the extra volume of blood.[2] When this test is positive, it may improve the diagnostic value of JVD. If the patient tenses or holds his or her breath during this procedure, a false positive may be elicited, because these maneuvers (tensing and breath holding) may increase venous return.

◆ **Thorax and abdomen.** The next and final areas of inspection are the thorax and the abdomen. Both the anterior and posterior thorax should be assessed for skeletal deformities (e.g., pectus excavatum, straight back) that may displace the heart and cause systolic murmurs.[1] The skin on the chest wall and the abdomen should be checked for scars, bruises, wounds, and bulges associated with pacemaker implants. Respiratory rate, pattern, and effort should also be observed and recorded.

Thoracic reference points. The thoracic cage is divided with imaginary vertical lines (sternal, midclavicular, axillary, vertebral, and scapular), and the intercostal spaces (ICSs) are divided with horizontal lines, to serve as reference points in locating or describing cardiac findings (Fig. 14-3). The ribs are numbered from 1 (the first rib below the clavicle) to 12. The intercostal space between each rib is numbered the same as the rib that lies above it. The second rib is the easiest to locate, because it is attached to the sternum at the angle of Louis. This angle (also called the *sternal angle*) is the bony ridge on the sternum that lies approximately 2 inches below the sternal notch (see Fig. 14-3, *A*). Once the second rib has been located, it can be used as a reference point to count off the other ribs and intercostal spaces.

Apical impulse. The anterior thorax must also be inspected for the apical impulse, sometimes referred to as the *point of maximal impulse (PMI).* The apical impulse occurs as the left ventricle contracts during systole and rotates forward, causing the left ventricular apex to hit the chest wall. The impulse is a quick, localized (2 × 2 cm), outward movement normally located just lateral to the left midclavicular line at the fifth intercostal space in the adult patient (Fig. 14-4). The apical impulse is the only normal pulsation visualized on the chest wall, and—if visible—the location, size, and character should be noted. The rest of the anterior thorax should be inspected for abnormal pulsations that

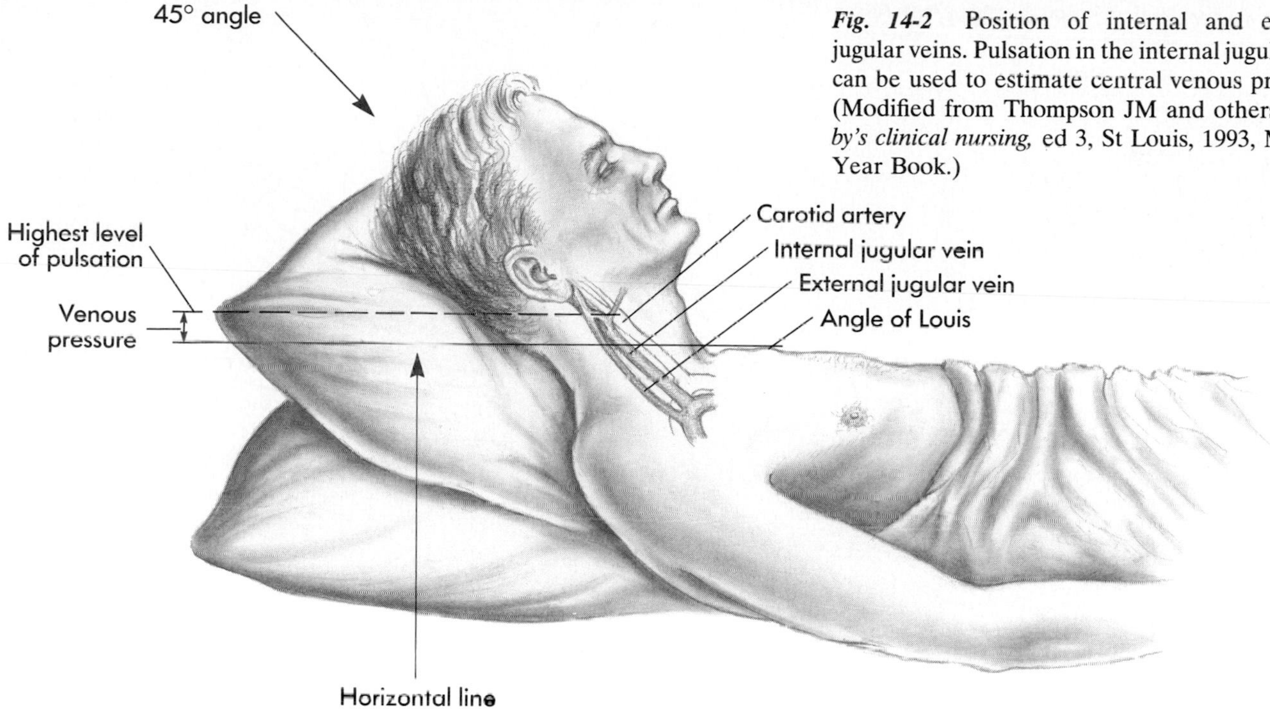

Fig. 14-2 Position of internal and external jugular veins. Pulsation in the internal jugular vein can be used to estimate central venous pressure. (Modified from Thompson JM and others: *Mosby's clinical nursing,* ed 3, St Louis, 1993, Mosby–Year Book.)

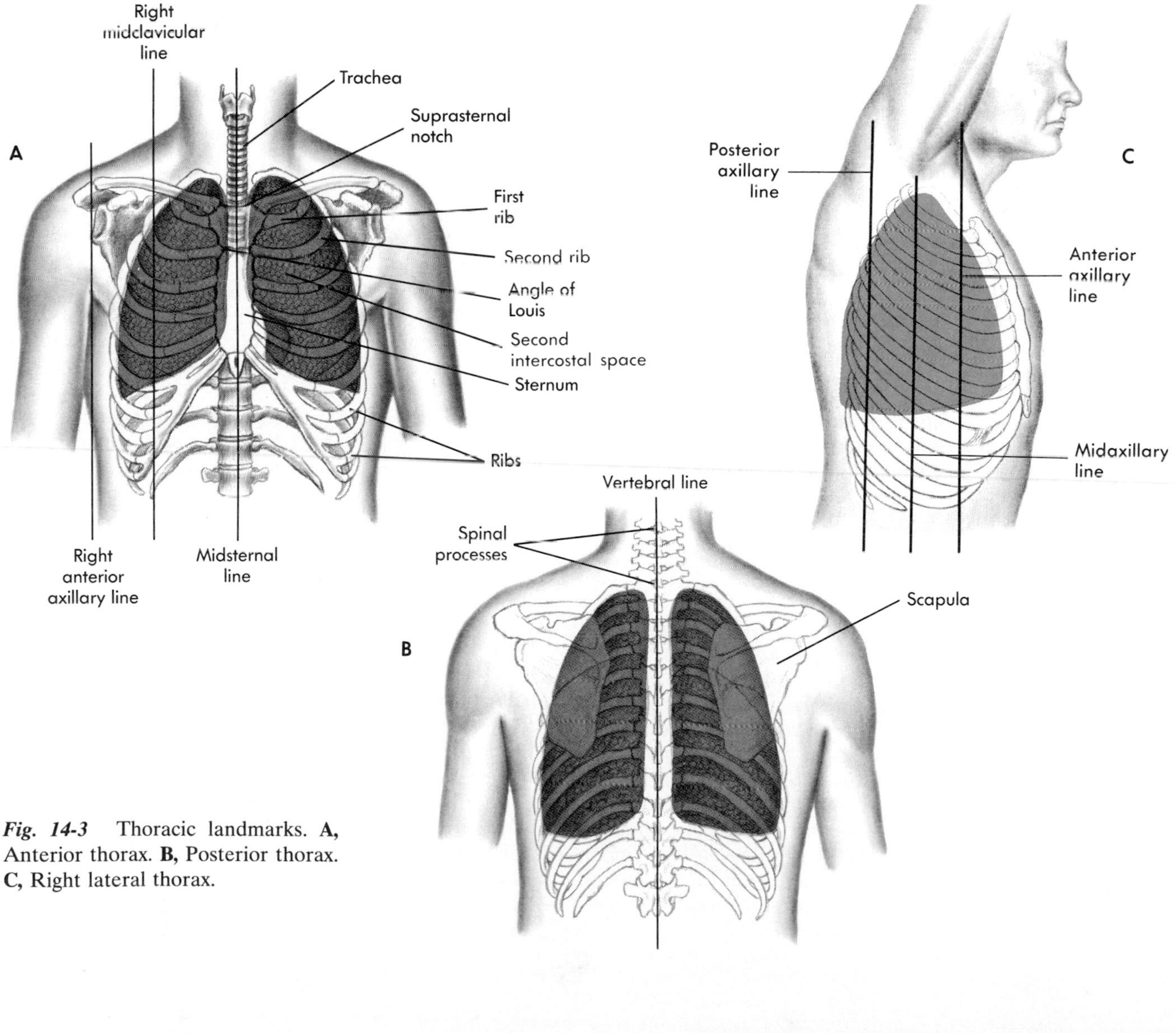

Fig. 14-3 Thoracic landmarks. **A,** Anterior thorax. **B,** Posterior thorax. **C,** Right lateral thorax.

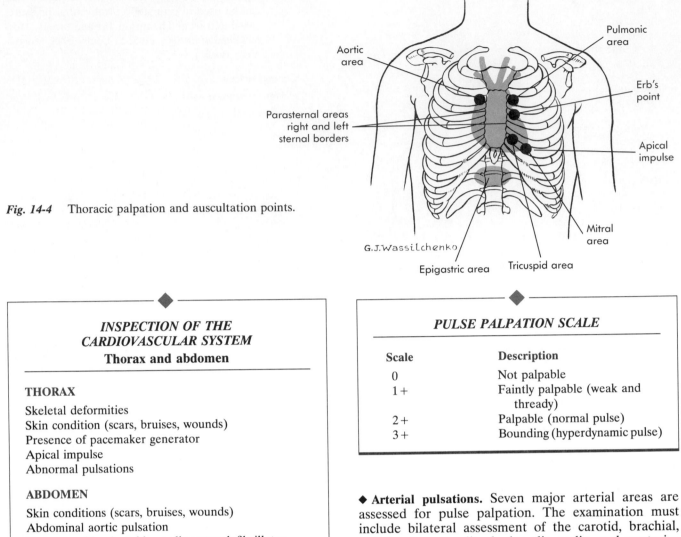

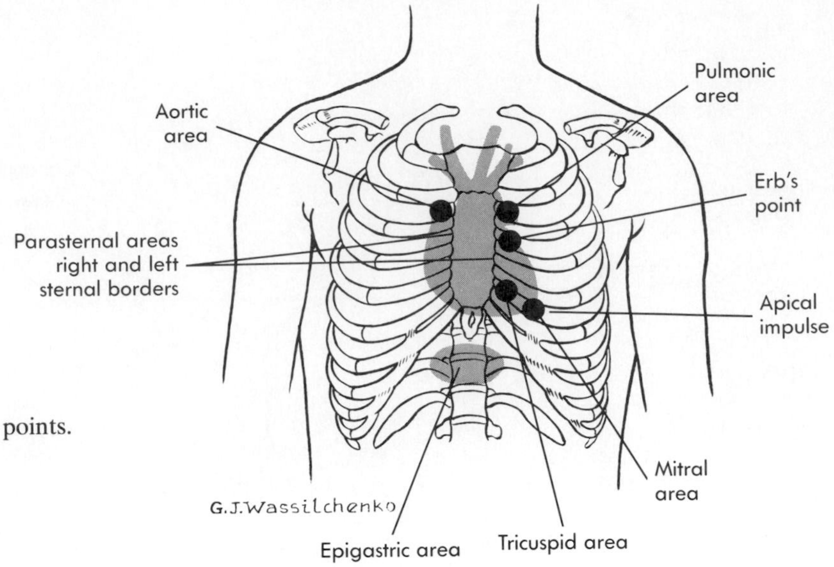

Fig. 14-4 Thoracic palpation and auscultation points.

INSPECTION OF THE CARDIOVASCULAR SYSTEM
Thorax and abdomen

THORAX

Skeletal deformities
Skin condition (scars, bruises, wounds)
Presence of pacemaker generator
Apical impulse
Abnormal pulsations

ABDOMEN

Skin conditions (scars, bruises, wounds)
Abdominal aortic pulsation
Presence of implantable cardiovertor defibrillator (ICD)

PULSE PALPATION SCALE

Scale	Description
0	Not palpable
1+	Faintly palpable (weak and thready)
2+	Palpable (normal pulse)
3+	Bounding (hyperdynamic pulse)

can indicate cardiac enlargement (e.g., a visible pulsation in the left parasternal region suggests right ventricular enlargement). The abdomen is also inspected for normal pulsations of the aorta, frequently seen in the epigastric area (Fig. 14-4). For a summary of the thoracic and abdominal areas of inspection, see the box above.

Palpation

Palpation is a technique that uses the sense of touch. The fingertips are sensitive to pressure, the backs of the fingers are sensitive to temperature, and the base of the fingers on the palmar side—as well as the lateral edge of the palm—are sensitive to pressure and vibrations. Palpation is done with a light touch and an unhurried, relaxed approach. Palpation is used to assess pulsations in the extremities, neck, thorax, and abdomen. Palpation is also used to assess the presence and amount of edema, the temperature of the skin, and capillary refill. The information obtained with palpation reinforces data collected with inspection and is especially important for the assessment of the vascular system.

◆ **Arterial pulsations.** Seven major arterial areas are assessed for pulse palpation. The examination must include bilateral assessment of the carotid, brachial, radial, ulnar, popliteal, dorsalis pedis, and posterior tibial arteries. The extremity pulses are assessed separately and compared bilaterally to check consistency. Pulse volume is graded on a scale of 0 to 3+ (see box above).

◆ **Upper extremities.** The radial and the brachial arteries are palpated for pulse quality in the upper extremities. These same arteries also are often punctured or cannulated for arterial blood gas specimens. It is imperative to assess frequently the pulse quality when the artery is cannulated, as well as the color, temperature, and pulse quality distal to the cannulated site. Occlusion of arterial blood flow is reflected by the absence of a pulse and/or coolness and pallor of the distal extremity.

Allen test. Before a radial artery is punctured or cannulated, the Allen test should be done to assess adequate blood flow to the hand through the ulnar artery. The Allen test is performed as follows:

1. The patient is requested to make a tight fist to squeeze the blood out of his or her hand.
2. The radial artery is compressed with firm thumb pressure by the examiner.
3. The patient is requested to open the hand, palm side up, while the radial artery is still occluded.
4. The time it takes for the color to return to the hand is noted.

If the ulnar artery is patent, the color will return within 3 seconds. Delayed color return (a "failed" Allen test) implies that the ulnar artery is occluded; therefore the radial artery is the only source of blood flow to the hand and should not be punctured or cannulated.

Capillary refill. Capillary refill assessment is a maneuver done on the nailbeds to evaluate arterial circulation to the extremity. The nailbed should be compressed to produce blanching, and release of the pressure should result in a return of blood flow and nail color in less than 3 seconds. The severity of arterial insufficiency is directly proportional to the amount of time necessary to reestablish flow and color.

◆ **Lower extremities.** The lower extremity pulses are the most difficult to locate – the popliteal pulses perhaps the most elusive. The popliteal pulses are found behind the knee, deep in the popliteal fossa, just lateral of the midline. The knee should be bent slightly to gain easier access to this area. The posterior tibial pulses are located behind the medial malleolus, and the dorsalis pedis pulses on the dorsal areas of the feet, usually just lateral to the extensor tendon of the great toe. The lightest touch, with at least three fingertips, and systematic movement across the top of the foot help to locate the dorsalis pedis. The dorsalis pedis and the posterior tibial pulses may be congenitally absent, but their presence is not entirely ruled out until they are checked with the patient's extremity in the dependent position.

Edema. Edema is fluid accumulated in the extravascular spaces of the body, such as the abdomen and the dependent tissues of the legs and sacrum. One must note whether the edema is dependent, unilateral or bilateral, and pitting or nonpitting (which indicates an arterial occlusion).[5] The amount of edema is quantified by measuring the circumference of the limb or pressing the skin of the feet, ankles, and shins against the underlying bone. If an impression is left in the tissue when the thumb is removed, it is called *pitting edema.* A patient with heart failure may gain 10 lbs or more of excess fluid before pitting is noted. Liver or renal failure and venous insufficiency with venous stasis can also cause pitting edema in the lower extremities (see box below).

Thrombophlebitis. The veins of the lower extremities are assessed with palpation, specifically for thrombophlebitis, which is an inflammation of the vein with thrombus formation. Venous thrombosis predisposes a patient to pulmonary emboli and chronic venous insufficiency. Embolization to the pulmonary tree is the most catastrophic sequela of deep vein thrombosis (DVT).[5] Squeezing or pressing the calves against the tibia may elicit pain, tenderness, increased firmness, or tension in the muscle. These signs suggest phlebitis and should alert the examiner to check other parameters that may aid in diagnosis, such as comparing leg circumferences and checking for increased heat in the extremity, unexplained fever, or tachycardia. Also, Homan's sign, in the presence of the other signs, can assist in the diagnosis of phlebitis.[2] To elicit Homan's sign, the examiner should flex the patient's knee and forcefully and abruptly dorsiflex the patient's foot. The sign is positive when pain is reported in the popliteal region and the calf. The box below lists the important points of palpation for upper and lower extremities.

◆ **Carotid pulses.** The carotid pulses are assessed by palpation for cardiac rate and rhythm and also for the amplitude and contour of the pulsation. Normally there is a swift upstroke to this pulse, with a slight rounded plateau at its peak and a gradual descent (Fig. 14-5). With an increased pulse pressure – such as occurs with such hyperdynamic states as fever, anxiety, hyperthyroidism, anemia, and exercise – the carotid pulse is large and "bounding," and the descending portion of the wave is as rapid as the upstroke. Aortic insufficiency can also cause this type of waveform because of the rapid run-off of blood through the incompetent valve. Decreased CO (such as occurs with aortic stenosis or heart failure) or hypotension will create a small wave with an upstroke as gradual as is the descent. If the carotid pulse is regular and alternates between large and small waves with every other wave being small, it is called *pulsus alternans.* Pulsus alternans is evidence of left-sided heart failure (see Fig. 14-5).

If blood flow through the carotid arteries is compromised at all by arteriosclerosis or plaque, palpation could easily cause total occlusion; thus only one carotid artery at a time should be palpated. Also, the carotid arteries

PITTING EDEMA SCALE

Scale	Description	Depth of indentation	Time to return to baseline
0	None present	0	–
1+	Trace	0 - ¼″ (0-0.5 cm)	Rapid
2+	Mild	¼ - ½″ (0.5-1.3 cm)	10-15 sec
3+	Moderate	½ - 1″ (1.3-2.5 cm)	1-2 min
4+	Severe	> 1″ (> 2.5 cm)	2-5 min

PALPATION OF THE CARDIOVASCULAR SYSTEM
Upper and lower extremities

UPPER EXTREMITIES

Brachial pulses
Radial pulses
Temperature
Capillary refill

LOWER EXTREMITIES

Popliteal pulses
Posterior tibial pulses
Dorsalis pedis pulses
Edema of feet, ankles, shins
Presence of phlebitis

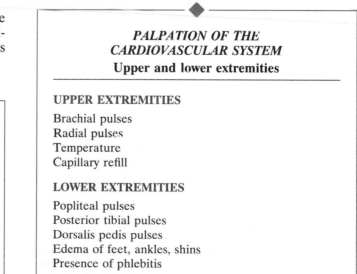

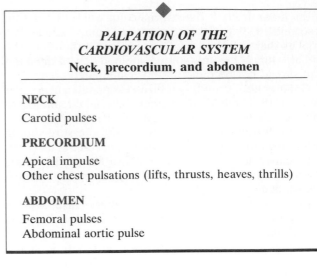

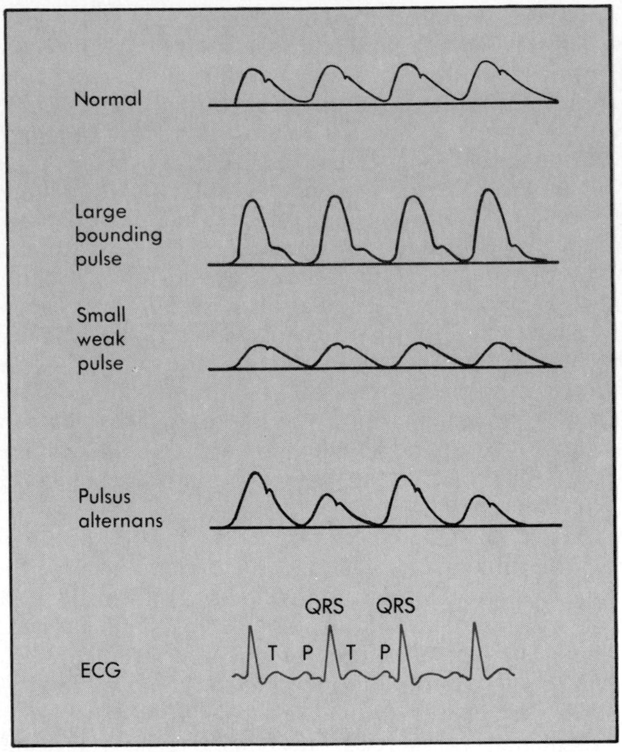

Fig. 14-5 The carotid pulse wave in relation to heart sounds and the ECG.

should be palpated in the lower half of the neck, well below the level of the carotid bodies, which—when stimulated—cause a decrease in heart rate.

◆ **Thorax.** The chest wall should be palpated for the apical impulse described previously. Its location, size, amplitude, and duration should be recorded. An enlarged left ventricle (left ventricular hypertrophy) is suspected when the apical impulse is enlarged (>2 cm) and is displaced laterally. When the apical impulse is difficult to locate, the patient can be turned to the left lateral decubitus position. This facilitates palpation of the impulse, because the left ventricle is against the chest wall in the left lateral position. Although this makes palpation of the apical impulse easier, it may also distort the placement and size of the impulse—limitations the examiner must consider. Once the apical impulse has been examined, the entire precordium (the chest area overlying the heart and great vessels) must be assessed for other pulsations. The precordial areas are labeled according to the underlying anatomy (see Fig. 14-4). Each area should be palpated in an orderly fashion.

The terminology used to communicate palpatory findings should describe as accurately as possible the sensation the examiner feels. Generally, accepted terminology refers to "thrusts" as localized and "heaves" or "lifts" as more diffuse movements. For example, right ventricular enlargement can cause a left parasternal "heave," and cor pulmonale—with both right atrial and right ventricular enlargement—can cause a sternal "lift." Left ventricular hypertrophy usually causes an

PALPATION OF THE CARDIOVASCULAR SYSTEM

Neck, precordium, and abdomen

NECK

Carotid pulses

PRECORDIUM

Apical impulse
Other chest pulsations (lifts, thrusts, heaves, thrills)

ABDOMEN

Femoral pulses
Abdominal aortic pulse

apical "thrust" as described. The paradoxical movement, or "heave," associated with ventricular aneurysm at the apex is often first detected by palpation. "Thrills" are vibrations that feel similar to a cat's purr and are associated with loud murmurs. Palpation of a thrill in the aortic area may indicate aortic stenosis or hypertension.

Description of location, amplitude, duration, direction (inward or outward), distribution (localized or diffuse), and timing in the cardiac cycle (systole or diastole) are helpful for determining the cause of a pulsation.

◆ **Abdomen.** The abdomen is palpated for the pulsations of the femoral arteries and the abdominal aortic artery. The femoral arteries are palpated by pressing deeply into the groin beneath the inguinal ligament, approximately midway between the anterior superior iliac spine and the symphysis pubis on both the right and left sides.

The aortic pulsation is normally located in the epigastric area (see Fig. 14-4) and can be felt as a forward movement by using firm fingertip pressure above the umbilicus. If the pulsation is prominent or diffuse or extends in the midline below the umbilicus, it may indicate an abdominal aneurysm. Refer to the box above for specifics of palpation of the neck, precordium, and abdomen.

Percussion

Percussion may be used in the cardiac physical examination to outline the left cardiac border. The apical impulse, however, located by inspection and palpation, is more reliable in determining the size of the left ventricle and is more quickly assessed.

Auscultation

Auscultation is used for blood pressure measurement, detection of carotid and femoral bruits, and assessment of normal and abnormal heart sounds and murmurs. Many good references are available for detailed study of heart sounds and murmurs.[1,2,6] The following information introduces the normal heart sounds and the ventricular filling sounds. Murmurs are presented in the broad categories of systolic and diastolic occurrence. The murmurs most commonly occurring subsequent to a myocardial infarction are discussed in more detail. The extracardiac murmur of the pericardial friction rub is also discussed, because it often occurs in the critical care setting and can be easily treated when properly identified.

◆ **Vasculature.** The carotid and femoral arteries should be auscultated for bruits. A bruit is an extracardiac vascular sound resulting from either (1) blood flow through a tortuous or a partially occluded vessel or (2) increased blood flow through a normal vessel. The sound is a high-pitched "sh-sh" sound that vacillates in volume with systole and diastole. Because the diaphragm of the stethoscope is usually too big to auscultate the carotid or femoral areas comfortably, the bell—pressed firmly enough into the skin to create a seal—will act as a good substitute. The skin, then, becomes a diaphragm and will transmit the high-pitched sound of the bruit. Light but firm pressure is the key when using the bell of the stethoscope to create a diaphragm.

◆ **Heart.** Auscultation of the heart can be the most challenging part of the cardiac physical examination. To summarize the advice given by most authors, the examiner must (1) discipline herself or himself to auscultate systematically across the precordium, (2) visualize the cardiac anatomy under each point of auscultation, expecting to hear the physiologically associated sounds, (3) memorize the cardiac cycle to enhance ability to hear the abnormal sounds, and (4) practice, practice, practice.

First and second heart sounds (S_1 and S_2). Normal heart sounds are referred to as *sound one (S_1)* and *sound two (S_2)*. S_1 is produced by the rapid deceleration of blood flow when the atrioventricular (mitral and tricuspid) valves close at the beginning of systole. S_2 is heard at the end of systole when the semilunar (aortic and pulmonic) valves reach closure. The actual sounds are caused not by the valve leaflets touching each other when they close, but by the vibrations created by the abrupt interruption of retrograde blood flow against the closed, tensed valve leaflets.[1,2] Both sounds are high-pitched and heard best with the diaphragm of the stethoscope. Each sound is loudest in an auscultation area located "downstream" from the actual valvular component of the sound (Fig. 14-6). For example, S_2—which is associated with aortic and pulmonary valve closure—can be heard best at the base of the heart, at the second ICS to the right and left of the sternum, in the areas labeled aortic and pulmonic. This is true because these areas overlie a section of vasculature "downstream" from the valves and in the same direction that sound travels. S_1 associated with closure of the mitral and tricuspid valves is heard best in the mitral and tricuspid areas. S_1 occurs immediately before the carotid upstroke. To identify it, if the heart rate is over 80 bpm, it may be helpful to simultaneously palpate the carotid artery pulsation while auscultating in the tricuspid or mitral area.

Both S_1 and S_2 are split sounds (Fig. 14-7) because of asynchronous left and right ventricular contraction. When there are no ventricular conduction blocks, the left side of the heart contracts milliseconds before the right. The left-sided heart valves, mitral and aortic, are the first heard components of each sound and are usually the loudest. The splits are best heard in the areas overlying the quieter components, the tricuspid and pulmonic valves. The S_2 is more obviously split, and the audible distance between the aortic and pulmonary components is increased with inhalation. This respiratory variation is called physiologic splitting and occurs because inspiration causes changes in pulmonary vascular impedence and in systemic and pulmonary venous return. These changes result in a lengthening of right ventricular ejection time and a corresponding shortening of left ventricular ejection time.[1,2] All the components of

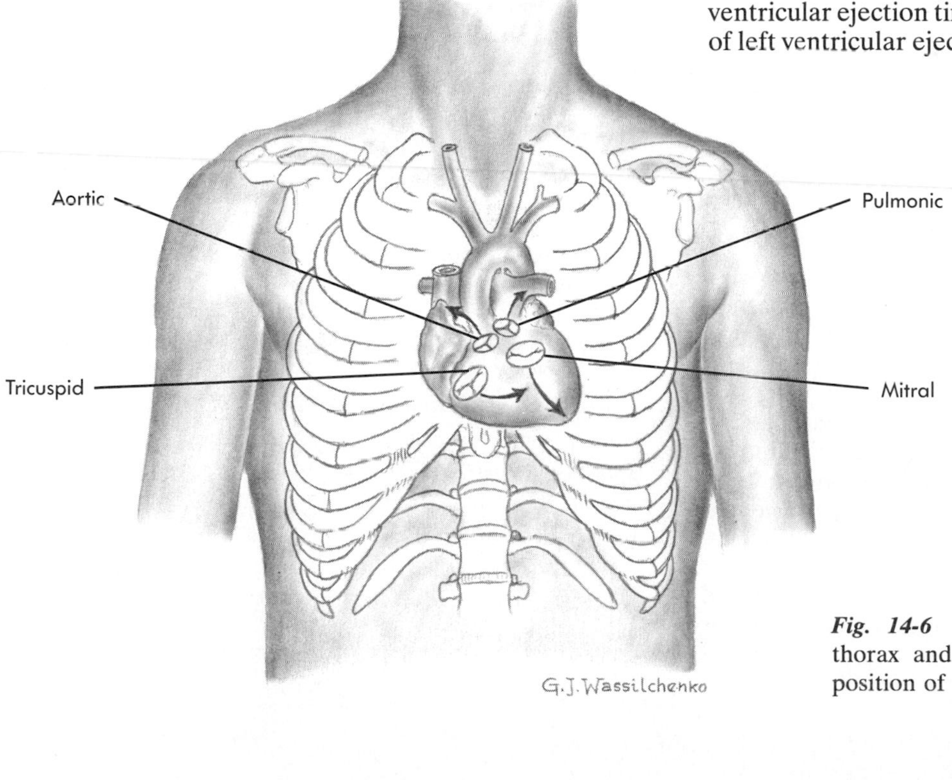

Fig. 14-6 Transmission of heart sounds to the thorax and their relationship to the anatomic position of the heart valves.

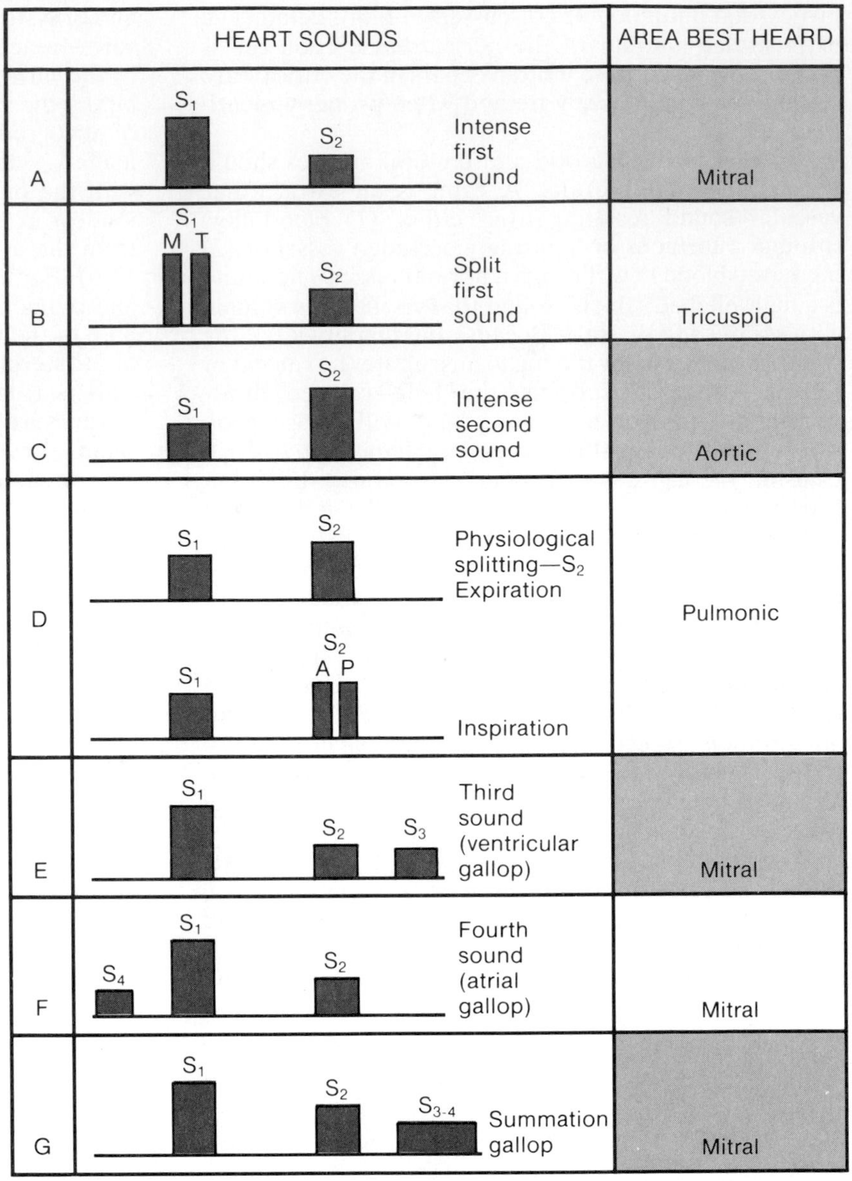

Fig. 14-7 Characteristics of normal and abnormal heart sounds and the auscultatory area where each is best heard.

the split sounds will be high-pitched and best heard with the diaphragm of the stethoscope. This information should help to differentiate the normal split sound from the ventricular filling sounds that may indicate pathology. See Table 14-2 for detailed characteristics of the normal heart sounds.

An advanced skill in auscultation is determining whether the S_1 and S_2 are louder or softer than normal. The intensity of the sounds vary with arrhythmias, hyperdynamic cardiac states, and the physical condition of the valves. Independent study, as well as practice and experience, prepare the novice to detect abnormal auscultation of S_1 and S_2.

Third and fourth heart sounds (S_3 and S_4). The abnormal heart sounds are labeled *sound three (S_3)* and *sound four (S_4)* and are referred to as *gallops* when auscultated during tachycardia. They are ventricular filling sounds,

Table 14-2 Characteristics of heart sounds one (S_1) and two (S_2)

S_1	S_2
High pitched	High pitched
Loudest in mitral area (apex)	Loudest in aortic area (base)
Normal split <20 msec	Normal split <30 msec
Split heard best in tricuspid area	Split heard best in pulmonic area
Important to differentiate between split S_1 and S_4	↑ Split with inhalation
Occurs immediately before carotid upstroke	↓ Split with exhalation

Table 14-3 Characteristics of heart sounds three (S_3) and four (S_4)

S_3	S_4
PHYSIOLOGIC CAUSES	
Related to diastolic motion and rapid filling of ventricles in early diastole	Related to diastolic motion and ventricular dilation with atrial contraction in late diastole
Can be normal in children and young adults (<40 yr)	May occur with or without cardiac decompensation
PATHOLOGIC CAUSES	
Ventricular dysfunction with an increase in end systolic volume (MI, heart failure, valvular disease, systemic or pulmonary hypertension)	Ventricular hypertrophy with a decrease in ventricular compliance (CAD, systemic hypertension, cardiomyopathy, aortic or pulmonary stenosis, ↑ in intensity with acute MI or angina)
Hyperdynamic states (anemia, thyrotoxicosis, mitral or tricuspid regurgitation)	Hyperkinetic states (anemia, thyrotoxicosis, arteriovenous fistula)
	Acute valvular regurgitation
RHYTHMIC WORD ASSOCIATION	
Ken....tuck..y	Ten..nes....see
S_1 S_2 S_3	S_4 S_1 S_2
SYNONYMS	
Ventricular gallop	Atrial gallop
Protodiastolic gallop	Presystolic gallop

occurring during diastole, and are low-pitched. One can differentiate between right and left ventricular gallops by location. Left ventricular S_3 and S_4 are heard best with the bell of the stethoscope positioned lightly over the apical impulse with the patient in the left lateral decubitus position, and right ventricular gallops are heard best at the left lower sternal border (LLSB). They are rhythmic (sounding similar to horses cantering) and have mimetic sounds as listed in Table 14-3. The sound of S_3 is similar to that of a stone dropping into water at the bottom of a well—dull and "thuddy." S_4 occurs at the end of diastole when the ventricle is full and is associated with the atrial contraction (kick). It is a hollow, snappy sound, as if the noncompliant ventricle cannot accept anymore volume unless it flows in hard and fast. The presence of S_3 is normal in persons younger than age 40 because of rapid filling of the ventricle and the motion it causes in the young, healthy heart.[7]

It is important to remember that both S_3 and S_4 are diastolic sounds. If extra sounds are heard, they can best be labeled as systolic or diastolic by using the "inching technique."[2] This means the aortic area, where S_2 is loudest, is auscultated first; then the stethoscope is "inched" across the pericardium toward the mitral area, where S_1 is loudest. It can then be determined whether the extra sound(s) is coming before S_2 (systolic event) or after S_2 (diastolic event). Once the timing is ascertained, the pitch should be assessed (high-pitched is a split S_1 or S_2, low-pitched is an S_3 or S_4). A useful test to differentiate between splits and ventricular filling sounds is to listen with the bell of the stethoscope. The examiner must press the bell down during auscultation, turning it into a diaphragm that accentuates only high-pitched sounds. If the extra sounds disappear, they may have been low-pitched S_3 or S_4.

CAUSES OF CARDIAC MURMURS

- ◆ An increased rate of flow through cardiac structures
- ◆ Blood flow across a partial obstruction or irregularity
- ◆ Shunting of blood through an abnormal passage from high to low pressure
- ◆ Backflow across an incompetent valve

GRADING OF CARDIAC MURMURS

Grade	Description
I/VI	Very faint, may be heard only in a quiet environment
II/VI	Quiet, but clearly audible
III/VI	Moderately loud
IV/VI	Loud; may be associated with a thrill
V/VI	Very loud; thrill easily palpable
VI/VI	Very loud; may be heard with stethoscope off the chest. Thrill palpable and visible

Murmurs. Heart murmurs are prolonged extra sounds that occur during systole or diastole. The sounds are vibrations caused by turbulent blood flow through the cardiac chambers. As indicated in the first box above, not all murmurs are caused by cardiac valvular disease. Some murmurs are caused by a high rate of blood flow through the ventricle, as occurs with fever, anemia, and exercise (high output states); other murmurs may be caused by such structural defects as patent foramen ovale (opening in the septum between the right and left atria). Murmurs are characterized by their timing (systolic/diastolic), location and radiation, quality (blowing, grating, harsh), pitch (high or low), and intensity (loudness graded on a scale of I to VI—the higher the number, the louder the murmur, as shown in the second box above). Table 14-4 describes the most common murmurs in terms of these characteristics.

In children or adolescents, systolic "high flow" murmurs are common and are a result of vigorous ventricular contraction. These murmurs have a low-to-medium pitch (heard best with the bell of the stethoscope), grade I to

Table 14-4 Characteristics of some murmurs

Defect	Timing in the cardiac cycle	Pitch, intensity, quality	Location, radiation
SYSTOLIC MURMURS			
Mitral regurgitation	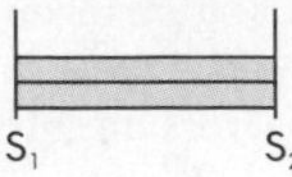	High Harsh Blowing	Mitral area May radiate to axilla
Tricuspid regurgitation	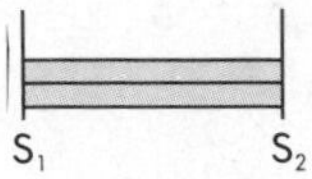	High Often faint, but varies Blowing	Tricuspid RLSB, apex, LLSB, epigastric areas Little radiation
Ventricular septal defect	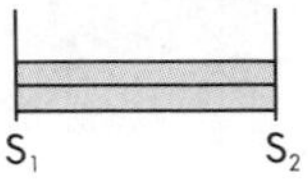	High Loud Blowing	Left sternal border
Aortic stenosis	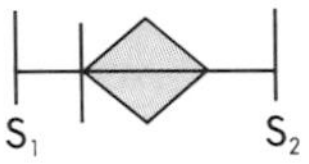	Chhhh hh Medium Rough, harsh	Aortic area to suprasternal notch, right side of neck, apex
Pulmonary stenosis	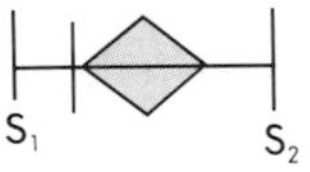	Low to medium Loud Harsh, grinding	Pulmonic area No radiation
DIASTOLIC MURMURS			
Mitral stenosis	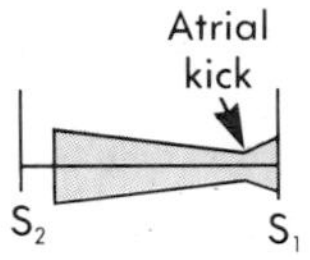	Low Quiet to loud with thrill Rough rumble	Mitral area Usually no radiation
Tricuspid stenosis	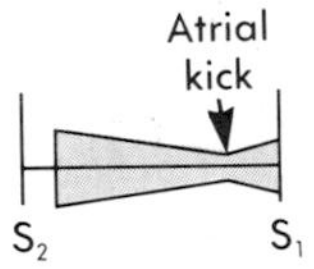	Medium Quiet; louder with inspiration Rumble	Tricuspid area or epigastrim Little radiation
Aortic regurgitation	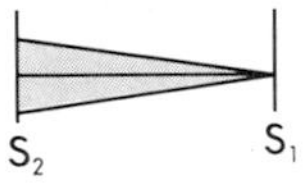	High Faint to medium Blowing	Aortic area to LLSB and aorta Erb's point
Pulmonic regurgitation	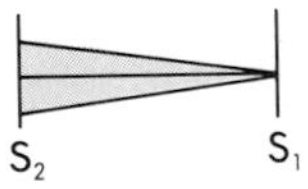	Medium Faint Blowing	Pulmonic area No radiation

RLSB, right lower sternal border; *LLSB*, left lower sternal border.

AUSCULTATION OF THE CARDIOVASCULAR SYSTEM
Precordium

AORTIC AREA

S_2 loud
Aortic systolic murmur

PULMONIC AREA

S_2 loud and split with inhalation
Pulmonic valve murmurs

ERB'S POINT

S_2 split with inhalation
Aortic diastolic murmur
Pericardial friction rub

TRICUSPID AREA

S_1 split
Right ventricular S_3 and S_4
Tricuspid valve murmurs
Murmur of ventricular septal defect

MITRAL AREA

S_1 loud
Left ventricular S_3 and S_4
Mitral valve murmurs

II intensity, and a blowing quality. They are often heard best in the tricuspid area and do not radiate.

When auscultating murmurs, the examiner should visualize the cardiac anatomy, specifically the location of the heart valves and the direction of sound transmission with valve closure and murmur. Generally the systolic valvular murmurs will radiate downstream from the valve that is narrowed (stenotic), and the diastolic valvular murmurs—indicating a backflow of blood through an incompetent valve—will be auscultated best directly over the area of the valve (Fig. 14-6). The box above reviews where sounds are best heard on the specific areas of the precordium.

◆ **Murmurs associated with myocardial infarction.** At the bedside, the nurse is often the first person to auscultate a murmur. The holosystolic or pansystolic murmurs that can occur during acute myocardial infarction are good examples. The auscultation of a new, high-pitched, holosystolic, blowing murmur at the cardiac apex heralds mitral valve regurgitation secondary to papillary muscle dysfunction. This murmur may be soft (I/VI or II/VI) and occur only during ischemic episodes when the papillary muscle contractility is impaired, but its presence is associated with persistent pain, heart failure, and higher mortality.[8] If the murmur is loud (V/VI or VI/VI), harsh, and radiating in all directions from the apex, the papillary muscle or chordae tendineae may have ruptured. This is an emergency situation requiring immediate medical and often surgical intervention.

Ventricular septal defect, or rupture, is another emergency situation. It creates the same type of harsh, holosystolic murmur, loudest along the left sternal border. The clinical picture associated with both the papillary muscle rupture and the ventricular septal defect is that of acute heart failure and cardiogenic shock. Immediate diagnosis and treatment are necessary to prevent deaths.

Pericardial friction rub. A pericardial friction rub is a sound that can occur within the first week of a myocardial infarction and/or cardiac surgery and is secondary to pericardial inflammation. Its appearance can indicate a pericardial effusion and warrants a cardiac ultrasound study.[9,10] It is a "to-and-fro," scratching sound that corresponds with cardiac motion within the pericardial sac (i.e., ventricular systole, ventricular diastole, and atrial systole), so it can be both a systolic and diastolic sound. It is high-pitched and best auscultated at Erb's point (the third ICS to the left of the sternum; see Fig. 14-4). It is often associated with chest pain, and it is important to differentiate pericarditis from myocardial ischemia. The detection of the pericardial friction rub can assist in the proper diagnosis and treatment.

REFERENCES

1. Braunwald E, editor: *Heart disease: a textbook of cardiovascular medicine,* ed 4, Philadelphia, 1992, WB Saunders.
2. Hurst J, editor: *The heart, arteries, and veins,* ed 7, New York, 1990, McGraw-Hill.
3. Anardi D: Assessment of right heart function, *J Cardiovasc Nurs* 6(1):12, 1991.
4. Clinical signs in heart failure, *Lancet* 2(8658):309, 1989.
5. Blank C, Irwin G: Peripheral vascular disorders: assessment and interventions, *Nurs Clin North Am* 25(4):777, 1990.
6. Leonard JJ and others: *Examination of the heart,* Dallas, 1974, American Heart Association.
7. Wilkin MK and others: Mechanism of disappearance of S_3 with maturation, *Am J Cardiol* 64(19):1394, 1989.
8. Barzilai B and others: Prognostic significance of mitral regurgitation in acute myocardial infarction, *Am J Cardiol* 65(18):1169, 1990.
9. Pierce CO: Acute post-MI pericarditis, *J Cardiovasc Nurs* 6(4):46, 1992.
10. Sugiura T and others: Clinical significance of pericardial rub with regional ventricular dilatation, *Chest* 100:128, 1991.

15

Cardiovascular Diagnostic Procedures

CHAPTER OBJECTIVES

- ◆ Describe the electrocardiographic changes that occur with hypokalemia and hyperkalemia.
- ◆ List important aspects of the normal chest radiograph with which the critical care nurse should be familiar.
- ◆ Describe proper placement of the electrodes for cardiac monitor leads II, MCL_1, and MCL_6 and for the 12-lead ECG.
- ◆ Explain the three methods for determining cardiac rate from an ECG.
- ◆ Explain the important electrocardiographic findings, assessment aspects, and nursing actions for each of the dysrhythmias described in the chapter.
- ◆ State the expected nursing actions for elevations in the central venous pressure and the pulmonary artery pressure and the pathologic conditions responsible for these elevations.

Information needed for assessment of the cardiovascular patient's status can be obtained through laboratory studies of blood serum. Accurate interpretation of these laboratory studies, along with the clinical picture, enables the critical care team to diagnose, treat, and assess the response to therapeutic interventions.

Laboratory studies of blood serum are performed to assess (1) other organ systems that reflect or secondarily affect cardiac status, (2) electrolyte levels that directly affect cardiac function, (3) enzyme levels that may reflect myocardial infarction, (4) hematologic status for determination of anemia or infection that may be a cause of cardiac disease or coagulation problems, and (5) serum lipid levels for treatment of a coronary artery disease risk factor.

LABORATORY ASSESSMENT

General Chemistry Studies

The routine chemistry studies performed in most hospital laboratories when a patient is admitted give information about glucose metabolism, kidney function, liver function, and electrolyte concentrations. The presence of increased glucose during a fasting state (serum drawn 12 hours after most recent ingestion of food or drink) may indicate diabetes mellitus, which is believed to accelerate atherosclerosis. Renal failure, assessed by determining increased levels of urea nitrogen and creatinine, may cause electrolyte imbalances of potassium and calcium, which affect cardiac conduction and contractility. Abnormal liver function tests may alert the medical team to liver dysfunction caused by failure of the right side of the heart that is not clinically evident. Liver function indexes seen on the chemistry report include alkaline phosphatase, bilirubin, aspartate aminotransferase (AST), and alanine aminotransferase (ALT). "Normal" laboratory values vary from institution to institution but should be readily available to the staff.

◆ **Potassium.** During depolarization and repolarization of nerve and muscle fiber, potassium and sodium exchange occurs intracellularly and extracellularly. Thus either an excess or a deficiency of potassium can alter cardiac muscle function. Too much potassium (hyperkalemia) will decrease the rate of ventricular depolarization, shorten repolarization, and also depress atrioventricular (AV) conduction. As the serum levels of potassium rise from the normal of 3.5 to 5.5 mEq/L, evidence of these phenomena can be seen on the ECG (Fig. 15-1). Tall, peaked T waves are usually, although not uniquely, associated with early hyperkalemia, followed by widening of the QRS complex and prolongation of the P wave and PR interval. If serum potassium levels rise above 10 to 14 mEq/L, depressed AV conduction (Fig. 15-2) will lead to cardiac standstill or ventricular fibrillation. Coexisting low serum sodium, calcium, or pH levels potentiate the cardiac effects of hyperkalemia.

A low serum potassium level (hypokalemia)—commonly caused by gastrointestinal losses, diuretic therapy with insufficient replacement, and chronic steroid therapy—is also reflected by the ECG (Fig. 15-3). Myocardial conduction is impaired, and ventricular repolarization is prolonged as evidenced by a prominent U wave. The U wave is not totally unique to hypokalemia, but its presence should alert the nurse to check the potassium serum level. Another ECG indicator of hypokalemia is the sudden occurrence of supraventricular and ventricular dysrhythmias. They result from the prolonged repolarization phase and can be evident in most patients with serum potassium levels below 2.6 mEq/L.[1] These rhythm disturbances are reversible with potassium replacement. (See box, p.185, for chemistry values that affect cardiac contractility.)

◆ **Calcium.** Maintaining a normal serum calcium (Ca^{++}) level is important because of its effect on myocardial contractility and cardiac excitability. The normal serum level ranges from 9 to 11 mg/dl. Increased amounts (hypercalcemia) strengthen contractility and shorten

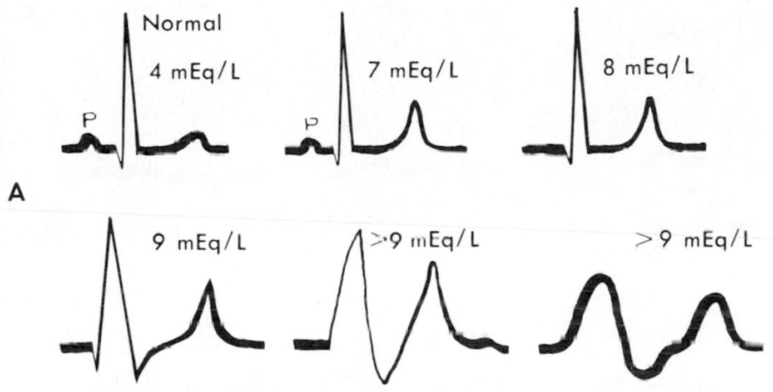

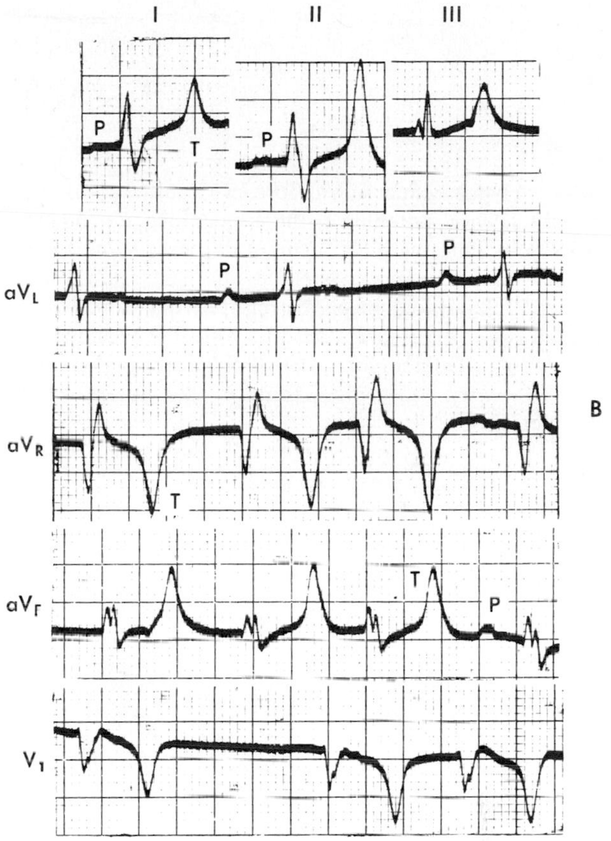

Fig. 15-1 Effects of hyperkalemia. **A,** The earliest electrocardiogram (ECG) change with hyperkalemia is peaking (tenting) of the T wave. With progressive increases in the serum potassium level, the QRS complexes widen, P waves disappear, and, finally, ventricular fibrillation develops. These changes do not necessarily occur with a specific serum potassium level. For example, some patients can have a normal ECG with a potassium level of 7 mEq/L, (patients with chronic renal failure), whereas other patients with an *acute* rise in serum potassium to a similar level will have ventricular fibrillation. **B,** Note the peaked T waves, widened QRS complexes, and prolonged PR intervals. Intermittently, a junctional rhythm is present with no P waves. (From Goldberger AL, Goldberger E: *Clinical electrocardiography: a simplified approach,* ed 4, St Louis, 1990, Mosby–Year Book.)

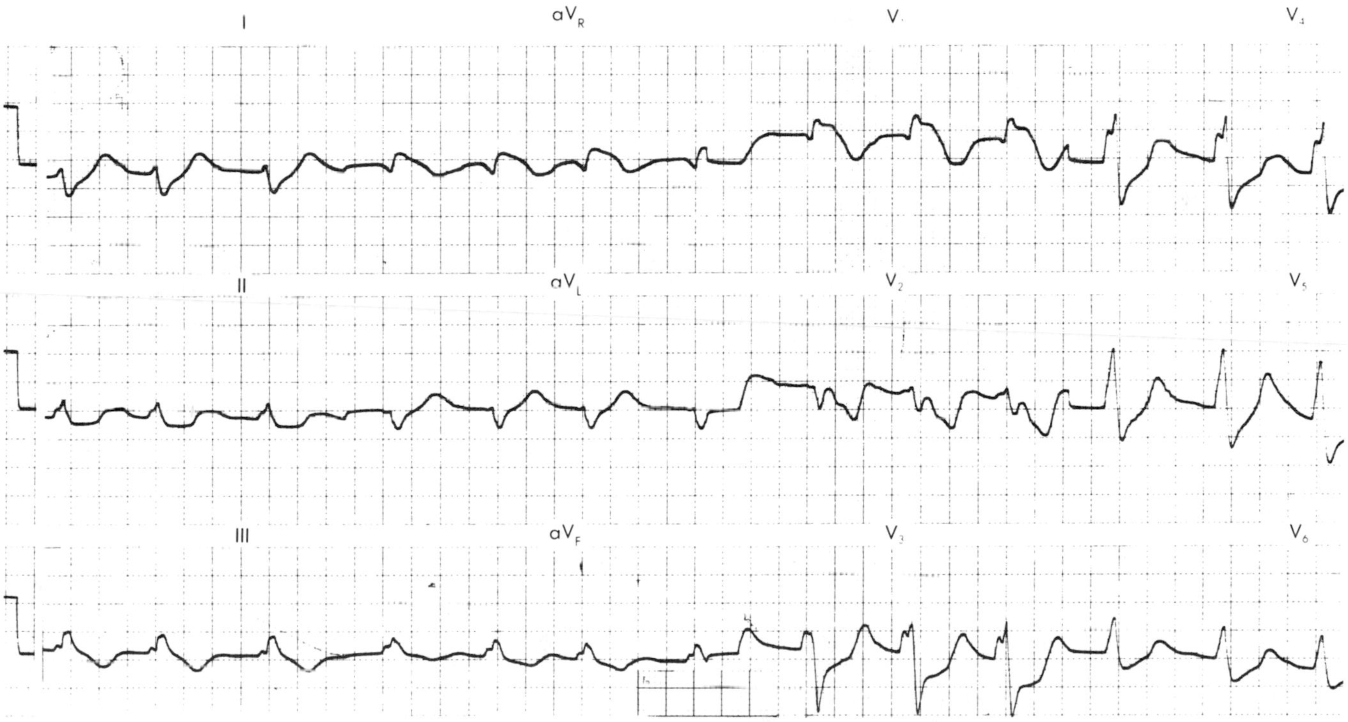

Fig. 15-2 Marked hyperkalemia. The potassium concentration is 8.5 mEq/L. Note the absence of P waves and the bizarre QRS complexes. (From Goldberger AL, Goldberger E: *Clinical electrocardiography: a simplified approach,* ed 4, St Louis, 1990, Mosby–Year Book.)

A

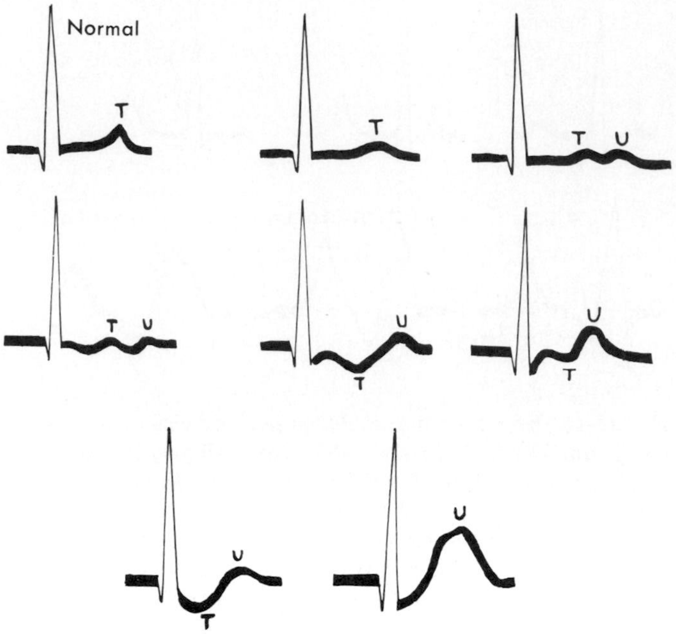

B

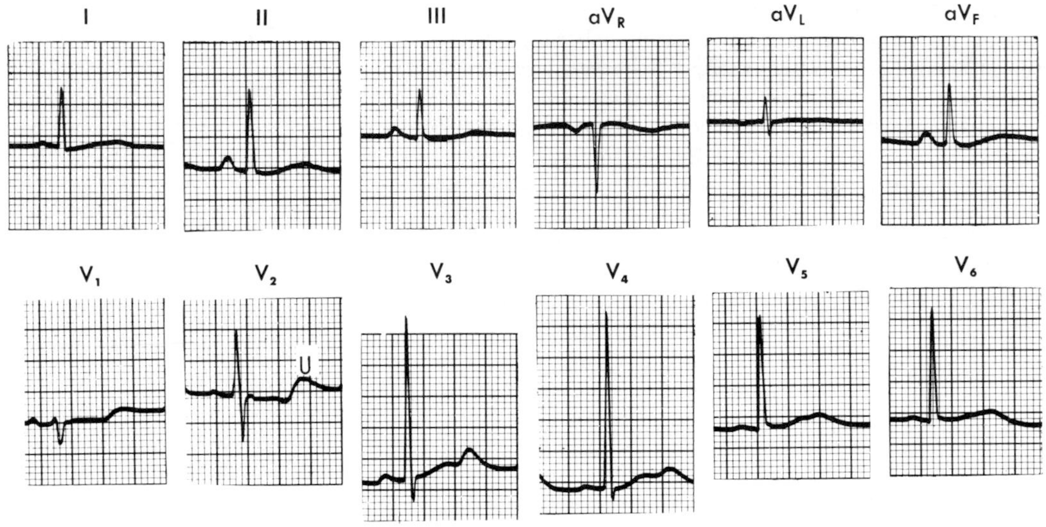

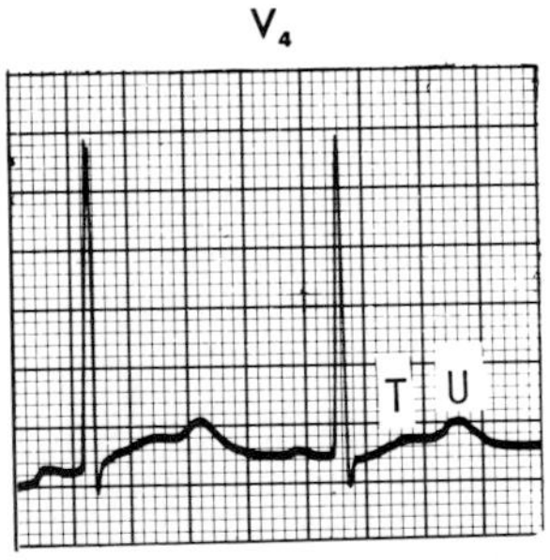

Fig. 15-3 Hypokalemia. **A,** Variable ECG patterns—ranging from slight T-wave flattening to the appearance of prominent U waves, sometimes with ST-segment depressions or T-wave inversions—may be seen with hypokalemia. These patterns are not directly related to a specific level of serum potassium. **B,** Serum potassium level is 2.2 mEq/L. Note the prominent U waves. (From Goldberger AL, Goldberger E: *Clinical electrocardiography: a simplified approach,* ed 4, St Louis, 1990, Mosby–Year Book.)

ventricular repolarization. The ECG demonstrates this shortened repolarization with a shortened QT interval. A low serum calcium level (hypocalcemia) has the opposite effect on the myocardium. The ECG shows a prolonged QT interval. Below a level of 6 mg/dl, QT prolongation is common, proportional to the amount of hypocalcemia, and reversed with infusion of calcium.[1]

Calcium levels are disrupted by tumors of the bone and lung, endocrine disorders, excessive intake or deficiency of vitamin D, intestinal malabsorption of calcium, kidney failure, and pancreatitis.

◆ **Magnesium.** Magnesium (Mg^{++}) is essential for many enzyme, protein, lipid, and carbohydrate functions in the body. In the bloodstream it is found predominantly within the cells, although an adequate serum level (extracellular) is essential to normal cardiac and skeletal muscle function. The normal serum range is from 1.5 to 2.5 mEq/L, and hypomagnesemia (< 1.5 mEq/L) is more commonly seen than elevated Mg^{++} levels. Hypomagnesemia can be caused by insufficient intake in the diet or in total parental nutrition (TPN), by chronic alcohol abuse, or by diuresis. In cardiac patients use of diuretics to treat heart failure (HF) or fluid overload after cardiopulmonary bypass (CPB) often contributes to low serum Mg^{++} levels. Cardiac consequences of hypomagnesemia are demonstrated on the ECG by tall T waves, inverted T waves, and depressed ST segments. In the acute cardiac patient ventricular dysrhythmias range from premature ventricular contractions (PVCs) to ventricular tachycardia (VT) and fibrillation (VF). In the critical care setting hypomagnesemia and hypokalemia often coexist in the same patient. Because these low electrolyte values are caused by similar factors (diuresis), the low Mg^{++} may be overlooked as a potential cause of ventricular dysrhythmias. The magnesium level is raised by administering IV magnesium sulphate or chloride, and the serum level is rechecked.

◆ **Cardiac enzymes.** Cardiac enzymes are proteins that are released from irreversibly-damaged myocardial tissue cells. The enzymes released by damaged myocardium include creatine kinase (CK) and lactate dehydrogenase (LDH). Other organs, when damaged or necrotic, will emit these same enzymes. Therefore, when measured as a whole, the enzymes are not cardiac specific. Each enzyme, however, can be broken into its component parts and labeled isoenzymes; the serum level of these cardiac-specific components will yield information of diagnostic value for cardiac disease. The typical sequence of appearance of each of the enzymes and its isoenzymes is listed in Table 15-1.

Both CK and LDH have isoenzymes that are cardiac-specific. CK has three isoenzymes composed of varying amounts of muscle (M) and brain (B) subunits. The brain and gastrointestinal tract contain high concentrations of CK-BB; skeletal muscle and myocardium contain CK-MM. Myocardial cells contain the CK-MB isoenzyme, which is only minimally found in any other tissue and appears in the serum only subsequent to myocardial cell death. CK-MB is, at present, the most specific and sensitive serum index for diagnosing myocardial infarction in patients evaluated within 24 hours of onset of chest pain.[2,3] It can be used to estimate infarct size.[3] Serial samples should be drawn during admission and 12 and 24 hours after admission to help establish or rule out the diagnosis of myocardial infarction. The serum specimens must be kept on ice if more than 2 hours will elapse between the draw and assay time, because time and heat will reduce the MB fraction.

LDH is composed of five isoenzymes (LDH_1, LDH_2, LDH_3, LDH_4, and LDH_5), and myocardial cells contain a majority of LDH_1 and LDH_2. Normal serum levels of LDH contain varying amounts of all five isoenzymes, with LDH_2 the dominant fraction, followed by LDH_1, LDH_3, LDH_4, and LDH_5, respectively. When myocardial infarction occurs, both the LDH_1 and the LDH_2 levels rise, and the $LDH_1:LDH_2$ ratio becomes greater than 1 (normally it is less than 1). In other words, the normal situation wherein LDH_2 levels are greater than LDH_1 levels is reversed. An LDH_1 level that is greater than the LDH_2 level can be diagnostic, especially if the patient is initially seen more than 24 hours after onset of symptoms and the CK-MB isoenzyme peak is missed. The $LDH_1:LDH_2$ ratio can flip back and forth, making it important to collect more than one specimen over time. False rises in the LDH_1 level can occur with hemolysis of red blood cells, so care must be taken in collecting the serum specimen.

It cannot be overemphasized that these enzymes are found in multiple other tissues and are released by these tissues in times of stress or tissue damage.[2,3] Therefore a diagnosis of myocardial infarction can be determined only after assessing the ECG changes and clinical manifestations, as well as the serum enzyme levels.

CHEMISTRY VALUES THAT IMPACT CARDIAC CONTRACTILITY

	NORMAL RANGE
Potassium (K^+)	3.5-5.5 mEq/L
Calcium (Ca^{++})	9-11 mg/dl
may also be reported in mEq/L	Total Ca^{++} 4.3-5.3 mEq/L Ionized Ca^{++} 1.9-2.25 mEq/L
Magnesium (Mg^{++})	1.5-2.5 mEq/L

Hematologic Studies

Hematologic laboratory studies that are routinely ordered for the management of patients with altered cardiovascular status are red blood cell (RBC or erythrocyte) level, hemoglobin (Hgb) level, hematocrit (Hct) level, erythrocyte sedimentation rate (ESR), white blood cell (WBC or leukocyte) level, and coagulation tests.

◆ **Red blood cells.** The normal amount of RBCs varies with age, gender, environmental temperature, altitude, and exercise. Males produce 4.5 to 6 million RBCs per cubic millimeter, whereas the normal level for females is 4 to 5.5 million per cubic millimeter. The major function of RBCs is to carry hemoglobin (Hgb), which transports and releases oxygen to the tissues of the body. Hgb levels

Table 15-1 Cardiac enzyme serum levels associated with myocardial infarction

Cardiac enzymes	Elevation (hours)	Peak (hours)	Duration (days)
Creatine kinase (CK)	4-8	12-24	3-4
Creatine kinase-MB (CK-MB)	4-8	12-20	2-3
Lactate dehydrogenase (LDH)	12-48	72-144	8-14
$LDH_1 : LDH_2$ (normally <1)	12-14 ($LDH_1 : LDH_2 > 1$)	72-144	14

range from 14 to 18 g/dl in males and from 12 to 16 g/dl in females. Hematocrit (Hct) is the volume percentage of RBCs in whole blood—40% to 54% for males and 38% to 48% for females. When the serum level of total RBCs falls, it is logical also to see a fall in Hgb and Hct levels. Anemia, a hematologic disorder of insufficient amounts of RBCs (and concurrently, decreased Hgb and Hct levels) can cause an increase in cardiac workload, cardiac dilation, and eventually cardiac failure. An increase in the number of RBCs (polycythemia) also results in increased levels of hemoglobin and hematocrit and often occurs as a response to tissue hypoxia. The erythrocyte sedimentation rate (ESR) is a measurement of how quickly RBCs separate from plasma in 1 hour. With injury (e.g., myocardial infarction), inflammation (e.g., endocarditis), or pregnancy, RBCs have higher globulin and fibrinogin levels, which cause faster precipitation and increase the sedimentation rate. Heart failure can decrease the ESR because of associated decreased levels of serum fibrinogen.

◆ **White blood cells.** Most inflammatory processes such as rheumatic fever, endocarditis, and myocardial infarction (producing necrotic tissue within the heart muscle) are reflected in an increased WBC level. The normal level of serum leukocytes for both genders is 5000 to 10,000 per cubic millimeter.

Blood Coagulation Studies

Coagulation studies are ordered, to determine serum clotting effectiveness. A patient who has stasis of blood (e.g., with atrial fibrillation or prolonged bed rest) or who has a history of thrombosis is at risk for developing a thrombus and may require anticoagulation. Heparin or oral anticoagulating drugs may be administered to prevent clot formation or extension of a clot, and coagulation studies will be ordered to guide dosage of these drugs. Most coagulation study results are reported as the length of time *in seconds* it takes for blood to form a clot in the laboratory test tube. (See the box below for normal values.) The *prothrombin time* (PT) is used to determine the therapeutic dosage of coumadin (warfarin sodium) necessary to achieve anticoagulation. The PT may be reported in seconds, in percents, or as a ratio. Increasingly, the PT is also being reported by use of the *International Normalized Ratio* (INR). The INR was developed by the World Health Organization (WHO) in an attempt to standardize PT results between clinical laboratories worldwide. The box illustrates target INR ranges for different cardiovascular conditions that require anticoagulation. The *partial thromboplastin time* (PTT) is used to measure the effectiveness of intravenous or subcutaneous heparin administration. An additional test of heparin effect is the *activated coagulation time* (ACT). The ACT can be performed outside of the laboratory setting in areas such as the cardiac catheterization laboratory or the operating room or in specialized critical care units. Normal and therapeutic values for all of these coagulation studies are shown in the box.

NORMAL AND THERAPEUTIC ADULT COAGULATION VALUES

Test	Normal Value	Therapeutic Value	
PT	11-16 sec*	1.5 to 2.5 times normal	
INR	<2.0	Chronic atrial fibrillation	2.0 to 3.0
		Treatment of DVT/PE	2.0 to 3.0
		Mechanical heart valve	3.0 to 4.5
aPTT	28-38 sec	1.5 to 2.5 times normal	
PTT	60-90 sec	1.5 to 2.5 times normal	
ACT	70-120 sec†	150-190 sec	

*PT normal value may vary by ± 2 sec between different laboratories.

†ACT normal value may vary with type of activator used.

PT = Prothrombin time; *INR* = international normalized ratio; aPTT = activated partial thromboplastin time; PTT = partial thromboplastin time; ACT = activated coagulation time; DVT = deep vein thrombosis; PE = pulmonary embolism.

Serum Lipid Studies

Four primary blood lipid levels are important in evaluating an individual's risk of developing and/or progressing coronary artery disease: total cholesterol; high-density lipoprotein—cholesterol (HDL); low-density lipoprotein—cholesterol (LDL); and triglycerides.

Table 15-2 Lipid profile studies for use in diagnosis of hyperlipidemia

Test	Normal values	Considerations
Total cholesterol	120-200 mg/dl	Desirable <200 mg/dl
Triglycerides	Men: 30-40 yrs: 46-316 mg/dl >50 yrs: 75-313 mg/dl Women: 30-40 yrs: 37-174 mg/dl >50 yrs: 52-280 mg/dl	Fasting 12-14 hours
LDL-cholesterol*	70-80 mg/dl	LDL/HDL ratio <3.0 High risk >160 mg/dl Desirable <130 mg/dl
HDL-cholesterol	Men: >26 yrs: 26-63 mg/dl Women: 30-40 yrs: 36-82 mg/dl >50 yrs: 37-92 mg/dl	Cholesterol/HDL ratio <4.5

From Schell M: *Focus on Critical Care AACN* 17(3): 203, 1990.

*If LDL value is not available, use this formula:

LDL = Total cholesterol − (triglycerides/5 + HDL-cholesterol)

Cholesterol and the lipoproteins that carry it are produced by the liver. Cholesterol in excess amounts (>200 mg/dl) in the serum forces the progression of atherosclerosis (see Table 15-2 for normal lipid levels). Of the total cholesterol, 70% is contained in LDLs and approximately 20% to 25% is in the HDLs. The remainder of total cholesterol and most of the triglycerides are found in *very* low-density lipoproteins (VLDL). The HDLs are associated with a decreased incidence of coronary artery disease, whereas the LDLs tend to deposit cholesterol on artery walls and increase the incidence of coronary artery disease.[4] When levels of cholesterol, LDLs, and triglycerides are elevated or the level of HDLs is low, it is a cardiac risk factor that needs to be addressed and modified in the rehabilitation setting.

DIAGNOSTIC PROCEDURES

Chest Radiography

◆ **Basic principles and technique.** Chest radiography is the oldest noninvasive method for visualizing images of the heart, yet it remains a frequently used and valuable diagnostic tool. Information about cardiac anatomy and physiology can be obtained with ease and safety at a relatively low cost. In the critical care unit, the nurse may be the first person to view the chest radiograph of an acutely ill patient. Nurses also have an important role in influencing the quality of the film through proper positioning and instruction of the patient. For these reasons, it is vital that critical care nurses gain a basic understanding of chest x-ray techniques and interpretation as they apply to the cardiovascular system.

Tissue densities. As x-rays travel through the chest from the emitting tube to the film plate, they are absorbed to a varying degree by the tissues through which they pass (Table 15-3). Very dense tissue, such as bone, will absorb almost all the x-rays, leaving the film unexposed, or white. The heart, aorta, pulmonary vessels, and the blood they contain are moderately dense structures, appearing as grey areas on the x-ray film. These vascular structures are surrounded by air-filled lung that allows the greatest penetration of x-rays, resulting in fully exposed (black) areas on the film. Thoracic structures can be studied best by examining their borders. Two structures with the same density, when located next to each other, will have no visible border. If a structure is located next to a contrasting density (e.g., vascular structures next to an air-filled lung), even subtle changes in size and shape can be seen.

Standard positions. In most institutions, a standard radiographic examination of the heart and lungs consists of posterioanterior (PA) and lateral films. Fluoroscopy is a simple and inexpensive tool for examination of the dynamics of cardiac contraction, but it has been replaced by two-dimensional echocardiography, which is more accurate. The major use of fluoroscopy currently is for guidance during catheterization and other instrumentation of the heart.

Ideally, the chest radiograph is taken in the x-ray department with the patient in an upright position; the film exposed during a deep, sustained inhalation; and the x-ray tube aimed horizontally 6 feet from the film. This is a PA film, because the beam traverses the patient from posterior to anterior. To understand why distance is important, place your hand between a light source (preferably a light bulb) and a piece of paper so that a shadow is cast. Try moving the light bulb closer, then farther away from your hand. As the light bulb is moved farther away, the shadow becomes smaller and sharper, with less distortion. In addition, the closer your hand is to the paper, the clearer the shadow becomes. In this illustration, the x-ray tube acts as the light bulb, providing the source of radiation. The film plate is the "paper" on which the shadow is cast.

Table 15-3 X-ray densities of intrathoracic structures

Metal or bone (white)	Fluid (gray)	Air (black)
Ribs, clavicle, sternum, spine	Blood	Lung
Calcium deposits	Heart	
Surgical wires or clips	Veins	
Prosthetic valves	Arteries	
Pacemaker wires	Edema	

Because most patients in critical care units are too ill to go to the x-ray department, chest radiographs are routinely obtained by using portable x-ray machines, with the patient either sitting upright or lying supine, depending on the patient's clinical condition and the judgment of the nurse. In both cases, the film plate is placed behind the patient's back and an anterioposterior (AP) projection is used, in which the x-ray beam enters from the front of the chest. In the supine film the x-ray tube can be only approximately 36 inches from the patient's chest because of ceiling height and x-ray equipment construction, resulting in an inferior quality film from a diagnostic standpoint, because the images of the heart and great vessels are somewhat magnified and not as sharply defined. Whenever possible, the upright (AP) film is preferred to the supine because it is quicker; it shows more of the lung, since the diaphragm is lower; and the images are sharper and less magnified.

A deep, sustained inhalation is important. During exhalation, the lungs appear to cloud and the heart appears larger, possibly leading to an erroneous diagnosis of congestive heart failure, diffuse atelectasis, or consolidation.[5] Alert patients will be encouraged by the radiology technician to take in a deep breath and hold it while the exposure is taken. With patients receiving mechanical ventilatory support, the exposure must be timed to coincide with maximal inhalation. Some patients will simply be unable to maintain a sustained inhalation on command, resulting in a distorted cardiac shadow and poor visualization of the lung fields. For this reason it is important to be able to compare and contrast serial chest films before determining that progress or deterioration has occurred.

◆ **Cardiac radiographic findings.** Diagnosis from cardiac x-ray film is twofold: it involves observation of anatomic structures and observation of the pulmonary vascular bed to infer physiologic data. Anatomic considerations center around evaluation of the size and shape of cardiac chambers and great vessels, as well as valve calcifications, if present. Physiologic observations are related to specific x-ray findings that suggest changes in pulmonary venous pressure, pulmonary artery pressure, or pulmonary blood flow.

Enlargement of the heart and great vessels. Four major factors can cause enlargement of the heart and great vessels (Table 15-4). One is pressure overload, which results from obstruction of outflow and can be either a gradual or a sudden process.

Chronic systemic hypertension is an excellent clinical example of gradual pressure overload. The left ventricle tends to hypertrophy without significant dilation of the chamber. Ventricular wall thickness may increase 2 to 3 times its original mass at the expense of internal cavity volume rather than increase in external size. Because most of the enlargement is internal, the severity of the problem does not correlate well with x-ray findings of only mild ventricular enlargement.[6] The atria can also experience hypertrophy because of gradual pressure overload, but because atrial walls are thin, dilation will occur, resulting in external enlargement and visualization on the x-ray film.

If the pressure overload is of sudden onset, there will not be time for hypertrophy to develop and the result will be primarily chamber dilation. A clinical example of sudden pressure overload is massive pulmonary emboli; high pulmonary pressures that result from obstruction (emboli) of pulmonary blood flow will cause marked right ventricular dilation, which can be seen on x-ray film.

A second factor resulting in heart and great vessel enlargement is volume overload, which results in dilation of all structures involved, usually without hypertrophy. The most common clinical example is heart failure. The severity of the volume overload usually correlates well with the severity of chamber enlargement as seen on the chest radiograph.

An abnormal cardiac muscle or vascular wall can also be responsible for cardiac enlargement seen on chest x-ray film. Cardiomyopathies are examples of abnormal cardiac muscle. Hypertrophic cardiomyopathy involves extreme wall thickening with little or no dilation and only mild external enlargement. Dilated cardiomyopathy, on the other hand, results in moderate-to-severe dilation, often with a very thin muscle wall and marked cardiac enlargement on x-ray film. A thoracic aortic aneurysm is an example of a vascular wall abnormality that results in enlargement of the aorta.

Poststenotic dilation applies only to arteries. It occurs because of turbulent flow distal to an obstruction. Clinical examples include pulmonic valve stenosis, resulting in dilation of the trunk of the pulmonary artery, and aortic valve stenosis, resulting in dilation of the middle ascending aorta.

Cardiothoracic ratio. Estimation of the cardiothoracic ratio (often abbreviated CT ratio) is a technique used to measure overall heart size, with some limitations (Fig. 15-4). It is done with an upright frontal view (AP or PA). The maximal cardiac diameter is measured and compared with the maximal thoracic diameter at the level of the diaphragm[3] measured to the inner border of the ribs.

Table 15-4 Factors affecting enlargement of the heart and great vessels

Physiologic factor	Clinical correlation
Pressure overload	
Gradual onset	Chronic hypertension
Sudden onset	Massive pulmonary emboli
Volume overload	Heart failure
Abnormal tissue	
Cardiac muscle	Cardiomyopathies
Vascular wall	Aortic aneurysm
Poststenotic dilation	Pulmonic or aortic valve stenosis

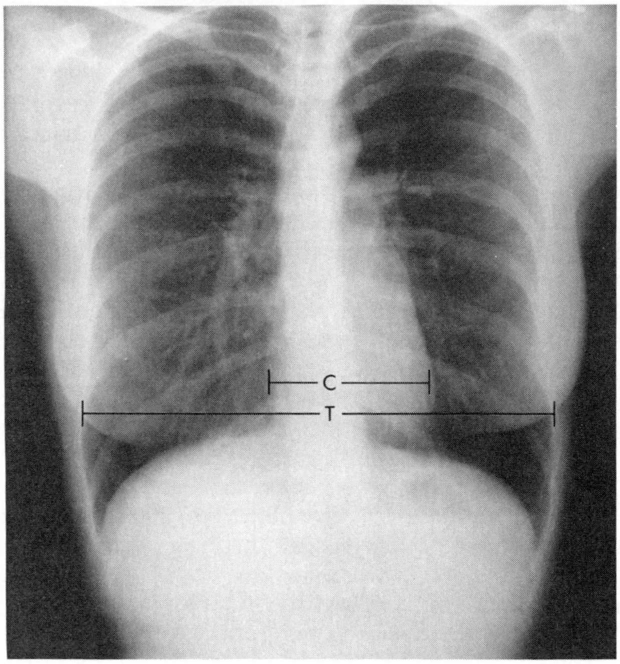

Fig. 15-4 Cardiothoracic (CT) ratio, a technique for estimating heart size on a PA chest film. Normally the cardiac diameter is 50% or less of the thoracic diameter when measured during full inhalation. *C,* Maximal cardiac diameter; *T,* maximal thoracic diameter measured to the inside of the ribs.

The CT ratio is considered abnormal if the cardiac diameter is greater than 50% of the total thoracic diameter. However, some false positives and some false negatives will occur using this criterion. It is most sensitive in detecting left ventricular enlargement, because the left ventricle enlarges toward the left chest wall. It is best to compare serial films, using the CT ratio to follow the progression of enlargement. One of the limitations of the CT ratio is that it may remain within normal limits in the presence of mild-to-moderate right ventricular or left atrial enlargement. Conditions that result in a falsely elevated CT ratio without actual cardiac enlargement include obesity, expiration or shallow inspiration (because of a high diaphragm position), chest wall deformity, and large pericardial fat pads. Because of these limitations, the CT ratio is most valuable when compared with a patient's previous films over time.

Assessment of chamber enlargement. Two basic principles apply to the assessment of cardiac enlargement through chest x-ray film: (1) in general, each chamber enlarges in a direction away from the remainder of the heart, and (2) if a particular chamber enlarges enough to come into contact with a rigid structure such as the spine or sternum, further enlargement will cause displacement and rotation of the entire heart.

In the frontal view of the chest, the right atrium composes the border of the right side of the heart, and the left ventricle represents the border of the left side (Fig. 15-5). Enlargement of either of these chambers can be seen and localized from this view. The right atrium enlarges to the right and causes increased fullness and convexity of the right cardiac border. Right atrial enlargement may be associated with superior vena cava and inferior vena cava dilation, causing widening of the right superior mediastinum. Left ventricular hypertrophy may not be clearly seen, and the CT ratio may remain normal. Rounding of the apex in comparison with previous films may be noted. If left ventricular dilation occurs as in congestive cardiomyopathy or volume overload, the CT ratio will increase to an above-normal level and the apex will be lower and laterally displaced.

In the lateral view of the chest (Fig. 15-6), the anterior border of the heart is formed by the right ventricle, which normally does not touch the sternum. The right ventricle initially enlarges anteriorly toward the sternum. As the right ventricle further enlarges, the whole heart rotates to the left and displaces the left ventricle posteriorly.

The upper posterior border of the heart is formed by the left atrium. The lower, more visible portion of the posterior border is composed of the left ventricle. Left atrial enlargement usually produces a double density behind the right atrial margin on a PA film. Other signs include upward and posterior displacement of the left main bronchus and displacement of the descending aorta.[7]

The superior vena cava forms the upper right border of the mediastinum on the frontal view. Because only the right border is defined (the left border blends in with the opacity of the rest of the mediastinal structures), the size of the superior vena cava cannot be measured accurately by chest x-ray film. The inferior vena cava is seen best in the lateral view. The posterior border is visible from where it leaves the diaphragm to where it enters the pericardial sac. The thoracic aorta lies within the mediastinum and is not clearly visible on either PA or lateral films if normal. When enlarged, the thoracic aorta rises out of the mediastinum and into contact with lung tissue, making it easier to visualize.

Pericardial effusions can sometimes be visible on a chest radiograph. A pericardial effusion will cause the entire outline of the heart to enlarge symmetrically. Occasionally, the separation of layers of epicardial fat from layers of extrapericardial fat by fluid can be seen on a lateral view just anterior to the right ventricle. Normally, this separation should be no greater than 2 mm; if it is greater, a pericardial effusion exists.[8] However, other noninvasive procedures, such as echocardiography, are much more specific in diagnosing and quantifying pericardial effusions.

◆ **Interpretation of pulmonary vascular patterns.** Under normal conditions the pulmonary arteries and veins are sharply defined, with a gradual decrease in blood vessel diameter from the center of the lungs to the periphery.

Pulmonary artery hypertension exists when pulmonary artery pressures are elevated because of obstruction at the pulmonary arteriolar level. This condition is seen clinically in patients who have chronic obstructive pulmonary disease and in those who have had multiple pulmonary emboli. The major vascular change visible on chest radiograph is dilation of the main pulmonary artery and its central hilar branches. The degree of dilation of the pulmonary arteries seen on x-ray film correlates closely with the degree and duration of pressure elevation. In addition, peripheral vessels may appear decreased in size, and, if chronic, tortuosity of lobar and segmental arterial branches occurs, along with "pruning" of the pulmonary arterial tree, which means that arterial branches become short and stumpy, not continuing to the periphery as they normally would.[9]

Pulmonary venous hypertension actually represents high pressures throughout the pulmonary circulation, beginning in the left atrium, being transmitted backward across the pulmonary veins, pulmonary capillaries, and pulmonary arteries, and resulting in right ventricular systolic hypertension. This entire sequence is caused by increased resistance to flow in the left side of the heart, either at the level of the mitral valve, as in mitral stenosis, or secondary to left ventricular failure.

Pulmonary venous pressure can be measured directly by a balloon-tipped pulmonary artery catheter wedged in the pulmonary capillary bed. As pulmonary venous congestion develops, pulmonary artery wedge pressure (PAWP) can be estimated from the venous markings on the chest x-ray film (Table 15-5).[10] Normal PAWP is 5 to 10 mm Hg. As the PAWP rises to 10 to 15 mm Hg, venous blood flow is redistributed so that upper and lower lung fields are perfused equally. Blood vessels in the apex of the lung, which were previously collapsed, now open as pressure within the vascular bed exceeds alveolar pressure.

With a further rise in PAWP to 15 to 20 mm Hg, upper lung fields are actually better perfused than are lower lung fields. On the chest x-ray film, pulmonary arteries and veins in dependent parts of the lung become smaller, mainly because of perivascular edema. When venous pressure, which is highest in the lower lobes of the lung because of gravity, exceeds plasma oncotic pressure (normally 20 to 25 mm Hg), fluid leaves the vascular bed and enters the interstitial space, causing edema. The edema surrounds and compresses arterioles and capillaries, increasing resistance to flow and decreasing size.

At PAWP of 25 to 35 mm Hg, edema of the interlobular septa occurs and can be seen on chest x-ray film. Known as *Kerley-B lines,* these fine, straight, linear shadows occur at right angles to the pleura and are

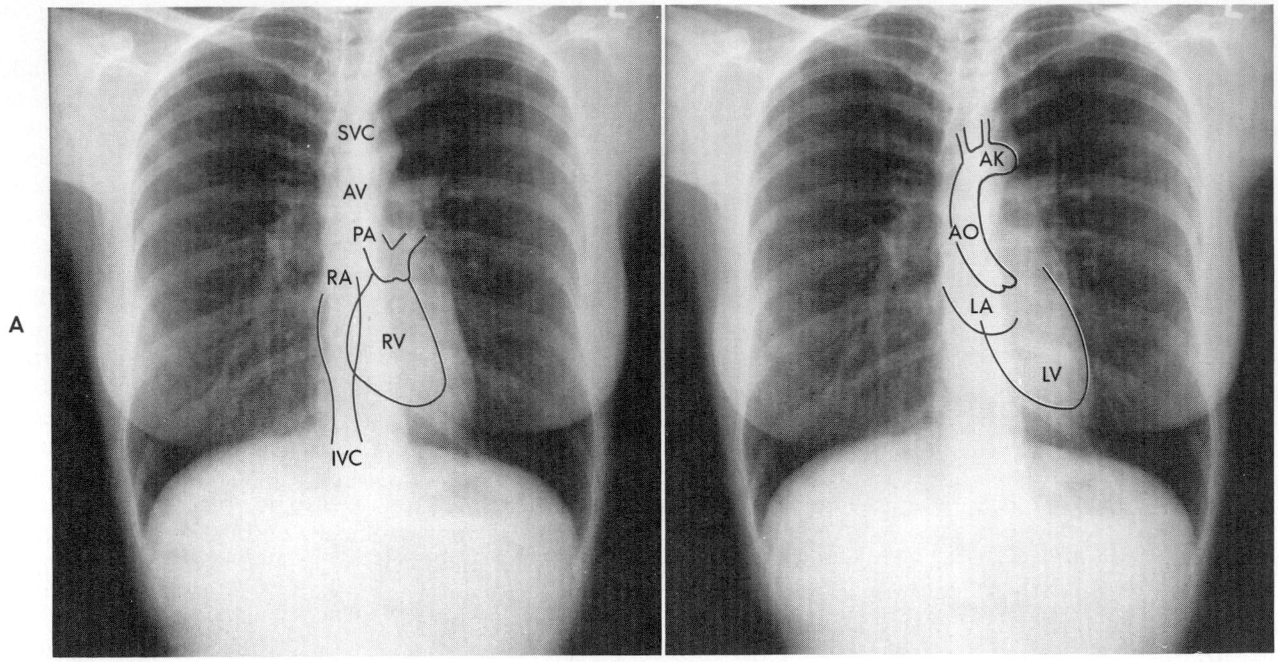

Fig. 15-5 Location of cardiac structures on a PA chest film. **A,** *AV,* Azygos vein; *SVC,* superior vena cava; *PA,* pulmonary artery; *RA,* right atrium; *RV,* right ventricle; *IVC,* inferior vena cava. **B,** *AO,* Aorta; *AK,* aortic knob; *LA,* left atrium; *LV,* left ventricle.

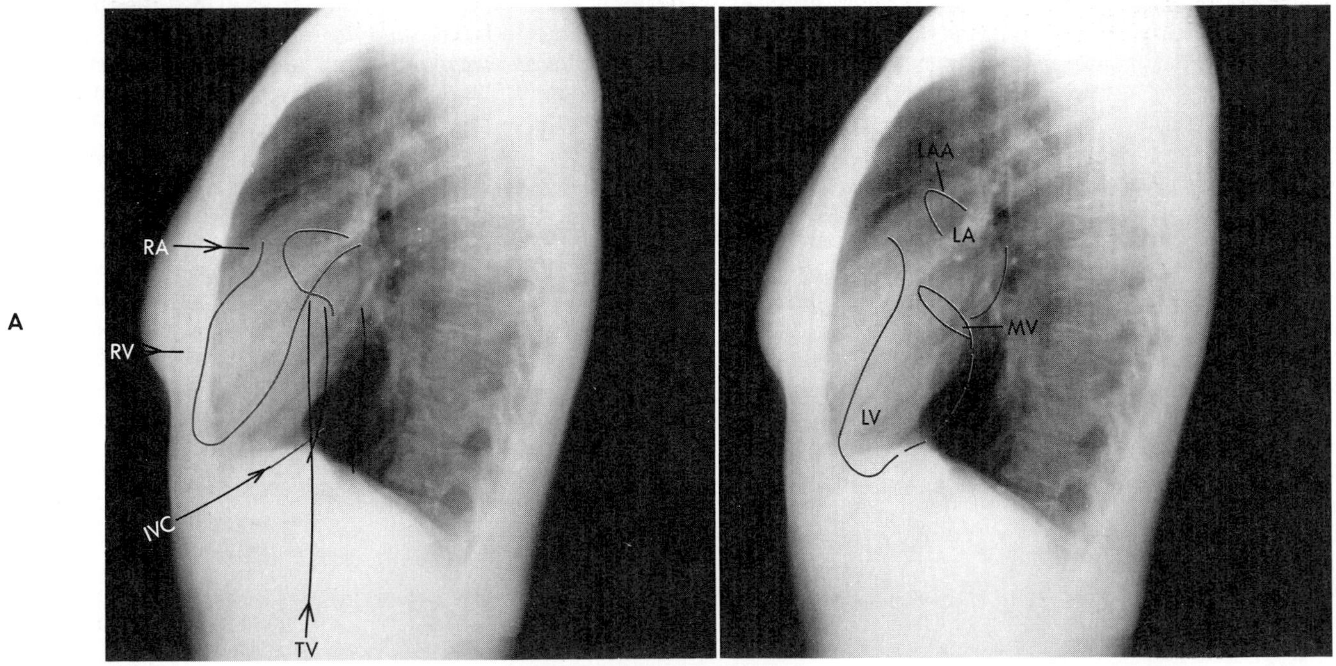

Fig. 15-6 Location of cardiac structures on a lateral chest film. **A,** *RV,* Right ventricle; *RA,* right atrium; *IVC,* inferior vena cava; *TV,* tricuspid valve. **B,** *LV,* Left ventricle; *MV,* mitral valve; *LA,* left atrium; *LAA,* left atrial appendage.

Table 15-5 Chest x-ray estimation of PAWP*

Pulmonary artery wedge pressure (mm Hg)*	Chest x-ray findings
5-10	Normal
10-15	Equal perfusion of upper and lower lung fields
15-20	Upper lung perfusion > lower lung perfusion
20-25	Interstitial edema in lower lobes
25-35	Kerley-B lines; increased size of main pulmonary artery and hilar branches; perihilar haze
>35	Diffuse perihilar infiltrates

*These PAWP values are guidelines. PAWP values may vary in individual patients.

approximately 1 to 2 cm long. They first appear in the dependent basilar area of the lung. The main pulmonary artery and hilar branches increase in size because of the elevation of pressure. As edema increases, clear definition of the hilar branches is lost and there is a faint, ill-defined increase in density around the hilum known as *perihilar haze.* Finally, as the PAWP exceeds 35 mm Hg, frank pulmonary edema ensues. The chest radiograph demonstrates these fluid-filled alveoli as diffuse infiltrates in the perihilar region.

The chest radiograph often continues to show evidence of pulmonary edema even after treatment has been initiated and pulmonary artery pressures have returned to normal. Interstitial fluid takes time to return to the vascular bed and be removed, which probably accounts for the time lag seen between the return of the PA pressures to normal and clearing on the x-ray film.

Coexisting conditions, such as pneumonia or atelectasis, will complicate chest film interpretation and render the chest radiograph less helpful in determining the extent of pulmonary edema. Although chest x-ray findings correlate reasonably well with pulmonary capillary wedge pressures in acute left ventricular failure, some evidence exists that this correlation is poor in chronic heart failure. Mahdyoon[11] studied 22 patients in severe end-stage congestive heart failure awaiting heart transplantation. These patients were all receiving maximal medical therapy, including digitalis, diuretics, and vasodilators. Among the group, the mean pulmonary capillary wedge pressure was 33 ± 6 mm Hg, and the mean cardiac index was 1.8 ± 0.5 L/min/m^2. Despite significant hemodynamic evidence of left-sided failure, 6 patients (27%) showed no x-ray evidence of pulmonary congestion; 9 patients (41%) showed redistribution of pulmonary blood flow but no evidence of interstitial edema; 6 patients (27%) showed redistribution of pulmonary blood flow and interstitial edema, but not alveolar edema; and only 1 patient showed classic redistribution of pulmonary blood flow, interstitial edema, and alveolar edema. Although the sample size was relatively small, this study raised the valid concern that the chest radiograph can significantly underrate the degree of pulmonary venous congestion in chronic left ventricular failure. In those cases, direct hemodynamic monitoring with a thermodilution pulmonary artery catheter would provide a more accurate assessment.

Electrocardiography

Electrocardiography is a complex subject about which much literature has been written and to which entire books have been devoted—and justifiably so. A detailed evaluation of a 12-lead electrocardiogram (ECG) can provide a wealth of cardiac diagnostic information and often provides the basis on which other definitive diagnostic tests are selected. This section provides a general understanding of dysrhythmias commonly encountered in clinical practice and a sound basis for understanding the value of the many clinical applications of electrocardiography.

◆ **Basic principles.** The ECG records electrical changes in heart muscle. It does not record mechanical contraction, which usually immediately follows electrical depolarization. However, a condition known as *electromechanical dissociation* occasionally occurs, in which the heart is mechanically at a standstill while rhythmic electrical impulses continue to be generated and then recorded on the ECG.

A review of the cardiac action potential illustrates electrical changes that occur (Fig. 15-7). During phase 0 *(depolarization),* the electrical potential changes rapidly from a baseline of −90 mV to +20 mV and stabilizes at about 0 mV. Because this is a significant electrical change, it appears on the ECG. Phases 1 and 2 represent an electrical plateau, during which time mechanical contraction occurs. Because there is no significant electrical change at this time, nothing shows on the ECG. During phase 3 *(repolarization),* the electrical potential again changes, this time a little more slowly, from 0 mV back to −90 mV. This is another major electrical event, and it is reflected on the ECG. Phase 4 represents a resting period, during which chemical balance is restored by the sodium pump, but since positively charged ions are exchanged on a one-for-one basis, there is no electrical activity and no visible change occurs on the ECG tracing.

Electrocardiographic leads. All electrocardiographs use a system of one or more *leads.* A lead consists of three electrodes: a positive electrode, a negative electrode, and a ground electrode. The function of the ground electrode is to prevent the display of background electrical interference on the ECG tracing. Leads do not transmit any electricity to the patient—they just sense and record it.

The positive electrode on the skin acts as a camera. If the wave of depolarization travels toward the positive electrode, an upward stroke, or *positive deflection,* is written on the ECG paper (Fig. 15-8, *A*). If the wave of depolarization travels away from the positive electrode, a downward line, or *negative deflection,* will be recorded on the ECG (Fig. 15-8, *B*). When depolarization moves perpendicularly to the positive electrode, a biphasic complex will occur. Sometimes the complex may even appear almost flat or isoelectric if the electrical forces

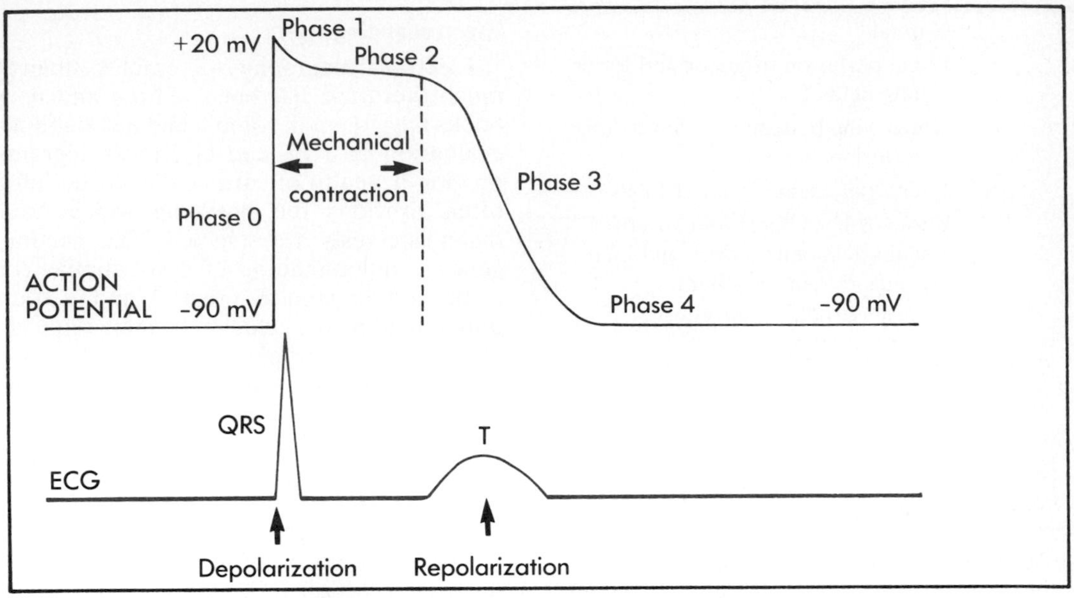

Fig. 15-7 Correlation of the action potential of a ventricular myocardial cell with the electrical events recorded on the surface ECG. Note that the ECG is "silent" during phase 2 of the action potential. Mechanical contraction is occurring, but there is no significant electrical activity.

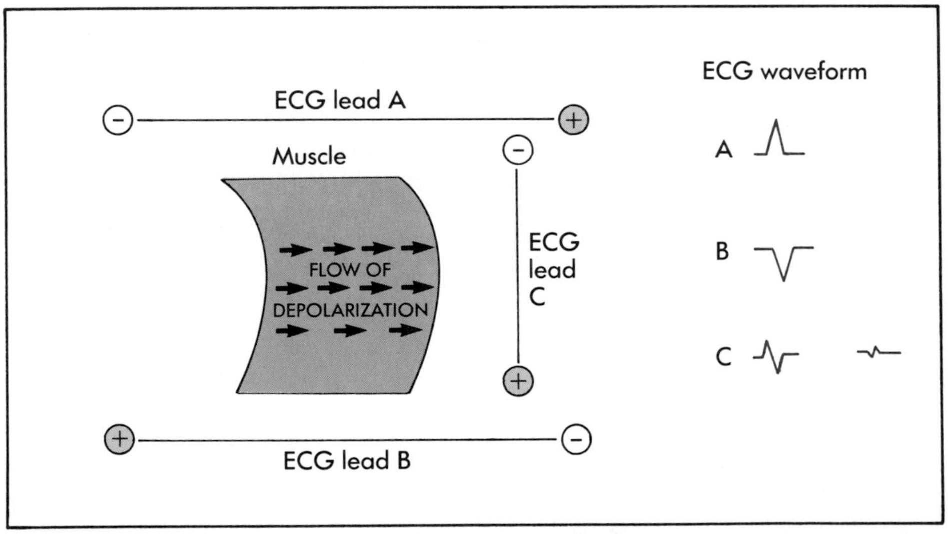

Fig. 15-8 Effect of lead position on the ECG tracing. *A,* Flow of depolarization toward the positive electrode will result in a positive deflection on the ECG. *B,* Flow of depolarization away from the positive electrode will result in a negative deflection on the ECG. *C,* Flow of depolarization perpendicular to the positive electrode will result in a biphasic or nearly isoelectric deflection on the ECG. This basic principle applies to both the P wave and the QRS complex.

traveling in opposite directions are equal and have the effect of canceling out each other (Fig. 15-8, *C*). The size of the muscle mass being depolarized also has an effect, with the larger muscle mass having a greater influence on the tracing.

The wave of ventricular depolarization in the healthy heart travels from right to left and head to toe. The appearance of the waveforms in different ECG leads will vary, depending on the location of the positive electrode. The standard 12-lead ECG provides a picture of electrical activity in the heart from the 12 different positions of the positive electrodes.

A standard 12-lead ECG consists of six limb leads and six chest leads (Fig. 15-9). The limb leads are obtained by placing electrodes on all four extremities. The exact location on the extremities does not matter, as long as skin contact is good and bone is avoided. The machine will interpret all extremity signals as coming from the connection of the extremity to the torso, that is, from the shoulder or groin.

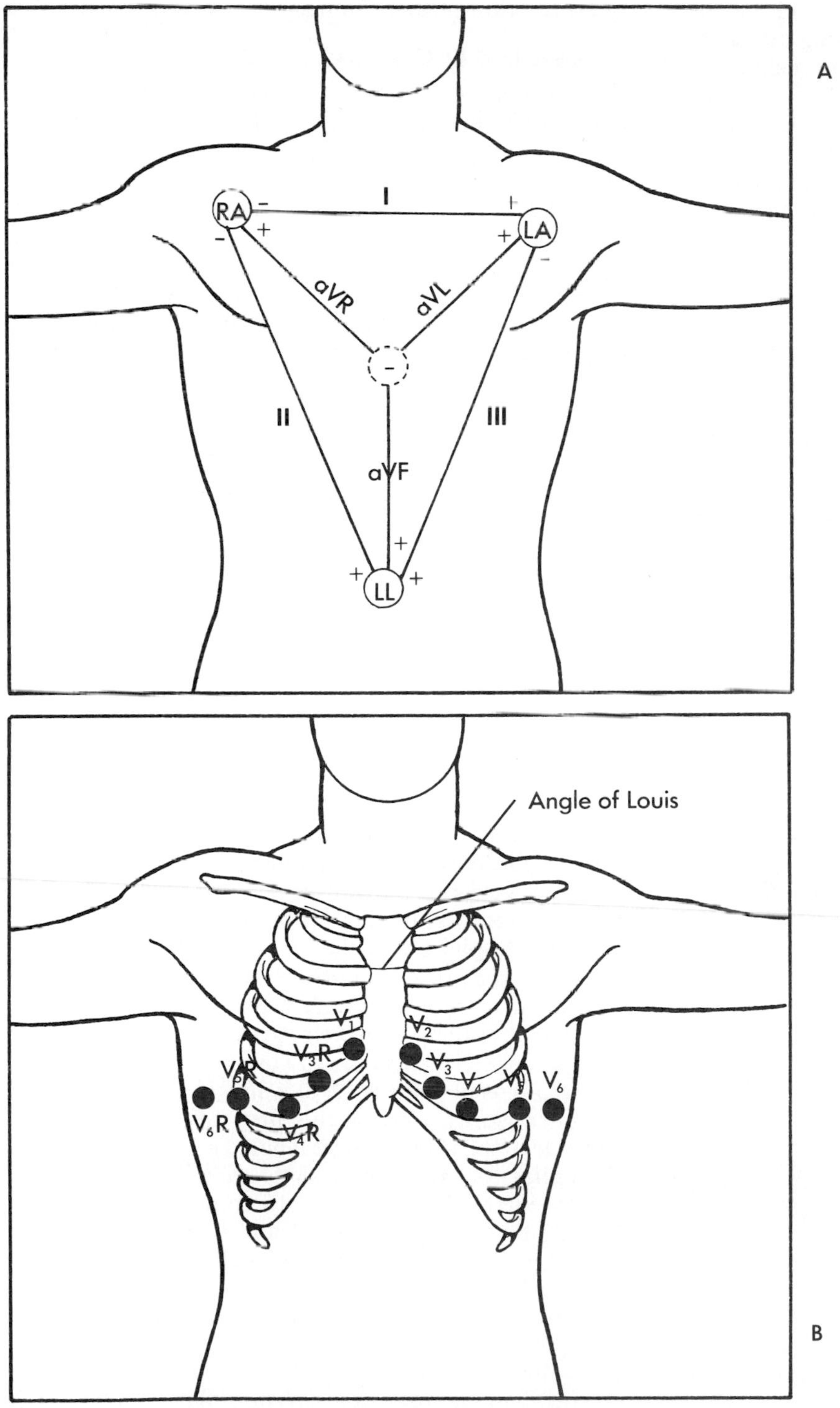

Fig. 15-9 **A,** Standard limb leads. Leads are actually located on the extremities. Leads I, II, and III are bipolar, using both a positive and a negative electrode. Leads aV_R, aV_L, and aV_F are augmented unipolar leads that use the calculated center of the heart as their negative electrode. **B,** Precordial leads. V_1 to V_6 are the six standard precordial leads and are placed as follows: V_1—fourth intercostal space, right sternal border; V_2—fourth intercostal space, left sternal border; V_3—equidistant between V_2 and V_4; V_4 fifth intercostal space, left midclavicular line; V_5—anterior axillary line, same horizontal level as V_4; V_6—midaxillary line, same horizontal level as V_4. In addition, the right precordial leads V_3R to V_6R are shown. They are not part of a standard 12-lead ECG but should be done whenever a right ventricular infarction is suspected. Their placement is identical to V_3 to V_6, except on the right side of the chest rather than on the left.

Leads I, II, and III are bipolar limb leads in that they consist of a positive and a negative electrode. The other three limb leads are labeled aV_R, aV_L, and aV_F, representing augmented vector right, left, and foot. These unipolar leads consist only of a positive electrode, with the negative electrode calculated within the machine at roughly the center of the heart. Under these circumstances the ECG tracing would ordinarily be very small, so the machine enhances, or *augments*, it. The term *vector* refers to directional force.

The six standard precordial chest leads are labeled "V" leads and are distributed in an arch around the left side of the chest. They are useful for viewing electrical forces traveling from right to left or front to back but are not helpful in evaluating vertical forces in the heart. For an accurate interpretation, all 12 leads must be considered. In addition, right-sided precordial chest leads can be placed for a closer look at electrical forces in the right ventricle. Labeled V_3R, V_4R, V_5R, and V_6R, they should be added to the standard 12-lead ECG whenever right ventricular infarction is suspected. A right ventricular infarction is most commonly associated with an inferior or posterior left ventricular infarction but has occasionally been noted in the setting of anterior infarction as well.[12]

Baseline distortion. It is important that the tracing have a flat baseline, which is that portion of the tracing that is between the various waveforms. Two forms of artifact can distort the baseline: 60-cycle interference and muscular movement. Sixty-cycle interference (Fig. 15-10, *A*) results from leakage of electrical current somewhere within the system and appears as a generalized thickening of the baseline. It can usually be resolved by ensuring that all electrical equipment at the bedside is well grounded. Occasionally, it may be necessary to unplug one piece of equipment at a time until the offending device is found. Muscular movement (Fig. 15-10, *B*) is displayed as a coarse, erratic disturbance of the baseline. In most cases, asking the patient to lie quietly while the ECG is being run is sufficient. If movement is caused by shivering or seizure activity, it is best to wait until the activity subsides before obtaining the 12-lead ECG. If tremor is caused by Parkinson's disease or other neuromuscular disorders, a resolution may not be possible. It should be remembered that the artifact will have an adverse effect on the accurate interpretation of the tracing.

A

B

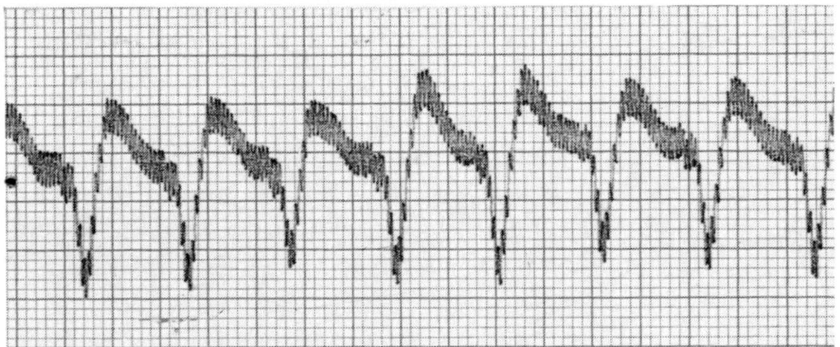

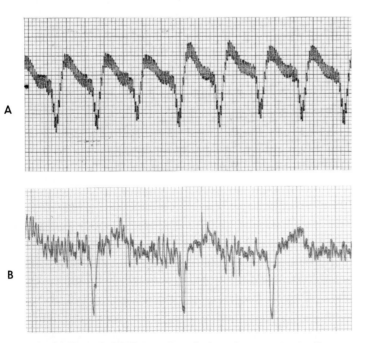

Fig. 15-10 **A,** Artifact – 60-cycle interference. **B,** Artifact – muscular movement.

◆ Twelve-lead ECG analysis

Specialized ECG paper. ECG paper records the speed and magnitude of electrical impulses on a grid composed of small and large boxes (Fig. 15-11). There are five small boxes in every large box. At a standard paper speed of 25 mm/second, one small box (1 mm) is equivalent to 0.04 second, and one large box (5 mm) represents 0.20 second. Distances along the horizontal axis represent speed and are stated in seconds rather than in millimeters or number of boxes. The vertical axis represents magnitude or strength of force. At standard calibration, one small box equals 0.1 mV, and one large box equals 0.5 mV. It is important to look for the standardization mark, which is usually located at the beginning of the tracing (Fig. 15-12, *A*). The mark indicates 1 mV and at standard calibration should go up two large boxes. Twelve-lead ECGs are sometimes run at different calibrations. If, at standard calibration, some complexes are so tall they run off the paper, the tracing should be repeated at half standard (Fig. 15-12, *B*), and the calibration mark will rise only one large box. If all of the complexes on a standard tracing are very small, it may be repeated at double standard, with the calibration mark going up four large boxes (Fig. 15-12, *C*). In any case, the calibration must be clearly marked on the tracing, because some diagnostic conclusions are based on the magnitude of specific portions of the ECG complex.

Waveforms. The analysis of waveforms and intervals provide the basis for ECG interpretation (Fig. 15-13). The P wave represents atrial depolarization. The QRS complex represents ventricular depolarization, corresponding to phase 0 of the ventricular action potential. It is referred to as a *complex* because it can actually consist of several different waves, depending on the placement of the positive electrode and the direction of the spread of electrical activity in the heart. Basically, the letter Q is used to describe an *initial* negative deflection; in other words, only if the first deflection from the baseline is negative will it be labeled a Q wave. The letter R applies to any positive deflection. If there are two positive deflections in one QRS complex, the second is labeled R′ (read "R prime") and is commonly seen in lead V_1 in right bundle branch block. The letter S refers to any subsequent negative deflections. Any combination of these deflections can occur and is collectively called the *QRS complex* (Fig. 15-14). The QRS duration is normally 0.10 second (2½ small boxes) or less.

The T wave represents ventricular repolarization,

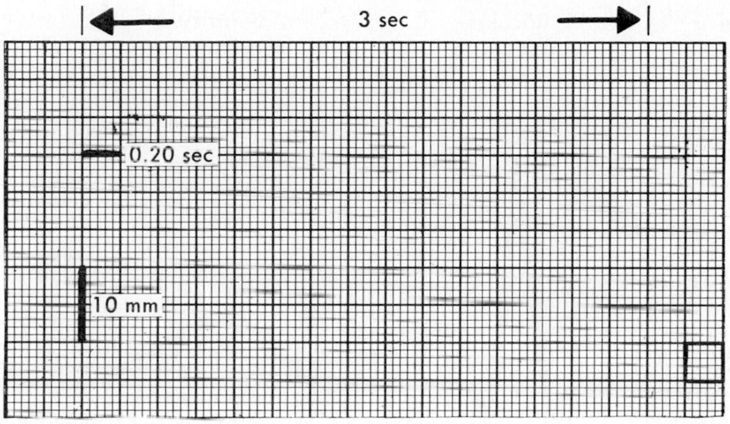

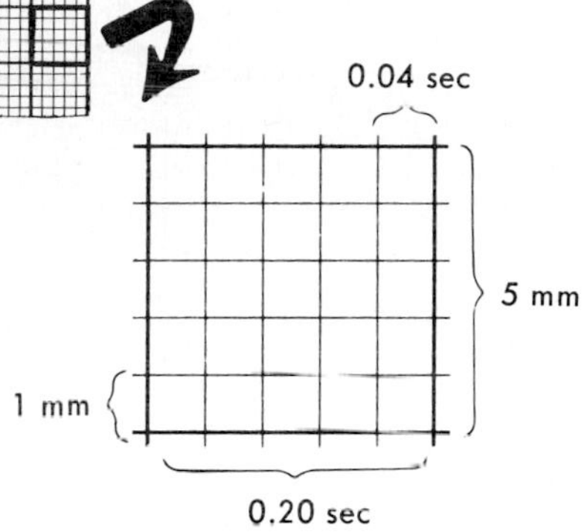

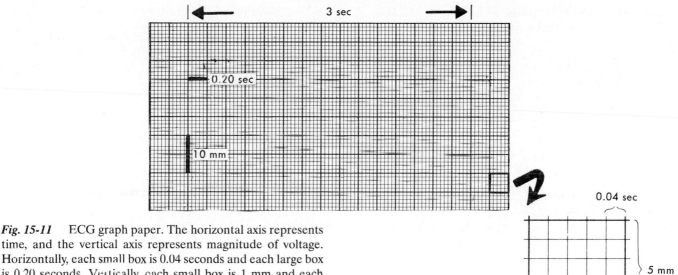

Fig. 15-11 ECG graph paper. The horizontal axis represents time, and the vertical axis represents magnitude of voltage. Horizontally, each small box is 0.04 seconds and each large box is 0.20 seconds. Vertically, each small box is 1 mm and each large box is 5 mm. Markings are present every 3 seconds at the top of the paper for ease in calculating heart rate. (From Goldberger AL, Goldberger E: *Clinical electrocardiography: a simplified approach,* ed 4, St Louis, 1990, Mosby–Year Book.)

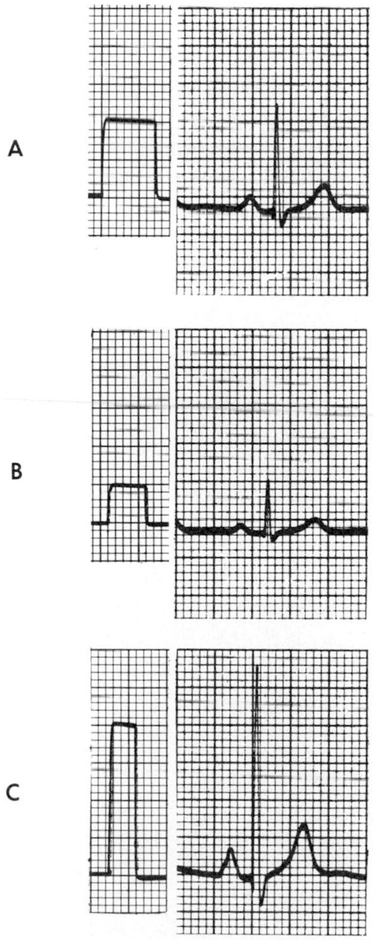

Fig. 15-12 **A,** Normal standardization mark, in which the machine is calibrated so that the standardization mark is 10 mm tall. **B,** Half standardization, used whenever QRS complexes are too tall to fit on the paper. **C,** Twice normal standardization, used whenever QRS complexes are too small to be adequately analyzed. (From Goldberger AL, Goldberger E: *Clinical electrocardiography: a simplified approach,* ed 4, St Louis, 1990, Mosby–Year Book.)

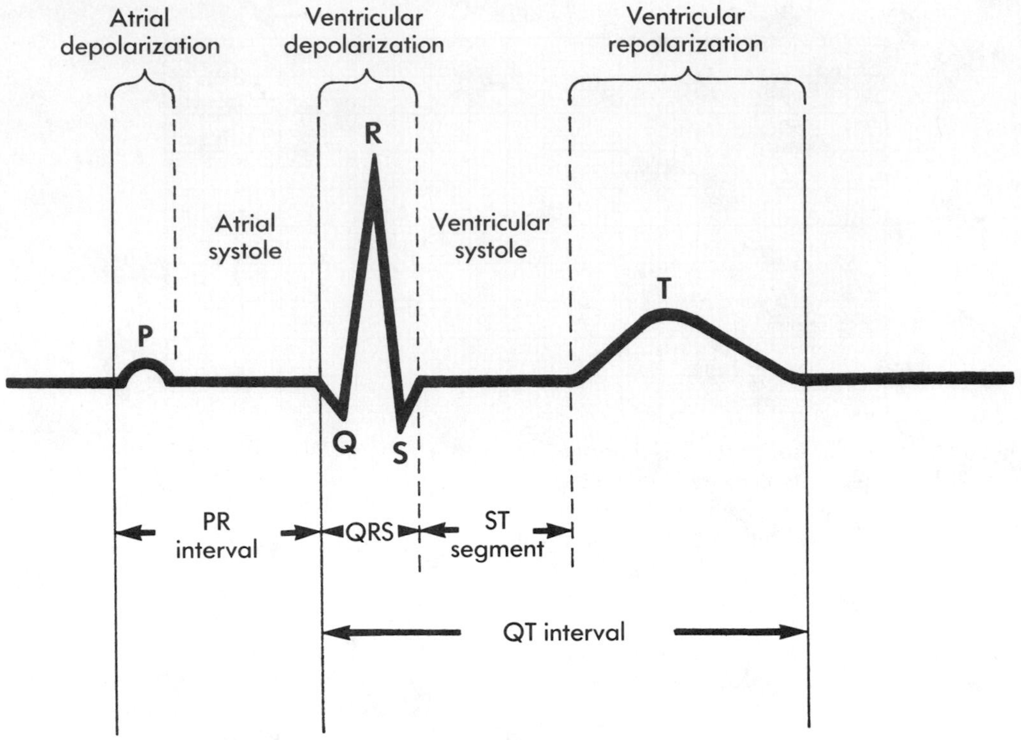

Fig. 15-13 Normal ECG waveforms, intervals, and correlation with events of the cardiac cycle. The P wave represents atrial depolarization, followed immediately by atrial systole. The QRS represents ventricular depolarization, followed immediately by ventricular systole. The ST segment corresponds to phase 2 of the action potential, during which time the heart muscle is completely depolarized and contraction normally occurs. The T wave represents ventricular repolarization. The PR interval, measured from the beginning of the P wave to the beginning of the QRS, corresponds to atrial depolarization and impulse delay in the AV node. The QT interval, measured from the beginning of the QRS complex to the end of the T wave, represents the time from initial depolarization of the ventricles to the end of ventricular repolarization.

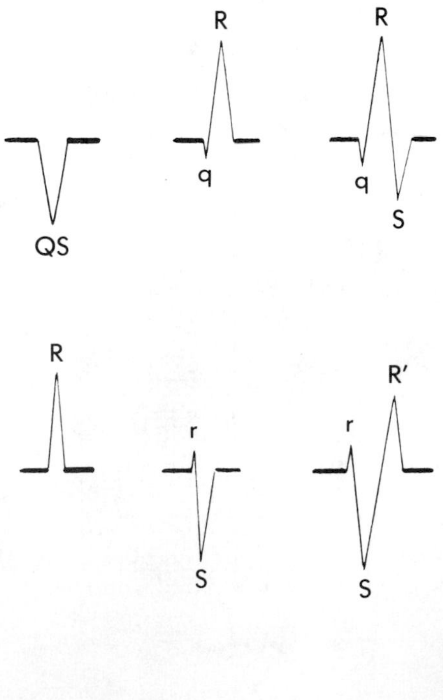

Fig. 15-14 Examples of QRS complexes. Small deflections are labeled with lowercase letters, whereas uppercase letters are used for larger deflections. A second upward deflection is labeled *R′* (read "R prime"). (Modified from Goldberger AL, Goldberger E: *Clinical electrocardiography: a simplified approach,* ed 4, St Louis, 1990, Mosby–Year Book.)

corresponding to phase 3 of the ventricular action potential. The onset of the QRS to approximately the midpoint or peak of the T wave represents an absolute refractory period, during which the heart muscle cannot respond to another stimulus no matter how strong that stimulus might be (Fig. 15-15). From the midpoint to the end of the T wave, the heart muscle is in the relative refractory period. The heart muscle has not yet fully recovered, but it could be depolarized again if a strong enough stimulus were received. This can be a particularly dangerous time for ectopy to occur, especially if any portion of the myocardium is ischemic, because the ischemic muscle will take even longer to fully repolarize. This sets the stage for the disorganized, self-perpetuating depolarizations of various sections of the myocardium that is known as *ventricular fibrillation.*

Intervals between waveforms. Intervals between waveforms are also evaluated (see Fig. 15-13). The PR interval is measured from the beginning of the P wave to the beginning of the QRS complex. Normally, the PR interval is 0.12 to 0.20 second in length and represents the time between sinus node discharge and the beginning of ventricular depolarization. Because most of this time period results from delay of the impulse in the AV node, the PR interval is an indicator of AV nodal function.

The portion of the wave that extends from the end of the QRS to the beginning of the T wave is labeled the *ST segment.* Its duration is not measured. Instead, its shape and location are evaluated. The ST segment should be flat and at the same level as the isoelectric baseline. Elevation or depression is expressed in millimeters and may indicate ischemia. The QT interval is measured from the beginning of the QRS complex to the end of the T wave and indicates the total time interval from the onset of depolarization to the completion of repolarization. At normal heart rates, the QT interval should be less than half of the RR interval (measured from one QRS complex to the next). However, the normal value of a QT interval is dependent on heart rate, so that a heart rate of 40 beats per minute (RR interval of 1.5 seconds), the normal QT interval is 0.50 second, only one third of the RR interval. Conversely, at a heart rate of 150 beats per minute (RR interval of 0.40 second), the normal QT interval is 0.25 second, fully 60% of the RR interval.

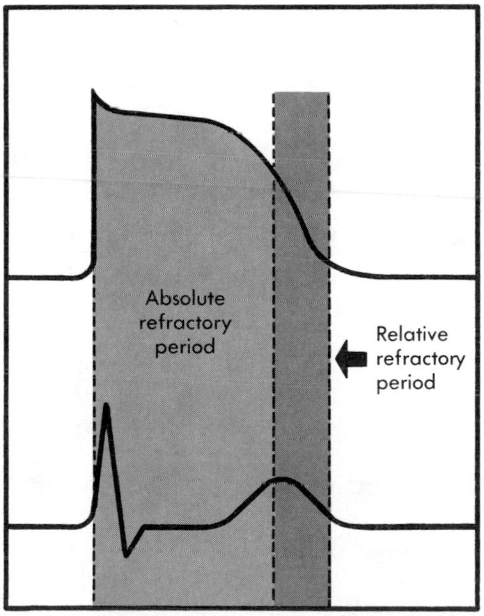

Fig. 15-15 Absolute and relative refractory periods correlated with the cardiac muscle's action potential and with an ECG tracing.

The most accurate method for evaluating a QT interval is to refer to a chart—available in most ECG textbooks—for its normal value at the specific heart rate. A prolonged QT interval is significant because it can predispose the patient to the development of a rapid form of ventricular tachycardia known as *torsades de pointes.* A long QT interval can be idiopathic (congenital) or can be acquired as a result of electrolyte imbalance or antidysrhythmic drug therapy. Quinidine is the antidysrhythmic drug most frequently responsible for the acquired form of prolonged QT interval. Although both forms of prolonged QT interval may produce similar dysrhythmias, there are distinct differences in their response to sympathetic nervous system stimulation and in their treatment. The acquired or drug-induced long QT syndrome is thought to arise from prolongation of the ventricular refractory period. Acute therapy is directed at increasing the heart rate, which will shorten the QT interval. Long-term management includes correction of the metabolic abnormality or removal of the responsible drug. In the idiopathic long QT syndrome, an autonomic imbalance exists, resulting in an enhanced response to sympathetic stimulation. Torsades de pointes usually occurs after some form of sympathetic discharge, such as sudden exertion, fright, emotional stress, delirium tremens, or cocaine use.[13] Therapy in that case is aimed at blocking beta adrenergic receptors with either medication (beta blockers) or surgery (left sympathectomy).

Although the ECG records only electrical events, it is helpful to understand the correlation of these intervals to the physiologic events of the cardiac cycle. Immediately after the P wave and during the PR interval, atrial systole occurs. Similarly, ventricular systole begins immediately after the QRS complex and continues until approximately the midpoint of the T wave (Fig. 15-13).

Ventricular axis. Electrical impulses spread through cardiac muscle tissue in many directions at once when the ventricular muscle is depolarized. All of these individual forces can be averaged to describe the overall direction that current is traveling, which is called the *mean vector.* The mean vector can be plotted on a circular graph known as the *hexaxial reference system* (Fig. 15-16), and a degree can be assigned to it. This degree represents the ventricular axis.

Normal range for ventricular axis varies slightly, but it is approximately −30 to +110 degrees. Right-axis deviation is present if the axis falls between +110 degrees and +180 degrees. Left-axis deviation is present if the axis falls between −30 and −90 degrees. If the axis

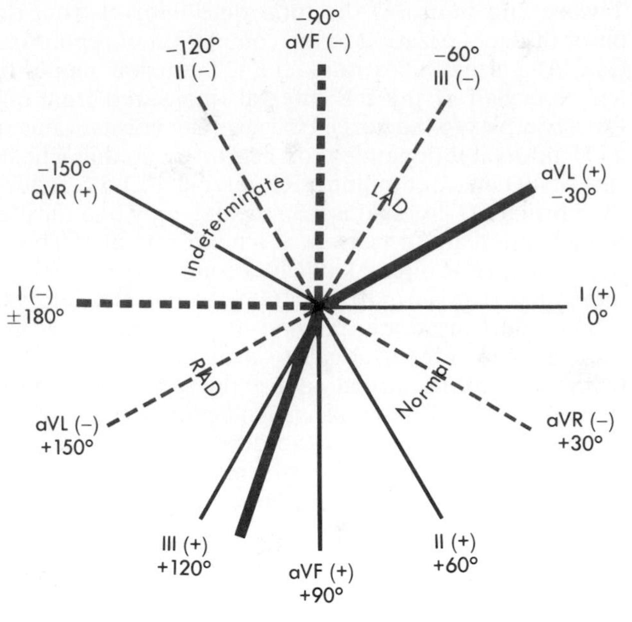

Fig. 15-16 Hexaxial reference system. *RAD,* right axis deviation; *LAD,* left axis deviation.

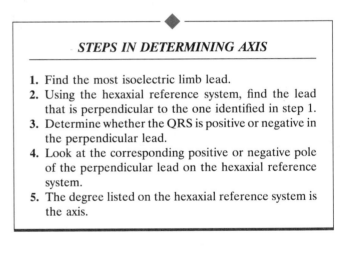

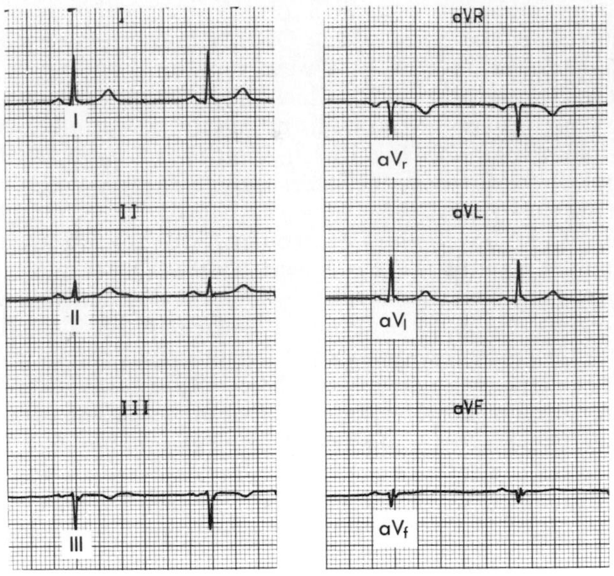

Fig. 15-17 Limb leads of normal ECG illustrating normal axis of 0 degrees.

plots in the upper left portion of the circle, it is called an *indeterminate axis* and can happen only if the wave of depolarization starts in the bottom of the ventricle and spreads upward toward the atria. Clinically, this can be seen in beats of ventricular origin, such as premature ventricular contractions (PVCs) and some pacemaker-initiated beats. To determine the frontal plane ventricular axis, the six limb leads are examined to find the lead with the smallest QRS complex, or the most equiphasic (equal portions above and below the baseline) if no complex is clearly the smallest. In Fig. 15-17, lead aV_F is the smallest. Next, using the hexaxial reference system (see Fig. 15-16), the lead is found that is perpendicular to the one that had the smallest complex. For example, perpendicular to lead aV_F is lead I, so the mean vector lies parallel with lead I. The third step is to determine if the QRS complex is positive or negative in the lead parallel to the mean vector (in this case, I). If the QRS is positive, the mean vector is directed toward the positive electrode. If the QRS is negative, the mean vector is directed away from the positive electrode. In Fig. 15-17, the QRS in lead I is upright, or positive. The positive pole of lead I is at the right midpoint of the hexaxial reference system and corresponds to a numeric degree of zero, which is normal (see box on right).

◆ **Cardiac monitor lead analysis.** During continuous cardiac monitoring, adhesive, pre-gelled electrodes are used to obtain an ECG tracing that is similar to one lead of a 12-lead ECG. At a minimum, this requires three electrodes: one positive, one negative, and one ground. In some clinical areas, five electrodes are used, either to monitor two leads simultaneously or to allow selection of several different leads at any time through a lead selector switch on the monitor. Typical placement of the five electrodes in a multilead system is illustrated in Fig. 15-18. Three leads—II, MCL_1, and MCL_6—are commonly used for continuous monitoring, although others may also be used.

Lead II. On a standard 12-lead ECG, lead II is formed by a positive electrode attached to the left leg, a negative electrode attached to the right arm, and a ground electrode on the right leg. It is not practical to connect electrodes to the arms and legs during continuous monitoring, but the general placement remains the same. The positive electrode is placed on the lower left torso, at least below the level of the sixth rib and preferably below the rib cage completely. The negative electrode is placed on the right shoulder, and the ground electrode is usually placed on the left shoulder (Fig. 15-19). The location of the ground is not significant. In patients with a normal electrical axis, this lead displays a waveform that is predominantly upright, has the greatest amplitude, and thus has the best signal-to-noise ratio. For this reason it is a popular monitoring lead and one that is often recommended by manufacturers of

◆

STEPS IN DETERMINING AXIS

1. Find the most isoelectric limb lead.
2. Using the hexaxial reference system, find the lead that is perpendicular to the one identified in step 1.
3. Determine whether the QRS is positive or negative in the perpendicular lead.
4. Look at the corresponding positive or negative pole of the perpendicular lead on the hexaxial reference system.
5. The degree listed on the hexaxial reference system is the axis.

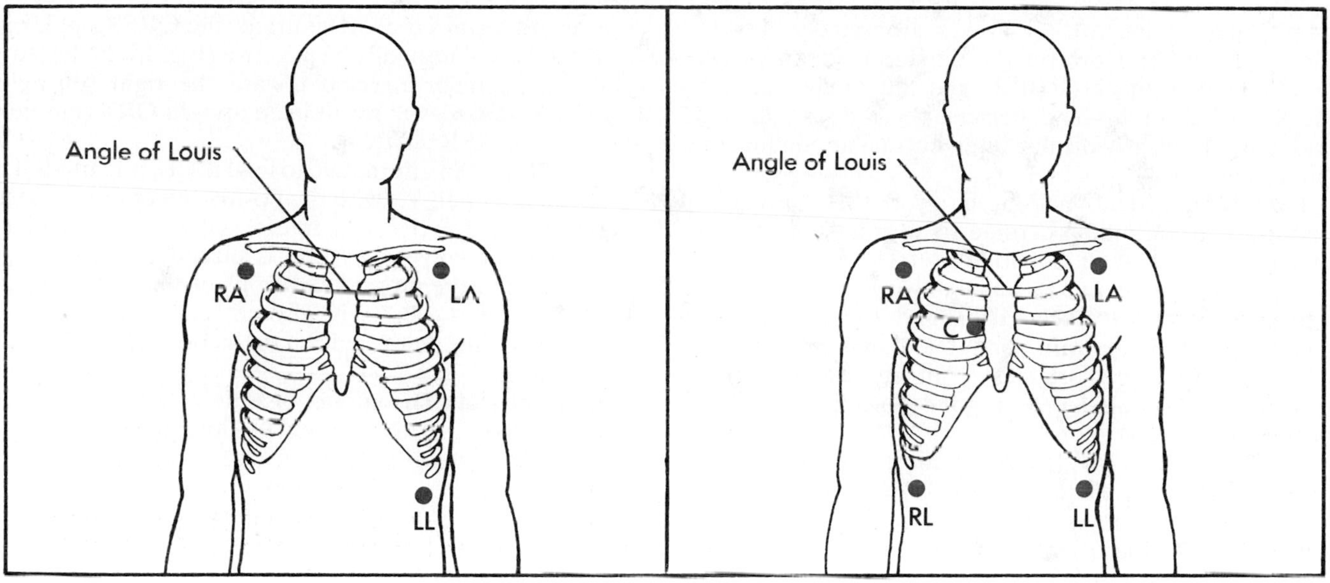

B

Fig. 15-18 **A,** Three electrodes and lead-wire cables allow monitoring of three of the limb leads (I, II, and III) and can also be rearranged to monitor MCL_1 and MCL_6 (see Fig. 15-20, A). **B,** Multilead monitoring system: five electrodes and lead-wire cables allow monitoring of any of the six standard limb leads (I, II, III, aV_R, aV_L, or aV_F) and any one precordial lead, usually V_1 or MCL_1. The cable attachments are color-coded for quick identification and placement. Accurate electrode placement is essential.

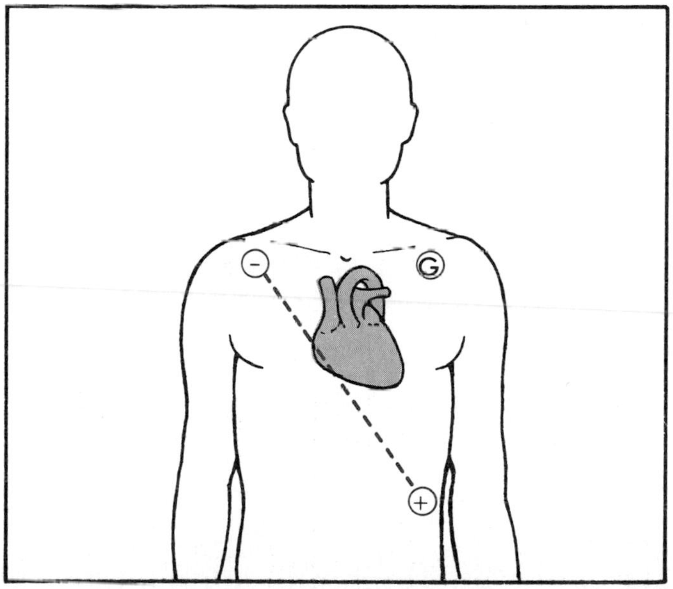

A

Fig. 15-19 Monitoring lead II. **A,** Electrode placement. The negative electrode is placed below the right shoulder; the positive electrode is placed on the lower left torso (preferably below the rib cage, but at least below the sixth rib); and the ground is usually placed below the left shoulder. **B,** Typical ECG tracing.

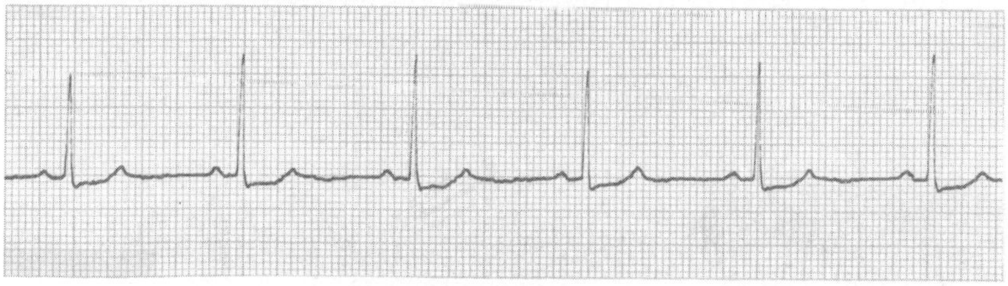

B

monitoring equipment.[14] P waves are usually easy to identify in lead II. However, it is difficult to identify right bundle branch block (RBBB) and left bundle branch block (LBBB) in this lead, because this is a vertical lead and does not clearly display interventricular conduction changes.

Lead MCL_1. Identification of an RBBB pattern is important in continuous cardiac monitoring, not only for diagnosing a new conduction defect, but also for verifying placement of a pacemaker wire, differentiating between ventricular tachycardia and supraventricular tachycardia with aberrant conduction, and determining whether PVCs are originating in the right or left ventricle. Lead MCL_1 is a good selection for this purpose.

"MCL_1" stands for "modified chest lead one." It is equivalent to a V_1 lead on a 12-lead ECG. The tracings are similar but not identical. In both, the positive electrode is at the fourth intercostal space just to the right of the sternum. It is extremely important for this electrode to be placed accurately.

With V_1 the ECG machine calculates the negative electrode at the center of the heart, whereas with MCL_1 the negative electrode is located just below the left shoulder. In MCL_1 the ground electrode is usually placed on the right shoulder but may also be placed in the V_6 position to allow changing to a lead MCL_6 with a lead selector switch, rather than changing electrode placement. Because the positive electrode is to the right of the heart and most of the electrical activity in the heart is directed toward the left ventricle, the QRS complex in lead MCL_1 will normally be negative (Fig. 15-20, B). Any abnormal activity directed toward the right ventricle, such as in RBBB, will result in an upright QRS complex, often in an RSR′ pattern.

Lead MCL_6. An alternative to lead MCL_1 is lead MCL_6. This is a modified V_6, with the positive electrode located in the V_6 position (left fifth intercostal space, midaxillary line). The negative electrode is placed below the left shoulder, and the ground can be placed below the right shoulder. Lead MCL_6 is also an adequate lead for monitoring interventricular conduction changes (see Fig. 15-20).

◆ **Lead selection for optimal bedside monitoring.** In the early years of critical care nursing, the primary goals of cardiac monitoring were heart rate surveillance, detection of "warning," dysrhythmias (mostly PVCs), and early detection of lethal dysrhythmias (ventricular fibrillation or asystole). Although these are still goals of ECG monitoring in the critical care unit today, several more complex issues are now of concern. It is now known that not all wide QRS complex tachycardias are ventricular in origin; sometimes they are supraventricular with aberrant ventricular conduction. Many patients are now undergoing reperfusion therapy involving balloon angioplasty or thrombolysis, and these patients require continuous monitoring for ST-segment changes that may represent ischemia even in the absence of clinical symptoms. It is now important that the nurse admitting a patient to the critical care unit or telemetry unit make a well-planned choice of monitoring lead(s) that is tailored to the clinical needs of that particular patient. In addition, accuracy of lead placement is extremely important if these leads are to be used for specialized diagnostic purposes.[14]

A

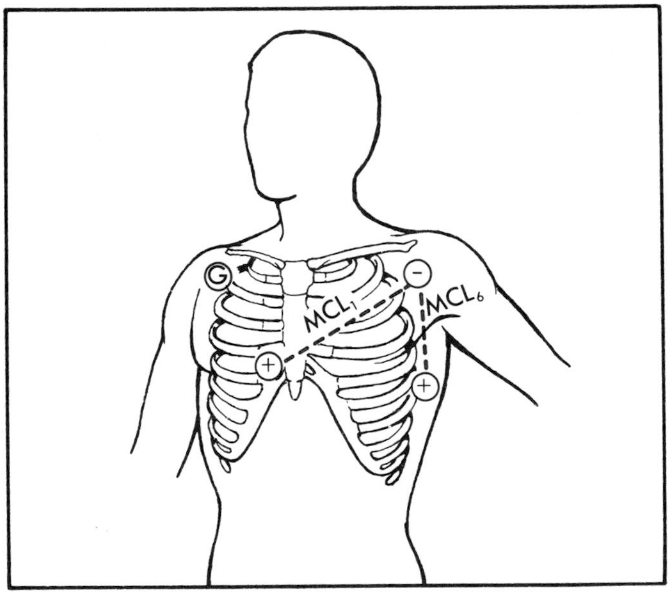

B

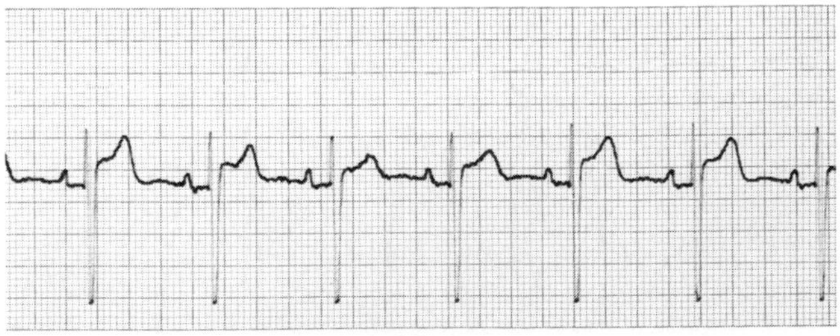

C

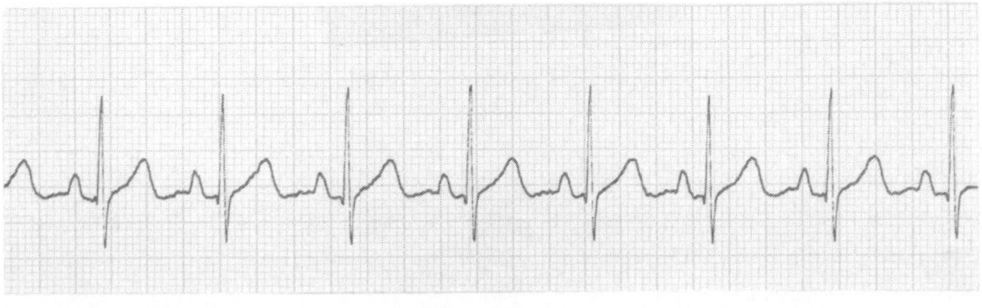

Fig. 15-20 **A,** Monitoring lead placement in MCL_1 and MCL_6. **B,** Typical ECG tracing in MCL_1. **C,** Typical ECG tracing in MCL_6.

Dysrhythmia monitoring. Patients with such serious cardiac diseases as acute myocardial infarction, heart failure, and cardiomyopathy are at high risk for the development of bundle branch blocks, complex ectopy, and wide complex tachycardias. These patients need to be monitored in a precordial lead that will document interventricular conduction changes.[14] This is lead MCL_1 or MCL_6 in a three-lead-wire system or V_1 or V_6 in a five-lead-wire system. Right and left bundle branch block cannot be accurately detected in lead II, because a portion of the wide QRS may be isoelectric, leading to the erroneous conclusion that the QRS duration is within normal limits. If only a single lead can be displayed, lead MCL_1 or V_1 is the best choice, with MCL_6 a good second choice if for some reason an electrode cannot be placed in the V_1 position (e.g., in patients with a sternal incision). If a second lead can be displayed simultaneously, lead MCL_6 or V_6 is the best choice, although this is difficult to obtain with current five-lead-wire systems because they include only one designated chest electrode. Instead, any one of the six standard limb leads will do as a second lead, and selection should be based on the patient's other monitoring needs, such as the need for ST-segment monitoring for ischemia. From a dysrhythmia standpoint, leads I or aV_F are also good second choices, because they can be used to identify a QRS axis diagnostic of ventricular dysrhythmias. (Both lead aV_F and lead I are required for this, but in a five-lead-wire system the critical care nurse can rapidly scroll through all six limb leads to obtain this information.) If three leads can be displayed simultaneously, lead MCL_1 or V_1 plus lead aV_F and lead I are the best choices.

ST-segment monitoring. In this era of thrombolytic therapy and percutaneous transluminal coronary angioplasty (PTCA), one of the major new responsibilities of the critical care nurse is monitoring for myocardial ischemia.[15] Myocardial ischemia may be accompanied by classic symptoms such as chest pain, or it may be "silent," without any clinical symptoms being recognized. Silent ischemia can often be detected by ST-segment changes in leads that are located directly over the ischemic area (ST elevation) or in leads that directly oppose that area (ST depression). Many cardiac monitoring systems are now equipped with an ST-segment monitoring option that allows parameters to be set and alarms to be triggered when ST deviation is noted. Even without this special program, ST changes can be detected visually in many cases. It must be remembered that the gain (calibration) on a bedside monitor is adjusted to maximize visibility of the tracing at a distance; as a result, the magnitude of ST-segment deviation is not accurate and must always be confirmed with a 12-lead ECG. In addition, ST-segment changes can sometimes occur as a result of position changes and be falsely interpreted as ischemia.[16] A 12-lead ECG is needed to confirm or refute the existence of true ischemic changes.

The best way to choose a lead for monitoring ST segments for ischemia is to look at the patient's 12-lead ECG during an episode of ischemia, if available. The standard 12-lead ECG obtained in an acute MI before thrombolytic therapy would reveal the leads that best demonstrated ischemia in that patient. Leads that showed ST-segment deviation during balloon inflation at the time of PTCA are the best leads to monitor after the procedure.[17] If this information is not available, leads to select for monitoring ischemic changes based on the coronary artery involved are given in Table 15-6.[18]

◆ **Hypertrophy.** Cardiac chamber enlargement can be suspected or diagnosed using the 12-lead ECG because muscle size will influence the ECG tracing. Atrial hypertrophy is identified by the size and shape of the P waves and is usually seen best in lead II. Wide m-shaped P waves are seen in left-atrial hypertrophy and are called *P-mitrale,* because left atrial hypertrophy is often caused by mitral stenosis (Fig. 15-21, *A*). Tall, peaked P waves occur in right atrial hypertrophy and are referred to as *P-pulmonale,* because this condition is often the result of chronic pulmonary disease (Fig. 15-21, *B*).

Ventricular hypertrophy is basically an increase in the size and muscle mass of one or both ventricles. Because a larger muscle is being depolarized, a greater amount of electrical activity is recorded on the ECG during

Table 15-6 Suggested leads for ST-segment monitoring

Coronary artery involved	Suggested lead to monitor
Left anterior descending	V_2 or V_3
Left circumflex	Lead III
Right coronary artery	Lead III or aV_F

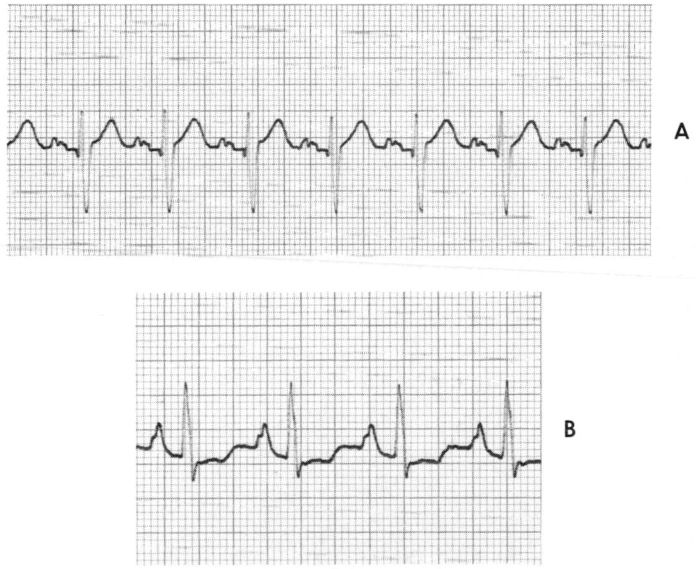

Fig. 15-21 Atrial hypertrophy. **A,** In left atrial hypertrophy the P wave is broad and notched and is sometimes called *P-mitrale* because it is often associated with mitral valve disease. **B,** In right atrial hypertrophy the P wave is tall and peaked and is sometimes called *P-pulmonale* because it is often associated with pulmonary disease.

depolarization. In ventricular hypertrophy, specific changes occur in the QRS complex.[19] Upright QRS complexes become taller, and negative QRS complexes become even more negative. Often the QRS becomes slightly wider, because it takes longer to depolarize a larger muscle. The QRS axis often shifts toward the enlarged ventricle, because a greater portion of the total electrical activity of the heart occurs there.

Because normal heart size varies from one individual to the next, certain criteria have been developed to evaluate ventricular hypertrophy (Table 15-7). Note that there are separate criteria for right ventricular hypertrophy and left ventricular hypertrophy.

◆ **Ischemia and infarction.** Ischemia occurs when the delivery of oxygen to the tissues is insufficient to meet metabolic demand. Cardiac ischemia can be the result of a sudden decrease in supply, such as when coronary artery spasm occurs, or can be the result of a sudden increase in demand, such as exercise. Ischemia is by nature a transient process. Either the balance of supply and demand is restored and the muscle tissue recovers or the imbalance becomes so great that the tissue can no longer survive and it becomes necrotic. Many nursing and medical interventions are directed toward saving as much ischemic tissue as possible. Infarction refers to the actual death and disintegration of muscle cells and their eventual replacement by scar tissue. Once infarction has occurred, that process cannot be reversed.

Both ischemia and infarction cause changes in the way cardiac muscle cells respond to electrical stimuli, and these changes can usually be seen in a 12-lead ECG tracing. The ECG changes that result from myocardial ischemia involve transient ST-segment and T wave abnormalities. ST-segment elevation will be seen when the positive electrode lies directly over an area of transmural ischemia (Fig. 15-22, *A*). If the reduction of blood flow is limited to the endocardium and some normal muscle tissue remains between the ischemic area and the positive electrode, ST-segment depression will be recorded.[20] In subendocardial ischemia, the ischemic area is closest to the inner cavity wall of the heart, and there is a layer of normal muscle tissue left surrounding it (Fig. 15-22, *B*). ST-segment depression would result, because the positive electrode is separated from the ischemic area by normal tissue. T waves most commonly flatten or become inverted, in part because of the influence of the depressed ST segment "dragging" them down. Occasionally, T waves that were inverted on a normal 12-lead ECG become suddenly upright on a tracing obtained during an ischemic episode. Essentially, a baseline ECG must be available for comparison, and any change in ST segment or T waves from that baseline is significant.

Infarction involves actual necrosis of muscle cells with eventual formation of scar tissue. These cells can no longer be depolarized when an impulse reaches them. If the infarction involves the epicardial (outer) layer of the heart muscle or the entire thickness of the heart wall, the QRS complex will change. Abnormal Q waves will develop in the leads overlying the affected area. Occasionally, the entire QRS complex just becomes smaller, without actual development of Q waves. If only the subendocardial layer of the heart muscle is infarcted, abnormal Q waves will not develop. In fact, there may be no change in the QRS complex. The diagnosis then depends on CK-MB or LDH_1 isoenzyme results and the clinical presentation. Initially, it was thought that non–

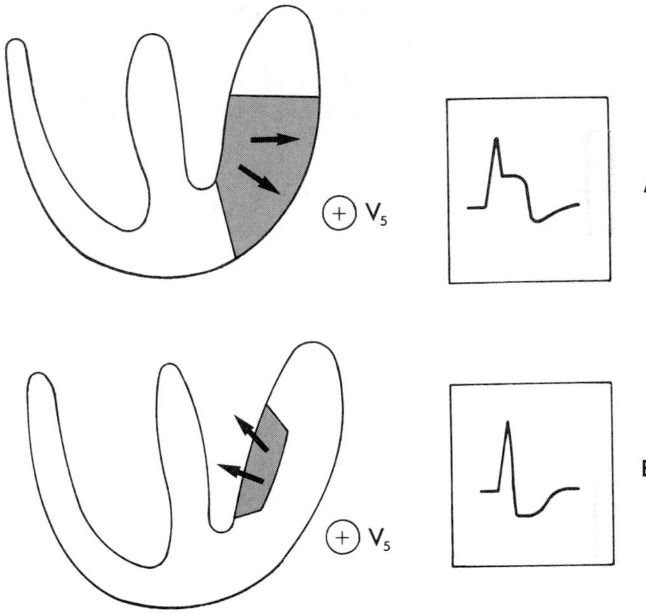

Fig. 15-22 **A,** Acute transmural ischemia. The electrical forces *(arrows)* responsible for the ST segment are directed outward through the entire thickness of the heart muscle wall, causing ST elevation in leads directly over the ischemic area. **B,** Acute subendocardial ischemia. The electrical forces responsible for the ST segment are deviated toward the inner layer of the heart, resulting in ST depression in leads directly over that area of the heart muscle wall.

Table 15-7 Criteria for evaluating ventricular hypertrophy

Left ventricle	Right ventricle
Presence of any one of the following:	Presence of any one of the following:
S wave in V_1 + R wave in V_5 or V_6 >35 mm	R : S ratio in lead V_5 or V_6 ≤1
Left atrial abnormality (broad, notched P waves)	S wave in V_5 or V_6 ≥7 mm
Intrinsic deflection (initial R or Q wave) in lead V_5 or V_6 ≥0.05 sec in duration	Right-axis deviation > +90 degrees
	P-pulmonale
NOTE: Sensitivity, 57%-66%; specificity, 85%-93%	NOTE: Sensitivity, 18%-43%; specificity, 83%-95%

Q-wave infarctions were relatively benign compared with Q wave or transmural infarctions. However, recent studies indicate that, although the extent of myocardial damage is less in patients with non–Q-wave infarction, these patients are very vulnerable to reinfarction. Mortality at the end of 3 years is the same for both groups.[2]

The location of the infarction can be roughly determined by noting the specific leads in which the ST segment and T wave changes are seen (Table 15-8). As a general guideline, the more leads that are involved, the larger the infarct. However, this guideline applies most accurately to anterior wall infarctions. When compared with serum enzyme (CK-MB) results, ECG estimates of the size of anterior wall infarctions correlated well with enzyme estimates. The same is not true of inferior wall infarcts, probably because of right ventricular involvement, which is difficult to assess on a standard 12-lead ECG.[22]

The relative age of the infarction can also be estimated. When blood flow in a coronary artery is occluded, the entire area of heart muscle normally perfused by that artery becomes ischemic. Collateral arterioles exist, which overlap and supply the perimeter of this area, and may prevent necrosis of some of the affected tissue. At the center of the ischemic area, collateral blood flow is minimal or does not exist at all. Within a few hours, this tissue begins to necrose, or die. On the ECG tracing, this process is illustrated as follows. Within minutes of the onset of infarction, ST-segment elevation occurs in the leads directly overlying the affected heart wall. This ST-segment elevation will persist for several days, gradually becoming less severe. Within the first few hours, T waves may become tall and symmetric. These are known as "hyperacute" T waves and also indicate acute ischemia. Meanwhile, usually within 4 to 24 hours from the onset of the infarction, abnormal Q waves begin to develop in the affected leads, and T waves begin to invert. Sometimes, instead of actual Q waves developing, the R waves just become smaller. This still indicates necrosis of muscle tissue. The ST segments become isoelectric again in several days or weeks, and the T wave becomes symmetric and deeply inverted in the affected leads. Occasionally, these T wave changes do not ever resolve. Usually, however, the T waves return to normal within several months. The Q waves usually persist for the remainder of the patient's life. Table 15-9 summarizes the timing of these changes.

Table 15-8 Location of ECG changes during myocardial infarction

Location of infarction	Leads involved
Anterior wall	I, aV_L, $V_{2\text{-}4}$
Inferior wall	II, III, aV_F
Ventricular septum	$V_{1\text{-}2}$
Lateral wall	$V_{4\text{-}6}$, I, aV_L
True posterior wall	Mirror-image changes in $V_{1\text{-}3}$
Right ventricle	V_4R, V_5R, V_6R

◆ **Ventricular conduction defects.** Intraventricular conduction defects are the result of an abnormal pathway of conduction through the ventricles. Normally, conduction spreads from the AV node to the bundle of His and from there down the right and left bundle branches. The right bundle branch is long and thin and terminates in a mass of Purkinje fibers, which spread the wave of depolarization to the surrounding right ventricular muscle. The left bundle branch divides after only a short distance into the left anterior fascicle, the left posterior fascicle, and the left septal fibers (Fig. 15-23). Each of these fascicles causes depolarization of separate areas of the left ventricle. If any part of the conduction system fails, the muscle cells in that area will still be depolarized, but not as quickly. Depolarization must then spread from cell to cell, a slower process than activation through specialized conduction pathways.

On the ECG, intraventricular conduction defects cause a widening of the QRS because of the slower spread of depolarization. The affected muscle tissue begins the slower cell-to-cell depolarization just as the other areas in the ventricle are almost finished. This later depolarization is then tacked onto the end of the normal QRS, making it prolonged and altering its shape.

Any part of the conduction system can be affected. The term *bundle branch block* refers to complete interruption of conduction through either the right bundle or the entire left bundle branch. In complete right or left bundle branch block, the QRS will always be 0.12 second or longer in duration. When only one fascicle of the left bundle branch is blocked, the QRS duration will be within normal limits, although usually more prolonged than before the conduction disturbance occurred.

Right and left bundle branch block. The chest leads are the most useful in identifying complete right and left bundle branch blocks. Specifically, V_1 and V_6 are the best leads from which to identify forces traveling in a horizontal direction, because they are located on the right and left sides of the heart, respectively. Fig. 15-24, *A* illustrates the normal sequence of ventricular activation and the usual shape of the QRS complex in V_1 and V_6.

In complete right bundle branch block (Fig. 15-24, *B*), the right ventricle is not activated through the rapid conduction system. Rather, it must be activated slowly, from one cell to the next. Electrical forces, not counter-

Table 15-9 Timing of ECG changes during myocardial infarction

Timing	Change
Immediate	ST-segment elevation in leads over the area of infarction
Within a few hours	Giant upright T waves
Several hours to 2 weeks	ST segment normalizes; T waves invert symmetrically
Several hours to days; usually remain for life	Q waves or reduced R-wave voltage

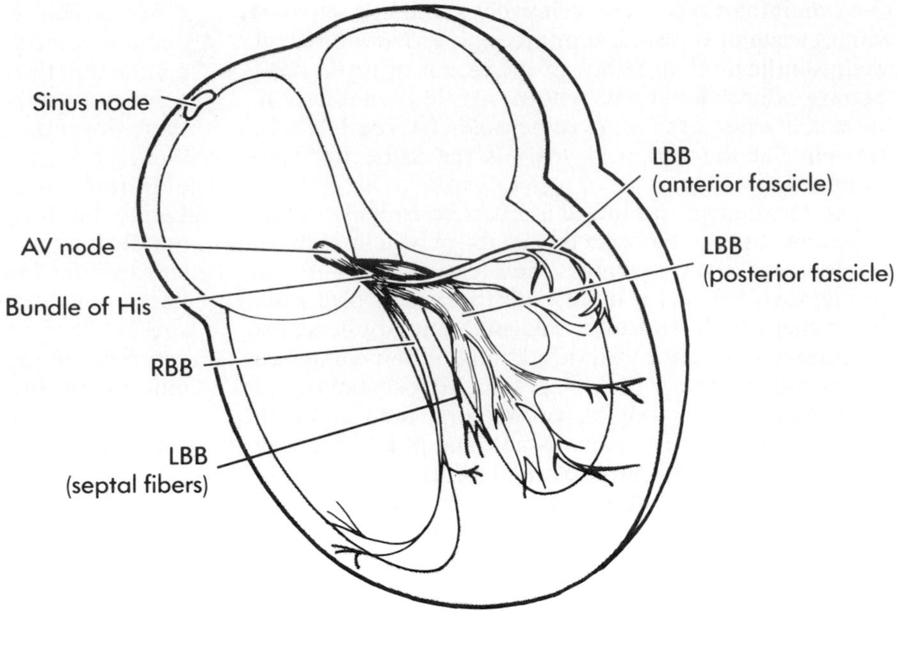

Fig. 15-23 Cardiac conduction system. (Modified from Conover MB: *Understanding electrocardiography: arrhythmias and the 12-lead ECG,* ed 6, St Louis, 1992, Mosby–Year Book.)

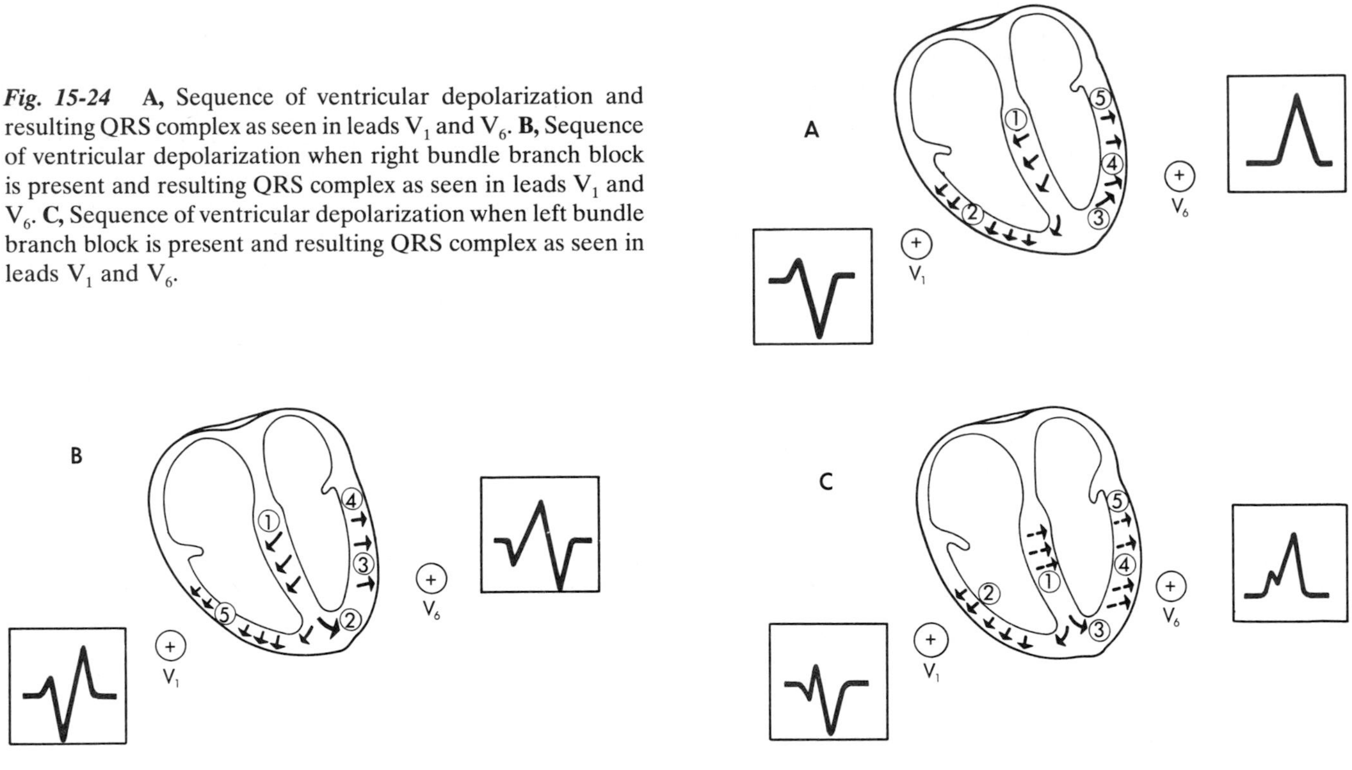

Fig. 15-24 **A,** Sequence of ventricular depolarization and resulting QRS complex as seen in leads V_1 and V_6. **B,** Sequence of ventricular depolarization when right bundle branch block is present and resulting QRS complex as seen in leads V_1 and V_6. **C,** Sequence of ventricular depolarization when left bundle branch block is present and resulting QRS complex as seen in leads V_1 and V_6.

balanced by opposing forces on the left, will be traveling toward the right at the end of the ventricular activation. The septum is depolarized first, in a normal manner from left to right. Next the wave of depolarization spreads through the left ventricle and is recorded in lead V_1 as a negative deflection. The final portion of the QRS complex is upright, indicating final forces traveling toward the right. This represents right ventricular depolarization that occurs after left ventricular depolarization is nearly complete. In lead V_6, the positive electrode is on the left side of the chest, so the waveforms are reversed. The final forces of the QRS are negative, because they are traveling toward the right and away from the positive electrode of V_6. Note that the final negative deflection in V_6 is smaller than the final upright deflection in lead V_1, because the positive electrode in V_6 is at a greater distance from the right ventricle.

In complete left bundle branch block (Fig. 15-24, *C*), the conduction through the left ventricle must spread from cell to cell. Because a portion of the common left bundle normally initiates depolarization of the septum, the septum also will be depolarized in an abnormal direction, from right to left. In lead V_1 this will be recorded as an initial negative deflection. Next, the right ventricle will be depolarized, seen as a small upright notch in the QRS as the forces travel briefly toward the positive electrode of V_1. Sometimes this notch will be absent. The sequence of events has not changed, but the left ventricle is already beginning to be depolarized cell to cell and may offset the rightward forces of right ventricular depolarization. The final forces travel toward the left as the left ventricle is being depolarized. The left ventricle is a very large muscle mass, so these final forces will be large and wide. In lead V_1 the final deflection will be a deep negative deflection (S wave), whereas in lead V_6 these final forces will inscribe a tall, upright deflection (R wave).

Bundle branch blocks can easily be diagnosed at the bedside if the patient is being monitored in lead MCL_1 or MCL_6, because these correlate closely with the precordial leads V_1 and V_6, respectively. A bundle branch block exists when the QRS complex is wider than 0.12 second (and the complex did not originate in the ventricles such as does a PVC or paced beat). To determine which bundle branch is blocked, examine the last part of the QRS just before it returns to the baseline in leads V_1 and V_6. If upright in V_1 and negative in V_6, a right bundle branch block exists. If negative in V_1 and upright in V_6, a left bundle branch block is present.

Hemiblocks. Hemiblocks involve conduction failure of only part of the left bundle branch. In left anterior fascicular block (also called *left anterior hemiblock*), left ventricular depolarization begins in the left posterior fascicle and spreads anteriorly through Purkinje fibers distal to the block. The QRS is only slightly prolonged, up to 0.02 second longer than the patient's previous QRS. However, the axis changes dramatically and becomes more negative than −30 degrees (left-axis deviation).[23] Other causes of left-axis deviation must be ruled out before a clinical diagnosis of left anterior hemiblock can be made (see first box on right). In left posterior fascicular block (also called *left posterior hemiblock*), the anterior portion of the left ventricle is depolarized first. Conduction then spreads slowly to the right, inferiorly and posteriorly. Once again the QRS is slightly prolonged. The axis then swings entirely the other direction and becomes greater than +110 degrees (right-axis deviation). Other causes of right-axis deviation must be ruled out before a clinical diagnosis of left posterior hemiblock can be made (see second box on right).

Bifascicular block. Blockage of any two branches of the ventricular conduction system constitutes bifascicular block. Any combination of these conduction disturbances can occur and can evolve into complete heart block. Development of right bundle branch block with left anterior fascicular block occurs in approximately 5% of patients with acute myocardial infarction, as does left bundle branch block. Right bundle branch block in combination with left posterior fascicular block is rare, probably because the left posterior fascicle is short and thick and has a dual blood supply from the left anterior descending and right posterior descending coronary arteries.

Bifascicular block that develops during an acute myocardial infarction warrants placement of a temporary pacemaker prophylactically in case complete heart block develops. When bifascicular block occurs in other patient populations, use of a pacemaker can be avoided if the patient is asymptomatic. However, most bifascicular block eventually progresses to complete heart block.

CAUSES OF LEFT-AXIS DEVIATION

Normal variation
Mechanical shifts: exhalation; high diaphragm caused by pregnancy, ascites, or abdominal tumor
Left anterior hemiblock
Left ventricular hypertrophy
Pulmonary emphysema (uncommon)
Wolff-Parkinson-White syndrome
Hyperkalemia
Cardiomyopathy

CAUSES OF RIGHT-AXIS DEVIATION

Normal variation
Mechanical shifts: inhalation, emphysema
Left posterior hemiblock
Right ventricular hypertrophy
Lateral wall myocardial infarction
Right bundle branch block
Dextrocardia

◆ **Dysrhythmia interpretation.** In clinical practice the terms *dysrhythmia* and *arrhythmia* often are used interchangeably. There may be discussion over which word is the most accurate. Both are correct, and either may be used in practice. In this textbook, dysrhythmia is the more commonly used term. A dysrhythmia is any disturbance in the normal cardiac conduction pathway. Dysrhythmias can be detected on a 12-lead ECG, but very often they occur only sporadically. For this reason patients in a critical care unit are monitored continuously, using a single or dual lead system, and rhythm strips are recorded routinely, as well as any time there is a change in the patient's rhythm. A systematic approach to evaluation of a rhythm strip is introduced first in this section, followed by specific criteria for common dysrhythmias encountered in clinical practice.

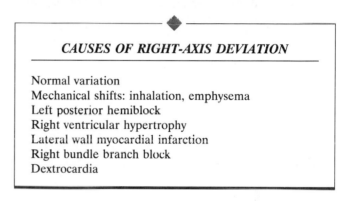

Heart rate determination. The first thing to assess when evaluating a rhythm strip is the ventricular rate. Regardless of the dysrhythmia involved, the ventricular rate holds the key to whether the patient will be able to tolerate the dysrhythmia, that is, maintain adequate blood pressure, cardiac output, and mentation. If the ventricular rate is consistently greater than 200 or less than 30, emergency measures must be started to correct the rate. A detailed analysis of the underlying rhythm disturbance can proceed later when the immediate crisis is over. There are three methods for calculating rate (Fig. 15-25, *A*):

1. Number of RR intervals in 6 seconds times 10 (NOTE: ECG paper is usually marked at the top in 3-second increments, making a 6-second interval easy to identify.)
2. Number of large boxes between QRS complexes divided into 300
3. Number of small boxes between QRS complexes divided into 1500

In the healthy heart, the atrial rate and the ventricular rate are the same. However, in many dysrhythmias the atrial and ventricular rates are different; thus both must be calculated. To find the atrial rate, the PP interval, instead of the RR interval, is used in one of the three methods listed for determining rate.

The choice of method for calculating the heart rate depends on the regularity of the rhythm. If the rhythm is irregular, the first method (RRs in 6 seconds × 10) is the only method that can be used (Fig. 15-25, *B*). If the rhythm is regular, it is more accurate to use the second or third method. The second method can be easier to use when two consecutive R waves fall exactly on dark lines, and it provides a rapid estimate of rate. The third method is recommended when both R waves do not fall exactly on dark lines.

Rhythm determination. The term *rhythm* refers to the regularity with which the P waves or R waves occur. Calipers assist in determining rhythm. One point of the calipers is placed on the beginning of one R wave, while the other point is placed on the very next R wave. Leaving the calipers "set" at this interval, each succeeding RR interval is checked to be sure it is the same width.

In describing the rhythm, three terms are used. If the rhythm is *regular*, the RR intervals are the same, ±10%. For example, if there are 20 small boxes in an RR interval, an R wave could be off by two small boxes, but the rhythm would still be considered regular.

If the rhythm is *regularly irregular,* the RR intervals are not the same, but some sort of pattern is involved, which could be grouping, rhythmic speeding up and slowing down, or any other consistent pattern (Fig. 15-26, *A*).

If the rhythm is *irregularly irregular,* the RR intervals are not the same, and no pattern can be found (Fig. 15-26, *B*).

P wave evaluation. The P wave should be analyzed by answering the following questions. First, is the P wave present or absent? Second, is it related to the QRS? It is hoped that one P wave will be in front of every QRS. Sometimes there may be two, three, or four P waves in front of every QRS. If this pattern is consistent, the P wave and QRS are still related, although not on a 1:1 basis.

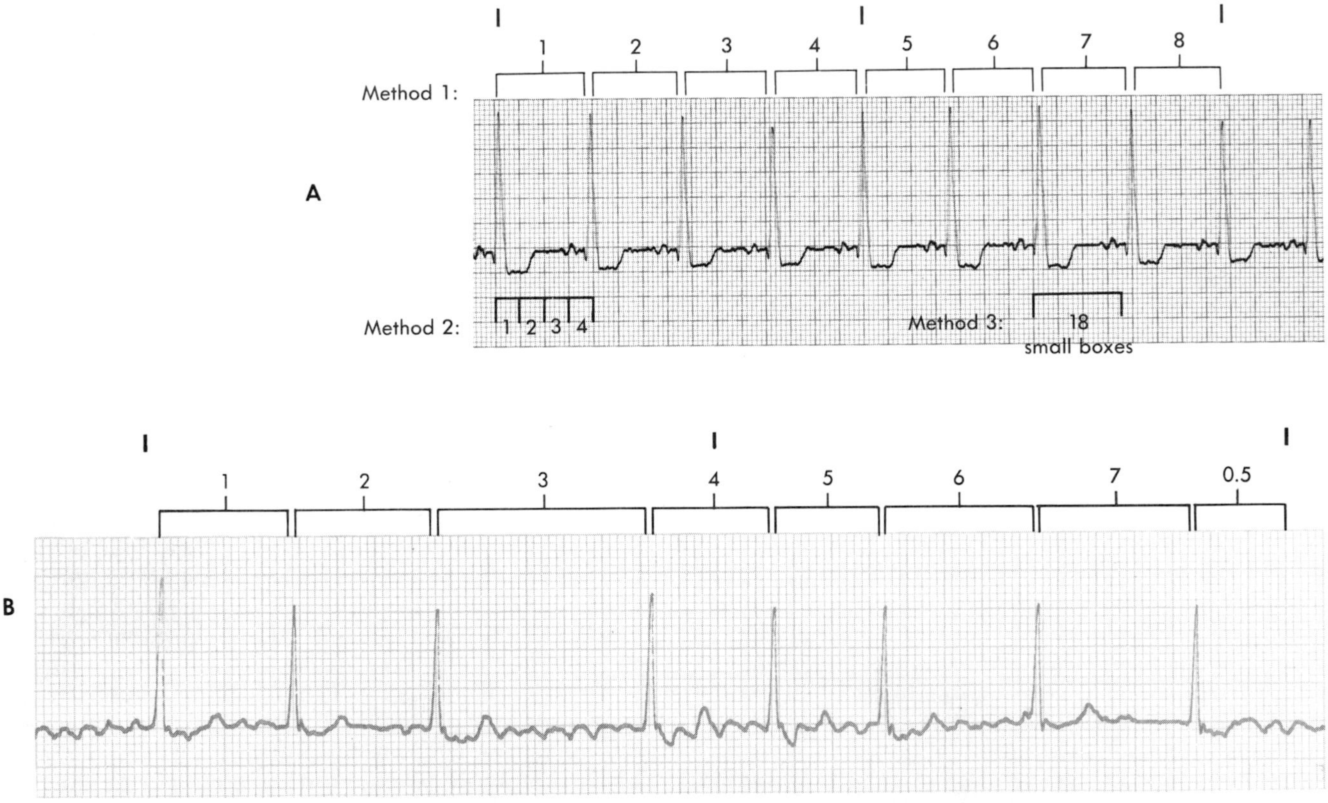

Fig. 15-25 **A,** Calculation of heart rate. *Method 1:* Number of RR intervals in 6 seconds multiplied by 10 (e.g., 8 × 10 = 80/min). *Method 2:* Number of large boxes between QRS complexes divided into 300 (e.g., 300 ÷ 4 = 75/min). *Method 3:* Number of small boxes between QRS complexes divided into 1500 (e.g., 1500 ÷ 18 = 84/min). **B,** Rate calculation if the rhythm is irregular. Only method 1 can be used (e.g., 7.5 intervals × 10 = 75/min).

A 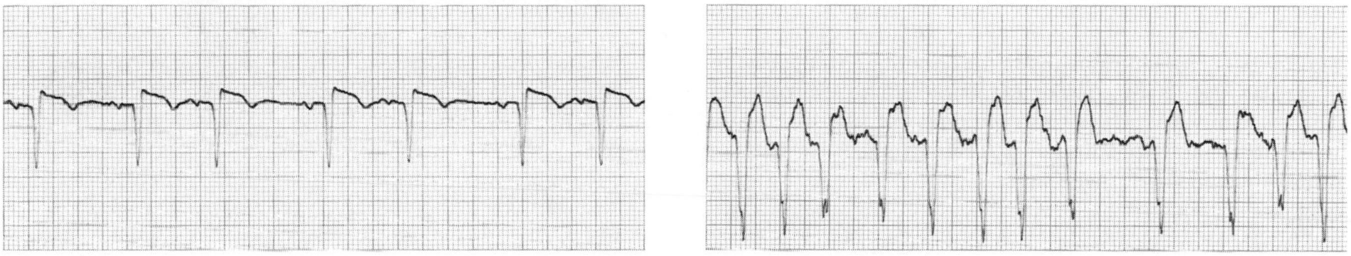 B

Fig. 15-26 **A,** Regularly irregular rhythm—irregular but with a consistent pattern, in that every other beat is premature. **B,** Irregularly irregular rhythm—irregular with no consistent pattern.

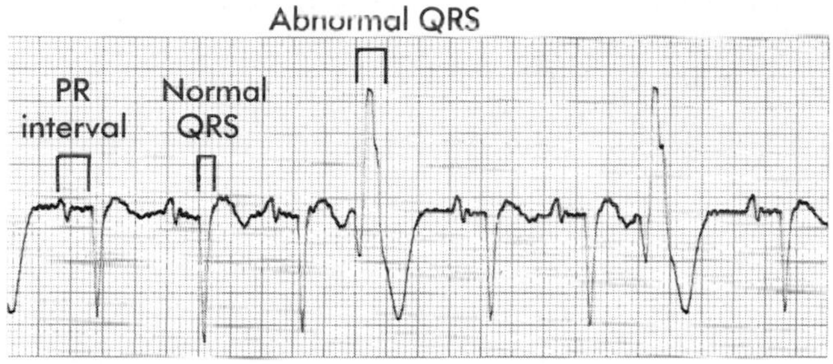

Fig. 15-27 PR interval measurement, from the beginning of the P wave to the beginning of the QRS complex. The PR interval on this tracing is 0.20 second. QRS duration illustrating both normal and abnormal intervals. The narrow QRS complexes measure 0.08 seconds, which is normal. The wide QRS complexes measure 0.20 second and are caused by ventricular ectopy.

PR interval evaluation. The duration of the PR interval, which normally is 0.12 to 0.20 second, is measured first. This is done by measuring from the start of a P wave to the beginning of the following QRS (Fig. 15-27). Next, all PR intervals on the strip are checked to be sure they are the same duration as the original interval.

QRS evaluation. The entire ECG strip must be evaluated to ascertain that the QRS complexes are consistently the same shape and width. The normal QRS duration is 0.06 to 0.10 second. If more than one QRS shape is on the strip, each QRS must be measured. The QRS is measured from where it leaves the baseline to where it returns to the baseline (see Fig. 15-27).

◆ Sinus rhythms. The cardiac cycle begins when an impulse originates in the sinus node. As the wave of depolarization spreads through the atria, a P wave is inscribed on the ECG. The impulse is delayed briefly in the AV node, which corresponds to the PR interval on the ECG. After leaving the AV node, the wave of depolarization spreads rapidly through the bundle of His and the bundle branches and causes ventricular depolarization, which is recorded as a QRS complex by the ECG. Contraction immediately follows depolarization. Contraction is terminated by repolarization, which is demonstrated as a T wave on the ECG.

Normal sinus rhythm. If all of the events just discussed occur in their normal sequence with normal rates and intervals, the patient is in normal sinus rhythm. Specifically, the following are the criteria for normal sinus rhythm:

1. Rate. The intrinsic rate of the sinus node is 60 to 100 beats per minute. *Intrinsic rate* is the normal rate at which a pacemaker site in the heart will depolarize automatically with no outside influences, such as drugs, fever, or exercise. In normal sinus rhythm, the rate must be whatever is "normal" for the sinus node, that is, 60 to 100 beats per minute.
2. Rhythm. The rhythm must be regular, plus or minus 10%.
3. P wave. P waves must be present, and one and only one must precede every QRS complex.
4. PR interval. This interval represents delay in the AV node. In normal sinus rhythm the PR interval is 0.12 to 0.20 second.
5. QRS. Size and shape does not matter in this complex, because it depends on lead placement and gain adjustments on the monitor. However, all QRS complexes should look alike. If conduction through the ventricles is normal, the QRS duration will be 0.06 to 0.10 second. Fig. 15-28 is an example of normal sinus rhythm in MCL_1.

Sinus bradycardia. Sinus bradycardia meets all of the criteria for normal sinus rhythm except that the rate is less than 60 (Table 15-10). It is normally seen in well-trained athletes at rest or in many other individuals during sleep. Other conditions in which sinus bradycardia occurs include vagal stimulation, increased intracranial pressure, drug therapy with digoxin or beta blockers, and ischemia of the sinus node caused by an acute inferior wall myocardial infarction. Sinus bradycardia is

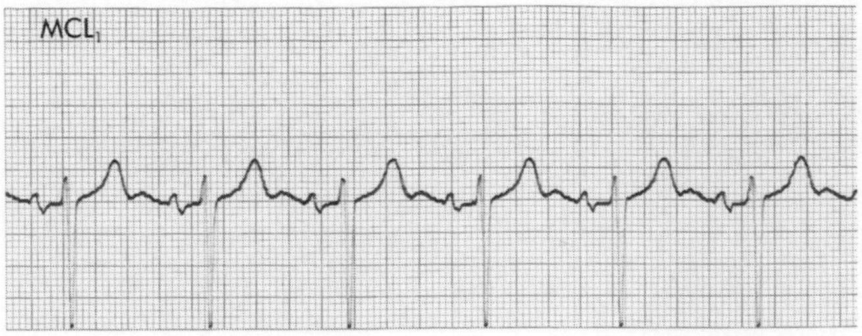

Fig. 15-28 Normal sinus rhythm. The rate is 70; the rhythm is regular. One P wave is present before each QRS complex. The PR interval is 0.18 second and does not vary throughout the strip. The QRS duration is 0.08 second. All evaluation criteria are within normal limits.

Table 15-10 Sinus rhythms

Parameters	Normal sinus rhythm	Sinus bradycardia	Sinus tachycardia	Sinus dysrhythmia
Rate	60-100/min	<60/min	>100/min	Variable
Rhythm	Regular	Regular	Regular	Irregular; respiratory variation
P wave	Present, with one per QRS	Present, with one per QRS	Present, with one per QRS	Present, with one per QRS
PR interval	0.12-0.20 sec and constant	0.12-0.20 sec and constant	0.12-0.20 sec and constant	0.12-0.20 sec and constant
QRS	0.06-0.10 sec	0.06-0.10 sec	0.06-0.10 sec	0.06-0.10 sec

generally not treated unless the patient displays symptoms of hypoperfusion, such as hypotension, dizziness, chest pain, or changes in level of consciousness.

Sinus tachycardia. Sinus tachycardia meets all the criteria for normal sinus rhythm except that the rate is greater than 100 beats per minute (see Table 15-10). Rates may be as high as 180 to 200 beats per minute in healthy, young adults with strenuous exercise. However, in the critical care setting, bed rest has been prescribed for most patients. It is wise to be skeptical of any "sinus tachycardia" with a rate greater than 150 and to search for a triggering focus other than the sinus node. For example, atrial flutter waves might be difficult to see at first glance because of baseline distortion caused by the high ventricular rate (Fig. 15-29).

Sinus tachycardia can be caused by a wide variety of factors, such as exercise, emotion, pain, fever, hemorrhage, shock, and congestive heart failure. Many drugs used in critical care can also cause sinus tachycardia, and common culprits are aminophylline, dopamine, hydralazine, beta stimulants such as epinephrine, and overzealous use of atropine. Tachycardia is detrimental to anyone with ischemic heart disease because it decreases time for ventricular filling, decreases stroke volume, and thus compromises cardiac output. In addition, tachycardia will increase heart work and myocardial oxygen demand while decreasing oxygen supply by decreasing coronary artery filling time.

If the cause of the tachycardia can be determined (e.g., fever or pain), the cause should be treated rather than trying to treat the heart rate directly. Several drugs are available to decrease the heart rate, and both calcium channel blockers and beta blockers are widely used for this purpose. However, a word of caution is warranted here. Cardiac output (CO) is determined by heart rate and stroke volume. If an injured heart can no longer maintain an adequate stroke volume, heart rate can be increased to maintain CO and supply an adequate blood flow to vital body tissues. If a drug is administered to force the sinus node to slow, severe and relatively immediate heart failure can result. The sinus node is controlled by many neural and humoral influences in the body, and the rate is set to try to meet the perceived demands; thus a close examination of the reason for the tachycardia is mandatory before treatment decisions are made.

Sinus dysrhythmia. Sinus dysrhythmia meets all of the criteria for normal sinus rhythm except that the rhythm is irregular (see Table 15-10). Usually this irregularity coincides with the respiratory pattern; heart rate increases with inhalation and decreases with exhalation (Fig. 15-30). Sinus dysrhythmia frequently occurs in children, and the incidence decreases with age. No treatment is required. To avoid being misled by other rhythm disturbances, one should examine all P waves closely to be sure that they are all the same shape and that the PR intervals are all constant.

◆ **Atrial dysrhythmias.** Atrial dysrhythmias originate from an ectopic focus in the atria, somewhere other than the sinus node. The ectopic impulse occurs prematurely before the normal sinus impulse is due to occur. Usually, the premature P wave initiates a normal QRS complex. However, some exceptions do occur. The early P wave usually looks different than the sinus P wave and often is inverted. The PR interval may be longer, shorter, or the same as the PR interval of a sinus beat.

Premature atrial contractions. Premature atrial contractions (PACs) are isolated, early beats from an ectopic focus in the atria. The underlying rhythm is usually sinus. The regular sinus rhythm is interrupted by an early,

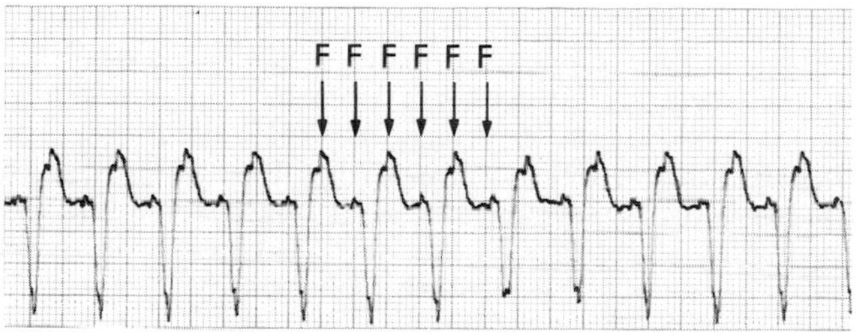

Fig. 15-29 Sinus tachycardia? In fact, this is atrial flutter with 2:1 conduction. Note how difficult it is to see the extra flutter waves *(F)* that are hidden in the QRS complexes.

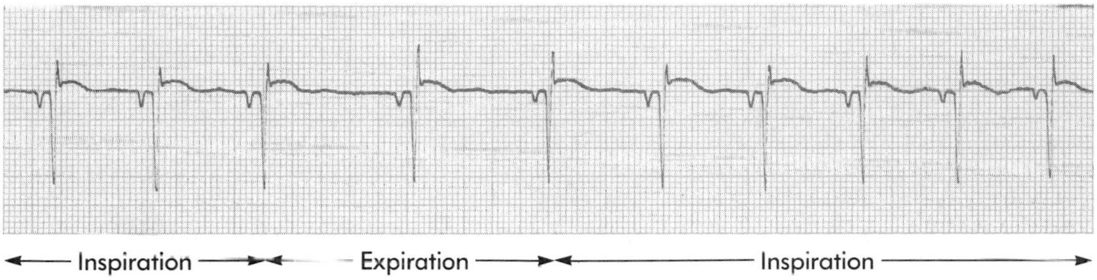

Fig. 15-30 Sinus dysrhythmia. Note the increase in heart rate during inspiration and decrease in heart rate during expiration.

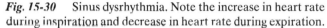

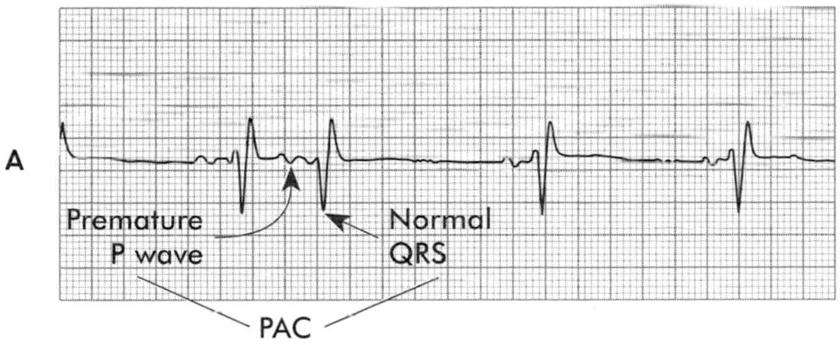

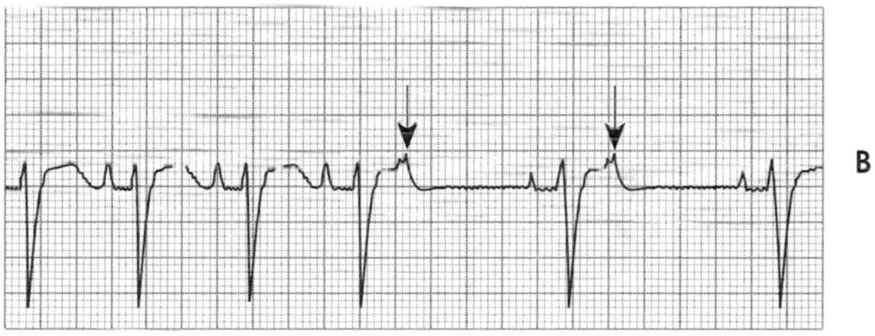

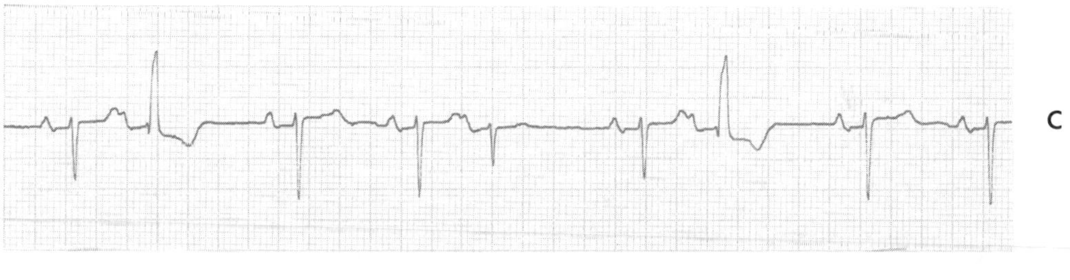

Fig. 15-31 Premature atrial contractions (PACs). **A,** Normally conducted PAC. The early P wave is indicated by the arrow, and the QRS that follows is of normal shape and duration. **B,** Nonconducted (blocked) PACs. The early P waves are indicated by arrows. Note how they distort the T waves, making them appear peaked, compared with the normal T waves seen after the third and fourth QRS complexes. **C,** Right bundle branch block aberration after a PAC.

abnormally shaped P wave. If the impulse arrives in the AV node after the AV node is fully repolarized, it will be conducted to the ventricles. If the ventricles are also fully repolarized, conduction through them will be normal and a normal QRS will be recorded on the ECG (Fig. 15-31, *A*).

Sometimes, the ectopic P wave arrives so early that the AV node is still in its absolute refractory period. In this case, the wave of depolarization will not move past the AV node and no QRS will follow. All that will be seen on the ECG is an early, abnormal P wave followed by a pause until the next sinus P wave occurs (Fig. 15-31, *B*). This is called a *nonconducted PAC.* Usually these P waves are so early that they are superimposed on the T wave of the previous beat, making them somewhat difficult to find. The pause that follows will still be clearly seen. Whenever an unexpected pause occurs in a rhythm, the T wave preceding the pause should be examined very carefully, comparing it with other T waves on the same strip and looking for distortions that may reveal a hidden, early P wave.

Occasionally, the early ectopic P wave can be conducted through the AV node, but part of this conduction pathway through the ventricles is blocked. Because the right bundle branch normally has the longest refractory period, it is usually the right bundle branch that is still blocked when the early impulse arrives. On the ECG, this will appear as an early, abnormal P wave, followed by an abnormally wide QRS, usually with a shape consistent with right bundle branch block (Fig. 15-31, *C*). Conduction through the ventricles that is different from normal is referred to as *aberrant*. Consequently, these early, abnormally conducted PACs are called aberrantly conducted PACs.

PACs can occur in normal individuals. They are accentuated by emotional disturbances, nicotine, tea, caffeine, and digitalis. Mitral valve prolapse is associated with an increased frequency of atrial dysrhythmias. Heart failure can also cause PACs because of increased pressure within the atria. As atrial pressure begins to rise, the atrial walls are stretched, causing irritability of atrial cells and the occurrence of PACs.

Paroxysmal supraventricular tachycardia. "Paroxysmal" means starting and stopping abruptly. Paroxysmal supraventricular tachycardia (PSVT) refers to the sudden interruption of sinus rhythm by an atrial ectopic focus that fires repetitively at a rate of 150 to 250 times per minute and eventually stops as suddenly as it began (Fig. 15-32). The rhythm of the PSVT is perfectly regular, because the same irritable ectopic focus in the atria is initiating each beat. Other common underlying mechanisms include circus-movement tachycardia and AV nodal reentry. P waves are present and abnormally shaped, although they may be difficult to identify because they often blend in with the previous T wave because of the rapid rate. It is most helpful if the beginning of the PSVT run is captured and recorded on ECG paper, because the early, abnormal P wave is often easiest to identify in front of the first beat of the run. The PR interval should be the same for each cycle in the run, but it will probably be different from the PR interval of the patient's own normal sinus rhythm. Just as with PACs, the QRS complex is usually normal, because once the impulse passes through the AV node, conduction through the ventricles follows the usual pathway (Table 15-11). However, aberrant conduction, often in the form of right bundle branch block, can occur. It will cause a wide QRS complex, leading to difficulty in differentiating this relatively benign dysrhythmia from its more serious counterpart, ventricular tachycardia. Further discussion of the difficulty of differentiating VT from PSVT is found on pp. 219-221. Sometimes, because of refractoriness in the AV node, not all of the ectopic P waves are conducted to the ventricles. Usually, at least every other P wave conducts a QRS, but occasionally the conduction ratio may drop to three P waves for every QRS.

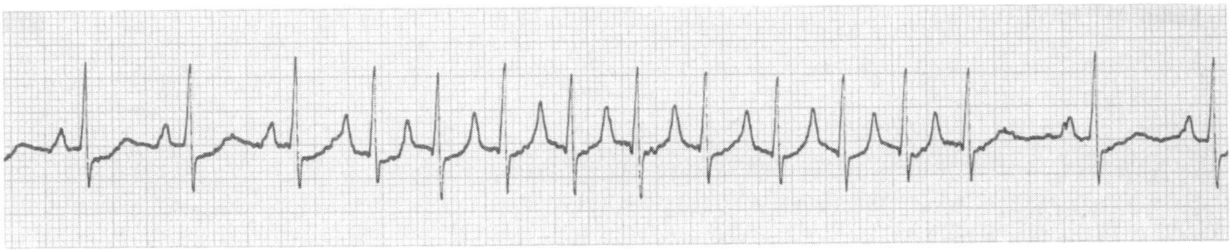

Fig. 15-32 Paroxysmal supraventricular tachycardia (PSVT). Note that the atrial rate during the tachycardia is 158 beats per minute. The run starts and stops abruptly.

Table 15-11 Atrial dysrhythmias

Parameter	Paroxysmal supraventricular tachycardia	Multifocal atrial tachycardia	Atrial flutter	Atrial fibrillation
Rate				
Atrial	150-250/min	100-160/min	250-350/min	>350/min (unable to count it)
Ventricular	Same or less	Same	Half or less	100-180/min (uncontrolled); <100/min (controlled)
Rhythm	Regular	Irregular	Atrial—regular; ventricular—may or may not be regular	Irregularly irregular
P wave	Present; abnormally shaped	Present; three or more different shapes	F waves	f waves
PR interval	May be normal or prolonged	Variable	Conduction ratio: flutter waves per QRS	Absent
QRS	0.06-0.10 sec	0.06-0.10 sec	0.06-0.10 sec	0.06-0.10 sec

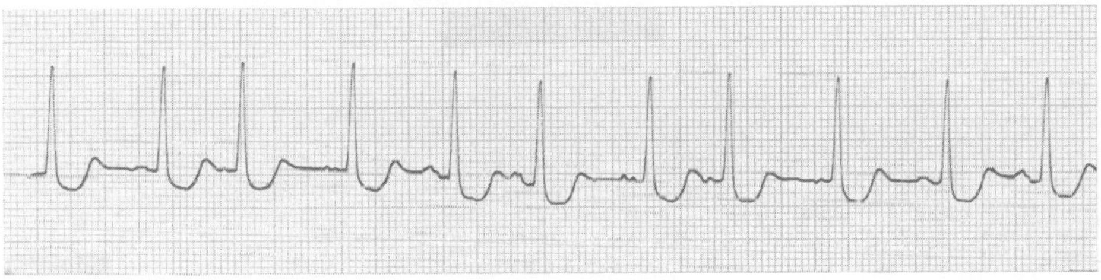

Fig. 15-33 Multifocal atrial tachycardia (MAT). Note that there are several differently shaped P waves and the PR intervals vary.

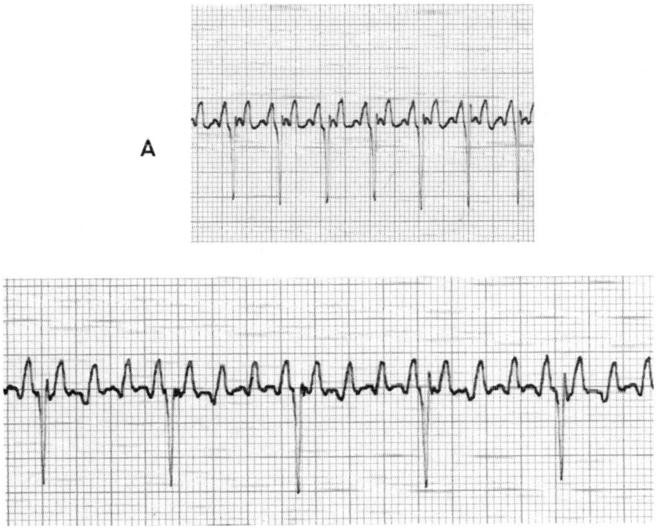

Fig. 15-34 **A,** Initial strip shows atrial flutter with 2:1 conduction through the AV node. **B,** During carotid sinus massage, the AV conduction rate is decreased, more clearly revealing the flutter waves.

PSVT has essentially the same causal factors as PACs. PSVT has greater clinical significance, because it may be sustained by reentry mechanisms for long periods and because it occurs at such a rapid rate. As stressed in the discussion of sinus tachycardia, rapid rates decrease ventricular filling time, increase myocardial oxygen consumption, and decrease oxygen supply. Heart failure, angina, or even myocardial infarction can result. PSVT usually responds rapidly to medical treatment, which may include the use of direct or indirect vagal maneuvers, intravenous calcium channel blocking agents, or electrical cardioversion. Intravenous adenosine is increasingly the drug of choice to slow conduction through the AV node, unmask the ectopic P waves, and restore normal sinus rhythm.[24]

Multifocal atrial tachycardia. Multifocal atrial tachycardia, sometimes referred to as *chaotic atrial tachycardia,* occurs when there are numerous irritable atrial foci that intermittently fire and generate an impulse (Fig. 15-33). The atrial rate is greater than 100 beats per minute but generally does not exceed 160. The distinguishing feature on the ECG is that there are at least three different P wave shapes, indicating at least three different irritable foci. This is most commonly seen in elderly patients with chronic obstructive pulmonary disease (COPD). COPD causes chronic pulmonary hypertension, which in turn causes chronically elevated right atrial and right ventricular pressures. The abnormally high right atrial pressure causes stretching of the right atrial muscle cells and chronic irritability. Because the underlying cause cannot be resolved, this dysrhythmia usually is refractory to any treatment.

Atrial flutter. Atrial flutter (AF) is believed to be caused by a steady circular pathway through which the wave of depolarization is continually moving. The loop is sufficiently large (or conduction through it sufficiently slow) that the current always finds the cells in front of it to be repolarized and ready to receive another stimulus. As a consequence, the current continually perpetuates itself. The atrial rate in atrial flutter is 250 to 350 beats per minute and is most often at 300 (see Table 15-11). At this rate, separate distinction of individual P waves is lost, and they blend together in a saw-tooth pattern (Fig. 15-34). In this state, P waves are more appropriately called *F waves* (flutter waves). Fortunately, the AV node does not allow conduction of all these impulses to the ventricles. When evaluating the rate of atrial flutter, one must calculate both atrial and ventricular rates.

The atrial rhythm will be perfectly regular, because the circuit is always the same length and therefore always requires the same time to complete. The ventricular rhythm will be regular if the same number of flutter waves occur between each QRS complex—in other words, if the degree of block at the AV node remains constant. Sometimes the refractoriness in the AV node changes from beat to beat, resulting in an irregular ventricular response. When describing atrial flutter, "PR interval" no longer applies; instead, it is a "conduction ratio," such as 3:1 or 4:1, that is used. In normal sinus rhythm, measuring the PR interval allows evaluation of the speed of conduction through the AV node; in atrial flutter, the number of flutter waves that bombard the AV node before one is allowed to pass through to the ventricles is a measure of AV nodal conduction. Once the impulse has passed the AV node, conduction through the ventricles is unaltered. The QRS duration should remain normal or at least the same as it was in normal sinus rhythm.

The major key to the clinical significance of atrial flutter is the ventricular response rate. If the atrial rate is 300 and the AV conduction ratio is 4:1, the ventricular response rate is 75 beats per minute and should be well tolerated. If, on the other hand, the atrial rate is 300 but the AV conduction ratio is 2:1, the corresponding ventricular rate of 150 may cause angina, acute heart failure, or other signs of cardiac decompensation. An atrial rate of 250 with a 1:1 AV conduction ratio yields

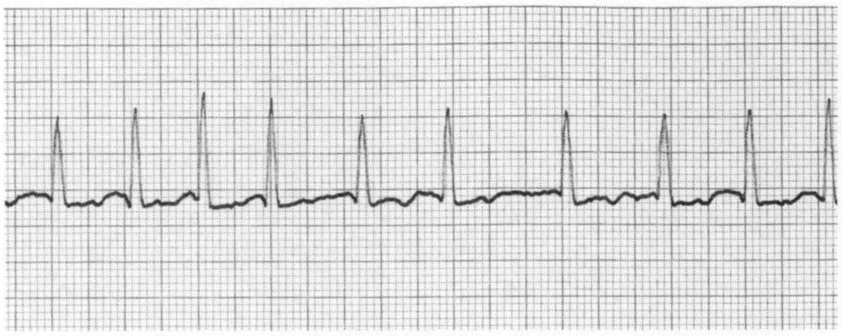

Fig. 15-35 Atrial fibrillation. Note the irregularly irregular ventricular rhythm.

a ventricular response rate of 250, and emergency measures are needed to decrease the ventricular rate.

Sometimes it is difficult to identify the flutter waves, especially if the conduction ratio is 2:1. Intravenous adenosine or vagal maneuvers can be useful diagnostic tools to increase briefly the refractory period of the AV node and allow better visualization of the F waves (Fig. 15-34). Only rarely do vagal maneuvers or IV adenosine terminate atrial flutter.[24] Usually atrial flutter can be converted back to sinus rhythm with the use of pharmacologic agents or cardioversion. If an adequate ventricular rate is all that is desired, administering a maintenance dose of digoxin or a calcium channel blocker usually suffices.

Atrial fibrillation. When numerous sites in the atria fire spontaneously and rapidly, an organized spread of depolarization can no longer take place, and atrial fibrillation (AF) results (Fig. 15-35). Small sections of atrial muscle are activated individually, resulting in quivering of the atrial muscle without effective contraction. The ECG tracing in atrial fibrillation is characterized by an uneven baseline without clearly defined P waves and an irregularly irregular ventricular rhythm. The QRS complex is usually normal, because the pathway through the ventricles is unchanged once the impulse leaves the AV node. The AV node acts as a filter to protect the ventricles from the 350 to 500 sporadic atrial impulses that are occurring each minute (see Table 15-11). In addition, the AV node itself does not receive all of the atrial impulses. When the atrial muscle tissue immediately surrounding the AV node is in a refractory state, impulses generated in other areas of the atria cannot reach the AV node, helping to explain the wide variation in RR intervals during atrial fibrillation.

A normal AV node conducts impulses to the ventricles at a rate of 100 to 180 times per minute. This rapid rate is not desirable, and a major therapeutic goal is to reduce the ventricular response rate to below 100 beats per minute. There are two ways to approach this goal: (1) convert the atrial fibrillation back to sinus rhythm using cardioversion or pharmacologic agents or (2) allow the atrial fibrillation to exist and use pharmacologic measures to control the ventricular response rate.

Electrical cardioversion may be successful in converting the rhythm to sinus if attempted within a few days or weeks of the onset of atrial fibrillation. Its success is less likely if the atrial fibrillation has existed for a long time. Cardioversion also carries with it the threat of precipitating emboli. During atrial fibrillation the atria do not contract; hence blood may pool in areas of the atrial walls. This pooling can promote thrombus formation (mural thrombi) within the atria. If cardioversion is successful and normal sinus rhythm is restored, the atria will again contract forcibly and, if thrombus formation has occurred, may send clots traveling through the pulmonary or systemic circulation. To prevent this, patients often receive anticoagulation therapy for several days or weeks before electrical cardioversion.

Sometimes patients will be in atrial fibrillation for only a few hours or days at a time and then convert back to sinus rhythm spontaneously. This is called *paroxysmal atrial fibrillation.* If it occurs often, these patients are also at risk for development of mural thrombi and subsequent emboli and should be on long-term anticoagulation therapy unless it is contraindicated.

Calcium channel blockers and digoxin are the most common chronically used drugs to control ventricular response rate in atrial fibrillation. The dosage is adjusted to keep the ventricular rate between 60 and 100 beats per minute. Beta blockers can also be used.

◆ **Junctional dysrhythmias.** Only certain areas of the AV node have the property of automaticity. The entire area around the AV node is collectively called the *junction;* hence impulses generated there are called *junctional.* After an ectopic impulse arises in the junction, it spreads in two directions at once. One wave of depolarization spreads upward into the atria and depolarizes them, causing the recording of a P wave on the ECG. At the same time, another wave of depolarization spreads downward into the ventricles through the normal conduction pathway, resulting in a normal QRS complex. Depending on timing, the P wave may be seen in front of the QRS but with a short PR interval, the P wave may be obscured entirely by the QRS, or the P wave may immediately follow the QRS. When atrial depolarization begins in the junction, the wave of depolarization spreads from the bottom of the atria upward, causing inversion of the P wave in lead II.

Premature junctional contraction. If only a single ectopic impulse originates in the junction, it is simply called a *premature junctional contraction.* On the ECG, the rhythm is regular from the sinus node except for one early QRS complex of normal shape and duration. The P wave can be entirely absent. If a P wave can be found, it very closely precedes or follows the QRS. In lead II, the P wave appears inverted (having a negative deflection), because the atria are being depolarized from the AV node upward, which is the opposite direction from the wave of depolarization that occurs when triggered by the sinus node. If the P wave appears before the QRS,

RESEARCH ABSTRACT

Accuracy of heart rate assessment in atrial fibrillation.

Sneed NV, Hollerbach AD: *Heart Lung* 21(5):427, 1992.

PURPOSE

The purpose of this study was to examine differences in accuracy of heart rate measurement in atrial fibrillation using different counting intervals.

DESIGN

Quasi-experimental, repeated measures factoral design

SAMPLE

The total sample consisted of 94 nurses from a large teaching hospital and an affiliated school of nursing: 29 registered nurses, 23 licensed practical nurses, 21 nursing students, and 21 registered nurses with advanced degrees. All subjects had experience taking apical and radial pulses of adult patients during the 2 months before the study and had no known hearing deficits.

INSTRUMENTS

A Hewlett Packard Model M1175A monitoring system with a dual-channel recorder was used. The monitor provided simultaneous ECG and plethysmograph (pleth) waveform recordings. All subjects used a standard stethoscope.

PROCEDURE

Data were collected in a quiet room on the clinical unit or in the school of nursing building. Each subject obtained six randomly-determined heart rate measurements using the 15-, 30-, and 60-second count for both apical and radial methods. Simultaneous ECG and pleth recordings were made, and ECG markings were made at both the beginning and the end of the count and at the end of 1 minute for the 15- and 30-second strips. The monitor was placed out of eyesight of the subjects. The investigator instructed the subjects when to start the count and timed the count with a stopwatch. To ensure interrater reliability for measures of the true heart rate, all r waves and pleth waves on the recordings were independently counted and recounted by two masters-prepared cardiovascular nurses until 100% agreement was obtained.

RESULTS

Of the 564 counts taken, 86% resulted in errors of underestimation, with only 10% errors of overestimation. Only 3% resulted in no error when compared with the ECG. Error tended to increase as the heart rate increased. Except for the 15-second radial count with the pleth standard, all counting interval and method errors were positively and significantly related to the rapidity of the heart rate (r = 0.29 to 0.69; p = .03 to .0001). Data from the pleth standard were usable only from patients whose heart rates were 80 or less (n = 48). Because of the difficulty in interpretation of the amplitude of the pleth waves, nearly half of the data were not included in analysis of the study. The greatest errors occurred when the radial pulse was compared with the ECG (71.3% to 77.7% for all three count intervals). Errors in apical counts when compared with the ECG ranged from 40.4% to 56.4%. Clinical significance in error was determined by expert cardiovascular nurses and cardiologists and was set at a 10% error. RNs and LPNs were significantly more accurate than were nursing students and RNs with advanced degrees in measuring radial pulses ($p < .05$); RNs and nursing students were significantly more accurate than were RNs with advanced degrees in measuring apical pulses ($p < .05$). The apical method was more accurate than was the radial method when either the ECG or the pleth was used as the standard ($p = < .04$). The 60-second count was significantly more accurate than was either the 15- or 30-second count ($p < .05$).

DISCUSSION/IMPLICATIONS

These findings indicate that the use of the apical pulse method using the 60-second counting interval is the most accurate for assessing heart rate in atrial fibrillation. Because errors increased as the heart rate increased, it appears to be important to use the 60-second count interval when heart rate is high. The nurses who were the most educated were the least accurate in counting heart rate. Accuracy appears to be related to the frequency, currency, and consistency of experience (skills are lost if practice is inconsistent). The plethysmograph proved to be an inaccurate method of measurement of the radial pulse in rapid atrial fibrillation. It is important that findings of this study be communicated to both student nurses and practicing nurses, so that accuracy of heart rate measurement is obtained. Future research should examine the variables that might affect accuracy of heart rate measurement in acutely ill patients. In addition, differing types of equipment used can be assessed for accuracy and best method.

the PR interval is less than 0.12 second. Premature junctional contractions have virtually the same clinical significance as do PACs. However, if the patient is receiving digoxin, digitalis toxicity should at least be suspected. Although digoxin slows conduction through the AV node, it also increases automaticity in the junction.

Junctional escape rhythm. Sometimes the junction becomes the dominant pacemaker of the heart (Table 15-12). Normally the intrinsic rate of the junction is 40 to 60 beats per minute. The intrinsic rate of the sinus node is 60 to 100 beats per minute. Under normal conditions the junction never has a chance to "escape" and depolarize the heart because it is overridden by the sinus node. However, if the sinus node fails, the junctional impulses can depolarize completely and pace the heart. This is called a *junctional escape rhythm* and is a protective mechanism to prevent asystole in the event of sinus node failure. Generally, a junctional escape rhythm (Fig. 15-36) is well tolerated, although efforts should be directed toward restoring sinus rhythm. Sometimes a pacemaker is inserted as a protective measure because of concern that the junction may also fail.

Junctional tachycardia and accelerated junctional rhythm. A junctional rhythm can also occur at a faster rate (see Table 15-12). As with sinus rhythm, the term *tachycardia* is reserved for rates greater than 100 per minute; thus junctional tachycardia is a junctional rhythm, usually regular, at a rate greater than 100. But what if the junctional rate is greater than 60 and less than 100 (faster than the intrinsic rate of the junction, yet not fast enough to be considered a tachycardia)? The phrase *accelerated junctional rhythm* applies to this situation. Accelerated junctional rhythm is usually well tolerated by the patient, mainly because the heart rate is within a reasonable range. Junctional tachycardia may not be tolerated as well, depending on the rate and the patient's underlying cardiac reserve. Once again, digitalis toxicity should be strongly suspected, because digoxin enhances automaticity of the AV node. If digitalis toxicity is present, the only treatment is to withhold digoxin until the dysrhythmia resolves.

◆ **Ventricular dysrhythmias.** Ventricular dysrhythmias result from an ectopic focus in any portion of the ventricular myocardium. The usual conduction pathway through the ventricles is not used, and the wave of depolarization must spread from cell to cell. As a result, the QRS complex is prolonged and is always greater than 0.12 second. It is the width of the QRS, not the height, that is important in diagnosing ventricular ectopy.

Premature ventricular contractions. A single ectopic impulse originating in the ventricles is called a *premature ventricular contraction (PVC)*. Some PVCs are very small in height but remain wider than 0.12 second. If in doubt, a different lead should be evaluated. The shape of the QRS varies, depending on the location of the ectopic focus. If the ectopic focus is in the right ventricle, the impulse spreads from right to left and the QRS resembles a left bundle branch block pattern, because the left ventricle is the last to be depolarized. In MCL_1, this is a wide, negative QRS (Fig. 15-37, *A*). If the ectopic focus is in the left ventricular free wall, the wave of depolarization spreads from left to right (Fig. 15-37, *B*).

Because the ectopic focus could be any cell in the ventricle, the QRS might take an unlimited number of shapes or patterns. If all of the ventricular ectopic beats look the same in a particular lead, they are called *unifocal,* which means that they probably all result from the same irritable focus (Fig. 15-38, *A*). Conversely, if the ventricular ectopics are of various shapes in the same lead, they are called *multifocal* (Fig. 15-38, *B*). Multifocal ventricular ectopics are more serious than unifocal ventricular ectopics because they indicate a greater area of irritable myocardial tissue and are more likely to deteriorate into ventricular tachycardia or fibrillation. In general, ventricular dysrhythmias have more serious implications than do atrial or junctional dysrhythmias and occur only rarely in healthy individuals.

A PVC originates in a ventricular cell that has become

Table 15-12 Junctional rhythms

Parameter	Junctional escape rhythm	Accelerated junctional rhythm	Junctional tachycardia
Rate	40-60/min	60-100/min	>100/min
Rhythm	Regular	Regular	Regular
P waves	May be present or absent; inverted in lead II	May be present or absent; inverted in lead II	May be present or absent; inverted in lead II
PR interval	<0.12 sec	<0.12 sec	<0.12 sec
QRS	0.06-0.10 sec	0.06-0.10 sec	0.06-0.10 sec

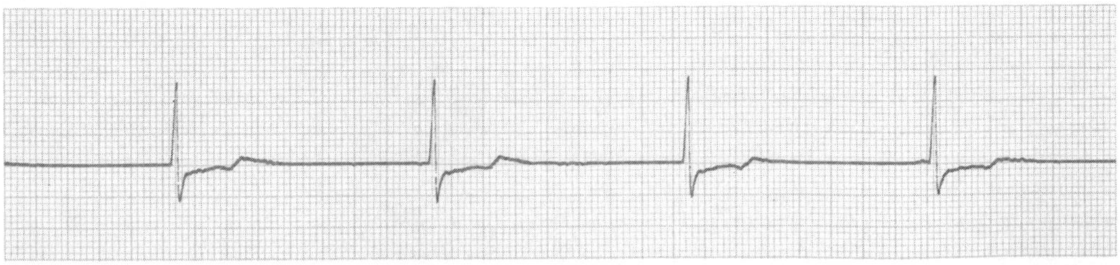

Fig. 15-36 Junctional escape rhythm. The ventricular rate is 38. P waves are absent, and the QRS is normal width.

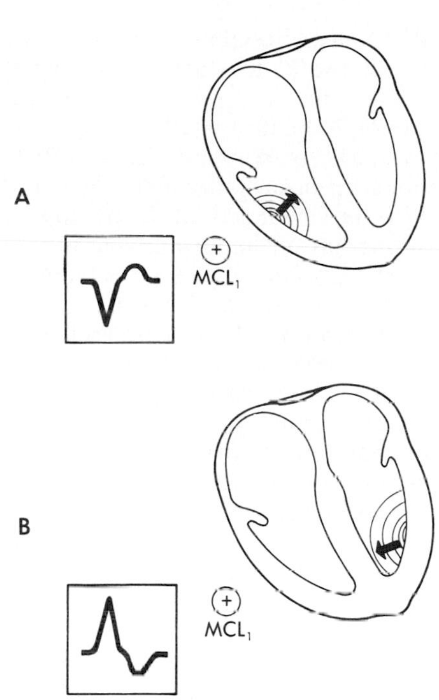

Fig. 15-37 **A,** Right ventricular premature ventricular contraction (PVC). The spread of depolarization is from right to left, away from the positive electrode in lead MCL_1, resulting in a wide, negative QRS complex. **B,** Left ventricular PVC. The spread of depolarization is from left to right, toward the positive electrode in lead MCL_1. The QRS complex will be wide and upright.

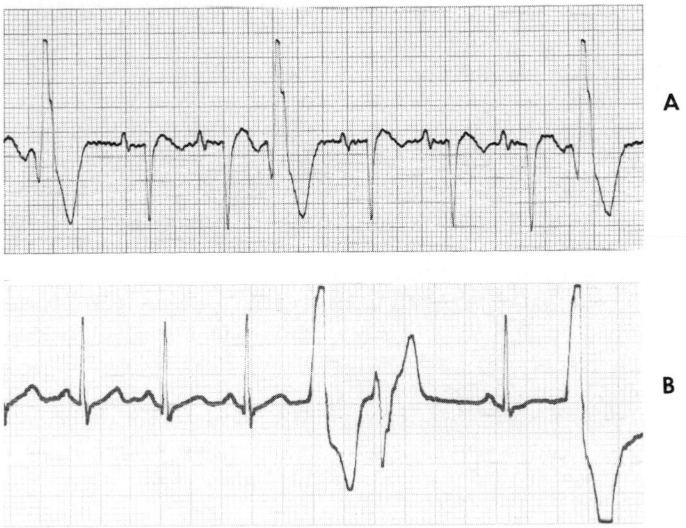

Fig. 15-38 **A,** Unifocal PVCs. **B,** Multifocal PVCs.

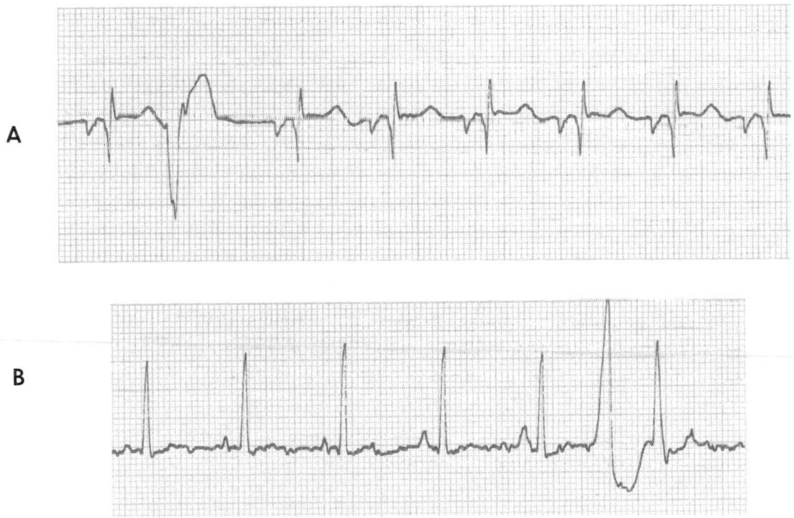

Fig. 15-39 **A,** PVC with a fully compensatory pause. The interval between the two sinus beats that surround the PVC (R_1 and R_2) is exactly 2 times the normal interval between sinus beats (R_3 and R_4). The fully compensatory pause occurs because the sinus node continues to pace despite the PVC. **B,** Interpolated PVC. The PVC falls between two normal QRS complexes without disturbing the rhythm. Note that the RR interval between sinus beats remains the same.

abnormally permeable to sodium, usually as a result of damage of one kind or another. Because of this new permeability to sodium, the cell reaches depolarization threshold before an impulse is received from the sinus node. Once depolarization threshold is reached, the cell automatically depolarizes, thus beginning total ventricular depolarization. Ordinarily, the ventricular impulse does not conduct back through the AV node; hence the sinus node is not disturbed and continues to depolarize the atria, resulting in a normal P wave. Conduction from the sinus node will not proceed into the ventricles if they are in a refractory state. The next sinus beat, assuming there is no further ventricular ectopy, will conduct normally through the AV node and into the ventricles.

COMPENSATORY PAUSE. If the interval from the last normal QRS preceding the PVC to the one following it is exactly equal to two complete cardiac cycles (Fig. 15-39, *A*), a compensatory pause is present. It does not usually occur in PACs or premature junctional contraction, so when present it is somewhat diagnostic of ventricular ectopy. If the normal sinus P wave that occurs immediately after the PVC finds the ventricles sufficiently recovered to accept another impulse, a normal QRS will result and the PVC will be sandwiched between two normal beats (Fig. 15-39, *B*). This PVC is referred to as *interpolated*, meaning "between." Interpolated PVCs usually occur when either the PVC is very early or the normal sinus rate is relatively slow.

Occasionally, the ventricular impulse spreads backward across the AV node to depolarize the atria. When this occurs, the sinus node is reset, and there is not a full compensatory pause.

DESCRIBING VENTRICULAR ECTOPY. PVCs can develop concurrently with any supraventricular dysrhythmia. Therefore it is not sufficient to describe a patient's rhythm as "frequent PVCs" or even "frequent unifocal PVCs." The underlying rhythm must always be described first, for example, "sinus bradycardia with frequent unifocal PVCs" or "atrial fibrillation with occasional multifocal PVCs." Timing of PVCs can also be described. When a PVC follows each normal beat, *ventricular bigeminy* is present (Fig. 15-40). If a PVC follows every two normal beats, it is called *ventricular trigeminy.*

The timing of PVCs can be important, especially if myocardial ischemia is present. The relative refractory period, represented on the ECG by the last half of the T wave, is a particularly vulnerable time for ectopy to occur because repolarization is not yet complete. Repolarization is even more delayed in ischemic tissue so that various portions of the ventricular muscle are not repolarized simultaneously. If a PVC occurs at this critical point when only a part of the muscle is repolarized, individual segments of muscle can depolarize separately from each other, resulting in ventricular fibrillation. This is called the *R-on-T phenomenon* (Fig. 15-41).

Two consecutive PVCs are described as a *couplet,* and three consecutive PVCs are called either a *triplet* or a *three-beat run of ventricular tachycardia.* More than three consecutive PVCs are considered ventricular tachycardia, but it is still useful to state how many beats of ventricular tachycardia occurred if the run was short, that is, fewer than 20 beats.

CAUSES OF PVCs. There are many causes of PVCs. They have been known to occur, although rarely, in healthy individuals with no evidence of heart disease. The critical care nurse has an important role in identifying factors that may be causing or at least contributing to the occurrence of PVCs. Acute ischemia is the most dangerous cause of ventricular ectopy. Ischemia causes cell membrane permeability to change, giving rise to early depolarization and the initiation of ectopic impulses. Ventricular ectopy that occurs during an acute ischemic event may require treatment with intravenous lidocaine or other antidysrhythmic drugs.

Metabolic abnormalities are frequent causes of the development of PVCs. Hypokalemia, hypoxemia, and acidosis predispose the cell membrane to instability and may cause ventricular ectopy. Treatment should be directed toward identifying the metabolic disturbance and correcting it. Arterial blood gas values and serum potassium and magnesium levels should be obtained if no recent results are available. The ability of oxygen and potassium values to change very rapidly in a critically ill patient must not be underestimated. If PVCs develop during suctioning of an intubated patient, a few additional breaths of 100% oxygen usually will be sufficient to restore adequate oxygenation and eliminate the ventricular ectopy.

Any form of heart disease can lead to the development of ventricular ectopy. Patients with cardiomyopathy or ventricular aneurysms can have chronic, severe ventricular ectopy, which may prove to be refractory to any antidysrhythmic agent. Invasive procedures, such as insertion of a Swan-Ganz catheter or cardiac catheterization, can cause PVCs by mechanically irritating the ventricular muscle. In these situations the ectopy will resolve with removal or advancement of the catheter. As a temporary measure, a one-time bolus of lidocaine can be used as a precaution against the development of a life-threatening dysrhythmia during these procedures.

Certain drugs can cause ventricular ectopy. Digitalis toxicity is often accompanied by PVCs, which are somewhat resistant to conventional antidysrhythmic therapy. Some antidysrhythmic drugs can actually cause more serious dysrhythmias than those they were intended to treat. This is called a *proarrhythmic effect* and can sometimes be fatal. Quinidine can prolong the QT interval by prolonging the ventricular refractory period

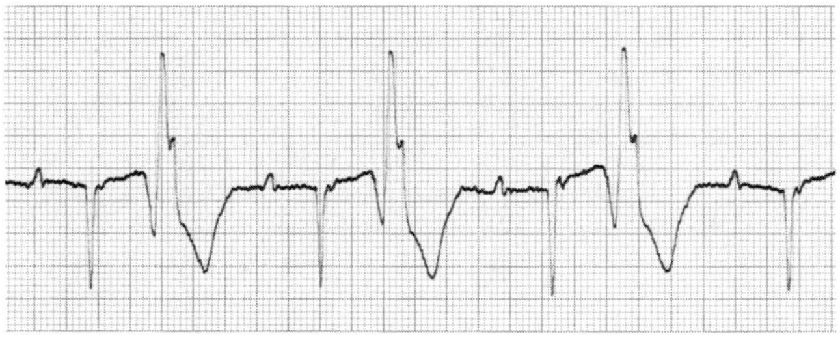

Fig. 15-40 Ventricular bigeminy.

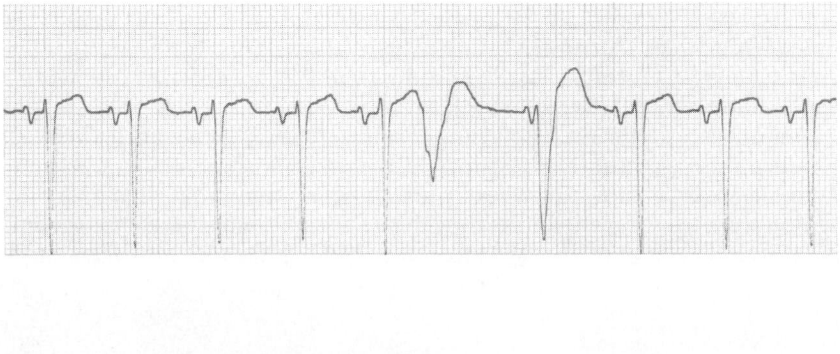

Fig. 15-41 R-on-T phenomenon.

to such an extent that a characteristic form of ventricular tachycardia, *torsades de pointes,* develops[13] (Fig. 15-42). In this dysrhythmia the ventricular tachycardia is very rapid and the QRS complexes appear to twist in a spiral pattern around the baseline. Clinically, torsades de pointes is poorly tolerated because of the extremely rapid rate. If not terminated, death will result. Sometimes torsades de pointes stops spontaneously, although the patient may experience a syncopal episode at the time of the dysrhythmia. Other antidysrhythmic drugs can also cause life-threatening dysrhythmias, although the exact mechanism involved is still unclear.

TREATMENT OF PVCs. Not all ventricular ectopy requires treatment. In individuals without significant underlying heart disease, PVCs do not represent an increased risk for sudden death and are considered benign. Approximately 30% of all patients with ventricular ectopic activity fall into this category.[25] If the patient complains of palpitations, therapy initially includes reassurance and elimination of such factors as caffeine or alcohol ingestion, emotional stress, and sympathomimetic drugs that increase ventricular irritability. If symptoms continue, mild tranquilizers can be administered, followed by beta blockers to reduce the response to sympathetic stimulation. Antidysrhythmic drugs should be used only as a last resort.

In patients with underlying heart disease, PVCs and/or episodes of nonsustained ventricular tachycardia are potentially malignant. Nonsustained ventricular tachycardia is defined as three or more consecutive premature ventricular beats at a rate faster than 110 per minute, lasting less than 30 seconds without hemodynamic collapse.[26] Approximately 65% of all patients with ventricular ectopic activity fall into this category.[25] In patients with only moderate left ventricular dysfunction (ejection fractions >30%), the risk of sudden death from a ventricular dysrhythmia is only modest, but in patients with severe left ventricular dysfunction (ejection fractions of <30%), the risk is high.

Because the occurrence of ventricular dysrhythmias in patients with heart disease has been shown to increase the risk of sudden death, these dysrhythmias have been treated aggressively with antidysrhythmic drugs for many years. However, until recently no well-controlled clinical trials had been performed to demonstrate that reduction of ventricular ectopics with antidysrhythmic drugs really improved morbidity and mortality statistics. In 1987 the National Institutes of Health began a randomized, double-blind study known as the *Cardiac Arrhythmia Suppression Trial (CAST)* to test the assumption that the treatment of ventricular dysrhythmias prolongs life. Patients with potentially malignant ventricular dysrhythmias were randomized into one of four groups: treatment with (1) encainide, (2) flecainide, (3) moricizine, and (4) placebo. These three drugs were chosen because they were the most effective in suppressing ventricular ectopics, as documented by Holter monitor recordings, and had the lowest incidence of side effects. The study was aborted, and interim results were released in 1989, when it was found that patients treated with encainide and flecainide had a significantly increased mortality over the placebo group, despite excellent suppression of ventricular ectopics and episodes of nonsustained ventricular tachycardia. What went wrong? The answer is not clear as yet. One possible explanation is that although most ventricular ectopic activity was suppressed by these drugs, the changes that they caused in the action potential may have altered the cell membrane in such a way that the likelihood of primary ventricular fibrillation was increased during episodes of transient ischemia or increased sympathetic nervous system activity.[25] Regardless of the mechanism, the results of this study have cast serious doubts on the efficacy of antidysrhythmic drug therapy in general. Until additional studies are done, antidysrhythmic drugs should be used with caution in this patient population, especially for long-term therapy. Beta blockers have been shown to decrease mortality by 26% to 48%, after a myocardial infarction,[27] and although they are only moderately effective in suppressing ventricular ectopic activity, they may be safer than are conventional antidysrhythmic drugs. Amiodarone also has been shown to decrease mortality after myocardial infarction but should be used with caution because of its potential for serious toxic side effects. Cardiovascular drugs and their side effects are discussed in greater depth in Chapter 17.

Patients who have already experienced sustained ventricular tachycardia or cardiac arrest are at especially high risk for sudden death. An extensive workup of these patients is warranted, including cardiac catheterization and electrophysiologic testing with programmed ventricular stimulation. Therapy is aimed at eliminating malignant ventricular ectopy and preventing recurrence of sustained ventricular tachycardia or ventricular fibrillation and may include treating the underlying cause, administering antidysrhythmic drugs, performing anti-

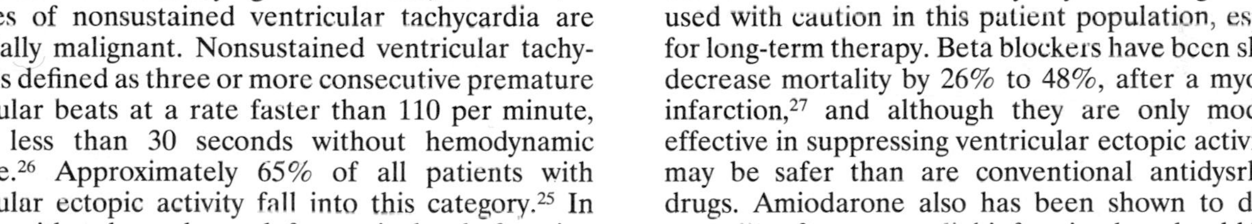

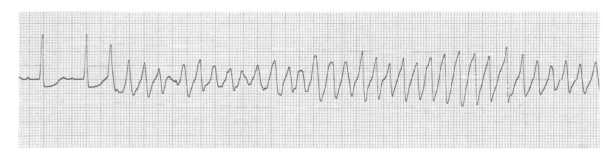

Fig. 15-42 Torsades de pointes.

dysrhythmic surgery, or implanting an antitachycardia pacemaker or an implantable cardioverter defibrillator (ICD).

IDIOVENTRICULAR RHYTHM. At times an ectopic focus in the ventricle can become the dominant pacemaker of the heart (Table 15-13). If both the sinus node and the AV junction fail, the ventricles will depolarize at their own intrinsic rate of 20 to 40 times per minute. This is called an *idioventricular rhythm* and is protective in nature. Rather than trying to abolish the ventricular beats, the aim of treatment is to increase the effective heart rate and reestablish a higher pacing site, such as the sinus node or AV junction. The heart rate may be increased pharmacologically with an infusion of isoproteronal (Isuprel). Or more commonly a temporary pacemaker is used to increase heart rate until the underlying problems that caused failure of the other pacing sites can be resolved.

An *accelerated idioventricular rhythm* occurs when a ventricular focus assumes control of the heart at a rate greater than its intrinsic rate of 40 per minute but less than 100 per minute (Fig. 15-43). Although relatively benign in and of itself, this rhythm must be closely observed for any increase in rate, or hemodynamic deterioration. Usually it is not treated pharmacologically if well tolerated, although a transvenous temporary pacemaker should be inserted electively as a precaution against sudden hemodynamic deterioration. Intravenous lidocaine should never be administered to a patient with an idioventricular rhythm, because it will suppress the ventricular pacemaker and convert the rhythm to asystole.

VENTRICULAR TACHYCARDIA. Ventricular tachycardia is caused by a ventricular pacing site firing at a rate of 100 times or more per minute (Fig. 15-44). The complexes are wide, and the rhythm may be slightly irregular, often accelerating as the tachycardia continues (see Table 15-13). In most cases the sinus node is not affected, and it will continue to depolarize the atria on schedule. P waves can sometimes be seen on the ECG tracing. They are not related to the QRS and may even conduct a normal impulse to the ventricles if their timing is just right. If the sinus impulse and the ventricular ectopic impulse meet in the middle of the ventricles, a fusion beat results. Fusion beats are narrower than are the ventricular beats and look like a cross between the patient's sinus QRS and the ventricular ectopic QRS (Fig. 15-45). When present, P waves and fusion beats are helpful in verifying the diagnosis of ventricular tachycardia.

Ventricular tachycardia can occur acutely in a variety of clinical settings, including myocardial ischemia, digitalis toxicity, electrolyte disturbances, and an adverse reaction of certain antidysrhythmic drugs. Patients with

Table 15-13 Ventricular rhythms

Parameter	Idioventricular rhythm	Accelerated idioventricular rhythm	Ventricular tachycardia	Ventricular fibrillation
Rate	20-40/min	40-100/min	>100/min	None
Rhythm	Usually regular	Usually regular	Usually regular	Irregular
P waves	Absent or retrograde	Absent or retrograde	Absent or retrograde	None
PR interval	None	None	None	None
QRS	>0.12 sec	>0.12 sec	>0.12 sec	Fibrillatory waves

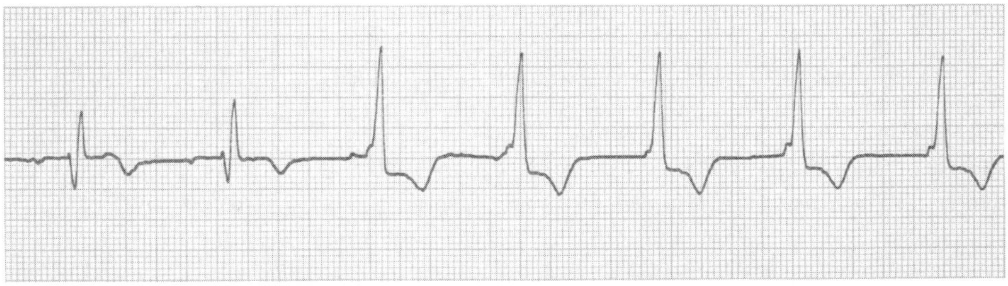

Fig. 15-43 Accelerated idioventricular rhythm (AIVR). The QRS duration is 0.14 second, and the ventricular rate is 65.

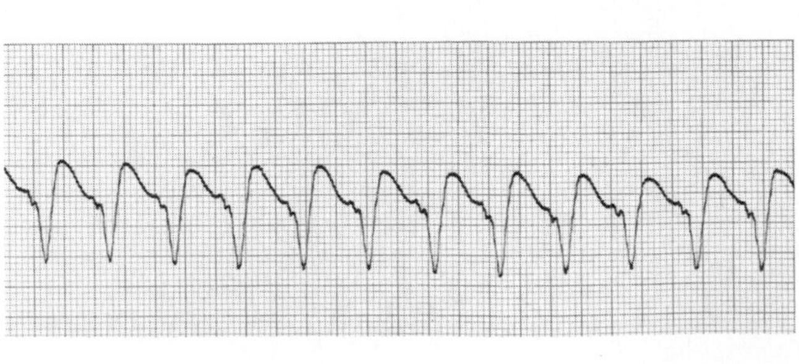

Fig. 15-44 Ventricular tachycardia.

chronic, severe heart disease, such as cardiomyopathy or ventricular aneurysm, may experience frequent episodes of ventricular tachycardia. Ventricular tachycardia is a serious dysrhythmia and must be treated quickly. Its rapid rate alone makes this dysrhythmia poorly tolerated. The benefit of the proper timing of atrial contraction, which would add volume to the ventricles just before contraction and enhance the force of contraction, is lost, thus greatly reducing cardiac output (CO). The fall in CO may cause the patient to lose consciousness. Finally, if not terminated quickly, ventricular tachycardia is very likely to degenerate into ventricular fibrillation and death.

VENTRICULAR FIBRILLATION. Ventricular fibrillation is the result of a rapid discharge of impulses from single or multiple foci in the ventricles, causing the ventricles to be unable to contract completely and effectively. The ventricles merely quiver, and there is no forward flow of blood. Without forward flow, there is no palpable pulse or audible apical heart tones. Clinically, ventricular fibrillation is indistinguishable from asystole (absence of electrical activity). On the ECG, ventricular fibrillation appears as a wavy baseline (Fig. 15-46), whereas in asystole the baseline is flat.

Ventricular fibrillation is sometimes further described as "coarse" or "fine." Coarse ventricular fibrillation is seen on the ECG as large, erratic undulations of the baseline, whereas in fine ventricular fibrillation the ECG baseline exhibits only a mild tremor. In either case, the patient does not have a pulse, no blood is being pumped forward, and defibrillation is the only definitive therapy. Generally, coarse ventricular fibrillation is more likely to be successfully defibrillated. Epinephrine can be used to try to change fine ventricular fibrillation to coarse ventricular fibrillation to facilitate defibrillation attempts. Antidysrhythmic drugs, such as intravenous lidocaine and bretylium, are also given if initial attempts at defibrillation fail. As with any cardiac arrest situation, supportive measures, such as CPR, intubation, and correction of metabolic abnormalities, are performed concurrently with definitive therapy. See Appendix B for Advanced Cardiac Life Support (ACLS) guidelines.

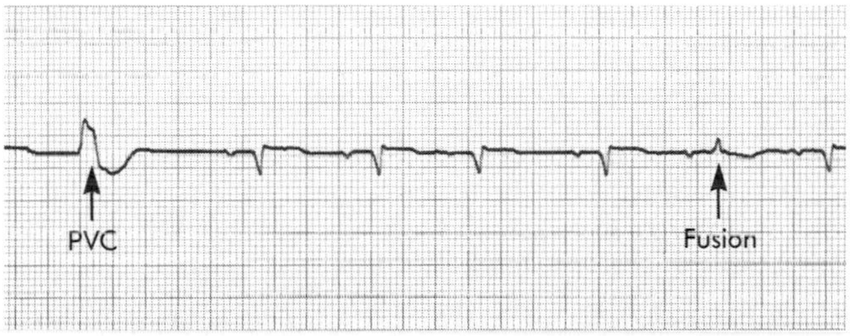

Fig. 15-45 Ventricular fusion beat *(arrows)*. The QRS duration is only 0.08 second, and the shape represents both the normal QRS and the previous PVC.

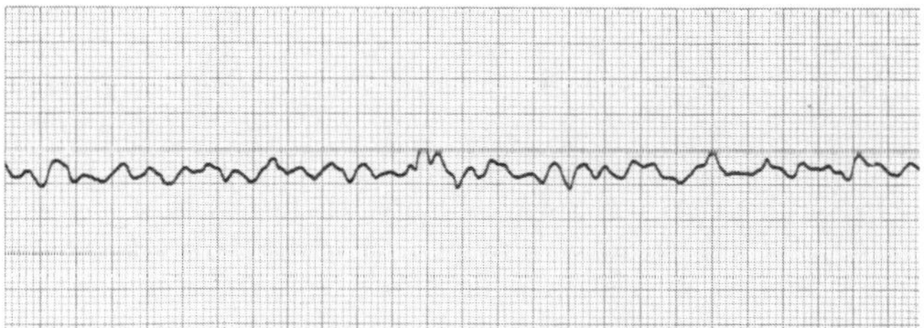

Fig. 15-46 Ventricular fibrillation.

Differential diagnosis of a wide QRS complex tachycardia. Tachycardias that are triggered by an ectopic atrial or junctional focus are called *supraventricular,* meaning that they come from an irritable site above the ventricles. Typical supraventricular tachycardia (SVT) has a narrow QRS complex (< 0.12 second), because the electrical impulse enters the ventricle through the AV node and still follows the normal conduction pathway via the bundle branches through the ventricles. Ventricular tachycardia (VT) always has a wide QRS complex (> 0.12 second), because the impulse begins somewhere within the ventricles and must spread slowly—cell to cell—without the benefit of the usual conduction system. Therefore it is easy to distinguish between typical SVT and ventricular tachycardia by QRS width alone.

Unfortunately, not all SVTs will result in a narrow QRS complex. There are three situations in which a supraventricular tachycardia has a wide QRS complex.[15]

1. The patient may already have a right or left bundle branch block, resulting in a wide QRS even during sinus rhythm. Understandably, if that patient develops an atrial or junctional tachycardia, the bundle branch block remains unchanged and the QRS complex is still wide.
2. A supraventricular impulse may arrive in the ventricles so early that only part of the conduction system is repolarized. One of the bundle branches is still refractory, causing the wave of depolarization to spread abnormally *(aberrantly)* through the ventricles and resulting in a wide QRS complex.
3. Occasionally an anatomic variant occurs in which the patient has a small strip of muscle tissue connecting the atria with the ventricles and bypassing the AV node. This is called *Wolff-Parkinson-White Syndrome,* or WPW. This is not a problem in normal sinus rhythm, although it sometimes causes subtle ECG changes that allow it to be detected. However, when rapid atrial dysrhythmias occur, they can be conducted directly to a portion of the ventricular myocardium without normal AV delay. Depolarization through the ventricles then proceeds from cell to cell rather than through the normal pathway of the conduction system, resulting in a wide QRS complex tachycardia that closely resembles ventricular tachycardia.

SIGNIFICANCE. Standard treatment for ventricular tachycardia includes administration of intravenous lidocaine, whereas supraventricular tachycardia is typically managed with intravenous verapamil.[28] If the diagnosis is incorrect and a supraventricular tachycardia is treated with lidocaine, the treatment is ineffective. If a ventricular tachycardia is mistakenly diagnosed as SVT and verapamil is given, the consequences can be disastrous. Buxton et al.[29] found that 11 of 25 patients (44%) with ventricular tachycardia who were given 5 to 10 mg of IV verapamil developed acute, severe hypotension or loss of consciousness requiring immediate cardioversion. In a group of 25 other patients with ventricular tachycardia who were treated with other antidysrhythmic drugs such as lidocaine and pronestyl, only one became hypotensive and none required emergency cardioversion. Therefore it is important in patients who are relatively hemodynamically stable to be sure of the mechanism of the tachycardia before treatment is initiated.

Regardless of the site of origin, a wide QRS complex tachycardia may not be well tolerated, mainly because of the rapid heart rate that prevents adequate ventricular filling during diastole, as well as increasing myocardial oxygen demand while decreasing time for coronary artery filling. Hemodynamic deterioration will be evidenced by syncope, severe hypotension, or symptoms of ischemia. In this case, emergency cardioversion needs to be performed regardless of whether the tachycardia is of ventricular or supraventricular origin.

Correct diagnosis of a wide QRS complex tachycardia may have an impact on the long-term management of a patient as well. If atrial flutter or fibrillation is determined to be the underlying mechanism, long-term treatment probably involves digoxin or a calcium channel blocker to reduce the heart rate response when these dysrhythmias occur. These drugs have little or no value in the long-term management of recurrent ventricular tachycardia. If ventricular tachycardia is determined to be the underlying mechanism in a patient without a history of ventricular dysrhythmias, a careful search for the cause (hypoxemia, electrolyte imbalance, excess sympathetic stimulation, or ischemia) is warranted. Depending on the clinical situation, the patient may require long-term antidysrhythmic therapy. If there is a history of ventricular tachycardia or "sudden death" and the patient is already on antidysrhythmic therapy, a recurrent episode of ventricular tachycardia indicates that the current treatment regimen is not effective and the therapy needs to be changed.

CLINICAL DIFFERENTIATION. Contrary to popular belief, hemodynamic stability or instability does not help to differentiate between ventricular tachycardia and SVT with a wide QRS complex.[30] In theory, a supraventricular tachycardia should be better tolerated, especially if atrial contraction is still occurring before each ventricular contraction (AV synchrony). However, clinically this is often untrue. Ventricular tachycardia may be well tolerated, especially if the rate is not greater than 150 per minute. Some patients can be in sustained VT for hours without significant hemodynamic compromise. Conversely, AV synchrony will still be lost in atrial fibrillation or atrial flutter, and the ventricular response rate may be very rapid, compromising ventricular filling and, in turn, cardiac output.

Careful physical examination can be of value in determining the source of the tachycardia. The jugular venous pulse should be assessed for the presence of *cannon "a" waves.* When the atria contract at the same time as ventricular systole, the AV valves are closed and the blood in the atria is forced to regurgitate into the venous system. This is seen as a very large pulsation in the jugular vein. If it occurs sporadically (i.e., not with every beat), it is a sign of *AV dissociation,* or independent beating of the atria and ventricles. Heart sounds provide another diagnostic clue. Variation of the intensity of the first heart sound (S_1) from beat to beat favors ventricular tachycardia, because this is also indicative of AV dissociation.

By far the most reliable means of diagnosing a wide QRS complex tachycardia is through careful analysis of the ECG. Heart rate and rhythm should be evaluated first, although they are not diagnostic by themselves. Rates of 130 to 170 per minute favor ventricular tachycardia. Rates greater than 170 per minute favor SVT with aberrant conduction, because healthy hearts can usually conduct impulses at rates less than 170 without altering the normal conduction pathway through the ventricles. Rates greater than 220 per minute, especially if accompanied by an irregular rhythm, favor atrial fibrillation with conduction around the AV node via a bypass tract.[31]

The QRS width should be measured in more than one lead, because the lead with the widest QRS complex is the most reliable indicator of true QRS duration. (It is assumed that some portion of the QRS complex is isoelectric in leads where the QRS appears to be more narrow.) QRS widths of <0.14 second favor SVT with aberrant conduction, whereas widths of >0.16 second favor ventricular tachycardia.[15]

The tracing should be examined closely for the presence of P waves. If P waves can be identified and they do not correlate on a 1:1 basis with the QRS complexes, AV dissociation exists and strongly suggests ventricular tachycardia. Although P waves may be found in any lead, they are most likely to be visible in V_1 or MCL_1.[15] If the sinus node remains in control of the atria and a ventricular ectopic focus is in control of the ventricles, it is likely that at some point the timing will be just right for the sinus impulse to conduct through the AV node and begin to depolarize the ventricles just as the ventricular ectopic focus fires. The resulting QRS complex is a fusion beat (see Fig. 15-45), which looks like a blend of the patient's normal QRS and the wide QRS complex of the ventricular dysrhythmia. Fusion beats also strongly suggest ventricular tachycardia.

Another helpful diagnostic criterion for ventricular tachycardia is a QRS axis in the northwest quadrant of -90 degrees to ± 180 degrees. An axis in this quadrant means that the wave of depolarization is directed upward and to the right, exactly the opposite of normal ventricular depolarization. Even when ventricular conduction is abnormal, as in bundle branch blocks, ventricular depolarization begins at the level of the AV junction and spreads downward toward the apex, although conduction disturbances direct the current flow more to the right or left than normal. Although not all ventricular tachycardias have an axis in the northwest quadrant, about one fourth of them do,[32] and when present, an axis in the northwest quadrant confirms the diagnosis of ventricular tachycardia. Fig. 15-47 illustrates how this abnormal axis can be rapidly identified from a five-lead-wire bedside monitor by noting the shape of the QRS in leads I and aV_F.

Finally, the shape of the QRS complex in the right precordial lead MCL_1 or V_1 and the left precordial lead MCL_6 or V_6 can be diagnostic of ventricular tachycardia or of SVT with aberrant conduction. Fig. 15-48 summarizes these QRS patterns. In addition, if the QRS complex is either entirely positive from V_1 through V_6 or entirely negative, the diagnosis is ventricular tachycardia. This phenomenon is known as *precordial concordance* and is also valid when only V_1 and V_6 are analyzed without the benefit of V_{2-5} as well. Using these criteria when examining both V_1 and V_6 (or MCL_1 and MCL_6) results in a diagnostic accuracy of 90%. If QRS axis is added to that (requiring examination of leads I and aV_F), the accuracy increases to 93%.[11]

IMPLICATIONS FOR CRITICAL CARE NURSING MANAGEMENT. Proper electrode placement and appropriate lead selection cannot be overemphasized. The diagnostic value of MCL_1 or MCL_6 is lost if the electrodes are not in the proper positions; even an error of one intercostal space can invalidate the usefulness of these leads. Lead selection is equally critical. Proper electrode placement is of little value if an unhelpful lead is chosen for monitoring. In a recent survey of critical care nurses, 74% chose to monitor their patients in a single lead II, despite the fact that lead II is almost useless in differentiating ventricular tachycardia from SVT with aberrant conduction.[14]

In addition to correct lead placement and selection, every effort should be made to record the wide QRS complex tachycardia on a standard 12-lead ECG. Certainly emergency treatment should not be delayed if the patient is hemodynamically unstable, but documenting the dysrhythmia by recording a "stat" 12-lead ECG should be given a high priority if time permits. Ventricular tachycardia and SVT are often nonsustained, and waiting for a physician's order or a technician to perform the test could result in failure to document the dysrhythmia at all, leaving the cause and subsequent therapy a mystery. Finally, if in doubt as to the origin of the wide QRS complex tachycardia, verapamil should be avoided because it has been known to cause rapid hemodynamic deterioration.

Atrioventricular conduction disturbance. Normally, the sinoatrial (SA) node triggers electrical depolarization in the heart. From there, the impulse travels through internodal tracts to the atrioventricular (AV) node. The impulse is delayed in the AV node to allow the atria to contract before the impulse is conducted to the bundle of His, bundle branches, and Purkinje fibers.

Clinically, the ability of the AV node to conduct is evaluated by measuring the PR interval and the relationship of P waves to QRS complexes (Table 15-14). The normal PR interval, measured from the beginning of the P wave to the beginning of the QRS complex, ranges from 0.12 to 0.20 second.

FIRST-DEGREE AV BLOCK. When all atrial impulses that should be conducted to the ventricles are conducted but the PR interval is greater than 0.20 second, a condition known as *first-degree AV block* exists (Fig. 15-49). First-degree AV block is not clinically significant by itself, but in a patient with an acute myocardial infarction, it may be a forerunner of more severe conduction disturbances and deserves close monitoring.

SECOND-DEGREE AV BLOCK. Second-degree AV block can be broadly defined as a condition in which one or more (but not all) atrial impulses that should be conducted fail to reach the ventricles. This very general description covers a wide variety of patterns with markedly variable clinical significance. Second-degree AV block can be divided into Mobitz type I (also known as Wenckebach), Mobitz type II, and high-grade AV blocks.

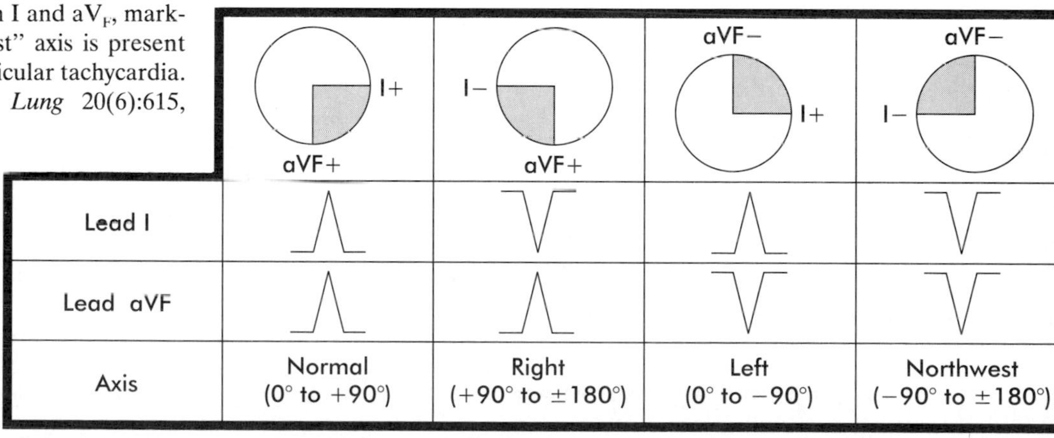

Fig. 15-47 Determination of QRS axis quadrant by noting predominant QRS polarity in leads I and aV_F. If QRS during tachycardia is primarily positive in both I and aV_F, axis falls within normal quadrant from 0 to 90 degrees. If complex is primarily negative in I and positive in aV_F, right axis deviation is present. If complex is predominantly positive in I and negative in aV_F, left axis deviation is present. Finally, if QRS is primarily negative in both I and aV_F, markedly abnormal "northwest" axis is present that is diagnostic of ventricular tachycardia. (From Drew B: *Heart Lung* 20(6):615, 1991.)

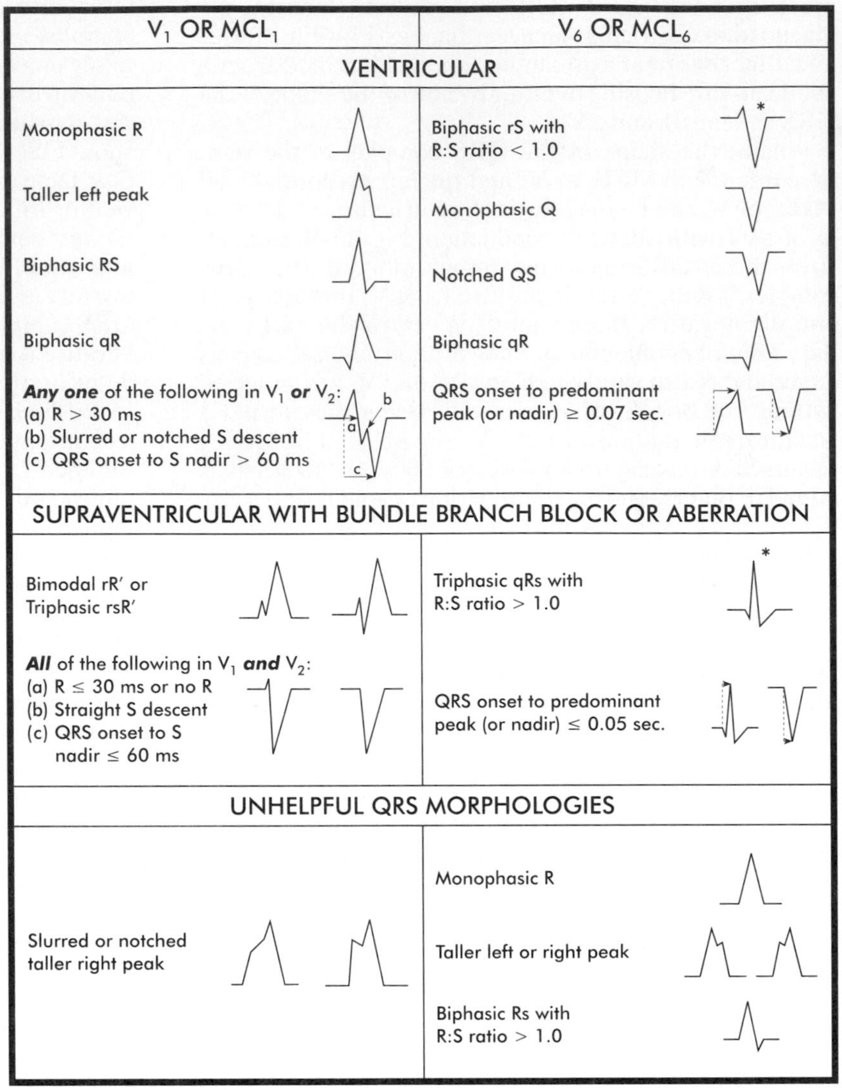

* Tachycardias with a right bundle branch block pattern in V_1 only

Fig. 15-48 Summary of morphologic clues in V_1 or MCL_1 *(left column)* and in V_6 or MCL_6 (*right column*) that are valuable in distinguishing supraventricular tachycardia with bundle branch block or aberration from ventricular tachycardia. If wide complex tachycardia with taller right peak pattern (i.e., unhelpful morphology) develops in a patient monitored with a single MCL_1 lead, the nurse should change leads to determine whether the wide complex falls into one of the diagnostic patterns in MCL_6. (From Drew B: *Heart Lung* 20(6):614, 1991.)

Table 15-14 Atrioventricular (AV) block

Parameter	First degree	Second-degree Mobitz I (Wenckebach)	Second-degree Mobitz II	Third degree (complete)
PR interval	>0.20 sec and constant	Increases with each consecutively conducted P wave	Constant	Varies randomly
P waves	1 P wave for each QRS	Intermittently not conducted, yielding more P waves than QRS complexes	Intermittently not conducted, yielding more P waves than QRS complexes	P waves independent and not related to QRS complexes
QRS	0.06-0.10 sec	0.06-0.10 sec	May be normal, but usually coexists with bundle branch block (>0.12)	0.06-0.10 sec if junctional escape pacemaker activates the ventricles >0.12 if ventricular escape pacemaker activates the ventricles

MOBITZ TYPE I. In Mobitz type I block, the AV conduction time progressively lengthens until a P wave is not conducted. Mobitz I is caused by an abnormally long relative refractory period. The rate of conduction depends on the moment of impulse arrival: the earlier the impulse arrives in the AV node, the longer it takes to conduct; the later it arrives, the shorter is the conduction time. Mobitz I second-degree AV block develops because each successive sinus impulse arrives earlier and earlier in the relative refractory period of the AV node until one sinus impulse finally arrives during the absolute refractory period and fails to conduct.

On the ECG, Mobitz type I AV block can be distinguished by PR intervals that progressively lengthen until a P wave finally is not conducted and is therefore not followed by a QRS (Fig. 15-50). If four P waves are conducted to the ventricles and the fifth one is not, a 5:4 conduction ratio is present (five P waves to four QRS complexes). The PR interval lengthening is usually greatest with the second beat of the cycle. The RR intervals become progressively shorter until the sinus P wave is not conducted. After that pause, the cycle repeats itself. It is useful to look at the RP interval to determine the earliness of the sinus impulse arrival in the AV node. The RP interval is measured from the beginning of the QRS to the beginning of the following P wave. As the RP interval decreases, the PR interval increases, and vice versa. This phenomenon is known as *RP-PR reciprocity* and always indicates Mobitz type I block.[33]

In Mobitz type I block the actual anatomic site of the block is at the level of the AV node itself. Usually, with an acute inferior wall infarction, the block is caused by ischemia and is transient. Still, the possibility of progression to a more serious conduction disturbance exists, warranting close observation and, occasionally, placement of a temporary pacemaker as a precautionary measure.

MOBITZ TYPE II. Mobitz type II block occurs in the presence of a long absolute refractory period with virtually no relative refractory period. This results in an "all or nothing" situation. Sinus P waves either will or will not be conducted. When conduction does occur, all PR intervals are the same. There is no RP-PR reciprocity. Usually, Mobitz II indicates block below the AV node, either in the His bundle or in both bundle branches. Most often, it occurs when one bundle branch is blocked and the other one is ischemic. Mobitz II block is more ominous clinically than is Mobitz I and often progresses to complete AV block. On the ECG the PR interval is constant (Fig. 15-51). If consecutive P waves are conducted, the difference between Mobitz I and Mobitz II second-degree AV block is apparent: in Mobitz I the PR interval gradually lengthens until finally a P wave is not conducted or is missed; in Mobitz II the PR intervals remain exactly the same, but suddenly a normal P wave (not premature) fails to conduct.

Occasionally, only every other P wave is conducted through the AV node (Fig. 15-52). This pattern could indicate either Mobitz I or II, because consecutive conduction of P waves—which would reveal either a lengthening or constant PR—does not occur. In Mobitz I the conduction ratios may have decreased from 4:3 to 3:2 to 2:1, yet the site and type of block have not changed. The change in conduction ratio may be caused by an increase in atrial rate, or it may change spontaneously.

In 2:1 conduction it is impossible to be certain whether the block is Mobitz type I or II from the surface ECG. If it occurs along with other Mobitz I ratios, it is probably still Mobitz I, and vice versa. If it is an isolated occurrence with no other strips for comparison, the QRS width and the PR interval offer valuable clues to the site of the block. In Mobitz I the QRS is usually normal and the PR interval is usually prolonged. In Mobitz II the QRS is usually wide and the PR interval is usually normal. Also, during an acute inferior myocardial infarction, Mobitz type I AV block with 2:1 conduction is much more common than is type II.[33]

HIGH-GRADE AV BLOCK. High-grade or advanced AV block is a form of second-degree AV block in which two

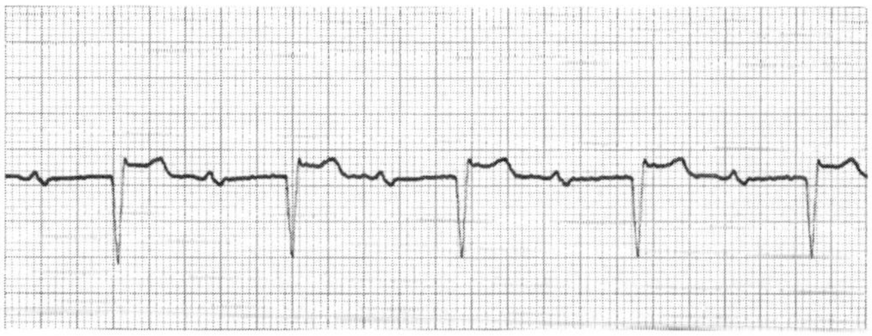

Fig. 15-49 First-degree AV block. The PR interval is prolonged to 0.44 second.

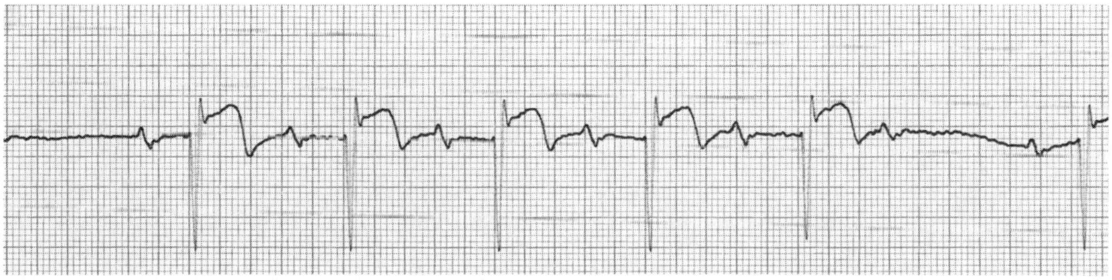

Fig. 15-50 Mobitz type I (Wenckebach) second-degree AV block. Note that the PR intervals gradually increase from 0.36 to 0.46 second until, finally, a P wave is not conducted to the ventricles.

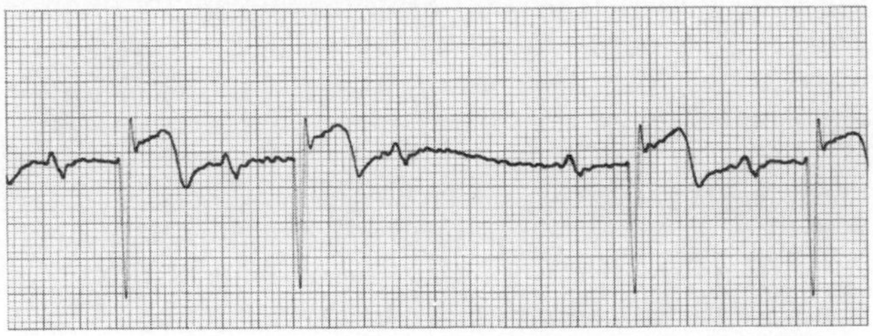

Fig. 15-51 Mobitz type II second-degree AV block. Note that the PR intervals remain constant.

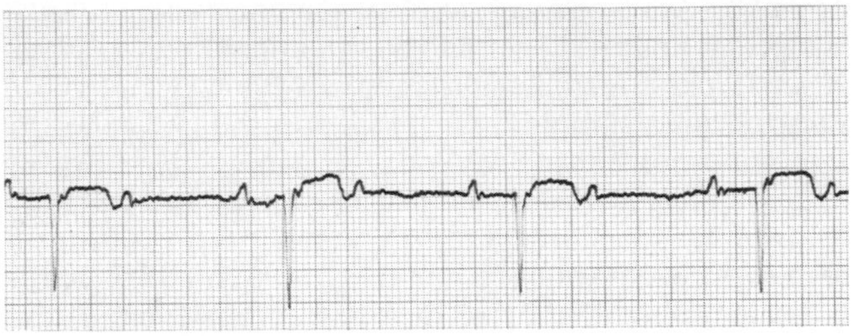

Fig. 15-52 2:1 AV block. Because no two consecutive P waves are conducted, it is not possible to determine with certainty whether this is Mobitz I or Mobitz II second-degree AV block.

or more consecutive atrial impulses fail to conduct through the AV node. On the ECG, several P waves occur before each QRS, but the PR intervals of all of the P waves that are followed by a QRS are the same. This is a severe form of second-degree AV block that is often followed by complete heart block.

In making this diagnosis, two important factors must be considered. First, the atrial rate must be reasonable—approximately 130 beats per minute or less. At high atrial rates, blocking of conduction at the level of the AV node is normal; in fact, it is crucial to protect the ventricles from dangerously high rates. In atrial flutter, with an atrial rate of 300 per minute, there is often 4:1 conduction, which yields a ventricular response rate of 75 per minute. This is desirable and is not high-grade AV block. Second, the failure of conduction must be caused by the existing block itself and not by a junctional or ventricular escape beat, which fires first and prevents conduction. If the sinus rate is 50 per minute and a junctional focus is firing at a rate of 60 per minute, many P waves do not have an opportunity to conduct because they occur shortly after the junctional beat and find the AV node or bundle branches still in the absolute refractory period. Marriott[34] coined the term "block-acceleration dissociation" for this condition. It can occur during mild or nonexistent AV block and yet can mimic complete AV block if not examined closely.

THIRD-DEGREE AV BLOCK. Third-degree, or complete, AV block is a condition in which no atrial impulses can conduct through the AV node to cause ventricular depolarization. The opportunity for conduction is optimal, yet none occurs. It is hoped that a junctional or ventricular focus will depolarize spontaneously at its intrinsic rate of 20 to 40 beats per minute and ventricular contraction will continue. If not, asystole occurs; there is no pulse, and death will result if intervention is not immediate.

On the ECG, P waves are present and usually occur at regular intervals. If a junctional focus is pacing the heart, normal QRSs are present but occur at a rate and timing interval totally independent of the P waves. The PR intervals vary widely, because the P wave and QRS are not related to each other. If a ventricular focus is pacing the heart, the QRS complex is wide and unrelated to the P waves (Fig. 15-53).

MEDICAL MANAGEMENT OF AV BLOCK. Clinically, the consequences of AV block range from benign to life-threatening. First-degree AV block is seldom of immediate concern but bears close observation for progression of the conduction disturbance. Second-degree Mobitz I (Wenckebach) is usually benign, especially during an acute ischemic episode. If hemodynamic compromise is present or deemed likely, a temporary pacemaker can be inserted prophylactically until the situation stabilizes or normal conduction is restored. Second-degree Mobitz II is more serious and often precedes complete AV block. Use of a temporary pacemaker is usually necessary, but its insertion can be elective if the patient remains hemodynamically stable. Complete heart block almost always requires use of a pacemaker. If the patient is hemodynamically unstable, an isoproterenol (Isuprel) drip or external pacemaker can be used to maintain an adequate ventricular rate until a temporary pacemaker can be inserted.

◆ Ambulatory electrocardiography

Definition and purpose. Ambulatory electrocardiography is a technique that records the ECG of patients while they perform their usual activities. It was designed to document, characterize, and quantify abnormal cardiac electrical activity (dysrhythmias or ischemic changes) that occurs at random during spontaneous activity or is induced by specific circumstances such as sleep, emotional stress, or physical activity.

Procedure. Two basic types of recording systems are available: continuous and intermittent. Although different in design, advantages, and limitations, each type can be used by ambulatory patients within or outside the hospital setting.

CONTINUOUS RECORDING SYSTEMS. Holter monitors are the oldest and most widely used continuous recording system. The patient wears skin electrodes and carries a box that contains an analog tape recorder, either with a shoulder strap or clipped to his or her belt or pocket. Usually the monitor is left on for 24 hours and then is returned to the hospital or clinic for reading. This is a totally noninvasive procedure with no immediate adverse effects.

When initially developed by Dr. Norman J. Holter in the 1930s more than 54 years ago, the equipment consisted of an 85-pound backpack with a short-range radio transmitter. The invention of the transistor in the 1950s reduced the recorder's weight to 6½ pounds, making it much more realistic for use on cardiac

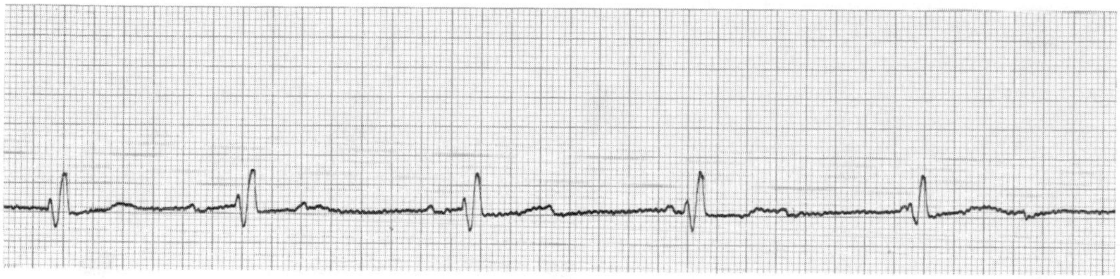

Fig. 15-53 Third-degree (complete) heart block.

patients. As technology has improved, the recording devices have become even smaller, so that at present a 4- × 6-inch recorder weighs less than 1 pound.

All Holter monitors record at least two leads, primarily to minimize inaccurate interpretation caused by artifact. Usually five electrodes are placed. Two of them are positive electrodes, corresponding approximately to the V_1 and V_5 positions on a standard 12-lead ECG. There are also two negative electrodes and one ground. Occasionally, additional electrodes are used to improve diagnostic capabilities. For example, a separate lead can be used to detect pacemaker spikes if the patient is being monitored for pacemaker dysfunction. The skin electrodes are disposable, pregelled, and self-adhering. They should be kept dry—not because of any electrical danger, but to prevent their falling off before the recording is completed. If skin irritation or hypersensitivity occurs, it can usually be relieved with hydrocortisone cream. The recorder is battery powered and can use either ¼-inch tape reels or ⅛-inch magnetic tape cassettes to record at very slow speeds, typically 0.0625 inches per second.[35] Reel-to-reel tapes have fewer technical problems and can provide a clearer recording, but cassette tapes are smaller and more convenient for the patient.

The tape saves all of the ECG tracings for a given time, usually 8 to 24 hours. The tape can correlate time with the tracing and display the time that an event occurred when the tape is decoded. Most also have an event marker, which the patient can press to indicate the onset of symptoms or another event that may be important. The patient is asked to keep a diary of his or her activities, symptoms, and any medications that are taken.

When the tape is returned to the hospital or clinic for reading, a technician places it in a machine that displays the tracing for review. The tracing is run at a faster speed than normal, or it would take 24 hours to read a 24-hour recording and the cost would be prohibitive. Usually the tape is run at 60 to 120 times normal speed, allowing a 24-hour report to be read in 15 to 30 minutes. Several techniques are used to aid the technician in interpretation of the tracing. One technique, audiovisual superimposition electrocardiographic presentation (AVSEP), places each QRS complex on top of the prior ones so that any that are abnormal stand out. R-to-R intervals are also measured by the machine, and a tone that varies in pitch—depending on the heart rate—is emitted. Using this system, a run of ventricular tachycardia would be both seen and heard by the technician.

Printed reports are also generated as the tape is read. Real-time printouts, at normal speed, can be run when any significant dysrhythmias are noted. A trend plot of heart rate, ST-segment level, or number of ectopics can also be printed. Most decoding machines count ectopics automatically, but it is up to the operator to validate that the decoder is really counting ectopy and not artifact. The final report is only as good as the technician scanning the data.

Continuous recording systems are the most thorough form of ambulatory electrocardiography because they record every heartbeat for 24 hours. They do not require the active participation of the patient (although a detailed patient log is helpful) and therefore do not miss asymptomatic ECG changes or dysrhythmias that may be accompanied by a loss of consciousness. When dysrhythmias occur that correlate with symptoms or symptoms occur in the absence of dysrhythmias, one of the primary goals of Holter monitoring has been achieved. Unfortunately, most patients do not have typical symptoms daily. If no significant dysrhythmias or symptoms occur during the 24-hour monitoring period, the test is completely useless. If dysrhythmias occur in the absence of symptoms, very little is gained, because people normally have asymptomatic dysrhythmias quite frequently and the dysrhythmias documented may or may not be the ones responsible for the patient's presenting symptoms. Rana et al.[36] examined 264 episodes of Holter monitoring in 252 elderly outpatients and found that the diagnostic yield was only 12%. Holter monitoring is quite expensive because of the sophisticated equipment required, especially for analysis of the recording, and the technician time involved. In this era of increasing health care costs, the expense of this test must be weighed against its potential benefits in individual cases.

Recently, digital continuous recording systems have been developed using very high-density semiconductor memory. The incoming signals are amplified, digitized, coded, and stored in solid state memory. Reports can then be printed, ranging from dysrhythmia summaries to "full disclosure" (tightly compressed printout of entire ECG tracing correlated with time markings). The digital systems have several advantages over the analog tape systems. They are smaller and have no mechanical parts (such as electrical tape drives and gears) that can fail. They use less energy and therefore require a smaller battery. The signal-to-noise ratio is improved, because there is no tape "noise" during recording or playback. In addition, some of these digital recorders have on-board intelligence that can analyze and process incoming data, classify complex dysrhythmias, track heart rate, and count PVCs. These specialized digital recorders are called *real-time analysis systems.* A built-in computer analyzes the ECG as it is recorded and stores only abnormal patterns.[35] The device weighs approximately twice as much as a standard Holter monitor because of the built-in computer. It also costs 3 to 5 times more, but this cost is offset by the decrease in hours needed for interpretation. This recording mode is very useful because the recorder can be used over a longer period (since the entire tracing is not stored) and interpretation is immediately available from the computer without needing an operator to decode it. Unfortunately, there are still some drawbacks. Accuracy is questionable, because events the computer considered insignificant are not stored. The computer's ability to analyze dysrhythmias is only as good as the algorithms with which it is programmed. In the rare event that battery failure occurs, all information can be lost. Human editing is still required to review computer-stored strips, to identify false-positive and false-negative events (dysrhythmia versus artifact), and to incorporate the information into a final report. This type of recording device stores approximately 120 10-second strips, which can be analyzed at a later time.

INTERMITTENT RECORDING SYSTEMS. A device similar to a Holter monitor that does not record the ECG continuously can be attached to the patient. When the patient is having symptoms, he or she presses a button to initiate the recording manually. Advantages of this mode center around the ability to leave the recorder on the patient for longer periods. With the intermittent recorder mode, the device can be worn for up to 96 hours and the patient can trigger active recording at the appropriate times. The disadvantage of this approach is that the ECG tracing just before the onset of symptoms is not recorded, leaving the precipitating factors a mystery. Also, the patient must be able to trigger the device; if loss of consciousness occurs rapidly, this is not possible and the dysrhythmia is not recorded. In addition, if the machine is used frequently by the patient in the initial hours of the recording or is left on by mistake, the memory may be full when an important symptomatic event occurs and no recording can be made.

Taking this concept a step further, *transtelephonic monitors* that are not attached to the patient at all have been developed. These monitors consist of a small box, about 4″ × 2½″ with four metal plates on the bottom. The box is issued to the patient for a specific time, often 1 month. The patient carries the box at all times. Whenever symptoms are experienced, the patient places the recording box in the center of the chest and places the four metal plates (electrodes) in firm contact with the skin. An alternative method, often preferred by patients, is to use two arm bracelets rather than direct chest placement. A button is then depressed to activate the recording, which lasts 1 to 2 minutes. The recording is stored until it is convenient for the patient to call a central analysis facility. At that time, the receiver of the patient's telephone is placed over a transmitter on the box and the recording is transmitted to the analysis facility, where it is printed out as a readable ECG tracing. A copy of the tracing is sent to the patient's physician, and the patient is advised if urgent medical attention is necessary. The center can contact the patient's physician or emergency medical personnel if the dysrhythmia is life-threatening. This system can be quite cost-effective, because it is less expensive than a continuous 24-hour Holter monitor and provides for a longer monitoring time, thereby increasing the chance that a recording will occur during symptoms. However, if symptoms are incapacitating, the patient may not be able to activate the system. Dysrhythmias that are asymptomatic are missed because the patient has no reason to activate the system.

Indications. Ambulatory electrocardiography is widely used in a variety of clinical situations (see box below). In 1989 the American College of Cardiology and the American Heart Association released a joint task force report outlining guidelines for the use of ambulatory electrocardiography.[37] Clinical indications were divided into three categories: those in which ambulatory monitoring has shown definite benefit, those in which ambulatory monitoring is of possible value, and those in which ambulatory monitoring is of little or no benefit. These recommendations are the basis for the following indications.

EVALUATION OF SYMPTOMS POSSIBLY RELATED TO DYSRHYTHMIAS. Palpitations, dizziness, and syncope are the clinical symptoms that are most effectively evaluated by ambulatory electrocardiography. Unless they occur daily, palpitations and dizziness are more likely to be detected with some type of intermittent recording device because of the longer monitoring time available. Syncope may incapacitate the patient before the recorder can be activated, justifying use of a continuous recording mode in that case. Shortness of breath, chest pain, and fatigue may also be caused by dysrhythmias. However, because these symptoms are more likely to be caused by other factors, use of ambulatory monitoring is of less certain value.

ASSESSMENT OF RR INTERVAL CHARACTERISTICS. Sleep apnea can be difficult to diagnose in the outpatient population. If it is suspected, a 24-hour ECG recording can be done to confirm the diagnosis. Sleep apnea causes a marked increase in vagal tone during the apneic phase, resulting in severe bradycardia. When breathing resumes, the heart rate increases again, creating a cyclic

CLINICAL USES OF AMBULATORY ECG MONITORING

- Evaluation of symptoms possibly related to dysrhythmias
- Assessment of RR interval characteristics
- Assessment of risk of future cardiac events
- Evaluation of efficacy of antidysrhythmic therapy
- Evaluation of pacemaker function
- Detection of myocardial ischemia

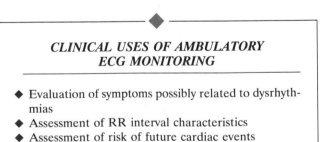

pattern of heart rate (RR interval) variation during sleep that is characteristic of sleep apnea. RR interval variation is also being investigated as a prognostic indicator in coronary artery disease, but more research is needed in this area before conclusions can be drawn.

ASSESSMENT OF RISK OF FUTURE CARDIAC EVENTS. When complex ventricular dysrhythmias occur in the setting of hypertrophic cardiomyopathy, the incidence of sudden death has been shown to increase. Likewise, PVCs and episodes of nonsustained ventricular tachycardia have been shown to be associated with a higher risk of sudden death in patients with left ventricular dysfunction after an acute myocardial infarction. In addition, ambulatory monitoring is a good prognostic indicator of the likelihood of developing symptomatic ischemia or congestive heart failure after myocardial infarction. Ouyang[38] studied a group of patients 4 to 5 days after an acute myocardial infarction and found that those who showed evidence of silent ischemia on the Holter monitor were at high risk to develop clinical angina or pulmonary edema. However, this was not significantly different from the predicted value of a predischarge exercise tolerance test.

Ambulatory electrocardiography is of less value in other patients with heart disease, because although ectopy will probably be found, it has not yet been shown to increase the risk of recurrent myocardial infarction, congestive heart failure, or sudden death. The possible exceptions are patients with variable threshold angina (angina in which the workload or circumstances necessary to provoke an attack change from day to day). When used in combination with exercise tolerance testing (ETT) in these patients, ambulatory monitoring can be of value in detecting ST-segment changes compatible with ischemia during daily activities that may have been missed on the ETT. Ambulatory monitoring has also been found to be a good prognostic indicator in fixed threshold angina, but not superior to ETT. It is the most sensitive in three-vessel disease or left main disease and less so in single or two-vessel disease.[39] In the past, Holter monitoring was used as a screening tool in asymptomatic individuals with known coronary artery disease or mitral valve prolapse or those without heart disease who wished to begin an exercise program or who had high-risk occupations (such as airline pilots), where a sudden dysrhythmia could threaten the lives of others. The ability of a 24-hour Holter recording to predict future dysrhythmic events in these individuals is extremely low, and it is not recommended for this purpose.

EVALUATION OF EFFICACY OF ANTIDYSRHYTHMIC THERAPY. Ambulatory monitoring is useful to assess drug response in patients who have frequent, reproducible, sustained, symptomatic PVCs; supraventricular dysrhythmia; or ventricular tachycardia. Antidysrhythmic drug effect can be clearly documented in these patients. Ambulatory monitoring can also be used in evaluating treatment of other dysrhythmias, such as paroxysmal atrial fibrillation, frequent PVCs, or infrequent short runs of ventricular tachycardia, supraventricular tachycardia, or Wolff-Parkinson-White syndrome. Side effects of medications can also be monitored, such as proarrhythmia or tachycardia, bradycardia, or conduction defects that may be drug-induced. However, even without a change in therapeutic regimen, DiMarco and Philbrick[40] found considerable day-to-day variability in dysrhythmias detected by ambulatory monitoring and warn that caution must be used in interpreting serial tests. Just because the number of ectopics is reduced after initiating therapy does not mean that the drug is effective, nor does an increase in ectopy necessarily indicate a prodysrhythmic effect.

EVALUATION OF PACEMAKER FUNCTION. Ambulatory monitoring is very useful in evaluating pacemaker function and malfunction, because it provides a window into the pacemaker's performance under various conditions of activity, rest, and sleep. Ambulatory monitoring is recommended for detection of myopotential inhibition, detection of pacemaker-mediated tachycardia, evaluation of antitachycardia pacing device function, and evaluation of the adequacy of rate response in a physiologic pacing system. Sometimes pacemakers can be falsely inhibited by *myopotentials,* which are electrical depolarizations of skeletal muscles that are sensed by the pacemaker as if they were cardiac in origin. The pacemaker will not pace while these depolarizations are being detected, and if the patient's underlying heart rate is very slow or absent, dizziness or syncope will result. Generally the skeletal muscles involved are those of the upper torso. Myopotential inhibition will not be detected on a routine ECG or pacemaker check in the clinic, because the skeletal muscles involved are at rest while the recording is taken.

Pacemaker-mediated tachycardia (PMT) is not exactly a pacemaker malfunction, but rather a situation in which a dual-chamber pacemaker is "tricked" into tracking itself at its maximal tracking rate (generally 120 to 130 beats per minute). Depending on the extent of their coronary artery disease, patients may experience palpitations, chest pain, shortness of breath, or fatigue. Even if a patient is able to check his or her pulse and report the rate, it is unclear once the episode is over whether the dysrhythmia was a simple supraventricular tachycardia, ventricular tachycardia, or PMT. An intermittent-recording device would be ideal in this situation, because it could be activated when symptoms occur and document the presence or absence of pacemaker spikes. If PMT is documented, simple reprogramming can solve the problem.

New antitachycardia-pacing devices are being developed that are able to deliver rapid "bursts" of pacing stimuli into either the atria or ventricles to convert an ectopic tachycardia back to normal sinus rhythm. Although the initial settings of these devices are usually based on individualized electrophysiologic studies, fine tuning can be based on ambulatory monitoring to tailor the function of the device to the actual dysrhythmias that occur during the course of the patient's daily activities.

Rate-responsive pacemakers are designed for patients in atrial fibrillation or for patients with sinus node dysfunction in which the heart rate does not increase appropriately when needed, such as during exercise. Rate-responsive pacemakers increase heart rate gradually to meet the perceived demand based on some type of sensing device. Adequacy of this rate response can be evaluated by correlating the heart rate trend on a 24-hour Holter monitor recording with the patient's activity diary.

Ambulatory monitoring may also be useful in routine pacemaker follow-up, which may include evaluating pacing and sensing immediately after implant, evaluating amount of pacemaker use in a 24-hour period, or evaluating rate variations and supraventricular dysrhythmias in patients with automatic implantable cardiac defibrillators. Ambulatory monitoring is not useful in further evaluation of pacemaker failure once it has already been documented by some other means, such as a routine pacemaker check.

DETECTION OF MYOCARDIAL ISCHEMIA. In most patients with known or suspected coronary artery disease, exercise tolerance testing is the preferred method of gauging presence and severity of coronary artery obstruction. However, patients with Prinzmetal's variant angina do not have exercise-induced ischemia. Their angina is caused by coronary artery vasospasm and can occur at any time, even during rest. ST-segment elevation is usually dramatic during the attack and can be quite reliably detected on a Holter monitor recording. Use of ambulatory monitoring for detection of ischemia (silent or symptomatic) based on ST-segment deviations in other patient populations remains controversial, because ST segments can be altered by such nonischemic factors as postural changes,[16] tachycardia, hypertension, adrenalin release, hyperventilation, left ventricular dimension and pressure changes, alterations in intraventricular conduction, and changes in drug levels.[37]

Nursing management. Nurses have a vital role in ensuring that patients receive maximal benefit from wearing a Holter monitor or using an intermittent-recording device. A well-informed patient can greatly enhance the quality of the recording.

Many patients' symptoms do not occur every day and may be missed during a random 24-hour recording. Often symptoms tend to occur in association with specific activities. The nurse should inquire about the types of activities that tend to provoke symptoms for a specific patient and encourage the patient to pursue those activities while wearing the monitor. In general, the patient is encouraged to be as active as possible. Keeping an accurate diary of activities is important, because it allows correlation of an identified dysrhythmia with a specific activity or symptom. Examples of items that the patient should record include medications, meals, exercise, emotional stress, arguments, smoking, bowel movements, urination, sexual intercourse, and sleep periods. In addition, any symptoms such as palpitations, lightheadedness, or chest pressure should be recorded.

The only activities that are restricted while wearing a Holter monitor are those that would get the chest electrodes or monitor wet, eliminating swimming and taking a shower or tub bath. Sponge baths are permitted as long as the chest electrodes are avoided. No activities are restricted when using a transtelephonic monitor, because it is not worn all the time.

◆ Exercise electrocardiography

Definition. Exercise electrocardiography consists of the recording of an ECG tracing during a period of stress on the heart muscle and its blood supply reserves to uncover and diagnose ischemia. Exercise places unique demands on the cardiovascular system. Systemic oxygen consumption increases markedly, requiring the heart to increase cardiac output (CO) to meet these demands. Myocardial contractility increases, resulting in greater stroke volume and systolic blood pressure. Heart rate is increased also as a result of circulating catecholamines. Normally, as heart rate and stroke volume rise, CO is increased dramatically and the tissue needs for oxygen are met. This enhanced myocardial performance is not without its price. Even at rest, the heart muscle extracts 70% of the oxygen available in the circulating blood. When the myocardial demand for oxygen increases during exercise, coronary blood flow must increase to maintain an adequate oxygen supply. In patients with coronary artery disease, coronary blood flow is not able to increase sufficiently to meet the high metabolic needs of the myocardium during exercise and ischemia results.

Indications. Exercise tolerance testing, or stress testing, is clinically useful in several settings. It helps evaluate the presence, absence, or severity of coronary artery disease, both in patients with known coronary heart disease and those initially seen with chest pain of unclear origin. Stress testing can evaluate the functional capacity of patients with or without heart disease and can be done serially to evaluate the effectiveness of medical or surgical therapy. Bogaty et al.[41] found that the workload achieved during stress testing correlated well with subsequent mortality but was not a good predictor of future myocardial infarctions. In patients who were able to complete only stage 1 of a Bruce protocol (5.1 METS), the 8-year survival rate was only 45%, whereas the 8-year survival rate was 93% among those patients able to complete stage 5 (10 METS).

Procedure. Originally exercise tests were conducted using a two-step platform that the patient climbed up and down repeatedly. This is called a *Master's two-step exercise test* and is still used in a few places because the cost of the equipment is minimal. The majority of exercise tests in the United States, however, are now performed using a treadmill on which both speed and slope can be varied, or a bicycle ergometer. A number of protocols have been developed using a treadmill. All reach virtually the same end point, but they vary the speed with which they approach that end point. Two popular ones are the Bruce protocol, in which both grade and speed are varied every 3 minutes, and the Balke protocol, in which speed remains constant and grade is gradually increased every minute.

Regardless of the protocol used, the ECG is printed at 1-minute intervals, as well as during any symptoms, visible ECG changes, or dysrhythmias. Blood pressure is also measured and recorded every minute.

The treadmill test is terminated when a desirable level, based on the patient's heart rate, is reached. A maximal stress test is one in which the predicted maximal heart rate for that patient is achieved. The maximal predicted heart rate can be estimated using the formula of 220 minus the patient's age. A goal of 85% to 90% of the predicted maximal heart rate is set for a submaximal test, and in most patients this level of exercise is sufficient to unmask any significant coronary artery disease. The test can also be aborted before that point for a number of reasons, which are listed in Table 15-15.[42] Blood pressure is expected to rise during exercise, but a systolic blood pressure greater than 220 mm Hg or a diastolic blood pressure greater than 110 mm Hg is considered high enough to stop the test.

A low-level stress test is sometimes performed before discharge from the hospital on patients who have had an acute myocardial infarction. In this case the heart rate is raised only to 120 or 130 beats per minute. Current results indicate that ST-segment depression or elevation that occurs during the predischarge low-level stress test is a reliable indicator of additional myocardium at risk. However, exercise-induced angina or abnormal blood pressure responses to exercise often do not appear during a low-level stress test, so a "normal" predischarge stress test must be followed later by a test closer to maximal level.[43]

PATIENT PREPARATION. The exercise test can be performed on an outpatient or inpatient basis. In either case, a physician must be present to supervise the test directly. As with any diagnostic procedure with inherent risks, the patient must be fully informed and consent obtained. It is ideal to conduct the exercise test in the morning after an overnight fast, because, after eating, blood is diverted from the general circulation to the gastrointestinal tract, especially the stomach, to facilitate absorption of nutrients during the digestive process, making less blood available to the coronary and systemic circulation. Logistically, however, exercise tests must be performed throughout the day. Patients are advised to eat a light meal no closer than 3 hours before the test is scheduled. They should dress comfortably in light clothing and wear comfortable shoes for brisk walking or running.

Table 15-15 Reasons for stopping the exercise ECG

Absolute	Relative
Acute MI	Marked ST or QRS changes
Severe angina	Increasing chest pain
Hypotension*	Fatigue and shortness of breath
Second- or third-degree AV block	Wheezing
Ventricular tachycardia	Leg cramps, claudication
Poor perfusion (pallor; cyanosis; cold, clammy skin)	Hypertension*
CNS symptoms (ataxia, vertigo, visual or gait disturbances, confusion)	Supraventricular tachycardia
Technical problems	
Patient's request	

*See text on this page for further description.

A brief history and physical examination of the patient should be obtained before beginning the exercise test to identify any contraindications to performing the test and to document medications the patient is taking that might interfere with test results. A 12-lead ECG is recorded at rest before beginning the exercise protocol, and another 12-lead ECG is usually recorded on completion of the test.

Various lead positions are used during the testing, depending on the number of leads that the equipment is able to monitor. Additional leads improve the accuracy of the test, because ischemia may be missed if a lead is not monitoring the particular portion of the myocardial wall that becomes ischemic. Some institutions use a six- or ten-lead system, but most use three leads, usually II, V_3, and V_5. Lead II will detect ischemic changes in the inferior wall, lead V_3 will show ischemia in the anterior wall, and lead V_5 will reveal ischemia in the lateral wall. Skin preparation for electrode placement is important, because the recording will be meaningless if an electrode falls off during exercise. Also, a blood pressure cuff is placed on one arm to measure the blood pressure response to exercise.

INTERPRETATION OF RESULTS. Considerable controversy exists about interpretation criteria for exercise ECG. ST-segment depression, either horizontal or downsloping, of 1 mm or more during or after exercise is the most diagnostic of coronary artery disease. Other criteria that are strongly suggestive of a positive result are found in Table 15-16.

ST-segment elevation, although a rare finding, is usually indicative of myocardial wall motion abnormalities such as an aneurysm, especially in patients who have had a previous myocardial infarction, and may actually be a more serious finding than ST depression.[44]

The point at which the end of the QRS complex intersects with the baseline is known as the *J-point* (Fig. 15-54, *A*). A certain amount of J-point depression (Fig. 15-54, *B*) is normal during exercise and is considered indicative of ischemia only if it is upsloping, greater than 2 mm below baseline, and greater than 0.08 second in duration.

Ventricular dysrhythmias are common in healthy individuals, especially at high levels of exercise. If they occur frequently at low levels or are multifocal or grouped, underlying heart disease is usually present.

Hypotension during exercise is defined as a drop in blood pressure of more than 10 mm Hg. Care must be taken to differentiate clinically significant hypotension from the physiologically normal drop in blood pressure that occurs during the first stage of exercise in an anxious patient. Pretest anxiety results in the release of excess catecholamines, which cause the blood pressure to rise before the test is begun. As exercise begins and the large blood vessels in the leg muscles dilate to increase blood flow, this elevated blood pressure will fall to normal. As exercise continues, however, an appropriate rise in systolic pressure should be expected. If the blood pressure falls as exercise increases—especially if accompanied by angina, ST-segment changes, or a drop in heart rate—the patient usually has severe three-vessel disease, global ischemia, and myocardial dysfunction.

Table 15-16 Criteria for positive exercise ECG test

Definitely positive	Strongly suggestive
Horizontal ST-segment depression of 1 mm or more during or after exercise	Horizontal or downsloping ST-segment depression of <1 mm during or after exercise
Downsloping ST-segment depression of 1 mm or more during or after exercise	Upsloping ST-segment depression of 2 mm or more beyond 0.08 sec from J-point during or after exercise
	Horizontal or upsloping ST-segment elevation of 1 mm or more during or after exercise
	ST-segment sagging 1 mm or more during or after exercise
	Hypotension
	Inverted U wave
	Frequent premature ventricular contractions (PVCs), multifocal PVCs, grouped PVCs, ventricular tachycardia provoked by mild exercise (70% or less of maximal heart rate)
	Exercise-induced typical angina, S_3, S_4, or heart murmur

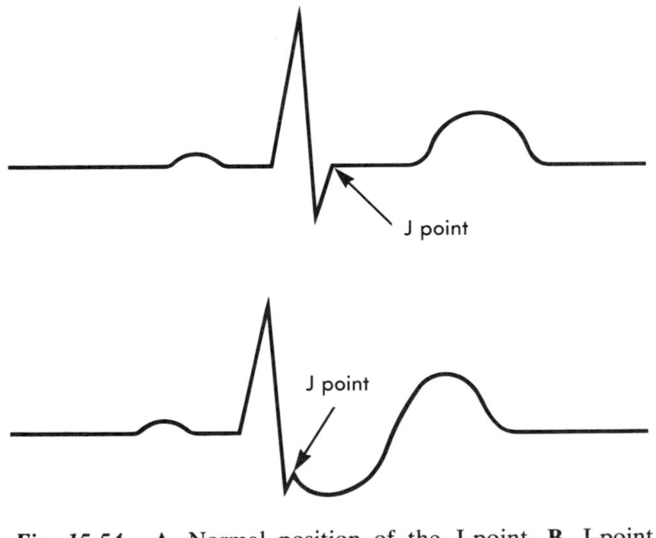

Fig. 15-54 **A,** Normal position of the J-point. **B,** J-point depression.

Many dysrhythmias and ECG changes during exercise are insignificant (see box, upper right). Hyperventilation can also cause ST-segment depression as a result of changes in vasomotor tone, and when this occurs, it is actually evidence against coronary artery disease. To rule out hyperventilation as a potential cause of ST-segment depression, the ECG tracing should be recorded during a brief period of hyperventilation before the test is begun.

INSIGNIFICANT EXERCISE ECG CHANGES

- Occasional unifocal premature ventricular contractions (PVCs)
- Atrial or junctional tachycardias
- First-degree or Wenckebach AV block
- Bundle branch block or hemiblock
- Alteration of T-wave shape
- Alteration of P-wave shape
- J-point ST depression less than 2 mm
- QT-interval change
- Prominent U waves

Drugs can sometimes influence the results of an exercise ECG test.[45] Digitalis causes ST-segment depression at rest, which is accentuated with exercise. In general, ST-segment depression of 4 to 5 mm almost always indicates ischemia. For those patients who experience mild ST-segment depression during exercise and who are also on digitalis, exercise test results will be inconclusive. In general, sensitivity of the test is decreased, but specificity remains unchanged. Beta blockers have the opposite effect. Because beta blockers decrease heart rate, blood pressure, and vascular response to circulating catecholamines, these drugs also blunt the normal response to exercise. Consequently, patients on beta blockers can usually exercise longer and have less ST-segment depression. However, if the test is continued until an adequate heart rate and blood pressure response are obtained, beta blockers do not significantly affect the accuracy of the test. Long-acting nitrates and calcium channel blockers do not adversely affect the test.

Unfortunately, both false-positive and false-negative exercise ECG interpretations occur. The incidence of false-positive results is high in asymptomatic, healthy individuals. The incidence of false-positive results is especially high in asymptomatic middle-aged women. As discussed, hyperventilation can cause false ST-segment depression, as can mitral valve prolapse syndrome, Wolff-Parkinson-White syndrome, and digitalis therapy.

False-negative results may be caused by early termination of the test for other reasons, such as fatigue or claudication before the level of imbalance between oxygen supply and myocardial oxygen demand is reached. Overly strict diagnostic criteria can cause real disease to be missed. The lead system used can result in certain areas of the myocardium not being represented, and ischemia in those areas will be missed. Antianginal drug therapy can also mask ischemia. False-negative results become less likely as the extent of disease increases (Table 15-17).

RECENT ADVANCES IN TEST INTERPRETATION. Recently work has been done using the ST-segment/heart rate slope to improve accuracy of the exercise tolerance test.[46] This technique normalizes the amount of ST-segment depression during exercise for changes in heart rate. The specificity reported with this technique is greater than 90%, with a sensitivity of 80%. This method also claims the ability to separate patients into categories of one-vessel, two-vessel, and three-vessel coronary artery disease. Because this is a relatively new approach to exercise ECG interpretation, more research is needed to determine in which patient populations this method is reliable and in which groups it is not. If a false-positive or false-negative result is suspected, exercise testing can be combined with thallium imaging for more definitive results.

COMPLICATIONS AND CONTRAINDICATIONS. Complications are rare during exercise testing, but they do occur. The mortality is 0.01% (1:10,000). Morbidity is 0.05% (5:10,000) and includes such adverse outcomes as myocardial infarction, cardiac arrest, and sustained ventricular tachycardia.[42] Cardiopulmonary resuscitation equipment must be readily available whenever exercise testing is done.

Contraindications to exercise testing can be divided into cardiac and noncardiac problems. Cardiac contraindications include acute myocardial infarction, acute heart failure, cardiogenic shock, unstable angina (as opposed to stable angina), severe aortic stenosis, and digitalis toxicity with its inherent increased risk of life-threatening dysrhythmias. Noncardiac contraindications include fever; acute illness such as hepatitis, renal failure, or pneumonia; pulmonary emboli; or severe physical disability.

Nursing management. Many patients are anxious about undergoing exercise testing, and the anxiety is often multifactorial. Patients without known heart disease may be afraid that they will "fail" the test, find they have heart disease, and perhaps need open heart surgery. If the patient generally follows a sedentary life-style, anxiety may be caused by the fear of "collapsing" on the treadmill or spending several days recovering from exhaustion. Some are afraid that they will be forced to go beyond their endurance. Often, low-level exercise testing is performed before discharge on patients who have been hospitalized for an acute myocardial infarction. These patients may be afraid that the strain on their heart is too great or that they will die during the test.

Proper patient teaching can do much to allay these fears. In addition to describing the procedure itself, the nurse should instruct the patient to fast for 3 hours before the test, refrain from smoking for at least 2 hours before the test, and wear comfortable shoes and loose-fitting clothes. The patient should be reassured that his or her heart will be monitored closely during the test and a physician will be standing by. Although the patient will be encouraged to continue as long as possible, the test will be stopped at the patient's request for symptoms such as fatigue, shortness of breath, or leg cramps. In addition, the staff will stop the test for significant ECG changes, blood pressure changes, or development of angina. The patient should also be told that the diagnostic value of the test is based on the maximal heart rate achieved, not on the length of time that he or she is able to remain on the treadmill. A well-trained athlete might be able to stay on the treadmill for 15 minutes, whereas an elderly or sedentary person may tolerate it for only 3 to 5 minutes; yet if 85% of the predicted maximal heart rate is achieved, both tests will have been equally diagnostic.

After the exercise test is completed, the patient will be assisted into a supine position. The ECG, pulse rate, and blood pressure will be monitored for at least 10 more minutes to detect dysrhythmias or signs of ischemia. The patient should be instructed to rest for the next 30 to 60 minutes after release from the exercise laboratory. Hot showers should be avoided for 3 to 4 hours to prevent development of orthostatic hypotension.

The nurse performing the test must be certain that emergency medications and a defibrillator are available in the test area and should be familiar with their use.

Table 15-17 Correlation of positive exercise ECG tests with location of coronary artery disease

Location of obstruction (>75% stenosis)	Incidence of positive exercise tolerance testing (%)
Single-vessel disease	
Right coronary artery	44
Left circumflex artery	44
Left anterior descending artery	77
Two-vessel disease	91
Three-vessel disease	100

From Chung K: *Manual of exercise ECG testing*, Stoneham, Mass, 1986, Butterworth Publishers.

◆ **Signal-averaged ECG.** The signal-averaged ECG is used to identify individuals at risk for sudden cardiac death from ventricular dysrhythmias. It is different from the 12-lead ECG, Holter monitoring, or a stress test and is used in the subset of patients predisposed to lethal ventricular dysrhythmias. This is a noninvasive test. The patient lies in a supine position and is asked to keep muscle movement to a minimum. Electrode leads are applied to the anterior and posterior chest wall, and the leads are connected to a signal-averaged ECG computer. This computer produces a high-resolution, high-magnification ECG signal. This "noise-free" ECG is then analyzed for both QRS duration and for the presence, duration, and measurement of late myopotentials.[47] After computer analysis, the signal-averaged ECG is described as either negative (normal) or positive (abnormal). A positive signal-averaged ECG is a predictor of increased risk for sudden cardiac death.

Myocardium that is damaged, either by myocardial infarction or by cardiomyopathy, produces late-activating myopotentials that may cause reentry ventricular dysrhythmias. The 12-lead ECG is not sufficiently sensitive to detect these low-amplitude, late potentials—hence the need for a high-resolution signal.

Many patients with a positive signal-averaged ECG (abnormal) will display a normal signal-averaged ECG when placed on antidysrhythmic medications. The signal-averaged ECG is not analyzed in isolation. It is used in conjunction with other cardiac diagnostic tests, including the electrophysiology study. It is a helpful adjunct to the electrophysiology study but does not replace it.[48]

◆ **Electrophysiology study.** The electrophysiology study (EPS) is an invasive diagnostic tool used to record intracardiac electrical activity. A person may have an EPS performed if he or she has a history of a syncopal episode (loss of consciousness), rapid wide complex tachycardia, or other cardiac electrical problems not diagnosed by the noninvasive diagnostic studies, such as the 12-lead ECG, treadmill stress test, signal-averaged ECG, or Holter monitoring.

Before the electrophysiology study, written and verbal education is given to the patient and family to increase their sense of security and to decrease stress and anxiety.[48] All antidysrhythmic medications are discontinued several days before the study so that any ventricular dysrhythmias may be readily induced during the EPS. Premedication is administered before the study to induce a relaxed state, and during the procedure the patient is conscious but receives sedation at regular intervals. The patient is fasting 6 hours before the EPS and remains supine throughout the procedure. A peripheral IV, radial arterial line, and surface ECG leads are placed. Then, electrophysiology catheters are inserted into the femoral vein and advanced to the right side of the heart under fluoroscopy. These catheters, similar to pacing catheters, are placed at specific anatomic sites within the heart to record the earliest electrical activity. These sites include the sinoatrial (SA) node, the atrioventricular (AV) node, the coronary sinus, the bundle of His, the bundle branches, and other selected areas of myocardium. Once the catheters are in position, a pacing technique known as *programmed electrical stimulation* is used to trigger the dysrhythmia. This technique delivers pulses of two to four early ventricular pacing beats, via the catheter, to the selected area of myocardium. Once the dysrhythmia is induced, it can convert to normal sinus rhythm spontaneously or be converted by rapid atrial pacing, cardioversion/defibrillation, or IV antidysrhythmic medications. During the EPS the electrophysiologist is looking for a site of early electrical activation that stimulates the myocardium before the SA node. At the end of the study all of the electrophysiology catheters are removed before the patient returns to the nursing unit.

After the EPS diagnosis, medical management is prescribed. Many of the possible interventions necessitate a return to the electrophysiology (EP) laboratory to monitor the effectiveness of the treatment. For example, if the diagnosis is Wolff-Parkinson-White (WPW) syndrome, the solution may be a catheter ablation of the accessory tract, with a follow-up EPS. If the diagnosis is reentry ventricular tachycardia, the treatment may be antidysrhythmic drugs or an implantable cardioverter defibrillator (ICD). In most cases, follow-up studies are performed as just described. However, with the latest generation of ICD generators, known as *tiered* therapy devices because of their three therapeutic components (pace termination, back-up bradycardia pacing, and cardioversion/defibrillation), it is not necessary for the patient to have EP catheters placed in the femoral vein. The EPS can be performed via the external ICD programmer in the EP laboratory. The ICD generator and leads can perform programmed electrical stimulation in a similar manner to a full EPS.

In summary, the electrophysiology study can provide valuable information about intracardiac electrical abnormalities and reveal specialized diagnostic clues that can be used to guide medical and nursing management of the patient with significant cardiac dysrhythmias.

◆ **Head-up tilt-table test.** A patient who is being evaluated for unexplained loss of consciousness (syncope) may undergo a head-up tilt-table test (HUTT) in addition to EPS and neurologic examination. If the neurologic examination is normal and the EPS is negative for dysrhythmias, the cause of loss of consiousness may be vasodepressor syncope (VDS), which is evaluated by a HUTT. VDS describes transient syncope caused by hypotension secondary to parasympathetic vasodilation and venous pooling.

The HUTT is usually conducted in the radiology department. The patient lies supine on a table and is connected to an ECG monitor. A noninvasive blood pressure cuff is applied, and an IV line is established. The table head is elevated to between 40 and 80 degrees following a standard protocol. Blood pressure and heart rate measurements are determined frequently. A positive VDS response occurs if the patient loses consciousness as the head of the table is raised. However, not all susceptible individuals experience syncope under resting conditions. In this situation, drugs such as isoproterenol (Isuprel) 1 to 8 mcg/min may be infused to increase heart rate and circulating catecholamines. If the patient has a HUTT-induced syncopal episode, secondary ventricular dysrhythmias may occur also. Therefore antidysrhythmic medications and a defibrillator must always be nearby.

Treatment of VDS varies according to the cause. If increased circulating catecholamine levels are the problem, beta blockers are used to decrease catecholamine effect. If increased vagal tone is the cause, atropine-like drugs that block the parasympathetic nervous system may be prescribed. Following treatment with appropriate medications, the HUTT is repeated. For the patient who has experienced syncope of unknown cause, the HUTT is a highly effective test if the EPS and neurologic examination are negative.

Cardiac Catheterization and Coronary Arteriography

◆ **Indications.** Cardiac catheterization and coronary arteriography are routine diagnostic procedures for patients with known or suspected heart disease. Clinical indications for cardiac catheterization include myocardial ischemia, unstable angina, evolving myocardial infarction, heart failure with a history that suggests coronary artery disease or valvular disease, and congenital heart disease. Cardiac catheterization is used both to confirm physical findings and to provide a baseline for medical or surgical therapy. During catheterization of the left side of the heart, hemodynamic pressure measurements are taken in the aortic root, the left ventricle, and the left atrium. Radiopaque contrast (dye) is used to visualize the left side of the heart (angiogram) and the coronary arteries (arteriogram). Catheterization of the right side of the heart is performed using a thermodilution pulmonary artery catheter.

Information obtained includes hemodynamic pressure measurements in the right atrium, right ventricle, pulmonary artery, and pulmonary capillary wedge position, as well as the measurement of cardiac output, calculated hemodynamic values, oxygen saturations, and an angiogram of the right-heart chambers using radiopaque contrast.

◆ **Procedure.** Before the catheterization the patient will meet with the cardiologist to discuss the purpose, benefit, and risks of the study. For many patients, cardiac catheterization is the first major procedure after a diagnosis of possible cardiac disease. The patient is often very anxious and has many questions. It is important that both nursing and medical staff fully answer patients' questions about the catheterization experience.

The morning of the procedure the patient fasts except for ingesting prescribed cardiac medications. Light premedication is given before the patient goes to the catheterization laboratory. If there is a history of allergy, an antihistamine or corticosteroid may be administered to prevent an anaphylactic reaction to the radiopaque contrast. Throughout the cardiac catheterization the patient remains awake and alert. He or she is positioned on a hard table with a C- or U-shaped camera arm overhead or to the side. This arm can be moved to view the heart from several different angles. Cardiac-catheterization catheters, available in a variety of designs and sizes, are placed in the groin area after the patient receives a local anesthetic. The choice of catheters is based on the cardiologist's experience and the diagnostic study required. The femoral artery is used to catheterize the left side of the heart, including the coronary arteries. The femoral vein is used to pass catheters to the right side of the heart. During the study the patient receives heparin systemically to reduce the risk of emboli. Many patients also receive nitroglycerin to control chest pain, particularly when the coronary arteries are full of contrast material during the coronary arteriographic procedure. At this time the patient may also experience bradycardia or hypotension. To move the contrast dye more quickly and minimize the vagal effect on heart rate and blood pressure, the patient may be asked to cough. If the bradycardia persists, atropine or—occasionally—a transvenous pacemaker may be used. If hypotension continues, IV fluids are administered as a bolus.

At the end of the study the heparin effect is reversed with protamine. The catheters are then removed, and pressure is applied to the groin area until bleeding has stopped. After catheterization the patient remains flat for 6 hours. Nursing care involves care of the groin site, which is checked frequently for evidence of bleeding or hematoma. Pedal and posterior tibial pulses are assessed every 15 minutes for the first hour after the catheterization and every 30 minutes to 1 hour thereafter. The patient is encouraged to drink large amounts of clear liquids, and the IV fluid rate is increased to 100 ml/hour. The additional fluid is given for rehydration because the radiopaque contrast acts as an osmotic diuretic. Patients who have elevated blood urea nitrogen (BUN) or creatinine levels before catheterization are at risk for renal failure from the dye. For these patients the quantity of contrast material is consciously limited to preserve kidney function. After the catheterization the cardiologist will meet with the patient and family to discuss the findings and plan of care.

Radionuclide Study: Thallium Scan

◆ **Indications.** The purpose of a thallium scan is to determine whether there is a perfusion defect in cardiac muscle. The study was developed as an adjunct to the exercise ECG stress test. A thallium scan is indicated for the patient with chest pain and known or suspected coronary artery disease and for the patient with a left bundle branch block (LBBB) or a permanent pacemaker in whom an ECG stress test may be difficult to interpret because of distortion of the QRS complex.

A thallium scan combines the techniques of both cardiology and radiology. In cardiology, coronary artery anatomy is important because regional myocardial blood supply is from specific coronary arteries and any blockage of an artery can lead to a discrete myocardial perfusion defect, meaning that the blood supply to this area is either decreased or absent. Although coronary arteriography will define the anatomy of the coronary arteries, it does not show whether the arteries perfuse the cardiac muscle. The radiology component involves the use of thallium 201 and a specialized perfusion-scanning camera. Thallium 201 is a low-energy radioactive isotope. It is an analog of potassium and acts like potassium when injected into the bloodstream. Because thallium is similar to potassium, it is absorbed from the bloodstream by cardiac muscle cells as part of the sodium-potassium adenosine triphosphatase (ATPase) pump. Thallium uptake depends on two factors: (1) the patency of the coronary arteries and (2) the amount of healthy myocardium with a functional sodium-potassium ATPase pump. If an area of myocardium is infarcted (dead), it will not take up thallium. Once thallium has been injected, a specialized scintillation camera and computer system can detect the areas of thallium concentration (uptake).

◆ **Procedure.** Before the thallium scan the patient should have the procedure fully explained, including a description of the equipment, since it may be overwhelming to some patients. The patient is usually fasting, because a thallium scan involves vigorous exercise. He or she should have a patent IV line inserted before the test. The thallium test takes place in a specialized laboratory that contains ECG monitoring equipment, cardiovascular exercise equipment (treadmill or stationary bicycle), and an Anger gamma scintillation camera. Once in the laboratory the patient is asked to exercise vigorously for up to 1 minute or longer or until angina or fatigue develops. At this point the thallium is injected into the bloodstream. After the injection the patient is asked to exercise vigorously for another minute to stress the heart and circulate the thallium. As soon as possible after exercise (within 10 minutes), the patient is asked to lie on the examination table for the first perfusion scan by the scintillation camera. The camera examines the heart from three angles: anterior, left anterior oblique, and left lateral oblique, to increase accuracy. On the camera screen the heart image looks like a circle with a hole. The myocardium appears, but the fluid-filled center does not. If no perfusion defect is seen, the test is complete for that patient. If a perfusion defect is noted, the patient is asked to return for a repeat scan in 4 hours. A perfusion defect present 4 hours later means the area is infarcted. If the perfusion defect has taken up thallium since the first test (redistribution), the area is ischemic.

Occasionally, a patient who cannot tolerate a thallium/ECG stress test will have a pharmacologic thallium test. In this case the patient is given dipyridamole (Persantine) to increase coronary artery blood flow, and the thallium test is then performed.

Phonocardiography

◆ **Definition.** Phonocardiography is the graphic display on paper of the sounds that occur in the heart and great vessels. The sounds are recorded from a transducer placed on the surface of the chest wall. The recording corresponds to the sounds heard during cardiac auscultation with a stethoscope.

◆ **Indications.** With practice, normal heart sounds can be heard quite clearly with a stethoscope, but low-frequency sounds, such as a S_4 or a soft murmur, can be more difficult to identify, especially if the patient has a tachycardia. Abnormal sounds may be too rapid or subtle for discernment by the senses. A graphic sound recording, or phonocardiogram, permits accurate timing of sounds and events and can reveal information about underlying hemodynamic events that is not obtainable through the physical examination alone. For example, the width of an S_2 split can be used as an index of severity in pulmonic stenosis.[49] The phonocardiogram can point out abnormalities of valve function or wall structure (such as idiopathic hypertrophic subaortic stenosis) and can actually improve results from subsequent cardiac catheterization by targeting specific areas for closer study.

Another advantage of a phonocardiogram over simple auscultation is that it provides a permanent, objective record of events. Subsequent comparisons can be made to evaluate progression of valvular dysfunction or to measure the degree of improvement after therapeutic interventions.

Phonocardiography can be combined with echocardiography to yield more information than either technique alone. The echocardiogram provides a time-frame reference for the phonocardiogram, allowing identification of sound components by their relationship to certain defined valvular motions (Fig. 15-55). At the same time, the phonocardiogram provides reference points for the echocardiogram, which improves the timing of certain phases of the cardiac cycle. The second heart sound, which represents the end of systole, is used most often in this regard. In aortic stenosis, the marked leaflet distortion prevents accurate estimates of the severity of obstruction by echocardiography alone. The phonocardiogram can provide an independent assessment of severity and can also follow the serial progression of the stenosis to help determine proper timing of intervention.

Several studies have been done using the phonocardiogram to correlate electrical and mechanical events in the heart. Inferences are then made regarding left ventricular filling pressures and hemodynamics. The C-point represents mitral valve closure on the echocardiogram and corresponds to the onset of systole (Fig. 15-56). The aortic component of the second sound on the phonocardiogram represents the end of systole. The distance between these two points indicates the duration of systole and can be used to estimate left atrial pressures noninvasively. This technique can be used clinically to determine which patient needs invasive pulmonary artery pressure monitoring. It can also replace pulmonary artery pressure monitoring in these patients for whom a high degree of accuracy is not critical.

By far the greatest value of phonocardiography at present is as a tool for teaching auscultation. After studying a phonocardiographic recording of a patient's heart sounds, students can return to the bedside and visualize each sound in their mind's eye. With practice, the ability to separate distinct sounds and quantify murmurs improves. Eventually, expert bedside auscultation replaces the need for the phonocardiogram except in rare instances.

◆ **Nursing management.** Patient teaching is important in relieving anxiety and eliciting cooperation. A quiet environment is desirable for proper recording of a phonocardiogram, because the equipment is very sensi-

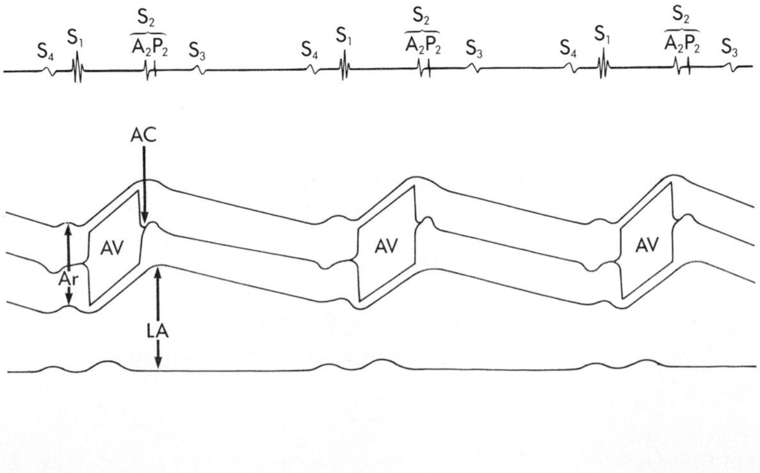

Fig. 15-55 Schematic drawing of a phonocardiogram and an echocardiogram at the aortic valve performed simultaneously; the sounds can be correlated with the actual valve motion. *Ar,* aortic root; *AV,* aortic valve in open position; *LA,* left atrium; *AC,* aortic valve in closed position.

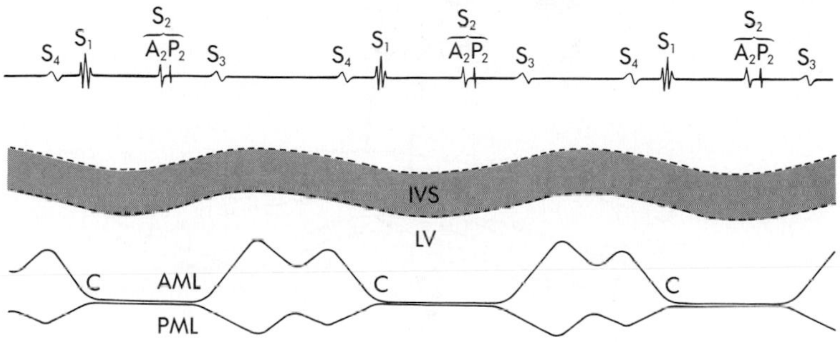

Fig. 15-56 Schematic drawing of a phonocardiogram and an echocardiogram at the mitral valve performed simultaneously. The C-point on the ECG occurs with the closing of the mitral valve and represents the onset of systole. The aortic component of the second heart sound (A_2) occurs with the closing of the aortic valve and represents the end of systole. *AML,* anterior mitral leaflet; *PML,* posterior mitral leaflet; *C,* closure of the mitral valve; *LV,* left ventricle; *IVS,* interventricular septum.

tive to sound waves. Several small microphones are placed on the patient's chest. In males, small areas of the chest may need to be shaved to improve skin contact with the microphones. The procedure is not uncomfortable and is usually completed in less than 20 minutes. When combined with echocardiography, which is often the case, the entire procedure may take as long as 45 minutes to 1 hour.

Echocardiography

◆ **Definition.** Echocardiography uses waves of ultrasound to obtain and display images of cardiac structures. Normal human hearing occurs at a sound frequency of 20 to 20,000 cycles per second (hertz). Ultrasound uses sound frequencies greater than 20,000 hertz (Hz). When used to image cardiac structures, the best results are achieved using 1.5 to 10 million hertz (mHz).[50] Usually 2.25 mHz are used with adults to allow optimal depth penetration, whereas 3 to 5 mHz are used in pediatrics to provide a clearer image of the smaller structures.

◆ **Indications.** Echocardiography is used to detect cardiac abnormalities such as mitral valve stenosis and regurgitation, prolapse of mitral valve leaflets, aortic stenosis and insufficiency, idiopathic hypertrophic subaortic stenosis, atrial septal defects, and pericardial effusions. Recent developments also allow detection of wall-motion abnormalities, estimation of ejection fraction and pulmonary artery pressures, and identification of intracardiac myomas. In the future, echocardiography may be able to detect and quantify coronary artery disease.

◆ **Procedure.** While the test is performed, the patient is in either a supine, left lateral, or semi-Fowler's position. Which position is used depends on the patient's clinical condition and on which position provides the best view of the structures examined. A transducer is placed on the skin, with lubricant between the transducer and the skin to improve contact and reduce artifact. The active element in the transducer is a piezoelectric crystal. *Piezoelectric* refers to the ability to transform electrical energy into mechanical (in this case, sound) energy, and vice versa. The transducer emits ultrasound waves and receives a signal from the reflected sound waves. Periods of sound transmission alternate with periods of sound reception.

Ultrasonic waves do not travel through air very well, and they are unable to penetrate very dense structures, such as bone; hence, in adults, the transducer is usually placed in the third or fourth intercostal space to the left of the sternum, because at that point the pericardium is in direct contact with the chest wall and the ultrasonic waves are not obstructed by either air or bone. Other positions are sometimes used if the standard location does not provide adequate visualization of the cardiac structures.

Ultrasound is reflected best at interfaces between tissues that have different densities. In the heart these are the blood, cardiac valves, myocardium, and pericardium. Because all these structures differ in density, their borders can be seen on the echocardiogram. In one type of echocardiography, a thin beam of ultrasound is directed through the heart (Fig. 15-57). Each interface is represented by a dot, and when recorded over time (like an ECG), each dot becomes a line on an oscilloscope. A strip-chart recording can be made of this tracing as the heart beats. Because this is a recording of heart motion over time, this technique is called an *M-mode* (motion-mode) echocardiogram. A typical M-mode echo is shown in Fig. 15-57.

M-mode echocardiogram. The M-mode echocardiogram is particularly useful for measuring cardiac wall thickness and chamber size, evaluating valve motion, and assessing contractile motion of certain portions of the heart wall. It provides a good view of the anterior interventricular septum, the left ventricular posterior wall from the base to the midportion, the aortic and mitral valves, and the left atrium. Areas that cannot be studied include the apex, lateral or free wall segments, and the true posterior and inferior wall of the left ventricle. Because all portions of the ventricular wall cannot be examined, it is difficult to determine the size of dyskinetic areas using this technique. Aneurysms are also hard to diagnose, depending on their location. If the heart muscle is contracting uniformly throughout, estimates of left ventricular function are quite accurate. However, if wall-motion abnormalities exist, this estimate of cardiac contractility will be unreliable. Estimates of left ventricular size and function are also unreliable if significant aortic regurgitation is present. M-mode echocardiograms are particularly useful in detecting small pericardial effusions and cardiac tamponade.[50]

Two-dimensional echocardiogram. Other techniques have been developed over the past several years to improve the accuracy of echocardiograms. One popular technique is the two-dimensional (2-D) echocardiogram. It uses numerous crystals in the transducer to create a

A

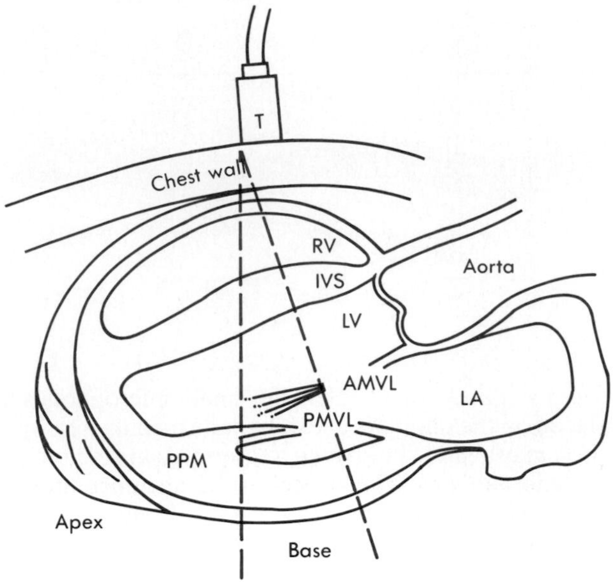

B

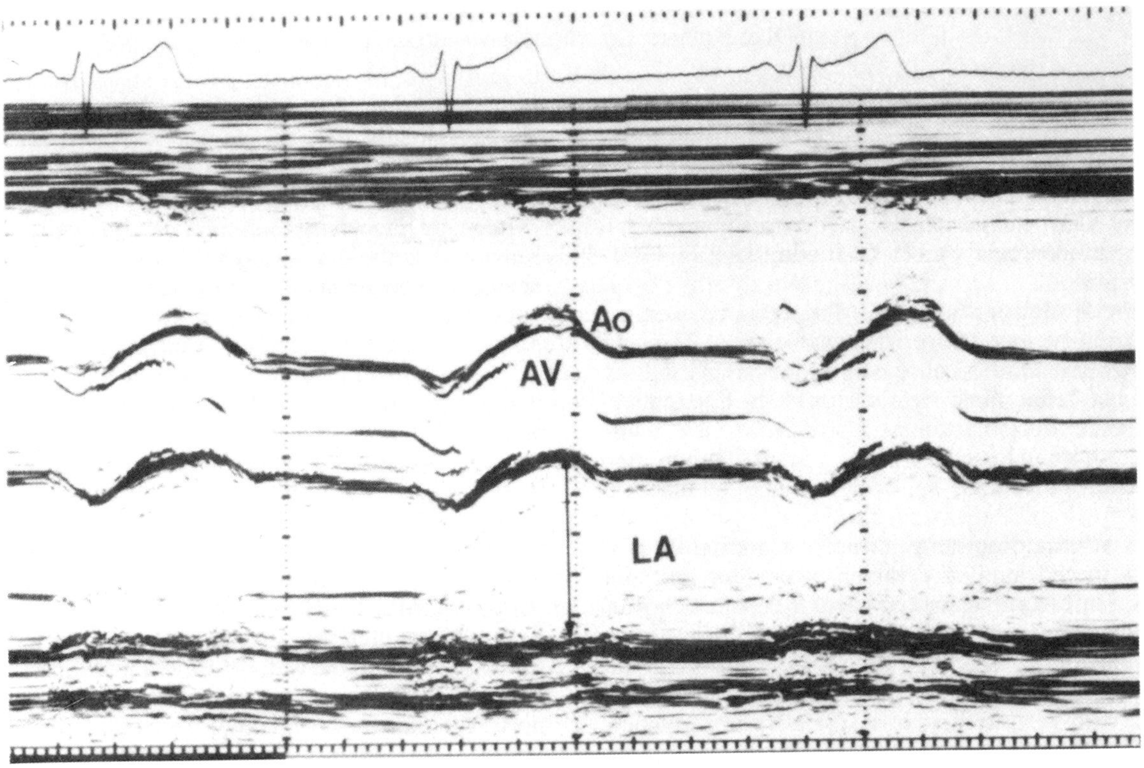

Fig. 15-57 **A,** Schematic presentation of cardiac structures transversed by two echobeams. **B,** Normal, M-mode echocardiogram at the level of the aorta, aortic valve leaflets, and left atrium. *RV,* right ventricle; *LV,* left ventricle; *IVS,* interventricular septum; *AMLV,* anterior mitral valve leaflet; *PMVL,* posterior mitral valve leaflet; *PPM,* posterior papillary muscle; *LA,* left atrium; *T,* transducer; *Ao,* aorta; *AV,* aortic valve. (**A** from Urden L, Davie J, Thelan, L: *Essentials of critical care nursing,* St. Louis, 1992, Mosby–Year Book; **B** from Kinney M and others: *Comprehensive cardiac care,* ed 7, St Louis, 1991, Mosby–Year Book.)

cross-sectional imaging plane. Sections of the heart are then viewed from a number of different angles (Fig. 15-58). The picture is displayed on an oscilloscope, and photographs are taken to serve as a permanent record. Because no timing markers are built into this technique, it is less accurate in measuring stroke volume when the rhythm is irregular and in detecting constrictive pericarditis and tamponade.[50] In many other ways it is superior to the M-mode echocardiogram. The 2-D echocardiogram provides better quantification of valvular stenosis and a greater ability to detect ventricular aneurysms. Because a whole "slice" of the heart is seen at once, the location of various structures in relationship to the rest of the heart is better appreciated, and the size of dyskinetic wall segments can be determined.

Several studies have shown that wall-motion abnormalities can be detected in nearly all patients within 4 hours after an acute myocardial infarction and the extent of muscle dysfunction is highly predictive of later complications. When wall-motion abnormalities exceed 20% of the size of the left ventricle, there is a substantial rise in in-hospital complications.[51] Based on this infor-

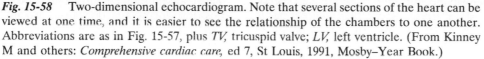

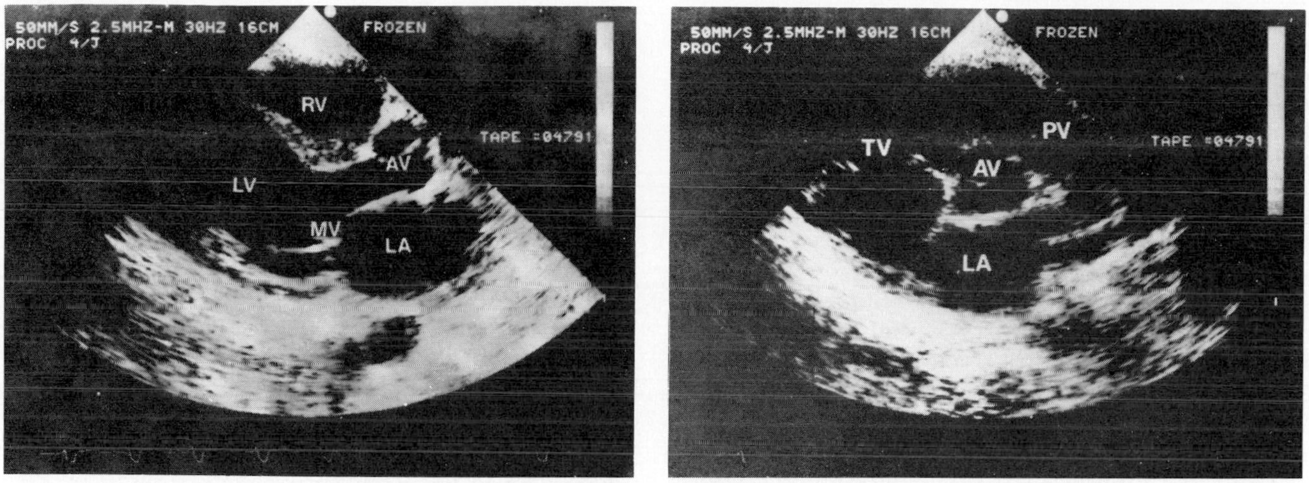

Fig. 15-58 Two-dimensional echocardiogram. Note that several sections of the heart can be viewed at one time, and it is easier to see the relationship of the chambers to one another. Abbreviations are as in Fig. 15-57, plus *TV,* tricuspid valve; *LV,* left ventricle. (From Kinney M and others: *Comprehensive cardiac care,* ed 7, St Louis, 1991, Mosby–Year Book.)

mation, the performance of an echocardiogram on all patients being evaluated for chest pain could help identify those patients who are likely to have had a myocardial infarction or who are at risk for complications and could benefit from admission to a coronary care unit.

Before the development of echocardiography, intracardiac myomas could be found only with angiography. M-mode echocardiograms could identify some intracardiac masses but could not define them clearly enough to differentiate myomas from clots or vegetations. Currently, the 2-D echocardiogram is able to locate and identify intracardiac masses and differentiate myomas from other causes of an intracardiac mass.

Doppler echocardiography. Doppler echocardiography provides a special kind of echocardiogram that assesses blood flow. It uses a pulsed or continuous wave of ultrasound that records frequency shifts of reflected sound waves, showing velocity and direction of blood flow relative to the transducer. Doppler echocardiography is especially useful in patients with valvular heart disease. Both regurgitation and stenosis can be detected and estimates made of their severity. When compared with cardiac catheterization results, Doppler echocardiography has been shown to predict accurately the pressure gradient across the affected valve.[52] When multiple valves are involved, the Doppler technique can clarify the extent of damage to the individual valves. Prosthetic valve function can also be evaluated, although this is best done in combination with phonocardiography because dysrhythmias or conduction disturbances can produce motion patterns that could mimic valve malfunction on the echocardiogram alone. Even normal prosthetic valves cause a small obstruction to forward flow and increase forward velocities. A trivial amount of regurgitation is also normal. It must be remembered that ultrasonic waves do not pass through metallic valves, so evaluation of flow behind the valve can be difficult. Repositioning the Doppler transducer under guidance from the 2-D echocardiogram may be helpful. Color-flow Doppler imaging is better than conventional Doppler recordings for evaluation of prosthetic valves because the regurgitant jets are often eccentric.[52] Other uses for Doppler echocardiography include evaluation of congenital anomalies, especially shunts and atresias; measurement of volume flow; and assessment of cardiac output. By measuring flow velocity in the right ventricular outflow tract, mean pulmonary artery pressure can be estimated with a high degree of reliability.[53]

Recently, Doppler signals have become available in color. Known as color-flow mapping or imaging, this technique analyzes Doppler signals from multiple intracardiac sites simultaneously. The Doppler tracing for each site is displayed in a color-coded format superimposed on a real-time 2-D echocardiographic image. Flow toward the transducer is displayed in one color, while flow away from the transducer is displayed in a contrasting color. The brightness of the color is varied to signify varying flow velocities.

Research is being conducted to determine whether echocardiography can be used to detect lesions in the coronary arteries. Contrast dye can be injected into the coronary arteries while the echocardiogram is being done, revealing underperfused areas. This technique is still under investigation. Even without contrast, high-intensity-echocardiograms can identify lesions in the walls of the left main and left anterior descending coronary arteries when significant obstruction is present. Compared with findings on cardiac catheterization, this technique yields 98% sensitivity and 67% specificity.[54] This could become a practical means of screening patients for left main coronary artery disease.

Transesophageal echocardiography. This is a relatively new technique in which the transducer (either M-mode, 2-D, Doppler, or a combination of these) is mounted on a flexible shaft similar to a gastroscope and advanced to various locations in the esophagus where images are examined. Because of the close anatomic relationship between the heart and the esophagus, transesophageal echocardiography (TEE) produces high-quality images of intracardiac structures and the thoracic aorta without the interference of the chest wall, bone, or air-filled lung.

The procedure is similar to an upper GI endoscopy. The patient should fast for a minimum of 6 hours before the procedure to prevent nausea and vomiting. Medication is usually given to reduce salivary secretions; sedation may be used, as well as antibiotic prophylaxis according to American Heart Association (AHA) recommendations, if any form of cardiac valve disease is present.[55] Next, the pharyngeal region is anesthetized with 2% viscous xylocaine and 10% xylocaine spray. The patient is placed in the left lateral decubitus position and a soft bite block is inserted between the teeth to prevent damage to the echoscope. As the echoscope is inserted, the patient is asked to swallow. The echoscope is advanced to 25 cm from the mouth, and imaging is begun.[56] Advancement to additional locations permits additional views (Fig. 15-59). TEE is also used intraoperatively, in which case sedation and local anesthetics are not required.

TEE is useful whenever the transthoracic approach is unsatisfactory, as in COPD and obesity and when chest wall changes caused by aging create obstacles to clear image visualization. In addition, TEE is superior to transthoracic echocardiography in a variety of situations. The entire thoracic aorta can be visualized clearly, and TEE is rapidly becoming the diagnostic procedure of choice in suspected dissecting aortic aneurysm, even surpassing aortic angiography.[56] Angiograms require the use of intravenous contrast agents (dye), which can cause further renal damage in patients who already have compromised renal function. TEE carries no such risk.

Both atrial chambers are well imaged with TEE, and the left atrial appendage is particularly well observed, making TEE the procedure of choice for detection of left atrial thrombus. Diagnosis and quantification of atrial septal defects can also be done with this method, and the addition of Doppler capabilities allows assessment of atrial shunting after percutaneous mitral valvuloplasty. Because of the ability to use higher-frequency ultrasonic waves than those used with transthoracic echocardiography, TEE is useful in evaluating patients with infective endocarditis to investigate the source of emboli, assess valve regurgitation, and identify valvular vegetations.[56] Both native and prosthetic mitral valves can be assessed for regurgitation or stenosis. Proximal coronary arteries and large pulmonary veins can also be imaged, although the value of this in relation to coronary angiography must be investigated further.

One other advantage of TEE over transthoracic echocardiography is that it is a convenient way to monitor cardiac function during open heart and general surgery. Transthoracic echocardiography was rarely used for this purpose, because it required manual placement of the transducer on the chest at all times. The transesophageal probe can be placed and left in position during the operative procedure. Global myocardial function can be monitored, new areas of dyskinesis (indicating ischemia) can be detected, and intracardiac air can be easily detected.

The risks involved in TEE are surprisingly low, even in unstable critically ill patients. The overall incidence of complications is less than 1%. Matsuzaki, Toma, and Kusukawa[56] reported complications of asymptomatic, nonsustained ventricular tachycardia; bradycardia; transient AV block; angina; bronchial asthma attack; and marked hypertension during initial insertion, which returned to near normal as the procedure continued. Zabalgoitia and others[55] also reported protracted nausea in one patient, sinus tachycardia in half of their

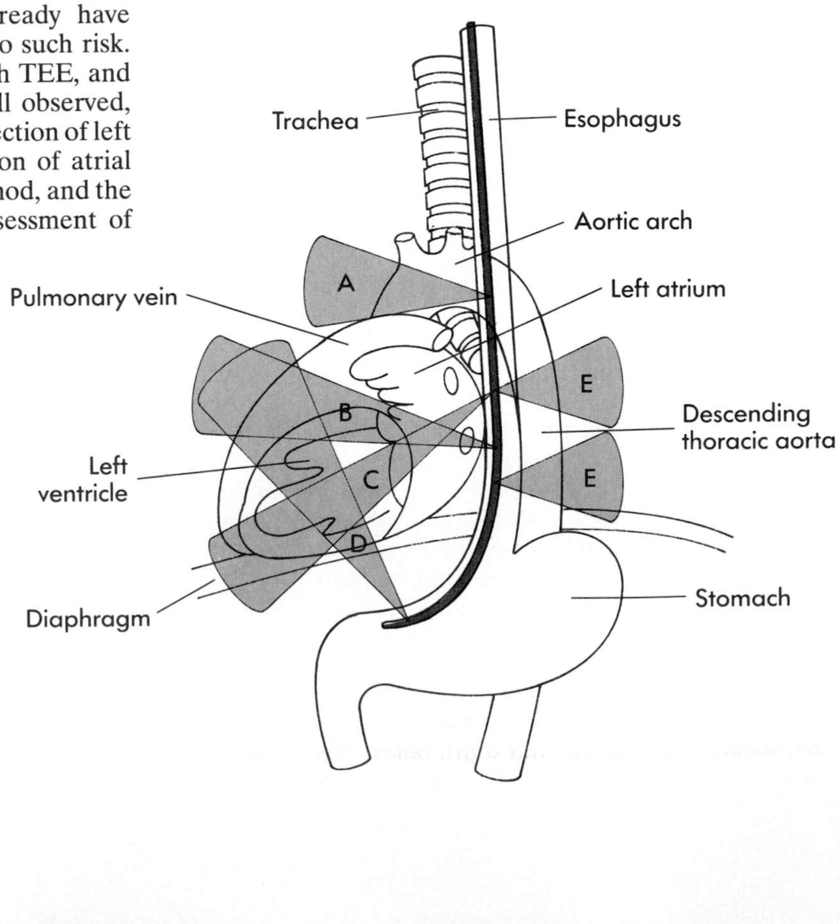

Fig. 15-59 Diagram of common scan planes during a transesophageal two-dimensional echocardiogram. **A,** Horizontal scan plane of aortic arch and distal portion of aorta. **B,** Basal short-axis (transverse), long-axis (sagittal) views, and short-axis views of both atria. **C,** Four-chamber and left atrioventricular long-axis views. Sagittal scan plane can image a cross section of the left ventricle. **D,** Transgastric short-axis of left ventricle and right ventricle. **E,** Transverse and sagittal scan sections of descending aorta.

patient group, and transient gagging during insertion in all. However, they did not mention anesthetizing the pharynx in their patients, which may have contributed to the high incidence of gagging. The most serious risk of the procedure is esophageal bleeding. This can occur during intraoperative use because of the large doses of heparin that are often administered during surgery. Patients with liver cirrhosis and/or esophageal varices are also at high risk for esophageal bleeding. The procedure should always be performed under constant monitoring, and if esophageal entry is difficult, it should not be forced.

◆ **Nursing management.** The echocardiograph can be brought to the bedside if necessary, but whenever possible the patient should be transported to the echocardiography laboratory. The room will be somewhat dark to improve the visual clarity of the images displayed on the screen. For transthoracic echocardiography, lubricant is placed on the patient's chest, and a transducer is placed in various positions to visualize cardiac and valvular structures. The procedure is not uncomfortable, but it may be tiresome for certain patients because of the length of the procedure, which is usually 30 to 60 minutes.

TEE is somewhat more uncomfortable, comparable to an upper GI endoscopy. Suction equipment should be available in the event that the patient vomits or has difficulty handling oral secretions.

Nuclear Magnetic Resonance

Nuclear magnetic resonance (NMR) is a noninvasive imaging technique that can obtain specific biochemical information from body tissue without the use of ionizing radiation. The procedure does not present any known hazard to living cells. In many respects, the image created is superior to both x-ray film and ultrasonography because bone does not interfere with magnetic resonance imaging.

◆ **Indications.** Currently, cardiac magnetic resonance imaging can provide information about tissue integrity, wall-motion abnormalities and aneurysms, ejection fraction,[57] cardiac output, and patency of proximal coronary arteries. In a recent study of 22 patients, the ejection fraction calculated from magnetic resonance imaging had an excellent linear correlation with the ejection fraction determined by left ventricular angiography ($r = 0.95$).[57] At present, however, the drawbacks to magnetic resonance imaging outweigh its advantages for most patients (Table 15-18), and it is currently not competitive with echocardiography and angiography.

Blood that is actively flowing does not emit a magnetic resonance signal; thus it provides a natural dark contrast material in the lumen of proximal coronary arteries. As a result, abnormalities of lumen size such as narrowing—which may provide evidence of obstruction—can be visualized.[58]

◆ **Procedure.** The method by which NMR scanning is performed is quite complex, but the basic concept is fairly simple. Certain atoms within molecules act as tiny bar magnets with north and south poles. The nuclei spin around this axis like a spinning top. Under normal conditions these small atomic magnets are arranged at random. If a patient is placed within a strong magnetic field, many of the nuclei line up in the same direction as the magnetic force. When a radio frequency wave is sent, some of the nuclei absorb this energy, causing them to fall out of alignment and wobble like a gyroscope that is winding down. This "wobbling" out of alignment is termed *resonance.* The process of returning to alignment with the magnetic field after the radio frequency signal is turned off is called *relaxation.* These energy changes can be detected and recorded by the scanner.

Table 15-18 Advantages and limitations of cardiac nuclear magnetic resonance imaging

Advantages	Limitations
Entirely noninvasive	Time-consuming
Does not involve ionizing radiation	Accurate gating limited to patients in normal sinus rhythm
Provides images in multiple planes with uniformly good resolution	Not widely available
	Expensive
Provides information about tissue characterization and blood flow	Cannot be used on critically ill patients because of access and equipment problems

From Stratemeier E and others: *Radiology* 158:775, 1986.

Each type of atom has its own unique resonance and relaxation pattern. The easiest one to record at present is the hydrogen ion, although other atoms such as phosphorus, sodium, and carbon are also being studied. Because there are two hydrogen ions per molecule of water, magnetic resonance imaging is especially sensitive to changes in tissue water content. Myocardial ischemic injury results in predictable increases in regional myocardial water content, allowing differentiation between normal and ischemic tissue. Infarction leading to myocardial scarring will result in tissue with a decreased water content, which can be identified on a magnetic resonance scan as an area of decreased signal intensity.

Magnetic resonance imaging works well for structures that have little or no motion, such as the brain. Cardiac applications have been limited because of the constant motion of the heart. In an attempt to overcome this limitation, various gating or slicing techniques have been used to time the images at exact phases of the cardiac cycle. The gating can be timed from the R wave of the ECG or from the arterial pulse tracing.[59] Either method is satisfactory as long as the patient is in normal sinus rhythm. With any irregularity of the rhythm, the gating technique becomes much less helpful.

◆ **Nursing management.** Magnetic resonance imaging is actually a very safe procedure. The main hazard is related to the presence of other metal substances in the environment. Because the magnetism used is approximately 40,000 times stronger than the magnetic field of the earth, metal objects such as IV poles or oxygen tanks can become projectiles if they come close enough to the magnet's pull. To avoid this, adequate security around the scanner is important, and many facilities use a metal detector to screen for metal objects on all people entering the area. This limitation also severely restricts the use of this technique in the critically ill patient.

Many patients have implanted metallic devices that have caused concern in the past. Laakman and others[60] tested 236 patients who had metallic implants and developed some guidelines about which implants are safe and which are not (Table 15-19). Neither a cardiac pacemaker nor an implantable cardioverter defibrillator (ICD) is safe because they may turn off or switch modes when exposed to a strong external magnetic field. Aneurysm clips are composed of ferromagnetic materials and could experience significant torque when exposed to the magnetic field.

Bedside Hemodynamic Monitoring

Invasive hemodynamic monitoring has become one of the major skill areas necessary for the critical care nurse. Using invasive catheters and sophisticated monitors, the nurse evaluates a patient's cardiac function, circulating blood volume, and physiologic response to treatment. Knowledge of the theoretic base that underlies hemodynamic monitoring will assist the clinician in developing decision-making skills to interpret and analyze trends and to formulate a nursing management plan appropriate for each individual patient.

◆ **Indications.** The range of medical diagnoses for which hemodynamic monitoring can be used is enormous. Most of these medical diagnoses are linked by three nursing diagnoses: (1) Alteration in Cardiac Output, (2) Alteration in Fluid Volume, and (3) Alteration in Tissue Perfusion. These nursing diagnoses are based on pathophysiologic processes that alter one of the four hemodynamic mechanisms that support normal cardiovascular function: preload, afterload, heart rate, and contractility. These mechanisms are described in Chapter 13, pp. 163-166. Treatment of alterations in cardiac output, fluid volume, and tissue perfusion will vary, based on the precipitating cause and medical diagnosis, as discussed later in this chapter in the section on pulmonary artery catheters. (pp. 254-260).

There are different levels of hemodynamic monitoring intensity, depending on the clinical needs of the patient. The simplest level includes monitoring heart rhythm, central venous pressure (CVP), and arterial blood pressure, a combination that is frequently used after uncomplicated general surgery or cardiac surgery. If the patient has a low cardiac output, such as might occur subsequent to an acute myocardial infarction, a more intense level of surveillance may be necessary. It might involve use of a thermodilution pulmonary artery catheter, which provides hemodynamic information that includes intracardiac pressures, direct measurement of CO, and—if necessary—continuous measurement of pulmonary arterial oxygen saturation (Svo_2). Another catheter used in critical care is the left atrial pressure line, which may be used in selected patients after cardiac surgery.

Table 15-19 Metallic implants in nuclear magnetic resonance imaging

Safe	Unsafe
Metallic orthopedic devices	Cardiac pacemaker
Surgical wires	Other electrical stimulating devices
Surgical clips	Aneurysm clips
Skin staples	Unknown types of metal implants in potentially vulnerable areas of the body
Central nervous system shunting devices	
Tantalum mesh	

From Laakman R and others: *Radiology* 157:711, 1985.

◆ Overview of hemodynamic monitoring

Equipment. A hemodynamic monitoring system has three component parts: (1) the invasive catheter and tubing connected to the patient, (2) the transducer, which receives the physiologic signal from the catheter and converts it into electrical energy, and (3) the amplifier/recorder, which increases the volume of the electrical signal and displays it on an oscilloscope and on a digital scale read in millimeters of mercury (mm Hg).

Although many different invasive catheters are inserted to monitor hemodynamic pressures, all catheters are connected to similar equipment. This consists of a bag of 0.9% normal saline solution, which will usually contain 0.25 to 2 units of heparin per milliliter,[61] a 300–mm Hg pressure infusion cuff, intravenous (IV) tubing; three-way stopcocks; and an in-line flush device for both continuous and manual fluid infusion. The addition of heparin to the IV setup is designed to maintain catheter patency. A multicenter nursing study has demonstrated that arterial monitoring lines maintained with a heparin flush solution have a greater probability of remaining patent than do lines maintained with nonheparinized solutions.[62] The tubing connects the invasive catheter to the transducer to avoid damping (flattening) of the waveform, which results in inaccurate pressure readings. The most frequently used transducers in clinical practice are disposable and use a silicon chip.

Calibration of equipment. To ensure accuracy of hemodynamic pressure readings, two baseline measurements are necessary: (1) calibration of the system to atmospheric pressure, and (2) determination of the phlebostatic axis for transducer height placement. To calibrate the equipment, the three-way stopcock nearest to the transducer is turned simultaneously to open the transducer to air (atmospheric pressure) and to close it to the patient and the flush system. The monitor is adjusted so that "0" is displayed, which equals atmospheric pressure. Then, using the monitor, the upper scale limit is calibrated while the system remains open to air. Standard scale limits for that monitor system are used. Finally, the stopcock is returned to its original position to visualize the waveform and hemodynamic pressures.[63]

The phlebostatic axis is a physical reference point on the chest that is used as a baseline for consistent transducer height placement. To obtain the axis, a theoretic line is drawn from the fourth intercostal space

RESEARCH ABSTRACT

Evaluation of the effects of heparinized and nonheparinized flush solutions on the patency of arterial pressure monitoring lines: The AACN Thunder Project.

The American Association of Critical-Care Nurses: Am J Crit Care 2(1):3, 1993.

PURPOSE

The purpose of this study was to evaluate the effects of heparinized and nonheparinized flush solutions on the patency of arterial pressure monitoring lines. Two specific questions were addressed: (1) Is there a significant difference in duration of patency (up to 72 hours) between arterial pressure monitoring lines maintained with heparinized flush solutions and those maintained with nonheparinized flush solutions?; and (2) What are the effects of potentially confounding variables on the duration of the patency of the two solutions?

DESIGN

Two-group randomized clinical trial design

SAMPLE

The sample consisted of 5139 subjects from 198 nationwide sites (52% community hospitals; 26% university affiliated; 8% federal; 2% military; 2% county; and 10% with other affiliations). A total of 412 critical care units were included, and bed size of the hospitals ranged from less than 300 (25%) to more than 800 (9%), with 41% having 300 to 500 beds and 25% listing 501 to 800 beds. Included in the sample were subjects who had an arterial line inserted for monitoring arterial pressure and/or blood drawing and subjects who had an arterial catheter connected to monitoring equipment that could display arterial waveforms. Patients were excluded from the study if they were pregnant, had known platelet counts below 100,000, were known to be sensitive to heparin, or had a physician order excluding heparin from the treatment plan. Of the study subjects, 51.1% were in the heparin group and 48.9% were in the nonheparin group. The mean age was 63 years and 67.2% were males. Of all subjects, 63.7% had an arterial line because of a surgical procedure. Most subjects (79.7%) had catheters 2 inches or less, and 85.7% of the catheters were 20- or 22-gauge. The radial artery was the most frequent insertion site (86.7%). The most frequently used base solution was saline (94.5%), followed by Ringer's solution (2.3%) and glucose (1.5%).

INSTRUMENT

Information regarding eligibility criteria, arterial catheter/monitoring, demographics, and comments were collected on four optically scannable pages.

PROCEDURE

The study was undertaken and coordinated by the American Association of Critical-Care Nurses and was entitled the "Thunder Project." Interested institutions were offered the opportunity to participate in the study if they indicated the ability to recruit a minimum of 30 subjects within a 6-month period, received human subjects approval from their institution, appointed a project site coordinator, and paid a participation fee. Of the 239 sites that originally enrolled, 198 (83%) completed data collection by the end of the study. Site coordinators directed the study within their institutions and were responsible for education and training of research associates and data collection and management. Subjects were randomly assigned in blocks of 30 to the heparin and nonheparin flush solution groups. Colored labels were affixed to the flush solution, flush solution bag, and arterial line to indicate the appropriate research protocol assignment. Patency checks were performed and recorded every 4 hours after arterial line insertion for 72 hours or until the line was removed. At each patency check period, the following were performed: pressure bag inflation check (if the proper inflation of 300 mm Hg or manufacturer recommendation was not attained, the pressure was corrected before the remainder of the procedure); square waveform test and backflow test; and the presence or absence of anticoagulants or thrombolytics from any other source in the preceding 4 hours were noted. When the arterial line was removed, the reason for the removal was recorded. Data were entered into the data base via the optical scan sheets; written comments were coded as to category and time.

RESULTS

Arterial pressure monitoring lines containing heparinized flush solutions demonstrated significantly greater ($p < .00005$) patency over time than lines containing nonheparinized flush solutions. Four additional variables significantly influenced the probability of patency: receiving other anticoagulants or thrombolytics; having a catheter longer than 2 inches; femoral insertion site; and male gender. The risk of nonpatency contributed by individual variables, as determined by the proportional hazards regression model, was greatest if heparin was not used in the flush solution, followed by not using a femoral line, not using other anticoagulants or thrombolytics, using a short line, and female gender.

DISCUSSION/IMPLICATIONS

The Thunder Project is an important landmark research study because it was initiated and coordinated by the American Association of Critical-Care Nurses,

Continued.

RESEARCH ABSTRACT—cont'd

using many nationwide data collection sites with a large number of subjects. The study addressed one of the most common nursing practice issues encountered in critical care units and the study findings are generalizable with multiple implications for clinicians. This project was an excellent example of research designed to answer questions surrounding daily critical care practice. Although these research findings indicated that heparin does significantly impact the patency of arterial pressure monitoring lines over time, heparinizing the flush solution does not guarantee patency of the line. Lines can be kept patent without heparin, and other individual variables also increase the probability of patency. In the end, the decision to use heparinized flush solutions needs to be determined by clinicians on an individual patient basis, with considerations for monitoring indications, diagnoses, prognoses, and risk factors.

where it joins the sternum to a midaxillary line on the side of the chest. This point approximates the level of the atria. If the transducer air-reference stopcock is level with this reference point, accurate hemodynamic pressure measurements can be obtained for most patients at various head-of-bed positions up to 60 degrees of elevation.[64-67] Patients do not have to be placed flat to obtain accurate PA pressure readings. Error in measurement can occur if the transducer is placed *below* the phlebostatic axis, because fluid in the system will weigh on the transducer and produce a false-high reading. If the transducer is placed *above* this atrial level, gravity and lack of fluid pressure will give an erroneously low reading. If several clinicians will be taking measurements, the reference point can be marked on the side of the patient's chest to ensure accurate measurements.

Intraarterial Blood Pressure Monitoring

◆ **Indications.** Intraarterial blood pressure monitoring is indicated for any major medical or surgical condition that compromises cardiac output, tissue perfusion, or fluid volume status. The system is designed for continuous measurement of three blood pressure parameters—systole, diastole, and mean arterial blood pressure (MAP). In addition, the direct arterial access is helpful in the management of patients with acute respiratory failure who require frequent arterial blood gas (ABG) measurements.

◆ **Catheters.** The size of the catheter used is proportionate to the diameter of the cannulated artery. In small arteries—such as the radial or dorsalis pedis—a 20-gauge, 3.8- to 5.1-cm, nontapered Teflon catheter is most often used. If the larger femoral or axillary arteries are used, a 19- or 20-gauge, 16-cm, Teflon catheter is used. Teflon catheters are preferred because of their lower risk of causing thrombosis.

The catheter insertion is usually percutaneous, although the technique varies with vessel size. Cannulas are most frequently inserted in the smaller arteries, using a "catheter-over-needle" unit in which the needle is used as a temporary guide for catheter placement. With this method, once the unit has been inserted into the artery, the needle is withdrawn, leaving the supple plastic cannula in place. Insertion of a cannula into a larger artery usually necessitates use of the Seldinger technique. This procedure involves (1) entry into the artery using a needle, (2) passage of a supple guidewire through the needle into the artery, (3) removal of the needle, (4) passage of the catheter over the guidewire, and (5) removal of the guidewire, leaving the cannula in the artery. If a cannula cannot be inserted into the artery using percutaneous methods, an arterial cutdown may be performed. This procedure is avoided if possible, because it involves a skin incision to expose the artery directly and is associated with a higher risk of infection.

◆ **Insertion.** Several major peripheral arteries are suitable for receiving a cannula and for long-term hemodynamic monitoring. The most frequently used site is the radial artery. If this artery is not available, the dorsalis pedis, femoral, axillary, or brachial arteries may be used. The major advantage of the radial artery is that collateral circulation to the hand is provided by the ulnar artery and palmar arch in most of the population; thus there are other avenues of circulation if the radial artery becomes blocked after catheter placement. Before radial artery cannulation, collateral circulation must be assessed, either by using the Doppler flowmeter or by the Allen test. In the Allen test the radial and ulnar arteries are compressed simultaneously. The patient is asked to clench and unclench the hand until it blanches. One of the arteries is then released, and the hand should immediately flush from that side. The same procedure is repeated for the remaining artery.

◆ **Nursing management.** Intraarterial blood pressure monitoring is designed for continuous assessment of arterial perfusion to the major organ systems of the body. Mean arterial pressure (MAP) is the clinical parameter most frequently used to assess perfusion, because MAP represents perfusion pressure throughout the cardiac cycle. Because one third of the cardiac cycle is spent in systole and two thirds in diastole, the MAP calculation must reflect the greater amount of time spent in diastole. The MAP formula when calculated by hand is as follows:

$$[(\text{Diastole} \times 2) \text{ plus } (\text{Systole} \times 1)] \text{ divided by } 3$$

Additional formulas for hemodynamic pressures are listed in Appendix C.

Thus a blood pressure of 120/60 mm Hg has a MAP of 80 mm Hg. However, the bedside hemodynamic monitor may show a slightly different digital number because most computers calculate the area under the curve of the arterial line tracing (Table 15-20). A MAP greater than

LEGAL REVIEW: Products liability

There are three theories of recovery for harm or injury suffered from defective medical products (drugs, diagnostic and treatment devices and equipment, and blood and blood components): (1) strict liability, (2) negligence, and (3) warranty.

Most states have adopted and codified the Restatement (Second) of Torts, Section 402A, definition of strict liability: One who sells a defective product that is unreasonably dangerous to the consumer is liable for harm to the consumer, even if the seller has exercised all possible care in the preparation and sale of the product and the consumer has not bought the product from the seller. The underlying public policy in this law is that consumers should be protected from the inevitable risks of harm brought about by mass production and marketing of products.

To prevail under this theory, the plaintiff must prove the defendant sold the product, the product was defective, the defect rendered the product unreasonably dangerous when used in a reasonably foreseeable manner, the defendant was in the business of selling the product and the defect existed at the time of the sale, the defect was the proximate cause of the damages, and the plaintiff suffered damages. However, under many state statutes, "sellers" may be immune from liability if the seller is not engaged in the assembly, design, or manufacture of the product and the defect originated in one of these areas of production.

There are three types of product defects: (1) defective manufacture, (2) defective design, and (3) inadequate or absent warnings (which are usually litigated under a negligence theory).

Under the negligence theory, the duty of reasonable care applies to the design, manufacture, and testing of the product to ensure safety. There is also a duty to provide adequate information and warnings to the consumer about the product. In strict liability the plaintiff's proof focuses on the condition of the product that is designed or manufactured in a certain way, whereas in negligence the proof focuses on the reasonableness of the defendant's conduct in designing, manufacturing, or selling the product and in providing product information and warnings.

Under the warranty liability theory, statements or representations about the character, fitness, condition, or quality of the product are at issue. Product warranties may be express or they may be presumed—that is, implied.

A hospital may be liable for negligence under corporate and respondeat superior theories for failure to monitor and maintain equipment safety and for failure to provide adequately trained staff to operate medical equipment and devices. Critical care nurses may be held personally liable for negligence or malpractice for using defective products or devices, for failure to properly monitor or use equipment, and for failure to comply with printed instructions for use.

Hospitals, doctors, and nurses frequently reuse medical devices (particularly heart catheters) for cost-containment reasons. In the event the reused device proves or becomes defective and causes injury, the hospital and staff—as well as the manufacturer and seller—may be liable under all three products liability doctrines.

In the Hawaii and Texas cases cited below, both states have "blood shield" statutes that bar certain claims against hospitals arising from a patient's contraction of acquired immunodeficiency syndrome from transfusion of contaminated blood. In *Gibson v. Methodist Hosp.*, the court held that blood was not a product for purposes of product liability and breach of warranty claims. In Hawaii, entities are statutorily exempt from strict liability for preparing or transfusing blood or blood components but are not exempt from liability for negligence. In the *Smith v. Cutter Biological, Inc.*, the court held that the Hawaii blood shield statute did not preclude negligence claims against four manufacturers of Factor VIII (antihemophilic factor concentrate) by a hemophiliac who became exposed to human immunodeficiency virus through Factor VIII injections, despite his inability to positively identify the actual tortfeasor (wrongdoer).

See Geddes A: Free movement of pharmaceuticals within the community: the remaining barriers, *Eur L Rev* 16:295, 1991; *Gibson v Methodist Hosp.,* 822 S.W.2d 95 (Tex. App. 1991); *Grubb v Albert Einstein Med. Center,* 387 A.2d 480 (Pa. 1978); Lynn JSR: Implantable medical devices: a survey of products liability case law, *Med Trial Tech Q* 38:44, 1991; *May v Broun,* 492 P.2d 776 (Or. 1972); *Phelps v Sherwood Med. Indus.,* 836 F.2d 296 (7th Cir. 1987); *Phillips v Medtronic, Inc.,* No. 86-4231-R (D. Kan. Feb. 23, 1990); Prosser WL and others: *Prosser and Keeton on the law of torts,* ed 5, St Paul, 1988, West; *Restatement (Second) of Torts* Sec. 402A; Shimm DS, Spece RG: Conflict of interest and informed consent in industry-sponsored clinical trials, *J Legal Med* 12:477, 1991; *Smith v Cutter Biological, Inc.,* 823 P.2d 717 (Haw. 1991).

Table 15-20 Hemodynamic pressures and calculated hemodynamic values

Hemodynamic pressure	Definition and explanation	Normal range*
Mean arterial pressure (**MAP**)	Average perfusion pressure created by arterial blood pressure during the complete cardiac cycle. The normal cardiac cycle is one-third systole and two-thirds diastole. These three components are divided by 3 to obtain the average perfusion pressure for the whole cardiac cycle.	70-100 mm Hg
Central venous pressure (**CVP**)	Pressure created by volume in the right side of the heart. When the tricuspid valve is open, the CVP reflects filling pressures in the right ventricle. Clinically, the CVP is often used as a guide to overall fluid balance.	2-4 mm Hg 3-8 cm water (H_2O)
Left atrial pressure (**LAP**)	Pressure created by volume in the left side of the heart. When the mitral valve is open, the LAP reflects filling pressures in the left ventricle. Clinically, the LAP is used after cardiac surgery to determine how well the left ventricle is ejecting its volume. In general, the higher the LAP, the lower the ejection fraction from the left ventricle.	5-12 mm Hg
Pulmonary artery pressure (PAP) (systolic, diastolic, mean) (**PA systolic [PAS]**, **PA diastolic [PAD]**, **PAP mean [PAP_M]**)	Pulsatile pressure in the pulmonary artery, measured by an indwelling catheter.	PAS 20-30 mm Hg PAD 5-10 mm Hg PAP_M 10-15 mm Hg
Pulmonary capillary wedge pressure or pulmonary artery wedge pressure (**PCW** or **PCWP** or **PAWP**)	Pressure created by volume in the left side of the heart. When the mitral valve is open, the PAWP reflects filling pressures in the pulmonary vasculature, and pressures in the left side of the heart are transmitted back to the catheter "wedged" into a small pulmonary arteriole.	5-12 mm Hg
Cardiac output (**CO**)	The amount of blood pumped out by a ventricle. Clinically, it can be measured using the thermodilution CO method, which calculates CO in liters per minute (L/min).	4-6 L/min (at rest)
Cardiac index (**CI**)	CO divided by body surface area (BSA), tailoring the CO to individual body size. A BSA conversion chart is necessary to calculate CI, which is considered more accurate than CO because it is individualized to height and weight. CI is measured in liters per minute per square meter BSA (L/min/m^2).	2.2-4.0 L/min/m^2
Stroke volume (**SV**)	Amount of blood ejected by the ventricle with each heartbeat. Hemodynamic monitoring systems calculate SV by dividing cardiac output (CO in L/min) by the heart rate (HR) then multiplying the answer by 1000 to change liters to milliliters (ml).	60-70 ml
Stroke volume index (**SI**)	SV indexed to BSA.	40-50 ml/m^2
Systemic vascular resistance (**SVR**)	Mean pressure difference across the systemic vascular bed, divided by blood flow. Clinically, SVR represents the resistance against which the left ventricle must pump to eject its volume. This resistance is created by the systemic arteries and arterioles. As SVR increases, CO falls. SVR is measured in either units or dynes/sec/cm^{-5}. If the number of units is multiplied by 80, the value is converted to dynes/sec/cm^{-5}.	10-18 units or 800-1400 dynes/sec/cm^{-5}

Systemic vascular resistance index (**SVRI**)	SVR indexed to BSA.	2000-2400 dynes/sec/ cm^{-5}/m^2
Pulmonary vascular resistance (**PVR**)	Mean pressure difference across pulmonary vascular bed, divided by blood flow. Clinically, PVR represents the resistance against which the right ventricle must pump to eject its volume. This resistance is created by the pulmonary arteries and arterioles. As PVR increases, the output from the right ventricle decreases. PVR is measured in either units or dynes/sec/cm^{-5}. PVR is normally one sixth of SVR.	1.2-3.0 units or 100-250 dynes/sec/cm^{-5}
Pulmonary vascular resistance index (**PVRI**)	PVR indexed to BSA.	225-315 dynes/sec/ cm^{-5}/m^2
Left cardiac work index (**LCWI**)	Amount of work the left ventricle does *each minute* when ejecting blood. The hemodynamic formula represents pressure generated (MAP) multiplied by volume pumped (CO). A conversion factor is used to change mm Hg to kilogram-meter (kg-m). LCWI is always represented as an indexed volume (BSA chart). LCWI increases or decreases because of changes in either pressure (MAP) or volume pumped (CO).	3.4-4.2 kg-m/m^2
Left ventricular stroke work index (**LVSWI**)	Amount of work the left ventricle performs with *each heartbeat*. The hemodynamic formula represents pressure generated (MAP) multiplied by volume pumped (SV). A conversion factor is used to change ml/mm Hg to gram-meter (g-m). LVSWI is always represented as an indexed volume. LVSWI increases or decreases because of changes in either pressure (MAP) or volume pumped (SV).	50-62 g-m/m^2
Right cardiac work index (**RCWI**)	Amount of work the right ventricle performs *each minute* when ejecting blood. The hemodynamic formula represents pressure generated (PAP mean) multiplied by volume pumped (CO). A conversion factor is used to change mm Hg to kilogram-meter (kg-m). RCWI is always represented as an indexed value (BSA chart). Similar to LCWI, the RCWI increases or decreases because of changes in either pressure (PAP mean) or volume pumped (CO).	0.54-0.66 kg-m/m^2
Right ventricular stroke work index (**RVSWI**)	Amount of work the right ventricle does *each heartbeat*. The hemodynamic formula represents pressure generated (PAP mean) multiplied by volume pumped (SV). A conversion factor is used to change mm Hg to gram-meter (g-m). RVSWI is always represented as an indexed value (BSA chart). Similar to LVSWI, the RVSWI increases or decreases because of changes in either pressure (PAP mean) or volume pumped (SV).	7.9-9.7 g-m/m^2

*The formulas for these hemodynamic values are listed in Appendix C.

60 mm Hg is necessary to perfuse the coronary arteries, brain, and kidneys. A MAP between 70 and 90 mm Hg is ideal for the cardiac patient to decrease LV work load. After a carotid endarterectomy or neurologic surgery, a MAP of 90 to 110 mm Hg may be more appropriate to increase cerebral perfusion pressure. Systolic and diastolic pressures are monitored in conjunction with the MAP as a further guide to the accuracy of perfusion. Should cardiac output decrease, the body will compensate by constricting peripheral vessels to maintain the blood pressure. In this situation the MAP may remain constant, but the pulse pressure (difference between systolic and diastolic pressures) will narrow. The following examples explain this point:

Mr. A: BP, 90/70; MAP, 76 mm Hg

Mr. B: BP, 150/40; MAP, 76 mm Hg

Both of these patients have a perfusion pressure of 76 mm Hg, but clinically they are very different. Mr. A is peripherally vasoconstricted, as is demonstrated by the narrow pulse pressure (90/70). His skin is cool to touch, and he has weak peripheral pulses. Mr. B has a wide pulse pressure (150/40), warm skin, and normally palpable peripheral pulses. Thus nursing assessment of the patient with an arterial line includes comparison of clinical findings with arterial line readings, including perfusion pressure and MAP.

Another clinical example of this hemodynamic nursing assessment is seen in patient JW 1 day after his coronary artery bypass graft (CABG) surgery. JW has recently been weaned from low-dose dopamine (Intropin) and sodium nitroprusside and has received a diuretic (20 mg of furosemide IV). He has voided 800 ml of urine via the Foley catheter during the last 2 hours. JW's MAP remains at 80 mm Hg, but his pulse pressure has narrowed by 30 mm Hg from 120/60 to 100/70. His heart rate has increased from 90 to 110 beats per minute (bpm). This clinical situation is not uncommon after furosemide administration, but the narrowed pulse pressure and increased heart rate may indicate hypovolemia. The nurse caring for JW is to monitor the *trend* of the MAP. If the MAP begins to decrease and JW shows signs of low CO, his physician should be notified. In most nonemergency situations, following the *trend* of the arterial pressure is more valuable than an isolated measurement.

The nurse caring for the patient with an arterial line must be able to assess whether a low MAP or narrowed perfusion pressure represents decreased arterial perfusion or equipment malfunction. Assessment of the arterial waveform on the oscilloscope, in combination with clinical assessment, will yield the answer. If air bubbles, clots, or kinks are in the system, the waveform will become damped, or flattened, and the troubleshooting methods described in Table 15-21 can be implemented. If the line is unreliable or becomes dislodged, a cuff pressure can be used as a reserve system. Slight differences exist between cuff and arterial pressures. These pressure differences are to be expected because the arterial catheter measures flow within the artery, whereas the mercury sphygmomanometer and stethoscope measure pressure from the outside.[68] Thus one technique measures flow and the other measures pressure. In the normovolemic patient, differences of 5 to 10 mm Hg do not affect clinical management. If the patient has a low CO or is in shock, the cuff pressure will be unreliable because of vasoconstriction and an arterial line should be inserted.

◆ **Arterial pressure waveform interpretation.** The arterial pressure waveform represents the ejection phase of left ventricular systole and is shown in Fig. 13-26. As the aortic valve opens, blood is ejected from the left ventricle and is recorded as an increase of pressure in the arterial system. The highest point recorded is called *systole.* After peak ejection (systole), force is decreased and pressure drops. A notch (the dicrotic notch) may be visible on the downstroke of this arterial waveform, representing closure of the aortic valve. The dicrotic notch signifies the beginning of diastole. The remainder of the downstroke represents diastolic runoff of blood flow into the arterial tree. The lowest point recorded is called *diastole.* A normal arterial pressure tracing is described in Fig. 15-60. Note that electrical stimulation (QRS) is always first and that the arterial pressure tracing follows the initiating QRS.

Specific problems with heart rhythm can translate into poor arterial perfusion if cardiac output falls. Poor perfusion may be seen as a single, nonperfused beat following a premature ventricular contraction (PVC) (Fig. 15-61) or as multiple, nonperfused beats (Fig. 15-62). In ventricular bigeminy, every second beat is poorly perfused (Fig. 15-63). A disorganized atrial baseline resulting from atrial fibrillation creates a variable arterial pulse because of the differences in stroke volume between each beat (Fig. 15-64). These cases illustrate that when two beats are close together, the left ventricle does not have time to fill adequately and the second beat is poorly perfused or is not perfused at all. If a stethoscope is placed over the apex of the heart, the beat can be heard, but it cannot be felt as a radial pulse. A pulse deficit occurs when the apical heart rate and the peripheral pulse are not equal. To determine whether a pulse deficit is significant, it is necessary to evaluate the clinical impact on the patient and whether there is any change in MAP or pulse pressure. Generally, the more nonperfused beats, the more serious the problem.

Pulsus paradoxus is a decrease of more than 10 mm Hg in the arterial waveform that occurs during inhalation (Fig. 15-61). It is caused by a fall in cardiac output as a result of increased negative intrathoracic pressure during inhalation. As pressure within the thorax falls, blood pools in the large veins of the lungs and thorax and stroke volume is decreased. This can be seen on an arterial waveform in a patient with cardiac tamponade, pericardial effusion, or constrictive pericarditis. It commonly occurs in hypovolemic patients who are mechanically ventilated, using large tidal volumes (12 to 15 ml/kg), or in patients who are spontaneously breathing very deeply. In pulsus alternans, every other arterial pulsation is weak. This sometimes occurs in patients with advanced left ventricular failure (see Fig. 15-62).

Table 15-21 Nursing measures to ensure patient safety and to troubleshoot problems with hemodynamic monitoring equipment

Problem	Prevention	Rationale	Troubleshooting
Overdamping of waveform	Provide continuous infusion of solution containing heparin through an in-line flush device (1 unit of heparin for each millimeter of flush solution).	To ensure that recorded pressures and waveform are accurate because a damped waveform gives inaccurate readings.	Before insertion, completely flush the line and/or catheter. In a line attached to a patient, back flush through the system to clear bubbles from tubing or transducer.
Underdamping, or "overshoot"	Use short lengths of noncompliant tubing. Use "square wave" test to demonstrate optimal system damping. Verify arterial waveform accuracy with the cuff blool pressure.	If the monitoring system is underdamped, both the systolic and diastolic values will be overestimated by both the waveform and the digital values. False high systolic values may lead to clinical decisions based on erroneous data.	Perform the "square wave" test to verify optimal damping of the monitoring system.
Clot formation at end of catheter	Provide continuous infusion of solution containing heparin through an in-line flush device (1 unit of heparin for each millimeter of flush solution).	Any foreign object placed in the body can cause local activation of the patient's coagulation system as a normal defense mechanism. The clots that are formed may be dangerous if they break off and travel to other parts of the body.	If a clot in the catheter is suspected because of a damped waveform or resistance to forward flush of the system, gently aspirate the line using a small syringe inserted into the proximal stopcock. Then flush the line again once the clot is removed and inspect the waveform. It should return to a normal pattern.
Hemorrhage	Use Luer-Lok (screw) connections in line setup. Close and cap stopcocks when not in use.	A loose connection or open stopcock will create a low-pressure sump effect, causing blood to back into the line and into the open air.	Once a blood leak is recognized, tighten all connections, flush the line, and estimate blood loss.
	Ensure that the catheter is either sutured or securely taped in position.	If a catheter is accidentally removed, the vessel can bleed profusely, especially with an arterial line or if the patient has abnormal coagulation factors (resulting from heparin in the line) or has hypertension.	If the catheter has been inadvertently removed, put pressure on the cannulation site. When bleeding has stopped, apply a sterile dressing, estimate blood loss, and inform the physician. If the patient is restless, an armboard may protect lines inserted in the arm.
Air emboli	Ensure that all air bubbles are purged from a new line setup before attachment to an indwelling catheter.	Air can be introduced at several times, including when central venous pressure (CVP) tubing comes apart, when a new line setup is attached, or when a new CVP or pulmonary artery (PA) line is inserted. During insertion of a CVP or PA line, the patient may be asked to hold his or her breath at specific times to prevent drawing air into the chest during inhalation.	Because it is impossible to get the air back once it has been introduced into the bloodstream, prevention is the best cure.

Continued.

Table 15-21 Nursing measures to ensure patient safety and to troubleshoot problems with hemodynamic monitoring equipment—cont'd

Problem	Prevention	Rationale	Troubleshooting
	Ensure that the drip chamber from the bag of flush solution is more than half full before using the in-line, fast-flush system.	The in-line, fast-flush devices are designed to permit clearing of blood from the line after withdrawal of blood samples.	If any air bubbles are noted, they must be vented through the in-line stopcocks and the drip chamber must be filled.
	Some sources recommend removing all air from the bag of flush solution before assembling the system.	If the chamber of the IV tubing is too low or empty, the rapid flow of fluid will create turbulance and cause flushing of air bubbles into the system and into the bloodstream.	The left atrial pressure (LAP) line setup is the only system that includes an air filter specifically to prevent air emboli.
Normal waveform with *low* digital pressure	Ensure that the system is calibrated to atmospheric pressure. Ensure that the transducer is placed at the level of the phlebostatic axis.	To provide a 0 baseline relative to atmospheric pressure. If the transducer has been placed *higher* than the phlebostatic level, gravity and the lack of hydrostatic pressure will produce a false *low* reading.	Recalibrate the equipment if transducer drift has occurred. Reposition the transducer at the level of the phlebostatic axis. Misplacement can occur if the patient moves from the bed to the chair or if the bed is placed in a Trendelenburg position.
Normal waveform with *high* digital pressure	Ensure that the system is calibrated to atmospheric pressure. Ensure that the transducer is placed at the level of the phlebostatic axis.	To provide a 0 baseline relative to atmospheric pressure. If the transducer has been placed *lower* than the phlebostatic level, the weight of hydrostatic pressure on the transducer will produce a false *high* reading.	Recalibrate the equipment if transducer drift has occurred. Reposition the transducer at the level of the phlebostatic axis. This situation can occur if the head of the bed was raised and the transducer was not repositioned. Some centers require attachment of the transducer to the patient's chest to avoid this problem.
Loss of waveform	Always have the hemodynamic waveform monitored so that changes or loss can be quickly noted.	The catheter may be kinked, or a stopcock may be turned off.	Check the line setup to ensure that all stopcocks are turned in the correct position and that the tubing is not kinked. Sometimes the catheter migrates against a vessel wall, and having the patient change position will restore the waveform.
Infection	Change the bag of flush solution every 24 hours. Change the line setup and the disposable transducer every 72 hours. Change the catheter insertion site dressing every 24 hours, and inspect the cannulation site for signs of infections. Apply antiseptic ointment and a sterile dressing to the catheter site.	These recommendations are provided by the Centers for Disease Control (CDC) and are based on research studies with hemodynamic monitoring equipment and on reports of infectious complications.	If local infection occurs, the catheter must be placed elsewhere by the physician, and the new insertion site must be dressed using antiseptic ointment and a sterile dressing. Sterile equipment must always be used, disposable equipment must not be reused, and nondisposable transducers must be sterilized after each patient usage. Hands should be washed before handling monitoring setup or dressings.

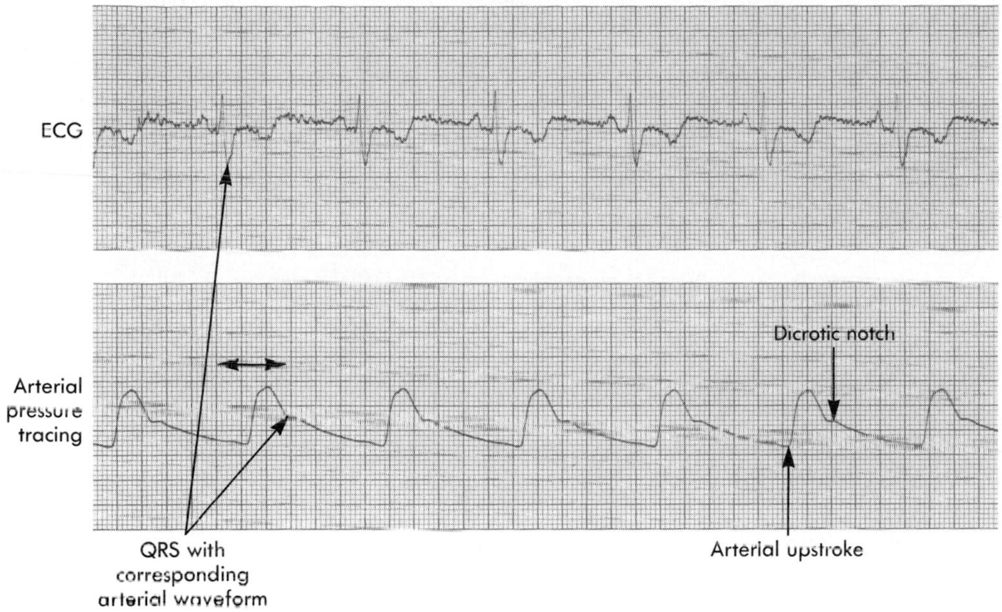

Fig. 15-60 Simultaneous ECG and arterial pressure tracings.

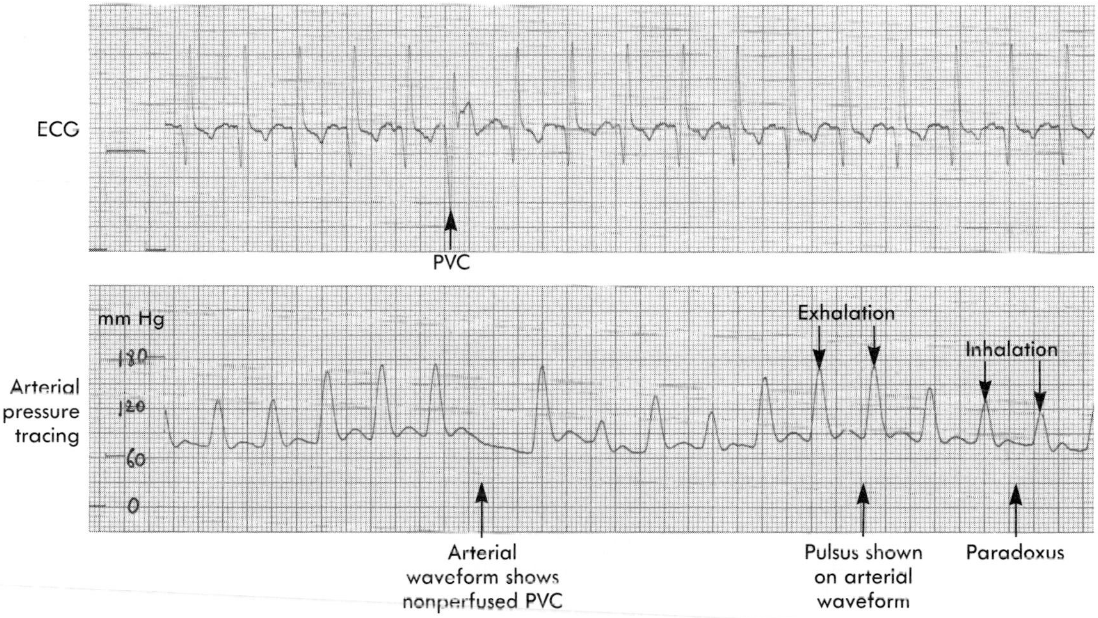

Fig. 15-61 Simultaneous ECG and arterial pressure tracings show normal arterial waveform with a nonperfused premature ventricular contraction (PVC). Arterial waveform also shows evidence of pulsus paradoxus in a patient who is mechanically ventilated.

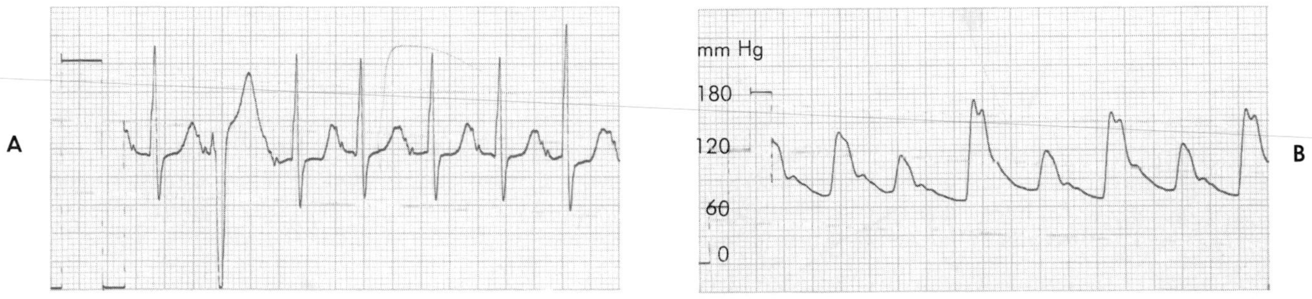

Fig. 15-62 Simultaneous **A,** ECG and **B,** arterial pressure tracings show pulsus alternans. A nonperfused PVC is also present.

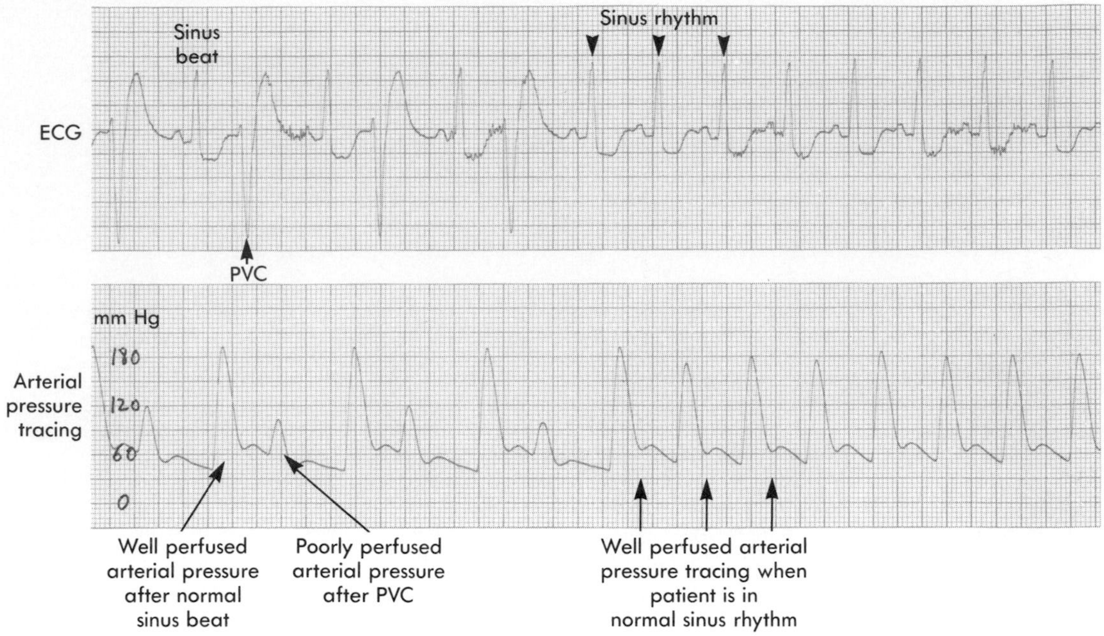

Fig. 15-63 Simultaneous ECG and arterial pressure tracings show ventricular bigeminy in which each ventricular beat is poorly perfused on the arterial pressure waveform in the first part of the tracing. In the second half of the tracing, there is a well-perfused arterial pressure tracing as the patient converts to normal sinus rhythm. .

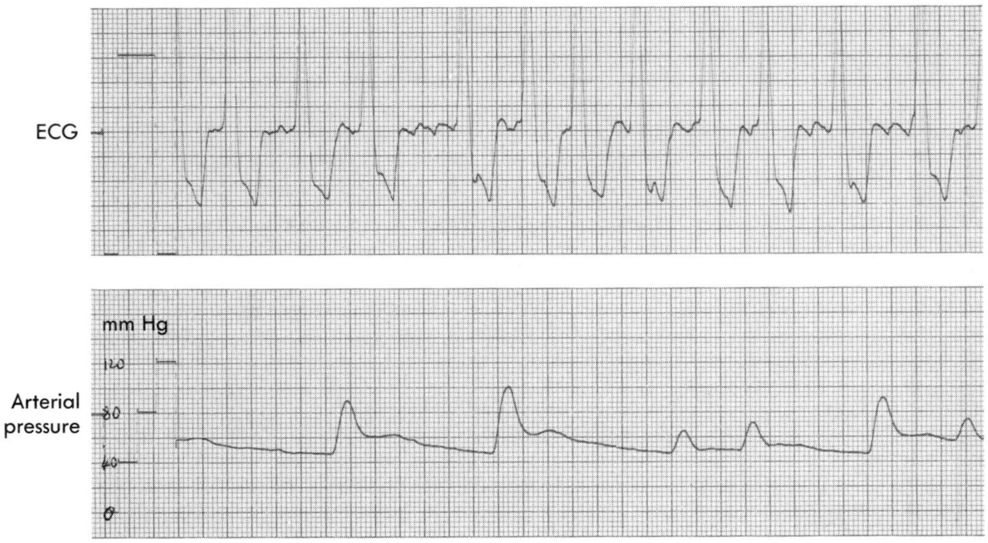

Fig. 15-64 Simultaneous ECG and arterial pressure tracings show atrial fibrillation, which results in irregular atrial pulsations. They create differences in beat-to-beat ventricular up-stroke volume, resulting in diminished or absent ventricular output as seen on the arterial waveform..

If the arterial monitor shows a low blood pressure, it is the responsibility of the nurse to determine whether it is a true patient problem or a problem with the equipment, as described in Table 15-21. A low arterial blood pressure waveform is shown in Fig. 15-65. In this case the digital readout correlated well with the patient's own cuff pressure, confirming that the patient was hypotensive. This arterial waveform is more rounded, without a dicrotic notch, when compared with the normal waveform in Fig. 15-60. A damped (flattened) arterial waveform is shown in Fig. 15-66. In this case the patient's cuff pressure was significantly higher than the digital readout, thus representing a problem with equipment. A damped waveform occurs when communication from the artery to the transducer is interrupted and produces false values on the monitor and oscilloscope.

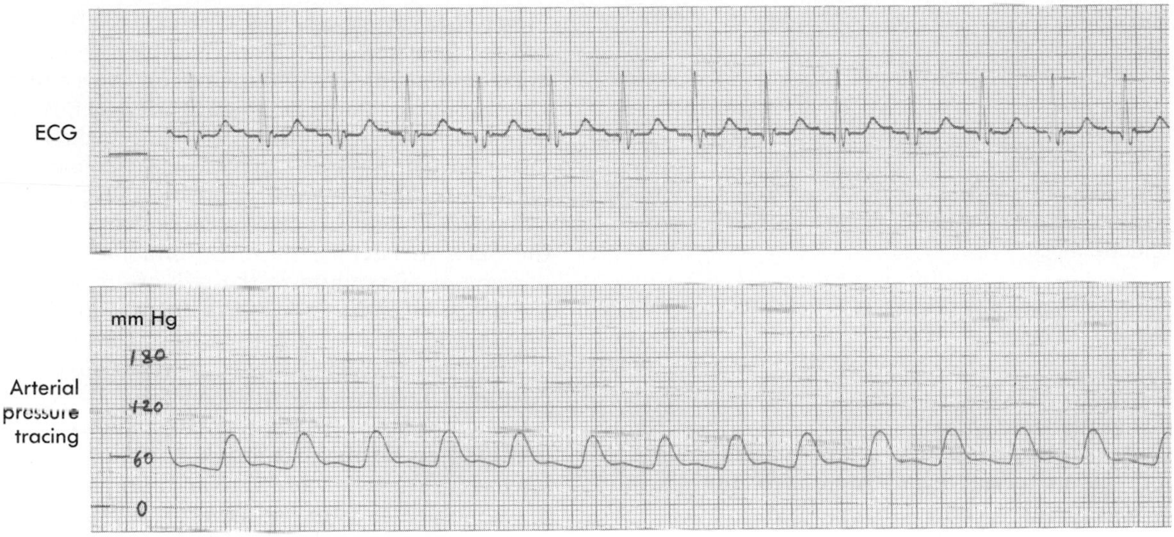

Fig. 15-65 Simultaneous ECG and arterial pressure tracings show a low arterial pressure waveform.

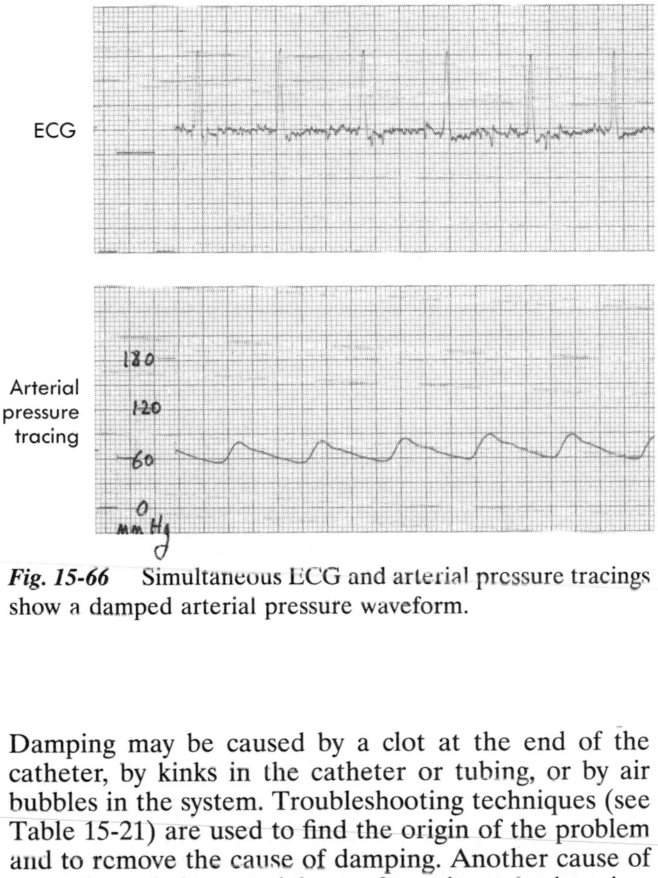

Fig. 15-66 Simultaneous ECG and arterial pressure tracings show a damped arterial pressure waveform.

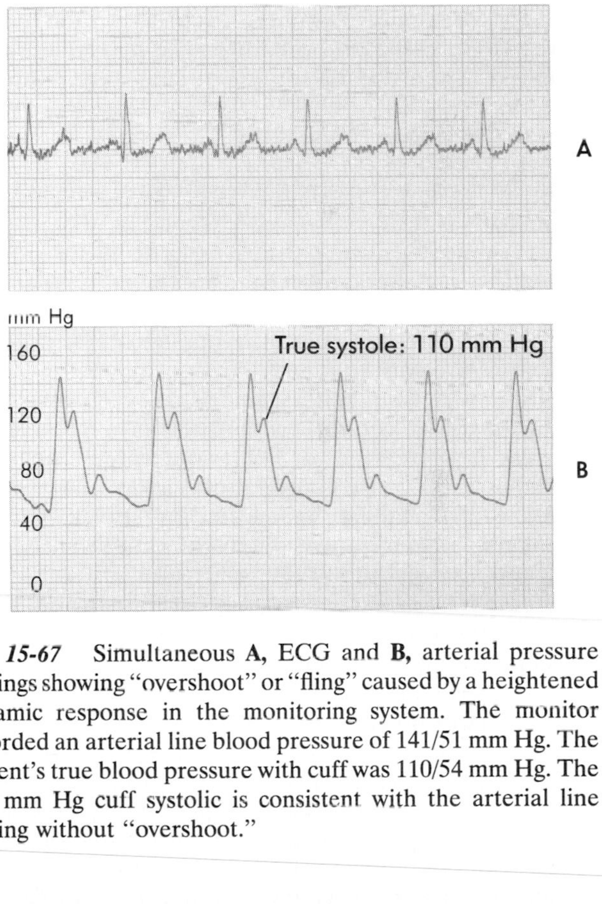

Fig. 15-67 Simultaneous **A,** ECG and **B,** arterial pressure tracings showing "overshoot" or "fling" caused by a heightened dynamic response in the monitoring system. The monitor recorded an arterial line blood pressure of 141/51 mm Hg. The patient's true blood pressure with cuff was 110/54 mm Hg. The 110 mm Hg cuff systolic is consistent with the arterial line tracing without "overshoot."

Damping may be caused by a clot at the end of the catheter, by kinks in the catheter or tubing, or by air bubbles in the system. Troubleshooting techniques (see Table 15-21) are used to find the origin of the problem and to remove the cause of damping. Another cause of distortion of the arterial waveform is underdamping, often called *overshoot* or *fling.* This is recognized by a narrow upward systolic peak that produces a false-high systolic reading when compared with the patient's cuff blood pressure as shown in Fig. 15-67. The overshoot is caused by increased dynamic response or oscillations within the system.[67,69] The monitoring system dynamic response can be checked at the bedside by performing the "square wave" or "frequency response" test. This test involves use of the manual flush system on the transducer. Normally the flush device allows only 3 ml of fluid per hour. With the normal waveform displayed, the manual fast-flush is used to generate a rapid increase in pressure, which is displayed on the monitor oscilloscope. As shown in Fig. 15-68, the normal dynamic response

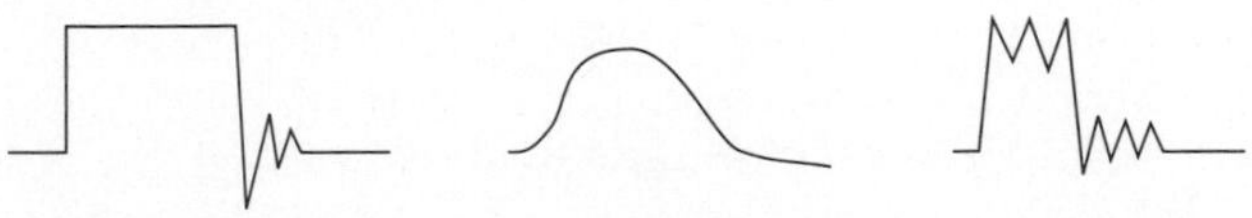

Fig. 15-68 Square wave dynamic frequency response test. **A,** Normal system dynamic response. **B,** System overdamped. **C,** System underdamped.

waveform shows a square pattern with one or two oscillations before the return of the arterial waveform. If the system is overdamped, a sloped—rather than square—pattern is seen. If the system is underdamped, there will be additional oscillations—or vibrations—seen on the "square wave."[69] See Table 15-21 for strategies to correct damping or overshoot in monitoring systems.

If either damping or overshoot is a consistent finding with a specific model of transducer or bedside monitor, the system should be serviced by the manufacturer. If there is any doubt about the accuracy of the arterial waveform, a cuff blood pressure reading should always be taken. As part of the routine nursing assessment, the cuff blood pressure is taken every shift and correlated with the intraarterial pressure.

Central Venous Pressure Monitoring

◆ **Indications.** Central venous pressure (CVP) monitoring is indicated whenever a patient has significant alteration in fluid volume (see Table 15-20). The CVP can be used as a guide in fluid volume replacement in hypovolemia and to assess the impact of diuresis after diuretic administration in the case of fluid overload. In addition, when a major IV line is required for volume replacement, a central venous line is a good choice because large volumes of fluid can easily be delivered.

◆ **Catheters.** Because many patients are awake and alert when a CVP catheter is inserted, a brief explanation about the procedure will minimize patient anxiety and gain cooperation during the insertion. This cooperation is important, because insertion is a sterile procedure and because the supine or Trendelenburg position may not be comfortable for many patients.

CVP catheters are available as single-, double-, or triple-lumen infusion catheters, depending on the specific needs of the patient. They are made from polyvinylchloride and are very soft and flexible. The catheters are designed for placement by percutaneous injection after skin preparation and administration of a local anesthetic. The standard CVP kit contains sterile towels, a needle introducer, syringe, guidewire, and catheter. The Seldinger technique, in which the vein is located by using a needle and syringe, is the preferred method of placement. A guidewire is passed through the needle, the needle is removed, and the catheter is passed over the guidewire. Once the catheter is correctly placed at the level of the right atrium, the guidewire is removed. Finally, an IV setup is attached and the catheter is sutured in place.

◆ **Insertion.** The large veins of the upper thorax (subclavian [SC] or internal jugular [IJ]) are most frequently used for percutaneous CVP line insertion. During insertion using the SC or IJ veins, the patient may be placed in a Trendelenburg position. Placing the head in a dependent position causes the internal jugular veins in the neck to become more prominent, facilitating line placement. To minimize the risk of air embolus during the procedure, the patient may be asked to "take a deep breath and hold it" any time the needle or catheter is open to air. The tip of the catheter should remain in the vena cava and not be permitted to migrate into the heart. After catheter placement, a chest radiograph may be obtained to verify placement and the absence of an iatrogenic hemothorax or pneumothorax. Other suitable insertion sites include the femoral and antecubital fossae veins. In the rare case that it is not possible to insert a CVP catheter percutaneously, a surgical cutdown may be performed.

◆ **Nursing management.** The CVP is used to measure the filling pressures of the right side of the heart. During diastole when the tricuspid valve is open and blood is flowing from the right atrium to the right ventricle, the CVP will accurately reflect right ventricular end-diastolic pressure (RVEDP). The normal CVP is 2 to 5 mm Hg (3 to 8 cm H_2O).

A low CVP often occurs in the hypovolemic patient and suggests there is insufficient blood volume in the ventricle at end-diastole to produce an adequate stroke volume. Thus to maintain normal cardiac output, the heart rate must increase.* This increase produces the tachycardia frequently observed in hypovolemic states and increases myocardial oxygen demand. An elevated CVP occurs in cases of fluid overload. To circulate the excess blood volume, the heart must greatly increase contractility to move a large volume of blood, again increasing the work load of the heart and increasing myocardial oxygen consumption.

The CVP is used in combination with the mean arterial pressure (MAP) and other clinical parameters to assess hemodynamic stability. In the hypovolemic patient, the CVP will fall before there is a significant fall in MAP because peripheral vasoconstriction will keep the MAP normal. Thus the CVP is an excellent early warning system for the patient who is bleeding, vasodilating, receiving diuretics, or rewarming after cardiac surgery. The CVP, however, is not a reliable indicator of left ventricular dysfunction. Left ventricular dysfunction, which can occur after an acute myocardial infarction, will increase filling pressures on the left side of the heart. The CVP, because it measures RVEDP, will remain normal until the increase in pressure from the left side is reflected back through the pulmonary vasculature to

*FORMULA: Heart rate times stroke volume equals cardiac output (HR × SV = CO). Thus any decrease in stroke volume must be balanced by an increase in heart rate to maintain cardiac output.

the right ventricle. In this situation a pulmonary artery catheter that measures pressures on the left side is the monitoring method of choice.[70]

To take CVP measurements the clinician has a choice of two methods: either a mercury (mm Hg) system, using a transducer and a monitor; or a water (cm H_2O) manometer system. If a patient changes from one system to the other, the CVP value will also change because mercury is heavier than water and 1 mm Hg is equal to 1.36 cm H_2O. To convert water to mercury, the water value is divided by 1.36 ($H_2O \div 1.36$). To convert mercury to water, the mercury value is multiplied by 1.36 (mm Hg $\times$ 1.36). To achieve accurate CVP measurements, the phlebostatic axis should be used as a reference point on the body and the transducer or water manometer zero must be level with this point. If the phlebostatic axis is used and the transducer or water manometer is correctly aligned, any head-of-bed position of up to 45 degrees may be accurately used for CVP readings for most patients.[71] Elevating the head of the bed is especially helpful for the patient with respiratory or cardiac problems who will not tolerate a flat position.

The risk of air embolus, although uncommon, is always present for the patient with a central venous line in place. Air can enter during insertion, through a disconnected or broken catheter, or along the path of a removed CVP catheter. This is more likely if the patient is in an upright position, because air can be pulled into the venous system with the increase in negative intrathoracic pressure during inhalation. If a large volume of air (200 to 300 cc) is infused rapidly, it may become trapped in the right ventricular outflow tract, stopping blood flow from the right side of the heart to the lungs. The patient may experience respiratory distress and cardiovascular collapse. Treatment involves administering 100% oxygen and placing the patient on the left side with the head downward (left lateral Trendelenburg position). This position displaces the air from the right ventricular outflow tract to the apex of the heart where it can be either resorbed or aspirated. Precautions to prevent an air embolism in a CVP line include using only Luer-Lok connections, avoiding long loops of IV tubing, and using screw caps on three-way stopcocks.[72]

◆ **CVP waveform interpretation.** The right atrial (CVP) waveform has three positive deflections—called *a, c,* and *v waves*—that correspond to specific atrial events in the cardiac cycle (Fig. 15-69). The *a wave* reflects atrial contraction and follows the P wave seen on the ECG. The downslope of this wave is called the *x descent* and represents atrial relaxation. The *c wave* reflects the bulging of the closed tricuspid valve into the right atrium during ventricular contraction. The *c wave* is small and not always visible but corresponds to the QRS-T interval on the ECG. The *v wave* represents atrial filling and pressure increase against the closed tricuspid valve in early diastole. The downslope of the *v wave* is named the *y descent* and represents the fall in pressure as the tricuspid valve opens and blood flows from the right atrium to the right ventricle. Certain heart rhythms can change the normal CVP waveform. In atrial fibrillation the CVP waveform has no recognizable pattern because of the disorganization of the atria. In a junctional rhythm or after a premature ventricular contraction (PVC), the atria are depolarized after the ventricles if there is retrograde conduction to the atria. This may be seen as a retrograde P wave on the ECG and as a large combined *ac wave* or *cannon wave* on the CVP waveform (Fig. 15-70). These cannon waves can be easily detected as large "pulses" in the jugular veins. Other pathologic conditions, such as advanced right ventricular failure or

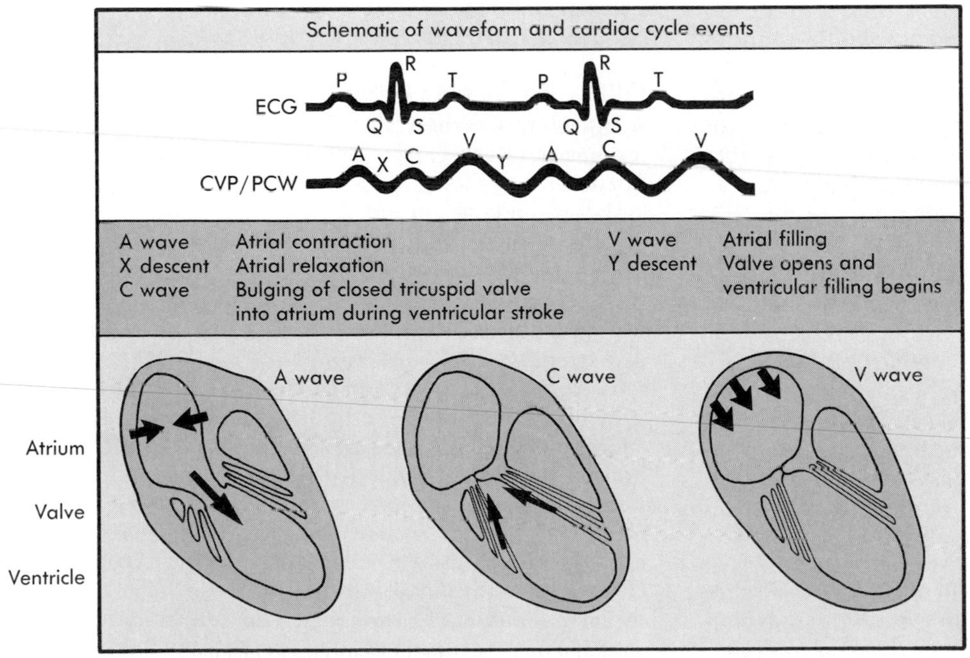

Fig. 15-69 Cardiac events that produce the CVP waveform with a, c, and v waves. A wave represents atrial contraction. X descent represents atrial relaxation. C wave represents the bulging of the closed tricuspid valve into the right atrium during ventricular systole. V wave represents atrial filling. Y descent represents opening of the tricuspid valve and filling of the ventricle.

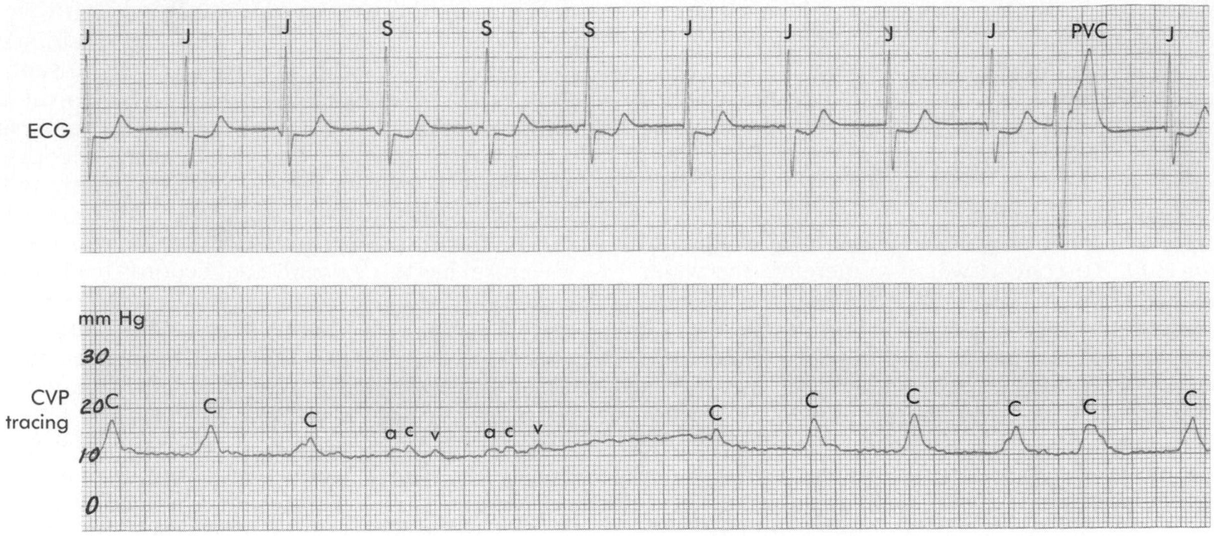

Fig. 15-70 Simultaneous ECG and CVP tracing. The CVP waveform shows large cannon waves (c waves) corresponding to the junctional beats or premature ventricular contractions *(strip above)*. As the patient converts to sinus rhythm, the CVP waveform has a normal configuration. *J,* Junctional rhythm followed by cannon waves on CVP waveform; *PVC,* premature ventricular contraction followed by cannon wave on CVP; *S,* sinus rhythm followed by normal CVP tracing with a, c, and v waves; *C,* cannon waves on CVP tracing; *ac,* normal right atrial pressure tracing.

tricuspid valve insufficiency, allow regurgitant backflow of blood from the right ventricle to the right atrium during ventricular contraction, producing large *v waves* on the right atrial waveform.

Left Atrial Pressure Monitoring

◆ **Indications.** Left atrial pressure (LAP) monitoring is used in selected cases after major cardiac surgery. Until the advent of the pulmonary artery catheter in the 1970s, LAP monitoring was used to assess hemodynamics on the left side of the heart. Today it is not used for routine monitoring. It is a clinical choice on rare occasions in the postoperative management of the cardiac surgery patient who has significant pulmonary hypertension.[73] In this situation, accurate left atrial pressures may be difficult to obtain with a pulmonary artery catheter.

◆ **Insertion.** The LAP catheter is inserted into the left atrium during open heart surgery. The single-lumen catheter exits through the chest wall and is attached to a routine hemodynamic monitoring setup that contains an in-line air filter.

◆ **Nursing management.** The placement of the LAP catheter directly into the left atrium places the patient at particular risk for air or tissue emboli. Nursing care is planned to reduce these equipment-related risks. An in-line air filter is added to the flush system that contains heparin to reduce the risk of air emboli. If the waveform becomes damped, noninvasive methods of troubleshooting—such as repositioning the patient—are performed. The catheter is not manually flushed, because to do so may increase the risk of emboli, resulting from clot formation at the tip of the catheter. Pericardial tamponade is a potential complication of LAP catheter removal. Therefore mediastinal chest tubes should be left in position until after the catheter is removed. Because of these risks, the LAP catheter is rarely left in place for more than 48 hours.

◆ **LAP waveform interpretation.** The LAP waveform consists of two positive deflections, which are termed the *a* and *v waves.* The *a wave* represents atrial contraction, and the *v wave* represents filling of the left atrium against a closed mitral valve. Normal LAP pressure ranges from 5 to 12 mm Hg and is elevated with mitral valve disease or severe heart failure on the left side.

Pulmonary Artery Pressure Monitoring

◆ **Indications.** When specific hemodynamic and intracardiac data are required for diagnostic and treatment purposes, a thermodilution pulmonary artery (PA) catheter may be inserted. This catheter is used for diagnosis and evaluation of heart disease, shock states, and medical conditions that compromise cardiac output or fluid volume. In addition, the PA catheter is used to evaluate patient response to treatment, as described in Table 15-22.

A significant advantage of the PA catheter over the previously described methods of monitoring is that it simultaneously assesses several hemodynamic parameters—including pulmonary artery systolic and diastolic pressures, the pulmonary artery mean pressure, and the pulmonary artery wedge pressure (PAWP)—and includes the capability of measuring cardiac output and of calculating additional parameters.

◆ **Cardiac output determinants.** The determinants of CO that can be measured by the PA catheter include *preload, afterload,* and *contractility* (see box, p. 256). The fourth

Table 15-22 Pulmonary artery catheters: selected indications for use and response to treatment

Diagnostic indications*	Possible cause	Associated clinical findings	Hemodynamic profile†	Treatment and expected response
Hypovolemic shock	Trauma Surgery Bleeding Burns Excessive diuresis	Cardiovascular (CV): sinus tachycardia, decreased blood pressure (BP) (systolic blood pressure [SBP] <90 mm Hg), weak peripheral pulses Pulmonary: lungs clear Renal: decreased urinary output Skin: normal skin temperature, no edema Neurologic: variable	Low cardiac output (CO) Low cardiac index (CI) (<2.2 L/min/m^2) High systemic vascular resistance (SVR) (>1600 dynes/sec/cm^{-5}) Low pulmonary artery pressure (PAP) Low pulmonary artery wedge pressure (PAWP)	Treatment: fluid challenge Expected hemodynamic response: Decreased heart rate (HR) Increased BP Increased PA Increased PAWP Increased central venous pressure (CVP) Increased CO/CI Decreased SVR
Early septic shock	Sepsis	CV: sinus tachycardia, decreased BP (SBP <90 mm Hg), bounding peripheral pulses Pulmonary: lungs may be clear *or* congested, depending on the origin of the sepsis Renal: decreased urinary output Skin: warm and flushed Neurologic: variable	High CO (>8 L/min) High CI Low SVR (<600 dynes/sec/cm^{-5}) Low PAP Low PAWP Low CVP	Treatment: IV fluid to maintain hemodynamic function Peripheral vasoconstricting agent (alpha) to increase SVR Antibiotics and laboratory cultures to find site of infection Expected hemodynamic response: Decreased HR Increased BP Increased PA pressures Increased PAWP/increased CVP Increased CO/CI Increased SVR
Advanced septic shock or multisystem failure shock	Sepsis Multiple Organ Dysfunction Syndrome (MODS)	CV: normal sinus rhythm or sinus tachycardia, decreased BP, weak peripheral pulses Pulmonary: lungs may be clear *or* congested, depending on the site of sepsis; acidosis based on arterial blood gas (ABG) values, may require mechanical ventilation Renal: decreased urinary output, may have increased blood urea nitrogen (BUN) and increased creatinine levels Skin: cool and mottled Neurologic: variable, depending on fluid status and drugs used in treatment	Low CO Low CI (<2.2 L/min/m^2) High SVR (>1600 dynes/sec/cm^{-5}) High or low PAP High or low PAWP High or low CVP	Treatment: Vasodilators to decrease SVR Antibiotics Support of body systems as necessary (e.g., mechanical ventilation or hemodialysis) Expected hemodynamic response: Decreased HR Increased BP Normal PA/PAWP/CVP pressures Decreased SVR, decreased pulmonary vascular resistance Increased CO/CI

*Patients undergoing major vascular or cardiac surgery may also have a PA catheter in situ to follow the trend of CO/CI, SVR/PVR, and fluid status during the first 24 hours after surgery.
†See Table 15-20 for definitions and Appendix C for normal values of hemodynamic parameters listed in this table.

Continued.

Table 15-22 Pulmonary artery catheters: selected indications for use and response to treatment—cont'd

Diagnostic indications*	Possible cause	Associated clinical findings	Hemodynamic profile†	Treatment and expected response
Cardiogenic shock	Left ventricular pump failure caused by acute myocardial infarction, severe mitral or aortic valve disease	CV: sinus tachycardia, possibly dysrhythmias, BP <90 mm Hg systolic, S_3 or S_4, weak peripheral pulses Pulmonary: lungs may have crackles or pulmonary edema Renal: decreased urinary output Skin: cool, pale, and moist Neurologic: may have decreased mentation caused by low BP and CO	Low CO Low CI (<2.2 L/min/m^2) High SVR (>1600 dynes/sec/cm^{-5}) High PAP High PAWP (>15 mm Hg) High CVP Low stroke volume index (SI) Low left cardiac work index (LCWI) Low left ventricular stroke work index (LVSWI)	Treatment: Inotropic drugs to increase left ventricular contractility Vasodilators or intraaortic balloon pump (IABP) to decrease afterload Diuretics to decrease preload Optimization of heart rate and control of dysrhythmias Expected hemodynamic response: Decreased HR Increased BP Decreased PAP Decreased PAWP Decreased CVP Decreased SVR Decreased PVR Increased CO/CI Increased SI Increased LCWI Increased LVSWI
Acute respiratory distress syndrome (ARDS) *or* noncardiogenic pulmonary edema	Trauma Sepsis Shock Inhaled toxins (smoke, chemicals, 100% oxygen) Aspiration of gastric contents Metabolic disorders	CV: sinus tachycardia, high or low BP, normal peripheral pulses Pulmonary: poor oxygenation and pulmonary edema, increased respiratory rate, or need for mechanical ventilation Renal: increased or decreased urinary output Skin: normal temperature Neurologic: anxiety or confusion associated with respiratory distress and poor oxygenation	Normal CO Normal CI Normal SVR Normal PAWP High PAP High PVR (>250 dynes/sec/cm^{-5}) Low right cardiac work index (RCWI) Low right ventricular stroke work index (RVSWI)	Treatment: Eliminate cause of ARDS Support pulmonary function as necessary Expected hemodynamic response: Decreased HR Normal BP Decreased PAP Decreased PVR Increased RCWI Increased RVSWI Normal CO/CI Normal SVR

DETERMINANTS OF CARDIAC OUTPUT

- Preload
- Afterload
- Contractility
- Heart rate

factor, *heart rate,* is not measured by the PA catheter. To assist in understanding the purpose and usefulness of the PA catheter, a review of the components of CO is presented here.

Preload. Clinicians frequently describe the hemodynamic numbers related to preload as "filling pressures." These numbers include pulmonary artery diastolic (PAD) pressure, left-atrial pressure (LAP), and pulmonary artery wedge pressure (PAWP), which measure preload in the left side of the heart, and CVP, which measures preload in the right side. Preload is the *volume* in the ventricle at end-diastole. Because diastole is the filling stage of the cardiac cycle, the volume in the ventricle at end-diastole represents the presystolic volume available for ejection for that cardiac cycle. It is not possible to measure left ventricular volume directly in the critical care unit. However, the presence of blood within the ventricle creates pressures that can be measured by the PA catheter and bedside monitoring computer. When the PA catheter is correctly positioned, the only valve between the PA catheter tip and the LV is the mitral valve. During diastole, when the mitral valve is open, there is no obstruction between the tip of the PA catheter and the left ventricle (Fig. 15-71). The LV preload volume creates *left ventricular end-diastolic pressure* (LVEDP). This is measured clinically by the *left atrial pressure* (LAP) or the *pulmonary artery wedge pressure* (PAWP). The PAWP is the value most frequently referred to in this chapter, because it is the value that is most often used in clinical practice. Normal LAP or PAWP is 5 to 12 mm Hg.

Clinically the PAWP has significance because a change in left ventricular volume (preload) will be reflected by a change in the measured PAWP. Change in preload relies on a concept known as *Starling's law of the heart*. This concept states that the force of ventricular ejection is directly related to two elements: (1) the volume in the ventricle at end-diastole (preload) and (2) the amount of myocardial stretch placed on the ventricle as a result. If the volume in the left ventricle is low, CO will also be suboptimal. If intravenous fluids (volume) are infused, CO will increase as LV volume and myocardial fiber stretch increase. This is true up to a point. Past this point, more fluid volume will overdistend the ventricle and stretch the myocardial fibers so much that cardiac output will actually decrease. This scenario is seen clinically in the setting of acute heart failure with pulmonary edema. The impact of preload on CO is represented in Figs. 15-72 and 15-73 using the Starling curve as a model.

The relationship of preload, PAWP, and CO is made more complex by the fact that not all preload volume is ejected with every heartbeat. The percentage of preload volume ejected from the left ventricle per beat is measured during cardiac catheterization and is described as the *ejection fraction* (EF). The volume ejected from the left ventricle with each beat is known as the *stroke volume* (SV) and can be measured at the bedside. In a patient with dilated cardiomyopathy, the preload volume might be 100 ml. However, the stroke volume ejected may be only 30 ml. The ejection fraction in this patient is 30%. The remaining preload volume (70 ml in this example) will significantly elevate PAWP. When the mitral valve opens at the beginning of diastole, the pressure in the left atrium (LA) needs to be slightly higher than pressures in the LV to allow filling. The 70 ml remaining in the ventricle will produce high LV diastolic pressures. This will elevate the LA filling pressure and consequently elevate PAWP. In this example the left ventricle is overstretched by excessive preload, and therefore CO will be below normal. A plan of care for this patient would include decreasing LV preload through restriction of IV/PO fluids, venodilation, and diuresis.

A significant relationship exists between LVEDP and myocardial dysfunction. As a general rule, the higher the LVEDP, the greater is the degree of myocardial dysfunction because the compromised ventricle is unable to eject all of the preload blood volume. A normal left ventricular EF is 70%. The greater the degree of myocardial dysfunction, the lower is the EF and the higher the preload and LVEDP.

LVEDP can be measured by two methods using a PA catheter. The most accurate is the PAWP. The second method involves using pulmonary artery diastolic (PAD)

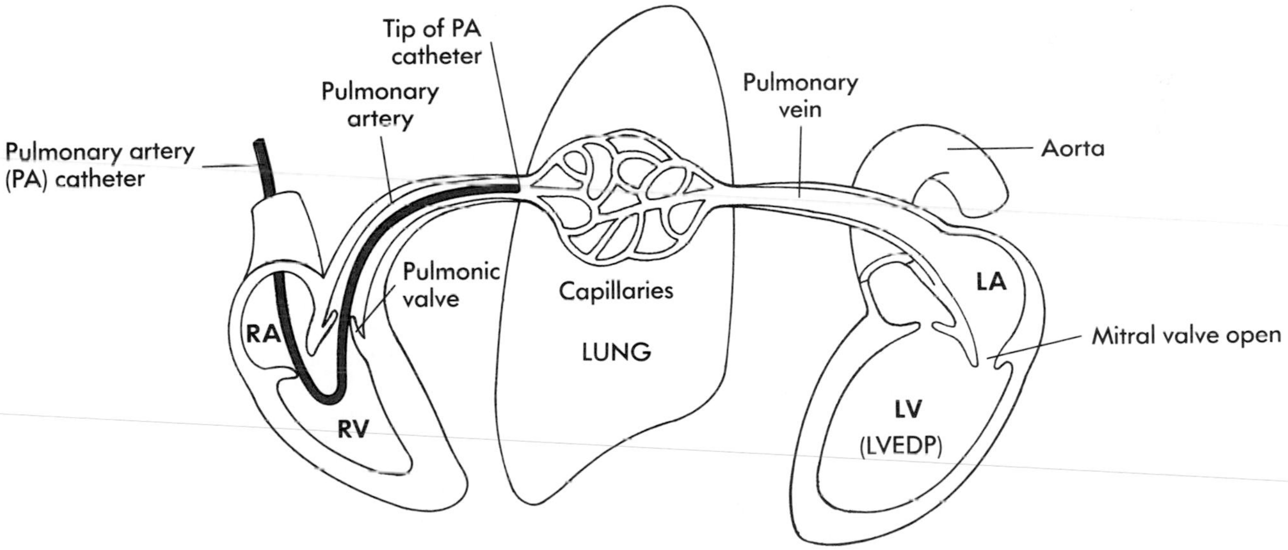

Fig. 15-71 Relationship of PAWP to LVEDP/preload. This diagram illustrates why, in the majority of clinical situations, the PAWP accurately reflects LVEDP or preload. During diastole, when the mitral valve is open, there are no other valves or other obstructions between the tip of the catheter and the left ventricle. Thus the pressure exerted by the volume in the LV is reflected back through the left atrium through the pulmonary veins and to the pulmonary capillaries.

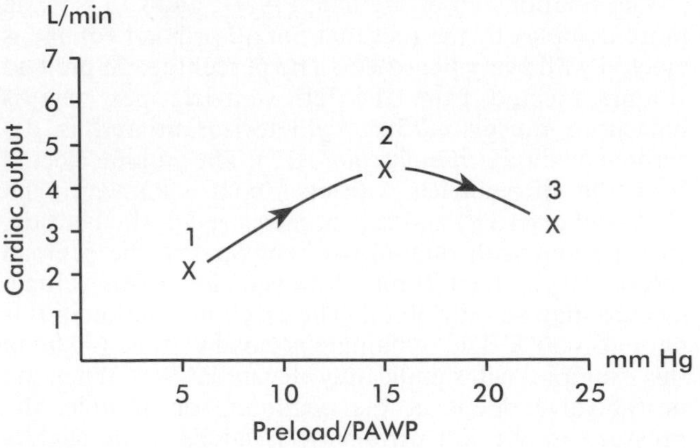

Fig. 15-72 Impact of preload on CO. *1,* Poor CO with low preload as a result of hypovolemia. *2,* Hypovolemia is corrected after the administration of 2 L of intravenous (IV) fluid. The preload volume in the ventricle is increased, and PAWP has risen. Because of the increased fiber stretch secondary to the increase in preload, CO has also risen. *3,* After the infusion of 2 more liters of IV solution, the myocardial fibers are overdistended, preload (PAWP) has increased, and CO has fallen as the volume in the left ventricle rises.

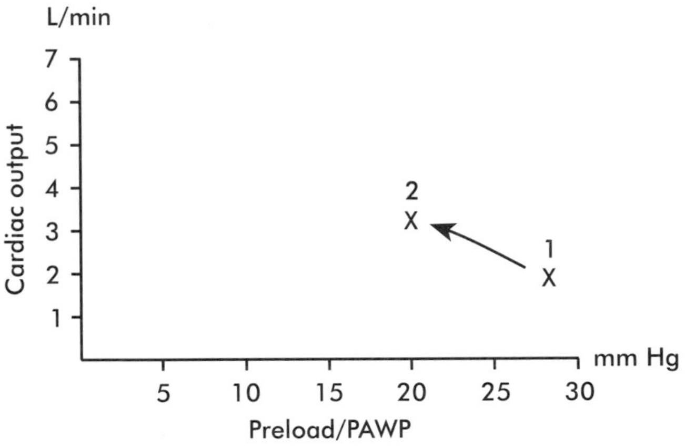

Fig. 15-73 Impact of preload and venodilation on CO. *1,* After an acute anterior wall myocardial infarction that has created significant left ventricular dysfunction, this patient has LV-pump failure with low CO and elevated filling pressures (↑ PAWP). One of the clinical problems faced by this patient is too much preload. *2,* After administration of diuretics to remove volume and nitroglycerin to dilate the venous system, preload is reduced and CO rises.

pressure, because during diastole in most patients, the PAD is equal to or 1 to 3 mm Hg higher than the mean PAWP and LVEDP. It is important to be aware that specific clinical conditions can alter the normal PAD/PAWP relationship. If the patient has lung disease that has elevated the PA pressures independently from the cardiac pressures, the PAD pressure will not accurately reflect function of the left side of the heart. The clinical conditions that cause PA pressures to rise but PAWP to remain normal are primary pulmonary hypertension and adult respiratory distress syndrome (ARDS). The difference between the PAD and the PAWP is called a *gradient.* Thus, when the PA catheter is inserted, if there is a large gradient between the PAWP and PAD pressure, the patient may have significant lung disease, (Table 15-23, *C*). In failure of the left side of the heart, both the PAWP and the PAD pressure will be elevated and approximately equal (see Table 15-22). It is physiologically impossible for the PAWP to ever be higher than the PAD pressure. The nurse should recalibrate and troubleshoot the monitoring system if this occurs (see Table 15-21).

Pathology of the mitral valve, either stenosis or regurgitation, alters the accuracy of PAWP and PAD pressures as parameters of left ventricular function. In mitral valve stenosis, left atrial pressure and PAWP are increased and cause pulmonary congestion; however, these values are *not* reflective of LVEDP because a stenotic mitral valve decreases normal blood flow from the left atrium to the left ventricle, decreasing left ventricular preload and consequently lowering LVEDP. Therefore a nonstenotic mitral valve is essential for accurate readings because a narrowed mitral valve increases PAWP and PAD pressure in the presence of a normal LVEDP. If mitral regurgitation (MR) is present, the mean PAWP reading is artificially elevated because of abnormal backflow of blood from the left ventricle to the left atrium during systole. This PAWP reading is distinguished by very large v waves on the PAWP tracing and may not be reflective of true LVEDP (Table 15-23, *F*).

The v waves can be dramatic in some patients. However, the size of the v wave is not related to the amount of mitral regurgitation, but to the compliance of the left atrium. If the mitral regurgitation is chronic and the left atrium is compliant, v waves may not be large. By contrast, in the setting of acute mitral regurgitation after infarction of a papillary muscle, the noncompliant atrium contributes to the large v waves.[74,75] Reading the PAWP tracing in the presence of mitral regurgitation is difficult. It has been suggested that if there are large v waves (acute MR), the trough of the x descent is the best predictor of LVEDP. If the v wave is small (chronic MR), the mean PAWP or LAP pressure can still estimate LV preload (LVEDP).[74,75]

Afterload. Afterload is defined as the pressure the ventricle has to generate to overcome the resistance to ejection created by the arteries and arterioles. It is a calculated measurement derived from information obtained from the PA catheter. As a response to increased afterload, ventricular wall tension rises. After a decrease in afterload, wall tension is lowered. Systemic or arterial afterload is measured by the *systemic vascular resistance* (SVR). Resistance of the right side of the heart is measured by the *pulmonary vascular resistance* (PVR). The PVR value is normally one sixth of the SVR. Normal SVR is 800 to 1200 dynes/sec/cm^{-5}, and normal PVR is 50 to 250 dynes/sec/cm^{-5}.

Pharmacologic manipulation of afterload to improve cardiac performance is frequently used with cardiac

Table 15-23 Clinical interpretation of pulmonary artery (PA) waveforms

PA pressure	Clinical interpretation	mm Hg	Waveform interpretation
Pulmonary artery systolic (PAS) pressure	PAS pressure reflects the systolic pressure in the pulmonary vasculature. See waveform A for normal waveform. It is elevated in pulmonary hypertension because of idiopathic causes, in some congenital heart defects, and in lung disease.		**Normal** 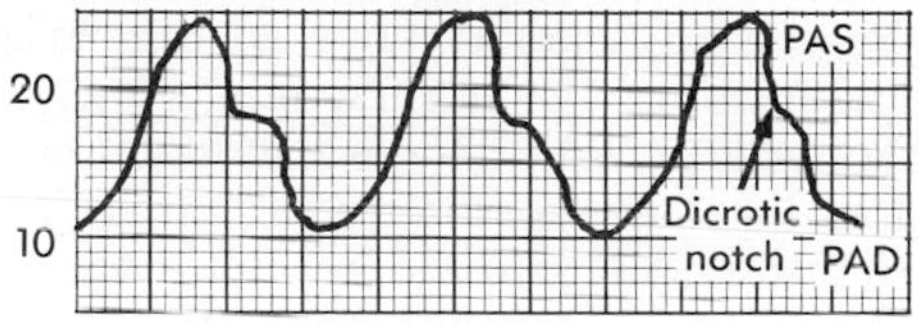 A
Pulmonary artery diastolic (PAD) pressure	In the patient with healthy lung vasculature, PAD pressure reflects left ventricular end-diastolic pressure (LVEDP), as shown in waveform B.		**PAD/PAWP Correlation in a Patient with Normal Lungs** 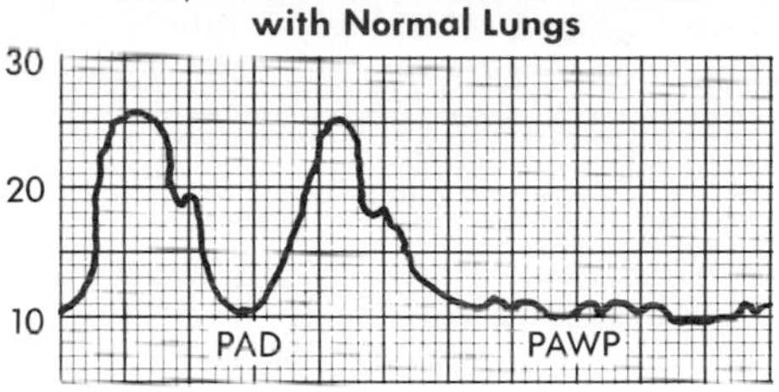 B
	In the presence of lung disease or pulmonary hypertension, PAD pressure is *not* an accurate reflection of pulmonary artery wedge pressure (PAWP), as shown in waveform C.		**Poor PAD/PAWP Correlation in a Patient with Lung Disease** 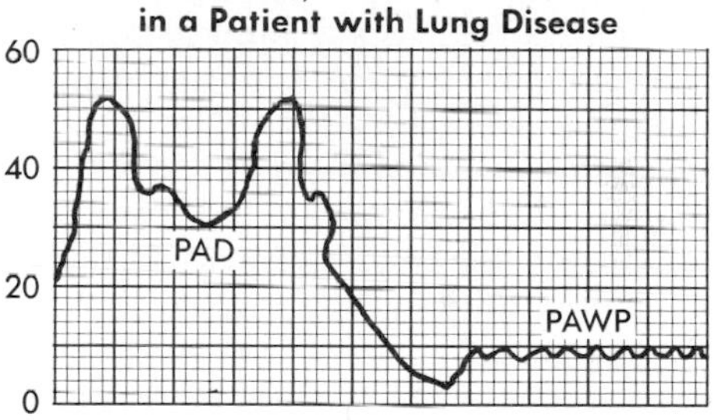 C
Mean pulmonary artery pressure (PAP mean or PAP_M)	PAP mean pressure is used in the calculation of pulmonary vascular resistance (PVR) and pulmonary vascular resistance index (PVRI) as described in Table 15-20. High mean pressures can be reflective of either cardiac or pulmonary disease. Low mean pressures are reflection of hypovolemia. See waveform D for PA mean placement.		**Placement of PAP Mean Value** 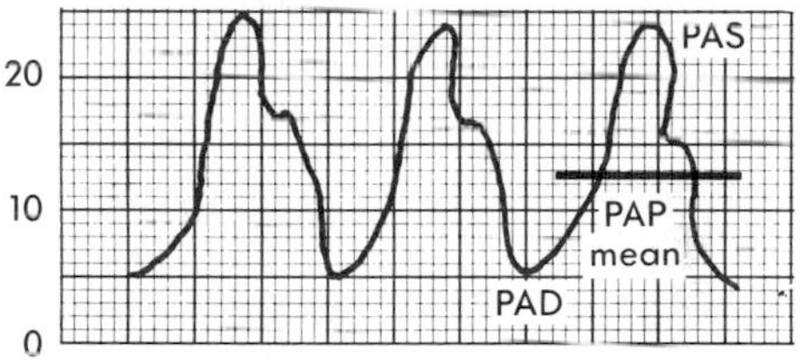 D
Pulmonary artery wedge pressure (PAWP) or pulmonary capillary wedge pressure (PCWP)	In the healthy patient, PAWP reflects blood in the left ventricle at end-diastole (LVEDP). The normal PAWP waveform is a left atrial waveform, as shown in waveform E.		**Normal PAWP Tracing with a and v Waves** 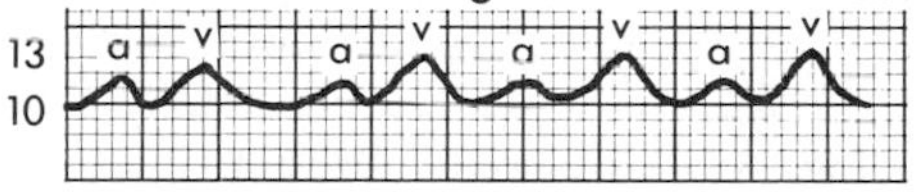 E
	If a patient has mitral valve regurgitation, the v waves are larger than normal, increasing PAWP and possibly not reflecting true LVEDP, as shown in waveform F.		**PAWP Tracing with Elevated v Waves caused by Mitral Valve Regurgitation** 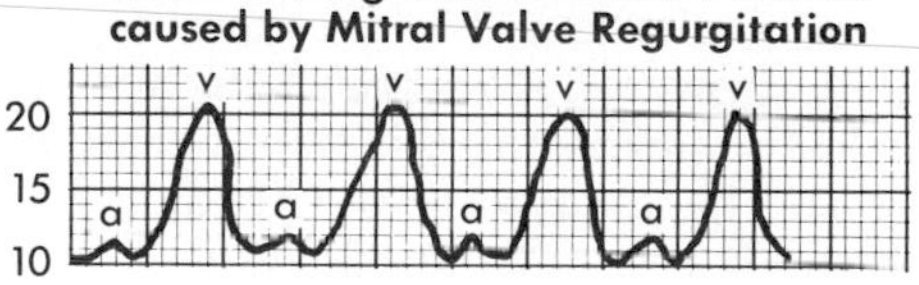 F
	PAWP is elevated in many cardiac disease states in which left ventricular function is compromised. PAWP is low in hypovolemic states.		

patients. For example, Mr. T had a large anterior wall myocardial infarction (MI) 2 days ago. As a result, he has symptoms of acute heart failure, an elevated SVR of 1840 dynes/sec/cm^{-5}, and a CO of 2.8 L/min. In a heart with decreased contractility after an MI, an afterload measurement above the normal range lowers cardiac output. To optimize Mr. T's cardiac function, systemic vasodilators or "afterload-reducing drugs" are prescribed to lower SVR into the normal range. After the administration of sodium nitroprusside 1 to 4 mcg/kg/min, Mr. T's SVR fell to 1070 and his CO increased to 3.9 L/min. In contrast, for the person with a normal heart without cardiac dysfunction, an elevated SVR may have minimal impact on CO. In summary, the importance of afterload on CO is related to the functional quality of the myocardium. Whether the heart muscle is globally damaged (cardiomyopathy) or regionally damaged (MI), small changes in SVR can produce significant changes in CO.

Contractility. Cardiac contractility, or inotropy, is the product of many factors that have an impact on myocardial muscle function. These factors can have either a positive inotropic effect and enhance contractility or a negative inotropic effect and decrease contractility. Significant factors related to contractility that can be measured by the PA catheter include preload filling pressures, afterload, CO, and left and right stroke work index values (LVSWI and RVSWI). LVSWI is a derived value that measures the force of cardiac contraction (see Table 15-20). Other factors that have an impact on contractility include myocardial oxygenation, electrolyte balance, positive and negative inotropic drugs, and the amount of functional myocardium available to contribute to contraction. Preload has an impact on contractility by Starling's mechanism. As volume in the ventricle rises, contractility increases. If the ventricle is overdistended with volume, contractility falls (see Figs. 15-72 and 15-73). Afterload alters contractility by changes in resistance to ventricular ejection. If afterload is high, contractility is decreased. If afterload is low, contractility is augmented. Hypoxemia also acts as a negative inotrope. The myocardium must have oxygen available to the cells to contract efficiently. In addition, specific electrolytes alter contractility—calcium is a positive inotrope, whereas hyperkalemia may result in asystole.

Intravenous drugs such as dopamine and dobutamine are prescribed for their positive inotropic effect, whereas beta blockers such as Inderal have a negative inotropic impact and lower CO. The nurse considers the impact of these pharmacologic agents on contractility when following the trend of the patient's hemodynamic profile. There is no single hemodynamic number that reflects contractility. However, if LV contractility is increased in response to treatment, this will be reflected by changes in PAWP and by an increase in CO and LVSWI.

◆ **Catheters.** The traditional pulmonary artery (PA) catheter, invented by Swan and Ganz, has four lumens for measurement of right atrial pressure (RAP or CVP), PA pressures, PAWP, and CO (Fig. 15-74, *A*). Multifunction catheters may have additional lumens, which can be used for IV infusion (Fig. 15-74, *B*), to measure continuous mixed venous oxygen saturation (Svo_2), right ventricular volume (Fig. 15-74, *C*), continuous cardiac output (Fig. 15-74, *D*), or to pace the heart using transvenous pacing electrodes.

The PA catheter is 110 cm in length, and it is made of polyvinylchloride. This supple material is ideal for flow-directional catheters. The most frequently used size is 7.5 Fr, although 5.0 and 7.0 Fr sizes are available. Each of the four lumens exits into the heart at a different point along the catheter length (see Fig. 15-74, *A*). The proximal (CVP) lumen is situated in the right atrium and is used for IV infusion, CVP measurement, withdrawal of venous blood samples, and injection of fluid for CO determinations. The distal (PA) lumen is located at the end of the PA catheter and is situated in the pulmonary artery. It is used to record PA pressures and can be used for withdrawal of blood samples to measure Svo_2. The third lumen opens into a latex balloon at the end of the catheter that can be inflated with 0.8 (7 Fr) to 1.5 (7.5 Fr) ml of air. The balloon is inflated during catheter insertion once the catheter reaches the right atrium, to assist in forward flow of the catheter and to minimize right ventricular ectopy from the catheter tip. It is also inflated to obtain PAWP measurements when the PA catheter is correctly positioned in the pulmonary artery.[75] The fourth lumen is a thermistor used to measure changes in blood temperature. It is located 4 cm from the catheter tip and is used to measure thermodilution CO. The connector end of the lumen is attached directly to the CO computer.

If continuous Svo_2 will be measured, the catheter will have an additional fiberoptic lumen that exits at the tip of the catheter (Fig. 15-74, *C*). If cardiac pacing will be used, two PA catheter methods are available. One type of catheter has three atrial (A) and two ventricular (V) pacing electrodes attached to the catheter so that when it is properly positioned, the patient can be connected to a pacemaker and AV paced. The other catheter method uses a specific transvenous pacing wire that passes through an additional catheter lumen and exits in the right ventricle if ventricular pacing is required. In addition, a right ventricular volumetric PA catheter is available that measures stroke volume in the RV. (Fig. 15-74, *C*).

◆ **Insertion.** If a PA catheter is to be inserted into a patient who is awake, some brief explanations about the procedure are helpful to ensure that the patient understands what is going to happen. The insertion techniques used for placement of a PA catheter are similar to those described in the section on CVP line insertion. In addition, because the PA catheter will be positioned within the heart chambers and pulmonary artery on the right side of the heart, catheter passage is monitored, using either fluoroscopy or waveform analysis on the bedside monitor (Fig. 15-75).

Before inserting the catheter into the vein, the physician—using sterile technique—will test the balloon for inflation and will flush the catheter with normal saline solution to remove any air. The PA catheter is then attached to the bedside hemodynamic line setup

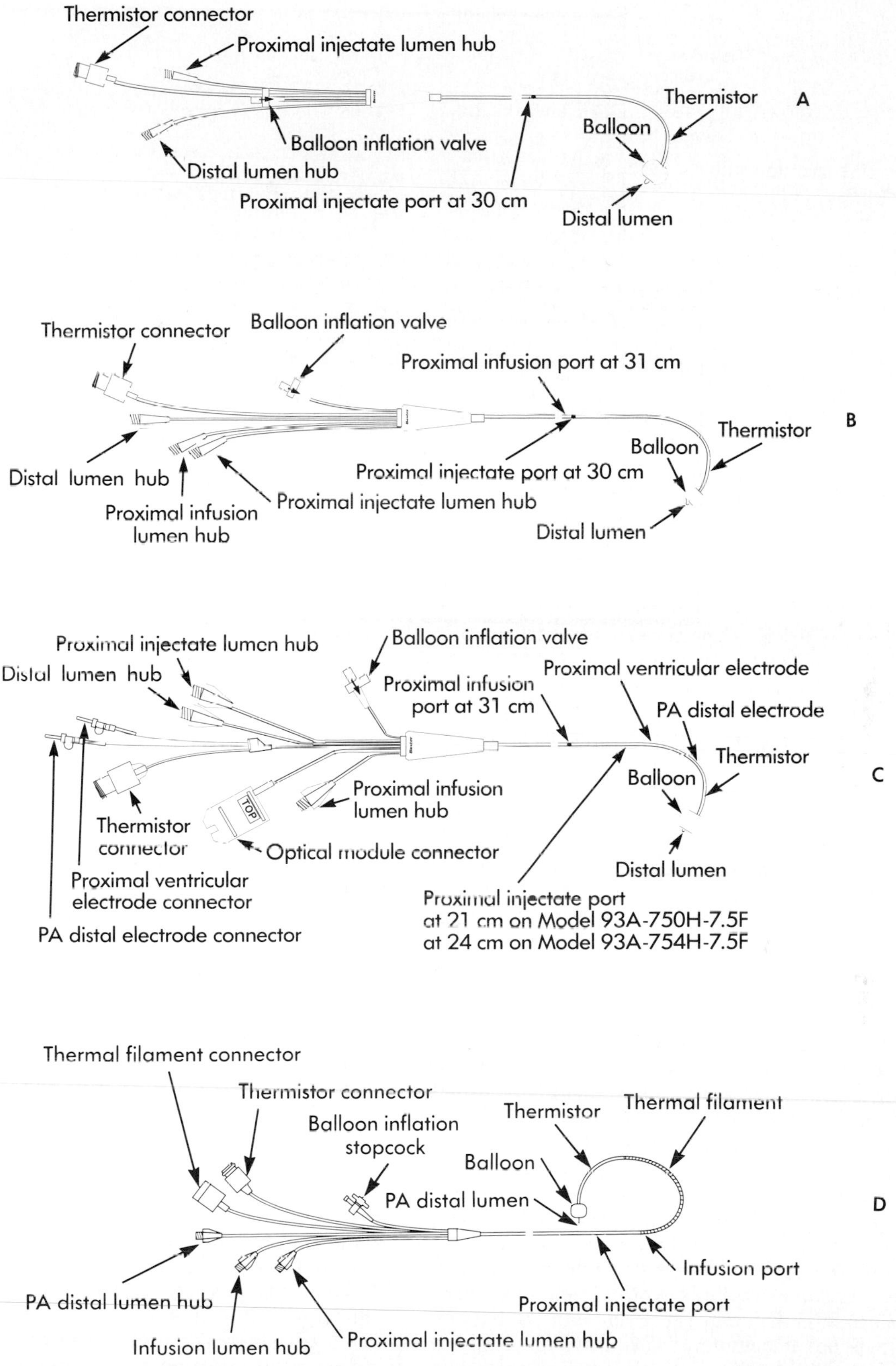

Fig. 15-74 Types of pulmonary artery catheters available for clinical use. **A**, Four-lumen catheter. **B**, Five-lumen catheter that includes an additional infusion lumen in the right atrium. **C**, Multifunction six-lumen catheter that combines an additional infusion lumen, right ventricular volume measurement, and continuous SvO_2 monitoring. **D**, Six-lumen catheter with continuous cardiac output capability. (Courtesy Baxter Healthcare Corporation, Edwards Critical Care Division.)

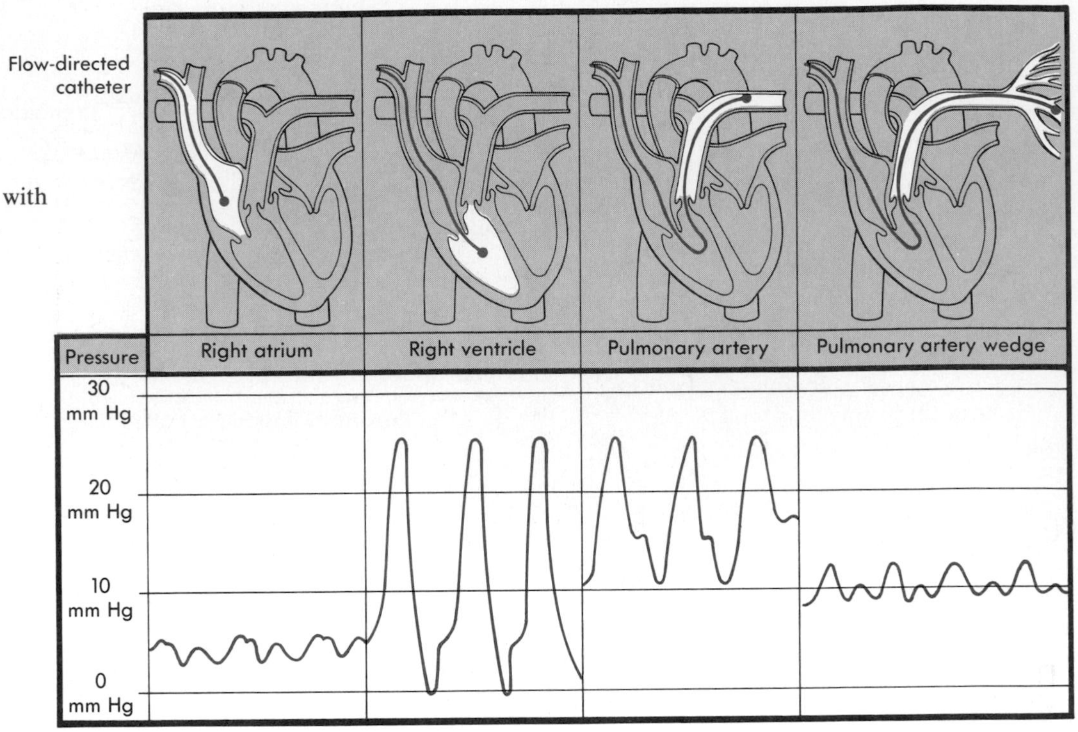

Fig. 15-75 PA insertion with corresponding waveforms.

and monitor, so that the waveforms can be visualized while the catheter is advanced through the right side of the heart (see Fig. 15-75). A larger introducer sheath (8.5 Fr), with the tip in the vena cava and an additional IV side-port lumen, is often used to cannulate the vein first. This remains in place, and the supple PA catheter is threaded through the introducer.

◆ **Pulmonary artery waveform interpretation.** As the PA catheter is advanced into the right atrium during insertion, a right atrial waveform should be visible on the monitor, with recognizable a, c, and v waves (see Fig. 15-75). The normal mean pressure in the right atrium is 2 to 5 mm Hg. Before passage through the tricuspid valve, the balloon at the tip of the catheter is inflated for two reasons. First, it cushions the pointed tip of the PA catheter so that if the tip comes into contact with the right ventricular wall, it will cause less myocardial irritability and consequently fewer ventricular dysrhythmias. Second, inflation of the balloon assists the catheter to float with the flow of blood from the right ventricle into the pulmonary artery. It is because of the features and balloon that PA catheters are described as flow-directional catheters. The right ventricular waveform has a saw-toothed pattern and is pulsatile, with distinct systolic and diastolic pressures. Normal right ventricular pressures are 20-30/0-5 mm Hg. Even with the balloon inflated, it is not uncommon for ventricular ectopy to occur during passage through the RV. All patients who have a PA catheter inserted must have simultaneous electrocardiographic monitoring, with defibrillator and emergency resuscitation equipment nearby.

As the catheter enters the pulmonary artery, the waveform again changes. The diastolic pressure rises. Normal PA systolic and diastolic pressures are 20- 30/10 mm Hg. A dicrotic notch, visible on the downslope of the waveform, represents closure of the pulmonic valve.

While the balloon remains inflated, the catheter is advanced into the wedge position. Here, the waveform decreases in size and is nonpulsatile—reflective of a normal left atrial tracing with *a* and *v wave* deflections. This is described as a *wedge tracing,* because the balloon is "wedged" into a small pulmonary vessel[76] (see Fig. 15-75). The balloon occludes the pulmonary vessel so that the PA lumen is exposed only to left atrial pressure and is protected from the pulsatile influence of the PA. When the balloon is deflated, the catheter should spontaneously float back into the PA. When the balloon is reinflated, the wedge tracing should be visible. The normal PAWP ranges from 5 to 12 mm Hg.

After insertion, the catheter is sutured to the skin, and a chest radiograph is taken to verify placement. If the catheter is advanced too far into the pulmonary bed, the patient is at risk for pulmonary infarction. If the catheter is not sufficiently advanced into the PA, it will not be useful for PAWP readings. However, in many critical care units, if the patient's PAD and PAWP values approximate (within 0 to 3 mm Hg), the PAD is reliably used to follow the trend of LV-filling pressure (preload). This avoids possible trauma from frequent balloon inflation. In this situation the PA catheter is consciously pulled back into a nonwedging position in the pulmonary artery. After insertion, a chest radiograph or fluroscopy is used to verify PA catheter position, to verify that it is not looped or knotted in the RV, and to rule out pneumothorax or hemorrhagic complications. A thin plastic cuff can be placed on the outside of the catheter when it is inserted to maintain sterility of that part of the PA catheter that exits from the patient. Then, if the catheter is not in the desired position or if it migrates out of position, the PA catheter can be repositioned. The plastic cuff is designed to keep the external catheter sterile for a short period after insertion.

◆ **Nursing management.** When caring for a patient with a PA catheter, the nurse must continuously monitor the PA tracing. A significant component of the nursing assessment involves evaluation of the PA waveform to ensure that the catheter has not migrated forward into the wedge position, because a segment of lung can be infarcted if the catheter occludes an arteriole for a prolonged period. For this reason, nurses' and physicians' accurate knowledge of differences in the PA versus PAWP waveform is vital in critical care units.[77,78]

Factors that affect PA measurement include normal fluctuations, head-of-bed position, and lateral body position relative to transducer height placement, respiratory variation, and positive end-expiratory pressure (PEEP).

Normal fluctuation. Some fluctuation in PA pressures over a 30-minute period is normal. A normal fluctuation range for PAD pressure and PAWP is 4 mm Hg. A normal fluctuation range for PAS is 5 mm Hg.[67] Therefore if a patient's PA pressures are 15/8 mm Hg with PAWP of 7 mm Hg and change to 19/10 mm Hg with a PAWP of 10 mm Hg, this may be normal. It is important to follow the trend of subsequent readings to see whether the values continue to rise or return to baseline.

Patient position. In the supine position, if the transducer is placed at the level of the phlebostatic axis, a head-of-bed position from flat up to 60 degrees is appropriate for most patients.[64-67,79,80] In the lateral position the fourth intercostal space and midsternum are suggested as the reference level.[79] However, nurse researchers differ in their findings as to whether PA and PAWP measurements are accurate with the patient in the lateral position.[64,67,79,80] At this point, if there is concern over the validity of pressure readings in a particular patient, it is more reliable to take measurements with the patient on his or her back, using up to 60 degrees head-of-bed elevation.

Respiratory variation. All PA and PAWP tracings are subject to respiratory interference, especially if the patient is on a positive-pressure, volume-cycled ventilator. During inhalation the ventilator "pushes up" the PA tracing to produce an artificially high reading (Fig. 15-76, *A*). During spontaneous respiration, negative intrathoracic pressure "pulls down" the waveform and can produce an erroneously low measurement[67] (Fig. 15-76, *B*). To minimize the impact of respiratory variation, the PAD should be read at end expiration, which is the most stable point in the respiratory cycle. If the digital number fluctuates with respiration, a paper readout can be obtained to verify true PAD.[81]

PEEP. Some clinical diagnoses, such as adult respiratory distress syndrome (ARDS), require the use of high levels of PEEP to treat refractory hypoxemia. If a PEEP of greater than 10 cm H_2O is used, PAWP and PA pressure will be artificially elevated. Because of this impact of PEEP, in the past, patients in some critical care units were taken off the ventilator to record PA pressure measurements. It has since been shown that this practice decreases the patient's oxygenation and may result in persistent hypoxemia.[67,82] Because patients remain on PEEP for treatment, they should remain on it during measurement of PA pressures. In this situation the trend of PA readings is more important than is one individual measurement.

Insertion and use of PA catheters is not entirely risk-free. Potential cardiac complications include ventricular dysrhythmias, endocarditis, valvular damage, cardiac rupture, and tamponade. Potential pulmonary complications include rupture of a pulmonary artery, pulmonary artery thrombosis, embolism or hemorrhage, and infarction of a segment of lung.[83] PA catheters are routinely removed by the critical care nurse without major complications. The most common incidents are ventricular dysrhythmias (5%) as the catheter is pulled through the RV.[83]

◆ **Cardiac output.** The PA catheter measures cardiac output (CO) with the bolus thermodilution method. This technique can be performed at the bedside and results in CO calculated in liters per minute. A known amount (5- or 10-ml bolus) of iced or room temperature normal saline solution is injected into the proximal lumen of the catheter. The injectant exits into the right atrium (RA) and travels with the flow of blood past the thermistor (temperature sensor) at the distal end of the catheter. Sometimes the right atrial (proximal) port is clotted off and not usable. Accurate COs can still be obtained using either a centrally placed introducer sheath,[84] an RA proximal infusion lumen,[85,86] or the right ventricular port of a specialized PA catheter.[87] See Fig. 15-74 for detailed diagrams of the location of these additional lumens on the different PA catheters.

The thermodilution CO method uses the indicator-dilution principle, in which a known temperature is the indicator, and it—in turn—is based on the principle that the change in temperature over time is inversely proportional to blood flow. Blood flow can be diagrammatically represented as a CO curve, on which temperature is plotted against time (Fig. 15-77, *A*). Many of the most recent hemodynamic monitors display this CO curve, which must then be interpreted to determine whether the CO injection is valid. The normal curve has a smooth upstroke, with a rounded peak and a gradually tapering downslope. If the curve has an uneven pattern, it may indicate faulty injection technique, and the CO measurement should be repeated. Patient movement or coughing will also alter the CO (Fig. 15-77, *B*).

Generally, three COs that are within a 10% mean range are obtained and are averaged to calculate CO. The CO is equally accurate whether iced or room temperature injectate is used.[88,89] To ensure accurate readings, the difference between injectant temperature and body temperature must be at least 10° C, and the injectant must be delivered within 4 seconds, with minimal handling of the syringe to prevent warming of the solution. This is particularly important if iced injectate is used. The closed injectate CO system is increasingly popular, because it is easy to use, decreases

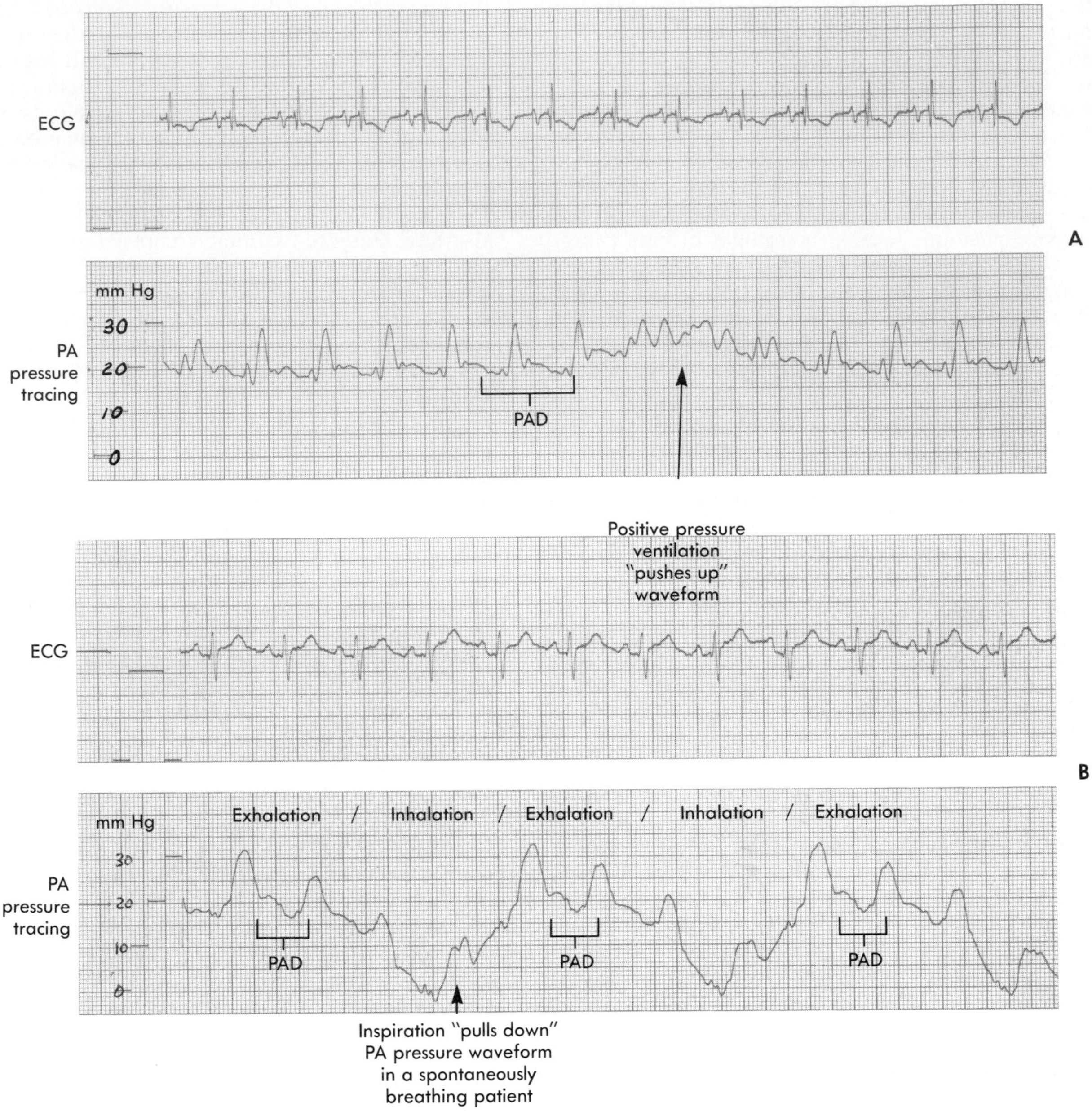

Fig. 15-76 PA waveforms that demonstrate the impact of ventilation of PA pressure readings. For accuracy, PA pressures should be read at end exhalation. **A,** Positive pressure ventilation: the increase in intrathoracic pressure during inhalation "pushes up" the PA pressure waveform, creating a false high reading. **B,** Spontaneous breathing: the decrease in intrathoracic pressure during normal inhalation "pulls down" the PA waveform, creating a false low reading.

the risk of infection associated with multiple syringes, and produces accurate CO measurements. With all delivery systems the injectant should be delivered at the same point in the respiratory cycle, usually end-exhalation. Reliable CO measurements can be obtained with the patient in a supine position with the head of bed elevated up to 30 degrees.[65]

Two clinical conditions will produce errors in the thermodilution CO measurement: tricuspid valve regurgitation and ventricular septal defect (VSD). If the patient has tricuspid valve regurgitation, the expected flow of blood from the right atrium to the pulmonary artery is disrupted by backflow from the right ventricle to the right atrium. This creates a lower CO measurement than the patient's actual output.[90,91] If the person has an intracardiac left-to-right shunt, such as occurs with a VSD, the thermodilution CO measures the large pulmonary volume and records a higher CO than the patient's true systemic output.[92]

At the present time the bolus thermodilution CO

RESEARCH ABSTRACT

Effect of backrest position on pulmonary artery pressure and cardiac output measurements in critically ill patients.

Cline JK, Gurka AM: *Focus Crit Care* 18(5):383, 1991.

PURPOSE

The purpose of this study was to determine the differences of cardiac output (CO) and pulmonary artery (PA) measurements relative to degree of head-of-bed (backrest) elevation.

DESIGN

Quasi-experimental comparative design

SAMPLE

A convenience sample of 12 subjects was drawn from the first admissions to the critical care unit who had a PA catheter in place and who were not undergoing medication-induced diuresis, receiving titrated medications that would affect the PA or CO measurements, or undergoing hemodialysis or peritoneal dialysis; who had no postural hypotension; and whose backrest elevation could not be altered for medical reasons. The seven men and five women ranged in age from 31 to 78 years. Admitting diagnoses varied, and four subjects were receiving mechanical ventilation with PEEP. PA lines had been in place 1 to 6 days.

INSTRUMENTS

A self-calibrating monitor (Model 514, Spacelabs, Inc., Redmond, WA) was used with a transducer (U-Onics Laboratories, Wayland, MA). The angle of backrest elevation was determined by using the calibrations on the bed (Hill-Rom, Batesville, IN). CO measurements were obtained using a CO computer model (Model COM 1, American Edwards, Santa Ana, CA).

PROCEDURE

Subjects were assigned to one of three groups, and each group was assigned a backrest position. The angle of backrest was determined and PA pressure was measured, with PA systolic and PA diastolic measured at end-expiration with the subject at rest. There was a 5-minute interval between position changes. Each injection for the CO measurement was accomplished in 4 seconds or less. The primary nurse researcher collected all data, and the technique and accuracy were validated by the observation of the second nurse investigator.

RESULTS

Four subjects had a variation in PA systolic (PAS) pressure of greater than 4 mm Hg with position change, whereas two subjects had a fluctuation in PA diastolic (PAD) pressure of greater than 4 mm Hg. The pulmonary capillary wedge pressure (PCWP) of all subjects fell within ±4 mm Hg. Some of the variations in PA and PCWP were statistically significant ($p < .05$); however, these were not determined to be clinically significant, requiring intervention. There was greater variability with backrest positions with CO measurements. For purposes of this study, a range of ±10% was considered to be an acceptable fluctuation in CO with backrest elevation. One subject showed a steady decrease with each backrest elevation, whereas another subject demonstrated a total CO decrease of 25% with 45-degree elevation. Yet another subject had a large degree of variation in CO in all backrest positions.

DISCUSSION/IMPLICATIONS

Findings from this study indicate that PA pressure and PCWP readings may be taken with backrest elevations ranging up to 45 degrees. However, CO measurements should be taken at elevations ranging only to 30 degrees. In addition, individual patient physiologic variables need to be considered when deciding elevation in relation to CO measurement. It is important to determine clinical significance in addition to statistical significance when analyzing data. This study had a small sample size and might be considered a pilot study for a larger study. The investigators point out that only two CO measurements were used to calculate the mean CO, instead of the customary three to five readings generally taken. Additional research on this topic might include the following: evaluation of the impact of various nursing care and medical treatments on CO and PCWP measurements; correlation of the CO and PCWP with physiologic patient variables; and determination of the effect of side-lying position with and without backrest elevation on CO and PCWP.

method is the only reliable measure of CO in the critical care unit setting. Other continuously monitored indicators related to oxygen use are not sufficiently reliable or consistent. Thus mixed venous oxygen saturation ($S\bar{v}O_2$)[93] and oxygen consumption[94] are not reliable indicators of CO in critically ill patients. However, considerable research is being conducted into the feasibility of continuously monitoring CO via a PA catheter setup. (Fig. 15-74, *D*) Two methods include ultrasound techniques, such as Doppler,[95,96] and a continuous thermodilution catheter using "heat pulses."[97] Researchers are also investigating whether CO can be assessed noninvasively by transthoracic electrical bioimpedance[98] and peripheral pulse contour CO.[97] At the present, few of these investigational methods are sufficiently reliable to replace the thermodilution CO in

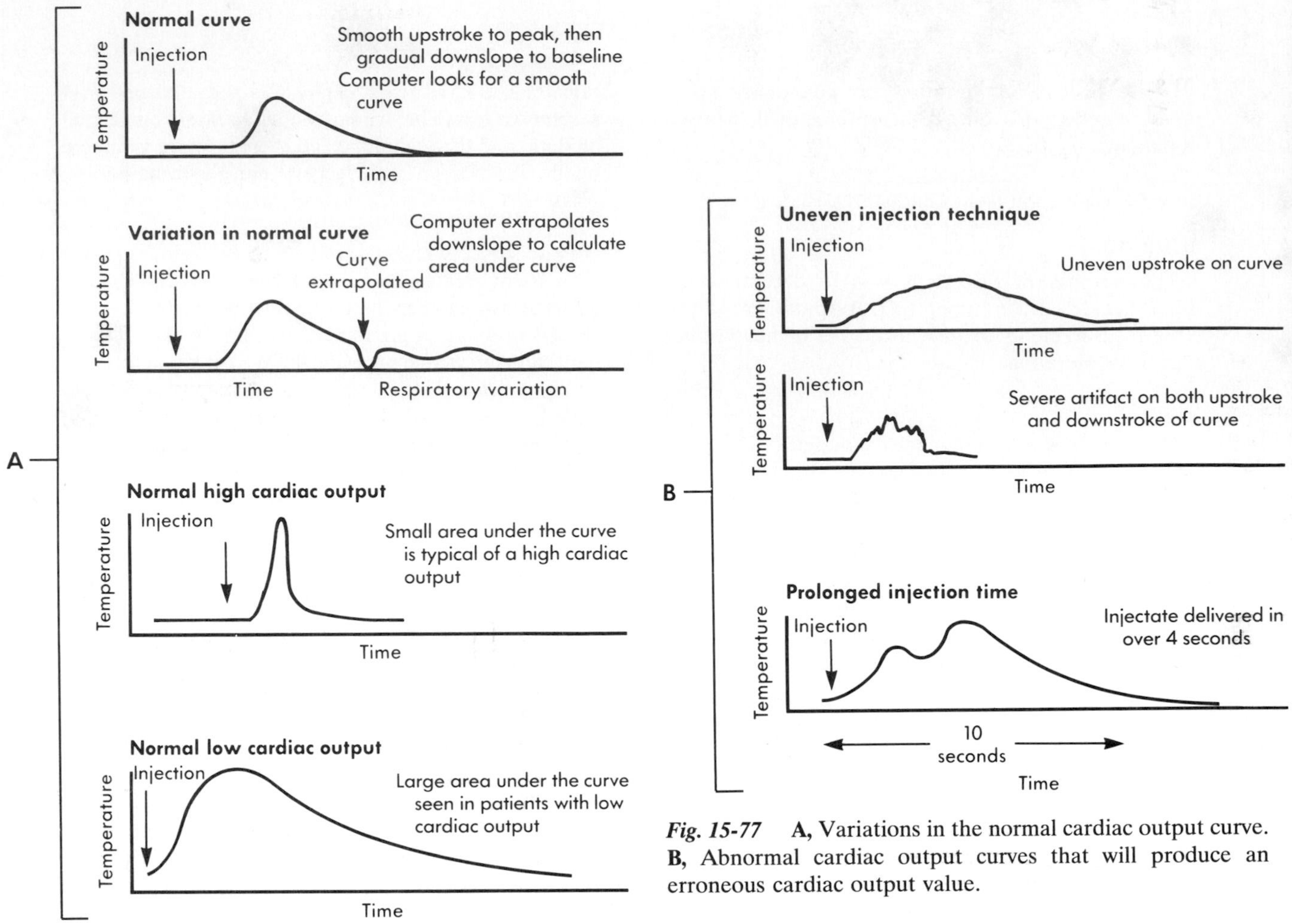

Fig. 15-77 **A,** Variations in the normal cardiac output curve. **B,** Abnormal cardiac output curves that will produce an erroneous cardiac output value.

the critical care unit. However, at some time in the future when this technology is feasible, the critical care nurse will be able to monitor a CO trend that is updated continuously the way heart rate, arterial pressure, and pulse oximetry are monitored today.

◆ **Calculated hemodynamic profiles.** For the patient with a thermodilution PA catheter in place, additional hemodynamic information can be calculated using routine vital signs, CO, and body surface area (BSA). These measurements are calculated using specific formulas that are indexed to a patient's body size, using either the DuBois Body Surface Chart or the computer program associated with the new generation of hemodynamic monitors.

The calculated hemodynamic profiles are described in Table 15-20. Clinical use of these profiles is described in two case studies. Case study 1 is a step-by-step interpretation of the hemodynamic profile to familiarize the reader with use of calculated values, and case study 2 uses only values indexed to body weight and illustrates the impact of treatment on these values over time (see boxes, pp. 267 and 268).

Continuous Monitoring of Mixed Venous Oxygen Saturation

◆ **Indications.** Continuous monitoring of mixed venous oxygen saturation (Svo_2) is indicated for the patient who has the potential to develop an imbalance between oxygen supply and metabolic tissue demand. This includes the patient in shock and the patient with severe respiratory compromise, such as adult respiratory distress syndrome (ARDS). Continuous Svo_2 monitoring measures the balance achieved between arterial oxygen supply (Sao_2) and oxygen demand at the tissue level by sampling desaturated venous mixed blood from the pulmonary artery (Svo_2). It is called *mixed venous blood,* because it is a mixture of all of the venous blood saturations from many body tissues. Under normal conditions the cardiopulmonary system achieves a balance between oxygen supply and demand. The four factors that contribute to this balance include cardiac output (CO), hemoglobin (Hgb), arterial oxygen saturation (Sao_2), and tissue metabolism (Vo_2). Three of these factors (CO, Hgb, and Sao_2) contribute to the *supply* of oxygen to the tissues. Tissue metabolism (Vo_2) deter-

HEMODYNAMIC PROFILE
CASE STUDY 1

Mr. SR has a medical history of cardiomyopathy and chronic obstructive pulmonary disease (COPD). He is admitted to a coronary care unit because of an exacerbation of his biventricular heart failure. He has been complaining of anginal pain and shortness of breath. His nursing diagnoses are Decreased Cardiac Output and Impaired Gas Exchange.

Height	163 cm	PAD	27 mm Hg	PVR	322 dynes/sec/cm^{-5}
Weight	79 kg	PAP_M	36 mm Hg	PVRI	612 dynes/sec/cm^{-5}/m^2
Body surface area (BSA)	1.9 m^2	PAWP	26 mm Hg	LCW	2.1 kg-m
		CVP	24 mm Hg	LCWI	1.1 kg-m/m^2
HR	104 bpm	CO	2.48 L/min	LVSW	2.4 g-m
ABP		CI	1.31 L/min/m^2	LVSWI	10.7 g-m/m^2
Systolic	88 mm Hg	SV	23.8 ml	RCW	1.21 kg-m
Diastolic	51 mm Hg	SI	12.5 ml/m^2	RCWI	0.64 kg-m/m^2
MAP	63 mm Hg	SVR	1257 dynes/sec/cm^{-5}	RVSW	11.7 g-m
PAS	55 mm Hg	SVRI	2388 dynes/sec/cm^{-5}/m^2	RVSWI	6.2 g-m/m^2

ANALYSIS OF HEMODYNAMIC PROFILE*

PROFILE	ANALYSIS
HR	Heart rate of 104 beats per minute (bpm) is above normal limits (normal, 60-100 bpm).
ABP (arterial blood pressure)	Narrow pulse pressure of 88/51 with a low mean arterial pressure (MAP) of 63 mm Hg (normal MAP, 65-90 mm Hg).
Pulmonary artery pressure	Pulmonary artery pressures are elevated (55/27 mm Hg), consistent with diagnosis of cardiomyopathy, failure of left side of heart, and COPD (normal PA, 25/10 mm Hg).
PAWP (pulmonary artery wedge pressure)	Elevated PAWP (26 mm Hg), consistent with diagnosis of cardiomyopathy and failure of left side of heart (normal PAWP, 5-12 mm Hg).
CVP (central venous pressure)	Elevated CVP (24 mm Hg), consistent with diagnosis of cardiomyopathy, failure of right side of heart, and COPD (normal CVP, 4-6 mm Hg).
CO (cardiac output) and CI (cardiac index)	Poor CO and CI (CO, 2.48 L/min; CI, 1.31 L/min/m^2). Both values are below normal (normal CO, 4-6 L/min; normal CI, 2.2-4 L/min/m^2).
SV (stroke volume) and SI (stroke volume index)	SV and SI are low (SV, 23.8 ml; SI, 12.5 ml/min/m^2). These results would be anticipated from the low cardiac output (normal SV, 60-70 ml; normal SI, 40-50 ml/min/m^2).
SVR (systemic vascular resistance) and SVRI (systemic vascular resistance index)	SVR and SVRI are at the upper normal range (SVR, 1257 dynes/sec/cm^{-5}; SVRI, 2388 dynes/sec/cm^{-5}/m^2). These values are not contributing to the low cardiac output at this time (normal SVR, 800-1400 dynes/sec/cm^{-5}; normal SVRI, 2000-2400 dynes/sec/cm^{-5}/m^2).
PVR (pulmonary vascular resistance) and PVRI (pulmonary vascular resistance index)	PVR and PVRI are elevated (PVR, 322 dynes/sec/cm^{-5}; PVRI 612 dynes/sec/cm^{-5}/m^2). High pulmonary vascular resistance may be contributing to the low cardiac output (normal PVR, 100-250 dynes/sec/cm^{-5}; normal PVRI, 225-315 dynes/sec/cm^{-5}/m^2).
LCWI (left cardiac work index) and LVSWI (left ventricular stroke work index)	Both LCWI and LVSWI are below normal (LCWI, 1.1 kg-m/m^2; LVSWI, 10.7 g-m/m^2), indicating that left-ventricular myocardial damage may be present. This is consistent with SR's diagnosis of cardiomyopathy (normal LCWI, 3.4-4.2 kg-m/m^2; normal LVSWI, 50-62 g-m/m^2).
RCWI (right cardiac work index) and RVSWI (right ventricular stroke work index)	RCWI is normal, but RVSWI is below normal (RCWI, 0.64 kg-m/m^2; RVSWI, 6.2 g-m/m^2), indicating that right-ventricular myocardial damage may be present. This is consistent with SR's diagnosis of cardiomyopathy and history of COPD (normal RCWI, 0.54-0.66 kg-m/m^2; normal RVSWI, 7.9-9.7 g-m/m^2).
Nursing impression	The hemodynamic data confirm the nursing clinical diagnosis of poor CO. The goal is to improve CO within the limits of SR's myocardial dysfunction and COPD. As CO improves and PA pressures decrease, the patient will have less pulmonary congestion, which will improve alveolar gas exchange.

*Formulas and normal values for the hemodynamic values are in Table 15-20 and Appendix C.

HEMODYNAMIC PROFILE
CASE STUDY 2

1. ADMISSION

Mrs. JL has been admitted to the critical care unit with pulmonary edema. She has a history of anterior wall myocardial infarction and severe chronic obstructive pulmonary disease (COPD).

Height	159 cm	MAP	106 mm Hg	SI	9.9 ml/m^2
Weight	45.8 kg	PAS	53 mm Hg	SVRI	5351 dynes/sec/cm^{-5}/m^2
Body surface area		PAD	27 mm Hg	PVRI	1046 dynes/sec/cm^{-5}/m^2
(BSA)	1.40 m^2	PAP_M	44 mm Hg	LCWI	1.9 kg-m/m^2
HR	131 bpm	PAWP	27 mm Hg	LVSWI	14.3 g-m/m^2
ABP		CVP	19 mm Hg	RCWI	0.78 kg-m^2
Systolic	160 mm Hg	CO	1.82 L/min	RVSWI	5.9 g-m/m^2
Diastolic	80 mm Hg	CI	1.3 L/min/m^2		

Analysis of hemodynamic profile 1*

In the above hemodynamic profile, note the fast heart rate; high MAP; high PA and CVP filling pressures; low CI, SI, LVSWI, and RVSWI; and high SVRI and PVRI. These values are consistent with a diagnosis of failure of the left side of the heart, causing pulmonary edema, which may lead to cardiogenic shock. Treatment focused on increasing the cardiac index by lowering SVRI and PVRI, using IV sodium nitroprusside and IV nitroglycerin in continuous infusion.

2. 3 HOURS LATER

Height	159 cm	MAP	83 mm Hg	SI	16.5 ml/m^2
Weight	45.8 kg	PAS	41 mm Hg	SVRI	3088 dynes/sec/cm^{-5}/m^2
Body surface area		PAD	26 mm Hg	PVRI	300 dynes/sec/cm^{-5}/m^2
(BSA)	1.40 m^2	PAM	33 mm Hg	LCWI	2.1 kg-m/m^2
HR	113 bpm	PAWP	26 mm Hg	LVSWI	18.6 kg-m/m^2
ABP		CVP	11 mm Hg	RCWI	0.84 kg-m/m^2
Systolic	104 mm Hg	CO	2.61 L/min	RVSWI	7.4 g-m/m^2
Diastolic	69 mm Hg	CI	1.86 L/min/m^2		

Analysis of hemodynamic profile 2

Results 3 hours later after sodium nitroprusside administration: note improving hemodynamics shown above as normal MAP and lower intracardiac filling pressures (PA and CVP). However, CI and SI remain low, and SVRI is above normal. Mrs. JL remains in severe left-ventricular failure because of her low CI.

3. THE NEXT DAY

Height	159 cm	MAP	77 mm Hg	SI	22.5 ml/m^2
Weight	45.8 kg	PAS	31 mm Hg	SVRI	2423 dynes/sec/cm^{-5}/m^2
Body surface area		PAD	15 mm Hg	PVRI	273 dynes/sec/cm^{-5}/m^2
(BSA)	1.40 m^2	PAP_M	23 mm Hg	LCWI	2.4 kg-m/m^2
HR	104 bpm	PAWP	15 mm Hg	LVSWI	22.9 g-m/m^2
ABP		CVP	4 mm Hg	RCWI	0.74 kg-m/m^2
Systolic	111 mm Hg	CO	3.28 L/min	RVSWI	7.1 g-m/m^2
Diastolic	60 mm Hg	CI	2.34 L/min/m^2		

Analysis of hemodynamic profile 3

The following day Mrs. JL's hemodynamics have improved with continued use of sodium nitroprusside and nitroglycerin. CI is in the low-normal range, and SVRI and PVRI are in the high-normal range. LVSWI remains low, reflecting the patient's compromised left ventricle from the previous anterior wall myocardial infarction.

*See previous box for explanation of abbreviations, and see Table 15-20 and Appendix C for explanation of hemodynamic values.

mines the quantity of oxygen extracted at tissue level or oxygen consumption and creates the *demand* for oxygen.

In addition to interpreting Svo_2, it is possible to calculate the quantity of oxygen that is provided by the cardiopulmonary system and the amount of oxygen consumed by the body tissues. These calculations are based on the principles of oxygen transport physiology and are the basis for calculation of Svo_2. These formulas are explained in greater detail in Table 15-24 and are listed in Appendix C.

◆ **Catheters.** In 1981 a fiberoptic PA catheter was designed that continuously monitors Svo_2. The catheter contains the traditional four lumens plus a lumen containing two or three optical fibers. The fiberoptics are attached to an optical module that is connected by a cable to a small bedside computer. The optical module

Table 15-24 Calculations and explanation of oxygen transport physiology

Name	Formula	Normal value	Explanation
Arterial oxygen saturation (Sao_2)	$\frac{HgbO_2}{(Hgb + HgbO_2) \times 100}$	>96%	Hgb, hemoglobin; $HgbO_2$, oxyhemoglobin. The arterial oxygen saturation represents the amount of oxyhemoglobin (oxygen bound to hemoglobin) divided by the total hemoglobin. Normally 96% of oxygen is bound to hemoglobin.
Blood oxygen content Cao_2 (arterial) Cvo_2 (venous)	(O_2 dissolved) + (O_2 saturation) ($Po_2 \times 0.0031$) + ($1.34 \times Hgb \times SO_2$)	19-20 vol % 12-15 vol %	Blood oxygen (O_2) content represents the amount of oxygen dissolved in 100 ml of blood. It can be calculated for both arterial blood (Cao_2) and for venous blood (Cvo_2) and is measured in volume percent (vol %). It is the combination of both dissolved O_2 (Pao_2) and O_2 saturation (Sao_2).
Blood oxygen transport	$CO \times Cao_2 \times 10$ (arterial) $CO \times Cvo_2 \times 10$ (venous)	1000 ml/min 750 ml/min	Oxygen transport represents the amount of oxygen transported to or from the tissues each minute in milliliters (ml/min). Arterial O_2 transport is a measure of the O_2 delivered to the tissues. Venous O_2 transport reflects the venous return to the right side of the heart. Oxygen transport is calculated by multiplying the cardiac output (CO) by the oxygen content (Cao_2 or Cvo_2) and by the number 10. The difference between normal arterial and normal venous O_2 return represents oxygen consumption by the tissues.
Tissue oxygen consumption (Vo_2)	Arterial O_2 transport minus venous O_2 transport ($CO \times Cao_2 \times 10$) − ($CO \times Cvo_2 \times 10$)	250 ml/min	Oxygen consumption represents the amount of oxygen consumed by the tissues in 1 minute. To calculate Vo_2, it is necessary to know both arterial oxygen transport and venous oxygen transport values, which are calculated in ml/min. The difference represents oxygen consumption.
Arterial venous oxygen difference (A-Vo_2 difference)	Arterial O_2 content minus venous O_2 content $Cao_2 - Cvo_2$	3.0-5.5 vol %	The arterial-venous oxygen difference represents the difference between the arterial oxygen content (Cao_2) and the venous oxygen content (Cvo_2). Because Cao_2 and Cvo_2 are measured in volume percent (vol %), A-Vo_2 difference is also measured in vol %.
Mixed venous oxygen saturation (Svo_2)	Arterial O_2 transport minus tissue consumption equals venous return ($CO \times Cao_2 \times 10$) − Vo_2	60%-80%	Mixed venous oxygen saturation (Svo_2) represents the venous oxygen return that is bound (saturated) with hemoglobin. Saturation is measured in percent (%). The Svo_2 value is a function of the amount of oxygen delivered to the tissues minus the amount of oxygen consumed by the tissues (Vo_2) in milliliters per minute. The higher the amount (ml) of oxygen in the venous return, the greater the hemoglobin saturation will be.

transmits a narrow band-width light. The light travels down one optical fiber, is reflected off the hemoglobin in the blood, and returns to the optical module through the receiving fiberoptic. The Svo_2 signal is averaged every 5 seconds and is recorded on a continuous display or printout.

The catheter is calibrated before insertion into the patient through a standard color reference system, which is part of the catheter package. Insertion technique and sites are identical to those used for placement of a conventional PA catheter. Waveform analysis and/or Svo_2 can be used for accurate placement. Once the catheter is inserted, recalibration is unnecessary unless the catheter becomes disconnected from the optical module. To calibrate when the catheter is inserted in a patient, a mixed venous blood sample must be withdrawn from the PA lumen and sent to the laboratory for analysis of oxygen saturation (Svo_2). To obtain accurate results, the laboratory should use a "reflectance" technique similar to the principle used in the fiberoptic catheter.

◆ **Nursing management.** Svo_2 monitoring provides a continuous assessment of the balance between oxygen supply and demand for an individual patient. Nursing assessment includes evaluation of the Svo_2 value and evaluation of the four factors (Sao_2, CO, Hgb, and Vo_2) that maintain the oxygen supply-demand balance.

Normal Svo_2 is 75%. For most critically ill patients, an Svo_2 value between 60% and 80% is evidence of adequate balance between oxygen supply and demand. If the Svo_2 value changes by more than 10% and this change is maintained for more than 10 minutes, the nurse should determine which of the four factors is affecting Svo_2.

Assessment of arterial oxygen saturation. The change in Svo_2 may be caused by a change in Sao_2. If the Sao_2 is increased because supplemental oxygen is being given, the Svo_2 will also rise. If the Sao_2 is decreased, Svo_2 will fall. Decreased Sao_2 can be caused by any action or disease that reduces oxygen supply, including ARDS, endotracheal suctioning, removing a patient from the ventilator, or removal of an oxygen mask. Fig. 15-78 shows a fall in Svo_2 after suctioning in a patient with ARDS. Transient decreases in Svo_2 related to a nursing action such as endotracheal suctioning are not usually a cause for concern. Some patients may be slow to resaturate up to the presuction level of Svo_2. In this case an appropriate nursing intervention is to wait until Svo_2 has again returned to baseline before initiating other nursing activities.

Assessment of cardiac output. A change in Svo_2 may also be caused by an alteration in cardiac output (CO). Four hemodynamic factors affect CO—preload, afterload, heart rate, and contractility. Changes in one or more of these individual factors will affect CO. Fig. 15-79 shows an improvement in a patient's Svo_2 from 70% to 80% after volume administration that increased preload *(point A)*. Later this patient's CO fell after a short run of ventricular tachycardia *(point B)*. Any major loss of heart rate will cause a decrease in CO. Alterations in contractility and afterload (systemic vascular resistance) also have the potential to alter CO. Because CO is an important component of the continuous Svo_2 value, several researchers questioned whether Svo_2 could be substituted for thermodilution CO as a monitoring tool. Studies of adult patients after cardiac surgery[93,99] and myocardial infarction[100] indicate that a sustained change in the Svo_2 value does not automatically mean there has been a change in CO. There was not a consistent or reliable correlation between Svo_2 and CO in these clinical studies. Rather, Svo_2 changes indicate a need to check a thermodilution CO at the bedside to determine the cause of the change in Svo_2. The Svo_2 measurement is very sensitive and serves as an early warning device for changes in patient condition, whether or not the change is the result of an alteration in CO.[101] Therefore Svo_2 monitoring is an additional level of hemodynamic monitoring but does not replace thermodilution CO.

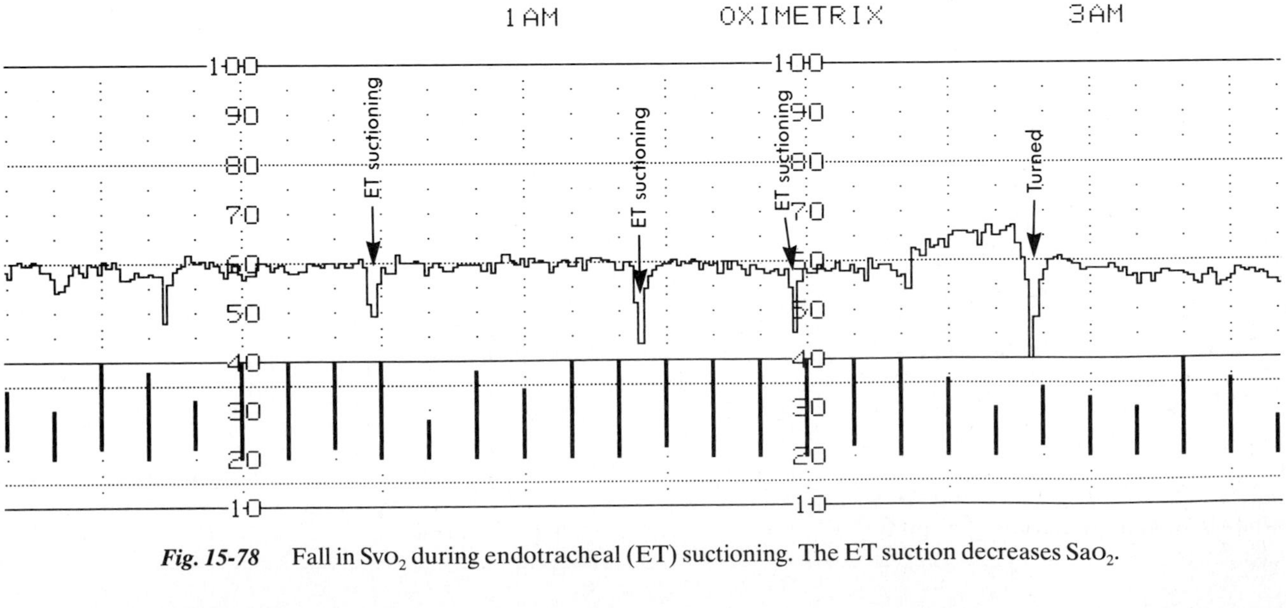

Fig. 15-78 Fall in Svo_2 during endotracheal (ET) suctioning. The ET suction decreases Sao_2.

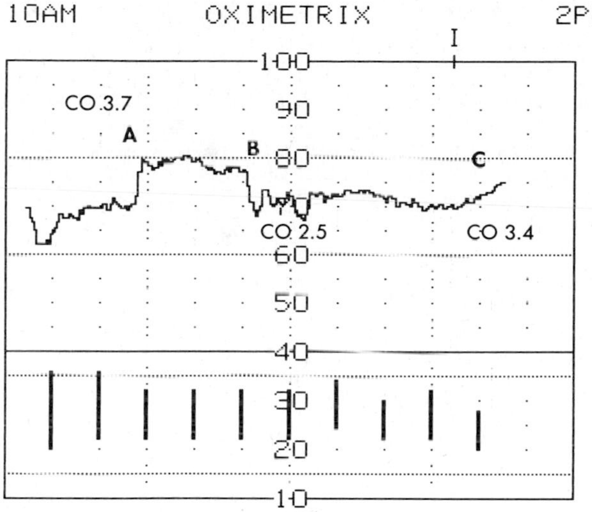

Fig. 15-79 Impact of changes in cardiac output (CO) on Svo_2 values. Point *A:* Just before point A, Svo_2 readings are low because CO and pulmonary artery pressures were low as a result of excessive diuresis. Infusion of 500 ml of colloid solution and 1000 ml of lactated Ringer's solution crystalloid increased the Svo_2 and improved the CO, which rose to 3.7 L/min. Point *B:* A short run of ventricular tachycardia caused the CO to fall to 2.5 L/min and decreased the Svo_2 value. Point *C:* The beginning of an upward trend in Svo_2 is related to administration of fluids and to improvement in CO and in filling pressures. CO is now 3.4 L/min. Graph represents a 4-hour printout; the space between each dotted line represents 20 minutes.

This principle is clearly illustrated in the case study on pp. 272-273, where an increase in Svo_2 is not associated with a significant rise in CO. The rationale and explanation for this finding are also discussed in the section on assessment of oxygen consumption.

Assessment of hemoglobin. Hemoglobin (Hgb) is the transport mechanism for oxygen in the blood. When oxygen is bound to Hgb, it is described as oxyhemoglobin ($Hgbo_2$). If the Hgb level falls as a result of bleeding or red cell destruction, the body maintains oxygen transport by increasing CO and using oxygen reserves in the venous blood return. Therefore the body can compensate efficiently for anemia. In the healthy person, Hgb must be extremely low before Svo_2 falls. However, in an anemic patient with a compromised cardiovascular system who cannot adequately increase CO, Svo_2 will decline as venous oxygen reserves are consumed by the body.

Assessment of oxygen consumption. Oxygen consumption (Vo_2) describes the amount of oxygen the body tissues consume for normal function in 1 minute. If the body's metabolic demands increase because of exercise or increased metabolic rate, the body will increase CO to augment oxygen supply and will also use reserve oxygen in the venous system. Normal oxygen delivery to the tissues is 1000 ml of oxygen per minute. At rest a person might consume one quarter of available oxygen or 250 ml of oxygen per minute. This leaves a venous oxygen reserve of 750 ml of oxygen per minute (Table 15-24). Thus for the normal individual, the combination of increased CO and use of considerable venous oxygen reserve provides adequate compensation for increased metabolic needs. However, for the critically ill patient with either cardiac or respiratory dysfunction, an increase in activity leading to increased oxygen consumption may overwhelm the cardiopulmonary system and oxygen reserves.

An example of the impact of increased oxygen consumption on Svo_2 is shown in the case study in the box on p. 273. Patient EH has just been admitted to the critical care unit and is cold and shivering after cardiopulmonary bypass and cardiac surgery. At point A, Svo_2 is low at 40%. This is caused by post–cardiopulmonary bypass shivering, which has greatly increased EH's oxygen consumption (Vo_2 is 322 ml/min). In addition, his low CO (3 L/min) and decreased arterial oxygen supply (505 ml/min) secondary to compromised cardiovascular function all contribute to the low Svo_2. At point B, the shivering has stopped after sedation; consequently, his tissue oxygen consumption (Vo_2) has decreased to 198 ml/min and Svo_2 has increased (60%). However, because of EH's compromised cardiovascular system, CO remains low with a low arterial oxygen transport. Thus the very low Svo_2 at point A is clearly caused by increased oxygen consumption in the presence of a compromised cardiovascular system and is not related to CO.[99-101]

In the critically ill patient, routine nursing procedures can increase Vo_2 by 10% to 36% (Table 15-25).[102] The bedside nurse can observe the effect of increased Vo_2 during routine nursing care and changes in patient position and in conditions that increase metabolic rate. Such activities as turning,[102-104] giving a backrub,[105] or getting a patient out of bed[106] are often accompanied by a sudden, temporary decrease in the patient's continuous Svo_2 reading. Once the movement is finished, most patients will resaturate up to their preactivity Svo_2 level within 4 to 5 minutes.[102-105,107] In critically ill patients it may take up to a full 5 minutes for resaturation (rise in Svo_2) to occur. In this situation the appropriate nursing action is to observe the patient clinically, in conjunction with monitoring Svo_2, and to postpone additional maneuvers until the Svo_2 has returned to baseline.[102]

Many clinical conditions that dramatically increase Vo_2 are frequently seen in critical care units. Such conditions as sepsis, multiple organ dysfunction syndrome (MODS), burns, head injury, and shivering can more than double normal oxygen tissue requirements (Table 15-25).[102,107] Such dramatic increases in Vo_2 will translate into a low Svo_2, even if the CO is normal (see case study, p. 272-273).

Assessment of Svo_2. If Svo_2 is within the normal range (60% to 80%) and the patient is not clinically compromised, one can assume that oxygen supply and demand are balanced for that individual. The situation becomes out of balance when there is either a decrease in oxygen delivery because of changes in Sao_2, CO, or Hgb or an increase in oxygen demand (increased Vo_2). If Svo_2 falls

HEMODYNAMIC PROFILE
CASE STUDY 3

Mr. EH has just been admitted to the cardiovascular critical care unit after open heart surgery. At point A, he has an extremely low mixed venous oxygen saturation (Svo_2) of 40%. An Svo_2 below 40% indicates that the oxygen supply is not adequate to meet the demands of the body tissues, resulting in metabolic acidosis. To determine the reason for the low Svo_2, one must know the hemoglobin (Hgb), the arterial oxygen saturation (Sao_2), the cardiac output (CO), and the tissue oxygen consumption (Vo_2). EH's Hgb value is 11.6 g/dl (normal male Hgb, 13.5-18.0 g/dl), which is acceptable after major surgery; the Sao_2 is 99.6% (normal, >97%), which is high because this patient is receiving mechanical ventilation with 70% oxygen immediately after surgery; and the CO is low at 3.15 L/min (normal, 4-6 L/min). EH is receiving dopamine 5 μg/kg/min for his low CO. He is shivering and cold because his body temperature is only 35.2° C after the surgery. Using the values described above—Hgb 11.6 g/dl; Sao_2, 99.6%; and CO 3.15 L/min—it is possible to calculate the Vo_2 for EH.

ARTERIAL SUPPLY	VENOUS RETURN
$CO (Pao_2 \times 0.0031) + (1.34 \times Hgb \times Sao_2)10$	$- \; CO (Pvo_2 \times 0.0031) + (1.34 \times Hgb \times Svo_2)10 = Vo_2$

(To calculate arterial oxygen supply, the oxygen in the venous return, Vo_2, and the difference between the arterial and venous oxygen content [A-Vo_2 difference], insert EH's values [in bold] into the above formula.)

ARTERIAL SUPPLY	VENOUS RETURN	*Vo_2*	*A-Vo_2 Difference*
$\mathbf{3.15}(\mathbf{354} \times 0.0031) + (1.34 \times \mathbf{11.6} \times \mathbf{0.99})10$	$- \; \mathbf{3.15}(\mathbf{20} \times 0.0031) + (1.34 \times \mathbf{11.6} \times \mathbf{0.38})10$		
3.15(1.0 + 15.3)10	3.15(0.06 + 5.90)10		
3.15(16.3)10	3.15(5.90)10		
505 ml/min	183 ml/min	= 322 ml/min	10.4 vol %

At point A the arterial oxygen supply to the tissues is 505 ml/min (normal, 1000 ml/min), whereas the oxygen returned in the venous blood is only 183 ml/min (normal, 750 ml/min). EH's Vo_2 is elevated at 322 ml/min (normal, 250 ml/min). The clinical goals for this patient would be to (1) increase the CO and (2) use sedation or muscle relaxants to decrease oxygen consumption by controlling the shivering. The difference between the oxygen content in the arterial and the venous blood (A-Vo_2 difference) is very large at 10.4 vol % (normal, 3.5-5.0 vol %). These calculated values confirm the nursing diagnosis of Altered Tissue Perfusion with a decreased cardiac output.

Two hours later, at point B, EH's Svo_2 has improved to a low normal value of 60%. Additional inotropic drugs have been administered. At this time the Hgb is 10.8 g/dl, Sao_2 is 99.6%, and CO remains low at 3.3 L/min. Thus the improvement in Svo_2 has not been caused by a dramatic increase in CO. When EH's oxygen consumption is calculated at point B, it becomes evident that the decrease in physical activity after sedation with morphine sulphate to reduce shivering has improved the Svo_2. EH's values are emplasized in bold.

ARTERIAL SUPPLY	VENOUS RETURN
$CO (Pao_2 \times 0.0031) + (1.34 \times Hgb \times Sao_2)10$	$- \; CO (Pvo_2 \times 0.0031) + (1.34 \times Hgb \times Svo_2)10 = Vo_2$

ARTERIAL SUPPLY	VENOUS RETURN	*Vo_2*	*A-Vo_2 Difference*
$\mathbf{3.3}(\mathbf{266} \times 0.0031) + (1.34 \times \mathbf{10.8} \times \mathbf{0.99})10$	$- \; \mathbf{3.3}(\mathbf{28} \times 0.0031) + (1.34 \times \mathbf{10.8} \times \mathbf{0.60})10$		
3.3(0.82 + 14.32)10	3.3(0.86 + 8.6)10		
3.3(15.1)10	3.3(9.4)10		
498 ml/min	300 ml/min	= 198 ml/min	5.7 vol %

At Point B, EH's arterial oxygen supply is still low at 498 ml/min, and the oxygen in his mixed venous blood return remains low at 300 ml/min. Vo_2 is now lower than normal (typical after sedation)—198 ml/min. At this time the A-Vo_2 difference is almost within normal limits at 5.7 vol %. These findings are confirmed by the low-normal Svo_2 value of 60% at point B. This case study illustrates the point that tissue oxygen consumption (O_2 demand) can be as important as cardiac output (CO) and oxygenation (O_2 supply) in determining mixed venous oxygen saturation (Svo_2) in the patient with a compromised cardiovascular system.

Continued.

HEMODYNAMIC PROFILE
CASE STUDY 3—cont'd

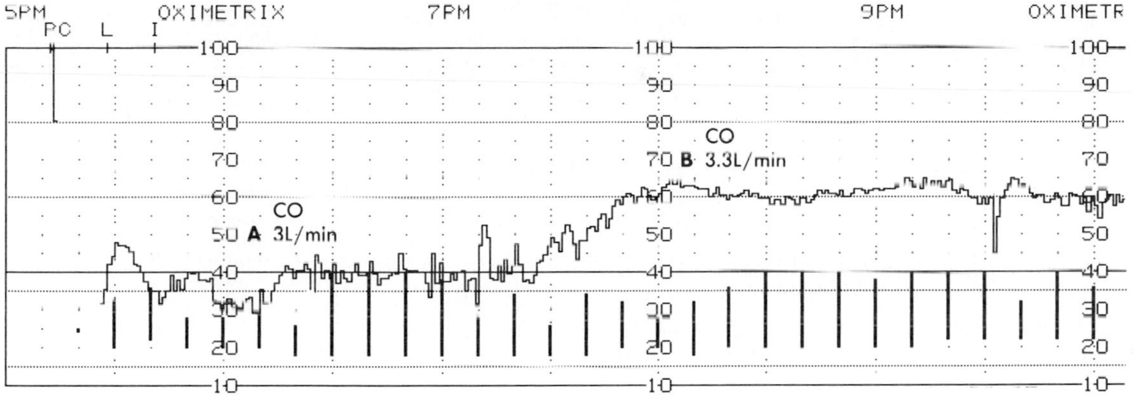

Table 15-25 Conditions and activities that alter oxygen consumption (Vo_2)

Condition or activity	% Increase over resting Vo_2	% Decrease under resting Vo_2
CLINICAL CONDITIONS THAT INCREASE Vo_2		
Fever	10% (for each 1° C over normal)	
Skeletal injuries	10%-30%	
Work of breathing	40%	
Severe infection	60%	
Shivering	50%-100%	
Burns	100%	
Routine postoperative procedures	7%	
Nasal intubation	25%-40%	
Endotracheal tube suctioning	27%	
Chest trauma	60%	
Multiple organ disfunction syndrome	20%-80%	
Sepsis	50%-100%	
Head injury, with patient sedated	89%	
Head injury, with patient not sedated	138%	
Critical illness in emergency department	60%	
NURSING ACTIVITIES THAT INCREASE Vo_2		
Dressing change	10%	
Electrocardiogram	16%	
Agitation	18%	
Physical examination	20%	
Visitor	22%	
Bath	23%	
Chest x-ray examination	25%	
Position change	31%	
Chest physiotherapy	35%	
Weighing on sling scale	36%	
CONDITIONS THAT DECREASE Vo_2		
Anesthesia		25%
Anesthesia in burned patients		50%

From White KM and others: *Heart Lung* 19(5):550, 1990.

Table 15-26 Clinical interpretation of Svo_2 measurements

Svo_2 measurement	Physiologic basis for change in Svo_2	Clinical diagnosis and rationale
High Svo_2 (80%-95%)	Increased oxygen supply	Patient receiving more oxygen than required by clinical condition
	Decreased oxygen demand	Anesthesia, which causes sedation and decreased muscle movement Hypothermia, which lowers metabolic demand (e.g., with cardiopulmonary bypass) Sepsis caused by decreased ability of tissues to use oxygen at a cellular level False high positive because PA catheter is wedged in a pulmonary capillary
Normal Svo_2 (60%-80%)	Normal oxygen supply and metabolic demand	Balanced oxygen supply and demand
Low Svo_2 (less than 60%)	Decreased oxygen supply caused by:	
	Low hemoglobin (Hgb)	Anemia or bleeding with compromised cardiopulmonary system
	Low arterial saturation (Sao_2)	Hypoxemia resulting from decreased oxygen supply or lung disease
	Low cardiac output (CO)	Cardiogenic shock caused by left ventricular pump failure
	Increased oxygen consumption (Vo_2)	Metabolic demand exceeds oxygen supply in conditions that increase muscle movement and increase metabolic rate, including such physiologic states as shivering, seizures, and hyperthermia and such nursing interventions as obtaining bed-scale weight and turning

below 60% and is sustained, the clinician must assume that oxygen supply is not equal to demand (see Table 15-24). It is helpful to assess the cause of decreased Svo_2 in a logical sequence that reflects knowledge of the meaning of the Svo_2 value.

1. To assess whether decreased Svo_2 is caused by decreased oxygen supply, verify the effectiveness of the ventilator or oxygen mask or check arterial oxygen saturation (Sao_2) by transcutaneous oximetry or from arterial blood gas values.
2. To assess cardiac function, perform a CO measurement.
3. To assess Hgb value, draw a blood sample for laboratory analysis.
4. Assess whether decreased Svo_2 is the result of a recent patient movement (Vo_2), a nursing action, or a clinical condition.

Always clinically assess the patient.

If Svo_2 falls below 40%, the balance of oxygen supply and demand may not be adequate to meet tissue needs at the cellular level. The cells change from an aerobic to anaerobic mode of metabolism, which results in the production of lactic acid and is representative of a shock state in which cellular injury or cell death may result. At this point every attempt should be made to determine the cause of the low Svo_2 and to correct the oxygen supply-demand imbalance.

In certain clinical conditions, Svo_2 may increase to an above-normal level (>80%), including times of low oxygen demand (decreased Vo_2) such as occurs during anesthesia (Tables 15-25 and 15-26) and in certain cases of sepsis in which the tissue cells cannot use the oxygen supplied to them and, as a consequence, venous oxygen reserve remains elevated and Svo_2 is higher than normal (see Table 15-23).

• • •

The range of diagnostic tools available to the bedside critical care nurse will continue to expand as we approach the end of the century. As critical care patient needs become more complex and nursing responsibilities increase, incorporation of appropriate diagnostic information into the nursing management plan will become even more vital.

REFERENCES

1. Goldberger AL, Goldberger E: *Clinical electrocardiography: a simplified approach,* ed 4, St Louis, 1990, Mosby–Year Book.
2. Henry JB: *Clinical diagnosis and management by laboratory methods,* ed 18, Philadelphia, 1991, WB Saunders.
3. Hurst JW: *The heart, arteries, and veins,* ed 7, New York, 1990, McGraw-Hill.
4. Schell M: Cholesterol, lipoproteins, lipid profiles: a Challenge in patient education, *Focus on Critical Care AACN* 17(3):203, 1990.
5. Mann H: Common errors in evaluating chest radiographs, *Postgrad Med* 87(1):275, 1990.
6. Dimmitt S: Limited value of chest radiography in uncomplicated hypertension, *Lancet* 2(8654):104, 1989.
7. Guthaner D, Breen J: Clinical aspects of chest roentgenology. In Marcus M, editor: *Cardiac imaging: a companion to Braunwald's heart disease,* Philadelphia, 1991, WB Saunders.
8. Heinsimer J and others: Supine cross-table lateral chest roentgenogram for the detection of pericardial effusion, *JAMA* 257(23):3266, 1987.

9. Stanford W: The radiology of right heart dysfunction: chest roentgenogram and computed tomography, *J Thorac Imaging* 4(3):7, 1989.
10. Pistolesi M and others: The chest roentgenogram in pulmonary edema, *Clin Chest Med* 6(3):315, 1985.
11. Mahdyoon H and others: Radiographic pulmonary congestion in end-stage congestive heart failure, *Am J Cardiol* 63(9):625, 1989.
12. McMillan J, Little-Longeway C: Right ventricular infarction, *Focus Crit Care* 18(2):158, 1991.
13. Schrem S and others: Cocaine-induced torsades de pointes in a patient with the idiopathic long QT syndrome, *Am Heart J* 120(4):980, 1990.
14. Drew B, Ide B, Sparacino P: Accuracy of bedside electrocardiographic monitoring: a report on current practices of critical care nurses, *Heart Lung* 20(6):597, 1991.
15. Drew B: Bedside electrocardiographic monitoring: state of the art for the 1990s, *Heart Lung* 20(6):610, 1991.
16. Kwan A, Nikolic G: Rapid cure of silent ischemia, *Heart Lung* 20(6):694, 1991.
17. Krucoff MW and others: Stability of multilead ST-segment "fingerprints" over time after percutaneous transluminal coronary angioplasty and its usefulness in detecting reocclusion, *Am J Cardiol* 61(15):1232, 1988.
18. Mizutani M and others: ST monitoring for myocardial ischemia during and after coronary angioplasty, *Am J Cardiol* 66(4):389, 1990.
19. Murphy M and others: Reevaluation of ECG criteria for left, right and combined cardiac ventricular hypertrophy, *Am J Cardiol* 53:1140, 1984.
20. Mirvis DM and others: Clinical and pathophysiologic correlates of ST-T wave abnormalities in coronary artery disease, *Am J Cardiol* 66(7):699, 1990.
21. Benhorin J: The prognostic significance of first myocardial infarction type (Q wave versus non-Q wave) and Q wave location, *J Am Coll Cardiol* 15(6):1201, 1990.
22. Hindman N and others: Relation between electrocardiographic and enzymatic methods of estimating acute myocardial infarct size, *Am J Cardiol* 58(1):31, 1986.
23. Spodick D: Left axis deviation and left anterior fascicular block, *Am J Cardiol* 61(1):869, 1988.
24. Sevenson AL, Meyer LT: Treatment of paroxysmol supraventricular tachycardia with adenosine: implications for nursing, *Heart Lung* 21 (4):350, 1992.
25. Morganroth J: Pharmacologic management of ventricular arrhythmias after the CAST, *Am J Cardiol* 65(22):1497, 1990.
26. Wood D: Potentially lethal ventricular arrhythmias: minimizing the danger, *Postgrad Med* 88(6):65, 1990.
27. Kuchar D, Thorburn C, Sammel N: Prediction of serious arrhythmic events after myocardial infarction: signal averaged electrocardiogram, Holter monitoring and radionuclide ventriculography, *J Am Coll Cardiol* 9(3):531, 1987.
28. American Heart Association Standards and guidelines for cardiopulmonary resuscitation and emergency cardiac care, *JAMA* 255(21):2841, 1986.
29. Buxton A and others: Hazards of intravenous verapamil for sustained ventricular tachycardia, *Am J Cardiol* 59(12):1107, 1987.
30. Cooper J, Marriott HJL: Why are so many critical care nurses unable to recognize ventricular tachycardia in the 12-lead electrocardiogram? *Heart Lung* 18:243, 1989.
31. Conover M, Marriott H: *Advanced concepts in arrhythmias,* ed 2, St Louis, 1989, Mosby–Year Book.
32. Akhtar M and others: Wide QRS complex tachycardia: reappraisal of a common clinical problem, *Ann Intern Med* 109:905-12, 1988.
33. Conner R: The Wenckebach phenomenon, *Heart Lung* 16(5):506, 1987.
34. Marriott HJL: AV block: An overdue overhaul, *Emerg Med* 13(6):85, 1981.
35. Ferraioli A and others: Electrocardiographic ambulatory monitoring with a real-time analysis system, *J Clin Monit* 6(4):307, 1990.
36. Rana M, Dunstan E, Allen S: Ambulatory electrocardiography in the elderly: an audit, *Br J Clin Pract* 43(9):341, 1989.
37. Knoebel S and others: ACC/AHA task force report: guidelines for ambulatory electrocardiography, *Circulation* 79(1):206, 1989.
38. Ouyang P: Frequency and importance of silent myocardial ischemia identified with ambulatory ECG monitoring in the early in-hospital period after acute MI, *Am J Cardiol* 65(5):267, 1990.
39. Hoberg E and others: Diagnostic value of ambulatory Holter monitoring for the detection of coronary artery disease in patients with variable threshold angina pectoris, *Am J Cardiol* 65(16):1078, 1990.
40. DiMarco J, Philbrick J: Use of ambulatory ECG (Holter) monitoring, *Ann Intern Med* 113(1):53, 1990.
41. Bogaty P and others: Prognosis in patients with a strongly positive exercise electrocardiogram, *Am J Cardiol* 64(19):1284, 1989.
42. Froelicher V: *Exercise and the heart: clinical concepts,* ed 3, St Louis, 1993, Mosby–Year Book.
43. Handler C, Sowton E: Stress testing predischarge and 6 weeks after myocardial infarction to compare submaximal and maximal exercise predischarge and to assess the reproducibility of induced abnormalities, *Int J Cardiol* 9(2):173, 1985.
44. Bruce R and others: ST segment elevation with exercise: a marker for poor ventricular function and poor prognosis, *Circulation* 77(4):897, 1988.
45. Detrano R and others: The diagnostic accuracy of the exercise ECG: a meta-analysis of 22 years of research, *Prog Cardiovasc Dis* 32(3):173, 1989.
46. Deckers J and others: A comparison of methods of analyzing exercise tests for diagnosis of coronary artery disease, *Br Heart J* 62(6):438, 1989.
47. Schactman M, Greene JS: Signal averaged electrocardiography: a new technique for determining which patients may be at risk for sudden cardiac death, *Focus Crit Care* 18(3):202, 1991.
48. Connelly AG: An examination of stressors in the patient undergoing cardiac electrophysiologic studies, *Heart Lung* 21(4):335, 1992.
49. Tavel M: *Clinical phonocardiography and external pulse recording,* St Louis, 1985, Mosby–Year Book.
50. Jawad I: *A practical guide to echocardiography and cardiac Doppler ultrasound,* Boston, 1990, Little, Brown.
51. Kloner R, Parisi A: Acute myocardial infarction: diagnostic and prognostic applications of two-dimensional echocardiography, *Circulation* 75(3):521, 1987.
52. Richards K: Doppler echocardiography in the diagnosis and quantification of valvular disease, *Mod Conc Cardiovasc Dis* 56(8):43, 1987.
53. Musewe N and others: Validation of Doppler-derived pulmonary arterial pressure in patients with ductus arteriosus under different hemodynamic states, *Circulation* 76(5):1081, 1987.
54. Presti C and others: Digital two-dimensional echocardiographic imaging of the proximal left anterior descending coronary artery, *Am J Cardiol* 60(6):1254, 1987.
55. Zabalgoitia M and others: Transesophageal echocardiography in the awake elderly patient: its role in the clinical decision-making process, *Am Heart J* 120(5):1147, 1990.
56. Matsuzaki M, Toma Y, Kusukawa R: Clinical applications of transesophageal echocardiography, *Circulation* 82(3):709, 1990.
57. Van Rossum A and others: Evaluation of magnetic resonance imaging for determination of left ventricular ejection fraction and comparison with angiography, *Am J Cardiol* 62(9):628, 1988.
58. Stratemeier E and others: Ejection fraction determination by magnetic resonance imaging: comparison with left ventricular angiography, *Radiology* 158:775, 1986.
59. Pohost G, Canby R: Nuclear magnetic resonance imaging: current applications and future prospects, *Circulation* 75(1):88, 1987.

60. Laakman R and others: Magnetic resonance imaging in patients with metallic implants, *Radiology* 157:711, 1985.
61. Bolgiano CS and others: The effect of two concentrations of heparin on arterial catheter patency, *Crit Care Nurse* 10(5):47, 1990.
62. American Association of Critical-Care Nurses: Evaluation of the effects of heparinized and nonheparinized flush solutions on the patency of arterial pressure monitoring lines: The AACN Thunder Project®, *Am J Crit Care* 2:3-15, 1993.
63. Dolter KJ: Increasing reliability and validity of pulmonary artery measurements, *DCCN* 8(3):183, 1989.
64. Lambert CW, Cason CL: Backrest elevation and pulmonary artery pressures: research analysis, *DCCN* 9(6):327, 1990.
65. Cline JK, Gurka AM: Effect of backrest position on pulmonary artery pressure and cardiac output measurements in critically ill patients, *Focus Crit Care* 18(5):383, 1991.
66. Dobbin K and others: Pulmonary artery pressure measurements in patients with elevated pressures: effect of backrest elevation and method of measurement, *Am J Crit Care* 1(2):61, 1992.
67. Bridges EJ, Woods SL: Pulmonary artery pressure measurement: State of the art, *Heart Lung* 22(2):99, 1993.
68. Hand HL: Direct or indirect blood pressure measurement for open heart surgery patients: an algorithm, *Crit Care Nurse* 12(6):52, 1992.
69. Quaal SJ: Quality assurance in hemodynamic monitoring, AACN Clinical Issues in Critical Care Nursing 4(1):197, 1993.
70. Rajacich N and others: Central venous pressure and pulmonary capillary wedge pressure as estimates of left atrial pressure: effects of positive end-expiratory pressure and catheter tip malposition, *Crit Care Med* 17(1):7, 11, 1989.
71. Cason CL, Lambert CW: Position and reference level of measuring right atrial pressure, *Crit Care Q* 12(4):77, 1990.
72. Thielen JB: Air emboli: a potentially lethal complication of central venous lines, *Focus Crit Care* 17(5):374, 1990.
73. Kelleher RM, Rose AA, Ordway L: Prostaglandins for the control of pulmonary hypertension in the postoperative cardiac surgery patient: nursing implications, *Crit Care Clin North Am* 3(4):741, 1991.
74. Haskall RJ, French WI: Accuracy of left atrial and pulmonary artery wedge pressure in pure mitral regurgitation in predicting left ventricular end-diastolic pressure, *Am J Cardiol* 61(1):136, 1988.
75. Pape LA and others: Relation of left atrial size to pulmonary capillary wedge pressure in severe mitral regurgitation, *Cardiology* 78:297, 1991.
76. Weed HG: Pulmonary "capillary" wedge pressure not the pressure in the pulmonary capillaries, *Chest* 100(4):1138, 1991.
77. Komodina KH and others: Interobserver variability in the interpretation of pulmonary artery catheter pressure tracings, *Chest* 100(6):1647, 1991.
78. Iberti TJ and others: A multicenter study of physicians' knowledge of the pulmonary artery catheter, *JAMA* 264(22):2928, 1990.
79. Cason CL and others: Effects of backrest elevation and position upon pulmonary artery pressures, *Cardiovasc Nurs* 26(1):1, 1990.
80. Groom L, Frisch SR, Elliott M: Reproducibility and accuracy of pulmonary artery pressure measurements in supine and lateral positions, *Heart Lung* 19(2):147, 1990.
81. Levine-Silverman S, Johnson J: Pulmonary artery pressure measurements, *West J Nurs Res* 12(4):488, 1990.
82. Lookinland S: Comparisons of pulmonary vascular pressures based on blood volume and ventilator status, *Nurs Res* 38(2):68, 1989.
83. Rountree WD: Removal of pulmonary artery catheters by registered nurses: a study in safety and complications, *Focus Crit Care* 18(4):313, 1991.
84. Hunn D and others: Thermodilution cardiac output values obtained by using a centrally placed introducer sheath and right atrial port of a pulmonary artery catheter, *Crit Care Med* 18(4):438, 1990.
85. Medley RS, DeLapp TD, Fisher DG: Comparability of the thermodilution cardiac output method: proximal injectate versus proximal infusion lumens, *Heart Lung* 21(1):12, 1992.
86. Pesola GR, Rostata HP, Carlon GC: Room temperature thermodilution cardiac output: central venous vs. right ventricular port, *Am J Crit Care* 1(1):76, 1992.
87. Pesola GR, Carlon GC: Thermodilution cardiac output: proximal lumen versus right ventricular port, *Crit Care Med* 19(4):563, 1991.
88. Bourdillon PDV, Fineberg N: Comparison of iced and room temperature injectate for thermodilution cardiac output, *Cathet Cardiovasc Diagn* 17:116, 1989.
89. Groom L, Elliott M, Frisch S: Injectate temperature: effects on thermodilution CO measurements, *Crit Care Nurse* 10(5):112, 1990.
90. Cigarroa RG and others: Underestimation of cardiac output by thermodilution in patients with tricuspid regurgitation, *Am J Med* 86:417, 1989.
91. Hamilton MA and others: Effect of tricuspid regurgitation on the reliability of the thermodilution cardiac output technique in congestive heart failure, *Am J Cardiol* 64:945, 1989.
92. Pearl RG, Siegel LC: Thermodilution cardiac output measurement with a large left-to-right shunt, *J Clin Monit* 7(2):146, 1991.
93. Halfmann SJ, Noll ML: Can continuous monitoring of mixed venous oxygen saturation be substituted for thermodilution cardiac output measurements? *Focus Crit Care* 17(2):157, 1990.
94. Lange RA and others: Limitations of the metabolic rate meter for measuring oxygen consumption and cardiac output, *Am J Cardiol* 64:783, 1989.
95. Perrino AC, Fleming J, LaMantia KR: Transesophageal Doppler ultrasonography: evidence for improved cardiac output monitoring, *Anesthesia Analog* 71:651, 1990.
96. Segal J and others: Instantaneous and continuous cardiac output in humans obtained with a Doppler pulmonary artery catheter, *Am Coll Cardiol* 16:1398, 1990.
97. Gillman PH: Continuous measurement of cardiac output: a milestone in hemodynamic monitoring, *Focus Crit Care* 19(2):155, 1992.
98. Woo MA and others: Comparison of thermodilution and transthoracic electrical bioimpedance cardiac outputs, *Heart Lung* 20(4):357, 1991.
99. Sommers M, Stevenson J, Hamlin R: SvO_2 and PVO_2 as predictors of cardiac index, *Heart Lung* 20(3):303, 1991.
100. Kyff JV and others: Continuous monitoring of mixed venous oxygen saturation in patients with acute myocardial infarction, *Chest* 95(3):607, 1989.
101. Copel LC, Stolanik A: Continuous SvO_2 monitoring: a research review, *DCCN* 19(4):202, 1991.
102. White KM and others: The physiologic basis for continuous mixed venous oxygen saturation monitoring, *Heart Lung* 19(5):548, 1990.
103. Winslow EH and others: Effects of a lateral turn on mixed venous oxygen saturation and heart rate in critically ill adults, *Heart Lung* 19(5):557, 1990.
104. Tidwell SL and others: Effects of position changes on mixed venous oxygen saturation in patients after coronary revascularization, *Heart Lung* 19(5):574, 1990.
105. Tyler DO and others: Effects of a 1 minute back rub on mixed venous oxygen saturation and heart rate in critically ill patients, *Heart Lung* 19(5):562, 1990.
106. Waite RM, Parsons D: Measurement of SvO_2, HR and MAP in myocardial revascularization patients upon initial postoperative activity, *Crit Care Nurse* 11(5):87, 1991.
107. White K: Using continuous Svo_2 to assess oxygen supply/demand balance in the critically ill patient, *AACN Clinical Issues in Critical Care Nursing* 4(1):134, 1993.

16

Cardiovascular Disorders

CHAPTER OBJECTIVES

- Describe the epidemiology and pathophysiology associated with coronary artery disease.
- Identify and describe the pathologic significance of nonmodifiable, minor modifiable, and major modifiable risk factors for the development of coronary artery disease.
- List the electrocardiographic, hemodynamic, and physiologic changes associated with myocardial infarction.
- List important aspects of the diagnosis and treatment of patients with heart failure, endocarditis, myocarditis, cardiomyopathy, valvular heart disease, hypertensive crisis, and peripheral vascular disease.
- List important aspects in the nursing assessment and care of patients with myocardial infarction, heart failure, endocarditis, myocarditis, cardiomyopathy, valvular heart disease, hypertensive crisis, and peripheral vascular disease.

Cardiovascular disease remains the leading cause of mortality in the United States. It claims more than 900,000 lives annually and places a heavy emotional and financial burden on society.[1] In 1968 a massive public health campaign was initiated to increase awareness of the risk factors attributed to the development of coronary artery disease. Since that time, mortality is steadily declining, and at least part of this positive effect is believed to result from changes in life-styles.[2] This is an encouraging trend, but enthusiasm must be tempered by the knowledge that the population is aging and cardiovascular disease is a progressive, degenerative process that is most prevalent in elderly persons.

CORONARY ARTERY DISEASE

Description

Coronary artery disease (CAD) is an insidious, progressive disease of the coronary arteries that results in their narrowing or complete occlusion. There are multiple causes for coronary artery narrowing (see box on right), but atherosclerosis is the most prevalent and affects the medium-sized arteries perfusing the heart, brain, kidneys, and extremities and the large arteries branching off the aorta. Atherosclerotic lesions may take different forms, depending on their anatomic location; the individual's age, genetic makeup, and physiologic status; and the number of risk factors present.

CAD has a long latent period. Fatty streaks appear within the aorta shortly after birth, but symptoms usually do not occur until late middle age when coronary artery lesions exceed 75% (i.e., 75% of the vessel lumen is occluded by atherosclerotic plaque).

Even though symptoms of atherosclerosis have been recognized in humans for thousands of years and lesions have been identified in mummies preserved from the fifteenth century BC,[3] the exact pathogenesis of atherosclerosis is not yet completely understood.

Etiology

Epidemiologic and actuarial data collected during the past 40 years have demonstrated an association between specific risk factors and the development of CAD. One of the most important epidemiologic studies is the Framingham Heart Study,[4] which began in 1948 and continues today with a second generation of subjects. Blood cholesterol levels are measured, smoking and activity histories are recorded, and blood pressure and electrocardiographic results are checked on a regular basis for participants in this study. As a result of this study and others like it, specific life-style habits have been identified that are associated with an increased probability of CAD development. These life-style habits are referred to as *coronary risk factors.* Several tools have been developed to assist the clinician in quickly and accurately identifying patients and populations at risk.

◆ **Risk factors.** Age, gender, and race influence the degree of risk for development of CAD. Factors that increase risk for development of CAD include elevated serum cholesterol levels, elevated blood pressure, cigarette smoking, abnormal glucose tolerance, sedentary life-style, stress, and type A behavior pattern. These factors are further delineated into nonmodifiable and major and minor modifiable factors (see box, p. 278).

ETIOLOGY OF CORONARY ARTERY DISEASE

Atherosclerosis
Thrombosis
Spasm
Coronary dissection
Aneurysm formation

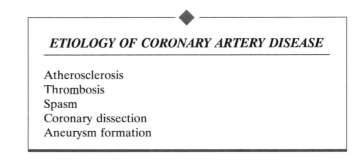

CORONARY ARTERY DISEASE RISK FACTORS

NONMODIFIABLE

Age
Gender
Family history
Race

MODIFIABLE

Major

Elevated serum lipids
Hypertension
Cigarette smoking
Impaired glucose tolerance
Diet high in saturated fat, cholesterol, and calories
Physical inactivity

Minor

Psychologic stress
Personality type

Nonmodifiable risk factors. CAD occurs approximately 10 years later in women than it does in men. After menopause, rates become the same for both genders. Family history is another significant risk factor. An individual has a positive family history if a close blood relative had a myocardial infarction or stroke before age 60 years. It is unclear whether the family history of CAD relates more to genetic predisposition or to family life-style habits. Since 1968 nonwhite populations of both genders have had higher CAD mortality rates than have white populations.[5]

Major modifiable risk factors

ELEVATED SERUM LIPIDS. Hyperlipidemia is a leading factor responsible for severe atherosclerosis. Cholesterol, triglycerides, and free fatty acids are all plasma lipids that are carried in the blood. Cholesterol is a steroid that is obtained endogenously by synthesis, especially in the liver, and exogenously from a diet high in saturated fats (see Chapter 50 for foods that may contribute to elevated serum cholesterol). Fatty acids are classified according to their level of saturation with hydrogen. Saturated fats (e.g., lard and butter) cannot absorb more hydrogen and tend to be solid at room temperature. Unsaturated fats can absorb additional hydrogen and usually are in soft or liquid form at room temperature. Triglycerides consist of three fatty acids connected to a glycerol molecule.

Serum cholesterol levels below 200 mg/dl are associated with minimal risk of CAD, whereas levels >270 mg/dl carry a fourfold increase in the risk.[5] (See Table 15-2 for desirable cholesterol lipid serum blood levels.) Cholesterol and triglycerides are transported in the blood by lipoprotein complexes, of which there are four major classes. These classes are distinguished by their protein density or by the percent of protein they carry. High density implies a high protein content, whereas low density indicates a low protein content. Chylomicrons, the first of these lipoproteins, are composed primarily of triglycerides. The second, very-low-density lipoproteins (VLDL), also known as B-lipoproteins, transport mainly triglycerides. The third, low-density lipoproteins (LDL), are B-lipoproteins, which are metabolized from VLDL and carry 60% to 75% of the total plasma cholesterol. The fourth, high-density lipoproteins (HDL), are composed of 50% protein, 25% phospholipid, 20% cholesterol, and 5% triglyceride. HDLs apparently clear cholesterol from the tissues and transport it to the liver. Children and premenopausal women often have an elevated HDL concentration, and both groups are considered at low risk for coronary disease. HDL levels are thought to increase in response to increased activity level and especially in response to aerobic exercises, weight loss, and cessation of cigarette smoking.[5]

HYPERTENSION. In the context of CAD, hypertension is the elevation of either systolic or diastolic pressure. Elevated systolic pressure is more predictive of risk, with levels consistently above 160 mm Hg of definite concern. The risk of CAD development in the presence of hypertension is proportional to the degree of blood pressure elevation. Hypertension is thought a risk factor because it causes damage to the vessel's endothelium and disrupts the antithrombogenic and permeability barrier.

Predisposing factors for hypertension are increased dietary sodium, obesity, sedentary life-style, excessive alcohol intake, oral contraceptives, and other medical problems that may influence the intrinsic mediators of blood pressure—the renin-angiotensin-aldosterone system and the sympathetic nervous system. Hypertension has a profound effect on the CAD risk profile in populations with elevated cholesterol levels (>160 mg/dl).

CIGARETTE SMOKING. Cigarette smoking is another major modifiable risk factor. Several studies indicate that the risk of CAD development is directly proportional to the number of cigarettes smoked per day. Those at highest risk are women smokers who also are using oral contraceptives, young men who smoke in excess of three packs per day, and middle-aged men with elevated cholesterol levels. Recent studies reveal that more women are smoking than ever before and that more teen-aged girls are starting to smoke than are teen-aged boys. Cigarette smoking unfavorably alters lipid levels, decreasing HDL levels and increasing LDL and triglyceride levels. Smoking results in cardiac electrical instability within cell membranes and impairs oxygen transport and use while increasing myocardial oxygen demand. Smoking also is thought to alter intimal endothelial permeability and to foster platelet agglutination. Fortunately, the damage from smoking is not unalterable, and after cessation the coronary risk falls rapidly, with a decrease of approximately 50% within 1 year.[6]

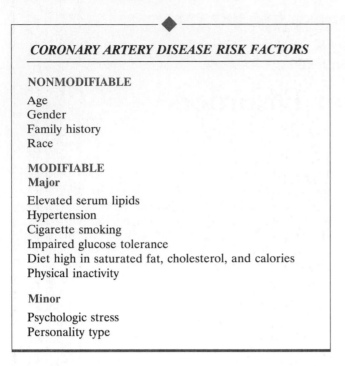

DIABETES MELLITUS. Diabetes mellitus is another potent risk factor. Women with diabetes mellitus are at greater risk for the development of CAD than are men with diabetes mellitus. Diabetes triples or quadruples a woman's risk, whereas a diabetic man's risk is increased by only 50%.[5] The younger the woman, the greater is her risk because diabetes negates the protective effect of estrogen.

The mechanism of how diabetes affects the coronary arteries is not well understood. However, it may alter platelet function or increase red blood cell adhesion. A positive association also exists between diabetes and hypertension, hypertriglyceridemia, and low levels of HDL. In addition, persons with diabetes tend to be more susceptible to both macrovascular and microvascular disease.

OBESITY. Obesity apparently affects the coronary artery risk profile by increasing susceptibility to the development of other risk factors, such as hypertension, impaired glucose tolerance, and hyperlipidemia, with increased LDL and decreased HDL levels. Obesity also is often associated with a sedentary life-style.

ORAL CONTRACEPTIVES. Oral contraceptives increase a woman's risk, especially after age 35 years, because oral contraceptives (1) alter blood coagulation, (2) alter platelet function, (3) alter fibinolytic activity, and (4) may inversely affect the integrity of vascular endothelium. This risk becomes significantly greater if the woman also smokes.

PHYSICAL INACTIVITY. Evidence continues to accumulate that a sedentary life-style increases the risk for CAD. A 20-year follow-up of 16,936 Harvard alumni demonstrated that those alumni who burned less than 2000 calories per week beyond their basal (minimal) level had a 64% higher risk for CAD.[6] Physical inactivity is also associated with lower HDL levels, higher LDL levels, hypertension, obesity, increased glucose intolerance, and elevated triglycerides .[6]

Minor modifiable risk factors

STRESS AND PERSONALITY. Researchers have been studying the effects of stress and personality on cardiac risk. The breakdown of families, poverty, stressful life events, and limited social support are being studied as potential precipitating factors. Certain behavioral characteristics were identified by Rosenman and Friedman[4,7] as associated with increased coronary risk. How stress or behavior influences the development of CAD is not well understood, but stress is associated with increased circulating catecholamines, which may precipitate hypertension, alteration in platelet function, increased fatty acid mobilization, and a resultant elevation of free fatty acids. These fatty acids may contribute to atherosclerotic plaque formation.

In summary, a great deal is still to be learned about atherosclerosis. One cannot pinpoint with absolute certainty the origins of atherosclerotic lesions. Further, researchers are uncertain why a risk factor in one individual may result in serious consequences but may not cause problems for another individual. Studies show that CAD is a multifactorial disease and the number of known risk factors increases the risk of developing the disease in an exponential rather than additive manner.[5]

Pathophysiology

Normal arterial walls are composed of three cellular layers: the intima, the innermost layer; the media, the middle layer; and the adventitia, the outermost layer (see Chapter 13, Fig. 13-11). The intima is the most susceptible to trauma; thus most primary lesions occur there, whereas the lesions that occur in the media are associated with more severe disease.

Three key elements that result in luminal narrowing or occlusions have been identified as follows[8]:

1. Smooth muscle proliferation
2. Formation of a connective tissue matrix composed of collagen, elastic fibers, and proteoglycans
3. Accumulation of lipids

◆ **Stages of plaque development.** Three stages of atherosclerotic plaque development have been identified (Fig. 16-1).[7,8] The first stage, *fatty streaks,* consists of broad-based lesions composed of lipid-laden macrophages and smooth muscle cells. Fatty streaks appear in the aorta soon after birth and at around age 15 years begin to develop in the coronary arteries, usually at bifurcation points. Remarkably, fatty streaks appear in all populations, even those with a low incidence of CAD; therefore the role they play as precursors of more complex lesions is unclear.

The second stage, the *fibrous plaque phase,* usually is identified by the occurrence of "classic" atherosclerotic plaques. Fibrous plaques are progressive lesions that begin to appear in young adults in their middle twenties. Changes that occur within the intima of the fibrous plaque include the key elements mentioned previously—proliferation of smooth muscle cells, the development of a connective tissue matrix, and the accumulation of intracellular and extracellular lipids.

The third stage, the *advanced (complicated) lesion phase,* consists of lesions usually seen with advancing age. The fibrous plaque undergoes several changes: (1) it becomes vascularized, (2) the core becomes calcified, and (3) the surface may desegregate and ulcerate, possibly resulting in (4) hemorrhage and thromboembolic episodes. Furthermore, the media may develop aneurysmal changes resulting from the decrease in smooth muscle cells.

◆ **Pathogenesis of plaque development.** Multiple theories exist about atheroma (plaque) formation, three of which are discussed here.

Response to injury. The response-to-injury hypothesis holds that the endothelium sustains some type of injury (either chemical or mechanical). As a result, structural and/or functional changes take place. The endothelium has two primary functions—first as a permeability barrier and second to provide a thrombo-resistant smooth surface. Injury disrupts the permeability barrier, allowing interaction between elements in the blood, such as between LDL and the wall of the vessel. The accompanying alteration in the thrombo-resistant surface may lead to platelet adherence, aggregation, and the release of platelet-derived growth factor, which usually is stored in the platelet.[8,9]

A pathophysiologic classification has been proposed to aid in the understanding of the pathogenesis of

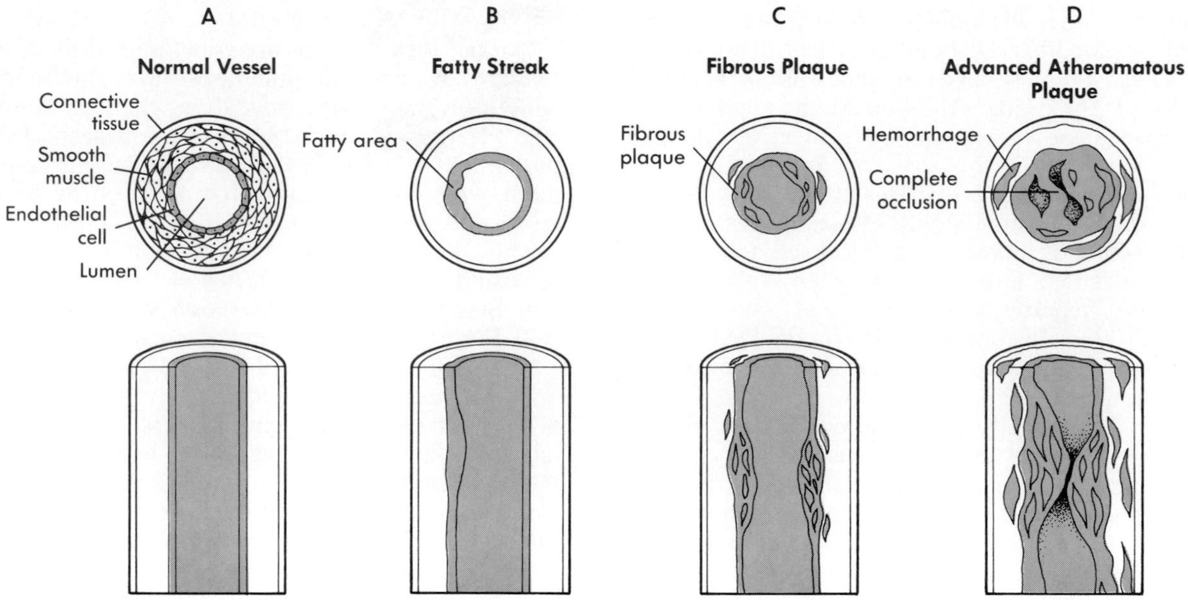

Fig. 16-1 The progression of atherosclerosis shown in both the longitudinal and the cross-sectional views. **A,** Normal vessel. **B,** First stage, fatty streaks. **C,** Second stage, fibrous plaque development. **D,** Third stage, advanced (complicated) lesions.

vascular injury. Type I injury consists of functional alterations of the endothelial cells without substantial morphologic changes; type II consists of endothelial denudation and intimal damage with intact internal elastic lamina; and type III reflects endothelial denudation with damage to both the intima and media.[10]

Monoclonal hypothesis. The monoclonal hypothesis put forth by Benditt and Benditt[11] proposes that each lesion has a common ancestral origin. Cell proliferation takes place because viruses or chemicals, such as hydrocarbons or cholesterol, alter the cellular genetic makeup, thereby producing a mutation. This mutation has a reproductive advantage over other cells and can reproduce at an enhanced rate. As a result the proliferating cells of an atherosclerotic plaque all stem from one mutated cell.

Thrombogenic hypothesis. The thrombogenic hypothesis, also known as the *encrustation theory,* relates closely to the injury hypothesis, which states that whenever there is endothelial injury, platelet agglutination and thrombus formation follow. Over time, platelet growth-promoting factor is released, resulting in proliferation of smooth muscle cells, which then become encased in connective tissue.[8] This is seen as the major mechanism for disease progression.[7]

A lipid lesion surrounded by a fibrotic cap can be easily disrupted, leading to type III vascular injury with thrombus formation. Small thrombi can then contribute to the growth of atherosclerotic plaque, whereas large thrombi may occlude, leading to unstable angina, myocardial infarction, and sudden ischemic death.[10-12]

◆ **Hemodynamic effect of CAD.** The major hemodynamic effect of CAD is the disturbance in the delicate balance between myocardial oxygen supply and demand. The three major determinants of this balance are heart rate, myocardial contractility, and myocardial wall tension. In healthy coronary arteries, myocardial oxygen extraction is almost maximal at rest, but it can increase fivefold with an increase in heart rate, blood pressure, or ventricular contractility. This increase in oxygen extraction occurs because healthy vessels can vasodilate in response to tissue hypoxia when oxygen demand increases.

Atherosclerosis alters the normal coronary artery's response to increased demand in two ways: (1) lesions that result in vessel-lumen occlusion of 75% or more restrict flow under resting conditions and (2) the vessels becomes stiff and lose the ability to dilate. The result is decreased driving pressure beyond the site of the lesion and less oxygenated blood available to the myocardial cells perfused by that vessel.[7] During ischemia (exercise or angina), the myocardium is forced to shift from aerobic metabolism to anaerobic metabolism, the consequences of which are (1) less efficient energy production, (2) lactic acid build-up, (3) intracellular hypokalemia, (4) intracellular acidosis, (5) intracellular hypernatremia, and (6) interference with the release of calcium from its storage sites in the sarcoplasmic reticulum.[3,7] The end result can be left ventricular dysfunction. This impaired left ventricular function results in decreased fiber stretch and contractility, decreased stroke volume, increased left ventricular end-diastolic volume (LVEDV), and increased left ventricular end-diastolic pressure (LVEDP). Further, the impairment of the calcium mechanism causes incomplete ventricular relaxation. This, in combination with poor ventricular emptying, may increase the LVEDP even more. Tissue hypoxia or ischemia is the end result of this process.

Angina. Angina is the sensory response to a transient lack of oxygen in the myocardium. It is not a disease, but rather a symptom of CAD. Angina has many characteristics (see box, below). The first description, a sensation of strangling in the breast, accompanied by anxiety or a fear of death, was published by Dr. William Heberden in 1772, and it is still accurate.[7]

Anginal pain may occur anywhere in the chest, neck, arms, or back, but the most common location is the retrosternal region. The pain frequently radiates to the left arm but also may radiate to both arms, the mandible, and/or the neck (Fig. 16-2). Levine's sign, a clenched fist placed over the sternum, frequently is demonstrated when patients indicate the location of their discomfort.[7]

Some relationship exists between the location of the chest pain and the site of the coronary occlusion. Patients with ischemic heart disease who report substernal or left-sided chest pain, with radiation to the left arm, usually have heart disease involving the left coronary artery, whereas those with epigastric pain radiating to the neck or jaw usually do not have disease of the left anterior descending coronary artery.[13]

Angina is classified as stable, unstable, and variant. *Stable angina* usually begins gradually and reaches maximal intensity during a matter of minutes before dissipating. It may be precipitated by activity, tachycardia, systemic hypertension, thyrotoxicosis, and sympathomimetic drugs, systemic illness, or anemia. Correction of the precipitating event, the administration of vasodilators, and life-style changes usually result in the termination of the angina. Stable angina often is managed medically for long periods.

Stable angina may be subdivided into *fixed threshold angina* and *varied threshold angina.* Fixed threshold angina is that which is predictable and caused by the same precipitating factors. It usually is the result of fixed lesions, with little acute vasoconstriction involved. Varied threshold angina is unpredictable. Patients may be able to walk two blocks pain-free some days, whereas on other days they may need to stop after only one block. Although a fixed lesion may be present, a dynamic component of coronary artery spasm also is present. Further, these patients may have more angina in the morning inasmuch as angiographic studies have shown smaller coronary arterial lumens in the morning hours than at other times of the day.[14]

Unstable angina is defined as a change in a previously established stable pattern or a new onset of severe angina. It usually is more intense than stable angina and often is described as pain rather than discomfort. Nitrates alone may no longer provide pain relief. Unstable angina also can be referred to as *preinfarction* or *crescendo angina, acute coronary insufficiency,* or *intermediate coronary syndrome*. It may be precipitated by the same events associated with stable angina or by (1) acceleration of atherosclerosis in multiple vessels, (2) left main coronary disease, (3) increase in localized platelet agglutination, (4) acute or chronic thrombosis, (5) plaque hemorrhage or fissure, or (6) acute vasoconstriction.[13]

Unstable angina may occur after a myocardial infarction as the result of mechanical problems, such as left ventricular aneurysm, mitral regurgitation secondary to ruptured papillary muscles, ventricular septal defect, or global left ventricular failure.[15] It usually is more intense, persists longer (up to 30 minutes), and may awaken patients from sleep.[7] The symptoms of unstable angina may be relieved only partially by rest or nitrates.

Variant, or *Prinzmetal's, angina* is caused by coronary artery spasm, which is defined as a reversible focal reduction in coronary artery diameter, leading to myocardial ischemia in the absence of preceding increases in myocardial oxygen consumption ($m\dot{V}O_2$) as reflected in elevation of heart rate or blood pressure. It is believed to result from spasm, with or without atherosclerotic lesion. Variant angina frequently occurs at rest and also can be cyclic, occurring at the same time every day. It usually is associated with ST segment elevation and

CHARACTERISTICS OF ANGINA PECTORIS

LOCATION

Beneath sternum, radiating to neck and jaw
Upper chest
Beneath sternum, radiating down left arm
Epigastric
Epigastric, radiating to neck, jaw, and arms
Neck and jaw
Left shoulder, inner aspect of both arms
Intrascapular

DURATION

0.5 to 30 minutes (stable)
Duration of longer than 30 minutes, without relief from rest or medication, indicates unstable or preinfarction symptoms

QUALITY

Sensation of pressure or heavy weight on the chest
Feeling of tightness, like a vise
Visceral quality (deep, heavy, squeezing, aching)
Burning sensation
Shortness of breath, with feeling of suffocation
Most severe pain ever experienced

RADIATION

Medial aspect of left arm
Jaw
Left shoulder
Right arm

PRECIPITATING FACTORS

Exertion/exercise
Cold weather
Exercising after a large, heavy meal
Walking against the wind
Emotional upset
Fright, anger
Coitus

MEDICATION RELIEF

Usually within 45 seconds to 5 minutes of sublingual nitroglycerin or nifedipine (Procardia) administration

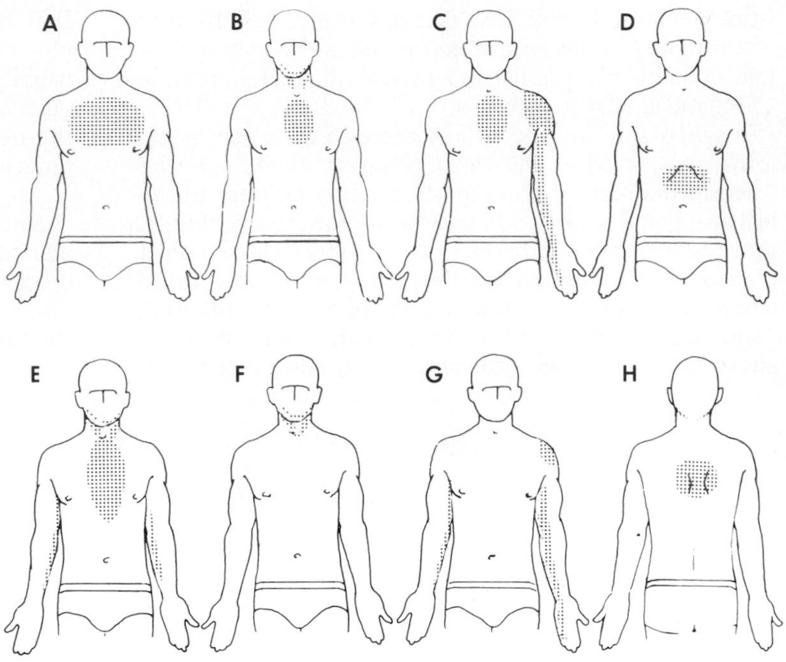

Fig. 16-2 Common sites for anginal pain. **A,** Upper part of chest. **B,** Beneath sternum radiating to neck and jaw. **C,** Beneath sternum radiating down left arm. **D,** Epigastric. **E,** Epigastric radiating to neck, jaw, and arms. **F,** Neck and jaw. **G,** Left shoulder. **H,** Intrascapular.

occasionally with transient abnormal Q waves.[7] Smoking tobacco and ingestion of alcohol and cocaine also may precipitate spasm.

Consequences of vasospasm include (1) a transient increase in myocardial oxygen demand over a fixed coronary reserve and (2) a transient decrease in myocardial oxygen supply.[10]

MEDICAL MANAGEMENT OF VARIANT ANGINA. Treatment of variant angina is aimed at decreasing the incidence of spasm and thereby reducing the risk of infarction or sudden death. Drugs of choice for the treatment of spasm are agents that vasodilate the coronary arteries, such as nitroglycerin (either sublingual, paste, patch, or spray); isosorbide dinitrate; or calcium channel blockers, such as nifedipine and diltiazem. Timing of administration is important because attacks of variant angina tend to be clustered between midnight and 8 AM. If a patient has a fixed atherosclerotic lesion, coronary artery bypass surgery may be indicated. Percutaneous transluminal coronary angioplasty (PTCA) or atherectomy may be performed with selected patients as long as extreme care is taken not to induce spasm.

Silent ischemia. Silent ischemia has been described in the literature for many years, but the incidence and mechanism have not been well understood.[16] Only during the past decade, with the advent of exercise stress testing and continuous ambulatory monitoring, has an awareness developed of the number of persons affected. Silent ischemia is defined as objective evidence of myocardial ischemia, without the patient experiencing any symptoms of angina.[16]

Silent ischemia is classified into three clinical types (see box, second column). Patients with type I ischemia are asymptomatic without signs or symptoms of cardiovascular disease, yet continuous monitoring or stress testing demonstrates myocardial ischemia. Frequently these patients are found to have multivessel CAD when later tested by coronary arteriography. As an example of the significance of this condition, in the Framingham heart study, one quarter of the patients had painless infarctions only detected by the presence of Q waves on the biannual electrocardiogram (ECG).[17] Type II patients are those who have had an acute myocardial infarction and demonstrate active ischemia but have no anginal symptoms. Patients with type III ischemia have some ischemic episodes that are accompanied by chest pain and other episodes without chest discomfort. Type III patients may or may not have had a prior infarction.

Several mechanisms may account for this phenomenon. The first is that the episodes of silent ischemia may demonstrate less severe ischemia, with less evidence of left ventricular dysfunction than ischemia with angina. The second is that Types I and II patients have higher pain thresholds. Smokers with CAD may have disturbance of regional myocardial perfusion and ST segment

SILENT ISCHEMIA

TYPE	CLINICAL CHARACTERISTICS
I	Objective evidence of myocardial ischemia without chest pain/symtoms
II	No anginal symptoms following a previous MI, but objective evidence of myocardial ischemia continues
III	Symptoms of angina with some episodes of ischemia, and asymptomatic with other ischemic events. May or may not have had a previous MI.

MI = Myocardial infarction.
Objective evidence of myocardial ischemia: ST segment changes seen on ECG monitoring.

depression during smoking. Mental stress also is believed to induce silent myocardial ischemia in patients with CAD.[17,18]

Once identified, silent ischemia usually is treated in the same manner as classic angina—with nitrates, beta blockers, calcium channel blockers, and life-style changes.

Medical Management

The major goals of medical therapy for CAD are to increase coronary perfusion and decrease myocardial work to prevent myocardial infarction (MI) and disability or death. Medical management depends on the frequency, severity, duration, and hemodynamic consequences of the angina. Pharmacologic therapy may include nitrates, beta blockers, and calcium channel blockers. CAD risk factors, such as hypertension or hyperlipidemia, should be treated aggressively. A low-sodium, low-cholesterol diet may be recommended. Activity will be restricted until episodes of angina are controlled. If pain persists despite maximal pharmacologic therapy and rest, an intraaortic balloon may be inserted to increase coronary artery perfusion pressure and to reduce afterload.

Tachycardias usually are treated with digoxin, calcium blockers, beta blockers, or antidysrhythmic agents. Hypertension is managed with diuretics or afterload reducers. Anemia may be treated with blood transfusions or iron supplements. For coronary spasm, nitrates or calcium blockers, or both, are used.

The change from stable to unstable angina represents a serious problem. The patient usually is admitted to a hospital, and bed rest is prescribed. It is important that any identified precipitating problems be treated. If the anginal pain continues, cardiac catheterization, intraaortic balloon support, thrombolytic therapy, PTCA, or coronary artery bypass surgery may be indicated.

Nursing Management

Nursing care of the patient admitted with angina focuses on continuous assessment and documentation of episodes of chest pain and on providing an environment that will help alleviate fear and anxiety and provide rest and security.

On admission, cardiac monitoring is instituted, a 12-lead ECG obtained, and any ongoing pain controlled. Then a systematic, holistic nursing assessment is performed, nursing diagnoses are identified and prioritized, and an individualized plan of care is developed.

Complaints of chest pain must be evaluated quickly. Chest pain in the patient with known or suspected coronary disease may represent myocardial ischemia, which must be treated while it is still reversible. See Chapter 17 for a full discussion of the range of therapies available for the treatment of acute or preinfarction angina. Assessment criteria include documentation of the characteristics of the pain, the patient's heart rate and rhythm, the presence of ectopic beats or conduction defects, the patient's mentation, and the overall status of his or her tissue perfusion (i.e., skin color, temperature, and pulses), and urine output.

NURSING DIAGNOSIS AND MANAGEMENT
Coronary artery disease/angina

- ◆ Acute Pain related to transmission and perception of cutaneous, visceral, muscular, or ischemic impulses secondary to myocardial ischemia, p. 566
- ◆ Activity Intolerance related to decreased cardiac output and/or myocardial tissue perfusion alterations, p. 366
- ◆ Anxiety related to threat to biologic, psychologic, and/or social integrity, p. 763
- ◆ Knowledge Deficit: ____(Specify) related to lack of previous exposure to information, p. 72
- ◆ Body Image Disturbance related to actual change in body structure, function, or appearance, p. 94
- ◆ Altered Sexuality Patterns related to fear of death during coitus secondary to myocardial infarction, p. 120

Smith[19] identified 11 factors that must be considered when assessing chest pain:

- ◆ Onset (either sudden or gradual)
- ◆ Precipitating factors (did visitors come or leave; was the patient up moving around?)
- ◆ Location (was it substernal; was it located in same area as previous pain?)
- ◆ Radiation (did it radiate to the jaw, neck, arm, or shoulder?)
- ◆ Quality (was it similar to previous anginal pain; was it less or worse?)
- ◆ Intensity (on a scale of 1 to 10, where would the patient rate it?)
- ◆ Duration (did it last seconds or minutes; how soon after onset did the patient call for help?)
- ◆ Relieving factors (what made it better—changing position, nitroglycerin, oxygen, the presence of the nurse?)
- ◆ Aggravating factors (did the environment, telephone calls, waiting for help worsen the pain?)
- ◆ Associated symptoms (was the pain accompanied by nausea, vomiting, diaphoresis, or dyspnea?)
- ◆ Emotional response (how did the patient feel about the pain; was he or she anxious, fearful, angry?)

MYOCARDIAL INFARCTION

With the advent of coronary care units in the late 1960s, great strides have been made in the treatment and survival rate of patients with myocardial infarctions. Today, almost 3 decades later, however, more than 500,000 persons per year still die of acute myocardial infarctions, with about 30% dying before reaching the hospital.[20] Of those who do receive treatment, approximately 80% survive.

Description

Myocardial infarction is the term used to describe irreversible cellular loss and myocardial necrosis that result from an abrupt decrease or total cessation of coronary blood flow to a specific area of the myocardium. Infarction is more prevalent in the left ventricle, and occlusions are most likely to cause myocardial necrosis when they occur in vessels that have not developed collateral flow. Infarction also occurs with more frequency in individuals with multivessel occlusions.

Etiology

Atherosclerosis is responsible for most myocardial infarctions because it causes luminal narrowing and reduced blood flow, resulting in decreased oxygen delivery to the myocardium. The three mechanisms that are primarily responsible for the acute reduction in oxygen delivery to the myocardium are (1) coronary artery thrombosis, (2) plaque fissure or hemorrhage, and (3) coronary artery spasm.

Coronary artery thrombi are now thought to be present in almost all acute occlusions. DeWood and others[7,8] found thrombus formation in 87% of patients who underwent cardiac catheterization within the first 4 hours after the onset of the symptoms of infarction. These thrombi, usually composed of platelets, fibrin, erythrocytes, and leukocytes, may be superimposed on a plaque or may align adjacent to a plaque. They release thromboxane A_2, serotonin, and thrombin, all vasoconstricting substances that compound the vessel narrowing and set up a vicious cycle of recurrent occlusion.[7,8]

Scientists have not determined the cause of thrombus formation, but plaque fissure or hemorrhage, or both, are thought to be predisposing events.[7,10,12] Plaques are classified according to their composition. Hard plaques are heavily calcified and fibrotic, whereas soft plaques are composed of cholesterol esters and lipids. Coronary artery thrombosis has been associated with rupture or cracks of the plaques and release of the plaque material into the vascular lumen. Plaque rupture can induce thrombosis by (1) forming a platelet plug, (2) releasing tissue thromboplastin from the plaque material that activates the clotting cascade, and (3) obstructing the vessel lumen with plaque components.

The role of coronary artery spasm in partial or complete coronary artery occlusion remains a mystery. Direct evidence has shown that vasospasm is present, but it is not known whether this results from hyperactive smooth muscle or whether it is a secondary response related to a plaque rupture and the release of vasoactive substances.

Pathophysiology

◆ **Zones of infarction, ischemia, and injury.** The area of cellular death and muscle necrosis in the myocardium is known as the *zone of infarction* (Fig. 16-3). On the ECG,

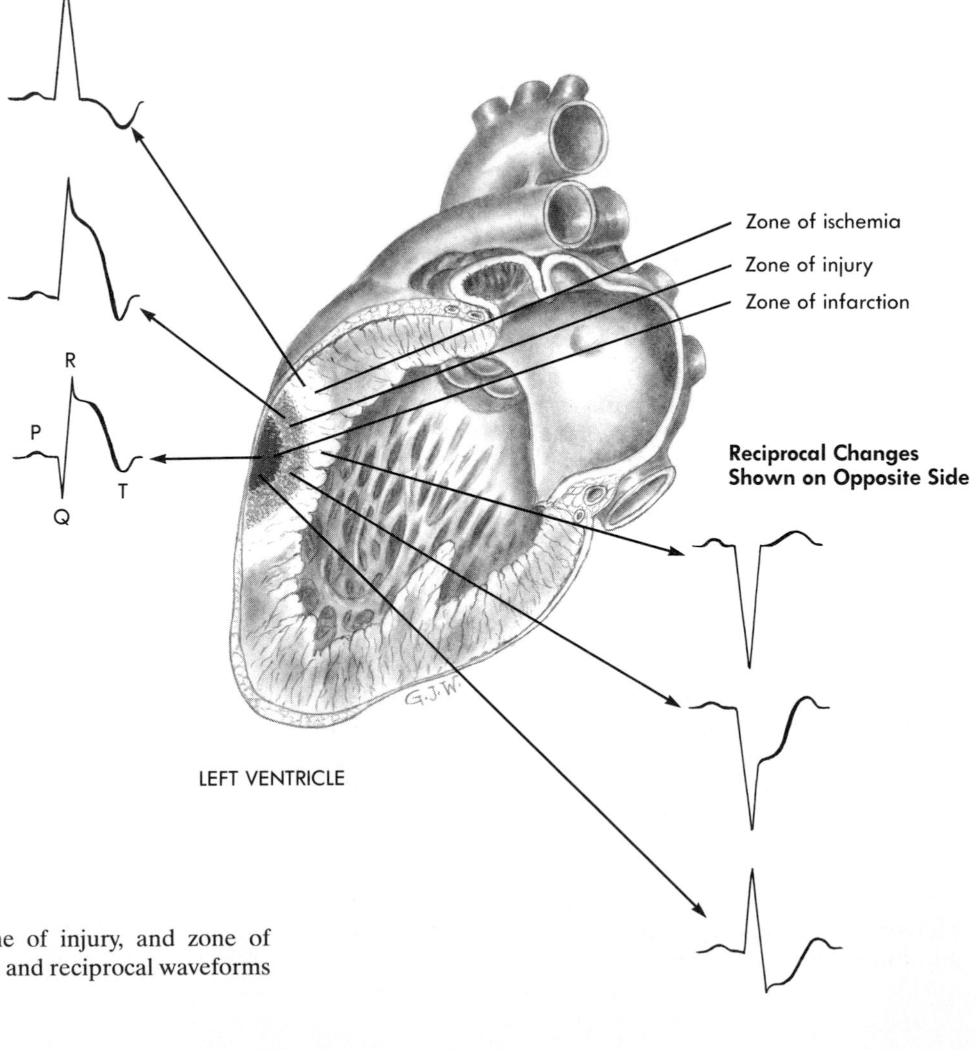

Fig. 16-3 Zone of ischemia, zone of injury, and zone of infarction, showing ECG waveforms and reciprocal waveforms corresponding to each zone.

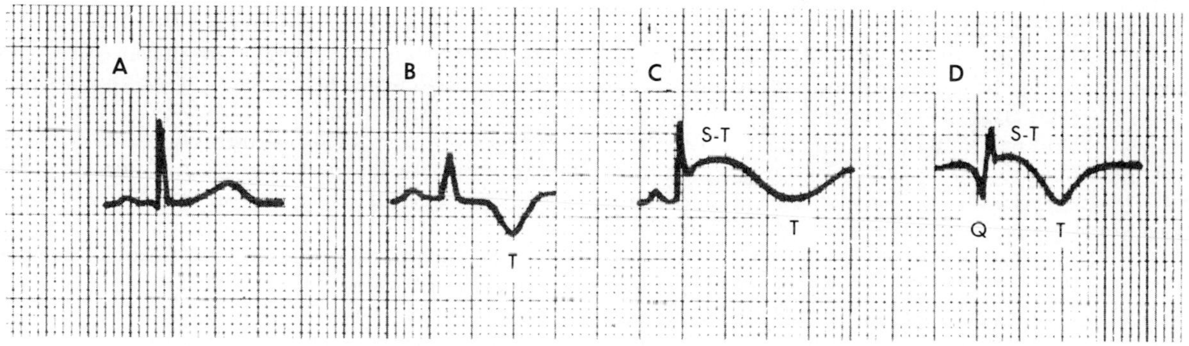

Fig. 16-4 ECG changes indicative of ischemia, injury, and infarction (necrosis) of the myocardium. **A,** Normal ECG. **B,** Ischemia indicated by inversion of the T wave. **C,** Ischemia and current of injury indicated by T wave inversion and ST segment elevation. The ST segment may be elevated above or depressed below the baseline, depending on whether the tracing is from a lead facing toward or away from the infarcted area and depending on whether epicardial or endocardial injury occurs. Epicardial injury causes ST elevation in leads facing the epicardium. **D,** Ischemia, injury, and myocardial necrosis. The Q wave indicates necrosis of the myocardium. (From Kinney M and others: *Comprehensive cardiac care,* ed 7, St Louis, 1991, Mosby–Year Book.)

evidence of this zone is seen by pathologic Q or QS waves, which reflect a lack of depolarization from the cardiac surface involved in the myocardial infarction (Fig. 16-4, *D*). As healing takes place, the cells in this area are replaced by scar tissue.

The infarcted zone is surrounded by injured but still potentially viable tissue in an area known as the *zone of injury* (see Fig. 16-3). Cells in this area do not fully repolarize because of the deficient blood supply. This is recorded as elevation of the ST segment (Fig. 16-4, *C*).

The outer region, as illustrated in Fig. 16-3, is the *zone of ischemia* and is composed of viable cells. Repolarization in this zone is impaired but eventually is restored to normal. Repolarization of the cells in this area manifests as T wave inversion (Fig. 16-4, *B*). This region also is the apparent site of many of the dysrhythmias associated with an infarction because of the impaired repolarization.

During the first 6 weeks after an infarction, the damaged myocardium itself undergoes many changes. Approximately 6 hours after the infarction, the muscle becomes distended, pale, and cyanotic. Over the next 2 days the myocardium becomes reddish purple, and an exudate may form on the epicardium. Leukocyte scavenger cells begin to infiltrate the muscle and carry away the necrotic debris, thereby thinning the necrotic wall. Approximately 3 to 4 weeks after the infarction, scar tissue begins to form and the affected wall becomes whiter and thicker.[7]

◆ **Classification of infarctions.** Myocardial infarctions frequently are classified according to their location on the myocardial surface and the muscle layers affected. A *transmural infarction* involves all three muscle layers—the endocardium, the myocardium, and the epicardium (Fig. 16-5). Transmural infarctions, because they result in full-thickness necrosis, have a higher incidence of left ventricular dysfunction. One method of determining left

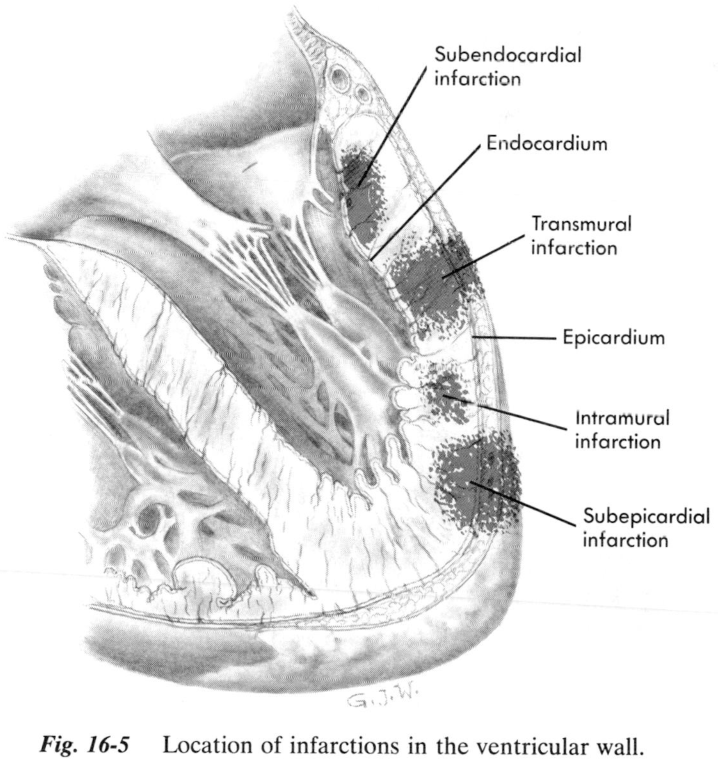

Fig. 16-5 Location of infarctions in the ventricular wall.

ventricular function involves calculating the ejection fraction. Ejection fraction is the volume of blood ejected with each contraction. The normal ejection fraction ranges from 63% to 70% and can be calculated noninvasively at the bedside by the Gated Blood Pool Scan. In the early postinfarction period an ejection fraction of 40% or more indicates a good prognosis, whereas an ejection fraction of less than 40%, and certainly less than 30%, suggests a poor prognosis.[21]

The electrocardiographic changes produced by a transmural infarction demonstrate alteration in both myocardial depolarization (QRS complex) and repolarization (ST-T complex). The change in depolarization is represented by the appearance of new Q waves. These Q waves are deeper (one-third to one-fourth the height of the R wave) and wider than normal (0.04 seconds or longer in duration).

The changes in repolarization involve ST-T changes that occur in two phases, the acute and the evolving. The acute-phase changes are reflected in ST segment elevation in the leads overlying the involved surface, with reciprocal ST changes in the leads reflecting the opposite surface. This ST elevation may be preceded by hyperacute T waves. During the evolving phase the elevated ST segments and hyperacute T waves become deeply inverted T waves.

Nontransmural infarctions are classified as either subendocardial, involving the endocardium and the myocardium, or subepicardial, involving the myocardium and the epicardium (see Fig. 16-5).

Because the endocardium has a much higher oxygen need than does the epicardium, subendocardial infarcions are the more common of the nontransmural infarctions. The most common electrocardiographic change seen with subendocardial ischemia is ST depression (Fig. 16-6). Generally, abnormal Q waves are not seen, and R wave progression is normal with a subendocardial infarction.

◆ **Location of myocardial infarctions.** The location and extent of a myocardial infarction depend on (1) the site and severity of coronary artery narrowing, (2) the presence, site, and severity of coronary artery spasm, (3) the size of the vascular bed perfused by compromised vessels, (4) the extent of collateral vessels, and (5) the oxygen needs of the poorly perfused myocardium.[18]

The location of infarction can be determined by correlating the ECG leads with Q waves and the ST segment T wave abnormalities (Table 16-1). Infarction most commonly occurs in the left ventricle and the interventricular septum; however, close to 25% of all patients who sustain an inferior myocardial infarction have some right ventricular damage.[22] Although rare, atrial infarcts also have been reported.

In examining an ECG, it is essential that groups of leads, rather than one lead at a time, be evaluated. Correlating a group of leads that display ECG change with the area of the heart reflected by the leads allows

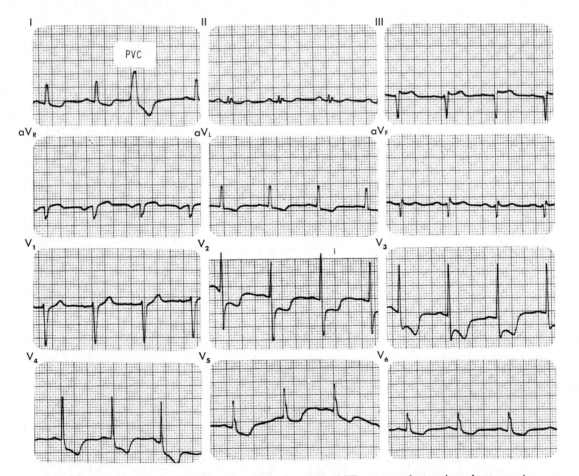

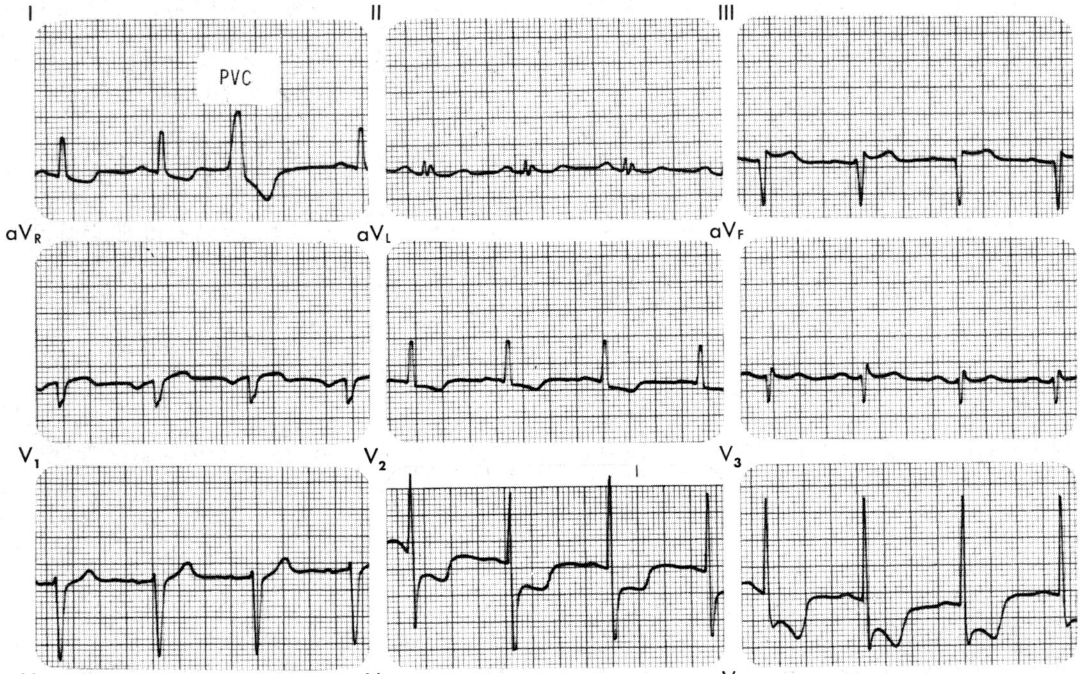

Fig. 16-6 Subendocardial infarction. Note the marked ST segment depressions, best seen in chest leads V_2 to V_5, consistent with subendocardial infarction. Slight ST segment elevations are seen in the reciprocal leads aV_r and III. (Modified from Goldberger AL, Goldberger E: *Clinical electrocardiography: a simplified approach,* ed 4, St Louis, 1990, Mosby–Year Book.)

(1) identification of the location of the infarction and (2) anticipation of potential electrical or mechanical complications. Remembering that the right coronary artery (RCA) perfuses the sinoatrial (SA) node, the proximal bundle of His, and the atrioventricular (AV) node and that an inferior wall infarction results from RCA occlusion will alert one to the conduction disturbances that are possible with an inferior wall myocardial infarction. Changes in the leads overlooking the anterior wall alert the observer to the possibility of mechanical problems or pump failure.

Table 16-1 Correlation between ventricular surfaces, ECG leads, and coronary arteries

Surface of left ventricle	ECG leads	Coronary artery usually involved
Inferior	II, III, aVF	Right coronary
Lateral	I, aVL	Left circumflex
Anterior	V_2-V_4	Left anterior descending
Septal	V_1-V_2	Left anterior descending
Apical	V_5-V_6	Left anterior descending
Posterior	V_1-V_2 (reciprocal changes)	Left circumflex

From Price SA, Wilson LM: *Pathophysiology: clinical concepts of disease processes*, ed 4, St Louis, 1992, Mosby–Year Book.

The three ECG manifestations used to diagnose infarction and to pinpoint the area of damaged ventricle are inverted T waves, indicative of myocardial ischemia; ST segment elevation, indicative of myocardial injury; and pathologic Q waves, indicative of cell death or infarction.

Anterior wall infarctions. Because the anterior surface is so large, it often is subdivided into anteroseptal, true anterior, and anterolateral sections.

Anteroseptal infarctions usually result from an occlusion of the left anterior descending coronary artery (LAD). Leads V_1 through V_4 reflect the electrical activity of the anteroseptal wall. On an ECG, a loss of septal depolarization is reflected as a loss of R wave progression in V_1 and V_2, leaving a QS complex. Q waves are seen in V_2 through V_4, and ST segment elevations and T wave inversions are seen in V_4 and V_5. Reciprocal changes usually are not seen with an anteroseptal myocardial infarction.

True anterior infarctions (Fig. 16-7, *A*) usually result from occlusion of the LAD and are seen on the ECG as loss of positive R progression in the chest leads (V_1 through V_6). ST segment elevation may be seen in leads V_1 through V_4, and T wave inversion may occur in leads I, aVL, and V_3 to V_5 (Fig. 16-7, *B*).

Anterolateral infarction occurs as a result of occlusion of the circumflex coronary artery. On ECG, Q waves and ST-T wave changes are seen in leads I and aV_l and in leads V_4, V_5, and V_6, which reflect lower lateral wall or left apical involvement. Reciprocal changes occur in the inferior leads II, III, and aV_F.

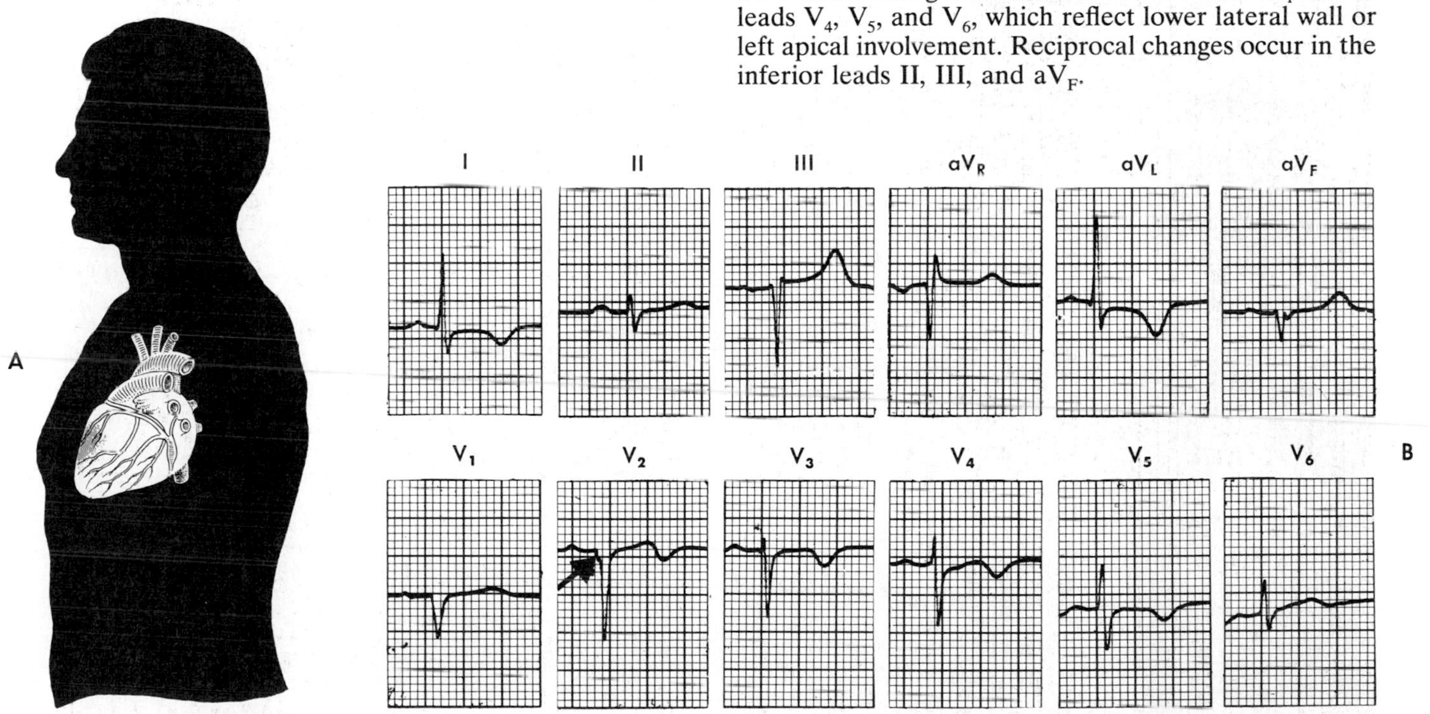

Fig. 16-7 **A,** Position of an anterior wall infarction. **B,** Anterior wall infarction. Note the QS complexes in leads V_1 and V_2, indicating anteroseptal infarction. There is also a characteristic notching (*arrow,* V_2) of the QS complex, often seen in infarctions. In addition, note the diffuse ischemic T wave inversions in leads I, aV_L, and V_2 to V_5, indicating generalized anterior wall ischemia. (From Goldberger AL, Goldberger E: *Clinical electrocardiography: a simplified approach,* ed 4, St Louis, 1990, Mosby–Year Book.)

Inferior wall infarctions. Inferior (diaphragmatic) infarctions (Fig. 16-8, *A*) occur with occlusion of the right coronary artery and are manifested by ECG changes in leads II, III, and aV_F. Reciprocal changes occur in leads I and aV_L (Fig. 16-8, *B*).

Posterior wall infarctions. Posterior infarctions (Fig. 16-9) occur with occlusion of the circumflex branch of the left coronary artery. Because the standard 12-lead ECG does not directly record activity on the posterior surface, a posterior wall myocardial infarction is documented by reciprocal changes seen as tall R waves and ST segment depression in leads V_1 and V_2.

The location of an infarction may be highly indicative of overall outcome. Anterior and anteroseptal infarctions, which result from occlusion of the LAD, are the least favorable types because of the serious left ventricular dysfunction that results. Anterior wall infarctions are associated with twice the mortality of inferior wall infarctions.[18,22]

Assessment and Diagnosis

The definitive diagnosis of myocardial infarction is based on the patient's clinical manifestations, electrocardiographic changes discussed in the previous section, and cardiac enzyme levels.

◆ **Clinical manifestations.** The most common clinical manifestation of infarction is prolonged severe chest pain, which frequently is associated with nausea, vomiting, and diaphoresis. This pain generally lasts 30 minutes or more and usually is located in the substernal or left precordial area. Unlike angina, which often is described as discomfort, the pain of infarction may be described as the most severe pain the individual has ever experienced. Descriptions used are "a heaviness," "like an elephant sitting on my chest," or a "viselike tightness." The pain may radiate to the back, the neck, the jaw, or the left arm, particularly down the ulnar aspect.[19] Neither rest nor nitrates relieve the pain. See the box on p. 289, left-hand column for other commonly occurring clinical manifestations of infarction.

◆ **Enzyme manifestations.** A complete discussion of the relationship of enzymes to diagnosis of myocardial infarction is presented in Chapter 15, p. 185. The reader is referred to that chapter for review.

Complications of Myocardial Infarction

Unfortunately, many patients experience complications occurring either early or late in the postinfarction course (see box, p. 289, top right). These complications may result from pumping or electrical dysfunctions. Pumping complications cause heart failure (HF), pulmonary edema, and cardiogenic shock. Electrical dysfunctions include bradycardia, bundle branch blocks, and varying degrees of heart block.[23]

◆ **Dysrhythmias.** Close to 95% of all patients who experience a myocardial infarction will have dysrhythmias. There are many potential causes such as those included in the box on p. 289, middle right, but ischemia of the pacemaker cells is the most common cause. Ischemia results in alterations in membrane excitability and in conduction and refractory periods, which in turn result in ST changes, enhanced automaticity, and reentry. Reentry is the reactivation of a tissue for the second time by the same impulse.

Sinus bradycardia (heart rate <60 beats/min) occurs in approximately 40% of all patients who sustain an acute myocardial infarction and is more prevalent with an

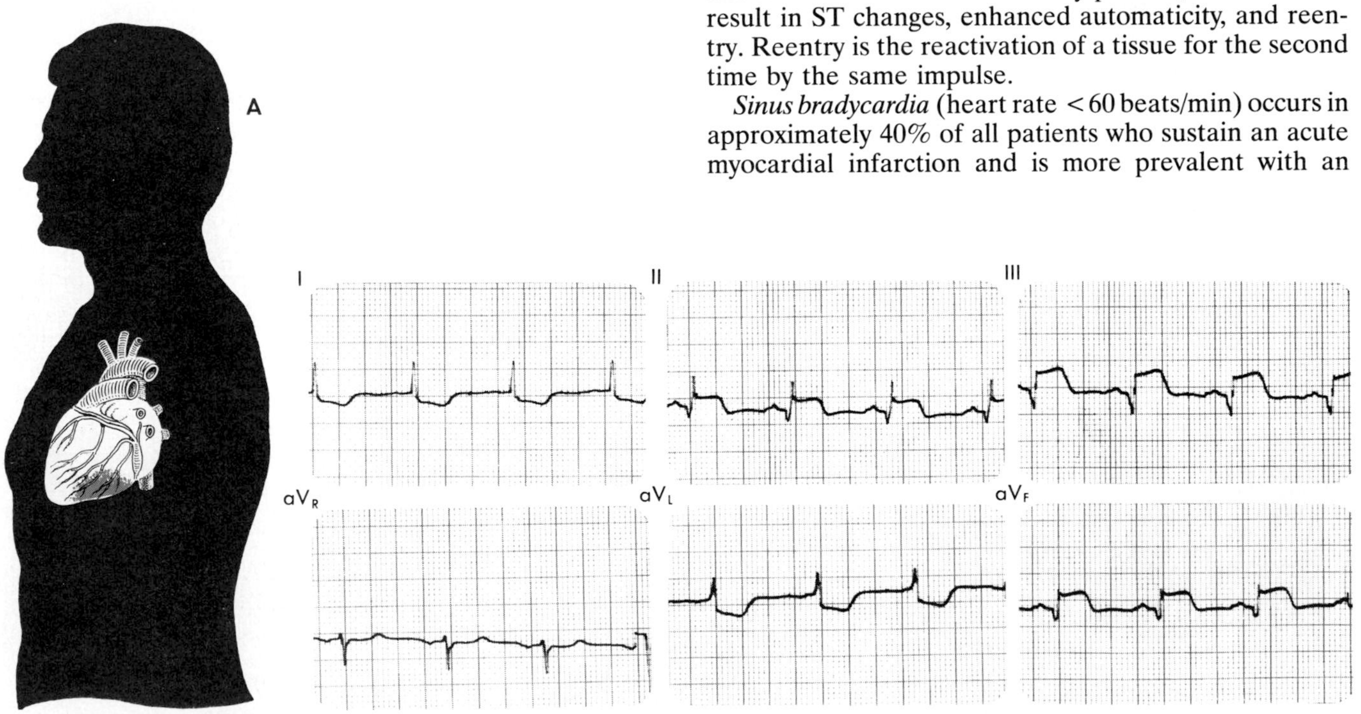

Fig. 16-8 **A,** Position of an inferior wall infarction. **B,** Acute inferior wall infarction. Note the ST elevations in leads II, III, and aV_R with reciprocal ST depressions in leads I and aV_L. Abnormal Q waves also are seen in leads II, III, and aV_F. (From Goldberger AL, Goldberger E: *Clinical electrocardiography: a simplified approach,* ed 4, St Louis, 1990, Mosby–Year Book.)

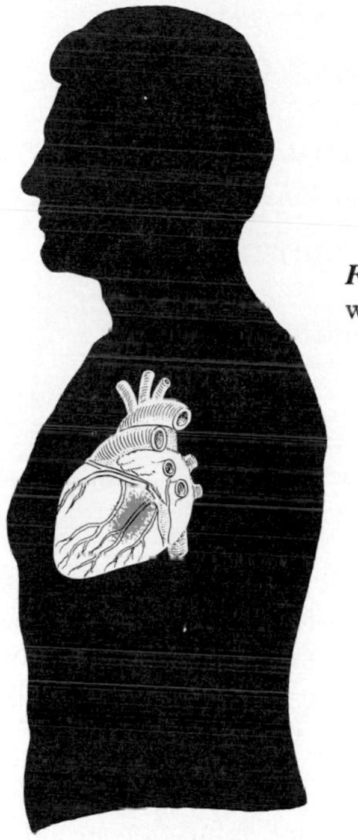

Fig. 16-9 Position of a posterior wall infarction.

CLINICAL MANIFESTATIONS OF ACUTE MYOCARDIAL INFARCTION

Tachycardia *with* or *without* ectopy
Bradycardia
Normotension or hypotension
Tachypnea
Diminished heart sounds, especially S_1
If left ventricular dysfunction present, may have S_3 and/or S_4
Systolic murmur
Pulmonary crackles
Pulmonary edema
Air hunger
Orthopnea
Frothy sputum
Decreased cardiac output
  Decreased urine output
  Decreased peripheral pulses
  Slow capillary refill
Restlessness
Confusion
Anxiety
Agitation
Denial
Anger

inferior wall infarction. Inferior wall myocardial infarctions usually are the result of a right coronary artery occlusion. The right coronary artery perfuses the SA and AV nodes in most people. Some bradycardia associated with an inferior wall myocardial infarction may be a compensatory response inasmuch as a slower heart rate

COMPLICATIONS OF MYOCARDIAL INFARCTION

Dysrhythmias
Ventricular aneurysms
Ventricular septal defect
Papillary muscle rupture
Pericarditis
Cardiac rupture
Sudden death
Heart failure
Pulmonary edema
Cardiogenic shock

ETIOLOGY OF DYSRHYTHMIAS IN MYOCARDIAL INFARCTION

Tissue ischemia
Hypoxemia
Autonomic nervous system influences
Metabolic derangements
  Acid-base imbalances
Hemodynamic abnormalities
Drugs (especially digoxin toxicity)
Electrolyte imbalances (e.g., hypokalemia, hypomagnesemia)
Fiber stretch
  Chamber dilation
  Cardiomyopathy

reduces myocardial oxygen demands. A slower heart rate, however, increases the risk for ectopic foci. Sinus bradycardia is seen most frequently in the immediate postinfarction period.

Sinus tachycardia (heart rate >100 beats/min) most often occurs with anterior wall myocardial infarctions. Anterior infarctions impair the left ventricular pumping ability, thereby reducing the ejection fraction and stroke volume. In an attempt to maintain cardiac output, the heart rate increases. Tachycardia must be corrected, not only because it greatly increases myocardial oxygen consumption, but because it shortens diastolic filling time, thereby decreasing stroke volume, systemic perfusion, and coronary artery filling.

Premature atrial contractions (PACs) occur in almost one half of all patients who sustain acute infarction.[7] PACs most commonly are caused by cell irritability resulting from distention of the left atrium secondary to increased left ventricular end-diastolic pressure and volume. The increase in volume and pressure of the left ventricle results from its poor contraction after the infarction.

Atrial fibrillation is a commonly seen atrial dysrhythmia associated with myocardial infarction and is more prevalent with an anterior wall infarction. It may occur spontaneously or be preceded by PACs or atrial flutter. With atrial fibrillation there is loss of atrial contraction, hence a loss of atrial kick and the extra stroke volume it carries. It is estimated that cardiac output can decrease by 30% when atrial kick is lost.[7] For this reason, atrial dysrhythmias are significant because of their ability to decrease cardiac output.

Within the first few hours after a myocardial infarction, almost all patients will have *premature ventricular contractions* (PVCs).[23] PVCs usually are controlled well by administering oxygen to reduce tissue hypoxia, correcting any acid-base or electrolyte imbalance, and administering intravenous lidocaine or other antidysrhythmic drugs.

PVCs and ventricular tachycardia occurring early (within the first few hours) in the postinfarction course usually are transient. When, however, these same dysrhythmias occur late in the course, they tend to be associated with high in-hospital mortality, because they usually are related to the cumulative loss of myocardium.[23,24]

AV heart block most frequently follows an inferior wall myocardial infarction. Because the right coronary artery perfuses the AV node in 90% of the population, occlusion of it leads to ischemia and infarction of the cells of the AV node.

The major goal of therapy for any dysrhythmia is preservation of cardiac output and tissue perfusion. Medications must be used with caution, particularly those that increase the cardiac workload or depress myocardial function.

◆ Sudden cardiac death

Description. An estimated 300,000 to 400,000 persons die a sudden cardiac death each year in the United States. This accounts for 50% or more of all cardiovascular deaths. The two major constructs are its suddenness and unexpectedness. On this basis a commonly used definition is that "sudden cardiac death (SCD) is natural death due to cardiac causes, heralded by abrupt loss of consciousness within 1 hour of the onset of acute symptoms, in a person with or without known preexisting heart disease, but in whom the time and mode of death are unexpected."[25]

Sudden cardiac death may be the initial symptom of coronary artery disease, occurring in approximately 25% of sudden death victims. A previous myocardial infarction, however, can be identified in as many as 75% of patients who die suddenly. Despite the unexpectedness of the event, a significant number of victims have nonspecific premonitory symptoms before arrest occurs. Patients who have been successfully resuscitated listed the presence of chest pain, dyspnea, indigestion, lightheadedness, and syncope in the hour before arrest. Fatigue was the most commonly reported symptom in the days and weeks before the event. Up to 40% of victims had been seen by their physicians in the preceding 4 weeks but only 12% because of cardiac symptoms.[26]

Etiology. The box above lists potential causes of sudden cardiac death. Most of these deaths occur in patients with preexisting ventricular dysfunction secondary to multivessel cardiac disease with or without a history of myocardial infarction. The sudden death episode usually begins as ventricular tachycardia (VT), which degenerates into ventricular fibrillation (VF)—events unassociated with either acute infarction or significant ischemia. Sudden death after a myocardial infarction usually occurs relatively early; then its incidence decreases with time. The first postinfarction year mortality from sudden cardiac death is about 6%, with 50% to 75% occurring within the first 6 months. Thereafter the total risk falls to about 2% to 3% per year. A sudden death episode, from which the patient was successfully resuscitated, even without myocardial infarction, places 50% of these survivors at risk for a second sudden death event within the following 2 years.[27,28]

Other SCD risk factors include primary myocardial disease such as dilated or hypertropic cardiomyopathy. This pathologic finding occurs in approximately 10% of sudden cardiac death victims.[26] Valvular heart disease, especially aortic stenosis, is the underlying cause of death in about 5% of cases. The exception is mitral valve prolapse, which is associated with a high incidence of cardiac dysrhythmias, but a low incidence of sudden cardiac death. Primary electrical disturbances, particularly AV block, ventricular preexcitation, and prolonged QT syndromes, account for about 2% of sudden cardiac deaths.[26]

Coronary risk factors, because of the role they play in the development of coronary artery disease (CAD) are all relevant, but some are more directly linked to risk of sudden cardiac death. Cigarette smoking disproportionately increases the risk of sudden death, especially in younger patients. This risk, which is proportional to the number of cigarettes smoked, appears to be transient and reversible and is diminished by cessation of smoking.[29]

Although the prevalence of sudden cardiac death increases with age, the percentage of deaths that are sudden actually decline as other morbid processes exact a greater toll with increasing age. Most victims of sudden death are between the ages of 45 and 69 years. Men are 3 times more likely than are women to die suddenly, and 70% to 90% of victims are men. Women

---

CAUSES OF SUDDEN CARDIAC DEATH (SCD)

MOST FREQUENT DYSRHYTHMIAS

Ventricular tachycardia → Ventricular fibrillation

UNDERLYING CARDIAC CONDITIONS

Heart failure
Idiopathic hypertrophic subaortic stenosis (IHSS)
Dilated cardiomyopathy
Myocardial infarction (MI)
Severe aortic stenosis

---

victims of sudden death have been noted to be more likely never to have married, to have a history of psychiatric treatment, to smoke, and to have greater alcohol consumption.[27,28]

Arterial hypertension may be the only risk factor identified in otherwise healthy persons. More than 25% of sudden cardiac death victims have a history of arterial hypertension that resulted in left ventricular hypertrophy and dysrhythmias.

The box on p. 290 identifies characteristics associated with highest risk for sudden cardiac death. The first is electrical instability. Frequent PVCs or complex (multifocal, couplets, short runs of VT or R-on-T) ventricular premature beats are clinical predictors of sudden cardiac death in patients with known CAD. However, in persons without demonstrated CAD, ventricular ectopy by itself appears to have little, if any, prognostic value.[26,28]

Pathophysiology. As indicated, extensive atherosclerosis is the most common pathologic finding in the arteries of victims of sudden cardiac death. Sites of 75% or more stenosis were present in three or four of the major vessels in 61% of hearts, and two vessels with at least 75% stenosis were found in 15% of victims.

A marked depression of the left ventricular ejection fraction is the most powerful predictor of sudden cardiac death in patients with chronic ischemic heart disease. An ejection fraction equal to or less than 30% is the single most powerful predictor for sudden cardiac death and is independent of dysrhythmias.

Again, conduction abnormalities such as prolongation of the QT interval, either as an inherited syndrome or drug-induced, increase risk for ventricular dysrhythmias. Syndromes such as Wolff-Parkinson-White, which utilize accessory pathways, bypassing the AV node, give rise to fast ventricular responses (190 to 300/min), resulting in a high incidence of these rhythms degenerating into ventricular fibrillation.

Medical management. Two major goals for the prevention of sudden death are the identification and treatment of high-risk patients. Survivors usually are placed on antidysrhythmic agents and overdrive pacing or, in some cases, may have an internal defibrillator unit implanted.[26,29]

◆ Postinfarction structural complications

Ventricular aneurysm. A ventricular aneurysm (Fig. 16-10) is a noncontractile, thinned left ventricular wall, which results in a reduction of the stroke volume. It occurs in approximately 12% to 15% of patients who survive acute transmural infarction.[23] A ventricular aneurysm most frequently occurs in the apical area and may develop within hours, or it may develop and enlarge over a period of weeks. A ventricular aneurysm may be (1) an anatomic lesion manifesting as cavity protrusion of the ventricular wall that is present during systole and diastole, or (2) a functional lesion—that is, ventricular protrusion that is present only during systole. The most common complications of a ventricular aneurysm are heart failure, ventricular tachycardias (VTs), and systemic emboli. Treatment usually is directed toward management of these complications and surgical repair by left ventricular aneurysmectomy.

The prognosis depends on the size of the aneurysm, overall left ventricular function, and the severity of coexisting CAD. Rupture of the aneurysm is rare, but nonetheless life-threatening, and usually occurs only if there is reinfarction of the border of the aneurysm.

Ventricular septal defect. When rupture of the ventricular septal wall (Fig. 16-11) occurs, it usually does so within the first week after the infarction.[7,23] This complication affects approximately 1% to 3% of the patients who sustain acute transmural infarction. It results from occlusion of either the anterior descending or posterior descending coronary artery, and the intraventricular septum will undergo ischemic necrosis if collateral circulation is inadequate. The rupture often is followed by acute heart failure and shock, the seriousness of which depends on the size of the defect.

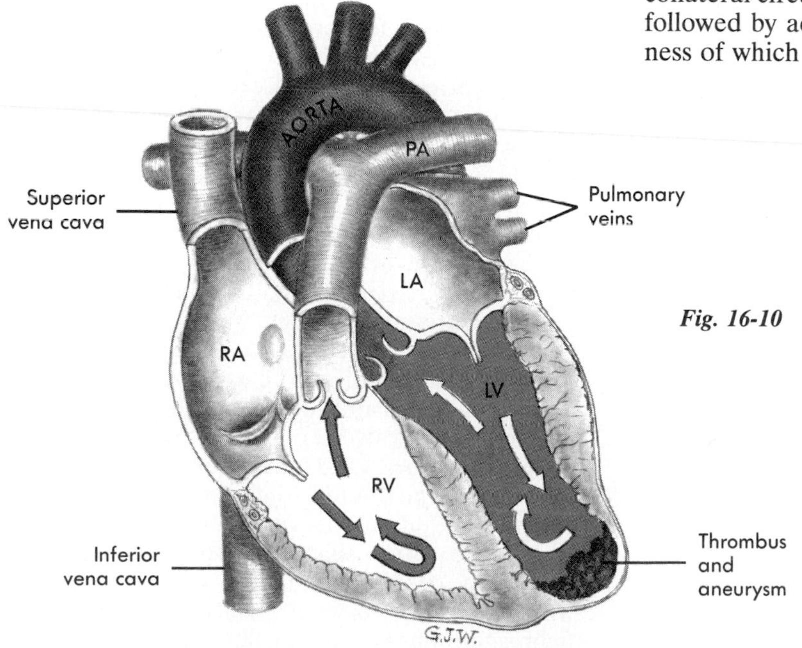

Fig. 16-10 Ventricular aneurysm.

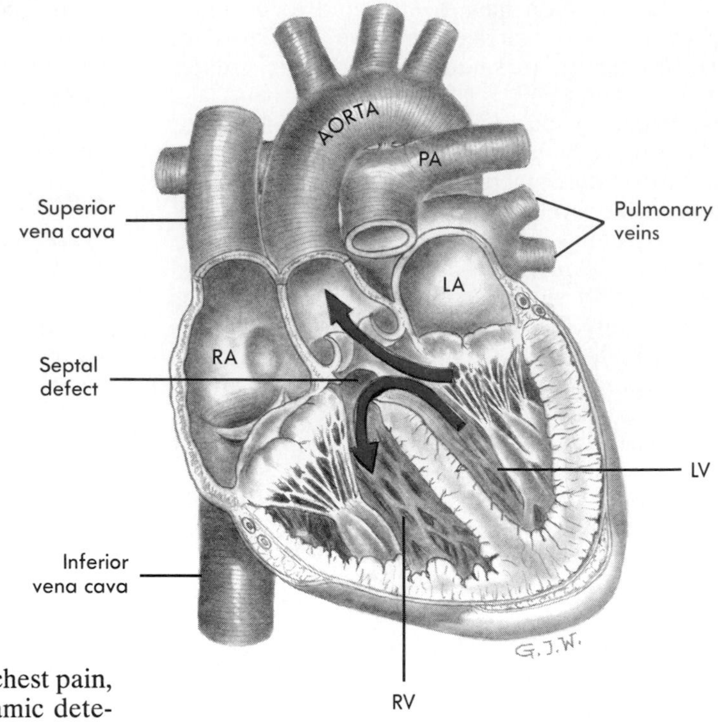

Fig. 16-11 Ventricular septal defect.

Rupture of the septum manifests as severe chest pain, syncope, hypotension, and sudden hemodynamic deterioration caused by shunting of blood from the left ventricle into the right ventricle through the septal opening. A new holosystolic murmur (accompanied by a thrill) can be auscultated and is best heard along the left sternal border. A definitive diagnosis of a ventricular septal defect (VSD) can be made at the bedside with use of a pulmonary artery catheter or transesophageal echocardiographic (TEE) examination. Blood samples drawn from both the distal pulmonary artery (PA) port and proximal central venous pressure (CVP) port will show an increase in oxygen saturation between the CVP and the distal PA sample, indicating that oxygen saturation increased in the right ventricle. This is physiologically impossible unless a VSD is present. Normally, oxygen saturation in the right ventricle is 75%; with a VSD the saturation level is increased to approximately 85%. The increase is the result of shunting of oxygenated blood from the left ventricle through the new defect into the right side of the heart. This is documented as the P/S ratio, or the ratio of blood going to the pulmonary circulation versus blood going to the systemic circulation. It is written, for example, as P/S 2:1, which means that for every liter of blood going into the systemic circulation, 2 liters are going into the pulmonary circulation.

Because rupture of the septum is a medical and surgical emergency, the patient's condition must be stabilized with vasodilators and an intraaortic balloon pump (IABP) to decrease afterload. The goal of afterload reduction in these patients is to decrease the amount of blood being shunted back to the right side of the heart and to increase the forward flow of blood to the systemic circulation. Mortality exceeds 80% with medical therapy alone; therefore most patients require emergency surgery to close the ventricular septum.

The surgical approach usually is through the left ventricle and frequently through the infarction itself. The septum is patched with a knitted Dacron velour patch, lined, if possible, with pericardium to make it immediately leakproof. If pericardium is not used, there may be residual shunting until platelets and fibrin agglutinate along the patch to seal it.

Papillary muscle rupture. Papillary muscle rupture can occur when the myocardial infarction involves the area around the mitral valve. This area has a high oxygen requirement because of tension generated during contraction. The usual blood supply source to this area is from more than one coronary artery; therefore ischemic injury suggests multivessel CAD. The papillary muscles function to keep the mitral valve closed tightly during ventricular systole. Infarction of the papillary muscles results in their inability to effect a mitral valve seal; consequently, blood is forced through the weakened mitral valve back into the lower-pressured left atrium during ventricular systole. The posteromedial papillary muscle has a single blood supply; therefore it has an increased incidence of rupture as compared with the anterolateral muscle, which has a dual blood supply.

The rupture may be partial or complete. Complete rupture is catastrophic and precipitates severe acute mitral regurgitation, shock, and death. Partial rupture (Fig. 16-12) also results in mitral regurgitation, but usually the condition can be stabilized with the intraaortic balloon pump and vasodilators before surgery, during which a mitral valve replacement will take place.

Cardiac rupture. Of deaths after myocardial infarction, 15% can be attributed to cardiac rupture, which often occurs in older patients who have systemic hypertension during the acute phase of their infarctions. Rupture frequently occurs around the fifth postinfarction day when leukocyte scavenger cells are removing necrotic debris, thinning the myocardial wall. Rupture commonly is preceded by infarct expansion, which is caused by the

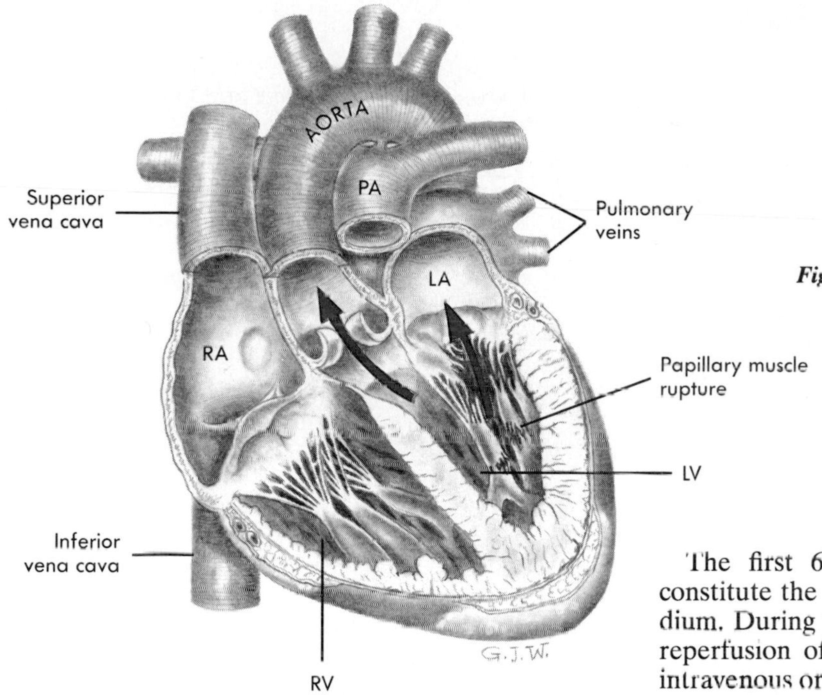

Fig. 16-12 Papillary muscle rupture.

regional thinning and dilation in the infarct zone without additional necrosis.

The onset usually is sudden. Bleeding into the pericardial sac results in tamponade, cardiogenic shock, electromechanical dissociation, and death. Survival is rare, and emergency pericardiocentesis is required to relieve the tamponade until a surgical repair can be attempted.

Pericarditis. Pericarditis is inflammation of the pericardial sac that occurs after acute myocardial infarction when the damage extends into the epicardial surface of the heart (as in transmural infarction). The damaged epicardium then becomes rough and tends to irritate and inflame the pericardium lying adjacent to it, precipitating the development of pericarditis.

Pain is the most common symptom of pericarditis, whereas the presence of a pericardial friction rub is the most common sign and is considered a clinical hallmark. Although the friction rub may not be audible at all times, it is best heard at the sternal border during inhalation and is described as a grating, scraping, or leathery scratching. Friction rubs often change from one examination to the next, thus complicating documentation. Pericardial pain, however, is aggravated by deep ventilations, change of position, swallowing, and coughing. Pericarditis *may* result in a pericardial effusion.[30]

Narcotics do not provide the relief achieved with aspirin, indomethacin, and either nonsteroidal antiinflammatory drugs or steroids such as dexamethasone and methylprednisolone. Long-term or high-dose steroids should be used with caution because they may impede tissue healing and scar formation.

Medical Management

The three principal goals of medical management for myocardial infarction are relief of pain, control of lethal dysrhythmias, and preservation of the myocardium.

The first 6 hours after the onset of chest pain constitute the crucial period for salvage of the myocardium. During this period it may be possible to achieve reperfusion of the infarcting myocardium with either intravenous or intracoronary thrombolysis, thrombolysis with percutaneous transluminal coronary angioplasty (PTCA), emergency PTCA, or emergency coronary artery bypass surgery (these therapies are discussed in Chapter 17). Studies show that myocardial tissue can be salvaged for at least 2 to 3 hours after the onset of symptoms, but in some patients this period may extend to 6 hours. Unfortunately, many persons do not seek treatment until this phase has passed.[31]

Pain control is a priority because continued pain is a symptom of ongoing ischemia, which places additional risk on noninfarcted myocardial tissue. Morphine remains the analgesic of choice; it decreases anxiety, restlessness, autonomic nervous system activity, and preload, thereby decreasing myocardial oxygen demands.

Intravenous nitrates, beta-blocking agents, and calcium channel blockers may be instituted to reduce myocardial oxygen demand by decreasing both preload and afterload or by direct effect on the coronary circulation. Beta-blocking agents may reduce infarct size by decreasing sympathetic tone, thus decreasing afterload.

Oxygen is used for a minimum of 24 to 48 hours after infarction to treat tissue hypoxia, which may be caused by left ventricular failure.

Because ventricular dysrhythmias are most prevalent in the early postinfarction period, the patient is monitored for heart rate and rhythm. Most patients also begin receiving intravenous lidocaine during this period.

Many times a pulmonary artery catheter is inserted, which allows correlation of chamber pressures to heart rate, blood pressure, urine output, and cardiac output. Thus pharmacologic and fluid replacement decisions can be based on concrete parameters of ventricular function as described in Chapter 15 in the section on PA catheters, pp. 254-266.

To decrease cardiac work and myocardial oxygen consumption, bed rest with commode privileges usually is prescribed for the patient during the first 24 to 48 hours. Stool softeners are used to decrease the risk of constipation from analgesics and bed rest and to decrease the risk of straining.

For the first 24 hours the patient may be placed on a liquid or soft diet to decrease the risk of aspiration should cardiac arrest occur during this time. Furthermore, liquids and soft foods are nonirritating and easily digested; therefore myocardial oxygen consumption and basal metabolic rate may decrease.

Anticoagulants sometimes are used to decrease the incidence of embolic complications from deep vein thrombosis and left ventricular thrombi, especially while bed rest is prescribed for the patient. Antiplatelet agents also may be started to decrease release from platelets of thromboxane A_2, which causes vasoconstriction and platelet aggregation. This therapy may be continued for an indefinite period of time inasmuch as recent studies have documented the beneficial antiplatelet effect of low-dose prophylactic aspirin.[32]

Diagnostic studies that assess left ventricular function (such as use of echocardiography and angiography) and studies that assess electrical function (such as 24-hour Holter monitoring and exercise stress testing) are all important in the decision-making process for risk assessment and both short-term and long-term management of acute myocardial infarction.

Nursing Management

The focus of the plan of care for the patient with a myocardial infarction must include (1) the recognition and treatment of potentially life-threatening complications, (2) the manipulation of the critical care environment so that it is calm and therapeutic, and (3) the identification of the psychosocial impact of the infarction on the patient.[33]

A considerable portion of time will be spent monitoring the patient for dysrhythmias and conduction defects and assessing vital signs for indications of shock, breath sounds for signs of pulmonary congestion, and heart sounds for abnormalities, such as an S_3, S_4, or a murmur.

Medications must be administered as prescribed, followed by assessment for side effects or toxic responses. If chest pain or dysrhythmias develop, it is important to record the onset in relation to the medication schedule. Sometimes medications must be given in smaller, more frequent doses to maintain a stable blood level and to avoid peaks and troughs in blood levels. If dysrhythmias continue, it is important to assess for noncardiac causes, such as fever, anxiety, tissue hypoxia, position of the pulmonary wedge catheter, and acid-base or electrolyte disturbances.

During the time bed rest is prescribed, it is important that the patient is in an upright or semi-Fowler's position to foster better lung expansion, thereby decreasing the risk of atelectasis. An upright position also decreases venous return, lowers preload, and decreases cardiac work.

The nurse controls the critical care unit environment to decrease noise, diminish sensory overload, and allow adequate rest periods.

NURSING DIAGNOSIS AND MANAGEMENT

Myocardial infarction and complications

- Acute Pain related to transmission and perception of cutaneous, visceral, muscular, or ischemic impulses, secondary to myocardial ischemia, p. 566
- Decreased Cardiac Output related to relative excess of preload and afterload secondary to impaired ventricular contractility, p. 358
- Decreased Cardiac Output related to supraventricular tachycardia, p. 358
- Decreased Cardiac Output related to ventricular tachycardia, p. 362
- Decreased Cardiac Output related to atrioventricular (AV) heart block, p. 359
- Activity Intolerance related to decreased cardiac output and/or myocardial tissue perfusion alterations, p. 366
- Sleep Pattern Disturbance related to fragmented sleep, p. 142
- Sensory/Perceptual Alterations related to sensory overload, sensory deprivation, and sleep pattern disturbance, p. 573
- Anxiety related to threat to biologic, psychologic, and/or social integrity, p. 763
- Ineffective Individual Coping related to situational crisis and personal vulnerability, p. 762
- Powerlessness related to health care environment or illness-related regimen, p. 98
- Altered Role Performance related to physical incapacity to resume usual or valued role, p. 97
- Body Image Disturbance related to actual change in body structure, function, or appearance, p. 94
- Sexual Dysfunction related to activity intolerance secondary to myocardial infarction, p. 118
- Altered Sexuality Patterns related to fear of death during coitus secondary to myocardial infarction, p. 120
- Altered Health Maintenance related to lack of perceived threat to health, p. 70
- Knowledge Deficit: Activity Restrictions, Fluid Restrictions, Medication, Reportable Symptoms related to lack of previous exposure to information, p. 72

HEART FAILURE

The most common cause of in-hospital mortality for patients with cardiac disease is heart failure (HF), also described as congestive heart failure (CHF).[34,35] Heart failure is responsible for one third of the deaths of patients with an acute myocardial infarction. It is the second most common complication of myocardial infarction, reflecting 20% to 25% involvement of the myocardium.

In 1983 it was estimated that 2.5 to 3 million Americans had been diagnosed with HF and that the incidence would increase by approximately 400,000 new cases per year because of the aging of the population.[35] The heart failure rate is higher in men than in women for all age-groups. The 5-year mortality in men is about 60%, whereas in women it is about 45%.

Description

Heart failure is a pathophysiologic state in which an abnormality of cardiac function is responsible for the failure of the heart to pump blood at a volume commensurate with venous return and/or with the requirements of the metabolizing tissues.[7,34,35] The basic function of the heart is to transfer blood coming into the ventricles from the lower pressure venous system into the higher pressure arterial system. Impaired cardiac function results in failure to empty the venous system and reduces delivery of blood to the pulmonary and arterial circulation—hence, heart failure.

◆ **Classifications of heart failure.** Heart failure can be classified in various ways. However heart failure is classified, it is important to remember that the cardiac chambers do not function in isolation. The ventricles, for example, have a common septal wall and are encircled and bound together by continuous muscle fibers; therefore any interruption or damage to one chamber eventually will affect all the chambers.

Failure of right side of heart. Failure of the right side of the heart is defined as ineffective right ventricular contractile function. Pure failure of the right side of the heart may result from an acute condition such as a pulmonary embolus or a right ventricular infarction, but most commonly it is caused by failure of the left side of the heart or the backing up of blood behind the left ventricle. Its common manifestations are weakness, peripheral or sacral edema, jugular venous distention, hepatomegaly, jaundice, liver tenderness, and elevated central venous pressure (CVP). If peripheral perfusion is greatly compromised, cyanosis may be present. Gastrointestinal symptoms include anorexia, nausea, and a feeling of fullness.[7,18]

Failure of left side of heart. Failure of the left side of the heart is defined as a disturbance of the contractile function of the left ventricle, resulting in pulmonary congestion and edema or decreased cardiac output, or both. Most frequently it occurs in patients with left ventricular infarctions, hypertension, and aortic and/or mitral valve disease. Over time with progression of the disease state, the fluid accumulation behind the dysfunctional left ventricle produces dysfunction of the right ventricle, resulting in failure of the right side of the heart and its manifestations.

Forward heart failure. Forward failure is defined as inadequate delivery of blood into the arterial system. It occurs when systemic resistance (afterload) is increased, producing decreased flow of blood out of the ventricles. This decrease results in a reduced cardiac output and hypoperfusion of vital organs. Forward failure frequently occurs with aortic stenosis or systemic hypertension.

Backward heart failure. Backward failure is defined as failure of the ventricle to empty. This results in an accumulation of fluid and an elevation of pressure in all the chambers and in the venous system behind the affected ventricle. It frequently occurs in conditions that result in a decreased systolic ejection, such as myocardial infarction and cardiomyopathy. When the left ventricle pumps ineffectively, blood pools within the chamber and left ventricular end-diastolic pressure (LVEDP) increases. As the mitral valve opens, the increased LVEDP results in increased atrial pressure, which is then transmitted back into the pulmonary circuit. The net effect is an increase in both the pressure and the fluid within and behind the affected ventricle.

Acute versus chronic heart failure. Acute versus chronic failure refers to the rapidity with which the syndrome develops, the presence and activation of compensatory mechanisms, and the presence or absence of fluid accumulation in the interstitial space. Any condition that results in a sudden drop in cardiac output also results in the manifestations of acute heart failure. The features of acute ischemic heart failure and chronic failure exhibit several important differences. First, patients with acute failure are normovolemic or hypovolemic as opposed to hypervolemic. Further, sodium and water retention, a feature of chronic failure, usually is not present in the initial days of acute heart failure, and structural chamber changes (dilation/hypertropy) have not yet occurred.[36,37]

Chronic failure may be abruptly exacerbated by the onset of dysrhythmias or by acute ischemia, which causes manifestations of acute failure. In summary, acute heart failure has a sudden onset, with no compensatory mechanisms. Chronic failure has a progressive onset, with symptoms that may be suppressed by medication, diet, and low activity level. A change to acute failure, however, can be precipitated by sudden illness or by cessation of medications. This may necessitate admission to a critical care unit.

Low ventricular versus high ventricular output failure. Low ventricular output failure is defined as a low ventricular output state that results in a decreased ejection fraction, which can be caused by infarction, hypotension, cardiomyopathy, or hemorrhage. Classic clinical manifestations are those of decreased peripheral perfusion, such as weak or diminished pulses, cool, pale extremities, and peripheral cyanosis. High ventricular output failure occurs in conditions that increase the cardiac output, such as thyrotoxicosis, anemia, and pregnancy. Peripherally, the pulse is strong and the extremities are warm and pink.[7]

◆ **Functional classification.** The New York Heart Association developed a method of classifying patients with heart disease on the basis of the activity level that initiates the onset of symptoms. The abbreviated functional classification is as follows:

Class I: Normal daily activity does not initiate symptoms.
Class II: Normal daily activities initiate onset of symptoms, but symptoms subside with rest.
Class III: Minimal activity initiates symptoms. Patients are usually symptom-free at rest.
Class IV: Any type of activity initiates symptoms, and symptoms are present at rest.

Etiology

Elderly persons, men, persons with hypertension, those with coronary artery disease, smokers, diabetics, and those with elevated cholesterol levels have been identified by the Framingham study as having high heart failure risk profiles.[7,35,36] Many precipitating causes of HF are listed in the box below.

A common precipitating cause is reduction or cessation of cardiac therapy, either pharmacologic or dietary. Patients with heart disease are usually on a regimen of multiple medications and may, at one time or another, question the financial burden or—when they are symptom-free—the need to continue therapy. Reduction or cessation of some therapy such as diuretics usually results in sodium and water retention, which may precipitate heart failure.

Dysrhythmias are another major precipitating or aggravating factor. Tachycardias reduce diastolic filling time, thereby decreasing stroke volume. They also increase myocardial oxygen demand and, by decreasing diastolic filling time, may precipitate angina. Atrial dysrhythmias may decrease cardiac output by approximately 30% through loss of the "atrial kick." Ventricular conduction defects, which result in loss of ventricular synchrony during ventricular contraction, also decrease stroke volume, thereby decreasing overall perfusion.[36]

Viral and bacterial infections and environmental, emotional, or physical stress that increases myocardial oxygen demands can precipitate heart failure. Other precipitating factors, such as bacterial endocarditis, myocarditis, and inflammation, decrease ventricular contractility. A noncardiac illness or a second form of heart disease, such as left ventricular failure secondary to a myocardial infarction in a patient with chronic hypertension and left ventricular hypertrophy, may cause ischemia, which will lead to decreased contractility and heart failure.

Pathophysiology

The two major determinants of cardiac output are heart rate and stroke volume; thus anything that affects one or both will affect cardiac output. Stroke volume, the volume of blood ejected with each systole, depends on three factors: (1) preload—the degree of fiber stretch at the end of diastole, (2) contractility—the change in the force of contraction, and (3) afterload—the pressure the ventricle must generate for ejection to occur. These three factors are the principal determinants of mechanical performance of the heart.

When the heart begins to fail and the cardiac output no longer is sufficient to meet the metabolic needs of the tissues, three major compensatory mechanisms are activated: the adrenergic system, the renin-angiotensin-aldosterone system, and the development of ventricular hypertrophy. These compensatory mechanisms maintain adequate perfusion pressure and enhance cardiac output by the manipulation of one or more of five factors: (1) heart rate, (2) stroke volume, (3) preload, (4) contractility, and (5) afterload.

The adrenergic compensatory mechanism is a result of increased sympathetic activity, which stimulates the release of catecholamines and increases the levels of circulating catecholamines, especially epinephrine. The increase in circulating catecholamines results in peripheral vasoconstriction, which leads to shunting of blood from nonvital organs, such as the kidneys and skin, to vital organs, such as the heart and brain. This, in turn, increases venous return, which increases preload.

Activation of the renin-angiotensin-aldosterone system results in constriction of the renal arterioles, decreasing the glomerular filtration rate and increasing the reabsorption of sodium from the proximal and distal tubules, which promotes fluid retention. Fluid retention also is augmented by the diminished hepatic metabolism of aldosterone secondary to systemic venous congestion and diminished hepatic perfusion. Severe heart failure increases the antidiuretic hormone level, enhancing the retention of water.

The final compensatory mechanism is the increase in ventricular wall thickness known as *ventricular hypertrophy.* An increase in systolic wall stress leads to replication of sarcomeres in parallel, which increases ventricular wall thickness in an arrangement known as *concentric hypertrophy.* An increase in volume or volume overload leads to replication of sarcomeres in series, resulting in fiber elongation and chamber enlargement known as *eccentric hypertrophy.* Myocardial hypertrophy increases the force of contraction. Therefore hypertrophy helps the ventricle overcome an increase in afterload.

In summary, the compensatory mechanisms may sustain cardiac function, especially at rest, but over a period of time may worsen the degree of failure as the retention of sodium and water leads to overdistention of the ventricles and a consequent decrease in the force of ventricular contraction.

Tachycardia eventually may become a negative factor because it increases myocardial oxygen demand while shortening coronary artery perfusion. This imbalance can lead to myocardial ischemia, which may decrease ventricular contraction, reduce ventricular filling, and necessitate a higher filling pressure. The end result may be both forward and backward failure. If heart failure progresses to the point where tissue perfusion is

PRECIPITATING CAUSES OF HEART FAILURE

Reduction or cessation of medication
Dysrhythmias
Systemic infection
Pulmonary embolism
Physical, environmental, and emotional stress
Pericarditis, myocarditis, and endocarditis
High ventricular output states
Development of serious systemic illness
Administration of a cardiac depressant or salt-retaining drug
Development of a second form of heart disease

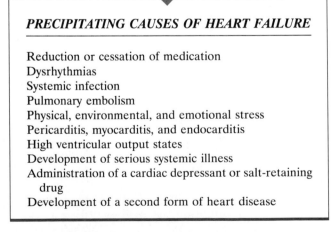

inadequate to meet the body's needs, the patient will be in *cardiogenic shock.* The pathophysiology and management of this condition are described on pp. 770-772.

Assessment and Diagnosis

The clinical manifestations of HF result from tissue hypoperfusion and organ congestion.[35] Symptoms can be cardiac or noncardiac in origin. Signs and symptoms frequently are described according to the form of failure; that is, forward failure manifests as fatigue and weakness, whereas backward failure manifests as pulmonary congestion and edema. Failure of the right side of the heart appears as systemic venous congestion and peripheral edema, whereas failure of the left side results in pulmonary venous congestion and pulmonary edema (Table 16-2).

The severity of clinical manifestations progresses as heart failure worsens. Initially signs and symptoms appear only with exertion but eventually occur at rest.

Dyspnea, which is labored breathing and frequently is described by patients as shortness of breath, results from pulmonary vascular congestion and decreased lung compliance. Dyspnea may then progress to orthopnea (difficulty breathing when supine) because of an increase in venous return (preload) that occurs in the supine position. Paroxysmal nocturnal dyspnea is a severe form of orthopnea in which the patient awakens from sleep gasping for air. Other respiratory symptoms include cardiac asthma (dyspnea with wheezing), a nonproductive cough, and pulmonary crackles progressing to the gurgling sounds of pulmonary edema.

◆ **Pulmonary edema.** Pulmonary edema (Fig. 16-13) inhibits gas exchange by impairing the diffusion pathway between the alveolus and the capillary. It is caused by increased left atrial and left ventricular pressure and results in an excessive accumulation of serous or serosanguineous fluid in the interstitial spaces and alveoli of the lungs. The most common causes are left ventricular failure resulting from acute myocardial infarction, acute myocardial ischemia, tight mitral stenosis, chronic mitral regurgitation (MR), acute MR from rupture of chordae tendineae and severe aortic regurgitation or aortic stenosis.

Two stages mark the formation of pulmonary edema. Stage I is characterized by interstitial edema, engorgement of the perivascular and peribronchial spaces, and

Table 16-2 Clinical manifestations of failure of right and left sides of heart

Left ventricular failure		Right ventricular failure	
Signs	**Symptoms**	**Signs**	**Symptoms**
Tachypnea	Fatigue	Peripheral edema	Weakness
Tachycardia	Dyspnea	Hepatomegaly	Anorexia
Cough	Orthopnea	Splenomegaly	Indigestion
Bibasilar crackles	Paroxysmal nocturnal dyspnea	Hepatojugular reflux	Weight gain
Gallop rhythms (S_3 and S_4)	Nocturia	Ascites	Mental changes
Increased pulmonary artery pressures		Jugular venous distention	
Hemoptysis		Increased central venous pressure	
Cyanosis		Pulmonary hypertension	
Pulmonary edema			

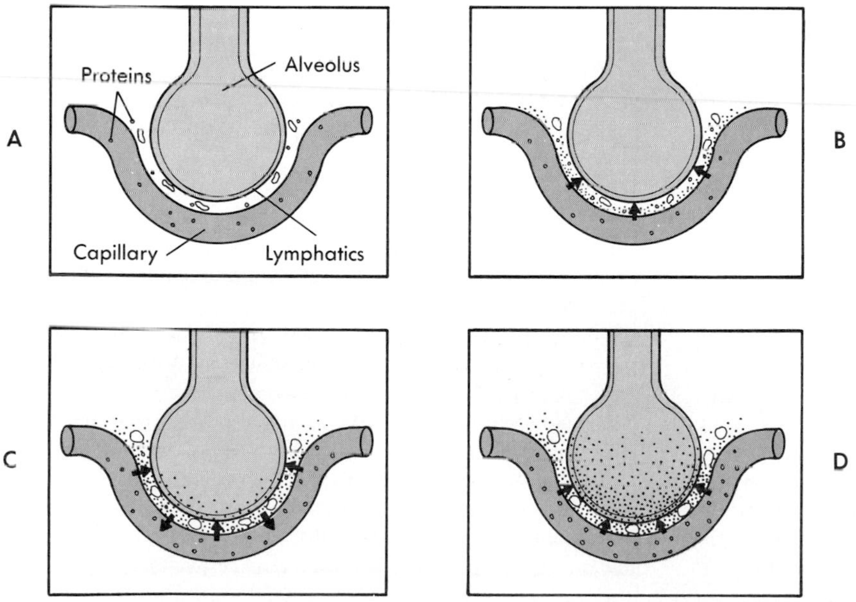

Fig. 16-13 As pulmonary edema progresses, it inhibits oxygen and carbon dioxide exchange at the alveolar capillary interface. **A,** Normal relationship. **B,** Increased pulmonary capillary hydrostatic pressure causes fluid to move from the vascular space into the pulmonary interstitial space. **C,** Lymphatic flow increases in an attempt to pull fluid back into the vascular or lymphatic space. **D,** Failure of lymphatic flow and worsening of left-sided heart failure results in further movement of fluid into the interstitial space and the alveoli.

increased lymphatic flow. Stage II is characterized by alveolar edema resulting from fluid moving into the alveoli from the interstitium. Eventually, blood plasma moves into the alveoli faster than the lymphatic system can clear it, interfering with diffusion of oxygen, depressing the arterial partial pressure of oxygen (Pao_2), and leading to tissue hypoxia. The sensation of suffocation that can occur at this time intensifies the patient's fright and elevates heart rate, further restricting ventricular filling. Increased discomfort and work of breathing place an additional load on the heart, and cardiac function becomes further depressed.

With acute onset, patients often are extremely breathless and anxious. They expectorate pink, frothy liquid, causing them to feel as if they are drowning. They may sit bolt upright, gasp for breath, or thrash about. The respiratory rate is elevated, and the use of accessory muscles of ventilation becomes apparent by nasal flaring and bulging neck muscles. Respirations are characterized by loud inspiratory and expiratory gurgling sounds. Diaphoresis is profuse, and the skin usually is cold, ashen, and cyanotic, reflecting low cardiac output, increased sympathetic stimulation, peripheral vasoconstriction, and desaturation of arterial blood.

Arterial blood gas values may be variable. In the early stage of pulmonary edema, respiratory alkalosis may be present because of hyperventilation. As the pulmonary edema progresses, however, and as gas exchange becomes impaired, respiratory acidosis and hypoxemia ensue. Laboratory studies also may document elevated liver function and elevated levels of bilirubin, liver enzymes, aspartate aminotransferase (AST, formerly SGOT), and alanine aminotransferase (ALT, formerly SGPT). Elevated blood urea nitrogen (BUN) and creatinine levels reflect renal hypoperfusion. Urine output is low and urine is concentrated, with low urine sodium and high urine osmolarity levels because of dilutional hyponatremia. The serum potassium level may vary, depending on the overall state of renal function and aggressiveness of diuresis.

The chest radiograph usually confirms an enlarged cardiac silhouette, pulmonary venous congestion, and interstitial edema. The interstitial edema markings on the chest radiograph are described as Kerley B lines.[36]

Medical Management

The goals of management of heart failure are threefold: (1) to identify and correct precipitating causes, (2) to relieve symptoms, and (3) to enhance cardiac performance.

In the acute phase the patient usually has a pulmonary artery catheter in place so that left ventricular function can be followed closely. Diuretics are administered to decrease preload and to eliminate fluid from the body. The intraaortic balloon pump and vasodilators, such as sodium nitroprusside and intravenous nitroglycerin, may be required to decrease afterload. The angiotensin-converting enzyme (ACE) inhibitors may alter chamber remodeling and slow the decline in contractility. Digitalis and positive inotropic agents, such as dopamine or dobutamine, may be administered to increase ventricular contractility. If pulmonary edema develops, morphine and diuretics will be used to remove excess fluid, to facilitate peripheral dilation, and to decrease anxiety. Only vasodilators have been shown to prolong life.

Hemodialysis or continuous arterial-venous hemofiltration with or without dialysis may be required to control sodium and water retention if HF-induced renal insufficiency is present.

Nursing Management

The focus of the plan of care for a patient with heart failure must include interventions that will decrease cardiac work, optimize cardiac function, and promote emotional and physical rest.

During periods of breathlessness, activity must be restricted; bed rest usually is prescribed for the patient, who is positioned with the head of the bed elevated to allow maximal lung expansion. The arms must be supported on pillows so there is no undue stress placed on the shoulder muscles. The legs may be placed in a dependent position to encourage venous pooling, thereby decreasing venous return.

Breath sounds should be auscultated frequently to determine adequacy of respiratory effort and to assess for onset or worsening of congestion. Oxygen through a nasal cannula may be administered to relieve dyspnea, blood should be evaluated, and diuretics or vasodilators may be administered. If the patient is not hypotensive, morphine may be administered to decrease hyperventi-

NURSING DIAGNOSIS AND MANAGEMENT
Chronic heart failure

- Impaired Gas Exchange related to ventilation/perfusion mismatch secondary to pulmonary vascular congestion, p. 470
- Decreased Cardiac Output related to relative excess of preload and afterload secondary to impaired ventricular contractility, p. 358
- Activity Intolerance related to decreased cardiac output and/or myocardial tissue perfusion alterations, p. 366
- Activity Intolerance related to postural hypotension secondary to prolonged immobility, narcotics, vasodilator therapy, p. 365
- Anxiety related to threat to biologic, psychologic, and/or social integrity, p. 763
- Sleep Pattern Disturbance related to fragmented sleep secondary to paroxysmal nocturnal dyspnea, p. 142
- Noncompliance: Medications, Fluid Restrictions, Activity Restrictions, Diet related to knowledge deficit and/or lack of resources, p. 71
- Altered Health Maintenance related to lack of perceived threat to health, p. 70

lation and anxiety. If the patient's ventilatory status worsens, the nurse must be prepared for endotracheal intubation and mechanical ventilation.

Patients in HF require aggressive pharmacologic therapy. The nurse must know the action, side effects, therapeutic levels, and toxic effects of the diuretics, the positive inotropic agents used to increase ventricular contractility, and vasodilators used to decrease preload. The patient's hemodynamic response to these agents, as well as to diuretic therapy and fluid restrictions, must be closely monitored.

The patient's ECG must be evaluated for any dysrhythmias that may be present or may develop as a result of drug toxicity or electrolyte imbalance. Patients in heart failure are prone to digoxin toxicity secondary to decreased renal perfusion, as well as to electrolyte (most frequently, sodium and potassium) imbalances.

The patient in heart failure may be prone to skin breakdown resulting from immobility, bed rest, inadequate nutrition, edema, and decreased perfusion to the skin and subcutaneous tissue. Frequent position changes and padding of dependent areas and bony prominences may be helpful.

Patients in failure frequently experience decreased appetite; therefore small, frequent meals may be more appropriate than the standard three large meals. Food should be as tasty as possible; favorite foods, as well as food from home, may be worked into the diet as long as the foods are compatible with nutritional restrictions.

Another major nursing function is to maintain an environment that fosters physical and emotional rest. The nurse needs to assess the patient's understanding of conservation of energy in planning activities and to collaborate with the patient in organizing the day's schedule. Rest periods must be carefully planned and adhered to, while independence within the patient's activity prescription is fostered. Vital signs should be recorded before an activity is begun, immediately on completion of the activity, and 5 minutes after completion. Signs of activity intolerance (i.e., dyspnea, fatigue, sustained increase in pulse, and onset of dysrhythmias) must be documented and reported to the physician. Activity must be gradually increased in a stepwise fashion. (A case study of cardiovascular physical assessment in heart failure is found on pp. 353-355.)

NURSING DIAGNOSIS AND MANAGEMENT
Acute heart failure and pulmonary edema

- ◆ Impaired Gas Exchange related to ventilation/perfusion mismatch secondary to pulmonary vascular congestion, p. 470
- ◆ Decreased Cardiac Output related to relative excess of preload and afterload secondary to impaired ventricular contractility, p. 358
- ◆ Activity Intolerance related to decreased cardiac output and/or myocardial tissue perfusion alterations, p. 366
- ◆ High risk for Infection risk factors: invasive monitoring devices, p. 366
- ◆ Sensory/Perceptual Alterations related to sensory overload, sensory deprivation, and sleep pattern disturbance, p. 573
- ◆ Anxiety related to threat to biologic, psychologic, and/or social integrity, p. 763
- ◆ Ineffective Individual Coping related to situational crisis and personal vulnerability, p. 762
- ◆ Sleep Pattern Disturbance related to circadian desynchronization, p. 143
- ◆ Knowledge Deficit: Medications, Fluid Restrictions, Activity Restrictions, Diet, Reportable Symptoms related to lack of previous exposure to information, p. 72

ENDOCARDITIS
Description

Infection by a microorganism of a platelet-fibrin vegetation on the endothelial surface of the heart results in infective endocarditis. It is a relatively uncommon disorder, which is seen more frequently in men than in women. In a study of 582 persons with infective endocarditis conducted by the Royal College of Physicians Research Unit, 137 had preexisting rheumatic heart disease, 108 had congenital heart disease, 145 had other cardiac abnormalities, chiefly mitral valve prolapse and calcific aortic valve disease, and 97 had prosthetic valves. Of these persons, 138 had previous attacks of infective endocarditis. The remaining 183 patients had no known cardiac history. Major predisposing factors are listed in the box below; however, no predisposing factor can be identified in 20% to 40% of patients with this disease.[38]

PREDISPOSING FACTORS IN ENDOCARDITIS

Rheumatic heart disease
Congenital heart disease
Mitral valve prolapse
Marfan's syndrome
Idiopathic hypertropic subaortic stenosis
Peripheral arteriovenous fistulas
Indwelling intravenous or intraarterial catheters
Cardiac and prosthetic valve surgery
Prosthetic aortic grafts
Degenerative heart disease
Alcoholism
Chronic hemodialysis
Intravenous drug abuse
Syphilitic aortic disease
Immunosuppression
Severe burns

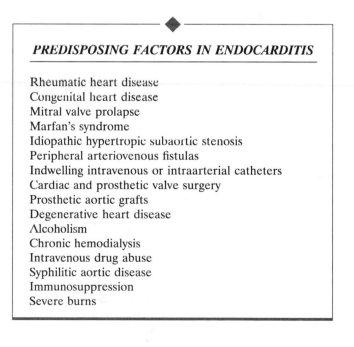

An additional group of patients at risk are those who have undergone valve replacement. In this setting valve infection is referred to as *prosthetic valve endocarditis* (PVE).

Etiology

The development of endocarditis depends on two factors: (1) there must be a susceptible lesion in the vascular endothelium and (2) there must be an organism to establish an infection.[18] The source of the organism may be unknown, or it may be traced to any type of invasive procedure, such as a biopsy, cannulation of the veins or arteries, urogenital procedures (especially if the patient has a urinary tract infection), dental work, or intravenous drug use.[7] Almost any bacteria or fungus can infect a susceptible site. In Western Europe and North America, streptococci and staphylococci account for approximately 90% of all endocarditis.

Endocarditis begins after the onset of bacteremia and the colonization of thrombotic vegetation. The bacteria is then encased in a platelet and fibrin shell, which protects it from destruction by phagocytic neutrophils, leading to a zone of localized agranulocytosis. It is because of this extensive protective mechanism and its ability to restrict the body's normal response to infection that antibiotic therapy must be so intensive and extensive.

Pathophysiology

Endocarditis may be classified as either acute or subacute. Acute infection develops on normal valves, progresses rapidly, causes severe destruction, and may be fatal if the patient is not treated. Subacute infection occurs on damaged heart valves and progresses much more slowly, and the outcome usually is positive with treatment. Survival may be possible even without treatment. The term *subacute bacterial endocarditis* (*SBE*) is not always accurate because, although most infections are bacterial, some are caused by yeast or fungus. It is much more useful to classify the disease according to causative microorganism. In cases of prosthetic valve endocarditis, surgical replacement of the valve is usually required.

Medical Management

Clinical manifestations of endocarditis are found in the box on this page. Treatment requires prolonged parenteral therapy with adequate doses of bactericidal antibiotics. An increasing number of patients are being discharged home to continue the parenteral therapy via a surgically implanted line such as a Port-A-Cath. These patients should be followed up closely to assess for acute valvular incompetence or acute onset of prosthetic valve dehiscence with accompanying heart failure, which will require emergency cardiac surgery.[7,18,38]

Nursing Management

The focus of nursing care for patients with infective endocarditis is resolution of infection, prevention of or early identification of complications, and preventive teaching.

CLINICAL MANIFESTATIONS OF ENDOCARDITIS

Fever
Splenomegaly
Hematuria
Petechiae
Cardiac murmurs
Easy fatigability
Osler's nodes (small, raised, tender areas most commonly found in pads of fingers and toes)
Splenic hemorrhages
Roth's spots (round or oval spots consisting of coagulated fibrin; seen in the retina and leads to hemorrhage)

Endocarditis requires a long course, usually 6 weeks, of intravenous antibiotics. During this time the patient must be continuously observed for any signs of worsening or recurrence of the infection. The patient's temperature must be monitored closely and any elevation reported to the physician. In addition, monitoring for subtle signs of infection, such as malaise, weakness, easy fatigability, and night sweats, is important.

Antibiotics must be administered as ordered and the patient assessed for signs and symptoms of side effects and drug toxicity. Intravenous access may become a problem, and the patency and integrity of the line must be ensured before and immediately after each antibiotic dose.

The nurse must be alert for clinical manifestations of heart failure caused by worsening valve dysfunction. Therefore the cardiovascular assessment should include the auscultation of heart sounds for the presence of or change in cardiac murmur.

A patient with infective endocarditis is at risk for embolic events, either cerebral or pulmonary. Therefore level of consciousness, any visual changes, or headache should be documented. Any shortness of breath or chest pain with hemoptysis also must be reported.

The patient must have adequate nutrition. Often small, frequent meals, which include favorite foods from home, are required. Obtaining daily weights is important until the weight stabilizes; then the daily weight is used in fluid management, and weekly weights are used for checking body weight.

During the most critical period, bed rest is prescribed for the patient. He or she requires range-of-motion exercises to maintain muscle tone and needs frequent turning and repositioning to prevent skin breakdown. Support and diversional activity also are important at this time, because depression related to a prolonged hospital stay commonly occurs.

As the patient recovers, he or she needs to know what signs and symptoms to report to the physician, how to take an oral temperature, activities that place him or her at risk for recurrence, and the necessity of letting other

NURSING DIAGNOSIS AND MANAGEMENT
Endocarditis

- ◆ Activity Intolerance related to decreased cardiac output and/or myocardial tissue alterations secondary to valvular dysfunction, p. 366
- ◆ High Risk for Infection risk factor: invasive monitoring devices, p. 366
- ◆ Altered Health Maintenance related to lack of perceived threat to health, p. 70

health care providers (e.g., dentist, podiatrist) know of the history of endocarditis. Before discharge from the hospital, the patient should carry a Medic Alert bracelet or emergency identification card.

MYOCARDITIS

Description

Myocarditis is an inflammatory process involving the myocardial wall. It can be a primary or secondary process, and the myocardial involvement can be focal or diffuse.

Etiology

Myocarditis is an insidious process that may take any one of three paths. Some patients have myocarditis, with no signs of heart failure; the second group frequently has a latent period of approximately 1 year before clinical manifestations of heart failure occur; and the third group is seen with rapid-onset heart failure.

Age, gender, and season may affect the incidence. Myocarditis occurs more frequently in men and in the spring and fall, seasons commonly considered "flu seasons." The first box, second column, lists the most common clinical manifestations of myocarditis.[39,40]

Myocarditis can result from a variety of viral, rickettsial, bacterial, and protozoal diseases. In the United States, however, viruses are the most common causative agents (see second box, second column). A definitive diagnosis can be made only by endomyocardial biopsy that reveals lymphocyte infiltration and myocyte necrosis.

Medical Management

No definitive therapy exists, and initial therapy usually is supportive and geared toward slowing the progression of the heart failure. Efforts are made to decrease cardiac work; therefore activity restrictions are placed on patients.

A regimen of afterload-reducing agents is combined with positive-inotropic agents and diuretics. The effects of immunosuppression therapy to decrease inflammation is being studied.[40]

Nursing Management

The focus of nursing care is similar to that for the patient with heart failure. Patients who undergo endomyocardial biopsy need to be assessed frequently for clinical manifestations of tamponade following the procedure. In addition, patients with myocarditis need emotional support and information to help them deal with the sudden onset and potentially life-threatening aspects of their disease process.[39,40]

CLINICAL MANIFESTATIONS OF MYOCARDITIS

Easy fatigability
Exertional dyspnea
Pericardial pain
Syncope
Sudden, unexplained heart failure

ENDOCARDITIS/MYOCARDITIS: MOST COMMON CAUSATIVE ORGANISMS IN UNITED STATES

RNA VIRUSES

Coxsackie A and B
Echovirus
Influenza A and B
Mumps

DNA VIRUSES

Varicella-zoster
Cytomegalovirus
Epstein-Barr

NURSING DIAGNOSIS AND MANAGEMENT
Myocarditis

- ◆ Acute Pain related to transmission and perception of cutaneous, visceral, muscular or ischemic impulses secondary to inflamed pericardium, p. 566
- ◆ Decreased Cardiac Output related to relative excess of preload and afterload secondary to impaired ventricular contractility, p. 358
- ◆ Decreased Cardiac Output related to decreased preload secondary to seticemia, p. 362

CARDIOMYOPATHY

Description and Etiology

Cardiomyopathies, which are diseases of the heart muscle, are classified as primary or secondary. Primary, or idiopathic, cardiomyopathy is defined as heart muscle disease of unknown cause, although both viral infections and autoimmunity are suspected causes.

Secondary cardiomyopathy is defined as heart muscle disease as a result of some other systemic disease, such as coronary artery disease, valvular disease, severe hypertension, alcohol abuse, or autoimmune disease.[18]

Pathophysiology

Cardiomyopathies are further classified into three main categories on the basis of abnormalities of structure and function. These categories include hypertrophic, restrictive, and congestive cardiomyopathy.

◆ **Hypertrophic cardiomyopathy.** Hypertrophic cardiomyopathy is a genetically transmitted autosomal dominant trait, which frequently appears in relatives who may be symptom-free. It is characterized by left ventricular hypertrophy and bizarre cellular hypertrophy of the upper ventricular septum, which may or may not result in outflow tract obstruction (Fig. 16-14). Frequently, septal hypertrophy pulls the papillary muscle out of alignment, which causes altered function of the anterior leaflet of the mitral valve and mitral regurgitation. The myocardial muscle becomes stiff and less compliant, resulting in increased resistance to blood entering the left atrium and an increase in diastolic filling pressures.

The most common symptom is exertional dyspnea related to elevated left ventricular diastolic pressure and increased wall stiffness, resulting in a decreased cardiac output. Syncope or "graying out" spells also are common because of the inability to increase the cardiac output with exertion.

Treatment is aimed at relaxing the ventricle and decreasing obstruction of the outflow tract. Most frequently used therapies are beta-blockers and calcium channel blockers.[41] It must be clearly stated in the patient's record that positive inotropic drugs should not be administered because of their propensity to increase ventricular contractility, thereby increasing outflow tract obstruction. These patients have an increased incidence of sudden death.

◆ **Dilated cardiomyopathy.** Dilated cardiomyopathy is characterized by grossly dilated ventricles without muscle hypertrophy (see Fig. 16-14). The muscle fibers contract poorly, resulting in global left ventricular dysfunction, low cardiac output, atrial and ventricular dysrhythmias, pooling of blood, which leads to embolic episodes, and eventually refractory heart failure and premature death.[42]

◆ **Restrictive cardiomyopathy.** Restrictive cardiomyopathy (see Fig. 16-14), which is the least common form of cardiomyopathy, is characterized by abnormal diastolic function. This cardiomyopathy results in ventricular wall rigidity as a direct consequence of wall fibrosis. The overall effect is to obstruct ventricular filling. Restrictive cardiomyopathy may be misdiagnosed as constrictive pericarditis.

Backward heart failure, low cardiac output, dyspnea, orthopnea, and liver engorgement are the most common clinical manifestations of restrictive cardiomyopathy. Treatment is directed toward the improvement of pump function, the removal of excess fluid, and administration of a low-sodium diet.

Medical Management

In recent years, with more widespread use of percutaneous endomyocardial biopsy, many patients originally diagnosed with idiopathic cardiomyopathy have been found to have active lymphocytic myocarditis. Treatment of idiopathic cardiomyopathy is not curative but is directed toward controlling symptoms. Treatment includes a decrease in activity and restriction of sodium intake; administration of diuretics, positive inotropic

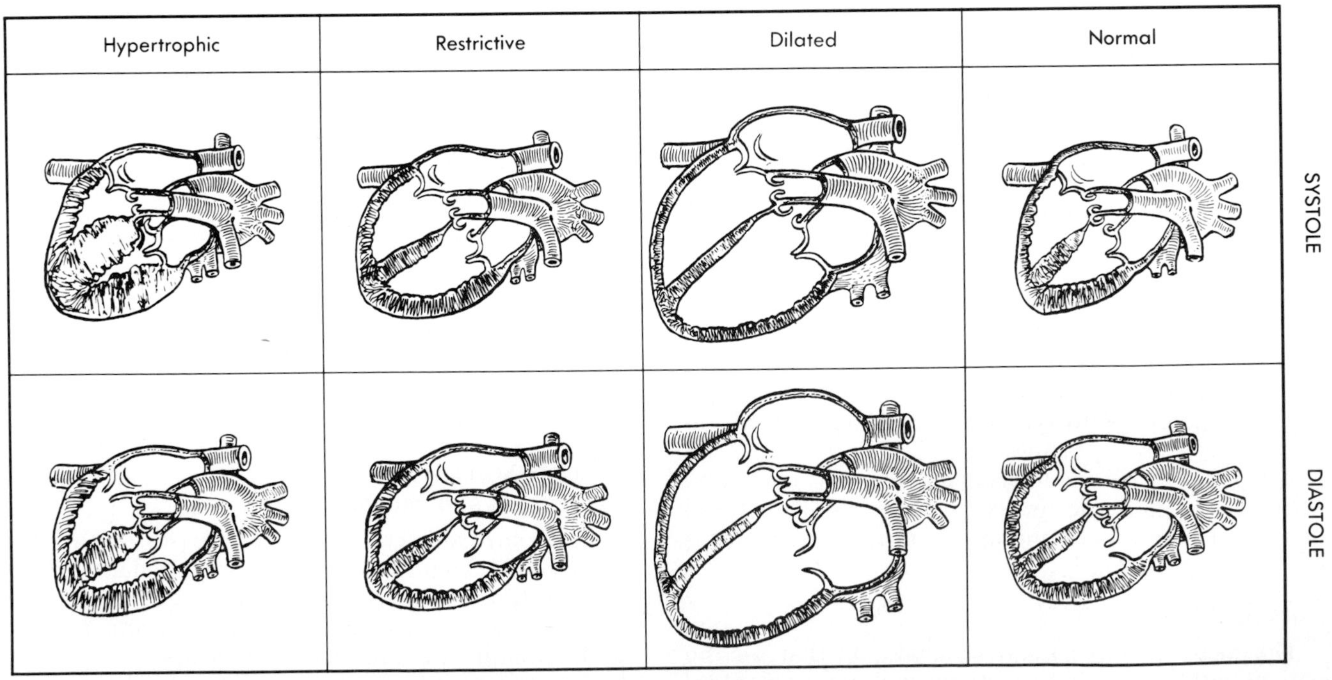

Fig. 16-14 Types of cardiomyopathies.

agents, vasodilators, and antidysrhythmic agents; and administration of oxygen during periods of acute exacerbations of heart failure; ultimately, heart transplantation may be the patient's only hope for survival. Information about the process of heart transplantation is found in Chapter 49, pp. 837-840.

Nursing Management

Many of the nursing interventions for the patient with cardiomyopathy are similar to those for the patient with heart failure. Patients must be monitored for clinical manifestations of worsening heart failure, that is, tissue edema, increased ventricular filling pressures, or neck vein engorgement, pulmonary congestion, weight gain, increased fatigue, and onset of gallop rhythms. Diuretics, medications to increase contractility, calcium channel blockers or beta blockers, and vasodilators to reduce preload should be administered as ordered and the patient's response to them assessed. Obtaining daily weights, maintenance of fluid restriction if ordered, and maintenance of accurate intake and output records are important. Patients with cardiomyopathy are prone to digoxin toxicity related to decreased excretion of the drug secondary to a decreased glomerular filtration rate.[43]

Nursing interventions also should be directed at maintaining the patient's current level of conditioning and toward collaborating with the physical therapist to maintain and, one hopes, to improve the patient's functional level. Activity plans need to reflect energy conservation; therefore activities should be clustered and include frequent rest periods.

The patient's understanding of this illness and his or her coping mechanisms and support systems must be assessed. Patients and families need to know what support services are available.

> ◆
>
> *NURSING DIAGNOSIS AND MANAGEMENT*
> **Cardiomyopathy**
>
> - ◆ Decreased Cardiac Output related to relative excess of preload and afterload secondary to impaired ventricular contractility, p. 358
> - ◆ Activity Intolerance related to knowledge deficit of energy-saving techniques, p. 365
> - ◆ Activity Intolerance related to decreased cardiac output and/or myocardial tissue perfusion alterations, p. 366
> - ◆ Anxiety related to threat to biologic, psychologic, and/or social integrity, p. 763
> - ◆ Powerlessness related to health care environment or illness-related regimen, p. 98
> - ◆ Powerlessness related to physical deterioration despite compliance, p. 99
> - ◆ Hopelessness related to perceptions of failing or deteriorating physical condition, p. 100
> - ◆ Sensory/Perceptual Alterations related to sensory overload, sensory deprivation, and sleep pattern disturbance, p. 573

VALVULAR HEART DISEASE

Description

Valvular heart disease is a cardiac dysfunction produced by structural and/or functional abnormalities of single or multiple cardiac valves. The result is alteration in blood flow across the valve.

Etiology and Pathophysiology

There are two types of lesions, *stenotic* and *regurgitant.* Valvular stenosis results in impeded flow across the valve, and valvular regurgitation results in bidirectional flow of blood across the valve. Valvular dysfunction affects overall cardiac function by increasing pressure work with stenotic lesions and by increasing volume work with regurgitant lesions. In an attempt to compensate for these dysfunctions, the myocardium either will dilate to accommodate an increased volume or will hypertrophy to increase contractility to maintain forward flow.[44]

In the past in the United States, most valvular lesions were rheumatic in origin; that is, damage was a direct result of group A beta-hemolytic streptococcal pharyngitis. Today, with the aging population, degenerative valve changes are equally important (see box below).

◆ **Mitral valve dysfunction.** *Mitral valve stenosis* (Table 16-3) is a progressive narrowing of the mitral valve orifice from 4 to 6 cm to less than 1.5 cm. This narrowing usually is caused by aging valve tissue or by acute rheumatic valvulitis, which results in diffuse leaflet thickening or fibrotic thickening of the margins of closure. The diffuse leaflet fibrosis and fusion of one or both commissures contributed to reduced leaflet mobility. The chordae tendineae also may be thickened, shortened, and fused, further contributing to the stenotic mitral orifice. As a result, the mitral valve no longer can open and close passively in response to chamber pressure changes; therefore blood flow across the valve is impeded.

Symptoms usually do not appear until the valve orifice is narrowed to 1.5 cm.[44] Early symptoms reflect failure of the left side of the heart, but as the dysfunction progresses, bilateral heart failure will be evidenced. Stenosis eventually produces a "fixed" cardiac output (CO). This is a CO that cannot increase in response to exercise. Once the valve orifice narrows to 1.5 cm, left atrial pressure increases in an attempt to force blood through the narrowed valve. This increase in pressure is followed by left atrial dilation, which distorts the

> ◆
>
> *ETIOLOGY OF VALVULAR HEART DISEASE*
>
> Rheumatic fever
> Infective endocarditis
> Inborn defects of connective tissue
> Dysfunction or ruptures of the papillary muscles
> Congenital malformations
> Aging valve tissue

Table 16-3 Valvular dysfunction

Pathophysiology	Clinical manifestations	Physical signs
MITRAL VALVE STENOSIS		
Left atrium must generate more pressure to propel blood beyond the lesion Rise in left atrial pressure and volume reflected retrograde into pulmonary vessels Right ventricular hypertrophy Right ventricular failure	Dyspnea on exertion Fatigue and weakness Pronounced respiratory symptoms—orthopnea, paroxysmal nocturnal dyspnea Mild hemoptysis with bronchial capillary rupture Susceptibility to pulmonary infections	Chest radiograph—pulmonary conges- tion, redistribution of blood flow to upper lobes ECG—atrial fibrillation and other atrial dysrhythmias Auscultation—diastolic murmur, accentuated S_1, opening snap Catheterization—elevated pressure gradient across valve; increased left atrial pressure, pulmonary artery wedge, pulmonary artery pressure; low cardiac output
MITRAL VALVE REGURGITATION		
Left ventricular dilation and hypertrophy Left atrial dilation and hypertrophy	Weakness and fatigue Exertional dyspnea Palpitations Severe symptoms precipitated by left ventricular failure, with consequent low output and pulmonary congestion	Chest radiograph—left atrial and left ventricular enlargement, variable pulmonary congestion ECG—P-mitrale, left ventricular hypertrophy, atrial fibrillation Auscultation—murmur throughout systole Catheterization—opacification of left atrium during left ventricular injection, V waves, increased left atrial and left ventricular pressures Variable elevations of pulmonary pressures
AORTIC VALVE STENOSIS		
Left ventricular hypertrophy Progressive failure of ventricular emptying Pulmonary congestion Failure of right side of heart, with systemic venous congestion Sudden death	Exertional dyspnea Exercise tolerance Syncope Angina Heart failure (left ventricular failure)	Chest radiograph—poststenotic aortic dilation, calcification ECG—left ventricular hypertrophy Auscultation—systolic ejection murmur Catheterization—significant pressure gradient, increased left ventricular end-diastolic pressure

Continued.

myocardial fibers, resulting in multiple ectopic atrial beats and the potential onset of atrial fibrillation. Atrial fibrillation further decreases the cardiac output and exacerbates the symptoms of heart failure and decreased perfusion. This combination of increased pressure and volume leads to pulmonary congestion, which may progress from mild congestion to pulmonary edema. As excess blood fills the pulmonary vasculature, the pulmonary vascular resistance increases, resulting in extra work by the right ventricle, which causes right ventricular hypertrophy. Because the right ventricle is ill-suited to function as a pump under these circumstances, the right side of the heart eventually fails, leading to systemic engorgement demonstrated by jugular venous distention, ascites, and peripheral edema. Failure of the right side of the heart may be compounded by functional tricuspid regurgitation secondary to the high pressure and volume on the right side.

Mitral valve regurgitation (see Table 16-3) can be secondary to rheumatic disease, or aging of the valve, or it can be caused by endocarditis, papillary muscle dysfunction, or a number of other events. In mitral valve regurgitation the valve annulus, leaflets, commissures, chordae tendineae, and papillary muscles may all be dysfunctional or the dysfunction may be isolated to just one component of the valve. The primary effects of mitral valve regurgitation result in thickening and retraction of a portion of the leaflet.

Mitral valve regurgitation results in retrograde flow of blood into the left atrium with each ventricular contraction. The left atrium dilates to accommodate this additional volume, whereas the left ventricle hypertrophies as it tries to maintain forward flow and an adequate stroke volume. Mitral valve regurgitation tends

Table 16-3 Valvular dysfunction—cont'd

Pathophysiology	Clinical manifestations	Physical signs
AORTIC VALVE REGURGITATION		
Increased volume load imposed on left ventricle Left ventricular dilation and hypertrophy	Fatigue Dyspnea on exertion Palpitations	Chest radiograph—boot-shaped elongation of cardiac apex ECG—left ventricular hypertrophy Auscultation—diastolic murmur Catheterization—opacification of left ventricle during aortic injection Peripheral signs—hyperdynamic myocardial action and low peripheral resistance
TRICUSPID VALVE STENOSIS		
Right atrium must generate higher pressure to eject blood beyond the lesion Right atrial dilation Systemic venous engorgement Increased venous pressures	Venous distention Peripheral edema Ascites Hepatic engorgement Anorexia	Chest radiograph—right atrial enlargement ECG—right atrial enlargement (P-pulmonale) Auscultation—diastolic murmur Catheterization—elevated right atrial pressure with large a waves; pressure gradient across the tricuspid valve
TRICUSPID VALVE REGURGITATION		
Right ventricular hypertrophy and dilation	Decreased cardiac output Neck vein distention Hepatic engorgement Ascites Edema Pleural effusions	Chest radiograph—right atrial and ventricular enlargement. ECG—right ventricular hypertrophy and right atrial enlargement, atrial fibrillation Auscultation—murmur throughout systole Catheterization—elevated right atrial pressure and V waves

to beget mitral valve regurgitation in that, as the volume and dimensions increase, the regurgitation worsens.[44] Once the left ventricle fails, the pulmonary venous pressure increases, leading to pulmonary congestion, increased pulmonary artery pressure, and right ventricular enlargement. Surgical intervention by either valve replacement or valvular reconstruction should occur before the patient reaches this stage. Reconstruction procedures include annuloplasty, with or without use of a prosthetic ring, or resection and repair of the valve.

Acute mitral valve regurgitation caused by papillary muscle rupture secondary to acute MI is a medical emergency that is not tolerated without aggressive medical therapy to stabilize the patient's condition, which frequently includes use of an intraaortic balloon pump. Once the patient has stabilized, he or she is taken to surgery for surgical replacement of the incompetent valve.

◆ **Aortic valve dysfunction.** *Aortic valve stenosis* (see Table 16-3) can result from aging, calcification of a congenital bicuspid valve, or rheumatic valvulitis. Irrespective of its cause, the effect is to impede ejection of blood from the left ventricle into the aorta, resulting in increased left ventricular systolic pressure, left ventricular hypertrophy, and eventually, at end-stage disease, left ventricular dilation. In addition, when the increase in volume and pressure is communicated back to the atrial and pulmonary vasculature, the result is an increase in left atrial pressure and volume, pulmonary venous pressure, and pulmonary congestion. In rare cases, if left untreated, right ventricular failure may develop. An incidence of sudden death is associated with aortic valve stenosis and usually occurs during exertion when demand acutely outstrips the heart's ability to provide an adequate cardiac output.

Aortic valve regurgitation (see Table 16-3) can occur as a result of rheumatic fever, systemic hypertension, Marfan's syndrome, syphilis, rheumatoid arthritis, aging valve tissue or discrete subaortic stenosis. Aortic valve regurgitation results in reflux of blood back into the left ventricle during ventricular diastole. To accommodate this extra volume, the left ventricle dilates. Over time, however, the left ventricle hypertrophies in an attempt to empty more completely and to meet the needs of the peripheral circulation.

◆ **Tricuspid valve dysfunction.** *Tricuspid valve stenosis* (see Table 16-3) is rarely an isolated lesion and usually occurs in conjunction with mitral or aortic disease, or both. Its origin most often is rheumatic fever. Tricuspid valve stenosis increases the pressure work of the usually low-pressure right atrium, resulting in right atrial hypertrophy. In addition, the right atrium dilates in an attempt to accommodate the residual right atrial volume and the incoming venous return. As a result, systemic venous congestion occurs, the consequences of which include jugular venous congestion, liver failure, hepatomegaly, ascites, and peripheral edema.

Tricuspid valve regurgitation (see Table 16-3) usually results from advanced failure of the left side of the heart or severe pulmonary hypertension.

◆ **Pulmonary valve dysfunction.** *Pulmonary valve disease* most often is related to congenital anomalies and produces failure of the right side of the heart. If untreated, it can result in severe irreversible pulmonary vascular changes.

◆ **Mixed valvular lesions.** Many persons have mixed lesions, that is, an element of both stenosis and regurgitation. Mixed lesions can accentuate the severity of a condition. For example, aortic stenosis and aortic regurgitation combined increase left ventricular volume and pressure and thereby multiply the degree of left ventricular work. On the other hand, mitral valve stenosis and aortic valve stenosis offer a protective combination. Mitral stenosis protects the left ventricle from the strain produced by aortic valve stenosis alone. Mitral valve stenosis, by decreasing forward flow from the left atrium to the left ventricle, reduces the residual volume in the left ventricle because of the aortic valve stenosis.[7,18,45] However, this combination will be poorly tolerated by the patient because of the low "fixed" cardiac output that results.

Nursing Management

The focus of care for the patient with valvular heart disease is to assess the patient's functional activity level and fluid volume status and to monitor for signs of heart failure, syncope, or anginal pain.

Patients with valvular heart disease frequently have decreased cardiac output because of decreased forward flow secondary to obstruction of flow through a stenotic valve or because of bidirectional flow across an incompetent valve. Positive inotropic and afterload-reducing agents should be administered as ordered and their effect carefully assessed and documented.

NURSING DIAGNOSIS AND MANAGEMENT
Valvular heart disease

- Decreased Cardiac Output related to relative excess of preload and afterload secondary to impaired ventricular contractility, p. 358
- Activity Intolerance related to decreased cardiac output and/or myocardial tissue perfusion alterations, p. 366
- Activity Intolerance related to postural hypotension secondary to prolonged immobility, narcotics, vasodilator therapy, p. 365
- High Risk for Altered Peripheral Tissue Perfusion risk factor: high-dose vasopressor therapy, p. 363
- Body Image Disturbance related to actual change in body structure, function, or appearance, p. 94

Vital signs are assessed frequently, and if the patient has indwelling catheters, hemodynamic parameters also are measured.

Activities are carefully planned to provide adequate rest periods to prevent fatigue.

Fluid status is assessed by auscultating breath and heart sounds. The appearance of pulmonary crackles or an S_3 may indicate fluid-volume overload. The jugular vein may be assessed for signs of increased distention, and diuretics and vasodilators are administered relative to fluid balance requirements. The patient is weighed daily, and fluid intake and output are accurately monitored.

Activities that precipitate anginal pain must be clearly documented. The patient may require oxygen and pain medication to treat the discomfort. Decreasing anxiety also may lessen the discomfort.

Patient teaching includes information related to (1) any diet and/or fluid restrictions, (2) actions and side effects of the medications, (3) prophylactic antibiotics before undergoing any invasive procedures such as dental work, and (4) when to call the physician about a change in heart status.

HYPERTENSIVE CRISIS

Description

Hypertensive crisis represents a clinical situation in which hypertension is associated with irreversible vital organ damage or a threat to life over a short period of time. The critical factor in hypertensive crisis is the accelerated rise of the blood pressure, which results in complications occurring over a period of hours or days rather than days to weeks.[46] A *diastolic* pressure greater than 130 mm Hg usually is labeled as severe hypertension.

Etiology

The overall incidence of hypertensive crisis is less than 1% of persons known to have hypertension. It usually is precipitated by noncompliance with medical therapy or diet, or both, or by inadequate treatment. Hypertensive crisis may be detected in patients with no history of the condition.

In patients with no history of hypertension, common causes of crisis include (1) acute or chronic renal disease, (2) acute central nervous system (CNS) events, (3) drug-induced hypertension, and (4) the ingestion of tyramine-containing foods or beverages (e.g., beer or cheese) during treatment with a monoamine oxidase inhibitor (MAOI). In addition, a state like that of catecholamine excess may follow the abrupt cessation of clonidine and guanabenz.[46]

Pathophysiology

The exact mechanism of hypertensive crisis is not known, but it is characterized by fibrinoid necrosis of the arterioles.

Assessment and Diagnosis

Hypertensive crisis is manifested by CNS compromise (headache, papilledema, coma), cardiovascular compro-

Table 16-4 Hypertensive emergencies

Emergencies	Examples of causes
CARDIOVASCULAR COMPROMISE	
Chest pain	Unstable angina, myocardial infarction, aortic dissection
Congestive heart failure	Myocardial infarction, severe hypertension, pheochromocytoma (very rare)
Hypertension after vascular surgery	Aortic aneurysmectomy, carotid endarterectomy, coronary artery bypass grafting
CENTRAL NERVOUS SYSTEM (CNS) COMPROMISE	
Papilledema	Increased intracranial pressure—mass lesion
	Malignant hypertension—any cause
Headache, agitation, lethargy, confusion	Hypertensive encephalopathy—any cause, subarachnoid hemorrhage, cerebrovascular accident (CVA)
Coma	CVA, advanced hypertensive encephalopathy, trauma, tumor
Seizures	Advanced hypertensive encephalopathy, CNS tumor, eclampsia, CVA (less common)
Focal neurologic deficit	CVA, CNS tumor, hypertensive encephalopathy
ACUTE RENAL FAILURE	Malignant hypertension, vasculitis, scleroderma, glomerulonephritis
CATECHOLAMINE EXCESS	Pheochromocytomas, MAOI in combination with certain drugs and foods, clonidine and guanabenz withdrawal

Modified from McRae RP, Liebson PR: *Med Clin North Am* 70(4):749, 1986.

mise (angina, myocardial infarction), acute renal failure, and a history consistent with catecholamine excess. Table 16-4 lists clinical findings that suggest hypertensive emergencies and gives examples of causes.

Medical Management

Hypertensive crisis necessitates admitting the patient to a critical care unit where antihypertensive therapy can be administered parenterally and blood pressure monitored continuously by means of an arterial line. Frequently used medications include furosemide, sodium nitroprusside, nitroglycerin, phentolamine, and labetalol.

Clonidine administered in hourly doses of 0.1 to 0.2 mg lowers severe hypertension. Other oral drugs that apparently are effective during crisis are guanabenz, minoxidil, nifedipine, and captopril. A loop diuretic and beta blocker usually are used concurrently to prevent reflex tachycardia and fluid retention, both of which may increase the blood pressure.[46,47,48]

It is important to remember that cerebral hypoperfusion can occur if mean blood pressure is lowered too rapidly. During the first 24 hours of treatment, it has been recommended that mean arterial pressure be decreased by no more than 20% to 30%.[48]

Hypertensive crisis with current therapy is associated with a 25% mortality at 1 year and 50% at 5 years. Most common causes of death are uremia, myocardial infarction, heart failure, and cerebrovascular accident.

> ◆
>
> ***NURSING DIAGNOSIS AND MANAGEMENT***
> **Hypertensive crisis**
>
> - ◆ Anxiety related to threat to biologic, psychologic, and/or social integrity, p. 763
> - ◆ Altered Cerebral Tissue Perfusion related to increased intracranial pressure secondary to brain trauma, hemorrhage, edema, infection, tumor, stroke, hydrocephalus, p. 560

Nursing Management

The focus of nursing care for the patient with hypertensive crisis is to return the blood pressure to the desired range and then to identify the factors that resulted in this life-threatening condition.

During the acute phase the patient must be closely observed for clinical manifestations of cardiac or neurologic compromise, such as cardiovascular collapse, ischemia, dysrhythmias, mental confusion, stupor, seizures, or coma.

Antihypertensive agents should be administered as ordered and the blood pressure closely monitored. If potent antihypertensive drugs such as nitroprusside or labetalol are being used, they should be infused through an infusion pump and an arterial line should be placed in the patient.

While obtaining the health history, the nurse needs to identify risk factors, to clarify any misconceptions the patient may have regarding hypertension and its treatment, and to identify learning needs.

AORTIC DISEASE

Aortic Aneurysm

◆ **Description.** An aneurysm is a localized dilation of the arterial wall that results in an alteration in vessel shape and blood flow. Fig. 16-15 displays the four types of aneurysms. Abdominal aortic aneurysm is 4 times more common than is thoracic aneurysm. Its incidence, which is higher in men than in women, is diagnosed most commonly after the fifth decade.

◆ **Etiology.** Most patients (90%) who are seen initially with an aneurysm have a history of systemic hypertension. Other causes of aneurysm include (1) atherosclerotic changes in the thoracic and abdominal aorta, (2) blunt trauma (deceleration injury), (3) cystic medial necrosis (Marfan's syndrome), (4) pregnancy, and (5) iatrogenic injury or dissection. Blunt trauma can cause rupture of the intimal and medial layers of the descending aorta at the ligamentum arteriosum. Increased blood volume and hypertension contribute to rupture of the aorta during pregnancy. Iatrogenic injuries may occur as

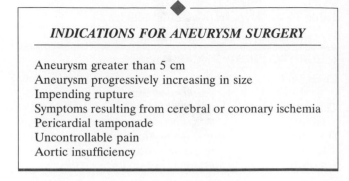

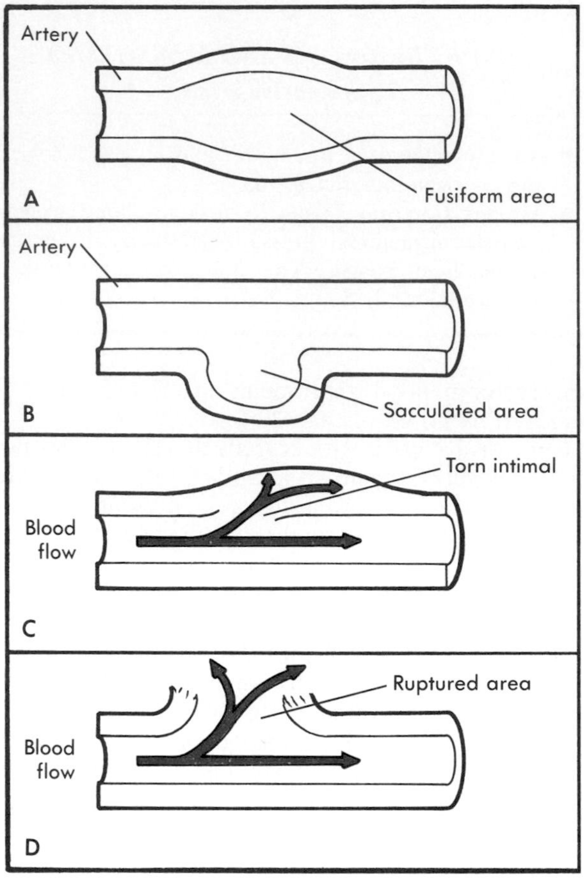

Fig. 16-15 Four basic types of aneurysms. **A,** Fusiform aneurysm, in which an entire segment of an artery is dilated, thus taking on a spindle or bulbous shape. Fusiform aneurysms occur most often in the abdominal aorta secondary to atherosclerosis. **B,** Sacculated aneurysm, which involves only one side of an artery and usually is located in the ascending aorta. **C,** Dissecting aneurysm, which occurs because of a tear in the intima, resulting in the shunting of blood between the intima and media of a vessel. **D,** Pseudoaneurysm, which results from a ruptured artery.

a result of the use of instruments during arteriography, cardiopulmonary bypass, intraaortic balloon procedures, and aortic surgery.

◆ **Pathophysiology.** Medial degeneration is the most common cause of aneurysm formation. Medial degeneration occurs as a normal part of the aging process and as a complication of Marfan's syndrome (Erdheim's cystic medial necrosis).

The ascending aorta and the aortic arch are the sites of the greatest hemodynamic stress and also are the most common sites of arterial dissection. Extensive medial degeneration frequently occurs in hypertensive patients and is a major contributing factor to aneurysmal risk.

◆ **Assessment and diagnosis.** For many years a person may be symptom-free or the aneurysm may be detected during routine abdominal examination as a palpable, pulsatile mass located in the umbilical region of the abdomen to the left of midline. A thoracic aneurysm may be identified on a routine chest x-ray film. Patients with an acute dissection or rupture, however, are seen initially with sudden onset of sharp, ripping or tearing pain located in the anterior chest, epigastric area, shoulders, or back.

INDICATIONS FOR ANEURYSM SURGERY

Aneurysm greater than 5 cm
Aneurysm progressively increasing in size
Impending rupture
Symptoms resulting from cerebral or coronary ischemia
Pericardial tamponade
Uncontrollable pain
Aortic insufficiency

Cardiovascular signs include severe hypertension, acute neurologic deficits, fleeting peripheral pulses, and a new murmur indicative of aortic insufficiency.

◆ **Medical management.** An aneurysm less than 4 cm in diameter can be managed medically with frequent monitoring of blood pressure and ultrasound testing to document any changes in size of the aneurysm. The patient is encouraged to lose weight if obesity is a factor, and blood pressure will be carefully monitored and hypertension treated to decrease hemodynamic stress on the site. An aneurysm greater than 5 cm usually is treated surgically (see box above).

Aortic Dissection

◆ **Description.** An aortic dissection occurs when there is separation of the vascular layers by a column of blood. This creates a false lumen, which communicates with the true lumen through a tear in the intima. This separation extends along the length of the vessel rather than coursing around the circumference.

◆ **Classification of dissections.** Aortic dissections are classified according to site of the tear. In the DeBakey classification system. Type I dissections extend from just above the aortic valve to the iliac bifurcation. Type II dissections are limited to the ascending aorta and most frequently are seen with Marfan's syndrome. Type III dissections begin in the descending aorta distal to the left subclavian artery and extend distally to the aortic bifurcation. Another classification, used by Dr. Shumway of Stanford University, classifies dissections into two groups: those that involve the arch of the aorta and place the patient at risk for tamponade (Type A); and those that involve the descending aorta only (Type B). In essence, Types I and II are similar to Type A (proximal aortic dissection); and Type III and Type B involve the descending or distal aorta (Fig. 16-16). Both classification systems are used in clinical practice (Fig. 16-16).

◆ **Assessment and diagnosis.** The classic clinical manifestation is the sudden onset of intense, severe, tearing pain, which may be localized initially in the chest, abdomen, or back. As dissection extends, pain radiates to the back or distally toward the lower extremities.

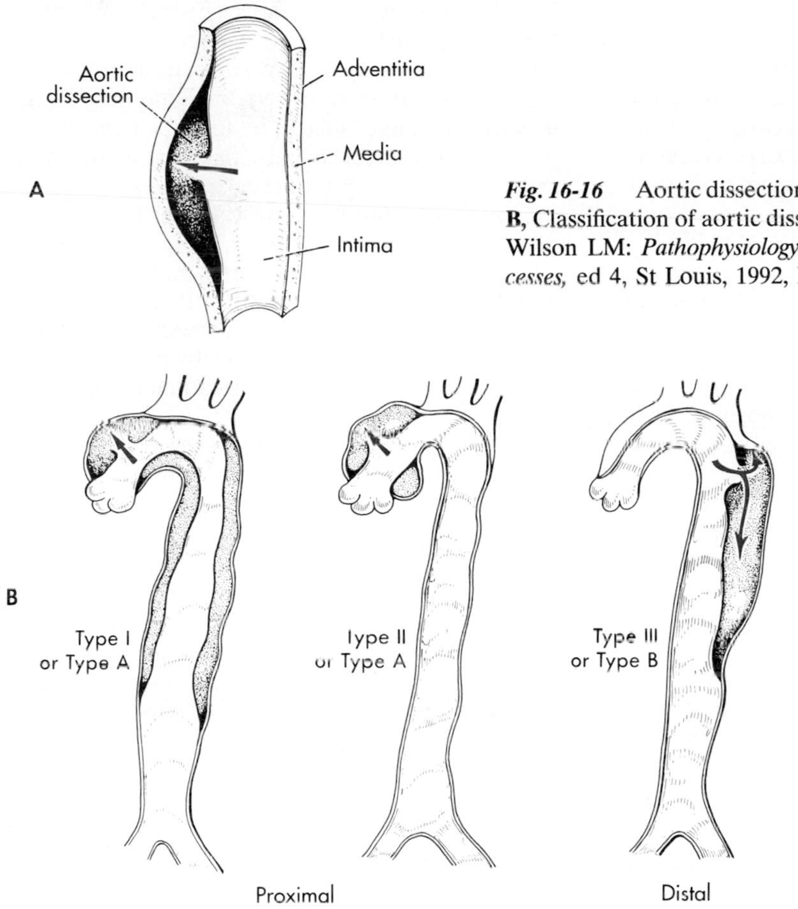

Fig. 16-16 Aortic dissection. **A**, Separation of vascular layers. **B**, Classification of aortic dissection. (Modified from Price SA, Wilson LM: *Pathophysiology: clinical concepts of disease processes,* ed 4, St Louis, 1992, Mosby–Year Book.)

Another cardiovascular sign may be a new murmur of aortic regurgitation if the dissection moves retrograde, extending back to the aortic valve. At this time the coronary arteries may be at risk, putting the patient in jeopardy of sustaining a myocardial infarction. Signs of shock may develop quickly with this type of lesion.

Patients usually exhibit severe hypertension and loss of peripheral pulses, and they may demonstrate acute neurologic deficits, which include syncope, altered level of consciousness, varying levels of paresthesia and paralysis, or possibly a cerebrovascular accident. Gastrointestinal symptoms include acute abdominal pain, melena, and hyperactive bowel sounds.

Renal symptoms include oliguria and hematuria. These symptoms usually occur with dissections that cause hypotension and those that involve the renal arteries.

The location of the dissection may be established by the site of pain. A distal dissection usually is accompanied by chest pain, which radiates to the back, abdomen, or legs. Central chest pain indicates an ascending dissection. Invasive diagnostic procedures that may be performed include aortogram (with radiopaque contrast), magnetic resonance imaging (MRI), or computed tomographic scan using contrast.

◆ **Medical management.** Medical management involves controlling hypertension and pain. Progression of the dissection is evaluated by the patient's report of worsening or new pain.

Surgical procedures include resection of the affected areas, followed by graft placement, repair or replacement of the aortic valve, and restoration of blood flow to major branches of the aorta.[51]

◆ **Nursing management.** The focus of nursing care for the patient with an aortic dissection is to lower and to maintain the blood pressure within prescribed parameters, to effect hemodynamic stability, and to control the pain.

The cardiovascular status should be assessed hourly, including monitoring blood pressure in both arms, checking peripheral pulses bilaterally, auscultating for an aortic murmur, and monitoring the ECG for ischemic changes or dysrhythmias, or both. Patients usually require an arterial line and receive potent vasodilators such as labetalol or sodium nitroprusside.

The patient's neurovascular status also is assessed hourly. Included in this assessment should be documentation of the presence and distribution of pain, pallor, paresthesia, paralysis, and pulselessness.

A quiet, nonstimulating environment is maintained to decrease stress, which can lead to increased levels of circulating catecholamines and consequent increases in heart rate and blood pressure. Analgesics also are useful in decreasing anxiety and increasing comfort. Because analgesics can mask the pain of further dissection, they are administered judiciously.

PERIPHERAL VASCULAR DISEASE

Description

Atherosclerosis is the most common cause of peripheral vascular disease. Alterations can occur in either the venous or arterial systems, with most occurring in the vessels of the lower extremities. Risk factors associated with peripheral vascular disease are the same as those for coronary artery disease.

Arterial Disease

◆ **Etiology and pathophysiology.** There are two major causes of occlusive arterial disease. The first is *arteriosclerosis obliterans,* a consequence of atherosclerosis. These lesions tend to occur at the origin or bifurcations of a vessel. The aortoiliac vessels, femoropopliteal vessels, and popliteal-tibial vessels are the most common sites for atherogenesis.

The second major cause of occlusive arterial disease is *thromboangiitis obliterans* (Buerger's disease), an occlusion caused by inflammation and thrombosis. Thrombi may originate in the left side of the heart as a consequence of atrial fibrillation or mitral stenosis. Thrombogenesis also occurs at the site of atherosclerotic plaque. Arterial occlusion obstructs blood flow to the distal extremity.

◆ **Assessment and diagnosis.** Intermittent claudication (cramping, aching pain during ambulation) usually is the first symptom of peripheral occlusive disease. This pain is relieved by rest, but as the disease progresses, the pain develops during rest. Relief may be obtained by placing the extremity in a dependent position. The site of the pain usually indicates the location of the lesion. Arterial pulses may be diminished, transiently present (vessel spasm), or absent distal to the site of occlusion.

Postural changes result in changes in skin color. With extremity elevation, the limb becomes pale. Dependency of the extremity yields a rubor or purplish discoloration.

Atrophic tissue changes include thickening of the nails and drying of the skin. Hair loss is common on the lower leg, dorsum of the feet, and toes. A temperature gradient usually is present as a line of demarcation between areas that are well perfused and those that are poorly perfused. There also may be wasting of muscle, as well as of soft tissue. As the disease progresses, it may result in ulcerations and gangrene.

Acute occlusions usually are seen initially with sudden onset of severe pain, loss of pulses, collapse of superficial veins, coldness and pallor, and impaired motor and sensory function.

◆ **Medical management.** Medical therapy is geared toward controlling or eliminating risk factors, providing good foot care, and suggesting alterations in life-style to promote rest and pain relief. Therapy also may include the use of anticoagulants, vasodilators, or antiplatelet drugs. If these therapies do not produce positive results, the patient may be a candidate for angioplasty.

Surgical therapy may be required if symptoms become disabling or threaten limb viability. Surgical procedures and the purpose of each include the following: (1) arterial reconstruction—to restore unimpeded flow and to redirect blood flow around the site of occlusion, (2) endarterectomy—to remove discrete plaque, and (3) lumbar sympathectomy—to decrease sympathetic tone and increase peripheral vasodilation. Severe occlusions may necessitate limb or partial limb amputation.

◆ **Nursing management.** The focus of nursing care for the patient with arterial insufficiency is to increase the arterial blood supply, decrease venous pooling, promote vasodilation, maintain tissue integrity, treat tissue hypoxia, and provide patient teaching.

The arterial blood supply may be increased by maintaining the extremity in a neutral (flat) or dependent position, encouraging ambulation (walking but not standing) as ordered, and performing active range-of-motion exercises when bed rest has been prescribed for the patient.

To decrease venous pooling, the patient should not sit or stand for long periods. If pooling does occur, the legs should be elevated to a neutral position. Walking should be encouraged.

The patient can promote vasodilation by keeping the extremity warm, ceasing smoking, and stopping the use of other vasoconstricting substances such as caffeine. He or she should not cross the legs when sitting or lying flat and should avoid anything that constricts blood flow, such as socks with tight-fitting elastic tops or garters.

Nursing interventions intended to preserve tissue integrity include (1) performing special foot care, which includes washing and carefully drying the feet each day, (2) having the patient wear cotton or wool stockings that are not mended and are seamless, and (3) having him or her wear protective footwear (i.e., a soft, flexible leather shoe with a closed, wide toe and a high toebox) whenever out of bed. Sandals, thongs, elastic bands over the instep, and pressure on the dorsum of the foot from tied laces are avoided. Skin color, temperature, and elasticity are checked. Adhesive tape is not applied directly to the skin. Any ulcerations are promptly identified and treated. The patient is encouraged to have a well-balanced diet to maintain tissue integrity and foster wound healing.

Tissue hypoxia may be treated by increasing blood flow to the extremity through walking or performing

---

NURSING DIAGNOSIS AND MANAGEMENT

Peripheral vascular disease

- ◆ Acute Pain related to transmission and perception of cutaneous, visceral, muscular, or ischemic impulses secondary to tissue ischemia, p. 566
- ◆ Anxiety related to threat to biologic, psychologic, and/or social integrity, p. 763
- ◆ Powerlessness related to physical deterioration despite compliance, p. 99
- ◆ Hopelessness related to failing or deteriorating physical condition, p. 100

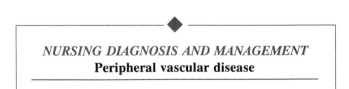

range-of-motion exercises. Tissue hypoxia is painful, and analgesics should be administered to allow the patient to achieve a comfort level that will foster his or her cooperation in ambulating.

Venous Disease

◆ **Description.** Venous disease occurs when there is alteration in the integrity of veins, resulting in decreased venous return or thrombosis.

◆ **Thrombolytic venous disease.** The most common form of venous disease usually manifests as thrombophlebitis. Thrombophlebitis is the formation of a thrombus, accompanied by inflammation, pain, tenderness, and redness at the site. The incidence is greatest in the lower extremity vessels, especially the saphenous, femoral, and popliteal veins. Thrombophlebitis can occur in either deep or superficial vessels and in upper or lower extremity vessels.

Etiology and pathophysiology. Stasis of blood, endothelial injury, and hypercoagulability of blood are referred to as *Virchow's triad.* Usually two of the three conditions must be present for thrombosis to occur.

Superficial thromboses. Superficial thromboses are characterized by cordlike veins that are readily palpable. The area surrounding the affected vessel often is tender to palpation, erythematous, and warm. The most common cause of superficial thromboses of the arms is intravenous therapy.

MEDICAL MANAGEMENT. Patients with superficial thromboses usually do not require anticoagulation therapy, and bed rest may be prescribed until the extremity is less tender and ambulation can be considered. Warm compresses may be used, along with elastic stockings. Superficial thromboses usually are not precursors of more serious conditions.

Deep vein thrombophlebitis. Obstruction of blood flow can occur within a deep vessel of the pelvis or lower extremity. This markedly increases the patient's risk of pulmonary embolism and long-term disability resulting from chronic venous insufficiency.

ASSESSMENT AND DIAGNOSIS. Development of deep vein thrombosis may be insidious. It occurs as a result of edema, causes of which include increased intravascular volume and increased intravascular pooling of blood. Pain is described as an aching or throbbing sensation, which worsens with ambulation. The presence of a positive Homans' sign, which is pain on dorsiflexion of the foot, heightens the suspicion of a deep vein thrombosis. Other manifestations include increased tissue turgor with swelling, increased skin temperature, dilation of superficial veins, and mottling and cyanosis caused by stagnant flow.

MEDICAL MANAGEMENT. Major therapeutic emphasis is placed on prophylaxis. The patient is confined to bed rest, along with elevation of the limb, anticoagulation therapy, and local applications of moist heat. Analgesics are prescribed to reduce discomfort. Measurement of both the affected calf and thigh should be done once a day. The measurement site should be marked on the extremity. Patients receiving anticoagulation therapy require careful assessment for bleeding tendencies, including obtaining frequent bleeding studies, testing stool and urine for occult blood, and inspecting gums for bleeding. Once the patient begins to ambulate, full-length, custom-fitted elastic stockings should be ordered. Complaints of or observation of dyspnea or chest pain must be evaluated to assess the risk of pulmonary embolism.

Medical management with anticoagulants is adequate for most patients; however, those at high risk for pulmonary embolism (i.e., patients with cancer, bleeding disorders, or spinal cord injury or patients who are comatose) may require surgical intervention. Possible procedures include venous thrombectomy, femoral vein interruption, inferior vena cava interruption, insertion of filtering devices, thrombolytic therapy, angioplasty, and laser treatment.

◆ **Chronic venous insufficiency.** Chronic venous insufficiency is produced by extensive deep vein thrombosis with resultant venous valve insufficiency. It usually is precipitated by chronic venous stasis and elevation of venous pressures, resulting in stretching and weakening of the valves. Over time, this condition may lead to the development of stasis ulcers.

◆ **Nursing management.** The focus of care for the patient with venous disease is to increase blood flow and to prevent complications from deep vein thrombosis or anticoagulant therapy.

During the acute phase, self-care activities are limited and bed rest maintained. The affected limb should be elevated above the level of the right atrium to decrease edema and venous stasis. Range-of-motion exercises can be performed with the unaffected leg. The patient is instructed to avoid use of the knee gatch on the bed because elevation of the knee impedes venous return. Warm, moist compresses may be applied, and calf and/or thigh measurements are obtained daily. Thigh-high or knee-high elastic stockings that have been custom fitted or Ace wraps can also be applied. The patient with a deep vein thrombosis is closely monitored for signs of pulmonary embolism and instructed to report immediately any chest pain, dyspnea, or tachypnea. Once the patient is ambulatory, walking is encouraged, but sitting or standing should be avoided. While the patient sits in a chair, low elevation of the affected extremity should be maintained.

Anticoagulant therapy is monitored by obtaining daily coagulation values. Bleeding is treated promptly. Stools are checked for occult blood. Mechanical trauma is avoided (e.g., the patient should use an electric razor, soft toothbrush, and unobstructed walkway).

REFERENCES

1. Alspach JG: The cost of cardiovascular disease: a life every 32 seconds, *Crit Care Nurse* 11(2):8, 1990.
2. Burke LE: Nursing grand rounds: risk-factor modification in the prevention of coronary artery disease, *J Cardiovasc Nurs* 1(4):67, 1987.
3. Benditt EP: The origin of atherosclerosis, *Sci Am* 236:74, 1977.
4. Kannel WB and others: A general cardiovascular risk profile: the Framingham study, *Am J Cardiol* 38:46, 1976.
5. McIntosh HD: Risk factors for cardiovascular disease and death: a clinical perspective, *J Am Coll Surgeons,* 14:24, 1989.
6. Paffenbarger RS and others: Physical activity as an index of heart attack risk in college alumni, *Am J Epidemiol* 108:161, 1978.
7. Braunwald E, editor: *Heart disease,* ed 4, Philadelphia, 1991, WB Saunders.
8. Ross R, Glomset JA: Atherosclerosis and the arterial smooth muscle cell, *Science* 180:1332, 1973.
9. Ross R, Glomset JA: The pathogenesis of atherosclerosis. I. *N Engl J Med* 295(7):369, 1976.
10. Fuster V and others: The pathogenesis of coronary artery disease and the acute coronary syndromes. II. *N Engl J Med* 326(5):310, 1992.
11. Benditt EP, Benditt JM: Evidence for a monoclonal origin of human atherosclerotic plaques, *Proc Natl Acad Sci* 70:1753, 1973.
12. Fuster V and others: The pathogenesis of coronary artery disease and the acute coronary syndromes. I. *N Engl J Med* 326(4):242, 1992.
13. Fruth RM: Differential diagnosis of chest pain, *Crit Care Nurs Clin North Am* 3(1):59, 1991.
14. Rocco MB and others: Circadian variation of transient myocardial ischemia in patients with coronary artery disease, *Circulation* 75:395, 1987.
15. Chambers CE, Leaman DM: Management of acute chest pain syndrome, *Crit Care Clin* 5(3):415, 1989.
16. Cohn PF: Silent ischemia, *Heart Disease and Stroke* 1(5):295, 1992.
17. Young AC and others: Silent ischemia after myocardial infarction, *Circulation* 82(3):suppl II-143, 1990.
18. Hurst W, editor: *The heart,* ed 7, New York, 1990, McGraw-Hill.
19. Smith CE: Assessing chest pain, *Nursing '88* 18(5):52, 1988.
20. Cupples LA and others: Long- and short-term risk of sudden coronary death, *Circulation* 85(1):suppl I-11, 1992.
21. Yusuf S and others: Routine medical management of acute myocardial infarction, *Circulation* 82(3):suppl II-117, 1990.
22. Hanisch PJ: Identification and treatment of acute myocardial infarction by electrocardiographic site classification, *Focus Crit Care* 18(6):480, 1991.
23. Mayberry-Toth B, Landron S: Complications associated with acute myocardial infarction, *Crit Care Nurs Q* 12(2):49, 1989.
24. Meldahl RV and others: Identification of persons at risk for sudden cardiac death, *Med Clin North Am* 72(5):1015, 1988.
25. Kremers MS: Sudden cardiac death: etiologies, pathologies, and treatment, *Diagnosis of the Month,* p 390, June 1988.
26. Hurwitz JL, Josephson ME: Sudden cardiac death in patients with chronic coronary heart disease, *Circulation* 85(1):suppl I-43, 1992.
27. Myerburg RJ and others: Sudden cardiac death: structure, function, and time-dependence of risk, *Circulation* 85(1):suppl I-2, 1992.
28. Wellens HJ and others: Sudden arrhythmic death without overt heart disease, *Circulation* 85(1):suppl I-92, 1992.
29. Waldo AL and others: General evaluation of out-of-hospital sudden cardiac death survivors, *Circulation* 85(1):suppl I-103, 1992.
30. Turk M: Acute pericarditis in the post-myocardial infarction patient, *Crit Care Nurs Q* 12(3):34, 1989.
31. Martin JS and others: Early recognition and treatment of the patient suffering from acute myocardial infarction: a description of the myocardial infarction triage and intervention project, *Crit Care Nurs Clin North Am* 2(4):681, 1990.
32. Rapaport E: Overview: rationale of thrombolysis in treating acute myocardial infarction, *Heart Lung* 20(5):538, 1991.
33. Gawlinski A: Nursing care after AMI: a comprehensive review, *Crit Care Nurs Q* 12(2):64, 1989.
34. Passmore JM, Goldstein RA: Acute recognition and management of congestive heart failure, *Crit Care Clin* 5(3):497, 1989.
35. Parmley WW: Pathophysiology and current therapy of congestive heart failure, *J Am Coll Cardiol* 13(4):771, 1989.
36. Sanders MR and others: The use of inotropic agents in acute and chronic congestive heart failure, *Med Clin North Am* 73(2):283, 1989.
37. Roberts R: Inotropic therapy for cardiac failure associated with acute myocardial infarction, *Chest* 93(1):suppl 22S, 1988.
38. Scrima DA: Infective endocarditis: nursing considerations, *Crit Care Nurse* 7(2):47, 1987.
39. Grady KL: Myocarditis: review of a clinical enigma, *Heart Lung* 18(4):347, 1989.
40. Owens-Jones S, Hopp L: Viral myocarditis, *Focus Crit Care* 15(1):25, 1988.
41. Courtney-Jenkins A: The patient with hypertrophic cardiomyopathy, *J Cardiovasc Nurs* 2(1):33, 1987.
42. Casey PE: Pathophysiology of dilated cardiomyopathy: nursing implications, *J Cardiovasc Nurs* 2(1):1, 1987.
43. Purcell JA: Advances in the treatment of dilated cardiomyopathy, *AACN Clin Issues Crit Care Nurs* 1(1):31, 1990.
44. Schakenbach LH: Physiologic dynamics of acquired valvular heart disease, *J Cardiovasc Nurs* 1(3):1, 1987.
45. Rahimtoola SH: Perspective on valvular heart disease: an update, *J Am Coll Cardiol* 14(1):1, 1989.
46. Houston MC: Pathophysiology, clinical aspects, and treatment of hypertensive crisis, *Prog Cardiovasc Dis* 32:99, 1989.
47. Winer N: Hypertensive crisis, *Crit Care Nurs Q* 13(3):23, 1990.
48. Fletcher AE, Bulpitt CJ: How far should blood pressure be lowered? *N Engl J Med* 326(4):251, 1992.
49. Crawford ES and others: Aortic dissection and dissecting aortic aneurysms, *Ann Surg* 208:254, 1988.
50. Dixon MB: Acute aortic dissection, *J Cardiovasc Nurs* 1(2):24, 1987.
51. Crawford ES and others: Surgical treatment of aneurysm and/or dissection of the ascending aorta and transverse aortic arch, *J Thorac Cardiovasc Surg* 98:659, 1989.

17

Cardiovascular Therapeutic Management

CHAPTER OBJECTIVES

- Discuss the prevention, identification, and management of pacemaker malfunction.
- Describe the immediate postoperative medical and nursing management of the adult cardiac surgical patient.
- Discuss the purpose and nursing and medical management of the patient with an implantable cardiovertor defibrillor (ICD).
- Summarize the nursing interventions pertinent to the patient undergoing percutaneous transluminal coronary angioplasty (PTCA), atherectomy, stent, or laser therapy.
- Describe the role of the critical care nurse during and after the administration of thrombolytic therapy.
- State the principal nursing management issues for safe care of the patient who requires a mechanical circulatory assist divice.
- Identify the major nursing implications related to the administration of antidysrhythmic and vasoactive drug therapy.

TEMPORARY PACEMAKERS

Pacemakers are electronic devices that can be used to initiate the heartbeat when the heart's intrinsic electrical system is unable to effectively generate a rate adequate to support cardiac output. Pacemakers can be used temporarily, either supportively or prophylactically, until the condition responsible for the rate or conduction disturbance resolves. Pacemakers also can be used on a permanent basis if the patient's condition persists despite adequate therapy. The use of temporary pacemakers as a diagnostic tool is gaining popularity.

This section emphasizes temporary pacemakers because the critical care nurse most often encounters them in critical care areas where the attending nurse is charged with the responsibility of preventing, assessing, and managing pacemaker malfunctions. References are made to permanent pacemakers where appropriate.

Indications

The clinical indications for instituting temporary pacemaker therapy are similar regardless of the cause of the rhythm disturbance that necessitates the placement of a pacemaker (see box). Such causes range from drug toxicities and electrolyte imbalances to sequelae related to acute myocardial infarction or cardiac surgery.

Dysrhythmias that are unresponsive to drug therapy and result in compromised hemodynamic status are a definite indication for pacemaker therapy. The goal of therapy in the case of bradydysrhythmia is to increase the ventricular rate and thus enhance cardiac output. Alternately, "overdrive" pacing can be used to decrease the rate of a rapid supraventricular or ventricular rhythm. This rapid pacing of the heart, or overdrive pacing, functions either to prevent the "breakthrough" ectopy that can result from a slow rate or "capture" an ectopic focus and allow the natural pacemaker to regain control.

After cardiac surgery, temporary pacing can be used to improve a transiently depressed, rate-dependent cardiac output. In addition, conduction disturbances that can occur after valvular surgery can be managed effectively with temporary pacing.

Several diagnostic uses for temporary pacing have evolved over the past several years. *Electrophysiology studies* (EPS) use special pacing electrodes to induce dysrhythmias in patients with recurrent symptomatic tachydysrhythmias. This allows the physician to closely evaluate the particular dysrhythmia and to determine appropriate therapy. For those patients whose tachydysrhythmia is found to be refractory to conventional antidysrhythmic therapy, *radiofrequency* (RF) *current catheter ablation* of the responsible tissue can be done safely and effectively in the electrophysiology laboratory. After a mapping procedure localizes the site of dysrhyth-

INDICATIONS FOR TEMPORARY PACING

Bradydysrhythmias
- Sinus bradycardia and arrest
- Sick sinus syndrome
- Heart blocks

Tachydysrhythmias
- Supraventricular
- Ventricular

Permanent pacemaker failure

Support cardiac output after cardiac surgery

Diagnostic studies
- Electrophysiology studies (EPS)
- Atrial electrograms (AEG)

mia formation, short bursts of radiofrequency current are delivered through the catheter, destroying the offending tissue with heat. Radiofrequency ablation appears more promising than its predecessor, direct current (DC) ablation, because it delivers a more precise localized ablation current that lowers the incidence of complications and does not require general anesthesia.[1-5]

The atrial electrogram (AEG) is simply an amplified recording of atrial activity that can be obtained through the use of atrial pacing wires and a standard electrocardiogram (ECG) machine. It often is used after cardiac surgery to facilitate the diagnosis of supraventricular dysrhythmias in patients with temporary atrial epicardial electrodes already in place.[6]

The Pacemaker System

A pacemaker system is a simple electrical circuit consisting of a pulse generator and a pacing lead (an insulated electrical wire) with either one or two electrodes.

◆ **Pacing pulse generator.** The pulse generator is designed to generate an electrical current that travels through the pacing lead and exits through an electrode (exposed portion of the wire) that is in direct contact with the heart. This electrical current initiates a myocardial depolarization. The current then seeks to return by one of several ways to the pulse generator to complete the circuit.

The power source for a temporary external pulse generator is the standard alkaline or mercury battery inserted into the generator. Implanted permanent pacemaker batteries are generally long-lived lithium cells.

◆ **Pacing lead systems.** The pacing lead used for temporary pacing may be bipolar or unipolar. In addition, leads are *transvenous* or *epicardial*. The bipolar lead used in transvenous pacing has two electrodes on one catheter (Fig. 17-1, D). The distal, or negative, electrode is at the tip of the pacing lead and is in direct contact with the heart, usually inside the right atrium or ventricle. Approximately 1 cm above the negative electrode is a positive electrode. The negative electrode is attached to the negative terminal, and the positive electrode is attached to the positive terminal of the pulse generator, either directly or via a bridging cable (Fig. 17-1). The epicardial lead system involves either one (unipolar) or

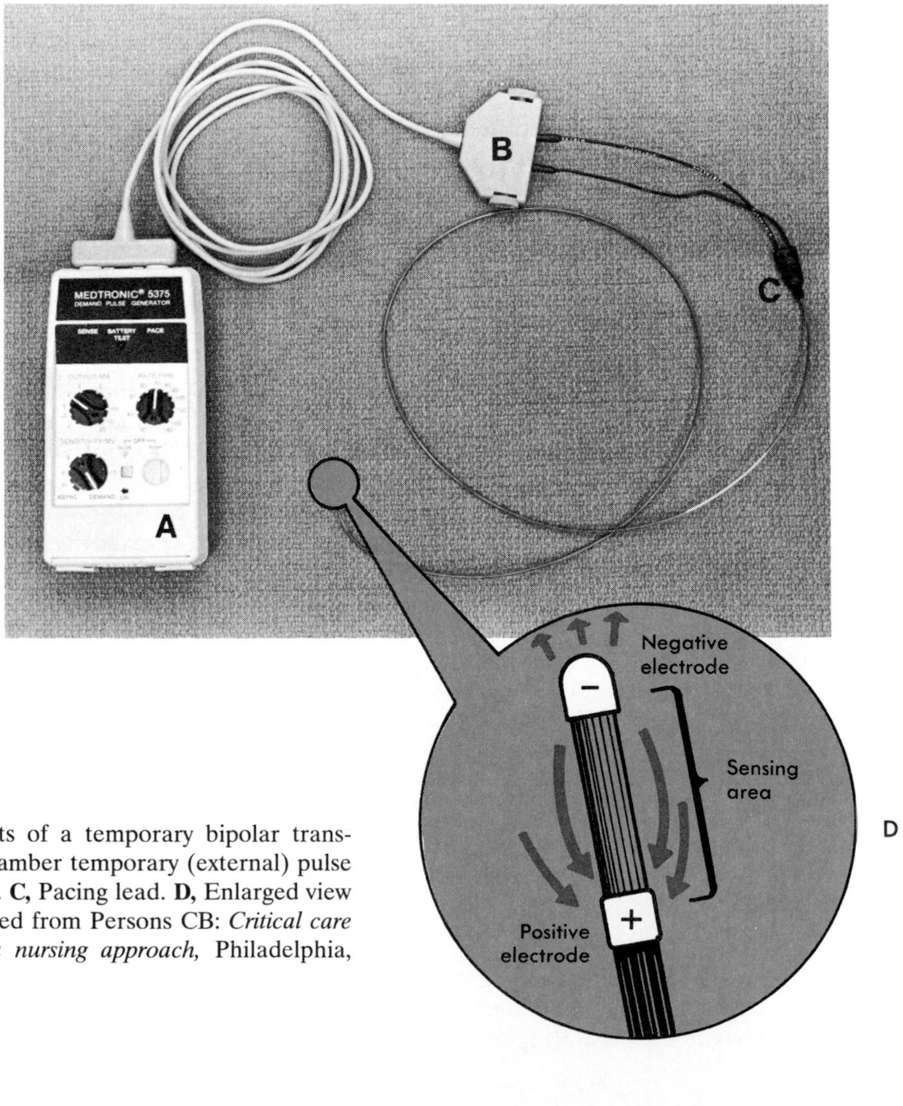

Fig. 17-1 The components of a temporary bipolar transvenous system. **A,** Single-chamber temporary (external) pulse generator **B,** Bridging cable. **C,** Pacing lead. **D,** Enlarged view of the components. (Modified from Persons CB: *Critical care procedures and protocols: a nursing approach,* Philadelphia, 1987, JB Lippincott.)

two (bipolar) pacing wires in direct contact with the heart. This method is frequently used for temporary pacing after cardiac surgery.

The bipolar epicardial lead system has two separate insulated wires (one negative and one positive electrode) loosely secured with sutures to the cardiac chamber to be paced and attached to the pulse generator as just described.

A unipolar pacing system (epicardial or transvenous) has only one electrode (a negative electrode) making contact with the heart. In the case of a permanent pacemaker, the positive electrode can be created by the metallic casing of the subcutaneously implanted pulse generator (Fig. 17-2). Or as is the case with a unipolar epicardial lead system, the positive electrode can be formed by a piece of surgical steel wire sewn into the subcutaneous tissue of the chest.

In both unipolar and bipolar systems the current flows from the negative terminal of the pulse generator down the pacing lead to the negative electrode and into the heart. The current is then picked up by the positive electrode and flows back up the lead to the positive terminal of the pulse generator.

There are advantages and disadvantages to both systems. Because the unipolar pacing system has a wide sensing area as a result of the relatively large distance between the negative and positive electrodes, it has better sensing capabilities than does a bipolar system. This feature, however, makes the unipolar system more susceptible to electromagnetic interference (EMI) or stray electrical impulses from the heart itself or from the critical care environment, such as intravenous infusion pumps that can adversely affect pacemaker function.

Pacing Routes

Several routes are available for temporary cardiac pacing (see box on right). Permanent pacing usually is accomplished transvenously, although in situations in which a thoracotomy is otherwise indicated, such as cardiac surgery, the physician may elect to insert permanent epicardial pacing wires.

Transcutaneous cardiac pacing is enjoying a revival of sorts, after having been abandoned many years ago because of the painful muscle contractions and soft tissue burns it caused. Transcutaneous cardiac pacing involves the use of two skin electrodes, one placed anteriorly and the other posteriorly on the chest, connected to an external pulse generator. It is a rapid, noninvasive procedure that nurses can perform in the emergency setting and has been gaining in popularity since improved technology has helped to minimize the problems associated with it.

Transthoracic pacing also is an emergency procedure that involves the insertion of a pacing wire into the ventricle through a needle inserted through the chest wall. This approach, however, is an invasive procedure associated with serious complications, such as pneumothorax and cardiac tamponade.

The insertion of temporary epicardial pacing wires has become a routine procedure during most cardiac surgical cases. Ventricular, and in many cases atrial, pacing wires are loosely sewn to the epicardium. The terminal pins of these wires are pulled through the skin before the chest is closed. If both chambers have pacing wires attached, the atrial wires exit subcostally to the right of the sternum and the ventricular wires exit in the same region but to the left of the sternum.[6] These wires can be

ROUTES FOR TEMPORARY PACING

Transcutaneous

Emergency pacing is achieved by depolarizing the heart through the chest by means of two large skin electrodes.

Transthoracic

A pacing wire is inserted emergently by threading it through a transthoracic needle into the right ventricle.

Epicardial

Pacing electrodes are sewn to the epicardium during cardiac surgery.

Transvenous (endocardial)

The pacing electrode is advanced through a vein into the right atrium, or right ventricle, or both.

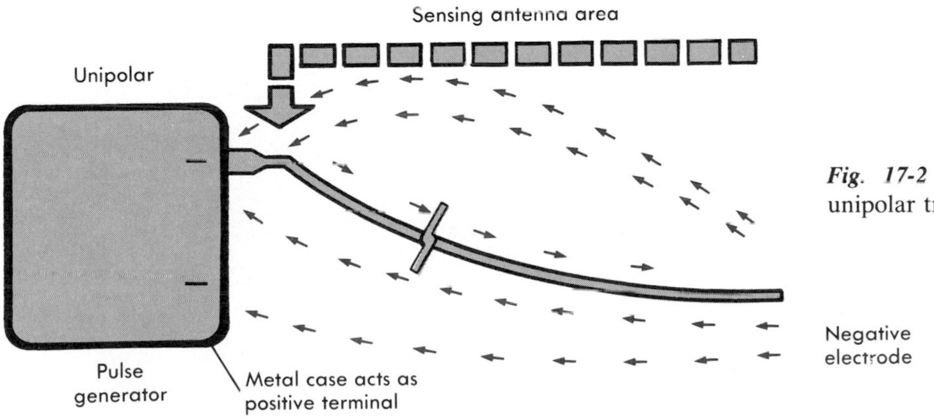

Fig. 17-2 The components of a permanent unipolar transvenous pacing system.

removed by gentle traction at the skin surface with minimal risk of bleeding.

Temporary transvenous endocardial pacing is accomplished by advancing a pacing electrode wire through a vein, often the subclavian or internal jugular, into the right atrium or right ventricle. Insertion can be facilitated either through direct visualization with fluoroscopy or by the use of the standard ECG.

Five-Letter Pacemaker Codes

In the 1960s, pacemaker terminology was limited to "fixed-rate" and "demand" pacing, followed by the introduction of "AV sequential" pacing in the early 1970s. Although these terms are still useful today for understanding pacemaker function (see box on right), the continued expansion of functional capabilities of pulse generators made it necessary to develop a more precise classification system. Therefore in 1974 the Inter-Society Commission for Heart Disease (ICHD) adopted a three-letter code for describing the various pacing modalities available. The code has since undergone several revisions, including the addition of two more letters representing programming characteristics and antitachycardia functions, to accommodate the development of newer devices that are rate-responsive or that combine pacing and shocking capabilities.[7] Based on the most recent revision of the ICHD code, a new generic pacemaker code was proposed and adopted for clinical use (see Table 17-1 for five-letter pacemaker code).[8] The original three-letter code, however, remains adequate to describe basic pacemaker function.

The original code is based on three categories, each represented by a letter. The first letter refers to the cardiac chamber that is paced. The second letter designates which chamber is sensed, and the third letter indicates the response to the sensed event. For example, a VVI pacemaker will pace the ventricle if the pacemaker fails to sense an intrinsic ventricular depolarization. Sensing of a spontaneous ventricular depolarization, however, inhibits ventricular pacing. On the other hand, a VAT pacemaker paces the ventricle at a fixed time after the sensing of a spontaneous atrial depolarization; that is, ventricular pacing is triggered by sensing of an atrial event. (See Table 17-2 for description of other three-letter pacemaker codes.)

PACEMAKER TERMINOLOGY

Fixed-rate (asynchronous)

Delivers a pacing stimulus at a set (fixed) rate regardless of the occurrence of spontaneous myocardial depolarizations.

Demand (synchronous)

Delivers a pacing stimulus only when the heart's intrinsic pacemaker fails to function at a predetermined rate; the pacing stimulus will be either inhibited or be triggered into the QRS complex when the intrinsic pacemaker functions.

Atrioventricular (AV) sequential (dual-chamber pacing)

Delivers a pacing stimulus to both the atrium and ventricle in proper sequence with sufficient AV delay to permit adequate ventricular filling.

Table 17-1 NASPE/BPEG generic (NBG) code

Position	I	II	III	IV	V
	Chamber(s) paced	Chamber(s) sensed	Response to sensing	Programmability	Antitachydysrhythmia function(s)
	0 = None	0 = None	0 = None	0 = None	0 = None
	A = Atrium	A = Atrium	T = Triggered	P = Simple programmability (rate, output, sensitivity)	P = Pacing (antitachydysrhythmia)
	V = Ventricle	V = Ventricle	I = Inhibited	M = Multiprogrammability	S = Shock
	D = Dual (A + V)	D = Dual (A + V)	D = Dual (T + I)	C = Communicating	D = Dual (P + S)
				R = Rate modulation (rate responsive)	
	S* = Single A or V)	S = Single (A or V)			

*Modified from Bernstein AD and others: The NASPE/BPEG generic pacemaker code for antibradycardia and adaptive rate pacing and antitachyarrhythmia devices, *PACE* 10:794, 1987.

*Used by manufacturer only.

NOTE: Positions I through III are used exclusively for antibradydysrhythmia function.

NASPE, North American Society of Pacing and Electrophysiology.

BPEG, British Pacing and Electrophysiology Group.

NBG, North American British Generic.

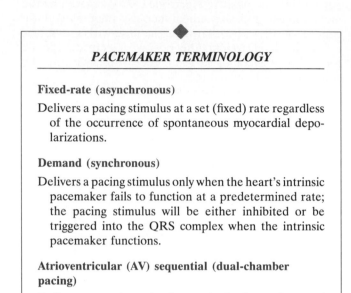

Table 17-2 Examples of three-letter pacemaker code

Pulse generator	Description
AOO	Atrial fixed rate Atrial pacing, no sensing
VOO	Ventricular fixed rate Ventricular pacing, no sensing
DOO	AV sequential fixed rate Atrial and ventricular pacing, no sensing
VVI	Ventricular demand Ventricular pacing, ventricular sensing, inhibited response to sensing
VVT	Ventricular demand Ventricular pacing, ventricular sensing, triggered response to sensing
AAI	Atrial demand Atrial pacing, atrial sensing, inhibited response to sensing
AAT	Atrial demand Atrial pacing, atrial sensing, triggered response to sensing
VAT	AV synchronous Ventricular pacing, atrial sensing, triggered response to sensing. The ventricular pacing stimulus will fire at a set time after sensing of a spontaneous atrial depolarization.
DVI	AV sequential Atrial and ventricular pacing, ventricular sensing, inhibited response to sensing. Both atrial and ventricular pacing are inhibited if spontaneous ventricular depolarization is sensed; if no spontaneous ventricular activity is sensed, then the atrium and ventricle will be paced sequentially.
VDD	Atrial synchronous, ventricular inhibited Ventricular pacing, atrial and ventricular sensing, inhibited response to sensing in the ventricle and triggered response to sensing in the atrium
DDD	Universal Both chambers are sensed and paced, inhibited response to sensing in the ventricle and triggered response to sensing in the atria

Pacemaker Settings

The controls on all external temporary pulse generators are similar, and their function should be thoroughly understood so that pacing can be initiated quickly in an emergency situation and troubleshooting can be facilitated should problems with the pacemaker arise.

The *rate control* (Fig. 17-3) regulates the number of impulses that can be delivered to the heart per minute. The rate setting depends on the physiologic needs of the patient, but in general it is maintained between 60 and 80 beats/min. Pacing rates for overdrive suppression of tachydysrhythmias may greatly exceed these values. If the pacemaker is operating in the atrioventricular (AV) sequential mode, the ventricular rate control also will regulate the atrial rate.

The *output dial* regulates the amount of electrical current (measured in milliamperes [mA]) that is delivered to the heart to initiate depolarization. The point at which depolarization occurs is termed *threshold* and is indicated by a myocardial response to the pacing stimulus (capture). Threshold can be determined by gradually decreasing the output from 5 mA until 1:1 capture is lost. The output setting is then slowly increased until 1:1 capture is reestablished; this threshold to pace should be less than 1.0 mA with a properly positioned pacing electrode. The output, however, should be set 2 to 3 times higher than threshold because thresholds tend to fluctuate. Separate output controls for both the atrium and the ventricle are used with an AV sequential pulse generator.

The *sensitivity control* regulates the ability of the pacemaker to detect the heart's intrinsic electrical activity. If the sensitivity is turned all the way up—that is, a setting of 1 mV (millivolts)—the pacemaker is maximally sensitive and can respond even to low-amplitude electrical signals coming from the heart. On the other hand, turning the sensitivity all the way down (adjusting the dial to a setting of 20 mV or to area labeled *async*) will result in the inability of the pacemaker to sense any intrinsic electrical activity and cause the pacemaker to function at a fixed rate. A sense indicator (often a light) on the pulse generator signals each time intrinsic cardiac electrical activity is sensed. A pulse generator may be designed to sense atrial or ventricular activity, or both. (See box, p. 318, for procedure for measuring sensitivity.) The sensitivity should be set 2 to 3 times higher than the measured sensitivity, usually at 3 mV. The pacemaker's sensing

A

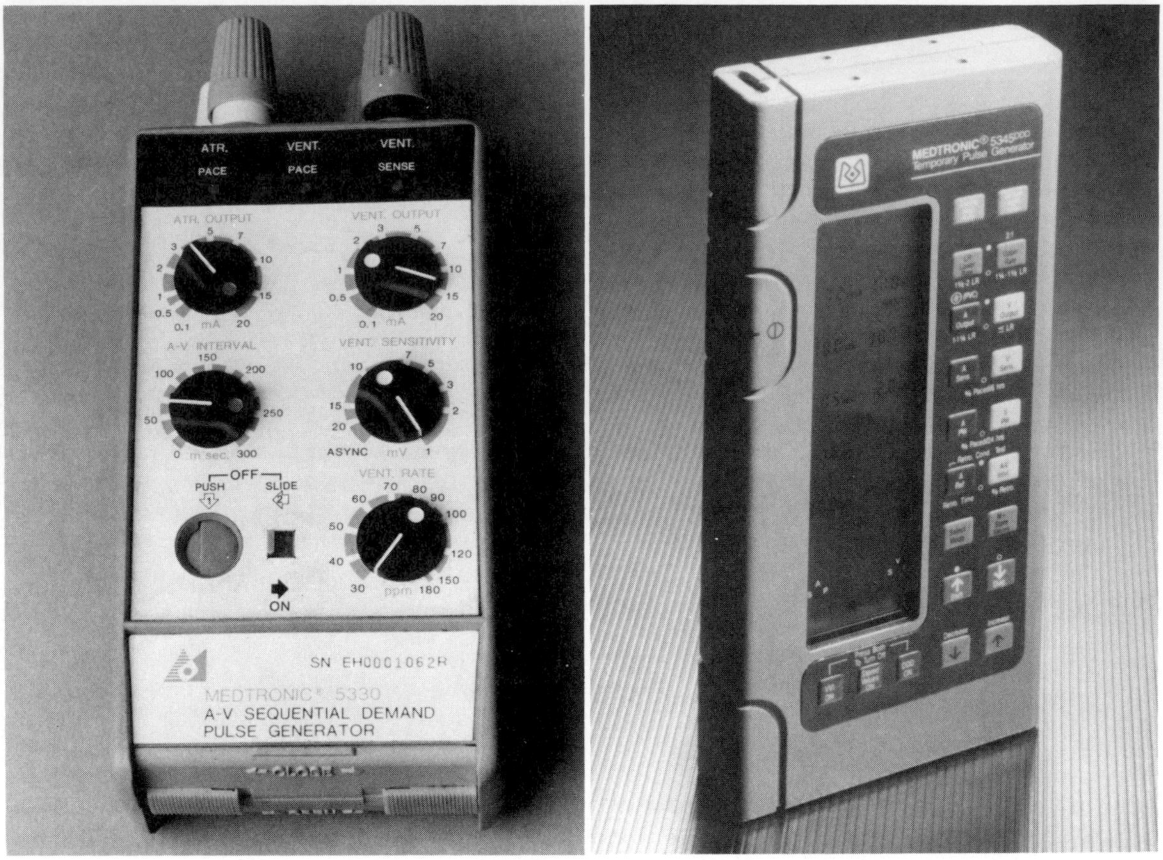

B

Fig. 17-3 Temporary dual-chamber pulse generators (external). (An example of a temporary single-chamber pulse generator is shown in Fig. 17-1.) **A,** AV sequential demand pulse generator. **B**, DDD pulse generator. (Courtesy Medtronic Inc., Minneapolis.)

TEMPORARY PACEMAKER SENSITIVITY SETTING

- Set sensitivity control between 1.5 and 3.0 mV.
- Adjust rate control to 10 beats/min below patient's intrinsic rate, and set the output dial at 5 mA. (The pacemaker should stop pacing and sensor lights begin flashing.)
- Gradually increase sensitivity until pacemaker begins to fire again. This is the sensitivity threshold.

ability can be quickly evaluated by observing for a change in pacing rhythm in response to spontaneous depolarizations.

The *AV interval* control (available only on AV sequential pacers) regulates the time interval between the atrial and ventricular pacing stimuli. Proper adjustment of this interval to between 150 to 250 msec preserves AV synchrony and permits maximal ventricular stroke volume and enhanced cardiac output.

The temporary DDD pacemakers have several other digital controls that are unique to this newer type of temporary pulse generator (Fig. 17-3, B). The lower-rate and higher-rate settings regulate the lowest and highest rate, respectively, at which the pacemaker can pace. The pulse width, which can be adjusted from 0.05 to 2.0 msec, controls the length of time that the pacing stimulus is delivered to the heart. There also is an atrial refractory period, programmable from 150 to 500 msec, which regulates the length of time after either a sensed or paced beat during which the pacemaker cannot respond to another stimulus.

Finally, an *on/off* switch is provided with a safety feature that prevents the accidental termination of pacing.

Pacing Artifacts

All patients with temporary pacemakers require continuous ECG monitoring. The pacing artifact is the spike that is seen on the ECG tracing as the pacing stimulus is delivered to the heart. A *P wave* should be visible after the pacing artifact if the atrium is being paced (Fig. 17-4, *A*). Similarly, a QRS complex should follow a ventricular pacing artifact (Fig. 17-4, *B*). With dual chamber pacing a pacing artifact precedes both the P wave and the QRS complex (Fig. 17-4, C).

Not all paced beats look alike. For example, the

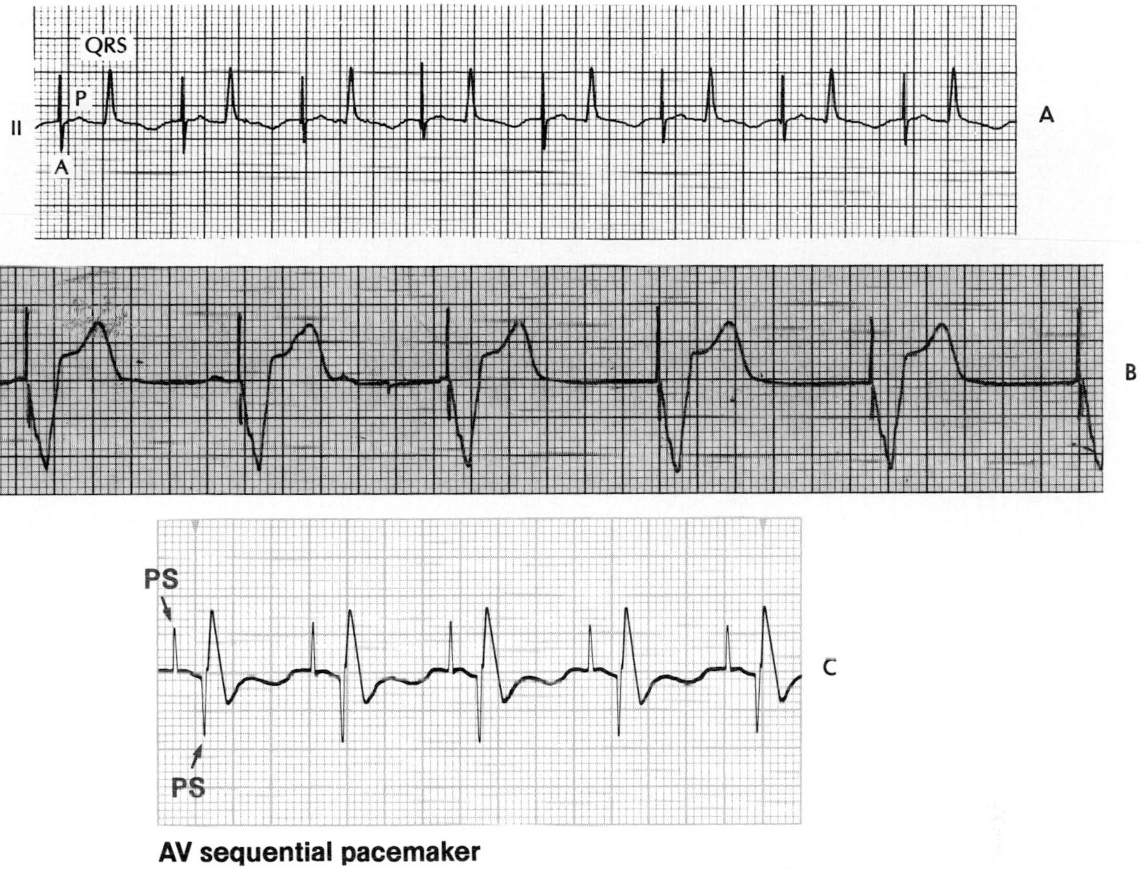

Fig. 17-4 **A,** Atrial pacing. **B,** Ventricular pacing. **C,** Dual chamber pacing. (**A** from Goldberger AL, Goldberger E: *Clinical electrocardiography: a simplified approach,* ed 4, St Louis, 1990, Mosby–Year Book. **B** from Conover MB: *Understanding electrocardiography: arrhythmias and the 12-lead ECG,* ed 6, St Louis, 1992, Mosby–Year Book; **C** from Huszar RJ: *Basic dysrhythmias: interpretation and management,* ed 2, St Louis, 1993, Mosby–Year Book.)

artifact produced by a unipolar pacing electrode is larger than that produced by a bipolar lead (Fig. 17-5). Furthermore, the QRS complex of paced beats will appear different, depending on the location of the pacing electrode. If the pacing electrode is positioned in the right ventricle, a left bundle branch block (LBBB) pattern will be displayed on the ECG. On the other hand, a right bundle branch block (RBBB) pattern will be visible if the pacing stimulus originates from the left ventricle.

Pacemaker Malfunctions

Most pacemaker malfunctions can be categorized as abnormalities of either pacing or sensing.

Problems with pacing can involve the failure of the pacemaker to deliver the following: the pacing stimulus, a pacing stimulus that depolarizes the heart, or the correct number of pacing stimuli per minute.

Failure of the pacemaker to deliver the pacing stimulus results in the disappearance of the pacing artifact, even though the patient's intrinsic rate is less than the set rate on the pacer (Fig. 17-6). This can occur either intermittently or continuously and can be attributed to failure of the pulse generator or its battery, a loose connection between the various components of the pacemaker system, broken lead wires, or stimulus inhibition as a result of EMI. Tightening connections, replacing the batteries or the pulse generator itself, or removing the source of EMI may restore pacemaker function.

If the pacing stimulus fires but fails to initiate a myocardial depolarization, a pacing artifact will be present but will not be followed by the expected P wave or QRS complex, depending on the chamber being paced (Fig. 17-7). This "loss of capture" most often can be attributed either to displacement of the pacing electrode or to an increase in threshold (electrical stimulus necessary to elicit a myocardial depolarization) as a result of drugs, metabolic disorders, electrolyte imbalances, and fibrosis or myocardial ischemia at the site of electrode placement. Repositioning the patient to the left side or increasing the output (milliamperes [mA]) may elicit capture.

Pacing also can occur at inappropriate rates. For

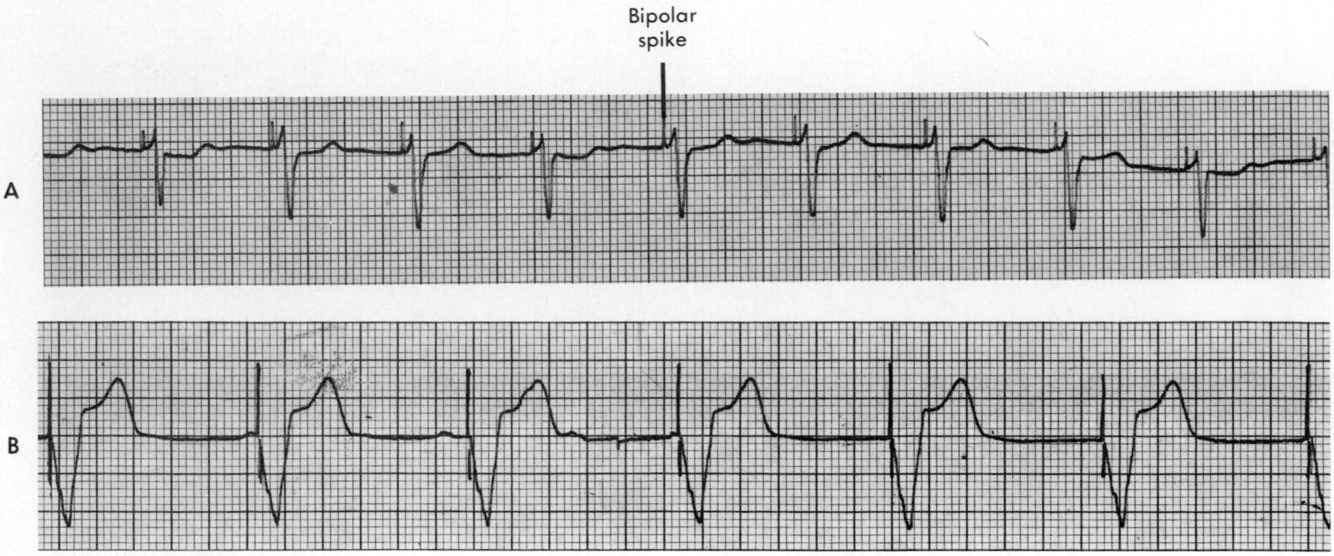

Fig. 17-5 **A,** Bipolar pacing artifact. **B,** Unipolar pacing artifact. (From Conover MB: *Understanding electrocardiography: arrhythmias and the 12-lead ECG,* ed 6, St Louis, 1992, Mosby–Year Book.)

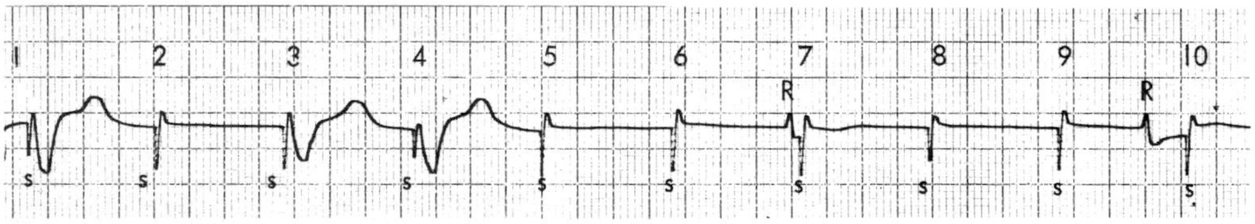

Fig. 17-6 Pacemaker malfunction: failure to pace. Notice that beats *1, 3,* and *4* show the pacemaker spikes *(s)* and normally paced QRS complexes and T waves. The remaining beats show only pacemaker spikes. *R* represents the patient's slow spontaneous QRS complexes. (From Goldberger E: *Treatment of cardiac emergencies,* ed 5, St Louis, 1990, Mosby–Year Book.)

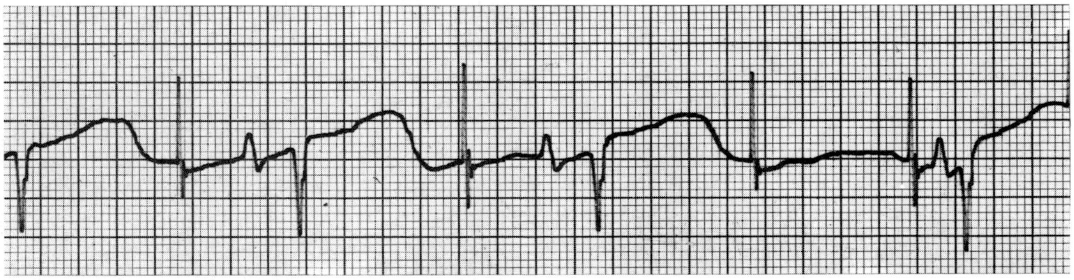

Fig. 17-7 Failure to capture. (From Conover MB: *Understanding electrocardiography: arrhythmias and the 12-lead ECG,* ed 6, St Louis, 1992, Mosby–Year Book.)

example, impending battery failure can result in a gradual decrease in paced rate or "rate drift." Another phenomenon, commonly referred to *runaway pacemaker,* will result in firing of the pacemaker stimulus at rates greater than the set rate. This malfunction, which is caused by failure of the pulse generator's circuitry, necessitates replacement.

Sensing abnormalities include both failure to sense and oversensing. Failure to sense is the inability of the pacemaker to sense spontaneous myocardial depolarizations. This results in competition between paced complexes and the heart's intrinsic rhythm. This malfunction can be demonstrated on the ECG by pacing artifacts that follow too closely behind spontaneous QRS

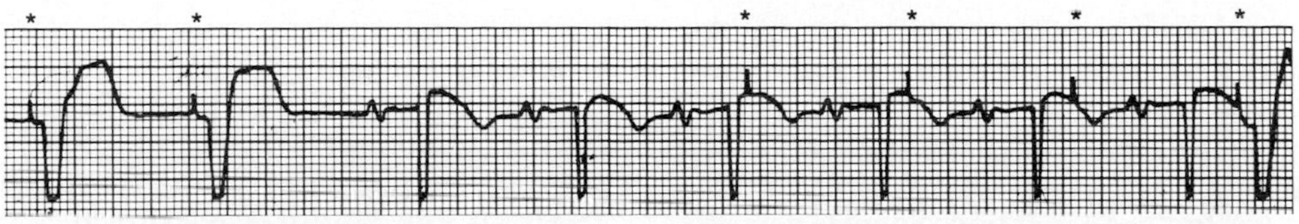

Fig. 17-8 Pacemaker malfunction: failure to sense. Notice that after the first two paced beats there is a series of sinus beats with first-degree AV block. Failure of the pacemaker unit to sense these intrinsic QRS complexes leads to inappropriate pacemaker spikes (*), which fall on T waves. Three of these spikes do not capture the ventricle because they occur during the refractory period of the cardiac cycle. (From Conover MB: *Understanding electrocardiography: arrhythmias and the 12-lead ECG,* ed 6, St Louis, 1992, Mosby–Year Book.)

complexes (Fig. 17-8). "R on T" phenomenon is a real danger with this type of pacer aberration; therefore the nurse must act quickly to determine the cause. Often the cause can be attributed to inadequate wave amplitude (or height of the P or R wave). If this is the case, the situation can be promptly remedied by increasing the sensitivity (moving the sensitivity dial toward its lowest setting). Other possible causes include lead displacement or fracture, pulse generator failure, or EMI-precipitated asynchronous pacing.

Oversensing results from the inappropriate sensing of extraneous electrical signals leading to unnecessary triggering or inhibiting of stimulus output, depending on the pacer mode. The source of these electrical signals can range from the presence of tall, peaked T waves to EMI in the critical care environment. Because most temporary pulse generators in use today are ventricular-inhibited, oversensing results in unexplained pauses in the ECG tracing as the extraneous signals are sensed and inhibit ventricular pacing. Often, simply moving the sensitivity dial toward 20 mV will stop the pauses.

Nursing Management

Myriad nursing responsibilities are associated with the care of a patient with a temporary pacemaker, but four major areas should be emphasized: surveillance for complications, protection against microshock, prevention of pacemaker malfunction, and patient teaching.

Infection at the lead insertion site is one complication associated with pacemakers. The site(s) should be carefully inspected for purulent drainage, erythema, or edema, and the patient should be observed for signs of systemic infection. Site care should be performed according to the institution's policy and procedure. Although most infections remain localized, endocarditis can occur in patients with endocardial pacing leads. A less frequent complication associated with transvenous pacing is myocardial perforation, which can result in rhythmic hiccoughs or cardiac tamponade.

Because the pacing electrode is in intimate contact with the heart, the nurse must take special care while handling the external components of the pacing system to avoid conducting stray electrical current from other equipment. Even a small amount of stray current could precipitate a lethal tachycardia. The possibility of "microshock" can be minimized by the wearing of rubber gloves when handling the pacing wires and by proper insulation of terminal pins of pacing wires when they are not in use. The latter can be accomplished either by using caps provided by the manufacturer or by improvising with a needle cover or section of disposable rubber glove. The wires should then be taped securely to the patient's chest to avoid accidental electrode displacement. Additional safety measures include using a nonelectric or a properly grounded electric bed, keeping all electrical equipment away from the bed, and permitting the use of only rechargeable electric razors.

Continuous ECG monitoring is essential to facilitate prompt recognition of and appropriate intervention for pacemaker malfunction; yet the nurse can do a great deal to prevent pacing abnormalities.

As mentioned, the temporary pacing lead and bridging cable should be properly secured to the body with tape to prevent the accidental displacement of the electrode, which can result in failure to pace or sense. The external pulse generator can be secured to the patient's waist with a strap or placed in a telemetry bag for the mobile patient. For the patient on a regimen of bed rest, the pulse generator can be suspended with twill tape from an intravenous (IV) pole mounted overhead on the ceiling, which not only will prevent tension on the lead while the

◆

NURSING DIAGNOSIS AND MANAGEMENT

Temporary pacemakers

- ◆ Decreased Cardiac Output related to atrioventricular heart block, p. 359
- ◆ High Risk for Infection risk factors: invasive monitoring devices, p. 366
- ◆ Knowledge Deficit: Position Restrictions related to lack of previous exposure to information, p. 72
- ◆ Body Image Disturbance related to functional dependence on life-sustaining technology, p. 95
- ◆ Self-Esteem Disturbance related to feelings of guilt about physical deterioration, p. 96
- ◆ Powerlessness related to health care environment or illness-related regimen, p. 98
- ◆ Anxiety related to threat to biologic, psychologic, and/or social integrity, p. 763

patient is moved (given adequate length of bridging cable) but also will alleviate the possibility of accidental dropping of the pulse generator.

It is important to be aware of all sources of EMI, which, within the critical care environment, could interfere with the pacemaker's function. Sources of EMI in the clinical area include electrocautery, defibrillation current, radiation therapy, magnetic resonance imaging devices, and transcutaneous electrical nerve stimulation (TENS) units. In most cases, if EMI is suspected of precipitating pacemaker malfunction, converting to the asynchronous mode (fixed-rate) will maintain pacing until the cause of the EMI can be removed. If the patient requires defibrillation, the pulse generator should be temporarily turned off during delivery of the shock to prevent possible damage to the pacemaker circuitry.

Finally, the nurse can inspect for loose connections between lead and pulse generator on a regular basis. In addition, replacement batteries and pulse generators should always be available on the unit. Although the battery has an anticipated life span of 1 month, it probably is sound practice to change the battery if the pacemaker has been operating continually for several days. The pulse generator should always be labeled with the date that the battery was replaced.

Patient teaching for the person with a temporary pacemaker emphasizes the same areas of prevention that the nurse normally would address. The patient is instructed not to handle any exposed portion of the lead wire and to notify the nurse should the dressing over the insertion site become soiled or dislodged. The patient also is advised not to use any electric devices brought in from home that could interfere with pacemaker functioning. Furthermore, patients with temporary transvenous pacemakers need to be taught to restrict movement of the affected extremity to prevent lead displacement.

Summary

The recent introduction of physiologic pacing (DDD), which is both rate-responsive (atrial sensing allows for increases in heart rate with exercise) and AV-synchronous, and the development of physiologic sensors that permit pacemaker autoregulation to maintain optimal physiologic function, demonstrates the complexities of present-day pacemaker technology.[9] Rate-responsive pacing capability is usually indicated by the addition of an "R" as a fourth letter, for example, DDDR. Table 17-3 describes the types of rate-responsive pacing generators currently in clinical use. The foregoing discussion has provided an introduction to the basic concepts of temporary pacemaker therapy. It is essential, however, that the nurse who cares for patients with either permanent or temporary pacemakers be intimately familiar with even the most sophisticated modes of pacemaker function. Only by keeping "pace" with current technology can the nurse accurately interpret pacer function and thereby safely and effectively care for these patients.

CARDIAC SURGERY

The nursing management of the patient undergoing cardiac surgery is demanding yet exciting work that requires the talents of an experienced team of critical care nurses. The following discussion introduces basic cardiac surgical techniques and principles of cardiopulmonary bypass and highlights the key points about postoperative care of the adult patient who requires either valve replacement or coronary revascularization.

Coronary Artery Bypass Surgery

Since its introduction more than 2 decades ago, coronary artery bypass surgery has been proved both safe and effective in relieving medically uncontrolled angina pectoris in most patients. With improved medical management of coronary artery disease (CAD), however, much debate has been generated regarding the efficacy of medical versus surgical therapy for CAD. The combined results of three major randomized trials continue to support the view that coronary artery bypass grafting (CABG) affords dramatic symptomatic improvement and an improved quality of life. CABG is more effective than medical therapy for improving survival in patients with left main or triple-vessel disease or with double-vessel disease involving the left anterior descending artery (LAD), as well as for relieving exercise-induced ischemia or chronic ischemia leading to left ventricular (LV) dysfunction. Medical therapy is recommended when ischemia is prevented by antianginal drugs that are well-tolerated by the patient.[10]

Table 17-3 Permanent pacemaker rate-responsive letter code

Pulse generator	Description
AAIR	AAI features plus rate-responsive pacing. It is used for patients with a symptomatic bradycardia with a paceable atrium and intact atrioventricular (AV) conduction.
VVIR	VVI features plus rate-responsive pacing. It is used for patients with an unpaceable atrium caused by chronic atrial fibrillation or other atrial dysrhythmia.
DDDR	DDD features plus rate-responsive pacing. It is used for patients with a symptomatic bradycardia in which the atrium is paceable but atrioventricular (AV) conduction is, or may become, unreliable.

Because these generators are rate responsive (R), they can increase (modulate) heart rate in response to a sensed physiologic variable, usually upper body movement.

Myocardial revascularization involves the use of a conduit or channel designed to bypass an occluded coronary artery. Currently, the two most successful conduits are the saphenous vein graft (SVG) and the internal mammary artery (IMA) graft. SVG involves the anastomosis of an excised portion of the saphenous vein proximal to the aorta and distal to the coronary artery below the obstruction (Fig. 17-9). The IMA, which usually remains attached to its origin at the subclavian artery, is swung down and anastomosed distal to the coronary artery (Fig. 17-10).

Both the right IMA (RIMA) and left IMA (LIMA) may be used as conduits. Of note, urgent coronary artery bypass surgery may preclude the use of the IMA in view of the extra time required to mobilize the artery, as well as the inability to effect cardioplegia through this conduit. Although only recently introduced, the IMA graft is gaining in popularity because it has demonstrated both short-term and long-term patency rates superior to those of the SVG.[11]

The right gastroepiploic artery recently has been introduced as an alternate conduit for CABG. Although

RESEARCH ABSTRACT

Effects of two types of head coverings in the rewarming of patients after coronary artery bypass graft (CABG) surgery.

Howell RD and others: *Heart Lung* 21(1):1, 1992.

PURPOSE

The purpose of this study was to examine the differences among the effects of two types of head covering (and no head covering) during the initial 8-hour postoperative phase after CABG surgery.

DESIGN

Experimental design

SAMPLE

The sample consisted of 81 subjects: group 1 (control group) had 28 subjects with no head covering; group 2 had 27 subjects with towel and disposable pad covering; and group 3 had 26 subjects with towel-only head covering. The mean age for all subjects was 61.2 years (group 1, 62.1; group 2, 58.6; group 3, 62.7). All subjects had undergone cardiopulmonary bypass (CPB)–induced hypothermia and general anesthesia during the CABG surgery and were receiving mechanical ventilation. Patients who had valvular surgical procedures and those who required more aggressive rewarming procedures were excluded from the study.

PROCEDURE

Subjects were randomly assigned to each of the three groups. An initial rectal temperature was taken within 5 minutes of the patient's arrival into the surgical intensive care unit (SICU), and the head covering (if any) was applied within 10 minutes after arrival. Bath blankets were placed on the patient within 20 minutes of arrival: one folded across the chest and two folded lengthwise across the abdomen and lower extremities. If the patient was assigned to one of the experimental groups, the head covering also was placed at this time. A second rectal temperature was taken 60 minutes after the initial measurement and every hour for a total of 8 consecutive hours. The room temperature was recorded hourly along with the rectal temperature. The blankets and head coverings (if any) were removed when the patient's temperature measured 98.4° F (36.9° C).

RESULTS

No statistically significant differences were found among the three groups in the mean length of time it took patients to reach normothermia and in the mean net temperature gain reached by patients. When the experimental groups (group 2 and group 3) were combined and compared with the control group (group 1), there were also no statistically significant differences. All subjects were recategorized into two groups: group A (50 subjects) had reached normothermia by the beginning of hour 5; and group B (31 subjects) took longer than 5 hours to reach normothermia. There were statistically significant differences ($p < .05$) between the two groups: group A was younger, the lowest induced operating room temperature was higher, and temperatures on SICU admission were warmer; in group B, durations of CPB were shorter.

DISCUSSION/IMPLICATIONS

Findings from this study indicate that no differences exist in rewarming of patients after CABG, either with the use of two types of head covering or with no head covering. Factors that prolong the hypothermic state, however—age, lowest induced operating room temperature, and length of CPB time—were identified. These factors will assist the critical care nurse to identify, on admission, patients at high risk for hypothermia related to CABG surgery. The study should be replicated with use of a larger sample; in addition, other physiologic variables that might affect the hypothermic state need to be examined. Further, other methods of rewarming should be examined so that the most appropriate interventions can be adopted.

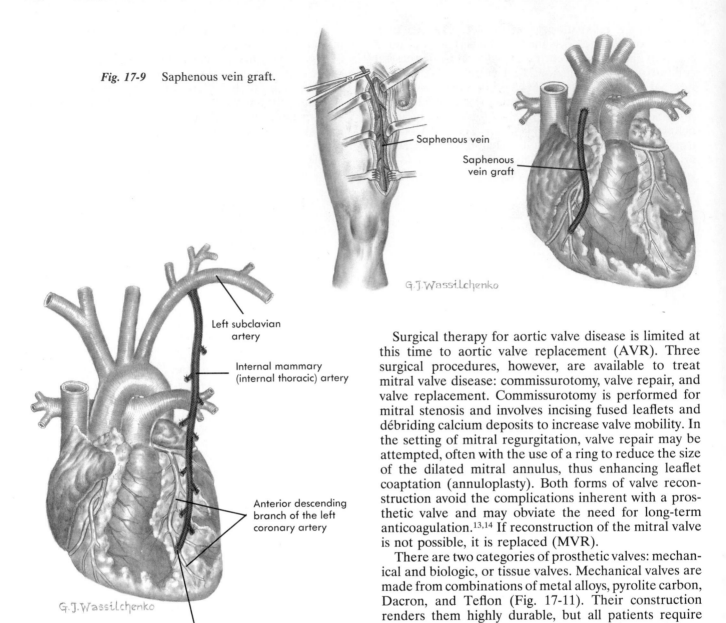

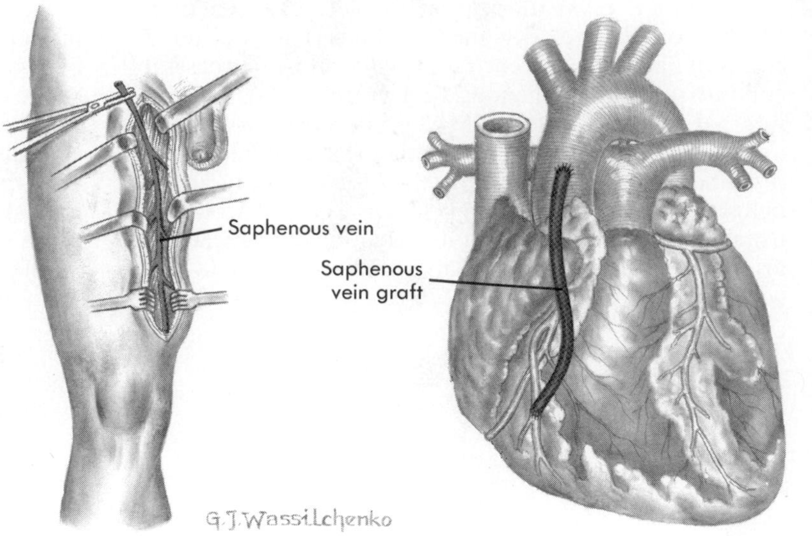

Fig. 17-9 Saphenous vein graft.

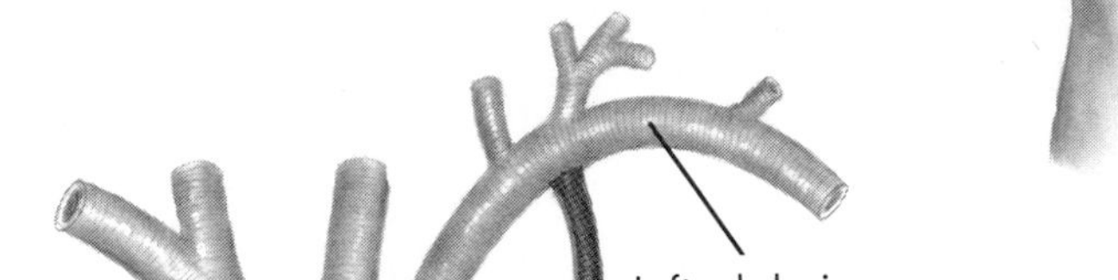

Fig. 17-10 Internal mammary artery graft.

it is a little smaller in diameter than the IMA, patency rates in the short-term follow-up available have been excellent.[12]

Valvular Surgery

Valvular disease results in various hemodynamic dysfunctions that usually can be managed medically so long as the patient remains symptom-free. There is reluctance to intervene surgically early in the course of the disease because of the surgical risks and long-term complications associated with prosthetic valve replacement. This consequence, however, must be weighed against the possibility of irreversible deterioration in left ventricular function that may develop during the compensated asymptomatic phase.

Surgical therapy for aortic valve disease is limited at this time to aortic valve replacement (AVR). Three surgical procedures, however, are available to treat mitral valve disease: commissurotomy, valve repair, and valve replacement. Commissurotomy is performed for mitral stenosis and involves incising fused leaflets and débriding calcium deposits to increase valve mobility. In the setting of mitral regurgitation, valve repair may be attempted, often with the use of a ring to reduce the size of the dilated mitral annulus, thus enhancing leaflet coaptation (annuloplasty). Both forms of valve reconstruction avoid the complications inherent with a prosthetic valve and may obviate the need for long-term anticoagulation.[13,14] If reconstruction of the mitral valve is not possible, it is replaced (MVR).

There are two categories of prosthetic valves: mechanical and biologic, or tissue valves. Mechanical valves are made from combinations of metal alloys, pyrolite carbon, Dacron, and Teflon (Fig. 17-11). Their construction renders them highly durable, but all patients require anticoagulation to reduce the incidence of thromboembolism. As a result of their low thrombogenicity, the biologic or tissue valves, usually constructed from animal or human cardiac tissue, offer the patient freedom from therapeutic anticoagulation. Their durability, however, is limited by their tendency toward early calcification. (See box, p. 325, for a description of various valvular prostheses.)

The choice of a valvular prosthesis depends on many factors. Because mechanical valves are more durable, for example, they may be chosen over a tissue valve for a young person who has a relatively long life span ahead. Similarly, a bioprosthesis (tissue valve) may be chosen for an older patient (older than 65 years of age); even though the valve has a reduced longevity, the patient has a decreased life expectancy. For patients with medical contraindications to anticoagulation or for patients whose past compliance with drug therapy has been questionable, a tissue valve should be selected. Technical considerations, such as the size of the annulus (or

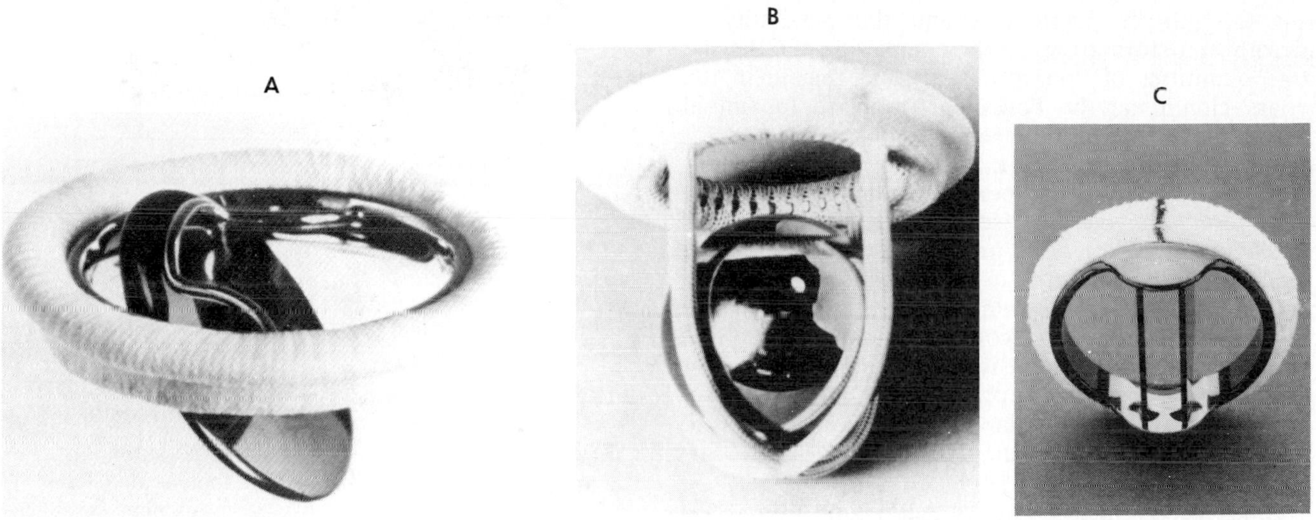

Fig. 17-11 **A,** The Bjork-Shiley tilting disk valve with pyrolytic carbon disk, stellite cage, and Teflon cloth sewing ring. The valve opens to 60 degrees. **B,** Starr-Edwards caged-ball valve model 6320 with completely cloth-covered stellite cage and hollow stellite ball, with specific gravity close to that of blood. **C,** The St. Jude Medical® mechanical heart valve, a mechanical central flow disk. (**A** and **B** from Eagle K and others: *The practice of cardiology,* ed 2, Boston, 1989, Little, Brown & Co; **C** courtesy St. Jude Medical, Inc, Copyright 1993, St Paul, Minn.)

anatomic ring in which the valve sits), also can influence the choice of valve (a bioprosthesis may be too big for a small aortic root).

Cardiopulmonary Bypass

Cardiopulmonary bypass (CPB) is a mechanical means of circulating and oxygenating a patient's blood while diverting most of the circulation from the heart and lungs during cardiac surgical procedures. The extracorporeal circuit consists of cannulas that drain off venous blood, an oxygenator that oxygenates the blood by one of several methods, and a pump head that pumps the arterialized blood back to the aorta through a single cannula. The patient is systemically heparinized before initiation of bypass to prevent clotting within the bypass circuit.

Systemic hypothermia during bypass can reduce tissue oxygen requirements to 50% of normal, which affords the major organs additional protection from ischemic injury. Lowering the body temperature to about 28° C (82.4° F) is accomplished through a heat exchanger incorporated into the pump. The blood is warmed back up to normal body temperature before bypass is discontinued.

The technique of hemodilution also is used to enhance tissue oxygenation by improving blood flow through the systemic and pulmonary microcirculation during bypass. Hemodilution refers to the dilution of autologous (patient's own) blood with the isotonic crystalloid solution used to prime the pump. Capillary perfusion is enhanced by hemodilution, because the reduced viscosity (stickiness) of the blood decreases both resistance to

---

CLASSIFICATION OF PROSTHETIC CARDIAC VALVES

MECHANICAL VALVES

Tilting-disk: a free-floating, lens-shaped disk mounted onto a circular sewing ring
- Bjork-Shiley
- Omniscience (Lillehei-Kaster)
- Medtronic-Hall (Hall-Kaster)

Caged-ball: a ball moves freely within a three- or four-sided metallic cage mounted on a circular sewing ring
- Starr-Edwards

Bileaflet: two semicircular leaflets, mounted on a circular sewing ring, that open centrally
- St. Jude Medical

BIOLOGIC TISSUE VALVES (BIOPROSTHESES)

Porcine heterograft: a porcine aortic valve mounted on a semiflexible stent and preserved with glutaraldehyde
- Hancock
- Carpentier-Edwards

Bovine pericardial heterograft: bovine pericardium fashioned into three identical cusps that are then mounted on a cloth-covered frame
- Ionescu-Shiley

Homograft: a human heart valve (aortic or pulmonic) harvested from a donated heart and cryopreserved; may or may not be mounted on a support ring

flow through the capillaries and the possibility of microthrombi formation. At the completion of CPB, the large quantities of "pump blood" that remain in the bypass circuit can be collected and used for initial postoperative volume replacement.

In response to findings that the low cardiac output syndrome often seen postoperatively might be a result of intraoperative myocardial ischemia or necrosis, efforts have been directed toward providing additional protection to the myocardium during bypass. At present, rapidly stopping the heart in diastole by perfusing the coronary arteries with a cold potassium cardioplegic ("heart-paralyzing") agent is the vehicle of choice for intraoperative myocardial protection. Cardioplegic solution is reinfused at regular intervals during bypass to keep the heart cold and still, which minimizes myocardial oxygen requirements.

Numerous clinical sequelae can result from CPB (Table 17-4). Knowledge of these physiologic effects allows the nurse to anticipate problems and intervene appropriately.

Table 17-4 Physiologic effects of cardiopulmonary bypass (CPB)

Effects	Causes
Intravascular fluid deficit (hypotension)	Third spacing Postoperative diuresis Sudden vasodilation (drugs, rewarming)
Third spacing (weight gain, edema)	Decreased plasma protein concentration Increased capillary permeability
Myocardial depression (decreased cardiac output)	Hypothermia Increased systemic vascular resistance Prolonged CPB pump run Preexisting heart disease Inadequate myocardial protection
Coagulopathy (bleeding)	Systemic heparinization Mechanical trauma to platelets Depressed release of clotting factors from liver as a result of hypothermia
Pulmonary dysfunction (decreased lung mechanics and impaired gas exchange)	Decreased surfactant production Pulmonary microemboli Interstitial fluid accumulation in lungs
Hemolysis (hemoglobinuria)	Red blood cells damaged in pump circuit
Hyperglycemia (rise in serum glucose)	Decreased insulin release Stimulation of glycogenolysis
Hypokalemia (low serum potassium) and Hypomagnesemia (low serum magnesium)	Intracellular shifts during bypass Postoperative diuresis secondary to hemodilution
Neurologic dysfunction (decreased level of consciousness, motor/sensory deficits)	Inadequate cerebral perfusion Microemboli to brain (air, plaque fragments, fat globules)
Hypertension (transient rise in blood pressure)	Catecholamine release and systemic hypothermia causing vasoconstriction

Postoperative Management

◆ **Cardiovascular support.** Postoperative cardiovascular support often is indicated because of a low output state resulting from preexisting heart disease, prolonged CPB pump run, and/or inadequate myocardial protection. Cardiac output can be maximized by adjustments in cardiac rate, preload, afterload, and contractility.

In the presence of low cardiac output, the heart rate can be appropriately regulated by means of temporary pacing or drug therapy. Temporary epicardial pacing usually is instituted when the heart rate of the adult patient who has had cardiac surgery drops below 80 beats/min. In the case of tachycardia, intravenous verapamil has proved quite effective when used to slow supraventricular rhythms with a ventricular response that exceed 110 beats/min. Because ventricular ectopy can result from hypokalemia, serum potassium levels are maintained in the high normal range (4.5 to 5.0 mEq/L) to provide some margin for error.

In most patients, reduced preload is the cause of low postoperative cardiac output. If a left atrial line has been inserted during surgery, monitoring left atrial pressure (LAP) can provide a more convenient and accurate guide to left ventricular preload than can the monitoring of the pulmonary capillary wedge pressure (PAWP). To enhance preload, volume usually is administered in the form of colloid or packed red cells. It is not uncommon to achieve greatest hemodynamic stability in these patients when filling pressures (LAP or PAWP) are in the range of 18 to 20 mm Hg (normally 5 to 12 mm Hg).

Partly as a result of the peripheral vasoconstrictive effects of hypothermia, many patients who have had cardiac surgery demonstrate postoperative hypertension. Although transient, postoperative hypertension can precipitate or exacerbate bleeding from the mediastinal chest tubes. In addition, the high systemic vascular resistance (afterload) resulting from the intense vasoconstriction can cause deterioration of cardiac performance. Therefore vasodilator therapy with intra-

NURSING DIAGNOSIS AND MANAGEMENT
Status post open heart surgery

- ◆ Decreased Cardiac Output related to hemopericardium secondary to open heart surgery, p. 360
- ◆ Decreased Cardiac Output related to supraventricular tachycardia, p. 358
- ◆ Decreased Cardiac Output related to atrioventricular heart block, p. 359
- ◆ Decreased Cardiac Output related to ventricular tachycardia, p. 362
- ◆ Decreased Cardiac Output related to decreased preload secondary to mechanical ventilation with or without PEEP, p. 359
- ◆ Decreased Cardiac Output related to relative excess of preload and afterload secondary to impaired ventricular contractility, p. 358
- ◆ Fluid Volume Deficit related to active blood loss, p. 639
- ◆ High Risk for Altered Peripheral Tissue Perfusion risk factor: high-dose vasopressor therapy, p. 363
- ◆ High Risk for Aspiration risk factors: impaired laryngeal sensation or reflex; impaired laryngeal closure or elevation; decreased lower esophageal sphincter pressure, p. 472
- ◆ Ineffective Airway Clearance related to impaired cough secondary to artificial airway, p. 466
- ◆ Ineffective Airway Clearance related to abdominal or thoracic pain, p. 466
- ◆ Ineffective Breathing Pattern related to abdominal or thoracic pain, p. 469
- ◆ Acute Pain related to transmission and perception of cutaneous, visceral, muscular, or ischemic impulses secondary to leg and/or sternotomy incision, p. 566
- ◆ High Risk for Infection risk factor: invasive monitoring devices, p. 366
- ◆ Activity Intolerance related to postural hypotension secondary to immobility, narcotics, vasodilator therapy, p. 365
- ◆ Sensory/Perceptual Alterations related to sensory overload, sensory deprivation, sleep pattern disturbance, p. 573
- ◆ Sleep Pattern Disturbance related to circadian desynchronization, p. 143
- ◆ Knowledge Deficit: Postoperative Exercise Regimen, Fluid Restrictions, Medication, Wound Care, Reportable Symptoms related to lack of previous exposure to information, p. 72
- ◆ Body Image Disturbance related to actual change in body structure, function, and appearance, p. 94
- ◆ Altered Sexuality Patterns related to fear of death during coitus secondary to myocardial infarction, p. 120

venous nitroprusside often is used to reduce afterload that will control hypertension and improve cardiac output.

If these adjustments in heart rate, preload, and afterload fail to produce significant improvement in cardiac output, contractility can be enhanced with positive inotropic support or intraaortic balloon pumping, thus augmenting circulation.

Nursing management. Hypothermia can contribute to depressed myocardial contractility in the patient who has had cardiac surgery. To prevent subsequent excessive temperature elevations while hyperthermia blankets are used to warm the patient, care should be taken to remove the blankets promptly when the temperature reaches 98.4° F (36.9° C).

◆ **Control of bleeding.** Postoperative bleeding from the mediastinal chest tubes can be caused by inadequate hemostasis, disruption of suture lines, or coagulopathy associated with CPB. Bleeding is more likely to occur with IMA grafts as a result of the extensive chest wall dissection required to free the IMA. If bleeding in excess of 150 ml/hr occurs early in the postoperative period, clotting factors (fresh-frozen plasma and platelets) and additional protamine (used to reverse the effects of heparin) may be administered along with prompt blood replacement. Recently, autotransfusion devices, which facilitate the collection and reinfusion of shed mediastinal blood, have become widely available.[15]

The use of prophylactic positive end-expiratory pressure (PEEP) in conjunction with mechanical ventilation may be helpful in controlling bleeding in some cases by increasing intrathoracic pressure enough to effect tamponade of oozing mediastinal blood vessels. Rewarming the patient will reverse the depressed manufacture and release of clotting factors that result from hypothermia. Persistent mediastinal bleeding, however—usually in excess of 500 ml in 1 hour or 400 ml/hr for 2 consecutive hours, despite normalization of clotting studies—is an indication for reexploration of the surgical site.

Nursing management. Chest tube stripping, to maintain patency of the tubes, is controversial because the high negative pressure generated by routine methods of stripping. It is believed to result in tissue damage that can contribute to bleeding. This risk, however, must be carefully weighed against the very real danger of cardiac tamponade if blood is not effectively drained from around the heart. Therefore chest tube stripping frequently is advocated in instances of postoperative bleeding. The technique of milking the chest tubes, however, may be advisable for routine postoperative care because this technique generates less negative pressure and decreases the risk of bleeding.

◆ **Pulmonary care.** Overnight intubation to facilitate lung expansion and to optimize gas exchange is common in patients who have had cardiac surgery. This is particularly advantageous for patients with IMA bypass, who tend to be more prone to postoperative pulmonary complications, such as atelectasis and pleural effusions, because the pleural space is entered during surgery. IMA bypass surgery also is associated with more postoperative pain than is SVG surgery. This postoperative chest pain can lead to shallow breathing, which if not corrected will aggravate atelectasis. Some patients who have underlying pulmonary disease related to long-term valvular dysfunction may require longer periods of mechanical ventilation. However, successful weaning from the ventilator within 4 to 12 hours after surgery is the usual occurrence.

◆ **Neurologic complications.** The transient neurologic dysfunction often seen in patients who have had cardiac surgery probably can be attributed to decreased cerebral perfusion and to cerebral microemboli, both related to the CPB pump run. Compounding these are environmental factors, such as sensory deprivation and sensory overload associated with being in a critical care unit. The term *postcardiotomy psychosis* has been used to describe this postoperative syndrome that initially may be seen as only a mild impairment of orientation but that may progress to agitation, hallucinations, and paranoid delusions.

Nursing management. Patients and family members need to be reassured that postcardiotomy psychosis is a temporary phenomenon that will resolve quickly. Meanwhile, every effort should be made to keep the patient informed of all that is going on in the surroundings so that unfamiliar sights, sounds, and smells are not overwhelming and confusing. Painful stimuli should be kept to a minimum, and meaningful stimuli, such as touching, should be encouraged. Nursing management should be organized to maximize optimal sleep patterns.

◆ **Infection.** Postoperative fever is fairly common after CPB. However, persistent temperature elevation above 101° F (37.8° C) should be investigated. Sternal wound infections and infective endocarditis are the most devastating infectious complications, but leg wound infection, pneumonia, and urinary tract infection also can occur.[16]

◆ **Renal involvement.** Hemolysis caused by trauma to the red blood cells in the extracorporeal circuit results in hemoglobinuria, which can damage renal tubules. Therefore small amounts of furosemide (Lasix) usually are given to promote urine flow if the urine output is low (less than 25 to 30 ml/hr) and "pink-tinged."

With advances in postoperative management, the average hospital stay is now 5 to 7 days after uncomplicated cardiac surgery.

Recent Advances

◆ **Surgical treatment of cardiac dysrhythmias.** In addition to intractable supraventricular tachydysrhythmias, malignant ventricular dysrhythmias, the major culprit in sudden cardiac death, can now be managed surgically when drug therapy has been unsuccessful or has produced intolerable side effects. Electrophysiologic testing and catheter mapping, are done before any decisions regarding surgical intervention. If catheter ablation of the dysrhythmia is not feasible or has proved ineffective, plans for surgical ablation can proceed.[17]

The origin of the dysrhythmia first is localized with specialized pacing electrodes during an open chest procedure (referred to as *intraoperative mapping*). The offending area of myocardium is then either excised or eliminated by cryosurgery (freezing) or laser.[17]

Coronary endarterectomy is having a modest revival as an adjunct to bypass procedures in patients with diffuse or small vessel disease. Laser technology has paved the way for investigation into intraoperative coronary laser recanalization.[18] The introduction of heart transplantation has generated much excitement and anticipation for patients who suffer from otherwise untreatable heart disease.

Although future trends in the surgical management of cardiac disease are difficult to predict, the critical care nurse must continue to be prepared to meet the challenge of providing a high level of nursing care at the bedside. A solid knowledge base and keen assessment skills are prerequisite for the accurate anticipation of problems and prompt intervention necessary to stabilize the patient and prevent the occurrence of life-threatening complications.

IMPLANTABLE CARDIOVERTER DEFIBRILLATOR

If a ventricular tachyrhythmia is not amenable to surgical ablation or to antidysrhythmic drugs, an implantable cardioverter defibrillator (ICD) may be inserted. The ICD is capable of identifying and terminating life-threatening ventricular dysrhythmias. The ICD system contains sensing electrodes to recognize the dysrhythmia, as well as defibrillation electrodes or patches that are in contact with the heart and can deliver a "shock."[19,20] These electrodes are connected to a generator that is surgically placed in the subcutaneous tissue in the upper left abdominal quadrant. (Fig. 17-12) The early-model generators could defibrillate or cardiovert only lethal dysrhythmias. Recent improvements in ICD treatment include the use of "tiered" therapy generators that incorporate antitachycardia pacing, bradycardia back-up pacing, low-energy cardioversion, and high-energy defibrillation options. With tiered therapy, antitachycardia pacing is used as the first line of treatment in some cases of ventricular tachycardia (VT). If the VT can be pace-terminated successfully, the patient will not receive a "shock" from the generator and may not even realize that the ICD terminated the dysrhythmia. If programmed bursts of pacing do not terminate the VT, the ICD will "cardiovert" the rhythm. If the dysrhythmia deteriorates into ventricular fibrillation (VF), the ICD is programmed to defibrillate at a higher energy. If the dysrhythmia terminates spontaneously, the device will not discharge.[21] (Fig. 17-12, C) Occasionally, the electrical rhythm may deteriorate to asystole or a slow idioventricular rhythm. In such cases the bradycardia back-up pacing function is activated.

The ICD has progressed not only in the area of programmable functions, but also in the insertion design. Initially, all ICDs were implanted surgically either during open heart surgery, with electrode patches sewn directly

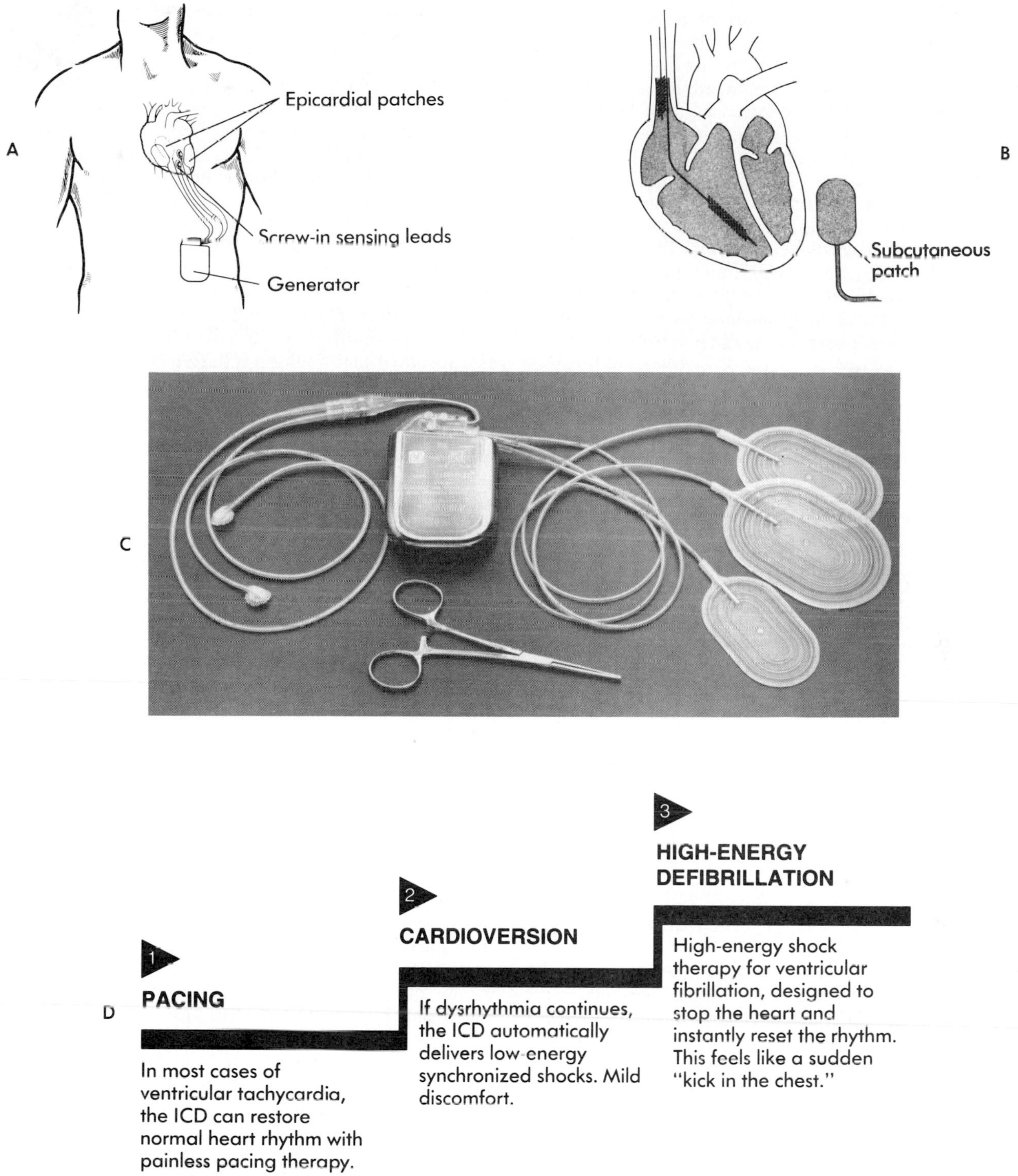

A
Epicardial patches
Screw-in sensing leads
Generator
B
Subcutaneous patch
C
D
1
PACING
In most cases of ventricular tachycardia, the ICD can restore normal heart rhythm with painless pacing therapy.
2
CARDIOVERSION
If dysrhythmia continues, the ICD automatically delivers low-energy synchronized shocks. Mild discomfort.
3
HIGH-ENERGY DEFIBRILLATION
High-energy shock therapy for ventricular fibrillation, designed to stop the heart and instantly reset the rhythm. This feels like a sudden "kick in the chest."

Fig. 17-12 **A,** Placement of an implantable cardioverter defibrillator (ICD) and epicardial lead system. The generator is placed in a subcutaneous "pocket" in the left upper abdominal quadrant. The epicardial screw-in sensing leads monitor the heart rhythm and connect to the generator. If a life-threatening dysrhythmia is sensed, the generator can pace-terminate the dysrhythmia or deliver electrical cardioversion or defibrillation through the epicardial patches. With this system, the leads/patches must be placed during open-chest (sternal or thoracotomy) surgery. **B,** In the transvenous lead system, open-chest surgery is not required. The pacing/cardioversion/defibrillation functions are all contained in a lead (or leads) inserted into the right atrium and ventricle. A subcutaneous patch may be placed under the skin. **C,** An example of an ICD tiered therapy generator (Medtronic PCD) with epicardial screw-in sensing leads and patches. **D,** Tiered therapy is designed to use increasing levels of intensity to terminate ventricular dysrhythmias. (Courtesy Medtronic Inc., Minneapolis.)

onto the epicardium or by means of a thoracotomy incision, with the patches attached to the outside of the pericardium. Currently, several new devices are being tested clinically that obviate the need for a thoracic surgical intervention. Transvenous electrode leads are inserted into the subclavian vein and advanced into the right side of the heart where contact with the heart endocardium is achieved. To improve defibrillation efficacy, an additional subcutaneous patch may be placed with some models. The endocardial leads are used for sensing, pacing, and cardioversion/defibrillation. They are connected to the generator by tunneling through the subcutaneous tissue; thus surgery is avoided. The advantage of using the endocardial lead system approach is that it is less invasive, less costly, and less traumatic for the patient and family.

Nursing Management

If the ICD system was implanted during open heart surgery, the postoperative care is similar to that for any patient undergoing cardiac surgery. If an endocardial lead system is implanted, the nursing management is less intense and hospital stay is shorter. In the case of a ventricular dysrhythmia, it is important to know the type of ICD implanted, how the device functions, and whether it is activated (i.e., *on*). Complications associated with the ICD include infection of the implanted system, broken leads, and the sensing of supraventricular tachydysrhythmias resulting in unneeded discharges.[21,22] To facilitate a positive psychologic adjustment to the ICD, education of the patient and family about the device is vital. Many centers also have successfully used family support groups for this patient population.

NURSING DIAGNOSIS AND MANAGEMENT
Implantable cardioverter defibrillator

- Decreased Cardiac Output related to ventricular tachycardia, p. 362
- Acute Pain related to transmission and perception of cutaneous, visceral, or ischemic impulses secondary to surgical incision(s) and ICD generator discharge, p. 566
- Knowledge Deficit: Preimplant and Postimplant Teaching, What ICD Does, and What Generator "Shock" Feels Like related to no previous exposure, p. 72
- Body Image Disturbance related to actual change in body structure and appearance secondary to implant of ICD generator and lead system, p. 94
- Altered Health Maintenance related to lack of perceived threat to health, p. 70
- Altered Sexuality Patterns related to fear of death during coitus secondary to myocardial infarction, p. 120
- If ICD was implanted during open heart surgery, see the Nursing Diagnosis and Management box on p. 327 for specific post–open heart surgery information.

CATHETER INTERVENTIONS FOR CORONARY ARTERY DESEASE

Percutaneous Transluminal Coronary Angioplasty

Percutaneous transluminal coronary angioplasty (PTCA) involves the use of a balloon-tipped catheter that, when advanced through an atherosclerotic coronary lesion (atheroma), can be inflated intermittently for the purpose of dilating the stenotic area and improving blood flow through it (Fig. 17-13). The mechanism of dilation originally was thought to be plaque compression that resulted in the immediate expression of plaque contents or its redistribution within the vessel wall. It is now believed, however, that the stretching of the vessel wall as a result of high balloon inflation pressures results in fracture of the plaque, which enlarges the vessel lumen.[23] PTCA provides an alternative to both traditional medical management of atherosclerotic heart disease and coronary artery bypass surgery, as well as a valuable adjunct to thrombolytic therapy in terms of reducing a severe stenosis that persists after thrombolysis.

Indications for Percutaneous Transluminal Coronary Angioplasty (PTCA)

Indications for PTCA have been considerably broadened since the initial application of this therapeutic technique. Whereas once only patients with single-vessel disease were considered for PTCA, now patients with multivessel disease, even those who have previously undergone saphenous vein and internal mammary artery (IMA) grafting, may be eligible for this procedure (see box, p. 331).

The restrictions regarding the characteristics of the lesion also have been loosened with improved technology. Left main coronary lesions have been successfully dilated under certain conditions. Also, no longer is the presence of an eccentric, (uneven distribution of plaque), moderately calcified, or nonproximal lesion an absolute contraindication to PTCA. Furthermore, it is now sometimes possible to traverse and dilate a totally occluded vessel.

The most significant advancement, however, has been the lifting of the requirement that only patients with disabling angina unresponsive to medical therapy be considered for PTCA. Clinical indications for PTCA have been expanded to include chronic stable angina, angina after coronary artery bypass grafting (CABG), both recent-onset and postinfarction unstable angina, and in acute myocardial infarction alone or in conjunction with thrombolytic agents. Even patients who are symptom-free but demonstrate evidence of ischemia during exercise testing (positive treadmill test result) may be considered as candidates for elective PTCA.[24]

Initially, most institutions required that patients preparing to undergo PTCA be candidates for coronary bypass surgery. Complications such as abrupt closure may arise during angioplasty, which necessitates immediate aortocoronary bypass grafting. Therefore it was the nurse's responsibility to provide the patient with some preoperative instruction before PTCA. Because urgent

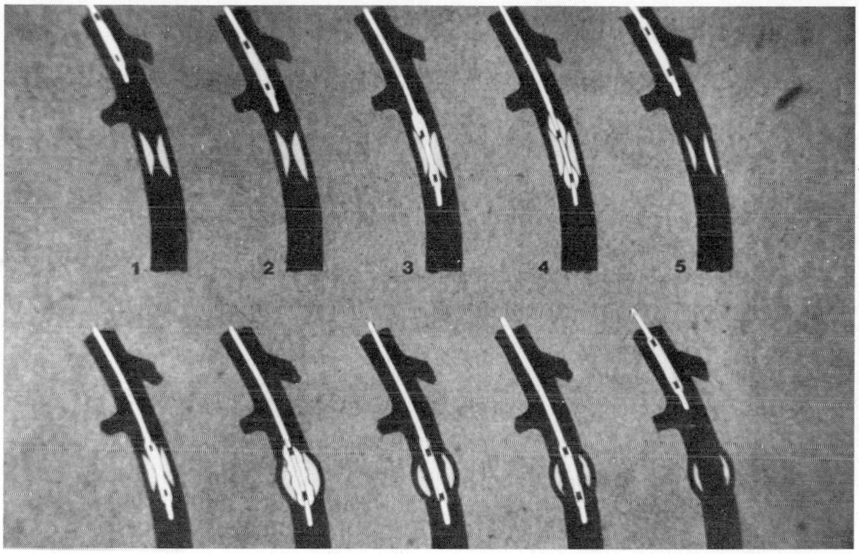

Fig. 17-13 Balloon compression of an atherosclerotic lesion. (From Kinney M and others: *Comprehensive cardiac care,* ed 7, St Louis, 1991, Mosby–Year Book.)

TRADITIONAL ELIGIBILITY CRITERIA FOR PTCA

Single vessel disease exclusive of left main lesions
Characteristics of the lesion
- Concentric
- Noncalcified
- Proximal
- Discrete (less than 1 cm length)
- No total occlusions

History of disease
- Short history of angina (less than 1 year)
- Inadequate control on medications

Normal ventricular function
Not in the setting of acute myocardial infarction
Must be a candidate for CABG

bypass surgery is required in only 1% to 3% of cases, a more selective surgical back-up plan is appropriate. Thus only those patients undergoing high-risk angioplasty, who are otherwise ideal surgical candidates, require formal surgical back-up support. Nevertheless, the availability of cardiac surgical services on site remains mandatory.

Procedure

PTCA is performed in the cardiac catheterization laboratory by means of fluoroscopy. Introducer sheaths are inserted percutaneously into the femoral artery and vein. The venous sheath can be used to perform a right ventricle catheterization with a pulmonary artery (PA) catheter or to insert a pacing catheter, or both. A catheter with pacing capabilities may be indicated if dilation of the right coronary artery or circumflex artery is anticipated because the blood supply to the conduction system of the heart may be interrupted, thus requiring emergency pacing. The pacing catheter also serves as an anatomic landmark for locating the lesions to be dilated. The patient is systemically heparinized to prevent clots from forming on or in any of the catheters. A special guiding catheter designed to engage the coronary ostia is inserted through the arterial sheath and advanced in retrograde manner through the aorta. Nitroglycerin or calcium channel blockers may be given at this time to prevent coronary artery spasm and to maximize coronary vasodilation during the procedure. A guidewire is then advanced down the coronary artery and negotiated across the occluding atheroma. The balloon catheter is advanced over this guidewire and positioned across the lesion. The balloon is inflated and deflated repetitively (each inflation not to exceed 90 seconds) until evidence of dilation is demonstrated on angiogram (Fig. 17-14). In cases that require prolonged balloon inflations, however, an autoperfusion angioplasty catheter is available with side holes that allow passive blood flow through the central lumen to distal coronary artery if adequate systemic blood pressure is present.[25]

The patient is transferred to the coronary care or angioplasty unit for overnight care and observation. The introducer sheaths are left in place for several reasons. First, the intravenous infusion of heparin is continued for 6 to 24 hours after PTCA to prevent clot formation on the roughened endothelium at the site of dilation.[23] Therefore removal of the sheaths during this time causes a predisposition to bleeding. Second, it allows for rapid vascular access should redilation become necessary. The arterial sheath must be attached to a continuous heparinized saline flush, however, and intravenous fluids must be infused through the venous sheath to maintain luminal patency. If the patient's postangioplasty course is uneventful, the sheaths usually are removed within 24 hours and the patient may be discharged to home 6 to 12 hours later.

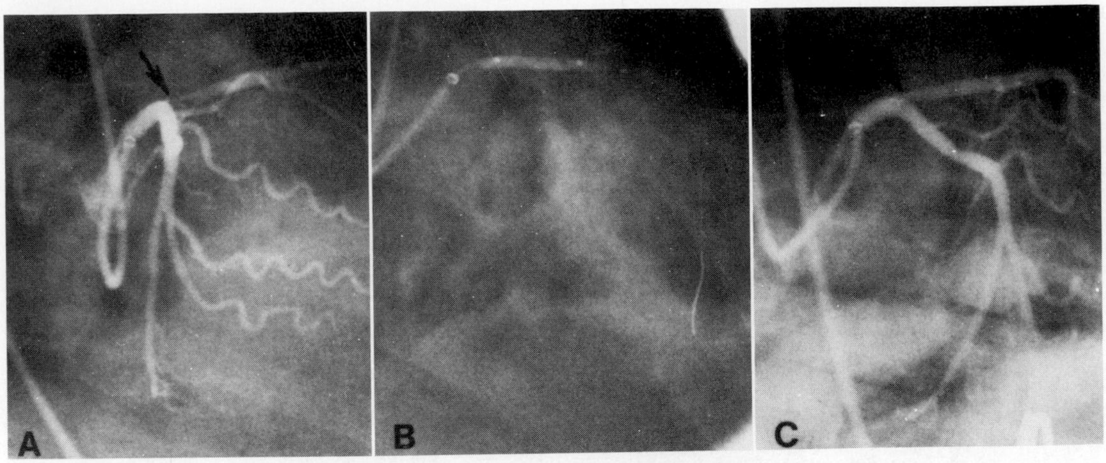

Fig. 17-14 Coronary arteriograms during PTCA. Arrows denote the lesion before dilation (**A**), with the balloon inflated (**B**), and after dilation (**C**). (From Kinney M and others: *Comprehensive cardiac care,* ed 7, St Louis, 1991, Mosby–Year Book.)

Complications

As stated earlier, serious complications can result from angioplasty that will necessitate emergency CABG surgery. These complications include persistent coronary artery spasm, myocardial infarction, and acute coronary occlusion. Other complications that can occur in the period immediately after angioplasty include bleeding and hematoma formation at the site of vascular cannulation, compromised blood flow to the involved extremity, allergic reaction to radiopaque contrast dye, dysrhythmias, and vasovagal response (hypotension, bradycardia, and diaphoresis) during manipulation or removal of introducer sheaths. Restenosis can occur up to 6 months after angioplasty; however, this late complication typically is amenable to repeat angioplasty. The mechanism involved in restenosis remains unclear, but it is thought to be related to intimal hyperplasia, as well as to platelet deposition and thrombus formation.[25] For this reason, patients are started on a regimen of antiplatelet drugs, for example, a combination of aspirin and dipyridamole.

Atherectomy, Lasers, and Stents

Coronary atherectomy, laser angioplasty, and placement of endovascular prostheses (stents) are new interventional technologies developed to address the problems of acute closure and restenosis associated with PTCA.[25]

◆ **Atherectomy.** Atherectomy is the excision and removal of the atherosclerotic plaque by cutting, shaving, or grinding; specialized coronary catheters are used to achieve a more controlled mechanism of injury, with the hope of fewer complications[27,28]

Three atherectomy devices are described in Table 17-5. At this writing, the Directional Coronary Atherectomy (DCA) device is the only one FDA-approved for use in the coronary arteries. The mechanism of action of the DCA catheter is shown in Fig. 17-15. The other two devices (Rotoblader and TEC) are in ongoing clinical trials. All three devices are FDA approved for use in peripheral arteries.

Table 17-5 Atherectomy devices

Device	Design	Uses
Directional atherectomy (Simpson Atherocath)	Rotating cup-shaped cutter within a windowed cylindric housing; plaque that protrudes into window is shaved off and collected within nose cone of cutter housing (Fig. 17-15)	Ostial lesions SVG Eccentric lesions in large vessels Proximal, discrete lesions
Rotational ablation (Rotablator)	A high-speed rotating diamond-studded bur; "sanding effect"; generates microparticles that pass distally into microcirculation	Distal lesions Long, diffuse lesions Tortuous vessels Calcified lesions Eccentric lesions Ostial lesions Small vessels
Transluminal extraction catheter (TEC)	Motorized cutting head with triangular blades; excised plaque removed by suction	Diffuse disease SVG

SVG, Saphenous venous graft.

The DCA catheter has presented a significant research advantage for understanding the pathogenesis of CAD and also the restenosis process after catheter interventions. Because DCA extracts pieces of atheroma that can be studied microscopically (rather like a biopsy

A

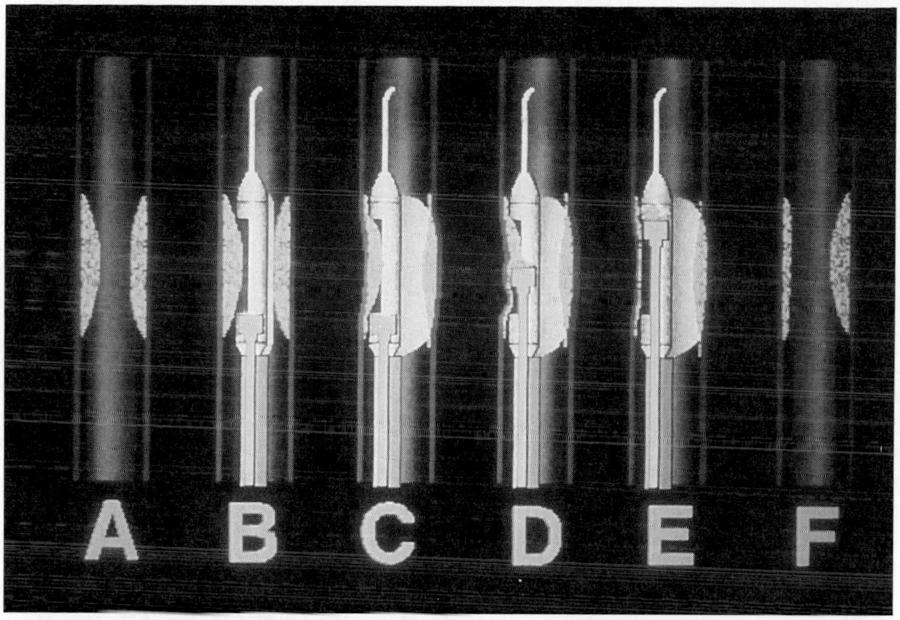

B

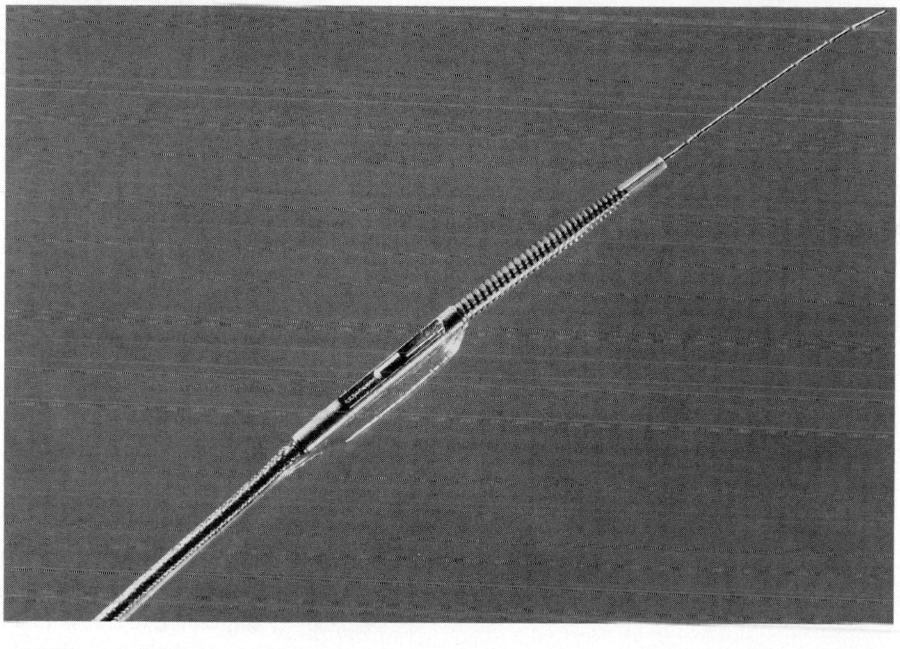

Fig. 17-15 **A,** Directional coronary atherectomy: *A,* atheroma (plaque) in vessel lumen; *B,* Simpson atherocath (DCA device) in position; *C,* inflation of low-pressure support balloon that pushes the plaque into the "window" of the device (the ability to turn the atherocath in different directions within the artery explains the name of the DCA device); *D,* the cutter begins to shear away plaque; *E,* the plaque is pushed into the nose cone (collection chamber) of the atherocath; *F,* vessel lumen shows decreased plaque after removal of catheter. **B,** Simpson atherocath.

specimen), progress has been made in the understanding of both CAD and the restenosis process caused by intimal hyperplasia.

◆ **Laser.** Laser plaque ablation in coronary arteries is being studied in clinical trials. During laser balloon angioplasty, heat and pressure are applied simultaneously to the coronary wall to create a less thrombogenic surface and to "weld" together the fractured intimal segment.[29] The excimer laser, which uses high-energy pulsed ultraviolet light—so-called cold laser—to vaporize plaque, is particularly suited for distal disease and occluded saphenous vein graft (SVG).[28]

◆ **Stent.** Another major coronary technology that has recently evolved is the coronary stent prosthesis. This is a self-expanding or balloon-expandable stent that is introduced into the coronary artery over a guidewire in a region that has been previously dilated with PTCA to prevent acute closure and restenosis, as well as to obtain a larger vascular lumen diameter.[28,30,31]

A stent is positioned at the target side, it is expanded, and the catheter is removed. Several types of stents are undergoing clinical trial. As shown by the examples in Fig. 17-16, stents have either thermal memory (Fig. 17-16, A), are self-expanding (Fig. 17-16, B), or are balloon expandable (Fig. 17-16, C).[31] At present, stents are not a routine procedure but are used where angioplasty or atherectomy has "failed."

Because the stent is a foreign object (generally made of stainless steel) in the bloodstream, the stent's presence in the coronary artery will activate the coagulation cascade. These patients are anticoagulated with IV heparin both during and after the procedure to prevent acute thrombosis of the stent. The efficacy of anticoagulation is assessed by the partial thromboplastin time (PTT) or activated clotting time (ACT) every 4 to 6 hours. (See Chapter 15, p. 186 for information on coagulation studies.) Subsequently Coumadin (warfarin sodium) is used to make the transition to oral anticoagulation. Bleeding is the major risk factor after a stent is placed. Nursing management focuses on prevention of bleeding complications, especially when the introducer sheaths are removed. Other drugs that are used to decrease platelet adhesiveness include IV Dextran infusion and oral aspirin and dipyridamole (Persantine). Conventional medications for treatment of coronary artery disease, such as IV nitroglycerin and calcium channel blockers, are also prescribed. The average hospital stay for a stent procedure is 5 to 7 days because of the intensive anticoagulation required. Within 3 to 6 weeks the stent surface will be covered by endothelium and anticoagulation will no longer be required.

The ideal stent should be flexible to go through small, tortuous coronary arteries, have low thrombogenesis, expand reliably in the artery, be radiopaque, and be made of biocompatible material.[31] Considerable research continues in the area of endovascular procedures. However, no one device is the answer. It is likely that stents will continue to be an adjunct to angioplasty, atherectomy, and thrombolytic drugs as part of an increasing number of interventional cardiology devices used to treat acute manifestations of coronary artery disease.

Nursing Management

Nursing management after angioplasty, atherectomy, or stent focuses on accurate assessment of the patient's condition and prompt intervention. The nurse is in the unique position at the bedside to continuously monitor for clinical manifestations of potential problems and take quick and appropriate action to minimize the deleterious effects of complications related to angioplasty.

It is essential that the nurse observe the patient for recurrent angina. Angina during angioplasty is an expected occurrence at the time of balloon inflation. It is caused by the temporary interruption of blood flow through the involved artery. It should subside, however, with deflation or removal of the balloon or the administration of nitroglycerin, or both. Angina after a coronary interventional procedure may be a result of transient coronary vasospasm, or it may signal a more serious complication. In any case the nurse must act quickly to assess for clinical manifestations of myocardial ischemia and initiate appropriate interventions as indicated. (See Chapter 16 on the care of the patient with acute myocardial infarction.) The physician usually orders intravenous nitroglycerin to be titrated to alleviate chest pain. Continued angina despite maximal vasodilator therapy generally rules out transient coronary vasospasm as the source of ischemic pain, and redilation or emergency coronary artery bypass surgery, or both, must be considered.

While the sheath is in place or after its removal, bleeding or hematoma at the sheath insertion site may occur as a result of the effects of heparin. The nurse observes the patient for bleeding or swelling at the puncture site and frequently assesses adequacy of circulation to the involved extremity. The nurse also assesses the patient for back pains, which can indicate retroperitoneal bleeding from oozing puncture sites. The patient should be instructed to keep the involved leg straight and not to elevate the head of the bed any more than 45 degrees while the sheath is in place (to prevent dislodgment) and for several hours after its removal (to prevent bleeding). Use of an Eggcrate mattress may help alleviate the lower back pain many patients experience while immobile after undergoing PTCA.[32] After sheath removal, direct pressure should be applied to the puncture site for 15 to 30 minutes; a sandbag may be ordered if direct pressure is inadequate for hemostasis. Patients usually are allowed to resume ambulation 6 to 8 hours later, depending on institutional protocol. Excessive bleeding or hematoma formation can become a serious problem because it may result in hypotension or compromised blood flow to the involved extremity, or both, thus necessitating surgical intervention in rare cases.

NURSING DIAGNOSIS AND MANAGEMENT
Post PTCA, coronary atherectomy, or stent

- ◆ Acute Pain related to transmission and perception of cutaneous, visceral, muscular, or ischemic impulses secondary to abrupt coronary artery closure, p. 566
- ◆ Fluid Volume Deficit related to active blood loss secondary to IV heparin therapy, p. 639
- ◆ High Risk for Altered Peripheral Tissue Perfusion risk factor: orthopedic injury or device applied to an extremity, p. 364
- ◆ Activity Intolerance related to postural hyypotension secondary to prolonged immobility, narcotics, vasodilation therapy, p. 365
- ◆ Altered myocardial tissue perfusion related to acute myocardial ischemia, p. 364
- ◆ Decreased Cardiac Output related to ventricular tachycardias, p. 362
- ◆ Anxiety related to threat to biologic, physiologic, and/or social integrity, p. 763

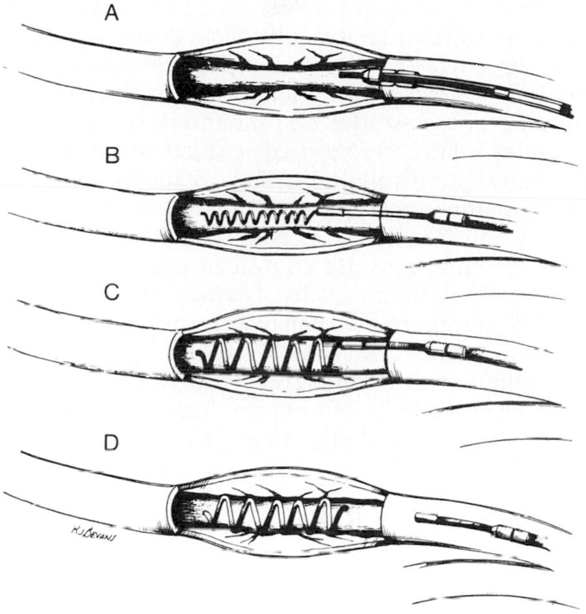

A. Stent is cooled with ice and straightened in catheter for placement.
B. Exposed to blood temperature, coil begins to expand.
C. Coil expands to full size in coronary artery.
D. Stent is released from delivery device and supports vessel. Catheter is removed from coronary artery.

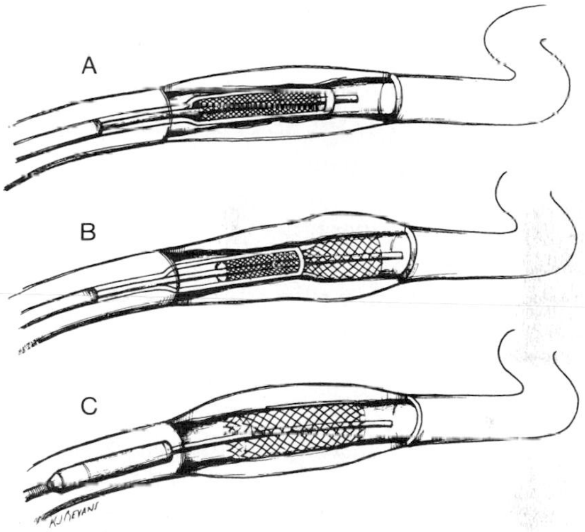

A. Stent is constricted in constraining catheter.
B. Stent is released from catheter.
C. Stent is fully expanded to support vessel. Catheter is removed from coronary artery.

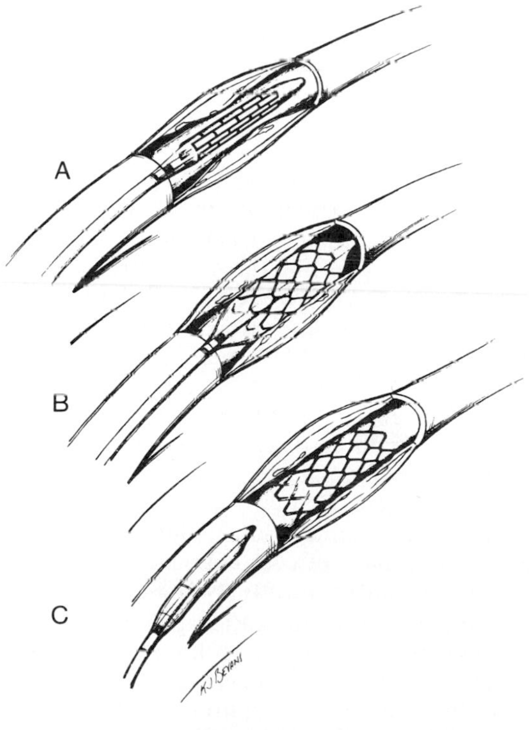

A. Stent is crimped onto balloon catheter for placement.
B. Stent is expanded against vessel wall.
C. Stent is supporting the vessel wall. Balloon catheter is withdrawn from coronary artery.

Fig. 17-16 Intracoronary stents. **Top,** Nitinol stent (heat sensitive). **Middle,** Medinvent stent (self-expanding). **Bottom,** Palmaz-Schatz stent (balloon expandable). (Modified from Bevans M, McLimore E: *J Cardiovasc Nurs* 7(1):34, 1992.

Typically, patients undergoing elective angioplasty are hospitalized for approximately 24 hours. Other catheter procedures may require a slightly longer hospital stay. Because these are only palliative procedures, these patients need education in risk-factor modification. Because of abbreviated hospital stay, the nurse often has insufficient time to do more than identify the offending risk factors and initiate basic instruction. Patients should be referred to local cardiac rehabilitation centers for more extensive teaching and follow-up to facilitate understanding and compliance with the therapeutic regimen.

Another teaching need that must be addressed is the patient's knowledge deficit related to discharge medications. As stated earlier, patients frequently are sent home on a regimen of antiplatelet drugs, as well as a nitrate such as a nitroglycerin preparation or isosorbide to promote vasodilation. In addition, if the patient has demonstrated evidence of a vasospastic component to the disease, calcium channel blockers will be prescribed. It is essential that the patient clearly understand the rationale for therapy, as well as potential side effects of each drug.

BALLOON VALVULOPLASTY

After the development of percutaneous balloon angioplasty for coronary artery disease, it became reasonable to consider adaptation of this technique as a nonsurgical intervention for stenotic cardiac valves. Although long-term results are not promising at this point, especially for aortic valvuloplasty, balloon valvuloplasty can provide palliation and short-term symptomatic relief in selected patient populations[34,35] (see box, below).

Balloon valvuloplasty is performed in the cardiac catheterization laboratory. The procedure is similar to a routine cardiac catheterization, including cannulation of the femoral artery and vein with percutaneous introducer sheaths. The balloon dilation catheter is then threaded over a guidewire across the stenotic valvular orifice.[36] The valves may be approached either retrograde via the aorta or antegrade across the interatrial septum. In the antegrade transseptal approach, the balloon catheter is passed across the interatrial septum, which results in the creation of a small atrial septal defect.[37] Subsequent inflations of the balloon increase the valve opening by separating fused commissures, cracking of calcified leaflets, and stretching of valve structures.[36,37] Inflations are continued until the disappearance of the balloon "waist," which indicates full inflation.[35] Regurgitant flow can result, particularly after mitral valvuloplasty.[36] The risks of balloon valvuloplasty, which are similar to those inherent in most catheterization procedures, include, but are not limited to, cardiac perforation, thromboembolic events, dysrhythmias, hypotension, and bleeding.[36]

INDICATIONS FOR BALLOON VALVULOPLASTY

AORTIC

- High risk for nonsurgical candidates with incapacitating symptoms
- Patients with aortic stenosis who require urgent noncardiac surgery
- Patients with severe heart failure or cardiogenic shock because of aortic stenosis whose conditions need to be stabilized until valve replacement is deemed safer
- Patients with poor left ventricular function, low cardiac output, and small gradient across a stenotic aortic valve whose need for aortic valve replacement requires assessment

MITRAL

- As an alternative to open mitral commissurotomy

THROMBOLYTIC THERAPY

Thrombolytic therapy is an important clinical intervention for the patient experiencing acute myocardial infarction (AMI). Before the introduction of streptokinase as a thrombolytic agent, the medical management of AMI focused on decreasing myocardial oxygen demands in an effort to minimize myocardial necrosis and thus preserve ventricular function. Recently, however, efforts to limit the size of infarction have been directed toward the timely reperfusion of the jeopardized myocardium. The use of thrombolytic therapy to accomplish this objective is predicated on the prevailing theory that the terminal event in most transmural infarctions is the rupture of an atherosclerotic plaque with thrombus formation.[38] The administration of a thrombolytic agent results in the lysis of the acute thrombus, thus recanalizing the obstructed coronary artery and restoring blood flow to the affected myocardium.

Thrombolytic Agents

◆ **Streptokinase.** Streptokinase (SK) is a thrombolytic agent derived from beta-hemolytic streptococci, which, when combined with plasminogen, catalyzes the conversion of plasminogen to plasmin, the enzyme responsible for clot dissolution in the body. SK can be administered either intravenously or by an intracoronary approach, which necessitates cardiac catheterization. The efficacy of both routes has been established, and both have been used in clinical practice. However, because of the significant lag time between onset of symptoms and the initiation of intracoronary SK, the intracoronary route is now considered obsolete.

The three major problems associated with the use of SK are its systemic lytic effects coupled with a long half-life, its potential antigenic effects if readministered, and hypotension. Because the anticoagulant action of SK is indiscriminate (non–clot-specific) and prolonged (half-life 20 to 25 minutes), bleeding is a common complication; thus the patient requires careful observation during the 12 hours immediately after administration (see first box, p. 337). In addition, because SK is a bacterial protein, it is strongly antigenic and can produce a variety of allergic reactions, including anaphylaxis,

SIGNS OF INADEQUATE HEMOSTASIS RELATED TO THROMBOLYTIC THERAPY

Bleeding or hematoma at puncture sites
Hematuria, hematemesis, hemoptysis, melena, epistaxis
Bruising or petechiae (pinpoint hemorrhages)
Flank ecchymoses with complaints of low back pain (suggestive of retroperitoneal bleeding)
Gingival bleeding
Change in neurologic status (intracranial bleeding)
Deterioration in vital signs, decreased hematocrit values (internal bleeding)

POSSIBLE ALLERGIC MANIFESTATIONS RELATED TO STREPTOKINASE THERAPY

Anaphylaxis	Flushing
Urticaria	Fever
Itching	Chills
Nausea	

especially when administered to a patient who either has received SK therapy previously or has had a recent streptococcal infection. It is necessary to be familiar with the possible allergic manifestations (see second box above), as well as cognizant of the fact that as a result of delayed antibody formation, symptoms may develop several days after infusion. Hypotension is sometimes associated with the rapid administration of SK. This fall in blood pressure usually responds to volume replacement but occasionally requires vasopressor support. SK is considerably more effective in lysine-fresh (less than 3 hours) thrombi as compared with older thrombi.[38]

◆ **Urokinase.** Urokinase (UK) is an enzymatic protein secreted by the parenchyma of the human kidney. Its thrombolytic effect results from the direct activation of plasminogen to form plasmin. This differs from SK, which first must form a complex with plasminogen that will activate plasmin to dissolve the clot (Fig. 17-17). UK also is non–clot-specific (activates circulating, non–clot-bound plasminogen, as well as clot-bound plasminogen) but has a shorter half-life than does SK. Although a systemic lytic state also may be produced, its administration is associated with fewer bleeding complications. Because UK is produced by the kidney, it is nonantigenic and thus well suited for use if subsequent thrombolytic therapy is indicated. Currently, however, it is difficult and expensive to produce, precluding extensive clinical use except in the setting of PTCA or atherectomy for acute ischemic syndromes, in which the use of adjunctive intracoronary UK to treat thrombus accumulation often results in maintained vessel patency.[39]

◆ **Tissue plasminogen activator.** Another mode of thrombolytic therapy is tissue plasminogen activator (t-PA). Marketed under the name Activase, t-PA is a naturally occurring enzyme (thus nonantigenic) that is clot-specific and has a very short half-life (5 to 10 minutes). It converts plasminogen to plasmin after binding to the fibrin-containing clot. This clot specificity results in an increased concentration and activity of plasmin at the site of the clot where it is needed (Fig. 17-18). It was hoped that this characteristic of t-PA would prevent the induction of a systemic lytic state that occurs with SK therapy. The results of recent studies comparing the adverse effects of SK and t-PA, however, show similar incidences of bleeding after administration.

◆ **APSAC.** Anisoylated plasminogen-streptokinase activator complex (APSAC; Eminase) is the newest thrombolytic agent approved by the Food and Drug Administration (FDA) (February 1990) for use in the treatment of acute myocardial infarction. Often referred to as a second-generation streptokinase, it has certain advantages over SK that are related specifically to duration of action, ease of administration, and fibrin selectivity.[40,41] Compared with SK, the duration of action has been quadrupled, and the time of administration has been reduced from 60 minutes to 2 to 5 minutes.[42] In addition, it is administered in an inactive form resistant to neutralization by plasmin inactivators. So although it is a non-clot-specific agent, there is enhanced binding to fibrin clots prior to activation because of its unique molecular structure. Disadvantages, which are similar to those of SK, include the potential for allergic reactions and hypotension. Evidence suggests, however, that the lytic state produced by APSAC and the other non–clot-specific agents (UK, SK) may account for the reduced tendency for thrombosis to recur after thrombolytic therapy.[44] APSAC is a promising therapeutic alternative that, along with SK and t-PA, is well suited for thrombolytic therapy.

Eligibility Criteria

Certain criteria have been developed, based on research findings, to determine the patient population that would most likely benefit from the administration of thrombolytic therapy. In general, patients with recent onset of chest pain (less than 6 hours' duration) are candidates. Research suggests that the earlier the treatment is instituted, the higher the likelihood of successful reperfusion. A large randomized study, however, demonstrated a reduction in mortality, even when thrombolytic therapy was begun between 6 and 24 hours after onset of chest pain.[45]

Patients with persistent ST segment elevation despite sublingual nitroglycerin or nifedipine, a sign of impending transmural infarction, are considered candidates for therapy. Patients with abnormal Q waves should not be excluded from therapy because this finding is not necessarily evidence of a completed infarction.

Other common criteria for the use of thrombolytic therapy are included in the first box, p. 338.

Evidence of Reperfusion

Several phenomena can be observed after the reperfusion of an artery that has been completely occluded by a thrombus (see second box, p. 338). Initially, there is an abrupt cessation of ischemic chest pain as blood flow is

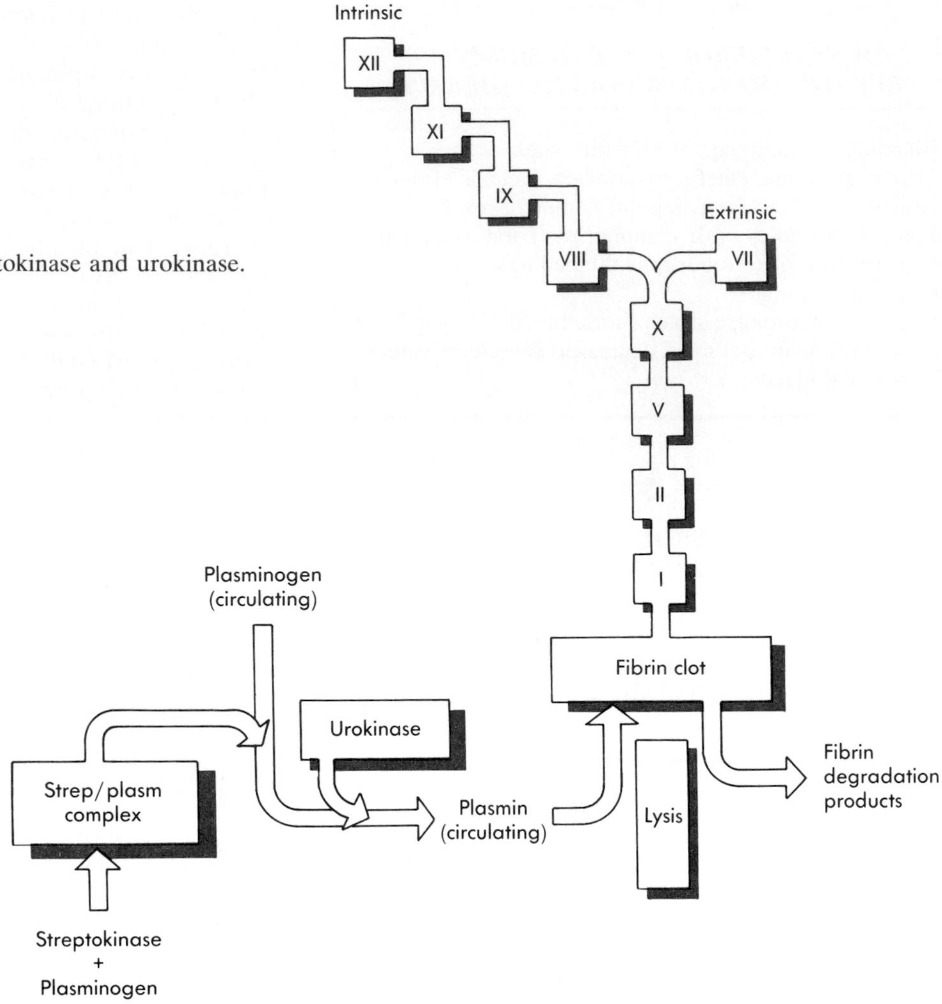

Fig. 17-17 Site of action of streptokinase and urokinase.

THROMBOLYTIC THERAPY SELECTION CRITERIA

- No more than 6 hours from onset of chest pain and less if possible
- ST segment elevation on ECG
- Ischemic chest pain of 30 minutes' duration
- Chest pain unresponsive to sublingual nitroglycerin or nifedipine
- Less than 76 years of age
- No conditions that might cause a predisposition to hemorrhage

NONINVASIVE EVIDENCE OF REPERFUSION

- Cessation of chest pain
- Reperfusion dysrhythmias primarily ventricular
- Return of elevated ST segments to baseline
- Early and marked peaking of creatine kinase (CK)

restored. Another reliable indicator of reperfusion is the appearance of various "reperfusion" dysrhythmias. Accelerated idioventricular rhythm (AIVR) is the most common reperfusion dysrhythmia, but premature ventricular contractions, bradycardias, heart block, ventricular tachycardia, and, rarely, ventricular fibrillation also may occur. The reason for the occurrence of these dysrhythmias remains unclear. Vigilant monitoring of the patient's ECG is essential, however, because a stable condition may deteriorate rapidly when recanalization occurs, and dysrhythmias should be treated appropriately.

Another noninvasive marker of recanalization is the rapid resolution of the previously elevated ST segments, which indicates restoration of blood flow to previously ischemic myocardial tissue. For this reason a monitoring lead should be chosen that clearly demonstrates ST elevation before initiation of therapy.[46]

The serum concentration of creatine kinase (formerly creatine phosphokinase) rises rapidly and markedly after reperfusion of the ischemic myocardium. This phenomenon is termed *washout,* because it is thought to result from the rapid readmission into the circulation of creatine kinase—an enzyme released by damaged myocardial cells—after restoration of blood flow to previously unperfused areas of the heart.

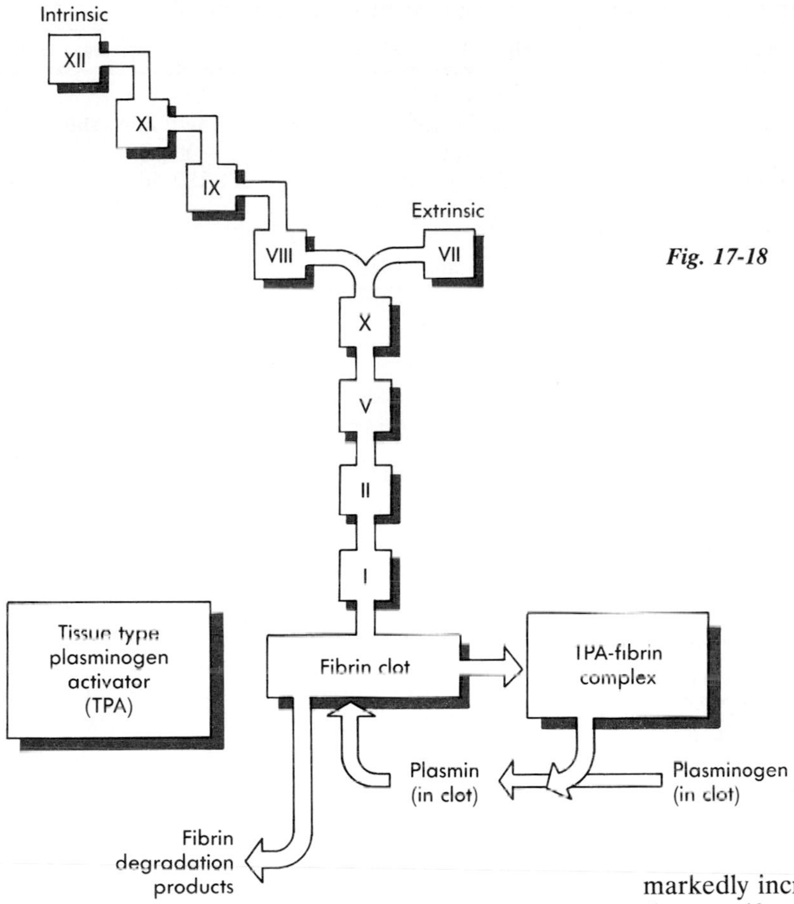

Fig. 17-18 Site of action of tissue plasminogen activator.

Recognition of these noninvasive markers of recanalization is essential for documenting the patient's response to thrombolytic therapy.

Administration

◆ **Streptokinase.** Intravenously administered SK, although not as effective in terms of recanalization as intracoronary streptokinase, has the advantage of being more practical in that it can be administered more rapidly after the onset of symptoms. Therefore SK is now routinely administered intravenously. The recommended dosage is 1,500,000 IU of SK administered intravenously over 60 minutes to achieve clot lysis.[46] The patient then undergoes IV heparinization to prevent early rethrombosis.[47]

◆ **Tissue plasminogen activator.** Tissue plasminogen activator was approved specifically for intravenous administration. The total dose of t-PA is 100 mg, with 60 mg administered over 1 hour (10 mg of which is administered as a bolus) to rapidly recanalize the infarct-related coronary artery. The remaining 40 mg is given over the next 2 hours, followed by a heparin drip to maintain patency of the recanalized artery and to prevent rethrombosis.[47]

◆ **APSAC.** Because it is inactive on administration, APSAC can be given rapidly as a bolus injection. The recommended dose is 30 units injected intravenously over 2 to 5 minutes. Because the half-life of APSAC is markedly increased (90 minutes), concomitant heparin therapy, if employed, should begin 4 to 6 hours after administration to decrease the risk of bleeding associated with the prolonged fibrinolytic activity[42] (Table 17-6).

Nursing Management

The most common complication related to thrombolysis is bleeding, not only as a result of the thrombolytic therapy itself but also because the patients routinely receive anticoagulation therapy for several days to minimize the possibility of rethrombosis. Therefore the nurse must continually monitor for clinical manifestations of bleeding (see box, p. 337, listing signs of inadequate hemostasis related to thrombolytic therapy). Mild gingival bleeding and oozing around venipuncture sites are common and not a cause of concern. Should serious bleeding occur, such as intracranial or internal bleeding, all fibrinolytic and heparin therapy should be discontinued and appropriate volume expanders or coagulation factors, or both, should be administered.

In addition to accurate assessment of the patient for evidence of bleeding, the nurse intervenes appropriately to prevent possible bleeding episodes. The nurse also avoids nonessential handling of the patient, keeps injections to a minimum, and remembers to provide additional pressure on injection, venipuncture, and particularly arterial puncture sites. Antacids can be given prophylactically, especially if the patient complains of gastric discomfort. The patient should be cautioned against vigorous toothbrushing and told to refrain from using straight-edge razors.

Table 17-6 Thrombolytic agents approved by the FDA for use in acute myocardial infarction

	Streptokinase*	Anistreplase (APSAC)	Alteplase (t-PA)
Fibrin-selective	No	Semiselective	Yes
Half-life	20-25 min (intermediate)	90 min (long)	5-10 min (short)
Dose	1.5 MU	30 units	100 mg
Duration of infusion	60 min constant infusion	2-5 min bolus	180 min complex infusion
Hypotension	+	+/−	−
Allergic reactions	+	+	−
Cost	Low	Moderately high	High

*Also approved for intracoronary use.
NOTE: Urokinase—approved only for intracoronary administration.
+ = Present; − = not present; +/− = may be present.

Summary

In most cases thrombolytic therapy has been determined to be successful in reopening occluded coronary arteries in the setting of acute myocardial infarction. This results in the salvage of myocardium by limiting infarct size, thus preserving left ventricular function and significantly reducing morbidity and mortality. When the three thrombolytic agents approved for intravenous use are compared in terms of reperfusion, t-PA and APSAC achieve higher, early patency rates. By 24 hours, however, all three agents have uniformly high patency rates.[38] In addition, the administration of heparin extends the anticoagulant effect of therapy beyond that of the thrombolytic agents and often is used 1 to 3 days, or more, after lytic therapy.[48] Also, the combined effects of aspirin's antiplatelet therapy have been shown to decrease mortality.

Finally, because the area of thrombolytic therapy is rapidly evolving, drug dose ranges and regimens are subject to change when research findings are updated. However, residual coronary stenosis resulting from the atherosclerotic process remains even after successful thrombolysis. This residual coronary stenosis can cause rethrombosis. Therefore thrombolytic therapy is recognized as an emergency procedure to restore patency until more definitive therapy can be initiated to effectively reduce the degree of stenosis (PTCA) or to bypass the offending occlusion (coronary artery bypass surgery). The optimal timing of these interventions is yet to be determined.

MECHANICAL CIRCULATORY ASSIST DEVICES

Intraaortic Balloon Pump

The intraaortic balloon pump (IABP) currently is the most widely employed temporary mechanical circulatory assist device used to support failing circulation (see second box on right). Its therapeutic effects are based on the hemodynamic principles of diastolic augmentation and afterload reduction.

The most commonly used intraaortic balloon consists of a single sausage-shaped polyurethane balloon that is wrapped around the distal end of a vascular catheter and positioned in the descending thoracic aorta just distal to the takeoff of the left subclavian artery. The second generation of intraaortic balloon catheters is more flexible and can be wrapped to a smaller diameter than their predecessors and therefore can be inserted into the femoral artery percutaneously rather than surgically. When attached to a bedside pumping console and properly synchronized to the patient's ECG pattern, the intraaortic balloon will inflate during diastole and deflate just before systole.

Initially, as the balloon is inflated in diastole concurrent with aortic valve closure, the blood in the aortic arch above the level of the balloon will be displaced retrograde (backward) toward the aortic root, augmenting diastolic coronary arterial blood flow and increasing myocardial oxygen supply (Fig. 17-19, *A*). The blood

NURSING DIAGNOSIS AND MANAGEMENT

Post-thrombolytic therapy

- High Risk for Fluid Volume Deficit risk factor: active blood loss secondary to decreased systemic fibrinogen and anticoagulation (heparin), p. 639
- Acute Pain related to transmission and perception of cutaneous, visceral, muscular, or ischemic impulses secondary to abrupt coronary artery closure, p. 566
- Altered Myocardial Tissue Perfusion related to acute myocardial ischemia, p. 364
- High Risk for Altered Peripheral Tissue Perfusion risk factor: orthopedic injury or device applied to an extremity (if thrombolytics administered via femoral sheath in cardiac catheterization laboratory, p. 364

INDICATIONS FOR THE USE OF INTRAAORTIC BALLOON PUMP

Left ventricular failure after cardiac surgery
Unstable angina refractory to medications
Recurrent angina after AMI
Complications of AMI
  Cardiogenic shock
  Papillary muscle dysfunction/rupture with mitral regurgitation
  Ventricular septal defect
  Refractory ventricular dysrhythmias

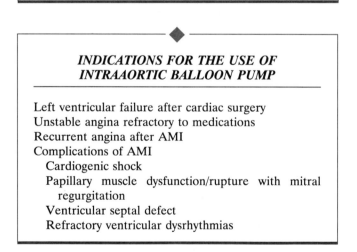

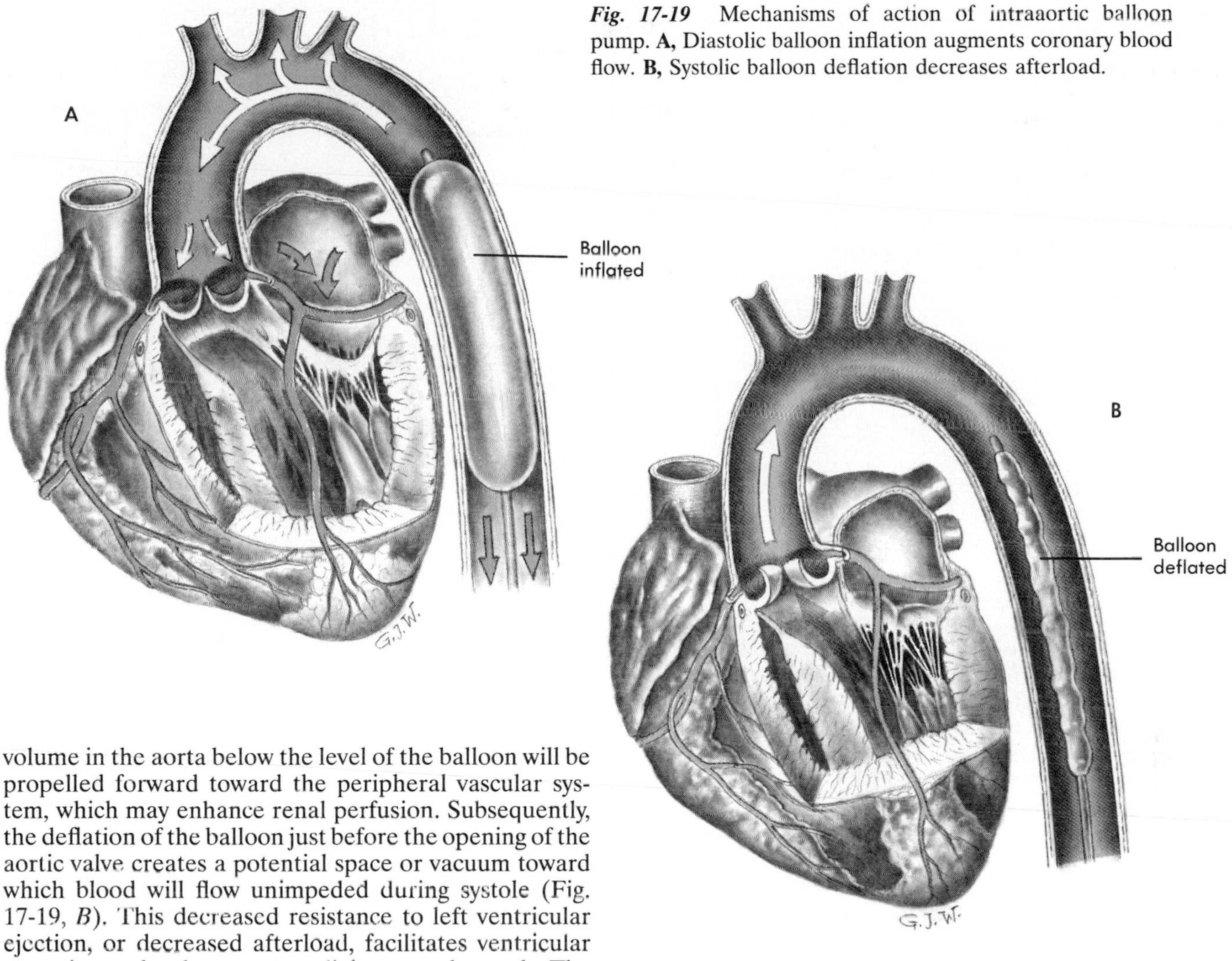

Fig. 17-19 Mechanisms of action of intraaortic balloon pump. **A,** Diastolic balloon inflation augments coronary blood flow. **B,** Systolic balloon deflation decreases afterload.

volume in the aorta below the level of the balloon will be propelled forward toward the peripheral vascular system, which may enhance renal perfusion. Subsequently, the deflation of the balloon just before the opening of the aortic valve creates a potential space or vacuum toward which blood will flow unimpeded during systole (Fig. 17-19, *B*). This decreased resistance to left ventricular ejection, or decreased afterload, facilitates ventricular emptying and reduces myocardial oxygen demands. The overall physiologic effect of IABP therapy is an improvement in the balance between myocardial oxygen supply and demand.[49] Contraindications to balloon pumping include aortic aneurysm, aortic valve insufficiency, and severe peripheral vascular disease.

Although the actual management of the pumping console and its timing functions may be delegated to specially trained personnel on the unit, several important nursing responsibilities relate to the care of the patient receiving IABP therapy.

The ECG and arterial pressure tracing should be constantly monitored to verify the timing and effect of balloon counterpulsations (Fig. 17-20). Dysrhythmias can adversely affect the timing of balloon inflation and deflation; thus rhythm disturbances must be detected and treated promptly.[50] In addition, balloon deflation can be accidentally triggered by pacemaker spikes that are mistaken for R waves. The resulting early deflation is not dangerous, but because it limits effective afterload reduction, an ECG lead that minimizes the pacing spike should be selected. Mean arterial pressure should be maintained at about 80 mm Hg with adequate pumping.

A major complication of IABP is ischemia of the involved limb secondary to occlusion of the femoral artery either by the catheter itself or by emboli from thrombus formation on the balloon. Consequently, the presence and quality of peripheral pulses distal to the catheter insertion site should be assessed frequently, along with color, temperature, and capillary refill of the involved extremity. Doppler localization of peripheral pulses may be required if pulses are difficult to palpate on the cannulated extremity. Signs of diminished perfusion must be reported immediately. Other vascular complications of IABP include acute aortic dissection and the development of pseudoaneurysms.[51]

In addition, the balloon catheter may migrate proximally, occluding the left subclavian artery or distally compromising renal circulation. Therefore careful assessment of the left radial pulse and urinary output is essential. Measures to avoid accidental displacement of the balloon catheter include ensuring that the patient observes complete bed rest, with the head of the bed elevated no more than 30 degrees, and prevents any flexion of the involved hip.

Log rolling is employed, moving the patient from side to side every 2 hours to maintain skin integrity and to prevent pulmonary atelectasis. The presence of the balloon pump should never be a deterrent to appropriate pulmonary toilet. Thrombocytopenia may occur as a result of mechanical destruction of the platelets by the

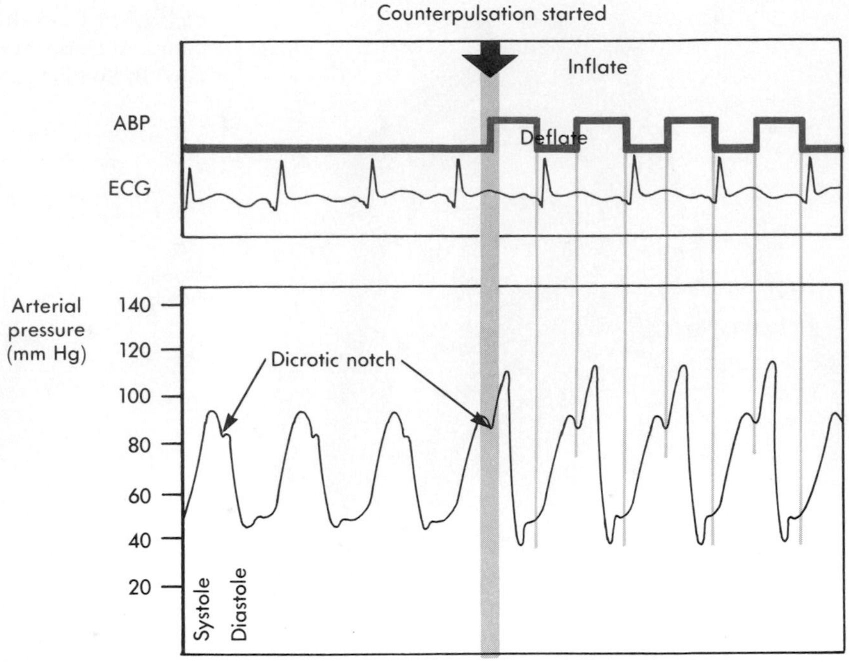

Fig. 17-20 The timing and effect of balloon counterpulsations. Timing is adjusted by synchronizing balloon inflation with the dicrotic knotch on the arterial waveform resulting in an elevated diastolic pressure. Inflation continues until the next R wave serves as a stimulus for balloon deflation. The arterial waveform exhibits a reduced systolic pressure during counterpulsation. (From Guzzetta CE, Dossey BM: *Cardiovascular nursing: holistic practice,* St Louis, 1992, Mosby–Year Book.)

pumping action of the balloon. Therefore platelet counts should be closely monitored, and the patient observed for evidence of bleeding. Because the groin insertion site is at high risk for contamination, a daily regimen of aseptic dressing changes with povidone-iodine (Betadine) should be strictly followed.

Finally, the psychologic needs of the patient must not be overlooked. Sleep deprivation is not at all uncommon, partly caused by the continuous nursing care requirements of the patient but also related to the noise level in the unit, including the sounds made by the balloon pumping device. In addition, these patients universally experience anxiety related to fear of not recovering and loss of control because of forced immobility.

Weaning from the balloon pump should be considered when hemodynamic stability has been achieved with no, or only minimal, pharmacologic support. One weaning procedure consists of slowly decreasing the pumping frequency from every beat down to every eighth beat as tolerated. To prevent thrombus formation on the balloon surface the IABP should remain at this minimal pumping ratio (or in a flutter mode) until its removal. Dependence on the balloon for over 48 hours, indicative of severe cardiac dysfunction, usually is associated with a poor prognosis.

External Counterpulsation

External counterpulsation (ECP) is a noninvasive method of diastolic augmentation in which the lower extremities are used as the pumping chambers. The system consists of two tapered, rigid cylinders that enclose the legs from ankle to thigh (Fig. 17-21). Between the leg and the rigid outer housing is a water-filled bag that obliterates the remaining space to form an airtight seal. Water is then pumped in and out of the bag in synchrony with the ECG to apply alternating positive and negative pressure to veins and arteries within the legs. During diastole, inflation of the bag forces both venous and arterial blood back toward the heart, increasing preload and coronary filling, respectively. To decrease afterload, negative pressure can be generated during systolic deflation to produce a vacuum effect similar to that seen with IABP.

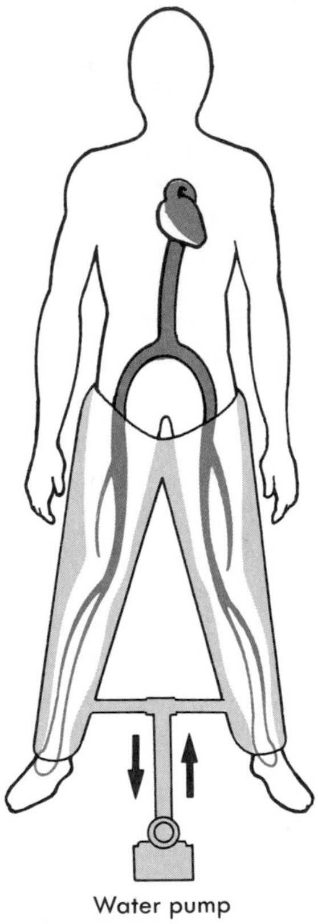

Fig. 17-21 External counterpulsation (ECP).

Compromised lower extremity circulation is the major complication associated with ECP. Patients frequently report pain, muscular cramping, and numbness and tingling in the lower extremities that in some cases may necessitate discontinuance of therapy. Prolonged periods of pumping should be interrupted for brief periods when possible to provide skin care and passive range of motion.

Indications for ECP are similar to those for IABP, with the obvious exceptions of patients who have undergone coronary revascularization with saphenous vein grafts. ECP has for the most part been replaced by other forms of circulatory support.

Ventricular Assist Devices

The ventricular assist device (VAD) is designed to support a failing natural heart by flow assistance. Diversion of varying amounts of systemic blood flow around a failing ventricle by means of an extracorporeal pump reduces cardiac workload while maintaining the circulation. VADs also can maintain adequate perfusion during periods of cardiac arrest.[52] Device selection is based on individual VAD capabilities and institutional preference (Table 17-7).

The VAD currently is indicated for two types of clinical applications. The first category of patients includes those who, despite aggressive medical therapy, continue to demonstrate persistent cardiac failure but who have the potential for regaining normal heart function if the heart is given time to rest. This category, termed *pending recovery,* consists of patients who either cannot be weaned from cardiopulmonary bypass or are in refractory cardiogenic shock after AMI. The second category, or *bridge to transplant,* includes those patients who need circulatory support until heart transplantation can be performed.[53]

The left ventricular assist device (LVAD) is used most commonly because LV failure occurs more frequently than does RV failure. Use of biventricular support (bi-VAD) is becoming more common because RV failure often follows LVAD placement.[54] Outflow cannulas that divert blood from the heart to the pump for LVAD are surgically placed in either the left atrium or LV apex depending on the indication for the device. For example, if the patient is "pending recovery" of the natural heart, preservation of LV function mandates left atrial cannulation. The right atrium is cannulated for outflow for right ventricular support. Inflow back to the heart from the pump is accomplished by cannulation of

Table 17-7 Ventricular assist devices

Type	Example	Use	Description	Insertion
Centrifugal	Biomedicus	Univentricular or biventricular support	Blood is diverted to a cone-shaped pump head where blades rotate and spin blood back through return cannula	Cannulate LA and aorta for LVAD Cannulate RA and PA for RVAD
Rotary	Hemopump	LV support	A propeller housed in the LV cannula draws blood from LV and propels it into the aorta	Via femoral artery, across aortic valve, and into LV
Pneumatic	Thoratec	Univentricular or bi-VAD support	External pulsatile pump that utilizes a pressurized air sac to eject blood through outflow cannula	Inflow through LA or RA and outflow to PA or aorta Inflow through ventricular apex when cardiotomy is expected
	TCI Heart-Mate	LVAD	A pneumatically driven, totally implantable pump with external drive console	Inflow from LV apex with outflow to aorta via graft
Electric	Novacor	LVAD	An electrically driven pulsatile pump that is implanted in an upper abdominal quadrant	Via LV apex and ascending aorta
Cardiopulmonary support	Bard CPS	Emergency resuscitation (e.g., supported angioplasty)	Femoral-femoral bypass; venous blood delivered to centrifugal pump that passes through normothermic heat exchanger to membrane oxygenator and back to patient	Percutaneous or cutdown insertion of catheters into femoral vein and femoral artery

LA, Left atrium; *LV*, left ventricle; *LVAD*, left ventricular assist device; *PA*, pulmonary artery; *RA*, right atrium; *RVAD*, right ventricular assist device; *VAD*, ventricular assist device.

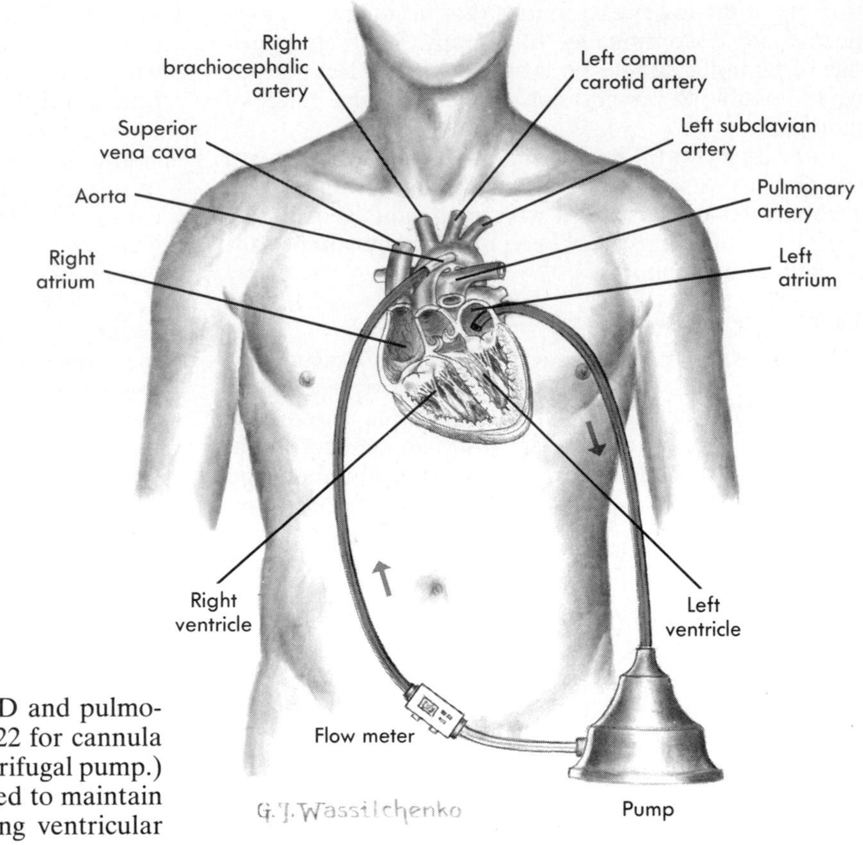

Fig. 17-22 Left centrifugal ventricular assist device (LVAD).

the aorta or femoral artery for the LVAD and pulmonary artery for the RVAD. (See Fig. 17-22 for cannula placement in LVAD configuration of centrifugal pump.) Flow rates between 1 and 6 L/min are used to maintain adequate cardiac output while decreasing ventricular workload.

Weaning is accomplished by gradually decreasing flow rates to allow the patient's ventricle to contribute more to total blood flow. Controversy exists with regard to anticoagulation; however, during weaning of VAD flow rates to less than 2 L/min, activated clotting times (ACT) should be maintained between 160 and 480 seconds with heparin, depending on institutional protocols. This minimizes the potential for thrombus formation in the extracorporeal circuit during weaning but also increases the risk of bleeding diathesis, which necessitates close monitoring.

EFFECTS OF CARDIOVASCULAR DRUGS

Multiple medications are used in the treatment of critically ill cardiovascular patients. The critical care nurse is responsible for preparation and administration of these drugs and often is required to titrate the dose on the basis of the patient's hemodynamic response. The medications used to treat cardiovascular disease are rapidly changing and expanding as more is learned about the pathophysiology of cardiac disease and improved formulas are developed by pharmaceutical companies. The critical care nurse with a general understanding of the mechanisms of action of the various drug classifications can readily apply this knowledge to new drugs within the same classification. The following discussion provides a concise review of drugs commonly administered to support cardiovascular function in the critical care setting. The emphasis is on intravenously administered medications that are used for the acute rather than the chronic management of cardiovascular conditions.

Antidysrhythmic Drugs

Antidysrhythmic drugs comprise a diverse category of pharmacologic agents used to terminate or prevent an array of abnormal cardiac rhythms. These drugs commonly are classified according to their primary effect on the action potential of cardiac cells (Fig. 17-23). Further discussion of the cardiac cell action potential is found in Chapter 13, pp. 159-162. The classification scheme shown in Table 17-8 is the most commonly used system. Classification of newer agents becomes more difficult because some of these agents have characteristics of more than one class and others have no characteristics of the current system.[55]

◆ **Class I drugs.** Class I agents are sodium channel blockers that decrease the influx of sodium ions through "fast" channels during phase 0 depolarization. This prolongs the absolute (effective) refractory period, thus decreasing the risk of premature impulses from ectopic foci. In addition, these drugs depress automaticity by slowing the rate of spontaneous depolarizations of pacemaker cells during the resting phase (phase 4).

Class I drugs can be further subdivided into three groups, according to their potency as sodium channel inhibitors and their effect on phase 3 repolarization.[56] Class IA agents—quinidine, procainamide, and disopyramide—block not only the fast sodium channels but also phase 3 repolarization and thereby prolong the action potential duration. Clinically this may result in measurable increases in the QRS duration and the QT interval. All class IA agents may depress myocardial

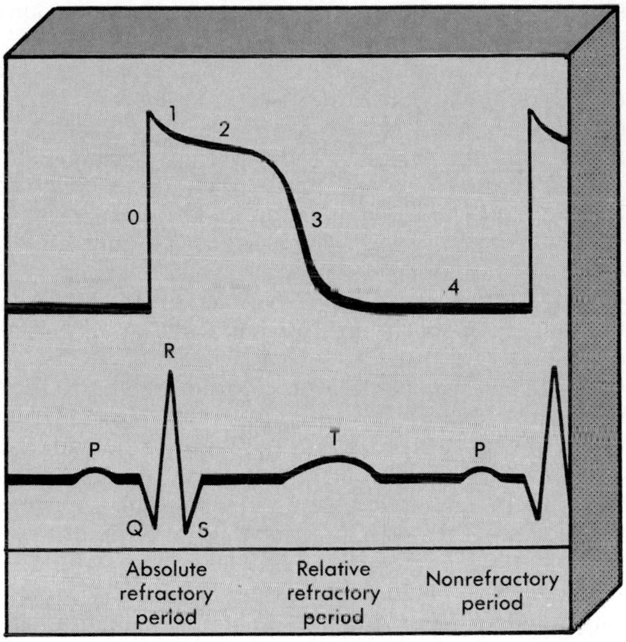

Fig. 17-23 The phases of the cardiac action potential and their relationship to the heart's refractory periods. *Phase 0,* Depolarization—rapid influx of sodium. *Phase 1,* Rapid repolarization—rapid efflux of potassium ions and decreased sodium conductance. *Phase 2,* Plateau—slow influx of sodium and calcium ions. *Phase 3,* Repolarization—continued efflux of potassium ions. *Phase 4,* Resting phase—restoration of ionic balance by sodium and potassium pumps.

Table 17-8 Classification of antidysrhythmic agents

Class	Action	Drugs
I	Blocks sodium channels ("stabilizes" cell membrane)	
IA	Blocks sodium channels and delays repolarization, thus lengthening the duration of the action potential	quinidine procainamide disopyramide
IB	Blocks sodium channels and accelerates repolarization, thus shortening the duration of the action potential	lidocaine mexiletine tocainide
IC	Blocks sodium channels and slows conduction through the His-Purkinje system, thus prolonging the QRS duration	flecainide encainide propafenone
II	Blocks beta receptors	acebutolol esmolol propranolol
III	Prolongs the duration of the action potential	amiodarone bretylium sotalol
IV	Blocks calcium channels	verapamil

contractility, with disopyramide having the most potent negative inotropic effect.[55] Drugs in class IB have only a moderate effect on sodium channels and actually accelerate phase 3 repolarization to shorten the action potential duration. Lidocaine, mexiletine, and tocainide belong to this group. Class IC agents are the most potent sodium channel blockers, with little effect on repolarization. Class IC drugs increase both the PR and the QRS intervals. Included in this group are encainide, flecainide, and propafenone. The results of the cardiac arrhythmia suppression trial (CAST) indicate that treatment with encainide and flecainide may be associated with increased mortality and have thus decreased the use of these agents in clinical practice.[57]

◆ **Class II drugs.** Class II drugs are beta-adrenergic blockers (beta blockers). These agents inhibit dysrhythmias mediated by the sympathetic nervous system by competing with endogenous catecholamines for available receptor sites. As a result, spontaneous depolarization during the resting phase (phase 4) is depressed and atrioventricular conduction is slowed. Drugs in this class can be further subdivided into cardioselective (those that block only $beta_1$) and noncardioselective (those that block both $beta_1$ and $beta_2$ receptors). Knowledge of the effects of adrenergic-receptor stimulation allows anticipation of not only the therapeutic responses brought about by beta blockade, but also the potential adverse effects of these agents (Table 17-9). For example, bronchospasm can be precipitated by noncardioselective beta blockers in a patient with chronic obstructive pulmonary disease (COPD) secondary to blocking the effects of $beta_2$ receptors in the lungs. Beta blockers also are negative inotropes and should be used cautiously in patients with left ventricular dysfunction.[58] Although numerous beta blockers are available, only acebutolol, propranolol, and esmolol are approved for the treatment of dysrhythmias. Esmolol (Brevibloc) offers advantages in the critically ill patient because of its short half-life (approximately 9 minutes). It is used in the treatment of supraventricular tachycardias, such as atrial fibrillation and atrial flutter.

◆ **Class III drugs.** Class III agents include amiodarone, bretylium, and sotalol. These agents markedly slow the rate of phase 3 repolarization, increasing the effective refractory period and the action potential duration.

Table 17-9 Effects of adrenergic receptors

Receptor	Location	Response to stimulation
alpha	Vessels of skin, muscles, kidneys, and intestines	Vasoconstriction of peripheral arterioles
$beta_1$	Cardiac tissue	Increased heart rate Increased conduction Increased contractility
$beta_2$	Vascular and bronchial smooth muscle	Vasodilation of peripheral arterioles Bronchodilation

Although their effect on the action potential is similar, these drugs differ greatly in their mechanism of action and their side effects. Bretylium is the only drug in this classification approved for intravenous use. It is used clinically in treating ventricular tachycardia that is refractory to other antidysrhythmic agents, such as lidocaine and procainamide.[59]

◆ **Class IV drugs.** Class IV agents are calcium channel blockers that inhibit the influx of calcium through slow calcium channels during the plateau phase (phase 2). This effect occurs primarily in tissue in which slow calcium channels predominate, primarily in the sinus and atrioventricular (AV) nodes and the atrial tissue. Verapamil (Calan, Isoptin) is the only drug in this category approved for use as an antidysrhythmic. It depresses sinus and AV node conduction and is effective in terminating supraventricular tachycardias caused by AV nodal reentry. Because accessory pathways are not affected by calcium channel blockade, verapamil should not be used in the treatment of Wolff-Parkinson-White syndrome.[55]

◆ **Adenosine.** Adenosine (Adenocard) is a newer antidysrhythmic agent that remains unclassified under the current system. Adenosine occurs endogenously in the body as a building block of adenosine triphosphate (ATP). Given in intravenous boluses, adenosine slows conduction through the AV node, causing transient AV block. It is used clinically to convert supraventricular tachycardias and to facilitate differential diagnosis of rapid dysrhythmias. Side effects are transient because the drug is rapidly taken up by the cells and is cleared from the body within 10 seconds.[60]

◆ **Side effects.** Antidysrhythmic drugs carry the risk of serious side effects, some of which may be life-threatening. The major side effects of the intravenous antidysrhythmic agents are listed in Table 17-10. The most severe complication is the potential for a "prodysrhythmic" effect. This may result in a worsening of the underlying dysrhythmia, the occurrence of a new dysrhythmia, or the development of a bradydysrhythmia. Torsades de pointes is a prodysrhythmia caused by class IA agents.[61] The development of a prodysrhythmia is unpredictable; thus the nurse plays an important role in evaluating ECG changes, monitoring drug levels, and assessing patient symptoms.

Inotropic Drugs

Critically ill patients with compromised cardiac function frequently require the use of medications to enhance myocardial contractility (positive inotropes). Clinically available inotropes include cardiac glycosides, sympathomimetics, and phosphodiesterase inhibitors. These agents increase myocardial contractility, resulting in improved cardiac output, more complete emptying of the ventricles, and decreased filling pressures.

Cardiac glycosides include digitalis and its derivatives. Although these drugs have been used for centuries, their slow onset of action and risk of toxicity make them more appropriate for the management of chronic heart failure.[62] Because digoxin also causes slowing of the sinus rate and a decrease in AV conduction, it may be administered in the acute care setting to control supraventricular dysrhythmias.

Sympathomimetic agents stimulate adrenergic receptors, thereby simulating the effects of sympathetic nerve stimulation. Included in this category are naturally occurring catecholamines (epinephrine, dopamine, and norepinephrine), as well as synthetic catecholamines (dobutamine and isoproterenol). The cardiovascular effects of these drugs, which vary according to their selectivity for specific receptor sites, may be dose-dependent as well.[63] Table 17-11 describes the cardiovascular effects of sympathomimetic drugs at various dosages.

◆ **Dopamine.** Dopamine hydrochloride (Intropin) is one of the most widely used drugs in the critical care setting. It is a chemical precursor of norepinephrine, which, in addition to both alpha and beta receptor stimulation, can activate dopaminergic receptors in the renal and mesenteric blood vessels. The actions of this drug are entirely dose-related.[59] At low dosages of 1 to 2 μg/kg/min, dopamine stimulates dopaminergic receptors, causing renal and mesenteric vasodilation. The resultant increase in renal perfusion increases urinary output. Moderate dosages result in stimulation of $beta_1$ receptors to increase myocardial contractility and improve cardiac output. At dosages greater than 10 μg/kg/min, dopamine predominantly stimulates alpha receptors, resulting in vasoconstriction that often negates both the beta-adrenergic and dopaminergic effects.

◆ **Dobutamine.** Dobutamine hydrochloride (Dobutrex) is a synthetic catecholamine with predominantly $beta_1$ effects. It also produces some $beta_2$ stimulation, resulting in a mild vasodilation. Dobutamine is more effective than is dopamine in increasing myocardial contractility, but it lacks the dopaminergic effects of that drug. Dobutamine is useful in the treatment of heart failure, especially in hypotensive patients who cannot tolerate vasodilator therapy.[59] The usual dosage range is 2.5 to 20 μg/kg/min, titrated on the basis of hemodynamic parameters.

◆ **Epinephrine.** Epinephrine (Adrenalin) is produced by the adrenal gland as part of the body's response to stress. This agent has the ability to stimulate both alpha and beta receptors, depending on the dose administered (see Table 17-11). At doses of 1 to 2 μg/min, epinephrine binds with beta receptors to increase heart rate, cardiac conduction, contractility, and vasodilation, thereby increasing cardiac output. As the dosage is increased, alpha receptors are stimulated, resulting in increased vascular resistance and blood pressure. At these doses epinephrine's impact on cardiac output depends on the heart's ability to pump against the increased afterload. Epinephrine accelerates the sinus rate and may precipitate ventricular dysrhythmias in the ischemic heart. Other side effects include restlessness, angina, and headache.

◆ **Norepinephrine.** Norepinephrine (Levophed) is similar to epinephrine in its ability to stimulate $beta_1$ and alpha receptors, but it lacks the $beta_2$ effects. At low infusion rates $beta_1$ receptors are activated to produce

Table 17-10 Pharmacology of selected antidysrhythmic agents

Drug	Indications	Dosage	Major side effects
Adenosine	Paroxysmal SVT	6 mg IV rapid push, repeat with 12 mg over 1-2 sec; follow with IV fluid (NS or D_5W)	Transient: flushing, dyspnea, hypotension
Lidocaine	Ventricular ectopy; PVC prophylaxis in AMI	50-100 mg bolus followed by continuous infusion of 1-4 mg/min	CNS toxicity
Procainamide	Ventricular ectopy resistant to lidocaine	50 mg IV q 1 min up to 1 g followed by infusion of 1-4 mg/min	Hypotension GI effects Widening of QRS and QT interval Drug-induced lupus syndrome
Propranolol	Supraventricular tachycardia	1-3 mg IV q 5 min not to exceed 0.1 mg/kg	Bradycardia Heart failure Heart block
Amiodarone	Life-threatening ventricular dysrhythmias	5-10 mg/kg slowly IV followed by an infusion of 10 mg/kg/day for 3-5 days	Corneal deposits Slate-gray or bluish skin Photosensitivity Pulmonary fibrosis Thyroid dysfunction
Bretylium	Refractory ventricular fibrillation	5 mg/kg IV bolus followed by 10 mg/kg dosages repeated at 15-30 min intervals for total of 30 mg/kg	Initially: hypertension, tachycardia, PVCs
	Ventricular tachycardia (second-line agent)	500 mg in 50 ml D_5W to infuse over 8-10 min, then continuous infusion at 1-2 mg/min	Subsequently: hypotension, bradycardia, nausea and vomiting
Verapamil	Supraventricular tachycardia	5-10 mg IV over 2 min followed 10 mg in 30 min if needed	Heart failure AV block Bradycardia Dizziness Peripheral edema
Esmolol	SVT	Loading dosage of 500 μg/kg/min over 1 min followed by infusion of 50 μg/kg/min for 4 min; repeat procedure q 5 min, increasing infusion by 25-50 μg/kg/min to maximum of 200 μg/kg/min	Hypotension Nausea

AV, Atrioventricular; *AMI*, acute myocardial infarction; *CNS*, central nervous system; *D_5W*, 5% dextrose in water; *GI*, gastrointestinal; *NS*, normal saline; *PVC*, premature ventricular contraction; *SVT*, supraventricular tachycardia.

increased contractility and thus augment cardiac output. At higher doses the inotropic effects are limited by marked vasoconstriction mediated by alpha receptors. Clinically norepinephrine is used most frequently as a vasopressor to elevate blood pressure in shock states.

◆ **Isoproterenol.** Isoproterenol hydrochloride (Isuprel) is a pure beta receptor stimulant with no alpha effects. It produces dramatic increases in heart rate, conduction, and contractility via $beta_1$ stimulation and vasodilation via $beta_2$ stimulation. Isoproterenol also produces vasodilation of the pulmonary arteries and bronchodilation. It greatly increases the automaticity of cardiac cells and frequently precipitates dysrhythmias, such as premature ventricular contractions and even ventricular tachycardia. These effects limit its usefulness in the compromised heart. Its most common use is as a temporary treatment for symptomatic bradycardia until a pacemaker is available.

◆ **Amrinone.** Phosphodiesterase inhibitors are a new group of inotropic agents that also are potent vasodilators. Drugs in this classification inhibit the enzyme phosphodiesterase, resulting in increased levels of cyclic adenosine monophosphate (AMP) and intracellular calcium. Amrinone (Inocor) is the first of these agents approved for use in the United States. Increases in cardiac output occur as a result of increased contractility (inotropic effects) and decreased afterload (vasodilative effects). Filling pressures tend to decrease, whereas the heart rate and blood pressure remain fairly constant. A loading dose of 0.75 mg/kg is given slowly over 2 to 3

Table 17-11 Physiologic effects of sympathomimetic agents

		Receptor activated				Cardiovascular effects		
Drug	**Dosage**	**alpha**	**beta$_1$**	**beta$_2$**	**dopa**	**CO**	**HR**	**SVR**
Dobutamine	<5 μg/kg/min	0	↑↑↑	↑	0	↑↑	↑	0/↓
	5-15 μg/kg/min	0	↑↑↑	↑↑	0	↑↑↑	↑↑	↓
	>20 μg/kg/min	0	↑↑↑	↑↑	0	↑↑↑	↑↑↑	↓↓
Dopamine	<3 μg/kg/min	0	↑	↑	↑↑↑	0/↑	0/↑	0
	3-10 μg/kg/min	↑	↑↑↑	↑	↑↑↑	↑↑↑	↑	↑
	10-20 μg/kg/min	↑↑↑	↑↑↑	↑	↑↑	↑↑	↑↑	↑↑↑
	>20 μg/kg/min	↑↑↑↑	↑↑	↑	↑	↑	↑	↑↑↑↑
Epinephrine	<2 μg/min	0	↑	↑↑	0	0/↑	0/↑	↓
	2-8 μg/min	↑↑	↑↑↑	↑↑	0	↑↑↑	↑	↑
	8-20 μg/min	↑↑↑	↑↑	↑↑	0	↑↑	↑↑	↑↑
Isoproterenol	1-7 μg/min	0	↑↑↑	↑↑↑	0	↑↑↑	↑↑↑	↓↓↓
Norepinephrine	<2 μg/min	↑↑↑	↑↑	0	0	↑	0/↓	↑↑↑
	2-16 μg/min	↑↑↑↑	↑↑	0	0	↓	↓	↑↑↑↑
Phenylephrine	10-100 μg/min	↑↑↑↑	0	0	0	0/↓	↓	↑↑↑

CO, Cardiac output; *HR*, heart rate; *SVR*, systemic vascular resistance.
0, No effect; ↑, increase; ↓, decrease.

minutes and is followed by a continuous infusion of 5 to 10 μg/kg/min. Because thrombocytopenia has occurred in a small percentage of patients receiving amrinone, platelet counts should be monitored and patients should be observed for hemorrhagic complications.[64]

Vasodilator Drugs

Vasodilators are pharmacologic agents that improve cardiac performance by various degrees of arterial or venous dilation, or both. The goal of vasodilator therapy may be a reduction of preload or afterload, or both. Afterload reduction is accomplished by vasodilation of arterial vessels. This results in decreased resistance to left ventricular ejection and may improve cardiac output without increasing myocardial oxygen demands. Reduction of preload is accomplished by dilating venous vessels to increase capacitance. This results in decreased filling pressures for a failing heart. These drugs may be classified into four groups on the basis of mechanism of action (Table 17-12).

◆ **Direct smooth muscle relaxants.** Direct-acting vasodilators include sodium nitroprusside (Nipride), nitroglycerin (Tridil), and hydralazine (Apresoline). These drugs produce relaxation of vascular smooth muscle, resulting in decreased peripheral vascular resistance. Hypotension may occur as a result of peripheral vasodilation, and headaches may be caused by cerebral vasodilation. Compensatory mechanisms can occur in response to the drop in blood pressure. These include baroreceptor activation that causes reflex tachycardia and activation of the renin-angiotensin system, with resultant sodium and water retention.[65]

Sodium nitroprusside (Nipride) is a potent, rapidly acting venous and arterial vasodilator, particularly suitable for rapid reduction of blood pressure in hypertensive emergencies and perioperatively. It also is effective for afterload reduction in the setting of severe heart failure. The drug is administered by continuous intravenous infusion, with the dosage titrated to maintain the desired blood pressure and systemic vascular resistance (SVR). Prolonged administration can result in thiocyanate toxicity, manifested by nausea, confusion, and tinnitus.[63]

Intravenous nitroglycerin (Tridil) causes both arterial and venous vasodilation, but its venous effect is more pronounced. It is used in the critical care setting for the treatment of acute heart failure (HF) because it reduces cardiac filling pressures, relieves pulmonary congestion, and decreases cardiac workload and oxygen consumption. In addition, nitroglycerin dilates the coronary arteries and is a useful adjunct in the treatment of unstable angina and acute myocardial infarction. The initial dosage is 10 μg/min, and the infusion is titrated upward to achieve the desired clinical effect: a reduction or elimination of chest pain, decreased pulmonary capillary wedge pressure, or a decrease in blood pressure. Nitroglycerin also is administered prophylactically to prevent coronary vasospasm after coronary angioplasty and atherectomy. The most common side effects of this drug include hypotension, flushing, and headache.[66]

Hydralazine (Apresoline) is a potent arterial vasodilator. It seldom is given as a continuous infusion, but rather in intravenously administered dosages of 5 to 10 mg every 4 to 8 hours. Occasionally, hydralazine is given as an intermediate drug in the transition between the weaning of a continuous infusion and the initiation of oral antihypertensive medications. The major side effect is reflex tachycardia mediated by the sympathetic nervous system. This may be diminished by the concomitant administration of beta blockers.

◆ **Calcium channel blockers.** Calcium channel blockers are a chemically diverse group of drugs with differing pharmacologic effects (Table 17-13). *Nifedipine* (Procardia) and other dihydropyridines are used primarily as arterial vasodilators. Nifedipine reduces the influx of calcium in the arterial resistance vessels. Both coronary and peripheral arteries are affected. It is used in the critical care setting to treat severe hypertension. It is available only in an oral form but frequently is prescribed sublingually. Although controversy exists over the absorption of sublingual nifedipine, studies indicate that if the drug is bitten before swallowing, the drug is absorbed more quickly.[67,68] Side effects of nifedipine are related to vasodilation and include hypotension, reflex tachycardia, flushing, headache, and ankle edema. *Verapamil* (Calan, Isoptin) and *diltiazem* (Cardizem) dilate coronary arteries but have little effect on the peripheral vasculature. These drugs are used in the treatment of angina, especially that which has a vasospastic component. Verapamil also is used as an antidysrhythmic in the treatment of supraventricular tachycardias.

◆ **ACE inhibitors.** Angiotensin-converting enzyme (ACE) inhibitors produce vasodilation by blocking the conversion of angiotensin I to angiotensin II. Because angiotensin is a potent vasoconstrictor, limiting its production decreases peripheral vascular resistance. In contrast to the direct vasodilators and nifedipine, ACE inhibitors do not cause reflex tachycardia nor induce sodium and water retention. These drugs may cause a profound fall in blood pressure, especially in patients who are volume-depleted. Blood pressure should be monitored carefully, especially during initiation of therapy.[69] *Captopril* (Capoten) and *enalapril* (Vasotec) are used in patients with heart failure to decrease SVR (afterload) and pulmonary capillary wedge pressure (preload). Captopril is available only in an oral form but has a relatively rapid onset of action (approximately 1 hour). Enalapril is available in an intravenous form and may be used to decrease afterload in more emergent situations.

◆ **Alpha-adrenergic blockers.** Peripheral adrenergic blockers block alpha receptors and veins, resulting in vasodilation. Orthostatic hypotension is a common side effect and may result in syncope. Long-term therapy also may be complicated by fluid and water retention.[68] *Labetalol* (Normodyne), a combined alpha and beta blocker, is used in the treatment of hypertensive emergencies. Because the blockade of $beta_1$ receptors permits the decrease of blood pressure without the risk of reflexive tachycardia and increased cardiac output, this drug also is useful in the treatment of acute aortic dissection.

Table 17-12 Characteristics of selected vasodilators

Classification/drug	Dosage	Effect (↓) Preload	Effect (↓) Afterload	Side effects
DIRECT SMOOTH MUSCLE RELAXANTS				
Sodium nitroprusside (Nipride)	0.25-6 μg/kg/min IV infusion	Moderate	Strong	Hypotension, reflex tachycardia, thiocyanate toxicity
Nitroglycerin (Tridil)	5-300 μg/min IV infusion	Strong	Mild	Headache, reflex tachycardia, hypotension
Hydralazine (Apresoline)	5-10 mg IV q 4 hr	None to mild	Moderate	Reflex tachycardia
CALCIUM CHANNEL BLOCKERS				
Nifedipine (Procardia)	10-30 mg SL	None	Strong	Hypotension, headache, reflex tachycardia
ACE INHIBITORS				
Captopril (Capoten)	6.25-100 mg PO q 8-12 hr	Moderate	Moderate	Hypotension, chronic cough, neutropenia
Enalapril (Vasotec)	0.625 mg IV over 5 min, then q 6 hr	Moderate	Moderate	Hypotension, elevation of liver enzymes
ALPHA-ADRENERGIC BLOCKERS				
Labetolol (Normodyne)	20-80 mg IV bolus q 10 min, then 1-2 mg/min infusion	Moderate	Moderate	Orthostatic hypotension, bronchospasm, AV block
Phentolamine (Regitine)	1-2 mg/min infusion	Moderate	Moderate	Hypotension, tachycardia

ACE, Angiotensin-converting enzyme; *SL*, sublingual.

Table 17-13 Physiologic effects of calcium channel blockers

Drug	Heart rate	Conduction	Contractility	Peripheral dilation	Coronary dilation
Nifedipine (Procardia)	0/↑	0/↑	0	↑↑↑	↑↑↑
Verapamil (Calan, Isoptin)	↓↓	↓↓↓	↓↓	↑	↑↑
Diltiazem (Cardizem)	↓	↓↓	↓	↑	↑↑

0, No change; ↓, decrease; ↑, increase.

Phentolamine (Regitine) is a peripheral alpha blocker that causes decreased afterload via arterial vasodilation. It is given as a continuous infusion at a rate of 1 to 2 mg/min and titrated to achieve the required reduction in blood pressure and SVR.[63] This drug also is used to treat the extravasation of dopamine. If this occurs, 5 to 10 mg is diluted in 10 ml normal saline and administered intradermally into the infiltrated area.

◆ **Vasopressors.** Vasopressors are sympathomimetic agents that mediate peripheral vasoconstriction through stimulation of alpha receptors (see Table 17-10). This results in increased systemic vascular resistance and thus elevates blood pressure. Some of these drugs (epinephrine and norepinephrine) also have the ability to stimulate beta receptors. Vasopressors are not widely used in the treatment of critically ill cardiac patients, because the dramatic increase in afterload is taxing to a damaged heart. Occasionally vasopressors may be used to maintain organ perfusion in shock states. For example, *phenylephrine hydrochloride* (Neo-Synephrine) or *norepinephrine* (Levophed) often is administered as a continuous intravenous infusion to maintain organ perfusion by increasing peripheral vascular resistance in the warm phase of septic shock.

REFERENCES

1. Jackman WM and others: Catheter ablation of accessory atrioventricular pathways (Wolff-Parkinson-White syndrome) by radiofrequency current, *N Engl J Med* 324:1605, 1991.
2. Grogan EW, Nellis SH, Subramanian R: Catheter ablation of ventricular endocardium using radiofrequency energy: determinants of lesion volume and shape, *J Electrophysiol* 3(4):243, 1989.
3. Goy JJ and others: Successful ablation of the AV conduction system with radiofrequency energy after failure of direct current shock catheter ablation, *J Electrophysiol* 3(1):70, 1989.
4. Oeff M and others: Effects of multipolar electrode radiofrequency energy delivery on ventricular endocardium, *Am Heart J* 119(3):599, 1990.
5. Kuck K-H and others: Radiofrequency current catheter ablation of accessory atrioventricular pathways, *Lancet* 337:1557, 1991.
6. Lynn-McHale DJ, Riggs KL, Thurman L: Epicardial pacing after cardiac surgery, *Crit Care Nurse* 11(8):62, 1991.
7. Catalano JT: Dual-chamber pacemaker rhythm, *Crit Care Nurse* 10(3):67, 1990.
8. Bernstein AD and others: The NASPE/BPEG generic pacemaker code for antibradycardia and adaptive rate pacing and antitachyarrhythmia devices, *PACE* 10:794, 1987.
9. Eckhard AH: Implantable devices—pending issues and future trends, *PACE* 13(9):1079, 1990.
10. Kirklin JW and others: ACC/AHA guidelines and indications for CABG surgery, *Circulation* 83:1125, 1991.
11. Green G: Use of internal thoracic artery for coronary artery grafting, *Circulation* 79 (suppl 1):130, 1989.
12. Foster ED, Kranc MAT: Alternative conduits for aortocoronary bypass grafting, *Circulation* 79 (suppl 1):I34, 1989.
13. Livesay JJ, Talledo OJ: The current preference for mitral valve reconstruction, *Texas Heart Institute J* 18(2):87, 1991.
14. Duran CMG, Gometza B, Devol EB: Valve repair in rheumatic mitral disease, *Circulation* 84(suppl 3):125, 1991.
15. Simpson GM: CATR: a new generation of autologous blood transfusions, *Crit Care Nurse* 11(4):60, 1991.
16. Gallo JA, Todd BA: Mediastinitis after cardiac surgery, *Crit Care Nurse* 10(6):64, 1990.
17. Grosso MA, Brown JM, Harken AH: Surgical treatment of cardiac arrhythmias, *Prim Cardiolo*, p . 51, June 1989.
18. Eagen JS: Lasers: applications in cardiovascular disease, *Crit Care Nurs Clin North Am* 1(2):311, 1989.
19. Moser SA, Crawford D, Thomas A: Caring for patients with implantable cardioverter defibrillators, *Crit Care Nurse* 8(2):52, 1988.
20. Brannon PHB, Johnson R: The internal cardioverter defibrillator: patient-family teaching, *Focus Crit Care* 19(1):41, 1992.
21. Akhtar M and others: Role of implantable cardioverter defibrillator therapy in the management of high-risk patients, *Circulation* 85 (suppl 1):I131, 1992.
22. Burke LR, Rodgers BL, Jenkins LS: Living with recurrent ventricular dysrhythmias, *Focus Crit Care* 19(1):60, 1992.
23. Vlietstra RE, Holmes DR: Percutaneous transluminal coronary angioplasty, *J Cardiac Surg* 3:56, 1988.
24. Ryan TJ and others: Guidelines for PTCA: a report of the ACC/AHA task force on assessment of diagnostic and therapeutic cardiovascular procedures (subcommittee on PTCA), *Circulation* 78(2):486, 1988.
25. Topol EJ: Emerging strategies for failed percutaneous transluminal coronary angioplasty, *Am J Cardiol* 63:249, 1989.
26. Safien RD and others: Coronary atherectomy—clinical, angiographic, and histological findings and observations regarding potential mechanisms, *Circulation* 82(1):69, 1990.
27. Good LP, Gentzler RD: Coronary atherectomy—an alternative to balloon angioplasty, *AORN J* 52(1):32, 1991.
28. Vlietstra RE, Brenner AS, Brown KF: Interventional cardiology techniques for coronary artery disease, *J Cardiac Surg* 6(3):415, 1991.
29. Spears JR and others: Percutaneous coronary laser balloon angioplasty: preliminary results of a multicenter trial, JACC 13(2):61A, 1989.
30. Halfman-Franey M, Levine S: Intracoronary stents, *Crit Care Nurs Clin North Am* 1(2):327, 1989.
31. Bevans M, McLimore E: Intracoronary stents: a new approach to coronary artery dilation, *J Cardiovasc Nurs* 7(1):34, 1992.
32. Beattie MS, Geden E: Reducing pain and discomfort following percutaneous transluminal coronary angioplasty, *Dimens Crit Care Nurs* 9(3):150, 1990.
33. TIMI Study Group: Comparison of invasive and conservative strategies after treatment with intravenous tissue plasminogen activator in acute myocardial infarction. Results of the thrombolysis in myocardial infarction (TIMI) phase II trial, *N Engl J Med* 320(10):618, 1989.

34. Ferguson JJ and others: Balloon aortic valvuloplasty, *Texas Heart Institute J* 17(1):23, 1990.
35. Barden C and others: Balloon aortic valvuloplasty: nursing care implications, *Crit Care Nurse* 10(6):22, 1990.
36. Russell AC, Blake SM: Aortic valvuloplasty: potential nursing diagnoses, *Dimens Crit Care Nurs* 8(2):72, 1989.
37. Kawaniski DT, Rahimtoola SH: Catheter balloon commissurotomy for mitral stenosis: complications and results, *JACC* 19(1):192, 1992.
38. Anderson JL: Therapeutic management of acute myocardial infarction, *Am J Hosp Pharm* 47 (suppl 2):S5, Sept 1990.
39. Schieman G and others: Intracoronary urokinase for intracoronary thrombus accumulation complicating PTCA in acute ischemic syndromes, *Circulation* 82(6):2052, 1990.
40. Pan M and others: Balloon valvuloplasty for mild mitral stenosis, *Cathet Cardiovasc Diagn* 24:1, 1991.
41. Saksena S, Parsonnet V: Implantation of a cardioverter defibrillator without thoracotomy using a triple electrode system, *JAMA* 259(1):69, 1988.
42. Sherry S: Unresolved clinical pharmacologic questions in thrombolytic therapy for acute myocardial infarction, *J Am Coll Cardiol* 12(2):519, 1988.
43. Kleven MR: Comparison of thrombolytic agents: mechanism of action, efficacy, and safety, *Heart Lung* 17(6) Part 2:750, 1988.
44. Sherry S: Pharmacology of Anistreplase, *Clin Cardiol* 13(3) Suppl V: V3, 1990.
45. ISIS-2 Collaborative Group: Randomized trial of intravenous streptokinase, oral aspirin, both or neither among 17,187 cases of suspected acute myocardial infarction, *Lancet* 2:349, 1988.
46. Briones TL: Tissue-plasminogen activator: nursing implications, *Dimens Crit Care Nurs* 8(4):203, 1989.
47. Stein B, Roberts R: Current status of thrombolytic therapy in acute myocardial infarction, *Texas Heart Institute J* 18(4):250, 1991.
48. Tiefenbrunn AJ: Clinical benefits of thrombolytic therapy in acute myocardial infarction, *Am J Cardiol* 69(2):3A, 1992.
49. Shoulders-Odom B: Managing the challenge of IABP therapy, *Crit Care Nurse* 11(2):60, 1991.
50. Smalling RW: The use of mechanical assist devices in the management of cardiogenic shock, *Texas Heart Institute J* 18(4):275, 1991.
51. Goran SF: Vascular complications of the patient undergoing intraaortic balloon pumping, *Crit Care Nurs Clin North Am* 1(3):459, 1989.
52. Quaal SJ: VADS: beyond intra-aortic balloon pumping, *Cardiovasc Nurs* 5(1):4, 1992.
53. Smith RG, Cleavinger M: Current perspectives on the use of circulatory assist devices, *AACN Clin Issues Crit Care Nurs* 2(3):488, 1991.
54. Emery RW, Joyce LD: Directions in cardiac assistance, *J Cardiac Surg* 6(3):400, 1991.
55. Stier F: Antidysrhythmic agents, *AACN Clin Issues Crit Care Nurs* 3(2):483, 1992.
56. Woosley RL, Funck-Brentano C: Overview of the clinical pharmacology of antiarrhythmic drugs, *Am J Cardiol* 61:61A, 1988.
57. Anderson JL: Reassessment of the benefit-risk ratio and treatment algorithms for antiarrhythmic drug therapy after the cardiac arrhythmia suppression trial, *J Clin Pharmacol* 30:981, 1990.
58. Weiner B: Hemodynamic effects of antidysrhythmic drugs, *J Cardiovasc Nurs* 5(4):39, 1991.
59. American Heart Association: *Textbook of advanced cardiac life support,* ed 2, Dallas, 1990, The Association.
60. McNulty SA: Pharmacological interventional testing for myocardial perfusion: a new application for adenosine, *Cardiovasc Nurs* 28(4):24, 1992.
61. Podrid PJ: Pharmacologic therapy for arrhythmias: attention to the benefit-risk ratio, *J Clin Pharmacol* 30:975, 1990.
62. Notterdam DA: Inotropic agents: catecholamines, digoxin, amrinone, *Crit Care Clin* 7(3):583, 1991.
63. Clements JV: Sympathomimetics, inotropics, and vasodilators, *AACN Clin Issues Crit Care Nurs* 3(2):395, 1992.
64. Budny J, Anderson-Drew K: IV inotropic agents: dopamine, dobutamine, and amrinone, *Crit Care Nurse* 10:54, 1988.
65. Deglin JH, Deglin S: Hypertension: current trends and choices in pharmacotherapeutics, *AACN Clin Issues Crit Care Nurs* 3(2):507, 1992.
66. Kuhn M: Nitrates, *AACN Clin Issues Crit Care Nurs* 3(2):409, 1992.
67. Kedas A, Shivley M, Burris J: Nursing delivery of sublingual nifedipine, *J Cardiovasc Nurs* 3(4):31, 1989.
68. Kaplan NM: Calcium entry blockers in the treatment of hypertension, 262:817, 1989.
69. Kuhn M: Angiotensin-converting enzyme inhibitors, *AACN Clin Issues Crit Care Nurs* 3(2):461, 1992.

18

Cardiovascular Nursing Diagnosis and Management

This chapter is designed to supplement the preceding chapters in the *Cardiovascular Alterations* unit by integrating theoretic content into clinically applicable case studies and nursing management plans.

The case study is designed to illustrate clinical problem solving and patient care management occurring in actual patients. The case, reviewed retrospectively, demonstrates how medical and nursing diagnoses may be effectively used in critical care. The case study also demonstrates revisions to the plan of care and the nursing and medical management outcomes that are apt to occur during the course of a complicated hospitalization as the patient responds physiologically to treatment. Often in a short case anecdote, such as presented in this chapter, the clinical answer may appear to be obvious from the day of admission. In practice, however, critical care patient management is sometimes investigative and the "correct" diagnosis for an individual patient may not become apparent until midway in the hospitalization. Or a patient with an apparently straightforward diagnosis may develop an unexpected complication, and the plan of care and potential outcomes will then require revision. Many of the case studies demonstrate this principle.

The nursing management plans, which—unlike the case study—are not patient-specific, provide a basis nurses can use to individualize care for their patients. In the previous *Cardiovascular Alterations* chapters, each medical diagnosis is assigned a Nursing Diagnosis and Management box. Using this box as a page guide, the reader can access relevant nursing management plans for each medical diagnosis. For example, nursing management of *endocarditis*, described on p. 300, may involve several nursing diagnoses and management plans outlined in this chapter and in other Nursing Diagnosis and Management chapters. Specific examples are (1) *Activity Intolerance related to decreased cardiac output secondary to valvular dysfunction*, on p. 366; (2) *High Risk for Infection risk factor: invasive monitoring devices,*, p. 366; (3) *Knowledge Deficit: Home Intravenous Medication Regimen related to lack of previous exposure to information*, on p. 72; and (4) *Altered Health Maintenance related to lack of perceived threat to health*, on p. 70. These examples highlight the interrelationship of the various physiologic systems in the body and the fact that pathology often has a multisystem impact in the critically ill.

Use of the case study and management plans can enhance the understanding and application of the *Cardiovascular* content in clinical practice.

CARDIOVASCULAR PHYSICAL ASSESSMENT CASE STUDY

CLINICAL HISTORY

Mrs. C is a 68-year-old white woman with history of coronary artery disease and hypertension. She has an 8-year history of exertional angina, which became unstable 3 weeks ago. A myocardial infarction (MI) was ruled out, and a cardiac catheterization procedure was performed, revealing significant obstruction in the left anterior descending (LAD) artery and in the right coronary artery (RCA) with an ejection fraction of 35%. She received coronary artery bypass grafting (CABG) to the LAD and RCA. Her postoperative course was uneventful until postoperative day 4.

She returned to the critical care unit from the medical/surgical ward, with acute shortness of breath and a rapid pulse reported to be 124 beats per minute.

CURRENT PROBLEMS

Mrs. C was lying in bed with the head of bed (HOB) elevated. Her expression was anxious. Her color was pale, and she was diaphoretic. She stated she felt extremely weak and in the past 12 hours became short of breath (SOB) with only mild exertion.

Clinical data were as follows: Ht., 5'8"; Wt., 160 lbs. (10 lbs. more than preoperative weight according to medical record); BP, 104/70; HR, 115/irreg; respiratory rate (RR), 28/min; assessment with HOB elevated to 30 degrees revealed jugular venous distention (JVD) and an estimated central venous pressure (CVP) of 12 cm H_2O by jugular venous pulsation.

Continued.

CARDIOVASCULAR PHYSICAL ASSESSMENT CASE STUDY—cont'd

Bilateral lower extremity edema was present. There was a surgical wound on the left leg, groin to ankle.

Lung sounds were decreased in the right lower lobe (RLL) and absent in the left lower lobe (LLL). There were no crackles and no production with coughing. Room air O_2 saturation was 90%.

Heart sounds S_1 and S_2 were normal; there was no S_3. No murmurs were heard; pericardial friction rub was present.

Laboratory data included the following: Hemogloblin (Hgb), 10.8 g/dl; Hematocrit (Hct), 31.3%; Sodium, 149 mEq/L; Potassium 4.4 mEq/L; Chloride 105 mEq/L; Bicarbonate 26 mEq/L; Urea nitrogen 17 mg/dl; Creatinine 1.2 mg/dl; and Glucose 98 mg/dl. Room air arterial blood gas (ABG) values were: pH 7.48; Po_2, 62 mm Hg; Pco_2, 47 mm Hg; bicarbonate, 25 mEq. 12-lead electrocardiogram (ECG) showed atrial fibrillation with ventricular response of 128 beats per minute. Chest X-ray examination demonstrated new pulmonary vascular congestion and large left pleural effusion since CABG.

MEDICAL DIAGNOSES

Heart failure
Atrial fibrillation

NURSING DIAGNOSES

- Decreased Cardiac Output related to relative excess of preload and afterload secondary to impaired ventricular contractility
- Impaired Gas Exchange related to ventilation/perfusion mismatch secondary to pulmonary vascular congestion
- Activity Intolerance related to decreased cardiac output and/or myocardial tissue perfusion alterations
- Anxiety related to threat to biologic, psychologic, and/or social integrity

◆ PLAN OF CARE

1. In collaboration with MD, administer diuretics to decrease preload and fluid volume excess and digoxin to decrease ventricular response rate to atrial fibrillation.
2. Decrease fluid intake; maintain strict I&O record.
3. Monitor vital signs and physical examination for response to treatment or continued deterioration.
4. Provide oxygen therapy with O_2 saturation monitoring to improve oxygenation without suppressing respiratory drive.
5. See that patient maintains strict bedrest in position of comfort to decrease energy expenditure.
6. Explain symptoms and management of care to reduce anxiety.

MEDICAL AND NURSING MANAGEMENT AND PATIENT OUTCOME

After 40 mg furosemide was given intravenously, the patient urinated 300 ml in the next hour. The atrial fibrillation converted to sinus tachycardia 110/min.

The physical examination revealed the following: BP, 80/60; HR, 110/regular; RR 28/min.

Patient continued to be diaphoretic with a change in mental status. Her lips appeared cyanotic.

She complained of SOB at rest and requested HOB to be elevated more.

JVD was present with HOB elevated to 45 degrees.

Hepatojugular reflux was present.

CVP was estimated at 18 cm H_2O using the internal jugular vein pulsation with the HOB elevated to 45 degrees.

Auscultation of breath sounds revealed crackles in lower one third of right lung.

O_2 saturation was 88% on 2 L O_2 via nasal prongs.

Heart sound S_1 and S_2 were normal; S_3 was present; no murmurs were heard. A pericardial friction rub was present.

MEDICAL DIAGNOSIS

Heart failure

NURSING DIAGNOSIS

- Decreased Cardiac Output related to excessive preload and afterload secondary to impaired ventricular contractility

◆ REVISED PLAN OF CARE

Insert pulmonary artery (PA) catheter.

CARDIOVASCULAR PHYSICAL ASSESSMENT CASE STUDY—cont'd

MEDICAL AND NURSING MANAGEMENT AND PATIENT OUTCOME

Pulmonary artery catheter readings were as follows: RA, 8; PA, 30/15; PAWP, 15 mm Hg. The catheter monitor readout showed good waveform for all pressures, but the pressures did not correlate with the physical assessment of JVD, estimated CVP of 18 cm H_2O, hepatojugular reflux, $+S_3$, and subjective symptoms. The height of the transducer was found to be higher than phlebostatic axis level. Once the transducer was lowered, the PA catheter readings were the following: RA, 13 mm Hg; PA, 60/26 mm Hg; PAWP 25 mm Hg.

Dopamine IV at 2 micrograms/kg/min and dobutamine IV at 5 micrograms/kg/min. were started. Urine output increased to 2500 ml over the next 8 hours, and the PA catheter readings were RA, 8; PA, 40/15; PAWP, 15 mm Hg. The patient's JVD disappeared, and subjectively she felt less SOB. Her ABGs with 2 L O_2 via nasal prongs were the following: pH, 7.44; Po_2, 86 mm Hg; Pco_2, 42 mm Hg; and bicarbonate, 26 mEq. Her cardiac rhythm remained in sinus with a ventricular rate of 96 beats per minute. The dobutamine was discontinued after 10 hours, and the patient was able to be weaned from the dopamine and oxygen within 24 hours. She left the critical care unit and continued postoperative CABG cardiac rehabilitation in preparation for discharge.

CARDIOVASCULAR SURGICAL CASE STUDY

CLINICAL HISTORY

Mr. H is a 70-year-old white man. He has a long history of coronary artery disease with associated ventricular dysrhythmias as described as follows:

1. Inferior wall myocardial infarction (MI) in 1955
2. Coronary artery bypass surgery (CABG) using vein grafts in 1980
3. Atherectomy to unblock one vein graft in 1988 (under investigational protocol)
4. Recurrent ventricular tachycardia (VT) at rate of 160/min in 1990; patient's VT poorly controlled on multiple antidysrhythmic medications
5. Development of first-degree heart block in 1990
6. Placement of implantable cardioverter defibrillator (ICD) in 1991 as protection against sudden cardiac death; the ICD device has antitachycardia capability in addition to cardioversion/defibrillation functions.

CURRENT PROBLEMS

Recently Mr. H developed unstable angina. He underwent a cardiac catheterization. This showed severe coronary artery disease in three native vessels, with progressive disease in the vein grafts and a posterior basilar aneurysm at the site of the old inferior MI. Because of his continued episodes of VT, Mr. H also underwent an electrophysiology (EP) study. The EP study included an endocardial catheter map of the ventricle to locate the focus of the VT. The EP study showed atypical left bundle/left axis VT arising from an area adjacent to the site of the inferior MI. The ICD also was tested and was functioning correctly.

MEDICAL DIAGNOSES

Coronary artery disease
Ventricular tachycardia

NURSING DIAGNOSES

- ◆ Acute Pain related to transmission and perception of cutaneous, visceral, muscular, or ischemic impulse secondary to ventricular tachycardia
- ◆ Anxiety related to threat to biologic, psychologic, and/or social integrity, secondary to VT and impending surgery

◆ PLAN OF CARE

Mr. and Mrs. H discussed with the cardiologist, surgeon, and electrophysiologist that Mr. H should be admitted to the hospital for a redo coronary artery bypass graft operation with a plan to use the internal mammary arteries. Because of the recurrent ventricular tachycardia and poorly controlled VT despite antidysrhythmic medications and ICD, Mr. H would also undergo ventricular cryoablation of the focus of his VT during the open heart surgery procedure.

Continued

CARDIOVASCULAR SURGICAL CASE STUDY—cont'd

MEDICAL AND NURSING MANAGEMENT AND PATIENT OUTCOME

Mr. H underwent open heart surgery with cardiopulmonary bypass (CPB) that involved CABG using both right and left internal mammary arteries and cryoablation of VT foci. Mr. H returned from the operating room to the critical care unit in stable condition after surgery. The nursing assessment revealed the following:

Neuro: Mr. H remained sedated and nonresponsive postanesthesia.

Resp: He was intubated and ventilated. Lungs were clear to auscultation, with bilateral breath sounds.

CV: Heart rate of 120, sinus tachycardia with occasional PVCs. Atrial and ventricular epicardial pacing wires were present. The wires were connected to a temporary pacemaker generator, which was turned off. (Temporary epicardial pacing wires are routinely inserted at the time of cardiac surgery). The ICD was programmed "on." The ICD will either pace, cardiovert, or defibrillate, depending on the specific dysrhythmia. There was a pulmonary artery catheter with side-port, a radial arterial line, and a peripheral IV in situ. His hemodynamics were stable: MAP, 60 mm Hg; CVP, 6 mm Hg; pulmonary artery wedge pressure (PAWP), 10mm Hg; cardiac output (CO), 2.9 L/min; cardiac index (CI), 1.87 L/min/m^2; systemic vascular resistance (SVR), 1659 dynes/sec/cm^{-5}.

Mr. H was bleeding via the mediastinal chest tubes (200 ml/hr).

Integument/Temp: Skin was cool and dry with palpable peripheral pulses. Initial core temperature was 35.3° C. (The low temperature was expected after cardiopulmonary bypass [CPB], and Mr. H was expected to rewarm and vasodilate in the next 6 to 8 hours.)

Medications: IV drips were dopamine at 3.0 mcg/kg/min; sodium nitroprusside (SNP) at 0.6 mcg/kg/min; and nitroglycerin at 66 mcg/min.

GI: Nasogastric tube was in place to decompress stomach; there was minimal bile-colored drainage. No bowel sounds were present.

GU: A large volume of dilute urine drained via the urinary catheter (400 ml/hr). This was secondary to diuretics given at the end of cardiopulmonary bypass.

Lab: Hematocrit (Hct), 28.9%; platelets, 98,000; glucose, 146 mg/dl; K^+, 3.2 mEq/L (replaced); magnesium, 1.9 mEq/L; prothombin time (PT), 15.9 secs or 47%; partial thromboplastin time (PTT), 38 seconds; and fibrinogen 129 mg/dl.

MEDICAL DIAGNOSES

CABG and ventricular cryoablation
ICD (previous surgery)

NURSING DIAGNOSES

- ◆ Hypothermia related to cold environment secondary to cardiopulmonary bypass and cardioplegia
- ◆ Fluid Volume Deficit related to active blood loss
- ◆ Decreased Cardiac Output related to surgery and high SVR
- ◆ High Risk for Decreased Cardiac Output related to ventricular dysrhythmias

◆ REVISED PLAN OF CARE

1. Increase body temperature by using warm blankets.
2a. (first intervention) Replace fluid lost as a result of bleeding, urine output, and rewarming, by CPB cell-saver, and plasmanate (blood not given at this time because Hct is greater than 25%).
2b. (second intervention) Slow bleeding by correcting prolonged coagulation times by administration of IV coagulation products: fresh frozen plasma, cryoprecipitate, and platelets.
3. Increase cardiac output by correcting the fluid volume deficit and decreasing SVR.
4. Continue to monitor for dysrhythmias.

CARDIOVASCULAR SURGICAL CASE STUDY—cont'd

MEDICAL AND NURSING MANAGEMENT AND PATIENT OUTCOME

Eight hours after return from surgery Mr. H was awake and had been medicated for incisional pain. His core temperature had risen to 38.3° C, and his periphery (hands and feet) was warm. Fluid volume replacement had been effective, and hemodynamic filling pressures had increased: MAP, 75-80 mm Hg; CVP, 18 mm Hg; PAWP, 22 mm Hg. In a patient with a previously damaged heart from an MI, higher filling pressures are often necessary to optimize contractility (Starling's law).

Four hours after surgery mediastinal bleeding had slowed to 50 ml/hr after administration of the IV coagulation products. Because of the clinical improvement, coagulation factors were not retested.

The cardiac output had increased to 5.12 L/min; cardiac index, 3.3 L/min/m^2; and SVR, 732 dynes/sec/cm^{-5}. The nurse had maintained the dopamine drip at a constant rate, but had increased the SNP to 1.2 mcg/kg/min. The increased SNP combined with rewarming had decreased SVR and raised CO effectively.

One hour after his return from surgery Mr. H's heart rate slowed to a sinus rhythm (79 bpm) with demonstration of his chronic first-degree heart block and bundle branch block. Because his cardiac output and peripheral perfusion remained stable, the nurse continued to monitor the situation. No treatment was given at that time. Two hours later Mr. H had a short burst of VT (6 beats). The VT was self terminating. The nurse informed the MD and continued to monitor the rhythm. No treatment was given at that time. Six hours later the heart rhythm deteriorated into a second-degree heart block, Mobitz type II. The nurse immediately turned on the temporary pacemaker generator that was connected to the epicardial pacing wires, and Mr. H was successfully AV-paced at a rate of 88 paced-bpm.

MEDICAL DIAGNOSES

CABG
Second-degree heart block
Ventricular dysrhythmias

NURSING DIAGNOSIS

◆ Decreased Cardiac Output related to second-degree AV heart block and ventricular tachycardia

◆ REVISED PLAN OF CARE

1. Maintain AV-paced rhythm while second-degree heart block is evaluted.
2. Continue to monitor cardiac rhythm while ventricular dysrhythmias are evaluated.

MEDICAL AND NURSING MANAGEMENT AND PATIENT OUTCOME

The remainder of Mr. H's stay in the ICU was uneventful. On the first postoperative day the endotracheal tube was removed without difficulty. His hemodynamics remained stable. IV drips were weaned off and were replaced by oral afterload-reducing medications. On the second postoperative day chest tubes were removed without problems and Mr. H was transferred out of the critical care unit to the telemetry cardiac surveillance unit the same day.

Because Mr. H's second-degree heart block persisted, he remained on the telemetry unit, AV-paced with a temporary generator. To protect Mr. H from the consequences of further deterioration in his conduction system, the cardiologist implanted a permanent, dual-chamber (DDD) pacemaker before Mr. H was discharged from the hospital.

MEDICAL DIAGNOSES

CABG
Ventricular dysrhythmias
Second-degree heart block
Permanent pacemaker

NURSING DIAGNOSIS

◆ Knowledge Deficit: Discharge for CABG, Permanent Pacemaker, and Antidysrhythmic Drugs related to lack of previous exposure to information

◆ REVISED PLAN OF CARE

Provide discharge teaching to Mr. H and his wife for his home care. Topics should include CABG surgery and cardiac risk factor modification, instructions on his pacemaker, and information on the effects of the antidysrhythmic drugs.

MEDICAL AND NURSING MANAGEMENT AND PATIENT OUTCOME

Mr. H received discharge teaching from both the CV nurse specialist and staff nurses in the days before his discharge from the hospital. The CABG was successful in eliminating Mr. H's angina. The ventricular dysrhythmias were more effectively controlled after the cryoablation. In addition, with the combination of the permanent pacemaker, the implantable cardioverter defibrillator, and adjusted antidysrhythmic medications, Mr. H's risk of sudden death caused by dysrhythmias was significantly decreased.

DECREASED CARDIAC OUTPUT RELATED TO SUPRAVENTRICULAR TACHYCARDIA

DEFINING CHARACTERISTICS

- Sudden drop in blood pressure
- Atrial and/or ventricular rate >100 bpm
- Decreased mentation
- Decreased urine output
- Chest pain
- Dyspnea

OUTCOME CRITERIA

- Systolic blood pressure (SBP) is >100 mm Hg.
- Mean arterial pressure (MAP) is >70 mm Hg.
- Ventricular heart rate is <100 bpm.
- Sensorium is intact.
- Urine output is >30 ml/hr.

NURSING INTERVENTIONS AND *RATIONALE*

1. Continue to monitor the assessment parameters listed under "Defining Characteristics."
2. Carefully distinguish supraventricular tachycardia from ventricular tachycardia. Monitoring the patient in lead V_1 or MCL_1, ***may assist in distinguishing ventricular ectopy from aberrancy.***
3. Follow critical care emergency standing orders regarding the administration of supraventricular antidysrhythmic agents, such as verapamil, quinidine, procainamide, propranolol, digoxin, and adenosine.
4. Consider positioning patient supine ***to increase preload.***
5. Identify precipitating factors when possible, such as emotional stress, caffeine, nicotine, and sympathomimetic drugs and intervene to reduce or eliminate their effect.
6. Assess apical-radial pulse ***to identify deficits indicating nonperfused beats.*** Monitor amplitude of peripheral pulses ***to ascertain perfusion to extremities.***
7. Monitor arterial blood pressure ***to determine symptomatic decompensation.***
8. With physician collaboration, consider carotid sinus massage or Valsalva maneuver, ***thereby increasing vagal tone.***
9. Anticipate possibility of synchronized cardioversion or overdrive pacing.
10. For atrial fibrillation that is either spontaneously, pharmacologically, or electrically converted, monitor for signs of cerebral, pulmonary, and/or peripheral thromboembolization as a result of liberation of mural thrombi.
11. If patient is hypoxemic or if dysrhythmia is suspected to be a result of or exacerbated by ischemia, administer oxygen observing the following principles:
    - Without physician collaboration, liter flow should be no greater than 2 L/min via nasal prongs in patients whose pulmonary history either is unknown or reveals a pattern of chronic CO_2 retention. ***Administration of oxygen at concentrations higher than 2 L/min via nasal prongs may induce CO_2 narcosis in patients who chronically retain CO_2.***
    - Oxygen should be administered with the goal of achieving ***an oxygen saturation (Sao_2) above 92% when measured by pulse oximetry or ABGs.***
    - Observe caution when administering oxygen at an FIo_2 greater than 40% ***in view of the higher risk for oxygen toxicity.***
12. Assess serum electrolyte levels, especially potassium and calcium, ***because increased or decreased electrolyte levels may exacerbate the dysrhythmia or may impair treatment of the dysrhythmia.***

DECREASED CARDIAC OUTPUT RELATED TO RELATIVE EXCESS OF PRELOAD AND AFTERLOAD SECONDARY TO IMPAIRED VENTRICULAR CONTRACTILITY

DEFINING CHARACTERISTICS

- Systolic blood pressure (SBP) <100 mm Hg
- Mean arterial pressure (MAP) <80 mm Hg
- Change in mentation
- Decreased urine output
- Cardiac index (CI) < 2.2 L/min/m^2
- Pulmonary artery wedge pressure (PAWP) >15 mm Hg
- Pulmonary artery diastolic pressure (PAD) >15 mm Hg
- Bibasilar fluid crackles
- Faint peripheral pulses
- Ventricular gallop rhythm (S_3)
- Skin cool, pale, moist
- Activity intolerance

OUTCOME CRITERIA

- Cardiac index is 2.2-4.0 L/min/m^2.
- SBP is >90 mm Hg.
- MAP is >80 mm Hg.
- PAWP and PAD are <15 mm Hg.

Relative excess of preload and afterload refers not to an actual increase in these volumes, but rather to the ability of the ventricle to handle normal volumes because of impaired ventricular function. Therefore the normal volumes become "excessive" to the poorly functioning ventricle.

DECREASED CARDIAC OUTPUT RELATED TO RELATIVE EXCESS OF PRELOAD AND AFTERLOAD SECONDARY TO IMPAIRED VENTRICULAR CONTRACTILITY—cont'd

NURSING INTERVENTIONS AND *RATIONALE*

The following interventions reduce preload

1. Continue to monitor the assessment parameters listed under "Defining Characteristics."
2. Implement fluid restriction.
3. Double concentrate intravenous drug drips when possible ***to decrease the amount of volume infused to the patient.***
4. Position patient with extremities dependent ***to pool blood in the extremities, thus decreasing preload.***
5. With physician collaboration, administer diuretics.
6. Titrate venous vasodilators and inotropic drips, per protocol, to desired SBP, MAP, PAWP, and/or PAD. Withhold and/or change drip rate when SBP, MAP, PAWP, and/or PAD begin to drop.

The following interventions reduce afterload

1. Intervene to reduce anxiety and ***thereby limit catecholamine release:*** administer intravenous MSO_4 per protocol and titrate to MAP or SBP, relaxation techniques, imagery (See care plan on Anxiety, Chapter 48).
2. Titrate arterial vasodilator drips to attain desired SBP, PAWP, and/or PAD. Change drip rate when SBP, PAWP, and/or PAD stabilize or begin to drop.
3. Anticipate possibility of intraaortic balloon pumping.

The following interventions reduce myocardial oxygen consumption

1. Absolute bed rest ***to decrease metabolic demand.***
2. Consider slackening activity restrictions if such restrictions precipitate anxiety. ***Anxiety stimulates the sympathetic outpouring of catecholamines and thereby increases myocardial oxygen consumption.***
3. Ensure that patient and family understand routine of critical care unit and explain all care given to patient ***to increase patient comfort level and to decrease catecholamine release associated with fear of being in an unknown environment.***

DECREASED CARDIAC OUTPUT RELATED TO DECREASED PRELOAD SECONDARY TO MECHANICAL VENTILATION WITH OR WITHOUT PEEP

DEFINING CHARACTERISTICS

- ◆ Sudden drop in SBP, PAWP, or PAD corresponding to the application of mechanical ventilation or PEEP, or changes in tidal volume delivery or level of PEEP.

OUTCOME CRITERIA

- ◆ SBP is >90 mm Hg; MAP is >70 mm Hg.
- ◆ PAWP, PAD are > 6 mm Hg.

NURSING INTERVENTIONS AND *RATIONALE*

1. Continue to monitor the assessment parameters listed under "Defining Characteristics."
2. Monitor vital organ perfusion (through assessment of urine output and mentation, for example) carefully, ***because some degree of reduction in cardiac output will coexist with the successful application of mechanical ventilation and/or PEEP.***
3. Position patient supine ***to increase preload and therefore cardiac output.***
4. With physician collaboration, consider increasing the administration of parenteral fluids to achieve ideal preload. (***The ideal preload may be that which existed before the application of mechanical ventilation and/or PEEP.)***

DECREASED CARDIAC OUTPUT RELATED TO ATRIOVENTRICULAR (AV) HEART BLOCK

DEFINING CHARACTERISTICS

- ◆ Systolic blood pressure (SBP) < 100 mm Hg
- ◆ Mean arterial pressure (MAP) < 80 mm Hg
- ◆ Ventricular rate < 60 bpm
- ◆ Decreased mentation or syncope
- ◆ Decreased urine output

OUTCOME CRITERIA

- ◆ Systolic blood pressure is > 90 mm Hg.
- ◆ MAP is >70 mm Hg.
- ◆ Ventricular rate is > 60 bpm.
- ◆ The patient is awake and responsive.
- ◆ Urine output is >30 ml/hr.

NURSING INTERVENTIONS AND *RATIONALE*

First-degree AV block

1. Continue to monitor the assessment parameters listed under "Defining Characteristics."
2. Monitor closely, measuring P-R intervals ***to determine further prolongation, which would suggest progression of heart block.***
3. With physician collaboration, consider withholding supraventricular antidysrhythmic agents such as digitalis, quinidine, beta blocking agents, and calcium channel blockers.

Continued.

DECREASED CARDIAC OUTPUT RELATED TO ATRIOVENTRICULAR (AV) HEART BLOCK—cont'd

Second-degree AV block—Mobitz I (Wenckebach pattern)

1. Continue to monitor the assessment parameters listed under "Defining Characteristics."
2. Monitor for symptomatic decompensation resulting from slow ventricular rate (rare).
3. While symptomatic, position patient supine ***to increase preload and therefore cardiac output.***
4. Monitor for progression to complete heart block.
5. With physician collaboration, consider withholding digitalis.
6. Eliminate sources of vagal stimulation. ***Vagal stimulation increases the delay in conduction at the AV node.***

Second-degree AV block—Mobitz II

1. Continue to monitor the assessment parameters listed under "Defining Characteristics."
2. Monitor closely for symptomatic decompensation as a result of slow ventricular rate (common).
3. While symptomatic, position patient supine ***to increase preload and therefore cardiac output.***
4. Monitor for progression of existing block, such as 2:1, 3:1, 4:1 conduction, and for progression to complete heart block.
5. Follow critical care emergency standing orders regarding the administration of positive chronotropic agents, such as atropine, or isoproterenol.
6. Anticipate possibility of temporary transvenous pacemaker insertion.

Third-degree (complete) AV block

1. Continue to monitor the assessment parameters listed under "Defining Characteristics."
2. Monitor closely for symptomatic decompensation resulting from slow ventricular rate (common).
3. While symptomatic, position patient supine ***to increase preload and therefore cardiac output.***
4. Follow critical care emergency standing orders regarding the administration of isoproterenol.
5. Anticipate the necessity of pacemaker insertion or use of external pacemaker (e.g., Pace-Aid).

DECREASED CARDIAC OUTPUT RELATED TO HEMOPERICARDIUM (TAMPONADE) SECONDARY TO OPEN HEART SURGERY

DEFINING CHARACTERISTICS

- Cardiac output (CO) < 5.0 L/min
- Cardiac index (CI) < 2.2 L/min/m^2
- Elevated PAWP, PAD, or CVP
- Narrowed pulse pressure
- Pulsus paradoxus
- Muffled heart sounds
- Distended neck veins
- Decreasing SBP or MAP
- Tachycardia
- Enlarged cardiac silhouette on chest film

OUTCOME CRITERIA

- Cardiac output is > 5.0 L/min.
- Cardiac index is > 2.2 L/min/m^2.
- PAWP, PAD, CVP are reduced to baseline.
- Crisp heart sounds are heard.
- SBP is > 100 mm Hg; MAP is > 70 mm Hg.
- Heart rate is reduced to baseline.
- Cardiac silhouette is reduced to baseline.

NURSING INTERVENTIONS AND *RATIONALE*

1. Continue to monitor the assessment parameters outlined under "Defining Characteristics."
2. Monitor mediastinal chest tube drainage for sudden cessation and/or increase. ***Either event is to be considered highly suggestive of impending cardiac tamponade.***
3. Milk mediastinal chest tubes per protocol ***to ensure continual patency.***
4. Titrate vasodilator drips ***to keep SBP below level at which graft(s) or anastomoses may leak or tear (usually SBP kept < 130 mm Hg).***
5. Anticipate the necessity of either bedside pericardiocentesis or return to surgery.

DECREASED CARDIAC OUTPUT RELATED TO DECREASED PRELOAD SECONDARY TO FLUID VOLUME DEFICIT

DEFINING CHARACTERISTICS

- CO < 5.0 L/min
- CI < 2.2 L/min/m^2
- PAWP, PAD, CVP less than normal or less than baseline
- Tachycardia
- Narrowed pulse pressure
- SBP < 100 mm Hg
- Mean arterial pressure (MAP) < 70 mm Hg
- Urine is < 30 ml/hr.
- Skin pale, cool, moist
- Apprehensiveness

OUTCOME CRITERIA

- CO is > 5.0 L/min.
- CI is > 2.2 L/min/m^2.
- PAWP, PAD, CVP are normal or back to baseline level.
- Pulse is normal or back to baseline.
- SBP is > 90 mm Hg.
- MAP is > 70 mm Hg.
- Urine is > 30 ml/hr.

NURSING INTERVENTIONS AND *RATIONALE*

For active blood loss

1. Continue to monitor the assessment parameters listed under "Defining Characteristics." In addition, a serum lactate level > 3 mosm is believed to represent cellular perfusion failure at its earliest stage.
2. Secure airway and administer oxygen.
3. Position patient supine with legs elevated ***to increase preload and therefore cardiac output.*** Avoid Trendelenburg's position ***because this position causes abdominal viscera to exert pressure against the diaphragm, thereby limiting diaphragmatic descent and inhalation.*** Consider low Fowler's position with legs elevated for patients with head injury ***to avoid increases in intracranial pressure.***
4. For fluid repletion use the 3 : 1 rule, replacing 3 parts of fluid for every unit of blood lost.
5. Administer solutions using the fluid challenge technique: infuse precise amounts of fluid (usually 5 to 20 ml/min) over 10-minutes periods and monitor cardiac loading pressures serially to determine successful challenging. If the PAWP or PAD elevates more than 7 mm Hg above beginning level, the infusion should be stopped. If the PAWP or PAD rises only to 3 mm Hg above baseline, or falls, another fluid challenge should be given.
6. Assess for signs and symptoms of fluid overload once fluid replacement has begun. These may include elevations above normal of PAP or CVP levels, pulmonary crackles, or dyspnea.
7. Replace fluids first before considering use of vasopressors, ***since vasopressors increase myocardial oxygen consumpton out of proportion to the reestablishment of coronary perfusion in the early phases of treatment.***
8. When blood available or indicated, replace with fresh packed red cells and fresh-frozen plasma ***to keep clotting factors intact.***
9. Move or reposition patient minimally ***to decrease or limit tissue oxygen demands.***
10. Evaluate patient's anxiety level and intervene via patient education or sedation ***to decrease tissue oxygen demands.***
11. Be alert to the possibility of development of adult respiratory distress syndrome (ARDS) and/or disseminated intravascular coagulation (DIC) in the ensuing 72 hours.

For dehydration

1. Continue to monitor the assessment parameters listed under "Defining Characteristics."
2. Position patient supine with legs elevated ***to increase preload and therefore cardiac output.*** Avoid Trendelenburg's position, because this position causes abdominal viscera to exert pressure against the diaphragm thereby limiting diaphragmatic descent and inhalation. Consider low Fowler's position with legs elevated for patients with head injury ***to avoid increases in intracranial pressure.***
3. Calculate the patient's 24-hour fluid requirements per BSA and replace with the appropriate electrolyte solution.
4. Administer solutions using the fluid challenge technique: infuse precise amounts of fluid (usually 5 to 20 ml/min) over 10-minute periods and monitor cardiac loading pressure serially to determine successful challenging. If the PAWP or PAD elevates more than 7 mm Hg above beginning level, the infusion should be stopped. If the PAWP or PAD rises only to 3 mm Hg above baseline, or falls, another fluid challenge should be given.
5. Assess for signs and symptoms of fluid overload once fluid replacement has begun. These may include, elevations of PAP or CVP to above normal levels, pulmonary crackles, or dyspnea.
6. Replace fluids first before considering use of vasopressors, ***since vasopressors increase myocardial oxygen consumption out of proportion to the reestablishment of coronary perfusion in the early phases of treatment.***

DECREASED CARDIAC OUTPUT RELATED TO VENTRICULAR TACHYCARDIA

DEFINING CHARACTERISTICS

- Sudden drop in blood pressure
- Syncope
- Loss of consciousness
- Faint or absent peripheral pulses

OUTCOME CRITERIA

- Systolic blood pressure (SBP) is > 90 mm Hg.
- Mean arterial pressure (MAP) is > 70 mm Hg.
- The patient is awake and responsive.
- Peripheral pulses are palpable.

NURSING INTERVENTIONS AND *RATIONALE*

1. Continue to monitor the assessment parameters listed under "Defining Characteristics."
2. Carefully distinguish ventricular tachycardia from supraventricular tachycardia. Monitoring the patient in lead V_1 or MCL_1, ***may assist in distinguishing ventricular ectopy from aberrancy.***
3. Monitor and treat the "warning dysrhythmias" (i.e., >6 premature ventricular contractions [PVCs] per minute, multifocal PVCs, R on T phenomenon, couplets, bursts of ventricular tachycardia, bigeminy, trigeminy).
4. Assess serum electrolyte levels (potassium/magnesium) and arterial blood gases (ABGs), ***because altered electrolytes, acid-base imbalance, and hypoxemia may exacerbate the dysrhythmia or may impair effectiveness of treatment.***
5. Follow critical care emergency standing orders regarding the administration of ventricular antidysrhythmic agents, such as lidocaine, bretylium, and procainamide.
6. For asymptomatic ventricular tachycardia, treat with lidocaine. For symptomatic ventricular tachycardia, treat with synchronized cardioversion. For pulseless ventricular tachycardia, treat as ventricular fibrillation and defibrillate. (See ACLS algorithms in Appendix B.)
7. Position patient supine ***to increase preload.***
8. Anticipate possibility that sporadic ventricular dysrhythmias may progress to ventricular tachycardia or ventricular fibrillation and be prepared to treat with implementation of synchronized cardioversion and defibrillation, respectively.
9. Anticipate possibility of cardiac standstill and activation of resuscitation protocol.
10. When safe rhythm is reestablished, carefully assess for femoral and carotid pulsations ***to rule out electromechanical dissociation.***
11. Identify precipitating factors when possible, such as hypoxia, electrolyte abnormalities, drug toxicity (especially amrinone, digitalis, quinidine, disopyramide, procainamide, phenothiazines, tricyclic and tetracyclic antidepressants), or recent MI, and intervene to reduce or eliminate their effect.

DECREASED CARDIAC OUTPUT RELATED TO DECREASED PRELOAD SECONDARY TO SEPTICEMIA

DEFINING CHARACTERISTICS

- Tachycardia > 100 bpm
- Skin dry, warm, flushed (early stage); cold, clammy, cyanotic (late stage)
- CO, CI, elevated (early stage); CO, CI, decreased (late stage)
- PA pressures decreased (early stage); elevated (late stage)
- SBP, MAP, less than normal or baseline (early); profound hypotension (late stage)
- Urine output < 30 ml/hr

OUTCOME CRITERIA

- Heart rate is normal or back to baseline.
- CO is > 5.0 L/min; CI is > 2.2 L/min/m²; SBP is > 90 mm Hg; MAP is > 70 mm Hg.
- Urine output > 30 ml/hr.

NURSING INTERVENTIONS AND *RATIONALE*

1. Continue to monitor the assessment parameters listed under "Defining Characteristics." In addition, a serum lactate level > 3 mosm is believed to represent cellular perfusion failure at its earliest stage.
2. Secure airway and administer oxygen.
3. Position patient supine with legs elevated ***to increase preload and therefore cardiac output in late-stage shock.***
4. Administer intravenous solutions as prescribed using the fluid challenge technique: infuse precise amounts of fluid (usually 5 to 20 ml/min) over 10-minute periods and monitor cardiac loading pressures serially to determine successful challenging. If the PAWP or PAD elevates more than 7 mm Hg above beginning levels, the infusion should be stopped. If the PAWP or PAD rises only to 3 mm Hg above baseline, or falls, another fluid challenge should be given.
5. Assess for signs and symptoms of fluid overload once fluid replacement has begun. These may include elevations above normal of PAP or CVP levels, pulmonary crackles, or dyspnea.
6. With physician collaboration, administer intravenous antimicrobials and closely monitor their effectiveness and specific side effects. Carefully assess patient for hypersensitivty reaction to antimicrobials.
7. With physician collaboration, administer vasopressor agents and positive inotropic drugs ***to maintain perfusion and cardiac output.***

DECREASED CARDIAC OUTPUT RELATED TO VASODILATION AND BRADYCARDIA SECONDARY TO SYMPATHETIC BLOCKADE OF NEUROGENIC (SPINAL) SHOCK AFTER SPINAL CORD INJURY ABOVE T6 LEVEL

DEFINING CHARACTERISTICS

- Postural hypotension, such as turning from supine to prone
- SBP < 90 mm Hg or below patient's norm
- Decreased PAP, PAD, and PAWP
- Decreased cardiac index
- Decreased SVR
- Bradycardia
- Cardiac dysrhythmias
- Decreased urinary output
- Hypothermia as a result of inability to retain body heat (See section on Neurological Alterations for the assessment and treatment of other neurological manifestations of spinal shock.)

OUTCOME CRITERIA

- SBP is > 90 mm Hg or within patient's norm.
- Fainting/dizziness with position change is absent.
- <10 mm Hg DBP drop with position change.
- HR is 60-100 beats/min.
- <20 beats/min HR increase with position change.
- CVP is 4 to 6 mm Hg.
- PAWP is 4 to 12 mm Hg.
- PAD is 8 to 14 mm Hg.
- SVR is 950 to 1300 dynes/sec/cm^{-5}.
- Cardiac index (CI) is 2.2 to 4.0 L/min/m^2.
- Urinary output is > 30 ml/hr.
- Body temperature is normal.

NURSING INTERVENTIONS AND *RATIONALE*

1. Continue to monitor the assessment parameters listed under "Defining Characteristics."
2. Implement measures ***to prevent episodes of postural hypotension.***
   - Change patient's position slowly.
   - Apply antiembolic stockings ***to promote venous return.***
   - Perform range-of-motion exercises every 2 hours ***to prevent venous pooling.***
   - Collaborate with physical therapy personnel regarding use of a tilt table ***to progress patient from supine to upright position.***
3. Administer crystalloid intravenous fluids using fluid challenge technique: infuse precise amounts of fluid (usually 5 to 20 ml/min) over 10-minute periods; monitor cardiac loading pressures serially to determine successful challenging.
4. Anticipate the administration of colloids.
5. Anticipate administration of vasopressors if fluid challenges ineffective.
6. Monitor cardiac rhythm. Be especially vigilant during vagal stimulating procedures such as suctioning ***because serious bradycardia can result.***
7. Administer atropine per critical care emergency standing orders for symptomatic sinus bradycardia.
8. Maintain normothermia by increasing temperature in patient's room and applying blankets. Avoid use of electric warming devices ***because of decreased peripheral blood flow and sensation.***

HIGH RISK FOR ALTERED PERIPHERAL TISSUE PERFUSION RISK FACTOR: HIGH-DOSE VASOPRESSOR THERAPY

RISK FACTORS

- Vasopressor therapy

DEFINING CHARACTERISTICS

- Pale or cyanotic digits
- Ischemic pain
- Delayed capillary refill
- Weak peripheral pulses

OUTCOME CRITERIA

- Digits are free from pallor or cyanosis.
- Ischemic pain is absent.
- Capillary refill is immediate.
- Peripheral pulses are full and equal.

NURSING INTERVENTIONS AND *RATIONALE*

1. Continue to monitor the assessment parameters listed under "Defining Characteristics."
2. Careful evaluation of the adequacy of peripheral perfusion is essential in patients receiving infusions of the following vasopressor drugs. In addition, ***extravasation of these agents into tissues results in localized ischemic necrosis and therefore the drugs are infused through central lines when possible.*** Dopamine infusions: at dosages >10 mcg/kg/min, alpha adrenergic receptors are stimulated ***producing moderate peripheral vasoconstriction;*** at dosages > 20 μg/kg/min, intense peripheral vasoconstriction results, ***producing serious perfusion alterations.*** Levarterenol bitartrate infusions: at all dosages alpha adrenergic receptors are stimulated ***producing the potential for perfusion alterations.***
3. Avoid high-dose vasopressor therapy. Titrate vasopressor drips to achieve and maintain SBP of 90 mm Hg or MAP above 70 mm Hg. Further augmentation of SBP or MAP should be accomplished by means of other modalities.
4. Immediate physician notification is indicated at the earliest sign of peripheral perfusion alterations.

HIGH RISK FOR ALTERED PERIPHERAL TISSUE PERFUSION RISK FACTOR: ORTHOPEDIC INJURY OR DEVICE APPLIED TO AN EXTREMITY

RISK FACTORS

- Orthopedic injury or manipulation of an extremity
- Orthopedic devices applied to an extremity

DEFINING CHARACTERISTICS

- Weak and/or unequal peripheral pulses
- Delayed capillary refill
- Ischemic pain distal to injury/manipulation/device
- Cool skin distal to injury/manipulation/device
- Paresthesias

OUTCOME CRITERIA

- Peripheral pulses are full and equal bilaterally.
- Capillary refill is equal bilaterally.
- There is no ischemic pain distal to injury/manipulation/device.
- There is equal skin temperature distal to injury/manipulation/device.
- Paresthesias are absent.

NURSING INTERVENTIONS AND *RATIONALE*

1. Continue to monitor the assessment parameters listed under "Defining Characteristics."
2. Elevate extremity above heart level ***to promote venous and lymphatic drainage, thereby reducing interstitial swelling.***
3. Apply ice over or bedside area of injury or manipulation for the first 24 hours. Follow a schedule of ice on 20 minutes, off 20 minutes, repeat. ***This optimizes the therapeutic effect of ice in prevention and/or reducing swelling.***
4. Maintain patency of wound drainage device ***to prevent excessive interstitial swelling or blood accumulation.***
5. Assess dressings for fit and loosen if constrictive to superficial blood vessels.

ALTERED MYOCARDIAL TISSUE PERFUSION RELATED TO ACUTE MYOCARDIAL ISCHEMIA SECONDARY TO CORONARY ARTERY DISEASE (CAD)

DEFINING CHARACTERISTICS

- Angina for more than 30 min but less than 6 hr
- ST segment elevation on 12-lead ECG
- Elevation of CK and CK-MB enzymes
- Apprehension

OUTCOME CRITERIA

- Systolic blood pressure (SBP) is >100 mm Hg.
- Mean arterial pressure (MAP) is >70 mm Hg.
- Ventricular heart rate is <100 bpm.
- PAP pressures are within normal limits or back to baseline.
- Cardiac index is >2.2 L/min/m^2
- Urine output is >30 ml/hr.
- 12-lead ECG is normalized without new q waves.
- Angina is absent.
- CK and CK-MB enzymes are within normal range.
- Patient and family are educated about coronary artery disease (CAD) risk factor modification.

NURSING INTERVENTIONS AND *RATIONALE*

Continue to monitor the assessment parameters listed under "Defining Characteristics."

The following interventions control pain.

1. In collaboration with the physician administer sublingual nitroglycerin (NTG) and start an intravenous (IV) NTG infusion. Titrate IV NTG ***to control pain.*** Maintain SBP >90 mm Hg.
2. Administer morphine sulfate IV.

The following interventions are to lyse clot in coronary artery.

1. In collaboration with physician, if appropriate for patient, infuse thrombolytic agent of choice ***to lyse clot in coronary artery.*** Maintain SBP at >90 mm Hg.
2. Infuse IV heparin and assess coagulation studies (ACT or PTT) per hospital protocol ***to prevent recurrent thrombosis.***
3. Administer low dose aspirin (80 mg to 325 mg) p.o.

Monitor hemodynamic/cardiac rhythm status.

1. Monitor cardiac rhythm for presence of dysrhythmias. Assess serum electrolytes (potassium and magnesium) and arterial blood gases (AGBs). Correct any imbalance. Administer lidocaine IV (1 mg/kg body weight) if PVCs are >6/min.
2. In case of cardiac/respiratory arrest, follow ACLS/hospital protocols. Have cardioversion/defibrillation equipment nearby.
3. Monitor SBP ***because many conditions (drugs, dysrhythmias, myocardial ischemi) may cause hypotension (SBP <90 mm Hg).***
4. If clinical condition deteriorates, a pulmonary artery (PA) catheter may be required. Be prepared to assist with insertion of PA catheter and to assess hemodynamic profile (PA pressures, PAWP, CO, and CI).
5. In collaboration with the physician, if appropriate for the patient, titrate additional vasodilator medications (sodium nitroprusside) or inotropic medications (dopamine, dobutamine) to maintain SBP >90 mm Hg and CI >2.2 L/min/m^2.

ACTIVITY INTOLERANCE RELATED TO POSTURAL HYPOTENSION SECONDARY TO PROLONGED IMMOBILITY, NARCOTICS, VASODILATOR THERAPY

DEFINING CHARACTERISTICS

- SBP drop > 20 mm Hg; heart rate increase > 20 bpm on postural change
- Vertigo on postural change
- Syncope on postural change

OUTCOME CRITERIA

- SBP drop is < 10 mm Hg; heart rate increase is < 10 bpm on postural change.
- Vertigo or syncope is absent on postural change.

NURSING INTERVENTIONS AND *RATIONALE*

1. Continue to monitor the assessment parameters listed under "Defining Characteristics."
2. ***To increase muscular and vascular tone,*** instruct and assist in the following bed exercises: straight leg raises, dorsiflexion/plantar flexion, and quadriceps setting and gluteal setting exercises.
3. Determine that the patient is hydrated to 24-hour fluid requirements per BSA ***to increase preload and thus stroke volume and cardiac output.*** Hydrate accordingly if not contraindicated by cardiac or renal disorders.
4. Assist with postural changes accomplished in increments:
   - Head of bed to 45 degrees and hold until symptom free
   - Head of bed (HOB) to 90 degrees and hold until symptom free
   - Dangle until symptom free
   - Stand until symptom free and ambulate
5. As soon as it is medically safe, assist patient to sit at bedside for meals.
6. When treating pain with narcotic analgesics, plan ambulation to occur well before peak action of drug.

ACTIVITY INTOLERANCE RELATED TO KNOWLEDGE DEFICIT OF ENERGY-SAVING TECHNIQUES

DEFINING CHARACTERISTICS

- Dyspnea on exertion
- Subjective fatigue on activity
- Heart rate elevations 30 bpm above baseline on activity; heart rate 15 bpm above baseline on activity for patients on beta blockers or calcium channel blockers

OUTCOME CRITERIA

- The patient has subjective tolerance of activity.
- Heart rate elevations are < 20 bpm above baseline on activity and are < 10 bpm above baseline on activity for patients on beta blockers or calcium channel blockers.

NURSING INTERVENTIONS AND *RATIONALE*

1. Continue to monitor the assessment parameters listed under "Defining Characteristics."
2. Teach and supervise energy-saving techniques based on the principle of performing work on exhalation, that is, standing up from a bed or chair, repositioning self in bed with or without help, reaching, washing face, brushing hair or teeth.
3. To the extent possible, have the patient perform work while seated.
4. Teach and supervise muscle-toning exercises, ***observing that a toned muscle uses less oxygen***, such as arm bends with elbows down, elbow bends with arms up, straight arm raises inward and outward, plantar flexion and dorsiflexion of the feet, straight leg raises.

ACTIVITY INTOLERANCE RELATED TO DECREASED CARDIAC OUTPUT AND/OR MYOCARDIAL TISSUE PERFUSION ALTERATIONS

DEFINING CHARACTERISTICS

- Heart rate elevations 30 bpm above baseline on activity; heart rate elevations 15 bpm above baseline on activity for patients on beta blockers or calcium channel blockers
- Heart rate elevations above baseline 5 minutes after activity
- Ischemic pain on activity
- Electrocardiographic changes on activity
- Subjective fatigue on activity

OUTCOME CRITERIA

- Heart rate elevations are <20 bpm above baseline on activity and are <10 bpm above baseline on activity for patients on beta blockers or calcium channel blockers.
- Heart rate returns to baseline 5 minutes after activity.
- Ischemic pain is absent on activity.
- The patient has subjective tolerance to activity.

NURSING INTERVENTIONS AND *RATIONALE*

1. Continue to monitor the assessment parameters listed under "Defining Characteristics."
2. Encourage active or passive range-of-motion exercises while the patient is in bed ***to keep joints flexible and muscles stretched.*** Teach patient to refrain from holding breath while performing exercises, ***avoiding Valsalva maneuver.***
3. Encourage performance of muscle-toning exercises at least 3 times daily, ***because a toned muscle uses less oxygen when performing work than an untoned muscle.***
4. Progress ambulation.
5. Teach patient pulse taking ***to determine activity tolerance:*** take pulse for full minute before exercise, then for 10 seconds and multiply by 6 at exercise peak.

HIGH RISK FOR INFECTION RISK FACTOR: INVASIVE MONITORING DEVICES

RISK FACTOR

- Invasive monitoring devices

DEFINING CHARACTERISTICS

- Fever of undetermined origin
- Tachycardia
- Elevated white blood cell count
- Reddened, inflamed catheter insertion sites
- Drainage from catheter insertion sites

OUTCOME CRITERIA

- Patient is afebrile.
- HR is within range of baseline.
- Catheter insertion sites are clear and dry.

NURSING INTERVENTIONS AND *RATIONALE*

NOTE: *The rationale for each of the following interventions is the avoidance of contamination and colonization of invasive lines and is based on national standards and supported with research.*

1. Continue to monitor the assessment parameters listed under "Defining Characteristics."
2. Practice handwashing—consisting of 15 seconds using mechanical friction and soap and water—before drawing blood or any line manipulation in which the closed system is interrupted.
3. Secure catheters to prevent piston movement (in and out).
4. Maintain an occlusive, sterile dressing. Gauze dressings over arterial lines are recommended.
5. Eliminate all nonessential stopcocks.
6. A different anatomic site should be selected for each catheter inserted.
7. Use uniform, prepackaged, sterile transducer/pressure monitoring and flush assembly.
8. A sterile gown should be worn when inserting central lines. For skin preparation, clean the skin with iodofor. Wear gloves, mask, and cap and use sterile drapes.
9. Use sterile normal saline as the flush solution.
10. To the extent possible, limit blood drawing by obtaining all specimens at the same time.
11. After obtaining a sample of blood, the stopcock should be flushed with saline to clear. All ports should be capped when not in use.
12. Transparent, occlusive dressings should be changed every 72 hours or when integrity is disrupted. Gauze dressings should be changed every 24 hours or sooner if soiled, saturated, or disrupted. Change IV tubing every 72 hours and IV fluids every 24 hours.
13. Catheters inserted in an emergency, without proper asepsis, should be removed and, if necessary, replaced under aseptic conditions.
14. At any sign of infection (localized pain, inflammation, sepsis, fever of undetermined origin), catheters should be removed and cultured.

V

PULMONARY ALTERATIONS

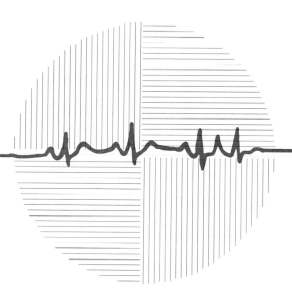

19

Pulmonary Anatomy and Physiology

CHAPTER OBJECTIVES

- Identify the anatomy of the thorax, conducting airways, and respiratory airways.
- Explain the pleural membranes and why the lungs stay inflated.
- Outline the organization of the pulmonary blood and lymph supply.
- Describe the process of ventilation and how it is regulated.
- Discuss the process of internal and external respiration.

The pulmonary system consists of the thorax, conducting airways, respiratory airways, and pulmonary blood and lymph supply. The primary function of the pulmonary system is gas exchange, that is, the movement of oxygen from the atmosphere into the blood stream and the movement of carbon dioxide from the blood stream into the atmosphere. The anatomic structures that constitute the pulmonary system are intimately related to function, and structural abnormalities can readily translate into pulmonary disorders; thus an applicable knowledge of anatomy and physiology is imperative in pulmonary care.

THORAX

The thorax contains the major organs of respiration. It consists of the thoracic cage, lungs, pleura, and muscles of ventilation. Together these structures form the ventilatory pump, which performs the work of breathing.

Thoracic Cage

The thoracic cage is a cone-shaped structure that is rigid but flexible. It must be somewhat rigid to protect the underlying structures, yet it also must be flexible to accommodate inhalation and exhalation. The cage consists of 12 thoracic vertebrae, each with a pair of ribs. Posteriorly each rib is attached to its own vertebra, but anteriorly attachment varies (Fig. 19-1). The first seven pairs of ribs are attached directly to the sternum. The eighth, ninth, and tenth pairs are attached by cartilage to the ribs above. The eleventh and twelfth ribs have no anterior attachment and for this reason they sometimes are referred to as *floating ribs.* The second rib is attached to the sternum at the angle of Louis, which is the raised ridge that can be felt just below the suprasternal notch.[1]

Lungs

The lungs are cone-shaped. The superior portion is known as the *apex* and the inferior portion is known as the *base.* The apical portion of each lung rises a few centimeters above the clavicle (see Fig. 19-1). Each lung is firmly attached to the thoracic cavity at the hilum and at the pulmonary ligament.[1]

The lungs are divided into lobes and segments. Lobes are separated by pleural membrane-covered fissures. The right lung, which is larger and heavier than the left, is divided into upper, middle, and lower lobes. The left lung is divided into only an upper and a lower lobe. A portion of the left lung, the lingula, corresponds anatomically with the right middle lobe. The horizontal fissure divides the right upper lobe from the right middle lobe. The oblique fissure divides the right upper and middle lobes from the lower lobe and the left upper lobe from the lower lobe. The lobes are divided into 18 segments, each of which has its own bronchus branching immediately off a lobar bronchus. Ten segments are located in the right lung and eight in the left lung.[1]

The area between the two lungs, the mediastinum, contains the heart, great vessels, lymphatics, and esophagus. A portion of the mediastinal area contains the hilum, also known as the *root* of the lungs, in which the visceral and parietal pleura form a sheath around the main-stem bronchi, the major blood vessels, and the nerves that enter and exit the lungs.[1]

Pleura

The pleura is a thin membrane that lines the outside of the lungs and the inside of the chest wall. The visceral pleura adheres to the lungs, extending onto the hilar bronchi and into the major fissures. The parietal pleura lines the inner surface of the chest wall and mediastinum. The two pleural surfaces are separated by the airtight pleural space, which contains a thin layer of lubricating fluid.[2]

Both the visceral and parietal pleurae have a blood and lymphatic supply through which they secrete and absorb fluid. Normally there is a continuous filtration of fluid from the capillaries of the parietal pleura into the capillaries of the visceral pleura (Fig. 19-2). At any one time only 3 to 5 ml remains within the pleural space because the fluid is constantly secreted and absorbed, with the excess fluid removed by the lymphatic system.[3] Approximately 1 to 2 L of fluid moves across the pleural space each day.[4] Pleural fluid allows the visceral and

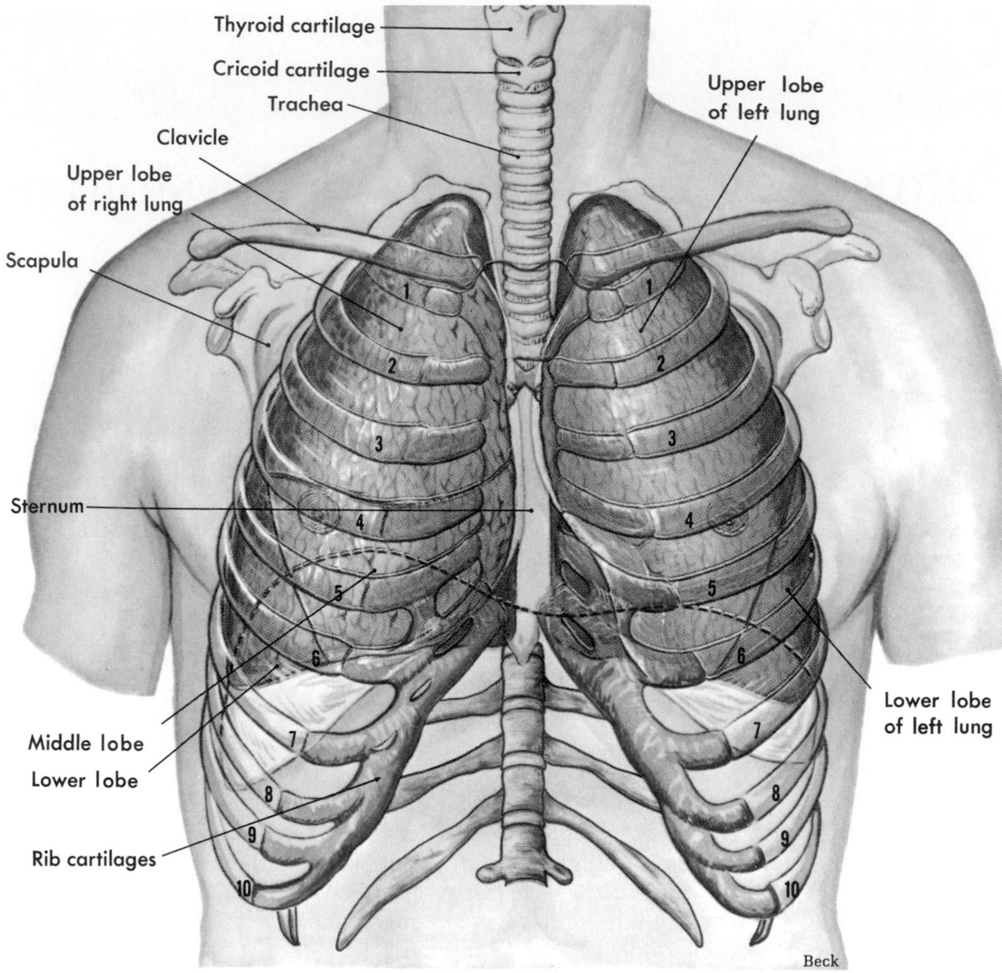

Fig. 19-1 Ventilatory structures of the chest wall and lungs, showing ribs (numbered) and lobes of the lungs. Each intercostal space takes the number of the rib above it. The dotted line indicates the location of the diaphragm at inhalation and exhalation. Note the apex of each lung rising above the clavicle. (From Thibodeau GA: *Anthony's textbook of anatomy and physiology,* ed 13, St Louis, 1990, Mosby–Year Book.)

parietal pleural membranes to glide against each other during inhalation and exhalation. Patients who have experienced a loss of pleural fluid or inflammation of the pleural space (pleuritis) often report severely painful breathing.

Two important characteristics distinguish the pleural space. First, the pleural space has a pressure within it termed *intrapleural pressure,* which differs in value from intraalveolar and atmospheric pressures. Second, the pleural space has the capacity to hold much more fluid than its normal volume of a few milliliters.

Normally, intrapleural pressure is less than intraalveolar pressure and less than atmospheric pressure. Intraalveolar pressure, also known as *intrapulmonary pressure,* reflects the pressure inside the lungs. Atmospheric pressure, in pulmonary physiology, is assigned a value of zero; any pressure less than atmospheric pressure is negative, and any pressure greater than atmospheric pressure is positive.[5] To simplify terminology, *zero* is used in reference to atmospheric pressure. Atmospheric pressure at sea level is approximately 760 mm Hg; intrapleural pressure and intrapulmonary pressure vary from slightly above to slightly below 760 mm Hg.[1,2]

Under normal conditions intrapleural pressure is less than atmospheric pressure, with a normal range of -4 cm H_2O to -10 cm H_2O during exhalation and inhalation, respectively (Fig. 19-3). A deep inhalation can generate intrapleural pressures of -12 to -18 cm H_2O. This negative intrapleural pressure results from forces within the chest wall that exert pressure to pull the parietal pleura outward and away from the visceral pleura while the elastic fibers within the lungs exert pressure to pull the visceral pleura inward away from the parietal pleura. The constant "pull" of the two pleural membranes in opposite directions from each other causes the pressure within the space to be subatmospheric.[6] It is the negative pressure in the pleural space that keeps the lungs inflated (see box, p. 373). If atmospheric pressure enters the pleural space, all or part of a lung will collapse, producing a pneumothorax.

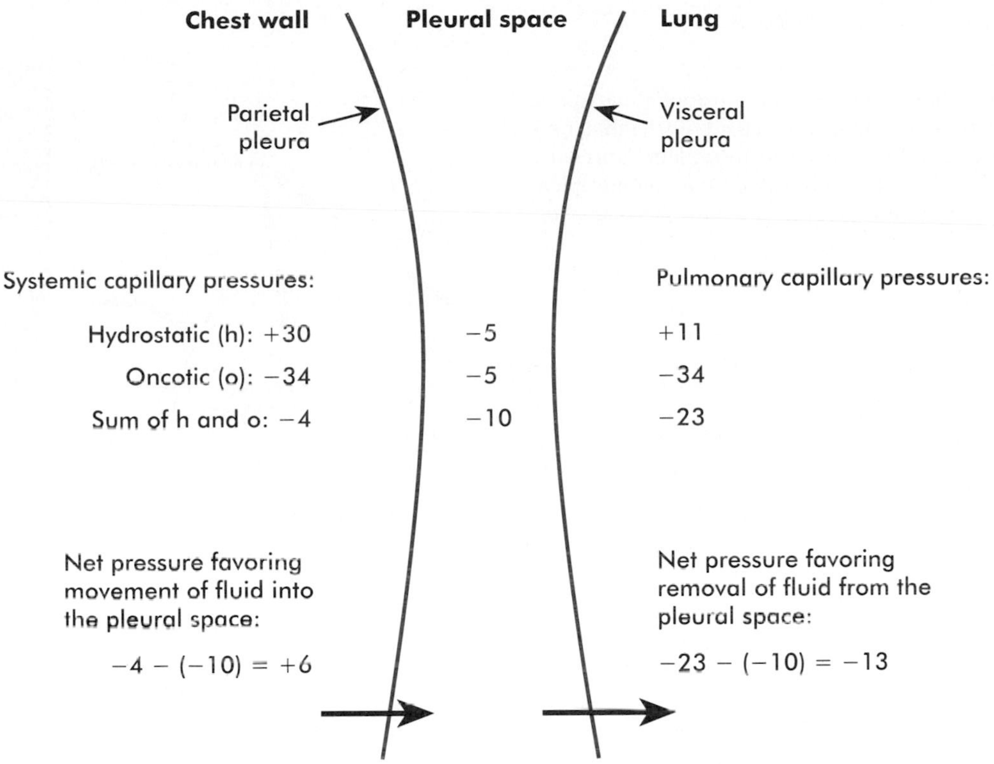

Fig. 19-2 Normal pleural fluid movement. A physiologic balance between the systemic and pulmonary capillaries provides continuous movement of fluid from parietal pleural capillaries into the pleural space and then into the visceral pleural capillaries. All pressures are in cm H_2O. Pressures that tend to force fluid out of the capillaries are shown with a plus (+) sign; pressures that tend to hold fluid in the capillaries or pleural space are shown with a minus (−) sign. A net +6 cm H_2O pressure favors fluid movement into the pleural space, and a net −13 cm H_2O pressure favors removal of fluid from the pleural space. In this diagram the two pleural membranes are shown apart, but in healthy persons the membranes touch, separated only by a thin (and radiologically invisible) film of pleural fluid. (From Martin L: *Pulmonary physiology in clinical practice: the essentials for patient care and evaluation,* St Louis, 1987, Mosby–Year Book.)

Muscles of Ventilation

The muscles of ventilation (Fig. 19-4) are governed by the regulatory activity of the medulla oblongata, which sends messages to the muscles to stimulate contraction and relaxation. This muscular activity controls inhalation and exhalation. Muscles that increase the size of the chest are termed *muscles of inhalation;* those that decrease the size of the chest are termed *muscles of exhalation.*

◆ **Muscles of inhalation.** The main muscle of inhalation is the diaphragm. The diaphragm is a dome-shaped fibromuscular septum that separates the thoracic and abdominal cavities. It is connected to the sternum, ribs, and vertebrae. During normal, quiet breathing the diaphragm does approximately 80% of the work of breathing. On inhalation the diaphragm contracts and flattens, pushes down on the viscera, and displaces the abdomen outward. Diaphragmatic contraction also lifts and expands the rib cage to some extent.[1,2,7]

The action of the diaphragm is governed by the medulla oblongata, which sends its impulses through the phrenic nerve. The phrenic nerve arises from the cervical plexus through the fourth cervical nerve, with secondary contributions by the third and fifth cervical nerves. For this reason and because the diaphragm does most of the work of inhalation, trauma involving C3 to C5 levels causes ventilatory dysfunction.[1]

Other muscles of inhalation include those that lift the rib cage. The most important of these are the external intercostal muscles, which elevate the ribs and expand the chest cage outward. In addition, the scalene, anterior serratus, and sternocleidomastoid muscles also participate to elevate the first two ribs and sternum.[1,6]

◆ **Muscles of exhalation.** Exhalation in the healthy lung is a passive event requiring very little energy. Exhalation occurs when the diaphragm relaxes and moves back up toward the lungs. The intrinsic elastic recoil of the lungs assists with exhalation.

Because exhalation is a passive act, there are no true muscles of exhalation other than the internal intercostal muscles, which assist the inward movement of the ribs. During exercise, however, exhalation becomes a more active event, requiring some participation of the acces-

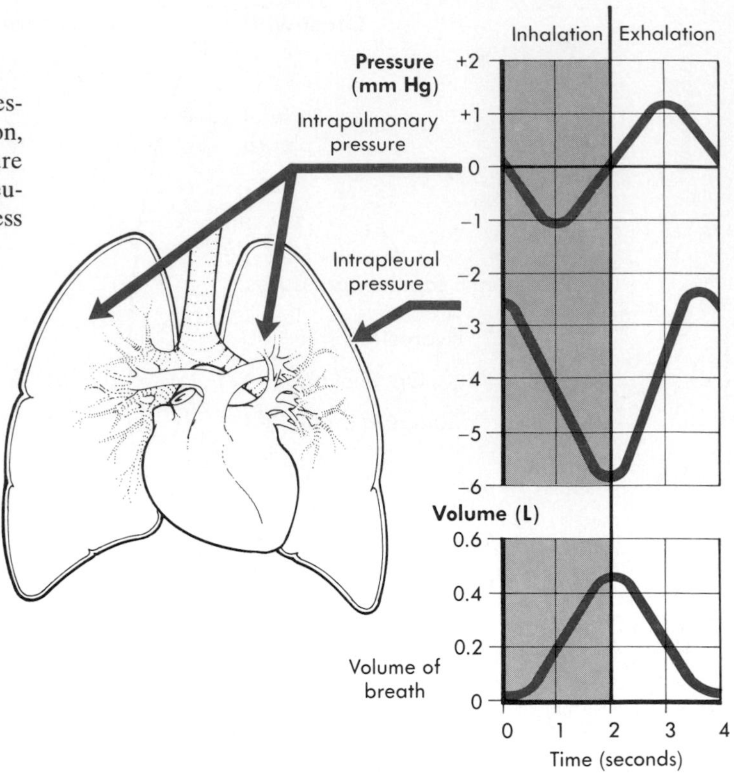

Fig. 19-3 Changes in intrapleural and intrapulmonary pressure during inhalation and exhalation. Just before inhalation, the intrapulmonary pressure falls and intrapleural pressure becomes more negative. Just before exhalation, the intrapleural pressure rises and intrapleural pressure becomes less negative.

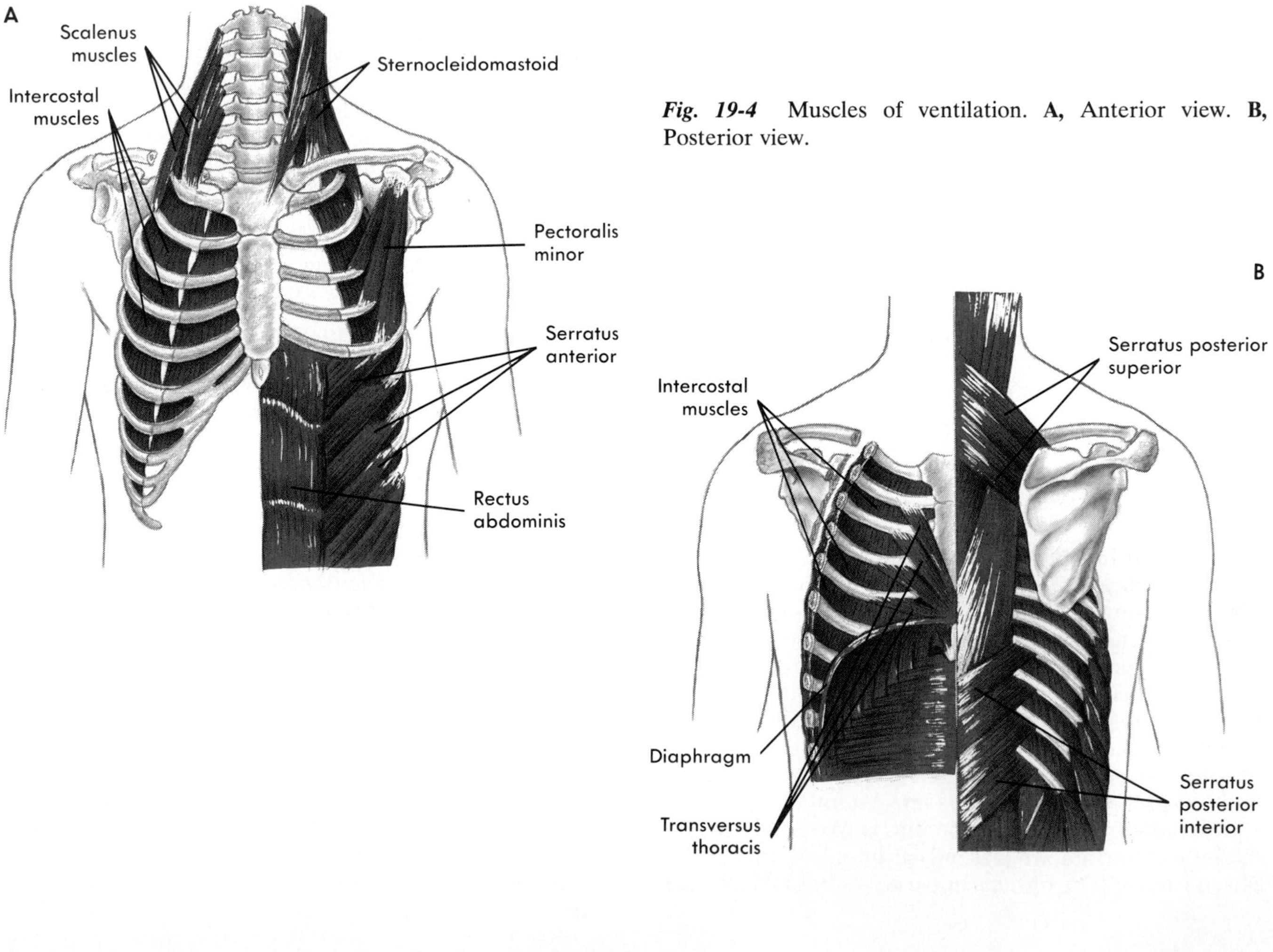

Fig. 19-4 Muscles of ventilation. **A,** Anterior view. **B,** Posterior view.

WHY THE LUNGS STAY INFLATED

The lungs stay inflated because the pressure surrounding them (intrapleural) is always less than the pressure within them (intrapulmonary).

WHY IS THE INTRAPLEURAL PRESSURE LESS THAN THE INTRAPULMONARY PRESSURE?

The intrapleural pressure is always (1) less than intrapulmonary pressure, (2) less than atmospheric pressure, and (3) considered negative because of the "pull" of the two pleural membranes in opposite directions. The parietal pleura is pulled outward by forces within the chest wall while the visceral pleural is pulled inward by the force of the elastic fibers within the lungs.

WHY DO THE TWO PLEURAL MEMBRANES "PULL" IN OPPOSITE DIRECTIONS?

The parietal pleura, attached to the chest, is pulled outward because the elastic fibers within the intercostal muscles exert outward pressure on the ribs. These fibers are in a relaxed state when the rib cage is fully expanded, such as during a deep inhalation. The visceral pleural, attached to the lungs, is pulled inward because the elastic fibers within the lungs, responsible for elastic recoil, exert pressure to make the lungs smaller. Elastic fibers in the lungs are in a relaxed position only when the lung is at its smallest configuration, such as occurs with a pneumothorax. Hence, because of the opposite pull of the chest wall and the lung and because the pleural membranes are attached to these structures, there is a constant pull of the two membranes in opposite directions. The subatmospheric pressure, which results within the pleural space, plus the greater than atmospheric intrapulmonary pressure within the lungs allow the lungs to remain inflated. Anything that causes the pressure within the pleural space to rise to atmospheric pressure or above will cause the lung(s) to collapse—a pneumothorax.

sory muscles of ventilation. Several muscles of the abdomen have long been thought to contribute to active exhalation.[2,6]

◆ **Accessory muscles of ventilation.** The accessory muscles of ventilation usually are considered those muscles that enhance chest expansion during exercise but that are not active during normal, quiet breathing. The accessory muscles include the scalene, sternocleidomastoid, and other chest and back muscles, such as the trapezius and pectoralis major. Use of the accessory muscles at rest, which is common in patients with chronic obstructive pulmonary disease, is hard work, inasmuch as the use of accessory muscles requires great amounts of energy and oxygen.[1] The accessory muscles sometimes are referred to as "oxygen robbers" because of the excessive amount of oxygen their use requires, depleting the amount available to other parts of the body.

CONDUCTING AIRWAYS

The conducting airways consist of the upper airways, trachea, and bronchial tree. The purpose of the conducting airways is threefold. The first is to warm and humidify the inhaled air. The second is to act as a protective mechanism that prevents the entrance of foreign matter into the gas exchange areas. The third is to serve as a passageway for air entering and leaving the gas exchange regions of the lungs.[1]

Upper Airways

The upper airways consist of the nasal and oral cavities, pharynx, and larynx. Their main contribution to ventilation is the conditioning of inspired air. Conditioned air is air that has been warmed, humidified, and cleaned of some irritants. Warming and humidifying, which are essential to achieving a nonirritant effect on the lower airways, occur mainly within the nose through a dense vascular network that lines the nasal passages. Many irritants are filtered by the coarse hairs that line the nasal passages.[1]

In addition, the epiglottis protects the lower airways by closing the opening to the trachea during swallowing, so that food passes into the esophagus and not the trachea. The epiglottis is a thin, leaf-shaped, elastic cartilage, located directly posterior to the root of the tongue, that is, attached to the thyroid cartilage. It opens widely during inhalation, permitting air to pass through the trachea into the lower airways.[1]

Trachea

The trachea is a hollow tube approximately 11 cm (4.5 inches) in length and 2.5 cm (1 inch) in diameter (Fig. 19-5). It begins at the cricoid cartilage and ends at the bifurcation (the major carina) from which the two main-stem bronchi arise. The carina is approximately at the level of the aortic arch,[2] the fifth thoracic vertebra,[8] or just below the level of the angle of Louis.[1] The trachea consists of smooth muscle supported anteriorly by 16 to 20 C-shaped, cartilaginous rings. These prevent tracheal collapse during bronchoconstriction and strong coughing. The posterior wall of the trachea lies contiguous with the anterior wall of the esophagus. Having no cartilaginous support, this wall is composed only of muscle tissue, which is separated from the anterior esophageal wall by loose connective tissue (see Fig. 19-5, *insert*).[1]

Bronchial Tree

The two main-stem bronchi are structurally different (see Fig. 19-5). The left bronchus is slightly narrower than the right, and because of its position above the heart, the left bronchus angles directly toward the left lung at approximately 45 to 55 degrees from the midline. The right bronchus is wider and angles at 20 to 30 degrees from the midline.[1] Because of this angulation and the forces of gravity, the most common site of aspiration of foreign objects is through the right main-stem bronchus into the lower lobe of the right lung.[2]

Each branching of the tracheobronchial tree produces a new generation of tubes (Fig. 19-6). The main-stem

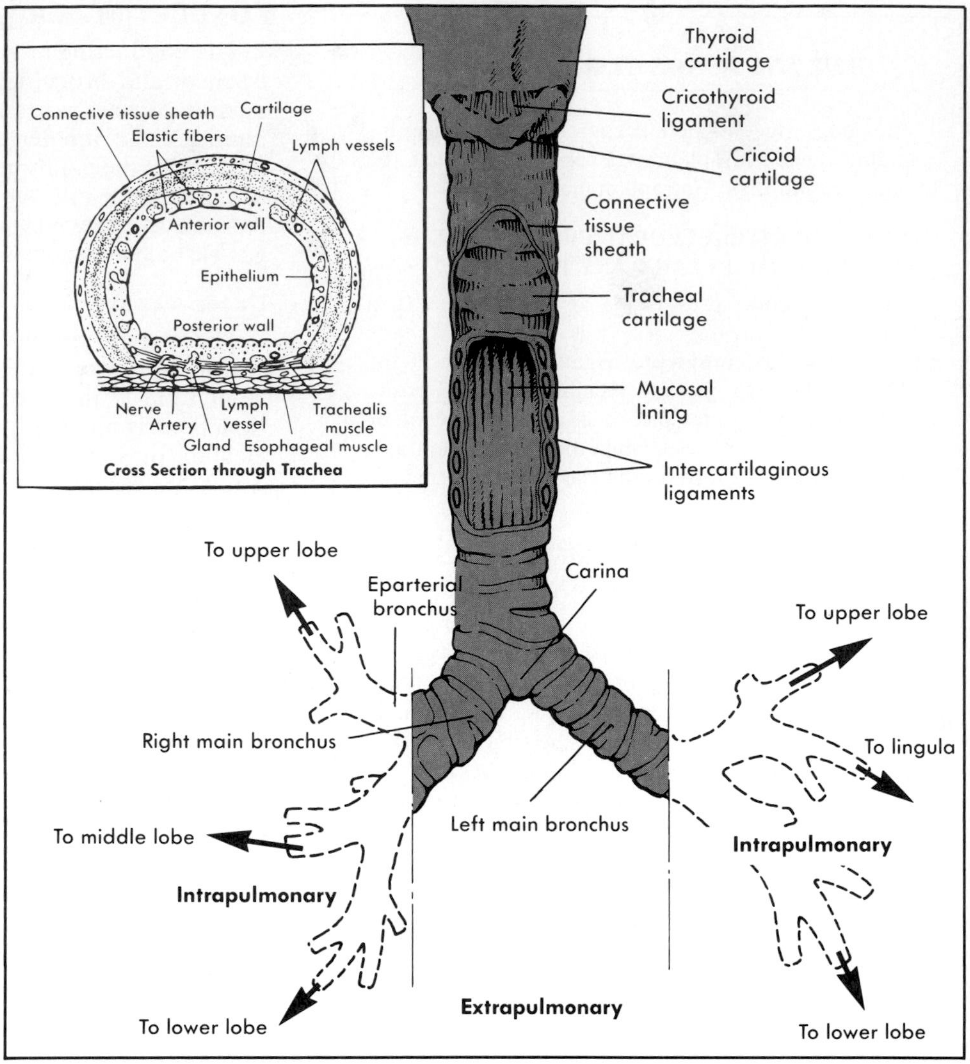

Fig. 19-5 Anterior view of the trachea and primary bronchi and a cross-section through a part of the trachea, including a C-shaped cartilaginous element. (From Martin DE: *Respiratory anatomy and physiology,* St Louis, 1988, Mosby–Year Book.)

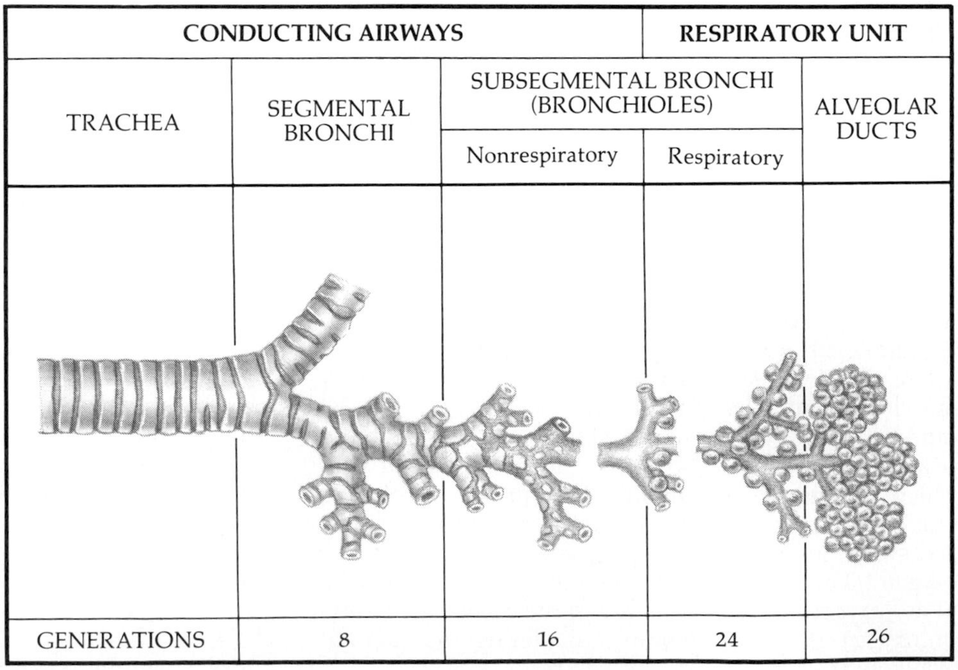
CONDUCTING AIRWAYS
RESPIRATORY UNIT
TRACHEA
SEGMENTAL BRONCHI
SUBSEGMENTAL BRONCHI (BRONCHIOLES)
Nonrespiratory
Respiratory
ALVEOLAR DUCTS
GENERATIONS
8
16
24
26

Fig. 19-6 Conducting and respiratory airways. (From Thompson JM and others: *Mosby's clinical nursing,* ed 3, St Louis, 1993, Mosby–Year Book.)

bronchi are the first generation; the next branch, the five lobar bronchi, is the second generation. The third generation includes the 18 segmental bronchi. The fourth through approximately the ninth generations are referred to as the *small bronchi,* beginning with the subsegmental bronchi. In these bronchi, diameters decrease; however, because the number of bronchi increases with each generation, the total cross-sectional area increases with each generation. The number of airways increase from 20 per generation at the fourth to approximately 1020 per generation at the tenth. The eleventh generation has approximately 7 times the cross-sectional area of the lobar bronchi. This great increase in the cross-sectional area of the lung is extremely significant in that it allows easy ventilation in spite of the small airway lumens through which air is passing.[1]

The final subdivision of the conducting airways is the bronchioles. These are tubes less than 1 mm in diameter and are distinguished by having a lack of connective tissue and cartilage within their walls. Their walls do, however, contain smooth muscle. When smooth-muscle constriction occurs, these airways may close completely from lack of structural support.[9] Some of the wheezing and dyspnea associated with asthma can be traced to bronchoconstriction of the bronchioles.[7] The terminal bronchioles form the last branch of the conducting airways, after which the gas exchange areas of the lungs begin. There are more than 32,000 terminal bronchioles.

The main defense system within the airways is the mucociliary escalator, or mucous blanket, a combination of mucus and cilia. The mucus, which floats atop the cilia (Fig. 19-7), traps foreign particles. Ciliary movement then propels the entire mucous blanket and any trapped particles upward toward the pharynx at an average speed of 1 cm/min.[6] Once the pharynx is reached, the mucus is either swallowed or cleared. The submucous glands of the airways produce approximately 100 ml of mucus per day, with all but about 10 ml reabsorbed through the bronchial lining.[10] The mucociliary escalator is so efficient that almost no particles larger than the size of 3 μm reach the alveoli.[2]

The cough reflex is another protective mechanism present in the lungs. Excessive amounts of foreign particles in the trachea and bronchi can initiate the cough reflex. Once initiated, the rapid expulsion of air carries any foreign particles with it.[6]

RESPIRATORY AIRWAYS

The respiratory airways consist of the respiratory bronchioles and the alveoli. The respiratory airways also are known as the *terminal respiratory units,* or the *acini.* It is in these regions of the lungs that gas exchange takes place. Gas exchange at this level is referred to as *external respiration.*

Respiratory Bronchioles

Each terminal bronchiole gives rise to an average of three respiratory bronchioles (Fig. 19-8). The respiratory bronchioles form the transition zone of the lungs. They act as both a conducting airway and a gas exchange unit. While they move air forward, alveolar outpouchings on their surfaces allow them to participate in gas exchange.[1]

Alveoli

Each respiratory bronchiole gives rise to several alveolar ducts. Alveolar ducts terminate in clusters of 10 to 16 alveoli. The alveolus is the primary site of gas exchange and the end point in the respiratory tract. Within the two lungs there are approximately 300 million alveoli.[1] The alveoli are composed of several types of cells, including type I and type II alveolar epithelial cells and alveolar macrophages.[1,2]

◆ **Type I alveolar epithelial cells.** Type I alveolar epithelial cells comprise approximately 90% of the total alveolar surface within the lungs (Fig. 19-9). They are the chief structural cells of the alveolar wall and play the major role in maintenance of the gas-blood barrier and in gas exchange. Type I cells are extremely susceptible to injury

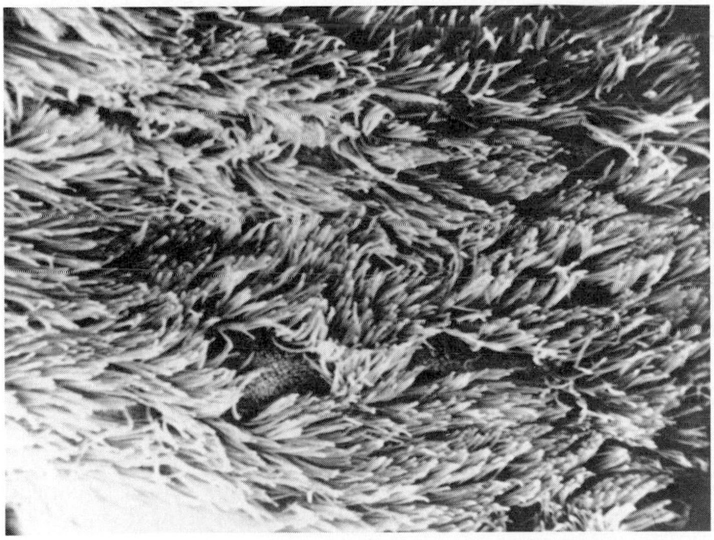

Fig. 19-7 Scanning electron micrograph of the luminal surface and cilia of a bronchiole from a normal adult male. (×2000.) (From Murray JF: *The normal lung,* ed 2, Philadelphia, 1986, WB Saunders, originally from Ebert RV, Terracio MJ: *Am Rev Resp Dis* 111:130, 1975.)

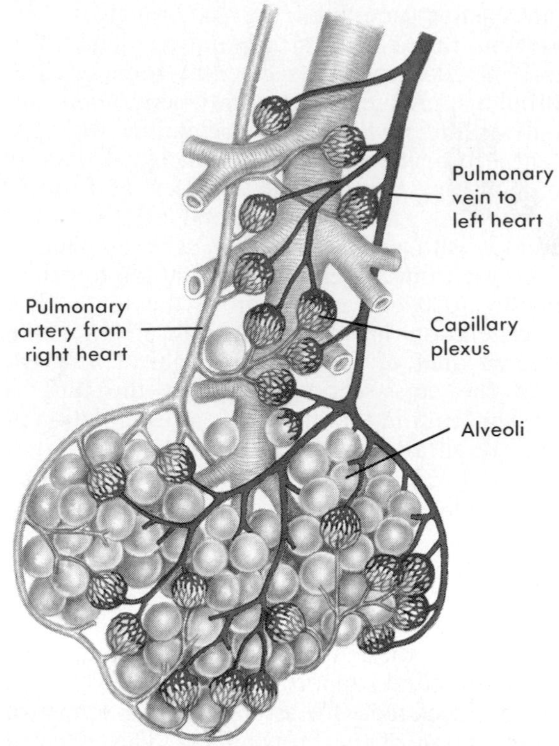

Fig. 19-8 Terminal ventilation and perfusion units of the lung. Pulmonary arterial blood is venous (dark gray) and pulmonary venous blood is oxygenated (red). (From Thompson JM and others: *Mosby's clinical nursing,* ed 3, St Louis, 1993, Mosby–Year Book.)

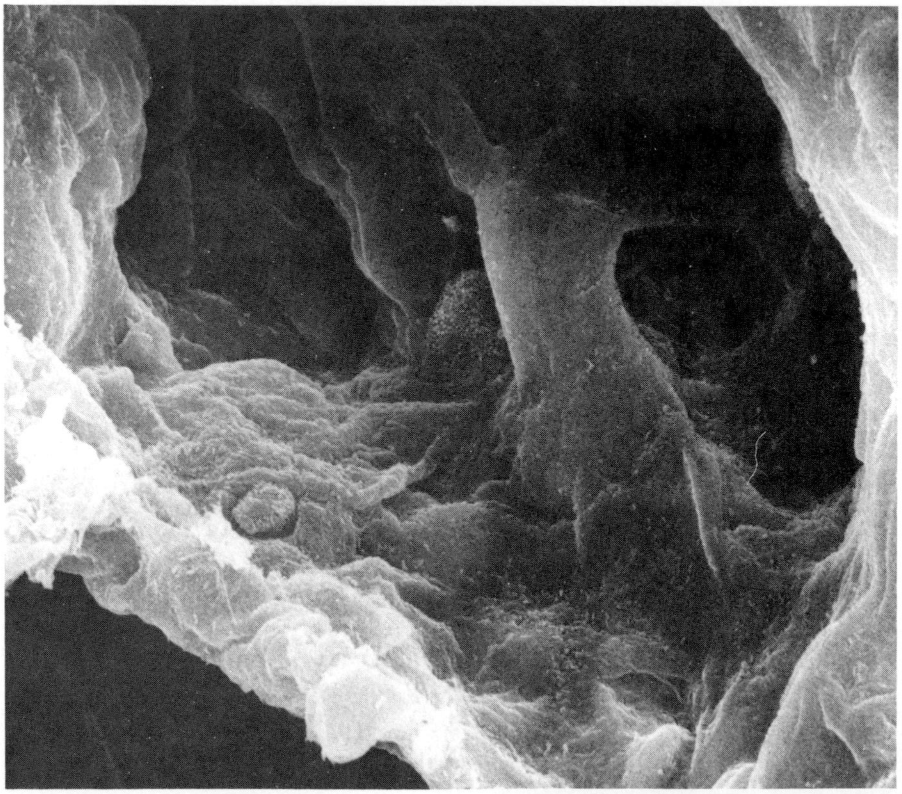

Fig. 19-9 Detail of an alveolar surface composed chiefly of type I alveolar epithelial cells. (Picture width – 1 cm equals 3.46 μm.) (From Martin DE: *Respiratory anatomy and physiology,* St Louis, 1988, Mosby–Year Book.)

and become inflamed when exposed to inhaled toxins. Research suggests that type II cells can regenerate and change to type I cells if necessary.[8]

Within the walls of the type I cells are the pores of Kohn (Fig. 19-10). These pores are believed to allow collateral movement of air between alveoli. The canals of Lambert are collateral air pathways that exist between type I cells and respiratory and terminal bronchioles. When a respiratory bronchiole is blocked or collapsed, gas may still be able to pass into alveoli distal to the

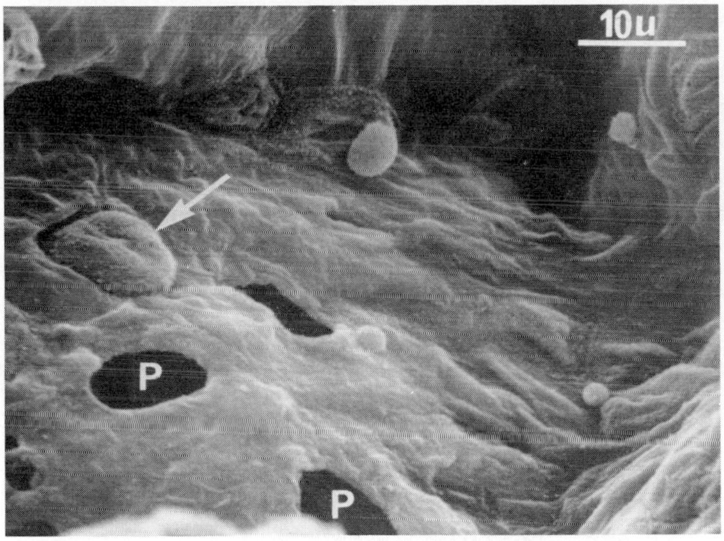

Fig. 19-10 Scanning electron micrograph of the surface of a human alveolus, showing pores of Kohn *(P)* and a macrophage *(arrow)*. (×1500.) (From Murray JF: *The normal lung,* ed 2, Philadelphia, 1986, WB Saunders; courtesy Dr MS Wang.)

blockage through the canals of Lambert. Thus collateral air passages are of significant benefit in any pathologic condition of the lung that results in obstruction of airflow into a portion of the lungs. In contrast, however, these pores and canals also allow the efficient movement of microorganisms through lung tissue.[1,7]

◆ **Type II alveolar epithelial cells.** Type II alveolar epithelial cells occur in much greater numbers than do type I cells, but because of their minute size, they comprise a smaller portion of the total alveolar wall. After injury to the alveolar wall, type II cells rapidly divide to line the surface; later they transform into type I cells. The most important function of the type II cells is their ability to produce, store, and secrete pulmonary surfactant (Fig. 19-11).[1,2]

Surfactant is a phospholipid composed of fatty acids bound to lecithin. Like other surfactants, such as detergents and soaps, pulmonary surfactant functions to lower surface tension of the alveoli. Whereas with detergents and soaps this decrease in surface tension cleans clothes, within the lungs it stabilizes the alveoli, increases lung compliance, and eases the work of breathing. When pulmonary disease disrupts the normal synthesis and storage of surfactant, the lungs become less compliant and the work of breathing increases. Severe loss of surfactant results in alveolar instability, collapse (atelectasis), and impairment of gas exchange. The classic example of this condition occurs in adult respiratory distress syndrome (ARDS).[7] Sighing is thought to contribute to the spread of surfactant throughout the lungs because the large volume of air generated by the sigh opens otherwise partially closed alveoli and spreads surfactant over their walls.[11]

Surfactant has a half-life of only 14 hours. This short time period accounts for the high metabolic activity of the type II cells. Thyroxine is thought to play a role in surfactant production because of its function in lipid metabolism. Studies in animals and humans have shown an increased production and storage of surfactant when thyroxine was administered. Acetylcholine, prostaglandins, and estradiol also are known to increase surfactant synthesis.[12]

◆ **Alveolar macrophages.** Alveolar macrophages are monocytes that originate in the bone marrow and are released into the blood stream (Fig. 19-12). On entering the pulmonary capillary circulation, they move through the capillary membrane wall into the interstitial space and the alveoli. Once in the alveoli, the monocytes transform into macrophages and assume a phagocytic role. They move from alveolus to alveolus through the pores of Kohn, keeping the alveoli clean and sterile through phagocytosis and microbial killing activity, which includes the secretion of hydrogen peroxide, lysozyme, and other substances that kill microorganisms.[2]

An increase or decrease in the number of alveolar macrophages is thought to be directly related to an individual's resistance to lung infection. Depression of macrophage activity can occur with the presence of cigarette smoke, hypoxia, hyperoxia, metabolic acidosis, uremia, ozone, and nitrogen dioxide; with ethanol and corticosteroid ingestion; and after viral infections.[8,13]

PULMONARY BLOOD AND LYMPH SUPPLY

Two vascular systems and one lymphatic system make up the pulmonary blood and lymph supply. The pulmonary circulation arises from the right side of the heart with the pulmonary artery and is the gas exchange network that surrounds the alveoli and empties into the left side of the heart. The bronchial circulation is the vascular system that perfuses the tracheobronchial tree.

Pulmonary Circulation

The pulmonary circulatory system begins at the pulmonary artery, which receives venous blood from the right ventricle. The pulmonary artery then divides into main-stem left and right branches and continues to branch until it forms the capillaries that surround the alveoli (see Fig. 19-8). Once blood is oxygenated, it returns to the left side of the heart through the pulmonary veins.[1,14]

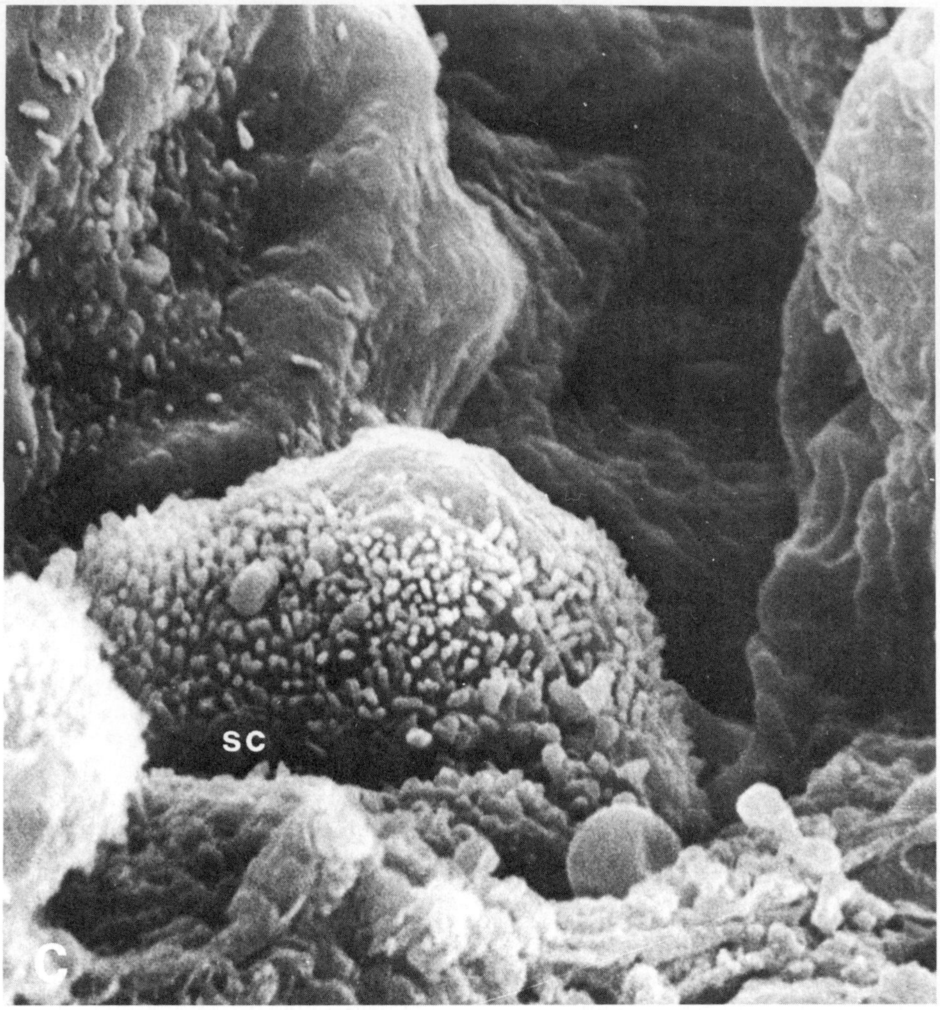

Fig. 19-11 Type II alveolar epithelial cell. Note the presence of brush microvilli on all except the bald top of the round luminal surface. Type II cells produce surfactant. (Picture width – 1 cm equals 0.85 μm.) (From Martin DE: *Respiratory anatomy and physiology,* St Louis, 1988, Mosby–Year Book.)

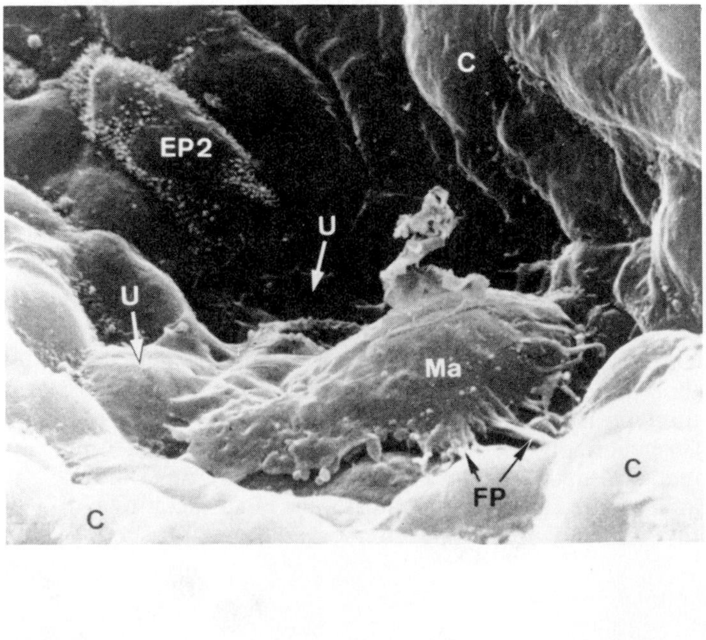

Fig. 19-12 Scanning electron micrograph of a healthy human lung, showing an alveolar macrophage *(Ma)* attached to the epithelium partly by filopodia *(FP)* and forming an undulating membrane *(U)* in the direction of forward movement to the left. Several capillaries *(C)* are evident, and a type II alveolar epithelial cell *(EP2)* can be seen in the background. (Original magnification ×3700.) (From Murray JF: *The normal lung,* ed 2, Philadelphia, 1986, WB Saunders; originally from Gehr P and others: *Respir Physiol* 32[2]:130, 1978.)

The pulmonary circulation is, by far, the largest vascular bed within the body and is the only one that receives the entire cardiac output. Just as the systemic circulation has a systolic and a diastolic blood pressure, so does the pulmonary circulation. Because of the relative lack of smooth muscle within the vessels of the pulmonary circulation, however, the pressures are vastly lower than within the systemic circulation.[1,14,15] Pulmonary artery systolic (PAS) pressure averages 25 mm Hg, pulmonary artery diastolic (PAD) pressure averages 10 mm Hg, and pulmonary artery mean (PAM) pressure is 15 mm Hg. Because of the low pulmonary artery pressures, right ventricular wall thickness needs to be only approximately one third of left ventricular wall thickness. However, just as hypertension can occur within the systemic circulation, it also can occur within the pulmonary circulation.[6,14]

Pulmonary hypertension is defined as increased pressure (PAS greater than 30 mm Hg and PAM greater than 18 mm Hg) within the pulmonary arterial system. Pulmonary hypertension can develop as a result of both cardiac and pulmonary abnormalities. Cardiac conditions include mitral stenosis, left ventricular failure, and congenital heart disease. Cardiac-generated pulmonary hypertension sometimes is called *passive pulmonary hypertension* because the rise in pressure is caused not by disease of the pulmonary vascular bed but by a rising left atrial pressure.[14]

The most common cause of pulmonary hypertension, however, is a pathologic condition of the lungs such as pulmonary embolism, as well as obliteration of the vascular bed associated with emphysema or hypoxic vasoconstriction (see box on right). The pulmonary hypertension resulting from hypoxic vasoconstriction, although caused in part by vasospasm, is largely a result of alterations in the structure of the blood vessels of the pulmonary circulation, which results in an increase in the medial thickness and a reduction in the size of the vascular lumen. Pulmonary hypertension increases the afterload of the right ventricle and, when chronic, can result in right ventricular hypertrophy.[16]

PATHOPHYSIOLOGY OF HYPOXIC VASOCONSTRICTION

Hypoxic vasoconstriction refers to vasoconstriction of any portion of the pulmonary-capillary bed that perfuses unventilated or underventilated alveoli. Although most blood vessels in the body dilate in response to hypoxia to deliver more blood flow to the hypoxic tissue, the pulmonary vessels do the opposite and constrict in response to hypoxia. Hypoxic vasoconstriction occurs in lung regions where the partial pressure of oxygen in alveolar gas (PA_{O_2}) falls below 60 mm Hg. Research indicates that the lower the PA_{O_2}, the greater will be the hypoxic vasoconstriction. The mediator of this response is as of yet unknown, but the vasoconstriction has the effect of directing blood flow away from the hypoxic alveoli to alveoli in which the PA_{O_2} is or might be normal.

The drop in PA_{O_2} can result from various conditions associated with chronic pulmonary disease, such as bronchoconstriction and chronic blockage of airways by mucus or from breathing low concentrations of oxygen, such as occurs in persons who live at a high altitude. Indeed, high altitude dwellers experience the same vascular changes in their pulmonary arterioles as do persons in whom hypoxic vasoconstriction develops as a result of chronic pulmonary disease.

Hypoxic vasoconstriction is not necessarily bad. When it occurs regionally within the lung, such as in atelectatic areas, it protects against severe hypoxemia by limiting shunt. When, however, hypoxic vasoconstriction becomes generalized throughout the lung, pulmonary hypertension will result.

Prolonged hypoxic vasoconstriction, such as commonly occurs in patients with chronic bronchitis, can lead to pulmonary hypertension and cor pulmonale. Pulmonary hypertension develops when the hypoxic vasoconstriction is diffuse and affects a significant amount of the pulmonary vascular bed.[16]

Alveolar-Capillary Membrane

The vessels of the alveolar-capillary membrane form a network around each alveolus that is so dense it forms an almost continuous sheet of blood covering the alveoli. The interior diameter of each capillary segment is approximately 10 μm, just large enough to allow red blood cells to squeeze by in single file so that their cell membranes touch the capillary walls (Fig. 19-13).[7] In this way, oxygen and carbon dioxide need not pass through significant amounts of plasma when diffusing into and out of the alveoli, making a highly efficient vehicle for gas exchange.

Each red blood cell spends approximately three fourths of a second in the alveolar-capillary network and is exposed to the alveolar gas of two or three alveoli.[2] In that short time hemoglobin is brought from its normal venous blood saturation level of 75% to its arterial saturation of more than 96%. Actually, hemoglobin levels have been shown to reach normal within only a 0.25 second exposure to alveolar gas; thus under conditions such as in tachycardia in which the red blood cells spend less time within the pulmonary capillary network, normal oxygenation can still occur.[2,6]

The alveolar-capillary membrane is composed of several layers of cells: the alveolar epithelium, the alveolar basement membrane, the interstitial space, the capillary basement membrane, and the capillary endothelium. Oxygen and carbon dioxide traverse easily across these layers, which present no barrier to diffusion because the membrane is only 4 to 8 μm thick.[2]

Distribution of Perfusion

The distribution of perfusion through the lungs is related to gravity and intraalveolar pressures. Because of the effects of gravity, the pressure in the capillaries in the lungs is higher in the bases than in the apexes. This promotes preferential blood flow to the gravity-

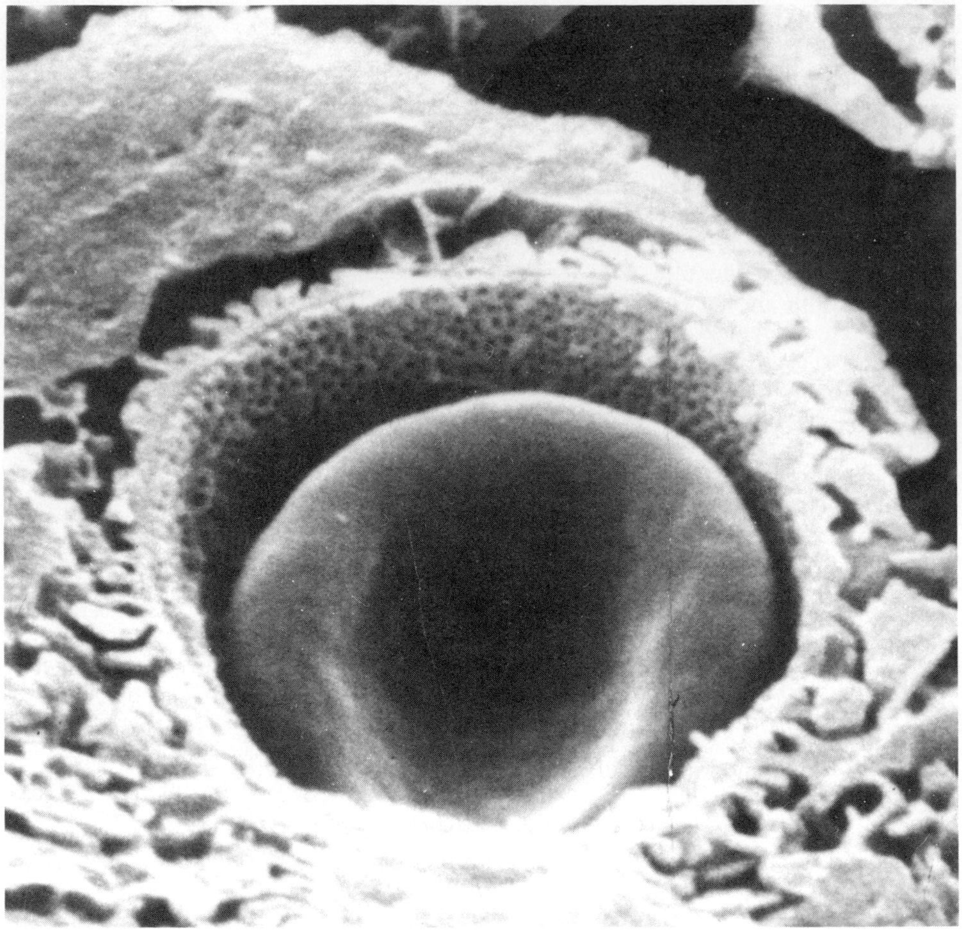

Fig. 19-13 Scanning electron micrograph of a red blood cell in a capillary. Note that the diameters of both are similar. In many instances the red blood cells course through even smaller capillaries, often through capillaries that are one half the diameter of the red blood cell. This is possible because the cells are pliable, mainly as a result of their biconcave disk shape. (From Martin DE: *Respiratory anatomy and physiology*, St Louis, 1988, Mosby–Year Book.)

dependent areas of the lungs. The intraalveolar pressures generally are equal throughout the various regions of the lungs. In some areas of the lungs the intraalveolar pressure has the potential of exceeding capillary hydrostatic pressure, resulting in an absence of blood flow to these areas.

On the basis of this concept the lung can be divided into three zones. Zone 1 is the nondependent portion of the lung, which has the potential of no perfusion. Zone 2 is the middle portion of the lung, which receives varying blood flow. Zone 3 is the gravity-dependent area of the lung, which receives a constant blood flow.[17,18]

Bronchial Circulation

The bronchial circulation, also known as the *systemic* blood supply to the lungs,[19] is the system that perfuses the tracheobronchial tree, visceral pleura, interstitial and connective tissue, some arteries and veins, lymph nodes, and the nerves within the thoracic cavity. The bronchial arteries that perfuse structures in the left side of the thorax branch off the aorta, and those that perfuse the right-sided structures branch from the intercostal, subclavian, or internal mammary artery. After perfusing the specific lung structures, most of the venous blood returns to the right side of the heart; however, some venous blood from the bronchial circulation returns directiy into the pulmonary veins and the left atrium.[15,19]

The left atrium normally contains pure oxygenated blood, with a hemoglobin saturation at 100%. The mixing of venous blood from the bronchial circulation with the oxygenated blood in the left atrium decreases the saturation of left atrial blood to a range between 96% and 99%. For this reason, while a person is breathing room air, the oxygen saturation of arterial blood is less than 100%. The dumping of venous blood into the left atrium is known as the *physiologic shunt.*[7] This term expresses two thoughts; physiologic means that this is a normal part of physiology, not a pathologic event, and shunt refers to the mixing of venous blood with arterial blood. Another system responsible for the addition of venous blood to the left atrium—thus contributing to the normal physiologic shunt—is the thebesian system, which perfuses the coronary arteries. These two systems constitute the normal physiologic shunt, which comprises approximately 3% to 5% of the total cardiac output.

Lymphatic Circulation

The lungs are more richly supplied with lymphatic tissue than is any other organ, perhaps because of their constant exposure to the external environment.[12] The lymphatic vessels parallel much of the pulmonary vasculature and the tracheobronchial tree to the level of the terminal and respiratory bronchioles. Lymphatic vessels also are located within the connective tissue of lung parenchyma and within the pleural membranes. These vessels eventually drain into the primary lymph nodes located at the hila of the lungs. The lymphatic system in the lungs serves two purposes. As part of the immune system, it is responsible for removing foreign particles and cell debris from the lungs and for producing both antibody and cell-mediated immune responses. It also is responsible for removing fluid from the lungs and for keeping the alveoli clear.[1,2]

VENTILATION

Ventilation—defined as the movement of air into and out of the lungs—is distinct from respiration, which refers to gas exchange, not movement of air. Air moves into and out of the lungs because of changes in the intrapulmonary pressure (pressure inside the lungs) compared with atmospheric pressure. When intrapulmonary pressure is less than atmospheric pressure, air will move from the area of higher pressure to the area of lower pressure. Thus when intrapulmonary pressure falls below atmospheric pressure, air will flow into the lungs (Fig. 19-3).[20] The movement of air into the lungs is known as *inhalation* whereas the movement of air out of the lungs is known as *exhalation*. Normal muscular action of the diaphragm, flexibility of the rib cage, elasticity of the lungs, and airway diameter are instrumental in allowing easy inhalation and exhalation (see box on right). Ventilation is regulated by the central nervous system.[6]

Inhalation

Intrapulmonary pressure falls below atmospheric pressure when the muscles of inhalation cause the chest and lungs to expand. As this expansion occurs, the volume of gas within the lungs moves into a larger space. When a fixed volume moves into a larger space, the pressure within the space will fall. Hence, at the command of the central nervous system, the muscles of ventilation contract, the thorax and lungs expand, and the intrapulmonary pressure falls. When the pressure falls below atmospheric pressure, air from the atmosphere will enter as an inhalation.[6,21]

Exhalation

Air moves out of the lungs because of the same principles that caused it to enter. When the intrapulmonary pressure is greater than the atmospheric pressure, air moves from the lungs into the atmosphere. Intrapulmonary pressure rises above atmospheric pressure when, just after inhalation, the muscles of ventilation relax, causing the thorax and ribs to lower and the lung to be compressed. This compression forces the gas within the lungs into a smaller area. When a fixed volume of gas is compressed into a smaller area, the pressure within the area rises. As the lungs are compressed, intrapulmonary pressure rises. When it rises above atmospheric pressure, exhalation occurs.[6,21]

HOW LUNG DISEASE CAN ALTER VENTILATION

Normal muscular action of the diaphragm, flexibility of the rib cage, elasticity of the lungs, and airway diameter are instrumental in allowing easy inhalation and exhalation. Any interference with these actions impairs normal ventilation. Pulmonary diseases can be categorized into obstructive or restrictive diseases, depending on how the underlying cause affects normal ventilation.

Restrictive diseases "restrict" lung or chest wall movement and include diffuse interstitial lung fibrosis, atelectasis, kyphoscoliosis, and severe chest wall pain. These conditions can be either acute or chronic, and because they restrict lung or chest wall expansion, or both, patients have smaller tidal volumes but an increased ventilatory rate to maintain minute ventilation.

Obstructive diseases result in obstruction to normal airflow. The classic examples are emphysema, in which airflow is decreased because of a decrease in lung recoil, and asthma, in which airflow is decreased because of diffuse airway narrowing. Emphysema results in lungs that inflate easily but, lacking the normal elastic recoil, do not compress to assist with exhalation. Patients with emphysema may have little difficulty inhaling but struggle to exhale.

Normal ventilation depends on many factors, the most important of which are flexibility of the rib cage and elasticity of the lungs, as well as normal action of the muscles of ventilation and normal airway diameter. When patients are critically ill with a disease that alters the function of any of these factors, assessment of the efficiency or inefficiency of ventilation is mandatory.

Work of Breathing

The work of breathing is the amount of work that must be performed to overcome the elastic and resistive properties of the lungs. The elastic properties are determined by lung recoil, chest wall recoil, and the surface tension of the alveoli. The resistive properties are determined by airway resistance.[9] Normally the work of breathing occurs during inhalation. Even exhalation, however, can be a strain when lung recoil, chest wall recoil, and/or airway resistance is abnormal, such as can occur in patients with emphysema, chronic bronchitis, asthma, pulmonary edema, and other pulmonary disorders.[6,9,21]

During normal, quiet ventilation only 2% to 3% of the total energy expended by the body is required by the pulmonary system.[6] During heavy exercise the amount of energy required by the pulmonary system can become progressively greater.[1] Thus the work of breathing can be a factor that limits exercise in the patient with pulmonary disease.[9]

Pathologic conditions of the pulmonary system can drastically change the energy requirement for ventilation. Pulmonary diseases that decrease lung compliance (atelectasis, pulmonary edema), decrease chest wall compliance (kyphoscoliosis), increase airway resistance (bronchitis, chronic obstructive pulmonary disease), or decrease lung recoil (emphysema) can increase the work of breathing so much that one third or more of the total body energy is used for ventilation.[6,9]

Pulmonary Volumes and Capacities

Pulmonary ventilation can be described in terms of volumes and capacities (Fig. 19-14). Tidal volume (V_T) is the amount of air inhaled and exhaled with each breath. Inspiratory reserve volume (IRV) is the maximum amount of air that can be inhaled over and above the normal tidal volume. Expiratory reserve volume (ERV) is the maximum amount of air that can be exhaled beyond the normal tidal volume. The residual volume (RV) is the amount of air left in the lungs after a complete exhalation. Inspiratory capacity (IC) is the sum of the tidal volume and the inspiratory reserve. Functional residual capacity (FRC) is the sum of the expiratory reserve volume and the residual volume. Vital capacity (VC) is the sum of the inspiratory reserve volume, the tidal volume, and the expiratory reserve volume. Total lung capacity (TLC) is the sum of all four volumes and represents the maximal amount of air that can be inhaled.[6,18,22]

Distribution of Ventilation

The distribution of ventilation throughout the lungs is not even. This is the result of a variety of factors, including the configuration of the thorax[22] and the effects of gravity on intrapleural pressure.[16,22] The thorax allows more lung expansion at the base than at the apex, which permits more ventilation to the base.[22] Gravity produces regional variations in pleural pressure. At rest the negative intrapleural pressure at the apex is greater than at the base. On inhalation the alveoli at the base expand more because they have less pressure to overcome.[16,22] In the upright person the base of the lung receives about 4 times more ventilation than does the apex.[22] In the supine person, gravity produces the same effects in the dependent zones of the lungs (posterior regions).[16,22]

Efficiency of Ventilation

The portion of total ventilation that participates in gas exchange is known as *alveolar ventilation.* The portion of ventilation that does not is known as *wasted ventilation.* The areas in the lungs that are ventilated but in which no gas exchange occurs are known as *dead space.* The conducting airways are referred to as *anatomic dead space* because they are ventilated but do not participate in gas exchange. In addition, some ventilation goes to unperfused alveoli. Without perfusion, gas exchange cannot take place and thus the ventilation is wasted. These unperfused alveoli are called *alveolar dead space.*

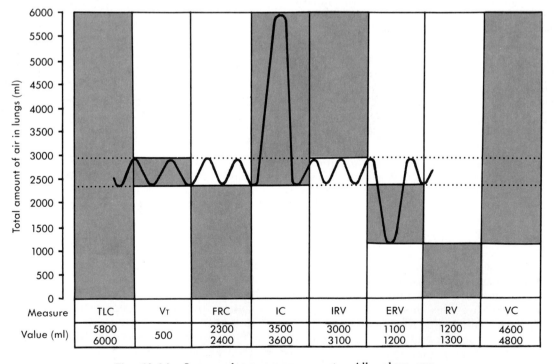

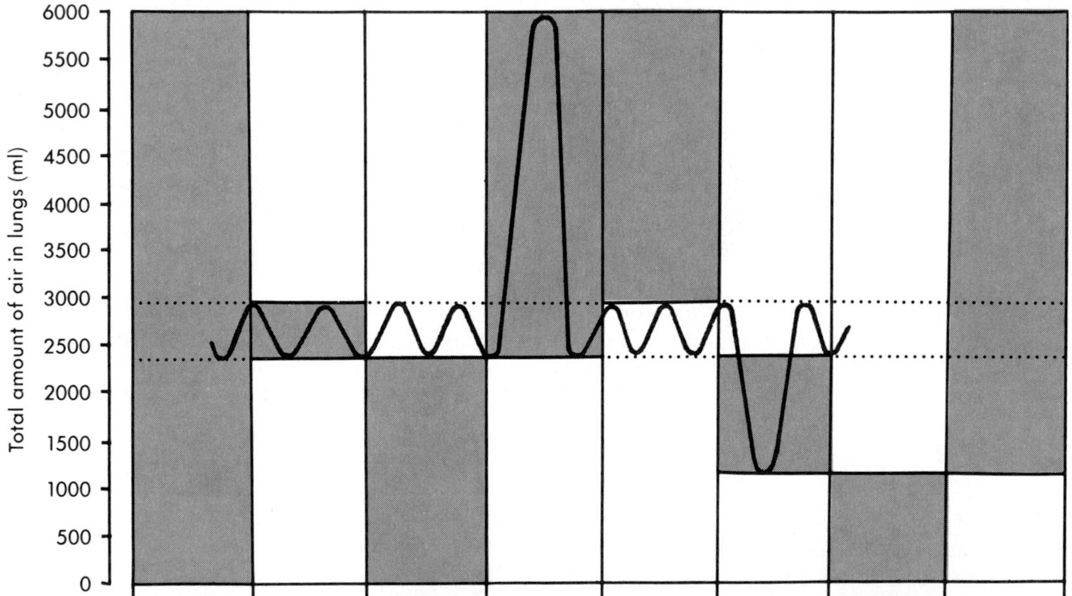

Measure	TLC	V_T	FRC	IC	IRV	ERV	RV	VC
Value (ml)	5800 6000	500	2300 2400	3500 3600	3000 3100	1100 1200	1200 1300	4600 4800

Fig. 19-14 Lung volume measurements. All values are approximately 25% less in women. *TLC,* Total lung capacity; *V_T,* tidal volume; *FRC,* functional residual capacity; *IC,* inspiratory capacity; *IRV,* inspiratory reserve volume; *ERV,* expiratory reserve volume; *RV,* residual volume; *VC,* vital capacity.

Anatomic dead space plus alveolar dead space is known as *physiologic dead space.*[9,22]

Regulation of Ventilation

Regulation of ventilation by the brain is complex and not completely understood. Ventilation is regulated by a triad comprising a controller (located within the central nervous system), a group of effectors (muscles of ventilation), and a variety of sensors that include chemoreceptors (central and peripheral) and mechanoreceptors (located in chest wall and lungs).[2] Efferent nerve fibers convey impulses from the controller to the effectors, whereas afferent nerve fibers carry impulses from some of the sensors to the controller (Fig. 19-15).[23]

◆ **Controller.** The central nervous system houses what is known as the *controller of ventilation.* Actually, the controller is not located in one specific area; rather, it is in several areas that work in conjunction to provide coordinated ventilation. The brainstem regulates automatic ventilation, the cerebral cortex allows voluntary ventilation, and neurons housed in the spinal cord process information from the brain and from the peripheral receptors, allowing them to send final information to the muscles of ventilation.[2]

In the brainstem, both the medulla oblongata and the pons are involved in ventilation. Four different groups of neurons are thought to participate in the regulation of inhalation and exhalation. The dorsal respiratory group, located in the medulla, is responsible for the basic rhythm of ventilation. Cells in this area are believed to automatically fire and trigger inhalation. The pneumotaxic center in the pons is responsible for limiting inhalation and thus triggering exhalation. This response also facilitates control of the rate and pattern of respiration. The ventral respiratory group, located in the medulla, is responsible for both inspiration and expiration during periods of increased ventilation. The ap-

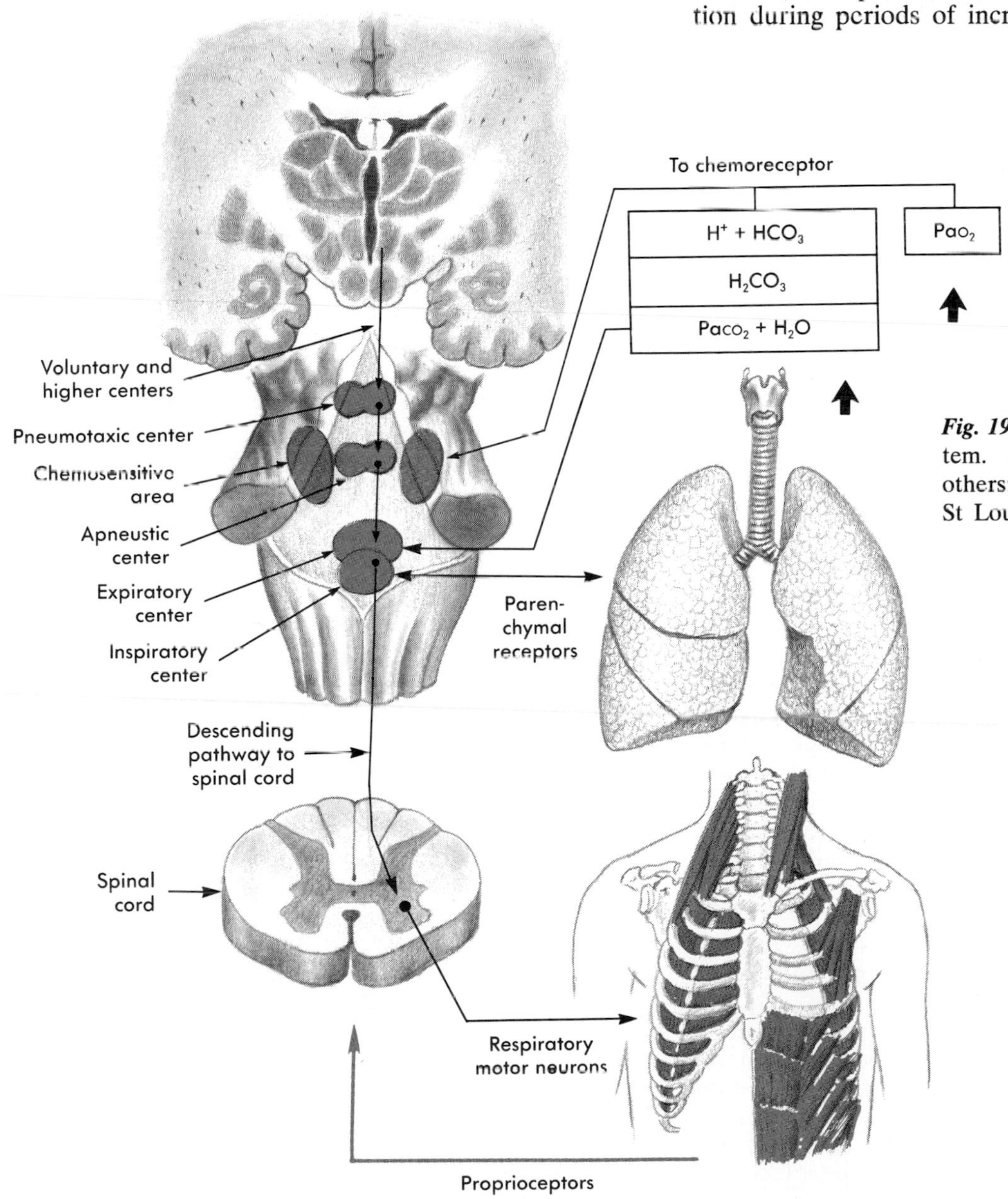

Fig. 19-15 Respiratory control system. (From Thompson JM and others: *Mosby's clinical nursing,* ed 3, St Louis, 1993, Mosby–Year Book.)

neustic center in the lower pons is thought to work with the pneumotaxic center to regulate the depth of inspiration.[6]

The cerebral cortex functions by allowing voluntary ventilation to override the automatic controls of the medulla and pons. Voluntary ventilatory control is most important during such behavioral states as crying, laughing, singing, and talking. During these states, voluntary control may override the automatic control, which responds chiefly to chemical stimuli and to changes in lung inflation.[9,12]

◆ **Effectors.** The effectors of ventilation are the muscles of ventilation. In considering their function in the control of ventilation, however, the most important issue is that they function in a coordinated fashion. The central nervous system regulates this function.

◆ **Sensors.** The main sensors for the regulation of ventilation are the central and peripheral chemoreceptors. These chemoreceptors respond to changes in the chemical composition of the blood or other fluid around them. Other sensors that are found in the lung include the irritant receptors, stretch receptors, and the juxtacapillary (J) receptors.

The central chemoreceptors are located near the ventral surface of the medulla oblongata. These chemoreceptors are surrounded by cerebral extracellular fluid, and they respond primarily to changes in the hydrogen ion concentration of that fluid. Ventilation is increased when the hydrogen ion concentration increases and is decreased when the hydrogen ion concentration falls. A rise in the plasma arterial carbon dioxide pressure ($Paco_2$) causes movement of carbon dioxide into the cerebrospinal fluid, stimulating the movement of hydrogen ions into the brain's extracellular fluid. These hydrogen ions then stimulate the chemoreceptors, and ventilation is increased. Consequently the increased ventilation causes exhalation of the excess carbon dioxide, the $Paco_2$ falls, and ventilation returns to normal. Central chemoreceptors are not affected by changes in arterial oxygen pressure (Pao_2).[6,9,23]

The peripheral chemoreceptors are located above and below the aortic arch and at the bifurcation of the common carotid arteries. The most important action of the carotid chemoreceptors is their response to changes in the Pao_2. The peripheral chemoreceptors are believed to be the only receptors that increase ventilation in response to arterial hypoxemia.[6] Thus immediate hyperventilation, one of the principal compensatory mechanisms in response to hypoxemia, is governed by these chemoreceptors.[7] It seems evident that the carotid bodies are responsible for this effect because it has been shown that patients have lost the ventilatory response to hypoxemia subsequent to bilateral carotid body resection or denervation.[12]

The peripheral chemoreceptors also respond to changes in $Paco_2$ and hydrogen ion concentration. An increase in either results in an increase in ventilation. Studies indicate that the peripheral chemoreceptors probably are more involved with short-term response to carbon dioxide, whereas the central chemoreceptors are responsible for the long-term response to carbon dioxide.[9]

Irritant receptors lie between airway epithelial cells and function to stimulate bronchoconstriction and hyperpnea in response to inhaled irritants.[2,9] Stretch receptors, which are located in the airways, are stimulated by changes in lung volume. They inhibit inhalation and are thought to protect the lung from overinflation (Hering-Breuer reflex).[2,9,23] Juxtacapillary (J) receptors lie in the alveolar walls close to the capillaries. They are stimulated by engorgement of the pulmonary capillaries and an increase in the interstitial fluid volume of the alveolar wall. Stimulation of the J receptors is thought to cause rapid, shallow breathing.[2,9]

RESPIRATION

Respiration refers to the movement of oxygen and carbon dioxide. Gas exchange that takes place at the lung level through the alveolar-capillary membrane is referred to as *external* respiration. The diffusion of gases in and out of the cells at the tissue level is referred to as *internal* respiration.[18]

All gases of concern in respiratory physiology are simple molecules free to move among each other in the atmosphere, where they remain in the gaseous state, and in tissue fluids, such as blood, where they remain in either a gaseous or a liquid state. These gases often are called *volatile* because of their unique ability to move from a liquid to a gaseous state and vice versa. An example can be seen with the change in oxygen as it moves from its gaseous state in the alveoli into its liquid state in the pulmonary capillaries.[6]

Diffusion

Oxygen and carbon dioxide move throughout the body by diffusion. Diffusion moves molecules from an area of high concentration to an area of low concentration. The difference in the concentrations of the gases is referred to as the *driving pressure.* Within the lungs diffusion occurs because of the driving pressure that is exerted by the concentration of each gas within the pulmonary capillaries and within the alveoli. Oxygen is in high concentration and thus exerts a high pressure within the alveoli as compared with the pressure it exerts within the pulmonary capillary. Therefore oxygen moves by diffusion from the alveoli into the pulmonary capillaries. On the other hand, carbon dioxide is in higher concentration within the pulmonary capillary than within the alveoli. Therefore carbon dioxide diffuses out of the capillaries into the alveoli where it is exhaled (Fig. 19-16, *A* and *B*).[6,9]

Several factors affect the rate of diffusion. These include the thickness of the alveolar-capillary membrane, the surface area of the membrane, the diffusion coefficient of the gas, and the driving pressure of the gases.[6] An increase in the thickness of the alveolar-capillary membrane will decrease the rate of diffusion. Pulmonary edema and fibrosis are two examples of situations in which this occurs.[6] A decrease in the surface area of the membrane also will decrease the rate of diffusion. This occurs with removal of a lung (pneumonectomy) or a portion of the lung (lobectomy) or in emphysema as a result of destruction of alveoli.[6] Sighing is an example of a temporary situation in which the surface area is expanded and diffusion is increased. The

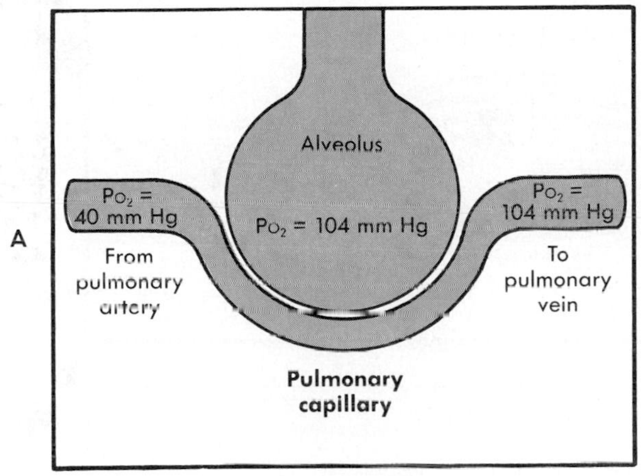

Fig. 19-16 **A,** Diffusion of oxygen from the alveolus into pulmonary capillary blood. The alveolar partial pressure of oxygen (PAO_2) of 104 mm Hg assumes room air has been breathed at sea level by a healthy subject. **B,** Diffusion of carbon dioxide from the pulmonary capillary blood into the alveolus. **C,** Diffusion of oxygen from the alveolus into pulmonary capillary blood. The PAO_2 is elevated because supplemental oxygen is being administered.

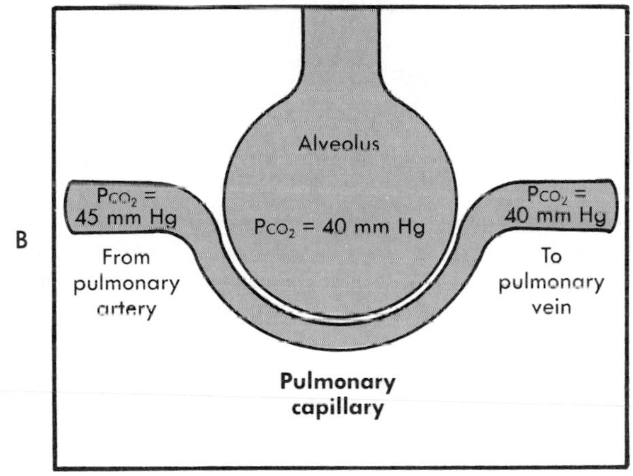

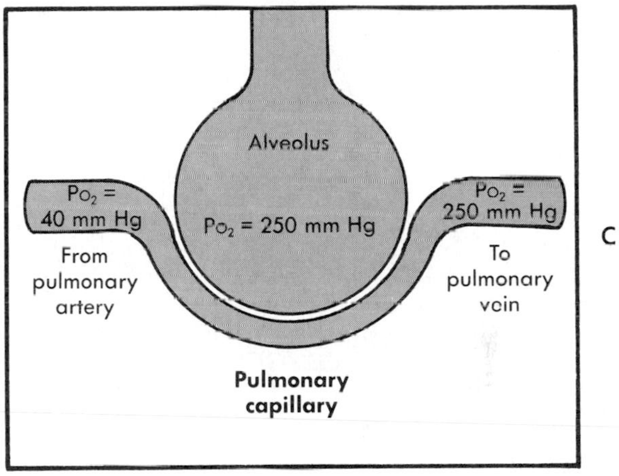

diffusion coefficient of each gas is determined by its solubility. Carbon dioxide diffuses 20 times more rapidly than does oxygen, and oxygen diffuses twice as fast as nitrogen.[6] The greater the driving pressure of the gas through the membrane, the greater the diffusion. The driving pressure is lower at higher altitudes because the effects of gravity on the gases are lessened.[23] The pressure difference is increased when supplemental oxygen is administered (Fig. 19-16, *C*).[24]

Ventilation/Perfusion Relationships

Ventilation and perfusion must be equally matched at the alveolar capillary membrane level for optimal gas exchange to take place. Because of regional variations in the distribution of ventilation and perfusion, the normal ventilation to perfusion ratio is 0.8.[24] A variety of factors can affect the matching of ventilation to perfusion in the lungs.

Ventilation/perfusion can be considered as a continuum. At one end there is the alveolus that is not receiving any perfusion, thus unable to participate in gas exchange. This situation is referred to as *alveolar dead space.* In this case the ventilation is not used or wasted. On the other end of the continuum, there is the alveolus that is not receiving any ventilation, thus unable to participate in gas exchange. This situation is referred to as *intrapulmonary shunting.* In this case the blood is returned to the left side of the heart unoxygenated.[9] Between these two extremes exist an infinite number of ventilation/perfusion mismatches. Although minor mismatching of ventilation may not significantly affect gas exchange, significant alterations in the relationship are detrimental.[17]

GAS TRANSPORT

Gas transport refers to the movement of oxygen and carbon dioxide to and from the tissue cells. The transportation vehicle is the blood stream, which is moved by the pumping action of the heart. At the tissue level, both oxygen and carbon dioxide move into and out of the cell by diffusion. Oxygen diffuses into the cell because of the pressure gradient that exists between oxygen in the capillary and oxygen in the cell (Fig. 19-17, *A*). Carbon dioxide diffuses into the capillary because of the pressure gradient that exists between carbon dioxide in the cell and carbon dioxide in the capillary[9] (Fig. 19-17, *B*). Changes in the pressure gradient can affect tissue oxygenation (see box, p. 386).

Oxygen Transport Within the Blood

Oxygen is transported to the tissues by the blood in two ways. It is either dissolved in plasma (Pao_2) or bound to hemoglobin molecules (oxygen saturation [Sao_2]). Most of the oxygen is transported by hemoglobin, with the portion of oxygen dissolved in plasma equal to approximately 3% of the total oxygen within the blood.[6]

The pressure exerted by the oxygen dissolved in plasma is important because this oxygen diffuses across

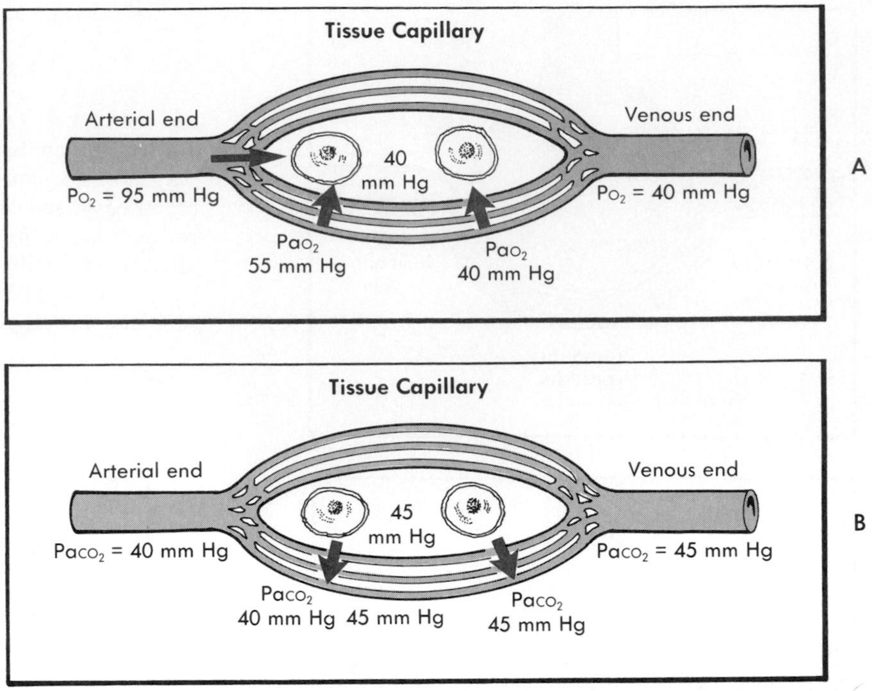

Fig. 19-17 **A,** Diffusion of oxygen from a tissue capillary into a tissue cell. **B,** Diffusion of carbon dioxide from a tissue cell into a tissue capillary.

◆

HOW CHANGES IN Pao_2 ALTER TISSUE OXYGENATION

Fig. 19-17 illustrates the pressure difference between the arterial partial pressure of oxygen (Pao_2) and the oxygen level of a tissue cell. (Intracellular oxygen levels vary widely from tissue to tissue, sometimes being much lower than the 40 mm Hg noted in Fig. 19-17). Oxygen diffuses because of the pressure gradient that exists between oxygen in the blood and oxygen in the cell. Suppose, because of pulmonary disease, the Pao_2 falls from 95 to 55 mm Hg. This causes the pressure gradient to be less, although diffusion still occurs. Now suppose the pulmonary disease worsens, causing the Pao_2 to fall further, severely compromising the pressure gradient. Tissue hypoxia results when the Pao_2 falls to the point at which a functional diffusion gradient no longer exists.

What happens when the Pao_2 is elevated above normal by the application of supplemental oxygen? The addition of supplemental oxygen may raise the Pao_2 to a level at which a more functional gradient exists. Considering Fig. 19-17 once more, it is easy to see that elevation of Pao_2 increases the gradient between oxygen in the arterial blood and oxygen in the tissue cell, thus improving diffusion.

the capillary membrane into the cells first and serves as the vehicle for the unloading of the oxygen from the hemoglobin molecule. As molecules of dissolved oxygen leave the plasma and diffuse into the cells, the molecules of oxygen move off the hemoglobin, dissolve into the plasma, and, in turn, diffuse into the cells.[23] For this process to begin, a pressure gradient must exist between the oxygen level in the capillary and the oxygen level in the cell.[9]

◆ **Oxyhemoglobin dissociation curve.** The relationship between dissolved oxygen and hemoglobin-bound oxygen is illustrated graphically as the oxyhemoglobin dissociation curve (Fig. 19-18). The sigmoid shape of the oxyhemoglobin dissociation curve illustrates several essential points about the relationship between the two ways oxygen is carried. The steep lower portion of the curve, at Pao_2 levels of 10 to 50 mm Hg, shows that the peripheral tissues can withdraw large amounts of oxygen from the hemoglobin molecule with only a small change in Pao_2, thus preserving the gradient for the continued unloading of hemoglobin.[23]

The area at Pao_2 levels of 60 to 100 mm Hg is called the *flat upper portion of the curve.* This portion shows that the saturation of hemoglobin remains high even as the Pao_2 declines. For example, in a healthy person, a Pao_2 of 60 mm Hg yields a saturation of 89%, whereas a Pao_2 of 100 mm Hg yields a saturation of 98%. The great drop in Pao_2 (from 100 to 60 mm Hg) causes only a small drop in oxygen saturation (from 98% to 89%).[24] For this reason, many patients with chronic lung disease manage quite well with a Pao_2 as low as 55 or 60 mm Hg. The ability of human beings to live comfortably at high altitudes is based on the unique relationship between dissolved oxygen and hemoglobin-bound oxygen. At high altitudes, because of the decreased barometric pressure, the Pao_2 will fall. There exists a wide range in which the Pao_2 can fall, yet loading of the hemoglobin molecule remains quite sufficient.[23]

Factors Affecting Oxygen Transport

Oxygen transport is determined by cardiac output, hemoglobin, and dissolved oxygen in the plasma (Pao_2).

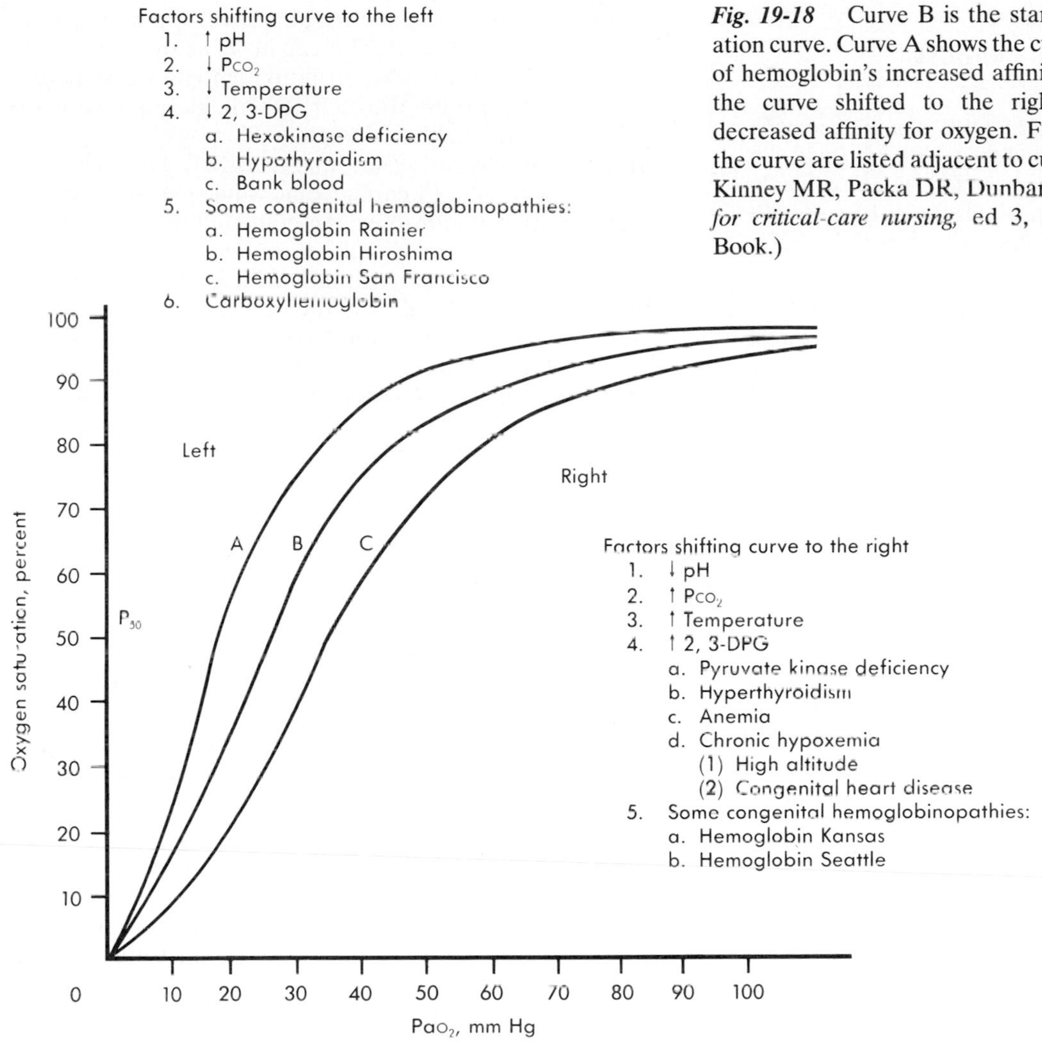

Fig. 19-18 Curve B is the standard oxyhemoglobin dissociation curve. Curve A shows the curve shifted to the left because of hemoglobin's increased affinity for oxygen. Curve C shows the curve shifted to the right because of hemoglobin's decreased affinity for oxygen. Factors responsible for shifting the curve are listed adjacent to curves A and C. (Modified from Kinney MR, Packa DR, Dunbar SB: *AACN's clinical reference for critical-care nursing,* ed 3, St Louis, 1993, Mosby–Year Book.)

Anything that affects these variables affects oxygen transport in the blood.[25] (Factors that affect cardiac output are not discussed here.)

◆ **Shifting of the oxyhemoglobin dissociation curve.** Under normal circumstances, hemoglobin has a steady and predictable affinity for oxygen. The combination of oxygen and hemoglobin based on this affinity is responsible for the position of the oxyhemoglobin dissociation curve wherein a given Pa_{O_2} yields a predictable oxygen saturation (Table 19-1).[23]

Occasionally events occur that alter the affinity hemoglobin has for oxygen. These events include changes in pH, Pa_{CO_2}, temperature, and 2,3-diphosphoglycerate (2,3-DPG) (see box, p. 388). Any time this affinity is altered, the position of the oxyhemoglobin dissociation curve shifts (Fig. 19-18). Shifts in the position of the curve mean there is a change in the way oxygen is taken up by the hemoglobin molecule at the alveolar level, as well as a change in the way oxygen is delivered at the tissue level.[9,24,26]

When the curve is shifted to the right (Fig. 19-18, *curve C*), there is a lower oxygen saturation for any given Pa_{O_2}; in other words, hemoglobin has less affinity for oxygen.

Table 19-1 Predictable relationship of Pa_{O_2} and Sa_{O_2} on the normal oxyhemoglobin dissociation curve

Pa_{O_2} (mm Hg)	Sa_{O_2} (%)
100	98
90	97
80	95
70	93
60	89
50	84
40	75
30	57
20	35
10	14

Although the saturation is lower than expected, a right shift enhances oxygen delivery at the tissue level because hemoglobin unloads more readily. Factors that cause this change in oxygen-hemoglobin affinity and shift the curve to the right include fever, increased Pa_{CO_2}, acidosis, and an increase in 2,3-DPG.[9,24,26]

WHAT IS 2,3-DPG?

2,3-Diphosphoglycerate (2,3-DPG), an organic phosphate found primarily in red blood cells, has the ability to alter the affinity of hemoglobin for oxygen. When the level of 2,3-DPG increases within the red blood cells, hemoglobin's affinity for oxygen is decreased (a shift in the oxyhemoglobin curve to the right), thus making more oxygen available to the tissues. Increased synthesis of 2,3-DPG apparently is an important component of the adaptive responses in healthy persons to an acute need for more tissue oxygen. Tissue hypoxia acts as the stimulus for production of 2,3-DPG, and increased amounts have been found in patients with anemia, right-to-left shunts, and congestive heart failure and in persons residing at high altitudes.[13]

A decrease in the amount of 2,3-DPG is detrimental to tissue oxygenation because this decrease causes hemoglobin's affinity for oxygen to increase (a shift in the oxyhemoglobin curve to the left). Situations resulting in decreased 2,3-DPG levels include hypophosphatemia, septic shock, and the use of banked blood. Blood preserved with acid citrate dextrose loses most of its red cell 2,3-DPG within several days. Blood preserved with citrate phosphate dextrose maintains its 2,3-DPG levels for several weeks. Transfusion of blood with low 2,3-DPG will not be beneficial for tissue oxygenation until the 2,3-DPG level is restored, which may take 18 to 24 hours.[26]

When the curve is shifted to the left (Fig. 19-18, *curve A*), quite the reverse occurs; there is a higher arterial saturation for any given Pao_2 because hemoglobin has an increased affinity for oxygen. Although the saturation is higher, oxygen delivery to the tissues is impaired because hemoglobin does not unload as easily. Factors that contribute to the effect include hypothermia, alkalemia, decreased $Paco_2$, and decreased 2,3-DPG.[9,24,26]

To assess whether the curve is shifted to the left or to the right, the Pao_2 at the 50% saturation level (P_{50} must be assessed. When the curve is in its normal position, a P_{50} is associated with a Pao_2 of 26.6 mm Hg (Fig. 19-18, *curve B*). If, when one looks at the P_{50}, the Pao_2 is higher, the curve is shifted to the right (Fig. 19-18, *curve C*). On the other hand, if, when one looks at the P_{50}, the Pao_2 is less than 26.6 mm Hg, the curve is shifted to the left (Fig. 19-18, *curve A*).[9,23,26] When working in a clinical situation in which a P_{50} is not available, one need only remember the aforementioned clinical situations that are responsible for left and for right shift of the curve.

◆ **Abnormalities of hemoglobin.** Hemoglobin carries approximately 97% of the total amount of oxygen held within the blood stream.[6] This great carrying capacity depends on hemoglobin that is normal in amount and molecular structure. Most hemoglobin abnormalities affect the oxygen-carrying capability of this molecule.[24]

The most common abnormality involving hemoglobin is a decrease in amount. This can be an acute or a chronic situation (anemia).[26] Abnormal hemoglobin structure also can pose problems, such as hemoglobin S, which is responsible for sickle cell anemia. Hemoglobin S has less affinity for oxygen than does normal hemoglobin.[24] Normal hemoglobin can become abnormal hemoglobin under certain conditions. Methemoglobin and carboxyhemoglobin are two such examples. Methemoglobin occurs when the iron atoms within the hemoglobin molecule are oxidized from the ferrous state to the ferric state. Methemoglobin does not carry oxygen. Carboxyhemoglobin occurs when carbon monoxide combines with hemoglobin. Carbon monoxide uses the same binding site as does oxygen and has a much greater affinity for hemoglobin.[9,24]

Carbon Dioxide Transport Within the Blood

Carbon dioxide, one of the end products of aerobic cellular metabolism, is produced continuously within the cells. On its way from the cells to the lungs, carbon dioxide is transported within the plasma and the erythrocytes. Carbon dioxide is transported, physically dissolved as the $Paco_2$ (5%), bound to blood proteins (including hemoglobin) in the form of carbaminohemoglobin compounds (5% to 10%), and combined with water to form carbonic acid (80% to 90%), some of which dissociates into hydrogen ions and bicarbonate.[6,9] In the lungs these methods of carbon dioxide carriage are reversed as the carbon dioxide leaves the plasma and erythrocytes for exhalation.[9,12,24]

REFERENCES

1. Tesoriero JV, Dail DH: Functional anatomy of the respiratory system. In Scanlan CL, Spearman CB, Sheldon RL, editors: *Egan's fundamentals of respiratory care,* ed 5, St Louis, 1990, Mosby–Year Book.
2. George RB, Chesson AL: Functional anatomy of the respiratory system. In George RB and others, editors: *Chest medicine: essentials of pulmonary and critical care medicine,* ed 2, Baltimore, 1990, Williams & Wilkins.
3. Sahn S: The pleura, *Am Rev Respir Dis* 138(1):184, 1988.
4. Kinasewitz GT, Fishman AP: Pleural dynamics and effusions. In Fishman AP: *Pulmonary diseases and disorders,* ed 2, New York, 1988, McGraw-Hill.
5. Martin L: *Pulmonary physiology in clinical practice: the essentials for patient care and evaluation,* St Louis, 1987, Mosby–Year Book.
6. Guyton AC: *Textbook of medical physiology,* ed 8, Philadelphia, 1991, WB Saunders.
7. Kinder RJ, Douce FH: Respiratory gas exchange mechanisms. In Burton GG, Hodgkin JE, Ward JJ, editors: *Respiratory care: a guide to clinical practice,* ed 3, Philadelphia, 1991, JB Lippincott.
8. Martin DE: *Respiratory anatomy and physiology,* St Louis, 1988, Mosby–Year Book.
9. Levitzky MG, Cairo JM, Hall SM: *Introduction to respiratory care,* Philadelphia, 1990, WB Saunders.
10. Cosenza JL, Norton LC: Secretion clearance: state of the art from a nursing perspective, *Crit Care Nurse* 6(4):23, 1986.
11. MacDonnell KF, Fahey PJ, Segal MS: *Respiratory intensive care,* Boston, 1987, Little, Brown.
12. Murray JF: *The normal lung: a basis for diagnosis and treatment of pulmonary disease,* ed 2, Philadelphia, 1986, WB Saunders.

13. Murray JF, Nadel JA: *Textbook of respiratory medicine,* Philadelphia, 1988, WB Saunders.
14. Matthay MA, Matthay RA: Pulmonary circulation. In George RB and others, editors: *Chest medicine: essentials of pulmonary and critical care medicine,* ed 2, Baltimore, 1990, Williams & Wilkins.
15. Gil J: The normal lung circulation: state of the art, *Chest* 93 (suppl 3):80S, 1988.
16. Thompson BT, Hales CA: Hypoxic pulmonary hypertension: acute and chronic, *Heart Lung* 15:457, 1986.
17. Reischman RR: Review of ventilation and perfusion physiology, *Crit Care Nurse* 8(7):24, 1988.
18. Shapiro B and others: *Clinical application of respiratory care,* ed 4, St Louis, 1991, Mosby–Year Book.
19. Deffebach ME and others: The bronchial circulation: small but a vital attribute of the lung, *Am Rev Respir Dis* 135(2):463, 1987.
20. Light RW: Mechanics of respiration. In George RB and others, editors: *Chest medicine: essentials of pulmonary and critical care medicine,* ed 2, Baltimore, 1990, Williams & Wilkins.
21. Ganong WF: *Review of medical physiology,* ed 15, Norwalk, Conn, 1991, Appleton & Lange.
22. Scanlan CL: Ventilation. In Scanlan CL, Spearman CB, Sheldon RL, editors: *Egan's fundamentals of respiratory care,* ed 5, St Louis, 1990, Mosby–Year Book.
23. Carpenter KD: Oxygen transport in the blood, *Crit Care Nurse* 11(9):20, 1991.
24. Gross GW, Scanlan CL: Gas exchange and transport. In Scanlan CL, Spearman CB, Sheldon RL, editors: *Egan's fundamentals of respiratory care,* ed 5, St Louis, 1990, Mosby–Year Book.
25. Ahrens TS: Concepts in the assessment of oxygenation, *Focus Crit Care* 14(1):36, 1987.
26. George RB: Alveolar ventilation, gas transfer, and oxygen delivery. In George RB and others, editors: *Chest medicine: essentials of pulmonary and critical care medicine,* ed 2, Baltimore, 1990, Williams & Wilkins.

20

Pulmonary Clinical Assessment

CHAPTER OBJECTIVES

- Explain the contents of a complete pulmonary history.
- Address inspection and palpation of the patient with pulmonary dysfunction.
- Discuss percussion and auscultation of the patient with pulmonary dysfunction.
- Describe the assessment findings associated with various pulmonary disorders.

Assessment of the patient with pulmonary dysfunction is a systematic process that incorporates both an inquiry into the chronology of the present illness, better known as a *history,* and an investigation of the current physical manifestations, better known as a *physical examination.* The purpose of the assessment is twofold: first, to recognize changes in the patient's pulmonary status that would necessitate nursing or medical intervention; and second, to determine the ways in which the patient's pulmonary dysfunction is interfering with his or her self-care activities.[1] Once completed, the assessment serves as the foundation for developing the management plan for the patient. The assessment process can be brief or can involve a detailed history and examination, depending on the nature and immediacy of the patient's situation. Whatever the setting, the nurse should develop and practice a sequential pattern of assessment to avoid omitting portions of the examination.[1]

HISTORY

Taking a thorough and accurate history is extremely important to the assessment process. The patient's history provides the foundation and direction for the rest of the assessment. The overall goal of the patient interview is to expose key clinical manifestations that will facilitate the identification of the underlying cause of the illness. This information will then assist in the development of an appropriate management plan.[2]

The initial presentation of the patient determines the rapidity and direction of the interview. For a patient in acute distress, the history should be curtailed to just a few questions about the patient's chief complaint and precipitating events. For a patient in no obvious distress, the history should focus on five different areas: (1) review of the patient's present illness, (2) overview of the patient's general respiratory status, (3) examination of the patient's general health status, (4) survey of the patient's family and social background, and (5) description of the patient's current symptoms.[1]

Present Illness

A review of the patient's present illness should be conducted in an attempt to elicit the clinical manifestations and problems in the order in which they occurred. Questions should include the following: (1) What brought you to the hospital? (2) What were the precipitating events? and (3) When did the problem start? As many details should be obtained as possible.[1,2]

Respiratory Status

An overview of the patient's general respiratory status also should be conducted to gather information about the patient's pulmonary history. Questions should include the following: (1) Do you currently have chronic lung disease, such as asthma, bronchitis, or emphysema? (2) Do you have a history of any lung disease, such as chronic respiratory infections or tuberculosis? and (3) Have you had any chest surgery? If the patient responds "yes" to any of these questions, further inquiry should be made as to the type, time of onset and duration of illness, major symptoms, and the patient's knowledge base about the disease.[1,3]

General Health Status

An examination of the patient's general health status should be conducted to gather information on the patient's past major and minor nonpulmonary illnesses. Questions should include the following: (1) Do you have any other chronic disease or illness? (2) Do you have a history of any other disease, illness, or surgery? and (3) Are you currently taking any medications, prescription or nonprescription? If the patient responds "yes" to any of these questions, further inquiry should be made as to the type, length, major symptoms, and the patient's knowledge base about the disease or medication.[1]

Life-style

A survey of the patient's social and occupational background should be performed to elicit information on the patient's life-style and exposure to occupational and environmental pollutants. Questions should include the following: (1) Do you smoke or have you smoked in the past? (2) Have you been exposed to "secondhand" smoke? and (3) Have you ever been exposed to lung irritants or cancer-causing agents, such as asbestos,

Table 20-1 Key symptoms in pulmonary disease

Symptoms	Possible respiratory causes
Dsypnea/shortness of breath, breathlessness, inability to catch breath, smothering tightness in chest, dyspnea on exertion, orthopnea	Airway obstruction, e.g., foreign body, bronchitis, mucus, asthma, chronic obstructive pulmonary disease (COPD), atelectasis, tumors, pneumothorax Altered mechanics of breathing, e.g., congestive heart failure (CHF), pulmonary embolism, pulmonary contusion, acute blood loss, anemia, splinting, chest wall deformity Hyperventilation syndrome
Chest pain accentuated by breathing, coughing, sneezing, laughing; usually sharp, knifelike burning quality to pain	Inflammation or trauma of ribs, muscles, nerves, and pleurae; pleurisy; rib fracture; costochondritis; intercostal myositis
Cough with or without sputum production	Exacerbation of COPD, pneumonia, interstitial lung disease, aspiration lung disorders, CHF, pulmonary embolism, noncardiogenic pulmonary edema, chronic irritation of respiratory mucosa

chemicals, fumes, beryllium, coal or stone quarry dust, or Agent Orange? If the patient responds "yes" to any of these questions, further inquiry should be made as to the type and duration of exposure.[1,3]

Symptoms

A description of the patient's current symptoms should be obtained, specifically regarding the presence of dyspnea, cough, and chest pain. During the discussion of symptoms, it is important to note the absence of a symptom from a usual cluster or grouping. For example, a cough is generally associated with pulmonary infection; absence of any cough would be noted as a significant negative in symptoms of this disorder and could help refine the list of possible causes. Table 20-1 outlines some of the possible pulmonary causes for these symptoms.

◆ **Dyspnea.** Dyspnea, or shortness of breath, is the most frequently reported complaint and most often the one that prompts the patient to seek assistance. Questions about dyspnea should center around the degree of breathlessness and functional impairment the patient is experiencing. Because dyspnea is a subjective complaint, its severity is difficult to assess. Often a patient's complaints of dyspnea do not correlate with the findings of pulmonary function tests, arterial blood gas (ABG) values, or other available objective measurements. Although a variety of methods are available to assess dyspnea, many of them are not practical for use in the critically ill patient.[4,5] One tool that can be used in this patient population is the Dyspnea Assessment Guide (DAG) (Fig. 20-1).[6]

The DAG is a three-part assessment tool. In the first section, the patient is asked to rate the degree of breathlessness he or she is experiencing, using the vertical analog dyspnea scale (VADS). The VADS consists of a vertical line with "shortness of breath as bad as can be" at the top and "no shortness of breath" at the bottom. Changes in severity or improvement can then be plotted along the continuum during the course of therapy. In the second section, the patient is asked to rate on a 5-point scale the subjective complaints of poor appetite, feeling worn out or weak, suffocation, tightness, congestion, and feeling of panic or anxiety. The scale ranges from 0 to 4, with 0 indicating no distress and 4 indicating much distress. In the third section, the nurse rates the degree of accessory muscle use by observing the rise of the patient's clavicle during inspiration. The rise of the clavicle is then classified as absent (not detected), mild (seen but not pronounced), or severe (pronounced).[6]

Table 20-2 Sputum characteristics seen in various pulmonary disorders

Appearance	Likely cause
Bloody, gelatinous sputum (currant-jelly sputum)	*Klebsiella pneumoniae*
Rusty sputum (prune-juice sputum)	Pneumococcal pneumonias
Thick, green sputum with blood streaking it	*Klebsiella pneumoniae*
Stringy, mucoid sputum	Asthmatic attack
Frothy sputum	Pulmonary edema
Purulent sputum of yellow, green, gray nature	Pneumonias

◆ **Cough.** Cough is another common complaint that requires further investigation. Questions about the patient's cough should center around onset, frequency, precipitating events, effort, and whether the cough is productive. If the cough is productive, the patient should be asked questions about the color, amount, odor, and consistency of the sputum.[1,7] Table 20-2 outlines the sputum characteristics seen in various pulmonary disorders.

◆ **Chest pain.** Another important symptom that should be completely investigated is the presence of chest pain. Questions should center around onset, duration, loca-

Direct Measure of Dyspnea

Indicate the amount of shortness of breath you are having at this time by marking the line.

Shortness of breath as bad as can be

No shortness of breath

Subjective Symptoms

On a scale of 0-4 with 0 indicating no distress and 4 indicating much distress, how much are you presently distressed by: (*circle answer*)

Poor appetite	0	1	2	3	4
Worn out or weak	0	1	2	3	4
Suffocation	0	1	2	3	4
Tightness	0	1	2	3	4
Congestion	0	1	2	3	4
A feel of panic or anxiety	0	1	2	3	4

Objective Sign

Rise of the clavicle during inspiration:

ABSENT = Not detected
MILD = Seen but not pronounced
SEVERE = Pronounced

Fig. 20-1 Dyspnea Assessment Guide (DAG). (From Gift AG: *Crit Care Nurs* 9(8):79, 1989.)

tion, quality, radiation, and associated, aggravating, and alleviating factors.[1] It is extremely important to differentiate the cause of the chest pain. Chest pain of cardiac origin is usually described as constricting, pressing, or sharp and is often associated with exertion, intense emotion, or eating a large meal. Chest pain of pulmonary origin is usually described as very sharp and is often associated with breathing.[7]

PHYSICAL EXAMINATION

Four techniques are used in physical assessment: inspection, palpation, percussion, and auscultation. Inspection is the process of looking intently at the patient. Palpation is the process of touching the patient to judge the size, shape, texture, and temperature of the body surface or underlying structures. Percussion is the process of creating sound waves on the surface of the body to determine abnormal density of any underlying areas. Auscultation is the process of concentrated listening with a stethoscope to determine characteristics of body functions.[8]

Inspection

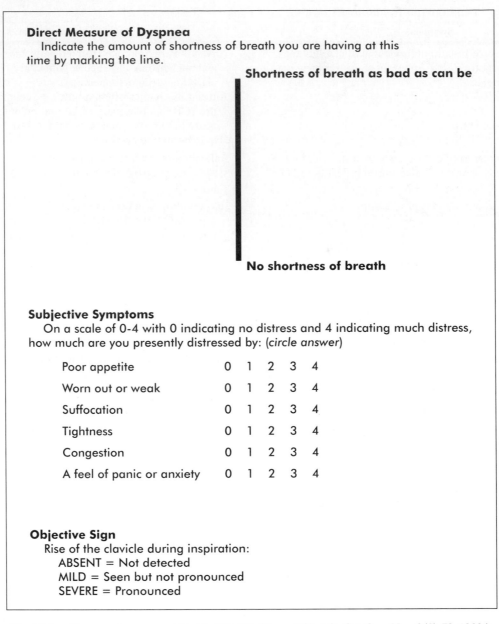

Inspection of the patient should focus on three different areas: (1) identification of general signs of pulmonary disease, (2) assessment of chest wall configuration, and (3) evaluation of respiratory effort. If possible, patients should be positioned upright, with their arms resting at their sides.[3] Inspection generally begins during the interview process.[1]

◆ **General signs.** Identification of general signs of pulmonary disease incorporates assessment of numerous items. This discussion focuses on assessment of mucous membranes and nailbeds. Assessment of the color of the mucous membranes is important in the identification of central cyanosis, which is manifested by a blue tint to the membranes. Central cyanosis is a sign of hypoxemia. Assessment of the shape of the nailbeds is also important in the identification of clubbing, which is manifested by an increase in the angle between the nail and the nailbed (Fig. 20-2). Clubbing occurs as the result of chronic tissue hypoxia and is associated with chronic obstructive pulmonary disease (COPD).[7]

◆ **Chest wall configuration.** Assessment of chest wall configuration incorporates observations about the size and shape of the patient's chest. Normally, the ratio of anteroposterior (AP) diameter to lateral diameter ranges from 1:2 to 5:7.[1,9] An increase in the AP diameter is suggestive of COPD.[1] The shape of the chest should be inspected for any structural deviations. Some of the more frequently seen abnormalities are pectus excavatum, pectus carinatum, barrel chest, and spinal deformities. In pectus excavatum (funnel chest), the sternum and lower ribs are displaced posteriorly, creating a funnel or pit-shaped depression in the chest. This causes a decrease in the AP diameter of the chest and may interfere with respiratory function. In pectus carinatum (pigeon breast), the sternum projects forward. This causes an increase in the AP diameter of the chest. The barrel chest is characterized by displacement of the sternum forward and the ribs outward. This also causes an increase in the AP diameter of the chest. Spinal deformities—such as kyphosis, lordosis, and scoliosis—may also be present and can interfere with respiratory function.[7,9,10]

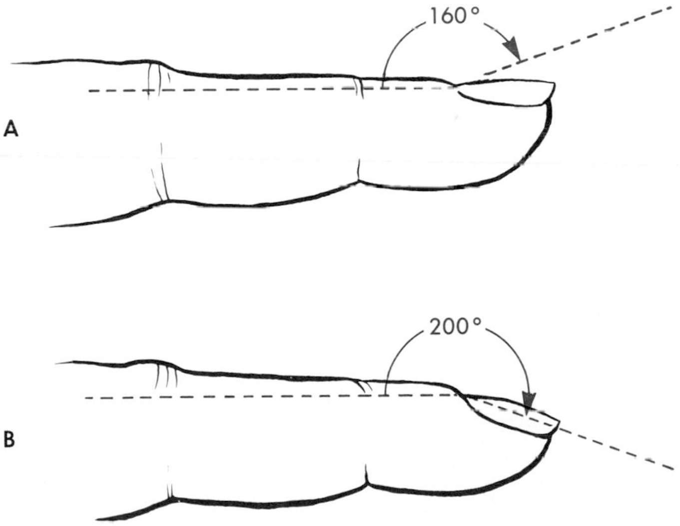

Fig. 20-2 Clubbing of the fingers. **A,** Normal. **B,** Loss of normal nail bed angulation. (From Kinney M and others: *Comprehensive cardiac care,* ed 7, St Louis, 1991, Mosby–Year Book.)

◆ **Respiratory effort.** Evaluation of respiratory effort incorporates observations on the rate, rhythm, symmetry, and quality of ventilatory movements.[1] Normal breathing at rest is effortless and regular and occurs at a rate of 12 to 20 breaths per minute.[3] There are a number of abnormal respiratory patterns (Fig. 20-3). Some of the more commonly seen patterns in patients with pulmonary dysfunction are tachypnea, hyperventilation, and air trapping. Tachypnea is manifested by an increase in the rate and decrease in the depth of ventilation. Hyperventilation is manifested by an increase in both the rate and depth of ventilation. Air trapping, also called *obstructive breathing,* usually occurs in the patient with COPD as a result of air trapping. As air becomes trapped in the lungs, ventilations become more shallow.[11]

Other areas that should be assessed are patient position, active effort to breathe, use of accessory muscles, presence of intercostal retractions, unequal movement of the chest wall, flaring of nares, and pausing midsentence to take a breath.[1] Normal, quiet breathing is relatively effortless and unlabored, whereas difficult breathing is quite labored. A classic example of extremely labored breathing is a patient suffering an exacerbation of COPD who sits in high-Fowler's position and leans forward, using the neck and chest accessory muscles to inhale and pursed-lip breathing to exhale. Gasps for air may make the distress readily apparent. The presence of other iatrogenic features, such as chest tubes, central venous lines, artificial airways, and nasogastric tubes, should be noted because they may affect assessment findings.

Palpation

Palpation of the patient should focus on three different areas: (1) confirmation of the position of the trachea, (2) assessment of respiratory excursion, and (3) evaluation of fremitus. In addition, the thorax should be assessed for any areas of tenderness, lumps, or bony deformities. The anterior, posterior, and lateral areas of the chest should be evaluated in a systematic fashion.[9,10]

◆ **Position of trachea.** Confirmation of the position of the trachea is performed to verify that the trachea is midline. It is assessed by placing the fingers in the suprasternal notch and moving upward. Deviation of the trachea to either side can indicate a pneumothorax, unilateral pneumonia, diffuse pulmonary fibrosis, a large pleural effusion, or severe atelectasis. With atelectasis the trachea shifts to the same side as the problem, and with pneumothorax the trachea shifts to the opposite side of the problem.[7,10]

◆ **Respiratory excursion.** Assessment of respiratory excursion involves measuring the degree and symmetry of respiratory movement. It is assessed by placing the hands on the anterolateral chest with the thumbs extended along the costal margin, pointing to the xiphoid process or on the posterolateral chest with the thumbs on either side of the spine at the level of the tenth rib (Fig. 20-4). The patient is instructed to take a few normal breaths, then a few deep breaths. Chest movement is assessed for equality, which signifies symmetry of thoracic expansion.[3,10] Asymmetry is an abnormal finding that can occur

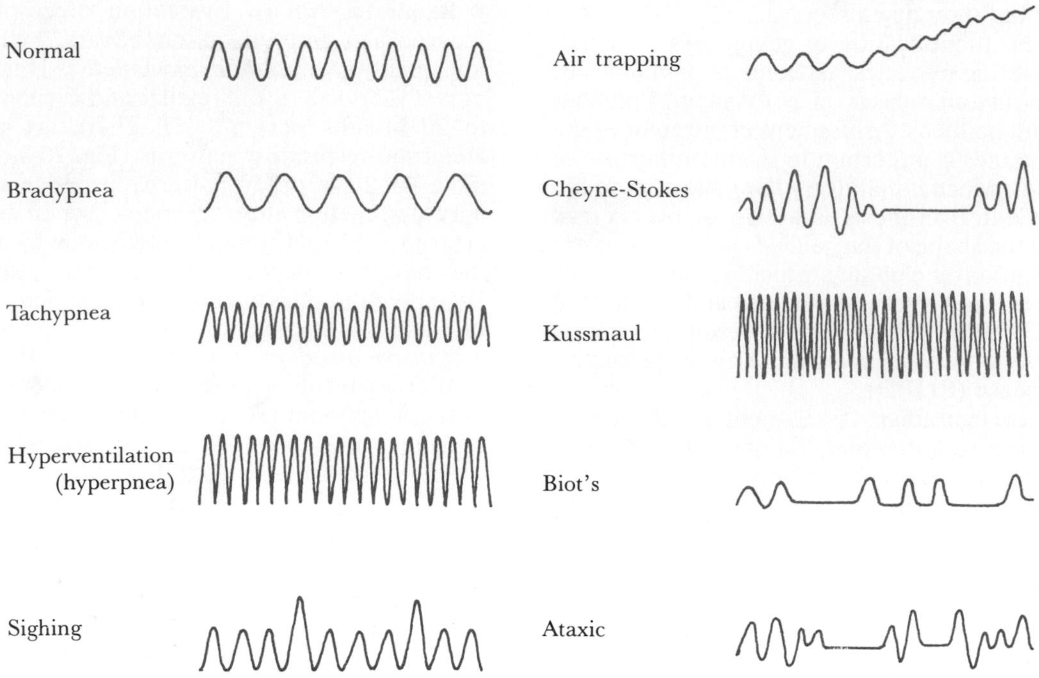

SOME INFLUENCES ON THE RATE AND DEPTH OF BREATHING

The rate and depth of breathing will

Increase with	**Decrease with**
Acidosis (metabolic)	Alkalosis (metabolic)
Anxiety	Central nervous system lesions (cerebrum)
Aspirin poisoning	Myasthenia gravis
Oxygen need (hypoxemia)	Narcotic overdoses
Pain	Obesity (extreme)
Central nervous system lesions (pons)	

Fig. 20-3 Patterns of respiration. The horizontal axis indicates the relative rates of these patterns. The vertical axis indicates the relative depth of respiration. (From Seidel HM and others: *Mosby's guide to physical examination,* ed 2, St Louis, 1991, Mosby–Year Book.)

with pneumothorax, pneumonia, or other disorders that interfere with lung inflation. The degree of chest movement is felt to ascertain the extent of lung expansion. The thumbs should separate 3 to 5 cm during deep inhalation.[10] Lung expansion of a hyperinflated chest is less than that of a normal one.[9]

◆ **Tactile fremitus.** Assessment of tactile fremitus is performed to identify, describe, and localize any areas of increased or decreased fremitus. Fremitus refers to the palpable vibrations felt through the chest wall when the patient speaks. It is assessed by placing the palmar surface of the hands against opposite sides of the chest wall and having the patient repeat the word "ninety-nine" (Fig. 20-5). The hands are moved systematically around the thorax until the anterior, posterior, and both lateral areas have been assessed. If only one hand is used, it is moved from one side of the chest to the corresponding area on the other side of the chest until all areas have been assessed.[10]

Fremitus varies from patient to patient and depends on the pitch and intensity of the voice. Fremitus is described as normal, decreased, or increased. With normal fremitus, vibrations can be felt over the trachea but are barely palpable over the periphery. With decreased fremitus, there is interference with the transmission of vibrations. Examples of disorders that decrease fremitus include pleural effusion, pneumothorax, bronchial obstruction, pleural thickening, and emphysema. With increased fremitus, there is an increase in the transmission of vibrations. Examples of disorders that increase fremitus include pneumonia, lung cancer, and pulmonary fibrosis.[3]

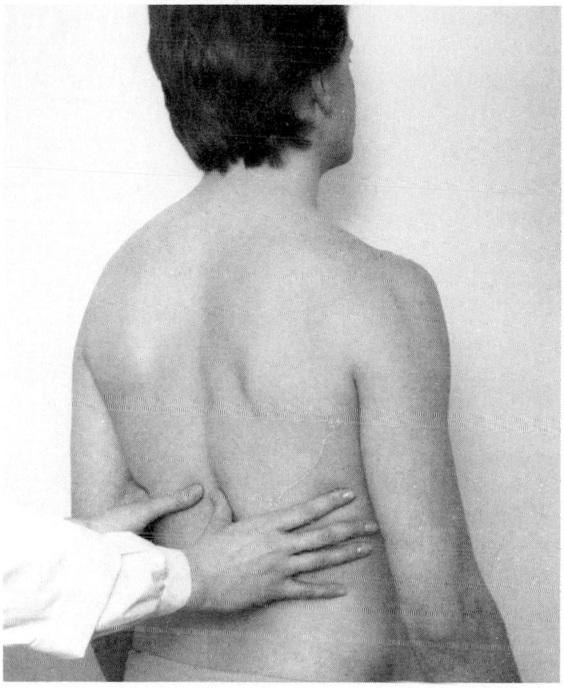

Fig. 20-4 Assessment of respiratory excursion. (From Malasanos L, Barkauskas V, Stoltenberg-Allen K: *Health assessment,* ed 4, St Louis, 1990, Mosby–Year Book.)

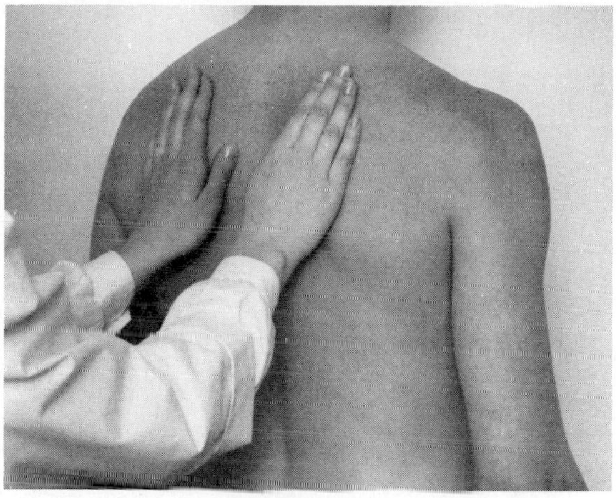

Fig. 20-5 Palpatation of fremitus, showing simultaneous application of the fingertips of both hands to compare sides. (From Malasanos L, Barkauskas V, Stoltenberg-Allen K: *Health assessment,* ed 4, St Louis, 1990, Mosby–Year Book.)

Percussion

Percussion of the patient should focus on two different areas: (1) evaluation of the underlying lung structure and (2) assessment of diaphragmatic excursion. Although not an often-used technique, percussion is a useful method for confirming suspected abnormalities.[7]

◆ **Underlying lung structure.** Evaluation of the underlying lung structure is performed to estimate the amounts of air, liquid, or solid material present. It is performed by placing the middle finger of the nondominant hand on the chest wall. The distal portion, between the last joint and the nailbed, is then struck with the middle finger of the dominant hand. The hands are moved side-to-side, systematically around the thorax, to compare similar areas, until the anterior, posterior, and both lateral areas have been assessed (Fig. 20-6). Five different tones can be elicited: resonance, hyperresonance, tympany, dullness, and flatness. These tones are distinguished by differences in intensity, pitch, duration, and quality. Table 20-3 describes the different percussion tones and their associated conditions.[1,9,11]

◆ **Diaphragmatic excursion.** Assessment of diaphragmatic excursion is accomplished by measuring the difference in the level of the diaphragm on inhalation and exhalation. It is performed by instructing the patient to inhale and hold the breath. The posterior chest is percussed downward, over the intercostal spaces, until the dull sound produced by the diaphragm is heard. The spot is marked. The patient is then instructed to take a few breaths in and out, exhale completely, and then hold his or her breath. The posterior chest is percussed again, and the new area of dullness over the diaphragm is then located and marked. The difference between the two spots is noted and measured. Normal diaphragmatic excursion is 3 to 5 cm.[7,9,10] It is decreased in such disorders or conditions as ascites, pregnancy, hepatomegaly, and emphysema. It is increased in pleural effusion or disorders that elevate the diaphragm, such as atelectasis or paralysis.

Table 20-3 Percussion tones and their associated conditions

Tone	Description	Condition
Resonance	Intensity—loud Pitch—low Duration—long Quality—hollow	Normal lung Bronchitis
Hyperresonance	Intensity—very loud Pitch—very low Duration—long Quality—booming	Asthma Emphysema Pneumothorax
Tympany	Intensity—loud Pitch—musical Duration—medium Quality—drumlike	Large pneumothorax Emphysematous blebs
Dullness	Intensity—medium Pitch—medium-high Duration—medium Quality—thudlike	Atelectasis Pleural effusion Pulmonary edema Pneumonia Lung mass
Flatness	Intensity—soft Pitch—high Duration—short Quality—extremely dull	Massive atelectasis Pneumonectomy

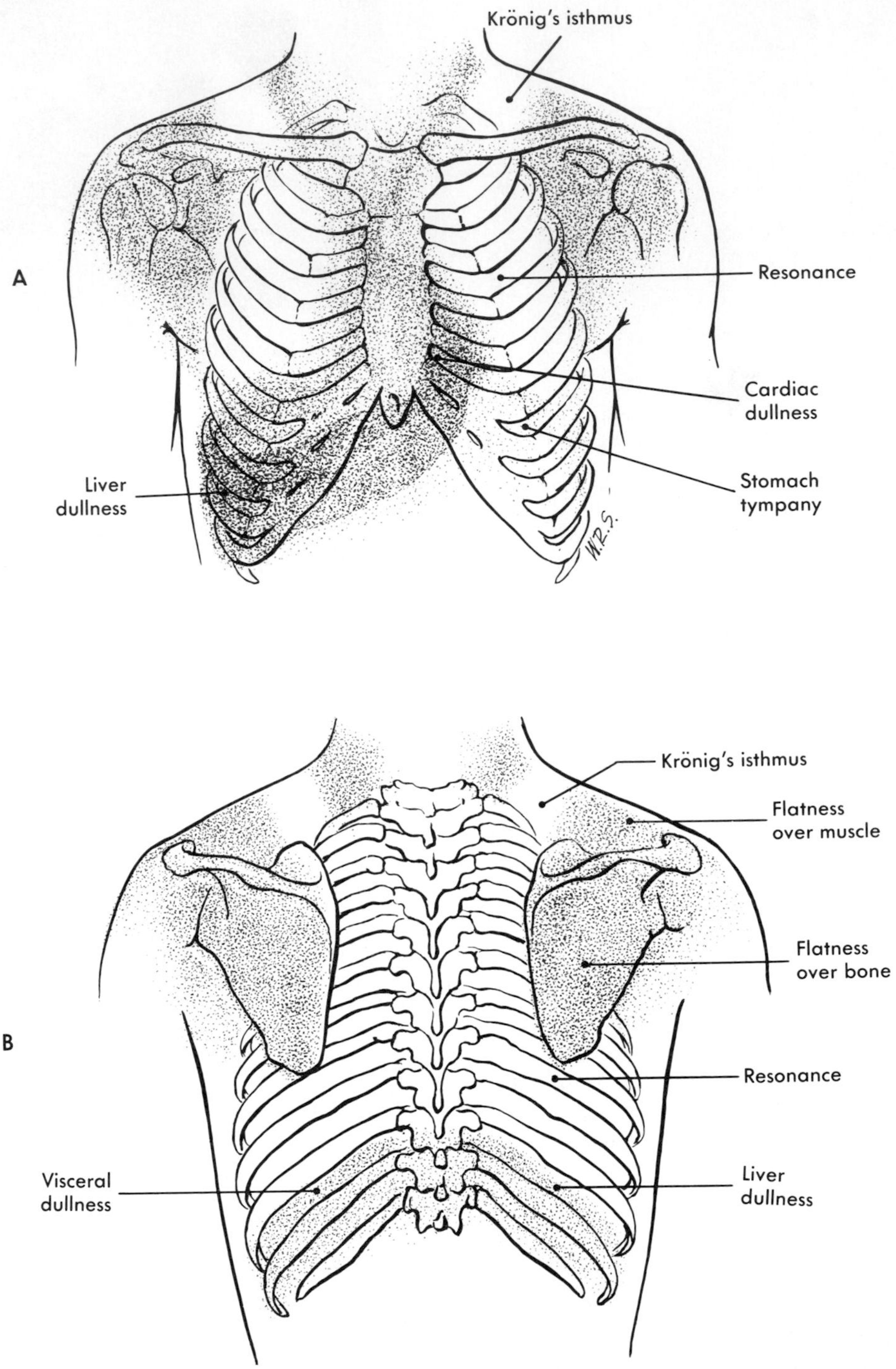

Fig. 20-6 Percussion sounds of the anterior, **A,** and posterior, **B,** thorax. (From Malasanos L, Barkauskas V, Stoltenberg-Allen K: *Health assessment,* ed 4, St Louis, 1990, Mosby–Year Book.)

Table 20-4 Characteristics of normal breath sounds

Sound	Characteristics	Findings
Vesicular	Heard over most of lung field; low pitch; soft and short exhalation and long inhalation	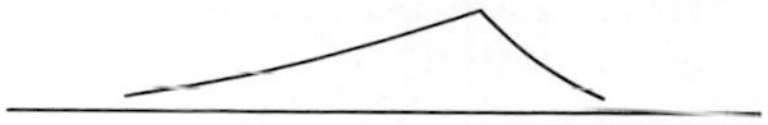
Bronchovesicular	Heard over main bronchus area and over upper right posterior lung field; medium pitch; exhalation equals inhalation	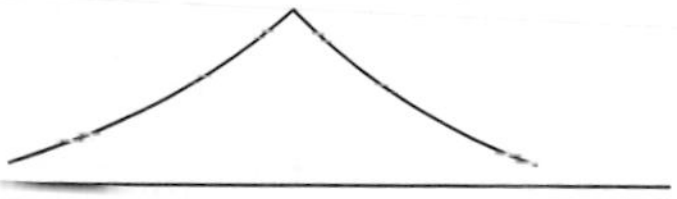
Bronchial	Heard only over trachea; high pitch; loud and long exhalation	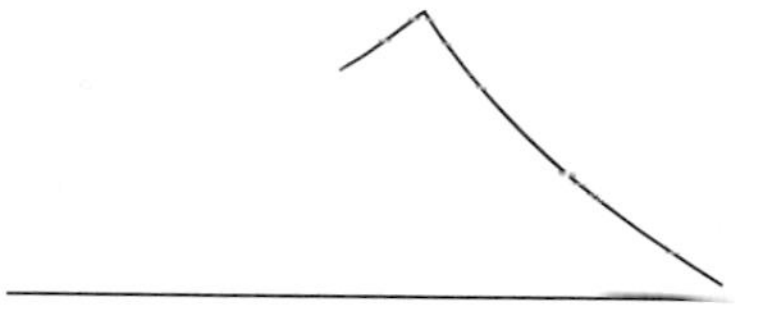

From Thomspon JM and others: *Mosby's clinical nursing*, ed 3, St Louis, 1993, Mosby–Year Book.

Auscultation

Auscultation of the patient should focus on three different areas: (1) evaluation of normal breath sounds, (2) identification of abnormal breath sounds, and (3) assessment of voice sounds. Auscultation requires a quiet environment, proper positioning of the patient, and a bare chest.[12] Breath sounds are best heard with the patient in the upright position.[7]

◆ **Normal breath sounds.** Evaluation of normal breath sounds is performed to assess air movement through the pulmonary system and to identify the presence of abnormal sounds. It is performed by placing the diaphragm of the stethoscope against the chest wall and instructing the patient to breathe in and out slowly with his or her mouth open. Both the inhalation and exhalation phases should be assessed. Auscultation should be done in a systematic sequence, side to side, top to bottom, anteriorly, posteriorly, and laterally.

Normal breath sounds are different, depending on their location. They are classified into three categories: bronchial, bronchovesicular, and vesicular. Table 20-4 describes the characteristics of normal breath sounds and their associated conditions.[3,9,11,12]

◆ **Abnormal breath sounds.** Identification of abnormal breath sounds occurs once the normal breath sounds have been clearly delineated. There are three categories of abnormal breath sounds: absent or diminished breath sounds, displaced bronchial breath sounds, and adventitious breath sounds. Table 20-5 describes the various abnormal breath sounds and their associated conditions.

An absent or diminished breath sound indicates that there is little or no airflow to a particular portion of the lung. It could be a small segment or an entire lung.[12] Displaced bronchial breath sounds are normal bronchial sounds heard in the peripheral lung fields instead of over the trachea. This condition is usually indicative of fluid or exudate present in the alveoli.[12] Adventitious breath sounds are extra or added sounds heard in addition to the other sounds already discussed. They are classified as crackles, rhonchi, wheezes, and friction rubs. Crackles (also called *rales*) are short, discrete, popping or crackling sounds produced by fluid in the small airways or alveoli. They are mainly heard on inhalation.[12] Crackles can be further classified as fine, medium, or coarse, depending on pitch.[3] Rhonchi are coarse, rumbling, low-pitched sounds produced by airflow over secretions in the larger airways or narrowing of the large airways. They are mainly heard on exhalation and sometimes can be cleared with coughing. Rhonchi can be further classified as bubbling, gurgling, or sonorous, depending on the characteristics of the sound.[12] Wheezes are high-pitched, squeaking, whistling sounds produced by airflow through narrowed small airways. They are mainly heard on exhalation but may be heard throughout the ventilatory cycle. Wheezes can be further classified as mild, moderate, or severe, depending on severity.[12] A pleural friction rub is a creaking, leathery, loud, dry, coarse sound produced by irritated pleural surfaces rubbing together. It is usually heard best in the lower anterolateral chest area during both inhalation and exhalation. Pleural friction rubs are caused by inflammation of the pleura.[3,10]

◆ **Voice sounds.** Assessment of voice sounds is particularly useful in detecting lung consolidation or lung compression. Three abnormal types of voice sounds are

Table 20-5 Abnormal breath sounds and their associated conditions

Abnormal sound	Description	Condition
Absent breath sounds	No airflow to particular portion of lung	Pneumothorax Pneumonectomy Emphysematous blebs Pleural effusion Lung mass Massive atelectasis Complete airway obstruction
Diminished breath sounds	Little airflow to particular portion of lung	Emphysema Pleural effusion Pleurisy Atelectasis Pulmonary fibrosis
Displaced bronchial sounds	Bronchial sounds heard in peripheral lung fields	Atelectasis with secretions Lung mass with exudate Pneumonia Pleural effusion Pulmonary edema
Crackles (rales)	Short, discrete, popping or crackling sounds	Pulmonary edema Pneumonia Pulmonary fibrosis Atelectasis Bronchiectasis
Rhonchi	Coarse, rumbling, low-pitched sounds	Pneumonia Asthma Bronchitis Bronchospasm
Wheezes	High-pitched, squeaking, whistling sounds	Asthma Bronchospasm
Pleural friction rub	Creaking, leathery, loud, dry, coarse sounds	Pleural effusion Pleurisy

bronchophony, whispering pectoriloquy, and egophony. Bronchophony describes a condition in which the spoken voice is heard on auscultation with higher intensity and clarity than usual. Normally the spoken word is muffled when heard through the stethoscope. It is assessed by placing the diaphragm of the stethoscope against the posterior side of the patient's chest and instructing the patient to say "ninety-nine." Bronchophony is present when the sound heard is clear, distinct, and loud. Whispering pectoriloquy describes a condition of unusually clear transmission of the whispered voice on auscultation. Normally the whispered word is unintelligible when heard through the stethoscope. It is assessed by placing the stethoscope against the posterior side of the patient's chest and instructing the patient to whisper "one, two, three." Whispering pectoriloquy is present when the sound heard is clear and distinct. Egophony describes a condition in which the voice sounds increase in intensity and develop a nasal bleating quality on auscultation. It is assessed by placing the stethoscope against the posterior side of the patient's chest and instructing the patient to say "e-e-e." Egophony is present when the "e" sound changes to an "a" sound.[10,12]

Table 20-6 presents a variety of common pulmonary disorders and their associated assessment findings.

REFERENCES

1. Rokosky JS: Assessment of the individual with altered respiratory function, *Nurs Clin North Am* 16:195, 1981.
2. Gehring PE: Physical assessment begins with a history, *RN* 54(11):26, 1991.
3. Brenner M, Welliver J: Pulmonary and acid-base assessment, *Nurs Clin North Am* 25:761, 1990.
4. Gift AG: Dyspnea, *Nurs Clin North Am* 25:955, 1990.
5. Gift AG: Clinical measurement of dyspnea, *Dimens Crit Care Nurs* 8:210, 1989.
6. Gift AG: A dyspnea assessment guide, *Crit Care Nurs* 9(8):79, 1989.
7. Levitzky MG, Cairo JM, Hall SM: *Introduction to respiratory care,* Philadelphia, 1990, WB Saunders.
8. Fitzgerald MA: The physical exam, *RN* 54(11):34, 1991.
9. King C: Examining the thorax and respiratory system, *RN* 45(8):55, 1982.
10. Malasanos L, Barkauskas V, Stoltenberg-Allen K: *Health assessment,* ed 4, St Louis, 1990, Mosby–Year Book.
11. Seidel HM and others: *Mosby's guide to physical examination,* ed 2, St Louis, 1991, Mosby–Year Book.
12. Boyda EK and others: *Pulmonary auscultation,* St Paul, 1987, 3M Health Care Group.

Table 20-6 Assessment findings frequently associated with common lung conditions

Condition*	Breath sound†	Description	Inspection	Palpation	Percussion	Auscultation
Healthy lung 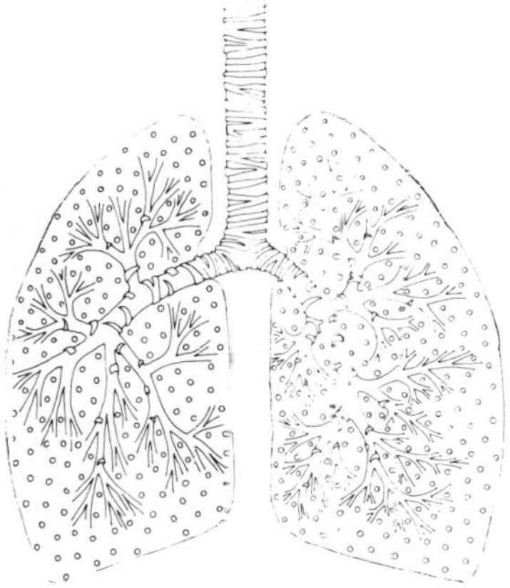	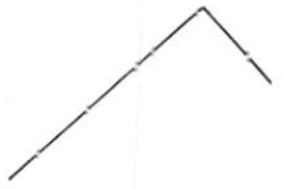	Tracheobronchial tree and alveoli are clear, pleurae are thin and close together: chest wall is mobile.	Symmetric rib and diaphragmatic movement – absence of accessory muscle activity Regular respiratory rhythm	Trachea – midline Expansion – equal bilaterally Tactile fremitus – present Diaphragmatic excursion – 3 to 5 cm	Resonant	Breath sounds – vesicular over periphery areas Voice sounds – normal Adventitious sounds – none except for a few transient crackles at the bases that clear with deep breathing
Asthma 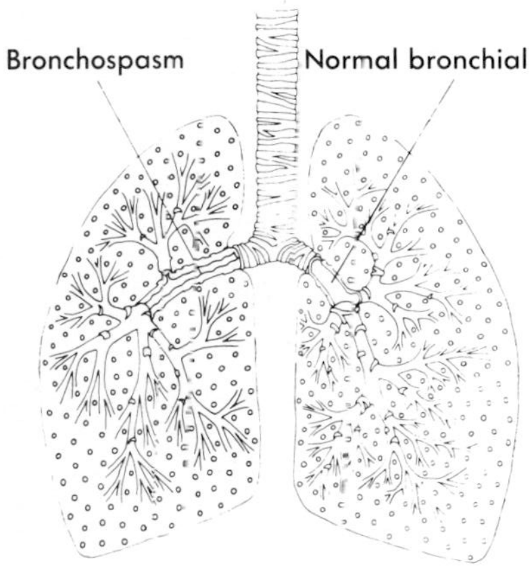	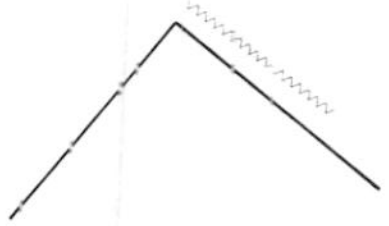	Asthma is characterized by intermittent episodes of airway obstruction caused by bronchospasm, excessive bronchial secretion, or edema of bronchial mucosa.	Central cyanosis Tachypnea with audible wheezing Use of accessory muscles of ventilation	Tactile fremitus – decreased	Hyperresonant	Breath sounds – distant, decreased Voice sounds – decreased Adventitious sounds- – wheezes

From Malasanos L and others: *Health assessment*, ed 4, St Louis, 1990, Mosby–Year Book.

*Although some disease conditions are bilateral, one diseased lung and one healthy lung are illustrated for each condition to provide contrast. Pathologic condition is illustrated on the left side, and the normal lung is on the right side.

† ⁘ denotes auscultation of crackles; ﹏ denotes auscultation of wheezes.

Continued.

Table 20-6 Assessment findings frequently associated with common lung conditions—cont'd

Condition*	Breath sound†	Description	Inspection	Palpation	Percussion	Auscultation
Atelectasis 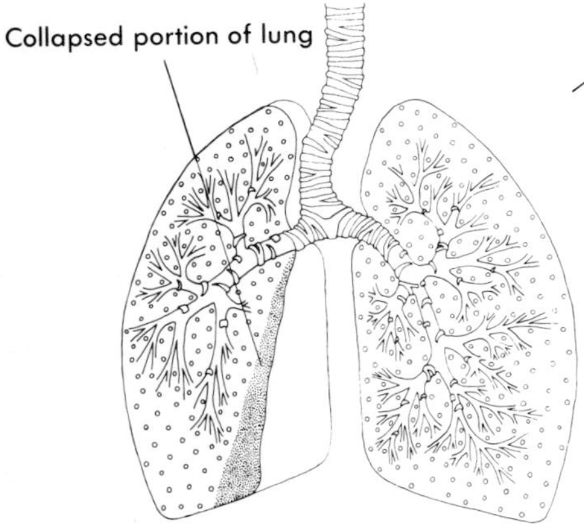	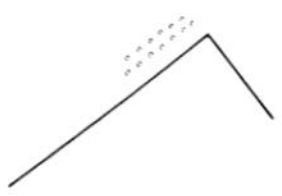	Atelectasis is the collapse of alveolar lung tissue, and findings reflect the presence of a small, airless lung; this condition is caused by complete obstruction of a draining bronchus by a tumor, thick secretions, or an aspirated foreign body, by persistent hypoventilation, and by lack of sighing.	Decreased chest motion on affected side Affected side retracted, with ribs appearing close together Cough may or may not be present Intercostal retraction on affected side during inhalation and bulging during exhalation	Trachea—shifted to affected side Expansion—decreased on affected side Tactile fremitus—decreased or absent over atelectasis	Dull to flat over affected area	Breath sounds—decreased or absent over affected area; high-pitched bronchial sounds when partial obstruction present Adventitious sounds—high-pitched; possible crackles during terminal portion of inspiration
Bronchiectasis 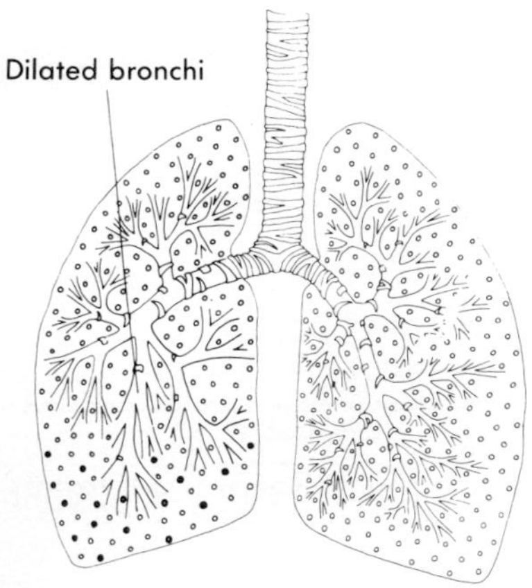	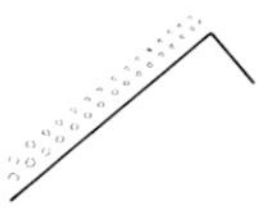	Bronchiectasis is abnormal dilation of the bronchi or bronchioles, or both. It results in copious amounts of thick mucus.	If mild, normal respirations; if severe, tachypnea Less expansion on affected side Cough with purulent sputum	Expansion—decreased on affected side Tactile fremitus—increased	Resonant or dull	Breath sounds—usually vesicular Voice sounds—usually normal Adventitious sounds—crackles

Bronchitis—chronic	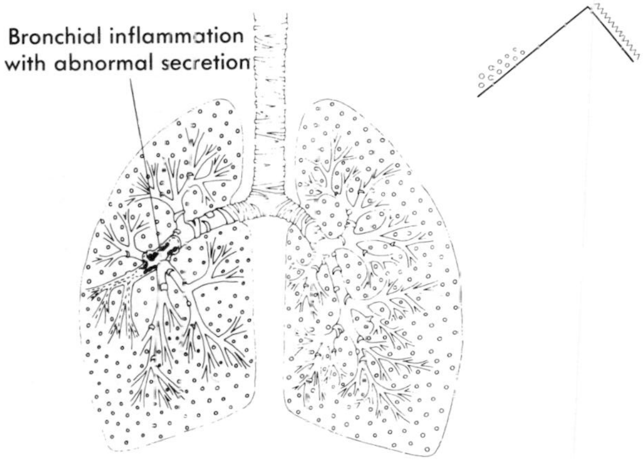	Chronic bronchitis is an inflammation of the bronchial tree characterized by partial airway obstruction or constrictions; it results in abnormal amounts of mucus, which—if not expectorated—causes abnormal ventilation/perfusion inequalities.	Rasping cough with mucoid sputum Central cyanosis Dependent edema	Tactile fremitus—normal or increased	Resonant or dull	Breath sounds—vesicular Adventitious sounds—localized crackles Wheezes Possibly decreased breath sounds if airways obstructed
Emphysema	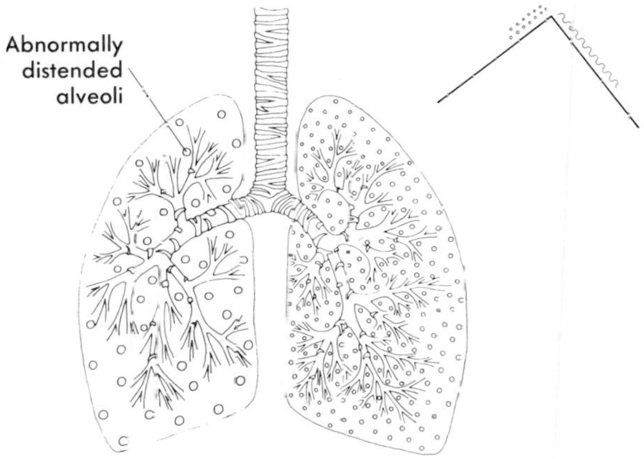	Emphysema is a permanent hyperinflation of the lung beyond the terminal bronchioles, with destruction of alveolar walls.	Dyspnea with exertion Barrel chest Tachypnea Use of accessory muscles of respiration Pursed-lip breathing High-Fowler's position, forward leaning shoulders, hunched position Possible clubbing of fingers	Expansion—diminished Tactile fremitus—decreased	Resonant to hyperresonant Diaphragmatic excursion—decreased	Breath sounds—decreased intensity; often prolonged exhalation Adventitious sounds—occasional wheeze, fine crackles during late inhalation

Continued.

Table 20-6 Assessment findings frequently associated with common lung conditions—cont'd

Condition*	Breath sound†	Description	Inspection	Palpation	Percussion	Auscultation
Pleural effusion and thickening Fluid in the pleural space 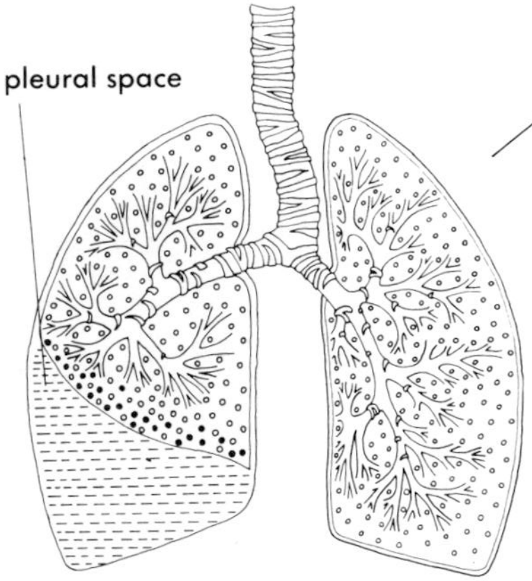	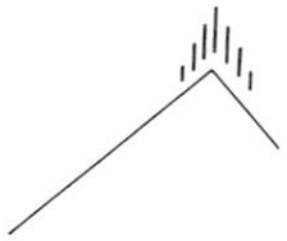	Pleural effusion is a collection of fluid in the pleural space; if pleural effusion is prolonged, fibrous tissue may also accumulate in the pleural space. The clinical picture depends on the amount of fluid or fibrosis present and the rapidity of development; fluid tends to gravitate to the most dependent areas of the thorax, and the adjacent lung is compressed.	Tachypnea Decreased chest expansion on the affected side (expansion may be normal when effusion is small)	Trachea—no deviation in small effusions; deviation toward normal side with large effusion Expansion—decreased on affected side with large effusions Tactile fremitus—decreased or absent	Dull to flat over effusion area	Breath sounds—decreased or absent over area involved in the effusion Adventitious sounds—sometimes pleural friction rub; possible crackles in thoracic area overlying effusion/normal lung interface
Pneumonia with consolidation Consolidation 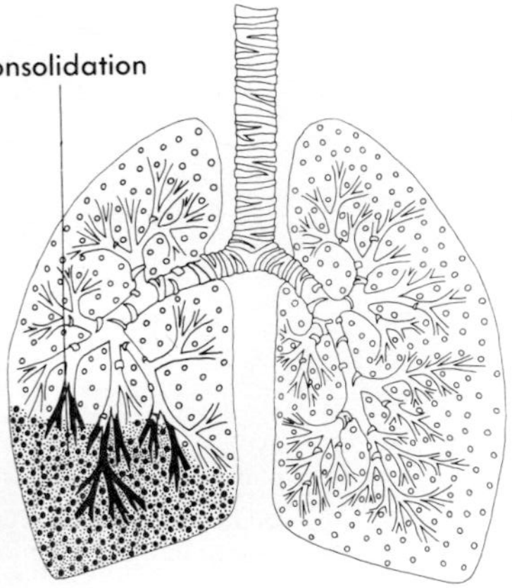	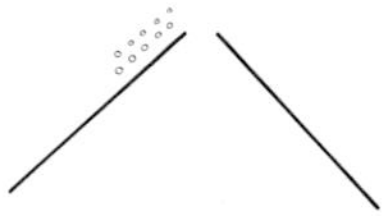	Pneumonia with consolidation occurs when alveolar air is replaced by fluid or tissue; physical findings depend on the amount of parenchymal tissue involved.	Tachypnea Guarding and less motion on the affected side or on both sides when bilateral pneumonia present Cough Possible sputum production	Expansion—limited on the affected side or bilaterally Tactile fremitus—usually increased but may be decreased if a bronchus leading to the affected area is plugged Trachea—no deviation or deviation to unaffected side in unilateral pneumonias	Dull to flat	Breath sounds—increased in intensity; bronchovesicular or bronchial breath sounds over affected area Voice sounds—increased bronchophony, egophony, whisper pectoriloquy Adventitious sounds—crackles when consolidation is small Changes may be minimal or absent

Pneumothorax 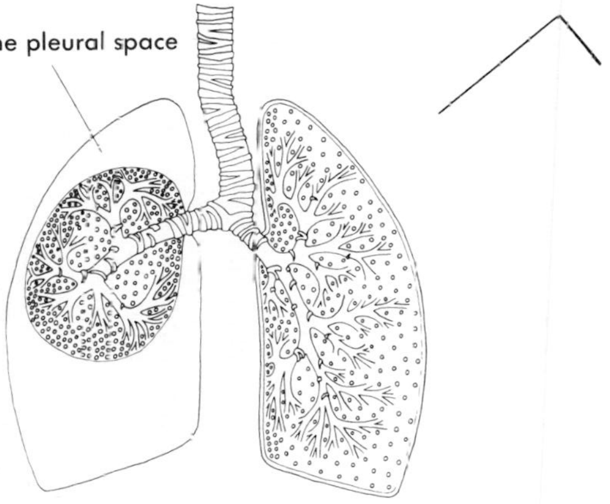 	Pneumothorax implies air in the pleural space. There are three types of pneumothorax: (1) closed – air in the pleural space does not communicate with the air in the lung; (2) open – air in the pleural space freely communicates with the air in the lung, and air in the pleural space is atmospheric; and (3) tension – air in the pleural space communicates with air in the lungs only during inhalation; air pressure in the pleural space is greater than atmospheric pressure. Physical signs depend on the degree of lung collapse and the presence or absence of pleural effusion.	Decreased chest wall motion If large, tachypnea and dyspnea Bulging of intercostal spaces on the affected side during exhalation Central cyanosis	Trachea – deviated toward normal side Expansion – decreased on affected side Tactile fremitus – absent over affected area Possible subcutaenous emphysema (crepitus)	Hyperresonant over affected area	Breath sounds – usually decreased or absent; if open pneumothorax, have an amorphic quality Voice sounds – decreased or absent Adventitious sounds – none Possible Hamman's sign (mediastinal crepitus)
Pulmonary fibrosis – diffuse 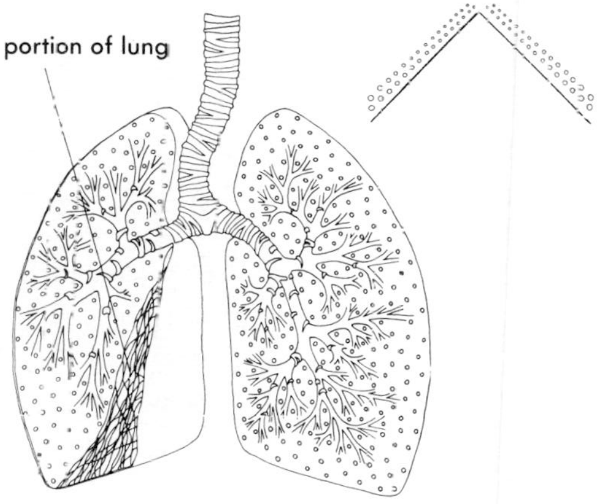 	Pulmonary fibrosis is the presence of an excessive amount of connective tissue in the lungs; consequently, the lungs are smaller than normal and less compliant; the lower lobes are usually the most affected.	Dyspnea on exertion Tachypnea Diminished thoracic expansion Central cyanosis	Trachea – deviated to most affected side	Resonant to dull	Breath sounds – reduced or absent, bronchovesicular or bronchial Vocal fremitus – increased; possible whisper pectoriloquy Adventitious sounds – crackles during inhalation and exhalation

21

Pulmonary Diagnostic Procedures

CHAPTER OBJECTIVES

- Outline the steps in analyzing an arterial blood gas level.
- Identify additional parameters that should be evaluated to assess total oxygenation of the blood.
- Describe the method for obtaining a sputum specimen from an endotracheal tube.
- Discuss the nursing care of patients undergoing pulmonary diagnostic procedures.

To complete the assessment of the critically ill pulmonary patient, a review of the patient's laboratory studies and diagnostic tests should be done. Although a large variety of procedures exist for diagnosing pulmonary disease, their application in the critically ill patient is limited. Only those studies and tests that are currently used in the critical care setting are presented here.

LABORATORY ASSESSMENT

Arterial Blood Gases

Interpretation of arterial blood gas levels can be difficult, especially if one is under pressure to do it quickly and accurately. One method that can help ensure accuracy when analyzing arterial blood gas levels is to follow the same steps of interpretation each time. A specific method to be used each time blood gas values must be interpreted is presented here (see box on right).

STEPS FOR INTERPRETATION OF BLOOD GAS LEVELS

STEP 1

Look at the Pao_2 level and answer the question, *"Does the Pao_2 level show hypoxemia?"*

STEP 2

Look at the pH level and answer the question, *"Is the pH level on the acid or alkaline side of 7.40?"*

STEP 3

Look at the $Paco_2$ level and answer the question, *"Does the $Paco_2$ level show respiratory acidosis, alkalosis, or normalcy?"*

STEP 4

Look at the Hco_3 level and answer the question, *"Does the Hco_3 level show metabolic acidosis, alkalosis, or normalcy?"*

STEP 5

Look back at the pH level and answer the question, *"Does the pH show a compensated or an uncompensated condition?"*

Step 1: Look at the Pao_2 and answer the question, "Does the Pao_2 show hypoxemia?" The Pao_2 is a measure of the partial pressure of oxygen dissolved in arterial blood plasma, with *P* standing for "partial pressure" and *a* standing for "arterial." Sometimes Pao_2 is shortened to Po_2. It is reported in millimeters of mercury (mm Hg).

The normal range in Pao_2 for persons breathing room air at sea level is 80 to 100 mm Hg. However, the normal range is age-dependent in two groups: infants and persons age 60 years and older. The normal level for infants breathing room air is 40 to 70 mm Hg.[1] The normal level for persons 60 years of age and older decreases with age as changes occur in the ventilation/perfusion (V/Q) matching in the aging lung.[2] The correct Pao_2 for older persons can be ascertained as follows: 80 mm Hg (the lowest normal value) minus 1 mm Hg for every year that a person is over the age of 60. Using this formula, it is found that a 65-year-old individual can have a Pao_2 as low as 75 mm Hg and still be within the normal range. (FORMULA for 5 years over 60 years of age: 80 mm Hg − 5 mm Hg = 75 mm Hg.) An acceptable range for an 80-year-old person is 60 mm Hg. (FORMULA for 20 years over the age of 60: 80 mm Hg − 20 mm Hg = 60 mm Hg.) At any age, a Pao_2 lower than 40 mm Hg represents a life-threatening situation that requires immediate action. In addition, a Pao_2 less than the predicted lowest value indicates hypoxemia, which means that a lower-than-normal amount of oxygen is dissolved in plasma.

Several reasons support analysis of the Pao_2 level before those of other blood gas components. First, a Pao_2 of less than 40 mm Hg severely compromises tissue oxygenation and calls for the immediate administration of supplemental oxygen and/or mechanical ventilation. Second, the test results for the Pao_2 level can be quickly analyzed. If the Pao_2 is above the lowest value for the patient's age, it is normal.

Step 2: Look at the pH level and answer the question, "Is the pH on the acid or alkaline side of 7.40?" The pH is the hydrogen ion (H^+) concentration of plasma. Calculation of pH is accomplished by using the partial pressure of carbon dioxide ($Paco_2$) and the plasma bicarbonate level (HCO_3^-). The formula used is the Henderson-Hasselbalch equation (see box on right).

The normal pH of arterial blood is 7.35 to 7.45, with the mean being 7.40. If the pH is less than 7.40, it is on the acid side of the mean. A pH less than 7.35 is known as *acidemia,* and the overall condition is called *acidosis.* If the pH is greater than 7.40, it is on the alkaline side of the mean. A pH greater than 7.45 is known as *alkalemia,* and the overall condition is called *alkalosis.*[3]

Step 3: Look at the $Paco_2$ and answer the question, "Does the $Paco_2$ show respiratory acidosis, alkalosis, or normalcy?" The $Paco_2$ is a measure of the partial pressure of carbon dioxide dissolved in arterial blood plasma, and it is reported in mm Hg. It is the acid-base component that reflects the effectiveness of ventilation in relation to the metabolic rate.[4] In other words, the $Paco_2$ value indicates whether the patient can ventilate well enough to rid the body of the carbon dioxide produced as a consequence of metabolism.

The normal range for $Paco_2$ is 35 to 45 mm Hg. This range does not change as a person ages. A $Paco_2$ of greater than 45 mm Hg defines respiratory acidosis, which is caused by alveolar hypoventilation. Hypoventilation can result from chronic obstructive pulmonary disease (COPD), oversedation, head trauma, anesthesia, drug overdose, neuromuscular disease, or hypoventilation with mechanical ventilation.[5]

Ventilatory failure results whenever the $Paco_2$ rises above 50 mm Hg. Acute ventilatory failure occurs when the $Paco_2$ is greater than 50 mm Hg and the pH is less than 7.30. It is referred to as *acute* because the pH is abnormal, thereby not allowing enough time for the body to compensate by returning the pH to the normal range. Chronic ventilatory failure is defined as a $Paco_2$ of greater than 50 mm Hg, with a pH of greater than 7.30.[1,2,6]

A $Paco_2$ value that is less than 35 mm Hg defines respiratory alkalosis, which is caused by alveolar hyperventilation. Hyperventilation can result from hypoxia, anxiety, pulmonary embolism, pregnancy, and hyperventilation with mechanical ventilation[5] or as a compensatory mechanism to metabolic acidosis.[4]

Step 4: Look at the HCO_3^- level and answer the question, "Does the HCO_3^- show metabolic acidosis, alkalosis, or normalcy?" The bicarbonate (HCO_3^-) is the acid-base component that reflects kidney function. The bicarbonate is reduced or increased in the plasma by renal mechanisms. The normal range is 22 to 26 mEq/L. A bicarbonate level of less than 22 mEq/L defines *metabolic acidosis,* which can result from ketoacidosis, lactic acidosis, renal failure, or diarrhea. A bicarbonate level that is greater than 26 mEq/L defines *metabolic alkalosis,* which can result from fluid loss from the upper GI tract (vomiting or nasogastric suction), diuretic therapy, severe hypokalemia, alkali administration, or steroid therapy.[4,5]

THE HENDERSON-HASSELBALCH EQUATION FOR BLOOD pH

The blood pH depends on the ratio of bicarbonate to dissolved carbon dioxide. As long as the ratio is 20:1, the pH will be 7.4.

$$pH = pK^* + \log \frac{\text{base}}{\text{acid}}$$

$$pH = pK + \log \frac{HCO_3^-}{CO_2}$$

$$pH = 6.1 + \log \frac{24 \text{ mEq/L}}{40 \times .03 \text{ mEq/L}}$$

$$pH = 6.1 + \log 20$$

$$pH = 6.1 + 1.3$$

$$pH = 7.4$$

*pK is the pH at which the substance is half dissociated and half undissociated—value here is 6.1; HCO_3^- normal is 24 mEq/L; CO_2 normal for arterial blood is 40 mm Hg and must be converted to mEq/L to be used in this equation. Therefore the 40 mm Hg is multiplied by .03 to convert to mEq/L.

Step 5: Look back at the pH level and answer the question, "Does the pH show a compensated or an uncompensated condition?" If the pH level is abnormal (i.e., less than 7.35 or greater than 7.45), the $Paco_2$, the HCO_3^-, or both also will be abnormal. This is an uncompensated condition, because there has not been enough time for the body to return the pH to its normal range.[3,5] Two examples of uncompensated ABGs follow:

1. Pao_2: 90 mm Hg
   pH: 7.25
   Pco_2: 50 mm Hg
   HCO_3^-: 22 mEq/L
   This is diagnosed as *uncompensated respiratory acidosis.*
2. Pao_2: 90 mm Hg
   pH: 7.25
   Pco_2: 40 mm Hg
   HCO_3^-: 17 mEq/L
   This is diagnosed as *uncompensated metabolic acidosis.*

If the pH is within normal limits and both the $Paco_2$ and the HCO_3^- are abnormal, the condition is compensated because there has been enough time for the body to restore the pH to within its normal range.[3,5] Two examples of compensated ABGs follow:

1. Pao_2: 90 mm Hg
   pH: 7.37
   Pco_2: 60 mm Hg
   HCO_3^-: 38 mEq/L
   This is diagnosed as *compensated respiratory acidosis with metabolic alkalosis.* The acidosis is considered the main disorder and the alkalosis the

compensating disorder, because the pH is on the acid side of 7.40.

2. $Pa{O_2}$: 90 mm Hg
   pH: 7.42
   $PC{O_2}$: 48 mm Hg
   HCO_3^-: 35 mEq/L
   This is diagnosed as *compensated metabolic alkalosis with respiratory acidosis.* The alkalosis is considered the main disorder and the acidosis the compensating disorder, because the pH is on the alkaline side of 7.40.

Other Considerations When Interpreting Arterial Blood Gases

In addition to the parameters discussed, a number of other factors should be considered when reviewing a patient's ABGs. These factors include oxygen saturation and content, expected $Pa{O_2}$, and base excess and deficit. In patients with hypoxemia, the alveolar-arterial oxygen tension difference and the arterial-alveolar oxygen tension ratio also should be calculated.

◆ **Oxygen saturation ($Sa{O_2}$).** Oxygen saturation is a measure of the amount of oxygen bound to hemoglobin, compared with hemoglobin's maximal capability for binding oxygen. It is reported as a percentage or as a decimal, with normal being greater than 95% on room air.[5] The $Sa{O_2}$ level cannot reach 100% (on room air) because of the normal physiologic shunting.[7] However, when supplemental oxygen is administered, the $Sa{O_2}$ level may approach 100% so closely that it is reported as 100%.

Proper evaluation of the $Sa{O_2}$ level is vital. For example, an $Sa{O_2}$ of 97% means that 97% of the available hemoglobin is bound with oxygen. The word "available" is essential to evaluating the $Sa{O_2}$ level, because the hemoglobin level is not always within normal limits and oxygen can bind only with what is available. A 97% saturation level associated with 10 g of hemoglobin does not deliver as much oxygen to the tissues as does a 97% saturation associated with 15 g of hemoglobin. Thus assessing only the $Sa{O_2}$ level and finding it within normal limits should not lead one to believe that the patient's oxygenation status is normal. The hemoglobin level must also be evaluated before a decision on oxygenation status can be made.[8]

◆ **Oxygen content.** Oxygen content ($Ca{O_2}$) is a measure of the total amount of oxygen carried in the blood, including the amount dissolved in plasma (measured by the $Pa{O_2}$) and the amount bound to the hemoglobin molecule (measured by the $Sa{O_2}$). $Ca{O_2}$ is reported in milliliters (ml) of oxygen carried per 100 ml of blood. The normal value is 20 ml of oxygen per 100 ml of blood. To calculate the oxygen content, the $Pa{O_2}$, the $Sa{O_2}$, and the hemoglobin level are used (see Appendix C). A change in any one of these parameters will affect the $Ca{O_2}$.[7]

The value of assessing the $Ca{O_2}$ is best illustrated by the examples in Table 21-1. Here, the ABG parameters that are most commonly used to evaluate oxygenation status ($Pa{O_2}$ and $Sa{O_2}$) are both normal. Assessing only the $Pa{O_2}$ and the $Sa{O_2}$ would lead to the invalid conclusion that Patient B's oxygenation status is normal. However, consideration of the hemoglobin and the $Ca{O_2}$ reveals that the oxygenation of Patient B's blood is significantly abnormal.

◆ **Expected $Pa{O_2}$.** When a patient receives supplemental oxygen, the $Pa{O_2}$ level is expected to rise. Knowing the level to which the $Pa{O_2}$ should rise in normal subjects on a given $FI{O_2}$ and comparing that with the level to which the $Pa{O_2}$ actually does rise in patients with pulmonary disease has value, because it illustrates how well the lung is functioning.

Calculating the expected $Pa{O_2}$ is accomplished by multiplying the $FI{O_2}$ value by 5.[1] Thus the expected $Pa{O_2}$ on an $FI{O_2}$ of 30% should be at least 150 mm Hg (30 × 5), whereas the expected $Pa{O_2}$ on an $FI{O_2}$ of 50% should be 250 mm Hg (50 × 5). These expected $Pa{O_2}$ values represent the oxygen level achievable with healthy lungs. Pulmonary disease can radically decrease the expected $Pa{O_2}$ level. It is impossible to apply the "$FI{O_2}$ value × 5" rule to achieve the expected $Pa{O_2}$ value when the patient is on a system that delivers oxygen by liters per minute. For these situations, Table 21-2 shows the

Table 21-1 Assessing oxygenation status

Patient	$Pa{O_2}$ level (mm Hg)	$Sa{O_2}$ level (%)	Hgb level (gm%)	$Ca{O_2}$ level (vol%)
A	100	97	15	19.8
B	100	97	10	13.3

Table 21-2 Guidelines for estimating $FI{O_2}$ with low-flow oxygen devices

100% O_2 flow rate (L)	$FI{O_2}$ (%)
NASAL CANNULA OR CATHETER	
1	24
2	28
3	32
4	36
5	40
6	44
OXYGEN MASK	
5-6	40
6-7	50
7-8	60
MASK WITH RESERVOIR BAG	
6	60
7	70
8	80
9	90
10	99+

From Shapiro BA, Harrison RA, Walton JR: *Clinical application of blood gases*, St Louis, 1989, Mosby–Year Book.
NOTE: Normal ventilatory pattern assumed.

FIO_2 levels that correspond to various oxygen delivery systems.

Table 21-3 illustrates three examples of what can occur when the expected PaO_2 level does not reach normal. Patient A shows a normal expected PaO_2; thus it is assumed that his or her lungs are performing normally. The fact that the expected PaO_2 has been reached means that he or she may not require supplemental oxygen. Patient B has not reached the expected PaO_2, but at least he or she is not hypoxemic; administration of supplemental oxygen will bring the PaO_2 above 80 mm Hg. However, because the expected PaO_2 has not been achieved, it should be assumed that removal of oxygen will result in hypoxemia.[1] Patient C has not reached the expected PaO_2, and he or she is therefore hypoxemic.

◆ **Base excess and base deficit.** Base excess and base deficit reflect the nonrespiratory contribution to acid-base balance and are reported in milliequivalents per liter above or below the normal range of −2 mEq/L to +2 mEq/L. A negative base level is reported as a base deficit, which correlates with metabolic acidosis, whereas a positive base level is reported as a base excess, which correlates with metabolic alkalosis.[3]

◆ **Alveolar-arterial oxygen tension difference.** The alveolar-arterial oxygen tension difference $(A\text{-}A)DO_2$, also written as $P(A\text{-}a)O_2$, is referred to as the *A-a gradient* (see Appendix C). It measures the difference between the oxygen tension within the alveolus *(A)* and the artery *(a)* and provides information on the efficiency of the transfer of oxygen into the blood at the alveolar-capillary level. Serial determinations of the A-a gradient provide clinically useful data on lung function in stable patients.[4]

The normal gradient for persons under 61 years of age is 10 to 15 mm Hg (measured while breathing room air).[8] However, the normal gradient is affected by age and supplemental oxygen administration. Age elevates the gradient, because the lungs develop V/Q mismatches as a normal part of aging, thereby resulting in less efficient oxygen exchange.[9] The use of supplemental oxygen elevates the gradient to an FIO_2 of at least 60%.[10] An elevated A-a gradient can result from V/Q mismatching or intrapulmonary shunting.[11] Table 21-4 illustrates the change in the A-a gradient in the hypoxemic patient.

◆ **The arterial-alveolar oxygen tension ratio.** The relationship between the PaO_2 and the PAO_2 can be expressed as a ratio PaO_2/PAO_2 or referred to as the *a/A ratio* (see Appendix C). The PaO_2/PAO_2 is not affected by supplemental oxygen administration and remains relatively stable when the FIO_2 changes, as long as the underlying lung condition is stable. The normal PaO_2/PAO_2 ratio is greater than 0.75 for any FIO_2.[8] A ratio of less than 0.75 indicates V/Q mismatching or intrapulmonary shunting.[12,13] Table 21-4 shows the change in the PaO_2/PAO_2 seen in a hypoxemic patient.

Table 21-3 The expected PaO_2 compared with the actual PaO_2

Patient*	FIO_2 level (%)	Expected PaO_2 level (mm Hg)	Actual PaO_2 level (mm Hg)
A	30	150	160
B	50	250	85
C	50	250	60

*Patients are all under 60 years of age.

Sputum Studies

Careful analysis of sputum specimens is crucial for the rapid identification and treatment of pulmonary infections. The most difficult aspect of sputum examination is proper collection of the specimen. In general, collection of a good sputum sample requires a conscious, cooperative, sufficiently hydrated patient.[14] When the patient has difficulty producing sputum, heated, nebulized saline may help to loosen secretions for expectoration. Chest physiotherapy combined with nebulization improve the success rate. Collection of a sputum specimen is best done in the morning, because there is a greater volume of secretions as a result of nighttime pooling.[15,16]

Many critically ill patients cannot cough effectively, and thus sputum collection by other means is required. These methods include tracheobronchial aspiration, transtracheal aspiration, and the use of a fiberoptic bronchoscopy with a protected brush catheter. Because

Table 21-4 The effects of increasing FIO_2 on PaO_2, PAO_2, $P(A\text{-}a)O_2$, and PaO_2/PAO_2, in a normal subject and a hypoxemic (right-to-left shunt) patient

FIO_2	PaO_2 (mm Hg)	PAO_2 (mm Hg)	$P(A\text{-}a)O_2$ (mm Hg)	PaO_2/PAO_2
NORMAL SUBJECT				
0.21	90	97	7	0.93
0.50	280	300	20	0.93
1.0	560	610	50	0.92
HYPOXEMIC PATIENT				
0.21	40	97	57	0.41
0.50	80	300	220	0.27
1.0	150	610	460	0.25

From Murray JF, Nadel JA: *Textbook of respiratory medicine*, Philadelphia, 1988, WB Saunders.

PROCEDURE FOR COLLECTION OF TRACHEAL OR ENDOTRACHEAL SPECIMEN

1. Clear the endotracheal or tracheostomy tube of all local secretions, avoiding deep airway penetration.
2. Attach a sputum trap to a sterile suction catheter, and advance the catheter into the trachea while trying to avoid contact with the endotracheal tube or tracheostomy tube.
3. After the catheter is fully advanced, apply suction until secretions return to the sputum trap. When enough secretions are collected, discontinue suctioning and remove the catheter.
4. Do not apply suction while the catheter is being withdrawn, because this can contaminate the sample with sputum from the upper airway. Do not flush the catheter with sterile water, because this dilutes the sample.
5. If the catheter becomes plugged with secretions, place it in a sterile container and send it to the laboratory. The specimen should be transported immediately or refrigerated if a delay is necessary.

each method has its own benefits and risks, the patient's clinical condition determines the appropriate technique.[17]

Many critically ill patients have endotracheal or tracheal tubes already in place. Collecting sputum specimens from these patients requires special attention to technique (see box above). Deep specimens should be obtained to avoid collecting specimens that contain resident upper airway flora that may have migrated down the tube. Colonization of the lower airways with upper airway flora can occur within 24 hours of intubation of tracheostomy.[18]

Once a sputum specimen is obtained, it is examined for volume, physical properties, mucopurulence, and color. Next, a microscopic examination is done to identify the source of the specimen. If a bacterial infection is suspected, a Gram stain followed by a culture and sensitivity (C&S) is performed.[14] The Gram stain should be performed first to evaluate whether the specimen is contaminated with oropharyngeal secretions.[17]

DIAGNOSTIC PROCEDURES

Bronchoscopy

Fiberoptic bronchoscopy is a relatively safe procedure that is most often used as both a diagnostic and therapeutic tool. Diagnostic indications include hemoptysis, infectious pneumonia, difficult intubation, pulmonary injury after chest trauma, acute burn inhalation injury, aspiration lung injuries, and acute upper airway obstruction. Therapeutic indications include the aspiration of foreign bodies, removal of obstructing secretions, atelectasis, difficult intubation, and resection of small, benign growths from the airway.[19,20]

Before the bronchoscopy, a complete patient history and examination, including a chest x-ray examination, should be performed.[21] Preoperative evaluation of the patient also should include clotting studies (PT, PTT, and platelet count) and evaluation of the arterial blood gas levels.[20] Hypoxemic patients will need supplemental oxygen during the procedure. The patient should have nothing by mouth for 6 hours before the bronchoscopy to reduce the risk of aspiration.[22,23]

Although a topical anesthetic can be used alone, it is generally supplemented by an intravenous sedative and/or analgesic. Diazepam (Valium) and midazolam HCl (Versed) are two agents frequently administered intravenously during the procedure. Preoperative medications for a diagnostic bronchoscopy may include atropine and intramuscular codeine. Atropine lessens the vasovagal response and reduces the secretions, whereas codeine decreases the cough reflex. When a bronchoscopy is performed therapeutically to remove secretions, medications other than analgesics are avoided because intratracheal topical anesthetics tend to decrease cough and impair secretion clearance.[24]

Complications to the procedure may be related to the procedure itself, the anesthetic, or an ancillary procedure. Minor complications include laryngospasm, epistaxis, fever, pulmonary infiltrates, altered pulmonary mechanics, and hemodynamic instability. Major complications include anaphylaxis, hypotension, cardiac dysrhythmias, bronchospasm, pneumothorax, hemorrhage, hypoxemia, and cardiopulmonary arrest.[19]

Thoracentesis

Thoracentesis is a simple, usually uncomplicated procedure for the removal of fluid or air from the pleural space. It is most frequently used as a diagnostic measure, although in rare circumstances it may be performed therapeutically, as in drainage of a pleural effusion or empyema.[25] No absolute contraindications to thoracentesis exist, although there are risks that generally contraindicate the procedure in all but emergency situations. These risk factors include unstable hemodynamics, coagulation defects, mechanical ventilation, the presence of an intraaortic balloon pump, or patients who are uncooperative. In most clinical situations, diagnostic thoracentesis can be delayed until these risk factors are eliminated.[18]

The patient should be placed in a sitting position with legs over the side of the bed and hands and arms supported on a padded overbed table. If the patient's condition precludes sitting, the side-lying position with the back flush with the edge of the bed can be used. The patient should be cautioned not to move or cough during the procedure.[18] During the thoracentesis, the site of the needle insertion is usually determined by previous chest x-ray examination, CT scan, or chest percussion. A local anesthetic is used to minimize patient discomfort during insertion of the thoracentesis needle.[25]

Complications associated with thoracentesis include pain, pneumothorax, and reexpansion pulmonary edema. Reexpansion pulmonary edema can occur when a large amount of effusion fluid is removed from the pleural space.[10,26] Removal of the fluid increases the negative intrapleural pressure, which can lead to edema when the lung does not reexpand to fill the space. The patient experiences severe coughing and shortness of breath. The onset of these symptoms is an indication to discontinue the thoracentesis. If the physician is measuring the negative pressure during the thoracentesis, withdrawal of fluid should stop when pressure exceeds −20 cm of water pressure.[18] The removal of a large amount of fluid has been associated with higher morbidity and decreased arterial oxygenation in association with reexpansion pulmonary edema. There is little evidence of improvement in a patient's condition with removal of large effusions, and subjective reports of dyspnea relief have varied.[26]

Pulmonary Function Tests

Pulmonary function tests (PFTs) are designed to quantify respiratory function and are an essential component of a thorough pulmonary evaluation. PFTs are used for a variety of purposes, including preoperative assessment, evaluation of lung mechanics, and diagnosis and tracking of pulmonary diseases. Variations in the normal pulmonary function occur with age, gender, and body size.[6]

Measurements can be taken to evaluate the various properties of the lung-thorax system. Static lung volumes provide a basic assessment of ventilatory function and are altered by abnormalities of the respiratory muscles, chest wall, lung parenchyma, and airways. These tests include measurement of tidal volume, inspiratory reserve volume, inspiratory capacity, expiratory reserve volume, vital capacity, residual volume, functional residual capacity, and total lung capacity (see box below).[21]

LUNG VOLUMES AND CAPACITIES

Tidal volume (VT): The volume of air exhaled after a normal resting inhalation. VT × respiratory rate = minute ventilation.

Inspiratory reserve volume (IRV): The amount of additional air that can be taken in after a normal inhalation.

Inspiratory capacity (IC): The maximal amount of air that can be inhaled after a normal exhalation.

Expiratory reserve volume (ERV): The additional amount of air that can be exhaled after a normal resting exhalation.

Vital capacity (VC): The maximal amount of air that can be exhaled after a maximal inhalation.

Residual volume (RV): The amount of air left in the lung after maximal exhalation.

Functional residual capacity (FRC): The amount of air left in the lung after a normal exhalation. The total of the ERV and RV.

Total lung capacity (TLC): The maximal volume of air in the lung after a maximal inspiration. The total of all lung volumes.

The elastic properties of the lungs and chest wall (pulmonary mechanics) can be evaluated through measurement of static and dynamic compliance (see Appendix C for formulas). Static compliance measures lung compliance, whereas dynamic compliance measures both lung and airway resistance. Normal static compliance is approximately 50 ml/cm H_2O. It decreases with any decrease in lung compliance, such as occurs with pneumothorax, atelectasis, pneumonia, pulmonary edema, and chest wall restrictions. Normal dynamic compliance is approximately 40 to 50 ml/cm H_2O. It decreases with any decrease in lung compliance or increase in airway resistance, such as occurs with bronchospasms and retained secretions. If both static and dynamic compliance change, lung compliance has changed. If static compliance remains the same while dynamic compliance changes, airway resistance has changed.[27]

Dynamic pulmonary function tests are designed to evaluate the function of the respiratory muscles, the thorax, and the lungs.[28] These tests are timed breathing studies that reflect the ease of ventilation and include forced vital capacity (FVC), forced expiratory flow at midpoint of vital capacity ($FEF_{25\%-75\%}$), forced expiratory flow at 1 and 3 seconds (FEV_1 and FEV_3), and maximal voluntary ventilation (MVV).[6]

In the critically ill patient, PFTs are usually done at the bedside using spirometry. These tests can be performed in the intubated or nonintubated patient. In the intubated patient, the spirometer is attached to the end of the endotracheal tube. In the nonintubated patient, a nose clip is placed on the patient and the patient is instructed to breathe through a spirometer tube. The patient should be seated on the side of the bed if possible.[6,29]

The spirometer can be used to measure both static and dynamic lung parameters except residual volume (RV) and functional residual capacity (FRC). Bedside PFTs usually include respiratory rate (f), tidal volume (VT), minute ventilation (VE), MVV, and FVC. Additional flow and pressure parameters that can be obtained include maximal inspiratory pressure (MIP), maximal expiratory pressure (MEP), and peak expiratory flow rate (PEFR), $FEF_{25\%-75\%}$, and FEV_1 and FEV_3.[6,29] Table 21-5 provides a description of each of these parameters.

Ventilation/Perfusion Scanning

Ventilation/perfusion scanning is indicated when a serious alteration of the normal ventilation/perfusion (V/Q) relationship is suspected. V/Q studies are most frequently ordered to diagnose and follow a suspected pulmonary embolus. V/Q scanning is approximately 90% accurate in determining this diagnosis. Comparing the perfusion scan with the results of a chest x-ray examination may improve these percentages somewhat.[30] Because results are less than 100% accurate in predicting pulmonary emboli, most V/Q scans will be interpreted in one of four ways[31]:

1. **Normal** This interpretation is used when the perfusion scan is normal and the probability of pulmonary embolism approaches zero.

Table 21-5 Bedside pulmonary function tests

Test	Description
Respiratory rate (f)	Number of breaths per minute
Tidal volume (VT)	Volume of air exhaled after a normal resting inhalation
Minute ventilation (VE)	Volume of air expired per minute (tidal volume × respiratory rate = minute ventilation)
Maximal voluntary ventilation (MVV)	Maximal amount of air that can moved into and out of the lungs in 1 minute
Forced vital capacity (FVC)	Maximal amount of air that can be forcefully exhaled from the lungs after maximal inhalation
Maximal inspiratory pressure (MIP)	Maximal negative pressure generated on inhalation
Maximal expiratory pressure (MEP)	Maximal positive pressure generated on exhalation
Peak expiratory flow rate (PEFR)	Maximal flow rate achieved during forced exhalation
Forced expiratory flow at midpoint of vital capacity ($FEF_{25\%-75\%}$)	Measure of the average flow rate during the middle 50% of exhalation
Forced expiratory flow at 1 and 3 seconds (FEV_1 and FEV_3)	Volume of air exhaled in first and third seconds of forced exhalation

2. **Low probability** This interpretation is used when there are small V/Q mismatches, when there are focal V/Q matches with no corresponding radiographic abnormalities, or when the perfusion defects are considerably smaller than the radiographic abnormalities.
3. **Intermediate or indeterminant probability** This interpretation is used when there are severe diffuse airflow obstructions, perfusion defects corresponding in size and position to radiographic abnormalities, and a single moderate V/Q mismatch without a corresponding radiographic abnormality.
4. **High probability** This interpretation is used when the perfusion defects are substantially larger than the radiographic abnormalities or when there is one or more large or two or more moderate V/Q mismatches with no corresponding radiographic abnormalities.

The V/Q scan consists of both a ventilation scan and a perfusion scan. The ventilation scan is performed by having the patient inhale a radiolabeled gas and air mixture through a mask. The perfusion scan is performed by intravenously injecting the patient with a radioisotope. Scintillation cameras record the gamma radiation images produced by the isotope as it is breathed or perfused into the lung. When an obstruction of the isotope's flow into an area of the lung occurs, the diminished radioactivity will be reflected in the camera image of that zone.[30]

STEPS FOR INTERPRETATION OF A CHEST X-RAY FILM

STEP 1

Look at the different densities (black, gray, and white), and answer the question, *"What is air, fluid, tissue, and bone?"*

STEP 2

Look at the shape or form of each density, and answer the question, *"What normal anatomic structure is this?"*

STEP 3

Look at both right and left sides, and answer the question, *"Are the findings the same on both sides or are there differences (both physiologic and pathophysiologic)?"*

STEP 4

Look at all the structures (bones, mediastinum, diaphragm, pleural space, and lung tissue), and answer the question, *"Are there any abnormalities present?"*

STEP 5

Look for all tubes, wires, and lines, and answer the question, *"Are the tubes, wires, and lines in the proper place?"*

Chest Radiography

Chest radiography is an important diagnostic procedure for any critically ill patient. Chest x-ray examinations aid in the diagnosis of various disorders and complications and assist in the evaluation of treatment.[32] See Chapter 15 for a discussion of the basic principles and techniques of chest radiography.

When interpreting a chest x-ray film, a systematic method is used for viewing it (see box above). Areas of the film that should be assessed include bones, mediastinum, diaphragm, pleural space, and lung tissue. See Fig. 21-1 for an example of a normal chest x-ray film.

◆ **Bones.** The clavicles, ribs, thoracic and cervical spine, and scapulae should be assessed. The clavicles should be symmetric, and the ribs should be an equal distance apart. The thoracic and cervical spine should be straight without signs of curvature. The scapulae usually appear as areas of added density in the upper lung fields. There should be no evidence of fractures, calcification and lesions (increased density), or demineralization (decreased density).[33,34]

◆ **Mediastinum.** The structures in the mediastinal area that should be assessed are the cardiac silhouette and the trachea. See Chapter 15 for a complete discussion of the cardiac silhouette. The trachea should be midline with a slight deviation to the right as it approaches the carina.[33,34] Shifting of the mediastinal structures can occur with atelectasis (toward the area of involvement), pneumothorax (away from the area of involvement),

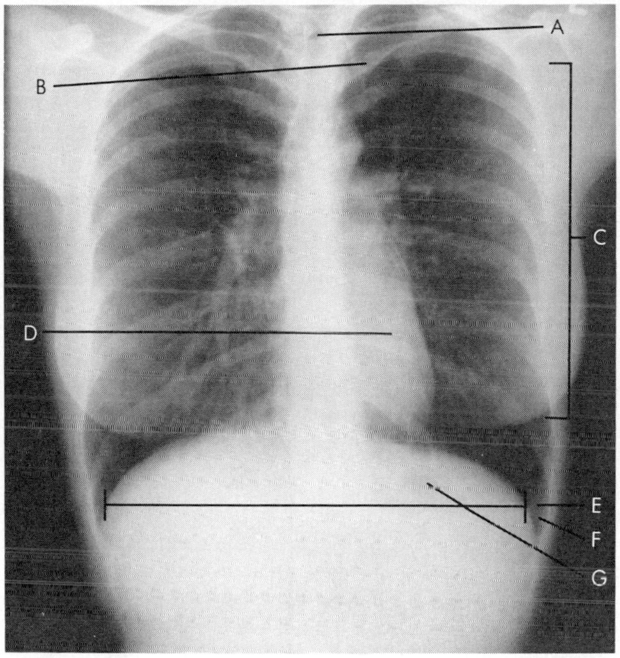

Fig. 21-1 Location of structures on normal PA chest film. **A,** Trachea. **B,** Clavicle. **C,** Ribs. **D,** Cardiac silhouette. **E,** Diaphragm. **F,** Costophrenic angle. **G,** Gastric air bubble.

pleural effusion, tumors, and removal of all or a portion of a lung.[34]

◆ **Diaphragm.** The diaphragm should be clearly visible with sharp costophrenic angles (where the chest wall and the tapered edges of the diaphragm meet).[34] The level of the diaphragm (on deep inspiration) should appear at the tenth or eleventh rib,[34] with the right side slightly higher than the left.[33] A gastric air bubble may be found under the left side of the diaphragm.[33,34] An elevated diaphragm may be seen in pregnancy, obesity, conditions that cause air or fluid to accumulate in the peritoneal space, intestinal obstruction, or splitting.[34] An elevated hemidiaphragm is associated with a number of conditions, including phrenic nerve injury, previous chest surgery, subphrenic abscess, trauma, stroke, tumor, pneumonia, and radiation therapy.[33] Flattening of the diaphragm can be a sign of increased air in the lungs, such as occurs with chronic obstructive pulmonary disease (COPD) or a pleural effusion.[32] Obliteration or "blunting" of the costophrenic angle can occur with pleural effusion, atelectasis, or pneumothorax.[33,34]

◆ **Pleural space.** Identification of the pleural space on a chest x-ray film is an abnormal finding. The pleural space is not visible unless air (pneumothorax) or fluid enters it (pleural effusion). As fluid accumulates in the pleural space, it surrounds the lung and eventually compresses it. With a pleural effusion, blunting of the costophrenic angle may be evident first, with flattening of the diaphragm and obscuring of the heart borders occurring as the effusion grows.[34] With a pneumothorax, the pleural edges become evident as one looks through and between the images of the ribs on the film. A thin line appears just parallel to the chest wall, indicating where the lung markings have pulled away from the chest wall.[33] In addition, the collapsed lung will be manifested as an area of increased density separated by an area of radiolucency (blackness).[34]

◆ **Lung tissue.** The lung tissue should be viewed for any areas of increased density or increased radiolucency that could indicate an abnormality. Increased density can be the result of accumulation of fluid in the lungs (e.g., water, pus, blood, edema fluid) or collapse of lung tissue (as occurs with atelectasis or pneumothorax). Increased radiolucency is caused by increased air in the lungs, as may occur with COPD. In some patients a fine line may be present on the right side at about the level of the sixth rib in the mid-lung field. This is a normal finding and represents the horizontal fissure, which separates the right upper lobe from the right middle lobe.[33]

◆ **Tubes, wires, and lines.** The chest x-ray film also should be assessed for proper placement of all tubes, wires, and lines. When properly positioned, an endotracheal tube should be 2 to 4 cm above the carina. The nasogastric tube should be run the length of the esophagus with the tip in the stomach. The pulmonary artery catheter should be viewed running through the right atrium and right ventricle into the pulmonary artery.[32,34] Additional items that may be present include temporary or permanent pacing wires, permanent pacing generator, automatic implantable cardioverter defibrillator (AICD), chest tubes (pleural or mediastinal), pulmonary artery catheter, central venous pressure (CVP) line electrocardiograph (ECG) electrodes, and surgical markers and clips.

Nursing Management of the Patient Undergoing a Diagnostic Procedure

The nursing management of a patient undergoing a diagnostic procedure involves a variety of interventions, which include preparing the patient psychologically and physically for the procedure, monitoring the patient's responses to the procedure, and assessing the patient after the procedure. Preparing the patient includes teaching the patient about the procedure, answering any questions, and positioning the patient for the procedure. Monitoring the patient's responses to the procedure includes observing the patient for signs of pain, anxiety, or respiratory distress and monitoring vital signs, breath sounds, and oxygen saturation. Assessing the patient after the procedure includes observing for complications of the procedure and medicating the patient for any postprocedure discomfort.[23]

REFERENCES

1. Shapiro BA, Harrison RA, Walton R: *Clinical application of blood gases,* St Louis, ed 4, 1989, Mosby–Year Book.
2. Klocke RA: Ventilation, pulmonary blood flow, and gas exchange. In Fishman AP, editor: *Pulmonary diseases and disorders,* ed 2, New York, 1988, McGraw-Hill.
3. Brenner M, Welliver J: Pulmonary and acid-base assessment, *Nurs Clin North Am* 25:761, 1990.
4. Shapiro BA: Arterial blood gas monitoring, *Crit Care Clin* 4:479, 1988.

5. Mims BC: Interpreting ABGs, *RN* 50(3):42, 1991.
6. Kersten LD: *Comprehensive respiratory nursing,* Philadelphia, 1989, WB Saunders.
7. Carpenter KD: Oxygen transport in the blood, *Crit Care Nurse* 11(9):20, 1991.
8. Reischman RR: Impaired gas exchange related to intrapulmonary shunting, *Crit Care Nurse* 8(8):35, 1988.
9. Murray JF: *The normal lung,* Philadelphia, 1986, WB Saunders.
10. Martin L: *Pulmonary physiology in clinical practice: the essentials for patient care and evaluation,* St Louis, 1987, Mosby–Year Book.
11. Mims BC: *Advanced pulmonary update,* Lewisville, Tx, 1990, Barbara Clark Mims Associates.
12. Ahrens TS, Rutherford KA: The new pulmonary math, *AJN* 87:337A, 1987.
13. Ahrens TS: Blood gas assessment of intrapulmonary shunting and deadspace, *Crit Care Clin North Am* 1:641, 1989.
14. Lekas NJ: Clinical microbiology: nosocomial infections and microbiologic procedures. In Victor LD, editor: *Manual of critical care procedures,* Rockville, Md, 1989, Aspen.
15. Murray JF, Nadel JA: *Textbook of respiratory medicine,* Philadelphia, 1988, WB Saunders.
16. Washington JA: Maximizing diagnostic yield from sputum examination, *J Resp Dis* 7:81, 1981.
17. Chodosh S: Sputum examination. In Fishman AP, editor: *Pulmonary diseases and disorders,* ed 2, New York, 1988, McGraw-Hill.
18. McDonnell K, Fahey P, Segal M: *Respiratory intensive care,* New York, 1987, Little, Brown.
19. Khawaja IT, Ebinger D, Cinquina L: Bronchoscopy in critically ill patients, *Postgrad Med* 88(8):109, 1990.
20. Krell WS: Bronchoscopy in the critically ill. In Victor LD, editor: *Manual of critical care procedures,* Rockville, Md, 1989, Aspen.
21. Baum G, Wolinsky E: *Textbook of pulmonary disease,* ed 4, Boston, 1989, Little, Brown.
22. Kaye W: Invasive therapeutic techniques, *Heart Lung* 12(3):122, 1983.
23. Kee JL: *Laboratory and diagnostic test with nursing implications,* ed 3, Norwalk, Conn, 1991, Appleton & Lange.
24. Haponik EF, Kvale P, Wang KP: Bronchoscopy and related procedures. In Fishman AP, editor: *Pulmonary diseases and disorders,* ed 2, New York, 1988, McGraw-Hill.
25. Talamonti WJ: Thoracentesis and chest tube insertion. In Victor LD, editor: *Manual of critical care procedures,* Rockville, Md, 1989, Aspen.
26. Sahn S: Pleural effusion: diagnosis and management, *Hosp Med* 24(8):77, 1988.
27. Mims BC: *Mechanical ventilation: process and practice,* Lewisville, Tx, 1989, Barbara Clark Mims Associates.
28. Williams D, Cugell D: Pulmonary function tests: indications and interpretation, *Hosp Med* 24(5):23, 1988.
29. Norton LC: Assessment of the adult. In Sexton DL, editor: *Nursing care of the respiratory patient,* Norwalk, Conn, 1990, Appleton & Lange.
30. Stratton MB: Ventilation-perfusion scintigraphy in diagnosis of pulmonary thromboembolism, *Focus Crit Care* 17:287, 1990.
31. Biello DR: Radiological (scintigraphic) evaluation of patients with suspected pulmonary thromboembolism, *JAMA* 257:3257, 1987.
32. Jaquith S: Chest x-ray interpretation: implications for nursing intervention, *Dimens Crit Care Nurs* 5:8, 1986.
33. Sheldon RL, Dunbar RD: Systematic analysis of the chest radiograph. In Scalon CL, Spearman CB, Sheldon RL, editors: *Egan's fundamentals of respiratory care,* ed 5, St Louis, 1990, Mosby–Year Book.
34. Sanches F: Fundamentals of chest x-ray interpretation, *Crit Care Nurse* 6(5):41, 1986.

22

Pulmonary Disorders

CHAPTER OBJECTIVES

- Describe the etiology and pathophysiology of various pulmonary disorders.
- Identify the clinical manifestations of various pulmonary disorders.
- Explain the treatment of various pulmonary disorders.
- Discuss the nursing management of patients with various pulmonary disorders.

ACUTE RESPIRATORY FAILURE

Description

Acute respiratory failure (ARF) is a clinical condition in which the pulmonary system fails to maintain adequate gas exchange.[1] It is probably the most prevalent problem seen in critical care today.[2,3] ARF can be classified as hypoxemic normocapnic respiratory failure (Type I) or hypoxemic hypercapnic respiratory failure (Type II), depending on the patient's arterial blood gases (ABGs). In Type I respiratory failure the patient presents with a low Pao_2 and a normal $Paco_2$, whereas in Type II respiratory failure Pao_2 is low and $Paco_2$ is high.[2,3]

Etiology

ARF results from a deficiency in the performance of the pulmonary system.[2,3] It usually occurs secondary to another disorder that has affected some portion of the system.[4] The cause of ARF is classified as extrapulmonary or intrapulmonary, depending on the component of the respiratory system that is affected. Extrapulmonary causes include disorders that affect the brain, spinal cord, neuromuscular system, thorax, pleura, and upper airways. Intrapulmonary causes include disorders that affect the lower airways and alveoli, pulmonary circulation, and alveolar-capillary membrane. Table 22-1 lists the different causes of ARF and their associated disorders.[5]

Pathophysiology

Hypoxemia is the result of impaired gas exchange and is the hallmark of acute respiratory failure. Hypercapnia may be present, depending on the underlying cause of the problem. The causes of hypoxemia include alveolar hypoventilation, right-to-left shunting, and ventilation/perfusion (V/Q) mismatching.[6] Type I respiratory failure results from V/Q mismatching and intrapulmonary shunting. Type II respiratory failure results from the same conditions that cause type I failure plus alveolar hypoventilation.[5]

Alveolar hypoventilation occurs when the amount of oxygen being brought into the alveoli is insufficient to meet the metabolic needs of the body.[5] The decrease in ventilation results in a decrease in oxygen available for gas exchange.[4] Hypoxemia caused by alveolar hypoventilation is often associated with hypercapnia and commonly results from extrapulmonary disorders.[5]

Right-to-left intrapulmonary shunting occurs when blood reaches the arterial system without passing through ventilated regions of the lungs. When the shunted blood mixes with the oxygenated blood, it lowers the average level of oxygen present in the blood.[5] Intrapulmonary shunting includes both physiologic shunting and pathologic shunting. Physiologic shunting occurs when the blood from the thebesian and bronchial veins returns to the left side of the heart after perfusing the heart and lungs, respectively.[7] Physiologic shunting composes 3% to 5% of the cardiac output (CO).[6] Pathologic shunts occur as a result of cardiac, pulmonary vascular, or pulmonary parenchymal shunting. Cardiac shunting occurs with such disorders as atrial and ventricular septal defects. Pulmonary vascular shunting occurs with such disorders as pulmonary arteriovenous fistulas and malformations. Pulmonary parenchymal shunting occurs when a portion of a lung is not ventilated as the result of alveolar collapse (e.g., atelectasis), alveolar consolidation (e.g., pneumonia), or excessive mucus accumulation (e.g., chronic bronchitis).[5]

Ventilation/perfusion (V/Q) mismatching occurs when ventilation and blood flow are mismatched in various regions of the lung in excess of what is normal. Blood passes through alveoli that are underventilated for the given amount of perfusion. The blood leaving these areas has a lower-than-normal amount of oxygen.[5] V/Q mismatching is the most common cause of hypoxemia and is responsible for most, if not all, of the hypoxemia of chronic obstructive pulmonary disease (COPD), interstitial lung disease, and pulmonary embolism.[8,9]

If allowed to progress, hypoxemia can result in a deficit of oxygen at the cellular level.[4] As the tissue demands for oxygen continue and the supply diminishes, an oxygen supply/demand imbalance occurs and tissue hypoxia develops. Decreased oxygen to the cells contributes to impaired tissue perfusion and the development of lactic acidosis.[1,10]

Table 22-1 Etiology of acute respiratory failure

Area of system affected	Disorder*
EXTRAPULMONARY	
Brain	Drug overdose Central alveolar hypoventilation syndrome Brain trauma or lesion Postoperative anesthesia depression
Spinal cord	Guillain-Barré syndrome Poliomyelitis Amyotrophic lateral sclerosis Spinal cord trauma or lesion
Neuromuscular system	Myasthenia gravis Multiple sclerosis Neuromuscular-blocking antibiotics Organophosphate poisoning Muscular dystrophy
Thorax	Massive obesity Chest trauma
Pleura	Pleural effusion Pneumothorax
Upper airways	Sleep apnea Tracheal obstruction Epiglottitis
INTRAPULMONARY	
Lower airways and alveoli	Chronic obstructive pulmonary disease (COPD) Asthma Bronchiolitis Cystic fibrosis Pneumonia
Pulmonary circulation	Pulmonary emboli
Alveolar-capillary membrane	Pulmonary edema Adult respiratory distress syndrome (ARDS) Inhalation of toxic gases Near-drowning

*Not an inclusive list.

Cerebral tissue hypoxia results in activation of the sympathetic nervous system (SNS). Stimulation of the SNS leads to an increase in respiratory rate and CO in an attempt to compensate for decreased tissue perfusion. In addition, blood is shunted away from nonessential areas of the body to priority areas in attempt to keep the major organs perfused.[4,11]

A number of complications are associated with ARF (see box, upper right). These complications may be the direct result of the effects of hypoxemia on the different organ systems or secondary to the management and treatment of the disorder. In addition, the development of one complication may precipitate the development of another.[12]

COMPLICATIONS OF ACUTE RESPIRATORY FAILURE (ARF)

PULMONARY
Pulmonary emboli
Barotrauma
Pulmonary fibrosis

CARDIOVASCULAR
Dysrhythmias
Decreased cardiac output (CO)

GASTROINTESTINAL
Decreased motility
Hemorrhage

RENAL
Fluid retention
Acute renal failure

INFECTIOUS
Nosocomial pneumonia
Sepsis

PSYCHOLOGIC
Anxiety
Depression
Confusion
Psychosis

OTHER
Malnutrition
Anemia
Disseminated intravascular coagulation (DIC)

Assessment and Diagnosis

The patient with ARF may experience a variety of clinical manifestations, depending on the underlying cause and the extent of tissue hypoxia. The clinical manifestations are related to the development of hypoxemia, hypercapnia, acidosis, and activation of compensatory mechanisms. Table 22-2 lists the clinical manifestations of ARF. Because the clinical symptoms are so varied, they are not considered reliable in predicting the degree of hypoxemia or hypercapnia.[4,11]

Diagnosing and following the course of respiratory failure is best accomplished by arterial blood gas (ABG) analysis. ABG analysis confirms the level of $Pa{CO_2}$, $Pa{O_2}$, and blood pH. ARF is generally accepted as being present when the $Pa{O_2}$ is <50 mm Hg and/or the $Pa{CO_2}$ is >50 mm Hg.[2,3,13] In patients with chronically elevated $Pa{CO_2}$ levels, these criteria must be broadened to include a pH <7.35.[14]

Medical Management

Medical management of the patient with ARF is aimed at treating the underlying cause, promoting

Table 22-2 Clinical manifestations of acute respiratory failure (ARF)

Organ system	Clinical manifestations
Neurologic	Restlessness Agitation Headache Disorientation Seizures Decreased level of consciousness
Cardiovascular	Increased heart rate Hypertension (early) Hypotension (late) Chest pain Dysrhythmias
Pulmonary	Increased respiratory rate Increased respiratory depth Increased respiratory effort
Renal	Decreased urine output Edema
Gastrointestinal	Decreased bowel sounds Nausea and vomiting Abdominal distention Bleeding
Integumentary	Cool, clammy, pale skin Decreased capillary refill

adequate gas exchange, and preventing multiple organ dysfunction syndrome (MODS). Medical interventions for promoting gas exchange include improving oxygenation and ventilation. Interventions for supporting organ systems include maintaining adequate hemodynamic and fluid balance to promote tissue perfusion and maintaining adequate nutrition.

Actions to improve oxygenation include supplemental oxygen administration and the use of positive pressure. The goal of oxygen therapy is to correct hypoxemia. Although the absolute level of hypoxemia varies in each patient, most treatment approaches aim to keep the oxygen saturation at 90% or above. The goal is to keep the tissues' needs satisfied but not produce carbon dioxide narcosis or oxygen toxicity.[2] Supplemental oxygen administration is effective in treating hypoxemia related to alveolar hypoventilation and V/Q mismatching.[5] When intrapulmonary shunting exists, supplemental oxygen alone is ineffective.[5,10] In this situation, positive pressure—in the form of constant positive airway pressure (CPAP) or positive end-expiratory pressure (PEEP)—is necessary to open collapsed alveoli and facilitate their participation in gas exchange. Because positive pressure is generally delivered via ventilator, patients who need positive pressure must usually be intubated and ventilated. In addition, patients whose hypoxemia is not quickly corrected by supplemental oxygen should also be intubated and ventilated.[15]

Administration of supplemental oxygen to patients with chronic hypercapnia may depress the ventilatory drive by removing the hypoxic stimulus to breathe. Consequently, hypoventilation and acidosis develop. Supplemental oxygen should be delivered to these patients in a controlled fashion using a low-flow device. These patients should be carefully monitored for signs of respiratory depression.[14]

Interventions to improve ventilation include intubation and mechanical ventilation. Intubation can be accomplished either orally or nasally. If prolonged intubation is required, a tracheostomy should be considered. Once intubated, the patient is placed on a positive-pressure ventilator. The selection of mode and settings depends on the patient's underlying condition, severity of respiratory failure, and body size.[15] In the patient with chronic hypercapnia, the settings should be adjusted to keep the pH normal, but not the $Paco_2$.[14]

Medications to facilitate removal of secretions and dilate airways may also be of benefit in the treatment of the patient with ARF. Mucolytics administered via nebulizer help liquefy secretions, which facilitates their removal. Bronchodilators aid in smooth muscle relaxation and are of particular benefit to patients with airflow limitations.[11,14] Xanthines, such as theophylline and aminophylline, are administered systemically. $Beta_2$ agonists such as isoetharine (Bronkosol), metaproterenol (Alupent, Metaprel), terbutaline (Brethine, Bricanyl), and albuterol (Proventil, Ventolin) are usually administered via nebulizer to the critically ill patient.[16]

Sedation is necessary in many patients to assist with maintaining adequate ventilation. It can be used to comfort the patient and decrease the work of breathing, particularly if the patient is fighting the ventilator.[4] Analgesics should be administered for pain control. In some patients, sedation does not decrease spontaneous respiratory efforts enough to allow adequate ventilation. Neuromuscular paralysis may be necessary to facilitate optimal ventilation.[17] Paralysis also may be necessary to decrease oxygen consumption in the severely compromised patient.[18] Three neuromuscular blocking agents commonly used are pancuronium (Pavulon), vecuronium (Norcuron), and atracurium (Tracrium).[17,18]

The maintenance of tissue perfusion is critical in preventing complications associated with hypoxemia and other medical therapies. Two major problems that can occur are hypovolemia and decreased CO. Hypovolemia is treated with fluid administration. Decreased CO is treated with vasoactive agents. The choice of agent depends on whether a problem exists with preload, afterload, or contractility. The patient should be continually monitored for signs of organ dysfunction.[12]

Nursing Management

Nursing management of the patient with acute respiratory failure incorporates a variety of nursing diagnoses. Nursing care is directed by the specific etiology of the respiratory failure, although some common interventions are used. The nurse has a significant role in optimizing oxygenation and ventilation, preventing infections, maintaining surveillance for complications of ARF, facilitating nutritional support (see Chapter 50), and providing comfort and emotional support (see

RESEARCH ABSTRACT

The association between interdisciplinary collaboration and patient outcomes in a medical critical care unit.

Baggs JG and others: *Heart Lung* 21(1):18, 1992.

PURPOSE

The purpose of this study was to examine the relationship between the amount of interdisciplinary collaboration involved in making a patient care decision and patient outcomes in the critical care unit.

DESIGN

Prospective descriptive design

SAMPLE

The staff sample consisted of 56 RNs (95% women) with an average age of 31.6 years who had worked as RNs an average of 9.6 years. Of these RNs, 43% had a diploma or associate degree in nursing, 46% were baccalaureate prepared, and 9% had a master's degree in nursing. The physician sample consisted of 31 resident physicians (35% women) with an average age of 27.9 years. Eighteen of the residents were in their first year of residency, with the remainder in their second year. The setting was a large, northeastern university medical center 17-bed medical critical care unit that admitted all critically ill patients, with the exception of surgical or burned patients.

INSTRUMENTS

The Decision About Transfer (DAT) scale was developed for this study and measured collaboration and satisfaction with respect to specific decisions. Responses to questions were in the Lickert format, and both face and content validity were reported by the investigators. The Collaborative Practice Scales (CPS) were given to residents and the Index of Work Satisfaction (IWS) was given to nurses to evaluate the criterion-related validity of the newly developed DAT. Both the CPS and IWS have previously established validity and reliability. The Acute Physiology and Chronic Evaluation (APACHE II)—which allocates points for degree of derangement of physiologic systems, age, and chronic disease—was used to measure severity of illness of patients in the medical critical care unit.

PROCEDURE

An experienced critical care nurse collected the APACHE II scores for all eligible patients for their first and last 24 hours in the medical critical care unit. During the shift when patients were designated for transfer, DAT questionnaires were administered to the nurse and residents responsible for the patient. All data were collected before the occurrence of any negative patient outcomes. For this study, negative outcomes were considered to be either readmission to the medical critical care unit or death during the same hospitalization.

RESULTS

The amount of interdisciplinary collaboration about the transfer, as reported by RNs, was significantly and positively related to patient outcomes, controlling for severity of illness ($p = .02$). As the amount of reported collaboration increased, incidence of negative outcomes decreased. There was no significant relationship between residents' reports of collaboration and patient outcomes. The APACHE II was a significant predictor of outcome ($p = .000$). The correlation between amount of collaboration reported by nurses and residents about the same decisions was low ($p = .056$). Collaboration was significantly positively associated with satisfaction about decision making for both residents and RNs ($p = .000$).

DISCUSSION/IMPLICATIONS

Findings from this study indicate that critical care nurses' perceptions of interdisciplinary collaboration on the decision to transfer patients from the critical care unit were positively related with patient outcomes. In addition, patient-predicted risk of negative outcomes decreased from 16% when the RN reported no collaboration in decision making to 5% when the process was fully collaborative. Although the sample size was small and findings cannot be generalized outside of the study population, important implications are to be drawn from this study. It appears that participation of both professions in the decision about the appropriateness of transfer leads to better patient outcomes. Collaboration is even more important when more alternatives are available in the decision-making process. Future research can focus on the following: larger samples in different settings using subjects with multiple diagnoses; fiscal implications of collaborative decision making; refinement of the newly developed instruments for this study; variables that contribute to the complexity of the decision-making process, such as patient or family anxiety about transfer; and clarification on the subject of collaboration among physicians and nurses.

NURSING DIAGNOSIS AND MANAGEMENT
Acute respiratory failure

- ◆ Impaired Gas Exchange related to alveolar hypoventilation secondary to *(specify)*, p. 471
- ◆ Impaired Gas Exchange related to ventilation/perfusion mismatch secondary to *(specify)*, p. 470
- ◆ Ineffective Breathing Pattern related to chronic airflow limitations, p. 467
- ◆ Inability to Sustain Spontaneous Ventilation related to respiratory muscle fatigue secondary to mechanical ventilation, p. 468
- ◆ Ineffective Airway Clearance related to excessive secretions, or abnormal viscosity of mucus, p. 464
- ◆ Ineffective Airway Clearance related to impaired cough secondary to artificial airway , p. 466
- ◆ High Risk for Aspiration risk factors: impaired laryngeal sensation or reflex; impaired laryngeal closure or elevation; decreased lower esophageal sphincter pressure, p. 472
- ◆ Decreased Cardiac Output related to decreased preload secondary to mechanical ventilation with or without PEEP, p. 359
- ◆ Altered Nutrition: Less Than Body Protein-Caloric Requirements related to lack of exogenous nutrients and increased metabolic demand, p. 673
- ◆ High Risk for Infection risk factor: invasive monitoring devices, artificial airway, p. 366
- ◆ Sensory/Perceptual Alterations related to sensory overload, sensory deprivation, sleep pattern disturbance, p. 573
- ◆ Sleep Pattern Disturbance related to fragmented sleep and/or circadian desynchronization, pp. 142 and 143
- ◆ Body Image Disturbance related to functional dependency on life-sustaining technology, p. 95
- ◆ Powerlessness related to health care environment or illness-related regimen, p. 98
- ◆ Ineffective Individual Coping related to situational crisis and personal vulnerability, p. 762

Chapter 8).[4,11] Nursing interventions to optimize oxygenation and ventilation include positioning, preventing desaturation during procedures, preventing hypoventilation, promoting secretion clearance, and administering sedation and neuromuscular-blocking agents as needed.

Positioning of the patient with ARF depends on the type of lung injury. The goal of positioning is to facilitate or optimize V/Q matching and thus help to alleviate hypoxemia. Patients with unilateral lung disease should be positioned with the good lung down. Patients with diffuse lung disease should be positioned prone with the right lung down and/or should be continuously turned. Some patients benefit from nonrecumbent positions, such as sitting or a semierect position.[19,20] Repositioning should be done at least every 2 hours.[20]

A number of activities can prevent desaturation from occurring during a procedure. These include performing the procedure only as needed, hyperoxygenating and hyperventilating the patient before pulmonary toilet, and providing adequate rest and recovery time between various procedures. During the procedure the patient should be continuously monitored with a pulse oximeter for signs of desaturation.[20,21]

Nursing management of the patient receiving a neuromuscular-blocking agent should incorporate a number of additional interventions. Because paralytic agents only halt muscle movement and do not inhibit pain or awareness, they should be administered with a sedative or anxiolytic agent. Three anxiolytic agents are commonly used: diazepam (Valium), lorazepam (Ativan), and midazolam (Versed). Pain medication should also be administered if the patient has a pain-producing illness or surgery. Frequently, reorientation and explanations for all procedures is critical because the patient can still hear but not move or see. The patient is also at high risk for developing the complications of immobility. Interventions related to the prevention of skin breakdown, atelectasis, and deep vein thrombosis should be implemented. Patient safety is another concern, because the patient cannot react to the environment. Special precautions should be taken to protect the patient at all times.[17,18]

ADULT RESPIRATORY DISTRESS SYNDROME

Description

Adult respiratory distress syndrome (ARDS) is a form of ARF that occurs secondary to another event. ARDS can be described as an "acute lung injury occurring in patients with identified risk factors to ARDS, characterized by the presence of refractory hypoxemia, diminished pulmonary compliance, radiographic evidence of pulmonary edema, and normal pulmonary capillary wedge pressure."[22] Mortality for ARDS ranges from 60% to 95%, depending on the initiating event and subsequent complications.[23]

Etiology

A wide variety of clinical conditions are associated with the development of ARDS (see box, p. 418). They can be divided into direct and indirect injuries, depending on the primary event or site of injury. Aspiration of gastric contents and sepsis are the two most commonly associated disorders with ARDS. Regardless of the cause, the outcome is stimulation of the inflammatory-immune system.[23,24]

CONDITIONS LEADING TO ARDS

DIRECT PULMONARY INJURY

Aspiration of gastric contents or other toxic substances
Near-drowning
Inhalation of toxic substances
Viral/bacterial pneumonia
Chest trauma
Embolism: fat, air, amniotic fluid
Oxygen toxicity
Radiation pneumonitis

INDIRECT PULMONARY INJURY

Sepsis—especially gram-negative
Severe pancreatitis
Multiple emergency blood transfusions
Multiple trauma
Disseminated intravascular coagulation (DIC)
Shock states
Nonpulmonary systemic diseases
Cardiopulmonary bypass
Anaphylaxis
Narcotic drug abuse

Pathophysiology

Recent studies are inconclusive on the sequence of events in the development of ARDS. It is generally believed that stimulation of the inflammatory-immune system initiates a pansystemic response that includes the sequestering of neutrophils in the lungs. Direct injury, complement activation, and stimulation of tissue macrophages and other mediators all play a role in attracting neutrophils to the lung interstitium. Once activated, the neutrophils release a variety of biochemical, humoral, and cellular mediators, which results in injury to the capillary endothelium. These mediators include oxygen-free radicals, proteases, interleukin 1, tumor necrosis factor (TNF), prostaglandins thromboxane A_2, leukotrienes, platelet-activating factor, bradykinin, and histamine.[23,25,26]

The cumulative effect of the mediators is increased capillary membrane permeability. Injury to the alveolar-capillary endothelium allows for increased amounts of not only fluid, but also proteins, to leak into the pulmonary interstitium. As the fluids accumulate in the interstitium, normal local controlling factors (e.g., oncotic pressure, capillary hydrostatic pressure, lymphatic drainage) are overwhelmed. Eventually, fluid and proteins enter the alveoli and damage the type II cells, resulting in impaired surfactant production. The alveoli collapse as a result of interstitial-intraalveolar edema and the loss of surfactant. Collapse of the alveoli results in intrapulmonary shunting, decreased functional residual capacity (FRC), and decreased lung compliance.[23,27]

In addition to increasing capillary permeability, the mediators cause bronchoconstriction, destruction of the elastin and collagen fibers of the lung parenchyma, pulmonary microemboli formation, and pulmonary artery vasoconstriction. Bronchoconstriction results in increased airway resistance, decreased lung compliance, and V/Q mismatching. Destruction of the lung parenchyma results in decreased lung compliance and diffusion defects. Pulmonary microemboli and pulmonary artery vasoconstriction result in pulmonary hypertension, increased pulmonary edema, and increased alveolar dead space. All of these consequences coupled with the effects of atelectasis lead to an increase in work of breathing and hypoxemia. Increased work of breathing leads to fatigue and hypoventilation, which further heighten hypoxemia.[23,27,28]

Complications of ARDS are numerous. They include sepsis, nosocomial pneumonia, airway trauma, gastrointestinal hemorrhage, and multiple organ dysfunction syndrome (MODS).[23] MODS is the primary cause of death in the patient with ARDS.[29] A number of theories postulate that ARDS is just part of a multisystem response to injury. Instead of organ failure's being related to impaired gas exchange from the pulmonary consequences of the disease, the new theories indicate that organ failure starts from the same inflammatory-immune–mediated response that initiated the ARDS. It is theorized that ARDS is apparent first because of the immediate nature of impaired gas exchange.[25,29]

Assessment and Diagnosis

The patient with ARDS may present with a variety of clinical manifestations, depending on the precipitating event. The clinical picture may be one of acute pulmonary edema, ARF, or gradually increasing respiratory insufficiency. Clinical manifestations generally include dyspnea, tachypnea, tachycardia, labored breathing, and change in mental status. As the disease progresses, diffuse fine crackles (rales) and wheezes may be heard.[23,27,28,30,31]

An analysis of ABGs reveals a low PaO_2, despite increases in supplemental oxygen administration (refractory hypoxemia). The $PaCO_2$ is low at first, as a result of hyperventilation. Eventually, the $PaCO_2$ increases as the patient fatigues. The pH is high initially but decreases as acidosis develops.[31]

Initially the chest radiograph may be normal, because the changes in the lungs do not become evident for 24 hours. As the pulmonary edema becomes apparent, diffuse patchy interstitial and alveolar infiltrates appear. This progresses to multifocal consolidation of the lungs.[32] Chest x-ray evaluation at this point may reveal a "white out" of the lung.

The actual diagnosis of ARDS is based on clinical, laboratory, and radiologic criteria. Clinical criteria include a history of a precipitating event associated with ARDS and presence of dyspnea, tachycardia, and tachypnea. Radiologic criteria include diffuse bilateral alveolar infiltrates on the chest x-ray film.[27] Laboratory criteria include evidence of hypoxemia, including a PaO_2 of <60 mm Hg on an FIO_2 of 40% or PaO_2/FIO_2 of <200,[27] shunt of $>20\%$, and an increase in the alveolar-arterial tension difference.[31] Pulmonary function studies reveal a decrease in static and dynamic compliance, decrease in FRC, decrease in vital capacity, and an increase in minute ventilation.[31] In addition, the patient should have a pulmonary capillary wedge pressure (PCWP) of <18 to rule out pulmonary edema of cardiac origin.[27,31]

Medical Management

Medical management of the patient with ARDS involves a multifaceted approach. This strategy includes treating the underlying cause, promoting gas exchange, supporting tissue oxygenation, and monitoring for complications. Medical interventions to promote gas exchange include supplemental oxygen administration, PEEP, intubation, and mechanical ventilation. Oxygen should be administered at the lowest level possible to support tissue oxygenation. Continued exposure to high levels of oxygen can lead to oxygen toxicity, which further perpetuates the entire process. The goal is to maintain a PaO_2 of 60 mm Hg with a FIO_2 of <.60.[23,27] Because the hypoxemia that develops with ARDS is often refractory to oxygen therapy, it is usually necessary to facilitate oxygenation with PEEP.

PEEP has several positive effects on the lungs. These include recruiting collapsed alveoli, increasing FRC, and redistributing fluid in the intraalveolar space to the interstitial space. Thus PEEP decreases intrapulmonary shunting, decreases V/Q mismatching, increases compliance, and improves gas exchange. PEEP also has several negative effects. These include decreasing cardiac output (CO) caused by decreasing venous return, ventricular dysfunction as a result of increasing pulmonary vascular resistance, and barotrauma. The amount of PEEP a patient requires is determined by considering both PaO_2 and CO.[27,33]

Intubation and mechanical ventilation are usually required to facilitate ventilation, particularly as fatigue develops and ventilatory failure occurs. During the acute phase of ARDS the patient should receive complete ventilator support. This allows the ventilator to do the majority of the work of breathing and the patient to rest. Ventilator support can be provided by a variety of modes, including assist-control (also called *continuous mandatory ventilation*), intermittent mandatory ventilation (IMV), synchronized intermittent mandatory ventilation (SIMV), pressure control ventilation (PCV), and pressure support ventilation (PSV).[23,33]

Other ventilatory modalities available are high-frequency jet ventilation (HFJV) and inverse ratio ventilation (IRV). These modes are usually employed when conventional ventilatory strategies are not working. HFJV uses small tidal volumes delivered at high rates to decrease inflation pressures. The advantages are decreased airway pressures, resulting in less hemodynamic compromise and a decreased risk of barotrauma. Recent studies indicate that HFJV does not improve oxygenation and that it is no better than conventional ventilation modes.[33]

IRV is another newer mode that is showing more promise in the treatment of ARDS than is HFJV. IRV prolongs the inspiratory (I) time and shortens the expiratory (E) time, thus reversing the normal I:E ratio. The effect is intentional air trapping, which increases FRC and alveolar recruitment while maintaining lower airway pressures. Disadvantages to IRV include the development of auto-PEEP, which can cause hemodynamic compromise and worsening gas exchange. In addition, patients on IRV usually require neuromuscular blockade and sedation to prevent them from fighting the ventilator.[33]

Interventions to support tissue perfusion include fluid administration, blood administration, and maintenance of CO. Fluid therapy is aimed at maintaining adequate intravascular volume to optimize preload and CO, yet minimize contribution to lung edema. Hemodynamic monitoring is recommended as a way to accurately assess fluid needs. A PCWP in the range of 10 to 12 mm Hg is desired, and the use of fluid challenges (or diuretics, depending on the direction of the pressure alteration) should be used to achieve this range. The type of fluid depends on the patient's underlying condition and

NURSING DIAGNOSIS AND MANAGEMENT

Adult respiratory distress syndrome

- ◆ Impaired Gas Exchange related to ventilation/perfusion mismatch secondary to *(specify)*, p. 470
- ◆ Inability to Sustain Spontaneous Ventilation related to respiratory muscle fatigue secondary to mechanical ventilation, p. 468
- ◆ Ineffective Airway Clearance related to impaired cough secondary to artificial airway, p. 466
- ◆ High Risk for Aspiration risk factor: impaired laryngeal closure or elevation secondary to tracheostomy or endotracheal tube, p. 472
- ◆ Decreased Cardiac Output related to decreased preload secondary to mechanical ventilation with or without PEEP, p. 359
- ◆ Altered Nutrition: Less Than Body Protein-Calorie Requirements related to lack of exogenous nutrients and increased metabolic demand, p. 673
- ◆ High Risk for Infection risk factors: invasive monitoring device, artificial airway, p. 366
- ◆ Sensory/Perceptual Alterations related to sensory overload, sensory deprivation, sleep pattern disturbance, p. 573
- ◆ Sleep Pattern Disturbance related to fragmented sleep and/or circadian desynchronization, pp. 142 and 143
- ◆ Hopelessness related to failing or deteriorating physical condition, p. 100
- ◆ Anxiety related to threat to biologic, psychologic, and/or social integrity, p. 763

severity of ARDS.[31] When hemoglobin is low, blood administration is beneficial to maximize oxygen-carrying capacity.[23] Vasoactive and inotropic agents may be necessary to maintain an adequate CO.[30]

A number of investigational studies of other therapies for the treatment of ARDS are underway. These therapies include drugs to block or neutralize the various mediators released as part of the inflammatory-immune response and methods to limit the damage to the lungs. A number of drugs are being tested, and these include nonsteroidal antiinflammatory drugs, oxygen-free radicals scavengers, platelet activation factor antagonists, and prostaglandin E_1. Methods to limit damage to the lungs include surfactant replacement and extracorporeal carbon dioxide removal.[23]

Nursing Management

Nursing interventions include optimizing oxygenation and ventilation, optimizing CO and tissue perfusion (see Chapter 17), preventing infections, maintaining surveillance for complications of ARDS, facilitating nutritional support (see Chapter 50), and providing comfort and emotional support (see Chapter 8).[23,31]

ATELECTASIS

Description

Atelectasis occurs as a result of collapse of the alveoli. It can occur in any portion of the lung and can involve any amount of lung tissue, including an entire lobe or lung.[8] Atelectasis develops because alveoli become underinflated or uninflated and is a common postoperative problem.[34]

Etiology

Atelectasis can be the result of a variety of abnormalities. These include airway obstruction, abnormal breathing patterns, compression of lung tissue,[6] and a lack of surfactant.[8] A number of disorders can cause these abnormalities (see box, upper right).

ETIOLOGY OF ATELECTASIS

AIRWAY OBSTRUCTION

- Mucus plug
  - Cystic fibrosis
  - Chronic obstructive pulmonary disease (COPD)
  - Bronchiectasis
  - Pneumonia
- Foreign object
- Airway tumor

ABNORMAL BREATHING PATTERNS

- Immobility
- Medications
  - Sedatives
  - Hypnotics
  - Tranquilizers
- Surgery and anesthesia
- Pain

COMPRESSION OF LUNG TISSUE

- Large pneumothorax
- Abdominal distention
- Pleural effusion
- Obesity
- Tumors
- Pneumatocele

LACK OF SURFACTANT

- Adult respiratory distress syndrome (ARDS)

Pathophysiology

Atelectasis occurs when the volume of air in the alveoli is less than the volume needed to keep the alveoli open. The amount of air left in the lungs at the end of exhalation is known as the *functional residual capacity* (FRC). The volume of air needed to keep the alveoli open is known as the *critical closing volume* (CCV). When the FRC is lower than the CCV, atelectasis occurs.[35,36]

An airway obstruction can lead to atelectasis as a consequence of a blockage that completely or partially occludes the entry of fresh air into the distal airways. Lack of new ventilation to these areas promotes the absorption of air (excluding nitrogen) distal to the blockage, and the volume of air in alveoli falls below the CCV. Subsequently, the collapse of lung tissue occurs. This phenomenon is known as *absorption atelectasis*[1,6,8] (see box, p. 421).

Abnormal breathing patterns result in atelectasis because of incomplete expansion of the lungs. Typically the breathing pattern causing the most risk is shallow monotonous breathing. This pattern reduces the amount of air in the lungs and facilitates collapse of the alveoli. Postoperative pain is one of the most common causes of abnormal breathing patterns in patients.[6]

Compression of lung tissue can lead to atelectasis as a result of an increase in pressure surrounding the alveoli. The pressure does not allow air to enter the alveoli, and they collapse.[6] This type of atelectasis is known as *compression atelectasis.*[1]

Atelectasis related to lack of surfactant occurs because the surface tension in the alveoli is increased. Normally, surfactant lines the alveoli, decreasing the surface tension within them and preventing collapse. A loss of surfactant greatly increases the surface tension inside the alveoli and promotes collapse.[8] Conditions that cause a surfactant deficiency include hypoxia, acidosis, cardiopulmonary bypass, pulmonary edema, pulmonary lavage, aspiration, asphyxia, and pulmonary emboli.[37]

Atelectasis results in areas of the lung that are not ventilated but are still perfused (intrapulmonary shunting). Hypoxemia develops as a consequence of intrapulmonary shunting. Hypoxemia is relatively uncommon when all cases of atelectasis are considered, and it occurs most often in acute atelectasis when one or more lobes are involved.[38]

ABSORPTION ATELECTASIS

According to Shapiro et al.[1]: "Absorption atelectasis is the most common type of acute lung collapse and is usually caused by retained secretions." Secretions that obstruct bronchi or bronchioles prevent air from entering the alveoli distal to the obstruction. This lack of fresh air with which to inflate the alveoli after each exhalation results in deflation of the alveoli and atelectasis. Collapse is not complete, however, because alveoli remain inflated with nitrogen from the atmosphere, since nitrogen does not diffuse into the pulmonary capillary.

Absorption atelectasis can also result from the administration of an oxygen concentration that is both too high and administered over too long a time. Normally, alveoli are held open because they are filled by atmospheric gas largely composed of nitrogen that remains within the alveoli after all of the oxygen has diffused into the pulmonary capillary. When a concentration of oxygen above the normal atmospheric level of 21% is administered, some of the nitrogen is "washed out" or replaced by oxygen. The higher the concentration of oxygen, the greater the amount of nitrogen washed out. When nitrogen is replaced by oxygen, alveoli do not remain well inflated, because all of the oxygen diffuses into the pulmonary capillary, leaving alveoli empty. Thus the higher the concentration of oxygen administered, the less well inflated will be the alveoli. This is referred to as "nitrogen wash out absorption atelectasis." Because of this pathology, it is not recommended that oxygen be administered at an FIo_2 above 40% to 50%.

Postoperative atelectasis is a major complication of surgery. It is related to a combination of the abnormalities just discussed. Patients undergoing thoracic and upper abdominal surgery are at the greatest risk, although atelectasis occurs to some extent after all surgeries.[39] It appears to be caused by a number of factors, including changes in chest wall mechanics, upward displacement of the diaphragm, absorption atelectasis, pain, and decreased removal of secretions.

Chest wall mechanics are altered by anesthesia. On induction of anesthesia, the inspiratory muscle tone is decreased while the expiratory muscle tone is increased. This leads to a reduction in FRC, which potentiates atelectasis. Upward displacement of the diaphragm is related to supine positioning, general anesthesia, and neuromuscular paralysis. The FRC declines as much as 30% with a position change from upright to supine; thus the lung is less well inflated when the patient is in the supine position. General anesthesia and neuromuscular paralysis increase intraabdominal expiratory muscle tone, resulting in an increase in intraabdominal pressure, which forces the diaphragm upward.[35,36] In addition, dysfunction of the diaphragm is thought to occur. It has been reported that a general anesthesia alone, regardless of the type of surgery performed, can result in 24 hours of impaired diaphragmatic activity.[39]

Assessment and Diagnosis

Symptoms resulting from atelectasis develop in proportion to the underlying respiratory impairment, the extent of the atelectasis, and the abruptness of onset. Atelectasis that develops slowly in a segment or lobe of an otherwise healthy patient generally causes few symptoms.[40] However, a patient who develops atelectasis and has an ongoing acute or chronic disease may exhibit severe symptoms.[34]

Physical signs of atelectasis vary, depending on the size of the affected area and the patency of the airways that lead into the atelectatic area. Crackles, bronchial breath sounds, and egophony may be present if the airways are open, whereas decreased breath sounds are found when the airways are occluded.[40] Crackles can be auscultated on the periphery of the atelectatic area, whereas decreased-to-absent breath sounds may be heard directly over the area. Large amounts of atelectatic lung tissue can produce tracheal deviation toward the affected side, dull percussion findings, and decreased chest excursion on the affected side.[41] ABG analysis may show a low Pao_2, indicating hypoxemia.

Atelectasis is often first noticed on a chest radiograph by such abnormalities as displacement of lobar fissures[40] (which occurs as a result of loss of lung volume); opacity of an area; obliteration of known borders, such as one of the cardiac borders;[38] or elevation of the diaphragm on the affected side. Atelectasis remains one of the many dysfunctions that is best confirmed by chest x-ray examination.

Medical Management

Medical management of atelectasis should focus on prevention of the disorder. In many instances, atelectasis can be prevented with delivery of inspiratory volumes that will adequately ventilate the lung on a regular basis, such as several times every hour. Many methods can be used to achieve adequate ventilation, including incentive spirometry (IS) (see the section on nursing management) and intermittent positive pressure breathing (IPPB). In the postoperative period, analgesics should be prescribed to control pain and facilitate breathing.[21]

Many patients are reluctant to use the incentive spirometer or perform deep breathing because of associated discomfort or pain. Analgesics should be prescribed, particularly if the patient has had surgery. Care must be taken to assess the level of analgesia necessary to relieve pain, yet allow maximal lung inflation without oversedation and the development of shallow ventilations.[36]

Interventions for the treatment of atelectasis include those just discussed plus the administration of bronchodilators and/or mucolytics, chest physical therapy (CPT) if secretion retention occurs, oxygen therapy for hypoxemia, and mechanical ventilation if respiratory failure occurs. IPPB is used more often as a treatment for atelectasis than it is as a prevention. It must be used correctly to be effective. This means that during the inhalation period of IPPB, air flow should be auscultated throughout all lung fields to ascertain the adequacy of ventilation. One of the major limitations of IPPB use occurs because patients are not supervised during the treatment. As a result of the discomfort associated with chest inflation, many patients stop air flow out of the machine before full lung inflation is achieved, thus negating the effectiveness of the treatment. IPPB treatments require supervision by a nurse or therapist who can instruct the patient about the depth of breath necessary to achieve maximal effect.[1]

Nursing Management

Nursing interventions can be extremely instrumental in preventing atelectasis. These interventions include proper patient positioning and early ambulation, deep breathing, incentive spirometry (IS), and patient education. The goal is to promote maximal lung ventilation and prevent hypoventilation.

When sitting at the bedside or ambulating, patients must be encouraged to keep the thorax in straight alignment while they breathe deeply. This position best accommodates diaphragmatic descent and intercostal muscle action. The sitting or standing position provides enhanced ventilation to areas of the lung that are dependent in the supine position, thus accommodating maximal inflation and—in some instances—gas exchange.[19,20] Frequent repositioning is essential, because it results in a change in ventilatory pattern and V/Q distribution and moves secretions. Repositioning should be done a minimum of every 2 hours while the patient is awake. Ambulation is essential in restoring lung function and should be initiated as soon as possible.[34]

Deep breathing with maximal inhalations held for approximately 3 seconds or longer should be incorporated into the management plans for any patient at risk for developing atelectasis. Both the duration and the depth of inflation, which should be at least twice the tidal volume, are important in preventing, as well as treating, alveolar collapse.[40] The chest should be auscultated during inflation to ensure that all dependent parts of the lung are well ventilated and to help the patient understand the depth of breath necessary for optimal effect. Coughing should be avoided unless secretions are present, because it may actually precipate atelectasis.[4]

Incentive spirometry involves having the patient take at least 10 deep, effective breaths per hour using an incentive spirometer. Ten breaths has been recommended, because research has shown it to be the average number of deep breaths (sighs) taken per hour by normal, healthy persons.[40] An hourly regimen of deep breathing is recommended, because studies have indicated that some alveoli remain open for only 1 hour after the onset of hypoventilation; thus hourly hyperventilation is mandatory.[1,21] Close supervision of patient compliance with the prescribed regimen is recommended, as is the auscultation for breath sounds during the patient's maximal inhalations.

Patient teaching cannot be overlooked in the prevention of atelectasis. All of the interventions just discussed require patient cooperation and thus should be incorporated into a patient teaching plan. Preoperative teaching is most effective and should include as many of these nursing interventions as time will allow, including practice with an incentive spirometer if postoperative orders will include its use.[34]

Nursing actions encompass all of the interventions just discussed plus maintaining surveillance for signs of respiratory decompensation (see box below). If secretions are present, coughing and suctioning may be necessary. Suctioning should be reserved for those patients who cannot raise their secretions with coughing.[4]

NURSING DIAGNOSIS AND MANAGEMENT
Atelectasis

- ◆ Ineffective Breathing Pattern related to abdominal or thoracic pain, p. 469
- ◆ Ineffective Airway Clearance related to excessive secretions or abnormal viscosity of mucus, p. 464
- ◆ Impaired Gas Exchange related to alveolar hypoventilation secondary to *(specify)*, p. 471
- ◆ Impaired Gas Exchange related to ventilation/perfusion mismatch secondary to *(specify)*, p. 470

MANIFESTATIONS OF RESPIRATORY DECOMPENSATION

INADEQUATE AIRWAY

Stridor
Noisy respirations
Supraclavicular and intercostal retractions
Flaring of nares
Labored breathing with use of accessory muscles

INADEQUATE VENTILATION

Absence of air exchange at nose and mouth (breathlessness)
Minimal/absent chest wall motion
Manifestations of obstructed airway
Central cyanosis
Decreased or absent breath sounds (bilateral, unilateral)
Restlessness, anxiety, confusion
Paradoxical motion involving significant portion of chest wall
Decreased Pa_{O_2}, increased Pa_{CO_2}, decreased pH

INADEQUATE GAS EXCHANGE

Tachypnea
Decreased Pa_{O_2}
Increased dead space
Central cyanosis
Chest infiltrates on x-ray evaluation

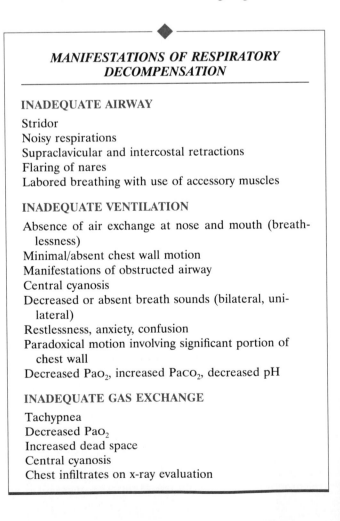

PNEUMONIA

Description

Once the leading cause of death, pneumonia continues to be a major health problem. Despite the use of antibiotics, it is still the most common cause of infectious mortality and remains the fifth leading cause of death in the United States.[42] Nosocomial pneumonias account for 17.8% of hospital-acquired infections, with the majority of cases occurring in the critical care area. Pneumonia has an overall mortality of 30% to 80%, making it the most common cause of death from a nosocomial infection.[43]

Etiology

A number of conditions predispose a patient to the development of pneumonia. These include depressed gag and cough reflexes, decreased ciliary activity, increased secretions, decreased lymphatic flow, atelectasis, fluid in the alveoli, abnormal phagocytosis and humoral activity, and impaired alveolar macrophages. Table 22-3 list these conditions and their causes.[44]

Pneumonias can be classified as community-acquired or hospital-acquired (nosocomial) infections. The most frequently seen community-acquired pneumonia is pneumococcal.[44,45] Other organisms commonly seen are *Legionella pneumophila,* viruses, *Mycoplasma pneumoniae,* and *Haemophilus influenzae.*[45] Hospital-acquired pneumonias are generally caused by gram-negative enteric bacteria. *Klebsiella, Enterobacter, Escherichia coli, Proteus, Pseudomonas,* and *Serratia* are those most frequently encountered. *Pneumocystis carinii* is the predominate cause of pulmonary infection in patients with AIDS (see box below).[46-48] Often, institutions have their own resident flora that predominate in nosocomial infections.

Table 22-3 Altered host defenses

Condition	Etiologies
Depressed epiglottal and cough reflexes	Unconsciousness, neurologic disease, endotracheal or tracheal tubes, anesthesia, aging
Decreased cilia activity	Smoke inhalation – smoking history, oxygen toxicity, hypoventilation, intubation, viral infections, aging, COPD
Increased secretion	COPD, viral infections, bronchiectasis, general anesthesia, endotracheal intubation, smoking
Atelectasis	Trauma, foreign body obstruction, tumor, splinting, shallow ventilations, general anesthesia
Decreased lymphatic flow	CHF, tumor
Fluid in alveoli	CHF, aspiration, trauma
Abnormal phagocytosis and humoral activity	Neutropenia, immunocompetent disorders, such as AIDS, patients receiving chemotherapy
Impaired alveolar macrophages	Hypoxemia, metabolic acidosis, cigarette smoking history, hypoxia, alcohol use, viral infections, aging

COPD, chronic obstructive pulmonary disease; *CHF*, congestive heart failure.

Pathophysiology

Development of acute pneumonia implies a defect in host defenses, a particularly virulent organism, or an overwhelming inoculation event. Bacterial invasion of the lower respiratory tract can occur by inhalation, aspiration, migration from adjacent sites or colonization, direct inoculation, and hematogenous seeding. The most common method appears to be microaspiration of bacteria colonized in the upper airway.[42,43]

The oropharynx has a stable population of resident flora that may be anaerobic or aerobic. When stress occurs – such as with illness, surgery, or a viral infection – pathogenic organisms replace normal resident flora. Previous antibiotic therapy affects the resident flora population, making replacement by pathologic organisms more likely. The pathogens are then able to invade the sterile lower respiratory tract. It has been demonstrated that 57% of critically ill patients have gram-negative bacteria present in the oropharynx. Disruption of the gag and cough reflexes, altered consciousness, abnormal swallowing, and artificial airways all predispose the patient to aspiration and colonization of the lungs and subsequent infection.[43]

Infection results in pulmonary inflammation, with or without significant exudates. V/Q mismatching and intrapulmonary shunting occur, resulting in hypoxemia as lung consolidation progresses. Untreated pneumonia can result in acute respiratory failure and septicemia. Mortality increases with associated disease states –

PNEUMOCYSTIS CARINII *PNEUMONIA*

Pneumocystis carinii pneumonia (PCP) is the most common pulmonary infection seen in the patient with AIDS. PCP is a protozoan infection that commonly occurs in childhood. This opportunistic infection lies dormant until the immunocompromised state of the patient allows its recurrence.

The onset of the pneumonia may be sudden or gradual with the clinical manifestations becoming apparent over weeks. Clinical manifestations include a dry cough, dyspnea, fever, and malaise. As the pneumonia progresses, the patient develops hypoxemic normocapnic respiratory failure.

The two drugs used for the treatment of PCP are trimethoprim-sulfamethoxazole (TMP-SMX) and pentamidine isethionate. Both drugs are given intravenously and are very toxic. Pentamidine also can be administered via aerosol. Adverse reactions to these drugs include high fever, nausea and vomiting, liver and renal dysfunction, neutropenia, and thrombocytopenia.

such as diabetes, malnutrition, immunosuppression, or chronic obstructive lung disorders—and patient age.[44]

Assessment and Diagnosis

The diagnosis of pneumonia is made on the basis of clinical manifestations, radiologic changes, and microbiologic data. Dyspnea is the primary symptom experienced in diffuse pneumonia. Coughing and wheezing with sputum production may be present. Often the patient complains of fever or chills, although these may occur less frequently in elderly and immunosuppressed patients. Pleuritic pain may be a prominent feature. Generally, the onset will be acute with the patient feeling quite unwell over a brief period. However, in the hospitalized patient the onset can also be insidious. In critically ill patients, many of whom have multiple-system problems and various invasive monitoring devices in place, the cause of an infection that has an indolent course can be easily obscured.[45]

Clinical examination reveals hyperpnea or tachypnea, possibly associated with crackles and wheezes over the area of involvement. Chest x-ray evaluation may show infiltrates, depending on the length of illness and absence of other lung problems. An elevated leukocyte count is seen in bacterial pneumonias. A normal or decreased white blood cell count in the presence of pneumonia suggests an overwhelming infection and a poor prognosis. Sputum cultures and blood cultures should be obtained to completely assess the patient's condition. Because of the difficulty involved with sputum collection and culture, the causative agent may not be identified. A Gram stain is very useful, because the results are immediately available and can indicate the probable bacteria.[42,43]

Medical Management

Medical management of the patient with pneumonia should include antibiotic therapy, oxygen therapy for hypoxemia, mechanical ventilation if acute respiratory failure (ARF) develops, fluid management for hydration, nutritional support, and treatment of associated medical problems and complications. For patients having difficulty mobilizing secretions, mucolytics and therapeutic bronchoscopy may be necessary.[42,45]

Although bacteria-specific antibiotic therapy is the goal, this may not always be possible because of the seriousness of the patient's condition and difficulties in identifying the organism. The time spent obtaining bacterial specimens should be balanced against the need to begin some treatment based on patient condition. Empiric therapy has become a generally acceptable approach. In this approach, choice of antibiotic treatment is based on the most likely etiologic organism, while avoiding drug toxicity or superinfection. If available, gram-stain results should be used to guide the choice of antibiotics.[42,45]

Antibiotics should be chosen that offer broad coverage against gram-negative and gram-positive organisms. Factors such as atypical features, COPD with high risk of *Haemophilus* infection, and other exposure risks should be considered when selecting the antibiotic. Efforts to isolate the particular organism should continue. Failure of the patient to improve or further worsening indicates the need to reevaluate therapy. A persistent fever in a patient who otherwise seems to be improving may represent drug fever and should be considered if other sources of infection have been excluded. The antibiotic therapy used should be refined as additional data are obtained. This helps reduce the unnecessary risks of toxicity or development of multiresistant bacteria. Care should always be given to antibiotic choice when renal, hepatic, or hematopoietic impairment exists.[42,45]

Selection of the antibiotic should reflect clinical efficacy, microbiologic activity, antibiotic penetration, metabolism, and side effects. With increasing awareness of the need to control the cost of medical care, the expense of an antibiotic can become a factor in selection. Recent literature has focused on the ability of antibiotics to penetrate the blood-bronchus barrier as a criterion for successful treatment of pneumonia in some populations. Generally, this becomes a concern in people with chronically damaged or hypersecreting bronchial systems.[42]

Antibiotic therapy is generally stopped when the patient has been afebrile for several days with a previously abnormal (elevated or depressed) white blood cell count close to or at normal levels. Reexamination of the sputum should demonstrate freedom from bacteria. Infiltrates can be evident on x-ray examination for extended periods after the pneumonia has resolved and should not be considered a reason to continue drug therapy. Critically ill patients may require a longer course of antibiotic therapy. Gram-negative pneumonias, *Legionella,* and staphylococcal pneumonia may require antibiotic treatment for as long as 3 weeks.[49]

Nursing Management

Nursing interventions for the patient with pneumonia include supporting oxygenation and ventilation, promoting secretion clearance, maintaining surveillance for

---

NURSING DIAGNOSIS AND MANAGEMENT
Pneumonia

- Ineffective Airway Clearance related to excessive secretions or abnormal viscosity of mucus, p. 464
- Impaired Gas Exchange related to alveolar hypoventilation secondary to *(specify),* p. 471
- Impaired Gas Exchange related to ventilation/perfusion mismatch secondary to *(specify),* p. 470
- Altered Nutrition: Less Than Body Protein-Calorie Requirements related to lack of exogenous nutrients and increased metabolic demand, p. 673
- Powerlessness related to health care environment or illness-related regimen, p. 98
- Anxiety related to threat to biologic, psychologic, and/or social integrity, p. 763

respiratory decompensation, and preventing the spread of infection. In addition, the patient's response to the antibiotic therapy should be monitored for adverse effects.

A variety of interventions promote secretion clearance. Actions to prevent secretion retention include providing adequate systemic hydration, humidifying supplemental oxygen, and preventing hypoventilation. In addition to those discussed previously, actions to facilitate secretion removal include suctioning (endotracheal or nasotracheal) and chest physical therapy (percussion, vibration, postural drainage, and coughing) (see Chapter 23).[21]

Prevention should be directed at eradicating pathogens from the environment and interrupting the spread of organisms from person to person. Significant progress has been made in removing contaminants from the patient environment through proper disinfection of respiratory equipment and increased use of disposable supplies. Other possible environmental sources of pathogens include suctioning equipment and indwelling lines. These invasive tools must be given proper aseptic care. Proper hand-washing technique is the single most important measure available to prevent the spread of bacteria from person to person.[43]

ASPIRATION LUNG DISORDER

Description

The presence of abnormal substances in the airways and alveoli as a result of aspiration is misleadingly called *aspiration pneumonia.* This term is misleading because the aspiration of toxic substances into the lung may or may not involve an infection. Aspiration lung disorder is a more accurate title, because injury to the lung can result from the chemical, mechanical, and/or bacterial characteristics of the aspirate.

Etiology

Aspiration has been recorded in as many as 77% of critically ill patients with artificial airways in place.[50] A number of factors have been identified that place the patient at risk for aspiration (see box below).[51] Some common causes of aspiration lung disorder in the critically ill patient are inert fluids, foreign bodies, oropharyngeal bacteria, and gastric contents. Table 22-4 describes the specific clinical entity each cause gives rise to.

RISK FACTORS ASSOCIATED WITH ASPIRATION

Impaired consciousness
Compromised glottal closure
Compromised cough reflex
Ileus or gastric dilation
Nasogastric feeding tubes (large or small bore)
Artificial airways
Disorders affecting pharyngeal or esophageal motility
Tracheoesophageal fistulas
General anesthesia
Cardiopulmonary resuscitation
Improper patient positioning during tube feeding
Esophageal strictures

Table 22-4 Clinical entities associated with aspiration lung disorder

Inoculum	Pulmonary sequelae	Clinical features	Therapy
Acid	Chemical pneumonitis, late bacterial infection possible	Acute shortness of breath, tachypnea, tachycardia; hypoxemia, bronchospasm, fever; sputum: pink, frothy; x-ray film: infiltrates in one or both lower lobes	Correct hypoxemia, administer intravenous fluids, monitor blood gases, administer antibiotics for associated bacterial infections
Oropharyngeal bacteria	Bacterial infection, lung abscess, empyema	Usually insidious onset, cough, fever, purulent sputum, leukocytosis; x-ray film: infiltrate involving dependent pulmonary segment or lobe ± cavitation	Antibiotics
Inert fluids (water, blood, barium)	Airway obstruction, reflex airway closure	Acute shortness of breath, cyanosis ± apnea, pulmonary edema, hypoxemia	Tracheal suctioning during or immediately after aspiration event, correct hypoxemia
Particulate matter, foreign bodies	Airway obstruction	Depends on level of obstruction: ranges from acute apnea and rapid death to irritating chronic cough ± recurrent infections	Extraction of large particulate matter via bronchoscopy, antibiotics for infections

From Baum G, Wolinsky E: *Textbook of pulmonary disease*, ed 4, Boston, 1989, Little, Brown.

Pathophysiology

The type of lung injury that develops after aspiration is determined by a number of factors, including the quality of the aspirate and the status of the patient's respiratory defense mechanisms. Aspirate qualities to be considered include volume, pH, and presence of bile, particulate matter, food, and bacteria.[52]

Aspiration of inert liquids and large foreign bodies may produce an airway obstruction. Smaller foreign bodies may block a portion of the lung, causing atelectasis, bronchospasm, or pneumonia. Aspiration of oropharyngeal secretions carries bacteria into the lower respiratory tract and can cause pneumonia (see section on pathophysiology of pneumonia, p. 423).

Aspiration of gastric contents results in the development of chemical pneumonitis. Aspirates with a pH of <2.5, a volume of 0.4 to 1.0 ml/kg,[50] or with food, particulate antacid, or fecal material increase the chance of damage to the lungs.[53] Initially, bronchospasm may occur secondary to reflex airway closure. Damage to the alveolar capillary membrane results in massive fluid leaks into the alveoli and the development of noncardiogenic pulmonary edema. The fluid decreases surfactant production, which results in atelectasis.[52,53] In addition, hypoxemia results from the intrapulmonary shunting and V/Q mismatching. Acute respiratory distress can develop in minutes. One third of the patients develop overwhelming pneumonia or adult respiratory distress syndrome (ARDS).[53]

Assessment and Diagnosis

Clinically, the patient presents with signs of respiratory distress. Initially, the patient may have shortness of breath, coughing, or wheezing, depending on his or her level of consciousness. Tachypnea, tachycardia, hypotension, fever, and rales also are present. Copious amounts of sputum are produced as pulmonary edema develops.

ABGs reflect hypoxemia and a widened alveolar-arterial oxygen tension difference, while an increased FIO_2 is needed to maintain satisfactory oxygenation. If bacterial infection becomes established, the white blood cell count may become elevated and sputum cultures positive. Chest x-ray film changes appear 12 to 24 hours after the initial aspiration. The validity of the chest x-ray examination in diagnosing aspiration lung disorder is related to the prior status of the patient. Patients with underlying lung involvement may already have significant pulmonary infiltrates present on the chest x-ray film, clouding the interpretation. In massive aspiration, diffuse bilateral infiltrates suggest pulmonary edema is present, whereas lesser aspirations show atelectasis in the early period. Later chest films show large, fluffy infiltrates.[54]

Medical Management

Management of the patient with aspiration lung disorder includes both emergency and follow-up treatment. When aspiration is witnessed, emergency treatment should be instituted to secure the airway and minimize pulmonary damage. The patient should be placed in a slight (6 to 8 inches head-down) Trendelburg's position and turned to the right lateral decubitus position to aid drainage and avoid involvement of other lung areas.[54] Oropharyngeal suctioning should immediately follow. Direct visualization by bronchoscopy is indicated when large particulate aspirate blocks airways. Bronchial and pulmonary lavage is not recommended, because studies have demonstrated that this practice disseminates the aspirate in lungs and increases damage.[52,54]

After airway clearance, attention should be given to supporting oxygenation and hemodynamics. Hemodynamic changes result from fluid shifts that can occur after massive aspirations, causing noncardiogenic pulmonary edema. Monitoring intravascular volume is essential, and judicious amounts of replacement fluids should be instituted to maintain adequate urinary output and vital signs. Hypoxemia should be corrected with supplemental oxygen or mechanical ventilation with PEEP, if necessary.[52]

Recent studies have been performed on the efficacy of prophylactic H^2 blockers such as ranitidine (Zantac), cimetidine (Tagamet), and famotidine (Pepcid) in lessening gastric acidity in patients before surgery. Results have shown that lessening of the acid level of gastric secretions minimizes lung injury when aspiration occurs. Metoclopramide hydrochloride (Reglan), a dopamine antagonist, has been shown to decrease gastric volume and increase upper gastrointestinal motility and gastric sphincter tone. It may be advantageous when given preoperatively.[53]

Nursing Management

Nursing management of the patient with aspiration lung disorder includes optimizing oxygenation and ventilation, preventing further aspiration events, and maintaining surveillance for respiratory decompensation. Interventions to prevent further aspiration events include careful monitoring of patients receiving tube

NURSING DIAGNOSIS AND MANAGEMENT
Aspiration lung disorder

- Impaired Gas Exchange related to ventilation/perfusion mismatch secondary to aspiration, p. 470
- Ineffective Airway Clearance related to excessive secretions or abnormal viscosity of mucus, p. 464
- High Risk for Aspiration risk factors: impaired laryngeal sensation or reflex; impaired pharyngeal peristalsis or tongue function; impaired laryngeal closure or elevation; increased gastric volume; decreased lower esophageal sphincter pressure; decreased antegrade esophageal propulsion, p. 472
- Hopelessness related to failing or deteriorating physical condition, p. 100
- Anxiety related to threat to biologic, psychologic, and/or social integrity, p. 763

feedings, maintaining elevation of the head of the bed, and frequent suctioning of the oropharynx of intubated patients to prevent secretions from pooling above the cuff of the tube.[51] In addition, meticulous oral care is critical in decreasing the bacterial colonization of the oropharynx.[43]

PULMONARY EMBOLUS

Description

A pulmonary embolus (PE) occurs when a clot from another site detaches and lodges in the pulmonary artery (PA), disrupting the blood flow to a region of the lungs. A submassive (acute) PE results in occlusion of <50% of the pulmonary vascular bed, whereas a massive PE results in occlusion of >50% of PA flow.[55,56] PE is the most common acute pulmonary disorder seen in hospitalized patients today.[55,57] It is also one of the most misdiagnosed disorders. Three of four patients with a PE either die within 1 hour or are not diagnosed as having a PE.[58]

Etiology

Pulmonary emboli arise from the venous system, with 90% to 95% coming from the deep leg veins and the rest from the right ventricle, upper extremities, and the renal, hepatic, and pelvic veins.[55,59] A number of predisposing factors and precipitating conditions put a patient at risk for developing a PE (see box on right).[56,59] Of the three predisposing factors (i.e., hypercoagulability, injury to vascular endothelium, and venous stasis [Virchow's triad]), venous stasis appears to be the most significant.[59]

Pathophysiology

A massive PE occurs with the blockage of a lobar or larger artery, resulting in occlusion of more than 50% of the pulmonary vascular bed. A submassive PE involves several smaller emboli that block the more distal branches of pulmonary circulation.[56] Blockage of the PA system has both pulmonary and hemodynamic consequences. The effects on the pulmonary system are an increase in alveolar dead space, pneumoconstriction, and loss of surfactant. The hemodynamic effects include an increase in pulmonary vascular resistance and right ventricular workload.[55,56]

An increase in alveolar dead space occurs because an area of the lung is receiving ventilation without being perfused. The ventilation to this area is known as *wasted ventilation,* because it does not participate in gas exchange. This effect leads to alveolar dead-space ventilation and an increase in the work of breathing. To limit the amount of dead-space ventilation, pneumoconstriction of the airways in the area involved occurs.[55,56]

Pneumoconstriction develops as a result of bronchoalveolar hypocarbia, hypoxia, and the release of humoral, cellular, and biochemical mediators. Bronchoalveolar hypocarbia occurs as a consequence of decreased carbon dioxide in the affected area and leads to constriction of the local airways, increased airway resistance, and redistribution of ventilation to perfused areas of the lungs. A variety of mediators are released from the site of the injury, either from the clot or the surrounding lung tissue, which further causes constriction of the airways.[55,56]

A loss of surfactant also occurs in the affected area. Surfactant serves to keep the alveoli from collapsing. A loss of surfactant leads to the development of atelectasis and transudation of interstitial fluid into the alveoli.[55,56]

Secondary to the development of these pathophysiologic responses is the development of dyspnea and hypoxemia. Dyspnea is thought to occur as a result of fluid in the alveoli stimulating the J receptors (juxtacapillary receptors are located in the walls of alveoli near the capillaries).[56] In addition, the increase in work of breathing needed to maintain adequate gas exchange adds to the feeling of dyspnea. Hypoxemia occurs as a result of V/Q mismatching.[55]

RISK FACTORS FOR PULMONARY THROMBOEMBOLISM

PREDISPOSING FACTORS

- Venous stasis
  - Atrial fibrillation
  - Decreased cardiac output (CO)
  - Immobility
- Injury to vascular endothelium
  - Local vessel injury
  - Infection
  - Incision
  - Atherosclerosis
- Hypercoagulability
  - Polycythemia

PRECIPITATING CONDITIONS

- Previous pulmonary embolus
- Cardiovascular disease
  - Congestive heart failure
  - Right-ventricular infarction
  - Cardiomyopathy
  - Cor pulmonale
- Surgery
  - Orthopedic
  - Vascular
  - Abdominal
- Cancer
  - Ovarian
  - Pancreatic
  - Stomach
  - Extrahepatic bile duct system
- Trauma (injury or burns)
  - Lower extremities
  - Pelvis
  - Hips
- Gynecologic status
  - Pregnancy
  - Postpartum
  - Birth control pills
  - Estrogen replacement therapy

The major hemodynamic consequence of a PE is the development of pulmonary hypertension, which is part of the effect of a mechanical obstruction when more than 50% of the vascular bed is occluded. In addition, the mediators released at the injury site and the development of hypoxia cause pulmonary vasoconstriction, which further exacerbates pulmonary hypertension. As the pulmonary vascular resistance increases, so does the work load of the right ventricle as reflected by a rise in PA pressures. Consequently, right ventricular failure occurs, which can lead to a decrease in left ventricular preload, decrease in cardiac output (CO), decrease in blood pressure, and shock.[55,56]

Assessment and Diagnosis

The patient with a PE may have any number of presenting clinical manifestations. Common symptoms include dyspnea, chest pain, apprehension, anxiety, cough, hemoptysis, diaphoresis, and syncope.[58,59] The chest pain is pleuritic in nature, with an abrupt onset and aggravated by deep breathing. The presence of hemoptysis usually indicates pulmonary infarction or atelectasis. Syncope is thought to occur secondary to the decrease in CO and blood pressure.[59]

Common signs include an increase in tachypnea, tachycardia, rales, decreased breath sounds over the affected side, wheezing,[56] and low-grade fever.[58] If right ventricular failure occurs, distended neck veins and an S_3 on auscultation may be present.[59] Additional signs that indicate right ventricular decompensation are fixed splitting of the second heart sound (P_2), resulting from delayed closure of the pulmonic valve,[56,59] and a diastolic murmur, caused by pulmonic insufficiency.[59]

Initial laboratory studies that may be done are an ABG analysis, electrocardiogram (ECG), and chest radiography. ABGs may show a low Pao_2, indicating hypoxemia; a low $Paco_2$, indicating hypocarbia; and a high pH, indicating a respiratory alkalosis. The hypocarbia with resulting respiratory alkalosis is caused by tachypnea.[60] Common ECG changes found are transient ST-T wave changes and sinus tachycardia. The classic findings of P-pulmonale, S wave in lead I, and Q wave with inverted T wave in lead III are associated with right ventricular failure and are seen in less than 20% of the patients.[55,59,60] Chest x-ray film findings vary from normal to abnormal with elevated hemidiaphragm, parenchymal infiltrates, and atelectasis.[55,59]

Differentiating a PE from other illnesses can be difficult, because many of its clinical manifestations are found in a variety of other disorders.[60] Thus a variety of other tests may be necessary, including a V/Q scan, pulmonary angiogram, and deep vein thrombosis (DVT) studies. A definitive diagnosis of a PE requires confirmation by a high probability V/Q scan, positive pulmonary angiogram, or strong clinical suspicion coupled with abnormal findings on lower extremity DVT studies.[58]

Medical Management

Medical management for the patient with a PE includes both prophylactic and definitive measures and the correction of the hypoxemia. Prophylactic interventions are focused on preventing the recurrence of a PE and include the administration of heparin and warfarin (Coumadin) and interruption of the inferior vena cava. Definitive actions are directed at treating the current PE and include the administration of thrombolytic agents and surgery to remove the clot. Measures to correct the hypoxemia include supplemental oxygen administration and intubation and mechanical ventilation.

Heparin is administered to the patient to prevent further clots from forming and has no effect on the existing clot. Generally 5000 to 10,000 units (U) is given by IV bolus and a continuous drip started at 1600 U/hr[58] or 15 to 25 U/kg/hr.[59] A partial thromboplastin time (PTT) is drawn 4 hours later to monitor the effects of the heparin. The heparin drip is titrated to keep the PTT 1.5 to 2 times normal.[59] The heparin drip should continue for 5 days, with warfarin given simultaneously. The patient should remain on warfarin for 3 to 6 months.[58] The warfarin should be regulated to keep the prothrombin time (PT) 1.3 to 1.5 times control,[58] or 15 to 18 seconds.[58,60]

Interruption of the inferior vena cava is reserved for patients in whom anticoagulation is contraindicated.[60] The procedure involves the placement of a multichanneled clip or an umbrella filter device in the vena cava. Neither device is completely effective in preventing the recurrence of a PE.[56]

The administration of thrombolytic agents in the treatment of PE has had limited success. Currently, thrombolytic therapy is reserved for use in patients with a massive PE and concomitant hemodynamic instability. Tissue plasminogen activator (tPA) is the thrombolytic agent of choice.[59]

Surgical embolectomy is considered a last resort measure that involves the extraction of the embolus from the pulmonary arterial system. It is reserved for the patient with a massive PE refractory to all other measures. It is an extremely risky surgery with an operative mortality of approximately 25%.[59]

To reverse the hemodynamic effects of pulmonary hypertension, additional measures may be taken. These include the administration of vasodilator and inotropic agents. Vasodilator agents have no effect on hypertension created by the mechanical obstruction, but they do reverse the vasoconstrictor effects of the mediators and hypoxia. Inotropic agents increase contractility to facilitate an increase in CO.[59]

Prevention of PE is the first line of treatment for the disorder. In one study the prophylactic use of low-dose subcutaneous heparin in surgical patients demonstrated a 66% reduction in deep vein thrombosis and a 50% reduction of PE. High-risk patients should receive 3500 U subcutaneously every 8 hours, with the dose adjusted to maintain a PTT in the high-to-normal range.[58]

Nursing Management

Nursing management of the patient with a PE should focus on optimizing oxygenation and ventilation, maintaining surveillance of anticoagulant/thrombolytic therapy, maintaining surveillance for respiratory decompen-

NURSING DIAGNOSIS AND MANAGEMENT
Pulmonary embolism

- ◆ Impaired Gas Exchange related to ventilation/perfusion mismatch secondary to *(specify)*, p. 470
- ◆ Acute Pain related to transmission and perception of cutaneous, visceral, muscular, or ischemic impulses secondary to (specify), p. 566
- ◆ Knowledge Deficit: *(specify knowledge)* related to lack of previous exposure to information, p. 72
- ◆ Anxiety related to threat to biologic, physiologic, and/or social integrity, p. 763

sation and shock, facilitating pain management, and providing patient education.

The patient receiving anticoagulant or thrombolytic therapy should be observed for signs of bleeding. The patient's gums, skin, urine, stool, and emesis should be screened for signs of overt or covert bleeding. The patient also should be assessed for signs of right and left ventricular failure, as evidenced by increased pulmonary vascular resistance, elevated PA pressures, elevated CVP, and decreased CO. Pain management should incorporate reassurance, relaxation, and analgesia. Patient education is extremely important, because the patient may be very anxious. All tests and procedures should be explained to the patient. Medication teaching for the patient going home while still receiving warfarin also is very important. In addition, the patient should be familiar with the clinical manifestations of thrombus formation.[56,57]

Prevention of PE should be a major nursing focus, because the majority of critically ill patients are at risk for this disorder. Nursing actions are aimed at preventing the development of DVT, which is a major complication of immobility and a leading cause of PE. These measures include the use of antiembolic stockings and/or pneumatic compression stockings, active/passive range of motion, and progressive ambulation. Patients at risk should be routinely assessed for signs of a DVT, specifically, deep calf pain (Homan's sign) (see Chapter 14).[56]

PNEUMOTHORAX

Description

The presence of air in the pleural space is known as a *pneumothorax.* A pneumothorax is referred to as "open" when there is a hole in the chest wall and "closed" when there is no opening to the outside. A tension pneumothorax is a type of pneumothorax in which the air in the pleural space is under pressure.[6]

Etiology

The three main causes of a pneumothorax are a perforation of the chest wall and parietal pleura that allows air to enter from the outside, perforation of the visceral pleura that allows air to enter from within the lung,[6,61] and formation of gas within the pleural space.[6] An open pneumothorax can be caused by a stab wound or gunshot wound to the chest. A closed pneumothorax can be caused by a wide variety of factors, including mechanical ventilation, blunt chest trauma, ruptured emphysematous bullae, chest wall defects, and central line insertions.[61] Gas can form in the pleural space as the result of an infection or empyema.[6]

Pathophysiology

An open pneumothorax occurs when a defect in the chest wall allows air to enter the pleural space from the outside. Immediately after the chest wall is opened, the pressure inside the chest and outside the chest equilibrate. As air enters the chest, the lung collapses. If the defect is greater than two thirds of the diameter of the trachea, air is sucked into the chest with each breath. This condition is often referred to as a *sucking chest wound.[61]*

A closed pneumothorax occurs when a defect in the visceral pleura allows air to enter the pleural space. As air accumulates in the space, it compresses the surrounding lung tissue, resulting in its collapse. A spontaneous pneumothorax is a form of closed pneumothorax that occurs without an inciting event, such as trauma or a central line insertion.[6]

A tension pneumothorax develops when air enters the pleural space from either the lung or the chest wall on inhalation and cannot escape on exhalation. A "one-way valve" effect is created, and the pressure inside the pleural space builds, collapsing the lung. The mediastinum and trachea are eventually displaced to the opposite side. This results in decreased venous return and compression of the opposite lung.[61]

Regardless of the underlying cause, once air enters the pleural space, the affected lung collapses. The collapsed lung, although not ventilated, is still perfused, resulting in intrapulmonary shunting. If the pneumothorax is large, hypoxemia and acute respiratory failure (ARF) can quickly develop.[61]

Assessment and Diagnosis

The clinical manifestations of a pneumothorax depend on the degree of lung collapse. When a pneumothorax is large, decreased respiratory excursion on the affected side may be noticed, along with bulging intercostal muscles. The trachea may deviate away from the affected side. Percussion reveals hyperresonance with decreased or absent breath sounds over the affected area.[41] As air escapes from the lung, it may leak into the surrounding tissue and subcutaneous emphysema develops. The patient should be assessed for crepitus, which is indicative of subcutaneous emphysema.[1] Distended neck veins may be present in a tension pneumothorax as a result of rising intrathoracic pressure. Knife wounds to the chest are readily visible, whereas bullet wounds may be recognized only by hearing the swish of air with ventilation. The pneumothorax is confirmed with a chest x-ray examination.[61]

Medical Management

A pneumothorax of less than 25% requires no treatment unless complications occur or underlying lung disease or injury is present. A tension pneumothorax is an emergency that requires immediate relief. A large-bore needle is inserted into the second intercostal space in the midclavicular line of the affected side. This relieves the pressure within the chest.[61,62] Sucking chest wounds require immediate treatment to prevent hypoxemia. The defect in the chest wall should be dressed with a sterile, occlusive dressing that allows air to escape on inhalation.[61]

Once stabilized, all tension pneumothoraces, open pneumothoraces, and large pneumothoraces (>25%) require intervention to evacuate the air from the pleural space and facilitate reexpansion of the collapsed lung. Interventions include needle aspiration of the air, placement of a percutaneous catheter attached to a one-way valve (Heimlich valve) or thoracic vent, and/or insertion of a chest tube with underwater seal suction drainage. A Heimlich valve is a small device that is easily secured to the chest, which allows air to escape from the pleural space but not enter. Chest tubes are usually inserted in the fourth or fifth intercostal space on the midaxillary line.[63] Once the tubes are inserted and connected to an underwater chest drainage system with at least 20 cm of suction, a chest x-ray examination should be performed to confirm reexpansion of the lung.[61]

Nursing Management

Nursing interventions for the patient with pneumothorax include optimizing oxygenation and ventilation, maintaining surveillance for respiratory decompensation, and maintaining the chest tube system (see Chapter 23).

NURSING DIAGNOSIS AND MANAGEMENT
Pneumothorax

- Ineffective Breathing Pattern related to abdominal or thoracic pain, p. 469
- Ineffective Breathing Pattern related to decreased lung expansion secondary to pneumothorax or pleural effusion, p. 468
- Impaired Gas Exchange related to alveolar hypoventilation secondary to thoracic pain, p. 471
- Acute Pain related to transmission and perception of cutaneous, visceral, muscular, or ischemic impulses secondary to surgery, p. 566
- Activity Intolerance related to knowledge deficit of energy-saving techniques, p. 365
- Knowledge Deficit: *(specify knowledge)* related to lack of previous exposure to information, p. 72
- Body Image Disturbance related to actual change in body structure, function, and appearance, p. 94
- Anxiety related to threat to biologic, psychologic, and/or social integrity, p. 763
- Altered Role Performance related to physical incapacity to resume usual or valued role, p. 97

THORACIC SURGERY

Types of Surgery

Thoracic surgery refers to a number of surgical procedures that involve opening the thoracic cavity (thoracotomy) and/or the organs of respiration. Indications for thoracic surgery range from tumors and abcesses to repair of the esophagus and thoracic vessels.[64] Table 22-5 describes a variety of thoracic surgical procedures and their indications. This discussion focuses only on the surgical procedures that involve the removal of lung tissue.

Preoperative Care

Before surgery, a complete evaluation of the patient is needed to determine the appropriateness of surgery as a treatment and to determine whether removal of lung tissue can be done without jeopardizing respiratory function. This is especially important when a lobectomy or pneumonectomy is being considered. When resection is being undertaken for tumor treatment, preoperative care includes evaluation of the type and extent of tumor and the physical condition of the patient.[65]

The evaluation of the patient's physical status should focus on the adequacy of cardiopulmonary function. The preoperative evaluation should include pulmonary func-

Table 22-5 Thoracic surgeries

Thoracic procedure	Definition	Indications
Segmental resection	Removal of segment of pulmonary lobe	Chronic, localized pyogenic lung abscess Congenital cyst or bleb Benign tumor Segment infected with pulmonary tuberculosis or bronchiectasis
Wedge resection	Excision of small peripheral section of lobe	Small masses that are close to pleural surface of lung, e.g., subpleural granulomas, small peripheral tumors (benign primary tumors)
Lobectomy	Excision of one or more lobes of lung tissue	Cancer Infections such as tuberculosis Miscellaneous benign tumors

Table 22-5 Thoracic surgeries—cont'd

Thoracic procedure	Definition	Indications
Pneumonectomy	Removal of entire lung	Malignant neoplasms Lung almost entirely infected Extensive chronic abscess Selected unilateral lesions
Decortication of lung	Removal of fibrinous, reactive membrane covering visceral and parietal pleura	Restrictive fibrinous membrane lining visceral and parietal pleura that limits ventilatory excursion; "trapped lung"
Thoracoplasty	Surgical collapse of portion of chest wall by multiple rib resections to intentionally decrease volume in hemithorax	Closure of chronic cavitary lesions and empyema spaces Closure of recurrent air leaks Reduction of open thoracic "dead space" after large resection
Thymectomy	Removal of thymus gland	Primary thymic neoplasm or myasthenia
Correction of pectus excavatum ("funnel chest")	Depression of sternum and costal cartilage corrected by moving sternum outward and realigning cartilage-sternal junction	Cosmesis and relief of cardiopulmonary compromise
Repair of penetrating thoracic wounds, drainage of hemothorax	Drainage of pleural cavity and control of hemorrhage	Hemorrhage produced by injury to thoracic vessels that causes blood loss, as well as compression of lung tissue and mediastinum, resulting in cardiopulmonary compromise
Excision of mediastinal masses	Removal of masses and cysts in upper anterior and posterior mediastinum	Mediastinal tumors (benign or malignant) Cysts Abscesses
Tracheal resection	Resection of portion of trachea, followed by primary end-to-end reanastomosis of trachea	Significant stenosis of tracheal orifice, usually related to mechanical pressure of cuffed tracheal tube; pressure produces tracheal wall ischemia, inflammation, and ulceration; these effects lead to formation of granulation tissue and fibrosis, which narrow tracheal orifice Tumors
Esophagogastrectomy	Resection of part of esophagus and at least cardial portion of stomach with primary anastomosis of proximal esophagus to remaining stomach	Carcinoma of esophagus anywhere from neck to esophagogastric junction Severe reflux esophagitis producing hemorrhage Extensive alkali burns of esophagus
Bullectomy	Removal by excision of cysts or pockets in lung, which result from confluence of many alveoli	Failure of medical therapy, such as antibiotics, and chest physiotherapy to control infection associated with such cysts or pockets Severe compression of tissue adjacent to pulmonary cysts or pockets
Closed thoracostomy	Insertion of chest tube through intercostal space into pleural space; chest tube is attached to water seal system, with or without suction	Provision of continuous aspiration of fluid from pleural cavity Prevention of accumulation of air in chest from leaks in lung or tracheobronchial tree
Open thoracostomy	Partial resection of selected rib or ribs, with insertion of chest tube into infected material to provide for continuous drainage	Drainage of empyemas when pleural space is fixed

From Johanson BC and others: *Standards for critical care*, ed 3, St. Louis, 1988, Mosby–Year Book.

tion tests to determine the patient's ability to lose lung tissue. Cardiac function also should be evaluated. Uncontrolled dysrhythmias, acute myocardial infarction, severe congestive heart failure, and unstable angina are all contraindications to surgery.[65]

Surgical Considerations

To provide adequate surgical exposure for a lung resection (pneumonectomy and lobectomy), the patient is usually placed in a lateral decubitus position during surgery. A posterolateral incision is made to permit upward displacement of the scapula. When a pneumonectomy or upper lobectomy is planned, an incision generally is made in the area of the fifth or sixth rib bed. When a lower lobectomy is planned, approach through the seventh rib area is more usual. Removing a rib and entering the thorax through the rib bed is preferred, because a tighter air seal is possible at closure.[65]

Special care is taken to avoid drainage of blood or secretions into the unaffected lung during surgery, because such an occurrence could cause hypoxemia and cardiac dysfunction. A double-lumen endotracheal tube is used during the surgery to protect the unaffected lung from secretions and necrotic tumor fragments. In addition, the deflated lung is suctioned and ventilated every 20 to 30 minutes during the procedure.[66]

After the pneumonectomy the mediastinal position requires evaluation. This is done on closure of the operative site and involves manometric measurement and a chest x-ray examination. With the patient lying in the supine position, pressure in the empty chest cavity should be -4 to -6 cm of H_2O pressure. When the pressure is abnormal, air or fluid can be added or withdrawn. If the abnormality is not corrected, a mediastinal shift can occur, resulting in hemodynamic compromise and cardiac dysfunction. A chest x-ray examination will show the location of the mediastinum.[65]

Careful evaluation of the mediastinal position is required regularly in the postoperative period also. The mediastinal position can be determined by palpating for tracheal deviation, palpating and auscultating the position of the apex of the heart, and performing a chest x-ray examination. If a mediastinal shift occurs, it should be corrected by injecting or withdrawing air or fluid.[67]

Complications and Medical Management

A number of complications are associated with a lung resection. These include acute respiratory failure, bronchopleural fistula, hemorrhage, and cardiovascular disturbances.

In the postoperative period, acute respiratory failure (ARF) may result from atelectasis, pneumonia, and/or adult respiratory distress syndrome (ARDS) (see the section on pathophysiology of acute respiratory failure, pp. 413-414). Atelectasis can occur as a result of anesthesia, the surgical procedure, immobilization, and pain (see section on pathophysiology of atelectasis, pp. 420-421). Treatment should be aimed at correcting the underlying problems and supporting gas exchange. Supplemental oxygen and mechanical ventilation with PEEP may be necessary.[67,68]

Development of a postoperative bronchopleural fistula is the chief cause of mortality after a lung resection.[67] A bronchopleural fistula develops when the suture line fails to secure occlusion of the bronchial stump and an opening develops. This can result from an imperfect stump closure, perforation of the stump (e.g., with a suction catheter), or high pressure within the airways (e.g., caused by mechanical ventilation).[69] During surgery, careful attention is given to isolating and closing the bronchus in an attempt to secure a lasting seal with subsequent stump healing.[67] In addition, early extubation is encouraged to eliminate the possibility of perforation of the stump and high airway pressures.[69] Clinical manifestations of a bronchopleural fistula include fever, purulent sputum, and massive bubbling of air through the chest tube system. The diagnosis is confirmed by bronchoscopy. Antibiotics should be prescribed if an infection is suspected. The fistula may close on its own, but occasionally surgery is necessary.[67]

The development of a bronchopleural fistula in a patient with a pneumonectomy can be life-threatening. The disruption of the suture line can result in flooding of the remaining lung, with fluid from the residual space producing aspiration. If this occurs, the patient should be placed with the operative side down (remaining lung up) and a chest tube should be inserted to drain the residual space.[67]

Hemorrhage is an early life-threatening complication that can occur after a lung resection. It can result from bronchial or intercostal artery bleeding or disruption of a suture or clip around a pulmonary vessel.[69] In all patients except those with a pneumonectomy, an increase in chest tube drainage can signal excessive bleeding. During the immediate postoperative period, chest tube drainage should be measured every 15 minutes and this frequency decreased as the patient stabilizes. If chest tube loss is >100 ml/hour, fresh blood is noted, or a sudden increase in drainage occurs, hemorrhage should be suspected.[66,67]

Cardiovascular complications after thoracic surgery include dysrhythmias and pulmonary edema. Resections of a large lung area or a pneumonectomy may be followed by a rise in central venous pressure. With the loss of one lung, the right ventricle must empty its stroke volume into a vascular bed that has been reduced by 50%. This means a higher pressure system is created, which increases right-ventricular work load precipitating right ventricular failure. Depending on previous heart function, acute decompensation of both ventricles can result. Measures are aimed at supporting cardiac function and avoiding intravascular volume excess. These measures include optimizing preload, afterload, and contractility with vasoactive agents (see Chapter 17).[67,69]

Postoperative Nursing Management

Nursing care of the patient with thoracic surgery incorporates a number of nursing diagnoses. Nursing management involves interventions aimed at optimizing

NURSING DIAGNOSIS AND MANAGEMENT
Thoracic surgery

- ◆ Ineffective Breathing Pattern related to abdominal or thoracic pain, p. 469
- ◆ Ineffective Airway Clearance related to abdominal or thoracic pain, p. 466
- ◆ Ineffective Airway Clearance related to excessive secretions or abnormal viscosity or mucus, p. 464
- ◆ Impaired Gas Exchange related to alveolar hypoventilation secondary to thoracic pain, p. 471
- ◆ Impaired Gas Exchange related to ventilation/perfusion mismatch secondary to *(specify)*, p. 470
- ◆ Acute Pain related to transmission and perception of cutaneous, visceral, muscular, or ischemic impulses secondary to surgery, p. 566
- ◆ Activity Intolerance related to knowledge deficit of energy-saving techniques, p. 365
- ◆ Knowledge Deficit: *(specify knowledge)* related to lack of previous exposure to information, p. 72
- ◆ Sleep Pattern Disturbance related to fragmented sleep, p. 142
- ◆ High Risk for Infection risk factor: invasive monitoring devices, p. 366
- ◆ Body Image Disturbance related to actual change in body structure, function, or appearance, p. 94
- ◆ Anxiety related to threat to biologic, psychologic, and/or social integrity, p. 763
- ◆ Altered Role Performance related to physical incapacity to resume usual or valued role, p. 97

oxygenation and ventilation, maintaining surveillance for complications, managing pain, and assisting the patient to return to an adequate activity level.[67]

Deep-breathing exercises should be performed regularly with patients who have undergone a thoracotomy. These exercises help reexpand collapsed lung tissue, thus promoting early resolution of the pneumothorax in patients with partial lung resections. Coughing, which should be encouraged only when secretions are present, assists in mobilizing secretions for removal. Because of intraoperative positioning and preoperative and perioperative medications, atelectasis and secretion pooling are common during the postoperative period. Furthermore, as a result of postoperative pain, the patient's ventilations may be shallow, thereby encouraging the development of atelectasis and secretion stasis. Respiratory infections can occur from retained secretions and incomplete lung expansion.[65-68]

The nurse should consider the surgical incision site and the type of surgery when positioning the patient. After a lobectomy the patient should be positioned with the unaffected (good) lung down (dependent) to promote V/Q matching. When the good lung is dependent, blood flow is greater to the area with better ventilation and V/Q matching is better. V/Q mismatching results when the affected lung is positioned down, because of the increase in blood flow to an area with less ventilation. The patient should be turned frequently to promote secretion removal but should have the affected lung dependent as little as possible.[69] The patient who has had a pneumonectomy should not be turned directly onto the unaffected side during the initial period, because the bronchial stump incision is fresh and there is an increased risk of disruption of the suture line. Tilting the patient slightly toward the unaffected side is possible, but the surgeon should indicate when free side-to-side positioning is safe.[65,66]

Chest tubes are placed after all thoracic surgery procedures (except a pneumonectomy) to remove air and fluid. During auscultation of the lungs, air leaks should be evaluated. In the early phase, an air leak is commonly heard over the affected area, because the pleura has not yet tightly sealed. As healing occurs, this leak should disappear. An increase in an air leak or appearance of a new air leak should prompt investigation of the chest drainage system to discover whether air is leaking into the system from outside or whether the leak is originating from the patient's incision (see Chapter 23). A significant air leak can result in a tension pneumothorax. Increased air leaks not related to the thoracic drainage system may indicate disruption of sutures.[65,66]

Pain can be a major problem after thoracic surgery. Pain can increase the work load of the heart, precipitate hypoventilation, and inhibit mobilization of secretions. Clinical manifestations of pain include tachypnea, tachycardia, elevated blood pressure, facial grimacing, splinting of the incision, hypoventilation, moaning, and restlessness.[70] There are several alternatives for pain management after thoracic surgery. The two most common methods are systemic narcotic administration and epidural narcotic administration. Systemic narcotics can be administered intravenously, intramuscularly, or via patient-controlled analgesia (PCA) method (see Chapter 30).[69] In addition, the patient should be assisted with splinting the incision with a pillow or blanket when deep breathing and coughing. Splinting stabilizes the area and reduces pain when moving, deep breathing, or coughing.[70]

Within a few days after surgery, range of motion to the shoulder on the operative side should be performed. The patient frequently splints the operative side and avoids shoulder movement because of pain. If immobility is allowed, stiffening of the shoulder joint can result. This is referred to as *frozen shoulder* and may require physical therapy and rehabilitation to regain satisfactory range of motion of the shoulder joint.[66]

Usually on the day after surgery, the patient is able to sit in a chair. Activity should be systematically increased, with attention to the patient's activity tolerance. With adequate pulmonary function before surgery and a surgical approach designed to preserve respiratory function, full return to previous activity levels is possible. This may take as long as 6 months to 1 year, depending on the tissue resected and the patient's general condition.[65]

REFERENCES

1. Shapiro BA and others: *Clinical application of respiratory care,* ed 4, St Louis, 1991, Mosby–Year Book.
2. Bone RC: Acute respiratory failure. In Burton GG, Hodgkin JE, Ward JJ, editors: *Respiratory care: a guide to clinical practice,* ed 3, Philadelphia, 1991, JB Lippincott.
3. Balk R, Bone RC: Classification of acute respiratory failure, *Med Clin North Am* 67:551, 1983.
4. Norton LC: Respiratory failure. In Sexton DL, editor: *Nursing care of the respiratory patient,* Norwalk, Conn, 1990, Appleton & Lange.
5. Pratter MR, Irwin RS: Extrapulmonary causes of respiratory failure, *J Intens Care Med* 1:197, 1986.
6. Kersten LD: *Comprehensive respiratory nursing,* Philadelphia, 1989, WB Saunders.
7. Kinder RJ, Douce FH: Respiratory gas exchange mechanisms. In Burton GG, Hodgkin JE, Ward JJ, editors: *Respiratory care: a guide to clinical practice,* ed 3, Philadelphia, 1991, JB Lippincott.
8. Guyton AC: *Textbook of medical physiology,* ed 8, Philadelphia, 1991, WB Saunders.
9. West JB: *Pulmonary pathophysiology,* Baltimore, 1987, Williams & Wilkins.
10. D'Alonzo GE, Dantzker DR: Respiratory failure, mechanisms of abnormal gas exchange, and oxygen delivery, *Med Clin North Am* 67:557, 1983.
11. Vaughan P: Acute respiratory failure in the patient with chronic obstructive lung disease, *Crit Care Nurse* 1(6):46, 1981.
12. Pingleton SK: Complications of acute respiratory failure, *Am Rev Respir Dis* 137:1463, 1988.
13. MacNee W: Treatment of respiratory failure: a review, *J R Soc Med* 78:61, 1985.
14. Rosen RL: Acute respiratory failure and chronic obstructive lung disease, *Med Clin North Am* 70:895, 1986.
15. Popovich J: The physiology of mechanical ventilation and the mechanical zoo: IPPB, PEEP, CPAP, *Med Clin North Am* 67:621, 1983.
16. Alfano SL: Drugs affecting respiratory function. In Sexton DL, editor: *Nursing care of the respiratory patient,* Norwalk, Conn, 1990, Appleton & Lange.
17. Halloran T: Use of sedation and neuromuscular paralysis during mechanical ventilation, *Crit Care Nurs Clin North Am* 3:651, 1991.
18. Davidson JE: Neuromuscular blockade, *Focus Crit Care* 18:513, 1991.
19. Castro MS, Everett B, deBolsblanc BP: Positioning patients with hypoxemia, *Crit Care Rep* 1:234, 1990.
20. Norton LC, Conforti C: The effect of body position on oxygenation, *Heart Lung* 14(1):45, 1985.
21. Cosenza JJ, Norton LC: Secretion clearance: state-of-the-art from a nursing perspective, *Crit Care Nurse* 6(4):23, 1986.
22. Murray J and others: An expanded definition of the adult respiratory distress syndrome, *Am Rev Respir Dis* 138:720, 1988.
23. Vaughan P, Brooks C: Adult respiratory distress syndrome: a complication of shock, *Crit Care Nurs Clin North Am* 2:235, 1990.
24. Mattay MA: The adult respiratory distress syndrome: definition and prognosis, *Clin Chest Med* 11:575, 1990.
25. Rinaldo JE, Heyman SJ: ARDS: a multisystem disease with pulmonary manifestations, *Crit Care Rep* 1:174, 1990.
26. Rinaldo JE, Christman JW: Mechanisms and mediators of the adult respiratory distress syndrome, *Clin Chest Med* 11:621, 1990.
27. Mims BC: *Advanced pulmonary update,* Lewisville, Tx, 1990, Barbara Clark Mims Associates.
28. Bradley RB: Adult respiratory distress syndrome, *Focus Crit Care* 14(5):48, 1987.
29. Dorinsky PM, Gadek JE: Multiple organ failure, *Clin Chest Med* 11:581, 1990.
30. Idell S: The deadly danger of ARDS, *Emerg Med* 21(7):67, 1989.
31. Roberts S: High-permeability pulmonary edema: nursing assessment, diagnosis, and interventions, *Heart Lung* 19:287, 1990.
32. Aberle DR, Brown K: Radiologic considerations in the adult respiratory distress syndrome, *Clin Chest Med* 11:737, 1990.
33. Stoller JK, Kacmarek RM: Ventilatory strategies in the management of the adult respiratory distress syndrome, *Clin Chest Med* 11:755, 1990.
34. McConnell EA: Minimizing respiratory problems, *Nurs '91* 21(11):35, 1991.
35. Foltz BD, Benumof JL: Mechanisms of hypoxemia and hypercapnia in the perioperative period, *Crit Care Clin* 3:269, 1987.
36. Fairshter RD, Williams JH: Pulmonary physiology in the postoperative period, *Crit Care Clin* 3:287, 1987.
37. Sexton DL: Anatomy and physiology. In Sexton DL, editor: *Nursing care of the respiratory patient,* Norwalk, Conn, 1990, Appleton & Lange.
38. Johnson NT, Pierson DJ: The spectrum of pulmonary atelectasis: pathophysiology, diagnosis, and therapy, *Respir Care* 31(11):1107, 1986.
39. Huddleston VB: Pulmonary problems, *Crit Care Nurs Clin North Am* 2:527, 1990.
40. Marini JJ: Postoperative atelectasis: pathophysiology, clinical importance and principles of management, *Respir Care* 29(5):516, 1984.
41. Malasanos L, Barkauskas V, Stoltenberg-Allen K: *Health assessment,* ed 4, St Louis, 1990, Mosby–Year Book.
42. Stratton CW: Bacterial pneumonias—an overview with emphasis on pathogenesis, diagnosis, and treatment, *Heart Lung* 15:226, 1986.
43. Craven DE, Regan AM: Nosocomial pneumonia in the ICU patient, *Crit Care Nurs Q* 11(4):28, 1989.
44. Chase RA, Gordon J: Overwhelming pneumonia, *Med Clin North Am* 70(4):945, 1986.
45. Niederman MS: Pneumonia: the ongoing challenge, *Emerg Med* 21(7):77, 1989.
46. Murray JF and others: Pulmonary complications of the acquired immunodeficiency syndrome: an update, *Am Rev Respir Dis* 134:504, 1987.
47. Meredith T, Acierno LJ: Pulmonary complications of acquired immunodeficiency syndrome, *Heart Lung* 17:173, 1988.
48. Rosen MJ: Intensive care of patients with AIDS, *Crit Care Rep* 1:224, 1990.
49. McDonnell K, Fahey P, Segal M: *Respiratory intensive care,* New York, 1987, Little, Brown.
50. Elpern EH, Jacobs ER, Bone RC: Incidence of aspiration in tracheally intubated adults, *Heart Lung* 16:527, 1987.
51. Methany NA, Eisenberg P, Spies M: Aspiration pneumonia in patients fed through nasoenteral tubes, *Heart Lung* 15:256, 1986.
52. DePaso WJ: Aspiration pneumonia, *Clin Chest Med* 12:269, 1991.
53. Saleh KL: Practical points in understanding aspiration, *J Post Anesth Nurs* 6:347, 1991.
54. Chokshi S, Asper R, Khandheria B: Aspiration pneumonia: a review, *Am Fam Physician* 33:195, 1986.
55. West JW: Pulmonary embolism, *Med Clin North Am* 70:877, 1986.
56. Roberts SL: Pulmonary tissue perfusion: altered: emboli, *Heart Lung,* 16:128, 1987.
57. Dickinson SP, Bury GM: Pulmonary embolism: anatomy of a crisis, *Nurs '89* 19(4):34, 1989.
58. Sherman S: Pulmonary embolism update, *Postgrad Med* 89:195, 1991.

59. Counselman FL: Best tests for pulmonary embolism, *Emerg Med* 22(21):66, 1990.
60. Schiff MJ: Finding and fighting pulmonary embolism, *Emerg Med* 21(7):47, 1989.
61. Committee on Trauma of the American College of Surgeons: *Advanced trauma life support,* Chicago, 1984, American College of Surgeons.
62. Zelenak MEC, Zelenak RR: Thoracentesis, thoracostomy, and thoracotomy in thoracic trauma, *Emerg Care Q* 4:55, 1988.
63. Kirby TJ, Ginsberg RJ: Management of the pneumothorax and barotrauma, *Clin Chest Med* 13:97, 1992.
64. Litwack K: Practical points in the care of the thoracic surgery patient, *Post Anesth Nurs* 5:276, 1990.
65. Simonson G: Cancer of the lung. In Sexton DL, editor: *Nursing care of the respiratory patient,* Norwalk, Conn, 1990, Appleton & Lange.
66. O'Byrne C: Postoperative care and complications in the thoracotomy patients, *Crit Care Q* 7(4):53, 1985.
67. Finkelmeier B: Difficult problems in postoperative management, *Crit Care Q* 9(3):59, 1986.
68. Forshag MS, Cooper AD: Postoperative care of the thoracotomy patient, *Clin Chest Med* 13:33, 1992.
69. Daitch JS: Post anesthesia care after thoracic surgery. In Frost EAM, editor: *Post anesthesia care unit current practices,* ed 2, St Louis, 1990, Mosby–Year Book.
70. Delgizzi L: Thoracic surgery. In Hathaway RG, editor: *Nursing care of the critically ill surgical patient,* Rockville, Md, 1988, Aspen.

23

Pulmonary Therapeutic Management

CHAPTER OBJECTIVES

- Describe nursing management of a patient receiving oxygen therapy.
- List the indications and complications of the different artificial airways.
- Outline the principles of airway management.
- Discuss the various modes of mechanical ventilation.
- Describe the management of a patient on mechanical ventilation.

OXYGEN THERAPY

Goals of Therapy

Normal cellular function depends on an adequate supply of oxygen to meet metabolic needs. The primary indications for oxygen administration are hypoxemia and tissue hypoxia. The goal of oxygen administration is to provide a sufficient concentration of inspired oxygen to permit full use of the oxygen-carrying capacity of the arterial blood, thus ensuring adequate tissue oxygenation if the cardiac output (CO) is adequate and if the hemoglobin (Hgb) concentration and structure are normal. Restoring adequate tissue oxygen tension eliminates the compensatory responses to hypoxia. Increased ventilatory work is a normal response to hypoxemia and/or tissue hypoxia, as is increased myocardial work. Appropriate oxygen therapy can decrease or prevent both of these increased work loads.[1,2]

Principles of Therapy

Oxygen is an atmospheric gas that must also be considered a drug, because—like most other drugs—oxygen has both detrimental and beneficial effects. Oxygen is one of the most commonly used and misused drugs. As a drug, it must be administered for good reason and in a proper, safe manner. Oxygen is generally ordered in liters per minute (L/min); as a concentration of oxygen expressed as a percent, such as 40%; or as a fraction of inspired oxygen (FIO_2), such as 0.4.[3]

The amount of oxygen administered depends on the pathophysiologic mechanisms affecting the patient's oxygenation status. In most cases the amount required should provide an arterial partial pressure of oxygen (PaO_2) of 60 to 90 mm Hg, so that a Hgb saturation of greater than 90% is achieved. The concentration of oxygen given to an individual patient is a clinical judgment based on the many factors that influence oxygen transport, such as Hgb concentration, CO, and the arterial oxygen tension.[2]

Once oxygen therapy has begun, the patient should continuously be assessed for level of oxygenation and the factors affecting it. The patient's oxygenation status should be evaluated several times daily until the desired oxygen level is reached and has stabilized. If the desired response to the amount of oxygen delivered is not achieved, the oxygen supplementation should be adjusted and the patient's condition reevaluated. It is important to use this dose-response method, so that the lowest possible level of oxygen is administered that will still achieve a satisfactory PaO_2.[3]

Methods of Delivery

Oxygen therapy can be delivered by many different devices. These devices are classified as either low-flow or high-flow delivery systems. A low-flow system supplies an amount of oxygen that is insufficient to meet all inspiratory volume requirements and depends on the existence of a reservoir of oxygen, dilution with room air, and the patient's ventilatory pattern. The anatomic reservoir in this case is composed of the nasopharynx and the oropharynx. As the patient's ventilatory pattern changes, the inspired oxygen concentration varies because of differing amounts of air mixing with the reservoir gas and the constant flow of oxygen. With a high-flow system, the oxygen flows out of the device into the patient's airways in amounts sufficient to meet all inspiratory volume requirements. This type of system is not affected by the patient's ventilatory pattern. Examples of low-flow systems are nasal cannulas, simple oxygen masks, partial rebreathing masks, and nonrebreathing masks. A Venturi mask is an example of a high-flow oxygen delivery system.[2,3]

◆ **Nasal cannula.** Low concentrations of oxygen can be successfully delivered through a nasal cannula, or prongs. The nasal cannula has the advantages of being lightweight, economic, disposable, and easily applied. Cannulas are generally well tolerated by patients and are one of the most commonly used devices for oxygen administration. However, nasal cannulas have the disadvantage of instability, resulting in displacement by a restless or unobservant patient. Such pathologic conditions as a deviated septum, mucosal drainage and edema, and nasal polyps can interfere with oxygen intake.[3]

The cannula is made of soft plastic and has two prongs that insert 1 cm into each naris. Oxygen flow from 1 to

15 L/min can be delivered comfortably, with the FIO_2 ranging from 24% to 50% (Table 23-1). Higher flows should be avoided because of the irritating and drying effect on the nasal mucosa.[2]

Because the nasal cannula is a low-flow system in which the oxygen concentration delivered is a mixture of ambient air and oxygen, the overall oxygen concentration will be altered by tidal volume and ventilatory pattern. For example, when a patient has a large tidal volume, the FIO_2 delivered to the alveoli is low because more air from the atmosphere mixes with the oxygen. Conversely, when the tidal volume is small, the FIO_2 is high. When a patient has a regular breathing pattern with consistent rate and tidal volume, cannulas can provide a relatively constant FIO_2.[1]

◆ **Simple masks.** The usual simple, open-face mask is a disposable plastic unit that does not have any valves or reservoir bag. It covers the nose and mouth, has vents for exhaled air, and delivers oxygen concentrations of up to 65% (see Table 23-1). Oxygen flow rates at a minimum of 5 to 6 L/min should be used to wash out the exhaled carbon dioxide that accumulates within the mask. The open-face mask is not recommended for controlled oxygen therapy, because it does not provide precise inspired oxygen concentrations. However, this mask is a convenient and relatively comfortable device for delivering moderate oxygen concentrations over short periods and thus is widely used. Limitations are similar to those of all masks and include discomfort and frequent removal of the mask for such activities as eating, expectorating, and coughing (see box, lower right).[2,3]

◆ **Partial rebreathing mask.** The partial rebreathing mask is a tight-fitting mask with a reservoir bag that is always open to the mask. The reservoir bag allows delivery of oxygen concentrations of greater than 60% at a flow rate of 10 L/min. The purpose of the mask is to conserve oxygen by having the patient rebreathe some of his or her exhaled air. The oxygen source flows into the neck of the mask, allowing oxygen to flow directly into the mask during inhalation and into the bag during exhalation. A flow into the bag of at least 5 to 6 L/min is required to prevent deflation of the reservoir bag. Because of the constant filling of the reservoir bag, only the first one third of the exhaled air volume enters the bag. This exhaled air is high in oxygen and low in carbon dioxide, because it is the volume of air that ventilated the anatomic dead space. Because minimal room air enters the mask, the concentration of delivered oxygen is fairly predictable, even if the patient's ventilatory pattern exceeds the flow rate of the oxygen source.[2,3]

◆ **Nonrebreathing masks.** The nonrebreathing mask is a mask and reservoir bag system similar to the partial rebreathing system. With this mask, however, a one-way valve is between the bag and mask, and no air enters the bag during exhalation. The exhaled air is diverted into the atmosphere through a flap valve in the face piece. If the oxygen source fails or the patient's needs suddenly exceed the flow of oxygen, a flap or spring-loaded valve either in the neck or in the mask itself permits the intake of room air. When the nonrebreathing mask has a tight seal over the face, it is designed to deliver 90% to 100% oxygen. However, in practice it usually delivers oxygen concentrations of 57% to 70%. Factors responsible for this decreased concentration of oxygen include entrainment of room air because of a loose-fitting mask and open exhalation ports that allow room air to dilute the oxygen from the reservoir bag.[3]

◆ **Venturi mask.** The most reliable control of FIO_2 can be achieved through use of a Venturi mask, which controls the oxygen concentration by flowing 100% oxygen at high velocity through a narrowed orifice or "jet." This high velocity causes entrainment of air at the orifice. The higher the velocity, the more the air is entrained; this is what is referred to as the *Bernoulli principle*, and it is one of the most accurate means of delivering a prescribed concentration of oxygen.[2,3] The FIO_2 can be varied by changing the orifice size. Venturi masks currently in use can deliver 24%, 28%, 35%, and 40% oxygen. The recommended flow rates for these percentages are, respectively, 4, 6, 8, and 8 L/min.[7]

Table 23-1 Estimation of FIO_2 with use of the nasal cannula and simple mask

Flow rate (L/min)	Estimate of FIO_2
NASAL CANNULA	
1-2	24%-28%
3-5	28%-35%
6-9	35%-45%
10-15	45%-50%
SIMPLE MASK	
6-8	35%-45%
8-10	45%-55%
10-12	55%-65%

OXYGEN MASKS

There are several different types of oxygen masks, which vary in construction and purpose. Most masks are made of soft plastic and are disposable. Masks can be uncomfortable because of the tight fit required on the face and because of the head strap that is necessary to hold the mask in place. Masks can also become hot because of the heat generated from the face around the nose and mouth. Some patients, especially those in severe respiratory distress, complain of claustrophobic feelings when wearing a mask. Despite the oxygen flow into the mask, patients feel "air hunger" because of the close fit of the mask and the heat trapped within it. Care and close observation should be used when masks are on patients who are likely to vomit, because the flow of vomitus can be blocked, thus increasing the chance of aspiration. Masks should also be used with care on the unconscious patient. An oral airway should always be in place to prevent airway obstruction by a flaccid tongue.

Venturi masks are especially efficacious in patients who are chronically hypoxemic and hypercapnic, such as occurs with chronic obstructive pulmonary disease (COPD). An excessive concentration of oxygen can cause respiratory depression in these patients, because their respiratory center is no longer responsive to hypercapnia and is dependent on a low Pa_{O_2} for stimulation to breathe. The Venturi mask can provide such a patient with a precise oxygen concentration that does not change with ventilatory pattern and hence offers more control for an oxygen-sensitive patient.[4]

Venturi masks have the same problems as do other masks and are also very wasteful of oxygen. The high air flow produced by the mask can be drying to the mucous membranes. Attempts to humidify the gas have not been very successful, because of the large amount of entrained air.[3]

Complications of Oxygen Therapy

Oxygen, like most drugs, has adverse effects and complications resulting from its use. The old adage "if a little is good, a lot is better" does not apply to oxygen. The lung is designed to handle a concentration of 21% oxygen, with some adaptability to higher concentrations, but adverse effects and oxygen toxicity can result if a high concentration is administered for too long.

◆ **Hypoventilation.** The first adverse effect of oxygen administration is hypoventilation. The hypoxemic, hypercapnic patient who has chronic lung disease is at risk of developing hypoventilation with oxygen supplementation. In this type of patient and those patients with a depressed respiratory drive (such as a patient with drug overdose), the administration of oxygen may actually cause abolition of the hypoxemia that is responsible for driving the ventilation, resulting in hypoventilation and an increase in the arterial partial pressure of carbon dioxide (Pa_{CO_2}). An elevated Pa_{CO_2} causes hyperventilation in most patients, because carbon dioxide is the stimulus to breathe. However, in patients who rely on hypoxemia as their main respiratory drive (e.g., patients with chronic hypercapnia), the Pa_{CO_2} may continue to rise as hypoventilation progresses. Eventually, the patient becomes somnolent and even obtunded because of carbon dioxide narcosis. Because of the risk of hypoventilation and carbon dioxide accumulation, all chronically hypercapnic patients require careful low-flow oxygen administration.[2,3]

◆ **Absorption atelectasis.** Another adverse effect of high concentrations of oxygen is absorption atelectasis. Breathing high concentrations of oxygen washes out the nitrogen that normally fills the alveoli. The higher the F_{IO_2} delivered to the alveoli, the lower will be the amount of nitrogen. Because nitrogen does not diffuse from an alveolus into the pulmonary capillary, it is responsible for holding open the alveolus. Therefore gradual shrinking of the alveolus can occur if a patient receives a high F_{IO_2} and is ventilating minimally. In this situation, oxygen in the alveolus is absorbed into the blood stream faster than it can be replaced by ventilation and collapse of the alveolus can result.[1]

◆ **Oxygen toxicity.** The most detrimental effect of breathing a high concentration of oxygen is the development of oxygen toxicity. It can occur in any patient breathing oxygen concentrations of greater than 50% for more than 24 hours. The patients most likely to develop oxygen toxicity are those who require intubation, mechanical ventilation, and high oxygen concentrations for extended periods.

Hyperoxia, or the administration of higher-than-normal oxygen concentrations, produces an overabundance of oxygen-free radicals. These radicals are responsible for the initial damage to the alveolar-capillary membrane. Oxygen-free radicals are toxic metabolites of oxygen metabolism. Normally, enzymes neutralize the radicals, which prevents any damage from occurring. During the administration of high levels of oxygen, the large number of oxygen-free radicals produced exhausts the supply of neutralizing enzymes. Thus damage to the lung parenchyma and vasculature occurs.[5]

The pathologic features of oxygen toxicity can be divided into an early exudative stage and a late proliferative stage. Within 24 to 48 hours of oxygen exposure, exudative changes appear. Initially, the capillary endothelial cells become damaged, and they leak serum protein and fluid into the interstitial space of the alveolar wall. This fluid is collected by the lymphatic system, which empties it into the general circulation. As the capillary damage progresses, the flow of fluid out of the capillaries increases and exceeds the lymphatic system's ability to drain it. With continued exposure to hyperoxia, the type I alveolar cells become damaged, allowing the escaped alveolar-capillary fluid to pass directly into the alveolar spaces and causing "flooding" of the alveoli and severe gas exchange impairment.[5]

The lung will respond with cellular proliferation if it survives the aforementioned process and the disease process originally responsible for the hypoxemia. Cellular proliferation occurs in an attempt to repair the alveolar damage, and the alveolar walls become filled with fibroblasts. Alveolar type II cells, which are relatively tolerant to hyperoxia, replicate and reestablish the damaged alveolar wall. Endothelial cell repair and replacement occurs, and the pulmonary edema is resorbed. The final result is irregular scarring that can lead to pulmonary fibrosis.[5]

A number of clinical manifestations are associated with oxygen toxicity. The first symptom is substernal chest pain that is exacerbated by deep breathing. A dry cough and tracheal irritation follow. Eventually, definite pleuritic pain occurs on inhalation, followed by dyspnea. Upper-airway changes may include a sensation of nasal stuffiness, sore throat, and eye and ear discomfort. Chest radiographs and pulmonary function tests show no abnormalities until symptoms are severe. Complete, rapid reversal of these symptoms occurs as soon as normal oxygen concentrations return.[5]

As oxygen toxicity progresses, objective pulmonary damage becomes evident. A chest radiograph reveals atelectatic streaks and patches of bronchopneumonia, and bronchoscopy reveals tracheobronchitis but no infection. As atelectasis develops, there is evidence of decreased vital capacity, decreased compliance, reduced functional residual capacity, and increased intrapulmonary shunting. These abnormalities are reversible several days after normal oxygen concentrations return. If high oxygen concentrations are still needed, permanent damage may occur.[3]

Nursing management of a patient receiving high concentrations of oxygen for more than 24 hours should involve the prevention, detection, and management of oxygen toxicity (see box below). Nursing actions to prevent oxygen toxicity include recognizing the limits of safe oxygen exposure, determining which patients are at risk, and minimizing the work of breathing. Interven-

PROTOCOL FOR PREVENTION OF OXYGEN TOXICITY

A. Prevention of toxic effects of oxygen
   1. Recognize guidelines of safe oxygen exposure.
      a. An FIO_2 of <50% can be tolerated for extended periods without obvious pathologic effects.
      b. With an FIO_2 of ≥50%, physiologic alterations may occur as early as 24 hours.
      c. An inspired gas of 100% oxygen for 24 to 48 hours will lead to exudative change within lung and microatelectasis caused by nitrogen washout.
   2. Determine which patients may have a disease state or physical condition that necessitates treatment with increasing oxygen concentrations.
      a. Individuals with hypoxia related to primary respiratory compromise (e.g., respiratory infection, adult respiratory distress syndrome [ARDS], pulmonary emboli, respiratory arrest)
      b. Individuals with hypoxia caused by a nonpulmonary process (e.g., cardiogenic shock, cerebrovascular accident [CVA], septic shock)
   3. Minimize work of breathing.
      a. Administer medications or treatments to resolve underlying disease process.
      b. Use an endotracheal or tracheostomy tube size 7 mm or greater to minimize resistance and work of breathing.
      c. Promote optimal pulmonary functioning through the following:
         (1) Optimal positioning to promote gas exchange
         (2) Providing for reexpansion or recruitment of alveoli by use of PEEP, inspiratory devices, and sigh mechanism and limited use of narcotics
         (3) Clearing secretions through coughing, turning, and deep breathing and suctioning as necessary
         (4) Preoxygenating before endotracheal suctioning to aid in preventing atelectasis and hypoxia
         (5) Preventing nosocomial infection
         (6) Providing sedation as necessary to improve oxygenation and allow patient to sleep
         (7) Providing nutritional support to maintain muscles, strength, and endurance
         (8) Maintaining fluid balance
         (9) Monitoring hemoglobin (Hgb) and hematocrit (Hct) whereby oxygen-carrying capacity may be optimized

B. Detection of adverse effects of oxygen
   1. Recognize clinical aspects of oxygen toxicity in setting of exposure of ≥50% oxygen for a period of 14 hours or longer.
      a. Report of substernal soreness, sore throat, painful inspiration, and nasal congestion
      b. Atelectasis precipitating a decrease in vital capacity and a decrease in diffusing capacity with prolonged exposure

C. Management of patients to minimize oxygen requirements
   1. Assess patient's oxygen requirements.
      a. Physical examination with particular emphasis on pulmonary examination and patient's strength and endurance
      b. Chest radiograph
      c. Ventilator management
         (1) Note ventilator setting FIO_2, tidal volume, and frequency
         (2) Use of PEEP to assist in preventing atelectasis
         (3) Calculation of lung expansibility or dynamic compliance by: Tidal volume/Peak airway pressure − PEEP
         In an intubated patient with normal lung function, expected value would be >30 cm H_2O.
         With a decrease in lung compliance, dynamic compliance will be <30 cm H_2O.
   2. Monitor laboratory data.
      a. Hgb and Hct: to determine patient's oxygen-carrying capacity
      b. Arterial blood gases
      c. Acid-base balance
   3. Recognize those factors that may influence susceptibility or resistance to pulmonary oxygen toxicity, including vitamins E and C, bleomycin, doxorubicin, hypothermia.

From Brown LH: *Focus Crit Care* 17(1):68, 1990.
FIO_2, Fraction of inspired oxygen; *PEEP*, positive end-expiratory pressure.

tions to minimize oxygen requirements include evaluating the patient's oxygen requirements, monitoring laboratory data, and recognizing factors that influence the development of oxygen toxicity.[5]

ARTIFICIAL AIRWAYS

Oropharyngeal and Nasopharyngeal Airways

Pharyngeal airways are made of rubber or plastic and are used to maintain airway patency by keeping the tongue from obstructing the upper airway. An oral airway is placed by inserting it upside down and rotating it 180 degrees as it is passed into the mouth. It should be used only in an unconscious patient who has an absent or diminished gag reflex. A nasal airway is placed by lubricating the tube and inserting it midline along the floor of the naris into the posterior pharynx. Respirations should be assessed after placement of either airway to ensure proper position. Complications of these airways include trauma to the oral or nasal cavity, obstruction of the airway, laryngospasm, and gagging and vomiting.[4,6,7]

Endotracheal Tubes

An endotracheal tube (ETT) is the most commonly used artificial airway for providing short-term airway management. Indications for endotracheal intubation include airway maintenance, secretion control, oxygenation, and ventilation.[7] An endotracheal tube may be placed through the orotracheal or nasotracheal route. In most situations involving emergency placement, the orotracheal route is used because the approach is simpler and affords use of a larger diameter endotracheal tube. Nasotracheal intubation provides greater patient comfort over time and is preferred in situations in which the patient has a jaw fracture. The advantages and disadvantages of orotracheal intubation and nasotracheal intubation are presented in Tables 23-2 and 23-3.[6]

Endotracheal tubes must meet certain standards for construction. These include specifications for materials, cuff characteristics, dimensions, markings, and packaging. The most common material used for ETTs is polyvinyl chloride. Any material may be used, as long as it is nontoxic to human tissue. The tube should also be smooth on the outside, be stiff enough to insert easily and not collapse with cuff inflation, and soften with body temperature to conform to the patient's airway. The cuff should gently conform to the trachea without permitting significant air leakage during ventilation. In addition, the cuff should inflate evenly, center itself in the trachea, allow for cuff pressure monitoring, and provide a system to indicate when it is inflated or deflated. Because of the high incidence of cuff-related problems, low-pressure, high-volume cuffs (soft cuffs) are preferred. ETTs are available in a variety of sizes, according to the internal diameter of the tube, and have a radiopaque marker either along the side of the tube or at the patient end of the tube.[8]

Before intubation, equipment should be organized to facilitate the procedure. Equipment that should be readily available includes a suction system with catheters and tonsil suction, a manual resuscitation bag (MRB) with a mask connected to 100% oxygen, a laryngoscope handle with assorted blades, a variety of sizes of ETTs, and a stylet. Before the procedure is initiated, all equipment should be inspected to ensure it is in working order. The patient should be prepared for the procedure if possible and have an intravenous catheter in place. The patient should be sedated before the procedure and a topical anesthetic applied to facilitate placement of the tube. In some cases a paralytic agent may be necessary if the patient is extremely agitated.[6,7]

The patient is positioned with the neck flexed and head slightly extended in the "sniff" position. The oral

Table 23-2 Orotracheal intubation: advantages and disadvantages

ADVANTAGES
Requires no surgical procedure for insertion
Does not damage nasal passage
Is not associated with sinusitis
Larger diameter, shorter tube is usually used, resulting in less resistance and mucous plugging, decreased work of breathing, and easier suctioning
Is easier to pass than nasotracheal tube during an emergency
DISADVANTAGES
May not be well tolerated, requiring more patient sedation
Is more difficult to stabilize than nasotracheal tube
Increases risk of unintentional extubation
May need oral airway to prevent tube biting
Patient may "tongue out" tube
Impairs oral hygiene
Cannot be used after major dental or mandibular surgery
Endobronchial intubation is possible

Table 23-3 Nasotracheal intubation: advantages and disadvantages

ADVANTAGES
Requires no surgical procedure for insertion
Tube is easily fixed
Is well tolerated by patient
Enables easy swallowing
Requires less sedation
Does not impair oral hygiene
Unintentional extubation is less likely
DISADVANTAGES
Smaller diameter, longer tube is used, resulting in greater resistance and mucous plugging, increased work of breathing, and more difficulty in suctioning and passing fiberoptic bronchoscope
May cause sinusitis
Cannot be used with nasal cerebrospinal fluid leaks or with sinus or nasal fractures
Endobronchial intubation is possible
May cause necrosis of intranasal septum

cavity and pharynx should be suctioned and any dental devices removed. The patient should be preoxygenated and ventilated using the MRB and mask with 100% oxygen. Each intubation attempt should be limited to 30 seconds. Once the ETT is inserted, the patient should be assessed for bilateral breath sounds and bilateral chest movement. The tube should then be secured and a chest radiograph obtained to confirm placement.[6,7] The tip of the endotracheal tube should be at least 2 cm above the carina but with the cuff below the cricoid cartilage.[9] Once final adjustment of the position is complete, the level of insertion (marked in centimeters on side of tube) should be noted.[7]

There are a number of complications with intubation. These include gastric intubation; right mainstem bronchus intubation; vomiting with aspiration; trauma to the mouth, nose, pharynx, trachea, esophagus, eyes, or facial tissue; laryngospasm; hypoxemia; and hypercapnia. Hypoxemia and hypercapnia can cause bradycardia, tachycardia, dysrhythmias, hypertension, and hypotension.[7,9]

A number of factors predispose a patient to the development of complications while he or she is intubated (see box on right). Complications that can occur include tube obstruction and displacement, sinusitis, nasal injury, and tracheoesophageal fistulas (Table 23-4). A number of complications can occur days to weeks after the ETT is removed. These include mucosal lesions, laryngeal and/or tracheal stenosis, and cricoid abscess (Table 23-4). Delayed complications usually require some form of surgical intervention to correct.[9]

Tracheostomy Tubes

A tracheostomy tube is the preferred method of airway maintenance in the patient requiring intubation for more than 21 days. It is also indicated in several other situations. These include upper airway obstruction or malformation, failed intubation, repeated intubations, presence of complications of endotracheal intubation, glottic incompetence, sleep apnea, and chronic inability to clear secretions.[6]

A tracheostomy tube provides the best route for long-term airway maintenance and avoids the oral, nasal, pharyngeal, and laryngeal complications of endotracheal intubation. The tube is shorter, of wider diameter, and less curved than is the endotracheal tube; thus the resistance to air flow is less, and breathing is easier. The tracheostomy has other advantages over endotracheal intubation, including easier secretion removal, increased patient acceptance and comfort, the possibility of the patient's eating and talking, and the facilitation of ventilator weaning, because a tracheostomy tube is easier to breathe through when the patient is off the ventilator. Table 23-5 presents a list of the advantages and disadvantages of a tracheostomy.[6,10]

Tracheostomy tubes may be single-lumen or double-lumen tubes. Single-lumen tubes consist of two parts: (1) the tube and a built-in cuff, which is connected to an air line for inflation purposes and (2) an obturator, which is used during tube insertion. The double-lumen tubes consist of the tube with the attached cuff, the obturator, and an inner cannula that can be removed for cleaning and reinserted or, if disposable, replaced by a new sterile inner cannula. The inner cannula can quickly be removed if it becomes obstructed, making the system safer for patients with significant secretion problems. Debate exists about the need for the inner cannula because of the development of newer tube materials and improved humidification systems. These advances decrease secretion adherence to the inside of the tube and may eliminate the need for a removable inner cannula. Single-lumen tubes provide a larger inside diameter for air flow than do double-lumen tubes, thus reducing air-flow resistance and allowing the patient to ventilate through the tube with greater ease.

Tracheostomy tubes are inserted via a tracheotomy procedure. Inoperative complications of a tracheotomy include hemorrhage, pneumothorax, pneumomediastinum, tracheoesophageal fistula, laryngeal nerve injury, and cardiopulmonary arrest. Immediate postoperative complications include hemorrhage, wound infection, subcutaneous emphysema, tube obstruction, and displacement of the tube (Table 23-6).[11] Later complications of a tracheotomy include tracheal stenosis, tracheoesophageal fistula, tracheoinnominate artery fistula, and tracheocutaneous fistula (see Table 23-6).[12]

NURSING INTERVENTIONS TO MINIMIZE COMPLICATIONS RESULTING FROM ARTIFICIAL AIRWAY PLACEMENT

- ◆ Stabilize the tube as much as possible to prevent movement within the larynx.
- ◆ Avoid frequent retaping, because this involves unnecessary manipulation of tube.
- ◆ Note the depth of the tube at placement and periodically thereafter to avoid displacement.
- ◆ Avoid overinflation of the cuff—maintain pressure at <25 mm Hg.
- ◆ Do not periodically deflate or inflate cuff.
- ◆ Use high volume–low-pressure cuffs.
- ◆ When nasotracheal intubation is present, inspect nares every day for signs of pressure necrosis.
- ◆ Provide frequent mouth care to decrease infection.
- ◆ Take measures to avoid traumatic extubation by patient (e.g., sedate or restrain).
- ◆ Follow strict aseptic technique when giving artificial airway care and when suctioning (use proper universal blood and body secretion precautions; gloves and goggles should be worn by all caregivers.
- ◆ Avoid excessive negative pressure during suctioning; use only amount necessary to remove secretions (i.e., keep below 120 mm Hg).
- ◆ Support ventilator tubing to avoid traction on the patient's airway tube.
- ◆ Take measures to avoid excessive movement by patient (e.g., repeated flexion and extension of head, coughing, chewing, tonguing the tube).

Table 23-4 Endotracheal tubes: complications, causes, and treatment

Complications	Causes	Prevention/treatment
Tube obstruction	Patient biting tube Tube kinking during repositioning Cuff herniation Dried secretions, blood, or lubricant Tissue from tumor Trauma Foreign body	*Prevention*: Place bite block. Sedate patient PRN. Suction PRN. Humidify inspired gases. *Treatment*: Replace tube.
Tube displacement	Movement of patient's head Movement of tube by patient's tongue Traction on tube from ventilator tubing Self-extubation	*Prevention*: Secure tube to upper lip. Restrain patient's hands. Sedate patient PRN. Ensure that only 2 inches of tube extend beyond lip. Support ventilator tubing. *Treatment*: Replace tube.
Sinusitis and nasal injury	Obstruction of the paranasal sinus drainage Pressure necrosis of nares	*Prevention*: Avoid nasal intubations. Cushion nares from tube and tape/ties. *Treatment*: Remove all tubes from nasal passages. Administer antibiotics.
Tracheoesophageal fistula	Pressure necrosis of posterior tracheal wall resulting from overinflated cuff and rigid nasogastric tube	*Prevention*: Inflate cuff with minimal amount of air necessary. Monitor cuff pressures every 8 hours. *Treatment*: Position cuff of tube distal to fistula. Place gastrostomy tube for enteral feedings. Place esophageal tube for secretion clearance proximal to fistula.
Mucosal lesions	Pressure at tube and mucosal interface	*Prevention*: Inflate cuff with minimal amount of air necessary. Monitor cuff pressures every 8 hours. Use appropriate size tube. *Treatment*: May resolve spontaneously. Perform surgical intervention.
Laryngeal or tracheal stenosis	Injury to area from end of tube or cuff, resulting in scar tissue formation and narrowing of airway	*Prevention*: Inflate cuff with minimal amount of air necessary. Monitor cuff pressures every 8 hours. Suction area above cuff frequently. *Treatment*: Perform tracheostomy. Place laryngeal stint. Perform surgical repair.
Cricoid abscess	Mucosal injury with bacterial invasion	*Prevention*: Inflate cuff with minimal amount of air necessary. Monitor cuff pressures every 8 hours. Suction area above cuff frequently. *Treatment*: Perform incision and drainage of area. Administer antibiotics.

Table 23-5 Tracheostomy: advantages and disadvantages

ADVANTAGES	DISADVANTAGES
Avoids complications of endotracheal tubes	Requires surgical procedure and anesthesia
Requires no endobronchial intubation	If extubation occurs during first 24 hours, possibly difficult to reinsert the tube
Does not impair oral hygiene and sinus drainage	Possible creation of false passage anterior to trachea in patients with thick necks
Speech is possible if appropriate device is used	Possible tearing of posterior tracheal membrane during tracheostomy tube insertion
Minimal resistance from short diameter, wide tube, and little mucous plugging during ventilation	Possible scar or persistent tracheocutaneous fistula after healing
Suctioning is easier and more effective	More expensive
Is better tolerated than orotracheal and nasotracheal tubes	Higher rate of complications
Is easily stabilized	More severe complications
Ventilator easily attached if acute respiratory distress occurs	
Reinsertion is easier	

Table 23-6 Tracheotomy: complications, causes, and treatment

Complications	Causes	Prevention/treatment
Hemorrhage	Vessels' opening after surgery Vessel erosion caused by tube	*Prevention*: Use appropriate size tube. Treat local infection. Suction gently. Humidify inspired gases. Position tracheal window not lower than third tracheal ring. *Treatment*: Pack lightly. Perform surgical intervention.
Wound infection	Colonization of stoma with hospital flora	*Prevention*: Perform routine stoma care. *Treatment*: Remove tube, if necessary. Perform aggressive wound care and debridement. Administer antibiotics.
Subcutaneous emphysema	Positive pressure ventilation Coughing against a tight, occlusive dressing or sutured or packed wound	*Prevention*: Avoid suturing or packing wound closed around tube. *Treatment*: Remove any sutures or packing if present.
Tube obstruction	Dried blood or secretions False passage into soft tissues Opening of cannula positioned against tracheal wall Foreign body Tissue from tumor	*Prevention*: Suction PRN. Humidify inspired gases. Use double-lumen tube. Position tube so that opening does not press against tracheal wall. *Treatment*: Remove/replace inner cannula. Replace tube.

Continued.

Table 23-6 Tracheotomy: complications, causes, and treatment—cont'd

Complications	Causes	Prevention/treatment
Displacement of tube	Patient movement Coughing Traction on ventilatory tubing	*Prevention*: Tie tapes to allow only one finger width between the tape and neck. Suture tube in place. Use tubes with adjustable neck plates for patients with short necks. Support ventilator tubing. Sedate patient PRN. Restrain patient PRN. *Treatment:* Cover stoma and manually ventilate patient via mouth Replace tube
Tracheal stenosis	Injury to area from end of tube or cuff, resulting in scar tissue formation and narrowing of airway	*Prevention*: Inflate cuff with minimal amount of air necessary. Monitor cuff pressures every 8 hours. *Treatment:* Perform surgical repair.
Tracheoesophageal fistula	Pressure necrosis of posterior tracheal wall resulting from overinflated cuff and rigid nasogastric tube	*Prevention*: Inflate cuff with minimal amount of air necessary. Monitor cuff pressures every 8 hours. *Treatment*: Perform surgical repair.
Tracheoinnominate artery fistula	Direct pressure from the elbow of the cannula against the innominate artery Placement of tracheal stoma below fourth tracheal ring Downward migration of the tracheal stoma resulting from traction on tube High-lying innominate artery	*Prevention*: Position tracheal window no lower than third tracheal ring. *Treatment*: Hyperinflate cuff to control bleeding. Remove tube and replace with endotracheal tube and apply digital pressure through stoma against the sternum. Perform surgical repair.
Tracheocutaneous fistula	Failure of stoma to close after removal of tube	*Treatment*: Perform surgical repair.

AIRWAY MANAGEMENT

The patient with an endotracheal or tracheostomy tube requires some additional measures to address the effects associated with tube placement on the respiratory and other body systems (see first box, p. 445). The tube bypasses the upper airway system. Therefore warming and humidifying of air must be performed by external means. Because the cuff of the tube can cause damage to the walls of the trachea, proper cuff inflation and management is imperative. In addition, the normal defense mechanisms are impaired and secretions may accumulate; thus suctioning may need to be performed to promote secretion clearance. Because the tube does not allow air flow over the vocal cords, developing a method of communication is also very important.

There is great potential for the development of a nosocomial pneumonia after the placement of an artificial airway. Once an artificial airway is placed, contamination of the lower airways follows within 24 hours. This results from a number of factors that directly and indirectly promote airway colonization (see second box, p. 445). The use of respiratory therapy devices (e.g., ventilators, nebulizers, and intermittent positive-pressure breathing machines) can also increase the risk of pneumonia. The severity of the patient's illness, presence of acute lung injury, or malnutrition significantly increases the likelihood that an infection will ensue. In addition, such therapeutic measures as nasogastric tubes, antacids, and histamine inhibitors facilitate the development of pneumonia. Nasogastric tubes promote aspiration by acting as a wick for stomach contents, whereas antacids and histamine inhibitors increase the pH level of the stomach, thus promoting the growth of bacteria that can then be aspirated.[13]

FACTORS THAT PREDISPOSE DAMAGE TO THE AIRWAYS BY ARTIFICIAL TUBES

GENERAL FACTORS

Prolonged intubation
Prolonged mechanical ventilation
Inadequate patient sedation
Repeated flexion and extension of the neck
Decerebrate or decorticate movements
Patient out of phase with controlled mechanical ventilation ("bucking" the ventilator)
Traction on the tube during turning, suctioning, and ventilator connection and disconnection
Previous prolonged intubation
Chronic airway or lung disease (especially sputum-producing disease) requiring frequent suctioning procedures
Airway infection
Hypotension

SITE-SPECIFIC FACTORS

Laryngeal

Multiple orotracheal or nasotracheal intubations
Inexperienced laryngoscopist, an emergency intubation, or self-extubation
Too large a translaryngeal tube

Tracheal

Cuff overinflation
Combination of high positive end-expiratory pressure (PEEP) and low lung compliance
Too small or large a cuff in relation to the tracheal size
Noncircular cross-sectional tracheal shape

HOW ARTIFICIAL AIRWAYS PROMOTE NOSOCOMIAL PNEUMONIA

Provide direct access to lower airways
Reduce local defenses by impairing cough and promoting mucociliary dysfunction
Fail to prevent aspiration
Act as a reservoir for bacterial growth
Increase mucus secretion
Promote stagnation of secretions
Induce airway inflammation, which promotes airway colonization
Cause tracheal epithelial cell damage

Humidification

Humidification of air normally is performed by the mucosal layer of the upper respiratory tract. When this area is bypassed, such as occurs in endotracheal intubation and tracheostomy or when supplemental oxygen is used, humidification by external means is necessary. Various humidification devices add water to inhaled gas to prevent drying and irritation of the respiratory tract, to prevent undue loss of body water, and to facilitate secretion removal.

Bubble diffusion humidifiers commonly are used to provide moisture to inhaled gas. They may be warm or cold humidifiers. With a cold humidifier, the gas diffuses out of a stem submerged in water, breaks into small bubbles, and vaporizes. At room temperature, the gas provides only approximately 50% of the humidification needed by the body. Therefore this method of humidification can lead to drying and irritation of mucous membranes when used for a significant time. Diffusion humidifiers cannot humidify gas adequately at higher rates of flow, making them more suitable for low-flow oxygen delivery over short time spans. Cold humidifiers are relatively simple and reliable devices and are available as disposable units, thus decreasing maintenance time and eliminating the potential for infection associated with reusable equipment. Warm humidifiers provide better humidification than do cold humidifiers, because warm humidification supplies both heat and moisture and breaks gas into smaller particles at higher flow rates. Heated cascade humidifiers are preferred for use with intubated patients, because 100% humidification of inhaled gas can be ensured.[14]

Aerosol Therapy

An aerosol is a liquid particle suspended in a gas. Distilled water or saline solutions often are used as liquid aerosol, but other solutions may be used. The inhalation of aerosols increases secretion clearance and liquifies mucus, but continuous administration of water aerosol can lead to water retention and fluid overload. Aerosol therapy should be used cautiously in patients with heart failure, respiratory distress, or decreased ability to clear secretions.[14]

The effects of aerosols on the respiratory tract depend on the level to which the aerosol penetrates the lungs. Penetration is related to particle size: particles of >30 microns in diameter are deposited in the upper airway, whereas particles of <5 microns can reach the smaller airways. The patient's breathing pattern can affect penetration. Slower breathing results in more fallout deposition in the upper airways, whereas larger tidal volumes and mouth breathing can encourage deeper aerosol penetration. Aerosol deposition increases with momentary breath holding at peak inhalation.[14]

Aerosols are cleared from the lungs by the mucociliary blanket or by phagocytosis. Nebulizers often are used to deliver aerosols to patients with a respiratory disease involving mucus production. Nebulizers are classified by power source, aerosol production, and water production. The two most commonly used nebulizers are the jet nebulizer and the ultrasonic nebulizer. These devices may become a source of bacterial contamination of the respiratory tract and therefore require disinfection between patient uses.[14]

Cuff Management

Because the cuff of the endotracheal or tracheostomy tube is a major source of the complications associated with artificial airways, proper cuff management is essential. To prevent the complications associated with cuff design, only low-pressure, high-volume cuffed tubes should be used in clinical practice. Even with these tubes, cuff pressures can be generated that are high enough to lead to tracheal ischemia and injury. Both cuff-inflation techniques and cuff-pressure monitoring are critical components to the care of the patient with an artificial airway.

Two different cuff-inflation techniques currently are being used—the minimal leak (ML) technique and the minimal occlusion volume (MOV) technique. The ML technique consists of injecting air into the cuff until no leak is heard and then withdrawing the air until a small leak is heard on inspiration.[15] Problems with this technique include difficulty maintaining positive end-expiratory pressure (PEEP),[6] aspiration around the cuff,[6,15] and increased movement of the tube in the trachea.[15] The MOV technique consists of injecting air into the cuff until no leak is heard, then withdrawing the air until a small leak is heard on inspiration, and then adding more air until no leak is heard on inspiration.[15] The problem with this technique is that it generates higher cuff pressures than does the ML technique.[16] The selection of one technique over the other should be determined for the individual patient. If the patient needs a seal to provide adequate ventilation and/or is at high risk for aspiration, the MOV technique should be used. If these are not concerns, the ML technique should be used.[16]

Cuff pressures should be monitored at least every 8 hours with a mercury or aneroid manometer.[6,15,16] Cuff pressures should be maintained at 18 to 22 mm Hg (25 to 30 cm H_2O), because greater pressures decrease blood flow to the capillaries in the tracheal wall and lesser pressures increase the risk of aspiration. Pressures in excess of 22 mm Hg (30 cm H_2O) should be reported to the physician. In addition, cuffs should not routinely be deflated, because this increases the risk of aspiration.[16]

One cuff on the market, made of foam, is self-inflating. It is deflated during tube insertion, after which the air line is opened to room air and the cuff self-inflates. It maintains a constant pressure of 20 mm Hg. Removal can be complicated if the plastic sheath covering the foam is perforated. When perforation occurs, the foam may not be deflatable because the air cannot be totally aspirated.[17]

Suctioning

Suctioning is often required to maintain a patent airway in the patient with an endotracheal or tracheostomy tube. Suctioning is a sterile procedure that should be performed only when the patient needs it and not on a routine schedule. A number of complications are associated with suctioning; including hypoxemia, atelectasis, bronchospasms, cardiac dysrhythmias, hemodynamic alterations, increased intracranial pressure,[18] and airway trauma.[6]

Hypoxemia can result from disconnecting the oxygen source from the patient and/or removing the oxygen from the patient's airways when the suction is applied.[18] Atelectasis is thought to occur when the suction catheter is larger than one half of the diameter of the ETT. Excessive negative pressure occurs when suction is applied, promoting collapse of the distal airways.[18] Bronchospasms are the result of the stimulation of the airways with the suction catheter.[18] Cardiac dysrhythmias, particularly bradycardias, are attributed to vagal stimulation.[19] Some hemodynamic alterations—such as increases in mean arterial pressure, cardiac output, and pulmonary artery pressure—are the result of lung hyperinflation during the procedure.[20] Airway trauma occurs with impaction of the catheter in the airways and excessive negative pressure applied to the catheter.[18]

A number of protocols regarding suctioning have been developed. Several different practices have been found helpful in limiting the complications of suctioning. Hypoxemia can be minimized by giving the patient three hyperoxygenation-hyperinflation breaths (breaths at 100% FIo_2 and 150% tidal volume), with either the ventilator or MRB, both before the procedure and after each pass of the suction catheter.[18,21] Atelectasis can be avoided by using a suction catheter with an external diameter less than one half of the internal diameter of the ETT. Using 100 mm Hg of suction or a flow rate of 15 to 20 L/min will decrease the chances of hypoxemia and airway trauma.[18] Limiting the duration of each suction pass to 10 seconds and the number of passes to only those necessary also will help minimize hypoxemia, airway trauma, cardiac dysrhythmias, and hemodynamic alterations.[18,21] The process of applying intermittent, instead of continuous, suction has been shown to be of no benefit.[22] In addition, the instillation of normal saline to help remove secretions has not proven to be of any benefit and the practice of normal saline lavage remains questionable.[23]

One of the newer devices to facilitate suctioning a patient on the ventilator is the closed tracheal suction system (CTSS). This device consists of a suction catheter in a plastic sleeve that attaches directly to the ventilator tubing. It allows the patient to be suctioned while remaining on the ventilator. Advantages of the CTSS include the maintenance of oxygenation and positive end-expiratory pressure (PEEP) during suctioning, the reduction of hypoxemia-related complications, and the protection of staff members from the patient's secretions. The CTSS is convenient to use, requiring only one person to perform the procedure. Concerns related to the CTSS include autocontamination, inadequate removal of secretions, and increased risk of unintentional extubation resulting from the extra weight of the system on the ventilator tubing. Autocontamination has been shown not to be an issue if the catheter is cleaned properly after every use and is changed every 24 hours. Inadequate removal of secretions may or may not be a problem, and further investigation is required to settle this issue.[24]

RESEARCH ABSTRACT

The effect of repeated endotracheal suctioning on arterial blood pressure.

Stone KS, Bell SD, Preusser BA: *Appl Nurs Res* 4(4):152, 1991.

PURPOSE

The purpose of this study was to examine the effects of three repeated lung hyperinflation-suction techniques on the mean arterial pressure (MAP) of patients after open-heart surgery.

DESIGN

Quasi-experimental repeated measure design

SAMPLE

The convenience sample consisted of 34 subjects (27 male and 7 female) at two large Midwestern hospitals. Excluded from the study were patients who had previous histories of chronic renal failure and/or chronic obstructive pulmonary disease (COPD). The mean age of all subjects was 55.2 years, and all were intubated and on a volume ventilator with a baseline FIo_2 of 0.40. Set tidal volumes ranged from 600 to 1200 cc; rates were set between 8 and 12 breaths/min. Endotracheal tube (ETT) size ranged from 7 to 9 mm.

INSTRUMENTS

Systolic and diastolic arterial blood pressures were measured by a polyethylene catheter in the radial artery connected to a Gould Statham P231D transducer (Spectramed, Oxnard, Calif.) and recorded on a Gould 2800, eight-channel direct writing recorder. The lung hyperinflation breaths were delivered by an MA1 ventilator (Puritan-Bennett, Overland Park, Kan.) that was primed to an FIo_2 of 1.0 verified by an in-line Hudson IL406 oxygen analyzer (Ventronics, Hudson Oxygen Therapy, Temecula, Calif.) and measured by an in-line Wright spirometer (Ferraris Development & Engineering Co., Ltd., Edmonton, England). A 14-French polyethylene Pharmaseal suction catheter (American Pharmaseal, Valencia, Calif.) was used for suctioning.

PROCEDURE

Baseline MAP data were obtained 1 minute before the procedure. The hourly protocol began with the delivery of three hyperinflation breaths delivered by a second ventilator (MA1) at an FIo_2 of 1.0 delivered at one of five randomly ordered volumes—one every 5 seconds, for a total of 15 seconds before suctioning. The ventilator flow rate was set at 55 L/min with an I:E ratio of 1:2. Immediately after the third hyperinflation breath, the subject was disconnected from the ventilator, the suction catheter was advanced down the ETT until resistance was met, and 10 seconds of continuous suction (16 L/min suction flow rate) was applied. The sequence of the procedure was repeated three times during each protocol and was timed using a stopwatch. After the last suction pass, the subject was placed back on the preprotocol ventilator and observed for 10 minutes after the procedure. The experimental protocol was repeated each hour until all five volumes were randomly tested in each subject.

RESULTS

Of the subjects, 94.2% were receiving intravenous medications and 53% were receiving nitroglycerine only. Fifteen subjects (44%) were receiving vasoactive medications titrated to maintain systolic blood pressure at 100 to 150 mm Hg. There was a statistically significant increase (p = .001) in MAP from baseline over the three lung hyperinflation-suction sequences; the increase in MAP was not volume dependent. There was an average increase in MAP of 13.72 mm Hg over the sequences. The largest increase in MAP occurred between lung hyperinflations two and three and between the first and second suction catheter passes (p = .05). MAP remained significantly elevated (p = .05) from baseline for 3 minutes during the postprotocol period; the MAP did not fall significantly below baseline at any time during the 10-minute postprotocol period.

DISCUSSION/IMPLICATIONS

The findings from this study indicate that MAP increases significantly over three hyperinflation-suction sequences and that these increases are cumulative with each successive sequence. Increases in MAP in patients after open-heart surgery may pose serious complications and should be avoided. The investigators recommend that the number of repeated lung hyperinflation-suction episodes should be limited to those necessary to maintain airway patency and to only those patients whose physiologic cues indicate the need for suctioning. The sample in this study was small, and the findings cannot be generalized outside of the sample population. Future studies can employ larger samples that are randomly selected and examine additional variables that might have an impact on MAP (i.e., vasopressors, blood volume status, and ventilator volumes and pressures). In addition, patients with other medical disorders should be studied for the relationship of these variables on their MAP.

Communication

One of the major stressors for the patient with an artificial airway is impaired communication. This is related to the inability to speak, insufficient explanations from staff members, inadequate understanding, fear of being unable to communicate, and difficulty with communication methods. A number of interventions can facilitate communication in the patient with an endotracheal or tracheostomy tube. These include performing a complete assessment of the patient's ability to communicate, teaching the patient how to communicate, using a variety of methods to communicate, and facilitating the patient's ability to communicate by providing the patient with his or her eye glasses or hearing aid.[25]

A number of methods are available to facilitate communication in this patient population. These include the use of verbal and nonverbal language and a variety of devices to assist the short-term and long-term ventilator-assisted patient. Nonverbal communication may include the use of sign language, gestures, lip reading, pointing, facial expressions, or eye blinking. Simple devices available include pencil and paper; magic slates; magnetic boards with plastic letters; picture, alphabet, or symbol boards; and flash cards. More sophisticated devices include typewriters, computers, talking tracheostomy and endotracheal tubes, and external handheld vibrators. Regardless of the method selected, the patient must be taught how to use the device.[25] Patients with ETTs should be encouraged to communicate in writing, because attempts at speech cause tube movement and increase tracheal injury.[6]

Extubation

Once the airway is no longer needed, it is removed. Extubation is a simple procedure that can be accomplished at the bedside. Before removal of the tube, the airway, mouth, and pharynx should be suctioned. All the air in the cuff of the tube is removed, as well as any tape or ties securing the tube. Before the procedure the patient is given several breaths using an MRB, and the tube is removed quickly after peak inflation.[6] After the removal of a tracheostomy tube, the stoma is covered with a dry dressing. The stoma should close within several days.[26] Complications of extubation include glottic edema, laryngeal dysfunction, sore throat and hoarseness, and vocal cord paralysis.

MECHANICAL VENTILATION

Indications

Mechanical ventilation is indicated in a variety of situations, including ventilatory failure, impaired gas exchange,[27,28] and some operative procedures, as well as prophylactically during impending collapse of other body systems.[28] Clinical indicators of mechanical ventilation include a respiratory rate of >35, maximal inspiratory pressure of <20 mm Hg, vital capacity of <10 ml/kg, minute ventilation of <3 or >20 L/min, $Paco_2$ of >50 mm Hg with a pH of <7.25, Pao_2 (with supplemental oxygen) of <55 mm Hg, or alveolar-arterial oxygen tension difference (with 100% oxygen) of >450 mm Hg.[28]

Types of Ventilators

The two main types of ventilators currently available are positive-pressure ventilators and negative-pressure ventilators. Negative-pressure ventilators are applied externally to the patient and decrease the atmospheric pressure surrounding the thorax to initiate a breath.[29] They are not commonly used in the critical care environment. Positive-pressure ventilators use positive pressure to deliver oxygen to the patient's lungs through an endotracheal or tracheostomy tube.[30] This process reduces the work of breathing and promotes gas exchange. There are three categories of positive pressure ventilators: volume-cycled, pressure-cycled, and time-cycled.[27]

Volume-cycled ventilators are designed to deliver a preset volume of gas to the patient. The machine can deliver the volume of gas despite changes in pressure within the patient's lungs. The major disadvantage to this type of ventilation is the increased risk of barotrauma. To avoid this complication, pressure limits are programmed into the ventilator. When the pressure limit is exceeded, the ventilator will "spill" the remaining volume of gas out of the system. This is the most commonly used type of ventilator in critical care.[27] Fig. 23-1 depicts three commonly used volume-cycled ventilators in critical care.

Pressure-cycled ventilators deliver gas until a preset pressure is reached. The disadvantage of this type of ventilation is that the volume of gas varies with the pressure in the patient's lungs. This type of ventilation can be useful in short-term ventilation situations.[27]

Time-cycled ventilators deliver gas over a preset time interval. The advantage of this type of ventilator is that the inspiratory phase can be held constant. The disadvantage is that pressure and volume change with each breath. This type of ventilation rarely is used in adults and more often is employed in neonates and children.[27]

Modes of Ventilation

The term *ventilator mode* refers to how the machine will ventilate the patient. In other words, selection of a particular mode of ventilation determines how much the patient will participate in his or her own ventilatory pattern. The choice depends on the patient's situation and the goals of treatment.[28] A large variety of modes are available (Table 23-7). Many of these modes may be used in conjunction with each other. Because brands of ventilators vary in their ability to perform certain functions, not all modes are available on all ventilators.

Ventilator Settings

A variety of settings on the ventilator allow the ventilator parameters to be individualized to the patient and the mode of ventilation selected (see box, p. 451). In addition, each ventilator has a patient-monitoring system that allows all aspects of the patient's ventilatory pattern to be assessed, monitored, and displayed. These monitoring capabilities include exhaled minute volume, exhaled tidal volume, total respiratory rate, peak pressure, plateau pressure, PEEP, mean airway pressure,

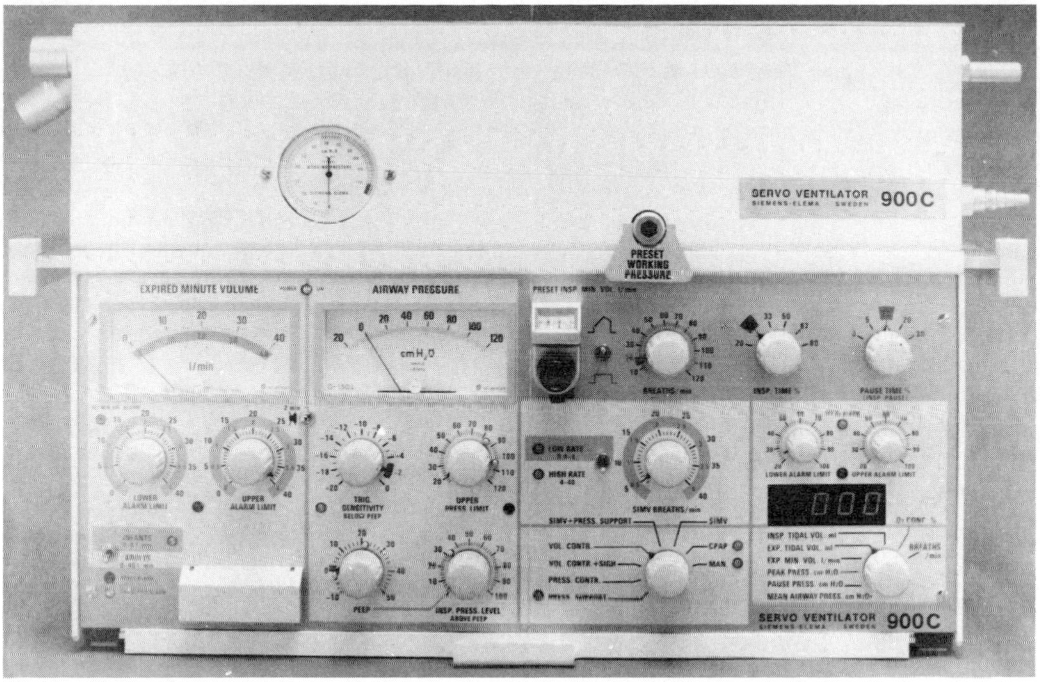

A

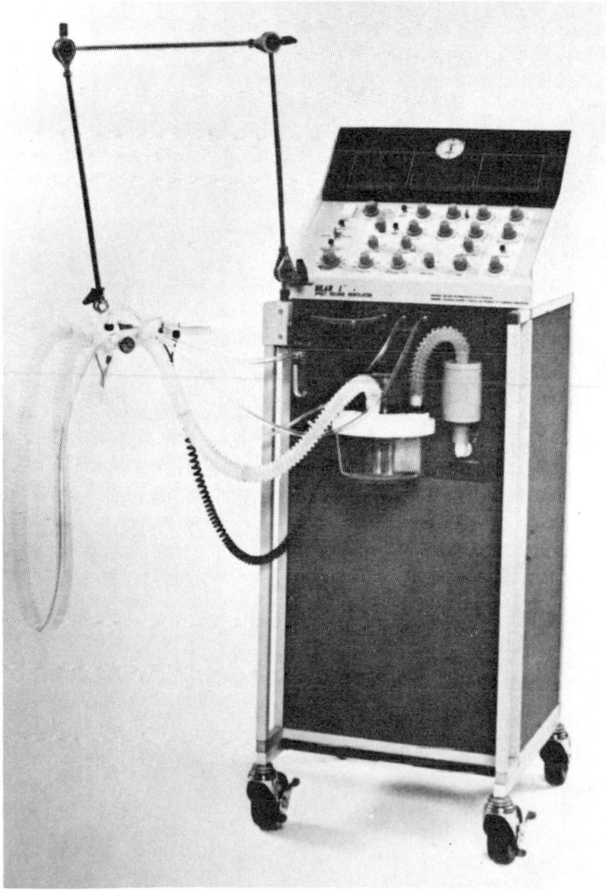

B

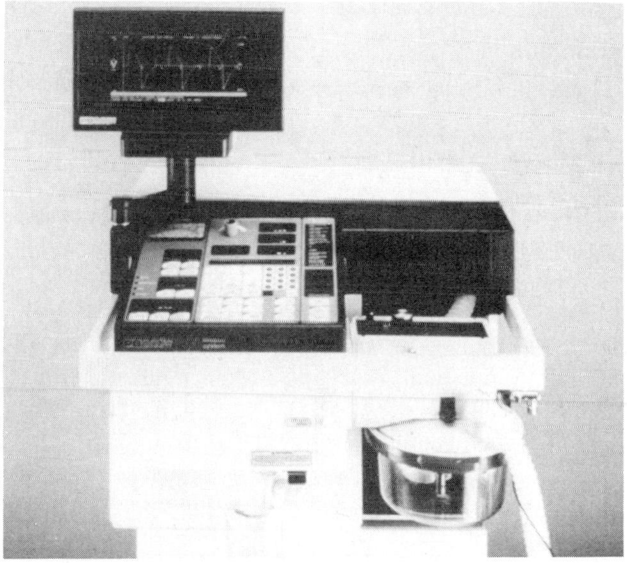

C

Fig. 23-1 Three types of volume-cycled ventilators. **A,** Servo 900C ventilator. **B,** Bear 1 adult volume ventilator. **C,** Puritan-Bennett 7200 microprocessor ventilator. (From Dupuis YG: *Ventilators: theory and clinical application,* ed 2, St Louis, 1992, Mosby–Year Book.)

Table 23-7 Modes of mechanical ventilation

Mode of ventilation	Clinical application	Nursing implications
Controlled ventilation (CV)—delivers gas at preset rate and tidal volume, regardless of the patient's inspiratory efforts[27, 30, 31]	CV is used as the primary ventilatory mode in patients who are apneic.[27, 31]	CV is used in patients unable to initiate a breath.[27] Spontaneously breathing patients must be sedated and/or paralyzed.[30]
Assist-Control ventilation (A/C)—delivers gas at preset tidal volume in response to patient's inspiratory efforts and will initiate breath if patient fails to do so within preset time[27, 30, 31]	A/C is used as primary mode of ventilation in spontaneously breathing patients with weak respiratory muscles.[27]	Hyperventilation can occur in patients with increased respiratory rates.[27, 30] Sedation may be necessary to limit the number of spontaneous breaths.[27]
Synchronous intermittent mandatory ventilation (SIMV)—delivers gas at preset tidal volume and rate while allowing patient to breathe spontaneously; ventilator breaths are synchronized to patient's respiratory effort[27, 30, 31]	SIMV is used both as primary mode of ventilation in a wide variety of clinical situations and as a weaning mode.[27, 31]	SIMV may increase the work of breathing and promote respiratory muscle fatigue.[27, 30]
Positive end-expiratory pressure (PEEP)—positive pressure applied during ventilator breaths Constant positive airway pressure (CPAP)—positive pressure applied during spontaneous breaths[31]	PEEP and CPAP are used in patients with hypoxemia refractory to oxygen therapy; they increase functional residual capacity and improve oxygenation by opening collapsed alveoli and preventing them from collapsing at end expiration.[31] PEEP is used with CV, A/C, or SIMV. CPAP is used as primary mode of ventilation.	Side effects include decreased cardiac output (CO), barotrauma, and increased intracranial pressure.[28, 31]
Pressure support ventilation (PSV)—preset positive pressure used to augment patient's inspiratory efforts; patient controls rate, inspiratory flow, and tidal volume[31-34]	PSV is used as the primary mode of ventilation in patients with stable respiratory drive, with SIMV to support spontaneous breaths, and as a weaning mode in patients who are difficult to wean.[31-34]	Advantages include increased patient comfort, decreased work of breathing and respiratory muscle fatigue, and promotion of respiratory muscle conditioning.[31-34]
Independent lung ventilation (ILV)—ventilation of each lung separately[31]	ILV is used in patients with unilateral lung disease, bronchopleural fistulas, and bilateral asymmetric lung disease.[35]	ILV requires double-lumen endotracheal tube, two ventilators,[30, 35] sedation, and/or pharmacologic paralysis.[30]
High-Frequency ventilation (HFV)—delivers a small volume of gas at a rapid rate Three different types: High-Frequency positive-pressure ventilation (HFPPV)—delivers 60-100 breaths/min High-Frequency jet ventilation (HFJV)—delivers 100-600 cycles/min High-Frequency oscillation (HFO)—delivers 900-3000 cycles/min[34]	HFV is used in situations in which conventional mechanical ventilation compromises hemodynamic stability, with bronchopleural fistulas, during short-term procedures, and with diseases that create a risk of barotrauma.[34]	Patients may need to be sedated. Inadequate humidification can compromise airway patency. Assessment of breath sounds is difficult.[33, 34]

Table 23-7 Modes of mechanical ventilation—cont'd

Mode of ventilation	Clinical application	Nursing implications
Mandatory minute volume (MMV)—allows patient to breathe spontaneously while ensuring delivery of constant minute volume if patient's minute volume falls below preset level[31]	MMV is used as a weaning mode[32] and with PSV as a backup in patients with unstable respiratory drives.[31]	MMV does not evaluate respiratory pattern. MMV may be achieved with rapid, shallow breathing.[31, 32]
Inverse ratio ventilation (IRV)—ventilation in which the proportion of inspiratory time to expiratory time is ≥1:1; can be initiated using pressure-controlled breaths (PC-IRV) or volume-controlled breaths (VC–IVR)[31, 36]	IRV is used in patients with hypoxemia refractory to PEEP, the longer inspiratory time increases functional residual capacity and improves oxygenation by opening collapsed alveoli, and the shorter expiratory time induces intrinsic PEEP (auto-PEEP) that prevents alveoli from recollapsing.[31, 36]	IRV requires sedation and/or pharmacologic paralysis because of discomfort. Increased intrathoracic pressure can result in excessive air trapping and decreased cardiac output (CO).[32]
Nocturnal nasal positive-pressure ventilation (NNPPV)—positive pressure delivered via a nasal mask with a volume ventilator[34]	NNPPV is used at night for patients with respiratory muscle weakness or nighttime hypoventilation.[34]	Mask should fit well and have soft padding. Equipment should be positioned to facilitate sleep.[34]

VENTILATOR SETTINGS

RESPIRATORY RATE (F)

Number of breaths the ventilator will deliver per minute.

TIDAL VOLUME (V_T)

Volume delivered to patient during a normal ventilator breath. Usual volume selected is 10 to 15 ml/kg.

OXYGEN CONCENTRATION (FIO_2)

Selects delivery of oxygen between 21% and 100%.

I:E RATIO

Ratio of inspiratory time to expiratory time. Determined by adjusting the inspiratory flow rate. Usually 1:2, unless inverse ratio ventilation is in use.

INSPIRATORY FLOW RATE (PEAK FLOW)

Flow of tidal volume delivery.

SENSITIVITY

Control that adjusts the ventilatory response to patient's respiratory effort. It determines the amount of effort the patient must generate to initiate a breath.

SIGHS

Allows periodic selection of a larger-than-normal tidal volume. Usual volume is 1½ to 2 times tidal volume, and usual rate is 4 to 5 times an hour.

PRESSURE LIMITS

Adjustable setting to regulate the maximal pressure the machine can generate to deliver the tidal volume. Once the pressure limit is reached, the ventilator will spill the undelivered volume into the atmosphere to protect the patient from barotrauma. The limit is usually set at 10 to 20 cm H_2O above the normal peak pressure.

spontaneous minute volume, spontaneous respiratory rate, circuit temperature, FIO_2, inspired tidal volume, pressure waveform, flow waveform, auto-PEEP, and respiratory mechanics. Monitoring capabilities vary slightly from one brand of ventilator to another.[37]

Complications

Mechanical ventilation is often lifesaving, but similar to other interventions, it is not without complications. Some complications are preventable, whereas others can be minimized but not eradicated. Physiologic complications associated with mechanical ventilation include decreased CO, unintentional acute respiratory alkalosis, increased intracranial pressure, massive gastric distention, impaired hepatic and renal function, and barotrauma.[38]

Positive-pressure ventilation increases intrathoracic pressure, which decreases venous return to the right side of the heart. Impaired venous return decreases preload, which results in a decrease in CO. Decreased CO is thought to be the mechanism of impaired hepatic and renal function. In addition, positive-pressure ventilation impairs cerebral venous return. Thus in patients with impaired autoregulation, positive-pressure ventilation can result in increased intracranial pressure. Unintentional respiratory alkalosis may occur secondarily to alveolar hyperventilation as a result of pain, anxiety, dyspnea, agitation, or inappropriate ventilator settings. Respiratory alkalosis can impair cerebral perfusion and predispose the patient to the development of cardiac dysrhythmias. Gastric distention occurs when air leaks around the endotracheal or tracheostomy tube cuff and overcomes the resistance of the lower esophageal sphincter. This problem can be prevented by inserting a nasogastric tube and ensuring appropriate cuff inflation.[38]

Barotrauma occurs in mechanically ventilated patients as a result of alveolar overdistention. This causes alveolar rupture and air leakage into the pulmonary interstitial space. Once in the space, the air travels out through the hilum and into the mediastinum, pleural space, subcutaneous tissues, pericardium, peritoneum, and retroperitoneum. This can result in a number of disorders, the most lethal of which is a pneumothorax.[38]

NURSING DIAGNOSIS AND MANAGEMENT
Controlled mechanical ventilation

- Inability to Sustain Spontaneous Ventilation related to respiratory muscle fatigue secondary to mechanical ventilation, p. 468
- Ineffective Airway Clearance related to impaired cough secondary to artificial airway, p. 466
- High Risk for Aspiration risk factors: impaired pharyngeal peristalsis or tongue function; impaired laryngeal closure or elevation, p. 472
- Decreased Cardiac Output related to decreased preload secondary to mechanical ventilation with or without PEEP, p. 359
- Sleep Pattern Disturbance related to fragmented sleep and/or circadian desynchronization, pp. 142 and 143
- Body Image Disturbance related to functional dependence on life-sustaining technology, p. 95
- Powerlessness related to health care environment or illness-related regimen, p. 98
- Ineffective Individual Coping related to situational crisis and personal vulnerability, p. 762
- Anxiety related to threat to biologic, psychologic, or social integrity, p. 763

Ventilator Management

Routine assessment of a patient on a ventilator includes monitoring the patient for both patient-related and ventilator-related complications. It should include a routine total assessment, with particular emphasis on the pulmonary system, placement of the endotracheal tube, and observation for subcutaneous emphysema and synchrony with the ventilator. Assessment of the ventilator should include a review of all the ventilator settings and alarms.[39]

Bedside evaluation of vital capacity, minute ventilation, arterial blood gas (ABG) values, and other pulmonary function tests may be warranted, according to the patient's condition.[40] The use of pulse oximetry can facilitate continuous, noninvasive assessment of oxygenation.[41] Static and dynamic compliance should also be monitored to assess for changes in lung compliance (see Appendix C).[40]

Some additional measures are required to maintain a trouble-free ventilator system. These include maintaining a functional MRB connected to oxygen at the bedside, ensuring that the ventilator tubing is free of water, positioning the ventilator tubing to avoid kinking, maintaining the patency of ventilator tubing and connections, changing ventilator tubing per hospital policy, and monitoring the temperature of the inspired air.[42] In addition, a clear understanding of the alarms and their related problems is important (Table 23-8).[43] If the ventilator malfunctions, the patient should be removed from the ventilator and ventilated manually with an MRB.

Weaning

Weaning should begin only after the original process requiring ventilator support for the patient has been corrected and patient stability has been achieved. Other factors to consider when weaning are length of time on ventilator, sleep deprivation, nutritional status, and psychologic readiness. Three areas that should be reviewed to determine readiness to wean are the patient's level of oxygenation, CO_2 elimination, and mechanical efficiency (see box on left, p. 453).[44-47]

Once readiness to wean has been established, the patient should be prepared for the process. The patient should be positioned upright to facilitate breathing and suctioned to ensure airway patency. In addition, the process should be explained to the patient and the patient offered reassurance. During the weaning process the patient should continuously be monitored for signs of weaning intolerance (see box on right, p. 453).[44]

A number of methods can be used to wean a patient from the ventilator. The method selected depends on the patient, his or her pulmonary status, and the length of time on the ventilator. The four main methods for weaning are T-tube, constant positive airway pressure (CPAP), intermittent mandatory ventilation (IMV), and pressure support ventilation (PSV).[44]

T-tube weaning consists of removing the patient from the ventilator and having him or her breathe spontaneously on a T-tube (T-piece). After a time, the patient is placed back on the ventilator. The goal is to progressively increase the time spent off the ventilator. During the weaning process the patient should be observed closely for respiratory muscle fatigue.[44,46] Extubation is considered once the patient is able to maintain adequate spontaneous respirations for at least 2 hours.[46] CPAP weaning is very similar to T-tube weaning, except the

Table 23-8 Troubleshooting the ventilator

Alarm	Causes	Nursing implications
Low exhaled volume	Cuff leak	Evaluate patency of cuff. Reinflate if necessary. If the cuff is ruptured, the tube will need to be replaced.
	Disruption in ventilatory tubing	Evaluate ventilator tubing and tighten or replace as necessary.
	Patient disconnected from ventilator	Reconnect to ventilator.
High pressure	Secretions in airway	Suction patient.
	Patient biting tube	Insert bite block.
	Tube kinked in airway	Reposition patient's head and neck.
	Cuff herniation	Deflate and reinflate cuff.
	Increased airway resistance/decreased lung compliance (e.g., caused by bronchospasm, pneumothorax, pulmonary edema)	Auscultate breath sounds. Notify physician if problem suspected. Evaluate static and dynamic compliance. Evaluate placement of tube on chest x-ray film (it may be touching the carina). Stabilize tube to prevent movement in airway.
	Patient coughing and/or fighting the machine	Explain all procedures to patient in calm, reassuring manner. Sedate patient as necessary.
Inoperative ventilator	Ventilator malfunction	Remove patient from ventilator, and ventilate manually with MRB. Call respiratory therapy.
Low oxygen pressure	Oxygen malfunction	Remove patient from ventilator, and ventilate manually with MRB. Call respiratory therapy.

WEANING CRITERIA

- FIO_2 of < 50%
- PEEP of <5 cm H_2O
- Respiratory rate <30 breaths/min
- Minute ventilation <10 L/min
- Static compliance >25-30 cm H_2O
- Maximal inspiratory pressure < −20 cm H_2O
- Vital capacity >10-15 ml/kg
- Spontaneous tidal volume >4-5 ml/kg
- Maximal voluntary ventilation > twice minute ventilation
- PaO_2 >60 mm Hg on an FIO_2 of <50%
- Shunt <15%-20%
- Alveolar-arterial oxygen tension difference <350 torr on an FIO_2 of 100%
- $PacO_2$ within patient's normal range

WEANING INTOLERANCE INDICATORS

- Dysrhythmias
- Increase or decrease in heart rate of >20 beats/min
- Increase or decrease in blood pressure of >20 mm Hg
- Increase in respiratory rate of >10 above baseline
- Tidal volumes of <250 ml
- Increase in minute ventilation of >5 L/min
- Diaphoresis
- Dyspnea
- Shortness of breath
- Restlessness
- Decrease in level of consciousness
- SpO_2 <90%
- PaO_2 <60 mm Hg
- Increase in $PacO_2$ with a decrease in pH of <7.35

patient is placed on the CPAP mode instead of a T-tube.[44]

Intermittent mandatory ventilation (IMV) weaning consists of placing the ventilator in the SIMV mode and slowly decreasing the rate until zero (or close) is reached. The rate is usually decreased one to three breaths at a time, and an ABG analysis is usually obtained 30 minutes afterward. This method allows the patient to gradually increase his or her spontaneous rate until support is no longer needed.[44,46]

Pressure support ventilation (PSV) weaning consists of placing the patient on the pressure support mode and setting the pressure support at a level that facilitates the patient's achieving a spontaneous tidal volume of 10 to 12 ml/kg. PSV augments the patient's spontaneous breaths with a positive-pressure "boost" during inspira-

paying particular attention to any tracheal deviation, asymmetry of chest movement, presence of subcutaneous emphysema, characteristics of breathing, quality of lung sounds, and presence of tympany or percussion sounds, which are indicative of pneumothorax.[54]

CHEST PHYSICAL THERAPY

Historically, chest physical therapy (CPT) has been used to supplement the patient's coughing effort or to substitute for it if cough is absent. CPT is directed at improving secretion clearance and airway function and includes various combinations of postural drainage, chest percussion and vibration, and cough enhancement. Recently, the efficacy of these techniques has been questioned. CPT has been found to benefit acutely ill patients with large volumes of secretions and lobar atelectasis. It has been found not to benefit patients with COPD who have small amounts of secretions, and it may cause bronchospasm and hypoxemia in acutely ill patients.[56]

Postural Drainage

Proper application of postural drainage requires knowledge of the anatomic arrangement of lung segments so that positioning for gravity drainage will result. The patient should be positioned with the area of lung to be drained uppermost and the airway as vertical as possible to facilitate movement of secretions. Postural drainage may be used alone or just before percussion and vibration and should be done early in the morning and at bedtime. Contraindications for postural drainage include increased intracranial pressure, recent myocardial infarction, spinal fractures, and within 1 hour after meals.[57]

Chest Percussion and Vibration

Chest percussion and vibration help dislodge secretions from airway walls, thereby enhancing removal by postural drainage and coughing. Percussion is performed by holding the hands in a cupped configuration and clapping rhythmically on the patient's chest wall. Vibration can be performed manually or with the aid of a machine. When manual vibration is performed, the nurse places her or his hands firmly against the patient's chest wall and as the patient exhales, the nurse shakes his or her arms, creating a gentle vibratory sensation in the chest. This technique is repeated two or three times in an area. Vibration is as effective as is percussion and may be better tolerated in some critically ill patients.[58] Contraindications for percussion and vibration include seizures, resectable lung cancer, obesity, pneumothorax (high risk for or actual), brittle bones, and hemorrhagic conditions.[57]

Cough Enhancement

Coughing is sometimes necessary for the removal of secretions from the tracheobronchial tree. To be effective, however, the cough must be a composite of several distinct and necessary phases, which are listed in Table 23-9. Effective coughing depends on (1) a deep inhalation, (2) strong contraction of the muscles of exhalation—in particular, the abdominal muscles, (3) a functioning glottis, and (4) airways that remain open during the terminal exhalatory phase of the cough. Abnormal functioning of any of these mechanisms decreases the effectiveness of coughing. An inability to take a deep breath; weak abdominal muscles; an unwillingness to use the abdominal muscles because of pain or poor positioning; and chronic, diffuse small airway collapse, such as can occur with COPD, can significantly reduce cough effectiveness. A reduction of cough effectiveness in the presence of mucus production will lead to ineffective airway clearance (see Table 23-9).[59]

The most effective position for coughing is upright in a sitting position, with the head and spine slightly flexed forward, the shoulders relaxed, and the knees flexed.[58,59] Lying supine or even in a semi-Fowler's position does not allow total lung inflation, diaphragmatic descent, or intercostal muscle action and thus decreases the efficiency of the cough. In addition, patients who have

Table 23-9 Factors that interfere with production of an effective cough

Components of an effective normal cough	Factors that interfere with an effective cough	Nursing action
Inhalation to near-total lung capacity	General weakness Inability to take a deep breath Positioning that impairs the deep breath	Consider teaching huff or augmented cough Position for effective cough
Closure of the glottis	Bypass of the glottis by artificial airway	—
Contraction of the abdominal muscles	Weak abdominal muscles Painful use of muscles Positioning that impairs use of the abdominal muscles	Huff cough Analgesics Position for effective cough
Sudden opening of the glottis with explosive exhalation	Inability to exhale with force Diffuse small airway collapse on exhalation Bypass of the glottis by artificial airway	Augmented cough Huff cough

abdominal incisions may experience less incisional pain when coughing while drawing their knees up toward the chest and/or by splinting the incision against a pillow. The feet should be braced against the mattress, so they can act as a support against which to generate greater abdominal muscle tension, producing a stronger cough.[58]

Taking an effective deep breath is another important part of cough enhancement. The patient should be encouraged to take several deep breaths before performing any coughing maneuvers. The nurse can encourage deep breathing by firmly (but not tightly) placing her or his hands on the lateral basal area of the patient's chest wall and asking the patient to push them out as far as the patient can while inspiring deeply.[59]

Several different coughing techniques are available to stimulate the cough reflex. These include the cascade (normal) cough, the huff cough, the end-expiratory cough, and the augmented cough. The cascade cough is performed by the patient's taking a deep breath and then doing a succession of coughs until the majority of air is out of his or her lungs. This action is then repeated several times until a productive cough is elicited, thereby facilitating the movement of secretions from the peripheral to the central airways.[59]

The huff cough (forced expiration technique) is similar to the cascade cough, except that the patient coughs with an open glottis. It produces a "huff" sound instead of a "cough" sound.[58,59] Huff coughing may be helpful for patients with COPD who have significant airway collapse on forced exhalation, because huff coughing is associated with higher flow rates than occur with the normal closed-glottis cough.[58] Furthermore, huff coughing may assist in moving secretions from the smaller airways into the main-stem bronchi or trachea, where the controlled cough technique can be used for effective expectoration.[59]

The end-expiratory cough is a coughing maneuver that can be used with patients with bronchiectasis. It promotes the emptying of secretions from bronchiectatic dilations of the airways. It is performed by instructing the patient to take three or four deep breaths, each followed by a prolonged slow exhalation. On the last breath the patient is instructed to exhale to a lung volume below the patient's resting lung volume and then cough without inhaling.[59]

The augmented cough is used for patients who cannot generate adequate expiratory muscle force. The patient is assisted to cough with a variety of techniques, depending of the etiology of his or her problem. For patients with muscle weakness, a lateral chest wall rib spring technique can be used. To perform this maneuver the hands are placed on the lateral chest wall and, as the patient coughs, the chest wall is abruptly compressed. For patients with abdominal wall weakness, the technique involves contracting the abdomen. To perform this maneuver, the palm of one hand is placed on the patient's upper abdomen (under the xiphoid process) and the other on the patient's shoulder. The patient is instructed to deep breathe and cough; as the patient coughs, the abdomen is abruptly compressed and the patient flexed forward.[59]

REFERENCES

1. Shapiro BA and others: *Clinical application of respiratory care,* ed 4, St Louis, 1989, Mosby–Year Book.
2. Levitzky MG, Cairo JM, Hall SM: *Introduction to respiratory care,* Philadelphia, 1990, WB Saunders.
3. Thalken FR: Medical gas therapy. In Scanlon CL, Spearman CB, Sheldon RL, editors: *Egan's fundamentals of respiratory care,* ed 5, St Louis, 1990, Mosby–Year Book.
4. Albarran-Solelo R and others: *Textbook of advanced cardiac life support,* ed 2, Dallas, 1987, American Heart Association.
5. Brown LH: Pulmonary oxygen toxicity, *Focus Crit Care* 17(1):68, 1990.
6. Stauffer JL: Medical management of the airway, *Clin Chest Med* 12:449, 1991.
7. Victor LD: Endotracheal intubation. In Victor LD, editor: *Manual of critical care procedures,* Rockville, Md, 1989, Aspen Publishers.
8. Colice GL: Technical standards for tracheal tubes, *Clin Chest Med* 12:433, 1991.
9. McCulloch TM, Bishop MJ: Complications of translaryngeal intubation, *Clin Chest Med* 12:507, 1991.
10. Wenig BL, Applebaum EL: Indications for and techniques of tracheotomy, *Clin Chest Med* 12:545, 1991.
11. Myers EN, Carrau RL: Early complications of tracheotomy: incidence and management, *Clin Chest Med* 12:589, 1991.
12. Wood DE, Mathisen DJ: Late complications of tracheotomy, *Clin Chest Med* 12:597, 1991.
13. Levine SA, Niederman MS: The impact of tracheal intubation on host defenses and risks for nosocomial pneumonia, *Clin Chest Med* 12:523, 1991.
14. Scanlan CL: Humidity and aerosol therapy. In Scanlan CL, Spearman CB, Sheldon RL, editors: *Egan's fundamentals of respiratory care,* ed 5, St Louis, 1990, Mosby–Year Book.
15. Goodnough SKC: Reducing tracheal injury and aspiration, *Dimens Crit Care Nurs* 7:324, 1988.
16. Tyler DO, Clark AP, Ogburn-Russell L: Developing a standard for endotracheal tube cuff care, *Dimens Crit Care Nurs* 10:54, 1991.
17. Bernhard W and others: Intracuff pressures in endotracheal and tracheostomy tubes: related cuff physical characteristics, *Chest* 87:720, 1985.
18. Stone KS: Endotracheal suctioning in the critically ill, *Crit Care Nurs Curr* 7:5, 1989.
19. Gunderson LP, Stone KS, Hamlin RL: Endotracheal suctioning-induced heart rate alterations, *Nurs Res* 40:139, 1991.
20. Stone KS and others: The effect of lung hyperinflation and endotracheal suctioning on cardiopulmonary hemodynamics, *Nurs Res* 40:76, 1991.
21. Stone KS: Ventilator versus manual resuscitation bag as the method of delivering hyperoxygenation before endotracheal suctioning, *AACN Clin Iss Crit Care Nurs* 1:289, 1990.
22. Czarnik RE and others: Deferential effects of continuous versus intermittent suction on tracheal tissue, *Heart Lung* 20:144, 1991.
23. Shekleton ME, Nield M: Ineffective airway clearance related to artificial airway, *Nurs Clin North Am* 22:167, 1987.
24. Noll ML, Hix CD, Scott G: Closed tracheal suction systems: effectiveness and nursing implications, *AACN Clin Iss Crit Care Nurs* 1:318, 1990.
25. Connolly MA, Shekleton ME: Communicating with ventilator dependent patients, *Dimens Crit Care Nurs* 10:115, 1991.
26. Godwin JE, Heffner JE: Special critical care considerations in tracheostomy management, *Clin Chest Med* 12:573, 1991.
27. Vasbinder-Dillon D: Understanding mechanical ventilation, *Crit Care Nurs* 8(7):42, 1988.
28. Grum CM, Morganroth ML: Initiating mechanical ventilation, *Intensive Care Med* 3:6, 1988.
29. Levine S, Levy S, Henson D: Negative-pressure ventilation, *Crit Care Clin* 6:505, 1990.

30. Luce JM: What to consider when choosing a positive-pressure ventilation mode, *Jour Crit Ill* 6:339, 1991.
31. Sassoon CSH, Mahutte K, and Light RW: Ventilatory modes: old and new, *Crit Care Clin* 6:605, 1990.
32. Weilitz PB: New modes of mechanical ventilation, *Crit Care Clin North Am* 1:689, 1989.
33. St John RE, Lefrak SS: Alternate modes of mechanical ventilation, *AACN Clin Iss Crit Care Nurs* 1:248, 1990.
34. Burns SM: Advances in ventilatory therapy, *Focus Crit Care* 17:227, 1990.
35. Simons B, Borg U: Independent lung ventilation, *Crit Care Rep* 1:398, 1990.
36. Marcy TW, Marini JJ: Inverse ratio ventilation in ARDS: rationale and implementation, *Chest* 100:494, 1991.
37. Kacmarek RM, Meklaus GJ: The new generation of mechanical ventilators, *Crit Care Clin* 6:551, 1990.
38. Pierson DJ: Complications associated with mechanical ventilation, *Crit Care Clin* 6:711, 1990.
39. Mims BC: *Mechanical ventilation: process and practice,* Lewisville, Tex, 1989, Barbara Clark Mims Associates.
40. Hess D: Bedside monitoring of the patient on a ventilator, *Crit Care Q* 6(2):23, 1983.
41. Hess D: Noninvasive respiratory monitoring during ventilatory support, *Crit Care Clin North Am* 3:565, 1991.
42. Landis K, Smith S: The mechanically ventilated patient: a comprehensive nursing care plan, *Crit Care Q* 6(2):43, 1983.
43. Grossbach I: Troubleshooting ventilator- and patient-related problems/Part 1, *Crit Care Nurs* 6:58, 1986.
44. Geisman LK: Advances in weaning from mechanical ventilation, *Crit Care Clin North Am* 1:697, 1989.
45. Bolgiano CS: Measure of bedside ventilatory parameters, *Crit Care Nurs* 10:60, 1990.
46. Tobin MJ, Yang K: Weaning from mechanical ventilation, *Crit Care Clin* 6:725, 1990.
47. Witta K: New techniques for weaning difficult patients from mechanical ventilation, *AACN Clin Iss Crit Care Nurs* 1:260, 1990.
48. Rutherford KA: Principles and application of oximetry, *Crit Care Nurs Clin North Am* 1:649, 1989.
49. Brown M, Vender JS: Noninvasive oxygen monitoring, *Crit Care Clin* 4:493, 1988.
50. Rueden KT: Noninvasive assessment of gas exchange in the critically ill patient, *AACN Clin Iss Crit Care Nurs* 1:239, 1990.
51. Talamonti WJ: Thoracentesis and chest tube insertion. In Victor LD, editor: *Manual of critical care procedures,* Rockville, Md, 1989, Aspen Publishers.
52. Carroll PF: *Understanding chest drainage,* Floral Park, NY, 1986, Pfizer Hospital Products Group.
53. Erickson RS: Mastering the ins and outs of chest drainage. Part 1, *Nursing* 19(5):37, 1989.
54. Erickson RS: Mastering the ins and outs of chest drainage. Part 2, *Nursing* 19(6):46, 1989.
55. O'Byrne C: Postoperative care and complications in the thoracotomy patient, *Crit Care Nurs Q* 7:53, 1985.
56. Kirilloff LH and others: Does chest physical therapy work? *Chest* 88:436, 1985.
57. Norton LC: Respiratory failure. In Sexton DL, editor: *Nursing care of the respiratory patient,* Norwalk, Conn, 1990, Appleton & Lange.
58. Scanlan CL: Chest physical therapy. In Scanlan CL, Spearman CB, Sheldon RL, editors: *Egan's fundamentals of respiratory care,* ed 5, St Louis, 1990, Mosby–Year Book.
59. Traver GA: Ineffective airway clearance: physiology and clinical application, *Dimens Crit Care Nurs* 4:198, 1985.

24

Pulmonary Nursing Diagnosis and Management

This chapter is designed to supplement the preceding chapters in the *Pulmonary Alterations* unit by integrating theoretic content into clinically applicable case studies and nursing management plans.

The case study is designed to illustrate clinical problem solving and patient care management occurring in actual patients. The case, reviewed retrospectively, demonstrates how medical and nursing diagnoses may be effectively used in critical care. The case study also demonstrates revisions to the plan of care and the nursing and medical management outcomes that are apt to occur during the course of a complicated hospitalization as the patient responds physiologically to treatment. Often in a short case anecdote, such as that which is presented in this chapter, the clinical answer may appear to be obvious from the day of admission. In practice, however, critical care patient management is sometimes investigative and the "correct" diagnosis for an individual patient may not become apparent until midway in the hospitalization. Or a patient with an apparently straightforward diagnosis may develop an unexpected complication, and the plan of care and potential outcomes will then require revision. Many of the case studies demonstrate this principle.

The nursing management plans, which—unlike the case study—are not patient-specific, provide a basis nurses can use to individualize care for their patients. In the previous *Pulmonary Alterations* chapters, each medical diagnosis is assigned a Nursing Diagnosis and Management box. Using this box as a page guide, the reader can access relevant nursing management plans for each medical diagnosis. For example, nursing management of *atelectasis*, described on p. 422, may involve several nursing diagnoses and management plans outlined in this chapter and in other Nursing Diagnosis and Management chapters. Specific examples are (1) *Ineffective Breathing Pattern related to abdominal or thoracic pain*, on p. 469; (2) *Ineffective Airway Clearance related to excessive secretions*, on p. 464; (3) *Impaired Gas Exchange related to alveolar hypoventilation secondary to (specify)*, on p. 471; and (4) *Impaired Gas Exchange related to ventilation/perfusion mismatch secondary to (specify)*, on p. 470. These examples highlight the interrelationship of the various physiologic systems in the body and the fact that pathology often has a multisystem impact in the critically ill.

Use of the case study and management plans can enhance the understanding and application of the *Pulmonary* content in clinical practice.

PULMONARY CASE STUDY

CLINICAL HISTORY

Mr. B is a 63-year-old obese man. He has a long history of chronic obstructive pulmonary disease (COPD) associated with smoking two packs of cigarettes a day for 40 years. During the past week Mr B has experienced a "flu-like" illness with fever, chills, malaise, anorexia, diarrhea, nausea, vomiting, and a productive cough with thick, brown, purulent sputum.

CURRENT PROBLEMS

Mr. B was admitted to the critical care unit from the emergency department with acute respiratory insufficiency. He sat up in bed, leaning forward, with his elbows resting on the overbed table. Mr B breathed through his mouth, taking rapid, shallow breaths, using his accessory muscles to ventilate. On inhalation, his nostrils flared and his intercostal muscles retracted. During exhalation, Mr. B used pursed-lip breathing and his intercostal muscles bulged. He appeared anxious and irritable and could speak only one or two barely audible words between each breath. Auscultation revealed crackles anteriorly and posteriorly in both right and left lower lung fields. Rhonchi were heard in the right upper lung field. His admission chest x-ray film revealed infiltrates in the right upper lobe, right middle lobe, right lower lobe, and left lower lobe. Gram stain of Mr. B's sputum contained numerous gram-positive diplococci. His baseline vital signs were: blood pressure (BP), 110/60; heart rate (HR), 114 (sinus tachycardia); respiratory rate (RR), 30; temperature (T), 101.3° F. His baseline arterial blood gas (ABG) values on a 50% nonrebreather mask were Po_2, 50 mm Hg; Pco_2, 33 mm Hg; pH, 7.42; HCO_3^-, 28 mEq/L; O_2 saturation, 88%.

Continued.

PULMONARY CASE STUDY—cont'd

MEDICAL DIAGNOSIS

Pneumococcal pneumonia

NURSING DIAGNOSES

- ◆ Ineffective Airway Clearance related to excessive secretions or abnormal viscosity of mucus
- ◆ Ineffective Breathing Pattern related to chronic airflow limitations
- ◆ Anxiety related to threat to biologic, psychologic, and/or social integrity

◆ PLAN OF CARE

1. Promote secretion clearance by humidifying supplemental oxygen, encouraging deep breathing, facilitating frequent position changes, providing chest physical therapy (postural drainage, chest percussion and vibration, and coughing techniques), ensuring adequate systemic hydration, and performing nasotracheal suctioning if necessary.
2. Promote an effective ventilatory pattern by encouraging pursed-lip and diaphragmatic breathing, positioning with the head of the bed up, and reducing energy demands.
3. Decrease anxiety by providing orientation and education to environment and illness, supporting existing coping mechanisms, speaking slowly and calmly, removing excess stimulation, and promoting presence of and comforting significant other.

MEDICAL AND NURSING MANAGEMENT AND PATIENT OUTCOME

Mr. B was started on antibiotic therapy and systemic and nebulized bronchodilators, his oxygen concentration was increased to 100%, and he was systemically hydrated with intravenous fluids. Six hours after admission Mr. B's condition continued to deteriorate. He was very confused and combative. Crackles and rhonchi were heard throughout both lung fields, respirations were shallow, and he no longer could produce an effective cough. Mr B was diaphoretic and had marked cyanosis around his lips. His vital signs were: BP, 90/60; HR, 130 (sinus tachycardia with occasional premature ventricular contractions); RR, 30; T, 103.1° F. His ABG values on a 100% nonrebreather mask were: Po_2, 40 mm Hg; Pco_2, 70 mm Hg; pH, 7.22; HCO_3^-, 28 mEq/L; O_2 saturation, 78%.

MEDICAL DIAGNOSIS

Acute respiratory failure

NURSING DIAGNOSES

- ◆ Impaired Gas Exchange related to ventilation/perfusion mismatch
- ◆ Inability to Sustain Spontaneous Ventilation related to respiratory muscle fatigue

◆ REVISED PLAN OF CARE

1. Support oxygenation by ensuring supplemental oxygen administration, preventing desaturation during procedures, encouraging deep breathing, facilitating frequent position changes, providing chest physical therapy, and suctioning nasotracheally if necessary.
2. Support adequate breathing by maintaining upper airway patency (positioning and use of an oropharyngeal or nasopharyngeal airway) and assisting with ventilation (using a manual resuscitation bag) if necessary.

PULMONARY CASE STUDY—cont'd

MEDICAL AND NURSING MANAGEMENT AND PATIENT OUTCOME

Mr B was intubated and placed on a ventilator with the following settings: mode, synchronized intermittent mandatory ventilation (SIMV); rate, 10; tidal volume (VT), 1100 ml; fraction of inspired oxygen (FIO_2), 100%, positive end-expiratory pressure (PEEP), 5 cm H_2O; pressure support (PS), 10 cm H_2O. ABG values on current ventilator settings were: PO_2, 80 mm Hg; PCO_2, 43 mm Hg; pH, 7.37; HCO_3^-, 28 mEq/L; O_2 saturation, 95%.

During the next 4 days Mr B was maintained on the ventilator. The FIO_2 was weaned down to 40% to maintain an O_2 saturation $>$90%. On the fifth day he was awake and alert and following commands appropriately. Lungs sounds were clear and with minimal secretions, and temperature was normal. Tube feedings were started at 50 ml/hr. The decision was made to wean Mr. B from mechanical ventilation. His weaning parameters were: minute ventilation (VE), 9 L/min; static compliance, 35 cm H_2O; maximum inspiratory pressure, −18 cm H_2O, vital capacity, 11 ml/kg; spontaneous tidal volume, > 3.5 ml/kg.

Weaning was initiated by decreasing the rate on the ventilator from 10 to 6 breaths per minute. Mr. B's baseline vital signs were: BP, 135/65; HR, 90 (sinus rhythm); spontaneous RR, 22; T, 98.4° F. Within one hour his vital signs were: BP, 165/75; HR, 115 (sinus tachycardia with premature ventricular contractions); spontaneous RR, 35. Mr. B was diaphoretic and restless and complained of dyspnea. His ABG values were: PO_2, 75 mm Hg; PCO_2, 60 mm Hg, pH, 7.33; HCO_3^-, 24 mEq/L; O_2 saturation, 93%. The weaning attempt was terminated, and his rate on the ventilator was increased back to 10. Over the next 5 days, three more unsuccessful attempts were made to wean Mr. B from the ventilator.

MEDICAL DIAGNOSIS

Chronic ventilatory failure

NURSING DIAGNOSES

- ◆ Dysfunctional Ventilatory Weaning Response (DVWR) related to inappropriate pacing of diminished ventilator support
- ◆ High Risk for Aspiration risk factor: impaired laryngeal closure or elevation

◆ REVISED PLAN OF CARE

1. Facilitate weaning by ensuring availability of energy substrates (oxygen and nutrition); promoting rest; using appropriate training techniques; teaching, modifying, and normalizing the environment; coaching and supporting all efforts; establishing trust; controlling and enhancing social support; and ensuring that staff and others respond appropriately to the patient's needs or wishes.
2. Prevent aspiration by maintaining the head of the bed elevated, frequently checking placement of nasogastric tube, checking amount of residual, and assessing bowel function.

MEDICAL AND NURSING MANAGEMENT AND PATIENT OUTCOME

On the tenth day Mr. B was taken to the operating room and a tracheostomy was performed. He was moved to the intermediate care unit for long-term ventilator management. During the next 3 days constant positive airway pressure (CPAP) weaning trials were successfully carried out. On the fourteenth day Mr. B was placed on a 40% humidified T-piece, with no signs of respiratory distress. On the fifteenth day Mr. B's tracheostomy tube was buttoned, and the following day the tracheostomy tube was removed. Mr. B was transferred to the pulmonary floor and entered a pulmonary rehabilitation program.

INEFFECTIVE AIRWAY CLEARANCE RELATED TO EXCESSIVE SECRETIONS OR ABNORMAL VISCOSITY OF MUCUS

DEFINING CHARACTERISTICS

- ◆ Abnormal arterial blood gas values
- ◆ Abnormal breath sounds
- ◆ Ineffective cough
- ◆ Dyspnea
- ◆ Verbal report of inability to clear airway

OUTCOME CRITERIA

- ◆ Cough produces thin mucus.
- ◆ Lungs are clear to auscultation.
- ◆ Arterial blood gas values are within patient's baseline.

NURSING INTERVENTIONS AND *RATIONALE*

1. Continue to monitor the assessment parameters listed under "Defining Characteristics."
2. In the absence of cardiac or renal dysfunction, hydrate the 24-hour fluid requirements per body surface area (BSA) ***to thin secretions. Adequate hydration is the most effective mucolytic.*** Avoid caffeinated beverages, ***because caffeine is a mild diuretic and can contribute to fluid loss.***
3. Monitor serum osmolality, ***considering that an elevation may indicate need for further hydration.***
4. Provide humidification to airways through mask, room vaporizer, other means ***to assist in thinning secretions.*** When artificial airway is present, ensure that humidification to airway is available and functioning properly. ***Thick, tenacious secretions may mean insufficient fluid intake and/or insufficient external humidification.***
5. Instruct and supervise controlled cough technique. If controlled cough technique is not possible, consider huff coughing or quad coughing techniques.

Controlled cough technique

a. Maximal inhalation—an effective cough is contingent on filling the lungs and airways distal to the mucus ***so that the succeeding forced exhalation will propel the mucus up to the airways. Maximal inhalation also increases airway caliber; as a result, it is more likely that the air will pass distal to partially obstructing mucus or foreign matter.***
b. Hold breath 2 seconds—***this step permits the patient to prepare for exhalation and allows distribution of the inhaled air to the lung's periphery.***
c. Cough twice—***the first cough will loosen mucus; the second will propel the mucus. Further coughing may use excessive oxygen and energy at a time when the lung volume has already been expelled with the first two coughs, and the effort is thus wasted.***
d. Pause—just long enough to regain control.
e. Inhale by sniffing—sniffing is recommended ***because a deep inhalation through the mouth may drive loose mucus back down into the airways.***
f. Rest.

Huff coughing

Huff coughing is a series of coughs produced with the glottis held open while saying the word "huff." The sharp sound of a cough should not be produced with a huff cough, but the sound should be that of forced exhalation. Huff coughing may be helpful for patients with COPD who have significant airway collapse on forced exhalation, ***because huff coughing is associated with higher flow rates in these patients than in the normal closed-glottis approach to coughing. Furthermore, huff coughing may assist in moving secretions from the smaller airways into the main-stem bronchi or trachea where the controlled cough technique can be used for effective expectoration.***

INEFFECTIVE AIRWAY CLEARANCE RELATED TO EXCESSIVE SECRETIONS OR ABNORMAL VISCOSITY OF MUCUS—cont'd

Quad coughing

Quad coughing is helpful in patients who have flaccid or weakened abdominal musculature. The most obvious example is the patient with paralysis or weakness caused by neuromuscular disorders. Quad coughing calls for the nurse to push upward and inward on the abdomen, toward the diaphragm, while the patient exhales.

a. Position for optimal coughing by placing patient either in high-Fowler's position with knees drawn up and a brace for his or her feet or on side with knees drawn up. ***High-Fowler's position promotes best diaphragmatic descent and maximal inhalation, which allow maximal cough. Drawn-up knees assist in abdominal muscle contraction, resulting in a stronger expulsive force and cough velocity.***
b. Assess sputum for color, consistency, and amount. ***Yellow or green mucus may mean chest infection; an increase in amount may mean a worsening condition.***
c. Assess for clinical manifestations of chest infection, such as fever, tachycardia, yellow or green mucus (culture and sensitivity may be necessary), leukocytosis, increase in pulmonary crackles or wheezes on chest auscultation, and chest radiograph consistent with alveolar infiltrates.
d. If patient is hypoxemic, administer oxygen, observing the following principles:
   - ◆ Without physician's collaboration, liter flow should be no greater than 2 L/min in patients whose pulmonary history is unknown or reveals a pattern of chronic carbon dioxide retention, ***because a high FIo_2 level in these patients may depress ventilatory drive.***
   - ◆ Oxygen should be administered with the goal of achieving a Pao_2 level no greater than 100 mm Hg. ***A higher Pao_2 level is of little value and may necessitate using an FIo_2 higher than 40%, which can precipitate oxygen toxicity.***
   - ◆ With physician's collaboration, consider the application of mechanical ventilation with positive end-expiratory pressure (PEEP) in patients whose hypoxemia is refractory to high concentrations of oxygen through mask or nasal prongs.

6. Reposition frequently (at least q 2 hr) and dynamically ***to mobilize secretions and to match ventilation with perfusion.***

7. With physician's collaboration, teach and supervise bronchial drainage with or without chest physiotherapy ***to assist with the expulsion of retained secretions.***

8. Consider suctioning nasopharyngeal airway or artificial tracheal airway when secretions are audible.

9. Allow rest periods between coughing sessions, chest physiotherapy, or other demanding activities.

10. Consider breathing exercise sessions that incorporate sustained maximal inhalation of at least 10 per hour with or without the use of an incentive spirometer ***to prevent atelectasis.***

INEFFECTIVE AIRWAY CLEARANCE RELATED TO IMPAIRED COUGH SECONDARY TO ARTIFICIAL AIRWAY

DEFINING CHARACTERISTICS

- Ineffective cough resulting from bypass of glottis with artificial airway
- Abnormal breath sounds

OUTCOME CRITERIA

- Cough produces thin mucus.
- Lung auscultation reveals mobilization of secretions with cough.

NURSING INTERVENTIONS AND *RATIONALE*

1. Continue to monitor the assessment parameters listed under "Defining Characteristics."
2. Ensure that the inspired air source (at *any* FIO_2) is humidified, ***because the artificial airway bypasses the body's normal humidification system.***
3. In the absence of cardiac or renal disease, hydrate to 24-hour fluid requirements per BSA ***to thin secretions.***
4. In patients with reduced vital capacity resulting from weak abdominal and/or diaphragmatic musculature, teach and supervise abdominal muscle-tightening exercises and diaphragmatic breathing.
5. Position for optimal coughing by placing patient either in high-Fowler's position with knees drawn up or on side with knees drawn up. ***High-Fowler's position promotes best diaphragmatic descent and maximal inhalation, which allow maximal cough. Drawn-up knees assist in abdominal muscle contraction, resulting in a stronger expulsive force and cough velocity.***
6. Suction artificial airway as necessary per unit standards.
7. Suction oropharyngeally and obtain frequent cuff pressure measurements ***to prevent aspiration of oropharyngeal secretions.***

INEFFECTIVE AIRWAY CLEARANCE RELATED TO ABDOMINAL OR THORACIC PAIN

DEFINING CHARACTERISTICS

- Abnormal breath sounds
- Weak, ineffective cough
- Presence of pain
- Tachypnea

OUTCOME CRITERIA

- Lungs are clear to auscultation.
- Cough produces thin mucus.

NURSING INTERVENTIONS AND *RATIONALE*

1. Continue to monitor the assessment parameters listed under "Defining Characteristics."
2. Treat pain according to its etiology. See "Acute Pain" in Chapter 28.
3. If patient is hypoxemic, administer oxygen, observing the following principles:
   - Without physician's collaboration, liter flow should be no greater than 2 L/min in patients whose pulmonary history is unknown or reveals a pattern of chronic carbon dioxide retention, ***because a high FIO_2 in these patients can depress ventilatory drive.***
   - Oxygen should be administered with the goal of achieving a PaO_2 no greater than 100 mm Hg. ***A higher PaO_2 is of little value and may necessitate using an FIO_2 higher than 40%, which can precipitate oxygen toxicity.***
4. In the absence of cardiac or renal dysfunction, hydrate to 24-hour fluid requirements per BSA ***to thin secretions and improve airway clearance.***
5. Emphasize deep breathing exercises with sustained maximal inhalation. ***They will stimulate an effective cough if, in fact, secretions are present in the airways. In addition, a more effective cough will be achieved because the high volumes of deep breathing will result in an increased velocity of expired air.***
6. Teach and provide incisional splinting, if appropriate, during breathing exercises in anticipation of cough stimulation and during coughing episodes.

INEFFECTIVE AIRWAY CLEARANCE RELATED TO NEUROMUSCULAR DYSFUNCTION AND IMPAIRED COUGH SECONDARY TO QUADRIPLEGIA, PARAPLEGIA, GUILLAIN-BARRÉ SYNDROME, MYASTHENIA GRAVIS, AND OTHERS

DEFINING CHARACTERISTICS

- ◆ Weak, ineffective cough
- ◆ Abnormal breath sounds

OUTCOME CRITERIA

- ◆ Cough is productive.
- ◆ Secretions are thin and clear.

NURSING INTERVENTIONS AND *RATIONALE*

1. Continue to monitor the assessment parameters listed under "Defining Characteristics."
2. If hypoxemic, administer oxygen, observing principles detailed under "Ineffective Airway Clearance related to excessive secretions or abnormal viscosity of mucus."
3. In the absence of cardiac or renal dysfunction, teach and provide hydration to 24-hour fluid requirements per BSA ***to thin secretions and facilitate airway clearance.***
4. Assist with quad coughing, ***since weakened or flaccid abdominal muscles will prevent effective cough.***
5. Position patient for most effective cough.
6. Consider chest physiotherapy (bronchial drainage and chest percussion) three to four times per day ***to assist with the expulsion of retained secretions.***
7. Change position at least q 2 hr ***to prevent stasis of secretions and to match ventilation with perfusion.***

INEFFECTIVE BREATHING PATTERN RELATED TO CHRONIC AIRFLOW LIMITATIONS

DEFINING CHARACTERISTICS

- ◆ Use of accessory muscles
- ◆ Dyspnea
- ◆ Nasal flaring
- ◆ Pursed-lip breathing
- ◆ Shortness of breath
- ◆ Tachypnea
- ◆ Increased AP diameter
- ◆ Assumption of 3-point position
- ◆ Altered inspiratory-to-expiratory ratio

OUTCOME CRITERION

- ◆ Patient demonstrates pursed-lip and diaphragmatic breathing regularly and during episodes of respiratory panic.

NURSING INTERVENTIONS AND *RATIONALE*

1. Continue to monitor the assessment parameters listed under "Defining Characteristics."
2. Teach and supervise pursed-lip breathing. ***Explain that this maneuver keeps airways open longer during exhalation and evacuates trapped air.*** The procedure for pursed-lip breathing should be used along with-diaphragmatic breathing during episodes of shortness of breath.
3. Teach and supervise diaphragmatic breathing. ***Explain that this maneuver saves energy (the diaphragm uses oxygen more efficiently than the accessory muscles) and retrains the diaphragm to assume its normal percentage of the work of breathing.*** Diaphragmatic breathing is useful in terminating episodes of acute shortness of breath but should *also* be incorporated into an hourly routine of muscle retraining.
4. During episodes of acute shortness of breath or dyspnea, it is useful for the nurse to actually *breathe with* the patient, using pursed-lip and diaphragmatic breathing techniques. It is *not* useful during such an episode to instruct or encourage the use of these techniques. Statements such as, "Now slow down your breathing" or "Take nice big breaths for me," ***do little to assist the patient in regaining control of his breathing pattern. In addition, concentration on techniques of breathing may serve the beneficial function of distracting the patient from fear and panic.***

INEFFECTIVE BREATHING PATTERN RELATED TO DECREASED LUNG EXPANSION SECONDARY TO PNEUMOTHORAX OR PLEURAL EFFUSION

DEFINING CHARACTERISTICS

- Tachypnea
- Abnormal breath sounds
- Unequal chest movement

OUTCOME CRITERIA

- Respiratory rate at rest is <20.
- Crackles are minimal or absent.
- Breath sounds are full and equal bilaterally.
- Chest expands symmetrically.

NURSING INTERVENTIONS AND *RATIONALE*

1. Continue to monitor the assessment parameters listed under "Defining Characteristics." In addition, check serial chest radiographs ***to monitor resolution of underlying disorder.***
2. Treat pain, if present, according to cause. See "Acute Pain" in Chapter 28.
3. If patient is hypoxemic, administer oxygen, observing the principles detailed under "Ineffective Breathing Pattern related to abdominal or thoracic pain."
4. Teach and supervise deep breathing with sustained maximal inspiration. ***In the patient with a pneumothorax and a chest tube, this maneuver reexpands the lung and evacuates air (and fluid) from the pleural space into the chest drainage system. In the patient with a pleural effusion, this maneuver may reexpand atelectatic portions of the lung overlying the pleural effusion.***
5. Reposition the patient q 2 hr, observing the "good lung down" principle ***to limit pain, as well as to better match ventilation with perfusion.*** Favor a head-of-bed up position ***to facilitate diaphragmatic descent.***
6. Avoid coughing exercises unless secretions are audible in the airways. ***Coughing is painful and, if performed unnecessarily (as in the absence of secretions), may promote airway collapse or atelectasis.***
7. For assessment and maintenance of chest tubes and closed chest drainage systems, see Chapter 21.

INABILITY TO SUSTAIN SPONTANEOUS VENTILATION RELATED TO RESPIRATORY MUSCLE FATIGUE SECONDARY TO MECHANICAL VENTILATION

DEFINING CHARACTERISTICS

- Dyspnea
- Increased restlessness
- Increased use of accessory muscles
- Decreased tidal volume during spontaneous breaths
- Increased P_{CO_2}

OUTCOME CRITERIA

- Tidal volume is greater than or equal to predicted.
- Breath sounds are clear from apices to bases.
- Normocapnia is present.

NURSING INTERVENTIONS AND *RATIONALE*

Continue to monitor the assessment parameters listed under "Defining Characteristics."

For mechanically ventilated patients

1. Assist the patient to distinguish spontaneous breaths from mechanically delivered breaths by helping him or her to identify the sensation of breathing ***(this is lost when air bypasses the nasooropharynx)*** through simple kinesthetic feedback: "The machine is giving you six breaths per minute; you are breathing on your own in between the machine breaths. Feel the difference between the machine's breaths and your own. You are working to make your own breaths as deep and full as the machine's."
2. Carefully snip excess length from the proximal end of the endotracheal tube ***to decrease dead space and thereby decrease the work of breathing. In similar fashion, ensure that ventilator circuit tubings impose no excess dead space.***
3. Collaborate with physician about the application of pressure support to the mechanical ventilator or about the use of a ventilator that will not increase the work of breathing during the IMV or SIMV breaths. ***There should be no excessive work of breathing on the part of the patient because of ventilator circuitry. Pressure support may decrease the work of breathing.***
4. Position patient in semi-Fowler's position ***for best use of ventilatory muscles and to facilitate diaphragmatic descent.***

INABILITY TO SUSTAIN SPONTANEOUS VENTILATION RELATED TO RESPIRATORY MUSCLE FATIGUE SECONDARY TO MECHANICAL VENTILATION—cont'd

5. Confront patient's fear and support his or her confidence; provide progress reports frequently: "The volume of your breaths is steadily increasing and this has made your lungs clearer. Your hard work is paying off."
6. Avoid pharmacologic sedation if possible. Consult with physician in selecting a sedative drug with minimal muscle relaxant effects.
7. With physician's collaboration, ensure that at least 50% of the diet's nonprotein caloric source is in the form of lipid (fat) versus carbohydrates ***to prevent excess carbon dioxide accumulation. Carbon dioxide is an end product of carbohydrate metabolism, and its excess accumulation in the blood stream falsely suggests a reduction in the patient's alveolar ventilation. In addition, excess carbon dioxide increases the patient's ventilatory workload.***

INEFFECTIVE BREATHING PATTERN RELATED TO ABDOMINAL OR THORACIC PAIN

DEFINING CHARACTERISTICS

- ◆ Abnormal breath sounds
- ◆ Abnormal blood gas values
- ◆ Unequal chest movement caused by splinting
- ◆ Tachypnea
- ◆ Presence of pain

OUTCOME CRITERIA

- ◆ Breath sounds are clear and equal bilaterally.
- ◆ Chest expands symmetrically.
- ◆ $Paco_2$ is 35 to 45 mm Hg.

NURSING INTERVENTIONS AND *RATIONALE*

1. Continue to monitor the assessment parameters listed under "Defining Characteristics."
2. Treat pain according to its cause. See "Acute Pain" in Chapter 28.
3. If patient is hypoxemic, administer oxygen, observing the following principles:
   - ◆ Without physician's collaboration, liter flow should be no greater than 2 L/min in patients whose pulmonary history is unknown or reveals a pattern of chronic carbon dioxide retention ***because a high FIo_2 in these patients may depress ventilatory drive.***
   - ◆ Oxygen should be administered with the goal of achieving a Pao_2 no greater than 95 mm Hg.
   - ◆ Observe caution when administering oxygen at FIo_2 greater than 40% ***in view of the higher risk for oxygen toxicity.*** With physician's collaboration, consider the application of mechanical ventilation with PEEP in patients whose hypoxemia is refractory to high concentrations of oxygen.

For thoracic pain

1. Carefully distinguish between chest wall pain and the pain of myocardial ischemia. For example, ask the patient if this pain is his "usual" chest wall or incisional pain, palpate the chest wall to elicit the pain, and have the patient take a deep breath to elicit the pain. ***These maneuvers will reasonably confirm the existence of chest wall or incisional pain versus the pain of myocardial ischemia. If any doubt exists, a 12-lead electrocardiogram (ECG) should be obtained.***
2. Teach and supervise deep breathing or incentive spirometry with sustained maximal inhalation. The emphasis with these modalities should be on the diaphragmatic breathing technique ***to increase abdominal expansion and decrease chest wall expansion, thereby decreasing pain.***
3. Reposition patient at least q 2 hr, observing the "good lung down" principle. ***This will result in decreased incidence of pain and better matching of ventilation with perfusion.***
4. Treat impaired coughing. See "Ineffective Airway Clearance related to abdominal or thoracic pain."

For abdominal pain

1. Teach and supervise deep breathing or incentive spirometry with sustained maximal inspiration. ***The emphasis for these maneuvers should not be diaphragmatic breathing but chest breathing to decrease the incidence of abdominal pain.***
2. Reposition patient frequently and dynamically. Favor semi-Fowler's to high-Fowler's position ***to maximize chest expansion.***

INEFFECTIVE BREATHING PATTERN RELATED TO MUSCULOSKELETAL IMPAIRMENT

DEFINING CHARACTERISTICS

- Unequal chest movement
- Decreased tidal volume
- Shortness of breath
- Dyspnea
- Use of accessory muscles
- Tachypnea
- Thoracoabdominal asynchrony

OUTCOME CRITERION

- Respiratory rate, depth, and timing are within patient's baseline.
- Use of accessory muscles is minimal or absent.

NURSING INTERVENTIONS AND *RATIONALE*

1. Continue to monitor the assessment parameters listed under "Defining Characteristics."
2. Prevent unnecessary exertion ***because the patient's ventilatory reserve is limited.*** Grade all activity to within the patient's tolerance as measured by heart rate elevations less than 30 beats above baseline with activity. Heart rate elevations less than 15 beats above baseline with activity indicates activity tolerance in patients receiving beta or calcium channel blockers.
3. If patient is hypoxemic, administer oxygen, observing the principles detailed under "Ineffective Breathing Pattern related to abdominal or thoracic pain." Ensure that oxygen is administered, especially during activity.
4. Teach and supervise energy-saving techniques.
5. Teach and supervise diaphragmatic breathing. ***Diaphragmatic breathing is especially effective in patients with unmodifiable chest wall restrictions because it allows an increase in the tidal volume through diaphragmatic descent, which is otherwise impossible through chest wall expansion.*** Incorporate the sustained maximal inspiration maneuver when possible.
6. Reposition patient dynamically q 2 hr, favoring semi-Fowler's to high-Fowler's position ***to facilitate diaphragmatic descent.***
7. Ideally, position the patient sitting at the bedside with arms resting on a pillow on the overbed table. ***This position eliminates splinting of the chest wall against any surface and thereby decreases chest wall restriction and work of breathing.***

IMPAIRED GAS EXCHANGE RELATED TO VENTILATION/PERFUSION MISMATCH SECONDARY TO (SPECIFY)

DEFINING CHARACTERISTICS

- Pao_2 <predicted for age
- $Paco_2$ >45 mm Hg
- SaO_2 < 90%
- Confusion
- Somnolence
- Restlessness
- Irritability
- Headache

OUTCOME CRITERIA

- Pao_2 is equal to predicted for age.
- $Paco_2$ is 35 to 45 mm Hg or back to baseline for patient.

NURSING INTERVENTIONS AND *RATIONALE*

1. Continue to monitor the assessment parameters listed under "Defining Characteristics." In addition, observe for physical clinical manifestations of tissue hypoxia (increased respiratory rate, visual disturbances, impairment of intellectual function, headache, lethargy, tachycardia, dysrhythmias).
2. Administer oxygen, observing the following principles:
   - Without physician's collaboration, liter flow should be no greater than 2 L/min in patients whose pulmonary history is unknown or reveals a pattern of chronic carbon dioxide retention, ***because a high FIo_2 in these patients may depress ventilatory drive.***
   - Oxygen should be administered with the goal of achieving a Pao_2 no greater than 100 mm Hg. ***A higher Pao_2 is of little value and may necessitate an FIo_2 higher than 40%, which can precipitate oxygen toxicity*** (see "Oxygen Toxicity" in Chapter 23).
   - With physician's collaboration, consider the application of CPAP or mechanical ventilation with PEEP in patients whose hypoxemia is refractory to high concentrations of oxygen. ***CPAP and PEEP accomplish alveolar hyperinflation, thereby increasing the surface area for gas exchange.***

IMPAIRED GAS EXCHANGE RELATED TO VENTILATION/PERFUSION MISMATCH SECONDARY TO (SPECIFY)—cont'd

3. In the absence of cardiac or renal dysfunction, hydrate to 24-hour fluid requirements per body surface area (BSA) ***to thin secretions. Adequate hydration is the most effective mucolytic. Avoid caffeinated beverages because caffeine is a mild diuretic and can contribute to fluid loss.***
4. Monitor serum osmolality, ***considering that an elevation may indicate need for further hydration.***
5. Provide humidification to airways through mask, room vaporizor, or other means ***to assist in thinning secretions.*** When artificial airway is present, ensure that humidification of airway is available and functioning properly. ***Thick, tenacious secretions may indicate insufficient fluid intake and/or a need for external humidification.***
6. Consider suctioning if mucus is suspected within the trachea. If mucus is suspected within the main-stem or segmental bronchi, assist in its passage into the trachea through cough or chest physiotherapy. ***Most studies show suctioning is effective only in evacuating mucus from the tracheal level; therefore every effort should be made to move mucus into the trachea before suctioning is attempted.*** Always preoxygenate and postoxygenate the patient's airways as part of the suctioning technique ***to prevent further decrease of the Pao_2 as a result of suctioning.***
7. For a patient with unilateral lung disease, position him or her with the good lung down because ***this will best match ventilation with perfusion and result in improved Pao_2.*** (Exception: place sick lung down in cases of lung abcess or unilateral interstitial pulmonary emphysema.)
8. For patient with bilateral lung disease, position with right lung down ***because this lung is larger than the left lung and affords a greater area for ventilation and perfusion. Further, the cardiac output may be enhanced in the right lateral position.***
9. Evaluate arterial blood gas values obtained with the patient in various positions so that the position that results in the best oxygenation may be revealed.
10. Change the patient's position at least q 2 hr, favoring those positions that allow the best oxygenation. Limit the time the patient spends in a position that compromises oxygenation. Avoid any position that seriously decreases the Pao_2.
11. When appropriate, instruct patient in controlled-cough technique or huff or quad cough techniques, depending on the patient's cough ability.
12. Instruct in the proper use of incentive spirometer ***as a means to prevent atelectasis, which can further complicate or worsen impaired gas exchange.***
13. Evaluate need for chest physiotherapy.

IMPAIRED GAS EXCHANGE RELATED TO ALVEOLAR HYPOVENTILATION SECONDARY TO (SPECIFY)

DEFINING CHARACTERISTICS

- $Paco_2$ > 45mm Hg
- Pao_2 < predicted for age
- Sao_2 < 90%

OUTCOME CRITERIA

- $Paco_2$ is 35 to 45 mm Hg.
- Pao_2 is within limits of norm for age.
- Sao_2 is greater than 90%.

NURSING INTERVENTIONS AND *RATIONALE*

1. Continue to monitor the assessment parameters listed under "Defining Characteristics." In addition, observe for physical clinical manifestations of tissue hypoxia (increased respiratory rate, visual disturbances, impairment of intellectual function, headache, lethargy, tachycardia, dysrhythmias).
2. Administer oxygen, observing the following principles:
   - Without physician's collaboration, liter flow should be no greater than 2 L/min in patients whose pulmonary history is unknown or reveals a pattern of chronic carbon dioxide retention ***because a high FIo_2 in these patients may depress ventilatory drive.***
   - Oxygen should be administered with the goal of achieving a Pao_2 no greater than 100 mm Hg. ***A higher Pao_2 is of little value and may necessitate an FIo_2 higher than 40%, which can precipitate oxygen toxicity (see "Oxygen Toxicity" in Chapter 21).***
   - With physician's collaboration, consider the application of continuous positive airway pressure (CPAP) or mechanical ventilation with positive end-expiratory pressure (PEEP) in patients whose hypoxemia is refractory to high concentrations of oxygen. ***CPAP and PEEP accomplish alveolar hyperinflation, thereby increasing the surface area for gas exchange.***
3. Intervene deliberately to resolve the specific cause of the alveolar hypoventilation.

HIGH RISK FOR ASPIRATION

RISK FACTORS

- ◆ Impaired laryngeal sensation or reflex
  - Reduced level of consciousness
  - Immediately postextubation
- ◆ Impaired pharyngeal peristalsis or tongue function
  - Neuromuscular dysfunction
  - Central nervous system dysfunction
  - Head or neck surgery
- ◆ Impaired laryngeal closure or elevation
  - Laryngeal nerve dysfunction
  - Artificial airways
  - Gastrointestinal tubes
- ◆ Increased gastric volume
  - Delayed gastric emptying
  - Tube feedings
  - Medication administration
- ◆ Increased intragastric pressure
  - Upper abdominal surgery
  - Obesity
  - Pregnancy
  - Ascites
- ◆ Decreased lower esophageal sphincter pressure
  - Increased gastric acidity
  - Gastrointestinal tubes
- ◆ Decreased antegrade esophageal propulsion
  - Position—trendelenburg, supine
  - Esophageal dysmotility
  - Esophageal structural defects or lesions

DEFINING CHARACTERISTICS OF AN ACTUAL PROBLEM

Early

- ◆ Hypoxemia

Later (6 hours after aspiration)

- ◆ Dyspnea
- ◆ Wheezing, crackles
- ◆ Cough with pink, frothy exudate, resembling cardiogenic pulmonary edema
- ◆ Fever
- ◆ Tachycardia
- ◆ Hypotension
- ◆ Radiologic: patchy alveolar infiltrates in portions of lung dependent at time of aspiration
- ◆ Evidence of gastric contents in lung secretions

OUTCOME CRITERIA

- ◆ Lungs are clear to auscultation.
- ◆ Pao_2 is proportional to that predicted for age and FIo_2.
- ◆ Lung secretions show no evidence of gastric contents.
- ◆ Patient is afebrile.

NURSING INTERVENTIONS AND *RATIONALE*

1. Continue to monitor the assessment parameters listed under "Defining Characteristics."
2. Auscultate bowel sounds and assess abdominal contour and girth. ***Rule out hypoactive peristalsis and abdominal distention with gastric contents, thereby avoiding the heightened risk of esophageal reflux.***
3. Position patient with 30-degree elevation of head of bed (lying on side ideally) ***to prevent gastric reflux through gravity.*** Whenever head elevation is contraindicated, a right lateral decubitus position is recommended ***because it facilitates passage of gastric contents across the pylorus.***
4. Suction and clear oropharyngeal secretions. For patients with cuffed tracheostomy or endotracheal tubes, suction oropharyngeally and obtain cuff pressure measurements ***to limit aspiration of oropharyngeal secretions.***
5. Maintain patency and functioning of nasogastric suction apparatus.
6. Treat nausea promptly; consider obtaining physician's order for antiemetic ***to prevent vomiting and resultant aspiration.***
7. With physician's collaboration, consider administration of oral antacids and H_2 receptor antagonists ***to increase gastric pH and thereby limit chemical burn to lung tissue should aspiration occur.***

HIGH RISK FOR ASPIRATION—cont'd

Additional interventions for patients receiving continuous or intermittent enteral tube feedings

1. Position patient with 45-degree head elevation at all times ***to prevent gastric reflux across an epiglottis held open by the gastric tube.*** If a head-down position becomes necessary at any time, interrupt the feeding 30 minutes to 1 hour before position change.
2. Check placement of feeding tube either by auscultation or radiographically at regular intervals (e.g., before administering intemittent feedings, after position changes, and after suctioning, coughing episodes, or vomiting). ***The feeding tube can migrate without demonstrating a change in its external position.***
3. Instill blue food coloring to feeding solutions ***to assist identification of gastric contents in pulmonary secretions. Green, red, or yellow food dye is unacceptable because each resembles other body substances.***
4. If possible, aspirate enteral contents through feeding tube and measure residual amounts before intermittent feedings and at regular during continuous feedings. Consider withholding intermittent feedings for residuals greater than 100 to 150 ml and interrupting continuous feedings for residuals greater than 20% of the hourly rate.
5. With physician's collaboration, consider administering metoclopramide (Reglan) ***to increase upper gastrointestinal motility and gastric sphincter tone and to decrease gastric volume.***

Additional interventions for patients with impaired swallowing

1. Assess for classic indicators of impaired swallowing—drooling (especially persistence of drooling with head reclined), food retained in mouth, poor head and neck control, tongue pumping or excess mouth movement before swallowing, coughing during or after eating, breathy or "gurgly" voice, and slurred speech.
2. Initiate consult with in-house "swallowing team." This team may consist of a speech pathologist, occupational therapist, physical therapist, dietitian, and/or physical rehabilitation nursing and medical staff members. ***Swallowing is not a reflex but a patterned response involving both voluntary and nonvolitional components. It may, in some instances be retrained after injury.***
3. Predict the patient's swallowing competence by assessing the symmetry and dynamics of tongue mobility. ***The swallowing response consists of coordinated movements of the tongue, palate, pharynx, larynx, and esophagus. This response is initiated by the tongue; therefore competence in initiating the swallow may be partially predicated.***
4. Predict airway protection by asking the patient to cough and clear the throat. ***A cough that is weak, "gurgly," or unobtainable indicates reduced airway closure, which is the reason for aspiration during the swallow.***
5. For the patient who is either being evaluated for swallowing difficulty or in whom swallowing is being reinitiated (e.g., after tracheal extubation or prolonged nothing-by-mouth status), observe swallowing competence by placing 3 ml of water on the patient's tongue. The swallow should be initiated within 1 second of introducing water to the oral cavity. If response is delayed or no response occurs after three attempts, consider formal evaluation by "swallowing team" and initiate NPO status. ***Water is hardest to swallow and easiest to aspirate; if swallowing is impaired sufficiently to result in pulmonary aspiration, the 3 ml of water is a safe medium with which to demonstrate this impairment.***
6. When reasonable swallowing competence has been established, provide foods with the consistency of yogurt, ice cream, pudding, or custard. ***Semisolids are more easily swallowed than either liquids or solids.***
7. Avoid introducing fluids into the patients's mouth with the use of a syringe. ***This maneuver partially bypasses the tongue, interfering with the swallowing response and therefore increasing the risk of aspiration.***

DYSFUNCTIONAL VENTILATORY WEANING RESPONSE (DVWR)

DEFINING CHARACTERISTICS

Mild DVWR

Responds to lowered levels of mechanical ventilator support with:

- ◆ Restlessness
- ◆ Slight increased respiratory rate from baseline
- ◆ Expressed feelings of: breathing discomfort; fatigue; warmth; increased need for oxygen
- ◆ Queries about possible machine malfunction
- ◆ Increased concentration on breathing

Moderate DVWR

Responds to lowered levels of mechanical ventilator support with:

- ◆ Slight increase from baseline blood pressure <20 mm Hg
- ◆ Slight increase from baseline heart rate <20 beats per minute
- ◆ Baseline increase in respiratory rate <5 breaths per minute
- ◆ Hypervigilence to activities
- ◆ Inability to respond to coaching
- ◆ Inability to cooperate
- ◆ Apprehension
- ◆ Diaphoresis
- ◆ Eye widening: "wide-eyed" look
- ◆ Decreased air entry on auscultation
- ◆ Slight respiratory accessory muscle use
- ◆ Color changes: pale, slight cyanosis

Severe DVWR

Responds to lowered levels of mechanical ventilator support with:

- ◆ Agitation
- ◆ Deterioration in arterial blood gases from current baseline
- ◆ Increase from baseline blood pressure >20 mm Hg
- ◆ Increase from baseline heart rate >20 beats per minute
- ◆ Respiratory rate increases significantly from baseline
- ◆ Profuse sweating
- ◆ Full respiratory accessory muscle use
- ◆ Shallow, gasping breaths
- ◆ Paradoxical abdominal breathing
- ◆ Uncoordinated breathing with the ventilator
- ◆ Decreased level of consciousness
- ◆ Adventitious breath sounds; audible airway secretions
- ◆ Cyanosis

RELATED FACTORS

- ◆ Ineffective airway clearance
- ◆ Sleep pattern disturbance
- ◆ Inadequate nutrition
- ◆ Uncontrolled pain or discomfort
- ◆ Knowledge deficit of the weaning process, patient role
- ◆ Patient perceived inefficacy about the ability to wean
- ◆ Decreased motivation
- ◆ Decreased self-esteem
- ◆ Anxiety: moderate; severe
- ◆ Fear
- ◆ Hopelessness
- ◆ Powerlessness
- ◆ Insufficient trust in the nurse
- ◆ Uncontrolled episodic energy demands or problems
- ◆ Inappropriate pacing of diminished ventilator support
- ◆ Inadequate social support
- ◆ Adverse environment (noisy, active environment; negative events in the room; low nurse-patient ratio; extended nurse absence from the bedside; unfamiliar nursing staff)
- ◆ History of ventilator dependence >1 week
- ◆ History of multiple unsuccessful weaning attempts

NURSING INTERVENTIONS AND *RATIONALE*

1. Ensure adequate oxygen supply and nutritional support.
2. Provide adequate rest periods.
3. Establish weaning plan with patient and other health care team members.
4. Set achievable goals for weaning; minimize setbacks.
5. Normalize surrounding environment by improving patient's appearance, assisting patient out of bed, and providing predictability to the patient's day.
6. Provide mastery experiences (slowing the pace of weaning and increasing chances of success).
7. Convey confidence regarding patient's ability to achieve the weaning goals.
8. Encourage feedback from the patient regarding state of comfort ***to teach awareness of the early onset of fatigue.***
9. Provide patient with feedback regarding the progress of the weaning goals; supply positive reinforcement and reassurance.
10. Stay with the patient; touch and hold hand.
11. Establish patient trust by maintaining calm approach, demonstrating confidence in patient's abilities, sharing information about oneself, and demonstrating nursing competence by explaining and acting with self-assurance.
12. Engage patient in collaborative activities (care planning).
13. Limit or expand family visiting as patient tolerates or desires.
14. Modify the environment by providing patient with personalized space and maintaining a quiet room.
15. Ensure that staff and others respond appropriately to the patient's needs or wishes.
16. Ensure consistency in nursing care givers during the weaning process.

VI

NEUROLOGIC ALTERATIONS

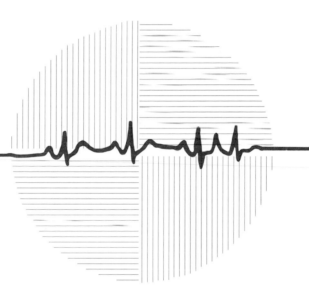

25

Neurologic Anatomy and Physiology

CHAPTER OBJECTIVES

- List the four protective mechanisms of the central nervous system.
- Describe the functions of the three portions of the brainstem.
- State two major functions of each of the four lobes of the cerebrum.
- Trace anterior and posterior cerebral circulation.
- Identify the major motor and sensory tracts of the spinal cord.
- Discuss the vascular supply to the spinal cord.

The nervous system is a unique, complex, and still somewhat mysterious network of fibers running throughout the body. It has the task of directing body systems and functions. Receiving thousands of bits of information each second from different sensory organs, this system transmits, analyzes, interprets, and integrates responses throughout the billions of nervous system cells. A basic understanding of the anatomy and physiology of the nervous system is essential to the delivery of quality critical care nursing. Although the roles and functions of the nervous system are diverse, a few principles and concepts apply to all. This chapter reviews the divisions of the nervous system and its microstructure or cellular level and functions. Mechanisms devised to provide protection to the nervous system also are presented. Finally, the anatomy and physiology of all components of the central nervous system are outlined.

DIVISIONS OF THE NERVOUS SYSTEM

The nervous system is the most highly organized system of the body, with all of its parts functioning as an inseparable unit. For review, this system may be classified in terms of location or according to function.

Anatomical Divisions

1. The central nervous system (CNS) comprises all the portions of the brain and spinal cord.
2. The peripheral nervous system (PNS) comprises the 12 pairs of cranial nerves plus the 32 pairs of spinal nerves and the peripheral nerves that connect the CNS with the body wall and the viscera.

Physiologic Divisions

1. The *somatic,* or *voluntary, nervous system* is composed of fibers that connect the CNS with structures of the skeletal muscles and the skin.
2. The *autonomic,* or *involuntary, nervous system* is composed of fibers that connect the CNS with smooth muscle, cardiac muscle, internal organs, and glands. It includes its sympathetic and parasympathetic branches.

Most activities of the nervous system originate from sensory receptors, such as visual, auditory, or tactile receptors. This sensory information is transmitted to the CNS by *afferent fibers* (sensory fibers). *Efferent fibers* (motor fibers) transmit the CNS response to the periphery to produce a motor response, such as contraction of skeletal muscles, contraction of the smooth muscles of organs, or secretion by endocrine glands. Transmission of both afferent (sensory) and efferent (motor) information in the CNS is performed by *internuncial fibers.* To better understand the macrostructure and functions of the nervous system it is essential to look first at the microstructure, or cellular level.[1]

MICROSTRUCTURE OF THE NERVOUS SYSTEM

The cellular units of the nervous system are the neurons and the neuroglia.[2,3] The neurons are the functional units of the nervous system and are responsible for conduction of nerve impulses, and the neuroglial cells provide support, repair, and protection for the delicate neurons.

◆ **Neurons.** More than 10 billion neurons are in the CNS alone. The cellular appearance of a neuron varies, depending on its specific function, but each cell contains three basic components (Fig. 25-1). The first component is the *cell body* (soma), which controls the metabolic activity of the cell. Inside the cell body is the nucleus, which stores ribonucleic acid (RNA) and deoxyribonucleic acid (DNA) and also contains the nucleolus for synthesis of RNA. Nissl bodies for storage of RNA and synthesis of protein, Golgi apparati for storage of protein and synthesis of cell membranes, neurofibrils for support, and lysosomes, which function as intracellular scavengers, are also contained in the cell body. An intact, well-nourished cell body is essential to the life of the neuron as a whole. If the cell body dies, the rest of the neuron also dies and cannot be replaced. These specialized cells cannot reproduce themselves; therefore cell bodies are grouped together in relatively protected areas. Cell bodies form the gray matter in the brain, the

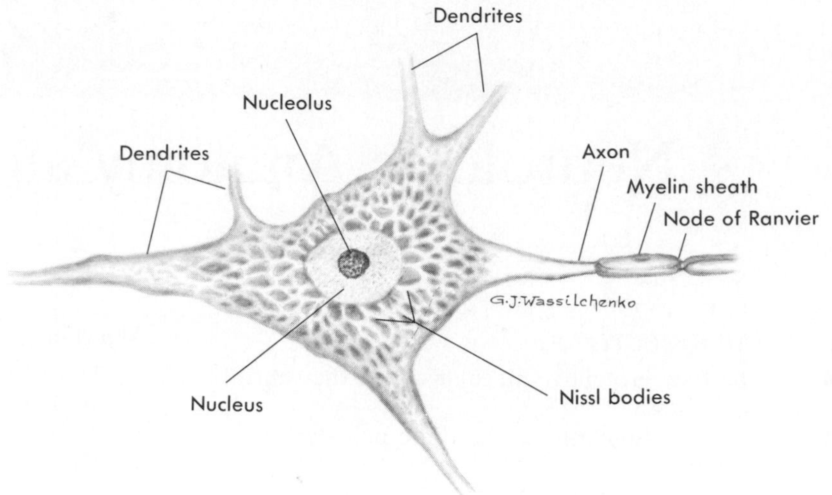

Fig. 25-1 Diagram of the neuron with composite parts.

brainstem, and the spinal cord. Ganglia, small nodules of nervous tissue lying close to the CNS, are cell bodies in the peripheral nervous system. The structural classification of neurons is as follows:

1. Unipolar: cell body with one process, which divides into a central branch—the axon—and a peripheral branch—the dendrite
2. Bipolar: cell body with two processes—one axon and one dendrite
3. Multipolar: cell body with one axon and several dendrites

Dendrites, the second component of a neuron, are branched fibers extending only a short distance from the cell body. Each neuron may have several dendrites, which carry impulses to the cell body. The third component of a neuron is the *axon.* Each neuron contains only one axon, which carries information away from the cell. Axons can be microscopic in length or extend up to 4 feet. Many axons are protected by a *myelin sheath,* which is a white protein-lipid complex laid down by Schwann cells in the PNS and by oligodendrocytes in the CNS. Myelin sheath acts as insulation for the conduction of nerve impulses. Fibers enclosed in the sheath are called *myelinated fibers;* those not enclosed are called *unmyelinated fibers.* The white matter of the CNS is composed of myelinated fiber tracts.

Myelin is not a continuous layer but has gaps called *nodes of Ranvier.* Nerve impulses are conducted from node to node; therefore conduction is more rapid. Loss of myelin sheath integrity disrupts nerve impulse transmission. Multiple sclerosis, for example, is a disease that causes degeneration of myelin.

◆ **Neuroglia.** Neuroglial cells are the support cells to the neuron. There are four types of neuroglial cells: astroglia, oligodendroglia, ependyma, and microglia (Fig. 25-2). These cells provide structural support, nourishment, and protection for the neurons (Table 25-1). In the nervous system there are 6 to 10 times more neuroglial cells than neurons. The clinical significance of neuroglia is its ability to retain mitotic abilities, as compared with neurons, which do not retain them. Therefore neuroglia can become the source of nonmetabolic CNS primary neoplasms.

Table 25-1 Types of neuroglial cells

Cell type	Function
Astroglia (astrocyte)	Supplies nutrients to neuron structure and to support framework for neurons and capillaries; forms part of the blood-brain barrier
Oligodendroglia	Forms the myelin sheath in the CNS
Ependyma	Lines the ventricular system; forms the choroid plexus, which produces CSF
Microglia	Occurs mainly in the white matter; phagocytizes waste products from injured neurons

Physiology of Nervous Tissue

The nervous system consists of chains of neurons with no actual anatomical continuity. Each neuron is a separate unit in contact with another neuron or target cell through *synapses* (Fig. 25-3).

The generation of a nerve impulse, as with other cells of the body, begins with the depolarization of the cell membrane. The speed of the impulse conduction depends on whether the nerve is myelinated or unmyelinated. In an unmyelinated nerve, depolarization must travel the entire length of the fiber. In myelinated nerves, impulses "jump" from one node of Ranvier to another. This node-to-node conduction, called *saltatory transmission,* increases the velocity of impulse transmission and decreases energy demands. Impulses are transmitted away from cell bodies by axons and pass from the axon of one cell body to the dendrite or cell body of another neuron through the synapse.

Actual synaptic transmission is a chemical process involving the release of neurotransmitters. Anatomically, a synapse travels from the *presynaptic terminal* or *knob* at the end of an axon, across the *synaptic cleft,* and to the *postsynaptic membrane.*

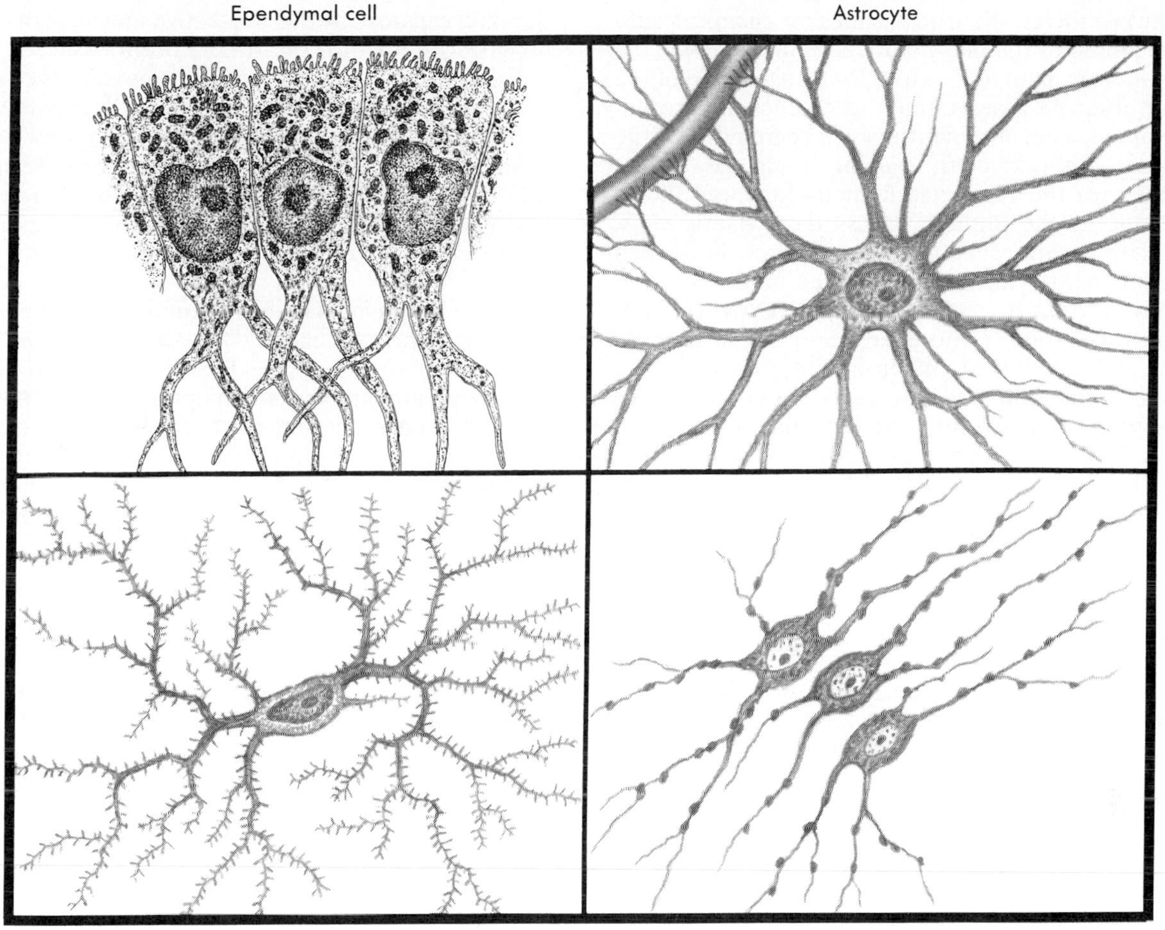

Fig. 25-2 Types of neuroglial cells. (From Thompson JM and others: *Mosby's clinical nursing,* ed 3, St Louis, 1993, Mosby–Year Book.)

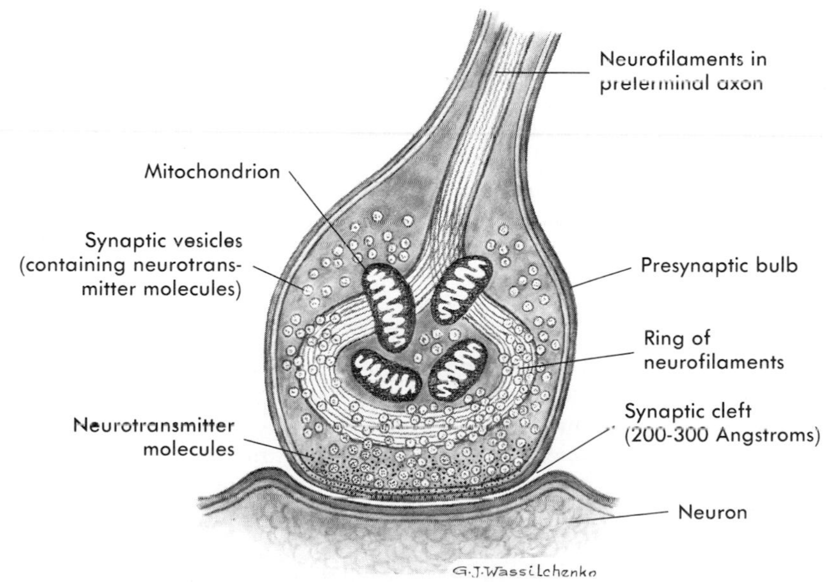

Fig. 25-3 Schematic diagram of a synapse.

◆ **Neurotransmitters.** Neurotransmitters, chemical substances secreted by the presynaptic terminal, provide the connection from axon to dendrite for transmission of the nerve impulse.[4] As a nerve impulse reaches the presynaptic terminal, neurotransmitters are secreted into the microscopic synaptic cleft, causing a change in the permeability of the postsynaptic membrane and therefore passage of the impulse across the synaptic cleft.

More than 30 different chemical substances have been identified as neurotransmitters and can be divided into two types—*excitatory* and *inhibitory.* Excitatory neurotransmitters promote the conduction of the impulse from one cell to the next. When inhibitory neurotransmitters are released, the neuron's internal charge becomes more negative and the resistance to depolarization is increased. The most common known neurotransmitters are acetylcholine, dopamine, norepinephrine, serotonin, γ-aminobutyric acid, glycine, and glutamic acid.

After synaptic transmission, binding of the neurotransmitters to the postsynaptic membrane continues until the neurotransmitter is inactivated by an enzyme (acetylcholine is inactivated by acetylcholinesterase), reabsorbed by the presynaptic terminal, or diffused away from the postsynaptic membrane.

Dysfunction of synaptic pathways results in poor or absent transmission of the nerve impulse. Parkinson's disease, resulting from the lack of dopamine in the basal ganglia, allows excitatory neurotransmitters to go unchecked. Symptoms of Parkinson's disease include tremors, rigidity of limbs, and difficulty initiating movement. Myasthenia gravis, a disease characterized by generalized weakness and fatigability of voluntary muscles, is caused by a reduction of acetylcholine receptors on the postsynaptic membrane.

CENTRAL NERVOUS SYSTEM

The CNS, composed of the spinal cord, brainstem, and brain, is the control unit for all physiologic functions. Review of the anatomy and physiology of the CNS begins with the most basic functions of the brainstem and progresses through the diencephalon to the highly developed cerebrum. The spinal cord is reviewed at the end of this section. Maintaining a healthy CNS is challenged by the delicateness of the nerves and tissues involved. Therefore several mechanisms are in place to provide protection and support to these fragile structures.

Protective Mechanisms

The brain and spinal cord have similar protective mechanisms,[5,6,7] but because of the distinct anatomic differences of these two portions of the CNS, each is discussed separately (see Spinal Cord section).

◆ **Bony structures.** The outermost protective measures underneath the integument are the bony structures that encase the CNS. The skull, or cranium, forms the bony container that surrounds the brain. Composed of eight flat, irregular bones fused through suture lines, the skull provides the brain protection from direct force or superficial trauma. Excessive force causing fracture of the skull can destroy this protective mechanism and push bony fragments into the fragile brain tissue.

Viewing the skull from the inside, the superior surfaces form a smooth inner wall, whereas the base of the skull, or basilar skull, contains ridges and folds with sharp edges, which provide structure for the support of different portions of the brain. Sharp blows to the head that cause shifting of intracranial contents can lead to brain tissue laceration and contusion across these sharp edges.

The cranium is an enclosed vault except for one large opening at the base called the *foramen magnum,* through which the brainstem projects and connects to the spinal cord. Several other very small openings in the base of the skull allow entrance and exit of blood vessels and cranial nerves.

◆ **Meninges.** Beneath the skull lies the second layer of intracranial protection, the meninges. The three layers of meninges are the dura mater, the arachnoid, and the pia mater (Fig. 25-4).

Dura mater. The first of the meninges beneath the skull is the dura mater. Consisting of two layers, this tough, fibrous membrane provides several functions. The outermost layer comprises the periosteum for the cranial bones and therefore adheres to the skull. The inner, meningeal layer of the dura extends into the cranial space. The four extensions of the dural layer are the falx cerebri, tentorium cerebelli, falx cerebelli, and diaphragma sellae.

The *falx cerebri* divides the right and left hemispheres of the brain vertically through the longitudinal fissures extending from the frontal lobe to the occipital lobe. The *tentorium cerebelli* forms a tent between the occipital lobes and the cerebellum and separates the cerebral hemispheres from the brainstem and cerebellum. Intracranial terminology labels all structures above the tentorium as supratentorial and all structures below as infratentorial. Structures below the tentorium are also located in the area referred to as the *posterior fossa.*

The *falx cerebelli* forms the division between the two lateral lobes of the cerebellum. The final compartment of the dura mater is the *diaphragm sellae,* which forms a roof over the sella turcica. Inside the sella turcica is the pituitary gland.

Further dural separations form the venous sinuses located throughout the intracranial space. These venous sinuses, which collect blood from intracerebral and meningeal veins, drain into the internal jugular vein to return venous blood to the heart.

Between the dura mater and the next meninges, the arachnoid, lies the subdural space. This narrow space has a large number of unsupported small veins connecting the arachnoid and dura, so this area is highly susceptible to injury. When the small vessels are stretched and torn, a subdural hematoma is formed.

Arachnoid membrane. The arachnoid membrane, the second meninges, is a delicate, fragile membrane that loosely surrounds the brain. Fine threads of elastic tissue called *trabeculae* connect the arachnoid to the pia mater, creating a spongy, weblike structure called the *subarachnoid space.* Located in the subarachnoid space are

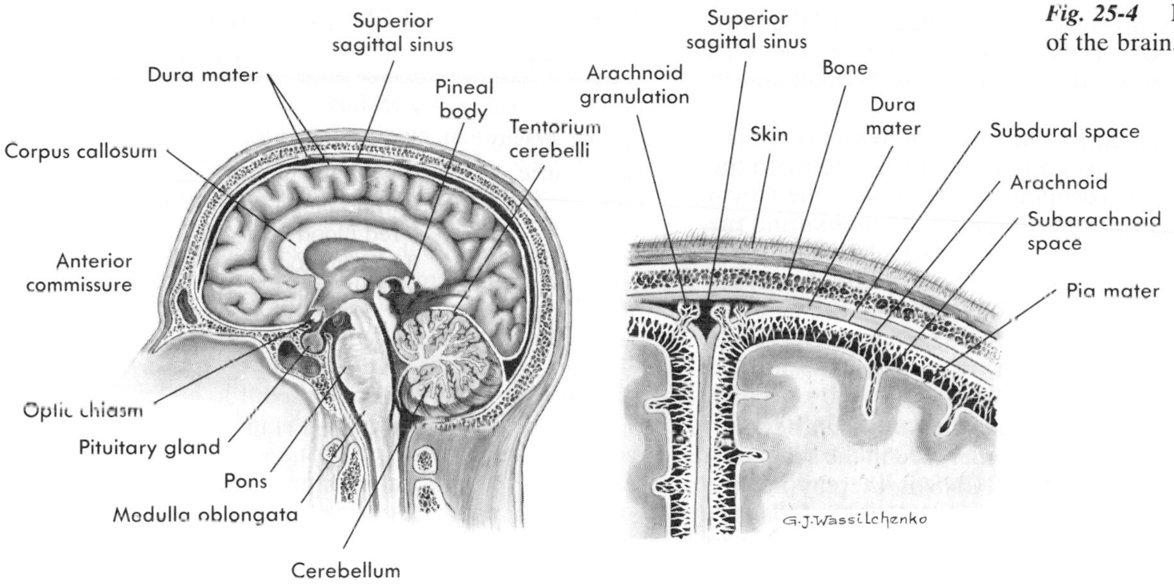

Fig. 25-4 Meningeal layers of the brain.

cerebrospinal fluid (CSF) and a variety of cerebral arteries and veins.

At the base of the brain, widened areas of subarachnoid space form cisterns, or pools, of CSF. The largest of these cisterns, the *cisterna magna,* lies between the medulla and the cerebellum and communicates with the fourth ventricle.

Tufts of arachnoid membrane, called *arachnoid villi,* or granulations, project into the superior sagittal and transverse venous sinuses. This communication between arachnoid villi and sinuses allows reabsorption of CSF from the subarachnoid space into the venous space. Several conditions, such as meningitis or subarachnoid hemorrhage, can obstruct these arachnoid villi and decrease the rate of CSF reabsorption. This arachnoid villi obstruction is termed *communicating hydrocephalus.*

Pia mater. The innermost delicate meninges is known as the *pia mater.* Rich in small blood vessels that supply a large volume of arterial blood to cerebral tissues, this membrane closely follows all folds and convolutions of the brain's surface. Tufts or folds of the pia mater in the lateral, third, and fourth ventricles form a portion of the choroid plexus that is responsible for the production of CSF.

◆ **Ventricular system.** A central CSF-filled core of the brain is called the *ventricular system* (Fig. 25-5). Made of four connected chambers lined with ependymal cells, the ventricles provide the anatomic structure around which the brain and brainstem are formed.

The two largest ventricles, one within each of the cerebral hemispheres, are called the *lateral ventricles.* Extending from the frontal lobe to the occipital lobe, they consist of a body and a frontal, temporal, and occipital horn. When cannulation of the ventricular system is required for drainage of CSF, that is, placement of an intracranial pressure monitor or CSF shunt, the frontal horn of the lateral ventricle is most often selected.

Connecting through the foramen of Monro, the two

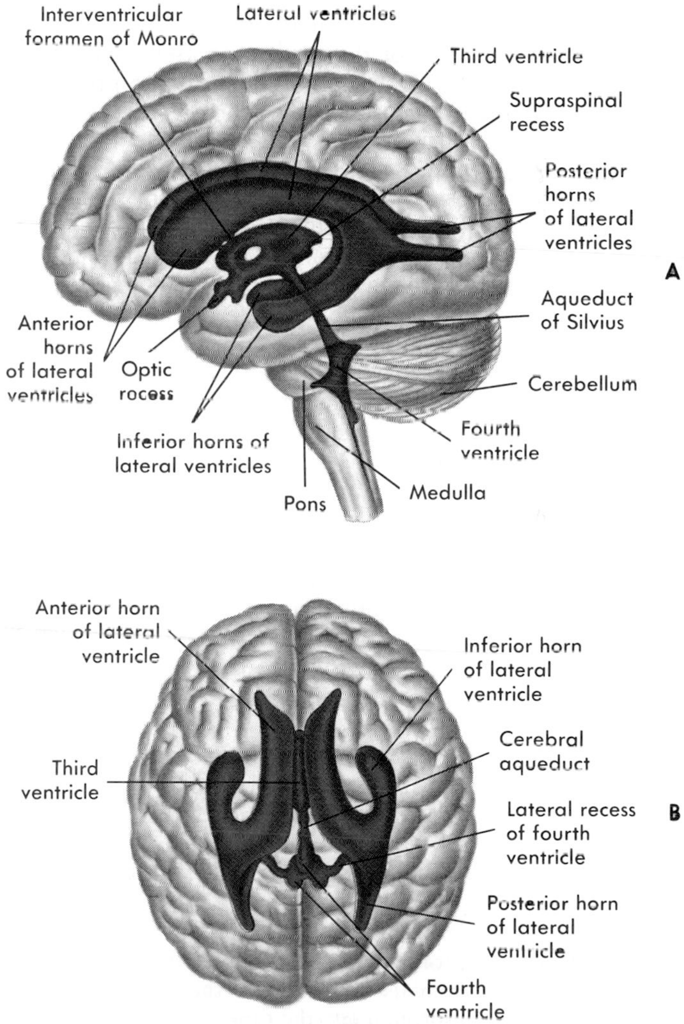

Fig. 25-5 Cerebral ventricles. **A,** Lateral view. **B,** Superior view. (From Thompson JM and others: *Mosby's clinical nursing,* ed 3, St Louis, 1993, Mosby–Year Book.)

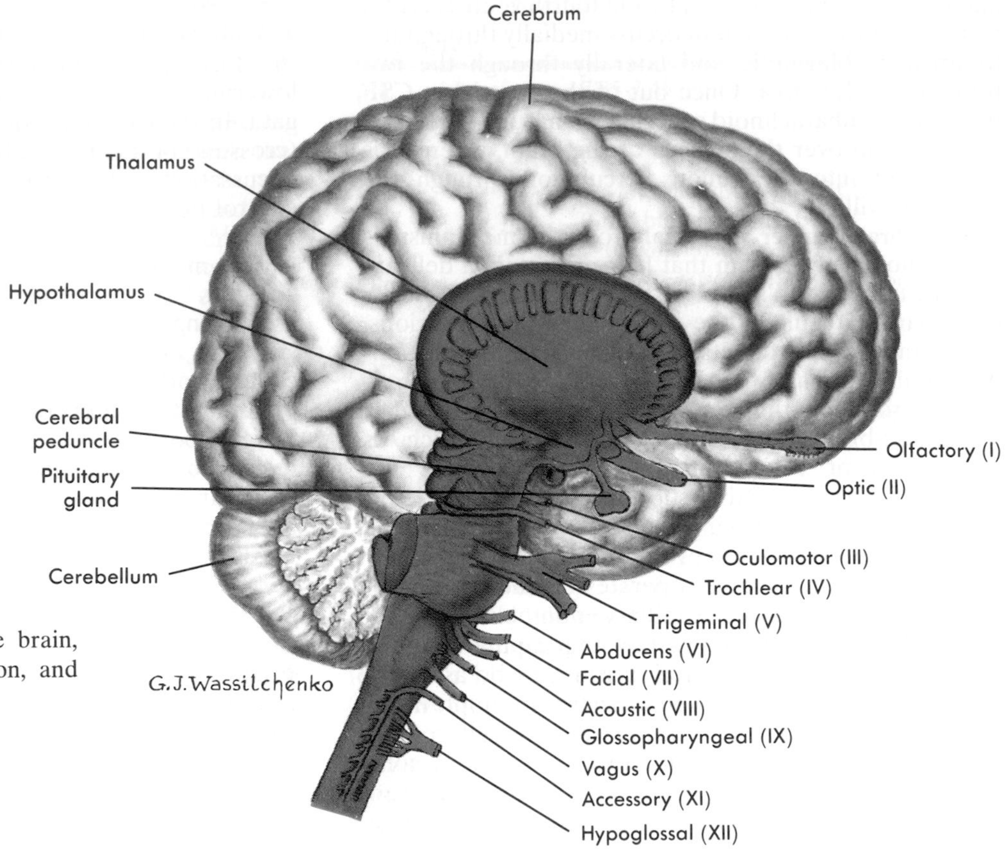

Fig. 25-7 Lateral view of the brain, showing brainstem, diencephalon, and cranial nerves.

Reticular Formation

The reticular formation is a diffuse set of neurons, both gray matter nuclei and white matter fiber tracts, that extend from the upper level of the spinal cord, through the medulla, pons, and midbrain into the thalamus and cerebral cortex.[4,6] Composed of both motor and sensory tracts, the reticular formation is closely tied to functions of the basal ganglia, thalamus, cerebellum, and cerebral cortex. This formation of neural fibers has many excitatory and some inhibitory capabilities, achieving the capacity to regulate the activity from the sources mentioned and to enhance, suppress, or modify impulse transmission. The main role of the reticular formation is to provide a balance between the excitatory and inhibitory stimuli to maintain normal muscle tone, which supports the body against gravity. Damage to the inhibitory areas above the reticular formation (cerebellum and basal ganglia) leads to an excitatory response of the body. Decorticate (abnormal flexion) or decerebrate (abnormal extension) posturing is a result of such an injury. Also located in the reticular formation are centers for blood pressure, respiration, and heart rate function.

◆ **Reticular activating system.** Located within the same region as the reticular formation is the reticular activating system (RAS). Also a diffuse network of fibers extending from the lower brainstem to the cerebral cortex, the RAS has two main levels. The lower portion of the RAS in the brainstem assists with the control of wake-sleep cycles and consciousness. The upper portion in the thalamus region allows the ability to focus attention on a specific task. When the upper RAS is damaged, the patient exhibits a vegetative state, exhibiting sleep-wake cycles and other brainstem functions but no upper levels of cerebration. Although the RAS is not the "center" of consciousness, communication between the cerebral cortex of the RAS is apparently necessary for consciousness to occur.[4,6]

Cerebellum

The cerebellum, separated from the cerebrum by the tentlike structure of the tentorium cerebelli, has also been called the "little brain" or the "hind brain." Approximately one-fifth the size of the brain, the cerebellum is composed of two lateral hemispheres and a central portion called the *vermis.* As is the cerebrum, the cerebellum is composed of a thin outer layer of gray matter, or cortex, and a core of white matter, or fiber tracts. Four pairs of nuclei are located deep in the white matter.

The cerebellum influences muscle tone associated with equilibrium, orientation in space, locomotion, and posture to ensure synchronization of muscle action. Input is received from sensory pathways of the spinal cord, the brainstem, and the cerebrum. Output is through descending motor pathways, such as the corticospinal, vestibulospinal, and reticulospinal tracts.

Cerebellar influences work through continual excitatory and inhibiting stimuli from deep nuclei of the white

Text continued on p. 489.

Table 25-3 Cranial nerves, origins, course, and functions

Cranial nerve	Origin and course	Function
I OLFACTORY		
Sensory	Mucosa of nasal cavity; only cranial nerve with cell body located in peripheral structure (nasal mucosa). Pass through cribiform plate of ethmoid bone and go on to olfactory bulbs at floor of frontal lobe. Final interpretation is in temporal lobe.	Smell. However, system is more than receptor/interpreter for odors; perception of smell also sensitizes other body systems and responses, such as salivation, peristalsis, and even sexual stimulus. Loss of sense of smell is termed *anosmia*.
II OPTIC		
Sensory	Ganglion cells of retina converge to the optic disc and form optic nerve. Nerve fibers pass to optic chiasm, which is above pituitary gland. Some fibers decussate; others do not. The two tracts then go to the lateral geniculate body near the thalamus and then on to the end station for interpretation in the occipital lobe.	Vision (Fig. 25-8).

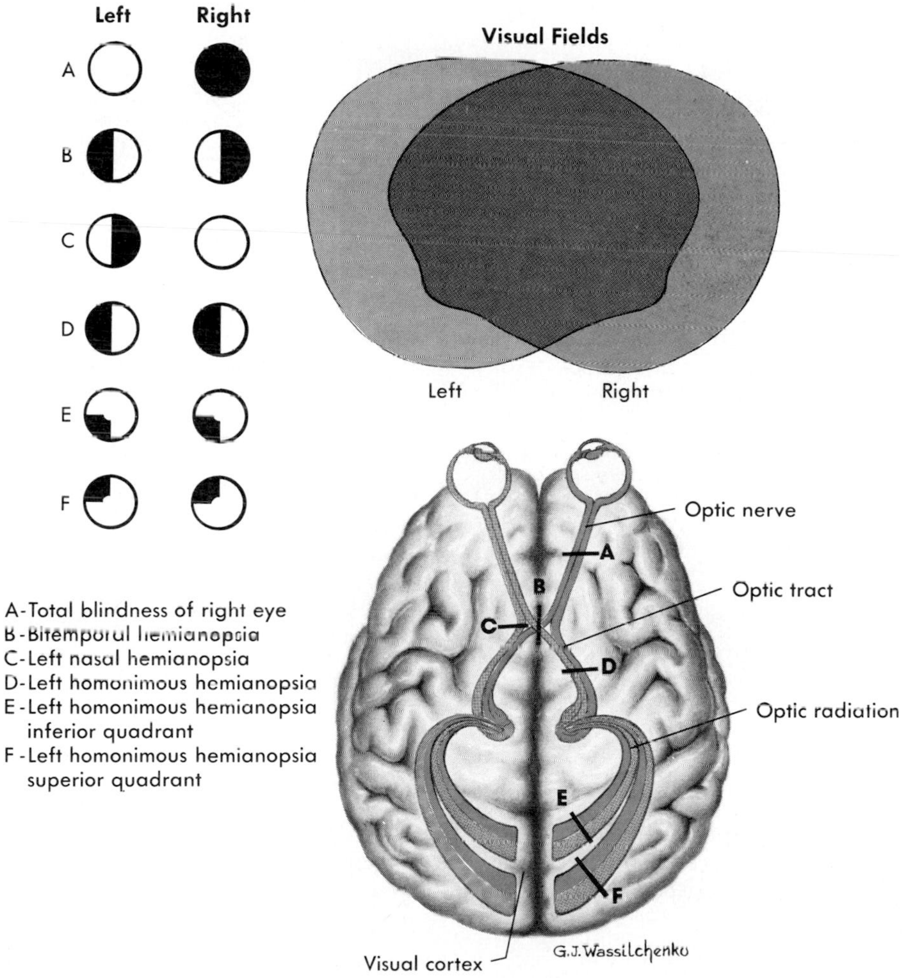

Fig. 25-8 Visual fields showing optic nerve, optic chiasm, optic tracts, and optic radiations. Examples of various visual field defects. (From Rudy E: *Advanced neurological and neurosurgical nursing,* St Louis, 1984, Mosby–Year Book.)

Continued.

Table 25-3 Cranial nerves, origins, course, and functions—cont'd

Cranial nerve	Origin and course	Function
III OCULOMOTOR		
	Originates in midbrain and emerges from brainstem at upper pons.	Extraocular movement of eyes (Fig. 25-9).
Motor	Motor fibers to superior, medial, inferior recti, and inferior oblique for eye movement; levator muscle of the eyelid.	Raise eyelid.
Parasympathetic	Parasympathetic fibers to ciliary muscles and iris of eye.	Constrict pupil; changes shape of lens.

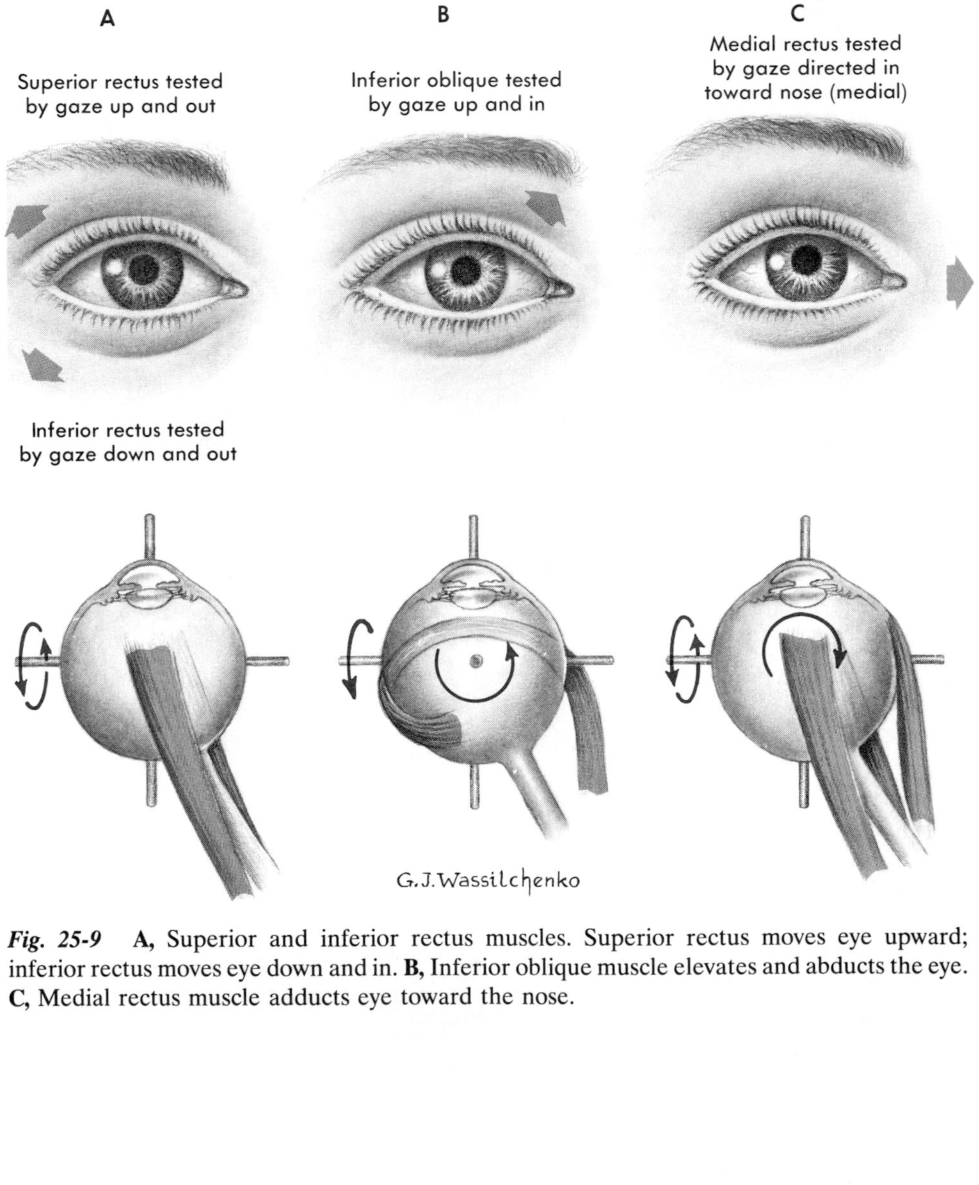

Fig. 25-9 **A,** Superior and inferior rectus muscles. Superior rectus moves eye upward; inferior rectus moves eye down and in. **B,** Inferior oblique muscle elevates and abducts the eye. **C,** Medial rectus muscle adducts eye toward the nose.

Table 25-3 Cranial nerves, origins, course, and functions—cont'd

Cranial nerve	Origin and course	Function
IV TROCHLEAR		
Motor	Midbrain origin near oculomotor, emerges at upper pons near cerebral peduncle. Motor fibers to superior oblique muscle of eyeball.	Extraocular movement of eyes (Fig. 25-10).
V TRIGEMINAL		
Sensory	Originates in fourth ventricle and emerges at lateral parts of pons. Has three branches to face: ophthalmic, maxillary, and mandibular.	*Ophthalmic branch:* Sensation to cornea, ciliary body, iris, lacrimal gland, conjunctiva, nasal mucosal membranes, eyelids, eyebrows, forehead, and nose. *Maxillary branch:* Sensation to skin of cheek, lower lid, side of nose and upper jaw, teeth, mucosa of mouth, sphenopolative-pterygoid region, and maxillary sinus. *Mandibular branch:* Sensation to skin of lower lip, chin, ear, mucous membrane, teeth of lower jaw and tongue.
Motor	Goes to temporalis, masseter, pterygoid gland, anterior part of digastric muscles (all for mastication), and the tensor tympani and tensor veli palatini muscles (clench jaws).	Muscles of chewing and mastication and opening jaw (Fig. 25-11).

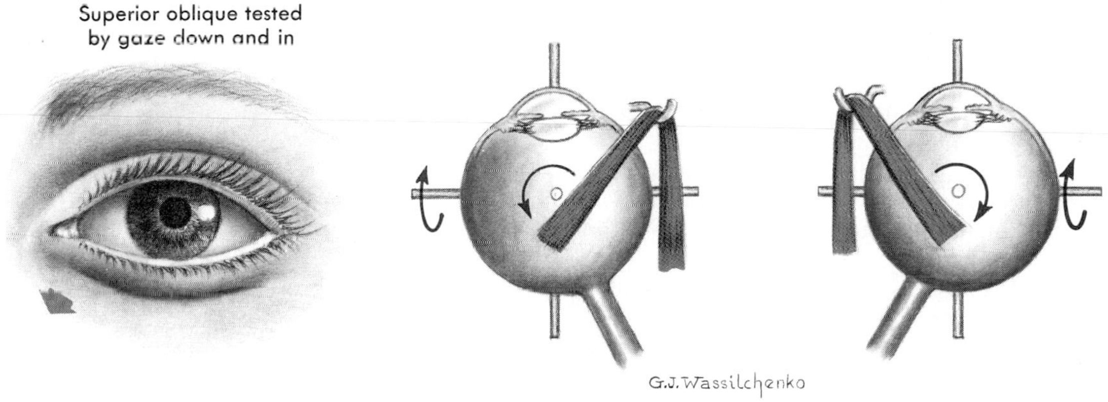

Fig. 25-10 Superior oblique muscle, which rotates the eye down and out at the same time it causes intorsion or inward rotation of the eyeball. The strongest primary action of this muscle is adduction; thus the gaze for testing this muscle is in and down.

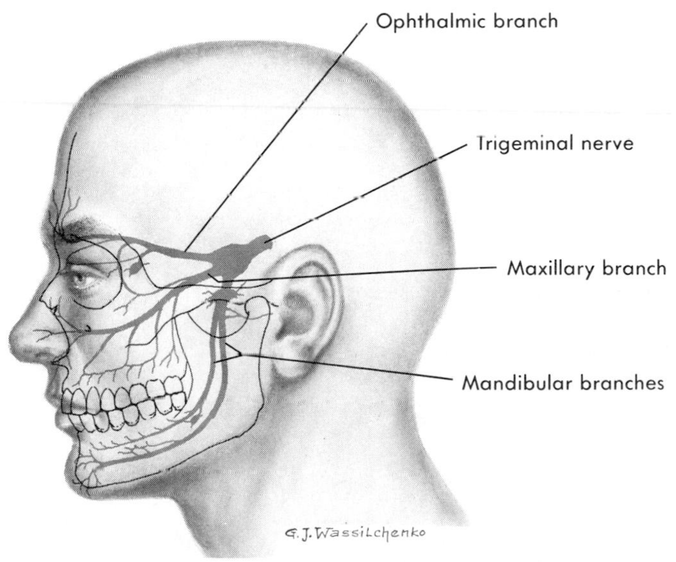

Fig. 25-11 Trigeminal nerve with innervation to face by ophthalmic, maxillary, and mandibular branches.

Continued.

Table 25-3 Cranial nerves, origins, course, and functions—cont'd

Cranial nerve	Origin and course	Function
VI ABDUCENS		
Motor	Posterior part of pons goes to lateral rectus muscle for eye movement.	Extraocular eye movement; rotates eyeball outward (Fig. 25-12).
VII FACIAL		
Sensory	Lower portion of pons goes to anterior two thirds of tongue and soft palate.	Taste in anterior two thirds of tongue. Sensation to soft palate.
Motor	Pons to muscles of forehead, eyelids, cheeks, lips, ears, nose, and neck.	Movement of facial muscles to produce facial expressions, close eyes.
Parasympathetic	Pons to salivary gland and lacrimal glands.	Secretory for salivation and tears.
VIII ACOUSTIC	Two divisions:	
Sensory	*Cochlear division:* Originates in spinal ganglia of the cochlea, with peripheral fibers to the organ of Corti in the internal ear. Goes to pons, and impulses transmitted to the temporal lobe.	Hearing.
	Vestibular division: Originates in otolith organs of the semicircular canals in the inner ear and in the vestibular ganglion. Terminates in pons, with some fibers continuing to cerebellum. The only cranial nerve that originates wholly within a bone, the petrous portion of the temporal bone.	Equilibrium.
IX GLOSSOPHARYNGEAL		
Sensory	Posterior one third of tongue for taste sensation and sensations from soft palate, tonsils, and opening to mouth in back of oral pharynx (fauces). Fibers go to medulla and then to the temporal lobe for taste and sensory cortex for other sensations.	Taste in posterior one third of tongue. Sensation in back of throat; stimulation elicits a gag reflex.
Motor	Medulla to constrictor muscles of pharynx and stylopharyngeal muscles.	Voluntary muscles for swallowing and phonation.
Parasympathetic	Medulla to parotid salivary gland via otic ganglia.	Secretory, salivary glands. Carotid reflex.

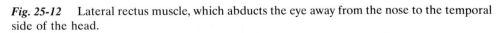

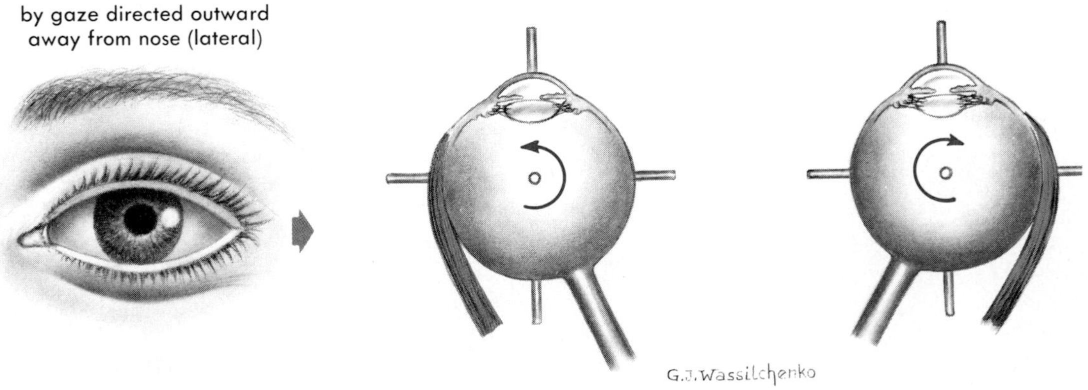

Fig. 25-12 Lateral rectus muscle, which abducts the eye away from the nose to the temporal side of the head.

Table 25-3 Cranial nerves, origins, course, and functions—cont'd

Cranial nerve	Origin and course	Function
X VAGUS		
Sensory	Sensory fibers in back of ear and posterior wall of external ear go to medulla oblongata and on to sensory cortex.	Sensation behind ear and part of external ear meatus.
Motor	Fibers go from medulla oblongata through jugular foramen with glossopharyngeal nerve and on to pharynx, larynx, esophagus, bronchi, lungs, heart, stomach, small intestines, liver, pancreas, kidneys.	Voluntary muscles for phonation and swallowing. Involuntary activity of visceral muscles of heart, lungs, and digestive tract.
Parasympathetic	Medulla oblongata to larynx, trachea, lungs, aorta, esophagus, stomach, small intestines, and gallbladder.	Carotid reflex. Autonomic activity of respiratory tract, digestive tract including peristalsis and secretion from organs.
XI SPINAL ACCESSORY		
Motor	This nerve has two roots, cranial and spinal. Cranial portion arises at several rootlets at side of medulla, runs below vagus, and is joined by spinal portion from motor cells in cervical cord. Some fibers go along with vagus nerve to supply motor impulse to pharynx, larynx, uvula, and palate. Major portion to sternomastoid and trapezius muscles, branches to cervical spinal nerves C2-C4.	Some fibers for swallowing and phonation. Turn head and shrug shoulders.
XII HYPOGLOSSAL		
Motor	Arises in medulla oblongata and goes to muscles of tongue.	Movement of tongue necessary for swallowing and phonation.

matter. The balancing of these two opposing forces results in smooth motor movements instead of rapid, jerky, erratic movements. This complex system in the cerebellum monitors and adjusts motor activity simultaneously with the performance of the activity.

Diencephalon

The diencephalon, the lowest structure of the cerebrum, lies at the top of the brainstem surrounding the third ventricle.[1,2,7] It is divided into four regions: the thalamus, hypothalamus, epithalamus, and subthalamus (see Fig. 25-7). Also located in this area are the pituitary gland and the internal capsule. The first two cranial nerves, I (olfactory) and II (optic), originate in the diencephalon region.

◆ **Thalamus.** The largest region of the diencephalon, the thalamus, consists of two connected ovoid masses of gray matter forming the lateral walls of the third ventricle deep in the cerebral hemispheres. The thalamus is a relay station for both motor and sensory activity, basic neuronal activity such as processing of brain activity (measured by electroencephalogram) and memory, thought, emotion, and complex behavior (Fig. 25-13).

The thalamus's role as a relay station for sensory input is a complex function coordinated with the parietal lobe of the cerebrum. All sensory pathways except olfactory communicate with some area of the thalamus. With the assistance of stimuli from the cerebral cortex, the thalamus sorts and sends sensory impulses to the appropriate area of the cerebral cortex for final processing.

The role of the thalamus in motor activity is to coordinate and integrate. It assists the cerebrum and cerebellum in providing a smooth, integrated motor response.

◆ **Hypothalamus.** The hypothalamus, located below the thalamus, forms the floor and anterior lateral walls of the third ventricle. Other landmarks around the hypothalamus are the optic chiasm, which is located behind the hypothalamus, and the pituitary gland, sitting below the hypothalamus in the sella turcica. The pituitary stalk connects the hypothalamus to the pituitary gland.

Functions of the hypothalamus include regulating and maintaining internal body environment and interacting with the limbic system to generate actual physical responses to emotions, such as blushing when embarrassed. Areas of the internal environment regulated and maintained by the hypothalamus include (1) temperature regulation, (2) autonomic nervous system responses, (3) regulation of food and water intake, (4) control of hormonal secretions of the pituitary, and (5) behavioral responses.

Temperature regulation. Temperature regulation is achieved by the anterior and posterior parts of the hypothalamus. As blood with increased temperature

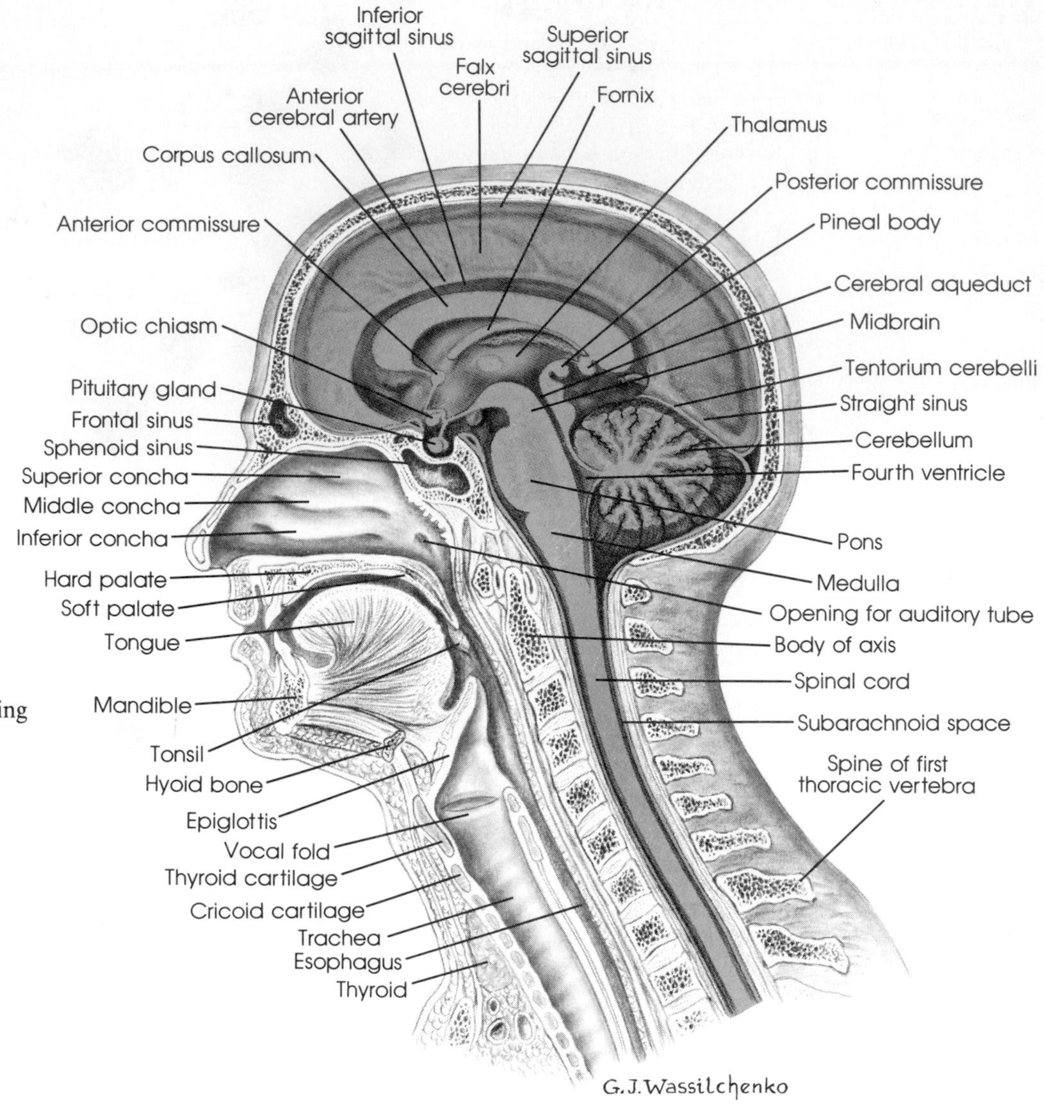

Fig. 25-13 Schematic drawing of sagittal section of head.

flows through the anterior region of the hypothalamus, stimuli travel to sweat glands to produce perspiration, to peripheral vessels to cause vasodilation, which allows heat loss through the skin, and to respiratory centers to increase respiratory rate. Low blood temperature stimulates the posterior region of the hypothalamus and causes vasoconstriction, piloerection, or "goose bumps," and shivering, which increases cell metabolism and produces heat.

Autonomic nervous system responses. The hypothalamus serves as the "brain" for the autonomic or involuntary nervous system. The parasympathetic (resting) system response is elicited by stimulation of the anterior region of the hypothalamus. The sympathetic (fight or flight) system responds when the posterior region of the hypothalamus is stimulated.

Regulation of food and water intake. Food intake is regulated by two centers: the *hunger center,* which causes the sensation of hunger when stimulated, and the *satiety center,* which decreases the desire for food when the stomach is full or blood glucose is high. Water intake is regulated through the secretion of *antidiuretic hormone* (ADH). A change in serum osmotic pressure is the stimulus for ADH response. An increase in serum osmotic pressure stimulates the release of ADH, and decreases in serum osmotic pressure depress the release of ADH (see Chapter 41).

Control of hormonal secretions by the pituitary gland. The interrelationships between the hypothalamus and the pituitary in the production, storage, and secretion of hormones are discussed in the section on the pituitary gland.

Behavioral responses. Behavioral responses influenced by the hypothalamus and interacting with the limbic system include behaviors associated with aggression, pleasure, punishment, and sexual activities.

◆ **Epithalamus.** Located in the dorsal portion of the diencephalon, the epithalamus contains the pineal gland, which is believed to play a role in physical growth and in sexual development. This gland often calcifies in early adulthood and can be identified on computed tomographic scan or radiographic films.

◆ **Subthalamus.** The subthalamus is located below the thalamus. It is integrated with extrapyramidal tracts of the autonomic nervous system and the basal ganglia.
◆ **Pituitary gland.** The pituitary gland, also known as the *hypophysis,* has been called the "master gland" because of its role in the regulation of hormone production of all other endocrine organs. Lying in the sella turcica, the pituitary gland is connected to the hypothalamus by the pituitary or hypophyseal stalk. The pituitary gland itself is divided into two lobes, the anterior (adenohypophysis) and the posterior (neurohypophysis). The anterior and posterior lobes of the pituitary are different and are described individually.

Anterior lobe. The anterior lobe constitutes 75% of the pituitary gland and is responsible for regulation of the majority of endocrine function. Hormone and other electrolyte levels in the blood are sensed by the hypothalamus. The hypothalamus then sends neurosecretory substances (releasing or inhibiting factors) through the blood supply of the pituitary stalk portal vein to the anterior pituitary. These neurosecretory substances cause the anterior pituitary gland to release or inhibit specific hormones. The seven major hormones of the anterior pituitary are adrenocorticotropic hormone (ACTH), thyroid-stimulating hormone (TSH), growth hormone (GH), prolactin (PRL), follicle-stimulating hormone (FSH), luteinizing hormone (LH), and melanocyte-stimulating hormone (MSH). Hormones are produced, stored, and then secreted from the pituitary when stimulated by the hypothalamus. Once the anterior pituitary hormone is released, it travels to the target endocrine gland and stimulates secretion of endocrine hormone, which then circulates through the blood supply back to the hypothalamus where an increased hormonal level is sensed. The hypothalamus stops the release of neurosecretory substances, and the stimulating cycle is broken. See the box (upper right) for an example of this cycle, using the thyroid gland and thyroxin.

Posterior lobe. The posterior lobe constitutes the other 25% of the pituitary gland and is directly connected to the hypothalamus by the pituitary stalk. The posterior lobe does not produce any hormones. However, the posterior lobe does secrete two hormones, ADH and oxytocin, which are produced by cells in the hypothalamus and trickle down fiber tracts through the pituitary stalk for storage in the posterior pituitary. When ADH or oxytocin release is required, the hypothalamus stimulates the pituitary to release these hormones rapidly in response to a variety of stimuli.
◆ **Internal capsule.** Fiber tracts from many portions of each half of the cerebrum converge in the area of the diencephalon on their way to the brainstem and spinal cord to form the internal capsule. The internal capsule contains both afferent and efferent fibers but is mainly considered a motor, or efferent, pathway (Fig. 25-14). All afferent (sensory) fibers traveling to the cortex travel through the internal capsule in the following succession: brainstem to thalamus to internal capsule to cerebral cortex. All efferent (motor) fibers leaving the cortex also pass through the internal capsule. Because of the collection of all major motor and sensory fibers through this small area, a tiny area of damage to the internal capsule causes major loss of motor and some sensory function on the opposite side of the body.

HORMONE-STIMULATING CYCLE

Thyroxin level is low in blood
↓
Hypothalamus senses low level
↓
Hypothalamus releases thyrotropin-releasing factor (TRF)
↓
TRF travels through portal venous system to anterior pituitary
↓
Anterior pituitary secretes thyroid-stimulating hormone (TSH) into blood
↓
TSH travels to thyroid gland and stimulates production of thyroxin
↓
Hypothalamus senses circulating amount of thyroxin
↓
TRF is not released

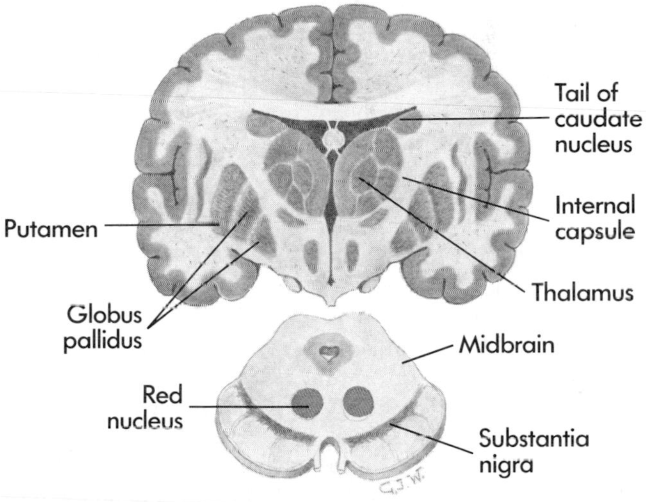

Fig. 25-14 Coronal section of brain.

Basal Ganglia

The main role of the basal ganglia is associated with motor function.[6,7] They provide a pathway and assist in processing information from the cerebral motor cortex and the thalamus. The basal ganglia are composed of several subcortical nuclei located deep within the white matter of the cerebral hemispheres. These paired sets of nuclei include the corpus striatum (composed of the caudate nuclei, the putamen, and the globus pallidus), the amygdala, the claustrum, the subthalamic nuclei, and the substantia nigra (Fig. 25-14).

Much of the basal ganglia's function is through the extrapyramidal (involuntary) motor pathways. It influences motor activity to integrate voluntary movement with associated movements and postural adjustments and suppresses skeletal muscle tone and postural reflexes. The basal ganglia also process input from visual, labyrinthine, and proprioceptive sources, resulting in smooth, coordinated movements of the body without loss of balance.

Cerebrum

The cerebrum is the largest portion of the brain, comprising 80% of its weight. It is composed of two cerebral hemispheres (right and left) incompletely divided by the longitudinal fissure. The cerebral hemispheres are connected at the base of the longitudinal fissure by the corpus callosum. The corpus callosum is a large tract of transverse or commissural fibers that provide a communication link between the two hemispheres.

The outside of the cerebrum is covered with a thin layer of gray matter (multiple layers of unmyelinated cell nuclei) called the *cerebral cortex.* Underneath the cerebral cortex are the white matter (myelinated) tracts, which communicate impulses from the cerebral cortex to other areas of the brain. Three types of fibers—commissural (transverse), projection, and association—are in the white matter and are named for the role they play in communication of information. *Commissural fibers* are tracts that communicate between corresponding parts of the two hemispheres. The corpus callosum is the largest of these fiber tracts. *Projection fibers* communicate between the cerebral cortex and lower regions of the brain and spinal cord. *Association fibers* communicate between various regions of the same hemisphere.

The cerebral hemispheres are divided into four surface lobes, based on anatomic divisions or fissures. The four paired lobes are the *frontal lobes,* the *parietal lobes,* the *temporal lobes,* and the *occipital lobes* (Fig. 25-15). Another area deeper inside the cerebrum can also be classified as a lobe and is called the *limbic lobe.*

Classification of different areas of the cerebral cytoarchitecture, based on minute histologic differences of the cell, is credited to Brodmann. More than 100 of these numbered areas have been identified (Fig. 25-16). See Table 25-4 (p. 494) for a summary of the cerebral lobes and their major functions.

◆ **Frontal lobe.** The largest of the four lobes of the cerebral hemispheres is the frontal lobe. The frontal lobe lies underneath the frontal bone of the skull and is separated posteriorly from the parietal lobe by the central fissure (fissure of Rolando) and inferiorly from the temporal lobe by the lateral fissure (Sylvian fissure). The major functions of the frontal lobe are voluntary motor function, higher mental functions, cognition, memory, personality, and language. Some of the higher control centers for autonomic nervous system function also lie in the frontal lobe.

The prefrontal area of the frontal lobe (areas 9 to 12) is concerned with the process of cerebration (or thought), affect, feeling, and emotion, as well as autonomic nervous system response in relation to emotional changes. The rationale behind the use of biofeedback techniques and relaxation techniques correlates with the prefrontal area's influence on the autonomic nervous system.

The premotor area (areas 6 and 8) is an association area for the motor area lying adjacent to it. When stimulated, the prefrontal area provides general body movements, such as turning the eyes and head and turning the trunk with the head. A connection exists between the premotor area and cranial nerves III, IV, VI, IX, X, and XII to allow coordination of the movements described.

The motor area, or motor strip (area 4), contains the cells for voluntary (pyramidal) motor functions of the opposite side of the body. The motor-strip functions are drawn spatially by the homunculus (Fig. 25-17, *A*). The appearance is of an upside-down man with a foot on the medial aspect of the frontal lobe. The knees, hips, trunk, and shoulders extend over the outer surface of the cortex and the hands, thumb, head, face, and tongue down the side to the lateral fissure, which is the border of the frontal lobe. The size of the area for each body part along this strip is proportional to the amount of dexterity associated with the body part's function. Therefore the large surface area of the trunk occupies a relatively small part of the motor strip. The smaller areas, such as the thumb or tongue, that involve a great deal of dexterity and fine motor movement occupy a larger area of this strip.

Broca's area (areas 44 and 45) is located at the inferior frontal gyrus. Part of the speech center, this area is responsible for the motor aspects of speech and is involved in coordination of activities for the formulation of verbal speech. Damage to this area results in an *expressive* or *nonfluent aphasia.*

◆ **Parietal lobe.** The parietal lobe is directly posterior to the frontal lobe on the other side of the central fissure. The posterior border of the parietal lobe is the parietooccipital fissure, which separates it from the occipital lobe. The inferior border is incompletely defined by the posterior portion of the lateral fissure. The main function of the parietal lobe is sensory, including integration of sensory information, awareness of body parts, interpretation of touch, pressure, and pain, and recognition of object size, shape, or texture.

The parietal lobe contains a sensory strip (areas 1, 2, and 3) that lies adjacent to the motor strip of the frontal lobe. Similar to the homunculus of the motor strip, the sensory homunculus re-creates a caricature of an upside-down man (Fig. 25-17, *B*). Sensory areas of body parts lie close to motor areas of the same parts. Also, areas of the body with greater tactile response occupy larger areas on the sensory strip. Fibers going to the sensory strip bring stimuli associated with cutaneous and deep sensibility sensations, as well as cutaneous sensation of touch, pressure, position, and vibration. Input from the thalamus also reaches the sensory strip.

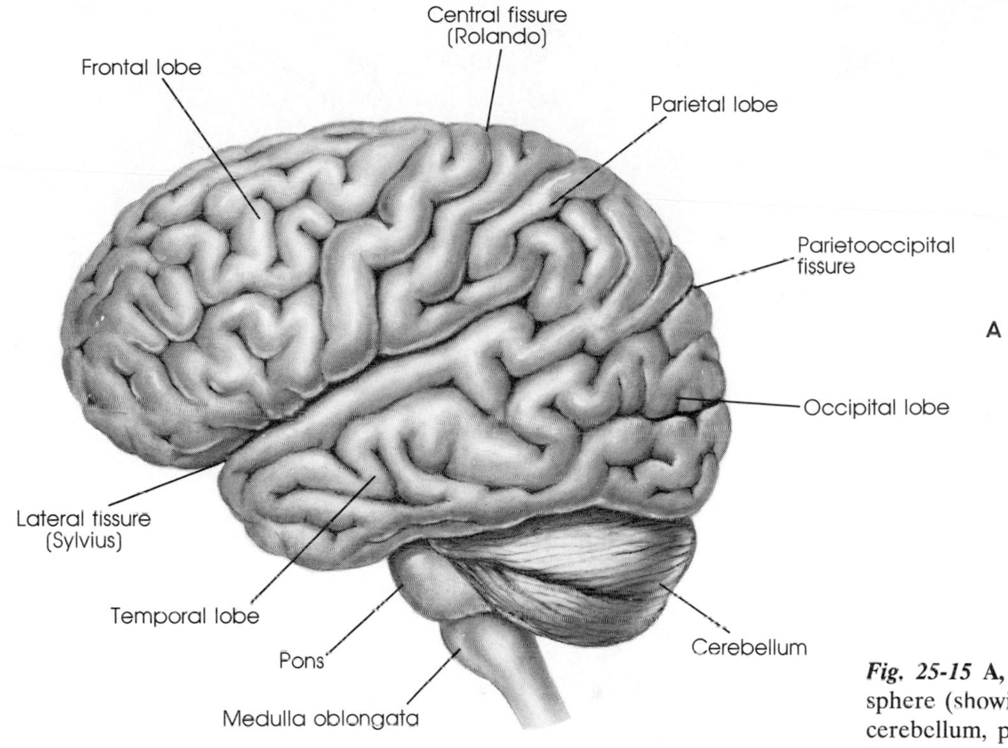

Fig. 25-15 **A,** Lateral view of cerebral hemisphere (showing lobes and principal fissures), cerebellum, pons, and medulla oblongata. **B,** Principal functional subdivisions of cerebral hemisphere.

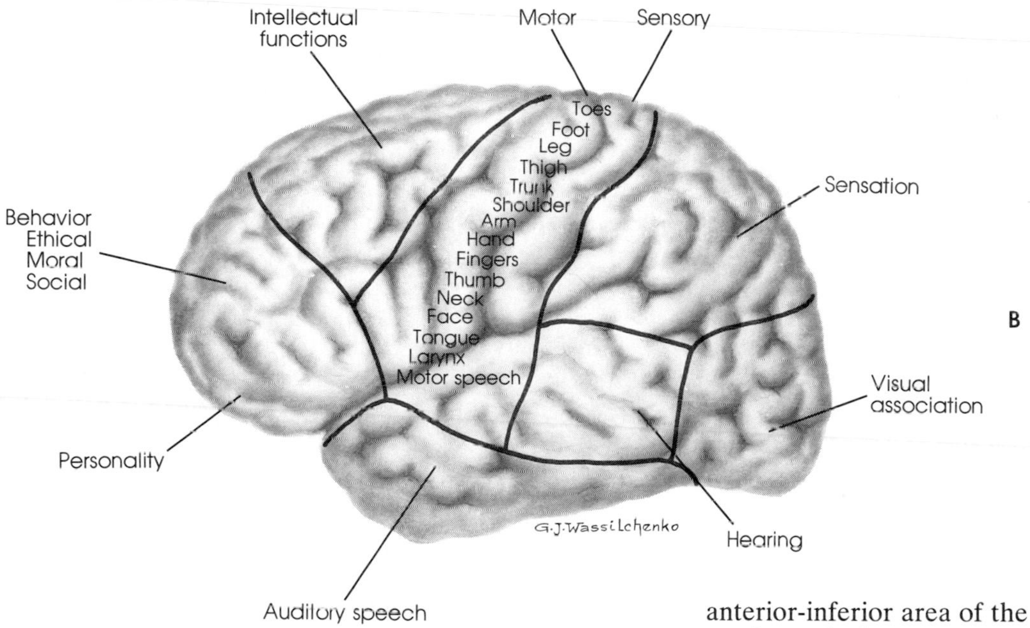

Associative areas of the parietal lobe (areas 5 and 7) interpret sensory input in terms of size, shape, texture, and weight. The parietal lobe provides the ability to localize a sensation and define it in terms of pressure, temperature, or vibration. Interpretive aspects of the parietal lobe's response to stimuli include awareness of body parts, orientation in space, and recognition of environmental spatial relationships.

A portion of the sensory aspect of speech and the understanding of the written word is located in the anterior-inferior area of the parietal lobe. Along with a portion of the temporal lobe, this area is called *Wernicke's area* (area 22).

◆ **Temporal lobe.** The temporal lobe lies beneath the temporal bone in the lateral portion of the cranium. The anterior, lower border of the temporal lobe is encased in the sphenoid wing. With a strong blow to the head the temporal lobe is easily contused and lacerated as it moves against this hard, irregular surface. Separated from the frontal and parietal lobes by the lateral fissure, this lobe has the primary functions of hearing, speech, behavior, and memory.

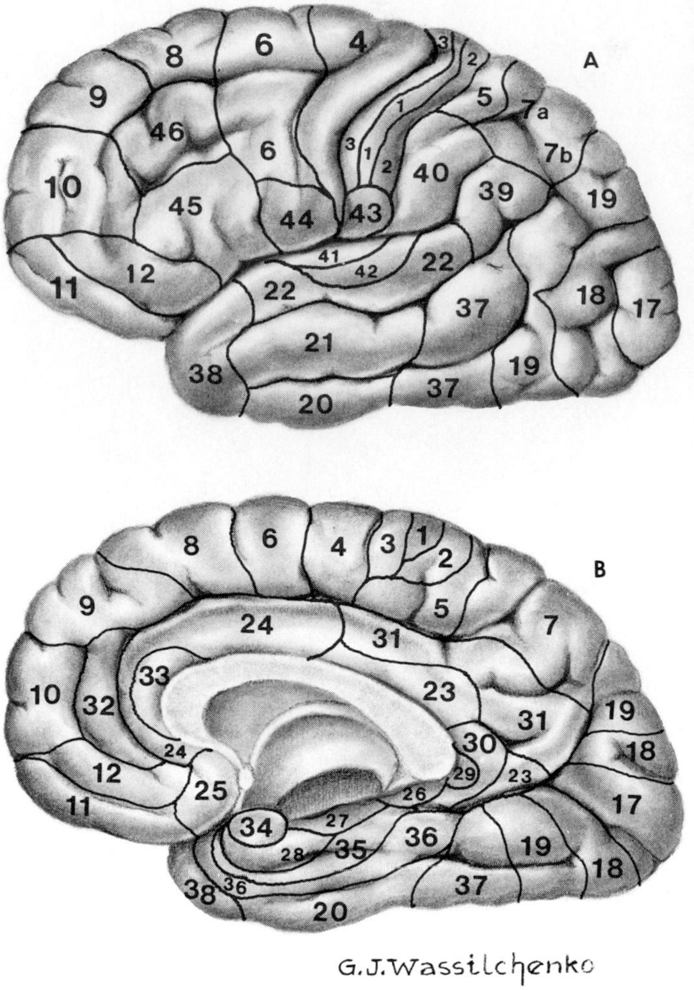

Fig. 25-16 Cytoarchitectural map of the lateral and medial surface of the human cortex according to Brodmann's map. **A,** Lateral surface. **B,** Medial surface.

Table 25-4 Cerebral lobes and their major functions

Cerebral lobes	Major functions
Frontal	Personality Moral, ethical, and social values Abstract thought Long-term memory Motor strip for opposite side of body
Parietal	Sensory strip for opposite side of body Two-point discrimination Recognition of object by size, shape, weight, or texture Body part awareness
Temporal	Hearing Special senses of taste and smell Interpretive area—integrates sounds, thoughts, and emotions
Occipital	Vision Visual recognition of objects Reading comprehension

The primary auditory areas (areas 41 and 42) receive sound impulses and assist in determining the source of the sound and interpreting the meaning of the sound. These areas are closely linked with Wernicke's area, which is located in both the parietal and temporal lobes. Responsible for the comprehension of both spoken and written language, Wernicke's area, in the dominant hemisphere, is called an *associative area.* Disruption of this area leads to *receptive (fluent) aphasia*—the individual can hear but is unable to interpret the message.

In the superior portion of the temporal lobe where the frontal, parietal, and temporal lobes meet is an essential *interpretive area* in which auditory, visual, and somatic association areas are integrated into complex thought and memory. Seizures in this region of the temporal lobe cause auditory, visual, or sensory hallucinations.

◆ **Occipital lobe.** The occipital lobe of the cerebrum forms the most posterior portion. It is separated from the cerebellum by the tentorium. Primary responsibility of the occipital lobe is vision and the interpretation of visual stimuli.

The primary visual cortex (area 17) receives impulses from projections of the optic tract. These impulses are then referred to the visual associative areas (areas 18 and 19) for interpretation and integration.

◆ **Limbic lobe.** One other cerebral section, which is anatomically part of the temporal lobe, is often separated from the temporal lobe for discussion of function and is called (although sometimes controversially) the *limbic lobe.* Also called the *rhinencephalon,* this lobe forms the border of the lateral ventricles and contains the hippocampus, the uncus, primary olfactory cortex, and the amygdaloid nucleus. The functions of the limbic lobe are self-preservation, primitive behavior, moods, the visceral processes associated with emotion, short-term memory, and the interpretation of smell.

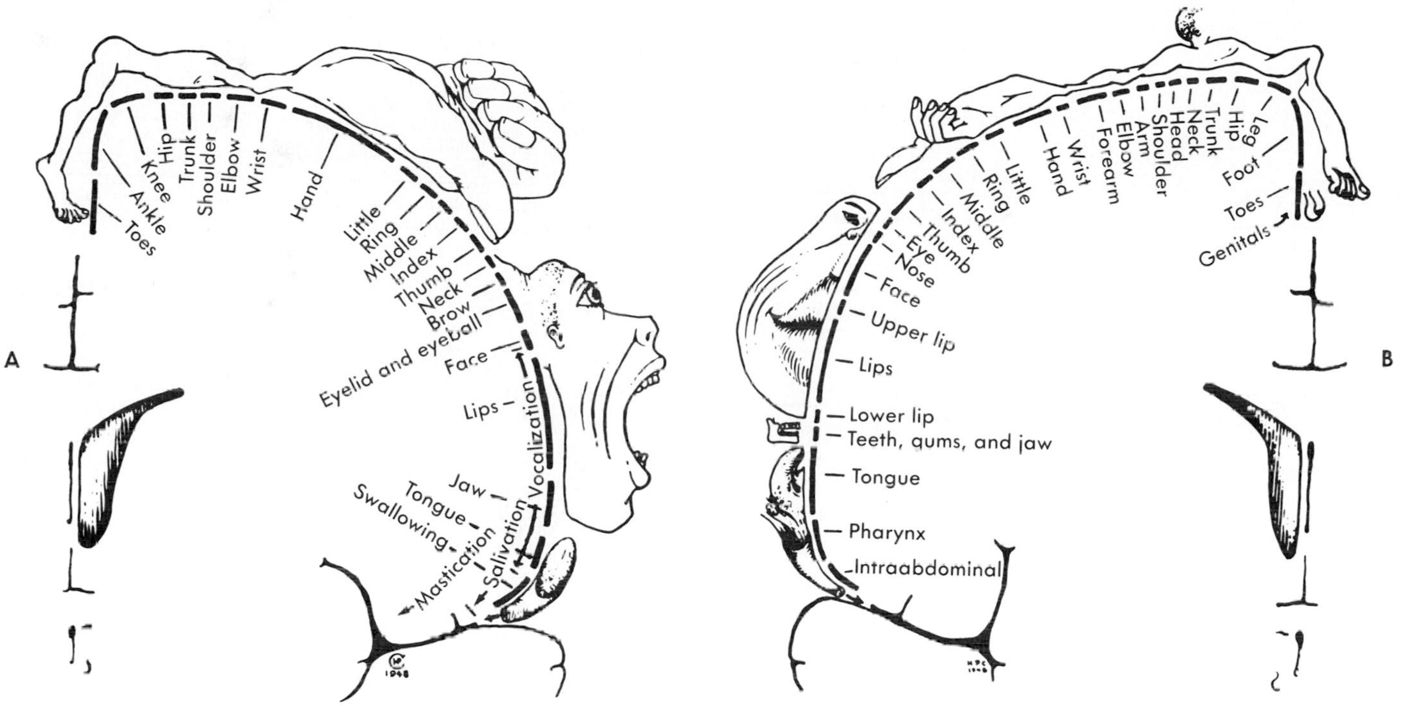

Fig. 25-17 Classic drawing of **A,** motor homunculus and **B,** sensory homunculus. (From Penfield W, Rasmussen T: *The cerebral cortex of man,* 1950, Macmillan; renewed 1978 by Theodore Rasmussen.)

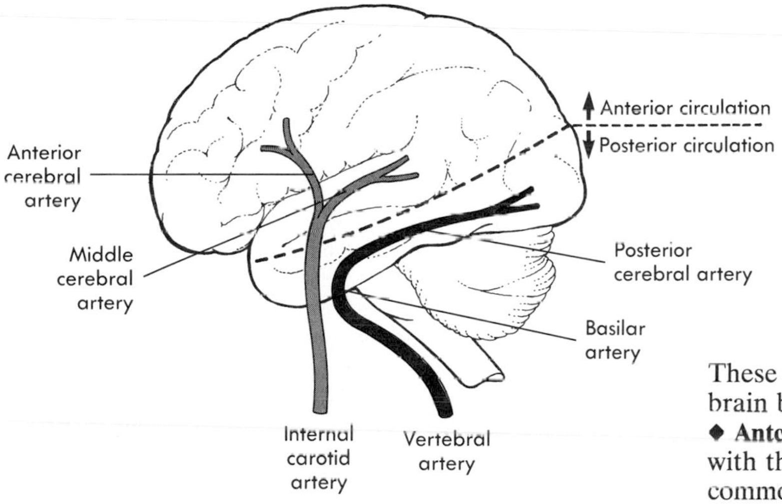

Fig. 25-18 Arteries of anterior and posterior cerebral circulation.

Cerebral Circulation

The brain constitutes 2% of the body's weight but uses 20% of the body's cardiac output. It requires approximately 750 ml of cerebral blood flow per minute. The role of cerebral circulation is to provide enough blood to supply oxygen, glucose, and nutrients to the cerebral tissues. There is no reserve of either oxygen or glucose in the cerebral tissues, and a lack or inadequate amount of either one rapidly disrupts cerebral function and produces irreversible damage. Two pairs of arteries, the internal carotids and the vertebral arteries, are responsible for supplying blood to the brain. Anatomically they can be separated into the arteries of the anterior circulation and the posterior circulation (Fig. 25-18).[5,6,7] These two circulations are connected at the base of the brain by the circle of Willis.

◆ **Anterior circulation.** The anterior circulation begins with the common carotid arteries (Fig. 25-19). The left common carotid originates from the arch of the aorta, and the right common carotid originates from the innominate artery. At the level of the crycothyroid junction, the common carotid splits to form the external and internal carotid arteries. The external carotid feeds the face, the scalp, and the skull and includes the branch called the *middle meningeal artery,* which lies between the skull and the dura. When the middle meningeal artery is torn or lacerated, the blood can develop into an epidural hematoma.

The internal carotid artery continues upward through the carotid siphon and enters the base of the skull through an opening in the petrous bone. At the base of the brain the internal carotid connects with the circle of Willis and then branches into the anterior and middle cerebral arteries, which are primarily responsible for

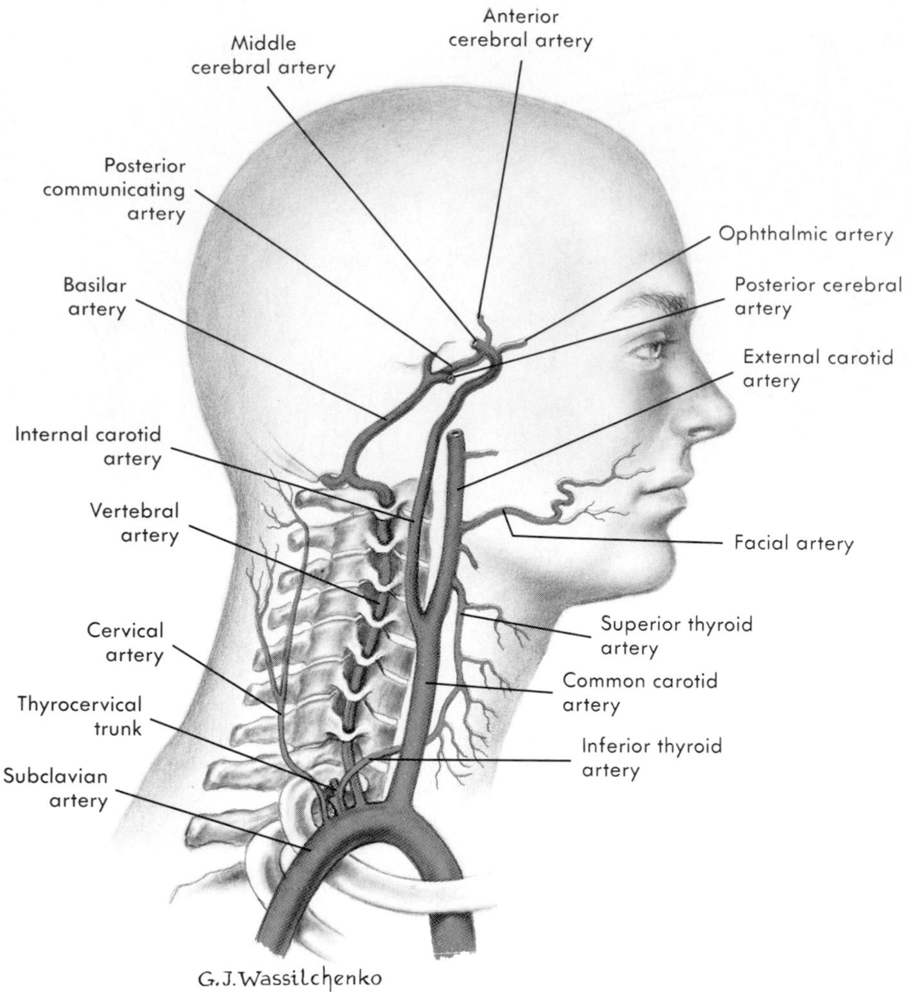

Fig. 25-19 Feeder arteries to the brain.

anterior circulation. One major branch of the internal carotid, the *ophthalmic artery,* exits before the circle of Willis and supplies blood to the optic nerve and eye.

◆ **Posterior circulation.** Posterior circulation begins with the two vertebral arteries, which originate from the subclavian arteries and travel posteriorly through small openings in the lateral spinous processes of the cervical spine. They enter the skull through the foramen magnum and at the level of the pons the two vertebrals join to form the *basilar artery.* Branches of the basilar artery feed the brainstem and the cerebellum. The basilar artery continues upward into the posterior portion of the circle of Willis and into the two posterior cerebral arteries.

◆ **Circle of Willis.** The circle of Willis is a vascular supply system unique to cerebral circulation (Fig. 25-20). Located in a small area above the optic chiasm in the subarachnoid space, the circle is fed by the internal carotid and basilar arteries. The three cerebral arteries (anterior, middle, and posterior) supplying each hemisphere are connected by communicating arteries to form a complete circle. The anterior communicating artery connects the right and left anterior cerebral arteries, and the two posterior communicating arteries connect the middle cerebral and posterior cerebral artery in each of the hemispheres.

In a normal situation the left internal carotid artery supplies blood to the left anterior and middle cerebral arteries, and the right internal carotid artery supplies blood to the right anterior and middle cerebral arteries, thus constituting anterior circulation. In the posterior circulation the basilar artery feeds both posterior cerebral arteries.

When an artery such as the right internal carotid is blocked with atherosclerotic material so that an inadequate amount of blood is flowing to the right anterior and middle cerebral arteries, blood from the left internal carotid will flow across the anterior communicating artery and assist with the vascular supply to the right hemisphere. Also, blood flow from the right posterior cerebral artery will flow through the right posterior communicating artery to supply blood to the right middle cerebral artery. Thus supply of oxygen and nutrients to the brain is not disrupted.

It is not unusual to have an anatomically incomplete circle of Willis. Autopsy and angiographic studies have supplied evidence that up to 50% of individuals have absent or hypoplastic communicating vessels.[6]

Anterior cerebral artery. The anterior cerebral artery runs anteriorly along the base of the brain and supplies the longitudinal fissure and therefore the medial surfaces of the frontal and parietal lobes. It also feeds the

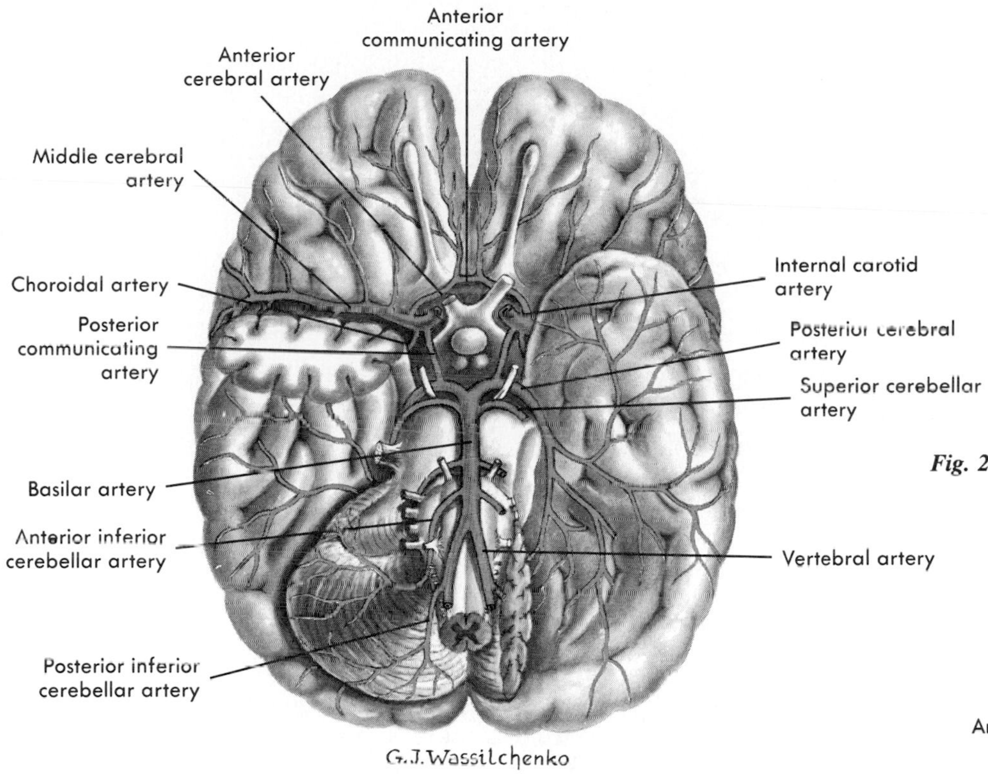

Fig. 25-20 Blood supply of the brain.

basal ganglia, portions of the internal capsule, and the corpus callosum.

Middle cerebral artery. The middle cerebral artery is the largest of the cerebral arteries. As a direct branch from the internal carotid, it travels laterally and feeds the surface of the frontal, parietal, and temporal lobes and the internal capsule.

Posterior cerebral artery. The posterior cerebral artery, a branch of the basilar artery, runs along the tentorium and feeds the occipital lobes and the medial and lateral aspects of the temporal lobe (Fig. 25-21).

♦ **Venous circulation.** Venous drainage is accomplished by the venous sinuses of the dura. Capillary flow moves to venules and then to cerebral veins, which empty into the sinuses located throughout the cranium. Blood from these sinuses empties into the internal jugular vein, which empties into the superior vena cava and then back into the right atrium.

Spinal Cord

The spinal cord is the extension of the medulla after its exit from the foramen magnum.[3,8] It is a long, ropelike structure composed of white and gray matter. The spinal cord itself tapers down to an end or *conus medullaris* at the level of the first or second lumbar vertebra. Exiting from the spinal cord are 31 pairs of spinal nerve roots, which travel through the intervertebral foramina. Because the spinal cord ends at L1 and the final nerve roots do not exit until the coccyx, long lengths of nerve roots, called the *cauda equina,* extend through the space in the lumbar and sacral regions. Most of the protective mechanisms for the cranium also exist, with slight modification, for the spinal cord.

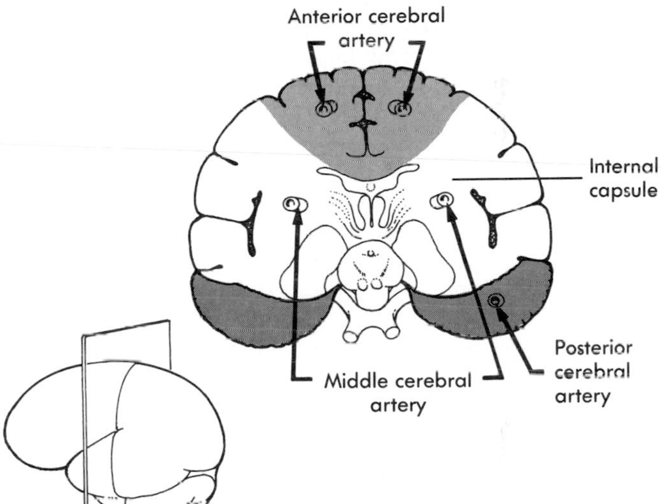

Fig. 25-21 Distribution of arterial blood supply.

♦ **Protective mechanisms**

Bony structures. The bony structure that encases the spinal cord is the vertebral column. Comprising 33 vertebrae and 24 intervertebral disks, this column, held together by ligaments and tendons, provides support and protection for the spinal cord plus structure and flexibility for body movement. The vertebrae are divided into sections in relation to their appearance. There are 7 cervical vertebrae, 12 thoracic vertebrae, 5 lumbar vertebrae, 5 sacral vertebrae (fused as 1), and 4 coccygeal vertebrae (fused as 1).

Although differences in vertebral appearance exist, the basic structure includes a vertebral body connected by two pedicles to the transverse processes (Fig. 25-22). Two laminae connect the transverse processes to the posterior segment of the vertebra, the spinous process,

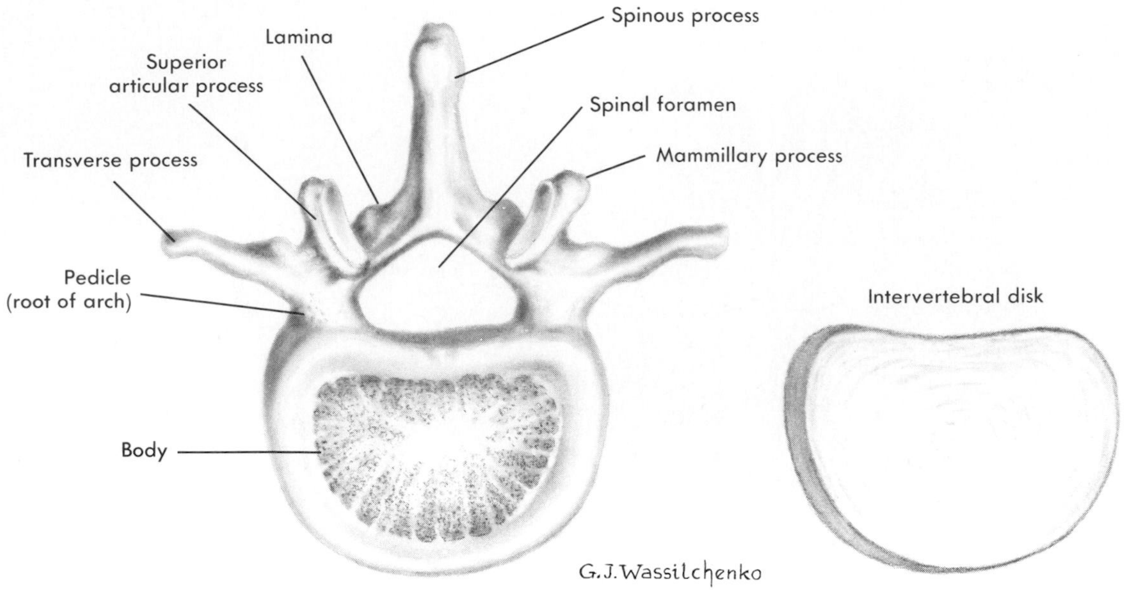

Fig. 25-22 Vertebra and intervertebral disk.

forming a ring. In the center of the spinal foramen is the canal, which houses the spinal cord.

Intervertebral disk. The bodies of the vertebrae are separated by an intervertebral disk. These fibrocartilaginous structures are between each vertebral body from the first cervical vertebrae to the beginning of the sacrum. The intervertebral disk is composed of two layers. The inner core, the nucleus pulposus, is a soft, gelatinous material, which assists in shock absorbancy along the spinal column. Surrounding the nucleus pulposus is the annulus fibrosus. This thick, tough outer layer provides firmer structure to assist the spinal column in supporting the weight of the body when upright.

When a patient suffering from severe back and leg pain is diagnosed as having a herniated disk, the annulus fibrosus has usually torn and a portion of the nucleus pulposus has herniated into the spinal foramen, pressing against the spinal nerve root as it exits the spinal cord across the pedicle. If surgery is required, a *laminectomy* or *diskectomy* is performed. It involves removal of one lamina to gain entrance to the spinal foramen. The herniated portion of the disk is then removed and pressure relieved.

Meninges. The meninges of the spinal cord are similar to those in the cranium (Fig. 25-23). The first meninges, the dura, is a continuation of the inner layer of the intracranial dura. Dura of the spinal cord encases the cord, the nerve roots, and the spinal nerves until they exit from the vertebral column. The dura extends to the level of the second sacral vertebra, even though the spinal cord itself ends at the L1 or L2 level.

The arachnoid membrane is the same weblike, delicate tissue that is in the cranium. Cerebrospinal fluid (CSF) flows in the subarachnoid space of the spinal cord also. Because the spinal cord terminates at L2 and the meninges continue to S2, a volume of CSF is contained in this space and can be tapped through a lumbar puncture procedure. The pia mater of the spinal cord is a thicker, firmer, less vascular membrane than that in the cranium.

◆ **Spinal nerves.** There are 31 spinal nerve pairs: 8 cervical, 12 thoracic, 5 lumbar, 5 sacral, and 1 coccygeal (Fig. 25-24).

In the cervical region the first seven pairs of nerves exit the cord above the corresponding vertebrae. The C8 nerve pair exits the spinal cord below the C7 vertebra. From this point on, all thoracic, lumbar, and sacral nerves exit below the corresponding vertebrae.

The spinal nerve has two roots: the dorsal root and the ventral root. The dorsal root is an afferent pathway and carries sensory impulses from the body into the spinal cord. The ventral root is an efferent pathway and carries motor information from the spinal cord to the body. The dorsal and ventral roots join together as they exit the spinal foramen and become a spinal nerve. Distribution of the sensory components of the spinal nerve has been well-defined. Displayed as sensory dermatomes, these diagrams allow identification of sensory innervation in the peripheral nervous system (Fig. 25-25).

◆ **Cross section.** The spinal cord is composed of both gray matter and white matter.[2,6] The central gray matter, which appears in the shape of an H, consists of cell bodies, small projection fibers, and glial support cells. The gray matter has been divided into areas based on the cell body type located within their boundaries. The three basic divisions are the anterior horn, the lateral horn, and the posterior horn. The anterior horn contains motor cells and is the final junction of motor information before it exits the CNS. The lateral horn contains preganglionic fibers of the autonomic nervous system: sympathetic fibers T1 to L2 and parasympathetic fibers S2 to S4. The posterior horn contains axons from the peripheral sensory neurons.

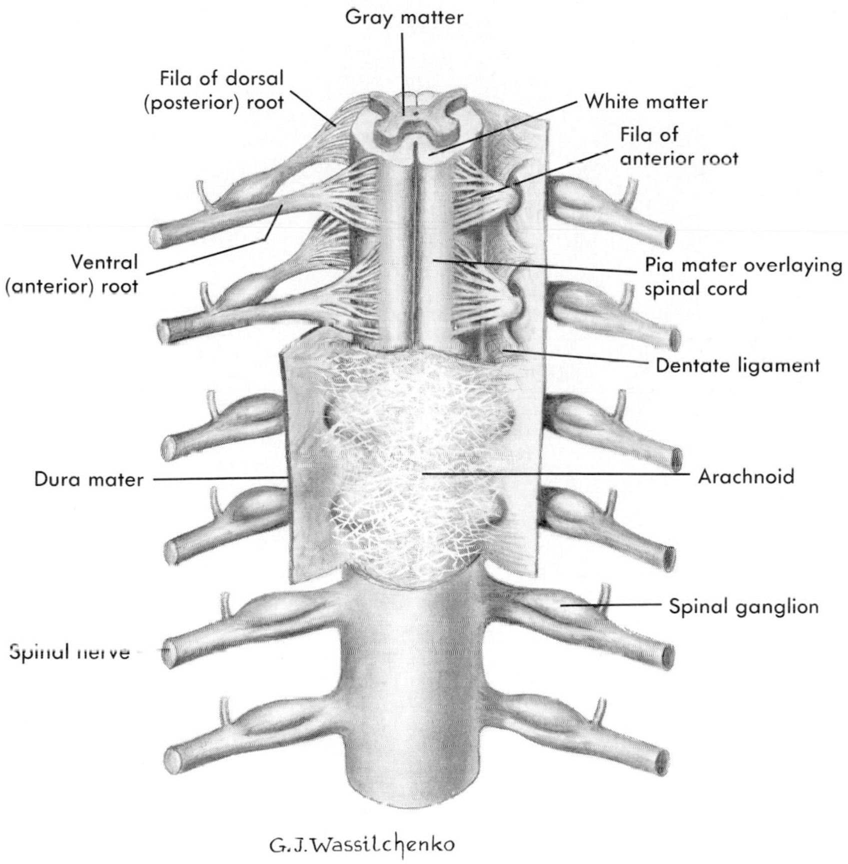

Fig. 25-23 Meningeal layers of the spinal cord. Segment of spinal cord is viewed from behind with portions of dura mater and arachnoid removed.

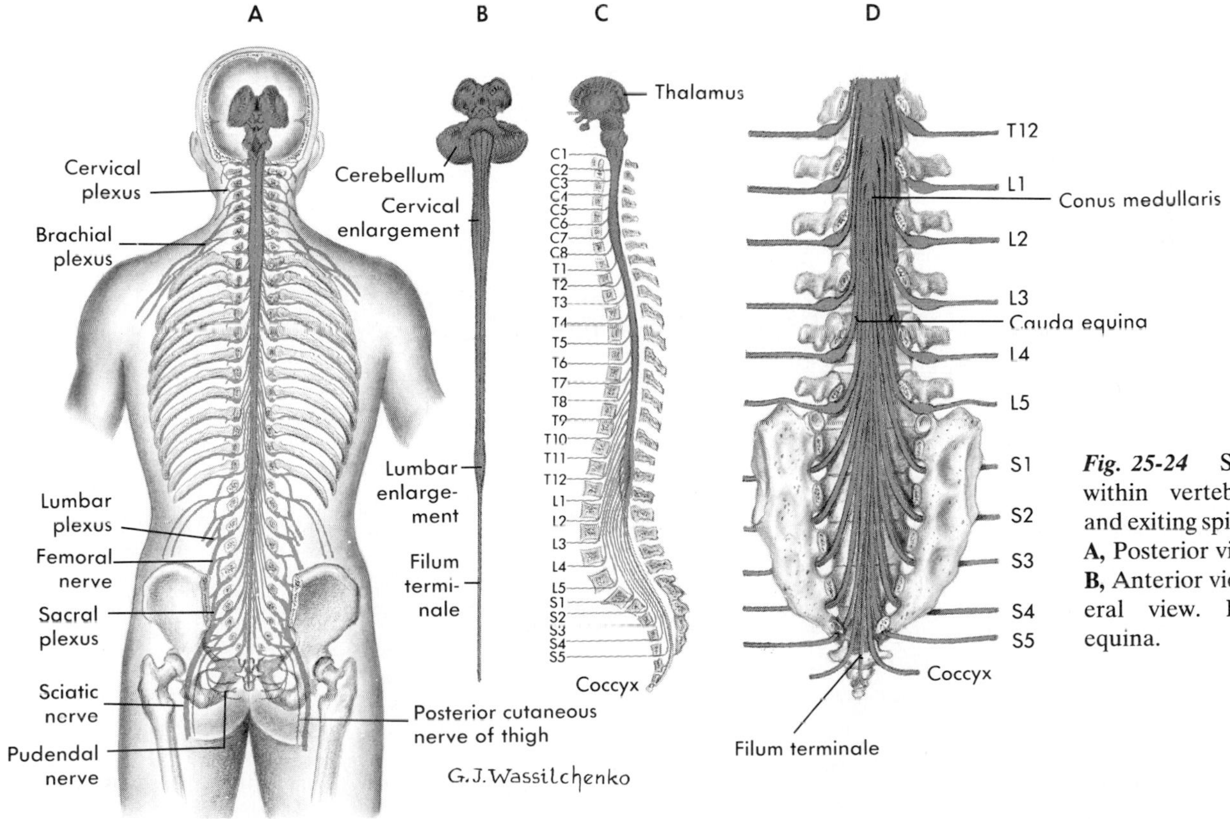

Fig. 25-24 Spinal cord within vertebral canal and exiting spinal nerves. **A,** Posterior view in situ. **B,** Anterior view. **C,** Lateral view. **D,** Cauda equina.

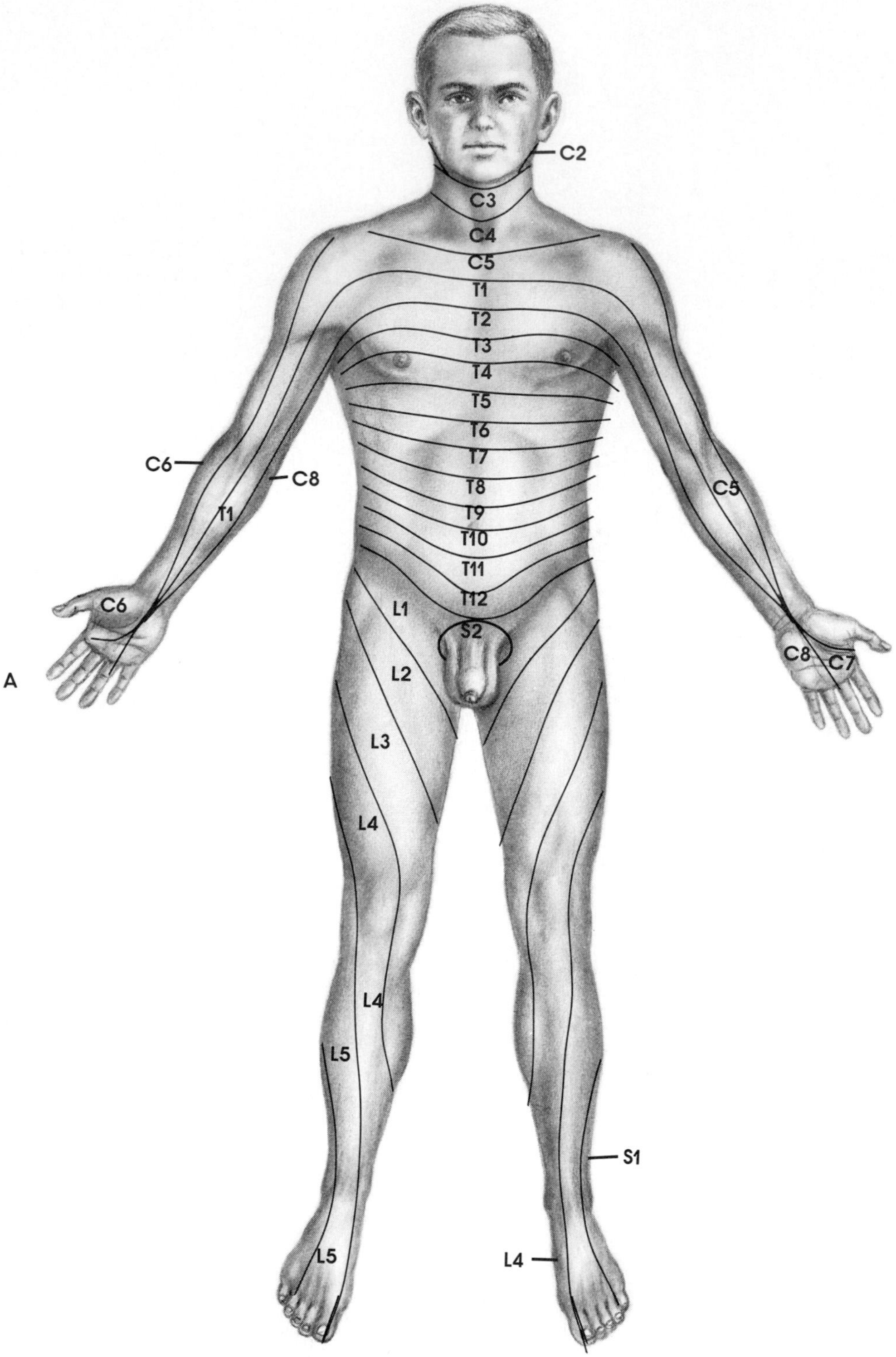

Fig. 25-25 Dermatomes. **A,** Anterior view. **B,** Posterior view.

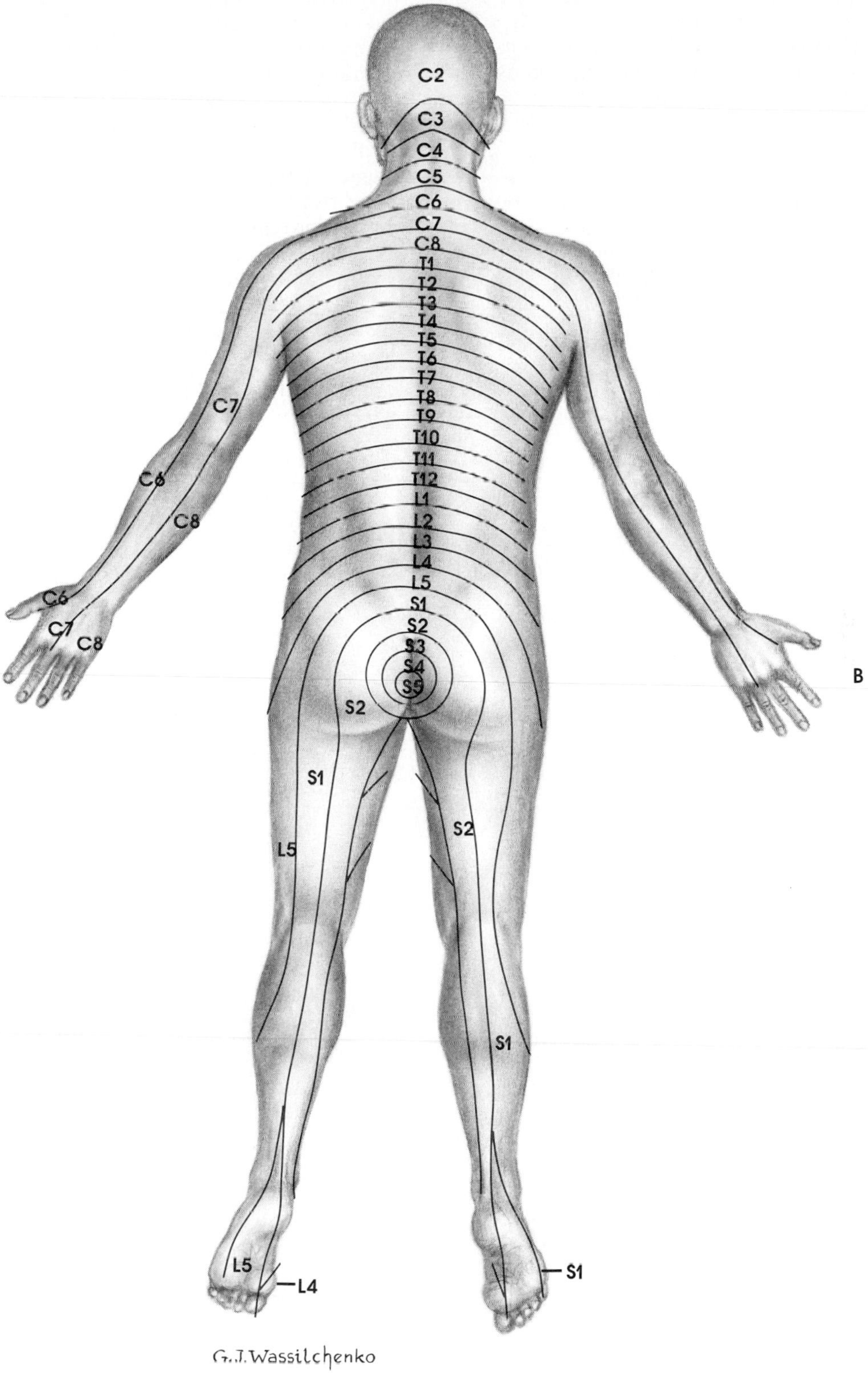

Fig. 25-25—cont'd For legend, see opposite page.

The white matter, which surrounds the gray matter, contains the myelinated ascending and descending tracts, which carry information to and from the brain (Fig. 25-26). Spinal tracts are named so that the *prefix denotes the origin of the tract and the suffix is the destination,* thus allowing easy identification of sensory or motor tracts. Sensory tracts begin with the prefix *spino* and motor tracts end with the suffix *spinal.*

Ascending or sensory tracts	*Descending or motor tracts*
Lateral spinothalamic tract: ascension of pain and thermal sensations	Ventral and lateral corticospinal tracts: descending voluntary motor tracts
Anterior spinothalamic tract: ascension of light touch and pressure sensation	Rubrospinal tract: originates in the nucleus of the midbrain; receives fibers from cerebellum and descends in the lateral and anterior funiculi; conveys impulses to control muscle synergy and tone
Posterior white columns: ascension of discriminatory touch	

Many other motor and sensory tracts are within the spinal cord, but only those presented here can be clinically tested.

◆ **Vascular supply.** Supply of arterial blood to the spinal cord comes from branches of the vertebral arteries plus small radicular arteries that enter at the intervertebral foramina. They combine to form the anterior spinal and two posterior spinal arteries. These three arteries, along with some additional radicular arterial flow from cervical, intercostal, lumbar, and sacral arteries, feed the entire length of the spinal cord (Fig. 25-27).

Arterial supply to the spinal cord is segmented at best; therefore certain portions of the spinal cord that receive their blood supply from two separate sources are vulnerable areas. These vulnerable areas are C2 to C3, T1 to T4, and L1 to L2. Evidence of this tenuous blood supply can occasionally be noted in a patient after open heart surgery or abdominal aortic aneurysm repair who becomes paraplegic because of loss of the small arterial feeders from the aorta responsible for spinal cord circulation.

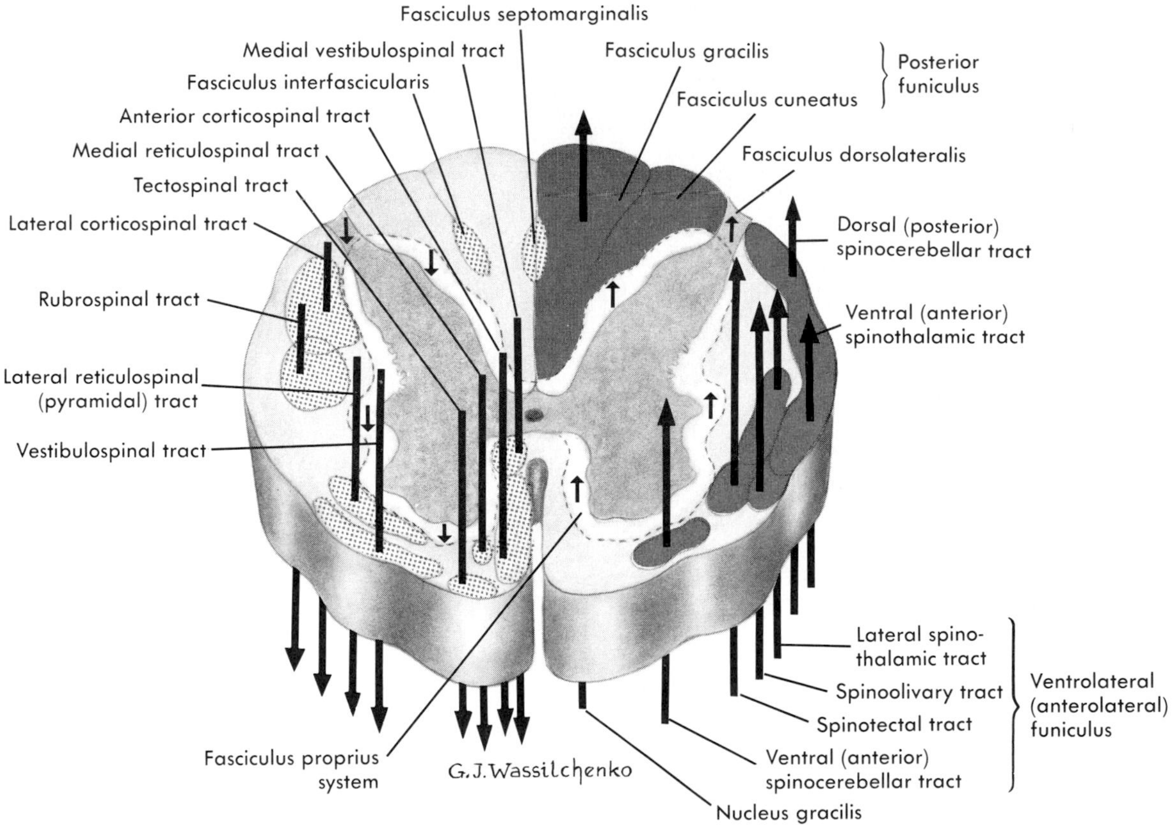

Fig. 25-26 Spinal cord tracts of the white matter.

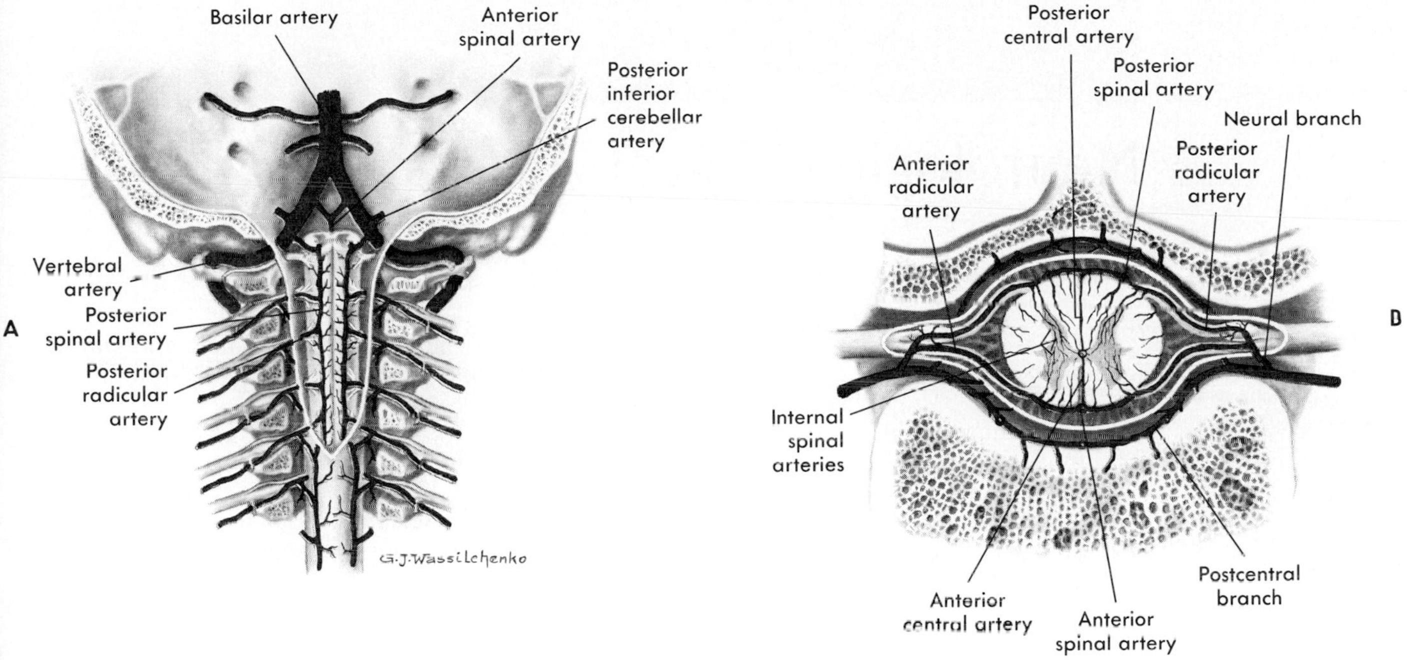

Fig. 25-27 Arteries of spinal cord. **A,** Cervical cord arteries. **B,** Vascular distribution in spinal cord.

REFERENCES

1. Guyton A: *Textbook of medical physiology,* ed 8, Philadelphia, 1991, WB Saunders.
2. Rudy EB: *Advanced neurological and neurosurgical nursing,* St Louis, 1984, Mosby–Year Book.
3. Snell R: *Clinical neuroanatomy for medical students,* ed 3, Boston, 1992, Little, Brown.
4. Hickey JV: *The clinical practice of neurological and neurosurgical nursing,* ed 3, Philadelphia, 1992, JB Lippincott.
5. Chusid JG: *Correlative neuroanatomy and functional neurophysiology,* ed 19, Los Altos, Calif, 1985, Lange Medical Publications.
6. Gilman S, Winans S: *Manter and Gatz's essentials of clinical neuroanatomy and neurophysiology,* ed 8, Philadelphia, 1992, FA Davis.
7. Williams PL, Warwick R, editors: *Gray's anatomy,* ed 37, New York, 1989, Churchill Livingstone.
8. Ricci MM: *American Association of Neuroscience Nurses core curriculum for neuroscience nursing,* ed 2, Chicago, 1984, AANN.

26

Neurologic Clinical Assessment

CHAPTER OBJECTIVES

- List the five components of the neurologic assessment.
- Discuss the acceptable and unacceptable methods of applying noxious stimuli.
- Describe the pathway of pupillary response.
- Define the respiratory patterns associated with neurologic deterioration.
- State the changes in vital signs associated with neurologic deterioration.
- Define brain death and persistent vegetative state.

Assessment of the patient with actual or potential neurologic dysfunction is the essential beginning point in the nursing process and forms the basis for nursing diagnosis. Only when the nurse is aware of all components of a patient's physiologic dysfunction can appropriate diagnosing, planning, intervention, and evaluation take place. This chapter presents a basic introduction to a neurologic examination in the critical care environment.

HISTORY

Neurologic assessment encompasses a wide variety of applications and a multitude of techniques. This chapter focuses on the type of assessment performed in a critical care environment. The one factor common to all neurologic assessments is the need to obtain a comprehensive history of events preceding hospitalization. An adequate neurologic history includes information about clinical manifestations, associated complaints, precipitating factors, progression, and familial occurrences. If the patient is incapable of providing this information, family members or significant others should be contacted as soon as possible. When someone other than the patient is the source of the history, it should be an individual who was in contact with the patient on a daily basis. Frequently, valuable information is gained, which directs the caregiver to focus on certain aspects of the patient's clinical assessment.

PHYSICAL EXAMINATION

Five major components make up the neurologic examination of the critically ill patient. They are evaluation of (1) level of consciousness, (2) motor movements, (3) pupillary function and eye movement, (4) respiratory patterns, and (5) vital signs. Until all five components have been assessed, a complete neurologic examination has not been performed.

Level of Consciousness

Assessment of the level of consciousness is the most important aspect of the neurologic examination. In most situations a patient's level of consciousness deteriorates before any other neurologic changes are noted. These deteriorations often are subtle and must be monitored carefully.

Level of consciousness assessment is a component of the mental status examination. Other components of the mental status examination include speech and language, memory, general information, calculation, and abstraction and judgment. In the critical care environment the assessment of these components may occur initially but usually is not a part of an ongoing evaluation.

◆ **Components of consciousness.** There are two major components of consciousness: *arousal or alertness* and *content of consciousness or awareness.*[1]

Arousal. Assessment of the arousal component of consciousness is an evaluation of the reticular activating system and its connection with the thalamus and the cerebral cortex. Arousal is the lowest level of consciousness, and observation centers on the patient's ability to respond to verbal or noxious stimuli in an appropriate manner.

Awareness. Content of consciousness is a higher-level function and is concerned with assessment of the patient's orientation to person, place, and time. Assessment of content of consciousness requires the patient to give appropriate answers to a variety of questions. Changes in the patient's answers that indicate increasing degrees of confusion and disorientation may be the first sign of neurologic deterioration.

◆ **Categories of consciousness.** The following categories, although vague, are often used to describe the patient's level of consciousness.[1]

Alert—Patient responds immediately to minimal external stimuli.

Lethargic—State of drowsiness or inaction in which the patient needs an increased stimulus to be awakened.

Obtunded—A duller indifference to external stimuli exists, and response is minimally maintained.

Stuporous—The patient can be aroused only by vigorous and continuous external stimuli.

Comatose—Vigorous stimulation fails to produce any voluntary neural response.

Frequently it is difficult to categorize patients under these descriptions. Also, the levels of consciousness are not defined in enough detail, and communication of patient condition often is misinterpreted. One clinician, for example, might describe a patient's response as *obtunded,* whereas the next clinician might describe the same response as *stuporous.* Because of this difficulty in communicating level of consciousness, a variety of assessment tools have been devised to assist in this evaluation.

◆ **Tools for assessment of consciousness.** The general rule for evaluation of an altered level of consciousness is to determine systematically the type and degree of noxious stimuli required to produce a response. This concept is incorporated into a variety of clinical assessment tools.

The most widely recognized level of consciousness assessment tool is the Glasgow Coma Scale (GCS).[2] This scored scale is based on evaluation of three categories: eye opening, verbal response, and best motor response (Table 26-1). The best possible score on the GCS is 15, and the lowest score is 3. Generally a score of 7 or less on the GCS indicates coma.

Originally the scoring system was developed to assist general communication concerning the severity of neurologic injury. Adapted and modified, this scale has become the basis of many neurologic assessment flow sheets. Several points should be kept in mind when the GCS is used for serial assessment. It provides data about level of consciousness only and never should be considered a complete neurologic examination. It is not a sensitive tool for evaluation of an altered sensorium. The GCS does not account for possible aphasia. The GCS is not a good indicator of lateralization of neurologic deterioration. Lateralization involves decreasing motor response on one side or changes in pupillary reaction.

Whatever assessment tool is chosen to measure level of consciousness, the goal is to identify subtle changes in consciousness responses. Communication of small signs of deteriorating consciousness may allow early intervention and thus prevent neurologic disaster.

Motor Movements

◆ **Levels of motor movements.** A simple way of organizing the assessment of motor movements is to use the categories defined in the Glasgow Coma Scale[2] as a guide. The difference in this part of the assessment is that now each extremity is evaluated and recorded individually.

Obeys commands—performs simple tasks on command and is able to repeat performance

Localizes to pain—organized attempt to localize and remove painful stimuli

Withdraws from pain—withdraws extremity from source of painful stimuli

Abnormal flexion—decorticate posturing spontaneously or in response to noxious stimuli

Extension—decerebrate posturing spontaneously or in response to noxious stimuli

Flaccid—no response to noxious stimuli; flaccid

In addition, a comparison of function is made with that of the opposite extremity. In the evaluation of a patient with spinal cord injury or dysfunction, a separate scale should be used with more detail about motor strength of particular muscle groups.

Table 26-1 Glasgow Coma Scale

Category	Score	Response
Eye opening	4	Spontaneous—eyes open spontaneously without stimulation
	3	To speech—eyes open with verbal stimulation but not necessarily to command
	2	To pain—eyes open with noxious stimuli
	1	None—no eye opening regardless of stimulation
Verbal response	5	Oriented—accurate information about person, place, time, reason for hospitalization, and personal data
	4	Confused—answers not appropriate to question, but use of language is correct
	3	Inappropriate words—disorganized, random speech, no sustained conversation
	2	Incomprehensible sounds—moans, groans, and incomprehensible mumbles
	1	None—no verbalization despite stimulation
Best motor response	6	Obeys commands—performs simple tasks on command; able to repeat performance
	5	Localizes to pain—organized attempt to localize and remove painful stimuli
	4	Withdraws from pain—withdraws extremity from source of painful stimuli
	3	Abnormal flexion—decorticate posturing spontaneously or in response to noxious stimuli
	2	Extension—decerebrate posturing spontaneously or in response to noxious stimuli
	1	None—no response to noxious stimuli; flaccid

◆ **Abnormal motor responses.** In the unconscious patient noxious stimuli may elicit an abnormal motor response (Fig. 26-1). These responses are identified as abnormal flexion (decorticate posturing) or extension (decerebrate posturing). The assessment of abnormal flexion and extension is an integral part of the motor component of the GCS. The exact anatomic location of these abnormal responses remains a mystery. Generally the severity of damage to the brain precludes localization of the lesion that causes these abnormal movements.[1]

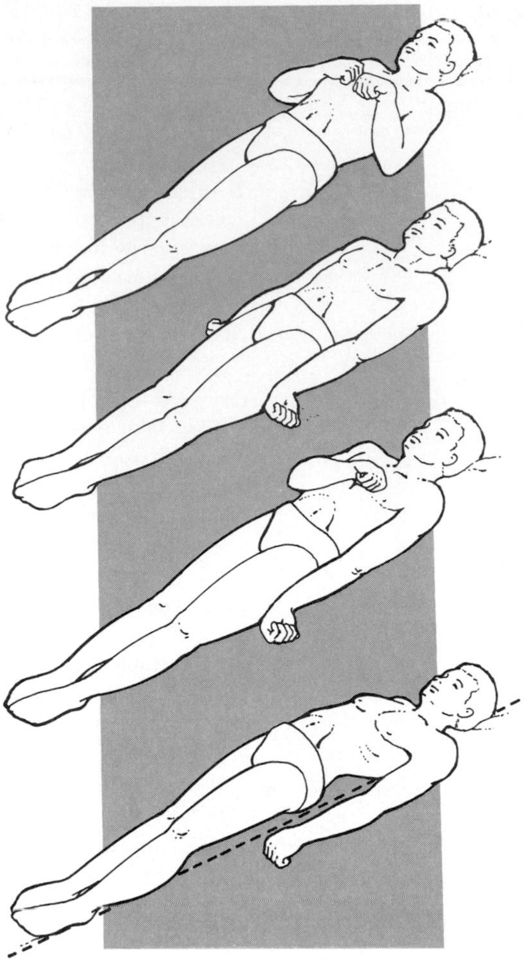

Fig. 26-1 Abnormal motor responses. **A,** Decorticate posturing. **B,** Decerebrate posturing. **C,** Decorticate posturing on right side and decerebrate posturing on left side of body. **D,** Opisthotonic posturing.

Abnormal flexion. Abnormal flexion also is known as *decorticate posturing.* In response to painful stimuli, the upper extremities exhibit flexion of the arm, wrist, and fingers with adduction of the limb. The lower extremity exhibits extension, internal rotation, and plantar flexion.

Extension. Extension also is known as *decerebrate rigidity,* or *posturing.* When the patient is stimulated, teeth clench and the arms are stiffly extended, adducted, and hyperpronated. The legs are stiffly extended with plantar flexion of the feet.

Because abnormal flexion and extension appear similar in the lower extremities, the upper extremities are used to determine the presence of these abnormal movements. It is possible for the patient to exhibit abnormal flexion on one side of the body and extension on the other. Outcome studies indicate that abnormal flexion or decorticate posturing has a less serious prognosis than does extension, or decerebrate posturing.[1]

◆ Motor assessment techniques

Obeys commands. Next to the assessment of orientation and awareness, the assessment of the patient's ability to follow commands is one of the highest levels of functioning evaluated. Several points must be recognized in assessing ability to follow commands. Commands given to a patient with an altered level of consciousness must be phrased in simple and direct statements, such as: "Show me your thumb." A common error made by clinicians in assessing the patient's ability to respond to commands is to include the simple command along with other verbal communication. To prevent sensory overload and therefore the patient's inability to respond to command, the command should not be included as part of any other conversation. An example of the inappropriate use of a simple command is: "Robert, your mother is here. Let's show her how much better you are doing. Robert, show her your thumb. Come on Robert, you did it for me an hour ago. Robert, show your mother your thumb. She will be very excited if she could see you do this. Robert, I know you can do it. Don't be stubborn." As a patient is emerging from an unconscious state, the brain is less capable of simultaneous processing and sorting of multiple stimuli. The key to assessment of the patient's ability to follow commands is to reduce surrounding stimuli or distractors and to keep the command simple and direct.

Another error commonly made in the assessment of the patient's ability to follow commands involves the type of command given. Appropriate commands are those that do not elicit random or reflex responses. "Squeeze my hand" is a common command used by caregivers and family alike. In low levels of consciousness, the reflex of hand grasp, if present, is initiated when the assessor's hand is placed within the patient's hand. If this is the case, it often is difficult to assess accurately whether the patient is responding to command or exhibiting a reflex response. Asking the patient to "Let go of my hand" after hand grasp also is difficult to assess accurately. Relaxation of the reflex can mimic the command: "Let go." Use of hand grasp in assessment of the patient's motor strength is separate from this discussion.

Acceptable commands include: "Show me your thumb" or "Stick out your tongue." When these commands are used, care must be taken that the command is not followed by visual or tactile stimuli. It is not uncommon to observe an assessment in which the nurse asks the patient to "show me your thumb" while tapping the patient's thumb. With this scenario it is impossible to determine whether the patient is following a verbal command or withdrawing from tactile stimuli.

Noxious stimuli. Once it has been determined that the patient is incapable of comprehending and following a simple command, the use of noxious stimuli is required to determine motor responses. A variety of acceptable ways of administering painful stimuli are presented here. Several commonly used but unacceptable means of delivering noxious stimuli also are discussed.

ACCEPTABLE

1. *Nail bed pressure* is an acceptable form of noxious stimuli. It requires use of an object such as a pen to apply firm pressure to the nailbed. Pressure applied to each extremity allows evaluation of individual extremity function. The patient's movement must not be inter-

rupted while the nurse is applying the nailbed pressure. Although this pressure is classified as noxious stimuli, if no response is elicited from nailbed pressure, other noxious stimuli measures should be employed.

2. *Trapezius pinch* is another acceptable method of delivering noxious stimuli. Performed by squeezing the trapezius muscle, this method allows for observation of total body response to stimuli. Trapezius pinch often is difficult to perform on large or obese adults.

3. *Pinching of the inner aspect of the arm or leg* is the final acceptable form of administering noxious stimuli. A small portion of the patient's tissue on the sensitive inner aspect of the arm or leg is pinched firmly, and each extremity is evaluated independently. Although this form of noxious stimuli is the most apt to cause bruising, it also is the most sensitive for eliciting a movement response.

UNACCEPTABLE

1. *Sternal rub* often is used as a form of noxious stimuli. Firm pressure is applied to the sternum in a rubbing motion, usually with the assessor's knuckles. If used repeatedly, the sternum could become excoriated, open, and infected. Open-handed firm patting of the sternal area to arouse the patient is acceptable.

2. *Supraorbital pressure* is another form of noxious stimuli that should be avoided. Patients with head injuries, frontal craniotomies, or facial surgery should not be evaluated with this method because of the possibility of underlying fractured or unstable cranium. Therefore it is better not to apply supraorbital pressure to deliver noxious stimuli.

3. *Nipple pinching and testicle pinching* has been used for many years. Although never described in texts as an acceptable method for delivering noxious stimuli, it often can be observed in the clinical setting. For obvious reasons this type of noxious stimuli is inappropriate and unnecessary.

◆ **Assessment of lateralizing signs.** Lateralizing signs are neurologic findings that occur only on one side of the body, such as unilateral deterioration in motor movements or changes in pupillary response. Lateralizing signs help to localize the lesion to one side of the brain. For example, a patient who was withdrawing to painful stimuli with both arms at the last examination is now withdrawing on the right but exhibiting abnormal flexion on the left. This change in response on the left side points to an expanding intracranial lesion on the right.

The occurrence of lateralizing signs indicates an emergency situation. Unilateral deterioration of motor movements and pupillary response may herald herniation. Notification of the physician and immediate intervention are imperative.

Pupillary Function and Eye Movement

The assessment of pupillary function and eye movement is an important component of the neurologic examination.[3] Especially in the unconscious patient or the patient receiving neuromuscular blocking agents and sedation, pupillary response is one of the few neurologic signs that can be assessed. Serial evaluation, appropriate technique, recognition of abnormalities, and good documentation are all important.

◆ **Anatomy of pupillary response.** Pupillary reaction is a function of the autonomic nervous system. Parasympathetic control of pupillary reaction occurs through innervation of the oculomotor nerve (cranial nerve [CN] III), which exits from the brainstem in the midbrain area. When the parasympathetic fibers are stimulated, the pupil constricts. Sympathetic control of the pupil originates in the hypothalamus and travels down the entire length of the brainstem. When the sympathetic fibers are stimulated, the pupil dilates (Table 26-2).

Pupillary changes provide a valuable tool to assessment because of pathway location (Fig. 26-2). The oculomotor nerve lies at the junction of the midbrain and the tentorial notch. Any increase of pressure that exerts

Table 26-2 Pathways of pupillary response

Sympathetic	Parasympathetic
Brainstem	CN III
Dilates	Constricts

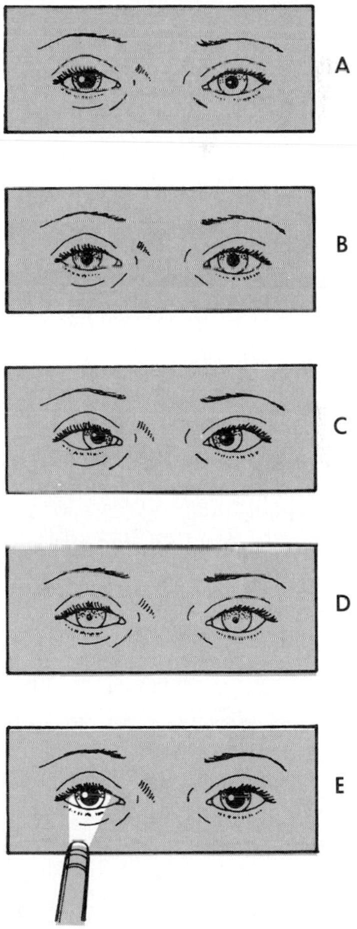

Fig. 26-2 Abnormal pupillary responses. **A,** Oculomotor nerve compression. **B,** Bilateral diencephalon damage. **C,** Midbrain damage. **D,** Pontine damage. **E,** Dilated, nonreactive pupils.

force down through the tentorial notch compresses the oculomotor nerve. Oculomotor nerve compression results in a dilated, nonreactive pupil. Sympathetic pathway disruption occurs with involvement in the brainstem. Loss of sympathetic control leads to pinpoint, nonreactive pupils. Pupillary reactivity also is affected by medications, particularly sympathetic and parasympathetic agents, direct trauma, and eye surgery. Pupillary reactivity is relatively resistant to metabolic dysfunction and can be used to differentiate between metabolic and structural causes of decreased levels of consciousness.

◆ **Anatomy of eye movement.** Control of eye movements occurs with interaction of three cranial nerves: oculomotor (CN III), trochlear (CN IV), and abducens (CN VI). The pathways for these cranial nerves provide integrated function through the internuclear pathway of the medial longitudinal fasciculus (MLF) located in the brainstem. The MLF provides coordination of eye movements with the vestibular and reticular formation (Fig. 26-3).

◆ **Assessment of pupillary response.** Evaluation of pupillary response includes assessment of size, shape (round, irregular, or oval), and degree of reactivity to light. The two pupils should be compared for equality. Any of these components of the pupil assessment could change in response to increasing pressure on the oculomotor nerve at the tentorium.

Pupil size should be documented in millimeters with the use of a pupil gauge to reduce the subjectivity of describing the pupil as small, medium, large, dilated, and so on. Although the pupils of most persons are of equal size, a discrepancy up to 1 mm between the two pupils is normal. Inequality of pupils is known as *anisocoria* and occurs in 15% to 17% of the human population.

Change or inequality in pupil size, especially in patients who previously have not shown this discrepancy, is a significant neurologic sign. It may indicate impending danger of herniation and should be reported immediately. With the location of the oculomotor nerve (CN III) at the notch of the tentorium, pupil size and reactivity play a key role in the physical assessment of intracranial pressure changes and herniation syndromes. In addition to CN III compression, changes in pupil size occur for other reasons. Large pupils can result from the instillation of cycloplegic agents, such as atropine or scopolamine, or can indicate extreme stress. Extremely small pupils can indicate narcotic overdose, lower brainstem compression, or bilateral damage to the pons.

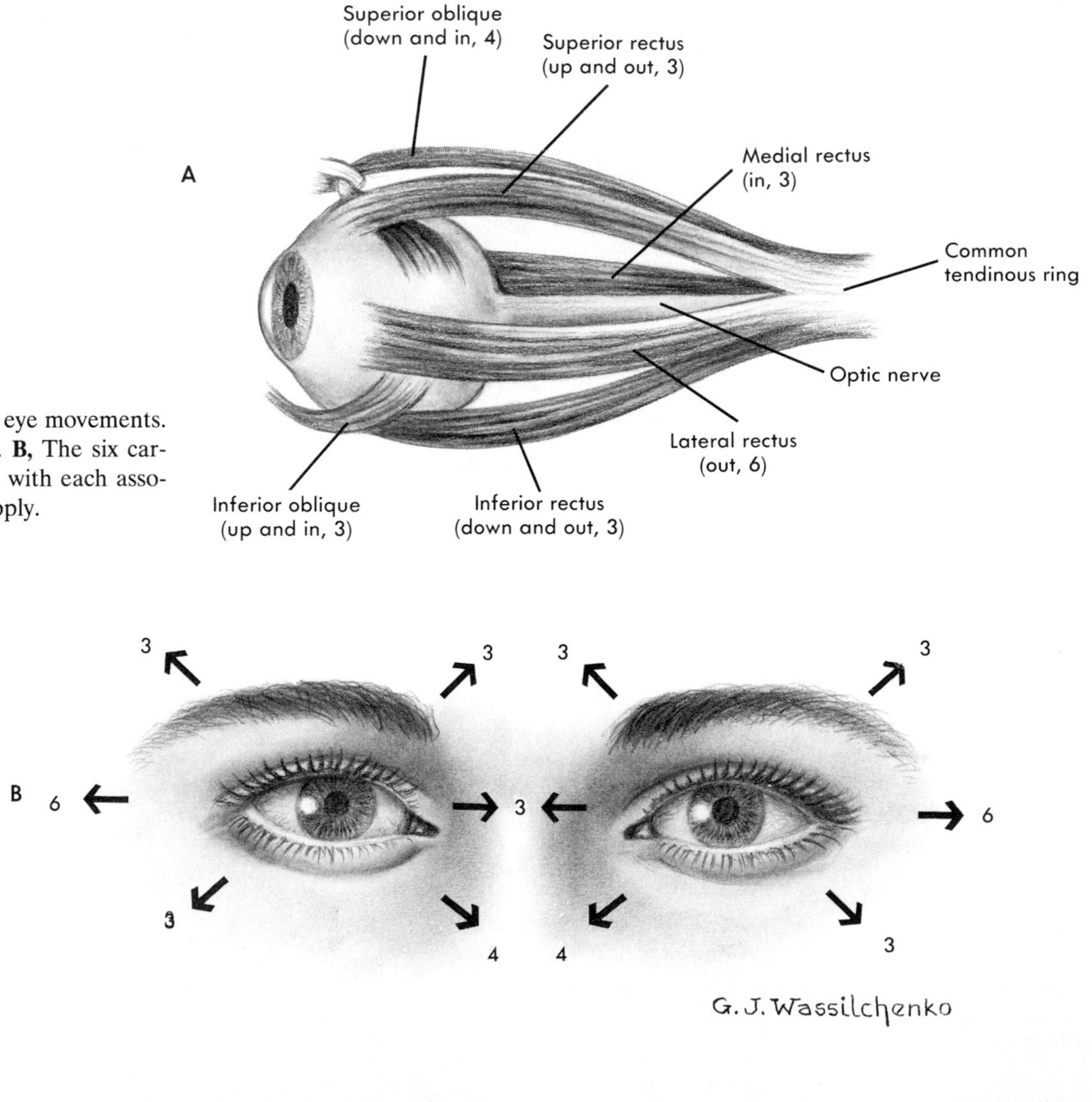

Fig. 26-3 Extraocular eye movements. **A,** Extraocular muscles. **B,** The six cardinal directions of gaze with each associated cranial nerve supply.

Pupil shape also is noted in the assessment of pupils. Although the pupil normally is round, an irregularly shaped or oval pupil may be noted in patients with elevated intracranial pressure. An oval pupil can indicate the initial stages of CN III compression. It has been observed that an oval pupil almost always is associated with an intracranial pressure (ICP) between 18 and 35 mm Hg.[4] The oval pupil appears to represent a transitional pupil that will return to normal size if ICP can be controlled but that will progress to dilation and unreactivity if ICP is not treated or cannot be controlled.[5]

The technique for evaluation of direct pupillary response to light involves use of a narrow-beamed bright light shone into the pupil from the outer canthus of the eye. If the light is shone directly onto the pupil, glare or reflection of the light may prevent the assessor's proper visualization. Concensual pupillary response is the constriction of the pupil in response to a light shone into the opposite eye.

◆ Assessment of eye movements

Extraocular movements. In the conscious patient the function of the three cranial nerves of the eye and their MLF innervation can be assessed by the nurse's asking the patient to follow a finger through the full range of eye motions. If the eyes move together into all six fields, extraocular movements (EOM) are intact.[6]

Oculocephalic reflex (doll's eyes). In the unconscious patient, assessment of ocular function and the innervation of the MLF is performed by eliciting the doll's eyes reflex. If the patient is unconscious as a result of trauma, the nurse should ascertain the absence of cervical injury before performing this examination.

To assess the oculocephalic reflex, the nurse should hold the patient's eyelids open and briskly turn the head to one side while observing the eye movements, then briskly turn the head to the other side and observe. If the oculocephalic reflex is intact, the doll's eyes reflex is present. The eyes deviate to the opposite direction in which the head is turned. If the oculocephalic reflex is not intact, the reflex is absent. This lack of response, in which the eyes remain midline and move with the head, indicates significant brainstem injury. If the oculocephalic reflex is abnormal, the doll's eyes reflex is abnormal. In this situation the eyes rove or move in opposite directions. Abnormal oculocephalic reflex indicates some degree of brainstem injury (Fig. 26-4).

Oculovestibular reflex (cold caloric test). The oculovestibular reflex usually is performed by a physician as one of the final clinical assessments of brainstem function. Twenty to 50 ml of ice water is injected into the external auditory canal. The normal eye movement response is a rapid nystagmus-like deviation toward the irrigated ear. This response indicates brainstem integrity. This test is an extremely noxious stimulation and may produce a decorticate or decerebrate posturing response in the comatose patient. This procedure is not recommended for use on a conscious patient (Fig. 26-5). An abnormal response is dysconjugate eye movement, which indicates a brainstem lesion, or no response, which indicates little to no brainstem function.

Respiratory Patterns

◆ Control of respirations. The activity of respiration is a highly integrated function that receives input from the cerebrum, brainstem, and metabolic mechanisms. A close correlation exists in clinical assessment among altered levels of consciousness, the level of brain or brainstem injury, and the respiratory pattern noted (Fig. 26-6).

Under the influence of the cerebral cortex and the diencephalon, three brainstem centers control respirations. The lowest center, the medullary respiratory center, sends impulses through the vagus nerve to innervate muscles of inspiration and expiration. The apneustic and pneumotaxic centers of the pons are responsible for the length of inspiration and expiration and the underlying respiratory rate.

◆ Respiratory patterns. Changes in respiratory patterns assist in identifying the level of brainstem dysfunction or injury. The respiratory patterns are defined in Table 26-3.

Evaluation of respiratory pattern also must include evaluation of the effectiveness of gas exchange in maintaining adequate oxygen and carbon dioxide levels. Hypoventilation is not uncommon in the patient with an altered level of consciousness. Alterations in oxygenation or carbon dioxide levels can result in further neurologic dysfunction. ICP increases with hypoxemia or hypercapnia.

Finally, assessment of the respiratory function in a patient with neurologic deficit must include assessment of airway maintenance and secretion control. Cough, gag, and swallow reflexes responsible for protection of the airway may be absent or diminished.

Several respiratory patterns have been noted to occur with metabolic disorders, such as Kussmaul's respirations. These respiratory patterns are initiated in the cerebral cortex in response to metabolic alterations and are a compensatory mechanism. Respiratory patterns of metabolic disorders are not identified in the same terms as the level of dysfunction of a structural injury.

Vital Signs

The final portion of the neurologic examination is the evaluation of vital signs. As a result of the brain and brainstem influences on cardiac, respiratory, and body temperature functions, changes in vital signs can indicate deterioration in neurologic status.

◆ Cardiac. The brain's tremendous metabolic demand requires an adequate supply of blood for continual perfusion of the brain. Evaluation of the cardiovascular system identifies inappropriate supply for the known cerebral demand.

Decreased cardiac output. For whatever reason (vasodilation, bradycardia, tachycardia, hypovolemia, or inadequate pump), decreased cardiac output leads to decreased perfusion of cerebral tissue, hypoxia, and neurologic injury. In the presence of increased ICP, decreased cardiac output is even more detrimental because low blood pressure must overcome the additional resistance of ICP to provide blood to the brain.

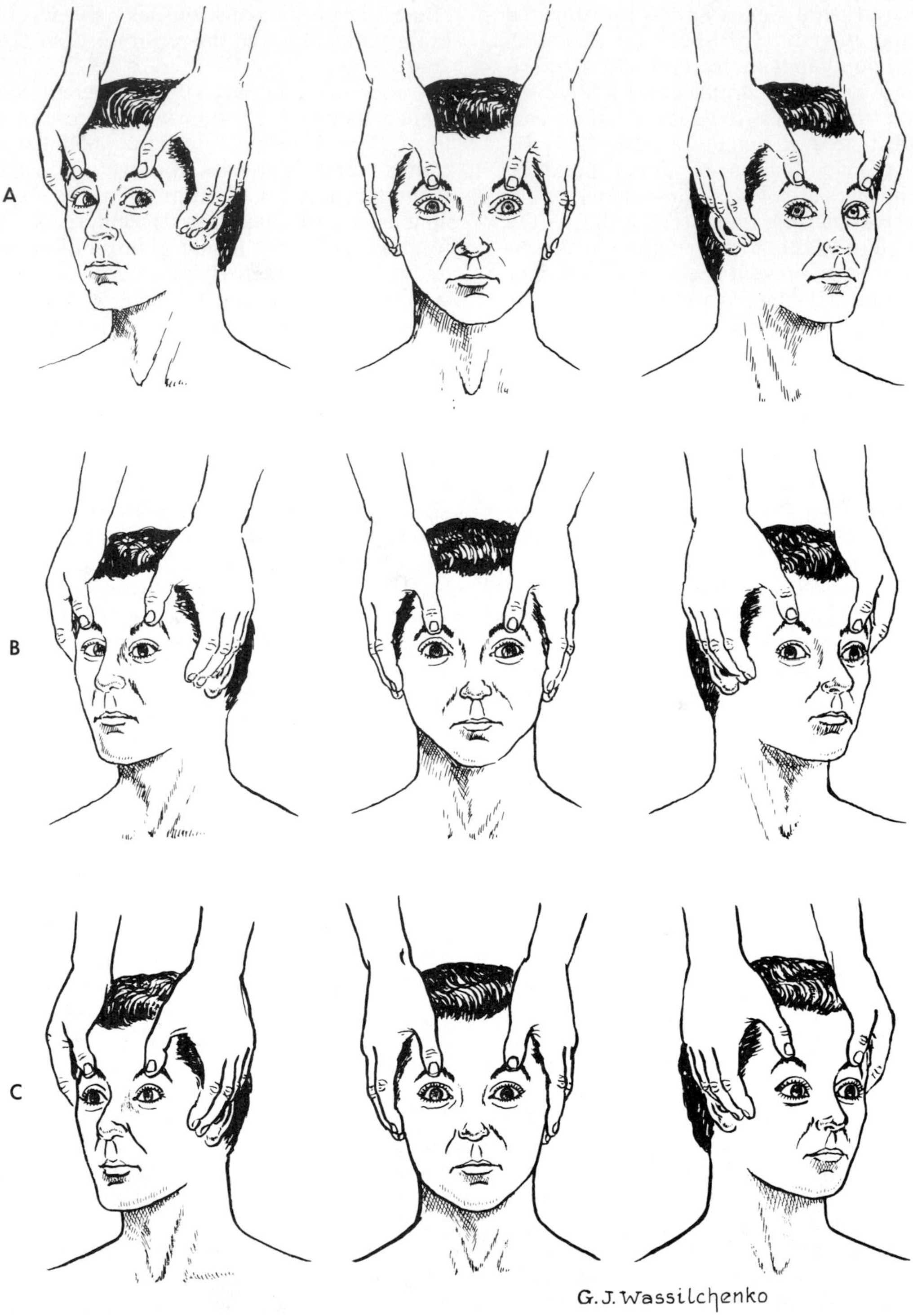

Fig. 26-4 Oculocephalic reflex (doll's eyes). **A,** Normal. **B,** Abnormal. **C,** Absent.

Table 26-3 Respiratory patterns

Pattern of respiration	Description of pattern	Significance
Cheyne-Stokes	Rhythmic crescendo and decrescendo of rate and depth of respiration; includes brief periods of apnea	Usually seen with bilateral deep cerebral lesions or some cerebellar lesions
Central neurogenic hyperventilation	Very deep, very rapid respirations with no apneic periods	Usually seen with lesions of the midbrain and upper pons
Apneustic	Prolonged inspiratory and/or expiratory pause of 2-3 sec	Usually seen in lesions of the mid to lower pons
Cluster breathing	Clusters of irregular, gasping respirations separated by long periods of apnea	Usually seen in lesions of the lower pons or upper medulla
Ataxic respirations	Irregular, random pattern of deep and shallow respirations with irregular apneic periods	Usually seen in lesions of the medulla

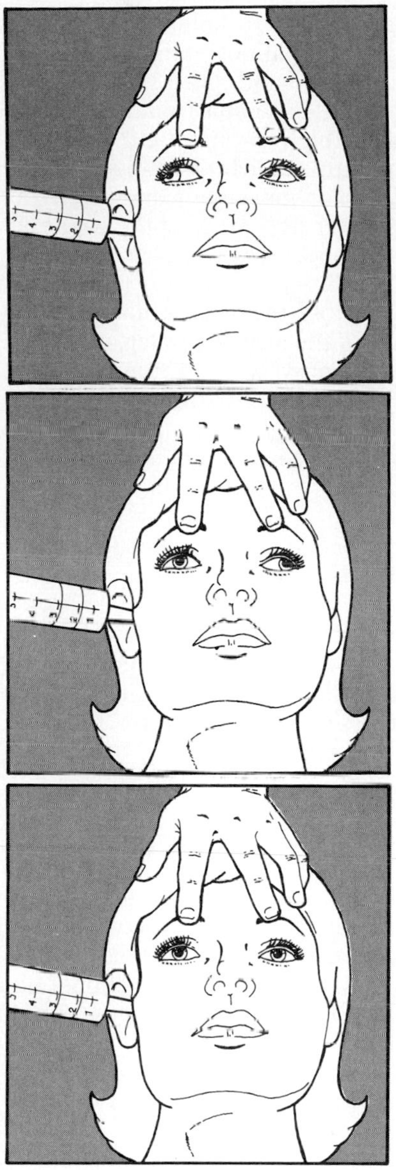
A
B
C

Fig. 26-5 Oculovestibular reflex (cold caloric test). **A,** Normal. **B,** Abnormal. **C,** Absent.

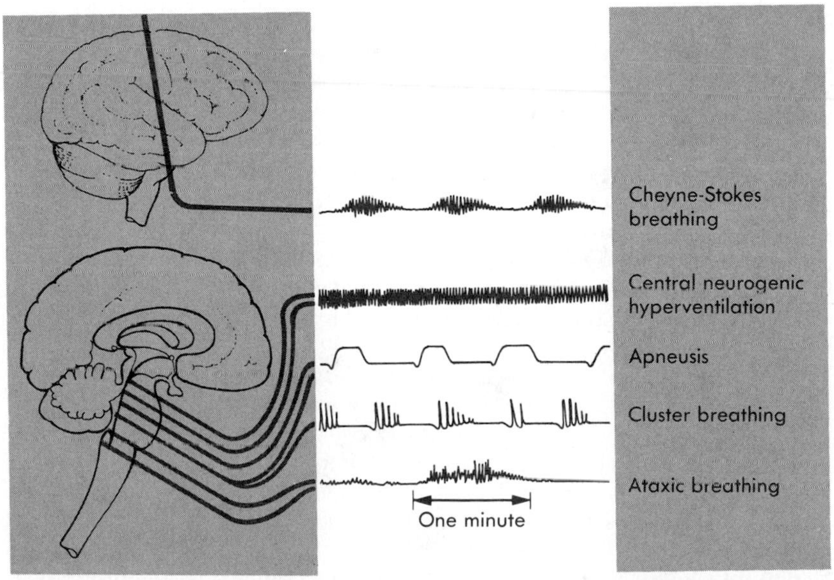

Fig. 26-6 Abnormal respiratory patterns with corresponding level of central nervous system activity.

Hypertension. A common manifestation of the intracranial injury is systemic hypertension. Cerebral autoregulation, responsible for the control of cerebral blood flow, frequently is lost with any type of intracranial injury. After cerebral injury the body often is in a hyperdynamic state (increased heart rate, blood pressure, and cardiac output) as part of a compensatory response. With the loss of autoregulation, as blood pressure increases, cerebral blood flow and cerebral blood volume increase, and therefore ICP increases. Control of systemic hypertension is necessary to stop this cycle.

Bradycardia. The medulla and the vagus nerve provide parasympathetic control to the heart. When stimulated, this lower brainstem system produces bradycardia. Increasing ICP frequently causes bradycardia. Abrupt ICP changes also can produce dysrhythmias, such as premature ventricular contractions (PVCs), atrioventricular (AV) block, or ventricular fibrillation.

Cushing's triad is a set of three clinical manifestations (bradycardia, systolic hypertension, and bradypnea) related to pressure on the medullary area of the brainstem. These signs often occur in response to intracranial hypertension or a herniation syndrome.

The appearance of Cushing's triad is a *late* finding that may be absent in neurologic deterioration. Attention should be paid to alteration in each component of the triad and intervention initiated accordingly.

RAPID NEUROLOGIC EXAMINATION

The Conscious Patient

An adequate neurologic examination should focus on covering all major areas of neurologic control. Any abnormalities identified can then be further evaluated and investigated. A neurologic examination should be organized, thorough, and simple so that it can be performed accurately and easily at each assessment point. The following steps provide an example of a rapid neurologic examination that can be performed in the critical care unit on a conscious patient with known or potential neurologic deficit.

1. *Level of consciousness.* Address the patient and ask a variety of orientation questions. Avoid the obvious, overused questions about name, date, and place, and focus on questions about recent and past events from the patient's experiences, such as spouse's name, home address, what was eaten at the previous meal. Be sure that, as examiner, you are aware of the correct answers to all questions asked.
2. *Facial movements.* During assessment of level of consciousness, observe the patient's facial movements for symmetry. Listen to speech patterns for evidence of slurred speech.
3. *Pupillary function and eye movements.* Perform pupil check and assess extraocular eye movements.
4. *Motor assessment.* Instruct patient to close eyes and to extend arms with palms upturned. Check for evidence of arm drift. This is a relatively sensitive evaluation of upper extremity weakness. Check hand grasp strength by placing two fingers in the palm of each of the patient's hands and instructing him or her to squeeze. (This hand grasp assessment is done to test upper extremity strength, not the patient's ability to follow simple commands.) Both hand grasps should be evaluated simultaneously for comparison of strength. Place hand on patient's thigh and instruct him or her to raise the leg straight up against resistance. Assess both lower extremities for movement and strength. Ask the patient to plantar flex (step on the gas) and dorsiflex (pull his or her toes toward his or her nose) against resistance.
5. *Sensory.* With a finger, stroke the patient bilaterally on the face, upper aspect of the arm, hand, leg, and foot. Ask the patient to identify what is touched and whether there is any difference in sensation between the two sides.
6. *Vital signs.* Note any increases in blood pressure, decreases in heart rate, or change in respiratory patterns.
7. Finally, ask the patient if he or she feels any differences between this and the previous examination.

This examination, which usually takes less than 4 minutes, is meant to provide a starting point. If any neurologic deficit is identified that is new or different from that of the last assessment, attention must be focused in more detail on that abnormality.

The Unconscious Patient

In the assessment of the unconscious patient, initial efforts are directed at achieving maximal arousal of the patient. Calling the patient's name, patting him or her on the chest, or shaking his or her shoulder accomplishes this task. Once the patient has been stimulated, the examiner can proceed with the neurologic examination.

1. *Level of consciousness.* Perform the Glasgow Coma Scale assessment.
2. *Pupillary assessment.* Perform pupillary assessment with special attention to size, reactivity, and shape of pupil in comparison with the opposite eye.
3. *Motor examination.* Assess each extremity individually by means of a predetermined coding score of motor movement.
4. *Respiratory pattern.* If the patient is not receiving mechanical ventilation, observe respiratory patterns for evidence of deteriorating level of function.
5. *Vital signs.* Include comparison of preassessment vital signs with postassessment vital signs, paying special attention to arterial blood pressure and ICP if these parameters are being monitored.

As in the assessment of the conscious patient, if any abnormalities or changes from previous assessment are noted, further investigation must occur. This assessment takes 3 to 4 minutes.

Neurologic Changes Associated with Intracranial Hypertension

Assessment of the patient for signs of increasing intracranial pressure is an important function of the critical care nurse. Increasing ICP can be identified by changes in level of consciousness, pupillary reaction, motor response, vital signs, and respiratory patterns.

LEGAL REVIEW: Coma, persistent vegetative state, and brain death

To maintain full consciousness, both the reticular activating system (RAS)—a brainstem regulatory system—and the cerebral hemispheres need to be reciprocally sustaining. Consciousness has two features: arousal and awareness.

Arousal is simply wakefulness and reflects activation of the RAS. It manifests by eye opening, either spontaneously or in response to stimuli. It may occur in the presence of complete destruction of the hemispheres.

Awareness implies functioning cerebral hemispheres and manifests by cognition of self and the environment. The patient demonstrates goal-directed or purposeful motor behavior and language.

Coma is a pathologic state in which neither arousal nor awareness is present. The patient maintains a sleeplike unresponsiveness from which he or she cannot be aroused. Nonpurposive, reflex movements, such as flexor (decorticate) or extensor (decerebrate) posturing, may be present.

In some cases after head trauma or ischemic-anoxic injury as a result of cardiac arrest, both hemispheres are severely damaged but the RAS is preserved. After a period of hours to days of coma, wakefulness returns without evidence of purposive behavior or cognition. This functionally decorticate state is distinct from coma and is known as the *vegetative state,* which may be persistent. Ventilation may remain spontaneous, and circulation is maintained. In the case of *In Re Quinlan,* Plum described a person in a chronic persistent vegetative state as one who retains the capacity to maintain the vegetative parts of neurologic function but no longer has any cognitive function.

However, Karen Ann Quinlan was not brain dead as defined by the ad hoc committee of the Harvard Medical School. The committee's definition included absence of response to pain or other stimuli; absence of pupillary, corneal, pharyngeal, and other reflexes; and absence of blood pressure and spontaneous respiration, as well as isoelectric or flat electroencephalograms, with testing repeated at least 24 hours later with no change.

Patients who are brain dead have irreversible loss of brain function and compose a small percentage of those who are comatose. In *brain death,* coma of established cause exists, with no evidence of cerebral function (absence of appropriate response to noxious stimulation and absence of decerebrate and decorticate reflex responses) or brainstem reflexes (pupils fixed in response to light stimulation, corneal blink reflex absent, doll's eyes reflex and ice-water caloric responses absent, and apnea without spontaneous ventilation) for 24 or more hours, with absent cerebral circulation and/or electrical activity confirmed by sequential angiography and/or electroencephalography.

A larger percentage of comatose patients are those with severe brain damage in whom prognosis is uncertain. For some of these persons the provision of comprehensive critical care ultimately promotes survival in a vegetative state, which may become persistent and chronic even as care is reduced to maintenance levels.

Most states have adopted statutes that define death and brain death. Similarly, most major medical institutions have hospital ethics committees (HECs) or institutional ethics committees (IECs) that (1) educate about medical-ethical issues, (2) develop the criteria, policies, and procedures that will be used to define, diagnose, and manage these various clinical conditions, and (3) resolve particular issues or cases. It is imperative for the critical care nurse to be intimately conversant with state law and the institution's established standards.

Ad Hoc Committee of the Harvard Medical School to Examine the Definition of Brain Death: *JAMA* 205:337, 1968; Bates D and others: *Ann Neurol* 2:211, 1977; Beresford HR. *Ann Neurol* 15(5):409, 1984; Caronna JJ: Approach to the patient with impairment of consciousness. In Kelley WN, editor: *Textbook of internal medicine,* Philadelphia, 1989, JB Lippincott; Cranford R: *Hastings Cent Rep* 18:27, 1988; Davis KM and others: *J Neurosci Nurs* 19(1):36, 1987; Fischer CM: *Acta Neurol Scand* 45(suppl 36):4, 1969; Fost N, Cranford R: *JAMA* 253:2687, 1985; *Idem.* APACHE II: *Crit Care Med* 13:818, 1985; *In Re Quinlan,* 70 NJ 10, 355 A2d 647, 654; *cert denied,* 429 US 922 (1976); Jennett B, Bond M: *Lancet* 1:480, 1975; Jennett B, Plum F: *Lancet* 7:734, 1972; Knaus WA and others: *Ann Surg* 202:685, 1985; Levy DE and others: *Ann Intern Med* 94:293, 1981, Longstreth WT Jr, Diehr P, Inui TS: *N Engl J Med* 308:1378, 1983; Medical consultants on the diagnosis of death to the President's Commission for the Study of Ethical Problems in Medicine and Biomedical and Behavioral Research: *JAMA* 246:2184, 1981; Murphy CA: *Specialty L Dig: Health Care* 158:7, Apr 1992; Narayan RK and others: *J Neurosurg* 54:751, 1981; Plum F, Posner JB: *The diagnosis of stupor and coma,* ed 3, Philadelphia, 1980, FA Davis; Teasdale G, Jennett B: *Lancet* 2:81, 1974; Ventura MG, Masser PG: Defining death: developments in recent law. In Rogers MC, Traystman RJ, editors: *Critical care clinics: symposium on neurologic intensive care,* vol 1, Philadelphia, 1985, WB Saunders; National Conference of Commissioners on Uniform State Laws: *Uniform brain death act,* 1978; National Conference of Commissioners on Uniform State Laws: 1978; Uniform determination of death act, 1980.

◆ **Level of consciousness.** As ICP increases, the level of consciousness deteriorates. Increased restlessness and confusion, agitation, or decreased responsiveness can all indicate deterioration in neurologic status. For the most part, level of consciousness is the first sign of deterioration in a conscious patient. Subtle changes that are identified and acted on may prevent the serious consequences associated with neurologic decline.

◆ **Pupillary reaction.** Any changes in pupillary size, shape, or reactivity are ominous signs. In the unconscious patient, pupils are the most sensitive indication that deterioration is in progress.

◆ **Motor response.** Deterioration in motor strength or the appearance of lateralizing signs may indicate increasing ICP. Even subtle changes in motor response can be highly predictive of neurologic deterioration.

◆ **Vital signs.** As described, vital signs play a variable role in the evaluation of deteriorating neurologic status. Increasing systolic blood pressure or development of bradycardia, or both, should signal the evaluator to further assess for potential deterioration in function.

◆ **Respiratory patterns.** Change in respiratory patterns can be a sensitive indicator of decreasing levels of function. The assessment of this parameter usually is lost, because most patients with critical neurologic injury are intubated and ventilated to prevent the serious neurologic damage caused by hypoxia and hypercapnia.

BRAIN DEATH AND PERSISTENT VEGETATIVE STATE

The subjects of brain death and patients in a persistent vegetative state (coma) remain controversial. For the nurse caring for patients in a persistent vegetative state, the situation often is physically and emotionally draining. These patients are totally dependent on continuous, labor-intensive care for maintenance of normal bodily function. Nutrition usually is provided by tube feeding or occasionally by hyperalimentation. Pulmonary care includes frequent suctioning, chest physiotherapy, and repositioning. Skin care involves frequent turning, positioning, and bathing to reduce the incidence of decubitus ulcers. At the same time the nurse expends a large amount of emotional energy dealing with family and friends of the patient.

When confronted with the challenge of caring for a patient in a persistent vegetative state, the nurse should use all resources available for support. Patient care conferences, physician-nurse discussions, and family meetings with physician, nurse, and social services should be standard procedures of care. It is important that all those involved with the patient have a realistic understanding of the patient's prognosis. If family, nursing staff, and physician are all aware of the severity of the illness and the limited potential for recovery, at least some of the stress and anxiety may be decreased.

REFERENCES

1. Plum F, Posner JB: *The diagnosis of stupor and coma,* ed 3, Philadelphia, 1980, FA Davis.
2. Teasdale G, Jennett W: Assessment of coma and impaired consciousness: a practical scale, *Lancet* 2:81, 1974.
3. Wilson SF and others: Determining interater reliability of nurses' assessment of pupillary size and reaction, *J Neurosci Nurs* 20(3):189, 1988.
4. Marshall LF and others: The oval pupil: clinical significance and relationship to intracranial hypertension, *J Neurosurg* 58:566, 1983.
5. Marshall SB and others: *Neuroscience critical care: pathophysiology and patient management,* Philadelphia, 1990, WB Saunders.
6. Bates B: *A guide to physical exam,* ed 5, Philadelphia, 1991, JB Lippincott.
7. Beresford HR: Severe neurologic impairment: legal aspects of decision to reduce care, *Ann Neurol* 15(5):409, 1984.
8. Steinbrook R: Artificial feeding—solid ground not a slippery slope, *N Engl J Med* 318(5):286, 1988.
9. Brophy vs New England Sinai Hospital, Inc: *J Am Geriatr Soc* 35(7):669, 1987.

27

Neurologic Diagnostic Procedures

CHAPTER OBJECTIVES

- ◆ Discuss the role of the nurse in diagnostic testing.
- ◆ State the complications associated with cerebral angiography.
- ◆ Describe the differences between cerebral angiography and digital subtraction angiography.
- ◆ State the differences between the two types of dye used in myelography.
- ◆ Explain the differences between electroencephalography and evoked potentials.
- ◆ Discuss the patient positioning required for lumbar puncture.

A wide array of diagnostic tests is available to assist the clinician in identifying the cause of neurologic dysfunction. Improved technology has increased the sophistication of assessment, especially in the area of radiographic procedures and electrophysiology studies. Neurodiagnostic testing is performed as an adjunct to a thorough neurologic examination. When clinical findings are identified on examination, the clinician begins the process of diagnosing the problem. Results of diagnostic testing should provide the examiner with data to further refine and locate the cause of the abnormality identified during the neurologic assessment of the patient. Management is based on clinical manifestations, pathologic conditions, and the results of the diagnostic tests.

The role of the nurse in neurologic diagnostic testing is varied, but three functions are always present: (1) patient/family education, (2) physical preparation, and (3) awareness of potential complications.

It is essential that the patient be aware of the reason for a procedure, the procedural process, and any preprocedure preparation. There also should be a discussion of the sensations and the level of discomfort involved. Once the physician has discussed the risks of the procedure with the patient, the nurse is available to listen to the patient's fears or concerns and attempt to lessen anxiety.

The nurse assists in the physical preparation by providing medications, scrubs, or dye solutions. During the procedure the nurse also might assist in maintaining patient position or compliance with procedure.

In addition to discussing concerns about risk factors, the nurse assesses the patient for potential development of any complications associated with the procedure. Proper observation and intervention, if necessary, are nursing responsibilities.

The goal of this chapter is to focus on the tests frequently performed on the critically ill patient rather than review all available diagnostic studies. Discussion of each test includes a definition and purpose of the test, a review of the procedure, and the patient care needs both before and after the procedure.

RADIOLOGIC PROCEDURES

Skull and Spine Films

The purpose of radiographs of the skull or spine is to identify fractures, anomalies, or possibly tumors. The role of skull radiographs in trauma has diminished with the advent of computerized axial tomography (CT). If the patient is to undergo a CT scan during the initial assessment process, a skull radiograph may not be necessary.

The procedure for obtaining skull and spine radiographs is relatively painless. Proper patient positioning is essential, especially for spine radiographs. In a search for spine fractures it frequently is difficult to obtain a clear view of C1-2 and C6-7. A C1-2 view is obtained by taking the x-ray through the open mouth of the patient (Water's view). Intubation, however, usually prevents this approach. Therefore spinal precautions—that is, cervical collar and strict maintenance of head alignment—must be maintained until the patient's condition allows for open mouth views. For C6-7 views, adequate visualization often requires the nurse or technician to pull down firmly on the patient's arms while the film is being taken.

Nursing care involves positioning of the patient to obtain adequate films. In any situation in which traumatic injury, especially head injury, is the cause of the patient's admission to the critical care unit, the cervical spine should be treated as unstable until proved otherwise.

Computerized Axial Tomography

CT scanning provides the clinician with a mathematically reconstructed view of multiple sections of the head and body. This is accomplished by passage of intersecting x-ray beams through the examined area and measurement of the density of substances through which the x-ray beam passes. The denser the substance through which the x-ray beam passes, the whiter it will appear on the finished film. The less dense a substance, the blacker it will appear. Therefore with normal findings in a CT scan of the head, bone appears white, blood appears off-white, brain tissue appears shaded gray, cerebral spinal fluid (CSF) appears off-black, and air appears black (Fig. 27-1).

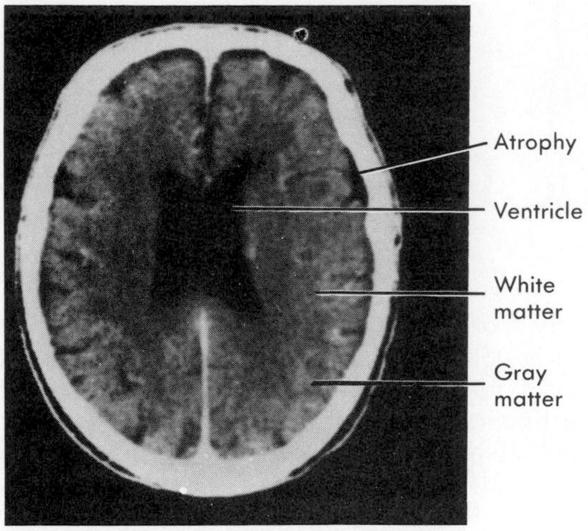

Fig. 27-1 CT scan image. (From Ballinger PW: *Merrill's atlas of radiographic positions and radiologic procedures,* ed 7, St Louis, 1991, Mosby–Year Book.)

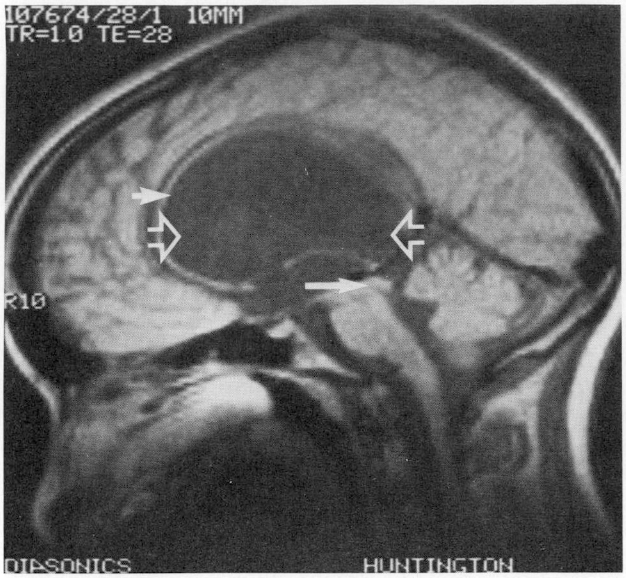

Fig. 27-2 Magnetic resonance image of the brain. Sagittal section demonstrating marked enlargement of the lateral ventricle *(open arrow)* with stretching of the corpus callosum *(arrowhead)* as a result of aqueductal stenosis *(arrow)* (SE 1000/28). (From Stark DD, Bradley WG: *Magnetic resonance imaging,* ed 2, St Louis, 1992, Mosby–Year Book.)

The purpose of the CT scan is to obtain rapid, noninvasive visualization of structures. CT scanning is indicated in the diagnostic work-up of severe headache, head trauma with associated loss of consciousness, seizures, hydrocephalus, suspicion of space-occupying lesions, hemorrhage, or vascular lesions and edema. There are two types of CT scans—contrast and noncontrast scans. The noncontrast scan is noninvasive, requires no premedication of the patient, and is good for analysis and location of normal brain structures. Noncontrast CT scans of the head are appropriate in trauma patients in whom the goal is to view the intracranial area for evidence of intracranial hemorrhage, cerebral edema, or shift of structures. Noncontrast CT scan is also appropriate in the diagnosis of hydrocephalus.[1,2]

The contrast CT scan involves the use of an intravenously injected contrast medium. The use of contrast enhances the vascular areas and allows for detection of vascular lesions or the further definition of lesions noted on a noncontrast scan.

Nursing care of the patient receiving a CT scan can be divided into two areas of focus: observation of patient tolerance of the procedure and observation of patient reaction to the dye in contrast scanning. Because of the associated activity and positioning, transporting and scanning of a critically ill patient with known or suspected intracranial hypertension can cause a deterioration in the patient's condition. The nurse must always remain with the patient during the CT scan and closely observe the neurologic status, vital signs, and, if monitored, intracranial pressure.

If the patient is to receive a contrast CT scan, questions about possible sensitivity to iodine-based dye should be ascertained beforehand if at all possible. During the infusion of the dye and for 10 to 30 minutes after, the patient should be observed closely for anaphylactic reaction. Of all patients receiving contrast CT scans, fewer than 1% per year have severe anaphylactic reactions, shock, or cardiac arrest.

Magnetic Resonance Imaging

Magnetic resonance imaging (MRI) is a relatively new procedure. The patient is placed in a large magnetic field. The nuclei of the atoms of the body are stimulated and momentarily absorb some of the energy generated by the magnetic field. Different tissue densities absorb and subsequently release differing amounts of energy. The release of the energy (resonance frequency) is then measured and plotted[3] (Fig. 27-2).

In MRI small tumors whose tissue densities differ from those of the surrounding cells can be identified before they would be visible by any other radiographic test. MRI also can identify small hemorrhages deep in the brain that are invisible on CT scan. Finally, MRI can detect areas of cerebral infarct within a few hours of the incident, as well as small areas of plaque in patients with multiple sclerosis.

Nursing management involves patient teaching and preparation. The procedure is lengthy and requires the patient to lie motionless in a tight, enclosed space. Many patients experience anxiety, panic, and an acute sense of claustrophobia. Mild sedation or a blindfold, or both, may be necessary. The neurologically impaired patient may not be able to comprehend the instructions, and sedation will be required. Removal of all metal from the patient's body and clothing is essential because the basis of MRI is a magnetic field. In the past it was believed that any metal material, such as dental filling, prostheses, or internal clips or staples, would prevent scanning. Further study and changes in the type of metals used for many procedures have made the test safer. Any questions about specific devices or metals should be directed to the neuroradiologist before testing. The test is considered relatively safe and noninvasive, but all risks have not yet been identified in this procedure.

Cerebral Angiogram

Cerebral angiography[1] involves the injection of radiopaque contrast medium into the intracranial or extracranial vasculature. With the use of serial radiologic filming, an angiogram traces the flow of blood from the arterial circulation through the capillary bed to the venous circulation. Cerebral angiography allows visualization of the lumen of vessels to provide information about patency, size (narrowing or dilation), any irregularities, or occlusion. The use of angiography is necessary in the diagnosis of cerebral aneurysm, arteriovenous malformation, carotid artery disease, and some vascular tumors. Information obtained from the angiogram guides the surgeon in choosing the operative approach or provides information on which to make medical management decisions other than surgery.

The procedure involves placement of a catheter in the femoral artery and threading it up the aorta and into the origin of the cerebral circulation. Other injection sites include a direct carotid or vertebral artery puncture or placement of a catheter in the brachial, axillary, or subclavian artery. Several views of vessels can be studied by means of angiogram. A four-vessel angiogram involves injections into the right and left internal carotid arteries and the right and left vertebral arteries. If the area of suspected disease already has been identified, a single vessel study may be all that is required. This is particularly true when angiography is used as a follow-up in the evaluation of intracranial vascular surgery. Also, if carotid artery disease is a working diagnosis, the angiogram may include views of the arch of the aorta, plus the external and internal carotid arteries.

Once the catheter is appropriately placed, the contrast medium is injected. Then a rapid succession of radiographs are taken as the contrast medium progresses through the cerebral circulation. Separate contrast medium injections are administered for each vessel being studied.

Nursing care associated with this invasive procedure is comprehensive. Patient instruction and education are essential to patient preparation. The patient's complete understanding of the role this procedure plays in diagnosis, as well as the process itself, relieves anxiety about the unknown and also ensures cooperation in what frequently is an uncomfortable procedure. Discomforts include the need to lie still on a cold, hard table and the possibility of pain during preparation and insertion of the groin catheter. The patient often experiences a hot, burning sensation when the contrast medium is injected, especially if it is injected into the external carotid system. Preparation of patients for this burning sensation assures them that it is not an abnormal occurrence. Finally, the patient must be aware of the postprocedure assessment.

Before and after the procedure, adequate hydration is necessary to assist the kidneys in clearing the heavy dye load. Inadequate hydration may lead to an acute tubular necrosis (ATN) and renal shutdown. If the patient is unable to tolerate oral fluids, an intravenous line should be placed before the procedure is begun.

Postprocedure assessment involves vital sign measurement, neurologic evaluation, observation of the injection site, and assessment of neurovascular integrity distal to the injection site every 15 minutes for the first 1 to 2 hours. Any abnormalities noted must be immediately reported.

Complications associated with cerebral angiography include (1) cerebral embolus caused by the catheter dislodging a segment of atherosclerotic plaque in the vessel, (2) hemorrhage or clot formation at the insertion site, (3) vasospasm of a vessel caused by the irritation of catheter placement, (4) thrombosis of the extremity distal to the injection site, and (5) allergic reaction to the contrast medium. With diagnostic cerebral angiography the risk of an intracranial vascular accident resulting in stroke is approximately 5/1000.[4]

Digital Subtraction Angiography

Digital subtraction angiography[1] is a newer method of visualizing the arteriovenous circulation of the intracranial space. Radiographic dye is injected into either the venous or the arterial circulation, but significantly less dye is necessary for this procedure than for arterial angiography. Films taken before and after dye injection are superimposed on each other and all matching images are subtracted. Thus only the dye-enhanced cerebral vessels are left for study and evaluation. Digital subtraction angiography eliminates the shadows and distortions of bone or other material that sometimes block the viewing of the cerebral vessels.

The major disadvantage of digital subtraction angiography involves the patient's ability to remain motionless during the entire procedure. Even swallowing interferes significantly with the imaging process. With venous injection of dye for the digital subtraction angiography, intracranial and extracranial vessels are enhanced. With arterial injection of dye, the same complications are possible as with cerebral angiography.

Interventional Angiography

Angiography recently has advanced from a purely diagnostic tool to an interventional tool. Interventional angiography results in the alteration of cerebral blood flow through vessels by two different methods, occlusion and dilation. Interventional angiography is used to alter the blood supply of a tumor or arteriovenous malformation by embolizing feeding vessels to reduce the size of the abnormal structure. This procedure involves the use of small beads of glue, absorbent gelatin sponge (Gelfoam), or muscle that are directed by the angiography catheter to the feeding vessels where they occlude blood flow. Recently a specially designed, detachable, inflatable balloon was developed that can be used to occlude surgically inaccessible aneurysms. These balloons are passed to the aneurysm through uniquely designed microcatheters that can enter vessels well under 1 mm in diameter. When the catheter enters the aneurysm, the balloon is inflated and detached.[4]

Dilation of cerebral vessels is accomplished in much the same manner as for cardiac vessels. Angioplasty and stent techniques, which are well established for the cardiac vasculature, are still under investigation for cerebral circulation. These techniques are limited to the carotid, internal carotid, and vertebral vessels; the greatest risk with the use of either angioplasty or stenting is the dislodging of debris that then could lodge distally in critical areas of the brain.

Nursing management after the patient has undergone interventional angiography is similar to that for diagnostic cerebral angiography. Because the risk of complications is greater with interventional angiography, the nurse should be especially meticulous and thorough in the postprocedure assessments.

Myelography

Myelography[2] is radiographic examination of the spinal cord and vertebral column after injection of a contrast material into the subarachnoid space by lumbar or cisternal puncture. Myelography allows visualization of the spinal canal, the subarachnoid space around the spinal cord, and the spinal nerve roots. Indications for myelography include identification of spinal canal blockage caused by herniated intervertebral disks, spinal cord tumors, bony fragments or growths, and congenital anomalies (Fig. 27-3).

The procedure involves a lumbar or cisternal puncture followed by an injection of contrast medium. It is performed fluoroscopically; the infusion of the dye is observed, and radiographic films are taken. Two basic types of contrast medium are used—an oil-based preparation (Pantopaque) or a water-based preparation (metrizamide). Use of an oil-based preparation, which is heavier than the CSF, allows the radiologist to place the patient in a variety of positions while observing the flow of dye through the spinal subarachnoid space. Disadvantages of the oil-based preparation include the lack of absorption of the dye from the subarachnoid space. Pantopaque must be removed at the end of the procedure. Use of an oil-based preparation is associated with a higher incidence of severe postprocedure headache as a result of CSF loss. Postprocedure care of a patient who has undergone Pantopaque myelogram involves keeping the patient flat in bed for 4 to 6 hours to prevent headache and CSF leak from the puncture site.

Use of the water-based preparation, which is lighter than CSF, allows for better visualization of nerve roots and projections off the spinal cord. Metrizamide is absorbed by the arachnoid system and therefore does not require removal after the procedure. Disadvantages to use of a water-based preparation include rapid dissolution of the dye into the subarachnoid space. The patient cannot be rolled into different positions to observe dye flow. Because of the potential toxicity of water-based preparations to the cerebral tissue, care must be taken to ensure that a large dye load does not reach the surface of the brain. This is accomplished by keeping the patient's head elevated 30 to 45 degrees after the procedure. Toxicity is evidenced by grand mal seizures. To assist the clearance of dye through the urine, adequate hydration is necessary for patients who undergo a metrizamide myelogram. Use of phenothiazines is to be avoided after a metrizamide myelogram because of the increase in symptoms of toxicity.

Possible risks involved with the use of myelography include injection of the dye outside the subarachnoid space, arachnoiditis as a result of irritation of the arachnoid membranes from a foreign material, allergic reactions to the dye that may cause confusion, disorientation, an anaphylactic reaction, headache, or grand mal seizure.[5]

CEREBRAL BLOOD FLOW STUDIES

The goal of cerebral blood flow studies[1] is to measure the amount of blood flow overall or in regions of the brain to detect areas of increased or decreased cerebral circulation. Normal cerebral blood flow values average 50 to 55 ml of flow per 100 g of cerebral tissue per minute. Studies to determine the actual amount of cerebral blood flow in the injured brain would be a valuable addition to the planning of interventions. Some techniques are available, but as yet none of the procedures has achieved wide acceptance in clinical practice.

Uses of cerebral blood flow studies include evaluation of cerebral vasospasm after subarachnoid hemorrhage; evaluation of cerebral blood flow during operative procedures that require extreme hypotension, such as aneurysm clipping; and evaluation of the changes in cerebral blood flow after cerebral vascular surgery, such as carotid endarterectomy, cerebral revascularization (superficial temporal artery–middle cerebral artery bypass), or arteriovenous malformation excision.

Methods of determining cerebral blood flow range from intracarotid or intravenous injection of radioisotopes to inhalation of isotopes or nitrous oxide. The most clinically acceptable method of cerebral blood flow analysis involves inhalation of xenon-133 for 3 to 5 minutes. Clearance of this isotope from brain tissue is then monitored by means of 16 to 32 probes that are placed externally around the head. Information from the probes is passed to a computer that calculates regional cerebral blood flow. This is the least invasive of all techniques. The difficulty with this method is that all body tissues take up xenon and then clear it, including the skin and muscles of the scalp under detectors. Although mathematic calculations are factored in, cerebral blood flow results are an estimated value at best. Further research and development are necessary to make this valuable diagnostic tool clinically acceptable and accurate.

DOPPLER ULTRASOUND

Ultrasound technology provides information about the flow velocity of blood through cerebral vessels using a noninvasive technique. A Doppler probe is placed externally over the vessel where ultrasonic waves are generated and blood flow velocities are calculated. As the diameter of the vessel changes, the velocity of the flow of blood through the vessel changes. The higher the flow velocity, the narrower the vessel. This narrowing can be the result of vasospasm or vessel plaque.

Extracranial Doppler Studies

Extracranial Doppler studies are used as a routine screening procedure for intraluminal narrowing of the

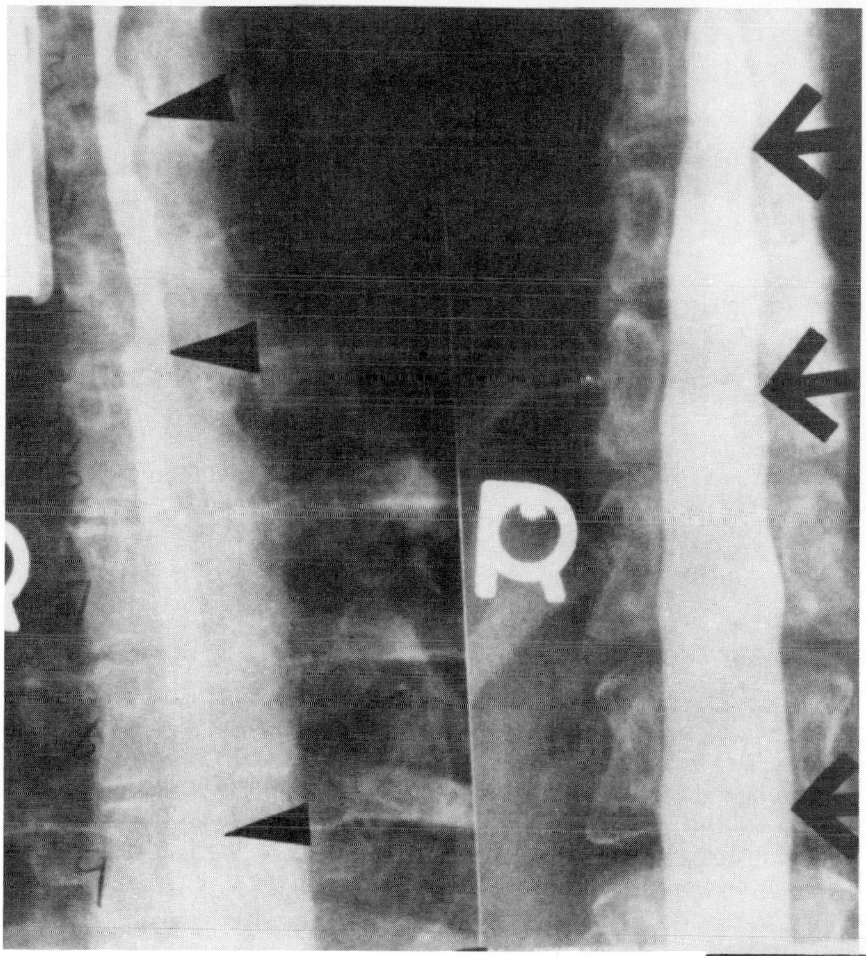

A

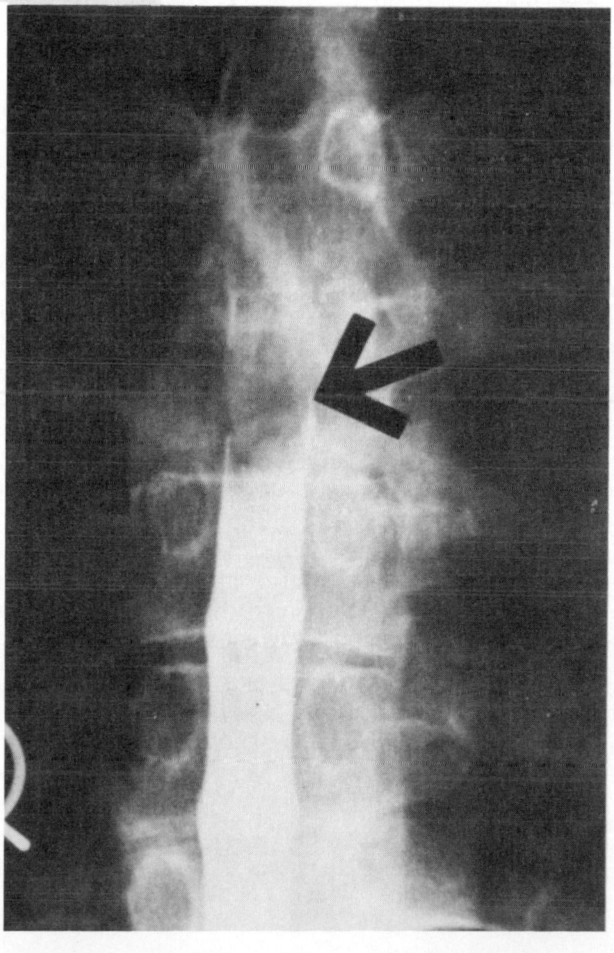

B

Fig. 27-3 **A,** Normal myelogram finding with dorsal thoracic view on left and lumbar view on right. Pointers and arrows indicate normal flow of radiographic dye (Pantopaque). **B,** Abnormal myelogram finding with obstruction of dye column caused by metastatic tumor compressing the canal. (From Pagana KD, Pagana TJ: *Diagnostic testing and nursing implications: a case study approach,* ed 3, St Louis, 1990, Mosby–Year Book.)

common and internal carotid arteries as a result of arteriosclerotic plaques or atheromata.[4] Extracranial Doppler studies are noninvasive, relatively inexpensive, and painless. When changes in flow velocities are noted that may indicate significant occlusion of the vessel, a cerebral angiogram often is indicated to verify the degree of severity of the narrowed vessel.

Transcranial Doppler Studies

Transcranial Doppler studies monitor cerebral blood flow velocity through cranial "windows" or thinned areas of the skull. One such area—the most popular—is the temporal bone. Depending on the angle of the Doppler probe, flow velocities can be measured in the anterior, middle, or posterior cerebral arteries. Current use of transcranial Doppler studies is mainly for postintracranial aneurysm rupture in which concern about vasospasm development is a factor. The noninvasive technique and portability of the equipment allow for frequent bedside monitoring of flow velocity and therefore vascular diameter. Use of serial transcranial Doppler studies for the detection of cerebral vasospasm greatly reduces the need for cerebral angiograms to verify and follow postsubarachnoid hemorrhage vasospasm.

ELECTROPHYSIOLOGY STUDIES

Two basic electrophysiologic studies are used in the critical care setting. Both studies can be performed intermittently to evaluate symptoms or review progress or used continuously to assist in ongoing assessment of neurologic function.

Electroencephalography

Electroencephalography (EEG)[3,6] is the recording of electrical impulses, commonly called *brain waves*, generated by the brain. This test has been in existence for many years and is well known to the general public. It is important for the nurse caring for a patient with a neurologic dysfunction to be aware of the appropriate indications for use of this testing procedure. The purpose of the EEG is to detect and localize abnormal electrical activity. This abnormal activity can be defined as slowing, which occurs in areas of injury or infarct, or as the spikes and waves seen in irritated tissue. Indications for the use of EEG include seizure focus identification, infarct, metabolic disorders, confirmation of brain death (electrocerebral silence), and some head injuries.

Noninvasive electrodes are placed on the head, and the electrical impulses detected are transferred to a central recording device that records the information in wave form. Five types of waves or rhythms may be present, as follows:

Alpha	8 to 13 cycles/second	Normal, relaxed state with eyes closed, seen often in occipital leads
Theta	4 to 7 cycles/second	Less common in adults than in children, characteristic of coma in brain injury
Beta	12 to 40 cycles/second	Fast waves indicating mental or physical activity
Sleep spindles	12 to 14 cycles/second	Seen in stage 2 sleep, not REM
Spike and wave	Variable	Seen in irritable brain tissue such as seizure

For further discussion of EEG, see Chapter 10.

In preparing the patient for an EEG, the nurse should stress the noninvasive aspects of this procedure. The awake patient may be asked to perform certain simple tasks during the procedure, such as blinking, closing the eye, or swallowing. Occasionally, testing needs to be performed during sleep or after a period of sleep deprivation.

Continuous monitoring of the EEG is becoming more common in the critical care environment. The goal of continuous EEG monitoring is to identify changes in electrical activity that could indicate inadequate vascular supply to an area or provide evidence of subclinical seizures. Subclinical seizures are evidenced by sharp spike and wave electrical activity that is not evident by visual observation of the patient. Subclinical seizures increase cerebral metabolic rate in response to the greatly increased cellular activity. This increased metabolic rate requires increasing supply of oxygen and nutrients to an already compromised vascular supply system. Detection and treatment of subclinical seizures may prevent secondary brain injury.

Evoked Potentials

Evoked potentials[2,3] involve the recording of electrical impulses generated by a sensory stimulus as it travels through the brainstem and into the cerebral cortex. Measuring evoked potentials is a sophisticated way of observing the status of sensory pathways as they enter the central nervous system, travel through the brainstem, and reach the cerebral cortex. Evoked potentials also can be used during therapeutically induced comas, such as barbiturate coma, inasmuch as these sensory pathways are unaffected by the depressive activity of such drugs. Another use of evoked potentials is in the determination of the existence of brainstem or spinal cord injury in the traumatically injured patient.

The three types of evoked potential tests are (1) visual evoked responses (VER), (2) brainstem auditory evoked responses (BAER), and (3) somatosensory evoked responses (SSER). VER involves monitoring of the visual pathways through the brainstem and cortex in response to the patient's viewing a shifting geometric pattern on a screen or placing a mask, which sends a flashing light stimulus, over the eye. BAER involves monitoring the auditory pathway through the brainstem and cortex in response to a rhythmic clicking sound sent through earphones placed over the patient's ears. SSER involves monitoring of sensory pathways from the extremities ascending the spinal cord through the brainstem and into the cortex. This is performed by administering a small electrical shock to a nerve root in the periphery, such as the ulnar or radial nerve.

Preparation of awake patients involves appropriate teaching so that they cooperate with the instructions for the procedure. No pain or discomfort is involved in the administration of these tests, except for the irritation of the small electrical shock used for SSER.

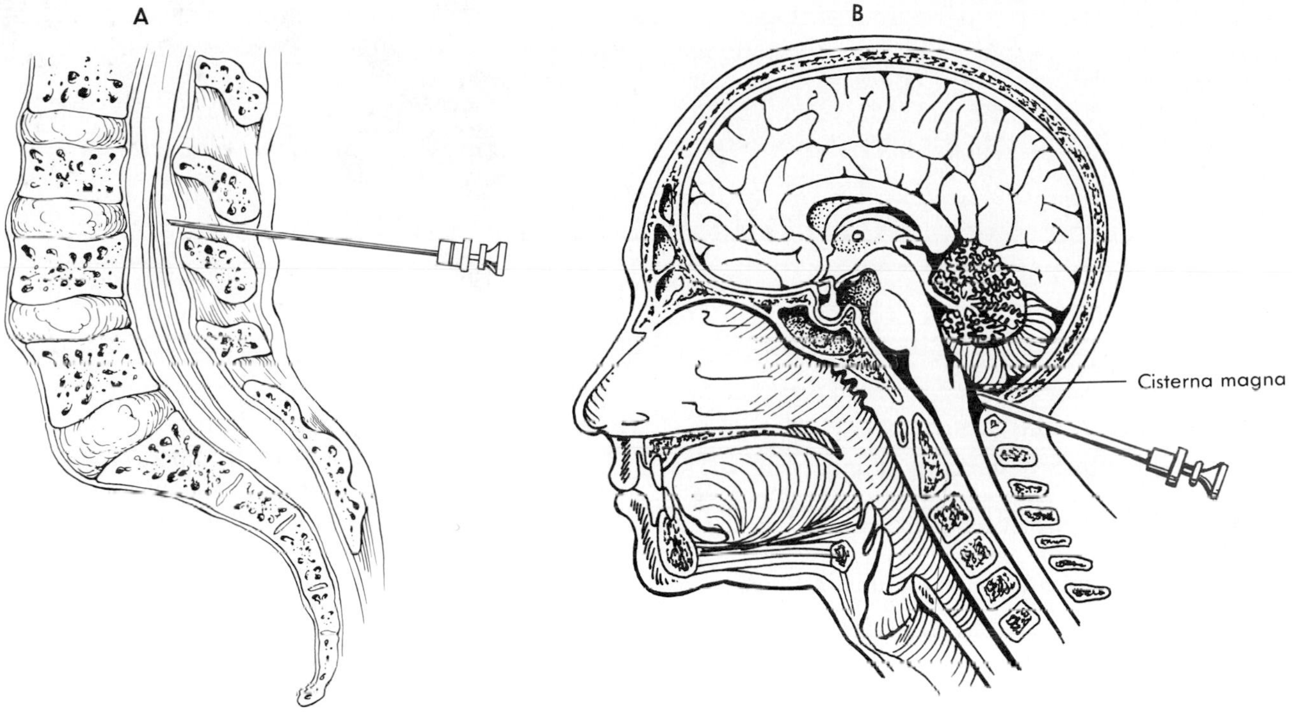

Fig. 27-4 **A,** Lumbar puncture. **B,** Cisternal puncture. (From Long BC, Phipps WJ: *Medical-surgical nursing: a nursing process approach,* ed 3, St Louis, 1993, Mosby–Year Book.)

LUMBAR PUNCTURE

The main purpose of lumbar puncture (LP) is to enter the subarachnoid space to obtain diagnostic information or to provide therapeutic intervention. Diagnostic information comes from samples of CSF evaluated for the presence of subarachnoid blood or infection, or for laboratory analysis. Pressure readings also are obtained for diagnostic use. Therapeutic modalities of an LP include removal of bloody or purulent CSF that the arachnoid villi are unable to clear, injection of medications into the subarachnoid space to bypass the blood-brain barrier (antibiotics or analgesics), or the introduction of spinal anesthesia.

An LP involves the introduction of an 18- to 22-gauge hollow needle into the subarachnoid space at L4-5 below the end of the spinal cord, which usually is at L1-2. The patient can be placed either in the lateral recumbent position with the knees and head tightly tucked or in the sitting position leaning over a bedside table or some other support (Fig. 27-4).

Risks associated with an LP include possible brainstem herniation if intracranial pressure is elevated or respiratory arrest associated with neurologic deterioration. During the procedure the nurse must monitor the patient's neurologic and respiratory status. Also, if the patient is not fully alert and cooperative, the nurse may need to assist the patient in maintaining the position necessary for performance of the LP.[6]

Cisternal puncture, which is the introduction of a needle into the cisterna magna at the C1-2 level, is another method for obtaining access to the subarachnoid space. Risks of cisternal puncture are slightly higher than those associated with an LP, but cisternal puncture is necessary if there is inability to enter the lumbar space because of scar tissue or some other physical barrier or if there is a total blockage of the CSF pathway somewhere along the spinal column.

REFERENCES

1. Cammermeyer M, Appeldorn C: *Core curriculum for neuroscience nursing,* Chicago, 1990, American Association of Neuroscience Nurses.
2. Hickey JV: *The clinical practice of neurologic and neurosurgical nursing,* ed 2, Philadelphia, 1986, JB Lippincott.
3. Borel C, Hanley D: Neurologic intensive care unit monitoring. In Rogers MC, Traystman RJ, editors: *Symposium on neurologic intensive care,* vol 1, Philadelphia, 1985, WB Saunders.
4. Marshall SB and others: *Neuroscience critical care: pathophysiology and patient management,* Philadelphia, 1990, WB Saunders.
5. Jones AG: Side effects following metrizamide myelography and lumbar laminectomy, *Neurosci Nurs* 19(2):90, 1987.
6. Rudy EB: *Advanced neurological and neurosurgical nursing,* St Louis, 1984, Mosby–Year Book.

28

Neurologic Disorders

CHAPTER OBJECTIVES

- Define the treatment dilemmas of aneurysm rupture associated with vasospasm and rebleeding.
- Define the concept of "malignant tumors" in the intracranial space.
- Discuss the pathophysiology of Guillain-Barré syndrome.

An understanding of the pathology of a disease, the areas of assessment on which to focus, and the usual medical management allows the critical care nurse to more accurately anticipate and plan nursing interventions. Although a wide array of neurologic disorders exists, only a few routinely require care in the critical care environment. This chapter presents a review of central nervous system tumors, cerebral vascular disease, Guillain-Barré syndrome, and acute pain.

CENTRAL NERVOUS SYSTEM TUMORS

Description

In the central nervous system (CNS), most primary neoplastic growths are a result of irregular mitosis of the support cells, the neuroglia. Neurons themselves have little ability to regenerate and minimal to no mitotic capability. Primary CNS tumors are classified as *benign* or *malignant,* but the definition of these terms varies from the tumor classification system of the rest of the body. Benign CNS tumors are those growths lying in accessible areas of the CNS, with slow growth and lack of invasiveness. These can be completely removed without significant neurologic deficit. Malignant tumors are neoplasms, such as glioblastoma multiforme, which have multiple fingerlike projections into normal tissue. Attempts to completely remove all of the tumor would cause unacceptable neurologic damage. Another type of CNS malignancy is the presence of a usually benign growth that lies deep in vital structures of the CNS where attempt at removal would cause severe neurologic deficit. It is malignant by location, not by histologic classification (Table 28-1).

Generally, CNS tumors do not metastasize outside the CNS. Metastatic cells from the body do reproduce in the CNS. Primary lesions of the lung, breast, and prostate contribute most significantly to metastatic lesions in the brain.

Incidence

The overall incidence of CNS tumors in the United States is 15,000 cases of brain tumors and 4000 cases of spinal cord tumors per year.[1] Most tumors occur in two age peaks. One peak is in childhood (ages 3 to 12) and the other in the later years (ages 50 to 70).

Etiology

Pediatric tumors vary in histology and other characteristics from tumors in the adult. A fairly common neoplastic disease in childhood, CNS tumors rank second only to the leukemias. More than two thirds of the pediatric lesions are in the posterior fossa (the cerebellum, midbrain, and brainstem region). The most common tumor in children is the medulloblastoma, which accounts for one quarter of the primary intracranial tumors in this age-group.[2] Other tumors of childhood are astrocytomas of the cerebellum, astrocytomas of the brainstem, and the malignant glioblastoma multiforme of both the cerebellum and the brainstem.[3]

In the adult population the most common tumor is glioblastoma multiforme, followed by meningioma and astrocytoma. Gliomas represent more than one half of all primary intracranial lesions.[4]

Pathophysiology

Basic to understanding the pathophysiology associated with any tumor of the brain or spinal cord are the accurate identification of the cell of origin and assessment of the aggressiveness of the cells of the tumor. A

Table 28-1 Benign versus malignant tumors in the central nervous system

Benign	Malignant
Encapsulated	Invades surrounding tissue
Well-differentiated cells—easily recognizable from normal brain tissue	Undifferentiated cells—difficult to distinguish from normal brain tissue
Surface access or easily accessible surgically	Difficult surgical access
Does not cause significant neurologic deficit	Surgical removal could cause significant neurologic deficit

variety of classification systems have been developed over the years to categorize CNS tumor cells. For discussion here, tumors are grouped by the "cell of origin" and order of frequency[5] (Table 28-2).

It must be remembered that tumors of the CNS are competing with normal tissue for space inside the enclosed environment of the cranium or spinal column. Malignancy of intracranial tumors can be viewed in terms of cytologic and biologic malignancy. Cytologic malignancy is based on cellular morphology, necrosis, mitosis, and invasiveness. In biologic malignancy the tumor probably will cause the patient's death.[1] Most cytologically malignant brain tumors also are biologically malignant. Because of the brain's sensitivity to increased pressure, some cytologically benign tumors are biologically malignant.

◆ Classification

Gliomas. Gliomas arise from the four neuroglial cells: astrocytes, oligodendroglia, ependymal cells, and microglia. Also considered a histologic cause for gliomas are neuroglial precursors. Gliomas compose more than 50% of all primary tumors of the CNS.

ASTROCYTOMAS. Astrocytomas are the largest group of neuroglial cells. They are believed to provide support and nutrients to the neuron. A range of tumors from benign to highly malignant arise from the astrocyte cell. These tumors are graded from I to IV. Astrocytoma grade I is a slow-growing tumor, which results in a life expectancy for the patient of up to 15 years. Astrocytoma grade II is a less well-differentiated cell that grows more rapidly, and the patient has a life expectancy of 8 to 10 years. Astrocytoma grade III has increasingly malignant cytologic features. Life expectancy of the patient with this tumor group is 2 to 5 years. The final, most severe astrocytoma, grade IV, also is known as *glioblastoma multiforme*. It is characterized by grossly undifferentiated cells, significant necrosis, and a high incidence of hemorrhage into the lesion. Life expectancy of the patient with glioblastoma multiforme is 6 to 18 months.[1]

Astrocytomas of the cerebellum and posterior fossa are most commonly seen in childhood and can range from grades I to IV. Because this usually is a slow-growing cystic tumor, the patient's life expectancy may be 10 years or longer with incomplete excision. Complete excision of these tumors often is possible.

OLIGODENDROGLIOMAS. Oligodendrogliomas arise from oligodendrocytes, which are responsible for myelination of nerve fibers in the CNS. Oligodendrogliomas, although usually benign, occasionally are malignant. They are slow growing, fairly solid, and discrete from surrounding brain tissue. Oligodendrogliomas are likely to have calcification as part of the mass. Frequently oligodendroglioma cells are found mixed with astrocytoma cells. The presence of a significant number of oligodendroglioma cells in an astrocytoma is a good prognostic sign.

EPENDYMOMAS. Ependymomas arise from the cells that line the ventricular cavities and the central canal of the spinal cord. Tumors arising from these cells are situated deep within the CNS. Usually a tumor of childhood, these tumors range from slow to rapid growth. Morbidity and mortality in this group of tumors are related to the rate of growth but also to the deep CNS location that makes accessibility to the lesion difficult.

Neuron tumors. Tumors arising from neuronal tissue are extremely rare because of the lack of mitotic ability of the neuron. Neuroblastoma, rarely a primary CNS lesion, and ganglioblastoma, tumors of ganglion cells, are two types most noted. These tumors occur in children and range from benign to malignant.

Meningiomas. Meningiomas arise from the cells of the pia and arachnoid, especially the arachnoid granulations. Most meningiomas are noninvasive and considered benign. They are encapsulated and well demarcated from surrounding tissue. Meningiomas most often are found around the venous sinuses, over the convexities of the brain, or on the sphenoid ridge. These extremely slow-growing tumors can become quite large before symptoms appear. Meningiomas are the most common extramedullary CNS tumor.

Acoustic neuromas or schwannomas. These tumors arise around cranial nerves, particularly the acoustic (VIII) nerve. They are from Schwann's cells, which are responsible for producing myelin in the peripheral nervous system. These tumors frequently are small and considered benign, but they grow in the brainstem area that is difficult to reach. Morbidity and mortality from these tumors usually are associated with pressure and damage to surrounding brainstem structures.

Pituitary tumors. Pituitary tumors comprise three types that arise from the adenohypophysis or anterior lobe of the pituitary. These three tumor types are chromophobe, eosinophil, and basophil adenomas.

The chromophobe adenoma responsible for 90% of pituitary tumors is a nonsecretory, space-occupying tumor. It produces its effect by placing pressure on surrounding secretory cells, which causes decreased production of stimulating hormones. This process results in symptoms of hypopituitarism: irregular menses, amenorrhea, decreased libido, impotence, decreased body hair, and decreased production of other stimulating hormones.

There are two recognized hormone-secreting pituitary tumors. Eosinophil adenomas secrete growth hormone (GH) that results in *giantism* before puberty and *acromegaly* after puberty. Basophil adenomas secrete adrenocorticotropic hormone (ACTH), which results in Cushing's syndrome. Further alteration of this classification system is required because it has become clear that other pituitary hormone–producing tumors, such as prolactin-secreting adenoma, also occur.

Two types of surgery are available for the removal of a pituitary tumor: transcranial hypophysectomy and transsphenoidal hypophysectomy (Fig. 28-1). The transsphenoidal approach has gained wide acceptance and is the surgery of choice unless the pituitary tumor has extended into the intracranial vault. Overall, the prognosis for persons with pituitary tumors that have not invaded surrounding structures of the CNS is excellent.

Table 28-2 Cerebral tumors

Type	Incidence	Etiology	Pathophysiology
MENINGIOMA	10%-15% of all intracranial tumors	Arise from the meninges and their derivatives; generally benign, malignant form rare	Highly vascular tumor that receives its blood supply from the meninges; slow-growing; firm, rubbery consistency that is easy to differentiate from normal tissue; most frequent location is the parasagittal region; may erode into bone of skull
GLIOMA			
Astrocytoma (grades I-IV)	30%-40% of intracranial tumors; 30% of tumors in children	Derived from astrocytes, which are the support framework for neurons and capillaries in the CNS	More rapid growing than meningiomas and not well-differentiated from edematous or necrotic brain; rarely metastasizes outside the CNS. Classified in ascending grades of malignancy; grade IV also known as *glioblastoma multiforme*
Oligodendroglioma	4%-5% of intracranial tumors	Arise from oligodendroglial cells, which are normally responsible for the myelin sheath in the CNS	May be slow-growing or a rapidly growing, highly malignant form. Well-defined, globular or cystic; can be soft, gelatinous, or mucinous. Located in the cerebral hemispheres, primarily frontal lobe, and occasionally in the ventricles
Ependymoma	5%-6% of intracranial tumors; most often seen in children or young adults	Arise from ependymal cells, which are responsible for the lining of the ventricular system and the choroid plexus	Slow-growing and usually benign histology but difficult to remove because of location in ventricles; fourth ventricle most common site. Causes obstruction of CSF outflow or erosion into the surrounding structures.
CRANIOPHARYNGIOMA	Small percentage of intracranial tumors (2%-4%); most common in 30-40 year age-group; may be seen in children	Arise from squamous cell nests	Benign, congenital, slow-growing tumor; largely cystic, solid; well-defined and firmly attached to surrounding brain tissue. Location usually is midline at the base of the brain near the pituitary stalk; often causes depressed anterior pituitary function. Could fill third ventricle, causing obstruction; could place pressure on optic chiasm or invade sella turcica, basal ganglia, or brainstem. Tends to recur because of embryonic remnants
PINEAL TUMOR	More common in men than in women between 20-30 years of age; may be called *teratoma*	Arise from primitive germ cells that migrate during fetal development	Most often located near the pineal gland; well-defined white-yellow or dark-brown cystic areas that contain remnants of bone, cartilage, teeth, or hair. Pinealoma also contains melatonin, which inhibits sexual development. Can extend and recur; can obstruct the cerebral aqueduct and third ventricle
PITUITARY TUMOR	8%-12% of all intracranial tumors	Arise from selected cells of the anterior pituitary gland	Causes endocrine system dysfunction resulting from dysfunction of pituitary hormone secretion through hypersecretion (eosinophilic or basophilic), hyposecretion, or disruption of function because of mass effect (chromophobic adenoma). Also can cause pressure on the optic chiasm, hypothalamic dysfunction, or erosion through sella turcica into nasal sinuses

Table 28-2 Cerebral tumors—cont'd

Type	Incidence	Etiology	Pathophysiology
VASCULAR TUMOR	Small percentage of intracranial tumors; more common in females	Called *hemangiomas* or *hemangioblastoma*; arise from abnormally developed blood vessels	Most located near skull or vertebral column; dura often involved; slow-growing mass, cavernous type; has a honeycomb appearance with irregular margins. Potential danger from this tumor type includes hemorrhage
METASTATIC TUMOR	Result in 10% of intracranial tumors	Arise from cells that have metastasized from primary site, particularly lung, breast, kidney, or melanoma	Metastasis that could appear anywhere in the intracranial space; single or multiple sites in brain. Usually well-defined, circumscribed, and solid; easy to distinguish from brain tissue. Can be area of initial symptoms before primary site is discovered.

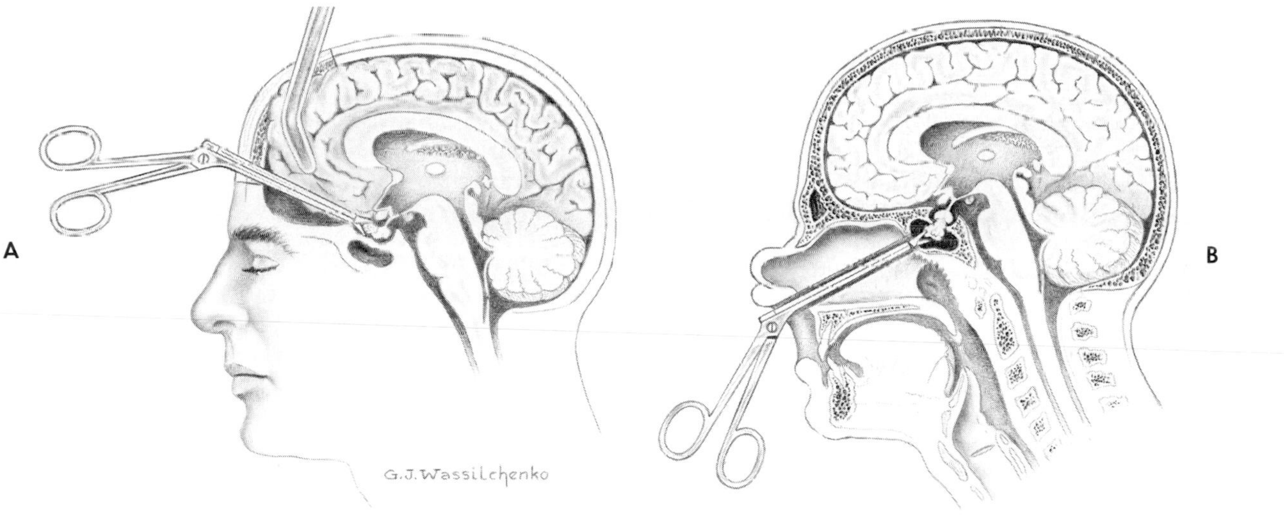

Fig. 28-1 **A,** Transcranial hypophysectomy. **B,** Transsphenoidal hypophysectomy.

Hypothalamic tumors. Hypothalamic tumors affect the functioning of the autonomic nervous system and the endocrine system. Thus they affect multiple diverse functions, such as gastrointestinal secretion and motility, blood pressure, sweating, sleep, response to pleasure and pain, and body temperature.

The hypothalamus acts as the thermostat to maintain body temperature. The "set point" of this thermostat can be changed in the following two ways. First, pyrogens, activating substances that produce fever, are released from damaged body tissues, from the destruction of leukocytes, or from invading pathogens themselves. These pyrogens in the blood stream cause the hypothalamic thermostat set point to rise. With the thermostat fixed on a higher-than-normal temperature, the rate of energy heat production is increased until the body temperature reaches this new set point. Second, the hypothalamic thermostat also can lower the set point in response to strong stimulation of skin temperature sensors. If the skin becomes overheated, the thermostatic set point is reduced a few tenths of a degree. The heat-losing activities of the hypothalamus are brought into play quickly before the excessive heat sensed by the skin can be transmitted to the interior of the body.[6]

Lesions of the more anterior portion of the hypothalamus lead to *hyperthermia,* which often is resistant to antipyretic drugs. Increased heat production—for example, from thyrotoxicosis—and impaired heat loss that occurs in decreased cardiac output states are some of the other causes of hyperthermia. In addition, extremes of environmental temperatures can lead to heat exhaustion or worse (heat stroke).

Malignant hyperthermia represents an extremely critical disorder of temperature regulation related to the reaction from potent anesthetic agents and depolarizing muscle relaxants that induce a hypermetabolic condition. It is an inherited disorder that affects males more often than females.[7] The triggering anesthetic releases calcium from the sarcoplasmic reticulum of muscle cells; for the muscle fibers to relax, calcium must be pumped back into the sarcoplasmic reticulum. This mechanism does not occur in malignant hyperthermia, and myoplasm calcium levels rise. Increased muscular contraction occurs, along with rigidity, and it and chemical events lead to increased heat production and oxygen consumption.[8] Temperatures can rise as high as 42.7° C (109° F). Potassium, magnesium, and phosphate leak into the extracellular fluid, and sodium moves into the cell. Dysrhythmias occur as a result of increased serum potassium, hypoxemia, and acidosis. Creatine phosphokinase (CPK) and myoglobin leak out of the muscle membrane and are excreted by the kidneys. Myoglobin can accumulate in the kidneys, leading to renal failure. In addition, altered platelet function can result in disseminated intravascular coagulation (DIC).[7]

Malignant hyperthermia should be suspected if intense muscle fasciculations and rigid masseter muscles are observed during anesthesia induction. Further clinical manifestations of malignant hyperthermia and its management are discussed in the nursing management plans on pp. 561 and 562.

Lesions in the more posterior parts of the hypothalamus may lead to *hypothermia* or *poikilothermia* (body temperature varies with that of the environment). Acute illnesses such as congestive heart failure, uremia, diabetes mellitus, drug overdose, and acute respiratory failure can cause severe failure of thermoregulation and lead to hypothermia. Hypothermia also can occur in a patient with a spinal cord injury that interrupts normal sympathetic outflow, but this hypothermia is not related to hypothalamic dysfunction. A better-known cause of hypothermia occurs from accidental exposure to excessively low environmental temperatures in which body heat is lost through conduction, convection, and radiation. In fact, 50% of the body's heat production can be lost through radiation from an uncovered head. Accidental hypothermia has been associated with myxedema, pituitary insufficiency, Addison's disease, hypoglycemia, cerebrovascular disease, cirrhosis, pancreatitis, and ingestion of drugs or alcohol.[8] A common scenario for hypothermia is to find an unconscious person lying on the ground in wintertime. Immersion in cold water creates an even more dramatic hypothermia because thermal conductivity of water is estimated to be 32 times that of thermal conductivity of air.[9]

Somnolence and hypotension often accompany hypothermia. Most deaths occur at body temperatures below 32° C and at environmental temperatures below 12° C. Asystole or ventricular fibrillation occurs at body temperatures of 20° C.[8] Treatment is aimed at preventing further heat loss and performing rewarming measures and advanced cardiac life support measures.

For the management of hyperthermia or hypothermia caused by primary brain abnormality that affects hypothalamic thermoregulation, the nurse cautiously tries to maintain normothermia, monitoring closely for rapid variations in body temperature. Guides to nursing interventions are noted in the neurologic management plans on hyperthermia related to pharmacogenic hypermetabolism and hypothermia related to environmental exposure, pp. 561 and 562.

Craniopharyngiomas. Craniopharyngiomas are tumors derived from remnants of embryonic tissue. They are found primarily in children. These tumors frequently are cytologically benign but biologically malignant because of the location or invasive potential.

Craniopharyngiomas are composed of epithelial-type cells that secrete a cholesterol-containing viscous fluid irritating to the CNS. Frequently the tumor portion is only a small part of the lesion, with the larger portion consisting of a fluid-filled cyst.[1]

Vascular tumors. Vascular tumors of the CNS include hemangioma, hemangioblastoma, and, in some classifications, arteriovenous malformation (AVM). A hemangioma is a closely packed group of abnormally dilated blood vessels. The hemangioblastoma contains a mixture of capillaries and large stromal cells. Both tumors usually are small and considered benign unless hemorrhage occurs. These lesions are found in both the brain and spinal cord.

The AVM is a tangled mass of arterial and venous vessels that may be seen initially as a mass lesion or CNS hemorrhage. AVMs are discussed in the section on cerebrovascular disease later in this chapter.

Metastatic lesions. Lesions that most commonly give rise to metastases in the CNS are lung and breast lesions. Tumor cells are spread by blood or the lymphatic system. Metastatic lesions generally are well circumscribed with a defined margin. Lesions, however, usually are multiple. The incidence of metastatic tumors of the CNS is increasing as therapy for limiting growth at other tumor sites improves.[1] Generally the blood-brain barrier remains intact with metastatic lesions so that treatment with chemotherapeutic agents is difficult.

Assessment and Diagnosis

Assessment of a suspected CNS tumor focuses on the patient's specific neurologic abnormalities. Possible neurologic dysfunctions are as varied as the different portions of the CNS. Patients initially may have focal neurologic deficit, history of increasing headaches that are worse in the morning than in the evening, seizure activity, hormonal changes, or personality changes.

Physical examination serves to further define the focal neurologic deficit. If the tumor is large enough to create a mass effect, papilledema may be found. Papilledema is present in 70% to 75% of all brain tumors.

Depending on the suspected abnormality, diagnostic work-up may include a CT scan, MRI, EEG, neuroendocrine tests, cerebral angiogram, chest x-ray examination, or bone scan. After a specific lesion has been identified, a biopsy specimen frequently is obtained for histologic examination. Once the type of tumor has been diagnosed, medical management can be planned.

Medical Management

Medical management of a CNS tumor centers on surgery, radiation, and chemotherapy. Depending on the type and location of the tumor, any or all of these treatment modalities may be employed.

If cerebral edema is a major factor associated with the

identified tumor, the use of steroids often is the beginning point of medical management. Steroid administration, particularly dexamethasone (Decadron), can result in a significant but temporary reversal of neurologic symptoms. Steroids, believed to reduce cerebral edema by strengthening the cell membrane, decrease neurologic deficit by reducing intracranial pressure.

◆ **Surgery.** Surgical removal of the entire lesion is the goal but not always the outcome. In benign, well-defined lesions, surgical removal may be the only treatment necessary. In invasive, poorly defined lesions, surgery is the beginning point of treatment. Even though it is well recognized that a craniotomy will not remove 100% of an invasive tumor, "debulking" of the tumor mass reduces pressure on surrounding structures and may slow the growth process.

◆ **Radiation.** With incompletely excised tumors, radiation often is the next step of medical management. Some tumors that occur in functionally critical areas, such as the brainstem, hypothalamus, or thalamus, are not surgically accessible without resulting in significant neurologic deficit. Radiation may be the primary medical management of these tumors. The goal of radiation is to destroy or retard the growth of tumor cells without damaging normal tissue. Histologic diagnosis of the tumor cell is essential in planning the type of radiation to be used. The total dose of radiation varies, depending on the tumor type, location, size of the field, and prior or concurrent chemotherapy. Generally it is not recommended to give more than 3500 to 5000 rads in total radiation treatment.

Use of stereotaxically placed radioactive-loaded catheters implanted into the tumor bed is a method currently being investigated. The patient undergoes catheter placement in the operating room and is admitted overnight to the critical care unit. The next day the catheters are loaded with radioactive material and the patient is transferred to a room equipped for handling radiation implants.

◆ **Chemotherapy.** Until recently, chemotherapy treatment was unavailable to patients with malignant brain tumors because it was believed that chemotherapeutic agents *did not cross the blood-brain barrier.* Although that is still of primary concern, other factors also limit the effects of chemotherapy on brain tumors. Tumors of the CNS are small by nature. Although mitosis of abnormal cells in the tumor bed is occurring, it may not occur at a fast enough rate for a course of chemotherapy to be effective.[10] Also, with further study it appears that the microenvironment of the tumor area is not heterogeneous and therefore not 100% sensitive to any one chemotherapeutic agent.[10]

In all considerations of chemotherapy, attention must be focused on protection of the normal delicate cerebral tissue.

◆ **Future treatment modalities.** Research and investigation in improved treatment of malignant CNS tumors continue in all the areas previously discussed. Microsurgical techniques and the use of laser surgery allow access to previously inoperable tumors and improved excision of invasive tumors. A variety of approaches in radiation therapy, including radionuclide seed implantation and the concurrent use of a variety of chemotherapeutic agents in conjunction with radiation, are under investigation. Advances in chemotherapy include the continued development of agents with greater specificity for CNS tumor cells.

A new concept for tumor management, which has been under clinical investigation, is stereotactic radiosurgery. Radiosurgery is performed through the use of a single high dose of ionizing radiation directed at a small, well-defined intracranial lesion without significantly affecting surrounding tissue. This technique is employed by use of a "gamma knife," or external high-energy photon beams from a linear accelerator.[11] Radiosurgery most often is used for histologically benign lesions, such as vascular malformations, acoustic neuromas, and pituitary adenomas. If the tumor volume is small, radiosurgery safely has caused tumor disappearance,

NURSING DIAGNOSIS AND MANAGEMENT

Cerebral tumors

- ◆ Altered Cerebral Tissue Perfusion related to increased intracranial pressure secondary to brain trauma, hemorrhage, edema, infection, tumor, stroke, hydrocephalus, p. 560
- ◆ Unilateral Neglect related to perceptual disruption secondary to stroke involving the right cerebral hemisphere, p. 564
- ◆ Impaired Verbal Communication: Aphasia related to cerebral speech center injury, p. 571
- ◆ High Risk for Aspiration risk factors: impaired laryngeal sensation or reflex; impaired pharyngeal peristalsis or tongue function; impaired laryngeal closure or elevation p. 472
- ◆ High Risk for Infection risk factor: invasive monitoring devices, p. 366
- ◆ Sleep Pattern Disturbance related to fragmented sleep, p. 142
- ◆ Sensory/Perceptual Alterations related to sensory overload, sensory deprivation, sleep pattern disturbance, p. 573
- ◆ Anxiety related to threat to biologic, psychologic, and/or social integrity, p. 763
- ◆ Ineffective Individual Coping related to situational crisis and personal vulnerability, p. 762
- ◆ Body Image Disturbance related to actual change in body structure, function, or appearance, p. 94
- ◆ Altered Role Performance related to physical incapacity to resume usual or valued role, p. 97
- ◆ Knowledge Deficit: Prognosis, Medications, Activity Restrictions, Reportable Symptoms related to lack of previous exposure to information, p. 72
- ◆ Hopelessness related to perceptions of failing or deteriorating physical condition, p. 100

shrinkage, or stabilization regardless of prior surgery, conventional irradiation, or tumor radioresistance.[12] The fact that radiosurgery often is performed with local anesthesia and without surgical incision makes radiosurgery a primary treatment alternative for patients who are elderly or medically infirm or who refuse microsurgical removal.[13]

Another concept in CNS tumor management currently is under clinical investigation. It involves the use of regional hyperthermia to destroy tumor cells. Hypoxia, poor blood flow, and acidic pH, common features in inner regions of many brain tumors, all enhance sensitivity to hyperthermia. Further clinical trials are needed to evaluate the efficacy of this therapy.[14]

Whatever the focus of the future, continued research for the treatment of malignant CNS tumors can only improve the outcome of this disease and its often tragic consequences.

Nursing Management

Most nursing management of the patient with a CNS tumor does not occur in the critical care environment. Generally, patients are in the critical care unit during the postoperative stage of craniotomy. With the advent of steroids, the cerebral edema associated with brain tumors and craniotomy virtually has been eliminated. Patients with an uncomplicated craniotomy for removal of a brain tumor often remain in the critical care unit only overnight, if at all. Patients who have had excision of a cervical or high thoracic spinal cord tumor will be in the unit postoperatively for close observation of respiratory status and motor/sensory function of the extremities.

The psychosocial aspects that face a patient with a CNS tumor must never be ignored, even in the immediate postoperative period. Support must be offered to the family or significant others, as well as to the patient.

CEREBROVASCULAR DISEASE

Cerebrovascular Accident

Cerebrovascular accident, commonly known as *stroke,* is a descriptive term for the onset of neurologic symptoms caused by the interruption of blood flow to the brain. There are two basic types of stroke: ischemic and hemorrhagic. Ischemic stroke is a stroke that produces symptoms resulting from an occlusion of a blood vessel. This can be either thrombotic or embolic in nature. Most thrombotic strokes are the result of the accumulation of atherosclerotic plaque in the vessel lumen, especially at bifurcations or curves of the vessel. An embolic stroke occurs when a small embolus from the heart or lower cerebral circulation travels distally and lodges in a small vessel, resulting in loss of blood supply. Hemorrhagic strokes are divided into intracerebral hemorrhage and subarachnoid hemorrhage. Intracerebral hemorrhage most often is caused by hypertensive rupture of a cerebral vessel. Subarachnoid hemorrhage can be caused by aneurysm rupture or arteriovenous malformation (AVM) rupture. In a prospective study of 694 patients hospitalized for stroke, 53% had thrombotic strokes, 31% had embolic strokes, 10% had intracerebral hematoma, and 6% had subarachnoid hemorrhage from aneurysm or AVM.[15]

◆ **Incidence.** Stroke is the third leading cause of death in the United States, preceded only by heart disease and cancer. Along with the high mortality associated with stroke, significant morbidity affects patients who survive. The Framingham study, an extensive 20-year follow-up of survivors of stroke in the 45- to 74-year age range, found that 31% needed assistance in self-care, 20% required assistance in ambulation, 71% had impaired vocational capacity 7 years after stroke, and 16% were institutionalized.[16] It is estimated that 1.6 million Americans have had strokes; 40% require special services and 10% total care.[17]

◆ **Risk factors.** The risk of a person having a stroke before reaching age 70 is 1 in 20.[18] The major risk factors for stroke are those that result in the development of atherosclerosis, such as hypertension, cardiac impairments, or diabetes mellitus.

Hypertension. By far the greatest risk factor of stroke is hypertension, and the risk is equal in men and women with comparable blood pressure. Hypertension is a factor in both ischemic and hemorrhagic stroke.

Hypertension leads to structural changes in cerebral arteries and accelerated atherogenesis. Over time, it also impairs cerebral autoregulation.

Cardiac impairments. Cardiac abnormalities, such as atrial fibrillation, coronary artery disease, or enlarged heart, are present in 75% of stroke patients. Atrial fibrillation, in particular, is associated with a high incidence of stroke. Blood pools in the poorly emptying atria of the heart. Tiny clots form in the left atrium, which then move through the heart and out into the cerebral circulation to cause embolic stroke.

Diabetes mellitus. Vascular disease in general is more prevalent in patients with diabetes mellitus. Thrombotic stroke from the accumulation of atherosclerotic plaque is the most common type of stroke in diabetic patients.

Minor risk factors. Other factors that have been linked less consistently with stroke are elevated blood lipids, obesity, smoking, stress, and family history.

The discussion of assessment, pathophysiology, diagnosis, and management of the aforementioned cerebrovascular disease processes is too large an undertaking for this chapter. Instead, focus is directed on the three pathologic conditions of hemorrhagic disease: aneurysm, arteriovenous malformation, and spontaneous hemorrhage. Because of the sudden onset and potential for mass effect of these hemorrhagic diseases, a critical care environment for stabilization and support is required more often than in the care of other types of cerebrovascular disease.

Cerebral Aneurysm

An aneurysm is an outpouching of the wall of a blood vessel that results from weakening of the wall of the vessel. Aneurysms can occur in vessels in other parts of the body from a variety of causes, but in this section the discussion centers on cerebral aneurysms. Most cerebral aneurysms are saccular or berrylike with a stem and neck. Aneurysms are usually small, 2 to 6 mm in diameter, but may be as large as 6 cm. Clinical concern arises if an aneurysm ruptures or becomes large enough to exert pressure on surrounding structures.

◆ **Incidence.** It is estimated that approximately 6% of strokes are caused by aneurysm rupture. The incidence of cerebral aneurysm has been estimated at 10 per 100,000 population.[19] It is possible for an individual to live a full life span with an unruptured cerebral aneurysm.

Subarachnoid hemorrhage (SAH) is usually the result of aneurysm rupture. Although there are other causes of SAH, aneurysm rupture is responsible for 70%.[20] Subarachnoid hemorrhage is a serious phenomenon with a mortality of 40% for the initial insult, and another 10% to 15% mortality is a result of complications such as rebleeding or vasospasm. Significant morbidity also is a major factor after SAH.[7] The peak incidence of aneurysm rupture is between 40 and 65 years of age. Few aneurysms rupture in persons younger than the age of 20.[21]

◆ **Etiology.** Ninety percent of aneurysms are congenital. The other 10% can be a result of traumatic injury (that stretches and tears the muscular middle layer of the arterial vessel), infectious material (most often from infectious vegetation on valves of the left side of the heart after subbacterial endocarditis) that lodges against a vessel wall and erodes the muscular layer, or of undetermined cause. Multiple aneurysms occur in 20% to 25% of the cases and often are bilateral, occurring in the same location on both sides of the head.

Aneurysms frequently occur at the base of the brain on the circle of Willis. The distribution is anterior communicating artery, 30%; posterior communicating artery, 25%; branching of the middle cerebral artery, 13%; and all other locations, 32% (Fig. 28-2). Most cerebral aneurysms, especially those that are congenital, occur at the bifurcation of blood vessels.

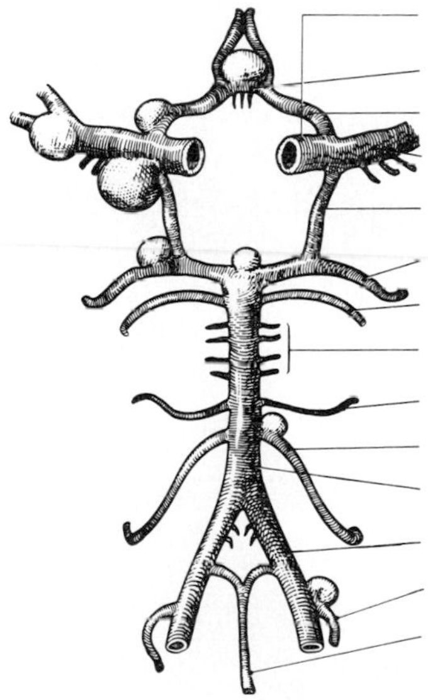

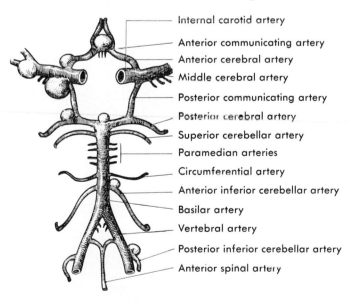

Fig. 28-2 The common sites of berry aneurysms. The size of the aneurysm in the drawing is proportional to the frequency of occurrence at the various sites. (From Wyngaarden JB, Smith LH, editors: *Cecil's textbook of medicine,* ed 16, Philadelphia, 1982, WB Saunders.)

◆ **Pathophysiology.** The cause of the defect in vessel development that occurs in the congenital aneurysm is unknown. A small portion of the inner muscular or elastic layer of the vessel is poorly developed, leaving a thin vessel wall. As the individual matures, blood pressure rises and more stress is placed on this thin vessel wall. Ballooning out of the vessel occurs, which gives the aneurysm its berrylike appearance.

The aneurysm becomes clinically significant when the vessel wall becomes so thin that it ruptures, sending arterial blood at a high pressure into the subarachnoid space. For a brief moment of aneurysm rupture, intracranial pressure is believed to approach mean arterial pressure and cerebral perfusion falls.[22] In other situations the unruptured aneurysm expands and places pressure on surrounding structures. This is particularly true with the posterior communicating artery aneurysm that puts pressure on the oculomotor nerve (CN III), causing ipsilateral pupil dilation and ptosis.

◆ Assessment and diagnosis

Initial presentation. The patient with an aneurysm usually is seen initially after subarachnoid hemorrhage. SAH becomes the working diagnosis until the cause of the hemorrhage is determined. Clinical manifestations of SAH range from sudden onset of the "worst headache of my life" to coma or death.

SAH has been divided into five grades for classification of severity of the neurologic deficits associated with the bleed[23]:

Grade I	Asymptomatic, minimal headache, slight nuchal rigidity
Grade II	Moderate to severe headache, nuchal rigidity, minimal neurologic deficit
Grade III	Drowsiness, confusion, mild focal neurologic deficit
Grade IV	Stupor, moderate to severe hemiparesis, early decerebrate posturing
Grade V	Comatose, decorticate or decerebrate posturing, moribund appearance

Of the patients who survive SAH, 45% report sudden, brief loss of consciousness followed by severe headache, 45% report severe headache associated with exertion but no loss of consciousness, and in 10% the bleeding was severe enough to cause loss of consciousness for up to several days.[24] Vomiting, nuchal rigidity (stiff neck), photophobia, seizure, hemiplegia, or other focal neurologic deficits are common.

A review of histories shows that the patient often reports one or more incidences of sudden onset of headache with vomiting in the weeks preceding major SAH. These are "warning leaks" of the aneurysm in which small amounts of blood ooze from the aneurysm into the subarachnoid space. The presence of blood is an irritant to the meninges, particularly the arachnoid membrane. This irritation causes headache, stiff neck, and photophobia. These small "warning leaks" seldom are detected because the condition is not severe enough for the patient to seek medical attention. If a neurologic deficit, such as third cranial nerve palsy, develops before aneurysm rupture, medical intervention is sought and the aneurysm may be surgically secured before the devastation of rupture can occur.

Diagnostic tests. Diagnosis of SAH is based on clinical presentation, as well as CT scan and lumbar puncture. When SAH is suspected, a CT scan is performed to identify subarachnoid blood. In 75% of the cases blood is present in the basal cisterns if the CT scan is performed within 48 hours of the hemorrhage. On the basis of the appearance and the location of the SAH, diagnosis of cause, such as aneurysm or AVM, may be made from the CT scan.

If results of the CT scan are unequivocal, a lumbar puncture is performed to obtain cerebrospinal fluid (CSF) for analysis. CSF after SAH is bloody in appearance with a red blood cell count greater than $1000/mm^3$. If lumbar puncture is performed more than 5 days after the SAH, CSF fluid is xanthochromic (dark amber) because blood products have broken down. Cloudy CSF usually indicates some type of infectious process, such as bacterial meningitis, not subarachnoid hemorrhage.

Once the SAH has been documented, a cerebral angiogram is necessary to identify the exact cause of the SAH. If a cerebral aneurysm rupture is the cause, angiogram also is essential to define the exact location of the aneurysm in preparation for surgery (Fig. 28-3).

◆ **Medical management.** Medical management of patients with SAH is complex. Decisions about surgical intervention and the timing of that intervention are based on the patient's clinical condition.

The two major complications after SAH from aneurysm rupture are rebleeding and vasospasm. To achieve a positive outcome after SAH, it is essential to preserve an adequate cerebral blood flow and to prevent a secondary aneurysmal rupture.[25]

Rebleeding. Rebleeding is the occurrence of a second SAH at any time in an unsecured aneurysm. The incidence of rebleeding is as great as 50% in the first few months, with the highest incidence being in the first few days after hemorrhage.[26] Mortality with rebleeding has been reported to be as high as 70%.[27] Definitive treatment for prevention of rebleeding is surgical clipping of the aneurysm. Because of the patient's clinical condition and the technical difficulty of the surgery, early surgical repair of the aneurysm is not always possible. Early surgery (within the first 48 hours after hemorrhage) is recommended for patients with a grade I or grade II SAH. In these patients the initial hemorrhage did not produce significant neurologic deficit, but the risk of rebleeding with a tragically high incidence of mortality is present until the aneurysm is secured.

For years the use of antifibrinolytic agents (aminocaproic acid) has been suggested in situations in which early surgery is not an option. Antifibrinolytic agents act by preventing the production of fibrin responsible for resolving the clot at the tip of the aneurysm. Controversy

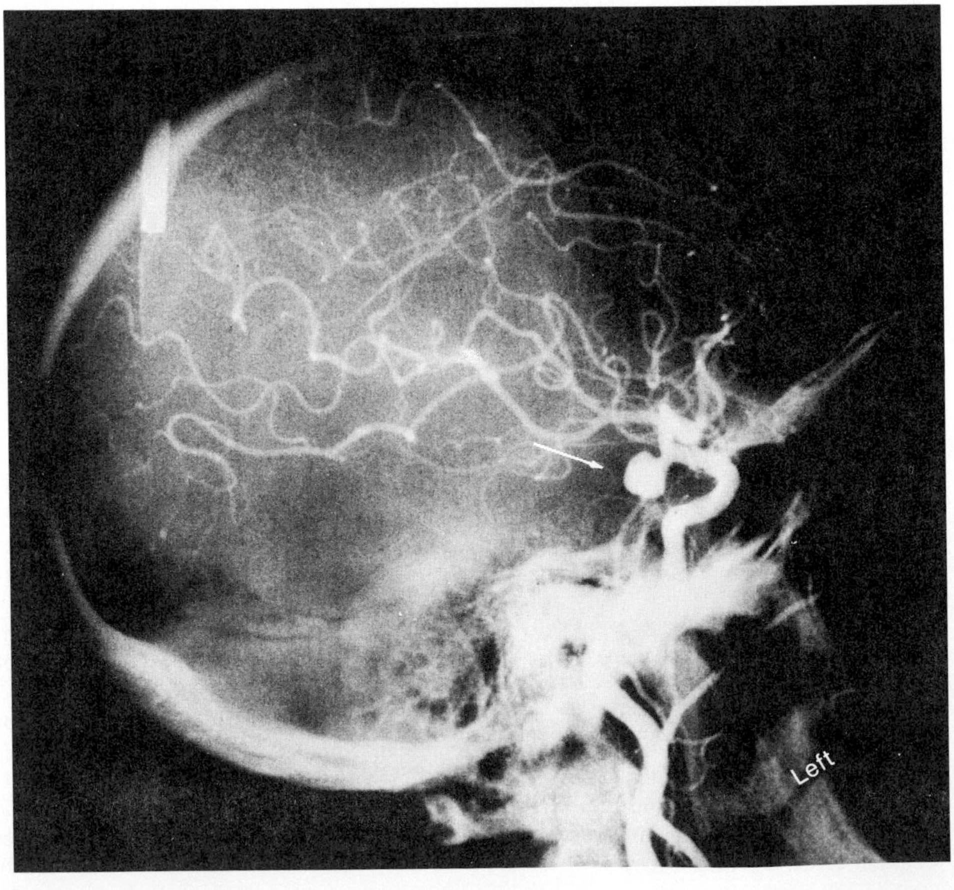

Fig. 28-3 Cerebral angiography showing location of aneurysm at posterior communicating artery. (From Tortorici M: *Fundamentals of angiography,* St Louis, 1982, Mosby–Year Book.)

continues to surround the use of these agents. Results of studies reporting the actual reduced incidence of rebleeding have been minimally positive. The main issue with the use of antifibrinolytic agents is the tendency of this drug to increase the incidence and severity of the other common SAH complication—vasospasm. Clinical trials continue to evaluate the efficacy of this treatment.[28,29]

Cerebral vasospasm. The presence or absence of cerebral vasospasm significantly affects the outcome after SAH. Vasospasm, which is the narrowing of the lumen of the vessel, is believed to be sustained arterial contraction as a response to subarachnoid blood clots coating the outer surface of the blood vessels,[19] and is a critical issue because of its location in the cerebral vasculature. Inasmuch as aneurysms occur at the circle of Willis, the major vessels responsible for feeding cerebral circulation are affected by vasospasm. Depending on the arterial vessels involved in the vasospasm reaction, decreased arterial flow occurs in large areas of the cerebral hemispheres. Ischemic stroke is the outcome of this decreased flow. The peak period for vasospasm is 7 to 14 days after rupture. Vasospasm begins around the third day after rupture and can last for 3 to 4 weeks. Vasospasm occurs in more than 30% to 40% of patients with SAH. In grades III and IV SAH, vasospasm has been reported in more than 65% of the patients.[30]

TREATMENT. A variety of therapies have been evaluated in an attempt to reverse or overcome the vasospasm. To date, two treatments seem to have potential benefit: induced hypervolemic hypertension and administration of calcium channel blockers.

Hypervolemic hypertension involves increasing the patient's blood pressure and cardiac output through the use of fluid and volume expanders, such as plasma. Systolic blood pressure is maintained between 150 and 160 mm Hg. This increase in volume and pressure forces blood at higher pressures through the vasospastic area. Many anecdotal reports exist of patients' neurologic deficits improving as systolic pressure increases from 130 to between 150 and 160 mm Hg. The obvious deterrent to use of induced hypertension is the risk of rebleeding in an unsecured aneurysm. This therapy can be used safely only after surgery for aneurysm clipping. The second complication associated with hypervolemic hypertension therapy is the risk of pulmonary edema associated with fluid overload. Careful monitoring of pulmonary artery wedge pressure, cardiac output, and oxygenation, as well as chest x-ray examination, is important.

The third significant complication possible with hypervolemic hemodilution is elevated intracranial pressure from the increased blood pressure and fluid load. Particularly if ischemic insult from vasospasm has already occurred, the introduction of a high volume of fluid is contraindicated.

The exact role of calcium channel blockers, which constitute the second regimen for the prevention and treatment of vasospasm, is unknown. Calcium channel blockers are believed to affect the influx of calcium, which occurs in an injured cell. Some calcium channel blockers (particularly nimodipine) have a selective cerebral vasodilator effect.[31]

Evidence is mounting in clinical research trials of the effectiveness of these agents if they are begun immediately after the initial hemorrhage.[28,30,31] Results of ongoing clinical trials indicate that treatment with calcium channel blockers is beneficial, both in terms of reduction of ischemic deficit attributable to vasospasm and in clinical outcome if given prophylactically. No apparent therapeutic benefit is evident once a neurologic deficit has developed.[32]

Timing of surgery is a key medical management issue. Historically, patients with aneurysm rupture were placed in a dark, quiet room for 10 to 14 days after SAH. Blood pressure was kept low, and sedation was used. If the patient survived the risk of rebleeding and the course of vasospasm, surgery was performed. The surgical outcome from this procedure was good, but many patients did not survive until the time of the surgery.

Since the introduction of microsurgery and improved surgical techniques, patients frequently are taken to the operating room within the first 48 hours after rupture. This early surgical intervention to secure the aneurysm eliminates the risk of rebleeding and allows hypertensive therapy to be used in the postoperative period for the treatment of vasospasm. Early surgery also allows the neurosurgeon to flush out the excess blood and clots from the basal cisterns (reservoir of CSF around the base of the brain and circle of Willis) to reduce the risk of vasospasm.

Early surgery is not recommended for all patients. Especially in those patients with grade IV or V SAH, early surgery may contribute to the morbidity or mortality. Careful consideration of each patient's clinical situation is necessary in determination of the timing of surgery.

Aneurysm clipping is the surgical procedure that is performed for repair of the aneurysm. This procedure involves a craniotomy to expose the area of aneurysm. The aneurysm itself is isolated, and a clip is placed over the neck of the aneurysm to eliminate the area of weakness. As stated earlier, this is a technically difficult procedure that requires the skill of an experienced neurosurgeon. It is not uncommon, particularly in early surgery, for the clot to break away from the aneurysm as it is surgically exposed. Extensive hemorrhage into the craniotomy site is the result, and cessation of the hemorrhage often causes increased neurologic deficits.

Development of hydrocephalus is a late complication that frequently occurs after SAH. Blood that has circulated in the subarachnoid space and has been absorbed by the arachnoid villi may obstruct these villi and reduce the rate of CSF absorption. Over time, increasing volumes of CSF in the intracranial space produce communicating hydrocephalus.

Treatment consists of placement of a drain to remove CSF. This can be a temporary measure, with a catheter placed into the lateral ventricle and attached to an external drainage bag, or permanent, with the placement of a ventriculoperitoneal shunt.

Arteriovenous Malformation

Arteriovenous malformation (AVM) is a tangled mass of arterial and venous blood vessels that shunt blood directly from the arterial side into the venous side, bypassing the capillary system. AVMs may be small, focal lesions or large lesions that occupy almost an entire hemisphere.

◆ **Incidence.** Although the incidence of AVM is not great, the management of a patient with an AVM is a medical challenge. Of all subarachnoid hemorrhages, 10% are caused by AVM.[20] In contrast to the middle-aged population with SAH from aneurysm, the AVM tends to bleed when the patient is younger. The peak age for AVM bleeding is 15 to 35 years. The mortality of the initial hemorrhage is approximately 20%. Risk of recurrent hemorrhage is about 20%, with an increase in mortality of 10% with each rebleeding episode.[21]

◆ **Etiology.** The cause of an AVM is always congenital. The exact embryonic reason for the development of this malformation is unknown. AVMs are not confined to the cerebral circulation. They occur also in the spinal cord and in the renal, gastrointestinal, or integumentary system; port-wine stains of the skin may be caused by small, superficial AVMs.

◆ **Pathophysiology.** Once the embryonic dysfunction that resulted in the AVM has occurred, the pathophysiologic features are related to the size and location of the malformation. The AVM can be fed by one or more cerebral arteries. Called *feeders,* these arteries tend to enlarge over time and increase the volume of blood shunted through the malformation, as well as increase the overall mass effect. Large, dilated, tortuous draining veins also develop as a result of the increasing flow of blood. Blood flowing into the venous side of the AVM does so at a higher than normal pressure. In a normal vascular flow, mean arterial pressure is 70 to 80 mm Hg, mean arteriole pressure is 35 to 45 mm Hg, and mean capillary pressure drops from 35 to 10 mm Hg as it connects with the venous side. Lack of this capillary bridge allows blood with a mean pressure of 35 to 45 mm Hg to flow into the venous system. Because there is no muscular layer in the vein as there is in the artery, veins become extremely engorged.

As a result of the shunting of blood through the AVM and away from normal cerebral circulation, poor perfusion occurs in the underlying cerebral tissues. This decreased perfusion produces a chronic ischemic state that results in cerebral atrophy.

◆ **Assessment and diagnosis.** Initial assessment of the patient's condition depends on the presenting symptoms. Although subarachnoid hemorrhage is one of the most common and severe presenting symptoms, other clinical manifestations also may occur before subarachnoid hemorrhage.

The onset of seizures frequently is the reason for the patient with an AVM to seek medical attention. As the mass of the AVM enlarges and the flow of blood increases, the pulsation of the blood vessel against the cerebral tissue surface causes a disturbance of the electrical activity of the area. Seizures can be focal or generalized.

Headaches are another common symptom of patients with an AVM. Headache may occur as a result of the increasing mass effect of the lesion or can be associated with vascular changes in response to the shunted blood. Headaches alone do not often trigger the suspicion of AVM because of the wide variety of reasons for headache.

A very small percentage of the patients demonstrate a bruit and report a constant swishing sound in the head with each heartbeat. In other patients the bruit can be auscultated with a stethoscope placed over the skull.

Other symptoms of AVM may include motor/sensory defects, aphasia, dizziness, or fainting. Because most patients are under the age of 30, symptoms such as these would not likely be attributed to atherosclerotic vascular disease.

Diagnostic evaluation includes CT scan, EEG, and angiogram. CT scanning is performed initially as a noninvasive study to begin the diagnostic process. If an AVM is suspected from the results of the noncontrast scan, a contrast scan is performed. An EEG is obtained to attempt to localize any seizure focus or to define areas of cortical injury caused by cerebral ischemia or atrophy.

Finally, for confirmation and definition of the AVM, an angiogram is performed. If surgical intervention is planned, an angiogram is required to identify the feeding arteries and draining veins of the AVM.

◆ **Medical management**

Surgical excision. Medical management traditionally has involved surgical excision of the AVM or conservative management of such symptoms as seizures and headache. The decision for surgical excision depends on the location and size of the AVM. Some malformations are located so deep in cerebral structures (the thalamus or midbrain) that attempts to remove the AVM would cause severe neurologic deficits. The history of previous hemorrhage, the age, and general condition of the patient also are taken into account in the decision about surgical intervention.

Reperfusion bleeding. Surgical excision of large AVMs includes the risk of reperfusion bleeding. As feeding arteries of the AVM are clamped off, the arterial blood that usually flowed into the AVM is now diverted into the surrounding circulation. In many cases the surrounding tissue has been in a state of chronic ischemia and the arterial vessels feeding these areas are maximally dilated. As arterial blood begins to flow at a higher volume and pressure into these dilated arteries, seeping of blood from the vessels may occur. The evidence of reperfusion bleeding in the operating room is an indication that no more arterial blood can be diverted from the AVM without risk of serious intracerebral hemorrhage. In the postoperative phase, low blood pressure is maintained to prevent further reperfusion bleeding. In large AVMs, two to four stages of surgery might be required over a 6- to 12-month period.

Embolization. Embolization is another method of reducing the size of an AVM. It also may be used on surgically inaccessible AVMs. Embolization is an interventional radiologic technique in which a catheter is placed in the groin or other site in a manner similar to that for an angiogram. Under fluoroscopy, the catheter is threaded up to the internal carotid artery. Small Silastic beads or a variety of other materials, such as glue, are then slowly introduced through the catheter. The increased flow to the AVM should carry the blocking material into the AVM. The purpose of this procedure is to block the feeding arterial portion of the AVM and therefore eliminate it. Frequently, embolization and surgery are combined. The patient undergoes one to three sessions of embolization to reduce the size of the lesion and then has a craniotomy for total excision.

Risks of the procedure include lodging of the substance in a vessel that feeds normal tissue. This occurrence creates an embolic stroke. Onset of neurologic symptoms is immediate. Another risk involves passage of the embolic substance through the lesion, out of the venous system, and into the lung. If this event should occur, a pulmonary embolus results.

Radiation therapy, particularly proton beam radiation, occasionally is used for large lesions that are not surgically accessible. The overall success of radiation therapy is unknown.

Intracerebral Hemorrhage

Intracerebral hemorrhage is the escape of blood into cerebral tissue. Causes of intracerebral hemorrhage are aneurysm or AVM rupture, trauma, or hypertensive hemorrhage. This section concentrates on hypertensive hemorrhage. Hemorrhage destroys cerebral tissue, causes cerebral edema, and increases intracranial pressure (ICP).

◆ **Incidence.** The incidence of hypertensive hemorrhage accounts for 2% of all deaths in the United States and is responsible for about 10% of the strokes and 15% of all intracranial hemorrhages.[15]

◆ **Etiology.** The cause of hypertensive stroke is largely a long-standing history of hypertension. Blood dyscrasia (leukemia, hemophilia, sickle cell disease), anticoagulation therapy, and hemorrhage into brain tumors are other possible causes of intracerebral hemorrhage. Frequently on questioning, the patient with a hypertensive hemorrhage will admit to having discontinued antihypertensive medication 2 to 3 weeks before the hemorrhage.

◆ **Pathophysiology.** The pathophysiology of intracerebral hemorrhage is caused by continued elevated blood pressure exerting force against smaller arterial vessels that have become damaged from arteriosclerotic changes. Eventually this artery breaks, and blood bursts from the vessel into the cerebral tissue, creating a hematoma. ICP rises precipitously in response to the increased overall intracranial volume.

◆ **Assessment and diagnosis.** Initial assessment usually reveals a critically ill patient who often is unconscious and requires ventilatory support. History from a relative or significant other describes a sudden onset of severe headache with rapid neurologic deterioration.

Vital signs usually reveal a severely elevated blood pressure (200/100 to 250/150 mm Hg), slow pulse, and deep, labored respirations. The patient arrives in the emergency room with many of the signs of increased ICP. ABCs should be addressed first to make sure airway is adequate, breathing patterns are acceptable, and circulation is present.

An antihypertensive medication usually is administered immediately to reduce the blood pressure to a relatively normal reading. If the hemorrhage is significant enough to cause increased ICP, the blood pressure should not be allowed to drop rapidly or too low. If blood pressure drops below 140 mm Hg systolic and ICP remains high, cerebral perfusion may be compromised.

◆ **Medical management.** Medical management of a hypertensive hemorrhage is similar to that for a traumatic hemorrhage. Surgical removal of the clot depends on the size and location of the clot, the patient's ICP, and other neurologic symptoms. If the hematoma is large and causes a shift in structures or ICP is elevated despite routine methods to lower it, a craniotomy for removal of the hematoma is performed. Nonsurgical management includes measures to maintain the ICP within normal limits and to support all other vital functions until the patient regains consciousness.

Nursing Management

Nursing management of the previously discussed cerebrovascular diseases requires that the nurse have a thorough knowledge of the pathophysiology of the disease, as well as a good understanding of the treatment plan. Accurate, detailed assessment is essential. Frequently the first sign of clinical deterioration is evidenced through subtle changes discovered in the neurologic examination.

Adequate blood pressure is necessary to continue to supply the brain with the appropriate amount of oxygen and nutrients. When, however, damage or disease of the cerebrovascular system is the cause of the patient's hospitalization, the actual level of blood pressure that is most appropriate for the patient depends on the underlying condition. After spontaneous intracerebral hemorrhage or initial subarachnoid hemorrhage, for example, it is important to keep the blood pressure relatively low. In vasospasm after subarachnoid hemorrhage, relatively high blood pressures are required for adequate perfusion. The nurse's role is to monitor blood pressure constantly, administer medications as necessary, and observe the patient's activities and interactions in response to blood pressure.

If the patient is comatose after the cerebrovascular insult, all interventions for caring for the immobile patient should be initiated. Because immobility is implicated in many patient complications, intervention to reduce the effects of immobility should begin as soon as possible.

Emotional support of the patient and family is, as always, important. Especially if the patient is dealing with a neurologic deficit, such as hemiplegia, aphasia, or any other significant neurologic problem, fears of dependency and of becoming a burden are issues that must be faced. Both the patient and family should be involved in all aspects of planning of care.

Two problems commonly found in the patient with

NURSING DIAGNOSIS AND MANAGEMENT
Cerebral vascular disease

- ◆ Altered Cerebral Tissue Perfusion related to increased intracranial pressure secondary to brain trauma, hemorrhage, edema, infection, tumor, stroke, hydrocephalus, p. 560
- ◆ Altered Cerebral Tissue Perfusion related to vasospasm secondary to subarachnoid hemorrhage after ruptured intracranial aneurysm or arteriovenous malformation, p. 558
- ◆ Unilateral Neglect related to perceptual disruption secondary to stroke involving the right cerebral hemisphere, p. 564
- ◆ Impaired Verbal Communication: Aphasia related to cerebral speech center injury, p. 571
- ◆ High Risk for Aspiration risk factors: impaired laryngeal sensation or reflex; impaired pharyngeal peristalsis or tongue function; impaired laryngeal closure or elevation; increased gastric volume; decreased lower esophageal sphincter pressure, p. 472
- ◆ High Risk for Altered Peripheral Tissue Perfusion risk factor: high-dose vasopressor therapy (vasospasm after cerebral artery aneurysm rupture), p. 363
- ◆ Impaired Gas Exchange related to alveolar hypoventilation secondary to decreased level of consciousness, p. 471
- ◆ Ineffective Breathing Pattern related to musculoskeletal impairment, p. 470
- ◆ Ineffective Airway Clearance related to impaired cough secondary to artificial airway, p. 466
- ◆ Activity Intolerance related to postural hypotension secondary to prolonged immobility, narcotics, vasodilation therapy, p. 365
- ◆ Altered Nutrition: Less Than Body Protein-Calorie Requirements related to lack of exogenous nutrients and increased metabolic demand, p. 673
- ◆ High Risk for Infection risk factors: invasive monitoring devices, p. 366
- ◆ Anxiety related to threat to biologic, psychologic, and/or social integrity, p. 763
- ◆ Ineffective Individual Coping related to situational crisis and personal vulnerability, p. 762
- ◆ Sensory/Perceptual Alterations related to sensory deprivation, sensory overload, sleep pattern disturbance, p. 573
- ◆ Sleep Pattern Disturbance related to fragmented sleep, p. 142
- ◆ Body Image Disturbance related to actual change in body structure, function, or appearance, p. 94
- ◆ Powerlessness related to health care environment and illness-related regimen, p. 98
- ◆ Altered Role Performance related to physical incapacity to resume usual or valued role, p. 97
- ◆ Self-Esteem Disturbance related to feelings of guilt about physical deterioration, p. 96
- ◆ Knowledge Deficit: Physical Rehabilitation, Medications, Reportable Symptoms related to lack of previous exposure to information, p. 72

cerebrovascular disease are detailed next: unilateral neglect and impaired communication.

◆ **Unilateral neglect.** Unilateral neglect, or *hemi-inattention,* is a perceptual neurologic defect characterized by an unawareness or denial of an affected half of the body. This neglect also may extend to extrapersonal space. This defect most often results from right hemispheric brain damage that causes left hemiplegia. Such a disorder of perception also may include disturbances of body image, spatial judgment, and sensory interpretation.[33] Perceptual defects are not as readily noticeable as are motor deficits but may be more debilitating to the patient and can lead to the inability to perform skilled or purposeful tasks. In addition to unilateral neglect, several other sensory/perceptual alterations that can occur with hemispheric damage are discussed here.

Lesions in the nondominant or right temporoparietal or parieto-occipital areas cause unilateral neglect more often than do left-hemispheric lesions. In most persons the left side of the brain is dominant for speech, analytic abilities, and verbal and auditory memory, and the right side specializes in spatial relations, perception, creativity, and nonverbal memory.

Stroke is a common cause of right hemispheric damage that can result in unilateral neglect. The blood supply to the parietal lobe is provided by all three major cerebroarterial distributions. The middle cerebral artery supplies the major portion of the parietal lobe, with the anterior cerebral artery supplying the anterior and medial parts and the posterior cerebral artery supplying a small posterior portion. Stroke in any of these vessels can damage the parietal lobe, resulting in perceptual impairments.[34]

Through the thalamus the parietal lobe receives sensory fibers that convey cutaneous and deep sensations arising from the opposite side of the body. Kinesthetic alterations in sensory perception include *hemianesthesia,* the loss of sensation in the affected side, and *paresthesias,* feelings such as heaviness, numbness, tingling, prickling, and a heightened sensitivity in the affected side. The loss of muscle-joint sense can lead to a loss of *proprioception,* or position sense, which affects the patient's balance and ability to ambulate.[34]

Some sensory data for vision are interpreted and integrated within the parietal lobe to establish an awareness of the body and its parts and a sense of spatial relationships. Defects in spatial orientation can interfere with the patient's ability to judge position, distance, movement, form, and the relationship of his or her body parts to surrounding objects. Patients may confuse such concepts as up and down and forward and backward. They may have difficulty following a route from one place to another and may even get lost in areas that were once familiar. Stroke patients may also experience reading and writing problems related to visual perception and visuospatial deficits. One type of spatial dyslexia is related to unilateral spatial neglect. The patient may not look at the beginning of a line of written material that appears on the left. Instead the patient fixes attention on a point to the right of the beginning of the line and reads to the end of the line. If asked to draw a design, the person completes only half a design or drawing.[35]

Some of these spatial-neglect problems are related to visual field defects. Visual field defects may accompany the unilateral neglect syndrome, although they do not cause it. A hemispheric lesion can interrupt the visual pathways, with the resulting visual defect dependent on the location and extent of the lesion. At the optic chiasm, nerve fibers coming from the nasal half of each retina cross to the opposite side, whereas fibers coming from the temporal half of each retina do not cross. This partial crossing allows binocular vision. In the optic chiasm, fibers from the nasal half of each retina join the uncrossed fibers from the temporal half of the retina to form the optic tract. Impulses conducted to the right hemisphere by the right optic tract represent the left field of vision, and those conducted to the left hemisphere by the left optic tract represent the right field of vision. Optic radiations extend back to the occipital lobes. Visual defects restricted to a single field, right or left, are termed *homonymous.* For example, a right-hemispheric lesion resulting in the loss of the left half of the visual field of each eye is called homonymous *hemianopsia.*

It is not uncommon for the patient experiencing unilateral neglect to have a significant visual field loss. The nurse may be the first person to detect that the patient has this defect. The patient with hemianopsia may neglect all sensory input from the affected side and initially may appear unresponsive if approached from the affected side. If the nurse approaches the patient from the healthy side, the patient actually may be quite alert. Another clue to hemianopsia is observing that the patient eats food only from one half of the tray.

Hemianopsia may recede gradually with time. Many patients can learn to scan their environment visually to compensate for the defect, although in the acute stage of stroke the patient may be too lethargic to follow instructions in methods of visual scanning. This visual defect can lead to fear and confusion and present a risk to the patient's safety. The nurse can lessen the detrimental effects of hemianopsia and unilateral neglect by making sure that the bed is positioned so the patient can see the door of the room and thus people coming and going. If the patient's "blind" side faces the door, the tendency to neglect the affected side will be accentuated. Once the patient is learning to scan visually, it may be advantageous to reverse this bed position to encourage interaction with the environment through visual scanning.[35,36]

Other specific syndromes resulting from right hemispheric lesions and associated with unilateral neglect include language problems—for example, difficulty understanding concepts such as proverbs and idioms. Patients may talk excessively but have difficulty getting to the point. Their voice and facial expressions may lack emotion (flat affect), and they may have difficulty understanding facial expressions and emotions in others.[37]

Body image often is disturbed after stroke. *Anosognosia* is the term used to denote varying degrees of denial of the affected side of the body. This denial may range from inattention to actual refusing to acknowledge a paralysis by neglecting the involved side or by denying ownership of the side, attributing the paralyzed arm or leg to someone else. This denial may cease as the acute cerebral condition and the patient's sensorium clear, although decreased motor ability or paralysis and decreased sensation in the affected side may persist.[33,38,39]

Perceptual disorders often include various *agnosias,* which are disturbances of the recognition or identification of objects that have been perceived by a single sense function—vision, hearing, or touch. Auditory agnosia and aphasia are discussed in detail in the following section on impaired communication.

In addition to visual field defects, some patients also may have visual agnosias. Some persons are unable to recognize objects or pictures of objects, whereas others cannot recognize faces and may have to rely on the voice or characteristic mannerisms of a familiar person to identify that person.[33,38,39]

Tactile agnosia, or *astereognosis,* is a perceptual disorder in which a patient is unable to recognize by touch alone an object that has been placed in his or her hand. This may occur even in the presence of an intact sense of touch. If allowed to see or hear the object, the person very likely recognizes it.

Lesions in the parietal lobe, as well as in other cortical structures, can result in *apraxia,* which is an inability to perform a learned movement voluntarily. Even though the patient may understand the task to be performed and may have intact motor ability, he or she is unable to perform the task and often fumbles and makes mistakes. The patient suffering from dressing apraxia, for example, may not be able to orient clothing in space and becomes tangled in the clothing when attempting to dress. In unilateral neglect the patient actually may fail to dress or groom the neglected half of the body.[33,38]

Patients with right hemispheric pathologic conditions may exhibit emotional lability, with periods of euphoria, impulsiveness, and inattention. A short attention span, lack of insight, and poor judgment may lead to injuries as the patient attempts to perform activities beyond his or her capabilities.[33,40]

Nurses tend to have higher expectations of patients with right hemispheric strokes because of their ability to speak. These patients, however, may have more difficulty returning to activities of daily living than do patients with aphasia from left hemispheric strokes.

The previous discussion has touched on some, but certainly not all, of the sensory/perceptual alterations that may accompany stroke. Clinically the stroke patient often has diffuse cerebrovascular disease and perhaps has experienced prior strokes. Perceptual defects are not always as readily apparent or as clear-cut as described here, underscoring the importance of ensuring that a comprehensive multidisciplinary neurologic evaluation of the stroke patient occurs within the critical care unit, using such team members as social workers, physical therapists, speech therapists, and occupational therapists. After this evaluation and with the physician's collaboration, a realistic determination of the patient's potential level of recovery should be made. This step is followed by formulating a multidisciplinary plan for comprehensive rehabilitation that can and should begin within the critical care unit.

◆ **Impaired communication.** Impaired communication is a condition that results from a person's difficulty in expressing and exchanging thoughts, ideas, or desires. Critical care nurses are acutely aware of the problems encountered in caring for patients with impaired communication. It is challenging enough to manage effective communication with intubated patients. But what of the brain-injured aphasic patient who may be unable to understand what is being said or written and/or who may be unable to express himself or herself verbally or in writing or even by gestures? Communication with such a patient can be frustrating and emotionally draining for the nurse, as well as the patient. Human beings operate primarily through the spoken and written word. It is said that when speech and language functions are disturbed as a consequence of brain disease, the resultant functional loss exceeds all others—even blindness, deafness, or paralysis—in gravity.[34]

Anatomy of language function. The posterior temporoparietal area contains the receptive speech center known as *Wernicke's area* (Fig. 28-4). The center for the perception of written language lies anterior to the visuoreceptive areas. Located at the base of the frontal lobe's motor strip and slightly anterior to it is *Broca's area,* also known as the *motor speech center.* These sensory and motor areas are connected by a large bundle of nerve fibers. Rather than receptive and motor language functions being entirely within discrete areas, it is believed that language is an integrated sensorimotor process, roughly located in these areas in the dominant cerebral hemisphere. It also is recognized that the elaborately complex functions of speech and language depend on other associative areas of the cerebrum and their thalamic connections. Consequently there is much inconsistency in the degree of communication impairment among patients with lesions located in the same area of the brain.[34,37,39]

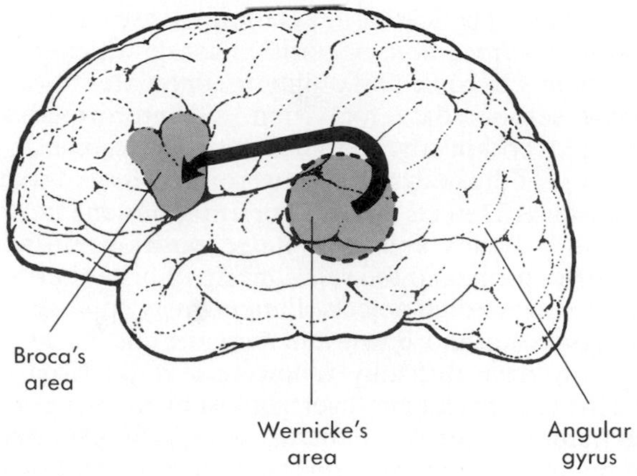

Fig. 28-4 Major areas of the cerebral cortex associated with speech. *Arrow* indicates interconnective fibers between the two speech areas.

Aphasia. Aphasia is a loss of language abilities caused by brain injury, usually to the dominant hemisphere. The left hemisphere is dominant for language function in 95% of the population. Most persons are right-handed and therefore left hemisphere–dominant. Not all left-handed persons, however, are right hemisphere–dominant; some remain left hemisphere–dominant.[38] The most common cause of aphasia is vascular disease involving the left middle cerebral artery. Other causes may be intracranial tumor or trauma in the frontal-parietal and frontotemporal area.

Aphasia involves more than just understanding speech or expressing oneself through verbal means. Language is a much broader term, referring to what the individual is attempting to interpret or convey through listening, speaking, reading, writing, and gesturing.[41] Most aphasias are partial rather than complete. The severity of the disorder depends on the area and the extent of the cerebral damage.

FLUENT APHASIA. Fluent aphasia, also referred to as *sensory, Wernicke's,* or *receptive aphasia,* occurs when the connection between the primary auditory cortex in the temporal lobe and the angular gyrus in the parietal lobe is destroyed. The patient's comprehension of speech is impaired, but he or she can still talk if the motor area for speech, Broca's area, is intact. The patient may in fact talk excessively, with many errors in the use of words. The patient is able to hear the examiner but cannot comprehend what is being said and cannot repeat the examiner's words. Such patients may talk nonsense, with rambling speech that gives little information. Patients with fluent aphasia also cannot read words, although they can see them. They cannot understand the symbolic content of printed or written symbols, a condition called *alexia.*[37,39,42]

In time, fluent aphasia usually improves to varying degrees. Some individuals improve to the point that it is difficult to detect the receptive deficit without special verbal and written tests. The most favorable outcomes are in those patients with the mildest forms of fluent aphasia.[34]

NONFLUENT APHASIA. Nonfluent aphasia, also known as *motor, Broca's,* or *expressive aphasia,* is primarily a deficit in language output or speech production. Depending on the lesion's size and exact location, a wide variation in the motor deficit can result. Nonfluent aphasia can range from a mild dysarthria (imperfect articulation as a result of weakness or lack of coordination of speech musculature), to incorrect tonation and phrasing, and, in its most severe form, to complete loss of all ability to communicate through verbal and written means. In this severe form of aphasia, there also is a loss of ability to communicate through conventional gestures, such as nodding or shaking the head for "yes" or "no." In most cases of nonfluent aphasia, the muscles of articulation are intact. If speech is possible at all, occasionally the words "yes" or "no" are uttered, sometimes appropriately. In some cases the words of well-known songs may be sung. Other patients, when excited or angered, may utter expletives.[34,37,38]

Some patients with nonfluent aphasia struggle or hesitate in trying to express words. They struggle to form words while using motor musculature (verbal apraxia), an articulatory disorder that is a feature of some nonfluent aphasias.[37] All these difficulties lead to exasperation and despair for the patient.

Most patients with nonfluent aphasia also have severely impaired writing ability. Even though penmanship may be intact, they are unable to express themselves through writing—a deficit termed *agraphia.* If the right hand is paralyzed, as is often the case, the patient still cannot write or print with the left hand.[34]

In the recovery phase of severe nonfluent aphasia, patients become able to speak aloud to some degree, although words are uttered slowly and laboriously. Many patients, however, are able to learn to communicate ideas to some extent.[34]

GLOBAL APHASIA. Global aphasia results when a massive lesion affects both the motor and sensory speech areas. The patient is unable to transform sounds into words and is unable to comprehend spoken words. All language modalities are affected, and impairment may be so severe that the patient may be unable to communicate on any level. These patients generally have severe hemiplegia and also homonymous hemianopsia. In these patients, language function rarely recovers to a significant degree unless the lesion is caused by some transient disorder, such as cerebral edema or a metabolic derangement.[34,39]

CONDUCTION APHASIA. Conduction aphasia occurs when a lesion disrupts the connection between Broca's and Wernicke's areas, although the anatomic basis is poorly defined. The features of conduction aphasia often resemble those of fluent aphasia. The patient may produce speech, but little of it conveys meaning. The patient's use of written language reflects the same problems as speech. These patients may be well aware of their deficit. They may be alert and able to comprehend everything they see and hear but remain incapable of self-initiated speech or repetition of words. They also have problems reading aloud, even though they may comprehend written words.[39]

Many other lesser-known and uncommon disorders of communication exist. This discussion explains only the most common forms of aphasia that the critical care nurse may encounter.

GUILLAIN-BARRÉ SYNDROME

Guillain-Barré syndrome (GBS), also known as *Landry-Guillain-Barré syndrome,* is a postinfectious peripheral polyneuritis characterized by a rapidly progressive ascending peripheral nerve dysfunction leading to paralysis. It is 90% to 100% reversible and is one of the most common peripheral nervous system diseases. Because of the ventilatory support required for these patients, GBS is one of the few peripheral neurologic diseases requiring a critical care environment.

Incidence

The annual incidence of GBS is 1.6 per 100,000 persons. It occurs 1.5 times more frequently in males than in females.[43] The incidence of GBS increased slightly for a period of time after the 1977 swine flu vaccinations.[44]

Etiology

The cause of GBS is unknown, but more than 50% of patients report a mild febrile illness, either respiratory or gastrointestinal, 1 to 3 weeks before the onset of clinical manifestations. The result is a possible autoimmune response of the peripheral nervous system.

Pathophysiology

This disease affects the motor and sensory pathways of the peripheral nervous system, as well as the autonomic nervous system functions of the cranial nerves. The major finding in GBS is a segmental demyelination process of the peripheral nerves. Inflammation around this demyelinated area causes further dysfunction.

The myelin sheath of the peripheral nerves is generated by Schwann's cells and acts as an insulator for the peripheral nerve. Myelin promotes rapid conduction of nerve impulses by allowing the impulses to jump along the nerve via nodes of Ranvier. Disruption of the myelin fiber slows and may eventually stop the conduction of impulses along the peripheral nerves. In GBS, the more thickly myelinated fibers of motor pathways and the cranial nerves are more severely affected than are the thinly myelinated sensory fibers of cutaneous pain, touch, and temperature. Symptoms of GBS include motor weakness, paresthesias and other sensory changes, cranial nerve dysfunction (especially the oculomotor, facial, glossopharyngeal, vagal, spinal accessory, and hypoglossal), and some autonomic nervous system dysfunction.

GBS is believed to be an autoimmune response to antibodies formed against the recent febrile illness, usually upper respiratory or gastrointestinal. Immune reactions from the T and the B cells of the lymphatic system set up a local inflammatory reaction that triggers further inflammation.

Once the temporary inflammatory reaction stops, myelin-producing cells begin the process of reinsulating the demyelinated portions of the peripheral nervous system. When remyelination occurs, normal neurologic function should return. In some instances the axon may be damaged during the inflammatory process. The degree of axonal damage is responsible for the degree of neurologic dysfunction that persists after recovery.

Assessment and Diagnosis

◆ **Clinical manifestations.** The usual course of GBS begins with an abrupt onset of lower extremity weakness that progresses to flaccidity and ascends over a period of hours to days. Motor loss usually is symmetric. In the most severe cases, complete flaccidity of all peripheral nerves, including spinal and cranial nerves, occurs.

Admission to the hospital occurs when lower extremity weakness prevents mobility. Admission to the critical care unit occurs when progression of the weakness threatens respiratory muscles. As the patient's weakness progresses, close observation is essential. Frequent assessment of the respiratory system, including ventilatory parameters such as inspiratory force and tidal volume, is necessary. The most common cause of death in patients with GBS is from respiratory arrest.

As the disease progresses and respiratory effort weakens, intubation and mechanical ventilation are necessary. Continued, frequent assessment of neurologic deterioration is required until the patient reaches the peak of the disease and plateau occurs.

◆ **Diagnostic findings.** The diagnosis of GBS is based on clinical findings plus CSF analysis and nerve conduction studies. CSF analysis demonstrates a normal protein initially, which elevates in the fourth to sixth week. No other changes in CSF occur. Nerve conduction studies that test the velocity at which nerve impulses are conducted show significant reduction, as would be expected with the demyelinating process of the disease.

Medical Management

The medical management of GBS is limited. No curative treatment exists for this disease. It simply must run its course, which is characterized by ascending paralysis that plateaus for 1 to 4 weeks. This stage is followed by descending paralysis and return to normal or near-normal function. The main focus of medical management is the support of bodily functions and the prevention of complications.

Some physicians support the use of steroids for their antiinflammatory effect. The effectiveness of steroids is difficult to assess. If steroids are prescribed, all usual precautions associated with steroid use should be followed.

The use of plasmapheresis also has been attempted. Plasmapheresis involves plasma exchanges or washes that remove the antibodies that cause the GBS. Plasmapheresis has achieved minimal acceptance in treatment. In a recently published study of 220 patients in a multicenter clinical trial, the long-term benefit of plasmapheresis demonstrated that 71% of the treatment group versus 52% of the control group ($P = .007$) had full muscular strength recovery at 1 year.[45]

Nursing Management

The nursing management of the patient with GBS is extensive. The goal of nursing management is to support all normal body functions until such time as the patient can do so on his or her own. Nursing management focuses on immobility, pulmonary care, nutritional support, pain management, and—very important—emotional support.

NURSING DIAGNOSIS AND MANAGEMENT
Guillain-Barré syndrome

- ◆ Ineffective Airway Clearance related to neuromuscular dysfunction and impaired cough secondary to quadriplegia, paraplegia, Guillain-Barré syndrome, myasthenia gravis, and others, p. 467
- ◆ Sensory/Perceptual Alterations related to sensory overload, sensory deprivation, sleep pattern disturbance, p. 573
- ◆ Acute Pain related to transmission and perception of cutaneous, visceral, muscular, or ischemic impulses secondary to reestablishment of myoneural activity, p. 566
- ◆ Ineffective Airway Clearance related to impaired cough secondary to artificial airway, p. 466
- ◆ Impaired Gas Exchange related to alveolar hypoventilation secondary to respiratory muscle paralysis, p. 471
- ◆ High Risk for Aspiration risk factors: impaired laryngeal sensation or reflex; impaired pharyngeal peristalsis or tongue function; impaired laryngeal closure or elevation; increased gastric volume; decreased lower esophageal sphincter pressure, p. 472
- ◆ Ineffective Breathing Pattern related to musculoskeletal impairment, p. 470
- ◆ Altered Nutrition: Less Than Body Protein-Calorie Requirements related to lack of exogenous nutrients, p. 673
- ◆ High Risk for Infection risk factors: invasive monitoring devices, p. 366
- ◆ Activity Intolerance related to postural hypotension secondary to prolonged immobility, narcotics, vasodilator therapy, p. 365
- ◆ Body Image Disturbance related to functional dependence on life-sustaining technology, p. 95
- ◆ Powerlessness related to health care environment and illness-related regimen, p. 98
- ◆ Anxiety related to threat to biologic, psychologic, and/or social integrity, p. 763
- ◆ Ineffective Individual Coping related to situational crisis and personal vulnerability, p. 762
- ◆ Knowledge Deficit: Course of Treatment, Prognosis related to lack of previous exposure to information, p. 72

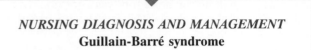

◆ **Immobility.** In patients with GBS, immobility may last for months. The usual course of GBS involves an average of 10 days for symptom progression and 10 days at maximum level of dysfunction, followed by 2 to 48 weeks of recovery. Although the condition is reversible, recovery from GBS is a long process.

◆ **Pulmonary care.** Total ventilatory support and pulmonary toilet are required at the peak level of the illness. As the patient's symptoms recede, weaning from the ventilator and initiation of coughing and deep breathing exercises are important in prevention of pulmonary complications.

◆ **Nutritional support.** Nutritional support should be implemented early in the course of the disease. Because it is known that GBS recovery is a long process, adequate nutritional support will be a problem for an extended period of time. Nutritional support usually is accomplished through the use of enteral feeding. The less invasive method of providing nutrition is preferable to the use of total parenteral nutrition because it reduces the risk of infection in a patient who is highly vulnerable.

◆ **Pain control.** Pain control is an important component in the care of patients with GBS. Although the patient has minimal to no motor function, most sensory functions are maintained. The patient feels considerable muscle ache and pain. Because of the lengthy nature of this illness, it is important to work closely with the physician and patient to identify a safe, effective, long-term solution to pain management.

◆ **Emotional support.** The emotional support required by these patients is extensive. Although the illness is almost 100% reversible, the total helplessness of the patient, the constant pain or discomfort, and the length of the course of the disease create difficulties in coping with this condition. It is important to remember that GBS does not affect the level of consciousness or cerebral function. Interaction and communication are necessary elements of the nursing management plan.

ACUTE PAIN

Pain is defined as "a state in which an individual experiences and reports the presence of severe discomfort or an uncomfortable sensation."[46] Pain is a protective mechanism for the body. It occurs when tissues of the body are damaged, causing the person to take some action to relieve it. Both human beings and animals are subject to feeling pain throughout their lives; it is a universally distressing feeling, whether acute or chronic. Relief of pain remains one of the major aspects of medical and nursing practice because fear of pain is second only to fear of death.

Unfortunately, undertreatment of pain occurs all too often in the American health care system. Physician and nurse ignorance abounds about the use of narcotics (opioids) for the treatment of pain. Much of this ignorance stems from misunderstandings about the differences among drug addiction, drug tolerance, and physical dependence[47,48] (see box, upper right). Reeducation of physicians and nurses must occur if this tragedy of pain undertreatment is to be avoided.

Controversy frequently arises between physicians and nurses about the adequacy of a patient's pain control regimen. Nurses often are denied the authority to adjust or titrate a patient's pain medication. The physician focuses on disease diagnosis and cure; the nurse focuses on care. McCaffery states, "The nursing profession must declare that pain control is a major nursing responsibility—and nursing education must make a commitment to provide knowledge at all levels of preparation that will enable nurses to present a case based on scientific knowledge and relevant observation of the individual patient."[49]

Critically ill patients, experiencing the acute pain of their disease process or surgical procedure, are particularly vulnerable. In addition, they often are subjected to painful invasive procedures for the purposes of monitoring, diagnosing, or treating their illness.

Acute pain usually is associated with body injury of some kind, with the pain disappearing when the injury heals. Chronic pain, on the other hand, persists beyond the expected healing time, lasts longer than 6 months, and often cannot be attributed to a specific injury.[50] Chronic malignant pain is associated with cancer or some other progressive disorder.

EFFECTS OF NARCOTICS

Narcotic addiction. A behavioral pattern characterized by compulsive drug-seeking behavior leading to an overwhelming involvement with the use and procurement of the drug for purposes other than medical reasons (i.e., pain relief)

Drug tolerance. Manifests as the clinical need to take more drug to achieve the original effect

Physical dependence. Manifests in withdrawal symptoms when the chronic use of opioids is abruptly discontinued or an opioid antagonist is administered

Signs of Acute Pain

Acute pain begins at a specific time and usually is accompanied by objective physical signs, which include the autonomic (sympathetic) responses of tachycardia, hypertension, diaphoresis, mydriasis, and pallor. Skeletal muscle reactions associated with acute pain include grimacing, clenching fists, pacing the floor, writhing, guarding, or splinting the affected part. Psychologic reactions may include distinct verbalizations of suffering and pleas for help and expressions of anger and crying. The person also may appear anxious, apprehensive, and fearful.

These objective physical signs are not always the most reliable indicators of the presence of pain. Pain has been described as a subjective experience, with the patient the only authority about the pain being experienced. McCaffery and Beebe[51] define pain as "whatever the experiencing person says it is, existing when he/she says it does." The nurse has the responsibilities of believing the patient and of seeking more information about the pain.

Pain Theories

Several complex theories of pain perception have been offered over the past 20 years. Older theories, such as the specificity theory and the pattern theory, rarely are mentioned in current literature because they are incomplete in explaining the phenomenon of pain. Yet they help the reader understand some of the complexities of pain and therefore are discussed briefly here.

The *specificity theory,* in brief, describes the transmission of pain impulses through special fibers to specific pain centers in the brain. Some afferent fibers go to motor fibers of the reflex arc in the spinal cord so that muscles respond immediately, for example, by pulling the hand away quickly when a finger touches a hot object. Other afferent fibers ascend through the spinothalamic tract to the thalamus where impulses are relayed to the cerebral cortex for processing. The spinothalamic tract is believed to carry sensory discriminative aspects of pain.[52]

The reticulospinal tract carries noxious sensations to the medullary and pontine reticular formation and terminates in the midbrain, thalamus, and hypothalamus. This tract is primarily responsible for poorly localized burning pain and visceral sensations.[52]

The phenomenon of phantom limb pain, postherpetic neuralgia, and causalgia are explained by the *pattern theory* of pain. The key concept of this theory is that after tissue injury, circuits that act as pattern-generating mechanisms can be established in the dorsal horns and possibly in other places along the sensory system, causing pain perception even though the stimuli that initiated pain are no longer present. Nonpainful stimuli, such as light touch or a breath of wind, can cause these reverberating pattern circuits to send impulses to the brain that are interpreted as pain. These same circuits sometimes fire spontaneously, even in the absence of peripheral stimulation.[53]

The specificity and the pattern theories do not adequately explain the pain process, however, because recent findings indicate that pain transmission can be modulated.

The *gate control theory* presented by Melzack and Wall in 1965 implies that these transmitted pain impulses can be modulated or altered through cortical and spinal influences. The potential blocking ability of certain cells along the transmission route can result in little or no pain perception, regardless of the intensity of the pain stimulus.

Small-diameter fibers of peripheral nerves conduct excitatory pain signals to the substantia gelatinosa in the dorsal horns of the spinal cord. If nothing blocks these impulses, they are transmitted to the ascending tracts that travel up the spinal cord to the brain where the pain is perceived. Large-diameter afferent fibers on the surface of the skin carry innocuous information that can, in effect, close the "gate" in the substantia gelatinosa, blocking the transmission of pain. These cutaneous large fibers can be stimulated by touch, vibration, rubbing, and scratching. Simply stated then, the gate is opened by activation of the small fibers but can be closed by stimulation of the large fibers. This excitation-inhibition is called the *gating mechanism.*[51]

Information from the brain also can increase or decrease the transmission of pain by relaying descending impulses that can open or close the gate. Information such as memories, emotions, and situations influence not only the perception of but the meaning attached to the pain impulse.[54] Decreased intensity or disappearance of pain can occur as a result of guided imagery, distraction, or anxiety reduction based on learning when the pain will end and how to relieve it.[25]

The gate control theory helps explain the effects of pain therapies such as relaxation techniques and cutaneous stimulation such as heat, cold, massage, and transcutaneous electrical nerve stimulation (TENS).

Other pain theories support the concept that pain impulses are mediated in the spinal cord before they reach the brain. The *endogenous opioid system* consists of biochemical substances known as endorphins. Endorphins are morphinelike peptides produced naturally in the body at various sites along neural synapses in the CNS. They modulate the transmission of pain perceptions by attaching to specific opioid receptors found in various regions of the brain and in the substantia gelatinosa of the dorsal horns of the spinal cord. Many of these opioid receptors in the brain are in areas associated with emotions. In addition to raising pain thresholds, endorphins, much like morphine, also produce sedation and feelings of euphoria. Like morphine, the pain-relieving actions of endorphins can be blocked by naloxone. Different levels of endorphins in different individuals may help explain differences in pain perception.[51]

It is believed that pain activates the endogenous opioid system. Other factors may also activate this system and include elevations of blood pressure, fear, stress, restraint, and hypoglycemia.[52] Endorphin levels also have been found elevated with exercise, noxious states, labor, and delivery. Endorphin release may explain why many individuals do not initially feel pain at the time of an accident or why a painful injury may be rendered painless during the heat of battle or sport. These persons experience a "stress analgesia." Endorphins might help explain the phenomenon of pain relief in some individuals after administration of placebos. Acupuncture and TENS use also may cause the release of endorphins, which add to the pain-relieving properties of these techniques. Increasing evidence indicates, too, that persons who experience chronic high levels of pain may be deficient in endorphins.[51,54]

Although endorphins are associated with pain inhibition, other neuropeptides are associated with pain transmission. The level of many neuropeptides—such as bradykinins, histamine, prostaglandins, serotonin, substance P—fluctuates throughout the day, possibly explaining why pain sensitivity seems higher (lower pain threshold) in the afternoon than in the morning. This fluctuation influences an individual's analgesic requirements at different times of the day.

The *multiple opioid receptor theory* implies that narcotics may bind to, or occupy, multiple opioid receptor sites on the ends of nerves in the spinal and supraspinal (brain) regions. These receptors are named mu (μ), kappa (κ), and sigma (σ). Certain drugs are highly site-specific. An agonist drug binds to an opioid receptor site, stimulates it, and induces an effect such as analgesia, sedation, respiratory depression, psychosis, or hallucinations, depending on which receptor types are stimulated. An antagonist drug such as naloxone binds to a specific receptor and blocks the activity of that receptor, or it displaces the agonist at the receptor site, thereby stopping the receptor activity. This may help explain how naloxone reverses the analgesic and CNS depressant effects of certain narcotics.[51]

Psychosocial Influences

Most body pain is a combination of mental events and physical stimuli. In fact, sustained anxiety, fear, and anger can even produce painful alterations in physiology such as muscle contractions and tension headaches.[39,42]

Pain is evaluated in higher brain centers in the cortex. People can experience different levels of pain in response to the same injury or insult. Physiologic differences such as endorphin levels help explain the phenomenon but not entirely. Pain tolerance differs among individuals and can vary within any individual in different situations. Personal factors such as knowledge of pain, its meaning and cause, the ability to control pain, and a person's stress level, as well as energy or fatigue levels, influence pain tolerance.[39,42]

Social and environmental factors such as interactions with others, responses of family and friends, stressors, and sensory overload or deprivation influence pain. A person's cultural background, beliefs, and past experiences also can influence pain. The situation in which pain occurs is significant. For instance, the pain associated with elective surgery may be perceived as more severe than that occurring from wounds incurred in battle, even if the latter involves a greater degree of tissue injury.[39,42]

Stress contributes to the severity of perceived pain. Persons who receive explanations of what they will feel in advance of painful procedures experience less stress than those who receive little or no explanation. A consequence of less stress may be an actual reduction in the severity of perceived pain.[39,42]

Cultural and societal influences on the expression of pain are great. For example, persons with stoic backgrounds tend to avoid verbal and nonverbal expressions of pain. Other cultures encourage outward displays of discomfort such as moaning and crying. These factors have great implications for nurses responsible for assessing and treating pain. The stoic individual actually is at risk for receiving inadequate pain relief measures. Health care workers must remember that these cultural differences affect only the expression of pain and not the differences in sensitivity to pain.[42]

Types of Acute Pain

Pain arising from different locations in the body and from underlying pathophysiologic processes accounts for some characteristic pain patterns. Superficial structures such as subcutaneous tissue, fascia, periosteum, ligaments, tendons, and parietal pleura are richly supplied with small pain fibers. Hence pain resulting from stimulation of these regions is relatively well localized and often is pricking and burning in nature. Conversely, visceral pain is poorly localized and often is referred to other areas, because the viscera and deeper somatic structures are more sparsely innervated with small pain fibers. Pain of visceral origin usually is felt somewhere within the segmental distribution of several nerve roots. The most common sites of pain from myocardial ischemia, for example, include the area behind the sternum, in the left pectoral region and shoulder, along the inner aspect of the left arm to the elbow, and occasionally in the back. All these sites are within the distribution of T1-3 nerve roots. Visceral pain usually is described as aching but may be sharp and penetrating (knifelike). Rarely, it is burning such as in the heartburn of esophageal irritation.[34,45]

When pain arises from a nerve root or trunk, its distribution follows the afferent distribution of the nerve. For example, the pain of a herniated intervertebral disk compressing the fifth lumbar nerve root causes deep as well as superficial pain extending down the lateral thigh and leg.[34]

Muscle cramps or spasms can provoke severe pain, and the muscles may be visibly and palpably taut. Massage and vigorous stretching are the most effective ways to stop the spasms. Muscle cramps can be caused by motor system disease, tetany, and dehydration after excessive sweating and salt loss. Metabolic diseases such as uremia, hypocalcemia, and hypomagnesemia also can cause muscle spasms.[55] Exactly why the muscle spasms cause pain is debatable, but it is probably because the overactive muscles demand more oxygen than can be supplied, resulting in ischemia with a build-up of ischemic metabolites.

The pain of muscle injury is similar to visceral pain in type, localization, and referral because deep skeletal pain and visceral pain are mediated through common deep sensory systems. In fact, chest wall pain often can mimic the pain of myocardial ischemia.[56]

Acute ischemic pain causes burning or aching pain in the tissues distal to a vascular occlusion. The pain possibly is caused by the release of metabolic factors related to tissue hypoxia and anoxia. Because exercise increases the metabolic demands of the tissues, pain from ischemia characteristically builds with the use of the involved muscles and initially is relieved by rest. Eventually, the ischemic pain is felt at rest, increases in intensity, and becomes aggravated by movement.[42,57]

Often the pain of an ischemic leg is aggravated by elevating the leg and lessened by dangling or lowering the leg. In addition, the extremity distal to the occlusion shows a loss of pulses, delayed capillary filling, and a decrease in skin temperature, eventually becoming cold and pale. Loss of skin sensation occurs within the first hour, with feelings of numbness reported. After approximately 6 hours, painful, ischemic muscle contractures develop.[42,57]

Evaluating Pain

Evaluating a patient's pain can be a difficult endeavor because pain is a subjective experience. If the adage that *pain is whatever the experiencing person says it is* is followed, then that person should be believed. Rather than spending time determining if someone actually has pain, the nurse can use time wisely by assessing the situation, determining the possible causes of the pain, and instituting measures to alleviate it.

Determining the cause of pain when it is not obvious can be critical to the patient's well-being. When a patient reports chest pain, for instance, it is vital that a differential diagnosis be made to confirm or reject the possibility of myocardial ischemia. Such a differental diagnosis is heavily influenced by the location, character, duration, and severity of the pain; what provokes it and makes it worse or better; the risk factor profile for coronary artery disease; and a past history of cardiovascular disease.[56] The need for a differential diagnosis of chest pain occurring in the patient after open heart surgery occurs with frequency. In these instances the presence of increased pain intensity during deep breathing and coughing helps distinguish chest wall pain from myocardial ischemic pain.

The nurse also assesses the behavioral aspects of pain such as moaning, crying, grimacing, restlessness, pacing, guarding, or withdrawal. These behavioral manifestations cannot be used as the only clues to the existence or severity of pain, however, because some individuals try hard not to show pain.

One of the best attempts to objectify the subjective is to ask the patient (if he or she is able) to rate the pain on a scale of 1 to 10. The nurse explains that a 0 means the absence of pain, 1 represents the least pain, and 10 represents the worst pain the person has ever experienced. Pain should be rated this way at its best, at its worst, and after pain relief measures to evaluate their effectiveness. This recorded response is used as a frame of reference to compare future episodes of pain.[39]

Critically ill adults with impaired verbal communication may not clearly communicate the psychologic reactions associated with acute pain. The nurse may then have to rely on the physical clues that can indicate pain, such as elevated blood pressure and pulse rate and changes in activity level.

Elderly persons represent another group at high risk for undertreatment of pain. Some of the following misconceptions contribute to this tragedy: (1) pain is a natural outcome of growing old; (2) pain perception decreases with age; (3) the potential side effects of narcotics makes them too dangerous to use; and (4) if the older person is depressed, especially if there is no known cause for the pain, depression is causing the pain (rather than the other way around). Cognitive and communication problems and inadvertent denial of pain (failing to use the word *pain*) can all add to the challenge of assessing pain in elderly persons. It is important to confer with family members of older patients who are unable to articulate their pain. Knowledge of the patient's usual manner of expressing pain is invaluable.[51]

Treating Pain

The treatment of pain has become much more sophisticated and efficient in recent years. In addition to the traditional oral, parenteral, and continuous intravenous (IV) infusion routes, patient-controlled analgesia (PCA), introduced in Europe in the 1970s, has steadily gained popularity in the United States.

The principle of PCA is a patient-titrated, self-administered narcotic analgesia by means of IV (most common) and epidural infusions.[58] Computerized PCA pumps deliver predetermined doses of medication into the patient's IV catheter when a control button (attached by a cord to the patient's gown) is pushed. Safeguards programmed into the pump, including a mandatory lockout interval between successive dosages, ensure that a safe dose is not exceeded. Advantages of this system include (1) significantly less narcotic medication to achieve satisfactory analgesia, (2) a reduced degree of sedation, (3) lowered patient anxiety associated with a sense of control, and (4) reduced demand on nursing time.[58,59] Lange et al.[59] also report improved pulmonary hygiene and increased and earlier mobility in those patients receiving PCA compared with a control group receiving periodic narcotic injections every 3 to 6 hours as needed.

Intravenous PCA is most widely used in the postoperative period. It is especially useful in thoracic, abdominal, and orthopedic postsurgical pain control. Stevens[60] reports that patients were most comfortable when use of the PCA device was initiated in the postanesthesia care unit (PACU) and then transported with them to the nursing unit. PCA applications are not limited to postoperative pain control; they can be used for control of pain in terminal cancer, sickle cell crisis, obstetric labor, acute traumatic injuries and burns, and myocardial ischemia. PCA also has been successfully used with children.[61]

Patients selected for PCA must be cooperative, able to understand and follow instructions, and feel confident handling their own analgesia. Preoperative teaching is recommended whenever possible.

Epidural analgesia also is becoming more popular and can be especially effective with thoracic, abdominal, and orthopedic surgery. Other methods of pain control include the transdermal route for administering fentanyl—used in cancer care—and injectable nonsteroidal anti-inflammatory agents such as ketorolac tromethamine (Toradol), often used for postoperative pain control.

REFERENCES

1. Kornblith PL, Walker MD, Cassady JR: *Neurologic oncology,* Philadelphia, 1987, JB Lippincott.
2. Farwell JR, Dohrmann GJ, Flannery JT: Medulloblastoma in childhood: an epidemiological study, *J Neurosurg* 61:657, 1984.
3. Albright AL, Price RA, Guthkelch AN: Brainstem gliomas of children: a clinicopathological study, *Cancer* 52:2313, 1983.
4. Schoenberg BS: Epidemiology of primary nervous system neoplasms. In Schoenberg BS, editor: *Advances in neurology,* vol 19, New York, 1978, Raven Press.
5. Zulch DJ: Principles of the new World Health Organization (WHO) classification of brain tumors, *Neuroradiology* 19:59, 1980.
6. Guyton AC: *Textbook of medical physiology,* ed 8, Philadelphia, 1991, WB Saunders.
7. Frederich C, Rosemann D, Austin M: Malignant hypothermia: nursing diagnosis and care, *J Post Anesth Nurs* 5(1):29, 1990.
8. Petersdorf RG: Hypothermia and hyperthermia. In Wilson J and others, editors: *Harrison's principles of internal medicine,* ed 12, New York, 1991, McGraw-Hill.

9. Matz R: Hypothermia: mechanisms and countermeasures, *Hosp Pract* 21(1):45, 1986.
10. Shapiro WR and others: Heterogeneous response to chemotherapy of human gliomas grown in mice, *Cancer Treat Rep* 65(suppl 2):55, 1981.
11. Mughmaw SB: An overview of methods in stereotactic surgery, *Radiol Tech* 63(6):402, 1992.
12. Coffey RJ, Lunsford LD, Flickinger JC: The role of radiosurgery in the treatment of malignant brain tumors, *Neurosurg Clin North Am* 3(1):231, 1992.
13. Stephanian E and others: Gamma knife surgery for sellar and suprasellar tumors, *Neurosurg Clin North Am* 3(1):207, 1992.
14. Welsh DM: Volumetric interstitial hyperthermia: nursing implications for brain tumor treatment, *J Neurosci Nurs* 20(4):229, 1988.
15. Jankovic J: Differential diagnosis of stroke. In Meyer JS, Shaw T, editors: *Diagnosis and management of stroke and TIAs,* Menlo Park, Calif, 1982, Addison-Wesley.
16. Gresham GE and others: Epidemiologic profile of long-term stroke disability: the Framingham study, *Arch Phys Med Rehab* 60:487, 1979.
17. Wolf P, Kannel W: Controllable risk factors for stroke: preventive implications of trends in stroke mortality. In Meyer JS, Shaw T, editors: *Diagnosis and management of stroke and TIAs,* Menlo Park, Calif, 1982, Addison-Wesley.
18. Kannel WB and others: Components of blood pressure and risk of atherothrombotic brain infarction: the Framingham study, *Stroke* 7:327, 1976.
19. Findlay JM, Macdonald RL, Weir BK: Current concepts of pathophysiology and management of cerebral vasospasm following aneurysmal subarachnoid hemorrhage, *Cerebrovasc Brain Metab Rev* 3(4):336, 1991.
20. Locksley HB: Natural history of subarachnoid hemorrhage, intracranial aneurysm and AVM. In Sachs AL and others, editors: *Intracranial aneurysms and subarachnoid hemorrhage: a cooperative study,* Philadelphia, 1969, JB Lippincott.
21. Tindall RSA: Cerebrovascular disease. In Rosenberg RN, editor: *Neurology,* New York, 1980, Grune & Stratton.
22. Normes H, Magnaes B: Intracranial pressure in patients with ruptured saccular aneurysm, *J Neurosurg* 36:536, 1972.
23. Hunt WE, Hess RM: Surgical risks as related to time of intervention in the repair of intracranial aneurysms, *J Neurosurg* 28:14, 1968.
24. Fisher CM: Clinical syndromes in cerebral thrombosis, hypertensive hemorrhage and ruptured aneurysm, *Clin Neurosurg* 22:117, 1975.
25. Cook HA: Aneurysmal subarachnoid hemorrhage, *AACN Clin Issues Crit Care Nurs* 2(4):664, 1991.
26. Jane JA, Winn HR, Richardson AE: The natural history of intracranial aneurysms: rebleeding rates during acute and long-term period and implication for surgical management, *Clin Neurosurg* 24:176, 1977.
27. Kassell NF, Haley EC, Torner JC: Antifibrinolytic therapy in the treatment of aneurysmal subarachnoid hemorrhage, *Clin Neurosurg* 33:137, 1986.
28. Beck DW and others: Combination of aminocaproic acid and nicardipine in treatment of aneurysmal subarachnoid hemorrhage, *Stroke* 19(1):63, 1988.
29. Kassell NF and others: Treatment of ischemic deficits from vasospasm with intravascular volume expansion and induced arterial hypertension, *Neurosurgery* 11(3):337, 1982.
30. Retruk KC and others: Nimodipine treatment in poor-grade aneurysm patients: results of a multicenter double blind placebo-controlled trial, *J Neurosurg* 68(4):505, 1988.
31. Adams HP: Early management of the patient with recent aneurysmal subarachnoid hemorrhage, *Stroke* 17(6):1068, 1986.
32. Robinson MJ, Teasdale GM: Calcium antagonists in the management of subarachnoid hemorrhage, *Cerebrovasc Brain Metab Rev* 2(3):205, 1990.
33. Olson E: Perceptual deficits affecting the stroke patient, *Rehabil Nurs* 16(4):213, 1991.
34. Adams RD, Victor M: *Principles of neurology,* ed 4, New York, 1989, McGraw-Hill.
35. Kalbach LR: Unilateral neglect: mechanisms and nursing care, *J Neurosci Nurs* 23(2):125, 1991.
36. Kelly K and others: Profound accidental hypothermia and freeze injury of the extremities in a child, *Crit Care Med* 18(6):679, 1990.
37. Pimental PA: Alterations in communication: biopsychosocial aspects of aphasia, dysarthria, and right hemisphere syndromes in the stroke patient, *Nurs Clin North Am* 21(2):321, 1986.
38. Dittmar S: *Rehabilitation nursing: process and application,* St Louis, 1989, Mosby–Year Book.
39. O'Brien MT, Pallett PJ: *Total care of the stroke patient,* Boston, 1978, Little, Brown.
40. Carpenito L: *Nursing diagnosis: application to clinical practice,* ed 3, Philadelphia, 1989, JB Lippincott.
41. Keller C and others: Psychological responses in aphasia: theoretical considerations and nursing implications, *J Neurosci Nurs* 21(5):290, 1989.
42. Luckmann J, Sorenson KC: *Medical-surgical nursing: a psychophysiologic approach,* ed 3, Philadelphia, 1987, WB Saunders.
43. Koobatian TJ and others: The use of hospital discharge data for public health surveillance of Guillain-Barré syndrome, *Ann Neurol* 30(4):618, 1991.
44. Keenlyside R, Brezman D: Fatal Guillain-Barré syndrome after the national influenza immunization program, *Neurology* 30:929, 1980.
45. French Cooperative Group on Plasma Exchange: Plasma exchange in Guillain-Barré syndrome one year follow-up, *Ann Neurol* 32(1):94, 1992.
46. Friedman L, Isselbacher K: Anorexia, nausea, vomiting and indigestion. In Wilson JD and others, editors: *Harrison's principles of internal medicine,* ed 12, New York, 1991, McGraw-Hill.
47. American Pain Society: *Principles of analgesic use in the treatment of acute pain or chronic cancer pain,* ed 2, Skokie, Ill, 1989, The Society.
48. World Health Organization: *Cancer pain relief and palliative care,* Geneva, 1990, The Organization.
49. McCaffery M: Pain control battle, *Am J Nurs* 91(11):15, 1991.
50. American Pain Society: Pain, *Am J Nurs* 88(6):816, 1988.
51. McCaffery M, Beebe A: *Pain: clinical manual for nursing practice,* St Louis, 1989, Mosby–Year Book.
52. Puntillo KA: The phenomenon of pain and critical care nursing, *Heart Lung* 17(3):262, 1988.
53. Numbers L: Pain: an introduction, *Nursing (Oxford)* 3(9):358, 1986.
54. Harrison M, Cotanch P: Pain: advances and issues in critical care, *Nurs Clin North Am* 22(3):691, 1987.
55. Griggs R: Pain, spasm, and cramps of muscle. In Wilson JD and others, editors: *Harrison's principles of internal medicine,* ed 12, New York, 1991, McGraw-Hill.
56. Goldman L, Braunwald E: Chest discomfort and palpitation. In Wilson JD and others, editors: *Harrison's principles of internal medicine,* ed 12, New York, 1991, McGraw-Hill.
57. Creager M, Dzau V: Vascular diseases of the extremities. In Wilson JD and others, editors: *Harrison's principles of internal medicine,* ed 12, New York, 1991, McGraw-Hill.
58. White P: Use of patient controlled analgesia for management of acute pain, *JAMA* 259(2):243, 1988.
59. Lange M, Dahn M, Jacobs L: Patient controlled analgesia versus intermittent analgesia dosing, *Heart Lung* 17(5):495, 1988.
60. Stevens J: Step-by-step implementation of PCA therapy, *Nurs Management* 20(12):35, 1989.
61. Schechter N, Berrien F, Katz S: The use of patient controlled analgesia in adolescents with sickle cell pain crisis: a preliminary report, *J Pain Symptom Management* 3:109, Spring 1988.

29

Neurologic Therapeutic Management

CHAPTER OBJECTIVES

- ◆ Discuss the concept of cerebral autoregulation.
- ◆ Diagram the volume-pressure curve.
- ◆ Calculate cerebral perfusion pressure.
- ◆ Describe the therapies commonly used to treat intracranial hypertension.
- ◆ Discuss the complications associated with high-dose barbiturate therapy.
- ◆ List the four supratentorial herniation syndromes.

Despite the diversity of neurologic abnormalities, one aspect of the critical care management of the neurosurgical patient is common to a wide variety of these pathologic conditions. This chapter focuses on the concepts of intracranial pressure (ICP) and the types of ICP monitoring. Also discussed are the therapies for management of intracranial hypertension.

ASSESSMENT OF INTRACRANIAL PRESSURE

Monro-Kellie Hypothesis

The intracranial space comprises three components: brain substance (80%), cerebrospinal fluid (CSF) (10%), and blood (10%). Under normal physiologic conditions the ICP is maintained below 15 mm Hg mean pressure. Basic to understanding the pathophysiology of ICP is the Monro-Kellie hypothesis.[1] This hypothesis proposes that an increase in volume of one intracranial component must be compensated by a decrease in one or more of the other components so that total volume remains fixed. This compensation, although limited, includes displacing CSF from the intracranial vault to the lumbar cistern, increasing CSF absorption, and compressing the low-pressure venous system.

Volume-Pressure Curve

When the brain is capable of compliance, significant increases in intracranial volume can be tolerated without much increase in ICP. The amount of intracranial compliance, however, is limited. Once this limit has been reached, a state of decompensation with increased ICP results. As the ICP rises, the relationship between volume and pressure changes, and small increases in volume may cause major elevations in ICP (Fig. 29-1). The exact configuration of the volume-pressure curve and the point at which the steep rise in pressure occurs vary with individual patients.[2] The configuration of this curve also is influenced by the cause and the rate of volume increases within the intracranial vault; for example, neurologic deterioration occurs more rapidly in a patient with an acute epidural hematoma than in a patient with a meningioma of the same size. Monitoring these changes in intracranial dynamics and continuous clinical assessment of the patient's neurologic status have proved beneficial in diagnosing and treating sustained rises in ICP. Such elevations of ICP often precede evidence of neurologic deterioration obtained through the clinical assessment.

Cerebral Blood Flow and Autoregulation

Cerebral blood flow (CBF) is proportional to meet the metabolic demands of the brain. Although the brain makes up only 2% of body weight, it requires 15% to 20% of the resting cardiac output and 15% of the body's oxygen demands.[3] In the past it was believed that CBF depended passively on arterial pressure. The normal brain, however, has a complex capacity to maintain a constant CBF despite wide ranges in arterial pressure—an effect known as *autoregulation* (Fig. 29-2). Mean arterial pressure (MAP) of 50 to 150 mm Hg

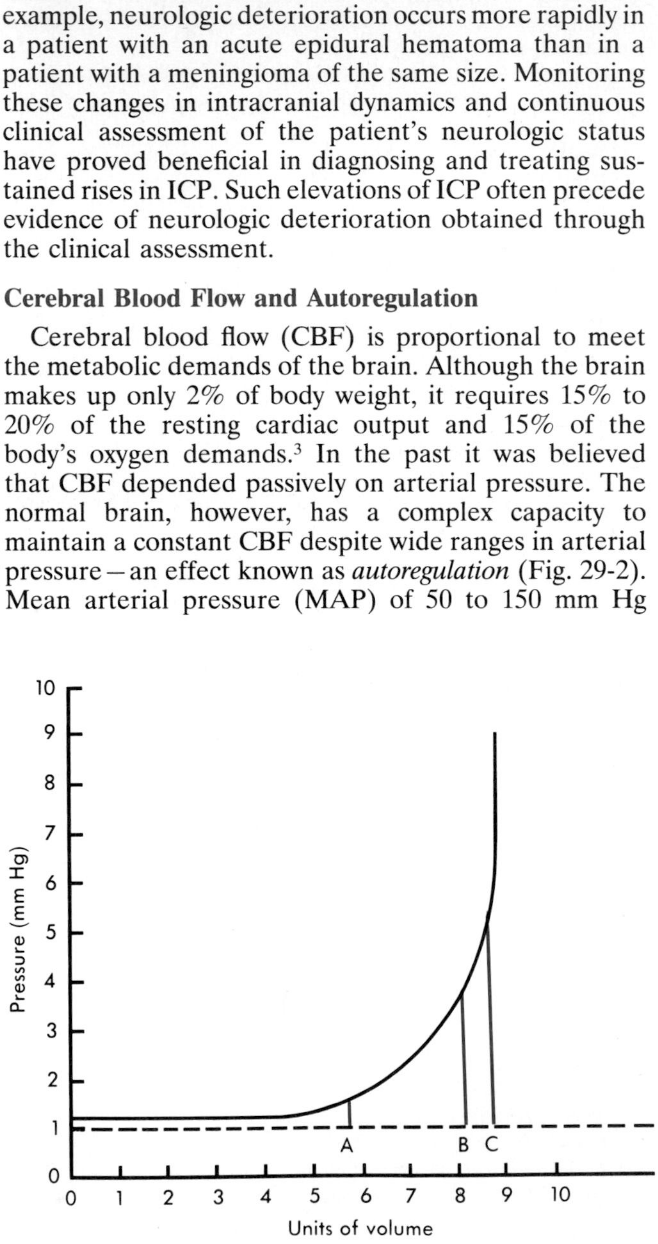

Fig. 29-1 Intracranial volume–pressure curve. **A,** Pressure is normal, and increases in intracranial volume are tolerated without increase in intracranial pressure. **B,** Increases in volume may cause increases in pressure. **C,** Small increases in volume may cause large increases in pressure.

RESEARCH ABSTRACT

The effects of familiar and unfamiliar voice treatments on intracranial pressure in patients with head injuries.

Treloar DM and others: *J Neurosci Nurs* 23(5):295, 1991.

PURPOSE

The purpose of this study was to examine the effect of familiar and unfamiliar stimulation on the intracranial pressure (ICP) of patients with head injuries.

DESIGN

Quasi-experimental, repeated-measures design

SAMPLE

The convenience sample consisted of 12 subjects (7 male, 5 female) in a surgical critical care unit of a tertiary medical center in the southeastern United States. Subjects admitted to the study were English-speaking; had no previous history of hydrocephalus, shunt placement, or hearing disorder; were not currently receiving intrathecal or intravenous medications; were not currently receiving mechanical ventilation with positive end-expiratory pressure greater than 10 torr; had ICP less than 40 torr; and Glasgow Coma Scale (GCS) score greater than 3. The mean age of the subjects was 31.5 years, with an average GCS of 7.8. All subjects had experienced closed-head injury and received mechanical ventilation with supplemental oxygen.

INSTRUMENTS

A Codman subarachnoid screw placed anteriorly to the coronal suture at the midpupillary line on the right side was used to measure ICP with a Mennon Horizon pressure-controlled patient monitor. Transducers were placed at the level of the middle external auditory canal. A General Electric battery-operated cassette tape recorder, model 3-50009B, was used for recording the taped message. The instrument used for adjusting decibel (dB) level of the taped message consisted of the Bruel and Kjaer sound meter, type 2330. A 60 dB level was used to simulate a normal conversation and control for sound intensity.

PROCEDURE

The closest relative or significant other whose voice the subject should easily recognize taped a message in a quiet area away from the critical care unit. The message lasted approximately 75 seconds and consisted of several general statements designed to promote comfort in the patient. The same message was recorded by the researcher. Before either message was played for the subject, a 10-minute baseline observation period occurred. The ICP for the last 60 seconds of this time was recorded as the baseline ICP. The recording of the familiar voice was played, during which ICP measurements were recorded at 5-second intervals for 1 minute, followed by measurements at 90, 120, and 180 seconds. The last ICP was recorded at 5 minutes from the time that the message first played. After the subject rested for 30 minutes, the procedure was repeated but with the message recorded in the researcher's voice.

RESULTS

No statistically significant differences were found between means obtained during the baseline period, the familiar voice period, and the unfamiliar voice period.

DISCUSSION/IMPLICATIONS

Findings from this study must be viewed cautiously because of the small sample size, and generalizations outside the study population are not applicable. Results of this study demonstrated minimal change in the ICP of patients with closed-head injuries who were exposed to the stimuli of familiar and unfamiliar voices. Subjects in this study all had normal baseline ICPs. Patients with greater than normal ICPs and decreased brain compliance might demonstrate a different response to verbal stimuli. A 75-second message may not have been enough time to elicit an auditory arousal response in the patients. Also, the specific location of injury and its effect on the auditory response was not known. Sequencing of the familiar and unfamiliar voice treatments was not randomized, which is a limitation of the study. Another limitation was the nonrandom selection of patients and the lack of controlled variables in terms of age, gender, type of injury, GCS scores, and ICP waveforms. Recommendations for future research include replication of the study with the use of a larger sample and correlating the effects of various physiologic variables.

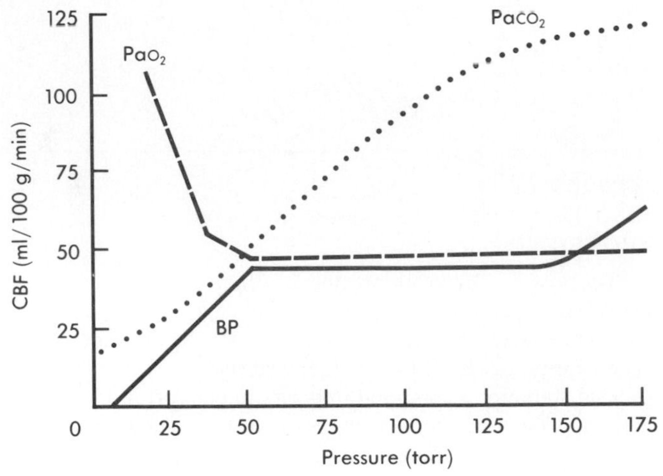

Fig. 29-2 Effects of arterial blood pressure, oxygen, and carbon dioxide on cerebral blood flow.

does not alter CBF when autoregulation is present.[3] Outside the limits of this autoregulation, CBF becomes passively dependent on the perfusion pressure. Factors other than arterial blood pressure that affect CBF are conditions that result in acidosis, alkalosis, and changes in metabolic rate.[9] Conditions that cause acidosis (hypoxia, hypercapnia, and ischemia) result in cerebral vascular dilation. Conditions causing alkalosis (e.g., hypocapnia) result in cerebral vascular constriction. Normally, a reduction in metabolic rate (e.g., from hypothermia or barbiturates) decreases CBF, and increases in metabolic rate (e.g., from hyperthermia) result in an increase in CBF.

Arterial blood gases exert a profound effect on CBF. Carbon dioxide, which affects the pH of the blood, is a potent vasoactive substance. Carbon dioxide retention (hypercapnia) leads to cerebral vasodilation, with increased cerebral blood volume, whereas hypocapnia leads to cerebral vasoconstriction and a reduction in cerebral blood volume. Hyperventilation therapy to induce hypocapnia often is used as a means of reducing ICP by reducing cerebral blood volume within the cranium. Prolonged hypocapnia, however, especially at an arterial partial pressure of carbon dioxide ($Paco_2$) less than 20 mm Hg, can produce cerebral ischemia.[4]

Low arterial partial pressure of oxygen (Pao_2), especially below 50 mm Hg, leads to cerebral vasodilation, which increases the intracranial blood volume and can contribute to increased ICP. The brain is thus exposed to ischemia directly through arterial hypoxemia, as well as through increased ICP. High Pao_2 has not been shown to affect CBF in either direction.

Cerebral blood volume may further be reduced through compression of the intracranial veins, expressing blood out of the brain. This is another compensatory mechanism of the brain for maintaining normal ICP.

Metabolic activity in the brain significantly influences CBF. Normally, when cerebral metabolic activity increases, a corresponding increase in CBF results to meet the demand.[4] Any pathologic process that decreases CBF could lead to a mismatch between metabolic demand and blood supply, resulting in cerebral ischemia. Barbiturate therapy is based on the principle of reducing cerebral metabolic rate in the presence of uncontrolled intracranial hypertension (prolonged increased ICP).

Cerebral Perfusion Pressure

Currently, it is difficult to measure CBF in the clinical setting. Cerebral perfusion pressure (CPP), an estimated pressure, is the blood pressure gradient across the brain and is calculated as the difference between the incoming MAP and the opposing ICP on the arteries[3,5]:

$$CPP = MAP - ICP$$

The CPP in the average adult is approximately 80 to 100 mm Hg, with a range of 60 to 150 mm Hg. The CPP should be maintained near 80 mm Hg to provide adequate blood supply to the brain. If the CPP drops below this point, ischemia may develop. A sustained CPP of 30 mm Hg or less usually will result in neuronal hypoxia and cell death. When the mean systemic arterial pressure equals the ICP, CBF may cease.

Assessment Techniques

◆ **Monitoring techniques.** Continuous measurement of ICP was first pioneered by Guillaume and Janny[6] in 1951 and was applied systematically to neurologically injured patients by Lundberg[7] in 1960. Lundberg also outlined criteria for the ideal ICP monitor. These criteria called for a procedure that would minimize the risk of trauma, intracranial infection, and CSF leakage, as well as provide continuous reliable pressure recording during diagnostic and therapeutic measures.

Since that time, much has been learned through the monitoring of ICP. However, there is still no agreement among neurosurgeons about which method is most appropriate. The common sites for monitoring ICP are the intraventricular space, the subarachnoid space, the epidural space, and the parenchyma.

The type of monitor placed in the ventricular system usually is a small catheter known as a *ventriculostomy catheter.* It is inserted through a burr hole with the patient under local anesthesia and usually is placed in the anterior horn of the lateral ventricle. If at all possible, the side chosen for placement of the ventriculostomy is the nondominant hemisphere (Fig. 29-3, *A*).

The second type of monitor frequently used is the subarachnoid bolt or screw. This small, hollow device is placed in a patient under local anesthesia through a burr hole, with the distal end lying in the subarachnoid or subdural space. The insertion of this device (Fig. 29-3, *B*)is easier than is the insertion of the ventriculostomy.

Another type of device commonly used is the epidural monitor. It too is placed through a burr hole while the patient is under local anesthesia. The physician must strip the dura away from the inner table of the skull before inserting the epidural monitor. The most common type of epidural monitor is the fiberoptic or pneumatic sensor, although other implantable epidural transducers often are used for long-term monitoring (Fig. 29-3, *C*).

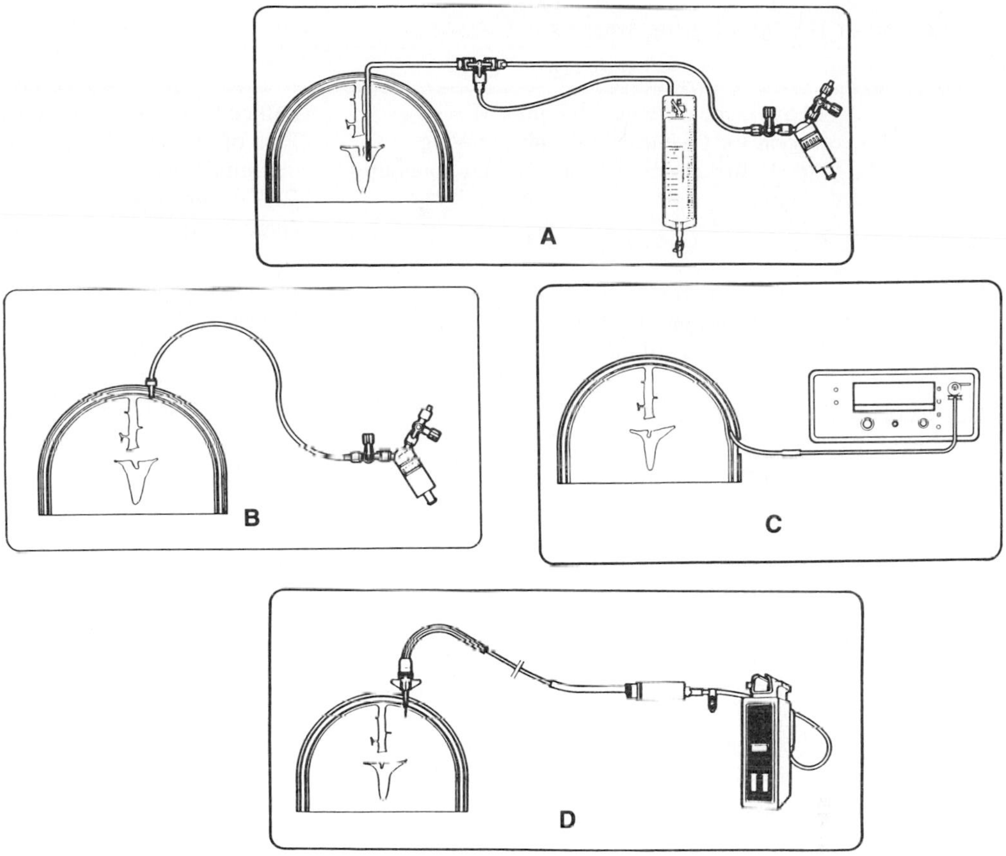

Fig. 29-3 **A,** Ventricular pressure monitoring system. **B,** Subarachnoid pressure monitoring system. **C,** Epidural pressure monitoring system. **D,** Intraparenchymal pressure monitoring system. (Courtesy Camino Laboratories, San Diego, Calif.)

The fourth type of ICP monitoring system is the fiberoptic transducer-tipped catheter (Fig. 29-3, *D*). This small (4F) catheter can be placed intraventricularly, intraparenchymally, in the subarachnoid space, or in the subdural space.

There are advantages and disadvantages to each of these systems for monitoring ICP[8] (Table 29-1). The type of monitor chosen depends on both the suspected pathologic condition and the physician's preference.

◆ **Intracranial pressure waves.** Since the beginning of ICP monitoring, clinicians have been interested in the waveforms associated with intracranial dynamics. As with arterial and pulmonary artery waves, the ICP wave has a systolic and a diastolic component (Fig. 29-4). Except in the research setting, little is being done in pulse-wave analysis of ICP waves, although recent reports have indicated that intracranial compliance may be assessable through the analysis of pulse waves. Instead, attention has focused on the ICP waveform *trend* or the trend of ICP over time. The three waves identified were first described by Lundberg[7] in the 1960s as A, B, and C waves (Fig. 29-5). These waves reflect spontaneous alterations in ICP associated with respiration, systemic blood pressure, and deteriorating neurologic status.

A waves, also called *plateau waves* because of their distinctive shape, are the most clinically significant of the three types. A waves usually occur in an already elevated baseline ICP (>20 mm Hg) and are characterized by sharp increases in ICP of 30 to 69 mm Hg, which plateau for 2 to 20 minutes and then return to baseline. The actual cause of A waves is unknown, but they may result from (1) vasodilation and increased CBF, (2) decreased venous outflow and therefore increased cerebral blood volume, (3) fluctuations in Pco_2 and therefore changes in cerebral blood volume, or (4) decreased CSF absorption. A waves frequently are preceded by B waves. Plateau waves are believed significant because of the reduced cerebral perfusion pressure associated with ICP in the 50 to 100 mm Hg range. Transient signs of intracranial hypertension such as a decreased level of consciousness, bradycardia, pupillary changes, or respiratory changes may accompany these waves. It has been suggested that prolonged increases in ICP associated with plateau waves could result in transient as well as permanent cell damage from ischemia. Management of A waves is directed at the reduction of the high pressure and prevention of other plateau waves.

B waves are sharp, rhythmic oscillations with a sawtooth appearance that occur every 30 seconds to 2

Table 29-1 Comparison of ICP monitoring systems

System	Advantages	Disadvantages
Ventricular catheter	Reliable measurement within CSF Access for CSF drainage and sampling Access for determination of volume-pressure curve	Difficulty locating lateral ventricle Risk of intracerebral bleeding or edema at cannula track Risk of infection Need for transducer repositioning with head movement
Subarachnoid bolt/screw	Useful if ventricles are small No penetration of brain Decreased risk of infection	Unable to drain CSF Unreliable pressure when high ICP herniates brain into bolt Requires intact skull Need for transducer repositioning with head movement
Epidural sensor	Ease of insertion No dural penetration Lower risk of infection No adjustment of transducer needed with head movement	Unable to drain CSF Unable to recalibrate or rezero after placement Questionable accuracy of sensing ICP through dura Separate large monitoring system required
Fiberoptic transducer-tipped catheter	Versatile system, which can be placed in ventricle, subarachnoid space, or brain tissue Able to monitor intraparenchymal pressure Access for CSF drainage with ventricular system No adjustment of transducer needed with head movement	Catheter relatively fragile Unable to recalibrate or rezero after placement Separate monitoring system required

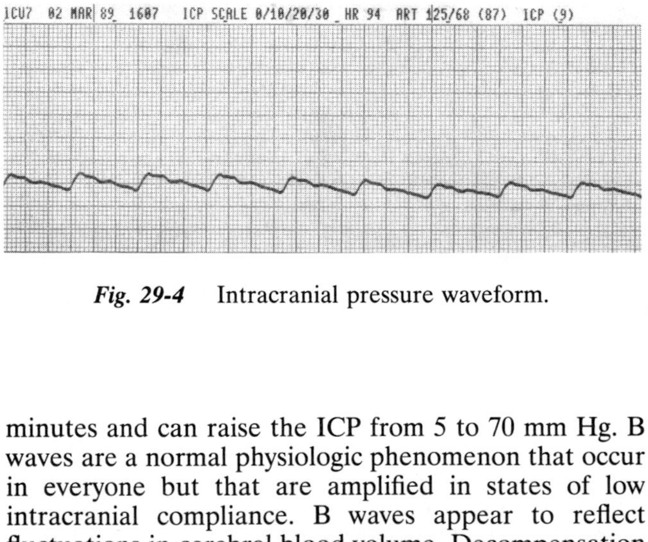

Fig. 29-4 Intracranial pressure waveform.

minutes and can raise the ICP from 5 to 70 mm Hg. B waves are a normal physiologic phenomenon that occur in everyone but that are amplified in states of low intracranial compliance. B waves appear to reflect fluctuations in cerebral blood volume. Decompensation of normal intracranial volume compensatory capacity is indicated by B waves with a high amplitude (> 15 mm Hg pressure change from peak to trough of wave).

C waves, smaller rhythmic waves that occur every 4 to 8 minutes, occur at normal levels of ICP. C waves are related to normal fluctuations in respirations and systemic arterial pressure.

MANAGEMENT OF INTRACRANIAL HYPERTENSION

Once intracranial hypertension is documented, therapy must be prompt to prevent secondary insults. Although the exact pressure level that denotes intracranial hypertension remains to be firmly established, most current evidence suggests that ICP generally should be treated when it exceeds 20 mm Hg.[9] All therapies are directed toward reducing the volume of one or more of the components (blood, brain, CSF) that lie within the intracranial vault. A major goal of therapy is to determine the cause of the elevated pressure and, if possible, remove the cause.[10] The use of computed tomography (CT) is invaluable in identifying mass lesions that can be surgically evacuated.[11] In the absence of a surgically treatable mass lesion, intracranial hypertension is treated medically. Nurses play an important role in rapid assessment and implementation of appropriate therapies for reducing ICP (see box, p. 550).

Patient Positioning

Positioning of the patient is a significant factor in both the prevention and treatment of elevated ICP. Positions that allow proper venous return are those that maintain the head and neck elevated 30 to 45 degrees and in a neutral position at all times. In these positions, gravity enhances venous drainage from the brain and head.[12,13]

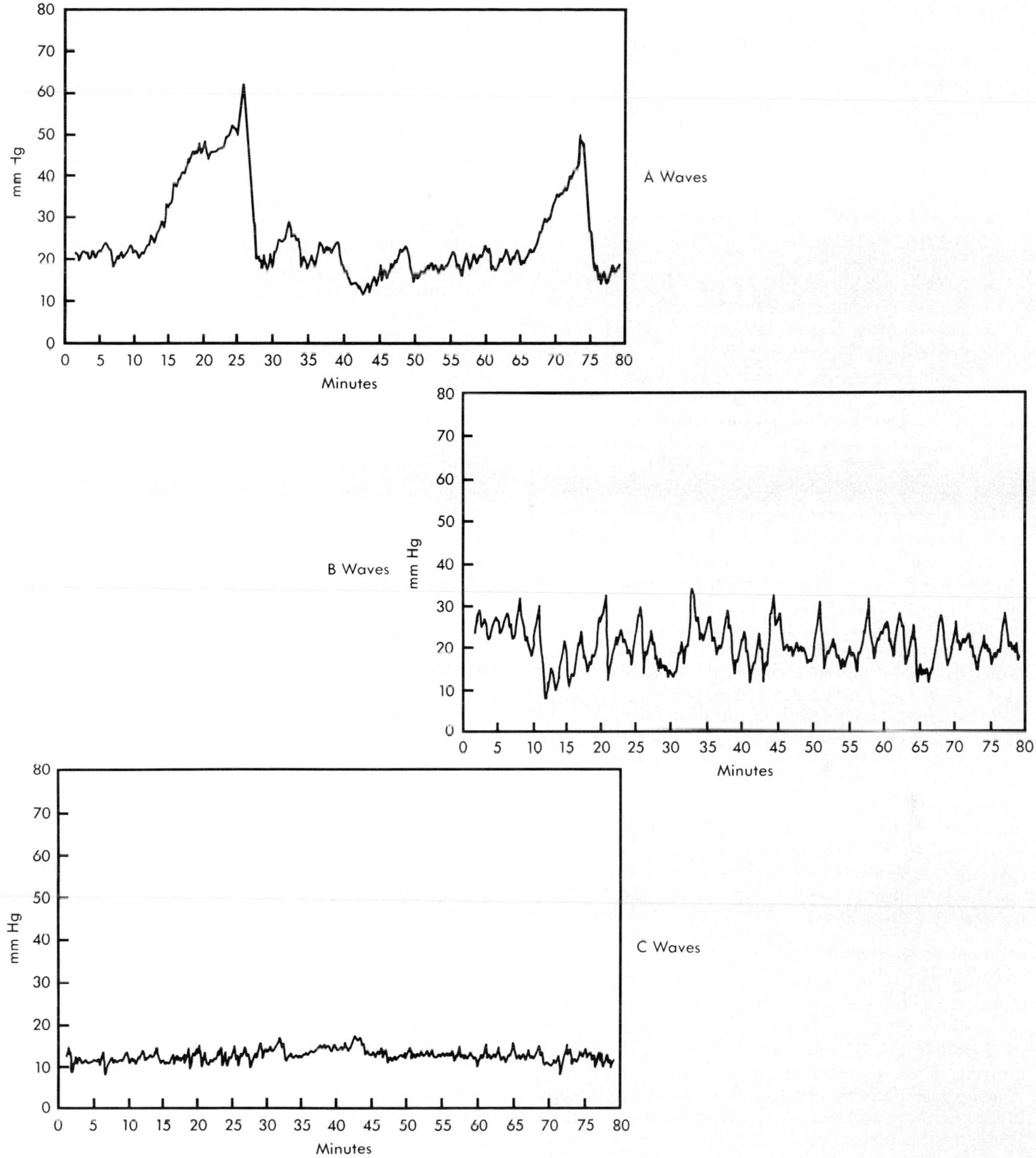

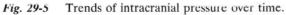

Fig. 29-5 Trends of intracranial pressure over time.

MANAGEMENT OF INTRACRANIAL HYPERTENSION

1. Keep patient's head elevated 30-45 degrees and in neutral plane.
2. Maintain controlled ventilation to an arterial partial pressure of carbon dioxide ($Paco_2$) of 25-30 torr with adequate sedation and neuromuscular blocking agents.
3. Maintain arterial partial pressure of oxygen (Pao_2) >70 torr.
4. Maintain systemic arterial pressure between 140 and 160 mm Hg systolic.
5. Maintain normothermia.
6. Use prophylactic anticonvulsants.
7. Perform ventricular drainage if possible.
8. Administer intravenous (IV) bolus of lidocaine as pretreatment for suctioning.
9. Administer mannitol (0.25-1 mg/kg) as needed.
10. Administer high-dose barbiturate therapy if all other conventional methods have failed.

Positions that impede venous return from the brain cause spikes in ICP. Obstruction of jugular veins or an increase in intrathoracic or intraabdominal pressure is communicated as increased pressure throughout the open venous system, thereby impeding drainage from the brain and increasing ICP. Positions that decrease venous return from the head (i.e., Trendelenburrg, prone, extreme flexion of the hips, and angulation of the neck) should be avoided if possible. If position changes such as Trendelenburrg's position are necessary to provide adequate pulmonary care, the critical care nurse must closely monitor ICP and vital signs. Mechanisms to reduce intracranial pressure (sedation, ventricular drainage) also may be employed during the time the patient is in Trendelenburrg's position.[14] Other impediments to cerebral venous drainage are positive end-expiratory pressure (PEEP) >5 to 10 cm H_2O pressure, coughing, suctioning, tight tracheostomy tube ties, and the Valsalva maneuver.

Controlled Ventilation

Controlled hyperventilation has been an important adjunct of therapy for the patient with increased ICP. If the carbon dioxide pressure (Pco_2) can be reduced from its normal level of 35 to 40 mm Hg to a range of 25 to 30 mm Hg in the patient with intracranial hypertension, vasoconstriction of cerebral arteries, reduction of cerebral blood flow, and increased venous return will result. Reducing the intracranial blood volume results in a general reduction in ICP.[9] Currently the use of controlled hyperventilation is under investigation. It is now believed that in certain situations of increased ICP, vasoconstriction of the cerebral vessels already has occurred. In these cases further application of controlled hyperventilation could cause vasoconstriction to such an extent that cerebral ischemia occurs.[15] It is well documented that high levels of Pco_2 cause cerebral vasodilation and contribute to elevated ICP. For this reason, Pco_2 levels greater than 40 mm Hg are considered dangerous.

The brain requires a constant supply of oxygen adequate to meet the demands of cerebral metabolism. Therefore maintaining uninterrupted oxygenation is of utmost importance in the management of brain injuries. In addition, hypoxia is a profound stimulus to increased cerebral blood flow and cerebral blood volume; therefore inadequate oxygenation in the presence of poor intracranial compliance will increase ICP.[16]

Although it is evident that hypoxemia should be avoided, no benefits can be gained from excessively high levels of oxygen. In fact, increasing inspired oxygen concentrations (FIo_2) above 60% may lead to toxic changes in lung tissue. With the increasing use of devices that monitor oxygen saturation (i.e., pulse oximeter and mixed venous oxygen saturation [Svo_2] monitors), there is greater awareness of the circumstances such as suctioning and restlessness that can cause oxygen desaturation and therefore elevate ICP.

Sedation and Neuromuscular Blocking Agents

Any treatment modality that increases the incidence of noxious stimulation to the patient carries with it the potential for increasing ICP. Such noxious stimuli include pain as a result of injuries sustained with the initial trauma, the presence of an endotracheal tube, coughing, suctioning, repositioning, bathing, and many routine nursing care procedures. Even patients who do not seem to move may respond to paralysis with decreased ICP, presumably because of improved chest wall compliance.[17]

To ensure adequate ventilation (Pco_2 of 25 to 30 and oxygen pressure [Po_2] >70) and in anticipation of the deleterious effects of noxious stimuli on ICP, sedatives alone or in combination with neuromuscular blocking agents may be used. Their use is recommended only in patients who have an ICP monitor in place, because sedation and especially neuromuscular blocking agents affect the reliability of neurologic assessment. Although sedation of the unconscious patient can obscure portions of the neurologic examination, its benefit may outweigh the risks.

The use of neuromuscular blocking agents without sedation is not recommended. Agents such as pancuronium bromide, for example, have no analgesic effect and do not adequately protect patients from pain and the physiologic responses that can occur from pain-producing procedures and, most important, from stimulation originating in the larynx. The need to have an endotracheal tube in place for long periods of time makes it necessary to sedate most and paralyze many of these patients.[18]

Temperature Control

Cerebral metabolic rate is directly proportional to body temperature, and it increases 5% to 7% per degree centigrade of increase in body temperature.[19] This fact is significant because as the cerebral metabolic rate increases, blood flow to the brain must increase to meet the tissue demands. To avoid the increase in blood volume that is associated with an increased cerebral metabolic rate, hyperthermia must be prevented in the patient with a brain injury. Antipyretics and cooling devices should be used when appropriate while the source of the fever is sought. Conversely, hypothermia reduces cerebral metabolic rate. At 30° C cerebral metabolic rate is decreased 50%. Maintenance of body temperature between 30° and 37° C may be beneficial if full cardiopulmonary support is given and if shivering, which greatly increases the body's metabolic requirements, is prevented. With the use of hypothermia, sedation and neuromuscular blocking agents or phenothiazines are administered to control shivering. Because of problems with intravascular hypovolemia, metabolic acidosis, and brain swelling associated with rewarming, the use of hypothermia for ICP control has not found wide acceptance.[16]

Persistent fluctuation and/or hypothermia or hyperthermia in conjunction with head injury is a grave prognostic sign and usually has been associated with death or a persistent vegetative state. These patients may represent a group with severe hypothalamic injury.[19]

Blood Pressure Control

Sustained systolic arterial hypertension (>160 mm Hg) in conjunction with elevated ICP should be vigorously treated. Control of systemic arterial hypertension may require nothing more than the administration of a sedative agent. Small, frequent doses may be sufficient to blunt noxious stimuli and prevent their triggering rises in blood pressure. In cases in which sedation has proved inadequate in controlling systemic arterial hypertension, primary antihypertensive agents are used. Care must be taken in choosing these agents because many of the peripheral vasodilators also are cerebral vasodilators (e.g., nitroprusside and nitroglycerin). It is believed, however, that all antihypertensives cause some degree of cerebral vasodilation. To reduce this vasodilating effect, it has been suggested that cotreatment with beta blockers (e.g., propranolol and labetalol) may be beneficial.[16]

Seizure Control

The incidence of posttraumatic seizures in the head-injured population has been estimated at 5%. Because of the risk of a secondary ischemic insult associated with seizures, many physicians prescribe anticonvulsant medications prophylactically. Seizures cause metabolic requirements to increase, which results in elevation of cerebral blood flow, cerebral blood volume, and ICP even in paralyzed patients. If blood flow cannot match demand, ischemia will develop, cerebral energy stores will be depleted, and irreversible neuronal destruction will occur.[16]

The usual anticonvulsant regimen for seizure control includes phenytoin or phenobarbital, or both, in therapeutic doses. The loading dosage for phenytoin is 15 to 18 mg/kg, and the loading dosage for phenobarbital is 4 to 8 mg/kg. Maintenance doses of phenytoin are administered to achieve a therapeutic blood level of 10 to 20 μg/ml. Maintenance doses of phenobarbital are administered to keep the blood level at 2 to 3 mg%.[20]

Intravenously administered phenytoin must be given with normal saline solution and infused slowly (less than 50 mg/min). Rapid IV administration has caused hypotension, premature ventricular contractions, and heart block. Intramuscular injection of phenytoin is not recommended because of its poor absorption from the tissues. Finally, when phenytoin is administered orally in conjunction with tube feedings, therapeutic levels should be closely monitored because absorption apparently is erratic. One recommendation to improve the absorption of phenytoin when it is given with enteral feedings is to discontinue the tube feeding 1 hour before the dose and reinstitute the feeding 1 hour after the dose. The effectiveness of this method in promoting the steady reabsorption of phenytoin needs substantiation through research. During administration of the phenobarbital loading dose, careful monitoring of the patient's vital signs is necessary to avoid a precipitous drop in blood pressure.

The question of the need for anticonvulsants after cerebral trauma remains unanswered. Studies of this issue, including the risks and benefits of anticonvulsant therapy, are currently being undertaken.

Lidocaine

Various forms of sensory stimulation (including tracheal intubation, laryngoscopy, and endotracheal suctioning) may provoke marked increases in ICP and MAP. One therapy used to prevent cerebral ischemia and acute intracranial hypertension has been the administration of lidocaine through an endotracheal tube or through intravenous infusion before nasotracheal suctioning.[9]

Lidocaine initially was introduced as a local anesthetic in 1948, and it is believed that its anesthetic properties make it efficacious in blunting ICP spikes secondary to tracheal stimulation. Studies have found that peak lidocaine concentrations are linearly related to the administered dose and that the rate of absorption depends on the vascularity of the site of administration.[9,16] It also has been documented that lidocaine is initially distributed to the lungs, then to the heart and kidneys, and then to muscle and adipose tissue.

The prophylactic administration of lidocaine before endotracheal suctioning has been widely practiced. In most cases, 50 to 100 mg is administered intravenously approximately 2 minutes before suctioning is performed. If the endotracheal route is chosen, 2 ml of 4% lidocaine is the preferred dose, and suctioning must be completed within 5 minutes of administering the drug. It is believed that adherence to this procedure protects the patient from the associated increases in ICP that occur with suctioning. A number of studies are in progress investigating the usefulness of lidocaine in this area.

Cerebrospinal Fluid Drainage

CSF drainage for intracranial hypertension may be used along with other treatment modalities. CSF drainage is accomplished by the insertion of a pliable catheter into the anterior horn of the lateral ventricle, preferably on the nondominant side. Such drainage can help support the patient through periods of cerebral edema by controlling spikes in ICP. One of the major advantages of the ventriculostomy is its dual role as both a monitoring device and a treatment modality. Because CSF provides a favorable medium for the development of infection, it is essential that flawless aseptic technique be followed during insertion and maintenance of the system. The ventricular system is connected to a drainage bag and is then maintained as a closed system for the period of time the ventriculostomy remains in place—usually 3 to 5 days.

When this system is used for treatment, there are two ways to accomplish removal of CSF: it can be removed intermittently when ICP becomes elevated, or it can be removed continuously, with the ventriculostomy bag at a predetermined level above the lateral ventricle. Intermittent drainage involves draining CSF for brief periods (30 to 120 seconds) when ICP exceeds the upper limits of normal. Frequent periods of drainage (more than four times per hour) should be reported to the physician. Continuous drainage is most often ordered when the patient has significant amounts of blood in the subarachnoid space (e.g., with a subarachnoid hemorrhage). The ventricular drainage bag is placed 10 to 15 cm above the level of the third ventricle so that if ICP exceeds 10 to 12 mm Hg, CSF will be shunted into the drainage bag. One very important concept to keep in mind is that when intracranial hypertension or a mass lesion is suspected, a lumbar puncture is contraindicated because of the risk of downward herniation.

Diuretics

◆ **Osmotic agents.** The effectiveness of osmotic agents in the reduction of ICP has been known for decades. The mechanism by which these diuretics reduce ICP continues as a subject of investigational interest. One belief is that these agents act by remaining relatively impermeable to the blood-brain barrier, thereby drawing water from normal brain tissue to plasma.[18,21] The direction of flow is from the hypoconcentrated tissue to the hyperconcentrated cerebral vasculature. If the situation becomes reversed and the tissue becomes hyperconcentrated in relation to the cerebral vasculature, a *rebound phenomenon* could occur. These agents have little direct effect on edematous cerebral tissue situated in an area of defective blood-brain barrier; instead, they require an intact blood-brain barrier for osmosis to occur.

The three best-known osmotic diuretics are urea, mannitol, and glycerol. Urea, the first osmotic diuretic widely accepted in the treatment of intracranial hypertension, was introduced by Javid[21] in the late 1950s. Although urea is still used in some clinical settings, mannitol has gained wide acceptance as the osmotic diuretic of choice. Mannitol, a larger molecule than urea, is retained almost entirely in the extracellular compartment and has little to none of the rebound effect noted with urea. It also has been suggested that mannitol in particular improves perfusion to ischemic areas of the brain, producing cerebral vasoconstriction and resulting in a reduction of ICP.[18] Glycerol, the effect of which is similar on the brain to that of mannitol, has the advantage of oral administration. It also apparently is a safe drug for long-term use. The fact that glycerol can be administered orally has no real benefit in the medical treatment of the patient with severe brain injury.

Perhaps the most frequent difficulty associated with the use of osmotic agents is the production of electrolyte disturbances. Careful attention should be paid to body weight and fluid and electrolyte stability. Serum osmolality should be kept between 300 and 320 mOsm/L. Hypernatremia and hypokalemia frequently are associated with repeated administration of osmotic agents. Central venous pressure readings should be monitored to prevent hypovolemia. The usual dosage of mannitol is 0.5 to 1.5 g/kg. Data suggest that small doses (0.25 g/kg) decrease ICP as rapidly and profoundly as higher doses (1 g/kg), but the effect is somewhat less prolonged (4 to 6 hours).[16] Smaller doses of mannitol simplify fluid and electrolyte management, and their use is encouraged whenever possible.[9,18]

◆ **Nonosmotic agents.** Nonosmotic diuretics also have been used to decrease ICP. Furosemide, one such nonosmotic diuretic, may act differently from osmotic agents by pulling sodium and water from edematous areas and, perhaps, by decreasing CSF production. One advantage of furosemide administration over the use of osmotic diuretics is that its effect is not generally associated with increases in serum osmolality. Therefore electrolyte imbalances may not be as severe with the use of nonosmotic diuretics.

Another diuretic in this category is acetazolamide. The action of this drug is to reduce the rate at which CSF is produced in the choroid plexus. Generally the use of acetazolamide in patients with head injuries is contraindicated because of its cerebral vasodilative effect.

High-Dose Barbiturate Therapy

Barbiturate therapy is a treatment protocol developed for the management of uncontrolled intracranial hypertension that has not responded to the conventional treatments previously described.[20] Uncontrolled ICP is described in the literature as follows[19,22,23]:

1. ICP >20 mm Hg for 30 minutes or more, with unresponsiveness to aggressive use of conventional therapies
2. ICP >40 mm Hg for 15 minutes or more or CPP <50 mm Hg, or both

In the early 1970s barbiturate therapy, which consisted of administering large doses of short-acting barbiturates to induce and maintain coma, was introduced.[24] Although the specific action of barbiturates in the reduction of ICP is unclear, several theories were developed to explain their effect on the central nervous system and the subsequent cerebral protection they provide. Barbiturates increase the cerebral vascular resistance and therefore decrease cerebral blood flow, resulting in a reduction in intracranial volume. Systemic blood pressure also is lowered, reducing hydrostatic pressure in the damaged cerebral tissue and helping arrest edema formation.[25] Barbiturates also slow cerebral metabolism by reducing the functional electrical generation of the neurons. This decreased cerebral metabolism thus lessens the glucose and oxygen demands of the brain.[25,26] Barbiturates also are effective anticonvulsants and may suppress subclinical seizure activities. Finally, it has been postulated that barbiturates are scavengers of free radicals and thereby prevent cell membrane damage and destruction.[26,27]

The two most commonly used drugs in high-dose barbiturate therapy are pentobarbital and thiopental. Pentobarbital, a longer-acting barbiturate, is administered in a loading dosage of 3 to 5 mg/kg of body weight over a 15-minute period, with a maintenance dosage of 1 to 2 mg/kg/hr. Thiopental, a shorter-acting barbiturate, is administered in a loading dosage of 1 to 5 mg/kg of body weight and a maintenance dosage of 1 to 3 mg/kg/hr. The goal with either of these drugs is a reduction of ICP to 15 to 20 mm Hg while maintaining a MAP of 70 to 80 torr. A therapeutic serum blood level for high-dose barbiturate therapy is 3 to 5 mg%. Patients are maintained on high-dose barbiturate therapy until ICP has been controlled within the normal range for 24 hours. Barbiturates should never be stopped abruptly but should be tapered slowly over approximately 4 days.[18]

The success of barbiturate therapy is directly proportional to the aggressiveness of the previously used conventional therapy. Therefore if hyperventilation, blood pressure control, and osmotic diuretics have not been used to their fullest extent, the addition of barbiturates will create a larger number of good outcomes in patients who might have done as well without their addition.[16] Because of the considerable resources required (extensive invasive monitoring and qualified medical and nursing personnel) and the risks of hypotension and infection, the indiscriminate use of barbiturates is not recommended.[20,27]

◆ **Complications of high-dose barbiturate therapy.** Complications of high-dose barbiturate therapy can be disastrous unless a specific and organized approach is used. The complications most frequently encountered are hypotension, hypothermia, and decreased cardiac output. If any occur and are allowed to persist unchecked, the consequences may lead to secondary insults to an already damaged brain. Hypotension, the most common complication, is a result of peripheral vasodilation and can be compounded in an already dehydrated patient who has received large doses of an osmotic diuretic in an attempt to control ICP. Careful monitoring of fluid status by central venous pressure or a pulmonary artery catheter can help in preventing this complication. Hypothermia results from a decrease in basal metabolic rate. This problem can lead to cardiac irritability and arrest if not reversed. To avoid these sequelae, the patient's temperature should be maintained between 33° and 37° C, and warming devices should be used if necessary. Decreased cardiac output results from hypotension or cardiac muscle suppression. It can be avoided by frequent monitoring of fluid status, cardiac output, and serum drug levels. If an adequate cardiac output cannot be maintained in the presence of normothermia, barbiturates must be reduced, regardless of serum levels.

NURSING DIAGNOSIS AND MANAGEMENT

Increased intracranial pressure

- ◆ Altered Cerebral Tissue Perfusion related to increased intracranial pressure secondary to brain trauma, hemorrhage, edema, infection, tumor, stroke, or hydrocephalus, p. 560
- ◆ Altered Cerebral Tissue Perfusion related to vasospasm secondary to subarachnoid hemorrhage after ruptured intracranial aneurysm or arteriovenous malformation, p. 558
- ◆ High Risk for Infection risk factors: invasive monitoring devices, p. 366
- ◆ High Risk for Aspiration risk factors: impaired laryngeal sensation or reflex; impaired laryngeal closure or elevation; increased gastric volume; decreased lower esophageal sphincter pressure, p. 472
- ◆ Ineffective Airway Clearance related to impaired cough secondary to artificial airway, p. 466
- ◆ Inability to Sustain Spontaneous Ventilation related to respiratory muscle fatigue secondary to mechanical ventilation, p. 468

The major unresolved issue in the use of high-dose barbiturates is their effect on outcome after head injury. Several laboratory and clinical trials have been undertaken to address this issue. Results of a multicenter randomized trial of barbiturates found that most elevations of ICP could be controlled with aggressive use of standard therapies of ICP management. For the small subset of patients in whom standard therapy fails to achieve ICP control, judicious, carefully monitored and administered high-dose barbiturate therapy is of benefit.[28]

HERNIATION SYNDROMES

The goal of neurologic evaluation, ICP monitoring, and treatment of increased ICP is to prevent herniation. Herniation of intracerebral contents results in the shifting of tissue from one compartment of the brain to another and places pressure on cerebral vessels and vital function centers of the brain. If unchecked, herniation rapidly causes death as a result of the cessation of cerebral blood flow and respirations.

Supratentorial Herniation

There are four types of supratentorial herniation syndrome: central or transtentorial, uncal, cingulate, or transcalvarial (Fig. 29-6).

◆ **Uncal herniation.** Uncal herniation is the herniation syndrome most often noted. In uncal herniation, a

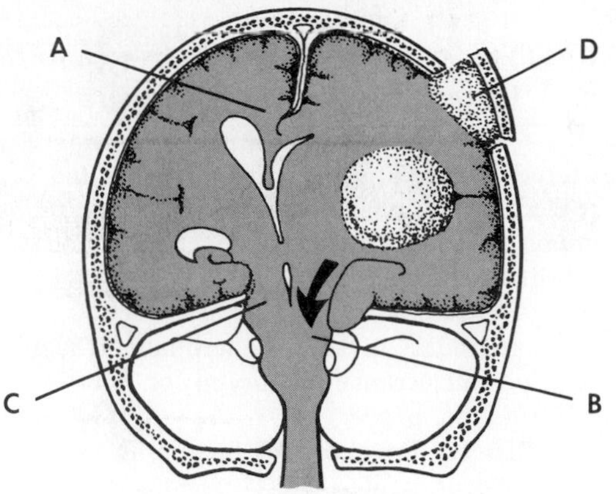

Fig. 29-6 Supratentorial herniation. **A,** Cingulate. **B,** Uncal. **C,** Central. **D,** Transcalvarial.

unilateral, expanding mass lesion, usually of the temporal lobe, increases ICP, causing the tip of the temporal lobe (uncus) to displace laterally. Lateral displacement pushes the uncus over the edge of the tentorium, puts pressure on the oculomotor nerve (cranial nerve III) and posterior cerebral artery ipsilateral to the lesion, and flattens the midbrain against the opposite side.

Clinical manifestations of uncal herniation include ipsilateral pupil dilation, decreased level of consciousness, respiratory pattern changes leading to respiratory arrest, and contralateral hemiplegia leading to decorticate or decerebrate posturing. If no intervention occurs, uncal herniation results in fixed and dilated pupils, flaccidity, and respiratory arrest.

◆ **Central or transtentorial herniation.** In central herniation an expanding mass lesion of the midline, frontal, parietal, or occipital lobes results in downward displacement of the hemispheres, basal ganglia, and diencephalon through the tentorial notch. Central herniation often is preceded by uncal and cingulate herniation.

Clinical manifestations of central or transtentorial herniation include loss of consciousness, small, reactive pupils progressing to fixed, dilated pupils, respiratory changes leading to respiratory arrest, and decorticate posturing progressing to flaccidity. In the late stages, uncal and central herniation syndromes are similar in their effects on the brainstem.

◆ **Cingulate herniation.** Cingulate herniation occurs when an expanding lesion of one hemisphere shifts laterally and forces the cingulate gyrus under the falx cerebri. Cingulate herniation occurs frequently. Whenever a lateral shift is noted on a CT scan, cingulate herniation has occurred. Little is known about the effects of cingulate herniation, and there are no clinical manifestations that assist in its diagnosis. Cingulate herniation is not life-threatening on its own, but if the expanding mass lesion that caused cingulate herniation is not controlled, uncal or central herniation will follow.

◆ **Transcalvarial herniation.** Transcalvarial herniation is the extrusion of cerebral tissue through the cranium. In the presence of severe cerebral edema, transcalvarial herniation occurs through an opening from a skull fracture or craniotomy site.

Infratentorial Herniation

There are two infratentorial herniation syndromes: upward transtentorial herniation and downward cerebellar herniation.

◆ **Upward transtentorial herniation.** Upward transtentorial herniation occurs when an expanding mass lesion of the cerebellum causes protrusion of the vermis (central area) of the cerebellum and the midbrain upward through the tentorial notch. Compression of the third cranial nerve and diencephalon occur. Obstruction of CSF flow occurs with blockage of the central aqueduct and distortion of the third ventricle. Deterioration occurs rapidly.

◆ **Downward cerebellar herniation.** Downward cerebellar herniation occurs when an expanding lesion of the cerebellum exerts pressure downward, sending the cerebellar tonsils through the foramen magnum. Compression and displacement of the medulla oblongata occur, rapidly resulting in respiratory and cardiac arrest.

The best treatment of any of these herniation syndromes is prevention. The goal of accurate assessment, evaluation, and intervention is the prevention of increasing pressure forces inside the cranium that would lead to herniation.

REFERENCES

1. Marmarou A, Tabaddor K: Intracranial pressure: physiology and pathophysiology. In Cooper PR, editor: *Head injury,* ed 2, Baltimore, 1987, Williams & Wilkins.
2. Mitchell PH, Amos D, Astley C: Nursing and ICP: studies of two clinical problems. In Miller JD, editor: *Intracranial pressure,* vol 6, New York, 1986, Springer-Verlag.
3. Rockoff MA, Kennedy SK: Physiology and clinical aspects of raised intracranial pressure. In Ropper AH, Kennedy SK, Zerfas NT, editors: *Neurologic and neurosurgical intensive care,* Baltimore, 1983, University Park Press.
4. Ward JD and others: Cerebral homeostasis and protection. In Wirth FP, Ratcheson RA, editors: *Neurosurgical critical care,* vol 1, *Concepts in neurosurgery,* Baltimore, 1987, Williams & Wilkins.
5. Hickey JV: *The clinical practice of neurological and neurosurgical nursing*, ed 3, Philadelphia, 1991, JB Lippincott.
6. Guillaume J, Janny P: Monometric intracranienne continue; interet physio-pathologique et clinique de la methode, *Presse Med* 59:953, 1951.
7. Lundberg N: Continuous recording and control of ventricular fluid pressure in neurosurgical practice, *Acta Psychiatr Neurol Scand Suppl* 149:1, 1960.
8. Hopkins CC: Infection: pathogenesis, prevention, and treatment. In Ropper AH, Kennedy SK, Zervas NT, editors: *Neurological and neurosurgical intensive care,* Baltimore, 1983, University Park Press.
9. Chesnut RM, Marshall LF: Management of head injury: treatment of abnormal intracranial pressure, *Neurosurg Clin North Am* 2(2):267, 1991.
10. Wrobel CJ, Marshall LF: Closed head injury management dilemmas. In Long DM, editor: *Current therapy in neurological surgery,* ed 3, St Louis, 1992, Mosby–Year Book.
11. Eisenberg HM, Weiner RN, Tabaddor K: Emergency care: initial evaluation. In Cooper PR, editor: *Head injury,* ed 2, Baltimore, 1987, Williams & Wilkins.

12. Mitchell PH: Intracranial hypertension: influence of nursing care activities, *Nurs Clin North Am* 21(4):563, 1986.
13. Snyder M: Relation of nursing activities to increases in intracranial pressure, *J Adv Nurs* 8:273, 1983.
14. Fontaine DK, McQuillan K: Positioning as a nursing therapy in trauma care, *Crit Care Nurs Clin North Am* 1(1):105, 1990.
15. Muizelaar JP and others: Adverse effects of prolonged hyperventilation in patients with severe head injury: a randomized clinical trial, *J Neurosurg* 75(5):731, 1991.
16. Rockoff MA, Ropper AH: Treatment of intracranial hypertension. In Ropper AH, Kennedy SK, Zervas NT, editors: *Neurologic and neurosurgical intensive care*, Baltimore, 1983, University Park Press.
17. Shapiro HM: Intracranial hypertension: therapeutic and anesthetic considerations, *Anesthesia* 43:445, 1975.
18. Marshall LF, Marshall SB: Medical management of intracranial pressure. In Cooper PR, editor: *Head injury*, ed 2, Baltimore, 1987, Williams & Wilkins.
19. Marshall LF, Smith RW, Shapiro HM: The outcome with aggressive treatment in severe head injuries, *J Neurosurg* 50:20, 1979.
20. Commission for the Control of Epilepsy and Its Consequences: Plan for nationwide action on epilepsy, vol 4, DHEW Pub No (NIH) 78-279, Bethesda, Md, 1978, National Institutes of Health.
21. Javid M: Urea in intracranial surgery: a new method, *J Neurosurg* 18:51, 1961.
22. Miller JD: Barbiturates and raised intracranial pressure, *Ann Neurol* 6(3):189, 1979.
23. Rudy EB: *Advanced neurological and neurosurgical nursing*, St Louis, 1984, Mosby–Year Book.
24. Shapiro HM, Wyte SR, Loeser J: Barbiturate-augmented hypothermia for reduction of persistent intracranial hypertension, *J Neurosurg* 40:90, 1974.
25. Anderson BJ: The metabolic needs of head trauma victims, *J Neurosci Nurs* 19(4):211, 1987.
26. Siesjo BK and others: Brain metabolism in the critically ill, *Crit Care Med* 4:283, 1976.
27. Swann KW: Management of severe head injury. In Ropper AH, Kennedy SK, Zervas NT, editors: *Neurological and neurosurgical intensive care*, Baltimore, 1983, University Park Press.
28. Eisenberg HM and others: High-dose barbiturate control of elevated intracranial pressure in patients with severe head injury, *J Neurosurg* 69:15, 1988.

30

Neurologic Nursing Diagnosis and Management

This chapter is designed to supplement the preceding chapters in the *Neurologic Alterations* unit by integrating theoretic content into clinically applicable case studies and nursing management plans.

The case study is designed to illustrate clinical problem solving and patient care management occurring in actual patients. The case, reviewed retrospectively, demonstrates how medical and nursing diagnoses may be effectively used in critical care. The case study also demonstrates revisions to the plan of care and the nursing and medical management outcomes that are apt to occur during the course of a complicated hospitalization as the patient responds physiologically to treatment. Often in a short case anecdote, such as presented in this chapter, the clinical answer may appear to be obvious from the day of admission. In practice, however, critical care patient management is sometimes investigative and the "correct" diagnosis for an individual patient may not become apparent until midway in the hospitalization. Or a patient with an apparently straightforward diagnosis may develop an unexpected complication, and the plan of care and potential outcomes will then require revision. Many of the case studies demonstrate this principle.

The nursing management plans, which—unlike the case study—are not patient-specific, provide a basis nurses can use to individualize care for their patients. In the previous *Neurologic Alterations* chapters, each medical diagnosis is assigned a Nursing Diagnosis and Management box. Using this box as a page guide, the reader can access relevant nursing management plans for each medical diagnosis. For example, nursing management of *cerebrovascular disease*, described on pp. 533-534, may involve several nursing diagnoses and management plans outlined in this chapter and in other Nursing Diagnosis and Management chapters. Specific examples are (1) *Ineffective Breathing Pattern related to musculoskeletal impariment,* p. 470; (2) *Ineffective Airway Clearance related to impaired cough secondary to artificial airway, on p. 466;* (3) *High Risk for Infection risk factors: invasive monitoring devices*, on p. 366; and (4) *Self-Esteem Disturbances related to feelings of guilt about physical deterioration*, on p. 96. These examples highlight the interrelationship of the various physiologic systems in the body and the fact that pathology often has a multisystem impact in the critically ill.

Use of the case study and management plans can enhance the understanding and application of the *Neurologic* content in clinical practice.

NEUROLOGIC CASE STUDY

CLINICAL HISTORY

Mrs. T is a 66-year-old white woman with a medical history of hypertension controlled by diet and medication. Her health otherwise has been good. Premorbid vital signs are not available.

CURRENT PROBLEMS

While leaving a grocery store with her husband, Mrs. T suddenly complained of severe headache and almost immediately collapsed to the floor. An ambulance transported her to the hospital. On arrival in the emergency department she was conscious, disoriented, and complaining of severe, diffuse headache. Her Glasgow Coma Scale (GCS) score was as follows: eye opening, 4; best verbal, 4; best motor, 6. The pupils were round and equal and reacted briskly to light. No nuchal rigidity was evident, and the motor examination was symmetrical. Her BP was 210/124; heart rate, 98 (NSR with occasional PVCs); and respiratory rate, 24 and regular.

NEUROLOGIC CASE STUDY—cont'd

MEDICAL DIAGNOSIS

Probable subarachnoid hemorrhage (SAH), grade II

NURSING DIAGNOSES

- ◆ Acute Pain related to transmission and perception of cutaneous, visceral, muscular, or ischemic impulses secondary to probable hemorrhagic cerebrovascular accident
- ◆ Altered Cerebral Tissue Perfusion related to increased intracranial pressure secondary to hemorrhage

◆ PLAN OF CARE

1. Perform a CT scan to definitively determine the nature of CVA.
2. Reduce blood pressure.

MEDICAL AND NURSING MANAGEMENT AND PATIENT OUTCOME

Procardia 10 mg was administered sublingually as Mrs. T was prepared for an emergency CT scan of the head. Her neurologic status rapidly deteriorated, she became stuporous and difficult to arouse, and her respirations became irregular. Her pupils were midposition and sluggish in reaction to light. Intubation, oxygenation, and manual hyperventilation were carried out, and she was transported to the CT scanner. Based on the results of the CT scan, the following diagnoses were made.

MEDICAL DIAGNOSIS

SAH extending into the ventricles with acute, obstructive hydrocephalus, grade IV

NURSING DIAGNOSES

- ◆ Altered Cerebral Tissue Perfusion related to increased intracranial pressure secondary to obstructive hydrocephalus
- ◆ High Risk for Impaired Gas Exchange risk factor: alveolar hypoventilation secondary to progressive transentorial brain herniation

◆ REVISED PLAN OF CARE

Mrs. T was taken directly to the OR for placement of a ventriculostomy for drainage of cerebrospinal fluid (CSF) to relieve the intracranial hypertension and to monitor the ICP.

MEDICAL AND NURSING MANAGEMENT AND PATIENT OUTCOME

Mrs. T was stable at the end of the procedure and was extubated in the OR. She was transferred to the critical care unit and was soon alert, but disoriented to time, and was experiencing short-term memory difficulty. Her GCS was 14. Pupils were equal and reactive to light, and the motor examination findings were symmetric. Her ICP was 10 cm H_2O; BP, 155/88; pulse, 85 (NSR); and respirations, 18 (regular). She was placed on nimodipine to lessen the potential for cerebral vasospasm, and precautions were taken to prevent subarachnoid rebleeding (bed rest, analgesics, stool softener, quiet, darkened room). An IV of $D_5\frac{1}{2}NS$ was maintained.

◆ REVISED PLAN OF CARE

The following day Mrs. T underwent cerebral angiography followed by a right frontal craniotomy for clipping of an anterior communicating artery aneurysm.

MEDICAL AND NURSING MANAGEMENT AND PATIENT OUTCOME

Mrs. T was continued on nimodipine postoperatively. Her BP averaged 150 to 160 mm Hg systolic, and ICP averaged 10 to 12 cm H_2O with bloody CSF drained in small amounts. Hydration was maintained with $D_5\frac{1}{2}NS$. Her serum Na^+ was 133 mEq/L, and other electrolytes, BUN, and creatinine were within normal limits. After 3 uneventful days the ventriculostomy was removed. Later that night Mrs. T became obtunded and developed a slight right lower facial droop and weakness of the left arm and leg. Because recurrent obstructive hydrocephalus was suspected, mannitol was administered. An emergency CT scan was done and revealed no recurrent hydrocephalus and no new bleeding. Her serum Na^+ at this time was 114 mEq/L.

Continued

NEUROLOGIC CASE STUDY—cont'd

MEDICAL DIAGNOSES

Cerebral vasospasm affecting both cereral hemispheres
Severe hyponatremia

NURSING DIAGNOSIS

◆ Altered Cerebral Tissue Perfusion related to (1) increased intracranial pressure secondary to brain hemorrage and (2) vasospasm secondary to subarachnoid hemorrage

◆ REVISED PLAN OF CARE

Hypertensive-hypervolemic therapy was warranted to combat the severe cerebral vasospasm, improve cerebral perfusion, and prevent cerebral infarction.

MEDICAL AND NURSING MANAGEMENT AND PATIENT OUTCOME

Nimodipine was continued. Mrs. T was placed with the head of bed elevated no higher than 10 degrees to improve cerebral perfusion. Her BP was maintained at 200 to 210 mm Hg systolic with IV crystalloids and colloids and a dopamine infusion. A pulmonary artery catheter was inserted to monitor and maintain the pulmonary capillary wedge pressure between 14 and 16 mm Hg. Hypertonic NaCl was administered IV to correct the severe hyponatremia, since fluid restriction is contraindicated in the presence of cerebral vasospasm. Mrs. T's Na^+ slowly rose to 132 mEq/L, and after several days of hypertensive-hypervolemic therapy she became more alert and was able to follow simple commands. The right facial droop persisted, and her left extremities were now flaccid, indicating that cerebral infarctions had occurred in both hemispheres. After 12 days this therapy was slowly withdrawn, and she was transferred from the critical care unit.

Two weeks later, while sitting in a chair, she became obtunded and aspirated. Right facial focal seizures were noted. Her serum Na^+ was again found to be 116 mEq/L. Her electrolyte imbalance was corrected, but she never fully regained consciousness. Mrs. T was later transferred to a skilled nursing facility. Her disease progression is unknown.

*ALTERED CEREBRAL TISSUE PERFUSION RELATED TO VASOSPASM SECONDARY TO SUBARACHNOID HEMORRHAGE AFTER RUPTURED INTRACRANIAL ANEURYSM OR ARTERIOVENOUS MALFORMATION**

DEFINING CHARACTERISTICS

Subarachnoid hemorrhage

◆ Aneurysm grading system according to Hunt and Hess[1]
- Grade I: minimal bleed
  - Asymptomatic or minimal headache
  - Slight nuchal rigidity
- Grade II: mild bleed
  - Moderate-to-severe headache
  - Nuchal rigidity
  - Minimal neurologic deficit (e.g., possible cranial nerve palsies—oculomotor [cranial nerve III] most common; unilateral pupillary dilation, ptosis, and dysconjugate gaze)
- Grade III: moderate bleed
  - Drowsiness
  - Confusion
  - Nuchal rigidity
  - Possible mild focal neurological deficits
- Grade IV: moderate-to-severe bleed
  - Very decreased level of consciousness, stupor
  - Possible moderate-to-severe hemiparesis
  - Possible early posturing (decorticate or decerebrate)
- Grade V: severe bleed
  - Profound coma
  - Posturing
  - Moribund appearance

*NOTE: Early management of subarachnoid hemorrhage also includes aggressive treatment to prevent or combat vasospasm. Therefore this care plan addresses the simultaneous management of subarachnoid hemorrhage and vasospasm.

ALTERED CEREBRAL TISSUE PERFUSION RELATED TO VASOSPASM SECONDARY TO SUBARACHNOID HEMORRHAGE AFTER RUPTURED INTRACRANIAL ANEURYSM OR ARTERIOVENOUS MALFORMATION—cont'd

- Pathologic reflexes resulting from meningeal irritation
  - Kernig's sign: resistance to full extension of the leg at the knee when the hip is flexed
  - Brudzinski's sign: flexion of the hip and knee during passive neck flexion
- Photophobia
- Nausea and vomiting

Vasospasm related to subarachnoid hemorrhage

- Worsening headache
- Confusion and decreasing level of consciousness
- Focal motor deficits, such as unilateral weakness of extremities, face
- Speech deficits, such as slurring, receptive or expressive aphasia
- Increasing BP, respiratory changes
- Homonymous hemianopsia

OUTCOME CRITERIA

- Patient is oriented to time, place, person, and situation.
- Pupils are equal and normoreactive.
- BP is within patient's norm.
- Motor function is bilaterally equal.
- Headache, nausea, and vomiting are absent.
- Patient has no clinical manifestations of increased ICP and herniation as evidenced by ICP 0-15 mm Hg and by above criteria.
- Patient verbalizes importance of and displays compliance with reduced activity.

NURSING INTERVENTIONS AND *RATIONALE*

1. Continue to monitor the assessment parameters listed under "Defining Characteristics." In addition, assess for indicators of increased ICP and brain herniation (see care plan, "Altered Cerebral Perfusion related to increased ICP"). ***ICP will increase during vasospasm only when caused by the edema resulting from brain ischemia or infarction.***
2. Anticipate early surgical intervention for patients with grade I, II, or III symptoms.
3. Maintain patent airway and adequate ventilation, and supply oxygen as ordered ***to prevent hypoxemia and hypercarbia.***
4. Monitor ABG values, and maintain $Pao_2 > 80$ mm Hg and $Paco_2 < 45$ mm Hg.
5. If hypertensive-hypervolemic therapy is prescribed, administer crystalloid, colloid, and plasma volume expander IV fluids and monitor pulmonary capillary wedge pressure (PCWP), pulmonary artery diastolic (PAD) pressure, systemic vascular resistance (SVR), and BP to achieve and maintain prescribed parameters preoperatively. Systolic blood pressure is usually maintained at 150-160 mm Hg.
6. Monitor lung sounds and chest x-ray reports ***because of the risk of pulmonary edema associated with fluid overload.***
7. Anticipate administration of calcium channel blockers such as nimodipine ***to decrease peripheral vascular resistance and cause vasodilation.***
8. For patients in severe vasospasm, anticipate barbiturate administration ***to decrease cerebral metabolic rate.***
9. Keep head of bed flat ***to optimize cerebral perfusion.***
10. Rebleeding is a potential complication of aneurysm rupture; to PREVENT REBLEEDING, the following interventions constitute subarachnoid precautions:
    - Ensure bed rest in a quiet environment ***to lessen external stimuli.***
    - Maintain darkened room ***to lessen symptoms of photophobia.***
    - Restrict visitors, and instruct them to keep conversation as nonstressful as possible.
    - Administer prescribed sedatives as needed ***to reduce anxiety and promote rest.***
    - Administer analgesics as prescribed ***to relieve or lessen headache.***
    - Provide a soft, high-fiber diet and stool softeners ***to prevent constipation, which can lead to straining and increased risk of rebleeding.***
    - Assist with activities of daily living (feeding, bathing, dressing, toileting).
    - Avoid any activity that could lead to increased ICP;
      ensure that the patient does not flex the hips beyond 90 degrees and avoids neck hyperflexion, hyperextension, or lateral hyperrotation ***that could impede jugular venous return.***

ALTERED CEREBRAL TISSUE PERFUSION RELATED TO INCREASED INTRACRANIAL PRESSURE SECONDARY TO BRAIN TRAUMA, HEMORRHAGE, EDEMA, INFECTION, TUMOR, STROKE, HYDROCEPHALUS

DEFINING CHARACTERISTICS

- ICP >15 mm Hg, sustained for 15-30 minutes
- Headache
- Vomiting, with or without nausea
- Seizures
- Decrease in Glasgow Coma Scale of two or more points from baseline
- Alteration in level of consciousness, ranging from restlessness to coma
- Change in orientation: disoriented to time and/or place and/or person
- Difficulty or inability to follow simple commands
- Increasing systolic BP of more than 20 mm Hg with widening pulse pressure
- Bradycardia
- Irregular respiratory pattern (e.g., Cheyne-Stokes, central neurogenic hyperventilation, ataxic, apneustic)
- Change in response to painful stimuli (e.g., purposeful to inappropriate or absent response)
- Signs of impending brain herniation, which, in addition to the above, may include the following:
  - Hemiparesis or hemiplegia
  - Hemisensory changes
  - Unequal pupil size (1 mm or more difference)
  - Failure of pupil to react to light
  - Dysconjugate gaze and inability to move one eye beyond midline if third, fourth, or sixth cranial nerves involved
  - Loss of oculocephalic or oculovestibular reflexes
  - Possible decorticate or decerebrate posturing

OUTCOME CRITERIA

- ICP is ≤15 mm Hg.
- CPP is >60 mm Hg.
- Clinical signs of increased ICP as described above are absent

NURSING INTERVENTIONS AND *RATIONALE*

1. Continue to monitor the assessment parameters listed under "Defining Characteristics."
2. Maintain adequate CPP.
   a. With physician's collaboration, maintain BP within patient's norm by administering volume expanders, vasopressors, or antihypertensives.
   b. Reduce ICP.
      - Elevate head of bed 30 to 45 degrees ***to facilitate venous return.***
      - Maintain head and neck in neutral plane (avoid flexion, extension, or lateral rotation) ***to enhance venous drainage from the head.***
      - Avoid extreme hip flexion.
      - With physician's collaboration, administer steroids, osmotic agents, and diuretics.
      - Drain CSF according to protocol if ventriculostomy in place.
      - Assist patient to turn and move self in bed (instruct patient to exhale while turning or pushing up in bed) ***to avoid isometric contractions and Valsalva maneuver.***
      - Avoid use of footboards if patient posturing; apply high-top tennis shoes instead: on 2 hours, off 2 hours.[2]
3. Maintain patent airway and adequate ventilation, and supply oxygen ***to prevent hypoxemia and hypercarbia.***
4. Monitor arterial blood gas (ABG) values, and maintain Pa_{O_2} >80 mm Hg, Pa_{CO_2} at 25-35 mm Hg, and pH at 7.35-7.45.
5. Avoid suctioning beyond 10 seconds at a time; hyperoxygenate and hyperventilate before and after suctioning.
6. Plan patient care activities and nursing interventions around the patient's ICP response. Avoid unnecessary additional disturbances, and allow patient up to 1 hour of rest between activities as frequently as possible. ***Studies have shown the direct correlation between nursing care activities and increases in ICP.***[3,4]
7. Maintain normothermia with antipyretic medications and external cooling or heating measures as necessary. Wrap hands, feet, and male genitalia in soft towels before cooling measures ***to prevent shivering and frostbite.***
8. With physician's collaboration, control seizures with prophylactic and as necessary (PRN) anticonvulsants. ***Seizures can greatly increase the cerebral metabolic rate.***
9. With physician's collaboration, administer sedatives, barbiturates, or paralyzing agents ***to reduce cerebral metabolic rate.***
10. Counsel family members to maintain calm atmosphere and to avoid disturbing conversation (e.g., condition, pain, prognosis, family crisis, financial difficulties).
11. If signs of impending brain herniation are present, do the following:
    - Notify physician at once.
    - Be sure head of bed is elevated 45 degrees and patient's head is in neutral plane.
    - Slow mainline intravenous (IV) infusion to keep-open rate.
    - If ventriculostomy catheter in place, drain CSF as ordered.
    - Prepare to administer osmotic agents and/or diuretics.
    - Prepare patient for emergency computed tomographic (CT) head scan and/or emergency surgery.

HYPERTHERMIA RELATED TO PHARMACOGENIC HYPERMETABOLISM (MALIGNANT HYPERTHERMIA)

DEFINING CHARACTERISTICS

Early signs

- BP >140/90
- Profuse diaphoresis
- Pulse rate >100
- Masseter and general skeletal muscle rigidity and fasciculations
- Tachypnea
- Decreased level of consciousness

Late signs

- Increasing core body temperature up to 42°-43° C (107.6°-109.4° F)
- Hot skin
- High-output left ventricular failure
  - Systemic blood pressure <90
  - Pulse rate >100 and ventricular dysrhythmias
  - Cardiac index >4.0 L/min/m²
  - PCWP and PAD >15 mm Hg; possible pulmonary edema
- Continued skeletal muscle rigidity and fasciculations
- Pao_2 <80 mm Hg
- Respiratory and metabolic acidosis
- Fixed, dilated pupils
- Seizures/coma/decerebrate posturing
- Urinary output <30 ml/hr; reddish-brown (myoglobinuria)
- Prolonged bleeding (DIC)

OUTCOME CRITERIA

- Core body temperature is below 38.3° C (101° F).
- Muscle rigidity and fasciculations are absent.
- Patient is alert and oriented.
- Pupils are normoreactive.

NURSING INTERVENTIONS AND *RATIONALE*

1. Continue to monitor assessment parameters listed under "Defining Characteristics."
2. Rapidly decrease metabolism.
   - It is recommended that health care institutions have an emergency malignant hyperthermia kit available that contains the items indicated below.
   - Administer dantrolene (Dantrium), ***which relaxes skeletal muscles by reducing the release of calcium from the sarcoplasmic reticulum.***
   - Observe for infiltration into surrounding tissues. ***Dantrolene is very alkaline and irritating to tissues.***
3. Initiate cooling measures.
   - Administer cold IV solutions (IV bag has been soaked in ice bath before administration).
   - Provide cool water sponge bath.
   - Apply cooling blanket until temperature within 1° to 3° F of desired level ***to avoid "overshoot" in which excessive cooling lowers the body temperature below the desired range.***
   - Institute iced saline solution lavages of stomach, rectum, and bladder.
   - Monitor core temperature continuously ***to avoid overcooling.***
4. Reverse metabolic and respiratory acidosis.
   - With physician's collaboration, administer sodium bicarbonate as necessary ***to treat metabolic acidosis.***
   - Initially hyperventilate patient with 100% oxygen; then ventilate with 15-20 ml/kg tidal volume at 15-20 breaths/min.
   - Assess ABG values frequently, and make ventilatory adjustments as necessary ***to remedy hypoxemia and hypercarbia.***
5. Provide adequate nutrients to the tissues, and correct electrolyte imbalances.
   - With physician's collaboration, administer 50% dextrose and regular insulin ***to increase glucose uptake into liver to meet hypermetabolic needs of body and enhance the movement of potassium from extracellular fluid back into the cells.***
   - Monitor serum electrolytes ***to assess efficacy of above action.***
   - Monitor blood urea nitrogen (BUN) and creatinine levels ***to evaluate for renal failure.***
   - Monitor serum enzyme levels, particularly CPK elevations, ***for indication of degree of muscle hyperactivity.***
6. Correct cardiovascular instability and dysrhythmias.
   - Titrate vasoactive and inotropic drips per protocol to desired systemic blood pressure, PCWP, and/or PAD.
   - Follow critical care emergency standing orders about the administration of antidysrhythmic agents.
7. Maintain a high urinary output (≥50 ml/hour). With physician's collaboration, perform the following:
   - Administer osmotic agents (mannitol) ***for excretion of excess fluid load and to increase urinary output to prevent renal failure.***
   - Administer diuretics (furosemide) ***to enhance secretion of myoglobin, potassium, sodium, and magnesium.***
   - Administer supplemental potassium chloride as indicated by serum potassium levels.
   - Possibly administer steroid (e.g., Solu-Cortef) ***for its mineralocorticoid effect of potassium excretion, to increase glomerular filtration rate, and to reduce cerebral edema.***
8. Correct hematologic abnormalities.
   - With physician's collaboration, administer heparin if DIC suspected.
   - Monitor coagulation studies ***for indications of DIC and for efficacy of heparin therapy.***
   - Assess stool/urinary/nasogastric (NG) drainage for occult blood.
9. Weigh patient daily ***to assist in assessment of hydration status.***

HYPOTHERMIA RELATED TO EXPOSURE TO COLD ENVIRONMENT, ILLNESS, TRAUMA (INCLUDING SPINAL CORD TRAUMA); OR DAMAGE TO THE HYPOTHALAMUS

DEFINING CHARACTERISTICS

- Core body temperature below 35° C (95° F)
- Skin cold to touch
- Slurred speech, incoordination
- At temperature below 33° C (91.4° F):
  - Cardiac dysrhythmias (atrial fibrillation, bradycardia)
  - Cyanosis
  - Respiratory alkalosis
- At temperatures below 32° C (89.6° F):
  - Shivering followed by muscle rigidity
  - Hypotension
  - Dilated pupils
- At temperatures below 28°-29° C (82.4°-84.2° F):
  - Absent deep tendon reflexes
  - Hypoventilation (3 to 4 breaths/min to apnea)
  - Ventricular fibrillation possible
- At temperatures below 26°-27° C (78.8°-80.6° F):
  - Coma
  - Flaccid muscles
  - Fixed, dilated pupils
  - Ventricular fibrillation to cardiac standstill
  - Apnea

OUTCOME CRITERIA

- Core body temperature is greater than 35° C (95° F).
- Patient is alert and oriented.
- Cardiac dysrhythmias are absent.
- Acid-base balance is normal.
- Pupils are normoreactive.

NURSING INTERVENTIONS AND *RATIONALE*

NOTE: Rapid rewarming of a chronically hypothermic patient by active external measures can lead to peripheral vasodilation, resulting in further loss of body temperature, mobilization of blood containing high potassium, low pH, high Pco_2, and low Po_2, profound hypotension, and fatal ventricular fibrillation. Keep in mind that children have been successfully resuscitated after immersion in cold water for 20 to 40 minutes.

1. Continue to monitor the assessment parameters listed under "Defining Characteristics." In addition, continuously monitor core body temperature with a low-reading thermometer.
2. Intubation and mechanical ventilation may be needed. Heated air or oxygen can be added ***to help rewarm the body core.*** Because carbon dioxide production is low, do not hyperventilate the hypothermic patient, ***because this action may induce severe alkalosis and precipitate ventricular fibrillation.***
3. Apply cardiopulmonary resuscitation (CPR) and advanced cardiac life support until core body temperature is up to at least 29.5° C before determining that patient cannot be resuscitated.
4. Monitor ABG values to direct further therapy, and be sure that the pH, Pao_2, $Paco_2$ are corrected for temperature.
5. For abrupt-onset hypothermia (e.g., immersion in cold water, exposure to cold, wet climate, collapse in snow) rewarming can take place rapidly ***because the pathophysiologic changes associated with chronic hypothermia have not had time to evolve.***
   - Institute rapid, active rewarming by immersion in warm water (38°-43° C).
   - Apply thermal blanket on top of patient at 36.6°-37.7° C. Some researchers suggest rewarming only the torso or trunk first, leaving the extremities exposed to room temperature. ***This is to prevent early peripheral vasodilation with abrupt redistribution of intravascular volume. This also prevents colder blood trapped in the extremities from returning to the body core before the heart is rewarmed.***[5]
   - Perform rapid core rewarming with heated (37°-43° C) IV infusion, hemodialysis, peritoneal dialysis, and colonic or gastric irrigation fluids.
6. Electrical defibrillation is usually successful in terminating ventricular fibrillation if the temperature is greater than 28° C.
7. Administer cardiac resuscitation drugs sparingly ***because as the body warms, peripheral vasodilation occurs. Drugs that remain in the periphery are suddenly released, leading to a "bolus effect" that may cause fatal dysrhythmias.***
8. Monitor peripheral circulation ***because gangrene of the fingers and toes is a common complication of accidental hypothermia.***
9. For chronic hypothermia, how aggressive the treatment is depends on the setting, the underlying disease, and the body temperature. Concurrent treatment of the underlying disease processes is indicated.
   - Core temperatures greater than 33° C may be rewarmed either slowly or rapidly.
   - Coma in a patient with a temperature greater than 28° C is probably not caused by hypothermia. Look for other causes, such as hypoglycemia, alcohol, narcotics, and head trauma, and treat accordingly.
   - If patient is hyperglycemic, remember that insulin is ineffective at body temperatures below 30° C.
   - Restore intravascular volume cautiously ***to avoid circulatory overloading of the hypothermic heart and to avoid precipitating pulmonary edema.*** As circulation and a more normal temperature are restored, the patient may require large volumes of crystalloid and colloid fluids ***to refill the dilated vascular bed.***

DYSREFLEXIA RELATED TO EXCESSIVE AUTONOMIC RESPONSE TO CERTAIN NOXIOUS STIMULI (E.G., DISTENDED BLADDER, DISTENDED BOWEL, SKIN IRRITATION) OCCURRING IN PATIENTS WITH CERVICAL OR HIGH THORACIC (T6 OR ABOVE) SPINAL CORD INJURY

DEFINING CHARACTERISTICS

NOTE: Anyone who has had dysreflexia knows how his or her body responds. Listen to the patient.

Major

- ◆ Paroxysmal hypertension (sudden periodic elevated BP greater than 20 mm Hg above patient's normal BP); for many spinal cord injury patients, a normal BP may be only 90/60
- ◆ Bradycardia (most common; pulse rate < 60 beats per minute) or tachycardia (pulse rate > 100 beats per minute)
- ◆ Diaphoresis (above the injury)
- ◆ Facial flushing
- ◆ Pallor (below the injury)
- ◆ Pounding headache (a diffuse pain in different portions of the head and not confined to any nerve distribution area)

Minor

- ◆ Nasal congestion
- ◆ Engorgement of temporal and neck vessels
- ◆ Conjunctival congestion
- ◆ Chills without fever
- ◆ Pilomotor erection (goose bumps) below the injury
- ◆ Blurred vision
- ◆ Chest pain
- ◆ Metallic taste in mouth
- ◆ Horner's syndrome (constriction of the pupil, partial ptosis of the eyelid, enophthalmos, and sometimes loss of sweating over the affected side of the face)

OUTCOME CRITERIA

- ◆ BP has returned to patient's norm.
- ◆ Pulse rate is > 60 or < 100 beats per minute (or within patient's norm).
- ◆ Headache is absent.
- ◆ Nasal stuffiness, sweating, and flushing above level of injury are absent.
- ◆ Chills, goose bumps, and pallor below level of injury are absent.
- ◆ Patient verbalizes causes, prevention, symptoms, and treatment of condition.

NURSING INTERVENTIONS AND *RATIONALE*

1. Continue to monitor the assessment parameters listed under "Defining Characteristics."
2. Place on cardiac monitor, and assess for bradycardia, tachycardia, or other dysrhythmias. ***Disturbances of cardiac rate and rhythm can occur because of autonomic dysfunction associated with dysreflexia.***
3. Do not leave patient alone. One nurse monitors the blood pressure and patient status every 3 to 5 minutes while another provides treatment.
4. Place patient's head of bed to upright position ***to decrease BP and promote cerebral venous return.***
5. Remove any support stockings or abdominal binder ***to reduce venous return.***
6. Investigate for and remove offending cause of dysreflexia.
   a. Bladder
      - ◆ If catheter not in place, immediately catheterize patient.
      - ◆ Lubricate catheter with lidocaine jelly before insertion.
      - ◆ Drain 500 ml of urine, and recheck BP.
      - ◆ If BP still elevated, drain another 500 ml of urine.
      - ◆ If BP declines after the bladder is empty, serial BP should be monitored closely ***because the bladder can go into severe contractions causing hypertension to recur.*** With physician's collaboration, instill 30 ml tetracaine through the catheter ***to decrease the flow of impulses from the bladder.***
      - ◆ If indwelling catheter in place, check for kinks or granular sediment that may indicate occlusion.
      - ◆ If plugged catheter is suspected, irrigate it gently with no more than 30 ml of sterile normal saline solution. If the bladder is in tetany, fluid will go in but will not drain out.
      - ◆ If unable to irrigate catheter, remove it, and prepare to reinsert a new catheter: proceed with its lubrication, drainage, and observation as stated above.
      - ◆ Atropine is sometimes administered ***to relieve bladder tetany.***

   b. Bowel
      - ◆ Using glove lubricated with anesthetic ointment, check rectum for fecal impaction.
      - ◆ If impaction is felt, ***to decrease flow of impulses from bowel,*** insert anesthetic ointment into rectum 10 minutes before manual removal of impaction.
      - ◆ A low, hypertonic enema or a suppository may be given ***to assist bowel evacuation.***

   c. Skin
      - ◆ Loosen clothing or bed linens as indicated.
      - ◆ Inspect skin for pimples, boils, pressure sores, and ingrown toenails and treat as indicated.
7. If symptoms of dysreflexia do not subside, have available the IV solutions and antihypertensive drugs of the physician's choosing (e.g., hydralazine, nifedipine, phentolamine, diazoxide, sodium nitroprusside). Administer medications and monitor their effectiveness. Assess BP, pulse, and subjective and objective signs and symptoms.
8. Instruct patient about causes, symptoms, treatment, and prevention of dysreflexia.
9. Encourage patient to carry medical bracelet or informational card to present to medical personnel in the event dysreflexia may be developing.

UNILATERAL NEGLECT RELATED TO PERCEPTUAL DISRUPTION SECONDARY TO STROKE INVOLVING THE RIGHT CEREBRAL HEMISPHERE

DEFINING CHARACTERISTICS

Major (must be present)

- Neglect of involved body parts and/or extrapersonal space
- Denial of the existence of the affected limb or side of body

Minor (may be present)

- Denial of hemiplegia or other motor and sensory deficits
- Left homonymous hemianopia
- Difficulty with spatial-perceptual tasks
- Left hemiplegia

OUTCOME CRITERIA

- Patient is safe and free from injury.
- Patient is able to identify safety hazards in the environment.
- Patient recognizes disability and describes physical deficits present (e.g., paralysis, weakness, numbness).
- Patient demonstrates ability to scan the visual field to compensate for loss of function or sensation in affected limb(s).

NURSING INTERVENTIONS AND *RATIONALE*

1. Continue to monitor the assessment parameters listed under "Defining Characteristics."
2. Maintain patient safety: ***because of the patient's usually brief stay within the critical care unit, the emphasis is placed on patient safety. Therefore the environment is adapted to the patient's deficit.***
   - Position the patient's bed with the unaffected side facing the door.
   - Approach and speak to the patient from the unaffected side. If the patient must be approached from the affected side, announce your presence as soon as entering the room ***to avoid startling the patient.***[6]
   - Position the call light, bedside stand, and personal items on the patient's unaffected side.
   - If the patient will be assisted out of bed, simplify the environment ***to eliminate hazards*** by removing unnecessary furniture and equipment.
   - Provide frequent reorientation of the patient to the environment.
   - Observe the patient closely, and anticipate his or her needs. In spite of repeated explanations, the patient may have difficulty retaining information about the deficits.
   - When patient is in bed, elevate his or her affected arm on a pillow ***to prevent dependent edema and support the hand in a position of function.***
3. Assist the patient to recognize the perceptual defect.
   - Encourage the patient to wear any prescription corrective glasses or hearing aids ***to facilitate communication.***
   - Instruct the patient to turn the head past midline to view the environment on the affected side.
   - Encourage the patient to look at the affected side and to stroke the limbs with the unaffected hand. Encourage handling of the affected limbs ***to reinforce awareness of the affected side.***
   - Instruct the patient to always look for the affected extremity or extremities when performing simple tasks ***to know where it is at all times.***
   - After pointing to them, have the patient name the affected parts.
   - Encourage the patient to use self-exercises (e.g., lifting the affected arm with the unaffected hand).
   - If the patient is unable to discriminate between the concepts of "right" and "left," use descriptive adjectives, such as "the weak arm," "the affected leg," or "the good arm" to refer to the body. Use gestures, not just words, to indicate right and left.

UNILATERAL NEGLECT RELATED TO PERCEPTUAL DISRUPTION SECONDARY TO STROKE INVOLVING THE RIGHT CEREBRAL HEMISPHERE—cont'd

4. Collaborate with the patient, physician, and rehabilitation team to design and implement a beginning rehabilitation program for use during critical care unit stay.

- ◆ Use adaptive equipment (braces, splints, slings) as appropriate.
- ◆ Teach the patient the individual components of any activity separately, then proceed to integrate the component parts into a completed activity.[7]
- ◆ Instruct the patient to attend to the affected side, if able, and to assist with the bath or other tasks.
- ◆ Use tactile stimulation ***to reintroduce the arm or leg to the patient.*** Rub the affected parts with different textured materials ***to stimulate sensations (warm, cold, rough, soft).***[8]
- ◆ Encourage activities that require the patient to turn the head toward the affected side, and retrain the patient to scan the affected side and environment visually.
- ◆ If patient is allowed out of bed, cue him or her with reminders to scan visually when ambulating. Assist and remain in constant attendance ***because the patient may have difficulty maintaining correct posture, balance, and locomotion.*** There may be vertical-horizontal perceptual problems, with the patient leaning to the affected side to align with the perceived vertical. Provide sitting, standing, and balancing exercises before getting the patient out of bed.
- ◆ Feeding: see "High Risk for Aspiration risk factors: impaired swallowing"
  - a. Avoid giving patient any very hot food items that could cause injury.
  - b. Place the patient in an upright sitting position if possible.
  - c. Encourage the patient to feed himself or herself; if necessary, guide the patient's hand to the mouth.
  - d. If the patient is able to feed himself or herself, place one dish at a time in front of the patient. When the patient is finished with the first, add another dish. Tell the patient what he or she is eating.[6]
  - e. Initially place food in the patient's visual field; then gradually move the food out of the field of vision and teach the patient to scan the entire visual field.[8]
  - f. When the patient has learned to visually scan the environment, offer a tray of food with various dishes.
  - g. Instruct the patient to take small bites of food and to place the food in the unaffected side of the mouth.
  - h. ***To eliminate retained food in the affected side of the mouth,*** teach the patient to sweep out these pockets of food with the tongue after every bite.[6]
  - i. After meals or oral medications, check the patient's oral cavity for pockets of retained material.

5. Initiate patient and family health teaching.

- ◆ Assess to ensure that both the patient and the family understand the nature of the neurologic deficits and the purpose of the rehabilitation plan.
- ◆ Teach the proper application and use of any adaptive equipment.
- ◆ Teach the importance of maintaining a safe environment, and point out potential environmental hazards.
- ◆ Instruct family members how to facilitate relearning techniques (e.g., cueing, scanning visual fields).

ACUTE PAIN RELATED TO TRANSMISSION AND PERCEPTION OF CUTANEOUS, VISCERAL, MUSCULAR, OR ISCHEMIC IMPULSES SECONDARY TO (SPECIFY)

DEFINING CHARACTERISTICS

Subjective

- ◆ Patient verbalizes presence of pain
- ◆ Patient rates pain on scale of 1 to 10

Objective

- ◆ Increase in BP, pulse, and respirations
- ◆ Pupillary dilation
- ◆ Diaphoresis, pallor
- ◆ Skeletal muscle reactions (grimacing, clenching fists, writhing, pacing, guarding or splinting affected part)
- ◆ Apprehensive, fearful appearance

OUTCOME CRITERIA

NOTE: Outcome is highly variable, depending on individual patient and pain circumstance factors.

- ◆ Patient verbalizes that pain is reduced to a tolerable level or is removed.
- ◆ Patient's pain rating on scale of 1 to 10 is lower.
- ◆ BP, heart rate, and respiratory rate return to baseline 5 minutes after administration of IV narcotic or 20 minutes after administration of intramuscular (IM) narcotic.

NURSING INTERVENTIONS AND *RATIONALE*

1. Continue to monitor the assessment parameters listed under "Defining Characteristics." In addition, monitor postural vital sign changes; determine hydration status and manage fluid volume deficit, if indicated, before administering narcotic analgesic.
2. Modify variables that heighten the patient's experience of pain.
   - ◆ Explain to the patient that frequent, detailed, and seemingly repetitive assessments will be conducted ***to allow the nurse to better understand the patient's pain experience, not because the existence of pain is in question.***
   - ◆ Explain the factors responsible for pain production in the individual. Estimate the expected duration of the pain if possible.
   - ◆ Explain diagnostic and therapeutic procedures to the patient in relation to sensations the patient should expect to feel.
   - ◆ Reduce the patient's fear of addiction by explaining the difference between drug tolerance and drug addiction. Drug tolerance is a physiologic phenomenon in which a drug dose begins to lose effectiveness after repeated doses; drug dependence is a psychologic phenomenon in which narcotics are used regularly for emotional, not medical, reasons.
   - ◆ Instruct patient to ask for pain medication when pain is beginning and not to wait until it is intolerable.
   - ◆ Explain that the physician will be consulted if pain relief is inadequate with the present medication.
   - ◆ Instruct patient in the importance of adequate rest, especially when it reduces pain ***to maintain strength and coping abilities and to reduce stress.***
3. Pharmacologic interventions.
   - ◆ For postsurgical or posttraumatic cutaneous, muscular, or visceral pain, perform the following:
     a. Medicate with narcotic maximally to break the pain cycle as long as level of consciousness and vital signs are stable: check patient's previous response to similar dosage and narcotic.

     NOTE: First dose received postoperatively is usually reduced by one half ***to evaluate patient's individual response to medication.***

     b. Continuous pain requires continuous analgesia.
        (1) Establish optimal analgesic dose that brings optimal pain relief.
        (2) Offer pain medication at prescribed regular intervals rather than making patient ask for it ***to maintain more steady blood levels.***

     c. If administering medication on prn basis, give it when patient's pain is just beginning, rather than at its peak. Advise patient to intercept pain, not endure it, or it may take several hours and higher doses of narcotics to relieve pain, leading to a cycle of undermedication and pain alternating with overmedication and drug toxicity.

     d. Perform rehabilitation exercises (turn, deep breathe, leg exercises, ambulate) shortly before peak of drug effect ***because this will be the optimal time for the patient to increase activity with the least risk of increasing pain.***

     e. When making the transition from one drug to another or from IM or IV to PO medications, the use of an equianalgesic chart, Table 30-1 is helpful. Equianalgesic means *approximately* the same pain relief. All IM and PO doses listed on Table 30-1 are considered equivalent and are compared with the analgesic standard, Morphine 10 mg IM. Many consider the IM and IV dose of medications equianalgesic; however, others recommend using one-half the IM dose for the IV dose. To effectively use analgesics, each patient requires an individualized choice of drug, dose, time interval, and route. Close monitoring of the patient's response is needed to determine if the right analgesic choice was made.[9,10]

     f. To assess effectiveness of pain medication, do the following:
        (1) Reevaluate pain 5 minutes after IV and 20 minutes after IM medication administration, observe patient's behavior, and ask patient to rate pain on scale of 1 to 10.

ACUTE PAIN RELATED TO TRANSMISSION AND PERCEPTION OF CUTANEOUS, VISCERAL, MUSCULAR, OR ISCHEMIC IMPULSES SECONDARY TO (SPECIFY)—cont'd

(2) Collaborate with physician to add or delete other medications that potentiate the action of analgesics, such as antiemetics, hypnotics, sedatives, or muscle relaxants.
(3) Observe for indicators of undertreatment: report of pain not relieved; observed restlessness, sleeplessness, irritability, and anorexia; decreased activity level.
(4) Observe for indicators of overtreatment: hypotension or bradycardia; respiratory rate < 10/min, excessive sedation.

g. If IV patient-controlled analgesia (PCA) is used, perform the following:

(NOTE: Patient-controlled analgesia allows patients to administer small doses of their prescribed medication when they feel the need. Constant levels of the drug in the bloodstream mean lower doses can be used to obtain analgesia. Pain control is improved because the patient is in control and experiences less fear of unrelieved pain. Reduced net narcotic use is noted, as is less sedation. Critical care patients appropriate for patient-controlled analgesia are those who are alert, such as burn patients, trauma patients without head injury, and some postoperative patients.)

(1) Instruct the patient on what the drug is, the dose, and how often it can be self-administered by pushing the button to activate the PCA machine. For example, "When you have pain, instead of asking the nurse to bring medication, push the button that activates the machine and a small dose of the pain medicine will be injected into your IV line. You can keep your pain under control by administering additional medicine as soon as your pain begins to return or increases. Also, push the button before undertaking a painful activity, such as ambulation. Try to balance your pain relief against sleepiness, and don't activate the machine if you start to feel sleepy. If your pain medicine seems to stop working despite pushing the button several times, call the nurse to check your IV. If you are not receiving adequate pain relief, the nurse will call your doctor."[9,11]
(2) Monitor vital signs, especially BP and respiratory rate, every hour for the first 4 hours, and assess postural heart rate and BP before initial ambulation.
(3) Monitor respirations every 2 hours while patient is on patient-controlled analgesia.
(4) If patient's respirations decrease to < 10/min or if patient is overly sedated, anticipate IV administration of naloxone.

h. If epidural narcotic analgesia is used, do the following:

(NOTE: The delivery of narcotics, such as morphine or fentanyl, by epidural route to specific receptors in the spinal cord selectively blocks pain impulses to the brain for up to 24 hours. Effective analgesia can be obtained without many of the negative side effects or serum narcotic concentrations. Critical care patients appropriate for epidural analgesia include postsurgical and trauma patients.)

(1) Keep patient's head elevated 30 to 45 degrees after injection ***to prevent respiratory depressant effects.***
(2) Observe closely for respiratory depression up to 24 hours after injection. Monitor respiratory rate every 15 minutes for 1 hour; every 30 minutes for 7 hours; and every 1 hour for the remaining 16 hours.
(3) Assess for adequate cough reflex.
(4) Avoid use of other CNS depressants, such as sedatives.
(5) Observe for reports of pruritus, nausea, or vomiting.
(6) Anticipate administration of naloxone for respiratory depression (and smaller doses of naloxone for pruritus).
(7) Assess for and treat urinary retention.
(8) Assess epidural catheter site for local infection. Keep catheter taped securely ***to prevent catheter migration.***

◆ For peripheral vascular ischemic pain (hypothetical vascular occlusion of leg), do the following:

a. Correctly identify and differentiate ischemic pain from other types of pain.
NOTE: Ischemic pain is usually a burning, aching pain made worse by exercise and lessened or relieved by rest. Eventually the pain occurs at rest. Coldness and pallor of extremity may be noted, especially if the limb is elevated above the heart level. Rubor and mottling of the skin may be evident from prolonged tissue anoxia and inability of damaged vessels to constrict. Eventually cyanosis and gangrenous tissue will be evident. Chronic ischemia leads to trophic changes in the limb, such as flaking skin, brittle nails, hair loss, leg ulcers, and cellulitis.
b. Administer pain medications and evaluate their effectiveness as previously described. Remember that the pain of ischemia is chronic and continuous and can make the patient irritable and depressed.
c. Treat the cause of the ischemic pain, and institute measures to increase circulation to the affected part (see nursing management plans, pp. 363 and 364).

Continued.

ACUTE PAIN RELATED TO TRANSMISSION AND PERCEPTION OF CUTANEOUS, VISCERAL, MUSCULAR, OR ISCHEMIC IMPULSES SECONDARY TO (SPECIFY)—cont'd

4. Nonpharmacologic interventions.
   ◆ Treat contributing factors (see "Theoretic Basis and Management"); provide explanations (see intervention number 2 at beginning of this care plan).
   ◆ Apply comfort measures, using gate control theory.
   a. See Appendix D for methods of therapeutic touch.
   b. Use relaxation techniques, such as back rubs, massage, warm baths. Use blankets and pillows ***to support the painful part and reduce muscle tension.*** Encourage slow, rhythmic breathing.
   c. Encourage progressive muscle relaxation techniques.
      (1) Instruct patient to inhale and tense (tighten) specific muscle groups, then relax the muscles as exhalation occurs.
      (2) Suggest an order for performing the tension-relaxation cycle (e.g., start with facial muscles and move down body, ending with toes).
   d. Encourage guided imagery.
      (1) Ask patient to recall an experienced image that is very pleasurable and relaxing and involves at least two senses.
      (2) Have patient begin with rhythmic breathing and progressive relaxation, then travel mentally to the scene.
      (3) Have the patient slowly experience the scene—how it looks, sounds, smells, feels.
      (4) Ask patient to practice this imagery in private.
      (5) Instruct the patient to end the imagery by counting to three and saying, "Now I'm relaxed." If person does not end the imagery and falls asleep, the purpose of the technique is defeated.
   e. If TENS unit is prescribed by physician, do the following:
      (NOTE: TENS is a battery-operated unit that serves as a nerve stimulator. It produces mild, tingling sensations as it blocks incisional pain messages to the brain. It is sometimes used as part of the pain relief program for the postsurgical patient.)
      (1) Take the TENS unit, patient pamphlet, and teaching electrodes to the patient before surgery to explain the process.
      (2) Apply electrodes to skin, and instruct patient in proper use of unit. Let patient experience how the TENS unit should feel when activated. Refer to manufacturer's directions for proper application and operation of TENS unit.
      (3) Electrodes are usually placed by the physician on the skin alongside the operative incision at the close of the surgical procedure in the operating room. The unit is usually used for 3 to 5 days as an adjunct to medications.
      (4) When the patient is awake and alert, readjust the amplitude or output of the TENS unit to the patient's comfort as necessary. Keep the TENS unit on continuously unless ordered otherwise. Occasionally, percutaneous epidural nerve stimulation is used when more than one nerve root is involved in producing pain. Again, patients are able to control their pain by adjusting the rate and frequency of a millivoltage electrical current stimulator affixed externally.
   f. Assist with biofeedback, which represents a wide range of behavioral techniques that provide the patient with information about changes in body functions of which the person is usually unaware. For example, information used to reduce muscle contraction is obtained by an electromyogram recorded from body surface electrodes. Changes in blood flow are produced by monitoring skin temperature changes. The person using biofeedback tries to change the display of information in the desired direction by actions such as reducing muscle tension or reducing or altering blood flow to a particular area. The critical care nurse should be familiar with the theoretic concepts of biofeedback and should support the patient in maximizing pain control through whatever techniques are successful for that patient.

Table 30-1 Equianalgesic Chart: Approximate Equivalent Doses of IM and PO Analgesics for Moderate and Severe Pain*

Analgesic	IM Route (mg)†	PO Route (mg)‡	Comments
Morphine	10	60 (30)§	Both IM and PO doses of morphine have a duration of action of about 4 to 6 hr. Sustained-release tablets, rectal suppositories, and preservative-free for spinal analgesia are also available. The PO dose is 3 to 6 times the IM dose. The lower PO dose is suggested by several clinicians (Lipman, 1980, 1982; Walsh, 1984) and is based on anecdotal evidence, not experimental research (Kaiko, 1986); it may be appropriate for some patients, especially elderly patients with chronic cancer pain. *All IM and PO doses in this chart are considered equivalent to 10 mg of IM morphine in analgesic effect*
Buprenorphine (*Buprenex*)	0.4 (0.3)	—	A narcotic agonist-antagonist that may precipitate withdrawal in patients *very* physically dependent on narcotics. Dose for the sublingual form (not available in the US) is 0.8 mg. Compared with morphine, this drug is longer acting and more likely to produce nausea and vomiting (Bradley, 1984). Respiratory depression is rare but serious because it is not readily reversed by naloxone ("Buprenorphine," 1986). Not available in Canada.
Butorphanol (*Stadol*)	2	—	A narcotic agonist-antagonist that may produce withdrawal in patients physically dependent on narcotics. May also produce psychotomimetic effects such as hallucinations. Not available in Canada.

Continued.

*The equianalgesic doses in this chart are based primarily on recommendations of the Analgesic Study Section, Sloan-Kettering Institute for Cancer Research, New York, based on double-blind analgesic research (Houde, 1979). This format is adapted from McCaffery, M: A practical, portable chart of equianalgesic doses, *Nursing* 17:56-57, Aug 1987.

†Based on clinical experience, many consider the IM and IV dose equianalgesic (Portenoy, 1987). However, some recommend using ½ the IM dose for the IV dose (American Pain Society, 1987).

‡Initial PO doses are usually lower than those listed here, especially for mild to moderate pain.

§Values in parentheses refer to differences of opinion among clinicians.

A guide to using the equianalgesic chart

- Equianalgesic means **approximately** the same pain relief. Onset, peak effect, and duration of analgesia of each drug often differ and may also vary with individual people.
- Variability among individuals may be due to differences in absorption, organ dysfunction, or tolerance to one narcotic and not to another.
- An equianalgesic chart is a *guideline*. The individual patient's response must be observed. Doses and intervals between doses are then titrated according to the individual's response.
- An equianalgesic chart is helpful when (1) switching from one drug to another or (2) switching from one route of administration to another.
- Dosages in this chart are *not* necessarily starting doses. They suggest the *ratio* for comparing the analgesia of one drug with another.
- Based on clinical experience, the IV dose is approximately the same as the IM dose. Dose adjustments are then made according to the individual's response. Some clinicians suggest approximately ½ the IM dose equals the IV dose.

Table references

American Pain Society: *Principles of analgesic use in the treatment of acute pain and chronic cancer pain: a concise guide to medical practice,* Washington, DC, 1987, The Society.
Beaver, W: Management of cancer pain with parenteral medication, *JAMA* 244:2653-2657, Dec 12, 1980.
Beaver, W, and Feise, G: A comparison of analgesic effect of oxymorphone by rectal suppository and intramuscular injection in patients with postoperative pain, *J Clin Pharmacol* 17:276-291, May/June 1977.
Bradley, J: A comparison of morphine and buprenorphine for analgesia after abdominal surgery, *Anaesth Intens Care* 12:303-310, Nov 1984
Buprenorphine, *Med Lett Drugs Ther* 28:56, May 23, 1986.
Houde, RW: Systemic analgesics and related drugs: narcotic analgesics. In Bonica, JJ, and Ventafridda, V, eds: *Advances in pain research and therapy*, vol 2, pp 263-273, New York, 1979, Raven Press.
Jaffe, J, and Martin, W: Opioid analgesics and antagonists. In Gilman, A, et al, eds: *The pharmacological basis of therapeutics*, ed 7, pp 491-531, New York, 1985, Macmillan Publishing.
Kaiko, R: Controversy in the management of chronic cancer pain: therapeutic equivalents of I.M. and P.O. morphine, *J Pain Sympt Manag* 1:42-45, Winter 1986.
Kaiko, R, et al: Central nervous system excitatory effects of meperidine in cancer patients, *Ann Neurol* 13:180-185, Feb 1983.
Kantor, T, et al: Adverse effects of commonly ordered oral narcotics, *J Clin Pharmacol* 21:1-8, Jan 1981.
Lipman, A: Comment on pain cocktail article, *Drug Intell Clin Pharm* 16:332, Apr 1982.
Lipman, A: Drug therapy in cancer pain, *Cancer Nursing* 3:39-46, Feb 1980.
McGee, J, and Alexander, M: Phenothiazine analgesia—fact or fantasy? *Am J Hosp Pharm* 36:633-640, May 1979.
Narcotic agonists and analgesics. In *Facts and comparisons: drug information*, 242b, Philadelphia, 1986, JB Lippincott.
Portenoy, RK: Continuous intravenous infusion of opioid drugs, *Med Clin North Am* 71:233-241, Mar 1987.
Romagnoli, A, and Keats, A: Ceiling effect for respiratory depression by nalbuphine, *Clin Pharmacol Ther* 27:478-485, Apr 1980.
Vernier, V, and Schmidt, W: The preclinical pharmacology of nalbuphine. In Gomez Q, ed: *Nalbuphine as a component of surgical anesthesia*, pp 1-9, Princeton, NJ, 1985, Excerpta Medica.
Walsh, T: Oral morphine in chronic cancer pain, *Pain* 18:1-11, Jan 1984.

Table 30-1 Equianalgesic Chart: Approximate Equivalent Doses of IM and PO Analgesics for Moderate and Severe Pain—cont'd

Analgesic	IM Route (mg)	PO Route (mg)	Comments
Codeine	130	200	Relatively more toxic in high doses than morphine, causing more nausea and vomiting and considerable constipation. The PO dose is about 1.5 times the IM dose.
Fentanyl (*Sublimaze*)	0.05	–	Most common use is for anesthesia, given IV. Onset of action when given IM is about 15 min; duration of action, about 90 min. Analgesic effect is not significantly increased by droperidol (Jaffe and Martin, 1985). Has been used as a substitute for high-dose IV morphine in terminally ill patients when morphine caused excitation. Used IV in neonates and for brief procedures.
Hydromorphone (*Dilaudid*)	1.5	7.5	Somewhat shorter acting than morphine. Also available as rectal suppository and in high-potency injectable form (10 mg/ml). The PO dose is 5 times the IM dose.
Levorphanol (*Levo-Dromoran*)	2	4	Longer acting than morphine when given in repeated, regular doses. Useful alternative to PO methadone. Careful titration required because drug accumulates; both dose and interval must be adjusted. Onset of action with PO dose occurs within 1½ hr. Because drug accumulates, analgesic effect may increase with repeated doses. *Initial* PO dose is twice the injectable dose. (The SC route is recommended over the IM route.)
Meperidine (*Demerol*)	75	300	Shorter acting (2 to 4 hr) than morphine. Watch for toxic effects on the central nervous system (CNS) caused by accumulation of the active metabolite normeperidine, which produces neuroexcitability. Use with caution in patients with renal disease. *Because of the risk to the CNS, 300 mg PO is not recommended.* Since normeperidine has a long half-life (15 hr or longer), decreasing the dose in patients exhibiting a toxic reaction may increase CNS excitability, causing seizures. Effects of normeperidine are increased (not reversed) by naloxone (Kaiko et al, 1983). The PO dose is 4 times the IM dose.
Methadone (*Dolophine*)	10	20	Longer acting than morphine when given in repeated, regular doses. Careful titration required because drug accumulates; both dose and interval must be adjusted. Onset with PO dose occurs within 1 hr. Because drug accumulates, analgesic effect may increase with repeated doses. *Initial* PO dose is twice the IM dose.
Methotrimeprazine (*Levoprome*)	20	–	A phenothiazine (nonnarcotic) drug. Duration of action is 4 to 5 hr. Common adverse effect is hypotension; not recommended for ambulatory patients (McGee and Alexander, 1979).
Nalbuphine (*Nubain*)	10 (20)	–	A narcotic agonist-antagonist that may produce withdrawal in patients physically dependent on narcotics. Longer acting and less likely to cause hypotension than morphine. In doses above 10 mg/70 kg, it causes no additional respiratory depression (Romagnoli and Keats, 1980; Vernier and Schmidt, 1985), so patient may be started on a high dose.
Opium (*Pantopon*, opium tincture)	20 (13.3)	(6 ml)	Infrequently used. Pantopon is the injectable form; opium tincture, the oral form. Pantopon, 20 mg, equals 10 mg of IM morphine (Beaver, 1980) or 15 mg of IM morphine ("Narcotic Agonists and Analgesics," 1986). Opium tincture contains 1% morphine, that is, 0.6 ml equals 6 mg of PO morphine. Therefore 6 ml equals 60 mg of PO morphine (Jaffe and Martin, 1985).
Oxycodone	–	30 (15)	Has faster onset and higher peak effect than most PO narcotics; duration of action is up to 6 hr. In one study of postoperative pain, a preparation similar to the old formulation of Percodan (containing oxycodone, aspirin, phenacetin, and caffeine) was more effective and caused fewer adverse reactions than 90 mg of PO codeine or 75 mg of PO pentazocine, and was almost equivalent to 12.5 mg of IM morphine (Kantor, et al, 1981).
Oxymorphone (*Numorphan*)	1 (1.5)	–	Also available as rectal suppository; 10 mg given rectally equals 10 mg if IM morphine (Beaver and Feise, 1977). Up to 1.5 mg IM is now recommended as equal to 10 mg of IM morphine (Jaffe and Martin, 1985).
Pentazocine (*Talwin*)	60	180	Narotic agonist-antagonist that may produce withdrawal in patients physically dependent on narcotics. Could produce psychotomimetic effects. The PO dose is 3 times the IM dose.
Propoxyphene HCl (*Darvon*)	–	500	The one recognized use is for mild to moderate pain unrelieved by nonnarcotics. *Never give as much as 500 mg PO*, only low PO doses (65 to 130 mg) are recommended. The IM form is not available in the United States.

IMPAIRED VERBAL COMMUNICATION: APHASIA RELATED TO CEREBRAL SPEECH CENTER INJURY

DEFINING CHARACTERISTICS

Major (must be present)
- Inappropriate or absent speech or responses to questions

Minor (may be present)
- Inability to speak spontaneously
- Inability to understand spoken words
- Inability to follow commands appropriately through gestures
- Difficulty or inability to understand written language
- Difficulty or inability to express ideas in writing
- Difficulty or inability to name objects

OUTCOME CRITERION
- Patient is able to make basic needs known.

NURSING INTERVENTIONS AND *RATIONALE*

1. Continue to monitor the assessment parameters listed under "Defining Characteristics."
2. Obtain a speech pathology evaluation (if available) ***to determine the extent of the patient's communication deficit (e.g., if fluent, nonfluent, or global aphasia is involved).***
3. Have the speech therapist post a list of appropriate ways to communicate with the patient in the patient's room ***so that all nursing personnel can be consistent in their efforts.***
4. Assess the patient's ability to comprehend, speak, read, and write.
   - Ask questions that can be answered with a "yes" or a "no." If a patient answers "yes" to a question, ask the opposite (e.g., "Are you hot?" "Yes." "Are you cold?" "Yes."). ***This may help determine if in fact the patient understands what is being said.***
   - Ask simple, short questions, and use gestures, pantomime, and facial expressions to give the patient additional clues.

   Stand in the patient's line of vision, giving a good view of your face and hands.
   - Have the patient try to write with a pad and pencil. Offer pictures and alphabet letters at which to point.
   - Make flash cards with pictures or words depicting frequently used phrases (e.g., glass of water, bedpan).[8]
5. Maintain an uncluttered environment, and decrease external distractions that could hinder communication.
6. Maintain a relaxed and calm manner, and explain all diagnostic, therapeutic, and comfort measures before initiating them.
7. Do not shout or speak in a loud voice. ***Hearing loss is not a factor in aphasia, and shouting will not help.***
8. Have only one person talk at a time. ***It is more difficult for the patient to follow a multisided conversation.***
9. Use direct eye contact, and speak directly to the patient in unhurried, short phrases.
10. Give one-step commands and directions, and provide cues through pictures or gestures.
11. Try to ask questions that can be answered with a "yes" or a "no," and avoid topics that are controversial, emotional, abstract, or lengthy.
12. Listen to the patient in an unhurried manner, and wait for his or her attempt to communicate.
    - Expect a time lag from when you ask the patient something until the patient responds.
    - Accept the patient's statement of essential words without expecting complete sentences.
    - Avoid finishing the sentence for the patient if possible.
    - Wait approximately 30 seconds before providing the word the patient may be attempting to find (except when the patient is very frustrated and needs something quickly, such as a bedpan).
    - Rephrase the patient's message aloud ***to validate it.***
    - Do not pretend to understand the patient's message if you do not.[6]
13. Encourage the patient to speak slowly in short phrases and to say each word clearly.
14. Ask the patient to write the message, if able, or draw pictures if only verbal communication is affected.
15. Observe the patient's nonverbal clues for validation (e.g., answers "yes" but shakes head "no").
16. When handing an object to the patient, state what it is, ***since hearing language spoken is necessary to stimulate language development.***
17. Explain what has happened to the patient, and offer reassurance about the plan of care.
18. Verbally address the problem of frustration over inability to communicate, and explain that patience is needed for both the nurse and the patient.
19. Maintain a calm, positive manner, and offer reassurance (e.g., "I know this is very hard for you, but it will get better if we work on it together").
20. Talk to the patient as an adult. Be respectful, and avoid talking down to the patient.
21. Do not discuss the patient's condition or hold conversations in the patient's presence without including him or her in the discussion. ***This may be the reason some aphasic patients develop paranoid thoughts.***

Continued.

IMPAIRED VERBAL COMMUNICATION: APHASIA RELATED TO CEREBRAL SPEECH CENTER INJURY—cont'd

22. Do not exhibit disapproval of emotional utterances or spontaneous use of profanity; instead, offer calm, quiet reassurance.

23. If the patient makes an error in speech, do not reprimand or scold but try to compliment the patient by saying, "That was a good try."

24. Delay conversation if the patient is tired. ***The symptoms of aphasia worsen if the patient is fatigued, anxious, or upset.***

25. Be prepared for emotional outbursts and tears in patients who have more difficulty in expressing themselves than with understanding. The patient may become depressed, refuse treatment and food, ignore relatives, and push objects away. Comfort the patient with statements such as, "I know it's frustrating and you feel sad, but you are not alone. Other people who have had strokes have felt the way you do. We will be here to help you get through this."[8,12,13]

SENSORY/PERCEPTUAL ALTERATIONS RELATED TO SENSORY OVERLOAD, SENSORY DEPRIVATION, AND SLEEP PATTERN DISTURBANCE

DEFINING CHARACTERISTICS

- Hallucinations
- Delusions
- Illusions
- Disorientation
- Short-term memory deficits
- Impaired abstraction

OUTCOME CRITERIA

- Patient has no evidence of hallucinations, delusions, or illusions.
- Results of reality testing are appropriate.
- Short-term memory is intact.
- Abstract reasoning is intact.

NURSING INTERVENTIONS AND *RATIONALE*

1. Continue to monitor the assessment parameters listed under "Defining Characteristics." Determine and document the patient's dominant spoken language, his or her literacy, and the language(s) in which he or she is literate. Determine and document his or her premorbid degree of orientation, cognitive capabilities, and any sensory-perceptual deficits. ***It is sometimes the case that people are not literate in their spoken language or, less frequently, that they are literate only in their second language. These situations can result in unfortunate errors in the appraisal of patients' ability to communicate in writing and in estimating the extent of their orientation. Similarly, assuming that the patients were or were not fully oriented before critical care admission bases the nurse's assessment on possibly erroneous assumptions.***

For sensory overload

1. Initiate each nurse-patient encounter by calling the patient by name and identifying yourself by name. ***This fosters reality orientation and assists the patient in filtering irrelevant or impersonal conversation.***
2. Assess the patient's immediate physical environment from his or her viewpoint, and explain equipment, its sounds, and its therapeutic purpose. Demonstrate audible and visual alarms, and explain the possible alarm conditions. ***This decreases alienation of the patient from the technologic environment and reduces the inherent sense of fear and urgency accompanying alarm conditions.***
3. For each procedure performed, provide "preparatory sensory information," i.e., explain procedures in relation to the sensations the patient will experience, including duration of sensations. ***Preparatory sensory information enhances learning and lessens anticipatory anxiety.***
4. Limit noise levels. Certainly, audible alarms cannot and should not be silenced, and many critical, albeit noisy, activities must take place in the critical care area. It has been shown, however, that noise levels produced by clinical personnel exceed those levels designated as "acceptable" and are often greater than those generated by technologic devices. Staff conversations should be kept soft enough that they are inaudible to the patient whenever possible. Critical care personnel should assume that everything said at or around a patient's bedside is intended for that patient's awareness and that it will be interpreted as pertaining to him or her. ***As in the discussion that follows, conversations about the patient but not to him or her foster depersonalization and delusions of reference.***
5. Well-enforced noise limits should exist for nighttime.
6. Readjust alarm limits on physiologic monitoring devices as the patient's condition changes (improves or deteriorates) ***to lessen unnecessary alarm states.***
7. Consider use of head phones and audio cassette with patient's favorite and/or subliminal or classical music. ***This can effectively filter out assaultive noise of the critical care environment and supplant it with familiar, soothing sounds and rhythms.***
8. Modify lighting. Day-night cycles should be simulated with environmental lighting. At no time should overhead fluorescent lights be abruptly turned on without either warning the patient, assisting him or her out of the supine position, and/or shielding his or her eyes with gauze or a face cloth. ***Continuous bright lighting sustains anxiety and promotes circadian rhythm desynchronization.***
9. To the extent possible, shield patients from viewing urgent and emergent events in the critical care unit. ***Resuscitation efforts, albeit difficult to conceal, engender fear in the patient and a sense of instability and vulnerability (e.g., "I'm next").*** When such an event occurs, the nurse should endeavor to elicit the patient's cognitive and emotional reaction; thoughts, impressions, and feelings should be shared and misconceptions clarified. A useful approach for the nurse in this interchange is that of emphasizing the differences between the patient at hand and the one resuscitated (e.g., "He was considerably older," "more unstable," "had serious lung disease").
10. Ensure patients' privacy, their modesty, and, at the very least, their dignity. Physical exposure and nudity, although seeming to pale in importance alongside such priorities as physiologic assessment and stabilization, are primal indignities in all individuals. Patients should be kept minimally exposed. When, in the course of assessment and intervention, it becomes necessary to expose the patient, the nurse should first verbally apologize for this necessity. ***To be naked is to feel vulnerable; to be vulnerable is to feel fearful. In this regard, fear is an emotion concomitant to critical care that is preventable through nursing intervention.***

Continued.

SENSORY/PERCEPTUAL ALTERATIONS RELATED TO SENSORY OVERLOAD, SENSORY DEPRIVATION, AND SLEEP PATTERN DISTURBANCE—cont'd

For sensory deprivation

1. Provide reality orientation in four spheres (person, place, time, and situation) at more frequent intervals than when testing. Convey this information in the context of routine conversation. SAMPLE STATEMENTS: "Mr. Clark, this is Tuesday morning and you're in University Hospital. Your heart surgery was yesterday morning, and you're doing well. My name is Joe, and I'm your nurse today." ***The patient is made to feel patronized by repetitions such as, "Do you know where you are?"*** Given the effects of general anesthesia, narcotic analgesics, sedatives, and sleep, it is fully expected that some degree of disorientation will exist normally.
2. Ensure the patient's visual access to a calendar. (Of interest, the design of most state-of-the-art critical care units now reflects many of the principles of sensory stimulation. One such coronary care unit was designed with a large wall clock facing the patient. A patient who had spent more than a week in this unit later reflected that one of the most "distressing, frustrating" aspects of his stay in the coronary care unit was the monotonous, inescapable attention to the clock and its painfully slow documentation of the passing of time.)
3. Apprise the patient of daily news events and the weather.
4. Touch patients for the express purpose of communicating caring. Hold their hands, stroke their brows, rub the skin on an aspect of their arms. ***Touch is the universal language of caring. In the setting of critical care, in which there is considerable physical body manipulation, it is useful and important to contrast assaultive touch with comforting touch.*** Touch can be used as a technique for distraction from painful stimuli when used in conjunction with uncomfortable procedures. See Appendix D, "Therapeutic Touch." (IMPORTANT: See discussion of the use of touch in "Management of the Patient Experiencing Hallucinations.")
5. Foster liberal visitation by family and significant others. Encourage significant others to touch the patient as consistent with their individual comfort level and cultural norms.
6. Structure and identify opportunities for the patient to exercise decision-making skills, however small. ***Although not so designated, patients with sensory alterations experience a type of "cognitive deprivation" as well.*** (See "Powerlessness," Chapter 47).
7. Assist patients to find meaning in their experiences. Explain the therapeutic purpose of all that they are asked to do for themselves and all that is done with them and for them. Avoid statements such as, "Will you turn to that side for me?" or "I need you to swallow this medication." ***These statements implicitly convey that the maneuver has some value for the nurses versus the patients.*** Similarly, use "thank you" judiciously. ***This simple salutation, when used indiscriminately, suggests something was done to benefit the nurses and not the patients.*** Patients need to find meaning and to identify their roles in the experience of critical illness and critical care. The sensations that constitute this experience and those that do not are made bearable and intelligible when attached to the larger picture of their conditions, treatment, and progress.

For sleep pattern disturbances. For excellent management strategies of sleep pattern disturbance, refer to Chapter 12, Sleep nursing management plans.

For management of the patient experiencing hallucinations

1. Approach the patient with a calm, matter-of-fact demeanor. ***The goal of this interaction is for the nurse to demonstrate external control. This helps decrease the anxiety and fear that generally accompany hallucinations and allows the patient to feel safe. Anxiety is transferable.***
2. Address the patient by name. ***This is a useful presentation of reality because self-identity is the last sphere of orientation to vanish.***
3. In responding to the patient's description of the hallucination, DO NOT deny, argue, or attempt to disprove the existence of the perceived event. ***Statements such as, "There are no voices coming from that air vent" or, "Look, I'm brushing my hand across the wall, and there are no bugs" confuse the patient further, because the hallucination, although frightening, is his or her perceived reality.***
4. Express to the patient that your experiences are dissimilar, and acknowledge how frightening his or hers must be. SAMPLE STATEMENT: "I don't hear (see, etc.) what you do, but I know how frightening such an experience must be to you. I'm Joe, your nurse, and I'm going to stay with you until the voices (etc.) go away." Remain with any patient who is experiencing a hallucination. ***Feelings of fear and anxiety often accelerate when a patient is left alone. He or she needs someone to represent a nonthreatening reality. In addition, validating the patient's feelings demonstrates acceptance and sensitivity to the experience and promotes trust.***

SENSORY/PERCEPTUAL ALTERATIONS RELATED TO SENSORY OVERLOAD, SENSORY DEPRIVATION, AND SLEEP PATTERN DISTURBANCE—cont'd

5. DO NOT explore the content of the hallucination with the patient by asking about its nature or character. ***The nurse is the patient's link with reality. Pursuit of a detailed description of a hallucination may signify to the patient that the nurse accepts his or her sensory distortion as factual. This may further confuse the patient and distance him or her more from reality.**** The nurse can help bridge the gap between the patient's misperception and reality by addressing the feelings (e.g., fear, anxiety) and/or meanings (e.g., danger, death) engendered by the hallucination. Determination of how the misperception affects the patient emotionally, acknowledgment of those feelings, and a calm, controlled, matter-of-fact approach will provide the trust and comfort he or she needs to tolerate this frightening experience. In other words, deal with the intent more than the content of the hallucination. ***The resultant decrease in anxiety will enable the patient to focus more accurately on his immediate environment.***
6. Talk concretely with the patient about things that are really happening. SAMPLE STATEMENTS: "How does your chest incision feel this afternoon, Mr. Clark?" "Your sister Kate was here to see you, but you were sleeping. She went down to the cafeteria and will be back." "Your secretions are a little easier for you to cough up today." ***Interpretation of reality-based stimuli by the nurse encourages the patient to focus on actual circumstances and discourages a preoccupation with sensory misperceptions.***
7. There may be circumstances in which it is appropriate for the nurse simply to distract the patient by changing the topic. This tactic is useful in situations of escalating anxiety and confusion or when all else fails. Topics should consist of basic themes that are universally understood and culturally congruent, such as music, food, or weather. They may also be topics of special interest to the patient, such as hobbies, crafts, or sports. Topics that evoke strong emotions, such as politics, religion, or sexuality, should be avoided with most patients. ***This is especially true of the patient with reality distortions; sometimes hallucinations and delusions are expressions of repressed conflicts associated with religious, sexual, or aggressive issues. Pursuit of such subjects could increase confusion and anxiety.***
8. The use of touch: ***Touch presents a nonthreatening external reality and can therefore be useful in the management of patients with sensory alterations. However, in the patient experiencing hallucinations (as well as delusions and illusions), touch can be readily misinterpreted as, for instance, aggression or pain, or it can actually provide the basis for a tactile illusion.*** Therefore the use of touch as an intervention strategy should be avoided in any patient who evidences escalating anxiety or paranoid, suspicious, or mistrustful thoughts.
9. Types of hallucinations include the following: auditory—voices or running commentaries, with self-destructive messages; visual—persons or images that appear threatening; olfactory—smells that may be interpreted as poisonous gases; gustatory—tastes that seem peculiar or harmful; and tactile—touch that feels unusual or unnatural.
10. Specific management strategies for patients experiencing hallucinations:

◆ Auditory hallucinations

a. Patient behaviors: Head cocked as if listening to an unseen presence; lips moving.

b. Therapeutic nurse responses: "Mr. Clark, you appear to be listening to something." If patient acknowledges voices: "I don't hear any voices, but I know this is troubling you. The voices will go away. Nothing is going to harm you. I'm Joe, your nurse, and I'll be here with you."

c. Nontherapeutic nurse responses: "Tell me about your conversations with these voices." "To whom do the voices belong—anyone you know?"

◆ Visual hallucinations

a. Patient behaviors: Staring into space as if focused on an unseen object; startled movements and anxious facial expression.

b. Therapeutic nurse responses: "Mr. Clark, something seems to be troubling you. Tell me what it is." If patient states he visualizes people, images, or the devil in his environment and implies a sense of danger, respond, "There are only nurses and doctors here, Mr. Clark. I know this must be upsetting, but these images will go away. We're here with you in the hospital. Nothing will happen to you."

c. Nontherapeutic nurse responses: "Describe the people you see. What are they wearing?" "What does the devil mean in your life? What about God?"

*An exception is the patient who the nurse suspects is experiencing auditory hallucinations, i.e., hearing "voice commands." To ascertain that the voices are not telling the patient to harm himself, it is appropriate for the nurse to ask simply and concretely, "What are the voices saying?"

Continued.

SENSORY/PERCEPTUAL ALTERATIONS RELATED TO SENSORY OVERLOAD, SENSORY DEPRIVATION, AND SLEEP PATTERN DISTURBANCE—cont'd

For management of the patient experiencing delusions

1. Explain all unseen noises, voices, and activity simply and clearly. ***They readily feed a delusional system.*** SAMPLE STATEMENTS: "That is Dr. Smith. He's come to see you and other patients here in the hospital." "The voices and activity you hear are from the bedside of the patient behind this curtain. He's being helped by one of the nurses."
2. Avoid the "negative challenge" (e.g., "Nobody here stole your belongings" or "Doctors and nurses do not harm people") of the patient's delusion. Similarly, avoid defending the referents of the patient's belief: "Nurses are good" and "Doctors mean well." ***Remember, a delusion is a belief, albeit false, that cannot be changed with logic. To attempt this change is to challenge the patient's belief system and thereby escalate his or her anxiety, further blurring the boundaries between reality and the patient's internally based "logic."***
3. For the patient with persecutory delusions who refuses food, fluids, or medications because of a belief they have been poisoned or tainted, permit the refusal unless it is a life-threatening event. Try again in 20 minutes; allow the patient to choose an alternate selection of food or to read the label on the unit's medication. Coercion, show of force, or engaging in complicated, logical justifications will only heighten the patient's suspiciousness and possibly reinforce the delusional belief. ***When the patient feels more in control, he or she need not rely on the "paradoxical" quality of the delusion to equip him or her with a false sense of power. His or her power instead is derived from making reality-based decisions.***
4. Staff members should be particularly careful not to engage in unnecessary laughter or whispering within view of the delusional patient. ***The delusional patient is hypervigilant, scanning the environment for evidence to corroborate or confirm his or her belief that staff members are colluding against him or her; clearly, laughter and whispers easily suggest this belief, this delusion of reference. This rationale pertains to the patient experiencing hallucinations and/or illusions as well.***
5. Observe the principles detailed in the third intervention under "Management of the Patient Experiencing Hallucinations."

For management of the patient experiencing illusions

1. As with the management of delusions, the nurse should simply and briefly interpret reality-based stimuli for the patient in a calm, matter-of-fact manner. ***Seen and unseen noises, voices, activity, and people can provide the stimulus for a sensory misinterpretation, an illusion.***
2. The immediate environment of the patient should provide as low a level of stimulation as possible. Nursing interventions detailed previously under "Sensory Overload" are especially relevant here.
3. The theme of the nurse's verbal approach to the patient experiencing illusions is similar to that outlined for hallucinations and delusions: address the feelings and meanings associated with the experience, not the content of the sensory misinterpretation.
   - Patient behaviors: Eyes darting, startled movements; frightened facial expression. "I know who you are. You're the devil come to take me to hell."
   - Therapeutic nurse responses: "I'm Joe, your nurse. I know this experience is troubling for you. You're in the hospital, and no one here will harm you."
   - Nontherapeutic nurse responses: "There are no such things as devils or angels." "Do you think the devil would be dressed in white?" ***The first nontherapeutic nurse response carries a parental tone (i.e., "you know better than that"), thus infantilizing the patient and adding to his or her feelings of powerlessness over the environment. The second nontherapeutic response reflects obvious logic, which is not in the patient's sensory domain; therefore it cannot be processed and only adds to his or her confused state.***
4. Observe the principles detailed under the fifth item in "Management of the Patient Experiencing Hallucinations."

REFERENCES

1. Hunt WE, Hess RM: Surgical risks as related to time of intervention in the repair of intracranial aneurysms, *J Neurosurgery* 28:14, 1968.
2. Andrus C: Intracranial pressure: dynamics and nursing management, *J Neuroscience Nurs* 21(4):85, 1991.
3. Rauch M, Mitchell P, Tyler M: Validation of risk factors for the nursing diagnosis decreased intracranial adaptive capacity, *J Neuroscience Nurs* 22(3):173, 1990.
4. Lee S: Intracranial pressure changes during positioning of patients with severe head injury, *Heart Lung* 18(4):411, 1989.
5. Matz R: Hypothermia: mechanisms and countermeasures, *Hosp Pract* 21(1):45, 1986.
6. O'Brien MT, Pallett PJ: *Total care of the stroke patient,* Boston, 1978, Little, Brown.
7. Dittmar S: *Rehabilitation nursing: process and application,* St Louis, 1990, Mosby–Year Book.
8. Carpenito L: *Nursing diagnosis: application to clinical practice,* ed 3, Philadelphia, 1989, JB Lippincott.
9. McCaffery M, Beebe A: *Pain: clinical manual for nursing practice,* St Louis, 1989, Mosby–Year Book.
10. American Pain Society: *Principles of analgesic use in the treatment of acute pain or chronic cancer pain,* ed 2, Skokie, Ill, 1989, The Society.
11. Grossmont District Hospital: *Patient controlled analgesia,* La Mesa, Calif, 1988.
12. Pimental PA: Alterations in communication: biopsychosocial aspects of aphasia, dysarthria, and right hemisphere syndromes in the stroke patient, *Nurs Clin North Am* 21(2):321, 1986.
13. Numbers L: Pain: an introduction, *Nursing (Oxford)* 3(9):358, 1986.

VII

RENAL ALTERATIONS

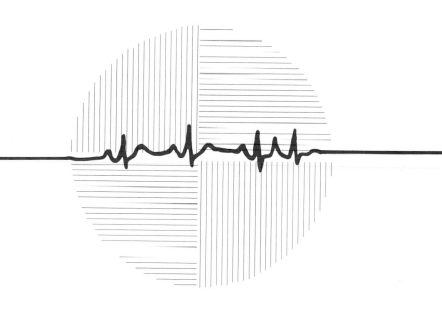

31

Renal Anatomy and Physiology

CHAPTER OBJECTIVES

- Identify and briefly describe the physiology of the normal anatomic structures of the kidney.
- Discuss important aspects of the following dynamics of fluid movement: osmosis, tonicity, diffusion, active transport, and filtration.
- Identify the pathway of renal filtrate.
- List and describe the functions of the kidneys.
- Discuss factors that control fluid volume excess and deficit.

Take a moment to stop and think about how many glasses of water you have consumed today. Estimating your water intake may be difficult. Water, the single most important compound to human existence, often is taken for granted. On the other hand, it is lauded in literature, promoted in advertising, fought over in the courts, and used in so many activities of daily life it boggles the mind.

Water in the human body not only provides a medium in which oxygen and nutrients dissolve and are used by the body but also regulates body temperature through insulation or evaporation and cushions body parts from injury. Dissolved within the body's water are substances such as potassium and sodium that are known as *electrolytes.* They are of critical importance in the maintenance of health.

KIDNEYS AND URINARY TRACT

Anatomy

The human kidneys are physiologic marvels in their ability to control and maintain fluid volume and electrolyte concentration precisely. This highly vascular pair of organs receives 25% of the cardiac output each minute[1] and efficiently separates the excesses of fluid, electrolytes, and metabolic by-products to produce urine. Because the kidneys function as primary regulators of fluid and electrolyte balance, a thorough understanding of their structure and function is central to any study of fluid and electrolytes.

◆ **Macroscopic structure.** The kidneys are bean-shaped organs that are approximately 12 cm long, 6 cm wide, and 2.5 cm thick.[2] The size of one kidney is comparable to the size of an adult male's fist. Each kidney weighs 4 to 6 ounces. A slight difference in kidney weight exists in females (closer to 4 ounces) and infants (kidneys are large in proportion to infant's size).

The kidneys' location is described as *retroperitoneal,* which means they are located outside and posterior to the abdominal cavity but lateral and anterior to the lumbar spine. Both are protected by the posterior rib cage, with the right kidney slightly lower than the left as a result of displacement by the liver.[2] This lesser amount of protection accounts for most traumatic kidney injuries that affect the right kidney.

Atop each kidney on the outer surface lies the adrenal gland. One function of these glands is to produce aldosterone, which allows the kidneys to control sodium and water balance.

An internal view of the kidney (Fig. 31-1) demonstrates the complexity of the filtering and collecting systems. The two distinct divisions of tissue within the kidney are known as the *cortex* and the *medulla.* Lying

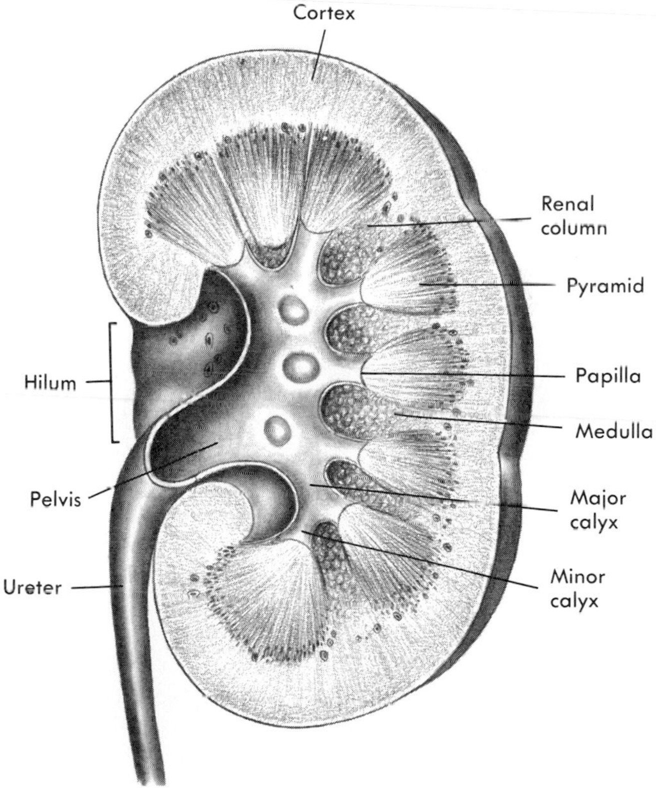

Fig. 31-1 Cross section of the kidney. (From Thompson JM and others: *Mosby's clinical nursing,* ed 3, St Louis, 1993, Mosby–Year Book.)

beneath the fibrous covering of each kidney, the cortical tissue contains the glomeruli and the proximal and distal tubules of the nephrons, which constitute the filtering mechanism of the kidney. The medulla comprises the innermost tissue layer of each kidney and is composed of the loops of Henle and the collecting ducts of the nephrons, which concentrate and collect the urine.

The renal pyramids are triangular divisions within the kidney that extend through both layers of tissue. The base of each pyramid is cortical tissue, and the apex of the pyramid contains collecting ducts, which converge to feed the urine into a canal known as a *calyx.*

As can be seen in Fig. 31-2, leading out of each kidney is a fibromuscular tube, the *ureter,* which is responsible for carrying the filtered and collected urine to the bladder. At the entrance to the bladder, each ureter implants posteriorly under the epithelium.[3]

The bladder is a muscular sac with a capacity of approximately 500 ml. The triple-layered musculature and specialized innervation control urine flow out of the body and prevent backflow.[3] As an extension of the bladder, the urethra, a hollow tube, provides the final conduit for urine to the outside.

The blood flow to the kidney begins with the abdominal aorta, from which the right and left renal arteries stem. Each renal artery further branches into anterior and posterior arteries to provide the blood supply to the entire kidney.[3]

Continuing to decrease in size but increasing in number, the anterior and posterior arteries become the interlobar arteries, which channel between the renal pyramids. The arterial divisions continue through two additional levels until, eventually, the afferent and efferent arterioles, which provide circulation to each of the millions of nephrons, are formed.

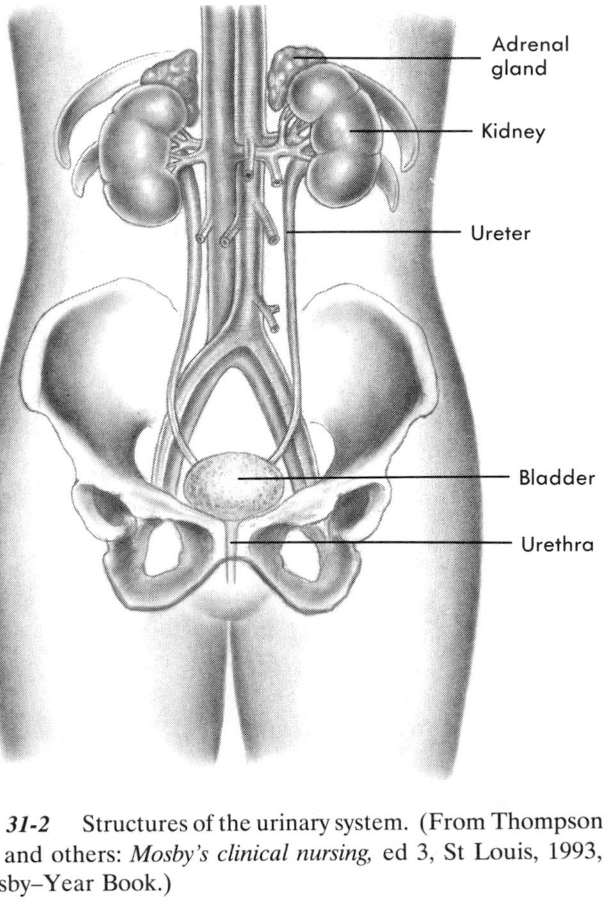

Fig. 31-2 Structures of the urinary system. (From Thompson JM and others: *Mosby's clinical nursing,* ed 3, St Louis, 1993, Mosby–Year Book.)

◆ **Microscopic structure.** The kidney tissue comprises approximately 1 to 1.5 million working units known as *nephrons.* Each nephron consists of the glomerulus, Bowman's capsule, proximal convoluted tubule, loop of Henle, distal convoluted tubule, and collecting duct. Not all of the nephrons function at the same level; some are held in reserve. This means the kidney can continue to function despite the loss of several thousand nephrons.

From the arterial circulation is formed a ball of capillaries known as the *glomerulus.* The glomerulus forms the beginning of each nephron and is the filtering point for the blood supply. As Fig. 31-3 indicates, the afferent arteriole leads into the glomerulus, and the efferent arteriole leads out of it. The sizes of the afferent and efferent arterioles are distinctly different, with the latter having the smaller lumen size. The size difference is of importance to glomerular filtration in that the larger afferent arteriole allows a greater flow of blood into the glomerulus. The smaller efferent arteriole offers resistance to the outflow of blood, thereby creating the high pressure in the glomerulus that facilitates the filtration of fluid out of the blood, into Bowman's capsule, and subsequently to the tubular network of the nephron.[4]

As the efferent arteriole leaves each kidney, it branches into a mesh of capillaries known as *peritubular capillaries.* The peritubular capillaries form a meshwork around the tubular structures of each nephron, providing further exchange of fluid, electrolytes, and essential nutrients between the intravascular volume and intratubular filtrate.

The glomerulus is surrounded by the tough, but membranous, tissue known as *Bowman's capsule.* The space between the capillary walls in the glomerulus and Bowman's capsule holds the initial filtrate from the blood. In other words, fluid, essential nutrients, and wastes are collected in the capsule space and begin to travel through a tubular network that forms the remainder of the nephron.

In the medullary tissue of the kidney, the peritubular capillaries become tiny venules and continue to enlarge until they form the right and left renal veins. This blood flow continues in the same fashion within and through each nephron.

◆ **Pathway of renal filtrate.** The excess fluid and solutes from the vascular volume filter through the glomerular capillary walls and form *filtrate,* which collects in Bowman's capsule. The filtrate travels through a tortuous section of tube known as the *proximal tubule.* The initial exchange of fluid and solutes between the intravascular volume and the intratubular filtrate occurs in this area.

The filtrate continues through a narrower, U-shaped area known as the *loop of Henle.* While it is contained in this area, concentration or dilution of the filtrate occurs, primarily as the result of gains and losses of sodium,

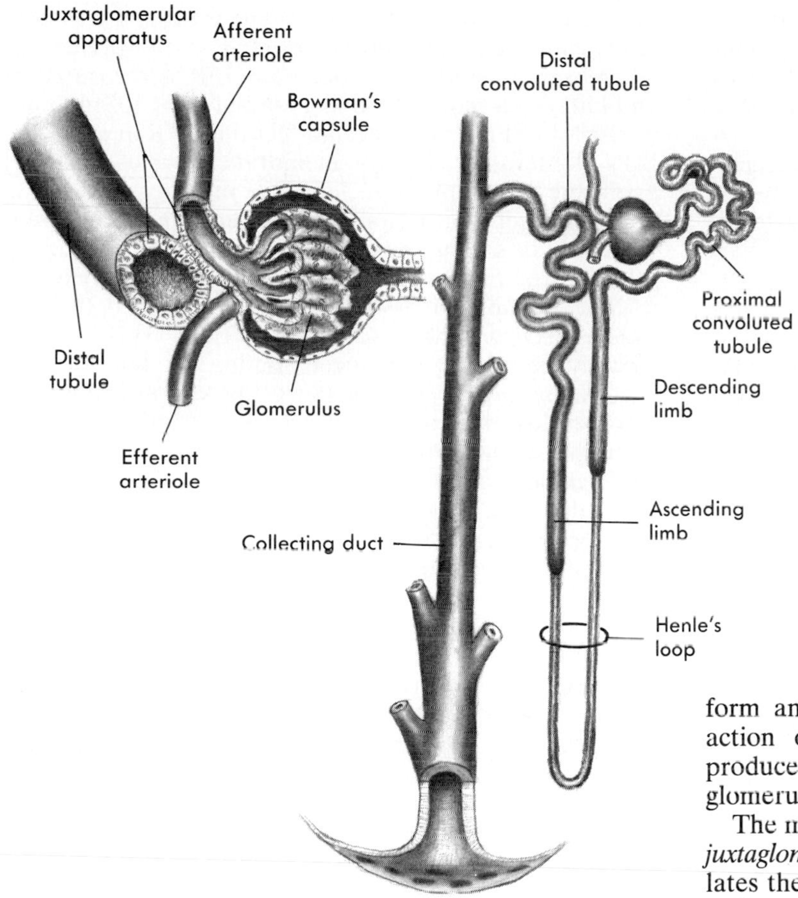

Fig. 31-3 Components of the nephron. (From Thompson JM and others: *Mosby's clinical nursing,* ed 3, St Louis, 1993, Mosby–Year Book.)

chloride, and water. At various locations along the loop of Henle, permeability to water, chloride, or sodium ions changes.

For example, the filtrate entering the descending portion of the loop of Henle is isotonic, but it quickly becomes hypertonic as the result of the loss of water to the hyperosmotic medullary interstitium and the reabsorption of sodium from the same area. As the filtrate flows through the ascending portion of the loop, sodium and chloride are lost to the interstitium, with water unable to enter the tubule because of the impermeability to water in this portion of the tubule. Thus as fluid enters the distal tubule, it is hypotonic.

The distal convoluted tubule is the site of potassium excretion, sodium reabsorption, and acid-base balance maintenance in the form of excretion of hydrogen ions and reabsorption of bicarbonate ions. Also, the distal tubule plays a small role in blood pressure regulation as the site for initiation of the renin-angiotensin-aldosterone system.

Specialized cells exist in the wall of the distal tubule at the point where the tubule touches the afferent arteriole. The cells, known as the *macula densa,* sense changes in filtrate flow and sodium concentration. The changes are transmitted to the *juxtaglomerular cells* in the afferent arteriole, and they release substances causing arteriolar constriction or dilation as necessary.[1]

These juxtaglomerular cells release renin, which helps form angiotensin II, a powerful vasoconstrictor. The action of angiotensin II on the efferent arteriole produces a rise in glomerular pressure and increases glomerular filtration.[1]

The macula densa and juxtaglomerular cells form the *juxtaglomerular apparatus,* a specialized area that regulates the renin-angiotensin feedback system.

From the distal tubule, the filtrate is pooled in areas known as *collecting ducts.* The collecting ducts allow the loss of water and urea, again resulting in a hypertonic urine. Several collecting ducts join to form the points of the renal pyramids and larger canals known as *calyces* (calyx–singular form). The calyces become larger still and unite in the renal pelvis, which then forms the ureters. Thus the urine flows from each collecting duct to the calyces and out through the ureters.

Continuing through the urinary tract, the urine is carried by peristalsis (a rhythmic contraction of the muscular ureters) to the bladder. When the bladder's capacity is reached, stimulation is initiated and the urine flows through the urethra to the outside.

◆ **Innervation.** The autonomic nervous system supplies the primary innervation to the kidneys and the urinary tract. The kidneys are supplied messages from the lowest splanchnic and inferior splanchnic nerves, which form the renal plexus. The inferior mesenteric plexus, the hypogastric plexus, and the pudic nerve from the sacral region serve the bladder, ureters, and urethra.[3,5]

An example of nervous control in the urinary tract is reflected in the process of micturition, or release of urine. Bladder fullness stimulates stretch receptors in the bladder wall and a portion of the urethra. Signals are sent through nerves in the sacral area and return as parasympathetic messages to contract the detrusor muscle that composes most of the bladder. With a full bladder, contractions usually are powerful enough to relax the external sphincter. Sympathetic stimulation returns the external sphincter to contraction after the urine is released. If insufficient urine has collected in the bladder to achieve release, the micturition reflex subsides but repeats regularly, with increasing force, over a period of time.[3]

Additional nervous control exists from the cerebral cortex and brainstem. The central nervous system regulates the micturition reflex, frequency, and external sphincter tone and allows conscious control over urinary release.

Functions of the Kidneys

Fluid and electrolyte balance depends critically on the continued efficient function of the kidneys. The renal system provides the primary route for reabsorption, excretion, and "fine tuning" of fluid and electrolyte balance and some acid-base balance.

◆ **Excretion of nitrogenous wastes.** Metabolic processes in the body produce certain waste products that are selectively filtered out of the circulation by the kidneys. Urea, uric acid, and creatinine are the most commonly measured by-products of protein metabolism that the kidneys filter out of circulation.

Clearance is defined as the ability of the kidney to clear certain substances from the plasma.[3] More specifically, clearance represents the volume of plasma that is cleared of a substance during a specific period of time. The unit of measurement representing clearance is milliliters per minute.

Clearance depends primarily on tubular reaction to substances in the glomerular filtrate. For example, the substance may be filtered by the glomerulus and then either reabsorbed or excreted partially or totally.[6] Many factors enhance or reduce clearance of substances through the kidney (see box below). Creatinine, a waste product of muscle metabolism, is produced in standard, predictable amounts by the body, and it is cleared from the blood in predictable amounts; therefore it is used as a standard for gauging the effectiveness of renal activity. The test for creatinine clearance requires that urine be collected for a 24-hour period and be analyzed for volume excreted and amount of creatinine present. At the same time, a blood sample is obtained for analysis of the amount of creatinine present.[7] A mathematic formula is used to calculate the rate of *creatinine clearance* and therefore to predict the adequacy of the kidneys' function. The normal creatinine clearance is roughly proportional to the glomerular filtration rate of 120 to 130 ml/min.

Closely allied with the concept of clearance is that of *glomerular filtration rate* (GFR). The GFR is the volume of plasma cleared of substances through the glomerular membrane per unit of time. The GFR is measured in milliliters per minute, with the normal GFR 125 ml/min.[4]

At least three factors can affect the GFR at any time: (1) glomerular capillary membrane permeability, (2) systemic blood pressure, and (3) the pressure of the blood (effective filtration pressure) entering the afferent arteriole or exiting the efferent arteriole. Any change in these three factors results in a change in the GFR.[6]

For example, if blood pressure is reduced through vasoconstriction of the afferent arteriole, GFR is significantly reduced. If vasoconstriction of the efferent arteriole occurs, the pressure increases inside the glomerulus and congestion occurs, forcing plasma out into the capsules and thereby reducing the GFR as well.[3]

◆ **Regulation of extracellular fluid volume.** The kidney has the unique ability to separate water regulation from electrolyte regulation in the nephron. Water is reabsorbed or excreted to maintain fluid balance. The maintenance of balance is primarily under the control of the *antidiuretic hormone* (ADH), produced by the posterior pituitary gland in the brain.

A multitude of factors, however, control water balance in the body. The conscious intake of fluids, for instance, provides the source of the fluid and the kidneys excrete the fluid. In large part body solute content determines this intake and output by stimulating various centers in the brain that regulate the body's water. For example, thirst is controlled by receptors in the vascular system that sense hypovolemia or by sensors in the cerebrum that sense sodium concentration.[8] Thirst, resulting from stimulation of these sensors, results in intake of fluids (if the individual is able). Water balance, however, is achieved primarily through the suppression or release of ADH and regulation of extracellular fluid (ECF) sodium levels.

ADH release results from signals of the osmoreceptors, baroreceptors, and stretch receptors located in the atria. The receptors send signals to the midbrain where ADH is manufactured and released into the general circulation, eventually resulting in increased fluid reabsorption by the renal tubules. Similarly, stretch receptors in the cardiac muscle sense hypervolemia, resulting in suppression of ADH release.[8]

◆ **Regulation of ECF electrolyte concentration.** The body controls electrolyte reabsorption in the renal tubules by providing a mechanism known as the *tubular maximum,* or *threshold.* Basically, the electrolytes and other substances reabsorbed are divided into threshold or nonthreshold substances. The substances and electrolytes useful to the body are reabsorbed in differing amounts to maintain normal plasma levels. For example, sodium, glucose, amino acids, calcium, and phosphorus are almost completely reabsorbed from the tubules.

Although potassium is needed, the amount present in the filtrate usually far exceeds the amount needed; therefore the excess is excreted. In other words, potassium reaches its tubular maximum and the excess is relinquished. Potassium also retains the distinction of being exchanged for sodium because it occurs in abundance in filtrate.[6]

FACTORS AFFECTING RENAL CLEARANCE

- Volume depletion
- Renal blood flow (hypoperfusion)
- Glomerular membrane permeability
- Blood pressure (hypertension or hypotension)
- Cardiac output (myocardial infarction, pericarditis)
- Aging

Nonthreshold substances usually are the waste products such as urea and creatinine that, although not actively reabsorbed, occur in low plasma levels because of passive diffusion into the peritubular network. Primary bulk reabsorption is performed in the proximal tubule, with the distal tubule the site for the fine tuning of, particularly, sodium, potassium, calcium, and phosphates.

◆ **Regulation of acid-base balance.** The nephron is involved in acid-base regulation by reabsorbing or excreting the various acids and bases.[1] Although the renal mechanism is not as swift in altering acid-base concentrations as that of the lungs, it is meant to regulate the day-to-day balance rather than to cope with the emergencies produced by excesses of either acids or bases.

Bicarbonate, the principal blood buffer, is reabsorbed from the tubules, and hydrogen is secreted into the tubules. Carbonic acid in the renal tubular cells splits and sends hydrogen ions (H^+) to the tubular lumen and bicarbonate (HCO_3^-) to the blood. Recombination and further dissociation of carbonic acid in the tubules produce carbon dioxide for perpetuation of the cycle and water for excretion. Hydrogen ions combine with either phosphates or ammonia and are transported into the tubular filtrate and eventually to the urine. Combination with either of these substances will release sodium and bicarbonate for reabsorption into the vascular system through the peritubular capillaries.[9]

FLUID COMPARTMENTS

Anatomy

The fluid of the human body is captured in distinct internal spaces referred to as *compartments.* Although the word *compartment* suggests that the fluid remains stationary within each space, the opposite is true. Fluid movement between compartments is dynamic and constant.

The compartments are separated from each other by thin sheets of tissue known as *membranes.* These membranes have openings (pores) that allow molecules of specific size and molecular weight to pass through while preventing larger, heavier molecules from doing so. This characteristic of the membrane is known as *semipermeability.*

Basically, the human body has two fluid compartments. The *intracellular* compartment refers to the fluids inside each of the body's cells. It is, by far, the larger compartment, accounting for 40% of a person's weight.

The remaining fluid is outside the cells in the spaces referred to as the *extracellular* compartment. This compartment is further divided into two subcompartments. The *intravascular* compartment, or blood supply, accounts for 5% of the body's weight. The tissue space, or *interstitial* compartment, is outside both the body cells and blood vessels and contains the remaining 15% of the body weight. Approximate amounts of fluid contained in each compartment are listed in Fig. 31-4, *A.*

The percentage of total body water varies slightly from individual to individual in relationship to age, gender, and body fat content. For instance, a lean adult male usually has a 60% body water content, whereas an adult female has closer to 50%. Infants have a body fluid content estimated at 77%; on the opposite end of the age continuum, body fluids decrease and may represent only 46% to 52% of body weight in elderly persons.[10] Also, with any increase in body fat, the body fluid percentage decreases because fat does not contain a significant amount of water.

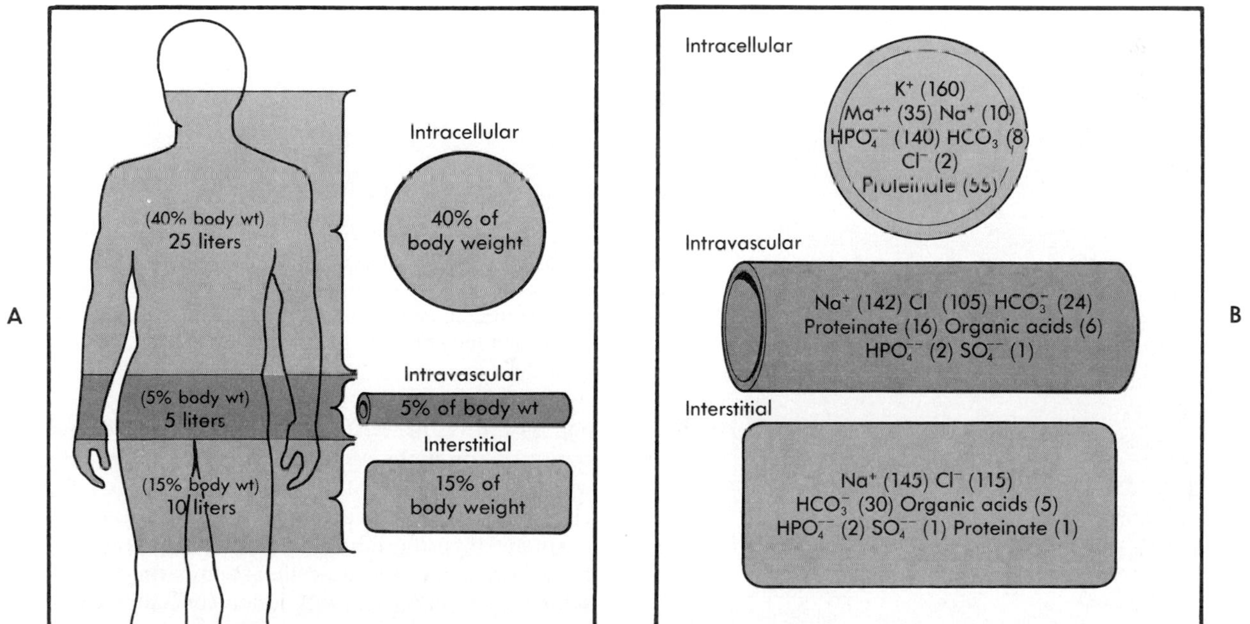

Fig. 31-4 **A,** Fluid compartments. **B,** Electrolytes by fluid compartment.

Composition

Any information about body fluids by necessity must involve a description of the substances contained within the fluids. In fact, movement of fluids within the body does not occur without simultaneous movement of these substances.

Electrolytes are elements or compounds that, when dissolved in water, dissociate into parts known as *ions* and give the fluid the ability to conduct an electrical current. The ions carry either a positive (+) or negative (−) charge. Positive ions are known as *cations,* and negative ions are known as *anions.* Electrolytes exist in differing amounts in each of the fluid compartments. The primary electrolytes and other substances of importance are listed by fluid compartment in Fig. 31-4, *B.*

A balance exists between cations and anions and other substances in the compartments. Maintaining this balance is of paramount importance to the normal function of all body systems. For example, the difference between the intravascular and interstitial compartments lies in the amount of proteinate in the vascular compartment.[11] This difference helps maintain a balance between these two compartments. Finally, there are obvious differences in electrolyte compositions between the intracellular and extracellular fluids.

Fluid and Electrolyte Physiology

An overall understanding is needed of both the structures containing or balancing electrolytes and the physiologic forces governing movement and balance. In addition, factors that inhibit or enhance the transfer of fluids and electrolytes are discussed.

◆ **Osmosis.** Osmosis is the movement of water through a semipermeable membrane from an area of dilution (greater quantity of water) to an area of concentration. For instance, if distilled water is contained on one side of a semipermeable membrane and a sugar-water solution is on the other, water will travel through the membrane to the sugar-water solution, as illustrated in Fig. 31-5. Osmosis is one of the forces that describes the physiologic shift of fluid from one compartment to another. For example, the intravenous infusion of a colloid solution results in an osmotic pull of fluid from the interstitial space into the intravascular space.

◆ **Tonicity.** *Isotonic, hypotonic,* and *hypertonic* all refer to tonicity, or the *osmolality* of body fluids. Basically, osmolality is defined as the measure of the number of particles in a solution. Osmolality is stated in *milliosmoles* and is derived by dividing the milligrams per liter of the substances by their atomic weight. The normal osmolality of body fluids is 275 to 295 mOsm/kg of body weight.[8]

Isotonic means that the number of particles in a solution contained on one side of a membrane or container approximates the number of particles in solution on the other side of the container or membrane. In humans, an isotonic solution is one that has roughly the same tonicity as blood plasma. Therefore cells bathed in an isotonic solution maintain consistency and do not lose fluid to their surroundings (Fig. 31-6, *A*). Care must be exercised to use *isotonic* solutions when their direct contact with the blood stream is necessary for more than short periods.

Hypertonic fluid contains a concentration of particles greater than that inside the cell (Fig. 31-6, *B*). When a hypertonic fluid is infused into the body for a prolonged time, fluid may be drawn out of the cells, causing a withering of the cell called *crenation.* If used appropriately, however, hypertonic solutions such as the osmotic diuretic *mannitol* can be effective in drawing excess fluid from the cells and interstitial spaces.

Hypotonic solutions contain fewer particles than does the solution inside the cell (Fig. 31-6, *C*). As a result, cells suspended in hypotonic fluid swell and burst, a condition known as *hemolysis.* In the event of dehydration, however, hypotonic solutions such as 0.45% saline replenish the fluids and some of the lost electrolytes.

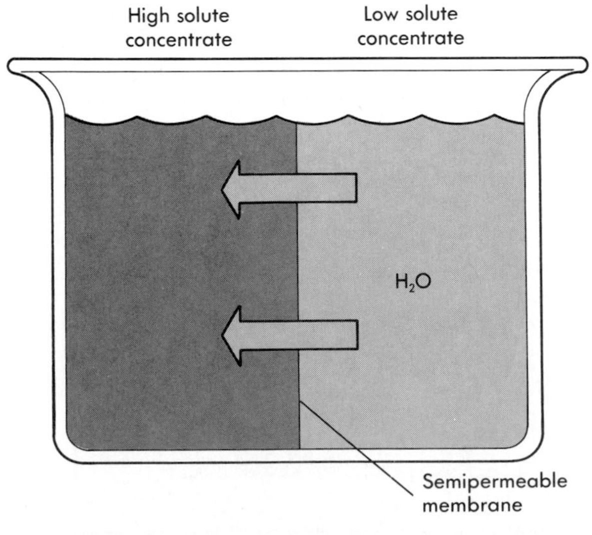

Fig. 31-5 Movement of water by osmosis.

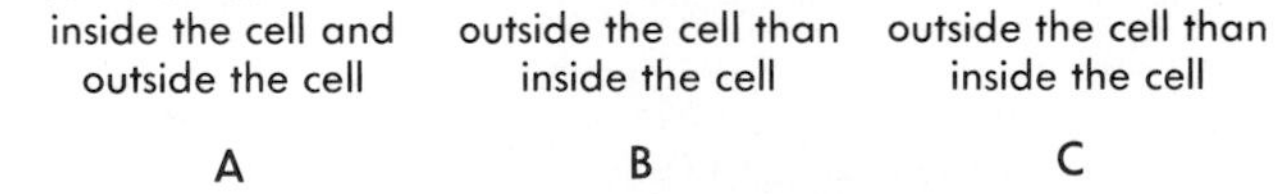

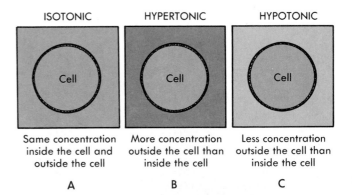

Fig. 31-6 **A,** Isotonic solution. The extracellular solution concentration is the same as the intracellular concentration, with no movement of water into or out of the cell. **B,** Hypertonic solution. The extracellular solution concentration is greater than the intracellular concentration. Water moves from the cell into the extracellular compartment. **C,** Hypotonic solution. The extracellular solution concentration is less than the intracellular concentration. Water moves from the extracellular compartment into the cell.

◆ **Diffusion.** Unlike osmosis, the process of diffusion is concerned with the solid particles suspended in the fluid. Diffusion is the movement of particles through a semipermeable membrane from an area of high concentration of particles to an area of low concentration of particles. The particles do not move in an orderly fashion but strike the membrane randomly and pass through it until equilibration is achieved on either side of the membrane.[10]

For example, urea particles suspended in glomerular filtrate travel through the renal tubules. As water is reabsorbed into the peritubular capillaries, the concentration of urea particles in the tubules rises. A concentration difference exists between the inside of the tubules and the tissue space outside. As a result, urea travels from the tubules into the tissue space and equilibrates the number of particles on either side of the tubular structure.[6]

A force that influences the diffusion of particles across the membrane is known as the *electrical gradient.* Ions carry a positive or negative charge and therefore interact on either side of the membrane by attracting substances with opposite charges or by repelling substances with like charges.[3]

Diffusion also depends on pore size versus molecular size of the particles of a substance. For instance, water molecules are small and diffuse easily, but glucose molecules are larger and pass with difficulty through membrane pores.

◆ **Active transport.** A concentration difference exists for various electrolytes on either side of the cell membrane. This concentration difference is called a *chemical* or *concentration gradient.* At times there is a need for an electrolyte such as potassium (K^+), which has a low concentration outside the cell, to move inside the cell to an area of high potassium concentration. To move against this chemical gradient (i.e., to move from an area of low concentration to an area of high potassium concentration), energy and a substance to carry the potassium are required. The process by which potassium moves against this chemical gradient is called *active transport.* At times sodium also moves by active transport.

Active transport has been likened to a pump by which the sodium and potassium are exchanged across the cell membrane and against the concentration gradient. Sodium combines with a carrier substance, a lipoprotein, and travels out of the cell, where it is released. The lipoprotein changes to accept the potassium ion, which is then transported into the cell and released. The system continues indefinitely under the influence of adenosine triphosphate (ATP), which provides the energy necessary for the carrier substances to travel.

The active transport mechanism changes the electrical charge on the cell membrane and gives the membrane the potential for accepting a message from the nervous system. This process allows contraction of skeletal muscle.

◆ **Filtration.** Filtration is defined as the movement of fluid and dissolved substances through a semipermeable membrane from an area of high pressure to an area of low pressure[10] (Fig. 31-7). The force of left-ventricular contraction pushes the blood through the circulatory system, causing exertion of pressure by the blood against the vessel walls. This force is known as *hydrostatic pressure.*

The hydrostatic pressure creates the tendency for fluids and dissolved substances to move into the interstitial spaces. If not for other forces counteracting the hydrostatic pressure, fluid would leave the intravascular space until it was depleted. However, whereas hydrostatic pressure creates fluid and electrolyte movement out of the intravascular compartment, the *colloid osmotic pressure* of the plasma tends to hold the fluid and substances in the intravascular space.[12] Colloid osmotic pressure is created by the presence of plasma proteins in the intravascular space.

◆ **Movement of water.** Forces generated by cardiac contraction, the plasma protein content in the vascular space, and the solute content of both the extracellular fluid (ECF) and intracellular fluid (ICF) result in a constant movement and balance of fluid content throughout the fluid compartments.

For example, fluid movement at the capillary level between the vascular and interstitial spaces is a function of protein content in the plasma (capillary colloid osmotic pressure) and the pressure generated through cardiac contraction, called *capillary hydrostatic pressure.* Similarly, solute and protein content of the tissue space result in generation of interstitial colloid osmotic pressure. Pressure generated through collection and emptying of the lymphatic system creates an interstitial hydrostatic pressure.

An increase in plasma volume results in increased capillary hydrostatic pressure, thereby forcing fluid into the interstitial space and creating edema. Conversely, a reduction in plasma volume causes movement of fluid from the interstitium to the vascular space as a result of the interstitial hydrostatic pressure's being greater than the capillary hydrostatic pressure. Also, a loss of plasma proteins in the vascular space lessens the capillary colloid osmotic pressure and results in movement of water to the interstitium.

Movement of fluid between the intracellular space and the extracellular space is primarily a function of the osmolality of the two spaces. For example, hyperosmolality of the ECF, although rare in persons able to obtain oral fluids, will result in movement of fluid from the intracellular space to the extracellular space (cellular dehydration).

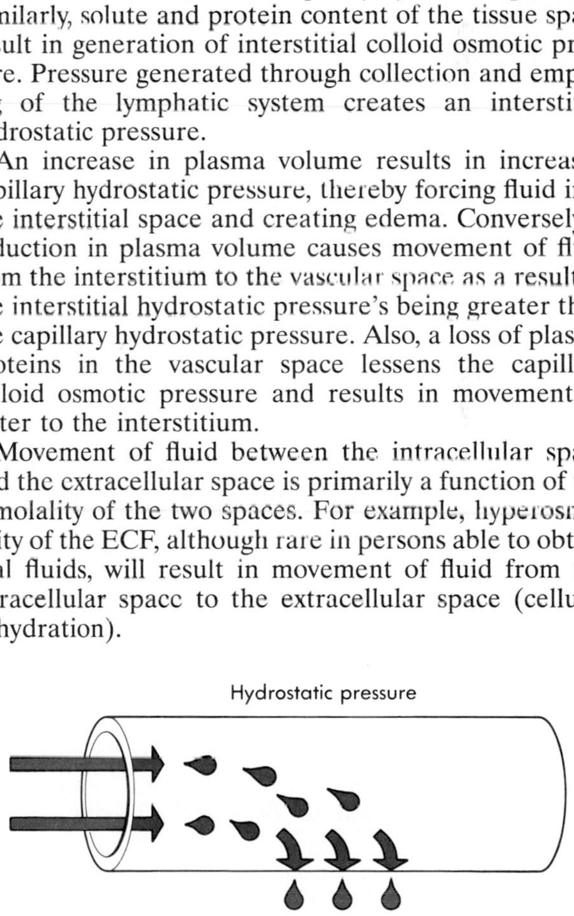

Fig. 31-7 Filtration. Hydrostatic pressure forces fluid out of the capillary into the interstitial space.

Functions of Electrolytes

The specific contributions of the electrolytes to the successful maintenance of overall body functioning are important. Very often, changes in the electrolytes can initiate serious organ dysfunction. Their replacement or reduction is required to restore the necessary equilibrium.

◆ **Potassium.** Although authorities disagree about which body electrolyte is most essential for normal cellular function, potassium always is ranked among the most important. Without this crucial element, for example, the heart muscle cannot function.

Potassium is the primary *intracellular* electrolyte. For this reason, it is difficult to measure true body stores. Changes in the intracellular potassium concentration, however, are quickly reflected by the measurement of the extracellular amount. For example, during tissue breakdown, potassium leaves the cells; thus the serum potassium level becomes elevated. The normal serum levels of potassium are 3.5 to 5.0 mEq/L.

Diffusion and active transport maintain the very narrow limits of potassium balance. Potassium leaves the cell by diffusion, moving toward the area of lesser concentration outside the cell, but it must be actively transported back into the cell to maintain cellular stability. With this movement, the cell membrane is made ready to accept neural messages, leading to one of the most important potassium functions in the body—that of aiding nervous impulse conduction and muscle contraction.

In addition to aiding nervous impulses and muscle contraction, potassium is responsible for enzyme activity that helps produce protein and carbohydrate metabolism for energy production. Also, because it is so abundant in the intracellular fluid, potassium primarily controls the maintenance of intracellular osmolality.

The gastrointestinal (GI) tract and skin excrete small amounts of potassium, but the major controllers of the body's potassium stores are the kidneys. Of the estimated 50 to 100 mEq/day ingested by an individual, 90% of the potassium will be reabsorbed before arriving at the distal convoluted tubule where the remainder usually is excreted. Reabsorption and secretion of potassium, however, are influenced by many factors,[13] which are presented in the first box, above right.

Potassium and sodium are in a constant state of competition within the body, despite the need for both electrolytes and despite their differing functions. The kidneys conserve sodium very carefully, whereas potassium is readily excreted. Potassium wasting may even continue despite the body's need for potassium, particularly when aldosterone levels are elevated.

A review of the normal values and functions of potassium appears in the second box, above right. Potassium is important not only to the human body but to the cells of other plant and animal life.

◆ **Sodium.** Sodium can easily be called the "great water regulator" because it is primarily responsible for shifts in body water and the amount of water retained or excreted by the kidneys. It is the most abundant extracellular electrolyte. The normal serum value for sodium is 135 to 145 mEq/L.

In addition to water regulation, sodium plays a role in transmission of nerve impulses through the "sodium pump," or active transport mechanism at the cellular level. Sodium also combines with either chloride or bicarbonate to maintain acid-base balance.

The body contains an incredibly complex system of safeguards and feedback mechanisms to protect the level of sodium in the ECF. The three organs responsible for regulating sodium balance are the kidneys, the adrenal glands, and the posterior pituitary gland.

Because of the extremely sensitive mechanism for retaining sodium, ingestion of large amounts of sodium is not necessary. In fact, for years the literature has indicated that excessive sodium ingestion is implicated in the development of hypertension and associated disorders. Functions of sodium are listed in the box on p. 587, left-hand column.

FACTORS AFFECTING REABSORPTION AND SECRETION OF POTASSIUM (K^+)

- ◆ Sodium balance: sodium deficit results in increased potassium loss.
- ◆ Acid-base balance: acidosis results in hydrogen movement into the cell and potassium movement out of it, and the potassium eventually is excreted in the urine.
- ◆ Use of diuretics (thiazides): their use results in increased distal tubular loss of potassium.
- ◆ Gastrointestinal (GI) disturbances: disturbances include vomiting and GI suctioning.
- ◆ Insulin: it promotes potassium's movement back into cells.
- ◆ Epinephrine: it enhances potassium's reabsorption from the distal tubule.

POTASSIUM

NORMAL SERUM VALUE

3.5-5.0 mEq/L

FUNCTIONS

Promotes transmission of nerve impulses
Maintains intracellular osmolality
Activates several enzymatic reactions
Aids in regulation of acid-base balance
Promotes myocardial, skeletal, and smooth muscle contractility

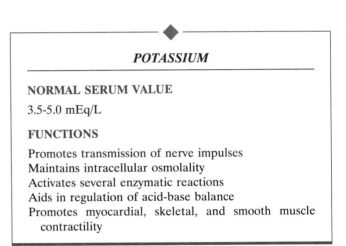

SODIUM

NORMAL SERUM VALUE

135-145 mEq/L

FUNCTIONS

Maintains extracellular osmolality
Maintains the active transport mechanism in conjunction with potassium
Controls body fluids (largely responsible for water movement and retention)
Aids in maintaining neuromuscular activity
Aids in some enzyme activities (helping to create energy)
Influences acid-base balance

CALCIUM

NORMAL SERUM VALUE

8.5-10.5 mg/dl or 4.5-5.8 mEq/L

FUNCTIONS

Maintains hardness of bone and teeth (crystalline in nature)
Contracts skeletal muscle
Coagulates blood
Maintains cellular permeability
Contracts heart muscle

◆ **Calcium.** When the word *calcium* is mentioned, the word *bone* immediately comes to mind. Indeed, 99% of the calcium in the body is contained in the bones. Calcium occurs in nature as a very hard crystalline element. It also is the electrolyte of greatest quantity in the human body, with stores estimated at 1200 g. The remaining 1% of the body calcium is contained primarily in the ECF or, specifically, in the blood stream.

The calcium contained within bone is essentially an inactive form that maintains bone strength and is a ready storehouse for mobilization of calcium to the serum in cases of depletion. The mobilization of calcium is accomplished through the influence of parathyroid hormone (PTH). Inasmuch as most calcium is contained within bone, it is inactivated for any other purpose. The calcium in the intravascular space is either bound to protein or floats freely in an ionized form, as do sodium and potassium.[14,15] The protein-bound calcium awaits usage during immediate crisis, whereas the ionized calcium is the active form, which functions in cell membrane stability, blood clotting, and other important functions.

In the ionized form, calcium plays an important role in maintaining the internal integrity of the cell. The amount of ionized calcium in the serum depends on changes in serum pH and on the availability of plasma protein, primarily albumin. Because changes in pH and albumin levels occur with relative frequency, measurement of the serum calcium often is deceptive.

For instance, a change in the serum albumin level affects the calcium level. As serum albumin levels rise, ionized calcium becomes bound to the newly available protein, thus lowering the ionized calcium. However, because total calcium is measured rather than the ionized fraction, the actual decrease in the ionized calcium may not be accurately reflected.

Conversely, should albumin levels fall, calcium is split free of the protein and creates an actual rise in the ionized calcium level. Under the influence of the hormone calcitonin, however, the ionized calcium may be returned to the bone, and the actual availability of the calcium again may not be accurately reflected.

The normal serum calcium level ranges from 8.8 to 10.5 mg/dl. For every increase or decrease in serum albumin of 1 g/dl, a change of 0.8 mg/dl occurs in the total serum calcium. Any serum calcium level should be accompanied by measurement of serum albumin.[15]

Calcium also is responsible for several critically important functions. Myocardial contractility is influenced primarily by calcium. Neuromuscular activity, cell permeability, thickness of cell membrane, coagulation of blood, and hardness of bones and teeth all depend on calcium levels. Functions of calcium are reviewed in the box above.

Calcium levels are highly dependent on individual dietary intake and a variety of physiologic mechanisms related to absorption. For example, the uptake of calcium is influenced by the level of phosphorus, the amount of vitamin D and its breakdown products, PTH, and the hormone *calcitonin.*[15] Other factors, such as changes in acid-base balance, change calcium levels in the ECF. For example, acidosis ionizes or splits calcium free from albumin, resulting in "ionized" hypercalcemia, whereas alkalosis enhances the binding of calcium to proteins, thereby creating a deficit of ionized calcium.[14,15]

◆ **Magnesium.** Magnesium is primarily an intracellular electrolyte; therefore, like potassium, it is measured solely by amounts in serum. Approximately 60% of the body's magnesium is located in bone.[16] Only approximately 1% is actually in the ECF, with the remainder in the ICF. In fact, other intracellular electrolytes, such as calcium and potassium, are affected by the level of magnesium present. For example, calcium and magnesium compete for absorption in the GI tract. If the dietary intake is higher in calcium than magnesium, calcium will be preferentially reabsorbed and vice versa.

Magnesium is found primarily in the ICF and helps maintain the correct potassium stores on either side of the cell membrane inasmuch as magnesium is required for appropriate function of the intracellular "carrier substances" that transport sodium and potassium across the cell membrane. A depletion of magnesium liberates potassium to the ECF and thereby increases renal excretion of potassium, resulting in hypokalemia.[17,18]

The normal value for magnesium in the serum is 1.3 to 2.1 mEq/L. The most important function of magnesium is ensuring the transportation of sodium and potassium across the cell membranes. In addition, magnesium plays roles in transmitting central nervous system (CNS) messages, maintaining neuromuscular activity, and activating enzymes for metabolism of carbohydrates and proteins. A summary of functions and factors affecting magnesium are listed in the box below.

◆ **Phosphorus.** Phosphorus often is omitted from texts when major electrolytes are considered. This intracellular anion, however, plays so many important roles in body function and maintenance that it cannot be ignored.

The normal serum phosphorus level is 2.5 to 4.5 mg%.[18] As with calcium and magnesium, however, the serum values of phosphorus represent a minute portion of actual body stores. Approximately 75% of the phosphorus is found in the bones, and part of the remaining amount is intracellular, thus rendering it difficult to measure. Serum phosphorus levels change frequently and dramatically, particularly in response to ingestion of phosphate-rich foods (milk, red meats, poultry, fish).[9]

The primary function of phosphorus is in the formation of ATP, which is the intracellular energy. The active transport mechanism cannot function without the energy provided by ATP. Additional functions of phosphorus are as follows: (1) maintenance of cell membrane structure, (2) maintenance of acid-base balance, (3) oxygen delivery to the tissues, (4) cellular immunity, and (5) maintenance of bone strength (see box, lower right).[18]

Absorption of phosphorus takes place in the GI tract, and excretion, for the most part, occurs in the kidney. At the level of the proximal renal tubule, phosphorus also is reabsorbed when body stores are low. Acid-base balance is, in a minor way, influenced by the availability of phosphorus. Phosphates, available in the renal tubular filtrate, combine with sodium and excess hydrogen ions to form sodium diphosphate (Na_2HPO_4). This complex then dissociates into sodium, which combines with the available bicarbonate and is reabsorbed into the peritubular capillary network. The remaining hydrogen and phosphates are excreted into the urine.[3]

An important reciprocal relationship exists between phosphorus and calcium; high levels of phosphorus result in low levels of calcium, and, conversely, high levels of calcium result in low levels of phosphorus. PTH secretion, vitamin D, and the renal tubules are all involved in this complex relationship.

◆ **Chloride.** Chloride rarely is found in the human body without being in combination with one of the major cations. Therefore changes in serum chloride levels usually indicate changes in the other electrolytes or in acid-base balance.

Inasmuch as chloride combines most frequently with sodium, it plays a major role in maintaining serum osmolality and, subsequently, water balance. Also, because it competes with bicarbonate for combination with sodium, it affects acid-base balance. In addition, chloride combines with hydrogen ions to form the hydrochloric acid present in gastric juice.

Red blood cell oxygenation and the transportation of carbon dioxide depend on adequate chloride levels. The dissociation of carbonic acid inside red blood cells creates hydrogen and bicarbonate ions. The hydrogen usually combines with hemoglobin, and the bicarbonate leaves the cell in exchange for the chloride ions moving into the cell (chloride shift).[3] Therefore carbon dioxide in the form of bicarbonate is liberated to travel to the lungs.

The normal serum chloride level is 98 to 106 mEq/L. It most often is ingested with sodium in the form of salt and, because of this combination with sodium, is reabsorbed or excreted in the renal tubules at the proximal tubular site. Chloride is actively transported out of the tubule into the renal medullary interstitium, again with sodium, to help maintain the high interstitial osmolality and the mechanism for concentrating the urine[6] (see box, p. 589, first box in left-hand column).

MAGNESIUM

NORMAL SERUM VALUE

1.5-2.5 mEq/L

FUNCTIONS

- Aids in neuromuscular transmission
- Aids in contraction of heart muscle
- Activates enzymes for cellular metabolism of carbohydrates and proteins
- Aids in maintaining the active transport mechanism at the cellular level
- Aids in transmission of hereditary information to offspring

PHOSPHORUS

NORMAL SERUM VALUE

2.7-4.5 mg/dl

FUNCTIONS

- Aids in structure of cellular membrane
- Helps deliver oxygen to the tissues
- Is integral part of intracellular energy production (ATP)
- Helps maintain bone hardness
- Aids in enzyme regulation (ATPase)

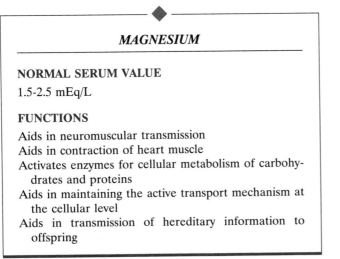

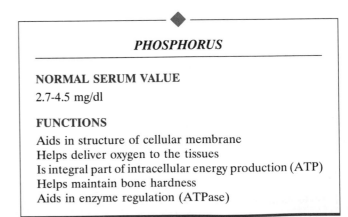

◆ **Bicarbonate.** Rarely does an electrolyte have a solitary purpose in the body. Bicarbonate, however, an anion present in ECF, performs the single, life-sustaining function of maintaining acid-base balance. Although bicarbonate is not solely responsible for acid-base balance, it is the major ECF buffer.

Bicarbonate (HCO_3^-) levels in the body are in balance with carbonic acid (H_2CO_3) levels; the ratio between the two must remain proportional (1 mEq H_2CO_3:20 mEq HCO_3^-), or acid-base disturbances result. When the carbonic acid level is elevated, the condition is known as *acidosis.* When the bicarbonate level is high, the condition is known as *alkalosis.* The normal serum level of bicarbonate is 24 to 28 mEq/L, and the normal value for carbonic acid is 1.2 to 1.4 mEq/L[12] (see second box below).

The amount of bicarbonate available in the ECF is regulated by the kidneys. Reabsorption of bicarbonate occurs primarily from the proximal tubule to the peritubular capillaries. Also, in response to acid-base balance and body requirements, bicarbonate is reconstructed in the distal tubule and reabsorbed into the blood. The kidneys either reabsorb or excrete bicarbonate in response to the number of hydrogen ions present.

◆ **Protein.** Although proteins are not electrolytes, the role they play in controlling body fluid movement and cell building maintenance cannot be minimized. Proteins are needed for basic cell structure and enzyme formation. When combined with other substances, proteins also can supply energy for body functions.

Protein, which is a nitrogen compound, is formed from amino acids that are stored in the liver in a process called *anabolism.* The subsequent breakdown of, for example, body tissues, food, and cellular structures is known as *catabolism.* Anabolism and catabolism usually are in dynamic balance within the body.

As stated, a secondary function of protein is maintenance of fluid balance, particularly between the intravascular and interstitial compartments. Contained within the intravascular compartment are the *plasma proteins:* albumin, globulin, and fibrinogen. These plasma proteins exert a pull on water molecules and therefore produce a force called *oncotic pressure,* or osmotic pressure, that retains fluid within the intravascular compartment. This force is maintained because proteins are large and cannot travel across the membrane unless the permeability of the membrane is changed in some significant way (e.g., by burns or infections). The normal total protein is 6.0 to 8.0 g/dl, of which 68% is albumin.[19]

A decrease in serum albumin lessens the oncotic pressure so that the tissue oncotic pressure is greater and pulls fluid from the vascular space into the interstitial space, causing edema. The effects of a low serum albumin level are exacerbated when the liver, in need of amino acids for anabolism, breaks down albumin.

With normal kidney function, intact proteins are not filtered through the glomerulus because of their large size. In disease states of the kidney, however, glomerular membrane permeability is altered, and protein molecules pass into the glomerular filtrate and appear in the urine. This appearance of protein in the urine is a cardinal sign of renal compromise and, if left unchecked, can result in severely depleted body protein stores.

CHLORIDE

NORMAL SERUM VALUE

98-106 mEq/L

FUNCTIONS

Maintains body osmolality (in conjunction with sodium)
Aids in body water balance (in conjunction with sodium)
Competes with bicarbonate for recombination with sodium to maintain acid-base balance
Maintains acidity of body fluids (gastric juice)

BICARBONATE

NORMAL SERUM VALUE

24-28 mEq/L

FUNCTIONS

Buffers the acidity of body fluids (controls the hydrogen ion concentration and combines with other body salts to maintain acid-base balance)

FACTORS CONTROLLING FLUID VOLUME DEFICIT AND EXCESS

Neurohormonal Control

Antidiuretic hormone (ADH or arginine vasopressin) is secreted by the posterior pituitary gland and functions as the primary controller of extracellular fluid (ECF) volume. Several mechanisms stimulate or inhibit the release of ADH in response to a wide array of stimuli (see box below). In addition to the usual stimuli, the presence of severe stress, either emotional or physical, is thought to initiate ADH release through the limbic system (surrounding the hypothalamus). This mechanism, however, is less defined as a source of stimulation than are the osmoreceptors in the hypothalamus.[8]

FACTORS STIMULATING RELEASE OF ADH

Hyperosmolality of ECF
Hypovolemia
Increased body temperature
Medications
- Narcotics
- Antineoplastics
- Oral hypoglycemics
- Beta-adrenergic drugs

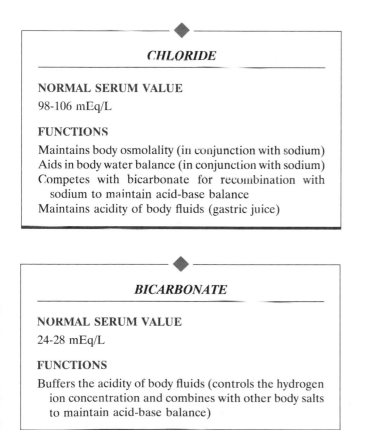

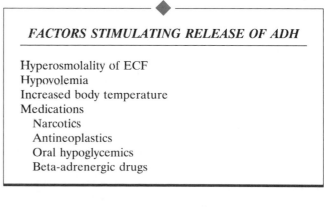

The strongest messages for release of ADH are sent by the osmoreceptors located in the hypothalamus. As serum osmolality rises above 385 mOsm/kg, ADH is released and carried through the circulation to the nephrons in the kidney. There ADH attaches to receptor sites in the loop of Henle, the distal convoluted tubule, and the collecting ducts. The action of ADH at these sites is to increase the permeability of the tubular structures to water. Water therefore can be reabsorbed into the circulatory system at a greater rate, leading to normalization of the serum osmolality and a steep rise in the urinary osmolality as less water in comparison to solute load is excreted.[8]

ADH can sustain the effect on the renal tubules only to a urinary osmolality of 1200 to 1400 mOsm/L. Therefore a secondary mechanism is required to maintain appropriate water reabsorption. That mechanism is thirst, which ensures that fluid will be consciously ingested to prevent water deficit.

◆ **Thirst.** The thirst center is located in the hypothalamus and is governed by the same osmoreceptors that stimulate ADH release. Two pathways exist for the stimulation of the thirst mechanism. First, hyperosmolality triggers osmoreceptors in the ventromedial nucleus of the hypothalmus to send impulses to the cerebral cortex. Second, hypovolemia leads to decreasing blood pressure, which stimulates baroreceptors in the chest, which in turn trigger thirst.[8] Control by the cerebral cortex makes thirst a mechanism that requires conscious effort to satisfy. To persons with limited ability to respond—such as adults who are comatose or disoriented, and infants—thirst may be stimulated in normal fashion but unsatiated; therefore fluid volume deficit may follow.[8]

ADH is easily inhibited by feedback mechanisms as discussed. The thirst mechanism, however, is less easily inhibited as is evidenced by patients' continued need to ingest fluid in the presence of edematous states, such as cardiac and renal failure.[8]

◆ **Renin-angiotensin-aldosterone system.** The inextricable relationship between sodium and water plays an important role in the influence of the renin-angiotensin-aldosterone system on body water regulation. As diagrammed in Fig. 31-8, a reduction in vascular volume stimulates the release of renin. Renin (in combination with angiotensinogen) splits the substance known as *angiotensin I* from the plasma globulins. Angiotensin I, in conjunction with converting enzymes in the lung, forms the powerful vasoconstrictor substance known as *angiotensin II.*

In turn, angiotensin II stimulates areas of the adrenal glands to secrete aldosterone (an adrenal mineralocorticoid), which acts on the renal tubules to reabsorb sodium into the circulation. When sodium is retained, so is water. Angiotensin II also constricts the renal vasculature, reducing renal blood flow and available glomerular filtrate, thus sending a signal to the posterior pituitary to release ADH. Frequently, in this way the two systems intertwine, not only to maintain fluid balance, but also to maintain electrolyte balance.[4]

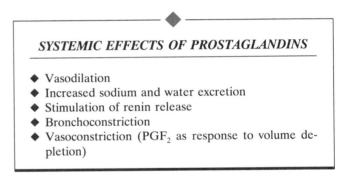

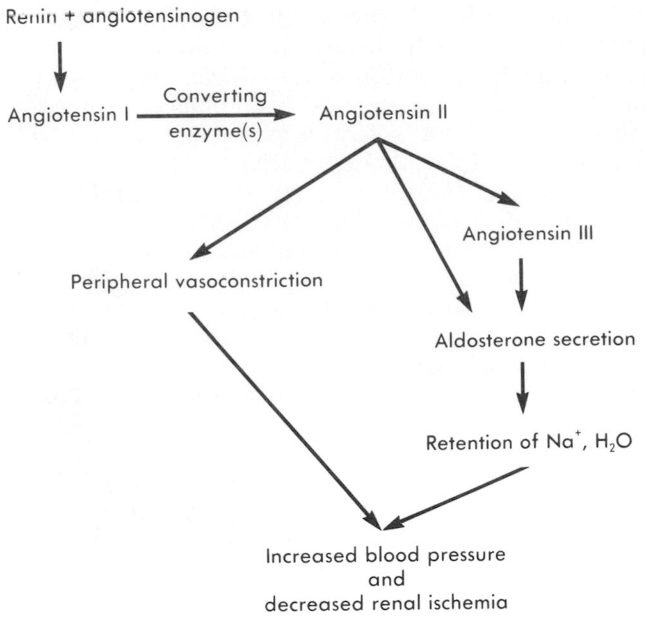

Fig. 31-8 The renin-angiotensin mechanism. (From Thompson JM and others: *Mosby's clinical nursing,* ed 3, St Louis, 1993, Mosby–Year Book.)

SYSTEMIC EFFECTS OF PROSTAGLANDINS

- Vasodilation
- Increased sodium and water excretion
- Stimulation of renin release
- Bronchoconstriction
- Vasoconstriction (PGF_2 as response to volume depletion)

◆ **Prostaglandins.** Prostaglandins play a pivotal role in the regulation of fluid and electrolyte balance. These localized hormonelike substances, which can be synthesized in many locations throughout the body, have very localized effects on those areas. Stimulation of prostaglandin production, however, may cause simultaneous changes in the kidneys, liver, and heart, resulting in widespread systemic changes.

Prostaglandins are produced in response to ECF volume overload or decreased perfusion of specialized tissues. The four distinct types of prostaglandins (PGE_2, PGF_{2a}, PGI_2, and PGD_2) exert such varied effects as vasodilation, increase in blood flow, increase in sodium and water excretion by the kidneys, and stimulation of the renin-angiotensin-aldosterone mechanism[20] (see box above).

At least two of the mechanisms that prostaglandins activate seem to oppose one another. In actuality, however, the opposition serves to fine-tune fluid and electrolyte balance. For example, prostaglandins directly affect the renal tubule to increase the rate of sodium and water excretion. At the same time, other prostaglandins stimulate the renin-angiotensin-aldosterone mechanism to favor sodium reabsorption. The opposition serves as a feedback mechanism to produce the appropriate type and amount of prostaglandins and, ultimately, to fine-tune water and sodium balance in the renal tubules.[20]

◆ **Atrial natriuretic peptide.** An additional influence on fluid and electrolyte regulation comes from the synthesis of atrial natriuretic peptide (ANP). This hormone is secreted from atrial cells through the coronary sinus in response to hypernatremia, hypervolemia, vasoconstriction, and decreased cardiac output. Atrial natriuretic hormone exerts many effects on sodium and water balance, among which are blocking aldosterone production, initiating vasodilation, and stimulating increased sodium and water excretion by the kidneys. Sites for stimulation of ANP production exist in the atrial walls, kidneys, lungs, vessel walls, eyes, brain, and adrenals. Production and release of ANP occur in response to the stimulation of stretch receptors that results from increased volume[21] (see box below).

Beneficial effects of ANP production include a reduction in fluid overload through diuresis, decreased cardiac workload, reduction in cardiac preload and afterload, and minor regulation of acid-base balance.[21] The primary effects of ANP delivery, however, appear to be circulatory volume control and blood pressure regulation.

Compartmental Fluid Shifts

Deficits and excesses of body fluids occur not through true gains or losses but through shifts between fluid compartments, leaving one compartment with a fluid deficiency and another with fluid overload. Osmotic and hydrostatic pressures influence the movement of fluids between the interstitial and intravascular compartments. A shift also may be the impetus for stimulating, through osmoreceptors or baroreceptors, the aforementioned sodium and fluid control mechanisms.

Colloid osmotic pressure is a pulling force generated by the plasma proteins. Because both the intravascular and interstitial compartments contain plasma proteins, colloid osmotic pressure is generated in both the intravascular and the interstitial space. Plasma colloid osmotic pressure maintains fluid in the intravascular compartment, and tissue colloid osmotic pressure maintains the fluid in the interstitial space. Albumin and, to a lesser extent, globulin generate this pulling force. Any condition that reduces the amount of albumin in the intravascular space (liver disease) or that changes the integrity of the membrane containing the proteins in the distinct compartments (burns) leads to fluid shifts. Although fluid shifts may not be considered true fluid deficits, the somatic responses to a deficit in one ECF compartment and an excess in the other are the same as for true loss of fluid from the body.[3]

Fluid balance depends on the relationship between the hydrostatic pressures in the tissue and vascular spaces and the osmotic pressures in the same spaces.

Hydrostatic pressure is produced through the action of the cardiovascular and lymphatic systems. Capillary hydrostatic pressure, on the other hand, is generated by the force of cardiac contraction. Tissue hydrostatic pressure is generated by the drainage of the lymphatic system.[3]

In addition to the differences in pressures, the membranes' permeability to solutes, water, and proteins and the surface area of the capillary endothelium affect water and solute movement.[3]

Renal Fluid Regulation

The dominant forces that regulate the renal response to fluid reabsorption and excretion are renal blood flow, glomerular filtration rate, and sodium regulation.[2,4] Secondary forces mediated by the circulatory system, sympathetic nervous system, and various hormones result in fine-tuning of fluid balance.

For example, inadequate renal blood flow reduces the pressure of the blood traveling into the glomerulus and elicits retention of sodium and water through renin release and the ADH mechanism. However, prolonged reduction in renal blood flow that impairs oxygen delivery produces tubular cell death, which begins to severely limit the ability of the tubules to accomplish excretion and reabsorption.

FACTORS STIMULATING RELEASE OF ATRIAL NATRIURETIC PEPTIDE

- Hypernatremia
- Hypervolemia
- Vasoconstriction
- Decreased cardiac output
- Increased cardiac preload and afterload
- Increased systemic vascular resistance

REFERENCES

1. Lancaster LE: Renal response to shock, *Crit Care Nurs Clin North Am* 2(2):221, 1990.
2. Chmielewski C: Renal anatomy and overview of nephron function, *ANNA J* 19(1):34, 1992.
3. Guyton AC: *Textbook of medical physiology,* ed 8, Philadelphia, 1991, WB Saunders.
4. Holechek MJ: Glomerular filtration and renal hemodynamics, *ANNA J* 19(3):237, 1992.
5. Ames SW, Kneisl CR: *Essentials of adult health nursing,* Menlo Park, Calif, 1988, Addison-Wesley.
6. Lancaster LE: Renal and endocrine regulation of water and electrolyte balance, *Nurs Clin North Am* 22(4), 1987.
7. Fischback FT: *A manual of laboratory diagnostic tests,* ed 4, Philadelphia, 1992, JB Lippincott.
8. Porth CM, Erickson M: Physiology of thirst and drinking: implication for nursing practice, *Heart Lung* 21(3):274, 1992.
9. Appel GB, Chase HS Jr: Diagnosis and treatment of acid-base disorders. In Askanazi J, Starker PM, Weissman C, editors: *Fluid and electrolyte management in critical care,* Boston, 1986, Butterworth Publishers.
10. Metheny NM: *Fluid and electrolyte balance – nursing considerations,* Philadelphia, 1987, JB Lippincott.
11. Oh MS, Carroll HJ: Regulation of extra- and intracellular fluid composition and content. In Arieff AI, Defronzo RA, editors: *Fluid electrolyte and acid-base disorders,* vol 1, New York, 1985, Churchill Livingstone.
12. Soltis B, Cassmeyer VL: Fluid and electrolyte imbalance. In Phipps WJ and others: *Medical-surgical nursing: concepts and clinical practice,* ed 4, St Louis, 1991, Mosby–Year Book.
13. Innerarity SA: Hyperkalemic emergencies, *Crit Care Nurs Q* 14(4):32, 1992.
14. Innerarity SA: Electrolyte emergencies in the critically ill renal patient, *Crit Care Nurs Clin North Am* 2(1):89, 1990.
15. Zaloga GP: Hypocalcemia in critically ill patients, *Crit Care Med* 20(2):251, 1992.
16. Kavanagh JM: Assessment of the cardiovascular system. In Phipps WJ and others: *Medical-surgical nursing: concepts and clinical practice,* ed 4, St Louis, 1991, Mosby–Year Book.
17. Thompson JM and others: *Mosby's clinical nursing,* ed 3, St Louis, 1993, Mosby–Year Book.
18. Workman ML: Magnesium and phosphorus: the neglected electrolytes, *AACN Clin Issues Crit Care Nurs* 3(3):655, 1992.
19. Kavanagh JM: Assessment of the cardiovascular system. In Phipps WJ and others: *Medical-surgical nursing: concepts and clinical practice,* ed 4, St Louis, 1991, Mosby–Year Book.
20. Spilman P, Whelton A: Nonsteroidal antiinflammatory drugs: effects on kidney function and implications for nursing care, *ANNA J* 19(1):19, 1992.
21. Birney MH, Penney DG: Atrial natriuretic peptide: a hormone with implications for clinical practice, *Heart Lung* 19(2):174, 1990.

32

Renal Clinical Assessment

CHAPTER OBJECTIVES

- Discuss the rationale involved in developing a consistent, sequential format for performing renal nursing assessment.
- Perform a thorough nursing assessment of a critically ill patient's renal system, and interpret the results.
- Identify methods for assessing normal skin turgor.
- Describe the pathophysiologic mechanism responsible for the development of edema and ascites, and identify the proper method for assessing each one.
- Describe the pathophysiologic mechanism responsible for orthostatic hypotension.

Understanding the anatomic location and physiologic workings of the body's fluids and electrolytes is of little or no value if the overt clinical manifestations of problems are not known or understood. The body presents a variety of clinical manifestations that demonstrate fluid and electrolyte disorders. A methodic examination furnishes data that help pinpoint the actual problem. The following section explains the process of taking a fluid and electrolyte history and assessing fluid and electrolyte balance. An outline of this information is presented in the box on p. 594.

HISTORY

A renal history should begin with a description of the chief symptom, written in the patient's own words. It is wise, however, to avoid accepting the patient's perception of what may have been the cause of the problem. Included in the description of the chief complaint should be its onset, location, and duration and factors that lessen or aggravate the problem.[1,2] Descriptions of any treatment sought by the individual, medications taken to alleviate symptoms, or procedures performed to ameliorate the problem often are helpful in delineating the extent of the current complaint.

Of particular concern in gaining a complete renal and fluid history is the patient's medical history. Similar symptoms, problems, or treatment for complaints in the past may give important clues to current treatment or may aid in establishing the cause of the problem. The patient and his or her family or significant other must provide as much detail as possible about the history.

The family history also may provide important information to aid in identifying and treating the patient's disorder. For example, the patient may reveal that one or two close family members have always had swelling of the extremities or high blood pressure. These symptoms might lead to questions about any history of kidney problems. A history is investigative and usually progressive in nature, with one question often leading to another.

PHYSICAL EXAMINATION

Inspection

Renal assessment begins with an inspection of the patient's neck veins. The supine position facilitates normal venous distention. In the absence of distention, the examiner suspects hypovolemia. Assessment continues with the head of the bed elevated to 45 to 90 degrees. If the veins remain distended more than 2 cm above the sternal notch when the bed is at 45 degrees, fluid overload may be suspected.[3]

The next step, hand vein inspection, is performed simply by observing for venous distention, which is the expected response when the hand is held in the dependent position. Venous filling that takes longer than 5 seconds suggests hypovolemia. When the hand is elevated, the distention should disappear within 5 seconds. If distention does not disappear within 5 seconds after the hand is elevated, fluid overload is suspected.

Inspection of the skin and mucous membranes provides readily visible signs of fluid alterations. When a fluid volume *deficit* exists, skin loses elasticity and mucous membranes become sticky. If a fluid volume *excess* exists, edema sometimes is present, particularly in dependent areas of the body. Without further assessment, however, the imbalance cannot be positively identified. Other disorders and contributing factors might lead to an inaccurate assumption of a fluid volume disorder. Mouth breathing, for instance, can dry the oral mucous membranes temporarily. A more accurate way to assess the fluid status of the oral cavity is to inspect the mouth with the use of a tongue blade. Stickiness of this area is more indicative of fluid volume deficit than are complaints of a dry mouth.[3]

Assessment of skin turgor provides additional data for identifying fluid-related problems. As the skin over the forearm is picked up and released, the rapidity of its return to its normal position should be observed. Normal elasticity and fluid status allow almost immediate return to shape once the skin is released. In fluid volume deficit,

IMPORTANT ASPECTS OF FLUID AND ELECTROLYTE ASSESSMENT

NURSING HISTORY

1. Chief complaint
2. History of present problem
   a. Onset
   b. Duration
   c. Clinical manifestations
   d. Medical management
   e. Medications
3. History of fluid or renal problems or familial history of fluid or renal problems
4. Dietary likes/dislikes/intake each day
5. Fluid likes/dislikes/intake each day
6. Dentures; if used, oral condition/hygiene
7. Cultural background
8. Educational background

NURSING ASSESSMENT

Fluid status (deficit/excess)

1. Skin turgor
2. Mucous membranes
3. Intake and output
4. Presence of edema/ascites
5. Diaphoresis
6. Low-grade fever
7. Neck and hand vein engorgement
8. Lung sounds—crackles
9. Dyspnea
10. Central venous pressure (CVP) <5 cm H_2O, >15 cm H_2O
11. Pulmonary capillary wedge pressure (PCWP) <10 mm Hg, >18 mm Hg
12. Tachycardia
13. Blood pressure (hypertension or hypotension)
14. Cardiac index (CI) <2 L/min/m^2
15. S_3, S_4 heart sounds
16. Headache
17. Blurred vision
18. Vertigo on rising
19. Papilledema
20. Behavioral and/or mental changes

Electrolyte status

1. Serum osmolality
2. Complete blood count (CBC)
3. Serum electrolyte level
4. Electrocardiogram (ECG) tracings (potassium, calcium, magnesium levels)
5. Behavioral and/or mental changes
6. Chvostek's, Trousseau's signs (calcium levels)
7. Changes in peripheral sensation (numbness, tremors)
8. Muscle strength
9. Gastrointestinal (GI) changes (nausea and vomiting)
10. Therapies that can alter electrolyte status (GI suction, diuretics, antihypertensives, calcium channel blockers)

however, the skin remains raised and does not return to its normal position for several seconds. Because of the usual loss of skin elasticity in elderly persons, this test is not accurate for fluid assessment of this age-group. Thus skin turgor can be assessed in the shoulder area, which retains elasticity.[3]

Changes in skin texture and overall appearance reveal much about fluid status. For example, the patient with renal failure has rough, dry skin and deposits of urate crystals on the skin, called *uremic frost.* These patients frequently have scratch marks because of the pruritus associated with renal failure.

Edema is defined as the presence of excess fluid in the interstitial space. The presence of edema, however, does not always indicate true fluid overload; a loss of albumin from the vascular space can cause peripheral edema, yet hypovolemia may be present.

Edema usually is assessed by applying fingertip pressure on the skin over a bony prominence, such as the ankles, pretibial areas (shins), and the sacrum. If the indentation made by the fingertip does not disappear within 30 seconds, "pitting" edema is present. Pitting edema indicates increased interstitial volume and is not evident until a weight gain of approximately 10% has occurred.[4] It is gauged by a subjective scale of 1 to 4, with +1 indicating only minimal pitting and +4 indicating severe pitting (see Table 32-1). Edema also may appear in hands and feet, around the eyes, and in the cheeks. Dependent areas, such as the sacrum, are the most likely to demonstrate edema in patients chronically confined to a wheelchair or bed. Skeletal muscles, which usually do not reveal changes in fluid status, reflect changes in electrolyte levels. A skeletal muscle change to weakness or paralysis usually signals a deficit of an electrolyte, particularly of a major cation (potassium and sodium). A calcium deficit, however, leads to the opposite extreme—severe cramping and muscle spasm.

Table 32-1 Pitting edema scale

Rating	Approximate equivalent
+1	5 mm depth
+2	8-10 mm depth
+3	>10 mm (lasting up to 30 sec)
+4	>20 mm (lasting longer than 30 sec)

Auscultation

Although auscultation is perhaps the most difficult area of assessment to master, it provides more accurate information about extracellular fluid (ECF) changes than the areas of assessment previously discussed. Listening for specific sounds in the heart and lungs provides information about the presence or absence of increased fluid in the interstitium or vascular space.

Auscultation of the heart requires not only assessing rate and rhythm but also listening for extra sounds, such as third and fourth heart sounds. Increased heart rate alone does not offer much data about fluid volume, but combined with a low blood pressure, it may indicate hypovolemia. Often hypertension is accompanied by a third or fourth heart sound, which may signal the presence of fluid overload. Caution should be exercised, however, in making assumptions about fluid status on the basis of a murmur, because murmurs also may be present in other cardiac disorders.[1]

Hypertension, which may indicate fluid overload, also can be caused by atherosclerotic or arteriosclerotic vessel changes. Blood pressure readings should be taken at rest with the patient lying, sitting, and standing. A comparison of the three readings should help establish a baseline from which to compare subsequent readings.

A drastic drop in pressure from lying to sitting or from sitting to standing represents an orthostatic drop known as *orthostatic hypotension.* A drop of 20 mm Hg in pressure, which can indicate a fluid volume deficit, occurs when the venous circulation is so volume-depleted that a sufficient preload is not immediately available after the position change. Orthostatic hypotension produces feelings of weakness or faintness. Peripheral vascular disease, however, which often damages the venous circulation of the lower extremities, may be responsible for orthostatic drops in the absence of hypovolemia.

Vascular sounds heard by auscultating major vessels are called *bruits* (Fig. 32-1). A bruit is a blowing or swishing sound, much like cardiac murmurs.[1,5] Fluid volume excess, coupled with stenosis or any impediment to vascular flow, produces a loud bruit.

Lung assessment is extremely important in gauging fluid status. Crackles indicate fluid volume excess. Dyspnea with any mild exertion or dyspnea at night that prevents sleeping in a supine position may indicate fluid overload. Shallow, gasping breaths punctuated by periods of apnea may reflect severe acid-base imbalances. Because the lungs are among the primary controllers of acid-base balance, it is important to identify the types of respiratory changes associated with each condition.

Palpation

Although palpation of the kidneys is not directly linked to fluid and electrolyte assessments, any subtle changes in kidney function can result in problems with fluids and electrolytes. Palpation of the kidneys is achieved through the bimanual capturing approach.

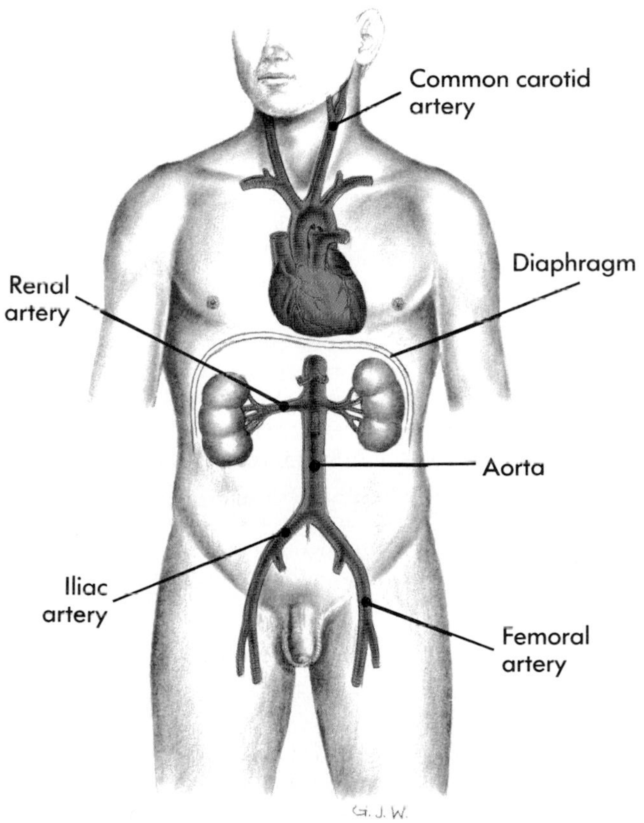

Fig. 32-1 Sites for auscultation of bruits.

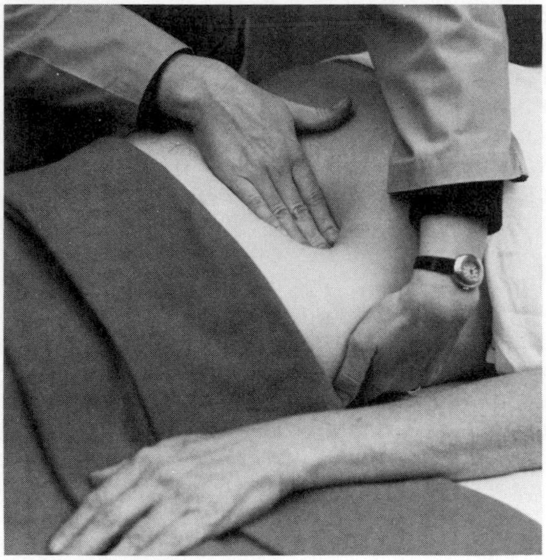

Fig. 32-2 Palpation of the kidney. (From Malasanos L, Barkauskas V, Stoltenberg-Allen K: *Health assessment,* ed 4, St Louis, 1990, Mosby–Year Book.)

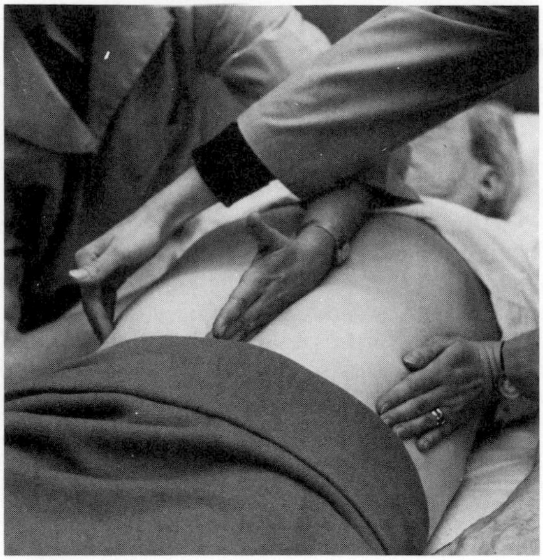

Fig. 32-3 Test for the presence of a fluid wave. (From Malasanos L, Barkauskas V, Stoltenberg-Allen K: *Health assessment,* ed 4, St Louis, 1990, Mosby–Year Book.)

Capturing is accomplished by placing one hand posteriorly under the flank of the supine patient with fingers pointing to the midline, while placing the opposite hand just below the rib cage anteriorly. The patient is asked to inhale deeply, while pressure is exerted to bring the hands together (Fig. 32-2). As the patient exhales, the examiner should feel the kidney between his or her hands. After each kidney is palpated in this manner, the two should be compared for size and shape. Each kidney should be firm, smooth, and of equal size.[4,5]

Problems should be suspected if an irregular surface is palpated, a size difference is detected, or the kidney extends significantly lower than the rib cage on either side. It should be remembered, however, that the right kidney does extend somewhat lower than the left as a result of its displacement by the liver.

Percussion

Percussion is performed to detect pain in the area of an organ or to determine excess accumulation of air, fluid, or solids in a body cavity. Although percussion of the kidneys per se does not give direct evidence of fluid and electrolyte level abnormalities, it can provide information about kidney location, size, and possible problems that could lead to future fluid and electrolyte level abnormalities.[2]

Percussion of the kidney is performed with the patient in a side-lying or sitting position, with the examiner's hand placed over the costovertebral angle (lower border of the rib cage on the flank). Striking the back of the hand with the opposite fist produces a dull thud, which is normal. Pain may indicate infection.

Observation and percussion of the abdomen also are of value in assessing fluid status. Percussing the abdomen (using the same procedure as for the kidneys but placing the patient supine) can result in a dull sound (solid bowel contents or fluid) or a hollow sound (gaseous bowel).[1,5]

Ascites, defined simply as severe fluid distention of the abdominal cavity, is an important observation in determining fluid imbalances. Differentiating ascites from distortion caused by solid bowel contents is accomplished by producing what is called the *fluid wave.* The fluid wave is elicited by exerting pressure to the abdominal midline while one hand is placed on the right or left flank. Tapping the opposite flank produces a wave in the accumulated fluid that can be felt under the hands (Fig. 32-3). Other signs of ascites are a protuberant, rounded abdomen and abdominal striae.

Ascites may or may not represent fluid volume excess. Severe ascites in persons with a compromised hepatic system actually may result from hypovolemia. The ascites occurs because the increased vascular pressure associated with hepatic dysfunction forces fluid and plasma proteins from the vascular space to the interstitial space and abdominal cavity. On the other hand, persons with renal failure may have ascites caused by true volume overload, which forces fluid into the abdomen because of increased capillary hydrostatic pressures.

Weight

One of the most important assessments of fluid status is the patient's weight. Significant fluctuations in body weight over a 1- to 2-day period indicate fluid gains and losses. This important sign often is forgotten or ignored, however, during assessment of the individual's renal and fluid status.

When possible, the patient should be weighed during admission to the critical care unit. It is important to note whether the current weight differs significantly from the weight 1 to 2 weeks before admission. Thereafter, the patient should be weighed daily for comparison with the previous day's weight. The weight should be obtained at the same time each day, with the patient wearing the same amount of clothing. One liter of fluid equals 1 kg, or approximately 2.2 pounds.

The individual's weight is of critical importance to the dialysis nurse caring for a patient with renal failure. The differences in weight from day to day are used in a mathematic formula for calculating the amount of fluid to remove during a dialysis treatment. Therefore setting the appropriate parameters for a safe, comfortable, yet effective hemodialysis treatment depends in large part on obtaining the patient's weight.

Intake and Output

Intake and output can be compared with the patient's weight to evaluate accurately the gain or loss of fluid. Urinary output plus insensible fluid losses (perspiration and water vapor from the lungs) can range widely from 750 to 2400 ml daily. When intake exceeds output, a positive fluid state exists. If disorders such as renal failure perpetuate the positive fluid gain, fluid overload results. Conversely, if output exceeds intake (fever, increased respiration, profuse sweating, vomiting, diarrhea, gastric suction), a negative fluid state exists.

Abnormal output of body fluids creates not only fluid imbalances but also electrolyte and acid-base disturbances. For example, gastrointestinal suction or loss by diarrhea can result in fluid deficit, sodium and potassium deficits, and metabolic acidosis (from excessive loss of bicarbonate). During a 24-hour period, fever can increase skin and respiratory losses by as much as 75 ml/1° F rise.[3]

In maintaining daily records of intake and output, all gains or losses must be recorded. A standard list of the fluid volume held in various containers (e.g., milk cartons and juice containers) expedites this process. Discussions about the importance of accurate intake and output with the patient and family or friends are necessary and can improve the accuracy of record keeping.

Hemodynamic Monitoring

Body fluid status is accurately reflected in measurements of cardiovascular hemodynamics. Measurements such as central venous pressure (CVP), pulmonary capillary wedge pressure (PCWP), left ventricular end-diastolic pressure (LVEDP), cardiac index (CI), and mean arterial pressure (MAP) provide for a clear picture of the increases or decreases in vascular volume returning and being ejected from the heart. Indeed, both volume depletion and overload can be easily detected by use of central vein or arterial catheters from which pressure measurements can be obtained (Table 32-2).

The CVP generally represents the filling pressures of the right atrium and thereby grossly represents a measurement of cardiac preload. Although CVP still is used in some cases, it can be altered by many factors, among which are patient position. A normal CVP is 5 to 15 cm H_2O.[6] In cases of volume depletion the CVP is less than 4 cm H_2O, whereas volume overload is reflected by readings of more than 15 cm H_2O.

Table 32-2 Hemodynamic assessment of fluid status

Measurement	Volume depletion	Volume overload
CVP	<4 cm H_2O	>15 cm H_2O
RAP	Normal or increased	Increased
PCWP	<4 mm Hg	>12 mm Hg
CI	<2.7 L/min/m^2	>4.3 L/min/m^2
MAP	Decreased or increased	Decreased or increased

The mean right atrial pressure (RAP) is more commonly used in the critical care area. This pressure represents the difference between the systolic and diastolic blood pressures in the right atrium. An acceptable RAP is up to 6 mm Hg.[7] In hypovolemic states the RAP may be normal, slightly elevated, or rapidly falling, depending on the degree of ongoing fluid loss and the presence of effects of compensatory mechanisms.[7] In fluid overload the RAP is increased.

The PCWP represents the left atrial pressure required to fill the left ventricle, whereas LVEDP represents the filling pressure of the left ventricle at the end of diastole.[8,9] In the healthy heart there is little impedence to equilibration of both the pressures. Therefore PCWP may be used to reflect LVEDP. If, however, barriers to flow exist, such as mitral valve disease or pulmonary vascular obstruction, the PCWP is greater than the LVEDP. The normal PCWP is 4 to 12 mm Hg.[7,9]

The CI represents the individual's cardiac output divided by the body surface area. This calculation, which demonstrates the cardiac output, or ejection volume of the left ventricle, is standardized for body size. The normal CI is 2.7 to 4.3 L/min/m^2. Compensatory mechanisms in early hypovolemic shock maintain the CI at or near normal. With prolonged loss, however, the CI falls. Fluid volume overload increases heart rate, which in turn increases cardiac output to a point. Pump failure may result from massive volume overload, in which case the CI falls.[7]

MAP is the product of systemic vascular resistance (SVR) times the cardiac output. This parameter represents an average of blood pressure within the cardiac system. Changes in SVR or cardiac output inevitably result in corresponding MAP changes. For example, an increase in SVR during the early stages of hypovolemic shock leads to elevation of the MAP. Ongoing losses eventually lead to a decreased cardiac output, which leads to a reduction in MAP.[7,9] (See Chapter 46 for more in-depth discussion of hemodynamic changes in hypovolemic shock.)

Other Clinical Observations

Disturbances in fluid and electrolyte levels often are accompanied by clinical manifestations less measurable than those previously mentioned but that, nonetheless, indicate serious change.

Changes in mental status, such as disorientation, often are caused by acidosis. Lethargy, coma, and confusion may result from sodium, calcium, or magnesium excess or deficit. Apprehension may be secondary to sodium deficit or to a shift of fluid from the plasma to the interstitium.[5] Also, persons with respiratory changes caused by fluid volume overload frequently are apprehensive.

Finally, apathy and withdrawal often accompany hypovolemic states.[5] Patients with renal failure with systemic increases in electrolytes, fluids, and nitrogenous waste products also can exhibit apathy, restlessness, confusion, and withdrawal. It often is difficult to separate the emotional component from the actual physiologic mechanism. Nonetheless, the importance of considering a fluid or electrolyte disorder as the cause of a mental or emotional change must be emphasized.

REFERENCES

1. Bates B: *A guide to physical examination,* ed 5, Philadelphia, 1991, JB Lippincott.
2. Baer CL, Lancaster LE: Acute renal failure, *Crit Care Nurs Q* 14(4):1, 1992.
3. Metheny NM: *Fluid and electrolyte balance—nursing considerations,* Philadelphia, 1987, JB Lippincott.
4. Grimes J, Burns E: *Health assessment in nursing practice,* ed 3, Boston, 1992, Jones & Bartlett.
5. Malasanos L, Barkauskas V, Stoltenberg-Allen K: *Health assessment,* ed 4, St Louis, 1990, Mosby–Year Book.
6. Pauley SY: Massive hemorrhage in trauma: the initial assessment, treatment, and monitoring, *NITA* 10(16):410, 1987.
7. Bustin D.: *Hemodynamic monitoring for critical care,* Norwalk, Conn, 1986, Appleton-Century-Crofts.
8. Zorb S: Care of the cardiac patient: assessment, evaluation, and nursing implications, *J Intravenous Nurs* 11(2):113, 1988.
9. Ley J: Fluid therapy following intracardiac operation, *Crit Care Nurse* 8(1):26, 1988.

33

Renal Diagnostic Procedures

CHAPTER OBJECTIVES

- Describe the effect of decreased serum albumin levels on fluid dynamics within the body.
- Identify how alterations of both the hemoglobin and the hematocrit levels can signal fluid volume deficit or excess.
- Explain why elevations of blood urea nitrogen and creatinine can signal renal dysfunction.
- Describe the relationship between serum osmolality and antidiuretic hormone.

A number of laboratory tests and diagnostic procedures are used to assess renal and fluid status. This chapter explains the most definitive tests.

LABORATORY ASSESSMENT

Serum

◆ **Albumin.** Slightly more than 50% of the total plasma protein is serum albumin. It is manufactured in the liver, and its normal blood levels are 3.5 to 5.5 g/dl. Albumin is primarily responsible for the maintenance of colloid osmotic pressure, which functions to hold fluid in the vascular space. The blood vessel walls, because of their impermeability to plasma proteins, prevent albumin from leaving the vascular space. But with third-degree burns (membrane destruction) or nephrotic syndrome (increased glomerular capillary permeability), albumin can escape from the vascular space and enter the interstitial space. In this process, the albumin carries along water, thereby creating a fluid shift.

Decreased albumin levels result in a plasma-to-interstitium fluid shift, which creates peripheral edema. A decreased albumin level can occur as a result of protein-calorie malnutrition in which available stores of albumin are depleted, oncotic pressure is decreased, and fluid is shifted from the vascular space to the interstitial space. Liver disease also can cause a fall in albumin levels as the diseased liver fails to synthesize sufficient albumin. Further, severe portal hypertension can force albumin and other plasma proteins into the abdominal cavity, creating ascites.

Increased albumin levels are rare. The body uses a fixed amount of protein for energy and body cell replacement and converts excess protein into stored fat. Most often if all plasma proteins are elevated, fluid volume deficit (hemoconcentration) is suspected.

◆ **Hemoglobin and hematocrit.** The hemoglobin (Hgb) and hematocrit (Hct) levels can indicate increases or decreases in intravascular fluid volume. Both Hgb and Hct values vary between genders, with the Hgb value in males normally 13.5 to 17.5 g/dl and in females 12 to 16 g/dl. The Hct value ranges from 40% to 54% in males and 37% to 47% in females. Hemoglobin transports oxygen and carbon dioxide; thus it maintains cellular metabolism and acid-base balance.

The hematocrit expresses the percentage of red blood cells (RBCs) in a volume of whole blood. An increase in the hematocrit often indicates a severe fluid volume deficit, which results in hemoconcentration—hence the elevated Hct level. Although rare, true disorders of RBC production, such as polycythemia, can result in an increased Hct level.

Conversely, a decreased Hct level can indicate fluid volume excess because of the dilutional effect of the extra fluid load. Decreases, however, also can result from anemias, blood loss, liver damage, or hemolytic reactions.[1] The history and bedside assessment aid in determining whether fluid imbalances or disease states, or both, are responsible.

◆ **Blood urea nitrogen and creatinine.** Blood urea nitrogen (BUN) and creatinine are both by-products of protein metabolism. The normal value for BUN is 9 to 20 mg/dl, and the normal value for creatinine is 0.7 to 1.5 mg/dl. The importance of these two serum tests is the disclosure of increased or decreased serum levels. Both BUN and creatinine levels become elevated when renal function deteriorates.

Creatinine is a by-product of normal cell metabolism and appears in serum in amounts proportional to the body muscle mass. Creatinine is easily excreted by the renal tubules. Tracing the amount of creatinine in the excreted urine and the amount of creatinine in the blood over 24 hours provides accurate information about kidney function.

Creatinine excess occurs most often in persons with renal failure in whom the diminished renal function impairs creatinine excretion. Muscle growth disorders such as acromegaly, however, can produce elevations through increased muscle mass. Also, malnutrition can result in transient increases in creatinine levels as the rapid muscle catabolism associated with malnutrition causes "dumping" of increased levels of creatinine into the circulation. Decreased levels of creatinine are rare and usually are associated with muscular dystrophy.[1]

BUN levels are not as accurate an indicator of renal failure as is the creatinine level because BUN levels fluctuate greatly with protein intake, whereas creatinine levels are relatively unaffected by protein intake. Elevations in the BUN level can be correlated with the clinical manifestations of uremia; as the BUN value rises, symptoms of uremia become more pronounced as a result of the irritation this metabolite produces on bodily membranes.

Increased levels of BUN (often called *urea*) also occur with fluid volume deficit (hemoconcentration), infection, medications, excessive protein intake, and renal failure. Decreased levels can result from fluid volume excess, liver failure, or protein malnutrition.[1]

◆ **Anion gap.** The anion gap is a calculation of the difference between the measurable cations (sodium and potassium) and the measurable anions (chloride and bicarbonate). The value represents the remaining unmeasurable anions present in the extracellular fluid (e.g., phosphates, sulfates, ketones, pyruvate, lactate). The following formula generally is used in the calculation of the anion gap:

$$Na^+ - (Cl^- + HCO_3^-)$$

Normal value is 10 to 12 mEq/L and should not exceed 14 mEq/L. An increased anion gap level reflects overproduction or poor excretion of acid products.[2,3]

Renal failure can increase the anion gap value because of retention of acids and altered bicarbonate reabsorption. Diabetic ketoacidosis results in ketone production, which also elevates the level of the anion gap. The measurement of the anion gap is a rapid, effective method for identifying acid-base imbalance, but it cannot be used to pinpoint the actual acid-base disturbance specifically.

◆ **Osmolality.** The serum osmolality level reflects the concentration or dilution of vascular fluid. The normal serum osmolality level is 275 to 295 mOsm/L.[1] Antidiuretic hormone (ADH) plays an important role in maintaining the serum osmolality level. When the serum osmolality level increases (e.g., with insufficient fluid intake), ADH is released from the pituitary gland and stimulates increased water reabsorption, which expands the vascular space and brings the serum osmolality level back to normal. A more concentrated urine also results. The opposite case occurs with a decreased serum osmolality level, which inhibits the production of ADH and results in increased excretion of water through the kidneys, producing dilute urine and bringing the serum osmolality level back to normal.

Urine

Urinary volume, contents, color, clarity, acidity, alkalinity, and odor provide excellent information about the patient's condition relative to fluids and electrolytes. Specific tests are presented in Table 33-1; several are discussed in greater detail to clarify certain disorders.

◆ **pH.** Urine pH indicates the acidity or alkalinity of the urine. The normal urinary pH level is 6.0, which is acidic, but it may range from 4.5 to 8.0. As the kidney regulates acid-base balance, far more hydrogen ions are excreted than bicarbonate ions, creating the acidity of the urine. Therefore changes in renal function produce changes in urinary pH value.

Table 33-1 Essential urinalysis tests for diagnosing renal disorders

Substance	Normal values
Specific gravity	1.003-1.030
Urinary osmolality	300-1200 mOsm/L
Urinary pH	4.5-8.0
Urinary electrolytes	
Sodium	80-180 mEq/24 hr
Potassium	40-80 mEq/24 hr
Chloride	110-20 mEq/24 hr
Calcium	50-300 mEq/24 hr

An increase in urinary acidity (decreased level of pH) indicates retention of sodium and acids by the body. Conversely, a decrease in urinary acidity (increased pH or more alkaline level) means the body is retaining bicarbonate. However, urinary pH levels are greatly affected by diet and medications. Certain food groups, such as citrus fruits and vegetables, lead to alkaline urine, whereas a diet high in protein can produce acid urine.

◆ **Specific gravity.** Specific gravity measures the density or weight of urine compared with that of distilled water. The normal urinary specific gravity level is 1.003 to 1.030 as compared with the normal specific gravity level of distilled water at 1.000. Because urine is composed of many solutes and substances suspended in water, its specific gravity level should always be higher than that of water, and it indicates the ability of the kidney to dilute or concentrate the urine.

Decreases in specific gravity values reflect inability of the kidneys to excrete the usual solute load into urine (less dense with fewer solutes). Increases in specific gravity values (a more concentrated urine) occur with a body fluid volume deficit as the result of fever, vomiting, or diarrhea. An increased specific gravity value also can occur with diabetes or glomerular membrane permeability changes, which allow glucose and protein in the urine, thereby increasing urine concentrations.[1,3]

◆ **Osmolality.** The urinary osmolality value more accurately pinpoints fluid balance than does the serum osmolality value, because the serum osmolality value is actually a reflection of serum sodium concentration and therefore is subject to far more influences than is the urinary osmolality value. The simultaneous measurement of both the serum and urinary osmolality levels, however, provides a more accurate assessment of fluid status. Normal urinary osmolality level is 300 to 1200 mOsm/kg and depends on reabsorption or excretion of water in the kidney tubules. The urinary osmolality level increases during fluid volume deficit because of the retention of fluid by the body. Conversely, the urinary osmolality level decreases during volume excess because fluid is excreted by the kidneys. In late renal failure, the urinary osmolality value usually is quite low because solutes and fluids are being abnormally retained.[4]

◆ **Glucose.** Glucose normally is reabsorbed by the renal tubules; therefore urine should be free of glucose. The appearance of glucose in urine, however, may be transient in nature, brought on by ingestion of a heavy carbohydrate load or caused by stress or the renal changes that accompany pregnancy.

Consistent appearance of glycosuria occurs during hyperglycemic episodes of diabetes when the renal threshold for glucose is exceeded and the excess glucose spills into the urine. When renal failure accompanies hyperglycemia, however, glycosuria cannot be considered indicative of the level of hyperglycemia because of the erratic excretion of glucose by the damaged nephrons.

◆ **Protein.** Protein, like glucose, normally is absent from urine because the large protein molecule cannot pass across the normal glomerular capillary membrane. Thus consistent appearance of protein in urine suggests compromise of the glomerular membrane and possible renal disease.

Transient appearance of protein in the urine can occur as the result of efferent arteriole constriction caused by stress, medications, extreme exercise, or extreme cold. Also, *proteinuria* can occur after ingestion of a high-protein meal or can accompany the renal changes associated with pregnancy.

Levels of proteinuria of 0.5 to 4.0 g/day indicate renal compromise, and the amount excreted directly correlates with the severity of the damage.[1]

◆ **Electrolytes.** Levels of urinary electrolytes are not as frequently measured as are serum electrolytes because of the lesser significance of urinary findings. To measure urinary electrolyte levels, a 24-hour urine sample is required. The electrolyte levels are highly variable, and the electrolytes depend on the kidneys for adequate excretion. Consequently, decreases in urinary electrolyte levels are highly suggestive of renal failure. The urinary sodium level, on the other hand, may increase because of the inability of aldosterone to effect sodium reabsorption in the damaged nephrons.[1]

◆ **Sediment.** The presence of epithelial cells and *casts* aids in identifying problems related to the kidneys. Casts are shells or clumps of cellular breakdown or proteinaceous materials that form in the renal tubular system and are washed out in the urinary flow. Although small numbers of epithelial cells normally appear in the urine and an occasional cast may be found, their consistent appearance is abnormal.

Consistent appearance of epithelial cells shed by the nephron may indicate *nephritis.* Casts differ in composition and size, and both characteristics correlate with the severity and type of renal damage. White blood cell casts indicate pyelonephritis and also occur during the exudative stage of acute glomerulonephritis. Red blood cell casts indicate glomerulonephritis, whereas hyaline casts are associated with renal parenchymal disease and glomerular capillary membrane inflammation.

DIAGNOSTIC PROCEDURES

Radiologic Assessment

Although laboratory assessment is used foremost in diagnosing renal and urologic problems, radiologic assessment confirms or clarifies causes of particular disorders. Radiologic assessment ranges from the simple to the sophisticated (Table 33-2) and provides informa-

Table 33-2 Renal imaging tests

Test	Comments
Kidney-ureter-bladder (KUB)	Flat-plate x-ray film of abdomen determines position, size, and structure of kidneys and urinary tract. KUB usually is followed by more sophisticated tests.
Intravenous pyelography (IVP)	Intravenous injection of contrast media plus x-ray film allows visualization of internal kidney (parenchyma, calyces, pelves, ureters, bladder). Timing of stages can delineate size and shape. Obstructions and tumors can be found. Drawback can be hypersensitivity to contrast medium.
Retrograde pyelography	Injection of iodine-based contrast medium through ureteral catheter into collection system (calyces, pelves, and ureters) allows visualization of clots, stones, and strictures. It may be useful when allergy to IVP dye exists (less chance of hypersensitivity in this test).
Renal angiography	Injection of contrast medium into arterial blood perfusing the kidney allows x-ray visualization of renal blood flow. Stenoses, cysts, clots, and tumors may be visualized, as may infarctions, traumas, and torn kidneys.
Renal computed tomographic (CT) scan	After administration of a radioisotope, which is absorbed by the kidneys, scintillation photography is performed in several planes. Density of the image helps determine tumor, cysts, hemorrhage, calcification, adrenal tumors, or necrosis. It may be used before or instead of renal biopsy.
Renal ultrasonography	High-frequency sound waves are transmitted to the kidneys and urinary tract and viewed on an oscilloscope. This type of test usually is used to search for fluid accumulation or obstruction.

Continued.

Table 33-2 Renal imaging tests—cont'd

Test	Comments
Magnetic Resonance Imaging (MRI)	A scanner produces three-dimensional images in response to the application of high-energy radiofrequency waves to the tissues. MRI produces clear images; the density of the image may indicate lesions, malformation of tissue, vessels, or tubules, and necrosis. MRI is more specific than renal ultrasonography or CT scan. It is helpful in the detection of renal masses, particularly in distinguishing simple cysts from those complicated by hemorrhage. MRI is noninvasive and painless, does not expose the patient to any known risks, and has no known complications.

tion about abnormal masses, abnormal fluid collection, congenital abnormalities, obstructions, and other disorders of the kidneys and urinary tract.[5]

Renal Biopsy

Renal biopsy is the definitive tool for diagnosing disease processes of the kidney. Two methods are used—closed biopsy and open biopsy. In either case, biopsy should be the last resort in diagnostic assessment because of the postprocedural risks of bleeding, hematoma formation, and infection.

Percutaneous needle biopsy (closed method) involves a flank introduction of a cannula (over an obturator) for obtaining a specimen containing both cortical and medullary kidney tissue. Open biopsy is actual surgical visualization of the kidney, at which time a tissue sample is obtained. Specimens are then examined in the laboratory. Biopsy determines the presence of diseases such as glomerulonephritis, amyloidosis, and lupus erythematosus and the cause of renal lesions.

REFERENCES

1. Fischbach F: *A manual of laboratory diagnostic tests,* ed 4, Philadelphia, 1992, JB Lippincott.
2. Narins RG Jr and others: Metabolic acid-base disorders: pathophysiology, classification and treatment. In Arieff AI, DeFronzo RA, editors: *Fluid, electrolyte and acid-base disorders,* vol 1, New York, 1985, Churchill Livingstone.
3. Tilkian SM, Conover MB, Tilkian AG: *Clinical implications of laboratory tests,* ed 4, St Louis, 1987, Mosby–Year Book.
4. Shorecki KL, Brenner BM: Edema forming states: congestive heart failure, liver disease, and nephrotic syndrome. In Arieff AI, DeFronzo RA, editors: *Fluid, electrolyte and acid-base disorders,* vol 1, New York, 1985, Churchill Livingstone.
5. Thompson JM and others: *Mosby's clinical nursing,* ed 3, St Louis, 1993, Mosby–Year Book.

34

Renal Disorders

CHAPTER OBJECTIVES

- List clinical manifestations of each of the serum electrolyte disturbances discussed in this chapter.
- Discuss nursing implications for the patient with an electrolyte disturbance.
- Differentiate bicarbonate and pH findings in metabolic acidosis and alkalosis.
- Describe the etiology of acute renal failure.
- Discuss the stages of acute renal failure.
- Describe important aspects of nursing management for the patient with acute renal failure.

ELECTROLYTE DISTURBANCES

Hypokalemia

Hypokalemia is a potassium deficit of the extracellular fluid (ECF), with a serum potassium level less than 3.5 mEq/L. Potassium deficit occurs as a result of the body's tendency to excrete potassium and is complicated by secondary conditions such as vomiting, gastric suction, and excess aldosterone production and by use of potent diuretics, which further increase potassium losses.[1]

Potassium in the ECF is constantly in a state of flux. The potassium filtered by the glomerulus is completely absorbed in the proximal tubule, secreted in the distal tubule, and either reabsorbed or secreted in the collecting ducts. Changes in renal tubular function or in the adrenal gland secretion of aldosterone (which causes potassium excretion) automatically result in potassium level changes (see box on right)

Clinical assessment of hypokalemia necessitates noting the serum potassium level inasmuch as it is impossible to look at actual total body stores of potassium. The most significant clinical sign related to potassium changes occurs in the electrocardiogram (ECG). Abnormal shifts of potassium in or out of cardiac muscle cells significantly alter the membrane potentials and subsequently influence conduction. Hypokalemia slows depolarization of the cells and thereby slows conduction velocity of the heart.[2] Hypokalemia also has been implicated in cases of sudden cardiac death in persons with cardiac compromise. See Fig. 15-3, *A* and *B,* for ECG changes associated with hypokalemia.

Persons with hypokalemia first have symptoms such as anorexia, fatigue, muscle weakness, dizziness, abdominal distention, decreased peristalsis, confusion, and weak irregular pulses.[3]

Hypokalemia is managed by oral or parenteral replacement. A diet rich in meats, fruits, and vegetables provides much potassium for the system, and potassium-rich salt substitutes also may be used to provide a source of replacement. Parenteral potassium replacement should not exceed 20 mEq/hr or 150 mEq/L/day in adults or 3 mEq/kg in children. In addition, potassium, *always* is diluted for parenteral use. Cardiac monitoring is indicated for high intravenous (IV) potassium therapy.

Potassium levels should be monitored carefully during potassium supplementation. Daily doses can be deter-

---

HYPOKALEMIA

DEFINITION

Deficit of potassium in the ECF

SERUM VALUE

Less than 3.5 mEq/L

ETIOLOGY

Metabolic alkalosis
Decreased potassium intake
Use of diuretics without potassium supplementation
Loss of gastrointestinal (GI) fluids (suction, nausea and vomiting, diarrhea)
Hyperaldosteronism (primary and secondary Cushing's syndrome)
Increased renin secretion
Prostaglandin secretion
Steroid use
Antibiotics

CLINICAL MANIFESTATIONS

Muscular weakness
Cardiac irregularities
Abdominal distention and flatulence
Paresthesia
Decreased reflexes
Anorexia, nausea, vomiting
Dizziness
Confusion
Increased sensitivity to digitalis
Electrocardiogram
  ST-segment depression
  Broad T waves
  U waves following or superimposed on the T waves

---

mined and adjusted according to dietary intake of potassium. Observation of renal function also is necessary to prevent hyperkalemia as a result of potassium retention.[1] Observation of IV sites for extrusion into the tissues is essential because potassium is highly caustic to the tissues.

Hyperkalemia

Hyperkalemia is an excess of potassium in the ECF, with a serum potassium level greater than 5.0 mEq/L. Most cases of hyperkalemia occur as a result of kidney failure. However, decreased aldosterone production, crushing injury, rapid administration of potassium solutions, and administration of potassium-sparing diuretics can result in elevation of serum potassium.[4,5] In addition, cell damage resulting from surgery, burns, or myocardial infarction releases potassium into the ECF[6,7] (see box below).

ECG findings in hyperkalemia also are of value in confirming a diagnosis of hyperkalemia. The appearance of tall, peaked T waves, a lengthening PR interval, widening QRS complexes, and flattening P waves indicate elevations of potassium[8] (see Figs. 15-1, *A* and *B*, and 15-2). Nausea and vomiting, diarrhea, numbness and tingling, weakness, and bradycardia also are signals to investigate the serum potassium level.[3]

Potassium supplementation should be discontinued. Administration of calcium parenterally temporarily blocks the effects of hyperkalemia in the heart muscle, but further measures are required to actually decrease serum levels, including sodium bicarbonate injection and the use of a mixture of hypertonic dextrose and insulin, which forces potassium back into the cells. Eventual excretion of potassium is necessary, however, particularly in the presence of renal failure. Consequently, cation-exchange resins (e.g., sodium polystyrene sulfonate [Kayexalate]) may be administered, and hemodialysis should be initiated.[6]

HYPERKALEMIA

DEFINITION

Excess potassium in the ECF

SERUM VALUE

Greater than 5.0 mEq/L

ETIOLOGY

Acute or chronic renal failure
Excess intake of potassium
Excess intake through infusions
Burns
Crushing injuries
Potassium-sparing diuretics (spironolactone [Aldactone], triamterene [Dyrenium])
Metabolic acidosis
Transfusions of old blood

CLINICAL MANIFESTATIONS

Irritability and restlessness
Anxiety
Nausea and vomiting
Abdominal cramps
Weakness
Numbness and tingling (fingertips and circumoral)
Cardiac irregularities (first tachycardia, then bradycardia)
Electrocardiogram
  Tall, peaked T waves
  Lengthening PR interval
  Widening QRS complex
  Flattened P waves

Hyponatremia

Hyponatremia is a deficiency of sodium in proportion to the water in the ECF. Hyponatremia can be deceptive because in several disorders there is not an actual deficit of sodium but an excess of water in relationship to the sodium. At least three scenarios offer further explanation of the possible alterations in sodium and ECF balance (see box, p. 605).

The first scenario is hyponatremia associated with an increase in the ECF volume. Commonly known as *water intoxication* or *dilutional hyponatremia,* this disturbance is associated with cardiac failure, liver disease, renal failure, and other disorders.[9] A concomitant inability to excrete the excess volume leads to dilution of the existing sodium.

In a person with renal compromise, for example, ingestion of water or infusion of IV solutions beyond the excretion capacity of the kidney results in dilutional hyponatremia. The decrease in glomerular filtration rate (GFR) is implicated as the primary mechanism for this occurrence.

Of particular interest to nursing is the care that must be exercised in monitoring the fluid status of the postoperative patient. Stress, pain, tissue hypoxia, mechanical ventilation, and certain drugs can stimulate the antidiuretic hormone (ADH) to conserve water in excess of desired quantities. In addition, replacement of fluid loss with dextrose in water (D_5W) leads to rapid metabolism of the glucose and can increase water load to the ECF compartment.[3]

Clinical findings include a serum sodium level below 135 mEq/L and a low serum osmolality (<285 mOsm/kg). Symptoms vary from mild to severe but may include fatigue, apprehension, abdominal cramps, nausea and vomiting, headache, and lethargy.[10]

A second picture of hyponatremia is a loss of both sodium and ECF. Implicated in the development of this disturbance are the loss of sodium-rich gastrointestinal (GI) fluids (e.g., from nausea and vomiting, diarrhea, GI suction), overuse of potent diuretics, and aldosterone insufficiency.

In the case of GI losses, not only sodium and water but also potassium are depleted. With less potassium avail-

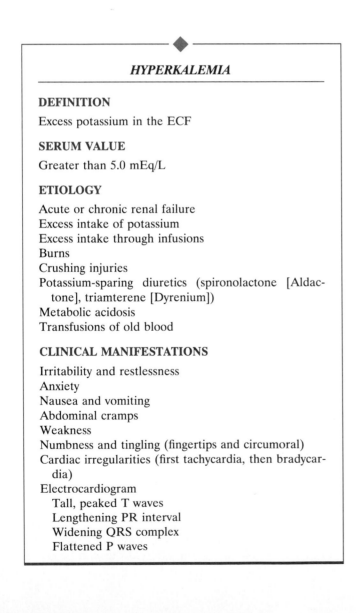

HYPONATREMIA

WATER INTOXICATION
Definition

Increased ECF volume, with inability to excrete the excess

Serum value

May be less than 125 mEq/L (very mild to severe); serum sodium value of 110-115 mEq/L known to occur

Etiology

Excess D_5W solution intravenously
Excess plain water intake
Renal failure

Clinical manifestations

Disorientation
Muscle twitching
Nausea and vomiting
Abdominal cramps
Headaches
Seizures

TRUE HYPONATREMIA
Definition

Actual deficit of body sodium

Serum value

Less than 135 mEq/L

Etiology

Gastric suction
Vomiting
Burns
Use of potent diuretics
Heat exhaustion (excessive sweating)
Loss from wounds and drainage
Diuretics
Use of tap-water enemas
Diarrhea
Adrenal insufficiency

Clinical manifestations

Apprehension
Dizziness
Postural hypotension
Cold, clammy skin
Decreased skin turgor
Tachycardia
Oliguria

HYPONATREMIA—cont'd

SYNDROME OF INAPPROPRIATE RELEASE OF ADH (SIADH)
Definition

Dilutional state plus sodium loss

Serum value

Less than 120 mEq/L

Etiology

Central nervous system (CNS) disorders
Major trauma (stress)
Malignancies (lung, pancreas, thymus)
Certain drugs (oral hypoglycemics, antineoplastics, diuretics, analgesics, bronchodilators)

Clinical manifestations

Anorexia
Nausea and vomiting
Abdominal cramps
Lethargy and withdrawal
Convulsions
Coma
Urinary osmolality greater than plasma (increased wasting of sodium)

able for excretion by the distal tubule, the stimulus to release aldosterone is partially lost and sodium is not sufficiently reabsorbed.[9]

Potent loop diuretics work to diminish the concentrating ability of the loop of Henle and therefore cause increased losses of both sodium and fluid. This hyponatremia is further complicated by a reduction in GFR brought on by the reduced vascular volume.

Medical management for both cases of hyponatremia involves treating the underlying conditions, administering IV sodium chloride solutions, and discontinuing diuretic therapy. Correction of the hyponatremic states with IV saline solutions may prevent the problem of fluid shifts from the ECF to the intracellular fluid (ICF) when sodium is lost.[1,11]

The critical care nurse must be cognizant of neurologic changes in the patient undergoing correction of hyponatremia. Rapid parenteral correction of hyponatremia initially may appear to be successful, with the subsequent appearance of transient unresponsiveness, swallowing difficulties, paresis, and eventual coma.[1] Studies have suggested that the brain adjusts to the hyponatremia over a period of time. Correction of the hyponatremia results in actual shrinkage of the brain tissue, resulting in severe neurologic signs and symptoms and even death.[12]

Finally, hyponatremia can result from the syndrome of inappropriate secretion of ADH (SIADH). Although SIADH is discussed at length in Chapter 43, it must be noted that a rather severe reduction of sodium without ECF loss can occur as a result of this disorder.

The condition results from oversecretion of ADH (vasopressin), which permits the continuous reabsorption of water from the renal tubular system. Sodium excretion is high in the urine, whereas large amounts of water are retained under the influence of ADH secretion. Fluid restriction, sodium replacement, mild diuretics, and drugs to control ADH secretion (demeclocycline) represent current treatment for the disorder.[13]

Hypernatremia

Sodium excess of the ECF is extremely dangerous but occurs rarely. Hypernatremia can arise from an actual increase in sodium or from losses of water. In all cases of hypernatremia, however, the increase in ECF sodium depletes the cells of fluid and leads to the symptoms commonly associated with this disorder (see box below).

Hypernatremia can occur with a loss of both ECF sodium and water, but the water loss far exceeds the amount of sodium loss. Watery diarrhea or profuse sweating can cause severe hypotonic fluid loss. Moderate-to-severe diarrhea can result in fluid losses of approximately 300 to 3000 ml/day.[14] The fluid loss concentrates the remaining sodium in the ECF, which, in turn, exerts an osmotic pull on the intracellular compartment and depletes the cells of fluid.

True hypernatremia can be caused by administration of (1) high sodium content tube feedings without sufficient water intake, (2) hypertonic saline solutions for correction of sodium imbalance, or (3) sodium bicarbonate during cardiac arrest.[10,15] Plumer and Cosentino[3] even suggest that dextrose in normal saline solution (D_5NS), infused in large quantities, can lead to hypernatremia. This occurrence, however, may be limited to elderly persons with decreased ability to excrete sodium and water or to postoperative patients with stress-induced renal disturbances.[3]

Finally, hypernatremia can result from water loss only, such as occurs with diabetes insipidus. This disorder is classified as either central diabetes insipidus (arising from central nervous system [CNS] causes) or nephrogenic diabetes insipidus, which results in a loss of the renal response to ADH, causing no reabsorption of water in the collecting ducts. As water is lost, sodium in the ECF rises.[1]

Regardless of the causes of hypernatremia, one particular characteristic remains common—thirst. Thirst is the main defense against hyperconcentration of the fluid compartments. The same osmoreceptors that trigger ADH release are responsible for stimulation of thirst and are stimulated when the serum osmolality rises to 294 mOsm/kg.[16] In patients with diabetes insipidus, an intense thirst is created by the rising serum osmolality, but water is not retained to maintain the fluid compartments. An enormous intake of fluid, however, helps maintain the serum osmolality near normal.

HYPERNATREMIA

DEFINITION

Excess sodium in the ECF

SERUM VALUE

Greater than 145 mEq/L

ETIOLOGY

Inability to respond to thirst (decreased fluid intake)
Heatstroke
Diarrhea (excess fluid loss)
Severe insensible loss (ventilation, sweating, burns)
Diabetes insipidus
Excessive administration of sodium solutions (e.g., hypertonic saline, sodium bicarbonate)
Hypertonic tube feedings without water supplement
NOTE: Hypernatremia usually is the result of dehydration of the ECF and subsequent hyperconcentration of the sodium.

CLINICAL MANIFESTATIONS

Extreme thirst
Fever
Dry, sticky mucous membranes
Altered mentation
Seizures (later stages)

Hypocalcemia

Calcium deficit can be misleading because of the three different ways calcium is held within the body. Of the calcium within the body, 98% to 99% is bound in bone and is not readily available. The remainder is either protein-bound (chelated by phosphate, sulfate, or citrate) or ionized in the blood stream.[17] Because serum calcium is primarily protein-bound, changes in serum protein values lead to changes in serum calcium values (1 g/dl protein relates to 0.8 mg/dl calcium).[18] Typically, a diagnosis of hypocalcemia means the serum calcium is less than 4.5 mEq/L, or 8.5 mg/dl.[19]

Serum calcium stores are replenished primarily through the action of the parathyroid hormone (PTH), which can mobilize calcium from the bone into the vascular space. Absorption of calcium from the intestinal tract, excretion from the kidneys, and constant bone rebuilding help maintain the available store. Disturbances in any of the three areas can result in a deficit or excess of calcium.[17]

A deficit of calcium, for instance, is possible when renal failure results in poor uptake of calcium in the GI tract, which occurs because the breakdown product of vitamin D, which is metabolized in renal cells, is not available in renal failure; thus the stimulus to reabsorb calcium from the intestines is lost, and the result is a decrease in serum calcium levels. In addition, hypoparathyroidism as a result of the removal of the parathyroid glands causes hypocalcemia. Of particular concern to the critical care nurse is the hypocalcemia resulting from the use of citrate anticoagulation of banked blood. The citrates tend to chelate the calcium, thereby lowering serum levels.[20]

The serum calcium level is affected by the inverse relationship that exists between calcium and phosphorus. When phosphorus levels are high, calcium absorption is inhibited; the reverse also is true.[19] Further, serum calcium levels are influenced by the pH of the arterial blood. In acidosis the lower pH results in the release of more calcium from protein binding, which elevates the ionized calcium. Conversely, an elevated pH results in calcium becoming more highly bound to protein, reducing the calcium.[17] Thus in correcting acidosis, care must be taken to monitor calcium and replace it as needed. Other causes of hypocalcemia can be seen in the box below.

The person experiencing hypocalcemia may display facial muscle twitching (Chvostek's sign) or carpophalangeal spasm (Trousseau's sign). Cardiac changes also are present with hypocalcemia and are reflected as prolonged QT segments on the ECG and decreased left-ventricular contractility.[17] Cardiac changes associated with hypocalcemia, however, are rare and occur at extremely low serum calcium levels.[20] Both problems result from the decreased availability of calcium to perform its role in cell depolarization and consequent neurotransmission. The degree of facial twitching can be directly correlated to the severity of the hypocalcemia. Mild twitching of the corners of the mouth, for instance, represents a mild reduction in serum calcium, whereas involvement of all branches of the facial nerve indicates markedly low serum levels.[20]

The symptomatology accompanying hypocalcemia can be somewhat insidious. Vague manifestations of nervousness, anxiety, syncope, paresthesias, or subtle behavioral changes should alert the caregiver to the possibility of hypocalcemia.[20]

Medical management of hypocalcemia depends on whether the disorder is acute or chronic. Acute hypocalcemia is treated with IV administration of calcium. An initial bolus of 200 mg is given over 10 minutes, followed by 1 to 2 mg/kg/hr until levels are normal (6 to 12 hours).[19] Successful treatment, however, often depends on normalizing the levels of other electrolytes. For example, the administration of calcium in the presence of hyperphosphatemia usually results in little success in correcting the original calcium imbalance. If magnesium levels are low, infusion of calcium results only in its excretion from the kidney in favor of magnesium retention. Drugs that cause predisposition to or that prolong hypocalcemia also should be discontinued.[19]

Chronic hypocalcemia such as that associated with renal failure can be treated with oral calcium and vitamin D preparations. The current recommendation is for vitamin D replacement in the form of dihydrotachysterol in daily doses of 0.5 to 1 mg.[20] As a preventive measure for persons with intact renal function, an oral calcium intake of 1 to 1.2 g/day has been recommended. Through the ingestion of milk, vegetables, oral calcium supplements, or bone meal, this level of intake can be achieved.[21]

HYPOCALCEMIA

DEFINITION

Deficit of calcium in the ECF

SERUM VALUE

Less than 8.5 mg/dl or 4.5 mEq/L

ETIOLOGY

Protein malnutrition (decreased albumin causes decreased calcium)
Decreased calcium intake
Burns or infection
Decreased parathyroid function (PTH controls serum calcium availability)
Decreased GI absorption of calcium (diarrhea)
Excessive antacid use (prevents absorption)
Renal failure (decreased vitamin D_3 available to stimulate absorption)
Diuretics
Hyperphosphatemia
Acute pancreatitis
Use of citrated banked blood
Anticonvulsant drugs

CLINICAL MANIFESTATIONS

Irritability
Muscular tetany
Muscle cramps
Decreased cardiac output (decreased contractions)
Bleeding (decreased ability to coagulate)
Fractures
Seizures
Laryngospasm
Syncope
Mental confusion
Paresthesias
Dry skin
Brittle nails and hair

Hypercalcemia

An excess of calcium in the ECF is known as *hypercalcemia.* Overstimulation of the parathyroid gland from a tumor, malignancies causing metastatic calcium release, and prolonged immobilization usually are implicated in the development of hypercalcemia. In fact, hypercalcemia is mediated almost exclusively from abnormalities in bone activity rather than absorption and release of calcium into the ECF.[1] The use of diuretics and drugs that stimulate PTH production can worsen existing hypercalcemia.[18] In addition, hyperthyroidism can stimulate increased bone production, and adrenal insufficiency can slow the renal excretion of calcium and speed the intestinal reabsorption.[20]

In patients with hypercalcemia, the serum calcium level is greater than 5.8 mEq/L, or 10.5 mg/dl. X-ray examination may demonstrate large areas of bone decalcification.[10] The affected person may experience deep bone pain, flaccid muscles, anorexia, nausea and vomiting, lethargy, confusion, headaches, and even pathologic fractures from the demineralization of the bone[1] (see box, p. 608, left-hand column).

Treatment of acute hypercalcemia involves dilution of the calcium by means of IV fluids and concomitant use

HYPERCALCEMIA

DEFINITION

Excess calcium in the ECF

SERUM VALUE

Greater than 10.5 mg/dl or 5.8 mEq/L

ETIOLOGY

Increased parathyroid activity (increases bone resorption of calcium)
Multiple fractures
Prolonged immobilization
Bone tumors
Other malignancies
Decreased phosphorus (inverse relationship between calcium and phosphate)
Hyperthyroidism
Adrenal insufficiency

CLINICAL MANIFESTATIONS

Deep bone pain
Excessive thirst
Anorexia, nausea, vomiting
Lethargy
Weakened muscles
Cardiac dysrhythmias
Dehydration
Confusion
Abdominal pain
Hypertension

of loop diuretics (furosemide) to enhance calcium excretion.[22] Thiazide diuretics inhibit excretion of calcium and should not be used in cases of hypercalcemia.[18] Oral phosphorus preparations may be given to increase bone deposition of calcium.[22] Phosphorus preparations, however, should not be given to those patients with renal failure. In addition, the diarrhea and/or constipation caused by phosphorus may be undesirable in some cases. IV phosphate administration is used as a last resort because of the potential for developing soft tissue calcification from calcium-phosphate precipitates.[18]

In patients with metastatic malignancies that cause hypercalcemia, drugs such as plicamycin (Mithracin) or the hormone calcitonin may be used. Plicamycin, a cytotoxic drug, is responsible for slowing bone resorption. Like many of the antineoplastic drugs, however, it also risks bone marrow depression and blood dyscrasias.[22] Calcitonin inhibits PTH activity and thereby slows loss of calcium from the bone.[18]

Hypomagnesemia

Magnesium is involved in enzymatic reaction, cellular permeability, and the maintenance of neuromuscular excitability. Conditions such as malnutrition, chronic alcoholism, prolonged diuresis, and severe diarrhea can lead to magnesium deficits. The main cause of magnesium deficit, however, involves loss from the GI tract[23] (see box above). The serum magnesium level will be less than 1.5 mEq/L.

HYPOMAGNESEMIA

DEFINITION

Deficit of magnesium in the ECF

SERUM VALUE

Less than 1.4 mEq/L

ETIOLOGY

Malnutrition
Chronic alcoholism (malnutrition)
Diuretics (prolonged use)
Severe diarrhea
Severe dehydration

CLINICAL MANIFESTATIONS

Choroid and athetoid muscle activity
Facial tics
Spasticity
Cardiac dysrhythmias:
  Premature ventricular contractions (PVCs)
  Ventricular fibrillation
Respiratory muscle depression
Confusion

Nutritional deficits such as result from administering parenteral nutrition or tube feedings that are magnesium-poor can lead to hypomagnesemia. The administration of loop diuretics such as furosemide also can increase magnesium losses. Magnesium losses, however, have most commonly been associated with chronic alcoholism, in which losses can stem from diarrhea and vomiting, as well as chronic malnutrition.

The clinical manifestations of hypomagnesemia involve the role magnesium plays in neuromuscular excitability. Severe respiratory muscle depression may occur, rendering the individual in need of mechanical ventilation. Mental apathy and confusion also may be present. Finally, life-threatening dysrhythmias can result from magnesium depletion.[23]

Treatment for hypomagnesemia usually involves IV replacement with magnesium sulfate. Before treatment is initiated, however, determination of adequate renal function should be undertaken. Patients with severe hypomagnesemia may be given 2 g as a 10% solution over 2 minutes, followed by 12 g in 1 L of fluid over 12 hours.[24] Moderate decreases may be treated with 24 to 40 mEq of magnesium sulfate administered parenterally daily for several days. Oral or nasogastric (NG) supplementation should approach 16 mEq/day.

Hypermagnesemia

The development of excess levels of magnesium in the ECF, although rare, goes hand in hand with chronic renal disease. The renal tubules can no longer excrete

HYPERMAGNESEMIA

DEFINITION

Excess of magnesium in the ECF

SERUM VALUE

Greater than 2.5 mEq/L

ETIOLOGY

Excessive intake of magnesium products (antacids and laxatives)
Renal failure
Severe dehydration if oliguria is present

CLINICAL MANIFESTATIONS

CNS depression (especially respiratory)
Lethargy
Coma
Bradycardia
Electrocardiogram
- Prolonged PR interval
- Wide QRS complex
- Tall T waves
- AV block
- PVCs

HYPOPHOSPHATEMIA

DEFINITION

Deficit of phosphate in the ECF

SERUM VALUE

Less than 3.0 mg/dl

ETIOLOGY

Diabetic ketoacidosis (renal wasting)
Malabsorption disorders
Renal wasting of phosphorus
Prolonged use of IV dextrose infusions
Low-phosphate diets in patients with renal failure
Phosphate-poor total parenteral nutrition solutions

CLINICAL MANIFESTATIONS

Hemolytic anemias
Depressed white cell function
Bleeding (decreased platelet aggregation)
Nausea, vomiting, and anorexia
Bone demineralization

magnesium, and dialysis is quite ineffective in removing magnesium.[23] Hypermagnesemia develops in persons with renal impairment who chronically take laxatives or antacids that contain magnesium. Temporary excesses of magnesium can occur as the result of ECF dehydration or its excessive administration for treatment of eclampsia.[10]

The clinical manifestations associated with hypermagnesemia demonstrate profound CNS involvement. The individual may exhibit muscle weakness, inability to swallow, hyporeflexia, hypotension, and cardiac dysrhythmias[23] (see box above). The plasma value typically is greater than 2.5 mEq/L, and the ECG demonstrates a prolonged PR interval, wide QRS complex, tall T waves, atrioventricular (AV) block, and premature ventricular contractions (PVCs).

Treatment for magnesium excess should be vigorous and immediate, with discontinuance of all magnesium-containing drugs, replacement of ECF volume (if a result of dehydration), and administration of calcium gluconate to counteract the effects of the magnesium.[10] Persons with severe hypermagnesemia may suffer from respiratory depression resulting from the effect of magnesium on the respiratory centers of the brain. Mechanical ventilation may become necessary to sustain ventilation until the excess is corrected.

Hypophosphatemia

Hypophosphatemia is a deficit of phosphorus in the ECF. Most phosphorus (85%) is held in the bone with calcium, 10% exists in the ECF, and the remainder is in the ICF, where it is responsible for energy formation (adenosine triphosphate [ATP]), nerve and muscle function, and the acid-base balance of the ECF. Phosphorus shares an inverse relationship with calcium. Losses or gains in either electrolyte cause the kidneys to retain or excrete the other. The serum level indicating hypophosphatemia is less than 2.5 mg/dl.[23]

Phosphorus loss occurs with conditions such as acute or chronic alcoholism, with excessive administration of electrolyte-poor IV solutions, and with overuse of antacids, which absorb phosphorus in the GI tract. Also implicated in hypophosphatemia are diabetic ketoacidosis and thermal burns[23] (see box above).

Alcoholism-induced hypophosphatemia is a multifaceted occurrence involving calcium, magnesium, and PTH. The chronically poor nutritional status of an alcohol-dependent person often results in deficiencies in vitamin D and intestinal irritability. Antacid ingestion to relieve the chronic GI irritability binds significant amounts of phosphate in the intestine. The twofold assault stimulates PTH for calcium reabsorption, which in turn leads to further excretion of phosphorus in the urine. Also, excessive use of electrolyte-free IV fluids such as D_5W leads to phosphorus' exiting the cells and its excretion in the urine.

Bleeding disorders from defective platelets and fragile red blood cell (RBC) membranes develop in the person with hypophosphatemia. Muscular weakness, paresthesia, and GI distress result from reduced energy and oxygen transport to cells, which phosphorus helps accomplish.[23]

Phosphorus stores generally are replaced very slowly because the actual serum level may not reflect a deficit in the intracellular compartment. Oral supplementation usually is achieved through ingestion of skim milk. Fleet's Phospho-Soda can be mixed in water and administered either orally or by NG or feeding tube. Parenteral phosphorus usually is not given unless the serum phosphorus reaches 1.0 mg/dl.[23] Parenteral preparations of phosphorus must be diluted, and care must be taken to monitor levels of phosphorus to prevent precipitation with calcium. Phosphate solutions should be administered in quantities no greater than 1 g over 24 hours.[25]

Hyperphosphatemia

Phosphorus excess of the ECF usually occurs in cases of chronic renal failure. The renal tubules no longer excrete phosphorus as before, but uptake continues in the GI tract. Hyperphosphatemia also can result from rapid cell catabolism that releases the cellular phosphorus stores into the ECF. Excessive oral intake of phosphates or intestinal reabsorption of phosphates from enemas can elevate the serum phosphorus. Elevations seldom become of concern, however, unless phosphate excretion through the kidney is reduced.[25]

The clinical manifestations of hyperphosphatemia (see first box on right) closely parallel those of hypocalcemia, inasmuch as these disorders are likely to occur simultaneously. Muscle tetany and soft tissue calcifications, however, usually are the more prominent signs of this disorder.[25]

Treatment for hyperphosphatemia may range from simple dietary restriction of phosphorus to ingestion of aluminum antacids, which bind phosphate in the intestine. Adequate hydration and correction of any existing hypocalcemia can enhance the renal excretion of the excess phosphate.[19]

Hypochloremia

Hypochloremia is a deficit of chloride in the ECF. Hypochloremia develops as a result of loss of fluids rich in chloride. These fluids also can be rich in sodium because chloride combines with sodium. Hypochloremia can be associated with acid-base disorders, particularly metabolic alkalosis inasmuch as the retention of bicarbonate, which occurs with metabolic alkalosis, leads to the excretion of chloride ions. Other causes of hypochloremia include vomiting, gastric suction, diarrhea, and overuse of potassium-wasting diuretics.[1,10]

In patients with metabolic alkalosis caused by gastric suctioning, chloride-rich gastric fluids are lost, concentrating the bicarbonate ions in the ECF. Overuse of diuretics leads to potassium wasting, which carries the chloride ions into the urine. The clinical manifestations of hypochloremia result primarily not from the loss of chloride but from the loss of potassium and ionized calcium[3] (see second box on right).

Treatment for hypochloremia usually involves chloride replacement with a variety of medications such as ammonium chloride tablets or a parenteral solution containing chloride.[3] Treatment of the causative disorder should proceed immediately.

Hyperchloremia

Hyperchloremia is an excess of chloride ions in the ECF. Just as a deficit of chloride is related to acid-base imbalance, so is hyperchloremia. In patients with metabolic acidosis in whom bicarbonate ions are lost excessively, chloride ions are retained. Severe diarrhea, excessive parenteral administration of isotonic saline solution, urinary diversions, and renal failure cause a predisposition to bicarbonate (HCO_3^-) loss and a concentration of existing chloride stores.[1]

HYPERPHOSPHATEMIA

DEFINITION

Excess of phosphate in the ECF

SERUM VALUE

Greater than 4.5 mg/dl

ETIOLOGY

Renal failure
Lactic acidosis
Catabolic stress
Chemotherapy for certain malignancies

CLINICAL MANIFESTATIONS

Tachycardia
Nausea
Diarrhea
Abdominal cramps
Muscle weakness
Flaccid paralysis
Increased reflexes

HYPOCHLOREMIA

DEFINITION

Deficit of chloride in the ECF

SERUM VALUE

Less than 98 mEq/L

ETIOLOGY

Loss of gastric contents (vomiting, suction)
Diarrhea (prolonged)
Excessive diuretic use
Excessive sweating
Prolonged use of IV dextrose (dilutes potassium and sodium, as well as chloride)
Metabolic alkalosis (more available bicarbonate, so chloride excreted)

CLINICAL MANIFESTATIONS

Hyperirritability
Tetany or muscular excitability
Slow respirations
Decreased blood pressure (with fluid loss)

In the person with hyperchloremia, initial weakness, lethargy, possible unconsciousness (in later stages), and deep rapid breathing are seen[3] (see first box on right). Serum chloride levels are greater than 108 mEq/L. Management of hyperchloremia is based on first treating the underlying cause and correcting the acidosis. In addition, parenteral administration of sodium bicarbonate can restore bicarbonate stores.[3]

Bicarbonate Deficit

A primary base bicarbonate deficit is referred to as *metabolic acidosis.* The arterial pH is decreased as a result of loss of bicarbonate. Causes include diarrhea, renal failure, tissue hypoxia, lactic acidosis, diabetic ketoacidosis, malnutrition, and salicylate overdose.[26]

Laboratory findings in patients with bicarbonate deficit include a plasma pH level below 7.35, a urinary pH level below 6, and a plasma bicarbonate level below 22 mEq/L.[3] Clinical manifestations usually include Kussmaul's respiration (deep, fast, rhythmic), weakness, disorientation, coma (in later stages), headache, and anorexia (see second box on right).

Bicarbonate deficit occurs in patients with renal failure because the GFR decreases and the available buffers are insufficient to allow acid secretion into the renal tubules. Therefore hydrogen ions are retained in place of bicarbonate, which is lost in the urine.[26] As bicarbonate levels in the ECF drop, potassium exits the cells and floods the ECF, leading to a hyperkalemic state.

Medical management of bicarbonate deficit is achieved by treating the cause and administering oral or parenteral bicarbonate.[3] Replacement of bicarbonate is calculated on the basis of body weight and the desired increment of increase in bicarbonate.[10]

Bicarbonate Excess

An excess of bicarbonate or excess loss of acid in the ECF is referred to as *metabolic alkalosis.* Retained bicarbonate is the result of disorders such as loss of acids from vomiting, gastric suction, hyperaldosteronism, or diuretic abuse.[26] Excessive ingestion of medications containing bicarbonate or use of parenteral solutions containing bicarbonate also can predispose a person to metabolic alkalosis. Potassium levels should be carefully monitored; metabolic alkalosis causes hydrogen ion release from the cells and a subsequent exchange for potassium, leading to potassium deficit of the ECF.

Metabolic alkalosis can develop from severe fluid and acid losses, causing the retention of bicarbonate, or it can develop from excessive addition of bicarbonate to the body. For instance, the removal of gastric acids through suction depletes the available hydrogen ions and predisposes the patient to an increase in bicarbonate ions.[26]

Clinical observations of bicarbonate excess include a urinary pH level greater than 7, plasma pH level greater than 7.45, and a plasma bicarbonate level greater than 26 mEq/L. Affected persons usually experience numbness and tingling of extremities, muscular hypertonicity, slow, shallow respirations with compensatory pauses, bradycardia, and tetany (see box, p. 612, left-hand column).

Treatment of bicarbonate excess primarily involves increasing excretion through the kidney. Further, if the patient is taking excessive bicarbonate-containing medications, withdrawal of these medications will be necessary. Also, if the cause is a loss in chloride, replacement of the chloride will produce bicarbonate excretion.

HYPERCHLOREMIA

DEFINITION

Excess of chloride in the ECF

SERUM VALUE

More than 108 mEq/L

ETIOLOGY

Severe diarrhea
Excessive parenteral administration of isotonic saline solution
Urinary diversions
Renal failure

CLINICAL MANIFESTATIONS

Weakness
Lethargy
Unconsciousness (in later stages)
Kussmaul's respiration

METABOLIC ACIDOSIS

DEFINITION

Bicarbonate deficit of the ECF

SERUM VALUE

Bicarbonate level less than 22 mEq/L
Partial pressure of carbon dioxide (Pco_2) normal or less than 35 mm Hg to compensate for the low bicarbonate level
pH below 7.35

ETIOLOGY

Diabetic ketoacidosis
Lactic acidosis
Uremia
Ingestion of acids (e.g., salicylates, alcohol, boric acid)
Starvation
Diarrhea
Some diuretics

CLINICAL MANIFESTATIONS

Kussmaul's respiration
Weakness
Dizziness
Rapid respirations
Coma (later stages)

METABOLIC ALKALOSIS

DEFINITION

Bicarbonate excess in the ECF

SERUM VALUE

Bicarbonate level greater than 26 mEq/L
Pco_2 level normal or greater than 45 mm Hg to compensate for the elevated bicarbonate level
pH level greater than 7.45

ETIOLOGY

Vomiting (with loss of chloride)
Excessive intake of alkalies
Primary aldosteronism (because of loss of potassium)
Diuretic use in patient with congestive heart failure (CHF) (on occasion)

CLINICAL MANIFESTATIONS

Hyperexcitability of muscles
Bradycardia
Bradypnea
Numbness and tingling

Hypoproteinemia

A reduction in protein of the ECF may be rapid or insidious and is a difficult-to-treat malady. Loss of protein can be sudden, such as with burns or surgery, or very slow and steady, such as with renal insufficiency (undetected), malnutrition, bleeding, or liver disease.[3] The serum albumin level is chronically less than 3.8 g (see box, right-hand column).

Initial symptoms may be weakness and fatigue, with a flatness of affect. Emotional depression, anorexia, flabbiness of muscles, weight loss, and edema of dependent areas also may be present.[10] Lesions may be unhealed because insufficient protein is available for wound repair. Traditionally, fluid imbalances related to decreased protein are discussed in relation to albumin, which accounts for 50% to 60% of total protein stores.

The edema associated with hypoproteinemia results from a plasma-to-interstitial fluid shift from a lack of oncotic pressure in the vascular space. For example, in patients with liver disease, insufficient amounts of albumin are produced, thereby lowering oncotic pressure within the vascular system. Portal hypertension increases albumin loss into the interstitium and creates increased edema.

Treatment is difficult because the patient may no longer be able to ingest orally the high amounts of protein needed to replace stores. NG feedings or total parenteral nutrition (TPN) can be used to replace stores, but the course of protein replacement often is lengthy. Human serum albumin can be used to treat hypoalbuminemia. Albumin must be administered slowly (2 to 3 ml/min), however, to avoid fluid overload as a result of normalizing oncotic pressure.[3]

HYPOALBUMINEMIA

DEFINITION

Deficit of protein in the ECF

SERUM VALUE

Less than 3.8 g/dl

ETIOLOGY

Protein-deficient diet
Burns
Starvation
Surgery (major, with prolonged recovery phase)
Digestive diseases

CLINICAL MANIFESTATIONS

Emotional depression
Muscle wasting
Peripheral edema (fluid shift)
Decreased resistance to infection
Poorly healing wounds

ACID-BASE ABNORMALITIES

Carbonic Acid Deficit in Extracellular Fluid

Carbonic acid deficit in the ECF usually is referred to as *respiratory alkalosis.* The deficit results from any condition that causes hyperventilation, such as pain, CNS lesions, fever, or assisted ventilation.[27]

The person who is hyperventilating loses carbon dioxide, which is required to formulate carbonic acid, but retains bicarbonate. The body attempts to compensate for the lost carbon dioxide by allowing excretion of bicarbonate through the kidneys, possibly inducing a deficit of bicarbonate.[27] Also, chloride may be exchanged for bicarbonate at the cellular level, thereby decreasing the available bicarbonate in the ECF.[27]

In addition to rapid breathing, the patient may experience tetany (because of the pH and calcium relationship), paresthesia, tingling and numbness (especially around the mouth), blurred vision, diaphoresis, dry mouth, and coma (later stages).[27] Laboratory findings reveal a serum pH level greater than 7.45 and Pco_2 level below 35 mm Hg.

Medical management is aimed at reducing the hyperventilation if the cause is known. For instance, sedating the patient may be helpful. Parenteral administration of chloride solutions is helpful in reducing the bicarbonate while the respiratory problem is treated.[26]

Carbonic Acid Excess in Extracellular Fluid

Carbonic acid excess is known commonly as *respiratory acidosis.* This disorder develops when the lungs fail to rid the body of the appropriate amount of carbon dioxide, resulting in formation of excess carbonic acid from the excess carbon dioxide. Hypoventilatory effort or obstruction to ventilations results in respiratory acidosis. Drugs, anesthetics, CNS damage, neurologic disease, or musculoskeletal diseases may be implicated in the development of this disorder. The kidneys compensate for the problem by excreting hydrogen, reabsorbing bicarbonate, and regenerating bicarbonate from the excess carbon dioxide. This process is slow, however (5 days for maximal effect), and other support measures usually are required.[27]

Treatment is aimed at correcting the cause of the hypoventilation or ventilatory distress. Oxygen or mechanical ventilation may be helpful.

ACUTE RENAL FAILURE

Description

Acute renal failure (ARF) can be defined as any rapid decline in glomerular filtration rate (GFR) with subsequent development of retention of metabolic waste products (azotemia). ARF usually is accompanied by oliguria or anuria[28] and is a short-term condition that lasts 10 to 25 days or longer.[29] If the appropriate treatment is not initiated or if the patient does not respond to treatment, the acute condition may lead to chronic renal failure.[30] ARF is a serious complication in the critically ill patient, and mortality remains high, ranging from 35% to 86% even with advanced critical care and dialysis techniques.[31] GI bleeding, sepsis, and CNS changes often are implicated in deaths related to ARF.[31]

Etiology

Causes of ARF are categorized into three areas: prerenal, intrarenal, and postrenal (see box, right hand column). *Prerenal* causes are associated with any insult that reduces vascular perfusion to the kidney. The GFR is decreased, leading to oliguria. The nephrons remain normal, and return to normal renal function is possible with prompt treatment of the underlying cause of the prerenal condition.[30]

Postrenal causes usually are obstructive disorders occurring beyond the kidney in the remainder of the urinary tract. As with prerenal conditions, prompt treatment aimed at alleviating the obstruction will restore normal kidney function and prevent permanent kidney damage.[30]

Intrarenal causes, also known as *intrinsic*, *primary*, or *parenchymal* damage, are insults to the kidney tissue such as infections, insults to the nephron such as glomerulonephritis, and scleroses from hypertension and diabetes mellitus. Damage from intrarenal conditions is primarily to the tubular component of the nephron.[30] The most common intrarenal condition is acute tubular necrosis,[28-30] which is discussed next.

ETIOLOGY OF ACUTE RENAL FAILURE

PRERENAL

Hemorrhage
Severe GI losses
Burns
Shock
Cirrhosis
Renal trauma
Volume depletion (actual loss or "third-spacing")
Congestive heart failure
Renal losses (diuretics, diabetes insipidus, osmotic diuresis)

INTRARENAL

Thrombus
Stenosis
Hypertensive sclerosis
Glomerulonephritis
Pyelonephritis
Acute tubular necrosis
Diabetic sclerosis
Toxic damage

POSTRENAL

Obstructions (stenosis, calculi)
Prostatic disease
Tumors

◆ Acute tubular necrosis (ATN)

Description. Acute tubular necrosis (ATN) refers to damage occurring within the epithelium of the tubular portions of the nephron. *ATN* sometimes is used synonymously with ARF but is, in fact, a cause of ARF; of all ARF, 75% to 90% is caused by ATN.[28] Damage to the cellular structures in this area prevents normal concentration of urine, filtration of wastes, and regulation of acid-base, electrolyte, and water balance. A number of disorders can result in ATN, and several contributing factors may work together to bring about tubular damage.[28]

Etiology. Common causes of ATN, listed in the box on p. 614, left-hand column, are divided into two categories—ischemic and toxic. Ischemic damage occurs irregularly along the tubular membranes, causing areas of tubular cell damage and cast formation. Toxic damage results from nephrotoxins, usually drugs, chemical agents, or bacterial endotoxins, which cause uniform, widespread damage. The renal tubular cells are constantly at risk for damage because of their normally high blood flows, high oxygen requirements, and the constant reabsorption and secretion of metabolites.

Pathophysiology. Several theories, often discussed and researched, explain the pathophysiology behind ATN. The *back-leak* theory suggests that tubular injury, whether ischemic or toxic, leads to return of metabolites (e.g., creatinine) to the peritubular circulation. This causes decreased urinary production with retention of wastes, water, and electrolytes.[32]

Another theory refers to *tubular obstruction* from interstitial edema or from an accumulation of casts and sloughing tissue that create an obstruction. Filtration ceases when tubular hydrostatic pressure reaches that of glomerular filtration pressure. This decreases the formation of urine because of the nonavailability of filtrate to process.[32]

The *vascular* theories suggest that damage to the tubules is mediated primarily by obstruction in the renal capillary beds. Prolonged ischemia results in afferent arteriolar constriction and a reduction of GFR, which decreases the available filtrate. The exchange between tubules and capillaries is obliterated, and tubular cells fail to receive the necessary blood flow and oxygen to sustain them.[32] *Decreased glomerular membrane permeability* is suggested as a fourth explanation. It restricts filtration but occurs at the cellular level and is independent of blood flow.

Finally, the last theory suggests that *vasoconstriction* reduces renal perfusion and reduces capillary flow in the cortical region of the kidney (site of most of the glomeruli), resulting in ATN.[32]

Phases. ATN typically has four phases.[30] The *onset (initiating) phase* is the period of time from which an insult occurred until cell injury. The phase lasts from hours to days, depending on the causative factor, with toxic factors lasting longer. If treatment is initiated during this time, irreversible damage can be alleviated.

The *oliguric/anuric phase,* the second phase of ATN, lasts 1 to 2 weeks. Oliguria is encountered more commonly in ischemic damage, whereas nonoliguria is seen most often in conditions in which toxic insults occurred to the kidneys.[30,33] The mortality rate in patients with nonoliguric ATN is 25%, whereas it is 66% if oliguria is present.[28] Anuria occurs more commonly in postrenal obstruction.[30] During this phase the GFR is significantly decreased, which leads to increased levels of blood urea nitrogen (BUN) and creatinine, to electrolyte abnormalities (hyperkalemia, hyperphosphatemia, hypocalcemia), and to metabolic acidosis.[28,30,33]

The third phase, the *diuretic phase,* lasts 7 to 14 days and is characterized by an increase in GFR and urine output, with as much as 2 to 4 L/day.[28,30] During this phase, tubular function returns slowly and tubular reabsorption may not be able to increase as quickly as GFR. The result in this inequality is sodium and water loss in the urine, which leads to volume depletion.[28]

The last phase of ATN is the *recovery* or *convalescent phase.* During this stage, renal function slowly returns to normal or near normal, with GFR 70% to 80% of normal within 1 to 2 years.[30] If significant renal parenchymal damage has occurred, BUN and creatinine levels may never return to normal.[28,30]

ETIOLOGY OF ACUTE TUBULAR NECROSIS

ISCHEMIC

Hemorrhage
Excessive diuretic use
Burns
Peritonitis
Sepsis
Congestive heart failure
Myocardial ischemia
Pulmonary emboli
Transfusion reactions
Obstetric complications (severe toxemia, abruptio placentae, placenta previa, uterine rupture)

TOXIC

Rhabdomyolysis
Hypercalcemia
Gram-negative sepsis
Nephrotoxic medications (aminoglycosides, cephalosporins, antimicrobials, antineoplastic agents, analgesics containing phenacetin)
Heavy metals
Radiocontrast media
Insecticides
Carbon tetrachloride
Methanol
Street drugs such as phencyclidine (PCP)

Assessment and Diagnosis

Assessment of ARF can be divided into laboratory (urine and blood), radiologic, and fluid areas. Table 34-1 summarizes assessment and findings in these three areas.

The laboratory assessment always includes a serum test of BUN and creatinine levels. BUN is neither the sole indicator of ARF nor the most reliable indicator of renal damage because, although it reflects cellular

Table 34-1 Assessment in acute renal failure

Assessment area	Findings
LABORATORY	
Blood	
Hgb and Hct	Decreased
Electrolytes	Increased potassium, decreased calcium, decreased sodium
Plasma osmolality	Variable, usually increased
BUN and creatinine	Increased
Urine	
Specific gravity	Decreased (fixed in chronic renal failure)
Urinary sediments	Normal to increased
Osmolality	Decreased
Creatinine clearance	Decreased
Sodium concentration	Decreased
RADIOLOGIC	
Renal scan	All radiologic findings depend on specific pathology findings
Intravenous pyelogram (IVP)	
Angiographies	
FLUID	
Urinary output	Decreased
Skin turgor	Variable
Edema	Usually present

damage, the BUN level is easily changed by protein intake, blood in the gastrointestinal tract, or cell catabolism. Creatinine, on the other hand, is an accurate reflection of renal damage because it is almost totally excreted by the renal tubules. Elevated levels of creatinine can reflect damage to as many as 50% of the nephrons. The creatinine level may not rise as rapidly as the BUN level, however, because creatinine is independent of urinary flow.[15]

The urinalysis can indicate problems with prerenal causes of failure specifically by demonstrating the presence of granular casts or cellular debris. The urinary osmolality level increases (>500 mOsm/L), and the specific gravity level increases (>1.020) as the kidneys conserve water and sodium as a result of decreased perfusion.[34] The urinalysis also can reveal intrarenal causes by demonstrating actual tubular epithelial cells, a decrease in osmolality (from retained solutes), and a high sodium content. Twenty-four hour clearances of BUN and creatinine are typically low.

Table 34-2 Urinalysis findings with acute tubular necrosis

Indicator	Value	Rationale
Volume	Decreased	Damaged tubules cannot excrete
Creatinine	60 mg/dl	Damaged tubules cannot excrete properly
Urea	300 mg/dl	Damaged tubules cannot excrete urea properly and urea may be reabsorbed
Potassium	21 mEq/24 hr	Decreased urine output and tubular dysfunction prevent K^+ from being secreted
Specific gravity	1.012 regardless of hydration	Damaged tubules cannot concentrate or dilute urine
Urine osmolality	250-350 mOsm/L regardless of hydration	Damaged tubules cannot concentrate or dilute urine
Casts	Present (epithelial)	From direct damage to the epithelium of the tubules
Red blood cells	Present	From glomerular and/or tubular damage
Cellular debris	Present	From tubular damage, actual sloughing of tubular walls may occur

Modified from Norris MK: *DCCN* (8)1:16, 1989.

Most of the electrolytes in the ECF will become increasingly elevated, depending on the cause of damage and length of time the damage has been present. As urinary output decreases, serum electrolyte levels increase. Typically, elevations of potassium and phosphorus and depression of sodium and calcium occur. Sodium will be depressed in the presence of retention of large amounts of fluids (dilutional effect).

Radiologic tests used in diagnosing renal disorders have become increasingly sophisticated and valuable tools. Sonography, tomography, and angiography can help pinpoint the causal mechanism and even help differentiate between acute disease and chronic renal failure (Table 33-2). Radiologic contrast media have been implicated, although rarely, in the development or worsening of renal disorders.[35]

Finally, general assessment can reveal the effects that renal failure has on other body systems. For instance, hemodynamic monitoring during treatment for prerenal causes is valuable in tracking fluid balance and the need for fluid removal (dialysis) or replacement (IV fluids). The remaining areas of assessment should include a general review of the body systems.

◆ **Acute tubular necrosis.** Assessment of ATN usually involves tracking the fluid losses, compartmental fluid shifts, and cardiovascular function and monitoring the patient's general physical condition. Because hypovolemia is the usual precursor of ischemic tubular damage, careful assessment of fluid losses from all potential sources is important. It can be accomplished through accurate intake and output measurements. The patient's weight also is indicative of fluid gains or losses over a 1- to 2-day period. Additional signs and symptoms, such as thirst, decreased skin turgor, and apathy, suggest ECF depletion.[28] Tables 34-2 and 34-3 summarize urinalysis and other common laboratory findings in ATN, and

Table 34-3 Other common laboratory findings with acute tubular necrosis

Indicator	Value	Rationale
Blood urea nitrogen	Elevated	Damaged tubules allow urea to be reabsorbed
Serum creatinine	Elevated	Damaged tubules cannot rid the blood of creatinine
Serum potassium	Elevated	Damaged tubules cannot excrete potassium to clear the blood
Serum pH	Usually lower	Damaged tubules cannot excrete hydrogen ions and save bicarbonate ions
Creatinine clearance	Decreased	Damaged tubules cannot excrete creatinine

Modified from Norris MK: *DCCN* (8)1:16, 1989.

clinical manifestations and related pathophysiology are noted in Table 34-4.

Monitoring blood pressures and hemodynamics is helpful in assessing the fluid changes associated with the progressive course of ATN. Measurement of the abdominal girth for ascites and testing for pitting edema over body prominences and in dependent body areas should be performed frequently. Finally, cardiac outputs and pulmonary artery pressure (PAP) measurements can indicate a fall in intravascular volume. Cardiac output can decrease with a severe initial insult (e.g., hemorrhage).

Toxic injury in ATN frequently is caused by bacterial sepsis. Gram-negative organisms produce toxins that have a direct, widespread necrotic effect on the tubular cells. If a hypovolemic state also exists, the toxins are further concentrated in the tubular filtrate, thereby increasing the risk of complicating the injury.[28]

Medical Management

Medical interventions for ARF are directed toward three basic goals: (1) correcting the causative mechanism, (2) promoting regeneration of the remaining functional renal capacity, and (3) preventing complications. Medical management is based on the three categories of causes of acute failure. Prerenal failure, involved with perfusion problems and often with fluid losses and shifts, requires two specific methods of management: fluid replacement and stimulation of output with diuretics. Also, the defect causing the initial perfusion problem must be corrected. Care must be taken in the use of diuretics to avoid creation of secondary electrolyte abnormalities.[36]

Intrarenal failure involves the introduction of increased amounts of water, solutes, and potential toxins into the circulation; thus prompt measures are needed to decrease their levels. Hemodialysis is the usual treatment of choice, particularly if volume overload creates pulmonary and cardiac compromise. Severe hyperkalemia almost always necessitates hemodialysis because of the life-threatening cardiac dysrhythmias resulting from hyperkalemia. Dialysis also may be initiated for cases of uremic pericarditis or severe azotemia in which other treatments are contraindicated.[29] A description of dialysis is found in Chapter 35.

Drugs, fluid restriction, and dietary control constitute a large part of the medical treatment for renal failure.

Table 34-4 Clinical manifestations and pathophysiology of acute tubular necrosis

Clinical manifestations	Pathophysiology
Fluid overload as manifested by: Hypertension Pulmonary edema Congestive heart failure Pneumonia Peripheral edema Periorbital edema Sacral edema Ascites	Decreased renal excretion of water, especially during oliguric phase of ATN
Hyperkalemia as manifested by ECG changes: Tall, tented T waves Depressed ST segment Prolonged PR interval Loss of P wave Wide QRS complex Cardiac arrest	Decreased renal excretion of potassium ions Acidosis Catabolism Bleeding Blood transfusions Dietary intake
Metabolic acidosis manifested by: Kussmaul's respirations Hyperkalemia Mental changes	Decreased renal hydrogen ion excretion Decreased renal absorption of sodium ions Decreased bicarbonate regeneration Decreased ammonia synthesis and ammonium excretion Decreased excretion of titratable acids Catabolism
Pericarditis as manifested by: *Classic triad* Fever Chest pain Pericardial friction rub *ECG changes* ST segment elevation with upward concavity Depressed PR interval Low QRS voltage	Pericardial membrane inflammation from uremic toxins

Modified from Lancaster L: *Crit Care Nurs Clin North Am* 2 (2):221, 1990.

Table 34-4 Clinical manifestations and pathophysiology of acute tubular necrosis—cont'd

Clinical manifestations	Pathophysiology
Pericardial effusion and tamponade as manifested by: Paradoxic pulse greater than 10 mm Hg Increased jugular venous pressure (JVP) with pulsations Decreased systolic blood pressure Narrow pulse pressure Muffled heart sounds Weak peripheral pulses Decreased level of consciousness	Bleeding and effusion of fluid into pericardial cavity caused by pericarditis
Hypertension (after shock syndrome is treated and ATN ensues)	Fluid overload and sodium retention Excess renin-angiotensin production
Hypotension (during shock syndrome and onset of ATN)	Hypovolemia Septicemia Excess dialysis and fluid removal
Anemia as manifested by: Decreased hematocrit Decreased hemoglobin Shortness of breath Decreased activity tolerance	Decreased renal erythropoeitin production Shortened RBC lifespan as a result of uremic toxins Altered folic acid action GI bleeding Hemodialysis blood loss
Potential for infection (NOTE: Urea is a hypothermic agent; therefore any temperature elevation in ATN is significant.)	Decreased macrophage activity as a result of uremic toxins Invasive lines and procedures Nosocomial and iatrogenic blood losses
Skin alterations as manifested by: Pale, yellow, dry, itching skin Purpura Uremic frost (only in terminally ill patients)	Uremic anemia Deposition of pigments, uremic toxins, and calcium phosphate in skin and irritation of peripheral nerves Capillary fragility and platelet dysfunction
Glucose intolerance	Decreased peripheral sensitivity to insulin but decreased half-life because of decreased renal excretion
Altered calcium and phosphate metabolism as manifested by: Hyperphosphatemia Hypocalcemia Metastatic calcifications Osteodystrophy (only if oliguric phase is very prolonged)	Decreased renal excretion of phosphate Decreased renal synthesis of vitamin D Excess parathyroid hormone Deposition of calcium phosphate crystals in skin, soft tissues, and other structures
Altered GI function as manifested by: Anorexia Nausea Vomiting Stomatitis Halitosis Gastritis with bleeding Diarrhea Constipation	Mucous membrane inflammation as a result of uremic toxins Decomposition of urea in GI tract and ammonia release, which irritates mucosa Capillary fragility and bleeding Electrolyte imbalances
Altered neuromuscular-mental function as manifested by: Drowsiness Confusion Irritability Coma Tremors Twitching Convulsions Peripheral neuropathy (restless legs syndrome) Decreased concentration Altered perception Decreased mentation	Uremic toxins' effect on nervous system Fluid and electrolyte imbalances

Fluid restriction is used to prevent circulatory overload and interstitial edema associated with ARF and is calculated on the basis of daily urinary volumes and insensible losses; thus obtaining daily weights and keeping accurate intake and output records become essential. Patients usually are restricted to 1 L of fluid if urinary output is 500 ml or less and insensible losses range from 500 to 750 ml/day. In the absence of oliguria, however, fluid intake may be liberalized on an individual basis, determined by matching the daily fluid output.[15]

Electrolyte levels require frequent observation, especially in the initial critical phases of failure. Potassium may quickly reach levels of 6.0 mEq/L and above. Other than through hemodialysis, hyperkalemia can be treated temporarily by IV infusion of insulin and glucose. An infusion of 100 ml of 50% dextrose accompanied by 20 units of regular insulin forces potassium back into the cells.[2] Sodium bicarbonate (40 to 160 mEq) may be infused to promote higher excretion of potassium in the urine.[2] Finally, sodium polystyrene sulfonate (Kayexalate), a cation-exchange resin, is mixed in water and sorbitol and given orally, rectally, or through an NG tube.[5] The resin captures potassium in the bowel, which eliminates it in the feces.

Dilutional hyponatremia, associated with renal failure, can be corrected with fluid restriction. If, however, sodium stores actually are depleted, 3% saline solution usually is administered intravenously as a replacement.[3] In addition, sodium levels may be raised during dialysis by changing the amount of sodium in the dialysate bath.

Calcium levels are reduced in renal failure, and, as previously described, the reduction is related to multiple factors, among which is hyperphosphatemia. Aluminum hydroxide preparations are administered to bind phosphorus in the bowel and thereby lower its level. Calcium also may be increased by use of calcium supplements, vitamin D preparations, and synthetic calcitriol (Rocaltrol).[19]

The nutritional aspect of renal failure may involve replacement, as well as restriction. With the availability of refined products, it has become easy to provide total parenteral nutrition (TPN) while the patient is undergoing dialysis. If the patient is anorexic and malnourished, TPN can be provided, and renal formulas are even available.

The renal diet prescription is quite restrictive. Protein, potassium, sodium, and phosphorus usually are limited. For instance, protein restriction may vary to limit azotemia.[34] Carbohydrates are encouraged, primarily to provide needed energy for healing. Refer to Chapter 50 for a more in-depth discussion of nutritional management of renal failure.

Nursing Management

Meticulous attention to fluid changes, cardiovascular problems, prevention of infection, and alleviation of symptoms provide more comfort and a better prognosis for the patient with ARF. In addition, providing teaching and emotional support for the patient and family becomes an integral part of the nursing care.

NURSING DIAGNOSES AND MANAGEMENT

Acute renal failure

- ◆ High Risk for Fluid Volume Excess risk factor: renal failure, p. 639
- ◆ Anxiety related to threatened biologic, psychologic, and/or social integrity, p. 763
- ◆ High Risk for Infection risk factors: protein-calorie malnourishment, invasive monitoring devices, p. 366
- ◆ Body Image Disturbance related to functional dependence on life-sustaining technology, p. 95
- ◆ Knowledge Deficit: Fluid Restriction, Reportable Symptoms, and Medications related to lack of previous exposure to information, p. 72
- ◆ Sensory/Perceptual Alterations related to sensory overload, sensory deprivation, and sleep pattern disturbance, p. 573
- ◆ Ineffective Individual Coping related to situational crisis and personal vulnerability, p. 762

The actual nursing management for the patient with ARF focuses on prevention or control of complications secondary to the disease process. In preventing infection, the nurse not only must frequently monitor for signs of infection but must maintain the patient's pulmonary hygiene, skin integrity, and nutrition. Consideration must be given to limiting invasive procedures and providing strict asepsis when dressing changes, catheterizations, or any such invasive procedures are required. Should the patient be immobile, frequent turning and observation of potential sites for skin breakdown enhance the chances of avoiding infection. If significant anasarca has developed, the use of a circulating air or air-fluid mattress may help prevent skin breakdown.

Frequent assessment of intake and output, particularly the output in response to any administered diuretics, is a necessary part of the nursing management for the patient in renal failure. Daily patient weights are correlated with the intake and output to confirm fluid overloads. The nurse should note the return of urinary output and seek replacement for the fluids and electrolytes that can be lost rapidly during this phase.

Hyperkalemia, hypocalcemia, hyponatremia, and hyperphosphatemia may all occur during ARF. The nurse must be aware of the clinical manifestations of these electrolyte imbalances and must prevent or control their associated side effects. The imbalances with the most potential hazard are hyperkalemia and hypocalcemia, which can result in life-threatening cardiac dysrhythmias. The nurse is involved not only in monitoring signs and symptoms of these imbalances but in teaching the patient and family ways to avoid imbalances and consequences of the imbalances.

Although the nurse can do little to prevent hyponatremia, nursing management must include frequent assessment for its clinical manifestations. The astute nurse also

LEGAL REVIEW: The law and regulation of medical records

Documentation in the patient's medical record must be (1) complete, (2) accurate, and (3) timely. The medical record provides legal proof of the nature and extent of care delivered to the patient. The critical care nurse has a legal duty to maintain the record in sufficient detail; insufficient or improper documentation may result in nursing liability or nonreimbursement by a third-party payer. The general rule, "What isn't in the medical record didn't occur," continues to prevail. The courts have held fairly consistently that failure to document care infers failure to provide care.

Federal regulations (including Medicare and Medicaid provisions under the Social Security Act), state laws and regulations (including hospital, medical, and nursing licensure statutes), accrediting organization (such as the Joint Commission on Accreditation of Healthcare Organizations) standards, professional organization standards, institutional policies and procedures, and custom all contribute to define documentation standards and to determine the form and content of the medical record.

As a general rule of law, the medical record is presumed to be accurate, absent evidence of tampering or fraud. Correcting an entry is lawful if the corrected portion remains legible; obliterating an entry may expose one to liability. Loss of the medical record raises a rebuttable presumption of negligence. Other documentation errors include factual omissions, unreasonably late entries, unauthorized entries, vague or ambiguous recordings, abbreviations not in common usage, personal opinions and subjectivity, failure to sign or time the record, and illegibility.

See *Battocchi v Wash. Hosp. Center,* 581 A 2d 759 (DC App 1990); *Brookover v Mary Hitchcock Memorial Hosp.,* 893 F. 2d 411 (1st Cir 1990); *Collins v Westlake Community Hosp.,* 312 NE 2d 614 (Ill 1974); *Joseph Brant Memorial Hosp. v Koziol,* 2 CCLT 170 (SCC 1978); Morrissey-Ross M: *Documentation: if you haven't written it, you haven't done it, Nurs Clin North Am* 23(2):363, 1988; Roach WH Jr: *Legal review: incentive for completing medical records–the legal risks, Top Health Rec Manage* 10 (3):78, 1990; *Rogers v Kasdan,* 612 SW 2d 133 (Ky 1981); *Stack v Wapner,* 368 A 2d 292 (Pa Super 1976); Staggers N: *Comput Nurs,* 6(4):164, 1988; *St. Paul Fire and Marine Ins. Co. v Prothro,* 590 SW 2d 35 (Ark App 1979); Tomes JP: *Healthcare records: a practical legal guide,* Westchester, Ill, 1990, Healthcare Financial Management Association; *Villetto v Weilbaecher,* 377 So 2d 132 (La App 1979); *Whalen v Roe,* 429 US 589, 97 S Ct 869 (1977).

must remember that as fluid overload worsens in the patient with oliguria, dilutional hyponatremia also may develop. Finally, hyperphosphatemia results most often in severe pruritus. Thus nursing care subsequently is directed at soothing the itching by performing frequent skin care with emollients, discouraging scratching, and administering phosphate-binding medications.

Care in preventing blood loss in the patient with renal failure centers on observation. Irritation of the GI tract from metabolic waste accumulation should be expected, and stools, NG drainage, and emesis should be tested for occult blood.

The nurse must give accurate, uncomplicated information to the patient and family about ARF, including its prognosis, treatment, and possible complications. The nurse should be aware that sleep-rest disorders and emotional upset can occur as complications of ARF and should encourage the patient and family to voice concerns, frustrations, and fears. Searching for ways to allow the patient to control some aspects of the acute care environment or treatment also is essential.

◆ **Acute tubular necrosis.** The nurse, who may provide additional preventive care for ATN alone, is in a unique position to identify patients at high risk for renal insult—for example, persons who have been exposed to toxins associated with ATN.

The nurse caring for the elderly postoperative patient must be aware that the GFR in this age-group may be decreased and that postoperative dehydration can result in hypoperfusion of the kidneys, with subsequent development of ATN. The critical care nurse must be vigilant of hemodynamic parameters (i.e., pulmonary artery pressure [PAP] and cardiac output) that provide early information about fluid balance and perfusion of the kidneys. The nurse must be alert not only for dehydration, but for fluid overload as well. Postoperative or trauma patients receiving fluid replacement require as strict attention to output as to intake. Subtle decreases in urinary output may not be observed unless comparisons of intake to output are made on a consistent basis.

REFERENCES

1. Innerarity SA: Electrolyte emergencies in the critically ill renal patient, *Crit Care Nurs Clin North Am* 2(1):89, 1990.
2. Commerford PJ, Lloyd EA: Arrhythmias in patients with drug toxicity, electrolyte, and endocrine disturbances, *Med Clin North Am* 68(6):1051, 1984.
3. Plumer AL, Cosentino F: *Principles and practice of intravenous therapy,* Boston, 1987, Little, Brown.
4. DeAngelis R, Lessig ML: Hyperkalemia, *Crit Care Nurse* 12(3):55, 1992.
5. Innerarity SA: Hyperkalemic emergencies, *Crit Care Nurs Q* 14(4):32, 1992.
6. Schwartz MW: Potassium imbalances, *Am J Nurs* 87(10):1292, 1987.
7. Weisberg LS, Szerlip HM, Cox M: Disorders of potassium homeostasis in critically ill patients, *Crit Care Clin* 5(4):835, 1987.

8. Huerta BJ, Lemberg L: Potassium imbalance in the coronary care unit, *Heart Lung* 14(2):193, 1985.
9. Aluis R, Geheb M, Cox M: Hypo- and hyperosmolar states: diagnostic approaches. In Arieff AI, DeFronzo RA, editors: *Fluid, electrolyte and acid-base disorders,* vol 1, New York, 1985, Churchill Livingstone.
10. Metheny NM: *Fluid and electrolyte balance: nursing considerations,* Philadelphia, 1987, JB Lippincott.
11. Cluitmans FH, Meinders AE: Management of severe hyponatremia: rapid or slow correction, *Am J Med* 88:161, 1990.
12. Tanneau RS and others: Deleterious effect of prolonged administration and fluid restriction after partial correction of severe hyponatremia, *Crit Care Med* 19(2):305, 1991.
13. Johndrow PD, Thornton S: Syndrome of inappropriate antidiuretic hormone—a growing concern, *Focus Crit Care* 12(5):29, 1985.
14. Starker PM, Gump FE: Gastrointestinal disorders. In Askanzi J, Starker PM, Weissman C, editors: *Fluid and electrolyte management in critical care,* Boston, 1986, Butterworth & Co.
15. Schrier R: *Renal and electrolyte disorders,* ed 3, Boston, 1986, Little, Brown.
16. Tonnensen AS: Water balance and control of osmolality. In Askanzi J, Starker, and Weissman C, editors: *Fluid and electrolyte management in critical care,* Boston, 1986, Butterworth & Co.
17. Desai TK, Carlson RW, Geheb MA: Hypokalemia and hypophosphatemia in acutely ill patients, *Crit Care Clin* 5(4):927, 1987.
18. Levine NM, Kleeman CR: Hypercalcemia: pathophysiology and treatment, *Hosp Pract* 22(7):93, 1987.
19. Zaloga GP, Chernow B: Hypocalcemia in critical illness, *JAMA* 256(4):1924, 1986.
20. Bybee DE: Saving lives in a parathyroid crisis, *Emerg Med* 19(15):62, 1987.
21. Spencer H and others: Calcium requirements in humans, *Clin Orthop* 184:270, 1984.
22. Coward DD: Cancer-induced hypercalcemia, *Cancer Nurs* 9(3):125, 1986.
23. Workman ML: Magnesium and phosphorus: the neglected electrolytes, *AACN Clin Issues Crit Care Nurs* 3(3):655, 1992.
24. Flink EB: Magnesium deficiency, *Hosp Pract* 15:1161, 1987.
25. Kurokawa K and others: Physiology of phosphorus metabolism and pathophysiology of hypophosphatemia and hyperphosphatemia. In Arieff AI, DeFronzo RA, editors: *Fluid, electrolyte and acid-base disorders,* vol 1, New York, 1985, Churchill Livingstone.
26. Appel GB, Stern L: Acute and chronic renal failure. In Askanzi J, Starker PM, Weissman C, editors: *Fluid and electrolyte management in critical care,* Boston, 1986, Butterworth & Co.
27. Laski ME, Kurtzman NA: Acid-base disturbances in pulmonary medicine. In Arieff AI, DeFronzo RA, editors: *Fluid, electrolyte and acid-base disorders,* vol 1, New York, 1985, Churchill Livingstone.
28. Douglas S: Acute tubular necrosis: diagnosis, treatment, and nursing implications, *AACN Clin Issues Crit Care Nurs* 3(3):688, 1992.
29. Baer CM, Lancaster LE: Acute renal failure, *Crit Care Nurs Q* 14(4):1, 1992.
30. Lancaster LE: Renal response to shock, *Crit Care Nurs Clin North Am* 2(2):221, 1990.
31. Jochimsen F and others: Impairment of renal function in medical intensive care: predictability of acute renal failure, *Crit Care Med* 18(5):480, 1990.
32. Norris MK: Acute tubular necrosis: preventing complications, *DCCN* 8(1):16, 1989.
33. Stark JL: Acute tubular necrosis: differences between oliguria and nonoliguria, *Crit Care Nurse Q* 14(4):22, 1992.
34. Sillix DH, McDonald FD: Acute renal failure, *Crit Care Clin 5(4):909, 1987.*
35. Sondheimmer JH, Migdal SD: Toxic nephropathies, *Crit Care Clin* 5(4):883, 1987.
36. Kellick KA: Diuretics, *AACN Clin Issues Crit Care Nurs* 3(2):472, 1992.

35

Renal Therapeutic Management

CHAPTER OBJECTIVES

- Describe the difference between crystalloid and colloid solutions.
- Name factors that determine the type, amount, and duration of intravenous therapy.
- Describe three types of intravenous volume expansion solutions.
- Identify and describe the various types of vascular access for hemodialysis.
- Describe the indications and contraindications to hemodialysis.
- Discuss the types of continuous renal replacement therapy.
- Discuss potential complications of the various types of dialysis and the associated nursing management.

VOLUME REPLACEMENT WITH INTRAVENOUS THERAPY

Myriad factors influence not only the need for intravenous fluids but also the type, amount, and duration of replacement. For example, factors such as type of fluid lost, urinary output, ongoing loss, "third spacing," and hemodynamic readings contribute to the initial and subsequent decisions to prescribe fluid replacement. The objectives of the fluid replacement are to replace losses of fluids and electrolytes and to prevent fluid imbalance in the face of ongoing loss.[1]

Maintenance fluid therapy is initiated only when oral fluid intake is inadvisable (postoperatively) or impossible.[1] Maintenance fluids are calculated with consideration for individual body surface area. Adults require approximately 1500 ml/m²/24 hr. Requirements may be affected by such factors as fever, burns, environmental temperature and humidity changes, and head injuries.[1] The rate of replacement depends on cardiac competency, adequacy of renal mechanisms, ongoing loss, and type of fluid required.

The debate regarding the use of crystalloid versus colloid solutions still rages.[2] In reality, both often are used with successful results. Crystalloid solutions, which are balanced salt solutions, are in widespread use for both maintenance infusions and replacement therapy. Colloids, which are salt solutions containing oncotically active particles, are employed most often in the later stages of loss to supplement volume and to achieve and maintain hemodynamic stability.[1,3]

Examples of crystalloid solutions are dextrose in water (D_5W, $D_{10}W$), normal saline (0.9% NaCl), half-strength saline (0.45% NaCl), and lactated Ringer's (LR). Dextrose in water is considered nearly isotonic and is used primarily for fluid maintenance or replacement and for provision of minimal calories. Normal saline is isotonic and is used for volume replacement, volume maintenance, or correction of hyponatremia, hypochloremia, and mild metabolic acidosis.[1,4]

Finally, LR, which contains several electrolytes and acid, is used to replace volume and electrolytes and to provide bicarbonate. LR, used frequently in the intraoperative environment, should be avoided in patients with renal failure. Other crystalloid solutions are described in Table 35-1.

Colloid solutions are used primarily for rapid volume expansion. The oncotically active particles (proteinate, synthetic polymers, or polysaccharides) pull fluid from the interstitium to expand circulating volume. A 10-ml infusion of albumin (25%), for example, pulls 350 ml into the vascular system. The volume expansion can last as long as 24 hours, with corresponding rises in pulmonary capillary wedge pressure (PCWP), mean arterial pressure (MAP), and cardiac index (CI).[4]

Hetastarch is a fluid and polymer combination that is isotonic in nature. Hetastarch, which provides sustained oncotic action (longer than 24 hours), has been implicated in the increase of prothrombin and partial thromboplastin times. Although this finding might indicate a tendency to cause bleeding, little evidence exists to substantiate any contraindication. Indeed, studies confirm the use of hetastarch in cardiac surgery with no difficulties with hemorrhage.[5]

On the other hand, the use of the polysaccharide volume expander *dextran* is contraindicated for patients with bleeding tendencies. Dextran has a sustained effect on clotting factors and platelets.[4]

Recent research showed that colloid therapy, after cardiac surgery, has permitted the use of smaller fluid volumes for the achievement and maintenance of hemodynamic stability. However, in situations in which capillary membrane permeability has been altered (e.g., burns, septic shock, anphylaxis), it has been suggested that colloids may cross into the interstitium and thereby create interstitial edema. Little evidence exists to support this hypothesis, but reluctance to use colloids frequently is based on the aforementioned assumption.[1]

Adequacy of intravenous fluid replacement depends on strict ongoing evaluation and frequent adjustment. Frequent monitoring of blood gases and electrolytes is

Table 35-1 Intravenous solutions

Name	Tonicity	Indication
CRYSTALLOIDS		
Dextrose in water (D_5W, $D_{10}W$)	Isotonic	To maintain volume To replace mild loss To provide minimal calories
Normal saline (0.9% NaCl)	Isotonic	To maintain volume To replace mild loss To correct mild hyponatremia
Half-strength saline (0.45% NaCl)	Hypotonic	For free water replacement To correct mild hyponatremia (when amount of Na^+ needed is unknown)
Multielectrolyte solution (Isolyte, Normosol)	Hypotonic	For free water and electrolyte replacement (used in fluid and electrolyte-restricted conditions)
Lactated Ringer's	Hypertonic	For maximum fluid and electrolyte replacement (contraindicated for patients with renal or liver disease or in lactic acidosis)
Hypertonic saline (3% and 5% NaCl)	Hypertonic	To correct severe hyponatremia (used only in situations of intensive monitoring)
COLLOIDS		
Salt-poor albumin (Plasmanate)	Hypertonic	For volume expansion For moderate protein replacement For achievement of hemodynamic stability in shock states
Hetastarch	Hypertonic	For volume expansion For long-term hemodynamic stability after cardiac surgery, burns, sepsis)
Dextran	Hypertonic	For volume expansion and support (contraindicated for patients with bleeding disorders)

required, and strictly regulated intake and output should be correlated with daily weight records. Finally, hemodynamic readings should be frequent and ongoing. Generally, minimal rises in central venous pressure (CVP) or the right atrial pressure (RAP) indicate the need for fluid replacement. Further decreases in CVP, PCWP, and CI indicate ongoing volume losses.[3,4] Significant rises in CVP and PCWP, with a fall in CI, may indicate hypervolemia, with underlying pump failure.[3,4]

DIALYSIS

A wide range of options is available for the treatment of acute renal failure: hemodialysis, peritoneal dialysis, and continuous renal replacement therapy.[6,7] A detailed discussion of each method follows.

Hemodialysis

Hemodialysis roughly translates as "separating from the blood."[8] As a treatment, hemodialysis literally separates and removes from the blood the excess electrolytes, fluids, and toxins. Although efficient in regulating chemicals, it does not remove all metabolites. Furthermore, electrolytes, toxins, and fluids increase between treatments, requiring performance of dialysis on a regular basis (3 to 4 hours three times per week). Indications and contraindications for hemodialysis[6,7,9] are listed in the box on p. 623.

The treatment works by circulating blood outside the body through synthetic tubing to a *dialyzer,* which consists of several membrane pockets (flat-plate type) or tubes (hollow-fiber type) (Fig. 35-1). While the blood flows through the membranes, which are semipermeable, a fluid known as the *dialysate bath* bathes the membranes and, through osmosis and diffusion, performs exchanges of fluid, electrolytes, and toxins from the blood to the bath.[9] The blood and bath are shunted in opposite directions (countercurrent flow) through the dialyzer to maintain the osmotic and chemical gradients at their highest.

To remove fluid, a positive hydrostatic pressure is applied to the blood and a negative hydrostatic pressure is applied to the dialysate bath. The two forces together, called *transmembrane pressure,* pull and squeeze the excess fluid from the blood. The difference between the two values (expressed in millimeters of mercury [mm Hg]) represents the transmembrane pressure and results in fluid extraction, known as *ultrafiltration,* from the vascular space.[10]

Heparin is added to the system just before the blood enters the dialyzer. Without the heparin, the blood would clot because its presence outside the body and its passage through foreign substances initiate the clotting mechanism. Heparin can be administered by bolus injection or intermittent infusion. Administration is

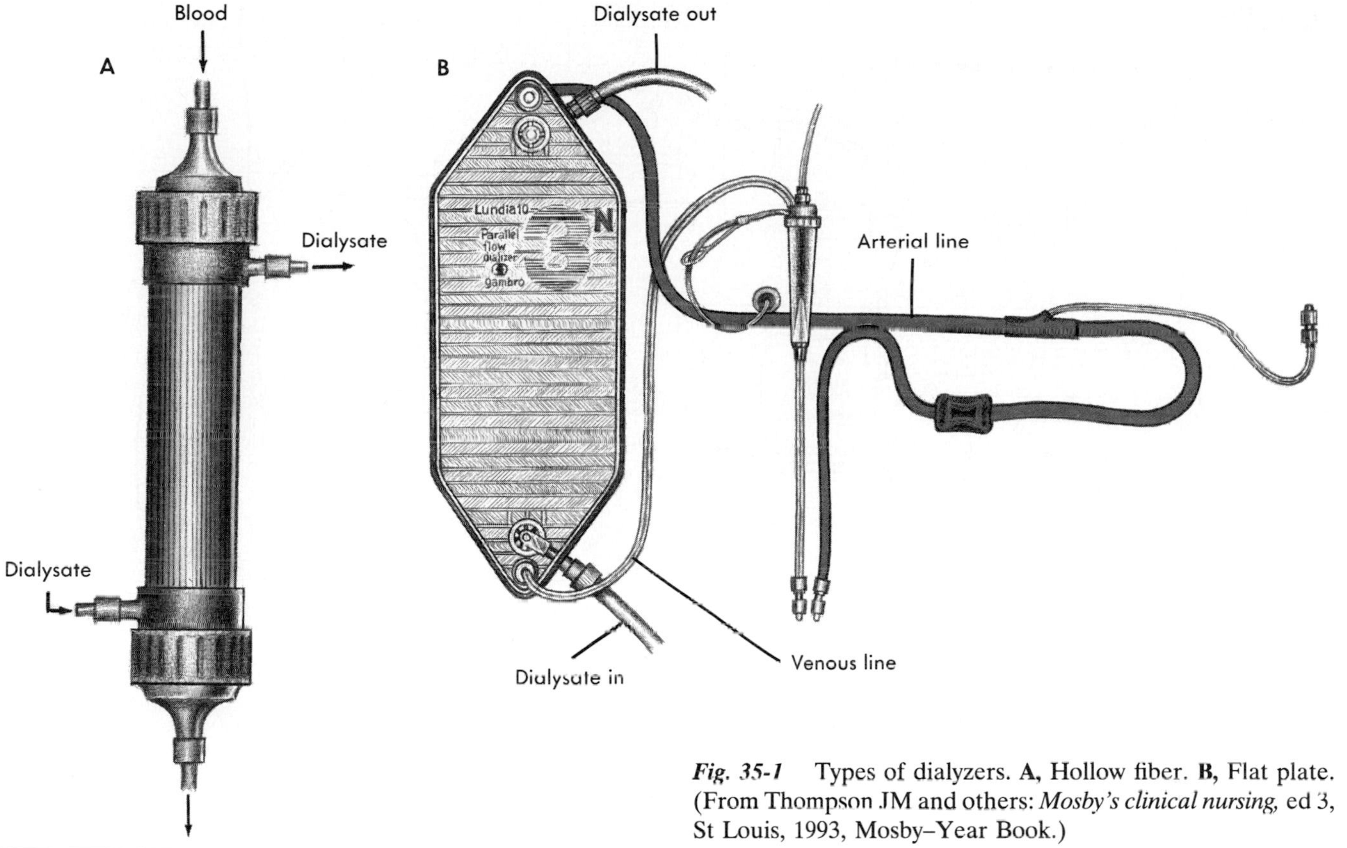

Fig. 35-1 Types of dialyzers. **A,** Hollow fiber. **B,** Flat plate. (From Thompson JM and others: *Mosby's clinical nursing,* ed 3, St Louis, 1993, Mosby–Year Book.)

INDICATIONS AND CONTRAINDICATIONS FOR HEMODIALYSIS

INDICATIONS

BUN >100 mg/dl
Serum creatinine >10 mg/dl
Hyperkalemia
Drug toxicity
Intravascular and extravascular fluid overload
Metabolic acidosis
Symptoms of uremia:
- Pericarditis
- GI bleeding
- Mental changes

Contraindications to other forms of dialysis

CONTRAINDICATIONS

Hemodynamic instability
Inability to anticoagulate
Lack of access to circulation

determined on the basis of an arbitrary dosage of units per kilogram of weight, followed by monitoring of the response to the particular dose by performing clotting times.[10] Heparin has a very short half-life; thus its effects subside within 2 to 4 hours. Also, the effects of heparin are easily reversed through the injection of protamine.

After leaving the dialyzer, the blood continues through synthetic tubing and is returned to the body. Because the systemic blood pressure is not sufficient to propel the blood through this *extracorporeal* (outside the vessels) circuit, a pump is used to provide a consistent flow of blood (200 to 400 ml/min) through the system. Various monitoring devices prevent blood loss, air embolus, access collapse, or high-pressure destruction of the dialyzer or access. The components of a hemodialysis system appear in Fig. 35-2.

The dialyzer, or artificial kidney, is designed as an attempt to mimic the action of the renal tubules. Active transport and other physiologic mechanisms, however, are not possible with synthetic membranes; thus the artificial kidney can provide for only partial normalization of the blood. There are two basic types of artificial kidneys—the plate dialyzer and the hollow-fiber dialyzer. No matter what the type of artificial kidneys, the process by which they function is the same.

The dialysis process moves blood through either microscopic hollow tubes or thin membranous pockets. The membranes have fixed-sized pores, which allow passage of small molecules (e.g., water, glucose, electrolytes) while preventing passage of some large molecules (e.g., red blood cells [RBCs], white blood cells [WBCs], viruses, bacteria).

The dialysate bath is composed of electrolytes, blood buffers, and water in quantities that create a diffusion

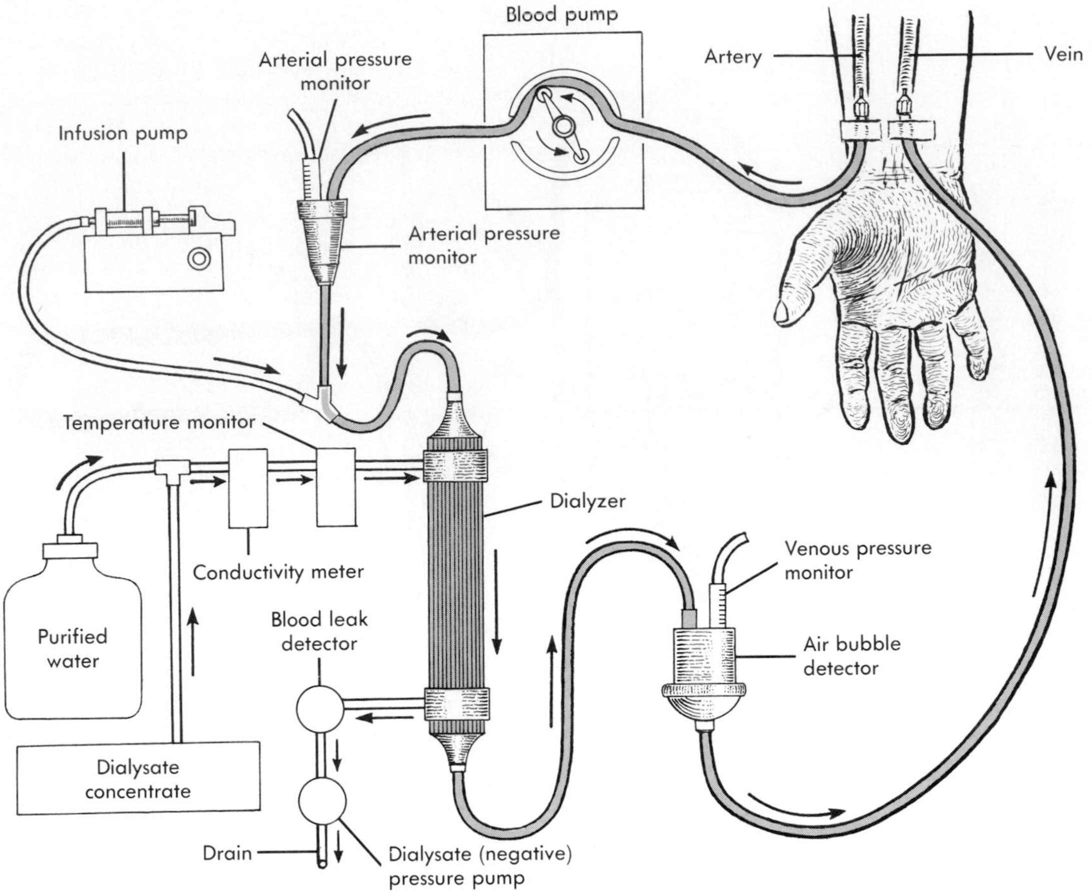

Fig. 35-2 Components of a hemodialysis system.

COMPOSITION OF DIALYSATE BATH

Purified water (reverse osmosis process)
Sodium chloride
Potassium chloride
Sodium bicarbonate (used frequently, although sodium acetate may be used as a substitute)
Calcium chloride
Magnesium chloride
Lactic acid

gradient across the membranes (see box above). For instance, the potassium content may be 2.0 mEq/L in the dialysate to enhance diffusion from the hyperkalemic blood of the renal patient to the dialysate. Calcium absorption also is enhanced by this process. Higher amounts of ionized calcium are placed in the dialysate than are present in the patient's serum. The calcium travels from the dialysate to the patient's vascular space, thereby improving calcium stores.

Several factors affect the efficiency of the dialysis treatment. Blood flow rate must be constant and sufficiently fast to provide the solute and fluid load that maintain the chemical and osmotic gradient on either side of the membrane. The dialysate flow rate should be 2 to 2½ times that of the blood.[10] The temperature of the dialysate should be comfortable (37° C plus or minus 3° C) to maintain blood temperature (98° to 101° F) and to maintain the ability of solutes to diffuse. The dialysate composition should maintain a concentration gradient between the dialysate and the fluid and solute-laden blood. In addition, the direction of flow of the dialysate should be countercurrent, with dialysate flowing in one direction and the blood in the opposite direction. Finally, differences in the pore size, membrane thickness, available membrane surface area, and composition of the membrane can affect the relative efficiency of the dialysis treatment (see box, p. 625).

Tap water is not safe for use in dialysis; the prevalence of calcium, magnesium, organic and inorganic matter, bacteria, and chloramines in tap water can jeopardize effective dialysis. Therefore purification methods must be undertaken to remove these materials, as well as salts contained in the tap water. Distillation, reverse osmosis purification, and carbon filtering are currently used methods for obtaining safe water for use in the dialysis treatment.[11]

◆ **Vascular access for hemodialysis.** Hemodialysis can be performed only by obtaining access to the blood stream.

FACTORS AFFECTING THE EFFICIENCY OF DIALYSIS

- Composition of dialysate
- Temperature of dialysate
- Dialyzer configuration (length of flow path)
- Membrane's thickness
- Membrane's pore size
- Flow rate of blood
- Flow rate of dialysate
- Actual treatment time
- Membrane's surface area

Over many years, various types of accesses, such as arteriovenous (A-V) fistulas, A-V shunts, A-V grafts, and femoral and subclavian catheters, have been created. The common denominator in most accesses is access to the arterial circulation and return to the venous circulation; femoral and subclavian catheters access the venous circulation only.

It is essential for the nurse to become familiar with each type of access, the potential problems that each can develop, and the nursing interventions each requires. The dialysis patient often is taught that the access is a "lifeline"; thus care on the part of patient and nurse can prevent complications.

A-V shunt. Because of the advent of subclavian and femoral catheters, A-V shunts are used infrequently today. If, however, the temporary catheters cannot be used, access can rapidly be obtained through an A-V shunt. The shunt consists of Teflon vessel tips, Silastic tubing, and a connection joint for creating the circuit between the arterial and venous tubing[12] (Fig. 35-3, *A*). The shunt requires a peripheral artery, usually radial or ulnar, and a peripheral vein, such as the cephalic or basilic. A cutdown is performed on each vessel, with the vessel tips inserted and sutured in place. Tubing extends from each vessel tip (outside the body) and is connected, when not being used for dialysis, by a straight connector or a heparin–T device. Blood flows in a U-shaped fashion from artery to vein. Shunts also may be inserted in the thigh or ankle areas. Complications common to A-V shunts are thrombosis, infection, and skin erosion. Nursing management considerations for A-V shunts are listed in Table 35-2.

A-V fistula. The A-V fistula is created by surgically visualizing a peripheral artery and vein, creating an opening in the artery and the vein, and anastomosing the two open areas. Anastomoses may be side-to-side, end-to-side, or end-to-end. The high arterial flow creates swelling of the vein, or a *pseudoaneurysm,* at which point (when healed) a large-bore needle can be inserted to obtain outflow. Inflow is accomplished through a second large-bore needle inserted into a peripheral vein distal to the fistula (Fig. 35-3, *B*).

If the patient's vessels are adequate, fistulas are the preferred mode of access because of the durability of the individual's own vessels and the relatively few complications in comparison to the other accesses. Development of sufficient flow to the fistula, however, may require weeks to months. Attempting to obtain flow from the underdeveloped fistulas often causes painful vascular spasm and reduced flow. In addition, internal accesses have the potential for creating arterial insufficiency because of the high arterial blood flow diverted for dialysis purposes. The arterial insufficiency produces a set of symptoms known as *vascular steal syndrome* (pale, cold distal extremity with severe spasmodic pain). Additional complications, such as thrombosis, infection (low rate), or venous hypertension, can occur with A-V fistulas.[13] The care of the fistula and nursing considerations are listed in Table 35-2.

A-V grafts. Currently, A-V grafts are, by far, the most frequently used access for treating chronic renal failure. Synthetic materials, such as Goretex, or biologic materials, such as human umbilical veins, provide a wide range of lumen sizes and graft lengths. The graft is a tube formed of the desired material (usually Goretex), which is surgically implanted in the limb. The area is surgically opened, and an artery and a vein are located. A tunnel is created (either straight or U-shaped) in the tissue in which the graft is placed. Anastamoses are made with the graft ends connected to the artery and vein. The blood is allowed to flow through the graft, and the surgical area is closed. The graft creates a raised area (looking like a vein) just under the skin and peripheral tissue layers (Fig. 35-3, *C*). Two large-bore needles are used for outflow and inflow to the graft. For both grafts and fistulas, after needle removal at the end of the hemodialysis treatment, pressure must be applied to stem bleeding. Nursing management and complications of the A-V graft are listed in Table 35-2.

Subclavian and femoral vein catheters. Subclavian and femoral vein catheters are used most often in cases of acute renal failure when short-term access is required or when vascular access is nonfunctional in a patient requiring immediate hemodialysis. Both subclavian and femoral catheters can be inserted at the bedside.

A dual-lumen subclavian catheter is the most commonly used form of vascular access for acute hemodialysis.[9] It has a central partition running the length of the catheter. The outflow catheter pulls the blood flow through openings that are proximal to the inflow openings on the opposite side. This design avoids dialyzing the same blood just returned to the area (recirculation), which can severely reduce the procedure's efficiency.

When a subclavian vein is not available, a shorter version of the catheter is used for quick placement into the femoral vein. In addition, a silicone rubber, dual-lumen catheter has been developed that is inserted into the subclavian or internal jugular vein. This newer catheter contains a Dacron cuff that decreases the incidence of catheter-related infection.[9]

The subclavian access must *always* be confirmed by chest x-ray film to evaluate the possibility of pneumothorax or hemothorax resulting from catheter insertion. Femoral catheter sites must be observed carefully for any signs of rapidly developing hematomas from femoral artery puncture.[12]

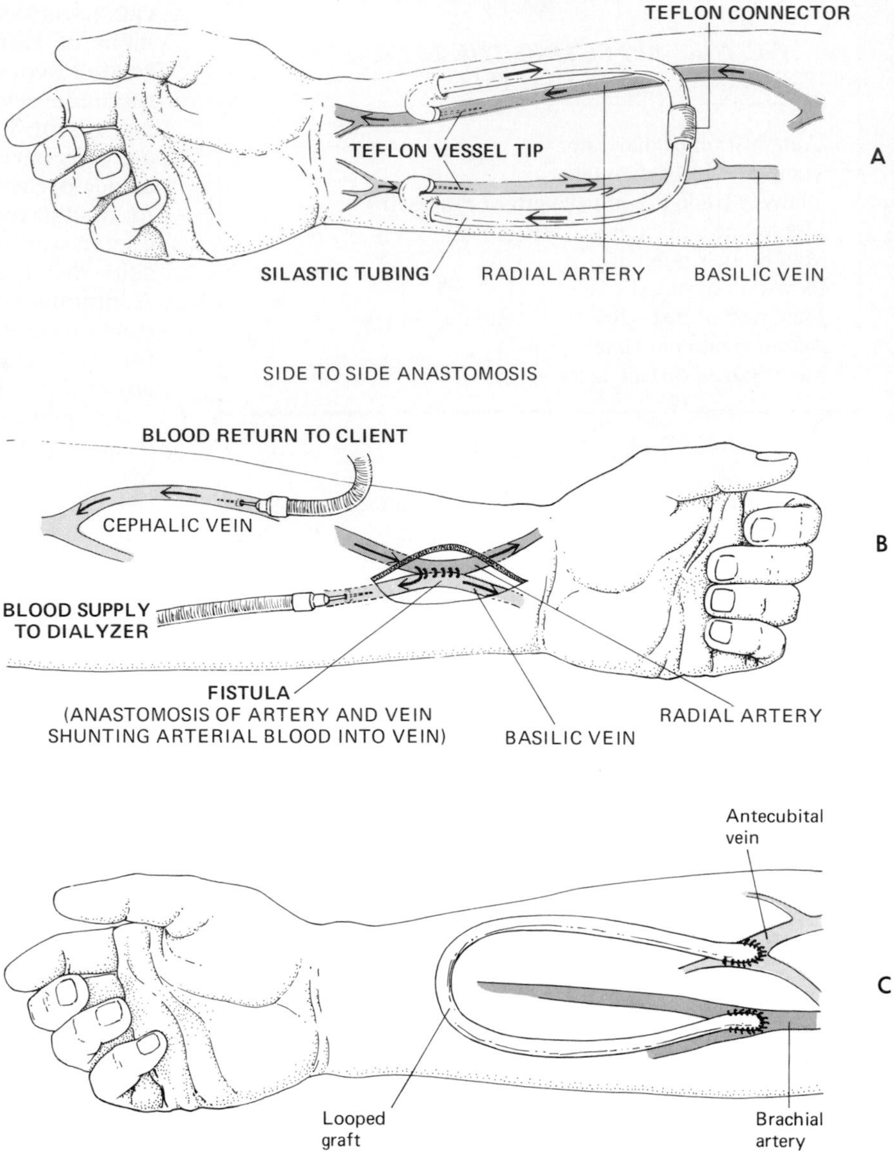

Fig. 35-3 Methods of vascular access for hemodialysis. **A,** External cannula or shunt. **B,** Internal A-V fistula. **C,** Looped graft in forearm. (From Kaga L: *Renal disease: a manual of patient care,* New York, 1979, McGraw-Hill.)

Peritoneal Dialysis

Peritoneal dialysis (PD) involves the introduction of sterile dialyzing fluid through an implanted catheter into the abdominal cavity. The dialysate bathes the peritoneal membrane, which covers the abdominal organs and overlies the capillary beds that support the organs. By the processes of osmosis, diffusion, and active transport, excess fluid and solutes travel from the peritoneal capillary fluid through the capillary walls, through the peritoneal membrane, and into the dialyzing fluid. After a selected time period, the fluid is drained out of the abdomen by gravity (Fig. 35-4). The process is then repeated. Indications and contraindications for PD[6,7] are summarized in the box on p. 628, upper left.

The peritoneal membrane's structure and capillary blood flow to the peritoneum account for the relatively slow nature of PD. The small capillary pores, the capillary membrane, the interstitium, the mesothelium of the peritoneum, and the fluid film layers in the capillary and the peritoneal cavity provide formidable barriers to fluid and solute passage.[14]

Much about the nature of the membrane is still a mystery, but several factors are implicated in changing the performance of the membrane. For instance, any change in the capillary blood flow changes solute removal but not to a great degree. This is probably a result of the relatively poor vasculature of the area in which not all capillaries are perfused at the same time and in which there exists resistance of the capillary membrane to solute transfer.[15]

The volume of dialysate instilled into the abdomen affects the clearance. Research has shown that during acute PD, 3.5 L/hr provides a urea clearance of 26 ml/min. During chronic, continuous PD, 2-L exchanges every 4 hours provide a clearance of 7 ml/min.[15] The dialysate should be instilled at body temperature to provide comfort, some vasodilation, and increased solute transport in the peritoneum.

The length of time the solution remains in the peritoneal cavity (dwell time) and the solution composition affect the outcome. The dwell time affects the

Table 35-2 Complications and nursing management of A-V shunt, A-V fistula, and A-V grafts

Type	Complications	Nursing management
A-V shunt	Clotting Dislodgment Skin erosion Infection Bleeding	1. Monitor for clinical manifestations of infection. 2. Monitor for clinical manifestations of thrombosis (darkening of blood, separation of serum or cellular compartment blood in tubing, decreased temperature of tubing). 3. Assess insertion site daily for erosion around insertion sites. 4. Use strict aseptic technique during dressing changes at insertion sites. 5. Teach patient to avoid sleeping on or prolonged bending of accessed limb. 6. Keep two shunt clamps attached to patient's clothing or access dressing at all times.
A-V fistula	Thrombosis Infection Pseudoaneurysm Vascular steal syndrome Venous hypertension Carpal tunnel syndrome Inadequate blood flow	1. Teach patient to avoid wearing constrictive clothing on limb containing access. 2. Teach patient to avoid sleeping on or prolonged bending of accessed limb. 3. Use aseptic technique when cannulating access. 4. Avoid repetitious cannulation of one segment of access. 5. Offer comfort measures, such as warm compresses or ordered analgesics, to lessen pain of vascular steal. 6. Teach patient to develop the blood flow in the fistulas through exercises (squeezing a rubber ball) while applying mild impedance to flow just distal to the access (at least once per day for 10 to 15 minutes).
A-V graft	Bleeding Thrombosis False aneurysm formation Infection Arterial or venous stenosis Vascular steal syndrome	1. Avoid too early cannulation of new access. 2. Teach patient to avoid wearing constrictive clothing on accessed limb. 3. Avoid repeated cannulation of one segment of access. 4. Use aseptic technique when cannulating access. 5. Monitor for changes in arterial or venous pressure while patient is on dialysis. 6. Provide comfort measures to reduce pain of vascular steal (e.g., warm compresses, analgesics as ordered).

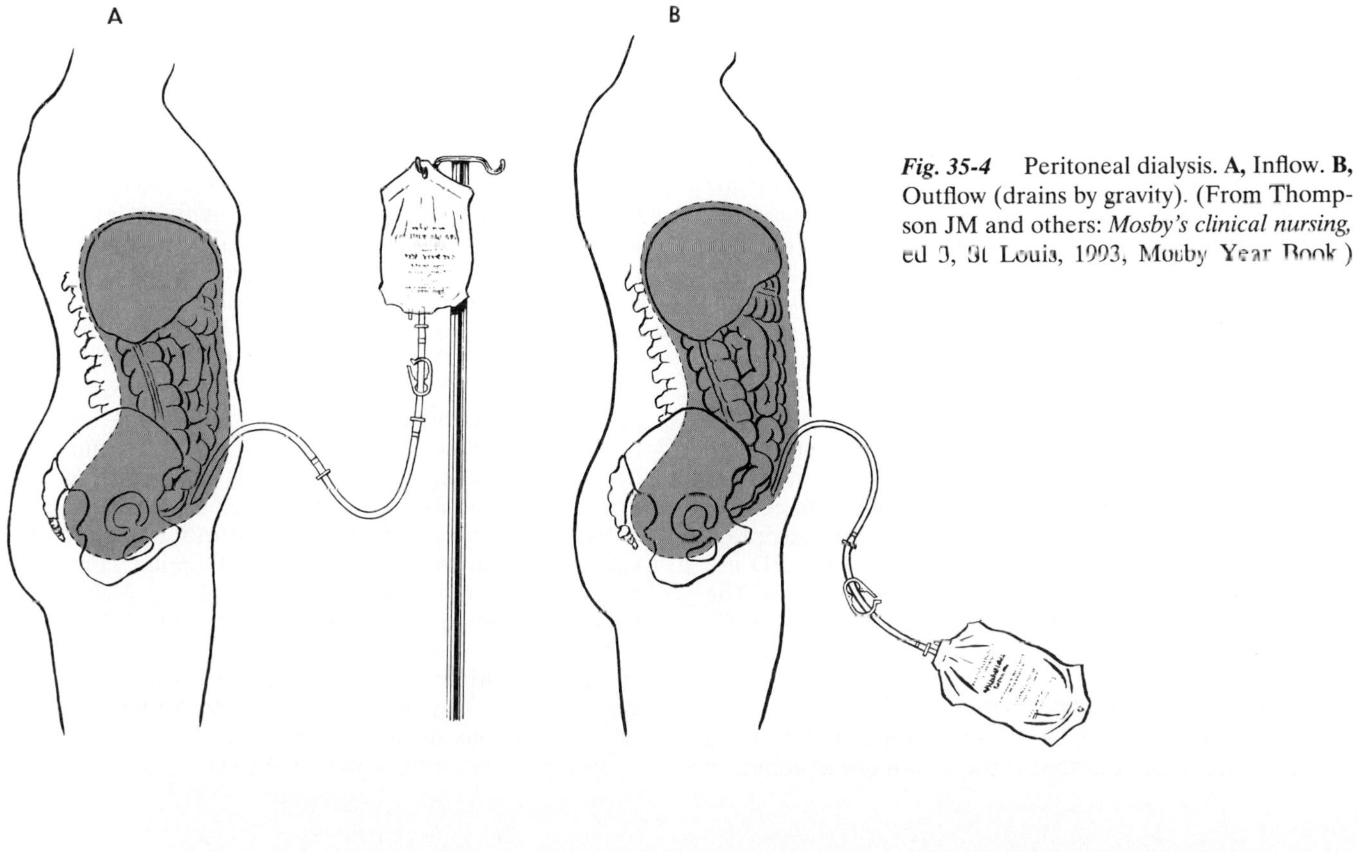

Fig. 35-4 Peritoneal dialysis. **A,** Inflow. **B,** Outflow (drains by gravity). (From Thompson JM and others: *Mosby's clinical nursing,* ed 3, St Louis, 1993, Mosby Year Book.)

INDICATIONS AND CONTRAINDICATIONS FOR PERITONEAL DIALYSIS

INDICATIONS
Uremia
Volume overload
Electrolyte imbalances
Hemodynamic instability
Lack of access to circulation
Removal of high-molecular-weight toxins
Patients with nonrenal critical illness who are receiving PD for chronic renal failure
Severe cardiovascular disease
Inability to anticoagulate
Contraindication to hemodialysis

CONTRAINDICATIONS
Recent abdominal surgery
History of abdominal surgeries with adhesions and scarring
Significant pulmonary disease
Need for rapid fluid removal
Peritonitis

Table 35-3 Dialysate concentrations for peritoneal dialysis (PD)

PD-1 solution	PD-2 solution	Low calcium solution
Na, 132 mmol/L	Na, 132 mmol/L	Na, 132 mmol/L
Ca, 3.5 mmol/L	Ca, 3.5 mmol/L	Ca, 2.5 mmol/L
Mg, 1.5 mmol/L	Mg, 0.5 mmol/L	Mg, 0.5 mmol/L
Cl, 102 mmol/L	Cl, 96 mmol/L	Cl, 95 mmol/L
Lactate, 35 mmol/L	Lactate, 40 mmol/L	Lactate, 40 mmol/L
Dextrose, 1.5%, 2.5%, 4.25%	Dextrose, 1.5%, 2.5%, 3.5%, 4.25%	Dextrose, 1.5%, 2.5%, 3.5%, 4.25%

Modified from Smith LJ: *AACN Clin Issues* 3(3):558, 1992.

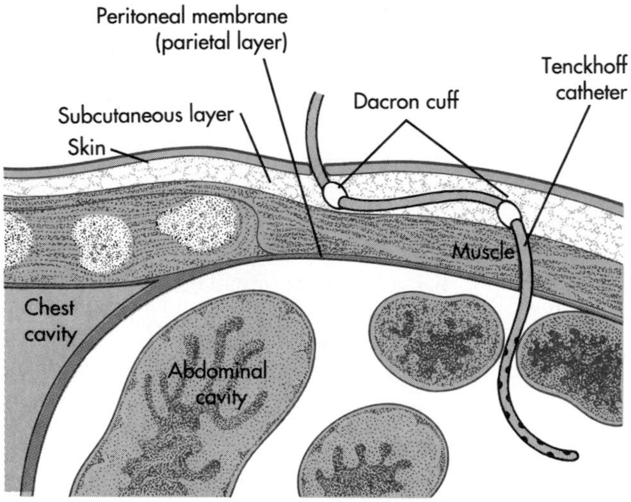

Fig. 35-5 Tenckhoff catheter used in peritoneal dialysis. (From Lewis SM, Collier IC: *Medical-surgical nursing assessment and management of clinical problems,* ed 3, St Louis, 1992, Mosby–Year Book.)

amount of fluid removed from the peritoneal capillaries, although a longer dwell time will not remove proportionately more fluid because of osmotic equilibration across the membranes. The various glucose concentrations of the dialysate provide for different rates of fluid removal. Dialysate concentrations are summarized in Table 35-3.

◆ **Catheter placement.** Two types of catheters are used for PD: the rigid stylet and the silicone catheter. The single-use *rigid stylet catheter* can be inserted at the bedside for immediate initiation of dialysis. Patient mobility is limited when the rigid stylet is in place because of the possibility of perforation.[14] The *silicone catheter* usually is inserted surgically, although it can be inserted at the bedside. This catheter is designed for multiple treatments over extended periods. Because the catheter is extremely flexible, the patient is able to move freely with minimal discomfort.[14]

Most catheters have an external segment, a tunnel segment that passes through subcutaneous tissue and muscle, a cuff for stabilization at the peritoneal membrane, and an external segment with numerous holes for fast delivery and drainage of dialysate (Fig. 35-5).

◆ **Complications.** Complications of PD can be numerous. The complications, which range from annoying to severe, require careful observation and intervention to control or even prevent further problems.[16] With the exception of peritonitis, however, the complications from PD are less severe than those associated with hemodialysis. The complications and nursing management related to PD are listed in Table 35-4.

Continuous Renal Replacement Therapy

Continuous renal replacement therapy (CRRT) is a newer mode of dialysis that is the treatment of choice in institutions where it is available.[17] CRRT is a continuous therapy lasting 12 hours or longer in which whole blood is circulated from an artery to a vein through a highly porous hemofilter.[6,17,18] The system allows for slow volume removal (5 to 15 ml/min) of dissolved noncellular components of the plasma, that is, urea, creatine, and electrolytes.[17,18] The hydrostatic pressure exerted by the patient's mean arterial pressure (MAP) forms the basis for continuous flow of blood through the hemofilter. To maintain this flow a MAP of greater than 70 mm Hg is necessary. The ultrafiltrate can be drained by gravity flow or by a suction-assisted collection system.[17]

Indications and contraindications for CRRT[6,7,18,19] are summarized in the box on p. 630. Because controlled removal and replacement of fluid are possible with CRRT, hemodynamic stability is maintained. This makes CRRT highly advantageous for use in the patient with myocardial failure, shock, or multiple organ dysfunction syndrome.[7,19] The three common forms of CRRT are slow continuous ultrafiltration (SCUF), continuous arteriovenous hemofiltration (CAVH), and continuous

Table 35-4 Complications and nursing management of peritoneal dialysis

Complications	Nursing management
Peritonitis	Assess for signs and symptoms: cloudy effluent, abdominal pain, rebound tenderness, nausea and vomiting, and fever. Obtain effluent sample for culture. Administer antibiotics as ordered. Teach patient and family signs and symptoms and their prevention.
Exit-site infection	Monitor site daily for signs and symptoms of infection: enduration, erythema, purulence, and hyperthermia. Increase daily cleaning of site. Apply topical antibiotics as ordered (this is a controversial practice). Teach patient and family to avoid agents such as creams and lotions around exit site.
Catheter-tunnel infection	Assess for signs and symptoms of infection: pain along tunnel, enduration for several centimeters away from catheter, erythema leading away from the exit site, and drainage at exit site or as tunnel is "milked" toward exit site. Teach patient and family signs and symptoms of infection. Teach patient and family to avoid pulls or tugs on the catheter or trauma to the exit site. Emphasize the need to maintain cleansing regimen at exit site.
Fluid obstruction	Change position of the patient (i.e., standing, lying, side-lying, knee-chest). Relieve patient's constipation. Irrigate the catheter. Ensure that sufficient fluid is in abdomen (sometimes requires a residual reservoir of approximately 50 ml).
Rectal pain	Ensure a sufficient reservoir of fluid. Use slow infusion rate.
Shoulder pain	Ensure that all air is primed from infusion tubing. Attempt draining the effluent with the patient in knee-chest position. Administer mild analgesics as ordered.
Hernias	Monitor for increase in size of or pain in area of hernia. Decrease volume of exchanges as ordered. Dialyze with the patient in the supine position. Use abdominal binder or support for the patient (as long as not binding on catheter exit site). Avoid initiation of PD until exit site healing has taken place (approximately 1 to 2 weeks) if possible.
Fluid overload	Increase use of hypertonic solutions. Decrease by mouth (PO) fluid intake. Shorten dwell times. Weigh patient frequently. Monitor lung sounds and peripheral edema.
Dehydration	Assess patient for decreased skin turgor, muscle cramps, hypotension, tachycardia, and dizziness. Discontinue hypertonic solutions. Increase PO fluid intake. Lengthen dwell times.
Blood-tinged effluent	Monitor for change in effluent color (clear yellow to pink or rusty). Administer heparin, as ordered, to avoid fibrin formation. Obtain patient history about catheter trauma and patient activity before appearance of complication.

arteriovenous hemodialysis (CAVHD). The decision as to which type of therapy to initiate is based on myriad factors, including clinical assessment, metabolic status, and severity of uremia.[17] A comparison of CRRT approaches is found in Table 35-5, and a discussion of each of these treatment modalities follows.

◆ **Slow continuous ultrafiltration (SCUF).** SCUF, as the name implies, slowly removes fluid, 100 to 300 ml/hr, through a process of convection.[6,18,19] This process consists of an exchange of solutes and solvents across a semipermeable membrane.[19] Because small amounts of fluid are removed via this process, it is the treatment of choice for patients with acute myocardial infarction with low renal perfusion and for those who have congestive heart failure with mild renal failure.[17]

The SCUF system setup is illustrated in Fig. 35-6, *A*.

The hemofilter and tubing are primed with a heparinized solution, which flows by gravity. Outflow ultrafiltrate is collected in a Foley or urometer bag.[19]

◆ **Continuous arteriovenous hemofiltration (CAVH).** CAVH is a process in which both fluid and solute are removed through convection in volumes of 500 to 800 ml/hr. In addition, large volumes of fluid replacement with appropriate and sufficient electrolytes are returned to the patient.[17,19] Replacement solutions may consist of standard solutions of bicarbonate or acetate and also include dextrose and electrolytes, such as potassium, magnesium, sodium, and calcium.[19] CAVH is indicated when the patient's clinical condition warrants moderate removal of fluid and solutes. Because large volumes are removed, fluid is replaced hourly with a continuous infusion. This is of particular importance to the patient with hemodynamic compromise who needs careful fluid monitoring. Fluid can be replaced as predilution or postfilter infusion.[17]

Hemofilters are designed to clear solutes and unbound molecules of up to 50,000 daltons. Typical hemodialysis can clear only particles of up to 10,000 daltons. Therefore the hemofilter clears many drugs that dialysis cannot remove, along with large amounts of fluids that cannot be removed in as great a quantity through hemodialysis. Hemofilters can remove fluid at the rate of 35 to 45 ml/mm Hg/hr.[20] Significant fluid removal alone can be accomplished by simply allowing the blood pressure to push the blood continuously through the circuit.

Ultrafiltration occurs through the combination of the hydrostatic pressure of the blood (blood pressure) and the negative hydrostatic pressure of the outflowing ultrafiltrate. The two pressures are opposed by the oncotic pressure created by the plasma proteins. Ultrafiltration is achieved as long as the oncotic pressure is overcome. Ultrafiltration can be supplemented by connection of the filtrate port to wall suction. Pressures of 100 to 150 mm Hg for patients with a hematocrit value greater than 30%, or 200 to 250 mm Hg for hematocrits less than 30%, should be applied.[20]

Fluid replacement is based on fluid losses and electrolyte values, with consideration given to achieving the desired reduction in the extracellular fluid volume.[20] Total output minus other intake (such as oral) minus the ordered hourly output equals the hourly replacement amount.[21] Replacement fluids may range from potassium-free lactated Ringer's solution to normal saline solution with a variety of additives (e.g., calcium chloride, magnesium sulfate, sodium bicarbonate) and D_5W.[20]

Anticoagulation is important because blood is traveling through an extracorporeal circuit. Commonly, a 2000-unit bolus of heparin is given before initiation of CRRT. Thereafter 5 to 10 U/kg/hr is infused throughout the treatment.[21] Clotting times frequently are determined to monitor anticoagulation.

The CAVH system setup is illustrated in Fig. 35-6, *B*. The system is the same as the SCUF with the addition of a replacement solution.[19]

◆ **Continuous arteriovenous hemodialysis (CAVHD).** The CAVHD method accomplishes both fluid removal and maximal removal of solutes. In addition, the process of conduction allows the passive diffusion of solutes across the semipermeable membrane so that solute removal is enhanced. This form of CRRT is similar to traditional

INDICATIONS AND CONTRAINDICATIONS FOR CONTINUOUS RENAL REPLACEMENT THERAPY

INDICATIONS

Need for large fluid volume removal in the hemodynamically unstable patient
Hypervolemic or edematous patients unresponsive to diuretic therapy
Patients with multiple organ dysfunction syndrome
Ease of fluid management in patients requiring large daily fluid volume, such as replacement for oliguria, TPN administration
Contraindications to hemodialysis and peritoneal dialysis
Inability to anticoagulate

CONTRAINDICATIONS

Hematocrit >45%
Lack of arterial access

Table 35-5 Comparison of continuous renal replacement therapy approaches

Type	Ultrafiltration rate	Fluid replacement	Indication
SCUF	100 to 300 ml/hr	None	Fluid removal
CAVH	500 to 800 ml/hr	Predilution or postdilution, calculating an hourly net loss	Fluid removal, moderate solute removal
CAVHD	500 to 800 ml/hr	Predilution or postdilution, subtracting the dialysate and then calculating an hourly net loss	Fluid removal, maximum solute removal

SCUF, Slow continuous ultrafiltration; *CAVH*, continuous arteriovenous hemofiltration; *CAVHD*, continuous arteriovenous hemodialysis.
Modified from Price CA: *AACN Clin Issues* 3(3):597, 1992.

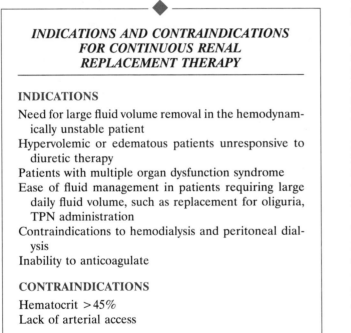

A

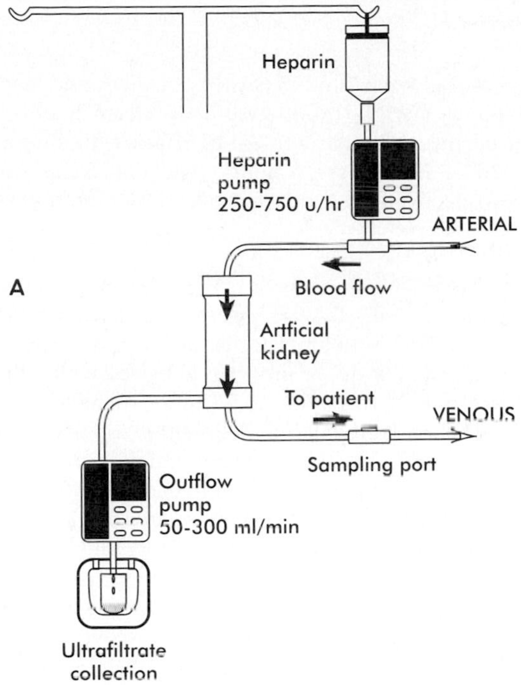

B

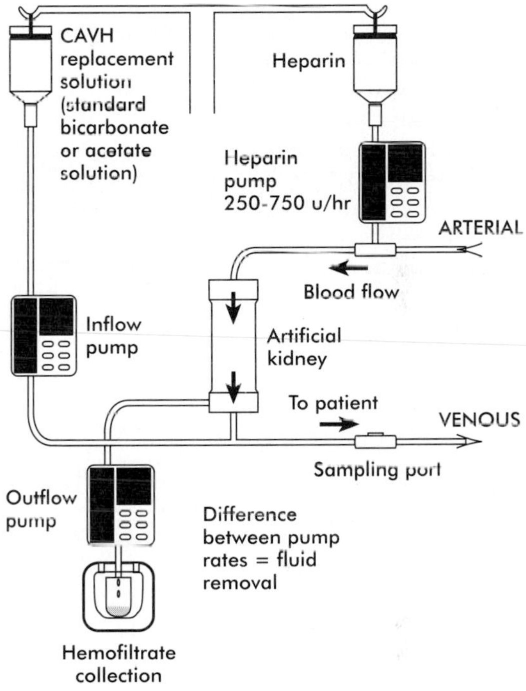

C

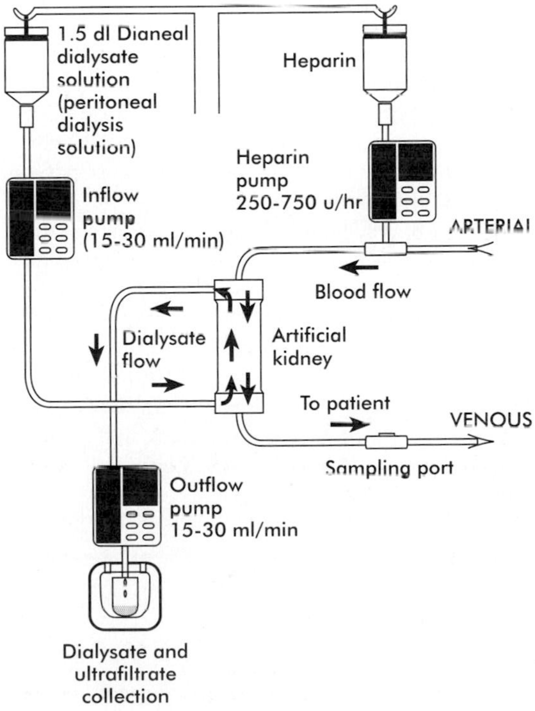

Fig. 35-6 **A,** SCUF system setup. **B,** CAVH system setup. **C,** CAVHD system setup. (Modified from Bosworth C: SCUF/SAVH/CAVHD: critical differences, *Crit Care Nurs Q* 14(4):45, 1992.)

RESEARCH ABSTRACT

Efficacy of continuous arteriovenous hemofiltration with dialysis in patients with renal failure.

Reynolds HN and others: *Crit Care Med* 19(11):1387, 1991.

PURPOSE

The purpose of this study was to describe the efficacy of continuous arteriovenous hemofiltration (CAVH) with dialysis in patients with renal failure without protein restriction.

DESIGN

Descriptive comparative survey design

SAMPLE

The convenience sample consisted of 28 patients (20 males, 8 females) with a mean age of 44.5 years, most of whom were admitted with diagnoses of multitrauma. The two most commonly associated causes of renal failure for the subjects were multiple organ dysfunction syndrome (MODS) (57%) and adult respiratory distress syndrome (ARDS) (25%). The mean duration of CAVH with dialysis was 10.9 days. For purposes of comparison, the subjects were divided into two groups: those in whom dialysis was begun when the blood urea nitrogen (BUN) value was <60 mg/dl ("early starters") and those in whom the BUN was >60 mg/dl ("late starters").

INSTRUMENTS

A CAVH with dialysis system (AN-69S, Hospal Industrie, Meyzieu, France) was used; the filter consisted of 15 parallel membranes made of polyacrylonitrile, each 22 μm in thickness, a total surface of 0.43 m^2, and an extracorporeal blood volume of 60 ml. Dialysate was delivered by a calibrated constant infusion pump (Travenol Flo-gard 800, Baxter Edwards Critical Care, Irvine, Calif.) in a direction countercurrent to the flow of blood. Either 1.5% Dianeal (Baxter Edwards Critical Care) or 0.9% saline was used as the dialysate.

PROCEDURE

Vascular access was obtained with femoral catheter kits (Desilet 11-cm CAVH, Vygon, Ecouen, France). Arterial access was always through the femoral arteries; venous access varied among femoral, subclavian, and internal jugular veins. The dialysate flow rate was typically 15 ml/min but may have been increased to 30 ml/min to achieve adequate urea clearance. Heparin was infused into the arterial side of the filter in amounts ranging from 300 to 1500 U/hr. Monitoring during the procedure consisted of hourly vital signs and laboratory studies (BUN, serum creatinine, electrolytes, glucose, calcium) and measurement of effluent fluid urea nitrogen at least every 6 hours. The data were obtained prospectively and collected over a 14-month period.

RESULTS

The BUN values of the two groups at the time of initiation of CAVH were statistically different ($p < .0001$), with lower BUN values in the early starters. Adequate control of urea was achieved with a dialysate flow rate of 15 ml/min in 24 of 28 subjects. The BUN level in both groups stabilized within a range of 40 to 75 mg/dl within 3 to 5 days. The initial daily urea clearance was significantly greater in the late-starter group ($p < .0001$), which also stabilized within 3 to 5 days of CAVH initiation. All subjects received alimentation within 24 hours of admission, either parenterally or enterally (mean protein load of 142 g/day). No statistically significant correlation was found between the daily urea creatinine clearance and the protein load. Five of the subjects survived (age 35 years or younger), four with MODS and all with ARDS, oliguric renal failure, and liver failure. All survivors had return of renal function and were able to be removed from renal support. Conversely, no subject survived who did not have return of renal function. Of the 16 patients classified as having MODS, 25% were survivors.

DISCUSSION/IMPLICATION

Dense oliguric or anuric renal failure developed in 12 of the 13 early starters, which supported the early prediction for prolonged renal support. Findings from this study indicate that stabilization of the BUN value and daily urea clearance occur within 3 to 5 days, which was achieved without any limitation of protein alimentation. Stabilization failed to occur in those subjects who were in a hypercatabolic state. The survival rate for the subjects in this study was 18%, and most patients who died did so within the first 10 days of CAVH. The investigators suggested that the subjects died of a process that is independent of the CAVH and that the deaths appear to be related to the underlying disease, that is, MODS or ARDS. The system of CAVH with dialysis appears to be efficacious in terms of control of BUN and clearance of urea. Future studies should include larger samples and might consider correlation of outcomes with physiologic variables, comparison of the various types of dialysis modalities, and experimental designs.

hemodialysis.[19] A peritoneal or custom dialysate solution is infused into the hemofilter to accomplish this removal of fluids. CAVHD is indicated in patients who require large-volume removal for severe uremia or severe acid-base imbalances. Although expensive, CAVHD is the most efficient form of CRRT.[17]

The system setup for CAVHD is illustrated in Fig. 35-6, *C*. Instead of a replacement fluid, the dialysate solution is added and infused through the hemofilter and removed with the ultrafiltrate.[19]

◆ **Vascular access for CRRT.** Single-lumen, large-bore catheters are placed into an artery and vein, with the femoral site the most common because of its large size and accessibility. Additional sites include the subclavian vein or a Scribner shunt.[19]

◆ **Complications of CRRT.** Although CRRT has been found to be a successful treatment for acute renal failure (ARF), potential complications are numerous (Table 35-6). The patient with ARF undergoing CRRT presents unique challenges to the critical care nurse. The nurse's role is crucial to early detection and treatment of any complications that result from CRRT therapy.[17,18,22-24] Table 35-8 describes problems, etiologies, clinical manifestations, and nursing management related to CRRT.

Table 35-6 Potential complications related to CRRT

Clinical finding	Potential rationales
Dehydration, hypotension	Incorrect intake/output calculations, inadequate prescription for fluid replacement
Electrolytes, acid-base abnormalities	Incorrect replacement fluids, incorrect dialysate, lactate intolerance
Hypothermia	Extracorporeal system, cool replacement fluids, cool dialysate
Hyperglycemia	High dextrose in dialysate
Decreased ultrafiltrate	Clotted hemofilter, poor blood flow through the hemofilter, need for predilution replacement fluid, hemoconcentration with hematocrit level above 35%, hypotension
Inadequate blood flow through the hemofilter	Clotted hemofilter, hypotension, kinked or positional catheters or tubing, too-small arterial and/or venous catheter
Clotted hemofilter	Improper heparinization, prolonged hypotension, poor blood flow rate, secondary to vascular accesses
Blood leak with blood in ultrafiltrate	Defective hemofilter, break in membrane integrity secondary to blunt trauma or high vacuum suction
Disconnection at catheter or hemofilter	Non-Luer-locked syringe connections, connections not secured with tape, patient out of bed

Modified from Price CA: *AACN Clin Issues* 3(3):597, 1992.

Table 35-7 Problems, etiologies, clinical manifestations, and nursing interventions related to CRRT

Problem	Etiology	Clinical manifestations	Nursing management
Decreased ultrafiltration rate	Hypotension Dehydration Kinked lines Bending of catheters Clotting of filter	Ultrafiltration rate decreases Minimal flow through blood lines	Observe filter and arteriovenous system. Control blood flow. Control coagulation time. Position patient on back. Lower height of collection container.
Filter clotting	Obstruction Insufficient heparinization As above	Ultrafiltration rate decreases, despite height of collection container being lower	Control heparinization. Maintain continuous heparinization. Call physician. Remove system. Prime catheters with heparin. Prime a new system and connect it. Start predilution with 1000 ml saline 0.9% solution per hour. Do not use three-way stopcocks.
Hypotension	Increased ultrafiltration rate Blood leak Disconnection of one of lines	Bleeding	Control amount of ultrafiltration. Control access sites. Clamp lines. Call physician.
Fluid and electrolyte changes	Too much/little removal of fluid Inappropriate replacement of electrolytes Inappropriate dialysate	Changes in mentation ↑ or ↓ CVP, PAWP ECG change ↑ or ↓ BP and heart rate Abnormal electrolyte levels	Observe for changes in central venous pressure or pulmonary capillary wedge pressure. Observe for changes in vital signs. Observe electrocardiogram for changes as result of electrolyte abnormalities. Monitor output values every hour. Control ultrafiltration.
Bleeding	System disconnection ↑ heparin dose	Oozing from catheter insertion site or connection	Monitor accelerated clotting time (ACT) no less than once every hour. Adjust heparin dose within specifications to maintain ACT. Observe dressing on vascular access for blood loss. Observe for blood in filtrate (filter leak).
Access dislodgment or infection	Catheter/connections not secured Break in sterile technique Excessive patient movement	Bleeding from catheter site or connections Inappropriate flow/infusion Fever Drainage at catheter site	Observe access site at least once every 2 hours. Ensure that clamps are available within easy reach at all times. Observe strict sterile technique when dressing vascular access.

Modified from Lievaart A, Voerman HJ: *Heart Lung* 20(2):152, 1991.

REFERENCES

1. Metheny NM: Why worry about IV fluids? *Am J Nurs* 90(6):50, 1990.
2. Kuhn MM: Colloids vs crystalloids, *Crit Care Nurse* 11(5):37, 1991.
3. Pauley SY: Massive hemorrhage in trauma: the initial assessment, treatment, monitoring, *NITA* 10(16):410, 1987.
4. Ley J: Fluid therapy following intracardiac operation, *Crit Care Nurse* 8(1):26, 1988.
5. Ley J and others: Crystalloid versus colloid therapy after cardiac surgery, *Heart Lung* 19(1):31, 1990.
6. Stark J: Dialysis options in the critically ill; hemodialysis, peritoneal dialysis, and continuous renal replacement therapy, *Crit Care Nurse* 14(4):40, 1992.
7. Baer CL, Lancaster LE: Acute renal failure, *Crit Care Nurs Q* 14(4):1, 1992.
8. Gutch CF, Stoner MH, Corea AL: *Review of hemodialysis for nurses and dialysis personnel,* ed 5, St Louis, 1993, Mosby–Year Book.
9. Pechman P: Acute hemodialysis: issues in the critically ill, *AACN Clin Issues Crit Care Nurs* 3(3):545, 1992.
10. Gutch FL, Keen M: Dialysis and delivery systems. In Cogan M, Garovoy M, editors: *Introduction to dialysis,* New York, 1985, Churchill Livingstone.
11. Easterling RE: Water treatment for in-center hemodialysis, including verification of water quality and disinfection. In Nissenson AR, Fine RN, editors: *Dialysis therapy,* St Louis, 1986, Mosby–Year Book.
12. Krupski WC and others: Access for dialysis. In Cogan M, Garovoy M, editors: *Introduction to dialysis,* New York, 1985, Churchill Livingstone.
13. Butt MH: Vascular access for chronic hemodialysis. In Nissensen AR, Fine RN, editors: *Dialysis therapy*, ed 2, St Louis, 1992, Mosby–Year Book.
14. Smith LJ: Peritoneal dialysis in the critically ill patient, *AACN Clin Issues Crit Care Nurs* 3(3):558, 1992.
15. Schonfeld P: Care of the patient on peritoneal dialysis. In Cogan M, Garovoy M, editors: *Introduction to dialysis,* New York, 1985, Churchill Livingstone.
16. Graham-Macaluso MM: Complications of peritoneal dialysis: nursing care plans to document teaching, *ANNA J* 18(5):479, 1991.
17. Price CA: Continuous renal replacement therapy: the treatment of choice for acute renal failure, *ANNA J* 18(3):239, 1992.
18. Price CA: An update on continuous renal replacement therapies, *AACN Clin Issues Crit Care Nurs* 3(3):597, 1992.
19. Bosworth C: SCUF/CAVH/CAVHD: critical differences, *Crit Care Nurs Q* 14(4):45, 1992.
20. Winkelman C: Hemofiltration: a new technique in critical care nursing, *Heart Lung* 14(3):265, 1985.
21. Palmer JC and others: Nursing management of CAVH for acute renal failure, *Focus Crit Care* 13(5):21, 1986.
22. Coloski D and others: Continuous arteriovenous hemofiltration patient: nursing care plan, *DCCN* 9(3):130, 1990.
23. Lievaart A, Voerman HJ: Nursing management of continuous arteriovenous hemodialysis, *Heart Lung* 20(2):152, 1991.
24. Pinson JM: Preventing complications in the CAVH patient, *DCCN* 11(5):242, 1992.

36

Renal Nursing Diagnosis and Management

This chapter is designed to supplement the preceding chapters in the *Renal Alterations* unit by integrating theoretic content into clinically applicable case studies and nursing management plans.

The case study is designed to illustrate clinical problem solving and patient care management occuring in actual patients. The case, reviewed retrospectively, demonstrates how medical and nursing diagnoses may be effectively used in critical care. The case study also demonstrates revisions to the plan of care and the nursing and medical management outcomes that are apt to occur during the course of a complicated hospitalization as the patient responds physiologically to treatment. Often in a short case anecdote, such as presented in this chapter, the clinical answer may appear to be obvious from the day of admission. In practice, however, critical care patient management is sometimes investigative and the "correct" diagnosis for an individual patient may not become apparent until midway in the hospitalization. Or a patient with an apparently straightforward diagnosis may develop an unexpected complication, and the plan of care and potential outcomes will then require revision. Many of the case studies demonstrate this principle.

The nursing management plans, which—unlike the case study—are not patient-specific, provide a basis nurses can use to individualize care for their patients. In the previous *Renal Alterations* chapters, each medical diagnosis is assigned a Nursing Diagnosis and Management box. Using this box as a page guide, the reader can access relevant nursing management plans for each medical diagnosis. For example, nursing management of *acute renal failure*, described on pp. 618-619, may involve several nursing diagnoses and management plans outlined in this chapter and in other Nursing Diagnosis and Management chapters. Specific examples are (1) *High Risk for Fluid Volume Excess risk factors: renal failure*, on p. 639; (2) *Anxiety related to threatened biologic, physiologic, and/or social integrity*, on p. 763; (3) *High Risk for Infection risk factors: invasive monitoring devices*, on p. 366; and (4) *Ineffective Individual Coping related to situational crisis and personal vulnerability*, on p. 762. These examples highlight the interrelationship of the various physiologic systems in the body and the fact that pathology often has a multisystem impact in the critically ill.

Use of the case study and management plans can enhance the understanding and application of the *Renal* content in clinical practice.

RENAL CASE STUDY

CLINICAL HISTORY

JT is a 55-year-old white man who was diagnosed with severe hypertension 3½ years ago. His medication regimen includes at least two potent antihypertensive drugs, as well as Lasix and a potassium supplement. He admits to frequent omissions of his medications because of a hectic work schedule. He weighs 235 lbs. and is at least 40 lbs. overweight. JT smokes at least one pack of cigarettes per day and drinks socially with clients several times each week.

CURRENT PROBLEMS

After a stressful day at work and several hundred miles of travel, JT arrived at his hotel room for the night. While sitting on the bed to remove his shoes, he experienced a sudden, intense midabdominal to lower abdominal pain. He began to feel faint and nauseated but was able to summon help. Paramedics arrived to find JT alert, ashen, and dyspneic. He complained of accelerating midabdominal pain radiating to his thoracic spine. Paramedics noted the following: BP, 88/40; P, 126; RR, 32 (despite receiving 6 L O_2; and tense, distended abdomen without bowel sounds.

EMERGENCY MEDICAL MANAGEMENT

En route to the hospital JT's systolic BP fell to 74 despite rapid IV infusion of lactated Ringer's solution. When the patient arrived at the hospital, an arterial line was placed, oxygen was continued, and a dopamine drip was initiated for blood pressure support at 90/50. Before dopamine initiation, JT's blood pressure was unstable for 45 minutes. A diagnosis of ruptured abdominal aortic aneurysm was made and immediate surgery was scheduled. Before surgery, JT received 1200 ml of IV fluids.

RENAL CASE STUDY—cont'd

MEDICAL DIAGNOSES

Ruptured abdominal aortic aneurysm
Class III hemorrhagic shock

NURSING DIAGNOSES

- ◆ Knowledge Deficit: Impending Surgery and Risks related to lack of previous exposure to information
- ◆ Fluid Volume Deficit related to active covert blood loss
- ◆ Acute Pain related to transmission and perception of visceral and ischemic impulses secondary to ruptured aneurysm
- ◆ Anxiety related to threat to biologic, psychologic and/or social integrity

◆ PLAN OF CARE

Surgery was scheduled to repair abdominal aortic aneurysm with synthetic graft.

MEDICAL AND NURSING MANAGEMENT AND PATIENT OUTCOME

During surgery JT experienced active blood loss of approximately 9 L, which was replaced with LR, Plasmanate, and whole blood. He returned to the critical care unit (CCU) in stable condition with the following assessment:

Neuro: Lethargic but responsive. Moves all extremities. Hand grasps equal but weak bilaterally, as are pedal pushes. PEERLA.

Resp: Rhythmic respirations at 26/min. Decreased excursion and diminished breath sounds throughout lung bases. O_2 continues per mask at 4 L/min. Po_2, 90 mm Hg; Pco_2, 40 mm Hg; pH 7.40; O_2 saturation, 96%.

CV: BP, 118/60; P, 98; mean arterial pressure (MAP), 80 mm Hg; RA, 4 mm Hg; cardiac output (CO), 6 L/min; pulmonary capillary wedge presure (PCWP), 8 mm Hg; systemic vascular resistance (SVR), 1014 dynes/sec/cm^5. Regular heart rate with no extra sounds. Peripheral pulses are 1+.

GI Integument/Temp: Skin cool and mottled over extremities, but upper body warm and dry. NG tube in right naris draining pink-tinged fluid. Abdomen soft and nondistended. Bowel sounds absent. Bulky dressing at midabdomen is clean, dry, intact.

GU: Foley catheter in place draining clear, dark amber urine. Approximately 500 ml urine in bag.

Lab: Hct, 28%; Hgb, 8.4 g/dl; Na, 136 mEq/L; K, 3.8 mEq/L; Cl, 108 mEq/L.

MEDICAL DIAGNOSES

S/P abdominal aortic aneurysm repair
Anemia

NURSING DIAGNOSES

- ◆ Hypothermia related to blood loss and physiologic shock compensation
- ◆ Fluid Volume Deficit related to active blood loss and ongoing NG losses
- ◆ Anxiety related to threat to biologic, psychologic, and/or social integrity
- ◆ Acute Pain related to transmission and perception of cutaneous, visceral, or muscular impulses secondary to surgical intervention

◆ REVISED PLAN OF CARE

1. Increase body temperature through the use of blankets.
2. Replace fluid through infusion of IV fluids as ordered.
3. Reposition patient frequently, and instruct and encourage him in the use of the incentive spirometer. Have patient perform passive and semiactive ROM.
4. Accurately measure and record I & O. Weigh patient daily. Monitor hemodynamic parameters hourly.
5. Explain surgery, CCU routine, and other care procedures. Encourage patient and family to ask questions.
6. Administer analgesics per physician order. Assess pain level every 2 to 3 hours. Assess response to all analgesics.

MEDICAL AND NURSING MANAGEMENT AND PATIENT OUTCOME

On the third postoperative day JT was transferred to the medical/surgical unit. On day 4 he began to experience decreased renal output to 50 ml/hr. Output continued to drop to 30 ml/hr. By day 5 his weight had increased 5½ lbs. 3+ edema was present in both lower extremities. JT complained of mild dyspnea and nausea. Despite Lasix administration, his renal output had not increased.

Laboratory values were as follows: K+, 5.4 mEq/L; Na, 138 mEq/L; Cl, 110 mEq/L; creatinine, 7.0 mg/dl; BUN 73 mg/dl. Cardiac tracings show peaked T waves. Kayexalate was administered, and a subclavian catheter was placed to initiate hemodialysis.

Continued.

RENAL CASE STUDY—cont'd

MEDICAL DIAGNOSES

S/P abdominal aortic aneurysm repair
Acute renal failure
Electrolyte imbalances
Anemia
Fluid overload

NURSING DIAGNOSES

- ◆ High Risk for Fluid Volume Excess risk factor: renal failure
- ◆ Altered Nutrition: Less than Body Requirements related to lack of exogenous nutrients
- ◆ Activity Intolerance related to decreased cardiac output secondary to unresolved anemia
- ◆ Acute Pain related to transmission and perception of cutaneous, visceral, and muscular impulses secondary to surgical incision and dialysis catheter
- ◆ Knowledge Deficit: Dialysis Initiation, Prognosis for Recovery, and Return to Previous Life-style related to lack of previous exposure to information

◆ REVISED PLAN OF CARE

1. Limit oral fluids to 1500 ml/24 hrs. Accurately measure and record I & O. Weigh patient before and after dialysis.
2. Assess for edema and changes in abdominal girth and circumferences of lower extremities.
3. Observe strict asepsis and monitor for clinical manifestations of infection.
4. Refer patient and family to dietician for instruction in fluid restriction and renal diet.
5. Structure treatment regimen to provide increased rest periods for patient.
6. Administer analgesics for pain relief, but instruct patient in use of adjunctive relief techniques (e.g., distraction, guided imagery, deep breathing, massage).
7. Involve hemodialysis staff and unit staff in educating patient regarding basic principles of dialysis treatment and self-care.

MEDICAL AND NURSING MANAGEMENT AND PATIENT OUTCOME

During the following 12 days, JT received 7 hemodialysis treatments. On the thirteenth postoperative day, he experienced a sudden, dramatic return of urinary output to 125 ml/hr by day's end. On day 18, JT was discharged to home with the following laboratory values: creatinine, 2.2 mg/dl; BUN, 36 mg/dl; Na, 140 mEq/L; K, 4.0 mEq/L. JT and his family received discharge teaching regarding nutritional intake, infection prevention, exercise, and relationship of life-style and adherence to medical regimen to subsequent health events.

FLUID VOLUME DEFICIT RELATED TO HYPONATREMIA (ABSOLUTE SODIUM LOSS)

DEFINING CHARACTERISTICS

- ◆ Central nervous system (CNS) symptoms: headache, lethargy, confusion, muscular weakness
- ◆ Postural hypotension
- ◆ Tachycardia
- ◆ Gastrointestinal (GI) symptoms: nausea, diarrhea, cramping
- ◆ Diaphoresis, cold and clammy skin
- ◆ Loss of skin turgor and elasticity
- ◆ Serum sodium <135 mEq/L
- ◆ Urinary specific gravity <1.010
- ◆ Elevated red blood cell and plasma protein levels

OUTCOME CRITERIA

- ◆ CNS symptoms (e.g., headache, lethargy) are absent.
- ◆ Blood pressure and heart rate return to baseline.
- ◆ Skin turgor is normal.
- ◆ Serum sodium and urinary specific gravity levels are normal.

NURSING INTERVENTIONS AND *RATIONALE*

1. Continue to monitor the assessment parameters listed under "Defining Characteristics."
2. With physician's collaboration, replace fluid and sodium loss with normal saline solution or with hypertonic saline solution (3% or 5%).
3. Provide oral fluids that are high in sodium, such as juice or bouillon.
4. Avoid the use of diuretics, especially thiazide and loop diuretics, ***because they will further decrease sodium.***
5. If patient is ambulatory, protect from falls until CNS symptoms and/or postural hypotension clears.
6. If performing nasogastric suctioning, irrigate tube with normal saline solution, not water. In addition, carefully restrict ice chip intake; consider using iced saline solution chips. ***Excessive intake of water dilutes serum sodium and can result in water intoxication.***

FLUID VOLUME DEFICIT RELATED TO ACTIVE BLOOD LOSS

DEFINING CHARACTERISTICS

- Cardiac output <5 L/min
- Cardiac index <2.5 L/min
- Pulmonary capillary wedge pressure (PCWP), PAD, central venous pressure (CVP) less than normal or less than baseline (PCWP <6 mm Hg)
- Tachycardia
- Narrowed pulse pressure
- Systolic blood pressure <100 mm Hg
- Urinary output <30 ml/hour
- Pale, cool, moist skin
- Apprehensiveness

OUTCOME CRITERIA

- Patient's CO is >5 L/min and CI is >2.5 L/min.
- Patient's PCWP, PAD, and CVP are normal or back to baseline level.
- Patient's pulse is normal or back to baseline.
- Patient's systolic blood pressure is >90.
- Patient's urinary output is >30 ml/hour.

NURSING INTERVENTIONS AND *RATIONALE*

1. Continue to monitor the assessment parameters listed under "Defining Characteristics." In addition, a serum lactate level >2 mOsm/L is believed to represent cellular perfusion failure at its earliest stage.
2. Secure airway and administer high flow oxygen.
3. Place patient in supine position with legs elevated ***to increase preload.*** Consider using low-Fowler's position with legs elevated for patient with head injury.
4. For fluid repletion use the 3:1 rule, replacing three parts of fluid for every unit of blood lost.
5. Administer crystalloid solutions using the fluid challenge technique: infuse precise aliquots of fluid (usually 5 to 20 ml/min) over 10-minute periods; monitor cardiac loading pressures serially ***to determine successful challenging.*** If the PCWP or PAD elevates more than 7 mm Hg above beginning level, the infusion should be stopped. If the PCWP or PAD rises only to 3 mm Hg above baseline or falls, another fluid challenge should be administered.
6. Replete fluids first before considering use of vasopressors, ***since vasopressors increase myocardial oxygen consumption out of proportion to the reestablishment of coronary perfusion in the early phases of treatment.***
7. When blood is available or its need is indicated, replace it with fresh packed red cells and fresh frozen plasma ***to keep clotting factors intact.***
8. Move or reposition patient minimally ***to decrease or limit tissue oxygen demands.***
9. Evaluate patient's anxiety level and intervene through patient education or sedation ***to decrease tissue oxygen demands.***
10. Be alert for the possibility of adult respiratory distress syndrome (ARDS) development in the ensuing 72 hours.

HIGH RISK FOR FLUID VOLUME EXCESS

RISK FACTOR

- Renal failure

DEFINING CHARACTERISTICS

- Weight gain that occurs during a 24- to 48-hour period
- Dependent pitting edema
- Ascites in severe cases
- Fluid crackles on lung auscultation
- Exertional dyspnea
- Oliguria or anuria
- Hypertension
- Engorged neck veins
- Decrease in urinary osmolality as renal failure progresses
- CVP >15 cm of H_2O
- PCWP 20-25 mm Hg

OUTCOME CRITERIA

- Weight returns to baseline.
- Edema or ascites is absent or reduced to baseline.
- Lungs are clear to auscultation.
- Exertional dyspnea is absent.
- Blood pressure returns to baseline.
- Neck veins are flat.

NURSING INTERVENTIONS AND *RATIONALE*

1. Continue to monitor the assessment parameters listed under "Defining Characteristics."
2. Promote skin integrity of edematous areas by frequent repositioning and elevation of areas where possible. Avoid massaging pressure points or reddened areas of skin ***because this results in further tissue trauma.***
3. Plan patient care to provide rest periods ***to not heighten exertional dyspnea.***
4. Weigh patient daily at same time in same clothing, preferably with the same scale.
5. Instruct the patient about the correlation between fluid intake and weight gain, using commonly understood fluid measurements (e.g., ingesting 4 cups [1000 ml] of fluid results in an approximate 2-pound weight gain in the anuric patient).

FLUID VOLUME DEFICIT RELATED TO DIARRHEA, WOUND DRAINAGE

DEFINING CHARACTERISTICS

- Dry mucous membranes and skin
- Weight loss in excess of 10%
- Acute thirst
- Hypotension
- Tachycardia
- Longitudinal wrinkling of the tongue
- Metabolic acidosis
- Serum electrolyte imbalances: hyperchloremia, hypokalemia
- Electrocardiogram (ECG) changes associated with hypokalemia

OUTCOME CRITERIA

- Mucous membranes are moist.
- The patient's weight returns to baseline.
- The patient's blood pressure returns to baseline.
- The patient's heart rate returns to baseline.
- Tongue is moist and nonwrinkled.
- The acid-base balance is normal.
- Serum electrolyte values are normal.

NURSING INTERVENTIONS

1. Continue to monitor the assessment parameters listed under "Defining Characteristics."
2. With physician's collaboration, replace base and electrolyte losses.
3. With physician's collaboration, replace fluid loss with intravenous isotonic saline solution or dextrose and one-half normal saline solution.
4. Provide oral fluids that are high in electrolytes, such as juices.
5. Provide oral potassium replacement according to serum potassium measurements as the metabolic acidosis is corrected.

FLUID VOLUME DEFICIT RELATED TO ACTIVE PLASMA LOSS AND FLUID SHIFT INTO INTERSTITIUM SECONDARY TO BURNS

DEFINING CHARACTERISTICS

- PCWP, PAD, CVP less than normal or less than baseline
- Tachycardia
- Narrowed pulse pressure
- Systolic blood pressure <100 mm Hg
- Urinary output <30 ml/hour
- Increased hematocrit level

OUTCOME CRITERIA

- The patient's PCWP, PAD, and CVP are normal or back to baseline.
- Systolic blood pressure is >90 mm Hg.
- Urinary output is >30 ml/hour.
- The patient's hematocrit level is normal.

NURSING INTERVENTIONS AND *RATIONALE*

1. Continue to monitor the assessment parameters listed under "Defining Characteristics." In addition, inspect soft tissues ***to determine the presence of edema.***
2. With physician's collaboration, administer intravenous (IV) fluid replacements (usually normal saline solution or lactated Ringer's solution) at a rate sufficient ***to maintain urinary output >40 ml/hour.*** Colloid solutions are avoided in the initial phases (but can be used later) because of the possibility of increased edema formation ***as a result of the increased capillary permeability.***

VIII

GASTROINTESTINAL ALTERATIONS

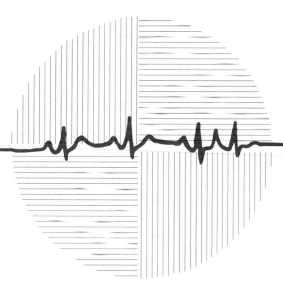

37

Gastrointestinal Anatomy and Physiology

CHAPTER OBJECTIVES

- Identify and briefly describe the physiology of the normal anatomic structures of the gastrointestinal tract.
- List and discuss the functions of the gastric secretions.
- Discuss the formation and function of bile.
- List and describe the exocrine functions of the pancreas, and discuss how pancreatic secretions promote digestion.
- Identify the most important functions of the large intestine, including actions of colonic bacteria.

The major function of the gastrointestinal (GI) tract is digestion—that is, to convert ingested nutrients into simpler forms that can be transported from the tract's lumen to the portal circulation and used in metabolic processes. The GI system also plays a vital role in detoxification and elimination of bacteria, viruses, chemical toxins, and drugs. Disturbances of the GI system itself or of the complex hormonal and neural controls that regulate it can severely upset homeostasis and compromise the overall nutritional status of the patient. Furthermore, any circumvention of the normal feeding mechanism (e.g., by mechanisms that bypass the oral route, such as tube and enteral feeding) can alter digestive processes or contribute to malabsorption.

Thus it is vital for the critical care nurse to have an active knowledge of the normal function of the GI tract to facilitate assessment, diagnosis, and intervention in patients with GI diseases.

ROLE OF THE BRAIN

Feeding actually begins with the sensation of hunger—the intrinsic desire for food—which is under the control of the feeding center in the lateral nuclei of the hypothalamus. Activation of the feeding center initiates a search for food. The satiety center, which provides the sensation of satisfaction and fulfillment after a meal and inhibits the feeding center, is located in the ventromedial nuclei of the hypothalamus. Thus the nutritional status of the body is a primary concern of the hypothalamus, which also excites the lower centers and the brainstem, in which the mechanics of feeding, such as chewing and mastication, are controlled.

MOUTH, ORAL CAVITY, AND PHARYNX

The mouth and accessory organs, which include the lips, cheeks, gums, tongue, palate, and salivary glands, perform the initial phases of digestion: ingestion, mastication, and salivation.

Ingestion and Mastication

The mouth is the beginning of the alimentary canal (Fig. 37-1) and is the means for ingestion and entry of nutrients. The teeth cut, grind, and mix food, transforming it into a form suitable for swallowing and increasing the surface area of food available to salivary secretions. Healthy dentition is vital for this process.

Mucous glands located behind the tip of the tongue and serous glands (Ebner's glands) located at the back of the tongue aid in the lubrication of food and in its distribution over the taste buds.

Salivation

Salivation has an important role in the first stage of digestion because saliva lubricates the mouth, facilitates the movement of the lips and the tongue during swallowing, and washes away bacteria. Saliva consists of approximately 99% water and 1% mucin and amylase (ptyalin). It also contains a large amount of ions, such as potassium and bicarbonate, as well as protein antibodies and thiocyanate ions, which are vital in destroying oral bacteria.

Approximately 1000 to 1500 ml of saliva is produced each day by three pairs of salivary glands: the submaxillary glands, the sublingual glands, and the parotid glands. Parotid gland secretions are enzymatic, containing amylase, which begins the chemical breakdown of large polysaccharides into dextrins and sugars.

The mouth and pharynx also are lined with small salivary glands that provide additional lubrication. Parasympathetic stimulation results in profuse secretions of watery saliva. Sympathetic stimulation causes release of small amounts of saliva with organic constituents from the submaxillary glands. Anticholinergic drugs reduce salivary secretion and a number of GI hormones, such as secretin, cholecystokinin, vasoactive intestinal peptide, and gastric inhibitory peptide.

ESOPHAGUS

The esophagus (gullet) is a collapsible tube that lacks cartilage. In adults it is 23 to 25 cm (9 to 10 inches) long and 1 to 2 cm (½ to 1 inch) wide. It is the narrowest part

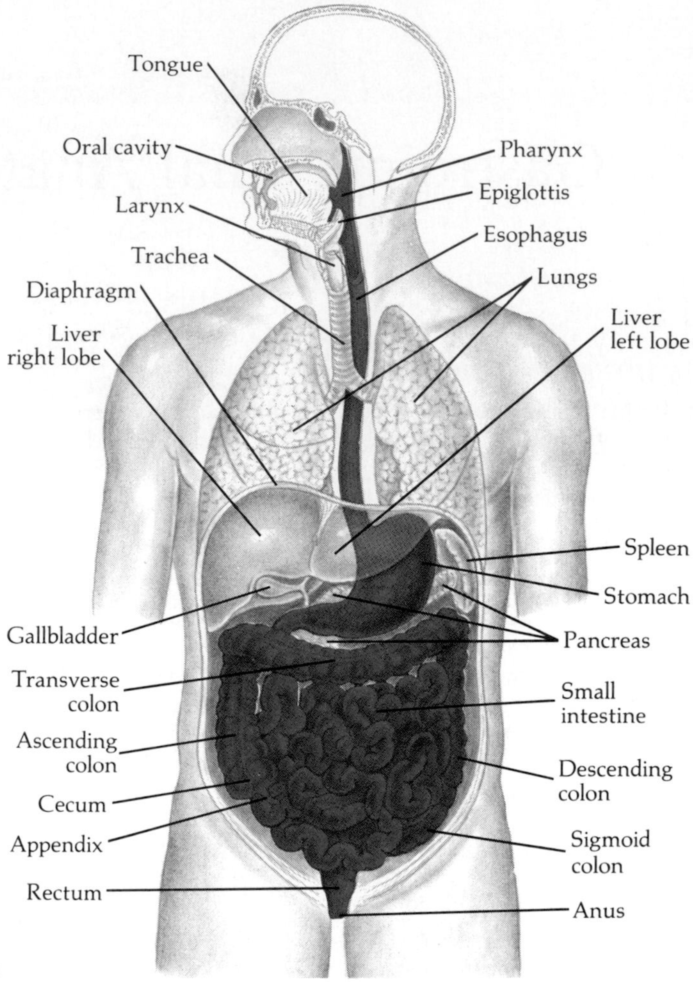

Fig. 37-1 Anatomy of the gastrointestinal system. (From Thompson JM and others: *Mosby's clinical nursing,* ed 3, St Louis, 1993, Mosby–Year Book.)

of the digestive tube and lies posterior to the trachea and heart, with attachments at the hypopharynx and at the cardiac portion of the stomach below the diaphragm. It begins at the level of the C6 to T1 vertebrae and extends vertically through the mediastinum and diaphragm to the level of T11.

The esophagus has two sphincters: (1) the hypopharyngeal, or the upper esophageal, sphincter, and (2) the cardiac, or lower esophageal, sphincter. The distal 3 to 5 cm of the esophagus constitutes the cardiac sphincter, which, although not grossly discernible, is an area of increased pressure. The stomach forms a 70- to 80-degree angle with the esophagus at this point.

The functions of the esophagus are to accept a bolus of food from the oropharynx, to transport the bolus through the esophageal body by gravity and peristalsis, and to release the bolus into the stomach through the cardiac sphincter. The esophagus also serves as an antireflex barrier and as a vent for increased gastric pressure.

The esophageal phase of deglutition is a visceral response and is reflex in nature. Peristalsis consists of waves of circular contractions and relaxations by which a bolus of food is propelled. A peristaltic wave takes 5 to 10 seconds to reach the stomach from the pharynx. Secondary peristalsis begins in the upper thoracic esophagus and is caused by distention from foods remaining in the esophagus. Body position (standing, recumbent), the acidity of the food bolus, pain, anxiety, and anger can affect transit time. Peristalsis is required for movement of liquids and semisolids in the recumbent position. Peristalsis declines with age.

At the cardiac sphincter a pressure of approximately +25 mm Hg is maintained, and it may reach 15 to 20 mm Hg higher than pressure in the fundus. This pressure difference normally prevents reflux of gastric contents and erosion of mucosa from acid-pepsin secretions. In addition, esophageal mucoid secretions provide lubrication and prevent mucosal excoriation caused by food entering proximally or by refluxing gastric contents distally.

ABDOMINAL ORGANS

The abdomen, the largest cavity in the body, contains the stomach, small and large intestines, liver, pancreas, kidneys, spleen, suprarenal glands, and uterus. The abdominal organs (see Fig. 37-1) are protected by the peritoneum, a serous membrane consisting of mesothelium and connective tissue.

Stomach

The stomach is an elongated pouch approximately 25 to 30 cm (10 to 12 inches) long and 10 to 13 cm (4 to 5

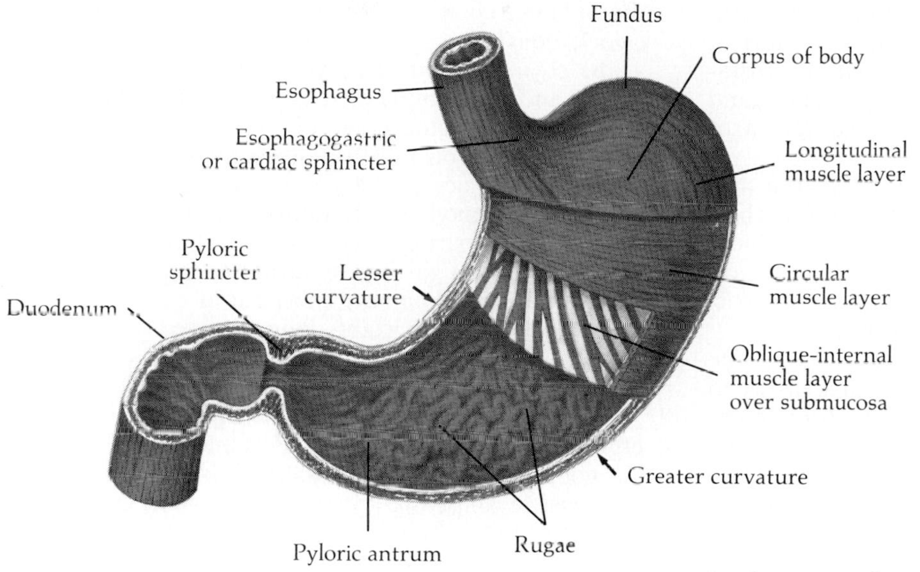

Fig. 37-2 Gross anatomy of the stomach. (From Thompson JM and others: *Mosby's clinical nursing,* ed 3, St Louis, 1993, Mosby–Year Book.)

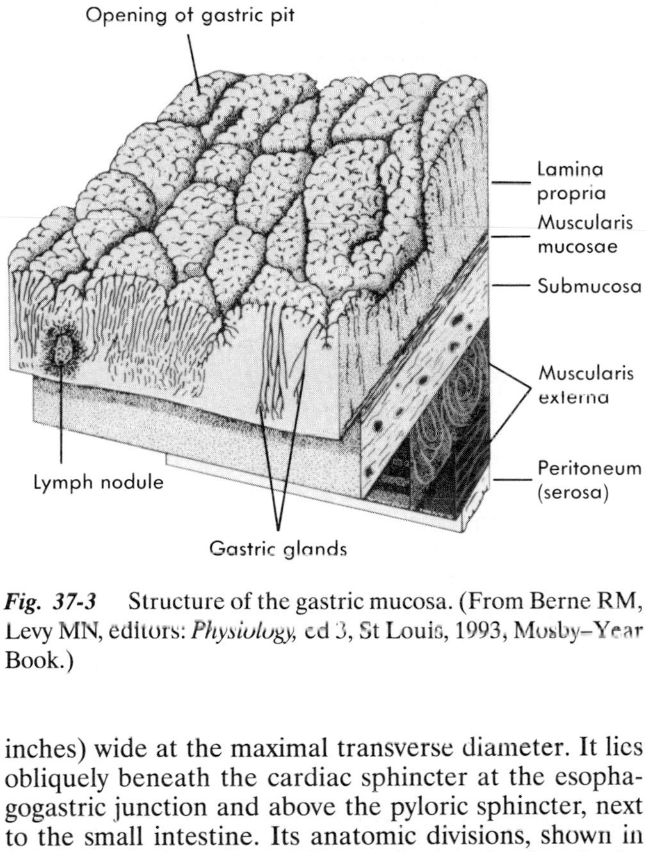

Fig. 37-3 Structure of the gastric mucosa. (From Berne RM, Levy MN, editors: *Physiology,* ed 3, St Louis, 1993, Mosby–Year Book.)

inches) wide at the maximal transverse diameter. It lies obliquely beneath the cardiac sphincter at the esophagogastric junction and above the pyloric sphincter, next to the small intestine. Its anatomic divisions, shown in Fig. 37-2, include the cardia at the proximal end; the fundus, which lies above and to the left of the cardiac sphincter; the body, the central portion; the antrum, an elongated constricted portion; and the pylorus, the distal end connecting the antrum to the duodenum. The greater curvature, which begins at the cardiac orifice and arches backward and upward around the fundus, is in contact with the transverse colon and the pancreas at the posterior edge. The lesser curvature extends from the cardia to the pylorus. Two sphincters control the rate of food passage: the cardiac at the esophagogastric junction and the pyloric at the gastroduodenal junction.

The shape and size of the stomach vary with body build, position, contents, digestive stage, development of gastric muscles, gender, posture, and condition of adjacent intestine. Its capacity is approximately 1 quart, or 1 L, of food or liquid. When distended, it may impede the descent of the diaphragm during inhalation.

The stomach wall has four layers[1,2] (Fig. 37-3):

1. The serous coat (tunica serosa), the outermost layer, consists of areolar tissue. It continues as a double fold from the lower edge of the stomach to cover the intestine.
2. The muscular coat (tunica muscularis) has three smooth muscle layers instead of the usual two: (a) an external, longitudinal layer, (b) a middle, circular layer, and (c) an inner, oblique layer, which extends from the fundus to the pyloric antrum.
3. The submucous coat (tunica submucosa) consists of loose areolar connective tissue, blood vessels, lymphatics, elastic fibers, and nerve plexuses.
4. The mucous coat (tunica mucosa), the innermost layer, consists of a muscular layer that is arranged in longitudinal folds, or rugae, that can expand. This layer contains 35 million glands that secrete up to 3000 ml of gastric juice per day.

◆ **Cytoprotective mechanisms of the gastric mucosa.** Epithelial cells of the gastric mucosa are very closely packed together and thus serve as a protective barrier, preventing diffusion of hydrogen ions into the mucosa. The surface epithelial cells produce alkaline mucus and secrete a bicarbonate-laden fluid. The mucus further protects the gastric mucosa by delaying back-diffusion of hydrogen ions and trapping them for neutralization by the secreted bicarbonate. In addition, gastric mucosal cells can compensate for cell destruction. Epithelial cells are in a constant state of growth, migration, and desquamation and are shed at a rate of one-half million per minute. The gastric mucosa also has the ability to increase blood flow; this provides an additional buffer for acid neutralization and aids in removing toxic metabolites and chloride ions from injured mucosa. Finally, the gastric mucosal cells synthesize a family of unsaturated fatty acids known as *prostaglandins.* Prostaglandins facilitate mucosal bicarbonate secretion and inhibit acid secretion by preventing the activation of parietal cells by histamine.[3-6]

Certain lipid-soluble substances can break the mucosal barrier and penetrate the cells, causing their destruction, edema, and bleeding. These substances include alcohol, lysolecithins, regurgitated bile acids, and other aliphatic acids, such as acetic, butyric, propionic, salicylic, and acetylsalicylic acids.

◆ **Circulation.** The large blood supply required for the motor and secretory activity of the stomach is provided by the celiac axis. Venous drainage occurs through the portal vein. Numerous lymphatic channels arise in the submucosa and terminate in the thoracic duct.

◆ **Motor functions.** Motor functions of the stomach include relaxation for storage, secretion, and digestion; peristaltic (mixing) activity; and emptying. These motor functions are regulated by (1) afferent and efferent fibers of the sympathetic and parasympathetic nervous systems, (2) reflexes operating through the celiac and intrinsic plexuses, and (3) gastric hormones.

◆ **Storage.** The stomach receives food from the cardiac sphincter, stores it for a period of time, and mixes it with gastric secretions. The food is then ground into a semifluid consistency called *chyme,* which is delivered via the pylorus to the duodenum.

◆ **Secretion and digestion.** The stomach has approximately 35 million glands of various types that secrete 1500 to 3000 ml of gastric juice into the lumen per day, depending on the diet and other stimuli. The major components of gastric juice are hydrochloric acid (HCl), pepsinogen, and mucus. Other components are intrinsic factor, inorganic salts such as potassium, gastric lipase, and protein.

Gastric juice has a pH near 1, but when mixed with food, its pH rises to 2 to 3. Peptic activity is optimal at a pH of 3.5. Gastric juice dissolves soluble foods, brings them close to the osmolarity of plasma, and also has bacteriostatic action.

The rate, amount, and type of gastric secretion are tightly controlled. The number of glands in the mucosa and the sensitivity of these glands to stimuli affect secretory activity, but the major stimuli are vagal (acetylcholine) activity, the antral hormone *gastrin,* and histamine.

Peristaltic activity. Only as much chyme is admitted as can be handled by the small intestine. Chyme, which has a high fat content, is slowed because bile secretion controls its accommodation. Regulation and coordination are provided by duodenal and jejunal enterogastrone. GI hormones—gastrin, secretin, cholecystokinin, somatostatin, and gastric inhibitory peptide (at nonphysiologic concentrations)—inhibit gastric emptying. Acid chyme is slowed until pancreatic enzymes and mucus neutralize the acidity. In contrast, vasoactive intestinal peptide increases gastric motility and relaxes the pyloric sphincter.

Emptying. The rate of gastric emptying is influenced by the volume, chemical composition, acidity, osmolality, caloric density, and temperature of the chyme. Highly acidic chyme inhibits emptying. Liquids empty before solids, and this emptying occurs faster in the sitting position or when the person is lying on the right side. Hyperosmolar and hypoosmolar solutions slow gastric emptying; fatty acids retard emptying. Unsaturated fatty acids retard emptying more than do saturated fatty acids. Temperature extremes (hot or cold) likewise retard emptying. Although the chemical and physical properties of the meal dominate the pace of emptying, other factors also are important. Pain, anxiety, sadness, and hostility inhibit emptying, whereas aggression accelerates emptying.

Narcotic analgesics also inhibit emptying. Anticholinergics can inhibit antral peristalsis and delay emptying, but not in conventional doses. Metoclopramide accelerates gastric emptying by facilitating acetylcholine release.

Gastric stasis occurs in numerous pathologic conditions, including iron-deficiency anemia, brain tumor, gastric carcinoma, hepatic coma, hypocalcemia, hypokalemia, irradiation, malnutrition, pancreatic disease, peritonitis, sepsis, uremia, and vagotomy.

Small Intestine

The small intestine, a coiled, folded tube approximately 7 m (22 to 23 feet) long, extends from the pyloric sphincter to the cecum and fills most of the abdominal cavity. It has three anatomic divisions:

1. The duodenum, shaped like the letter C, begins at the pyloric sphincter of the stomach. It is 25 cm (10 inches) long and 4 cm (1 to 1½ inches) wide.
2. The jejunum, the middle portion, lies in the left iliac and umbilical regions. It is 250 cm (8 to 9½ feet) long and 4 cm (1 to 1½ inches) wide.
3. The ileum, the terminus, lies in the hypogastric, right iliac, and pelvic regions. It is 375 cm (12 feet) long and 2.5 cm (1 inch) wide.

Although the demarcating line between the jejunum and the ileum is somewhat arbitrary, the ileum is narrower than the jejunum. The ileocecal valve, located at the terminal end of the ileum at the junction of the cecum and colon, controls the flow of small bowel contents into the large intestine and prevents reflux.

The mucous and submucous layers of the small intestine (Fig. 37-4) are arranged in visible circular folds, which are largest and most numerous in the distal duodenum and proximal jejunum and disappear in the lower ileum. These folds are covered by a second series of folds called *villi,* which are projections, 0.5 to 1.5 mm in length, that are in constant motion—constricting, lengthening, and shortening. The 4 to 5 million villi (see Fig. 37-4) give the intestine a velvety appearance. They are more numerous and larger in the jejunum than in the ileum. Villi contain a network of capillaries and blind lymphatic vessels called *lacteals.* The core of the villus also contains smooth muscle strands and free cells, such as lymphocytes, plasma cells, and granular leukocytes. The outer layer of the villus is composed of microvilli. The circular folds of the small intestine, along with the

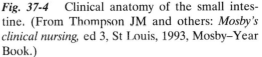

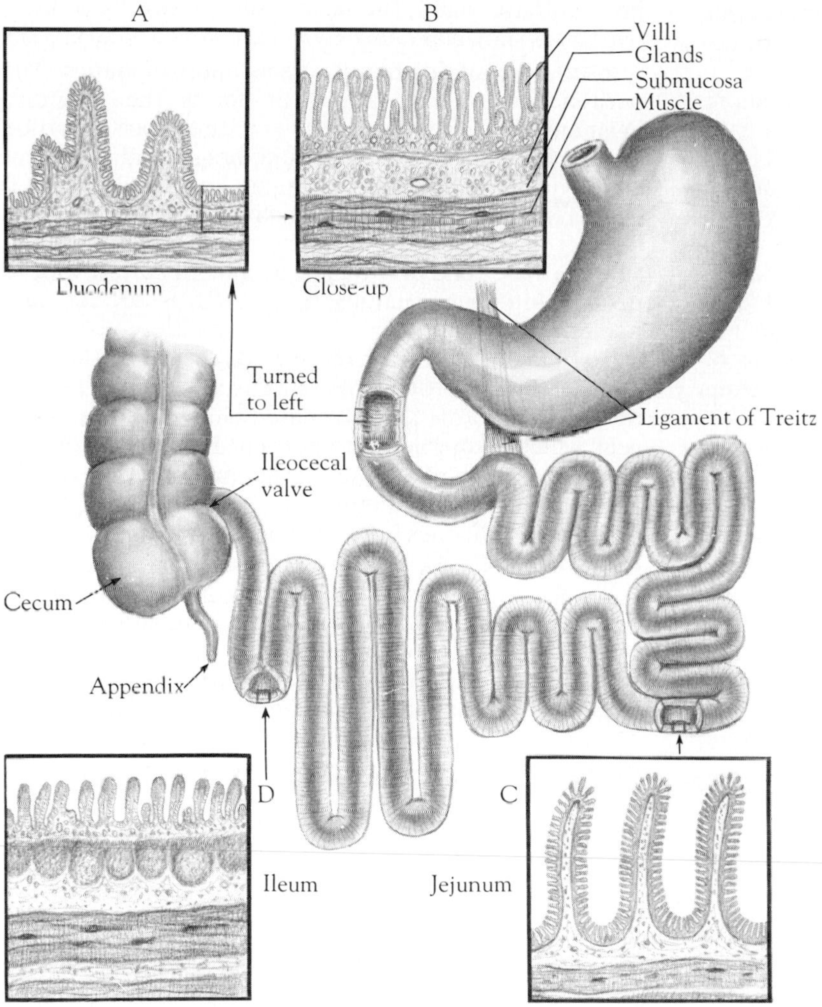

Fig. 37-4 Clinical anatomy of the small intestine. (From Thompson JM and others: *Mosby's clinical nursing,* ed 3, St Louis, 1993, Mosby–Year Book.)

villi and microvilli, increase the digestive-absorptive surface of the small intestine 600 times.

The lymphatic system in the mucosa of the jejunum and ileum includes (1) solitary nodules, which are supplied by one vein and one artery each and their own capillary cystem and (2) aggregated, circular-shaped lymph nodes (Peyer's patches), which consist of groups of 20 to 30 nodes and occur only in the ileum.

Extrinsic innervation is provided by both the sympathetic and parasympathetic systems. Sympathetic stimuli (epinephrine and norepinephrine) inhibit motility. Parasympathetic fibers of the vagus nerve (through acetylcholine) increase tone and motility and regulate intestinal reflexes. Resection of the vagus nerve has minimal effect on the small bowel. Intrinsic innervation, which initiates motor functions, is provided by two plexuses (Auerbach's and Meissner's) in the intestinal wall.

The functions of the small intestine include peristalsis, secretion, digestion, and absorption. As chyme enters the duodenum, it encounters secretions derived from the pancreas, liver, gallbladder, and small bowel.

◆ **Peristalsis.** Peristalsis in the small intestine is characterized by circular muscular contractions, the purpose of which is to continue the mixing of food and digestive juices. Peristalsis is controlled by Auerbach's plexus and occurs when a portion of the intestinal wall is distended with chyme. This distention initiates contractions along the intestine, giving the small bowel the look of a chain of sausage links. Peristalsis and villous movement facilitate the mixing of secretions with chyme. Large molecules of food are thus broken down to smaller ones, and water-insoluble substances are made soluble so that they can be better absorbed. Peristaltic waves move chyme 2 to 25 cm (1 to 10 inches) per minute toward the ileocecal valve.

◆ **Secretion.** The small intestine has two major types of glands, Brunner's glands and intestinal glands. Brunner's glands lie in the mucosa of the duodenum and secrete mucus, an alkaline fluid (pH of 9) that neutralizes chyme and protects the mucosa. Intestinal glands are found in pits of the mucosa and are called the *crypts of Lieberkühn.* These crypts secrete 2 to 3 L per day of yellow fluid containing enzymes that assist in nutrient digestion.

GI hormones influence the release of secretions from the stomach and other organs emptying into the duodenum. They also regulate small bowel motility, the osmolality of luminal contents, and the duodenal pH (maintained between 7 and 9). The two families of intestinal hormones are (1) the gastrin type, which includes gastrin and cholecystokinin and (2) the secretin type, which includes secretin, gastric inhibitory peptide, vasoactive intestinal peptide, and enteroglucagon.

◆ **Digestion and absorption.** The process of digestion, which involves breaking down larger molecules into small ones, is essential for most nutrients absorbed from the small intestine. Optimal conditions for digestion are maintained through pH and osmolality controls within the small intestine. The entry of chyme into the duodenum stimulates the production of secretin, which in turn stimulates the pancreas to secrete a highly alkaline fluid into the duodenum. As chyme enters the duodenum, it is mixed with the combined secretions of the duodenal mucosa and pancreas and with bile from the liver and gallbladder.

The small intestine absorbs up to 8 L of fluid per day, passing only a small part of this fluid into the large intestine. Carbohydrates, fats, amino acids, electrolytes, and water constitute the absorbed fluid. In addition, components of saliva, gastric juice, bile, and intestinal and pancreatic secretions also are absorbed. Absorption of nutrients occurs by a variety of mechanisms, depending on the physiochemical properties, the molecular weight, and the osmolality of the nutrient.

Liver

The liver is the largest internal organ in the body. Weighing 1200 to 1600 g (3 to 4 pounds), it is friable, dark red, and of a soft-solid consistency. Located in the right upper abdominal quadrant, it fits snugly against the right interior diaphragm. The liver is surrounded by connective tissue known as *Glisson's capsule,* which is covered by serosa and contains blood vessels and lymphatics. The peritoneum covering the liver forms the falciform ligament, which attaches the liver to the anterior portion of the abdomen between the diaphragm and umbilicus and divides the liver into two main lobes, right and left (Fig. 37-5). The right lobe, which is 6 times larger than the left, has three sections: the right lobe proper, the caudate lobe, and the quadrate lobe. The left lobe is divided into two sections. Each lobe is divided into numerous lobules.

◆ **Circulation.** The liver receives one third of the total cardiac output from two major sources: the hepatic artery, which provides oxygenated blood; and the portal vein, which is supplied with nutrient-rich blood from the gut, pancreas, spleen, stomach, and mesentery. The portal vein, which accounts for 75% of the total liver blood flow, branches into sinusoids to transport blood to each lobule. Unlike capillaries, sinusoids lack a definite cell wall but contain a lining of phagocytic (Kupffer's) cells and some nonphagocytic cells of modified epithelium. Sinusoids empty blood into an intralobular vein in the center of the lobule. Intralobular veins empty into larger veins and finally into the hepatic vein, which empties on the posterior surface of the liver and eventually into the vena cava. The hepatic artery also divides and subdivides between the lobules, supplying sinusoids with oxygenated blood before emptying into the hepatic vein.

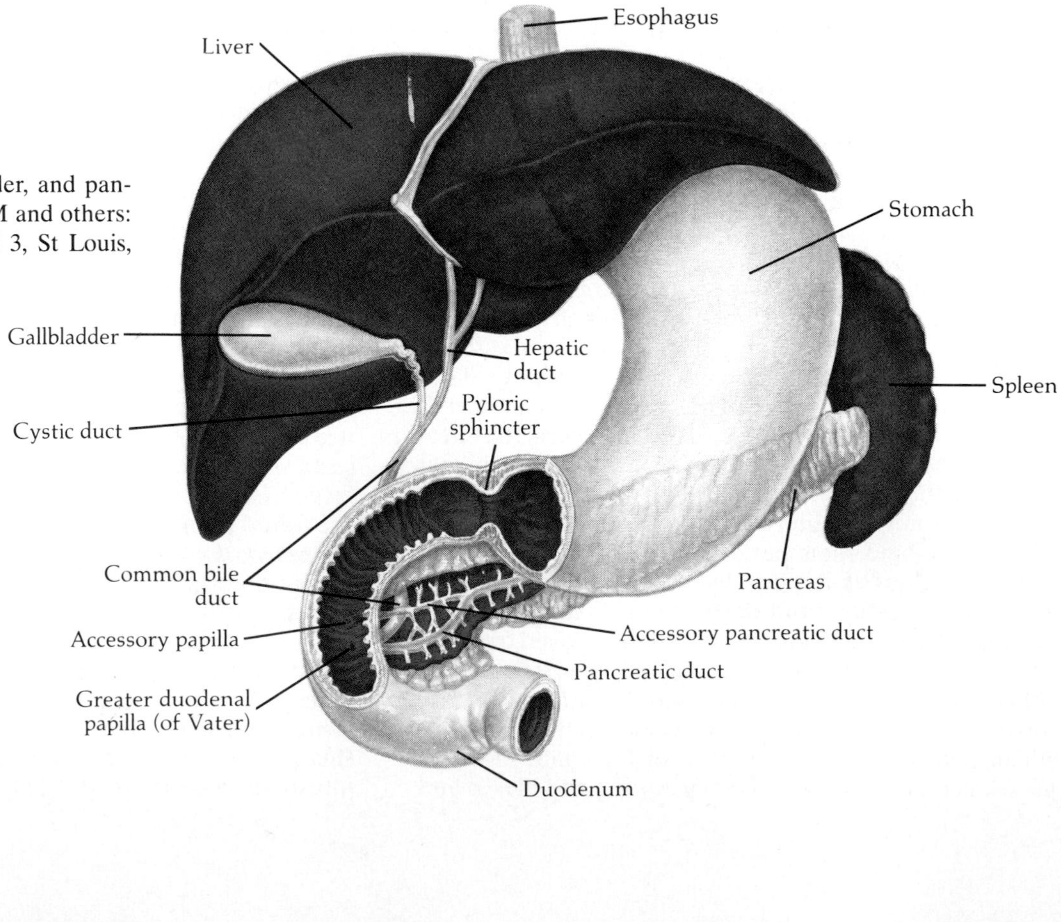

Fig. 37-5 Liver, gallbladder, and pancreas. (From Thompson JM and others: *Mosby's clinical nursing,* ed 3, St Louis, 1993, Mosby–Year Book.)

Lymphatic spaces are between liver cells. Lymph drains into lymphatic vessels that surround the hepatic vein and bile ducts. The liver's parenchymal cells (hepatocytes) have a variety of nondigestive functions that are beyond the scope of this text.

◆ **Digestive functions.** The liver plays a key role in metabolizing and storing carbohydrates, fats, proteins, and vitamins. Glycogen, the stored form of glucose, can be synthesized from glucose or from protein, fat, or lactic acid. Glycogen is broken down to glucose by the liver to maintain normal blood glucose levels. The liver also has a vital role in amino acid metabolism and can synthesize amino acids from metabolites of carbohydrates and fats. The liver synthesizes plasma proteins, such as globulins and albumin, important in maintaining the normal osmotic balance of blood, and also synthesizes the clotting factors *fibrinogen* and *prothrombin.* The liver deaminates amino acids to produce ketoacids and ammonia, from which urea is formed. In fat metabolism, the liver hydrolyzes triglycerides to glycerol and fatty acids in the process of ketogenesis and synthesizes phospholipids, cholesterol, and lipoproteins. Steroid hormones are conjugated, and polypeptide hormones are inactivated by the liver. In addition, the liver stores fat-soluble vitamins, vitamin B_{12}, and the minerals *iron* and *copper.* Finally, detoxification of drugs and toxins and degradation of worn red blood cells occur in the liver's Kupffer's cells, which belong to the reticuloendothelial system.

◆ **Bile.** The production of bile makes the liver a vital organ in digestion and absorption. The major components of bile are bile pigments, bile salts, cholesterol, neutral fats, phospholipids, inorganic salts, fatty acids, mucin, conjugated bilirubin, lecithin, and water, with traces of albumin, gamma globulin, urea, nitrogen, and glucose. The principal electrolytes of bile are sodium chloride and bicarbonate, and the major pigment is bilirubin.

Bile functions to emulsify fat globules, which facilitates digestion by lipases, as well as fat digestion and absorption of fat-soluble vitamins. Bile salts also serve as an excretion route for bilirubin, cholesterol, and various hormones (sex, thyroid, and adrenal). Approximately 80% of bile salts are reabsorbed actively in the distal ileum and are recycled to the liver through the enterohepatic circulation; only 20% are lost in the feces.

Bilirubin, the primary bile pigment, is formed from the heme portion of hemoglobin during the degradation of red blood cells by Kupffer's cells. When released into the blood stream, bilirubin binds to albumin as fat-soluble, unconjugated (indirect) bilirubin. Taken up by liver hepatocytes, indirect bilirubin is conjugated with glucuronic acid to form water-soluble, conjugated (direct) bilirubin, which is then excreted through hepatic ducts into the large intestine. If the amount of bilirubin sent to the liver is in excess, the ability of the liver to conjugate the bilirubin may be taxed; thus free, unconjugated indirect bilirubin will appear in the blood. High levels of indirect (unconjugated) bilirubin in the blood suggest hepatocellular dysfunction, whereas high levels of direct (conjugated) bilirubin suggest biliary tract obstruction.

Biliary System

The biliary system (Fig. 37-5) consists of the gallbladder and its related ductal system, including the hepatic, cystic, and common bile ducts.

◆ **Ductal system.** Bile, continuously formed in the liver, is excreted into the hepatic duct, which transports bile to the gallbladder. The hepatic duct then joins the cystic duct, forming the common bile duct, which empties into the duodenum. The common bile duct is surrounded by Oddi's sphincter, which pierces the wall of the duodenum and controls the flow of bile into the duodenum.

◆ **Gallbladder.** The gallbladder is a pear-shaped organ 7 to 10 cm (3 to 4 inches) long and 2.5 to 3.5 cm (1 to 1½ inches) wide, lying on the underside of the liver (see Fig. 37-5). It is attached to the liver by connective tissue, peritoneum, and blood vessels.

The main functions of the gallbladder are to collect, concentrate, acidify, and store bile entering it through the cystic duct from the hepatic duct. It can store up to 50 to 60 ml of bile from which approximately 90% of the water is removed so that bile is concentrated approximately 15 to 29 times. Cholesterol and pigment are likewise concentrated. Bile, which is golden or orange-yellow in the liver, becomes dark brown when concentrated in the gallbladder. By altering its shape and volume, the gallbladder regulates pressure within the extrahepatic biliary system. Relaxation of Oddi's sphincter, which surrounds the common bile duct as it enters the duodenum, is coordinated with gallbladder contraction through the regulatory action of cholecystokinin. Psychic factors, such as the sight, smell, and taste of food, can stimulate gallbladder contraction, whereas fear or excitement decreases contraction. After a meal the amount of bile entering the duodenum increases as a result of enhanced liver secretion and gallbladder contraction. Intestinal secretion of cholecystokinin and secretin, high levels of bile salts in the blood, and vagal stimulation increase biliary secretion.

Pancreas

The pancreas is a soft, lobulated, fish-shaped gland lying beneath the duodenum and the spleen (see Fig. 37-5). It is pinkish-yellow, 10 to 22 cm (5 to 10 inches) long, and 5 cm (1 to 1½ inches) wide. Its anatomic divisions include the head, which lies in the C-shaped curve of the duodenum to which it is attached; the body, the main part of the gland, which extends horizontally across the abdomen and is largely hidden behind the stomach; and the tail, a thin, narrow portion in contact with the spleen.

The main pancreatic duct, the duct of Wirsung, traverses the entire length of the organ. Wirsung's duct empties exocrine secretions into the ampulla of Vater, which is the same lumen draining the common bile duct, at the entrance to the duodenum. (In 40% of humans, the pancreatic duct and common bile duct empty separately into the duodenum. Approximately 15% of humans have an accessory duct, the duct of Santorini, which empties into the duodenum above the ampulla of Vater.)

The internal structural unit of the exocrine pancreas,

the lobule, consists of numerous small alveoli lined with secretory cells called *tubuloacinar cells* (i.e., shaped like tiny tubes and grapes). Each acinus has a small duct that empties into lobular ducts. Lobules are joined by connective tissue into lobes, which unite to form the gland. Likewise, the ducts from each lobule empty into the duct of Wirsung.

◆ **Exocrine functions.** Exocrine functions of the pancreas are limited to digestion. Acinar cells secrete pancreatic juice, which consists of water, sodium bicarbonate, and electrolytes (sodium and potassium) at a highly alkaline pH. Enzymes produced in the pancreas include the following: (1) proteolytic endopeptidases (i.e., trypsin, chymotrypsin, and carboxypeptidase), which are secreted as inactive precursors, and aminopeptidase, which is secreted in the active form; (2) deoxyribonuclease and ribonuclease; (3) amylase; and (4) lipase and cholesterol esterase. Within the secretory cells of the pancreas, a trypsin inhibitor prevents activation of trypsinogen, thus inhibiting autodigestion, the underlying cause of acute pancreatitis.

Pancreatic exocrine function is regulated by hormonal and neural signals. Hormonal signals are provided primarily by the intestinal hormones secretin and cholecystokinin, which are released from the duodenum and jejunum in response to stimulation by chyme in the intestine. Absorbed by the portal system, these hormones are transported to the pancreas. Secretin causes the pancreas to produce a high volume of fluid rich in water and bicarbonate, whereas cholecystokinin causes it to produce a juice rich in enzymes but low in volume. The two hormones potentiate each other's effects on the pancreas.

Although hormonal controls of the exocrine pancreas are believed only supplemental to vagal regulation, hormonal regulation of the exocrine pancreas is apparently more complex. In addition to secretin, vasoactive intestinal peptide also may mediate an increase in pancreatic fluid and bicarbonate secretion. In contrast to these hormones, which are stimulatory, somatostatin, vasopressin, and calcitonin have inhibitory functions in the exocrine pancreas.

In the duodenum, pancreatic sodium bicarbonate reacts with hydrochloric acid to produce carbonic acid. This is carried to the lungs, from which it is excreted as carbon dioxide and sodium chloride.

Parasympathetic stimulation of the pancreas increases exocrine secretions and blood flow to the pancreas. Anticholinergics decrease enzyme production, volume output, and ductal pressure. Alcohol and histamine, by stimulating gastric hydrochloric acid production, indirectly cause an increase in pancreatic secretions. Sympathetic stimulation is inhibitory.

◆ **Endocrine functions.** Endocrine tissue consists of spherical islets called *islets of Langerhans,* which are embedded within the lobules of acinar tissue throughout the pancreas, especially in the distal body and tail. Endocrine products include insulin (produced in beta cells), glucagon (produced in alpha cells), and gastrin; all of these hormones are secreted directly into the blood stream. Further discussion of the endocrine functions of the pancreas is included in Chapter 41.

Large Intestine (Colon)

The large intestine, or colon, is approximately 150 cm (5 feet) long and extends from the ileocecal valve to the anus. The divisions of the colon are the ascending colon, hepatic flexure, transverse colon, splenic flexure, descending colon, sigmoid colon, rectum, and anal canal. The caliber of the colon decreases as it proceeds distally and averages 1½ to 2 inches in width.

◆ **Colonic layers.** As with the small intestine the colon has four layers. Beginning with the outermost layer, they are the serosa, muscular layer, submucosa, and mucosa. The serosa is formed from the visceral peritoneum and covers most of the colon, with the exclusion of the distal rectum.

The muscular layer contains two smooth muscles: the circular and the longitudinal. These muscles work together to propel fecal matter through the colon and also to "knead" the stool into a compact bolus. The longitudinal muscle consists of three muscular bands (taeniae coli) that stretch from the cecum to the distal sigmoid colon. These muscular bands create sacculations of haustra, important clinical features that normally are apparent on a barium enema radiograph. Haustra aid segmentation so that absorption of fluid from the fecal bolus is achieved. The absence of haustra is associated with severe inflammation of the mucosal layer and may extend into the serosal layer.

The longitudinal muscle and the circular muscle work together to produce two primary types of colonic movement. Segmentation, which is the alternate contraction and relaxation of haustral folds, involves the circular muscle and facilitates (1) the grinding of food masses, and (2) fluid absorption. Peristalsis, the second type of movement, is produced primarily by the longitudinal muscles and propels the fecal bolus forward. Mass peristalsis is a strong, slow contraction in which the distal left colon contracts en masse to move the fecal bolus into the rectum.

The submucosa contains small arteries, veins, and lymphatic vessels and connects the muscular layer to the inner mucosal layer. The innermost layer of the colon, the mucosa, is lined with simple columnar epithelial cells and contains deep crypts of Lieberkühn (or intestinal) glands that are lined with mucus-producing goblet cells. Mucus is produced to ease the passage of the fecal material and to protect the mucosal surface from trauma. Water and electrolytes also are absorbed through the mucosa.

◆ **Rectum.** The rectum begins midsacrum, is 12 to 15 cm (5 inches) long, and is quite angulated. These angles, also known as *Houston's valves,* are important in the defecation process because they tend to slow the passage of fecal material in the rectal vault, thus assisting the continence mechanism.

◆ **Innervation.** The colon has an intrinsic nervous system, which consists of the myenteric plexus (located between muscle layers) and the submucosal, or Auerbach's, plexus (located in the submucosa). These nerves control colonic movement and secretion of mucus, respectively.

Both the sympathetic and parasympathetic branches of the autonomic system innervate the colon. Sympathetic stimulation inhibits colonic activity and relaxes the anal sphincters. Parasympathetic stimulation increases colonic activity and secretion but relaxes the anal sphincter.

◆ **Functions.** The major functions of the colon are as follows:

1. Reabsorption of water, sodium, chloride, glucose, and urea
2. Dehydration of undigested residue
3. Putrefaction of contents by bacteria
4. Movement of the fecal bolus through the colon
5. Elimination of the fecal mass

The colon receives approximately 600 to 1000 ml of fluid per day. All but 100 to 150 ml of it is absorbed in the ascending and transverse colon.

Potassium is secreted into the colonic lumen in the potassium-rich mucus secreted by goblet cells. Bicarbonate is secreted by the colon, creating an alkaline fecal matter with a pH of 7.8.

The colon contains billions of anaerobic bacteria that serve the following three functions:

1. To putrefy remaining proteins and indigestible residue
2. To synthesize folic acid, vitamin K, nicotinic acid, riboflavin, and some B vitamins
3. To convert urea salts to ammonium salts and ammonia for absorption into the portal circulation

Common colonic bacteria are *Escherichia coli, Aerobacter aerogenes, Clostridium perfringens,* and *Lactobacillus bifidus.*

Colonic gas is a normal product of swallowed air, diffusion from the blood, and bacterial action. The composition of intestinal gas is oxygen, nitrogen, carbon dioxide, methane, hydrogen, and trace gases. Fecal odor is a consequence of the trace gases. Feces is expelled from the colon through the defecation process, a complex act involving both autonomic and voluntary efforts. The stimulus for evacuation is distention of the rectum.

REFERENCES

1. Powell LW, Piper DW: *Fundamentals of gastroenterology,* ed 5, 1991, McGraw-Hill.
2. Guyton AC: *Textbook of medical physiology,* ed 8, Philadelphia, 1991, WB Saunders.
3. Kim MS: Physiologic responses in health and illness: an overview, *Ann Rev Nutr Res* 5:79, 1987.
4. Moran JR, Greene HL: Digestion and absorption. In Rombeau JL, Caldwell MD, editors: *Enteral and tube feeding, clinical nutrition,* vol 2, ed 2, Philadelphia, 1990, WB Saunders.
5. Ropka M: Alimentation. In Abels L, editor: *Critical care nursing: a physiologic approach,* St Louis, 1986, Mosby–Year Book.
6. Rowlands BJ, Miller TA: The physiology of eating. With particular reference to the role of gastrointestinal hormones in the regulation of digestion. In Rombeau JL, Caldwell JD, editors: *Enteral and tube feeding: clinical nutrition,* vol 1, ed 2, Philadelphia, 1990, WB Saunders.

38

Gastrointestinal Clinical Assessment and Diagnostic Procedures

CHAPTER OBJECTIVES

- Discuss the rationale involved in developing a consistent, sequential format for performing a gastrointestinal nursing assessment.
- Perform a thorough nursing assessment of the gastrointestinal system in a critically ill patient and interpret the results.
- Outline important diagnostic procedures for detection of various gastrointestinal disorders.

CLINICAL ASSESSMENT

History

An integral part of nursing care is use of information obtained from the patient or family, or both, during an initial interview. The health history of a patient in the critical care unit may be obtained by other health care clinicians (e.g., a resident or a paramedic) and is very abbreviated because of the rapidly changing status of critically ill patients.

The health history of patients with suspected or confirmed gastrointestinal (GI) disorders should be reviewed for the following[1]:

1. Past health history, including any surgery, diseases, or hospitalizations
2. Potential nonspecific problems that may affect the GI system—changes in weight, appetite, or activity level
3. Location and description of symptoms, including the site, pain characteristics, and temporal relationship to events (e.g., food intake, time of day)
4. Intake and output (food elimination)—diet (food patterns), nutritional status, bowel characteristics (stool descriptions), use of medication and alcohol, dependence on laxatives or enemas

To help ascertain the nutritional status of a patient, the nurse should review the history, focusing on weight loss, edema, anorexia, vomiting, diarrhea, decreased or unusual food intake, and chronic illness.

It is important to be aware of the nonspecificity of symptoms as they relate to the GI system; that is, some systemic manifestations of GI disorders occur, as do other systemic disorders that have a GI manifestation. The patient's history should be examined for information about multiple drug intake, GI alterations potentially caused by normal aging, and changes in psychosocial conditions that could result in physical problems (e.g., lack of money for dentures causing symptoms of dysphagia).

Physical Examination

The clinical assessment helps establish baseline data about the physical dimensions of the patient's situation.[1] In adapting the assessment of the critically ill patient with a GI disorder, the nurse should do the following:

1. Use the classic four approaches of inspection, palpation, percussion, and auscultation
2. Modify technique, extent, and frequency of assessment on the basis of the patient's pain level and whether abnormal results are obtained
3. Use assessment standards established for elderly persons when reviewing their physical findings (see box, pp. 653-654)

The assessment should proceed when the patient is as comfortable as possible and is in a supine position; however, the position may need readjustment if it elicits pain. To prevent stimulation of GI activity, the order for the assessment should be changed to inspection, auscultation, percussion, and palpation. Although assessment of the GI system classically begins with inspection of the abdomen, the patient's oral cavity also must be inspected to determine any unusual findings.

Percussion and palpation elicit information about deep organs, such as the liver, spleen, and pancreas. Because the abdomen is a sensitive area, muscle tension may interfere with assessment. Percussion often helps relax tense muscles and so is performed before palpation. Percussion, in the absence of any disease, is most helpful in delineating the position and size of the liver and spleen. With percussion, fluid, gaseous distention, and masses in the abdominal region can be detected. Palpation is the technique most useful in detecting abdominal pathologic conditions. The box on pp. 653-654 provides a review of the clinical assessment, along with normal and abnormal findings and additional related information.

LABORATORY ASSESSMENT

The value of various laboratory procedures used to diagnose and treat diseases of the GI system has often been emphasized. No single test, however, provides an overall picture of the various organs' functional state. Also, no single value is predictive by itself. More than 100

CLINICAL ASSESSMENT OF THE ADULT GASTROINTESTINAL SYSTEM

INSPECTION

Procedure

Perform in warm, well-lighted environment with patient in comfortable position with abdomen exposed; view from slightly above and to one side of patient's abdomen.

Observe skin (pigmentation, lesions, striae, scars, dehydration, venous pattern), contour, movement (respiratory, symmetry, peristalsis).

Normal findings

Skin: pigmentation varies considerably within normal because of race, ethnic background, occupation exposure; however, abdomen generally is lighter in color than other exposed areas.

Contour: slightly concave or slightly round appearance.

Movement: symmetric; no visible pulsations or peristaltic waves.

Abnormal findings

Skin: jaundice, skin lesions, tenseness, glistening, stretch marks, scars (keloids), masses.

Contour: distended (asymmetric/generalized).

Related information

Chart findings, using one of two anatomic maps (four quadrants or nine sections).

Geriatric

Connective tissue changes and lower total body water make determining dehydration through skin assessment difficult.

AUSCULTATION

Procedure

Listen below and to the right of umbilicus for bowel sounds; proceed methodically through all quadrants, lifting and placing diaphragm of stethoscope lightly.

Normal findings

Sounds in small intestine are high pitched and gurgling; colonic sounds are low pitched and have a rumbling quality.

Bowel sounds occur at a rate of 5 to 35/min.

Abnormal findings

Lack of bowel sounds throughout 5-minute period, extremely soft and widely separated sounds, and increased sounds with characteristically high-pitched, loud rushing sound (peristaltic rush).

Bruits, peritoneal friction rubs, venous hums.

Related information

Normal venous hum is audible at times but is abnormal when heard in periumbilical region and accompanied by a palpable thrill.

Decreased bowel sounds are not significant without added data (e.g., nausea, vomiting, digestion).

Geriatric

Pediatric chest piece on stethoscope is useful with emaciated patient.

Aging leads to lessened peristalsis (listen for full 5 minutes) and diminished mucus secretion in esophagus ("popping" sound as food is pushed down dry esophagus).

Laxative intake can cause loud gurgling sounds.

Bell of stethoscope is used to listen to vascular sounds; not uncommon to hear cardiac murmurs over abdominal area.

Because of decreased secretion of digestive enzymes, normal bowel sounds may sound "less combustible."

PERCUSSION

Procedure

Proceed systematically to percuss lightly the entire abdomen, including the liver and spleen.

Normal findings

Stomach: tympanic when empty.

Intestine: tympanic or hyperresonant.

Liver and spleen: dull.

Abnormal findings

Flatness over stomach.

Solid masses and distended bladder: dull sound.

Liver and spleen: dull sounds beyond anatomic borders.

Related information

Geriatric

Upper liver border usually is found in fourth or fifth intercostal space (adults) but in elderly persons drops to fifth to seventh intercostal space; liver span shrinks to 6 to 12 cm.

Changes in tonal quality in elderly persons are caused by changes in connective tissue and diminished muscle mass.

PALPATION

Procedure

Perform both light (tender) and deep palpation of each organ and each quadrant of abdomen.

Light: assesses depth of skin and fascia (depth approximately 1 cm).

Deep: assesses beneath rectus abdominis muscle; perform bimanually (4 to 5 cm deep).

Examine last any areas in which patient complains of tenderness.

Normal findings

No areas of tenderness or pain.

No bulges, masses, or hardening.

Continued.

CLINICAL ASSESSMENT OF THE ADULT GASTROINTESTINAL SYSTEM—cont'd

Abnormal findings

Rebound tenderness, rigidity.

If enlarged, gallbladder (right upper quadrant) palpable as small mass attached to liver.

Spleen palpable only if enlarged.

Related information

Liver sometimes cannot be palpated in healthy adult; however, in extremely thin but healthy adult, it may be felt at the costal margin.

Geriatric

Palpation of abdominal organs is easier because of relaxed abdominal musculature.

Loss of muscle tone is apparent, especially in diaphragm and costal margin.

Abdomen is preferred site for palpating skin to assess hydration because of wrinkling and loss of turgor elsewhere.

laboratory tests have been proposed for the study of the liver and biliary tract alone.

In a patient with cirrhosis, for example, prothrombin time, bilirubin, alkaline phosphatase, alanine aminotransferase (ALT), and aspartate aminotransferase (AST) values all show elevation, but hemoglobin and hematocrit values drop (a result of red blood cell destruction or GI bleeding, or both). In a patient with hepatitis, serum transaminase values rise early, then fall as bilirubin rises. Jaundice occurs as the total bilirubin value goes above 2.5 mg/dl. Mild prolongation of prothrombin time and elevation of alkaline phosphatase may occur. With hepatic coma, in addition to those values that reflect the underlying liver disease, a plasma aminogram shows altered amino acid patterns and serum ammonia levels rise but do not correlate well with the level of encephalopathy. Common laboratory tests used in the assessment of GI disorders[2] are found in Table 38-1.

DIAGNOSTIC PROCEDURES

Endoscopy

Several forms of fiberoptic endoscopy are available for the direct visualization and evaluation of the GI tract. The main difference between them is the length of the anatomic area that can be examined. Endoscopy is the procedure of choice for the diagnosis of upper GI (UGI) bleeding, having replaced barium contrast studies. Colonoscopy allows for diagnostic evaluation of lower GI (LGI) bleeding.

In addition to diagnostic accuracy, endoscopy provides therapeutic benefit in a variety of conditions. Specifically, endoscopy is used to achieve hemostasis in patients with UGI bleeding. Several endoscopic techniques are available to achieve hemostasis. Thermal techniques utilize laser photocoagulation or electrocoagulation to control bleeding. Topical or injectable techniques involve the use of sclerotherapy to control bleeding. Mechanical methods, such as endoscopic stapling or band ligation, also may be used to control bleeding.[3] There is no consensus as to whether any one particular endoscopic modality is preferable to another.

Invasive tests may present risks for the patient. Although rare, potential complications include bowel perforation (abdominal pain and distention, rectal bleeding, fever, mucopurulent drainage), hemorrhage, vasovagal stimulation, and oversedation.

Angiography

In performing GI angiography, the physician directly catheterizes the vessel supplying a particular portion of the UGI tract (e.g., the left gastric artery for gastroesophageal bleeding or the gastroduodenal artery for pyloroduodenal hemorrhage).[4] The purpose of most angiographic procedures performed today is not to locate a bleeding site, but rather to achieve transcatheter control of bleeding. Angiography is used in the diagnosis of UGI bleeding only when endoscopy fails,[5] and it is used to treat those patients (approximately 15%) whose GI bleeding is not stopped with medical measures or endoscopic treatment.[4]

Plain and Abdominal X-Ray Studies

Numerous radiologic studies are available to investigate large bowel disease further. The most noninvasive studies are the plain films, such as the chest and the abdominal x-ray. Air in the bowel serves as a contrast medium to aid in the visualization of the bowel. Gas patterns (the presence of gas inside or outside the bowel lumen and the distribution of gas in dilated and nondilated bowel) are best revealed by plain films. These studies detect bowel obstruction, perforation, foreign bodies, and calcifications. When a patient is unable to sit or stand for erect films, a left lateral decubitus radiograph is a good substitute. No special preparation is required for plain films.

Liver Biopsy

Liver biopsy is a bedside procedure, usually performed for diagnosis of primary liver disease. Morphologic, biochemical, bacteriologic, and immunologic studies can be performed on the tissue sample. The biopsy also can yield information about the progression of the patient's disease and response to therapy. It is performed less frequently for diagnosis of metabolic disease or malignancy or in patients with multiple organ dysfunction

Table 38-1 Common laboratory tests used in the assessment of gastrointestinal disorders

Test	Normal levels	Clinical significance
LIVER FUNCTION		
Serum bilirubin		
Total	0.0-1.0 mg/dl	Elevated in hepatocellular disease
Direct	0.0-0.4 mg/dl	Elevated in biliary disease
Indirect	0.0-0.6 mg/dl	Elevated in hepatocellular disease
Serum alkaline phosphatase		
Female	30-100 U/L	Elevated in biliary obstruction
Male	45-115 U/L	
Amino transferases		
AST		
Female	9-25 U/L	Elevated in hepatocellular disease
Male	10-40 U/L	
ALT		
Female	7-30 U/L	Elevated in hepatocellular disease
Male	10-55 U/L	
GGT	1.0-60.0 U/L	Elevated in acute liver disease, biliary obstruction, and acute pancreatitis
LDH	110-210 U/L	Elevated in hepatocellular disease
Serum total protein	6.0-8.0 g/dl	Decreased in hepatocellular disease
Serum albumin	3.1-4.3 g/dl	Decreased in catabolic states, such as cirrhosis
Serum globulin	2.6-4.1 g/dl	Elevated in chronic liver disease
Plasma ammonia	12-55 mmol/L	Elevated in hepatic failure, hepatic encephalopathy, cirrhosis
PANCREATIC EXOCRINE FUNCTION		
Serum amylase	53-123 U/L	Elevated in acute pancreatitis, biliary obstruction
Serum lipase	4-24 U/dl	Elevated in acute pancreatitis, biliary obstruction

AST, Aspartate aminotransferase (formerly SGOT); *ALT*, alanine aminotransferase (formerly SGPT); *GGT*, Gamma-glutamyltransferase; *LDH*, lactic dehydrogenase.

syndrome. The procedure requires patient compliance if performed without significant sedation. Generally it involves the following:

1. Anesthetizing the pericapsular tissue
2. Inserting either a coring or suction needle between the eighth and ninth intercostal space while the patient either breathes lightly or holds his or her breath
3. Withdrawing the needle with the sample
4. Positioning the patient on the right side for several hours (he or she must remain flat for 24 hours after the procedure)

The procedure is brief; however, it is not uncommon for the patient to experience some pain as a result of irritation to the liver tissue. Abdominal or radiating pain from the epigastric area should be reported immediately. Hemorrhage is a rare but serious complication, thus requiring monitoring of vital signs every 30 minutes for 4 hours and every hour for the next 8 hours. Other complications include damage to neighboring organs, bile peritonitis, infection at the needle site, and shock. This procedure generally is not undertaken if the patient is severely debilitated, is unable to cooperate, or has bleeding tendencies or sepsis or if liver dullness cannot be detected. Because of the invasive nature of liver biopsy, possible complications, limited total organ assessment ability, and the requirement of patient involvement, other techniques (liver scans, endoscopy), which partially replace the biopsy, have evolved.

Liver Scans

Liver scans currently are used in assessing a patient's hepatic status. A liver-spleen scan involves intravenous (IV) injection of radioisotopes, the uptake of which is primarily in the liver and spleen, with little or no uptake occurring in patients with cirrhosis or splenomegaly secondary to portal hypertension. A liver scan yields information about the size, vascularity, and blood flow of the organs. The scan requires IV injection of radionuclides. These short-lived isotopes concentrate in the bile, allowing visualization of the biliary system and gallbladder, along with emptying into the duodenum; nonvisualization indicates obstruction. The patient is not sedated but must be able to lie flat for 30 to 90 minutes during the scanning. Uptake results can indicate cirrhosis, hepatitis, tumors, abscesses, and cyst.

Ultrasound

Ultrasound plays a key role in the diagnosis of many acute abdominal conditions because it is sensitive in detecting obstructive lesions, as well as ascites. Ultrasound is easily performed and is well-tolerated by bedridden patients.

Computed Tomography

Computed tomography (CT) scan is a radiographic examination that provides cross-sectional images of internal anatomy. It detects mass lesions more than 2 cm in diameter and allows visualization and evaluation of many different aspects of GI disease,[6] such as acute pseudocyst of the pancreas, abdominal abscesses, biliary obstruction, and a variety of GI neoplastic lesions.[7]

Magnetic Resonance Imaging

Magnetic resonance imaging (MRI) is a radiologic examination that provides multiplanar images of the internal anatomy. This technique is based on the emission or absorption of electromagnetic radiation by nuclei when exposed to particular magnetic fields. Because MRI involves use of a powerful magnet, patients with metal implants or cardiac pacemakers cannot undergo this examination.

REFERENCES

1. Bates B: *A guide to physical examination,* ed 5, Philadelphia, 1991, JB Lippincott.
2. Normal reference values, *N Engl J Med* 327(10):718, 1992.
3. Kovacs TOG, Jensen DM: Therapeutic endoscopy for upper gastrointestinal bleeding. In Taylor MB, editor: *Gastrointestinal emergencies,* Baltimore, 1992, Williams & Wilkins.
4. Porter DH, Kim D: Angiographic intervention in upper gastrointestinal bleeding. In Taylor MB, editor: *Gastrointestinal emergencies,* Baltimore, 1992, Williams & Wilkins.
5. Elta GH: Approach to the patient with gross gastrointestinal bleeding. In *Textbook of gastroenterology,* vol 1, Philadelphia, 1991, JB Lippincott.
6. Dobranowski J and others: *Procedures in gastrointestinal radiology,* New York, 1990, Springer-Verlag.
7. Eisenberg RL: *Gastrointestinal radiology,* ed 2, Philadelphia, 1990, JB Lippincott.

39

Gastrointestinal Disorders and Therapeutic Management

CHAPTER OBJECTIVES

- Discuss the high-risk causes, medical treatment, and nursing management for patients with acute gastrointestinal bleeding.
- Describe the pathophysiology and nursing management for patients with acute pancreatitis.
- Describe the pathophysiology and nursing management for patients with acute intestinal obstruction.

ACUTE GASTROINTESTINAL BLEEDING

Description

Gastrointestinal (GI) hemorrhage is a medical emergency that accounts for nearly 1 billion dollars of current national health care expenditure[1] and results in almost 300,000 hospital admissions yearly.[2] Despite advances in medical knowledge and nursing care, the mortality for acute GI bleeding has not changed in more than 50 years[2,3]; it remains approximately 10%. Most cases of GI hemorrhage result from bleeding in the upper GI tract.[3] Although bleeding from lower GI tract lesions can be quite brisk and threatening, bleeding from colon cancer and hemorrhoids usually is slow and intermittent and does not require hospitalization.[3]

Although GI hemorrhage, if unrecognized or treated too late, can lead to hypovolemic shock and ultimately death (Fig. 39-1), studies have found that the most common cause of death in GI hemorrhage actually is the result of exacerbation of underlying disease rather than intractable hypovolemic shock.[1,4] Gogel and Tandberg[1] point out that patients with a history of previous upper gastrointestinal (UGI) hemorrhage have a better prognosis than do those with no previous bleeding, perhaps because they have proved their ability to tolerate severe blood loss. Acute GI perforation, peritonitis, and sepsis are rare complications of GI hemorrhage.[1]

Patients at highest risk for death from UGI bleeding are those who fit any one of the following criteria:

1. More than 60 years of age
2. Disease in three organ systems
3. Required transfusion of 5 or more units of blood
4. Concomitant lung or liver disease
5. Recent major operation, trauma, or sepsis
6. Immunosuppression
7. Shock

Etiology

◆ Stress ulcer

Description. The term *stress ulcer* (erosive gastritis) covers a spectrum of diseases ranging from superficial mucosal erosions to discrete, mature ulcers. Stress ulcers, which almost always are limited to the stomach, are lesions that produce diffuse mucosal oozing. Such bleeding does not often cause massive GI hemorrhage and generally is attributed to superficial capillaries. Overt bleeding occurs in 2% to 15% of critically ill patients, typically those who have not received stress ulcer prophylaxis.[5-8]

Patients at risk include those in high physiologic stress situations, such as occur with thermal injury, head trauma, extensive surgery, shock, or acute neurologic disease (see box, p. 658, upper left).

Curling's ulcer is the term used for stress ulceration of the stomach and duodenum after burn injury; it occurs in approximately 12% of all patients hospitalized for burns. Histologic findings may indicate that Curling's ulcers are deep, with chronic inflammatory changes. Curling's ulcers are an uncommonly seen form of stress ulceration compared with diffuse mucosal oozing,[4] which occurs more frequently in critically ill patients.

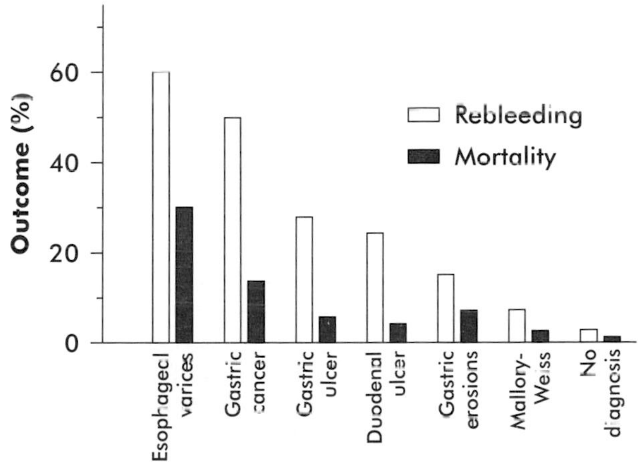

Fig. 39-1 Etiology of upper GI hemorrhage. (Modified from Lichtenstein DR, Berman MD, Wolfe MM: Approach to the patient with acute upper gastrointestinal hemorrhage. In Taylor MB, editor: *Gastrointestinal emergencies,* Baltimore, 1992, Williams & Wilkins, p 92.)

RISK FACTORS FOR STRESS ULCERATION

- Large (>50%) body surface area burns
- Intracranial lesions associated with coma
- Major trauma
- Fulminant hepatic failure
- Shock
- Sepsis
- Acute respiratory failure requiring prolonged mechanical ventilation
- Acute renal failure
- Coagulopathy

From Zuckerman G, Benitez J, Cort D: Medical therapy of nonvariceal upper gastrointestinal hemorrhage. In Taylor MB, editor: *Gastrointestinal emergencies,* Baltimore, 1992, Williams & Wilkins, p 121.

ETIOLOGY OF STRESS ULCERS

PRECIPITATING FACTORS

Patient's increased stress level (alteration in equilibrium)
Increased acid level in lumen of stomach (pH <3.5)

COFACTORS

Mucosal ischemia
Hydrogen-ion back diffusion (gastric barrier)
Gram-negative septicemia
Drug intake (e.g., steroids and catecholamines in patients with head trauma)

CLINICAL SUMMARY OF STRESS ULCERATION

- Between 5% and 20% of ICU patients not receiving prophylactic therapy will develop stress ulcer, manifested clinically by painless upper gastrointestinal bleeding.
- These lesions are multiple and are located in the gastric fundus or body.
- Endoscopic findings consist of multiple superficial erosions or ulcers with or without associated fresh or old blood.
- Prospective endoscopic studies show that gastric mucosal abnormalities develop within hours after admission in 75% of medical ICU patients and between 75% to 100% of patients with severe head trauma.
- Stress ulceration generally is not associated with high rates of gastric acid secretion except in the case of intracranial lesions associated with coma.
- ICU patients with stress-related bleeding have an overall greater mortality than similarly ill patients without stress bleeding.

From Zuckerman G, Benitez J, Cort D: Medical therapy of nonvariceal upper GI hemorrhage. In Taylor MB, editor: *Gastrointestinal emergencies,* Baltimore, 1992, Williams & Wilkins, p 122.

Erosions or ulcers that occur after intracranial operations or trauma are termed *Cushing's ulcers.* These ulcers occur less commonly in critically ill patients than does diffuse mucosal oozing.[4] They are associated with increased acid secretion and tend to bleed more often than do other types of stress erosions.[9]

Pathophysiology. Several pathophysiologic mechanisms have been implicated in stress ulcer formation (see box, upper right). The onset can be rapid (2 to 10 days), and hemorrhage can begin without pain. If hemorrhage goes untreated, mortality can exceed 50%. Patients at risk for development of stress ulcers should be assessed for the presence of hematemesis (red blood or coffee-ground emesis), bloody nasogastric aspirate, and melena (black or dark-red stools). A summary of clinical findings associated with stress ulceration is presented in the box, middle right.

Medical management. Pharmacologic gastric acid neutralization is the accepted treatment for stress ulcers and also may be used prophylactically in high-risk settings. A common regimen includes administering liquid antacids (30 to 60 ml every 4 hours) in an attempt to establish and maintain an alkaline gastric environment. At a pH of 5.0, 99.9% of the gastric acid is neutralized and pepsin activity is essentially nonexistent. Gastric pH should be monitored frequently, with an attempt made to maintain the pH above 3.5.[10] Although antacids are effective in preventing stress ulceration, they may be inconvenient to administer and can result in diarrhea and metabolic abnormalities.[11] It is especially important to avoid giving magnesium-containing antacids to patients with renal failure, because these agents can lead to magnesium intoxication. Antacids frequently will plug small feeding tubes; therefore a patient may require a 14-French or larger nasogastric tube when antacid administration becomes necessary.

Sucralfate, a weak antacid with antipepsin activity, also is effective prophylactic therapy for stress ulceration. It stimulates gastric cytoprotective mechanisms such as prostaglandin synthesis, and it protectively coats inflamed mucosal areas. Sucralfate's therapeutic advantage is that the incidence of nosocomial infections associated with its use is lower than has been documented in patients receiving high-dose acid suppression therapy.[10] Sucralfate's disadvantages are that it can be administered only orally and may cause constipation in some patients.[10]

Finally, courses of intravenous hydrochloric acid blockers (antagonists to histamine H_2 receptors), such as cimetidine or ranitidine, may be administered either by bolus or by continuous infusion. Histamine blockers prevent stress ulceration by increasing gastric mucosal blood flow and gastric cytoprotection via stimulation of mucus and prostaglandin synthesis.

◆ Peptic ulcer

Description. Peptic ulcer disease is the leading cause of UGI hemorrhage, accounting for approximately 50% of cases.[2] The term *peptic ulcer* refers to erosions located primarily in the gastric antrum and duodenum. Such erosions are deep, unlike stress ulcers, which tend to be superficial.

Pathophysiology. Peptic ulcer can be represented by the ulcer equation: acid + pepsin vs. mucosal resistance. This equation implies that the pro-ulcer forces (acid and pepsin) normally are held in check by the opposing forces of gastric mucosal resistance. Peptic ulcer results from an interaction between acid and peptic activity, concomitant with a breakdown in the gastroduodenal mucosal defense barrier.[11-14]

Normally, protection of the gastric mucosa from the powerful digestive effects of the pro-ulcer forces is accomplished in several ways. First, the gastroduodenal mucosa is coated by a glycoprotein mucus. The mucus forms a gel that prevents diffusion of pepsin and helps to maintain a mucosal-luminal pH gradient. Second, gastroduodenal epithelial cells secrete bicarbonate, which augments the actions of the glycoprotein mucus in maintaining this pH gradient. Finally, gastroduodenal epithelial cells are protected structurally against damage from acid and pepsin inasmuch as they are connected by tight junctions that help prevent such acid penetration.[11] Through these mechanisms, gastroduodenal mucosal pH is maintained above 6, even when the luminal pH is as low as 1.5.[11] Peptic ulceration results when these normally protective mechanisms cease to function, thus allowing gastroduodenal mucosal breakdown by the pro-ulcer forces of acid and pepsin.

Other mechanisms that influence ulcer formation include cigarette smoking, familial and genetic factors, emotions, stress, and sociocultural factors.[12,15]

◆ Nonspecific erosive gastritis

Description and pathophysiology. Of all UGI hemorrhages, 5% to 25% are the result of nonspecific erosive gastritis, which may be caused by a variety of different agents and disorders (see box, upper right), and are characterized by a wide spectrum of histologic appearances, including inflammation and ulceration.

Approximately 200,000 hospitalizations for GI bleeding and 10,000 to 20,000 deaths per year may be attributable to nonsteroidal anti-inflammatory drug (NSAID)–induced gastroduodenal mucosal damage,[16,17] which falls into the category of gastritis.[2] As the country's population ages, so do the ages of patients who are hospitalized in the nation's intensive care units; therefore nurses should be aware that the GI complications of NSAIDs[2,13,14,16-22] seriously affect millions of elderly patients with rheumatoid arthritis.

ETIOLOGY OF NONSPECIFIC EROSIVE GASTRITIS

Stress-related erosive syndrome (SRES)
Drug-induced
- Ethanol
- Nonsteroidal anti-inflammatory drugs
- Iron
- Potassium chloride
- Hepatic arterial chemotherapy
- Corrosives

Prolapse gastropathy
Ischemia
Vasculitis
Occlusive disease
Emboli
Postgastrectomy
Varioliform gastritis
Portal hypertension ("congestive gastropathy")
Radiation
Mechanical (instrumentation, nasogastric tube)

From Lichtenstein DR, Berman MD, Wolfe MM: Approach to the patient with acute upper gastrointestinal hemorrhage. In Taylor MB, editor: *Gastrointestinal emergencies,* Baltimore, 1992, Williams & Wilkins, p 104.

◆ Esophageal varices

Description. Investigators estimate that 19% to 57% of patients with cirrhosis and esophageal varices experience at least one GI hemorrhage. Significantly, this first bleeding episode is fatal in 28% to 66% of patients.[27] Esophageal variceal hemorrhage carries a poor prognosis—only 10% to 20% of these patients are alive 4 years later after their first bleeding episode from esophageal varices.[28]

Pathophysiology. Engorged and distended esophageal blood vessels are referred to as *esophageal varices.* Bleeding from such varices is a frequent and significant complication of cirrhosis, a disease that damages the liver sinusoid system. Without adequate sinusoid function, hepatic circulation is impaired and liver pressures are altered. This leads to a rise in portal venous pressure, causing collateral circulation to divert portal blood from high-pressure areas to adjacent low-pressure areas. The tiny esophageal vessels that receive this diverted blood lack sturdy mucosal protection, and as they become engorged and form varices, they become vulnerable to damage from gastric secretions, with subsequent rupture and hemorrhage[24-26] (Fig. 39-2).

Medical Management

The initial treatment priority for patients with acute GI bleeding is the control of bleeding and the restoration of adequate circulating blood volume,[1] usually by intravenous infusions of crystalloids and packed red blood cells. To this end a pulmonary artery catheter should be

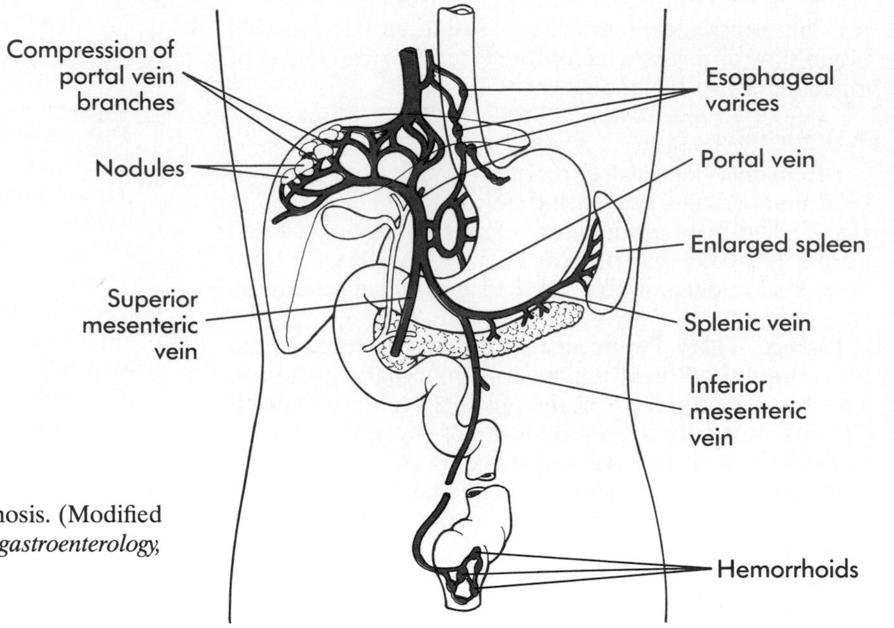

Fig. 39-2 Esophageal varices caused by cirrhosis. (Modified from Powell LW, Piper DW: *Fundamentals of gastroenterology,* Sydney, 1991, McGraw-Hill, p 141.)

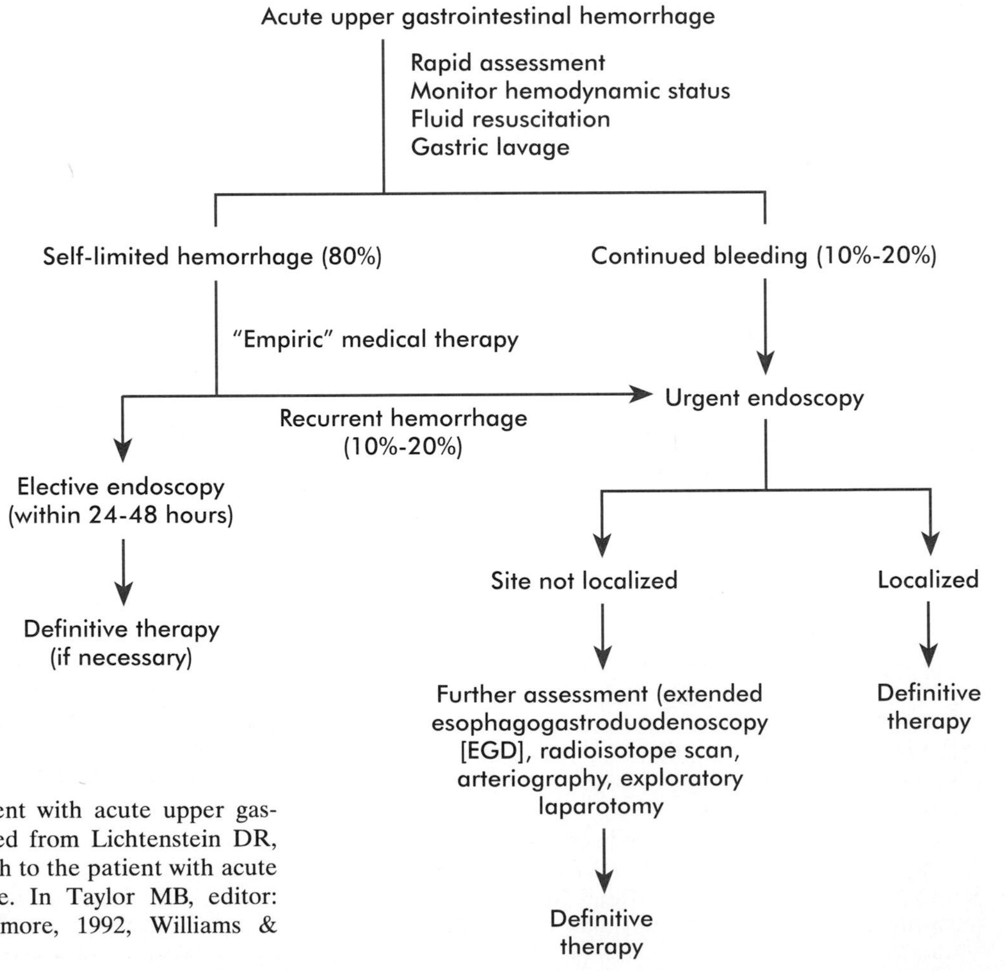

Fig. 39-3 Approach to the patient with acute upper gastrointestinal hemorrhage. (Modified from Lichtenstein DR, Berman MD, Wolfe MM: Approach to the patient with acute upper gastrointestinal hemorrhage. In Taylor MB, editor: *Gastrointestinal emergencies,* Baltimore, 1992, Williams & Wilkins, p 93.)

placed to more decisively guide fluid replacement therapy. Gastric lavage is then begun. Additional treatments include intravenous administration of vasopressin, endoscopic hemostasis, and/or interventional angiography. The patient who remains hemodynamically unstable despite volume replacement needs urgent surgery[1,29] (Fig. 39-3). For acute variceal hemorrhage, control of bleeding may be accomplished by endoscopic sclerotherapy (the endoscopic injection of a sclerosing agent into the bleeding varix), vasopressin infusion,[1] or balloon tamponade, such as with the Sengstaken-Blakemore, Linton, or Minnesota tube.[30]

Nursing Management

An accurate nursing assessment provides the foundation for nursing care of patients with GI bleeding. Postural vital sign changes are indicative of hypovolemia and should alert the nurse that severe blood loss has occurred. Hypovolemia from severe blood loss results in peripheral vasoconstriction and cool extremities; thus, palpating the distal extremities can be likened to a "poor person's Swan Ganz catheter."[32] Although an acute bleeding episode, of necessity, reduces the time available for obtaining the patient's health history, this assessment should not be totally eliminated. The nurse must determine any coexisting illnesses and obtain a list of the patient's current medications, including both prescription and nonprescription drugs, inasmuch as certain drugs and conditions are known to alter typical responses of vital signs to hemorrhage.[1] Mental confusion, pallor, and peripheral cyanosis signal the occurrence of a life-threatening bleeding episode.[1]

Hematemesis (red blood or coffee-ground emesis), bloody nasogastric aspirate, and melena (black or dark-red stools) are hallmark manifestations of GI bleeding. The effect of blood on stool character is shown in Table 39-1. It may be difficult to estimate the amount of blood in emesis or stool; in these cases a description of the sample and the patient's clinical profile can provide the initial sources for a nursing diagnosis.

Laboratory tests can help determine the extent of bleeding, although it is important for the nurse to realize that the patient's hematocrit value is a poor indicator of the severity or rapidity of an acute bleeding episode. That is, whole blood is lost, and if a hematocrit value is 45% and the patient loses a third of his or her blood volume in 5 minutes, the hematocrit will still be 45%. Studies have shown that the hematocrit may take as long as 72 hours to equilibrate after an episode of blood loss.[32] Measurement of arterial blood gases can help in detecting metabolic acidosis associated with severe hypovolemia. Electrolytes also should be assessed because severe hypokalemia and hyponatremia can develop in patients with hypovolemia.

Measurement of the prothrombin time, the partial thromboplastin time, and the total platelet count may help in guiding blood and blood product replacement therapy.[1] Diagnostic procedures such as endoscopy and arteriography can aid in establishing the site of the bleeding, although these procedures carry a higher risk when performed on an emergent basis.[1] Important nursing assessment responsibilities include the monitoring and reporting of laboratory results, as well as preparing the patient and family for interventional procedures.

Key nursing goals for the patient with acute GI bleeding include maintenance of adequate tissue oxygenation, prevention of fluid volume deficit related to blood loss, and optimization of hemodynamic status.

Regardless of what has caused the GI hemorrhage, the nurse first must see that venous access is achieved, so that fluid and blood resuscitation therapy can begin. Ensuring adequacy of intravenous infusions remains a nursing priority for the duration of treatment for acute GI bleeding.

To maintain adequate gas exchange and tissue oxygenation, the following interventions should be undertaken quickly:

1. Ensure open airway, and administer supplementary oxygen.
2. Initiate continuous monitoring for cardiac dysrhythmias.
3. Prepare for insertion of pulmonary artery catheter; record and monitor cardiac filling pressures once placement has been achieved.

Table 39-1 Effect of gastric blood loss on stool characteristics

Volume lost	Stool characteristics
20 ml	Normal appearance, occult-positive
100-200 ml	Melena
1000 ml (<4-hr transit)	Bloody
1000 ml (>4-hr transit)	Melena

From Gogel HK, Tandberg D: *Am J Emerg Med* 4(2):153, 1986.

NURSING DIAGNOSIS AND MANAGEMENT
Acute gastrointestinal bleeding

- ◆ Fluid Volume Deficit related to active blood loss, p. 639
- ◆ High Risk for Infection risk factor: invasive monitoring devices, p. 366
- ◆ High Risk for Aspiration risk factors: impaired laryngeal closure or elevation; decreased lower esophageal sphincter pressure, p. 472
- ◆ Anxiety related to threatened biologic, psychologic, and/or social integrity, p. 763
- ◆ Sensory/Perceptual Alterations related to sensory overload, sensory deprivation, and sleep pattern disturbance, p. 573
- ◆ Ineffective Individual Coping related to situational crisis and personal vulnerability, p. 762

◆ **Gastric lavage.** Management of gastric lavage is the next key nursing intervention for the patient with acute bleeding from the GI tract. Gastric lavage is used to decrease gastric mucosal blood flow, to evacuate blood and clots from the stomach, and to decrease hemorrhage. It may reduce vomiting and lessen the risk of aspiration, and some clinicians find gastric lavage a useful technique for monitoring the rate of bleeding and for preparing patients for endoscopy.[1]

Gastric lavage is initiated with the insertion of a large-bore nasogastric tube, commonly a Ewald tube. Gogel and Tandberg[1] claim that small-bore tubes are ineffective in removing clots and may be diagnostically misleading, because clots that cannot be aspirated will stain the return and create the false impression of continued bleeding. Therefore, before placement, additional holes should be cut in the proximal 6 to 8 cm of the Ewald tube to expand its drainage capacity.[1]

The nurse begins gastric lavage by instilling irrigation solution into the stomach and, subsequently (either by gravity or low suction), removing the fluid from the stomach into a collection basin. Use of a gastric lavage kit (Fig. 39-4) can greatly facilitate this process.

To use the kit, the nurse opens the top clamp, allowing irrigant to flow into the stomach by gravity. Approximately 500 to 700 ml of solution should be instilled at a time.[2] The nurse then reverses the clamp positions so that gravity (or low suction) acts to drain the stomach. Ensuring proper irrigant flow and adequate gastric drainage are key nursing responsibilities. The nurse must be alert to potential problems in the system; for example, blood clots may block portals in the Ewald tube and/or the tube may be "positional."[2]

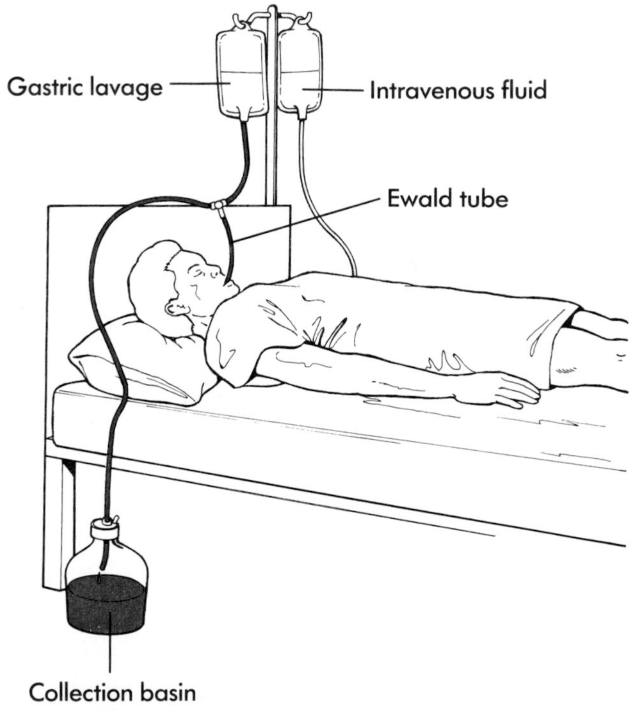

Fig. 39-4 Schematic depicting gastric lavage being performed using an Ewald tube connected to modified gastric lavage kit. (Modified from Lichtenstein DR, Berman MD, Wolfe MM: Approach to the patient with acute upper gastrointestinal hemorrhage. In Taylor MB, editor: *Gastrointestinal emergencies,* Baltimore, 1992, Williams & Wilkins, p 97.)

Historically, iced saline was favored as a lavage irrigant. Research has shown, however, that low-temperature fluids such as iced saline shift the oxyhemoglobin dissociation curve to the left and create adverse effects; these problems can include decreased oxygen delivery to vital organs and prolongation of bleeding time and prothrombin time.[2] Therefore room-temperature water or saline is the currently preferred irrigant for use in gastric lavage.[1,2]

◆ **Therapeutic effect tubes.** For the patient with acute bleeding from esophageal varices, therapeutic effect tubes, such as the *Sengstaken-Blakemore tube* or the *Linton tube,* may be needed. These tubes compress bleeding varices and stop acute variceal hemorrhage 75% of the time.[1] Here the nurse's responsibility is to stay with the patient and assist with insertion.

The most commonly used tube is the four-lumen Sengstaken-Blakemore tube (Fig. 39-5). Two of the lumina inflate the gastric and esophageal balloons, while the other two provide suction of the stomach and the esophagus.[33,35] The gastric balloon is inflated with 250 to 275 ml of air, and the esophageal balloon is distended to reach a pressure of 40 to 50 mm Hg.[34] Because the esophagus is totally occluded and rupture of the gastric balloon may result in complete airway obstruction (i.e., the tube rises into the nasopharynx), rupture of the esophagus and pulmonary aspiration are the potentially fatal complications of the Sengstaken-Blakemore tube.[34] Continuous monitoring for such complications is a nursing responsibility (see box, p. 663).

The Linton tube is a modification of the Sengstaken-Blakemore tube. It is designed with a single gastric balloon and one lumen for aspiration that ends in the stomach and another lumen that ends in the esophagus. In addition, its gastric balloon applies pressure to the intragastric veins because of its larger size; thus esophageal compression is not necessary. The Linton tube is as effective as the Sengstaken-Blakemore tube for controlling bleeding from esophageal varices[33]; however, it is more effective in controlling bleeding in patients with gastric varices.[1,33] The method of monitoring for complications is similar to that the nurse uses for the Sengstaken-Blakemore tube.

◆ **Vasopressin administration.** Another treatment modality used to control variceal bleeding is *intravenous vasopressin.*[32] Vasopressin reduces portal venous pressure and slows blood flow by constricting the splanchnic arteriolar bed.[35,36] It also causes significant systemic vasoconstriction and can lead to such complications as chest pain or cardiac ischemia, hypertension, congestive heart failure, dysrhythmias, phlebitis, bowel ischemia, and cerebral vascular accident.[33] Nursing responsibilities with use of this therapy include maintenance of a patent infusion and continuous monitoring for the aforementioned vasoconstrictive complications of therapy.[33]

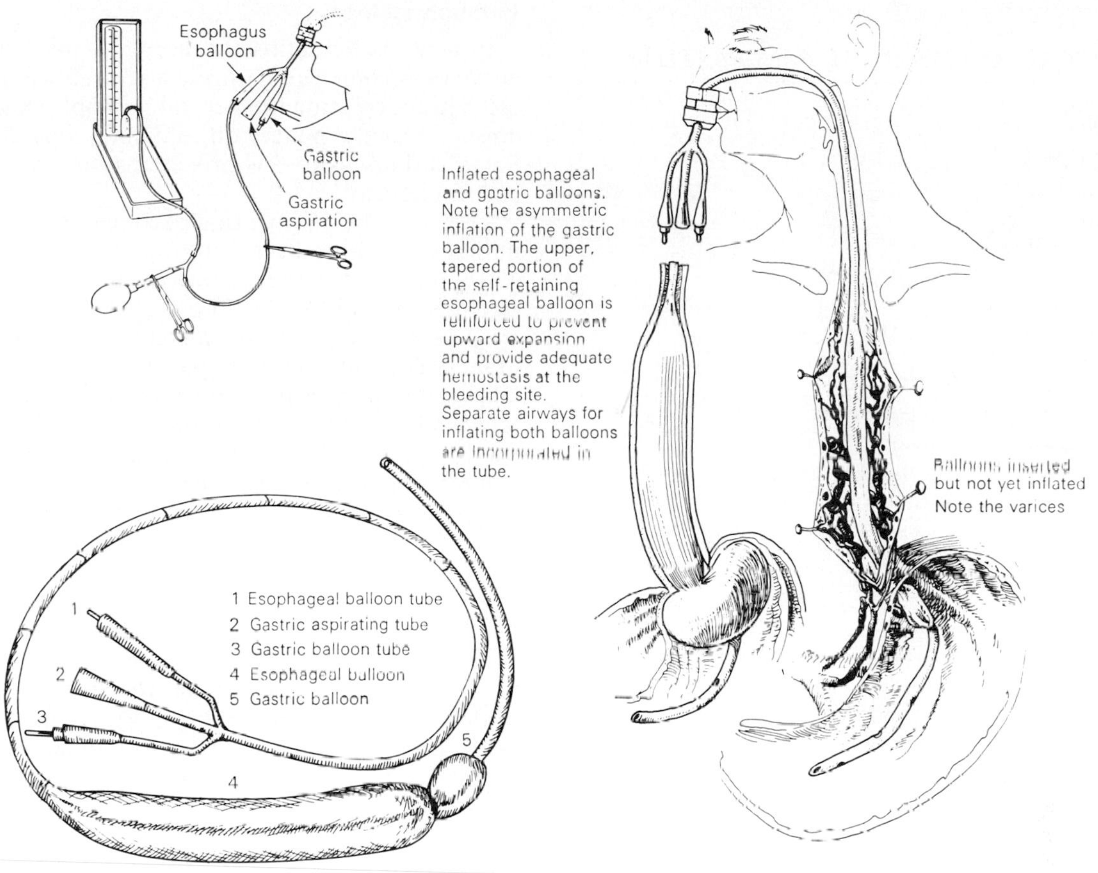

Fig. 39-5 Esophageal tamponade accomplished with Sengstaken-Blakemore tube. (Courtesy Davol Rubber Co, Providence, RI.)

• • •

The nurse monitors the patient's responses to the treatment just described for GI bleeding and continuously observes for complications of acute bleeding. Gastric perforation, although a rare complication, constitutes a surgical emergency. The patient reports sudden, severe, generalized abdominal pain, with significant rebound tenderness and rigidity. Perforation should be suspected when fever, leukocytosis, and tachycardia persist despite adequate volume replacement.[2] Prompt nursing recognition of the patient's changing status is vital.

ACUTE PANCREATITIS

Description

Pancreatitis is an inflammation of the pancreas that produces exocrine dysfunction. Infectious complications account for 80% of deaths in patients with acute pancreatitis.[37-44] Other complications of acute pancreatitis affect every organ system and include acute renal failure, myocardial depression, adult respiratory distress syndrome (ARDS), and disseminated intravascular coagulation (DIC) (see box, p. 664).

Because of improvements in fluid resuscitation and more sophisticated critical care nursing care, fewer patients today die of hypovolemia[45-49] than in the past.

COMPLICATIONS OF THE SENGSTAKEN-BLAKEMORE TUBE

- Aspiration
- Airway occlusion
- Esophageal perforation
- Death
- Cardiac dysrhythmias
- Pulmonary edema
- Bronchopneumonia
- Pressure effects
  - Laceration, ulceration of the stomach
  - Pressure necrosis of the hypopharynx
- Chest pain
- Hiccoughs

From Terblance J: Esophagogastric varices. In Taylor MB, editor: *Gastrointestinal emergencies,* vol 1, Baltimore, 1992, Williams & Wilkins, p. 36.

COMPLICATIONS OF ACUTE PANCREATITIS

Respiratory

Early hypoxemia
Pleural effusion
Atelectasis
Pulmonary infiltration
Adult respiratory distress syndrome
Mediastinal abscess

Cardiovascular

Hypotension
Pericardial effusion
ST-T changes

Renal

Acute tubular necrosis
Oliguria
Renal artery or vein thrombosis

Hematologic

DIC
Thrombocytosis
Hyperfibrinogenemia

Endocrine

Hypocalcemia
Hypertriglyceridemia
Hyperglycemia

Neurologic

Fat emboli
Psychosis
Encephalopathy

Ophthalmic

Purtscher's retinopathy—sudden blindness

Dermatologic

Subcutaneous fat necrosis

Gastrointestinal/hepatic

Hepatic dysfunction
Obstructive jaundice
Erosive gastritis
Paralytic ileus
Duodenal obstruction
Pancreatic
  Pseudocyst
  Phlegmon
  Abscess
  Ascites
Bowel infarction
Massive intraperitoneal bleed
Perforation
  Stomach
  Duodenum
  Small bowel
  Colon

From Ranson JHC: Complications of pancreatitis. In Taylor MB, editor: *Gastrointestinal emergencies,* Baltimore, 1992, Williams & Wilkins, p. 181.

Pathophysiology

In acute pancreatitis the normally inactive digestive enzymes become prematurely activated within the pancreas itself, creating the central pathophysiologic mechanism of acute pancreatitis, namely *autodigestion.*[31,37] Some authors liken this process to the occurrence of a chemical burn.[37]

Trypsin is the enzyme that becomes activated first and initiates the autodigestion process by triggering the secretion of proteolytic enzymes phospholipase A, elastase, and kallikrein. Phospholipase A, in the presence of bile, digests the phospholipids of cell membranes. This causes severe pancreatic parenchymal and adipose tissue necrosis, with subsequent release of free fatty acids.[39] Elastase activation causes dissolution of the elastic fibers of blood vessels and ducts, leading to hemorrhage. Kallikrein activation causes the release of bradykinin and kallidin, resulting in decreased peripheral vascular resistance, vasodilation, and increased vascular permeability.

Together these proteases and phosopholipases cause pancreatic inflammation and swelling. Extravasation of plasma and red blood cells in the area surrounding the pancreas causes fluid to be redistributed from the intravascular space to the retroperitoneum and bowel.[43] With large amounts of plasma volume sequestration, hypovolemia and hypotension occur and the patient goes into shock.[44]

Etiology

The two most common causes of acute pancreatitis are biliary disease (gallstones) and alcoholism.[38-40] Other much less common causes include peptic ulcer disease, surgical trauma, hyperparathyroidism,[39] vascular disease, and the use of certain drugs[39,41,42] (see box below). In 10% to 25% of patients with acute pancreatitis, no etiologic factor can be determined.[39,41]

DRUGS ASSOCIATED WITH ACUTE PANCREATITIS

DEFINITE	
Azathioprine	Sulfonamides
Thiazide diuretics	Tetracycline
Furosemide	Estrogens
Ethacrynic acid	Valproic acid
PROBABLE	
Chlorthalidone	Iatrogenic hypercalcemia
Procainamide	L-Asparaginase
Methyldopa	
EQUIVOCAL	
Acetaminophen	Corticosteroids
Isoniazid	Propoxyphene
Rifampin	

From Steer ML: Acute pancreatitis. In Taylor MB, editor: *Gastrointestinal emergencies,* Baltimore, 1992, Williams & Wilkins, p. 173.

Medical Management

The immediate treatment strategy is to administer intravenous fluids to prevent hypovolemic shock and to maintain hemodynamic stability. In severe forms of the disease the use of a pulmonary artery catheter guides such fluid management. To place the pancreas "at rest" a nasogastric tube is inserted and gastric suction is begun. Total parenteral nutrition should be started as soon as possible for patients with severe pancreatitis who show two or more adverse prognostic factors (see box below). Pain relief is another treatment priority, as are recognition and treatment of complications.[45,47]

Nursing Management

The initial nursing priority is a baseline nursing assessment of all organ systems with respect to hemodynamic status, tissue oxygenation, and gas exchange.[46,48] Vital signs should be taken frequently. Hypotension, tachycardia, low urine output, decreased pulse volumes, and increased capillary refill time should signal the nurse that circulatory perfusion is not adequate. A third heart sound may be heard upon cardiac auscultation, indicating heart failure and myocardial depression. Respiratory assessment may reveal tachypnea, cyanosis, and adventitious breath sounds, and blood gases may show decreased levels of arterial oxygen saturation. Neurologic and renal status also may be impaired if cardiac output is too low. The results of GI auscultation vary according to the presence or absence of bowel sounds; abdominal palpation reveals tenderness and guarding.

Uncommon inspection findings seen in acute pancreatitis include Grey Turner sign (gray-blue discoloration of the flank) and Cullen's sign (discoloration of the umbilical region).[39] Neuromuscular irritability may result from electrolyte deficiencies, but although muscle weakness or tremors may appear, tetany rarely develops.[39] Assessment of laboratory data usually demonstrates elevated levels of serum amylase and lipase. Leukocytosis, hypocalcemia, hyperglycemia, hyperbilirubinemia, and hypoalbuminemia also may be present (Table 39-2).

Pain assessment is another key nursing priority. Epigastric to midabdominal pain may vary from mild and tolerable to severe and incapacitating. Patients often report a "boring" sensation that radiates to the back. Nausea or vomiting, or both, may accompany the pain. The patient may obtain some comfort by leaning forward or by lying down with knees drawn up.

Nursing management goals include optimizing the patient's hemodynamic status, promoting gas exchange and tissue oxygenation, correcting fluid and electrolyte imbalances, relieving pain, and recognizing and treating complications.

Assisting with insertion of a pulmonary artery catheter and/or central venous catheter to guide fluid replacement therapy is an important nursing function, as are the continuous assessment and monitoring of pressure waveforms once the catheter is in place. Correction of fluid and electrolyte imbalances by administering intravenous infusions is another key nursing task.

Although analgesics should be liberally provided, the nurse should keep in mind that high doses of analgesic may impair the ventilatory pattern. Therefore the nursing objective regarding pain control should be to achieve pain relief while maintaining ventilations at normal depth and rate. Meperidine (Demerol) is the preferred agent because morphine may produce spasms at Oddi's sphincter.[31] Measures used to rest the pancreas, the NPO status, and gastric suctioning also assist in pain control. Relaxation techniques may augment analgesia.

The nurse must attend to a number of other details relating to the patient's condition. Abnormal results in laboratory data must be observed and reported so that

FACTORS ADVERSELY INFLUENCING SURVIVAL IN ACUTE PANCREATITIS

AT ADMISSION

Age >55 years
Hypotension
Abnormal pulmonary findings
Abdominal mass
Hemorrhagic or discolored peritoneal fluid
Increased serum LDH levels (>350 IU/L)
AST >250 U/dl
Leukocytosis ($>16,000/mm^3$)
Hyperglycemia (>200 mg/dl; no diabetic history)
Neurologic deficit (confusion, localizing signs)

DURING INITIAL 48 HOURS OF HOSPITALIZATION

Fall in hematocrit $>10\%$ with hydration or hematocrit $<30\%$
Necessity for massive fluid and colloid replacement
Hypocalcemia (<8 mg/dl)
Arterial Po_2 <60 mm Hg with or without adult respiratory distress syndrome
Hypoalbuminemia (<3.2 mg/dl)
Base deficit >4 mEq/L
Azotemia

From Latifi R, McIntosh JK, Dudrick SJ: *Surg Clin North Am* 71(3):583, 1991.

Table 39-2 Clinical findings in acute pancreatitis

Observation	Incidence (%)
Abdominal pain	95
Pain radiating to back	50
Abdominal guarding	50
Nausea/vomiting	80
Distention	75
Hypertension	10
Abdominal mass	15
Jaundice	20
Hematemesis	3
Melena	4

From Steer ML: Acute pancreatitis. In Taylor MB, editor: *Gastrointestinal emergencies*, Baltimore, 1992, Williams & Wilkins, p. 174.

NURSING DIAGNOSIS AND MANAGEMENT
Acute pancreatitis

- ◆ Acute Pain related to transmission and perception of cutaneous, visceral, muscular, or ischemic impulses secondary to acute pancreatitis, p. 566
- ◆ Ineffective Breathing Pattern related to abdominal or thoracic pain, p. 469
- ◆ Fluid Volume Deficit related to diarrhea, wound drainage, p. 640
- ◆ Altered Nutrition: Less Than Body Protein-Calorie Requirements related to lack of exogenous nutrients and increased metabolic demand, p. 673
- ◆ Anxiety related to threatened biologic, psychologic, and/or social integrity, p. 763
- ◆ Sensory/Perceptual Alterations related to sensory overload, sensory deprivation, and sleep pattern disturbance, p. 573
- ◆ Ineffective Individual Coping related to situational crisis and personal vulnerability, p. 762

favorable electrolyte balance may be attained. Cardiac dysrhythmias resulting from electrolyte imbalances should be promptly recognized and treated. Parenteral nutrition is needed for prolonged cases of pancreatitis in which NPO status must be maintained (usually longer than 5 days). A thorough review of the nursing interventions associated with parenteral nutrition is presented in Chapter 50.

The evaluation phase of the nursing process is directed toward evaluating the effects of nurse-administered treatments. Optimally, the aforementioned nursing interventions should normalize hemodynamics, gas exchange, and fluid and electrolyte levels, as well as provide pain relief for the patient.

The nurse must recognize complications of pancreatitis and treat them promptly. Septic complications are most common; Ranson[41] states that virtually all patients with fever or leukocytosis, or both, after 21 days of continuous treatment have pancreatic infection. Sepsis without manifestations of leukocytosis or fever can occur, which may require the use of antibiotics.[47,49-51]

Accurate pulmonary assessment is vital because abdominal pain often results in shallow, rapid breathing, which can precipitate respiratory depression. Pulmonary crackles, previously not found, may mean development of atelectasis, pneumonia, or ARDS; mechanical ventilation may be indicated. Chest auscultation of breath sounds remains essential. Further information on how the breathing pattern affects lung function is found in Chapter 22 in the discussions of atelectasis and ineffective breathing patterns.

ACUTE INTESTINAL OBSTRUCTION

Description

Acute intestinal obstruction occurs when bowel contents fail to move forward. Functional obstruction, also known as *paralytic ileus,* results from the absence of peristalsis and often occurs with hypokalemia. Mechanical obstruction results from occlusion of the bowel lumen and usually is the result of neoplasms.[51] The box above lists examples of both types of obstruction.

ETIOLOGY OF INTESTINAL OBSTRUCTIONS

FUNCTIONAL OBSTRUCTION

Prolonged intestinal distention
Hypokalemia
Peritonitis
Narcotic use
Intestinal ischemia
Sepsis

MECHANICAL OBSTRUCTION

Contained within lumen

Intussusception
Large gallstones
Meconium
Bezoars
Neoplasms

Extending into bowel wall

Congenital atresia
Congenital stenosis
Inflammatory bowel disease
Diverticulitis
Radiation
Neoplasms

Outside the bowel

Adhesions
Hernias
Neoplasms
Abscesses
Volvulus
Stomal stenosis

Pathophysiology

The obstructed bowel lumen accumulates fluid and gas proximal to the point of obstruction. Trapped fluids cause bowel distention, which triggers the secretion of fluid and electrolytes into the lumen and perpetuates the distention. Large losses of sodium, potassium, and chloride occur, as well as loss of hydrogen ions from the stomach.[52] As the obstruction continues, the vascular space becomes rapidly depleted and results in dehydration, hypotension, and hypovolemic shock. If intestinal distention progresses, the bowel wall edema can ultimately impede venous and arterial supply and can cause bowel necrosis and perforation. Once the bowel perforates, peritonitis and sepsis ensue.

Only minimal forewarning may occur with intestinal obstructions. Typically, patients are seen initially in acute distress, with abdominal distention, nausea and vomiting, obstipation, constipation, cramping abdominal pain, and high-pitched bowel sounds.[52]

Medical Management

Diagnosis of intestinal obstruction is aided by radiologic examination. A chest x-ray film and serial abdominal flat-plate films taken with the patient standing or sitting and supine reveal dilated loops of gas-filled bowel. Barium or meglumine diatrizoate (Gastrografin) enemas are used to locate the exact site and the degree of obstruction.

Medical interventions include replacement of fluids and immediate decompression of the obstruction with nasogastric suction. Use of long GI tubes is contraindicated for colonic obstruction. A sigmoid volvulus can be nonsurgically reduced by insertion of a rectal tube during sigmoidoscopy or barium enema, thus relieving the obstruction. Because the volvulus can recur, elective resection at a later date is desirable.

Surgical intervention is required when the obstruction fails to resolve within 24 hours. When the patient is not acutely ill, surgical resection can be a one-stage procedure with reanastomosis of the bowel, therefore eliminating the need for a temporary colostomy. More often a two- or three-stage procedure is used and a temporary colostomy created.

Nursing Management

The patient should be observed for clinical manifestations of bowel obstruction, such as abdominal distention, nausea, vomiting, and elevated blood phosphorous or amylase levels. Bowel sounds may be absent or faint and tinkling, depending on the extent of the obstruction. A nasogastric tube should be inserted for decompression. Placement and patency should be checked as needed (PRN) to ensure adequate decompression. Outputs greater than 1000 ml/8 hours can occur; therefore the patient should be monitored for electrolyte imbalance (hyponatremia and hypokalemia) and fluid volume deficit. Accurate intake and output must be maintained. Intravenous fluid and electrolyte solutions should be administered to prevent dehydration and replace lost electrolytes. Administration of antipyretics is necessary for treatment of fever.

Bowel necrosis and perforation are potential complications of colonic obstruction, and both can progress to sepsis. Bowel necrosis occurs as a result of impaired circulation associated with volvulus and closed-loop obstruction and with sustained excessive intraluminal pressure. Bowel perforation often results from overdistention of the bowel lumen and also is a sequela to bowel necrosis. These complications carry a high mortality and can be avoided by astute nursing observations, followed by prompt surgical intervention.

NURSING DIAGNOSIS AND MANAGEMENT

Acute intestinal obstruction

- ◆ Acute Pain related to transmission and perception of cutaneous, visceral, muscular, or ischemic impulses secondary to acute intestinal obstruction, p. 566
- ◆ Ineffective Breathing Pattern related to abdominal or thoracic pain, p. 469
- ◆ Decreased Cardiac Output related to decreased preload secondary to fluid volume deficit, p. 361
- ◆ Decreased Cardiac Output related to decreased preload secondary to septicemia, p. 362
- ◆ High Risk for Aspiration risk factors: impaired laryngeal closure or elevation; increased gastric volume; decreased lower esphageal sphincter pressure, p. 472
- ◆ Anxiety related to threatened biologic, psychologic, and/or social integrity, p. 763
- ◆ Ineffective Individual Coping related to situational crisis and personal vulnerability, p. 762

Therapeutic Management

Because GI intubation is so commonly used in critical care units, it is important for nurses to know the clinical indications and responsibilities inherent in their use. The four categories of GI tubes are based on function: nasogastric suction tubes, long intestinal tubes, therapeutic effect tubes (discussed previously), and feeding tubes (discussed in Chapter 50).

◆ **Nasogastric suction tubes.** Nasogastric suction tubes (Levin, Salem sump) remove fluid regurgitated into the stomach, prevent accumulation of swallowed air, may partially decompress the bowel, and reduce the patient's risk for aspiration. The tube is passed through the nose into the nasopharynx and then down through the pharynx into the esophagus and stomach. The length of time the nasogastric tube remains in place depends on its use. Nursing care should prevent the complications common to this therapy, which include the following: ulceration and necrosis of the nares, esophageal reflux, esophagitis, esophageal erosion and stricture, gastric erosion, and dry mouth and parotitis from mouth breathing; interference with ventilation and coughing; and loss of fluid and electrolytes (see box, p. 668).

◆ **Long intestinal tubes.** Miller-Abbott, Cantor, Johnston, and Baker tubes are examples of long intestinal tubes that are placed either preoperatively or intraoperatively. The long length allows removal of contents from the intestine that cannot be accomplished by a nasogastric tube. These tubes also can decompress the small bowel. In addition, they can splint the small bowel intraoperatively or postoperatively. Because progression of the tubes depends on bowel peristalsis, their use is contraindicated in patients with paralytic ileus and severe mechanical obstruction. In addition to monitoring for the complications associated with nasogastric tubes, the nurse should observe the patient for gaseous distention of the balloon section, which makes removal difficult; rupture of the balloon or spillage of mercury into the intestine; overinflation of the balloon, which can lead to intestinal rupture; and reverse intussusception if the tube is removed rapidly.

SELECT PATIENT PROBLEMS ASSOCIATED WITH NASOGASTRIC TUBES

NASOPHARYNGEAL DISCOMFORT

Etiology: absence of chewing, which is the normal stimulus to salivary secretions; mouth breathing as a result of the tubes being in place.

Clinical manifestations: sore throat, difficulty with swallowing, hoarseness, thirst, dry mucous membranes.

Plan: lubricate lips, chew sugarless gum, gargle with warm water and a mouthwash solution, use physiologic saliva or analgesic and/or anesthetic lozenges for severe discomfort (anesthetic lozenges may decrease swallowing or gag reflexes).

Prevention: symptoms decreased or absent with use of soft, small-bore tubes; use of therapeutic nursing measures.

NASAL EROSIONS AND NECROSIS

Etiology: pressure on nasal ala from tube.

Clinical manifestations: erosion of nasal ala.

Plan: tape tube so that no pressure is exerted against nasal ala; apply tincture of benzoin to area in which tape will be applied.

Prevention: use of soft, small-bore tube; tape properly.

ACUTE OTITIS MEDIA

Etiology: pressure from the nasoenteric tube at the opening of the eustachian tube, with entry of pathogenic bacteria into the middle ear.

Clinical manifestations: severe, dull, throbbing ear pain, fever, chills, slight dizziness, nausea, and vomiting; a child may pull on affected ear.

Plan: change nasoenteric tube to other nostril; administer antibiotic therapy if appropriate; perform myringotomy if severe.

Prevention: use of soft, small-bore tubes.

HOARSENESS

Etiology: irritation of laryngeal mucous membranes from presence of nasoenteric tube.

Clinical manifestations: hoarseness.

Plan: use soft, small-bore tube, steam or aerosol therapy, warm gargle, anesthetic lozenges.

Prevention: use soft, small-bore tube, adequate hydration, mouth care.

INABILITY TO WITHDRAW THE TUBE

Etiology: tube possibly lodged within folds of mucosa or "stuck" to gastric wall.

Clinical manifestations: tube does not respond to gentle pulling motions.

Plan: place the patient in a side-lying position and flush the tube with 20-50 ml of water; then pull back gently on the tube. If unsuccessful, repeat flushing of tube with patient in Trendelenburg's position (if not contraindicated). If both measures are unsuccessful, the tube should be cut, allowing evacuation of the lower portion through the rectum.

Modified from Bernard M, Forlaw L. In Rombeau J, Caldwell M, editors: *Clinical nutrition,* vol 1, *Enteral and tube feeding,* Philadelphia, 1984, WB Saunders.

REFERENCES

1. Gogel HK, Tandberg D: Emergency management of upper gastrointestinal hemorrhage, *Am J Emerg Med* 4(2):150, 1986.
2. Lichtenstein DR, Berman MD, Wolfe MM: Approach to the patient with acute upper gastrointestinal hemorrhage. In Taylor MB, editor: *Gastrointestinal emergencies,* Baltimore, 1992, Williams & Wilkins.
3. Elta GH: Approach to the patient with gross gastrointestinal bleeding. In Yamada T, editor: *Textbook of gastroenterology,* vol 1, Philadelphia, 1991, JB Lippincott.
4. Gogel HK. Personal communication, 1992.
5. Peura DA: Stress-related mucosal damage: an overview, *Am J Med* 83(6A):3, 1987.
6. Peura DA: Prophylactic therapy of stress-related mucosal damage: why, which, who, and so what? *Am J Gastroenterol* 85(8):935, 1990.
7. Konopad E, Noseworthy T: Stress ulceration: a serious complication in critically ill patients, *Heart Lung* 17(4):339, 1988.
8. Zuckerman GR, Shuman R: Therapeutic goals and treatment options for prevention of stress ulcer syndrome, *Am J Med* 83(6A):29, 1987.
9. Isenberg JI and others: Acid-peptic disorders. In Yamada T, editor: *Textbook of gastroenterology,* vol 1, Philadelphia, 1991, JB Lippincott.
10. Pilchman J, Lefton HB, Braden GL: Cytoprotection and stress ulceration, *Med Clin North Am* 75(4):853, 1991.
11. Mertz HR, Walsh JH: Peptic ulcer pathophysiology, *Med Clin North Am* 75(4):799, 1991.
12. Katz J: The course of peptic ulcer disease, *Med Clin North Am* 75(4):831, 1991.
13. Soll AH: Pathogenesis of peptic ulcer and implications for therapy, *N Engl J Med* 322(13):909, 1990.
14. Ohning G, Soll A: Medical treatment of peptic ulcer disease, *Am Fam Physician* 39(4):257, 1989.
15. Schindler BA, Ramchandani D: Psychologic factors associated with peptic ulcer disease, *Med Clin North Am* 75(4):865, 1991.
16. Agrawal N: Risk factors for gastrointestinal ulcers caused by nonsteroidal anti-inflammatory drugs (NSAIDs), *J Fam Pract* 32(6):619, 1991.
17. Silverstein F: Nonsteroidal antiinflammatory drugs and peptic ulcer disease, *Postgrad Med* 89(7):33, 1991.
18. Peterson WL: Peptic ulcer—an infectious disease? *West J Med* 152(2):167, 1990.
19. Price AH, Fletcher M: Mechanisms of NSAID-induced gastroenteropathy, *Drugs* 40(suppl 5):1, 1990.
20. Malagelada JR, Ahlquist DA, Moore SC: Defects in prostaglandin synthesis and metabolism in ulcer disease: *Dig Dis Sci* 31(suppl 2):20S, 1986.
21. Semble EL, WU WC: NSAID-induced gastric mucosal damage, *Am Fam Physician* 35(6):101, 1987.
22. Holt S, Saleeby G: Gastric mucosal injury induced by nonsteroidal anti-inflammatory drugs, *South Med J* 84(3):355, 1991.
23. Reference deleted in proofs.
24. Solomon J, Harrington D, Gogel HK: When the patient suffers from esophageal bleeding, *RN,* p. 24, Feb 1987.
25. Quinless FW: Severe liver function: client problems and nursing actions, *Focus Crit Care* 12(1):24, 1985.
26. Powell LW, Piper DW: *Fundamentals of gastroenterology,* Sydney, 1991, McGraw-Hill.
27. Andreani T and others: Preventive therapy of first gastrointestinal bleeding in patients with cirrhosis: results of a controlled trial comparing propranolol, endoscopic sclerotherapy and placebo, *Hepatology* 12(6):1413, 1990.
28. Christensen E and others: Prognosis after the first episode of gastrointestinal bleeding or coma in cirrhosis, *Scand J Gastroenterol* 24:999, 1989.
29. Sachdeva AK, Zaren HA, Sigel B: Surgical treatment of peptic ulcer disease, *Med Clin North Am* 75(4):999, 1991.
30. Snow ND, Almon M, Baillie J: Minnesota tube placement using a guide wire, *Gastrointest Endosc* 36(4):420, 1990.
31. Brown A: Acute pancreatitis: pathophysiology, nursing diagnoses, and collaborative problems, *Focus Crit Care* 18(2):121, 1991.
32. Laine L: Upper gastrointestinal tract hemorrhage, *West J Med* 155(3):274, 1991.
33. Terblance J: Esophagogastric varices. In Taylor MB, editor: *Gastrointestinal emergencies,* vol 1, Baltimore, 1992, Williams & Wilkins.
34. Meeroff JC: Management of massive gastrointestinal bleeding. II. *Hosp Pract* 21(5):93, 1986.
35. Ready JB, Robertson AD, Rector WG: Effects of vasopressin on portal pressure during hemorrhage from esophageal varices, *Gastroenterology* 100(5):1411, 1991.
36. Ohnishi K, Sato S: Effects of vasopressin on left gastric venous flow in cirrhotic patients with esophageal varices, *Am J Gastroenterol* 85(3):2933, 1990.
37. Poston GJ, Williamson RCN: Surgical management of acute pancreatitis, *Br J Surg* 77(1):5, 1990.
38. Steer ML: Acute pancreatitis. In Taylor MB, editor: *Gastrointestinal emergencies,* Baltimore, 1992, Williams & Wilkins.
39. Potts JR: Acute pancreatitis, *Surg Clin North Am* 68(2):281, 1988.
40. Singh M, Simsek H: Ethanol and the pancreas, *Gastroenterology* 98(4):1051, 1990.
41. Ranson JHC: Complications of pancreatitis. In Taylor MB, editor: *Gastrointestinal emergencies,* Baltimore, 1992, Williams & Wilkins.
42. Clavien PA, Burgan S, Moossa AR: Serum enzymes and other laboratory tests in acute pancreatitis, *Br J Surg* 76(12):1234, 1989.
43. Smith A: When the pancreas self-destructs, *Am J Nurs* 91(9):38, 1991.
44. Frey CFF, Bradley EL, Beger HG: Progress in acute pancreatitis, *Surg Gynecol Obstet* 167(4):282, 1988.
45. Steinberg WM, Schlesselman SE: Treatment of acute pancreatitis. Comparison of animal and human studies, *Gastroenterology* 93(6):1420, 1987.
46. Stanten R, Frey CF: Comprehensive management of acute necrotizing pancreatitis and pancreatic abscess, *Arch Surg* 125(10):1269, 1990.
47. Byrne JJ, Treadwell TL: Treatment of pancreatitis. When do antibiotics have a role? *Postgrad Med* 85(4):333, 1989.
48. Horton JW, Burnweit CA: Hemodynamic function in acute pancreatitis, *Surgery* 103(5):538, 1988.
49. Bradley EL: Antibiotics in acute pancreatitis. Current status and future directions, *Am J Surg* 158(5):472, 1989.
50. Lumsden A, Bradley EL: Secondary pancreatic infections, *Surg Gynecol Obstet* 170(5):459, 1990.
51. Holder WD: Intestinal obstruction, *Gastroenterol Clin North Am* 17(2):317, 1988.
52. Buechter KJ and others: Surgical management of the acutely obstructed colon, *Am J Surg* 156:163, 1988.

40

Gastrointestinal Nursing Diagnosis and Management

This chapter is designed to supplement the preceding chapters in the *Gastrointestinal Alterations* unit by integrating theoretic content into clinically applicable case studies and nursing management plans.

The case study is designed to illustrate clinical problem solving and patient care management occuring in actual patients. The case, reviewed retrospectively, demonstrates how medical and nursing diagnoses may be effectively used in critical care. The case study also demonstrates revisions to the plan of care and the nursing and medical management outcomes that are apt to occur during the course of a complicated hospitalization as the patient responds physiologically to treatment. Often in a short case anecdote, such as presented in this chapter, the clinical answer may appear to be obvious from the day of admission. In practice, however, critical care patient management is sometimes investigative and the "correct" diagnosis for an individual patient may not become apparent until midway in the hospitalization. Or a patient with an apparently straightforward diagnosis may develop an unexpected complication, and the plan of care and potential outcomes will then require revision. Many of the case studies demonstrate this principle.

The nursing management plans, which—unlike the case study—are not patient-specific, provide a basis nurses can use to individualize care for their patients. In the previous *Gastrointestinal Alterations* chapters, each medical diagnosis is assigned a Nursing Diagnosis and Management box. Using this box as a page guide, the reader can access relevant nursing management plans for each medical diagnosis. For example, nursing management of *acute gastrointestinal bleeding* , described on pp. 661-663, may involve several nursing diagnoses and management plans outlined in this chapter and in other Nursing Diagnosis and Management chapters. Specific examples are (1) *High Risk for Infection risk factors: invasive monitoring devices*, on p. 366; (2) *Anxiety related to threatened biologic, physiologic, and/or social integrity*, on p. 763; (3) *Fluid Volume Deficit related to active blood loss*, on p. 639; and (4) *Ineffective Individual Coping related to situational crisis and personal vulnerability*, on p. 762. These examples highlight the interrelationship of the various physiologic systems in the body and the fact that pathology often has a multisystem impact in the critically ill.

Use of the case study and management plans can enhance the understanding and application of the *Gastrointestinal* content in clinical practice.

GASTROINTESTINAL CASE STUDY

CLINICAL HISTORY

Mrs. M is a 47-year-old Native American woman about whom little is known.

CURRENT PROBLEMS

Mrs. M was brought by automobile to the hospital because she vomited blood earlier in the day. She was intoxicated on arrival at the hospital. Her friends, who were also intoxicated, left immediately. The patient promptly vomited more blood in the emergency room and became hypotensive. During the brief period when the patient could give a history, she said she had been in the hospital earlier and someone had put a tube in her stomach. No other direct medical history was available.

MEDICAL DIAGNOSES

Acute upper GI bleed
Hypovolemic shock

NURSING DIAGNOSES

- Fluid Volume Deficit related to active blood loss
- Sensory/Perceptual Alterations related to sensory overload, sensory deprivation, and sleep pattern disturbance
- High Risk for Aspiration risk factor: increased intragastric pressure

GASTROINTESTINAL CASE STUDY—cont'd

◆ PLAN OF CARE

1. Admit patient to the critical care unit (CCU) for medical and nursing management of acute upper GI bleeding.
2. Achieve hemostasis.
3. Replace lost blood volume.
4. Correct hypovolemic shock.
5. Maintain adequacy of oxygenation status.

MEDICAL AND NURSING MANAGEMENT AND PATIENT OUTCOME

To deal with a presumed variceal bleed, Mrs. M was started on intravenous vasopressin at 0.4 units per minute. A Sengstaken-Blakemore tube was inserted, and after an x-ray film was obtained, both gastric and esophageal balloons were inflated with 40 mm Hg pressure. Because Mrs. M's systolic blood pressure decreased to 50 mm hg, fluid resuscitation was begun. She received a total of 8 units of packed red blood cells, 4 units of fresh frozen plasma, and 7 liters of crystalloid solution (lactated Ringer's and normal saline). Dopamine infusion at 2-5 mcg/kg/min was initiated to help raise her blood pressure. Because of massive vomiting of blood and hypotension, Mrs. M was intubated to protect her airway. After initiation of these treatments, the nursing assessment revealed the following:

Neuro: Mrs. M was very agitated while being ventilated and was given a sedative and paralytic agent. She was able to move all extremities before a paralytic state was induced.

Resp: She was intubated and ventilated. Lungs remarkable for crackles at both bases. Ventilator settings: FIO_2, 40%; tidal volume, 900 cc; IMV mode, respiratory rate, 8; no PEEP or PSV.

CV: Sinus tachycardia with rate of 140. Blood pressure up to 136/80 after fluid resuscitation. Extremities without edema. Heart without murmur, gallop, rub, or click. Large-bore IV in the right femoral venous position.

Integument/Temp: Skin cool and dry with palpable peripheral pulses. No jaundice. Rectal temperature 100° F.

Medications: Because Mrs. M's blood pressure rose so quickly after fluid resuscitation, dopamine was weaned off. After insertion of the Sengstaken-Blakemore tube, bleeding seemed stopped; therefore, vasopressin infusion was also weaned off. Because of mild pulmonary congestion after fluid administration, Mrs. M was given 20 mg of intravenous furosemide to promote diuresis.

GI: Sengstaken-Blakemore tube in place. Abdomen soft, bowel sounds present. No stigmata of chronic liver disease.

GU: Foley catheter intact, draining 20 to 30 ml per hour of clear, amber-colored urine.

Lab: Blood alcohol level, 130 mg/dl; prothrombin time, 15.1 seconds with an international normalized ratio (INR) of 1.9; potassium, 3.1 mEq/L (replaced); O_2 saturation, 96%; hematocrit, 46% (hematocrit takes up to 72 hours to equilibrate after an acute bleeding episode.)

MEDICAL DIAGNOSES

Acute upper GI bleed (resolving)
Volume overload

NURSING DIAGNOSIS

◆ Fluid Volume Deficit related to active blood loss

◆ REVISED PLAN OF CARE

1. Discontinue the Sengstaken-Blakemore tube.
2. Continue to monitor for fluid volume and electrolyte imbalances, and replace fluids and electrolytes as needed.
3. Localize the site of bleeding by endoscopy, and provide endoscopic sclerotherapy if necessary.
4. Monitor for delirium tremens (DTs) related to alcohol withdrawal.
5. Ensure adequacy of oxygenation via monitoring of respiratory status and ventilator settings.

MEDICAL AND NURSING MANAGEMENT AND PATIENT OUTCOME

Sixteen hours after CCU admission, Mrs. M's Sengstaken-Blakemore tube was removed without difficulty. No further bleeding ensued. Endoscopy verified esophageal varices. No other bleeding sites were found. She received sclerotherapy (9.5 ml of 5% sodium morrhuate) to prevent further bleeding. Fluid volume balance was maintained effectively, with urine output 50 to 100 ml per hour and electrolytes within normal limits. BUN and creatinine also were within normal limits. Mrs. M still required quite a bit of sedation while she was on the ventilator; she demonstrated agitation and thrashing about in bed as the sedation wore off. Although vital signs were stable (BP, 102/47; RR, 14; P, 114), Mrs. M's rectal temperature rose to 100.4° F and rhonchi were audible in both lung fields. White blood cell count was 11,000, and arterial blood gases measured as follows: pH, 7.52; PCO_2, 36 mm Hg; PO_2, 69 mm Hg; O_2 saturation, 96%.

Continued.

GASTROINTESTINAL CASE STUDY—cont'd

MEDICAL DIAGNOSES

Acute GI bleed (resolving)
Pneumonia
Delirium tremens/alcohol withdrawal syndrome

NURSING DIAGNOSES

- Impaired Gas Exchange related to alveolar hypoventilation secondary to pneumonia
- Sensory/Perceptual Alterations related to alcohol withdrawal

◆ REVISED PLAN OF CARE

1. Culture sputum, urine, and blood.
2. Remove right femoral IV and start new IV.
3. Begin empiric antibiotic therapy.
4. Continue to provide sedation as needed until delirium tremens lessen.
5. Continue ventilatory support until respiratory status more stable.

MEDICAL AND NURSING MANAGEMENT AND PATIENT OUTCOME

The remainder of Mrs. M's stay in CCU was uneventful. Her urine culture was positive for *Escherichia coli*, blood culture was positive for *Staphylococcus aureus*, and sputum culture was positive for *S. aureus*, as well as *Haemophilus influenzae*. She was started on antibiotics and was given aggressive pulmonary toilet by her nurses. A new triple-lumen central venous catheter was placed without difficulty. Sedation was decreased, and ventilatory support was lessened. On day 4, agitation was decreasing, allowing less sedation. Mrs. M was effectively coughing up copious pulmonary secretions, temperature had decreased to 100° F, and she was placed on a T-tube with 40% oxygen. On day 5, Mrs. M continued to need less sedation and was demonstrating less agitation. Temperature was down to 99.8° F, and she was extubated without difficulty. With no further evidence of GI bleeding, she was transferred to the stepdown unit.

ALTERED NUTRITION: LESS THAN BODY PROTEIN-CALORIE REQUIREMENTS RELATED TO OVERFEEDING OF EXOGENOUS NUTRIENTS AND/OR ORGAN DYSFUNCTION

DEFINING CHARACTERISTICS

Carbohydrate related

- Blood glucose >150 mg/dl
- Glycosuria >3+
- Increased urinary output with low specific gravity
- Progressive clinical manifestations: thirst, diuresis, weight loss, clouded sensorium, nausea, headache, poor skin turgor, hypotension, convulsions, coma
- Increased minute ventilation compared with baseline (increased arterial partial pressure of oxygen [Pa_{O_2}])
- Increased arterial partial pressure of carbon dioxide (Pa_{CO_2}) compared with baseline before nutritional support was instituted
- Measured respiratory quotient >1
- >50% of nonprotein calories in nutritional support solution supplied as carbohydrate in a ventilator-dependent patient

Protein related

- Blood urea nitrogen (BUN) greater than baseline
- BUN:creatinine ratio greater than 10:1
- Diuresis or oliguria
- Greater than normal levels of potassium, magnesium, or phosphate, indicative of renal dysfunction

Lipid related

- Lipemia
- Hyponatremia without other cause
- Serum triglyceride level >250 mg/dl
- Decreased platelets without other cause
- Use of fat emulsions at >2-4 mg/kg/hr
- Clinical complaints of nausea, vomiting, headache, altered taste, allergic response

OUTCOME CRITERIA

Carbohydrate related

- Blood glucose is <150 mg/dl.
- Glycosuria is <2+.
- Fluid balance is evident.
- Clinical manifestations of progressive hyperglycemia are absent.
- Pa_{CO_2} level of ventilator-dependent patients is in normal range.
- 30%-50% of nonprotein calories are administered as fat emulsion.
- Measured respiratory quotient is <1

ALTERED NUTRITION: LESS THAN BODY PROTEIN-CALORIE REQUIREMENTS RELATED TO OVERFEEDING OF EXOGENOUS NUTRIENTS AND/OR ORGAN DYSFUNCTION—cont'd

Protein related

- BUN is within normal limits.
- BUN:creatinine ratio is within normal limits.
- Urinary output is at least 30 ml/hr.
- Serum and urinary levels of potassium, phosphate, and magnesium are normal.

Lipid related

- There is no evidence of lipemia.
- Serum triglycerides <250 mg/dl.
- Serum sodium level >130 mg/dl.
- Platelets are within normal limits for patient.
- Infusion of fat emulsion is in range of 2-4 mg/kg/hr.
- Patient has no clinical complaints.

NURSING INTERVENTIONS

Carbohydrate related

1. Assess serum glucose level on a daily basis; every-6-hour fingersticks for glucose may be needed.
2. Perform urinary testing for sugar every 6 hours.
3. Maintain infusion control of TPN or enteral infusion nutritional support infusion rates.
4. Maintain accurate intake and output, with tracking of fluid balance.
5. Observe and document clinical signs of progressive hyperglycemia.
6. Supplement with exogenous regular insulin as ordered.
7. Carefully observe and document ventilator-dependent patients' attempts at weaning.
8. Identify patients at risk early (e.g., septic, diabetic, hypermetabolic, or elderly patients, renal or pancreatic insufficiencies, use of steroids).
9. Obtain daily weights.
10. Gradually increase formula's or solution's hourly rates based on documented patient tolerance.

Protein related

1. Monitor serum values of BUN, creatinine, potassium, phosphate, magnesium.
2. Maintain accurate intake and output and measurement of fluid balance.
3. Obtain daily weights.
4. Perform daily assessment of sensorium.

Lipid related

1. Monitor laboratory values (triglycerides, platelets).
2. Control infusion of fat emulsion at a rate no greater than 125 ml/hr for 10% solutions and 62 ml/hr for 20% solutions.
3. Observe patient for nausea, vomiting, altered taste, headache, allergic response.

ALTERED NUTRITION: LESS THAN BODY PROTEIN-CALORIE REQUIREMENTS RELATED TO LACK OF EXOGENOUS NUTRIENTS AND INCREASED METABOLIC DEMAND

DEFINING CHARACTERISTICS

- Unplanned weight loss of 10% of body weight within the past 6 months
- Serum albumin <3.5 g/100 ml
- Total lymphocytes <1500 mm³
- Anergy
- Negative nitrogen balance
- Fatigue; lack of energy and endurance
- Nonhealing wounds
- Daily caloric intake less than estimated nutritional requirements
- Presence of factors known to increase nutritional requirements (e.g., sepsis, trauma, multiple organ disfunction syndrome [MODS])
- Maintenance of NPO status for >7-10 days
- Long-term use of 5% dextrose intravenously
- Documentation of suboptimal calorie counts
- Drug or nutrient interaction that might decrease oral intake (e.g., chronic use of bronchodilators, laxatives, anticonvulsives, diuretics, antacids, narcotics)
- Physical problems with chewing, swallowing, choking, salivation, and presence of altered taste, anorexia, nausea, vomiting, diarrhea, or constipation

OUTCOME CRITERIA

- Patient exhibits stabilization of weight loss or weight gain of ½ pound daily.
- Serum albumin is >3.5 g/dl.
- Total lymphocytes are >1500 mm³.
- Patient has positive response to cutaneous skin antigen testing.
- Patient is in positive nitrogen balance.
- Wound healing is evident.
- Daily caloric intake equals estimated nutritional requirements.
- Increased ambulation and endurance are evident.

Continued.

ALTERED NUTRITION: LESS THAN BODY PROTEIN-CALORIC REQUIREMENTS RELATED TO LACK OF EXOGENOUS NUTRIENTS AND INCREASED METABOLIC DEMAND—cont'd

NURSING INTERVENTIONS AND *RATIONALE*

1. Continue to monitor the assessment parameters listed under "Defining Characteristics."
2. Document factors that identify patients at risk for nutritional deficits.
3. Assess patient during physical care for signs of nutritional deficiencies.
4. Measure admission height and weight.
5. Weigh patient daily.
6. Ensure that specimens for biochemical tests of nutritional status are collected properly and on time.
7. Accurately collect blood samples through multilumen catheter.
8. Administer parenteral and enteral solutions as prescribed.
9. Control infusion rate of parenteral and enteral solutions through infusion control devices and check rate every hour.
10. Flush enteral feeding tubes every 4 hours *to maintain patency.*
11. Document oral intake through calorie counts.
12. Perform serial assessments of patient's strength, endurance, conditions of wounds.

HIGH RISK FOR INFECTION

RISK FACTORS

- ◆ Malnutrition and immunodeficiencies
- ◆ Invasive techniques of nutritional support
- ◆ Total lymphocytes <2000 mm^3
- ◆ White blood cell count greater than normal
- ◆ Anergy
- ◆ Temperature $>40°$ C
- ◆ Positive blood cultures, with organism same as identified from central venous catheter tip culture
- ◆ Clinical manifestations of sepsis without other cause identified
- ◆ Erythema, tenderness, or drainage around skin at site of access device

OUTCOME CRITERIA

- ◆ Total lymphocytes are >2000 mm^3.
- ◆ White blood cell count is within normal limits.
- ◆ Positive response to delayed cutaneous hypersensitivity is >5 mm.
- ◆ Temperature is normal.
- ◆ Blood culture is negative.
- ◆ No clinical manifestations of sepsis are evident.
- ◆ Skin integrity surrounding access device is uncompromised.

NURSING INTERVENTIONS AND *RATIONALE*

1. Monitor total lymphocyte counts, WBC, differential.
2. Follow directions for the placement of intradermal skin tests.
3. Monitor vital signs every 4 hours and urinary sugar levels or Accucheks every 6 hours.
4. Perform daily assessment for signs of infection and sepsis.
5. Maintain optimal aseptic environment during access-device insertion.
6. Use aseptic technique during manipulation of nutritional support system.
7. Perform daily inspection of access device insertion site for erythema, induration, drainage, tenderness, phlebitis.
8. Maintain sterile occlusive dressing over access device according to hospital protocol.
9. Protect access device site from potential sources of contamination (e.g., ostomies, draining wounds).
10. Refrigerate compounded nutritional support solutions and enteral formulas before use.
11. Maintain a closed sterile nutritional support system using Luer-Lok connections.

IX

ENDOCRINE ALTERATIONS

41

Endocrine Anatomy and Physiology

CHAPTER OBJECTIVES

- Briefly describe the physiology of the endocrine organs discussed in this chapter.
- List the target tissues for antidiuretic hormone (ADH), the effect of ADH on the target tissues, and the stimulus for release and inhibition of ADH.
- Describe the function of ADH in the maintenance of serum osmolality and blood volume.
- Discuss why the hypothalamus-hypophyseal system is vulnerable in traumatic head injuries.
- Describe the functions of insulin and glucagon in the maintenance of normal serum glucose.
- Identify the components of the negative feedback system used to stimulate production and release of thyroid hormones, and correlate their activities.

Maintaining the dynamic equilibrium among the various cells, tissues, organs, and systems of the human body is a highly complex and specialized process. Two systems regulate these critical relationships: the nervous system and the endocrine system. The nervous system communicates through nerve impulses that control skeletal muscle, smooth muscle tissue, and cardiac muscle tissue. The endocrine system controls and communicates through the distribution of potent hormones throughout the body (Fig. 41-1 lists the endocrine glands, hormones, target tissue, and action). When stimulated, the endocrine organ secretes hormones into surrounding body fluids. Once in circulation, these hormones travel to a specific target tissue where they exert a pronounced effect on specialized cells. Receptors found on the cell surfaces or within the cells are equipped with molecules that recognize and bind the hormone to the cell and produce a specific response.

Endocrine hormones may have a direct effect on body functioning, such as prolactin and the maintenance of milk production for breast-feeding. The effect of endocrine hormones may be more generalized, as with thyroxin and the rate of metabolism in the body. Diseases that affect the endocrine glands usually do not require emergency critical care interventions. When an endocrine crisis does occur, however, it often brings with it life-threatening consequences.

Diabetic ketoacidosis (DKA) is an endocrine emergency. It is perhaps the most common endocrine disorder for which the patient is admitted to the critical care unit. Hyperglycemic hyperosmolar nonketotic coma (HHNC), a potentially lethal metabolic disorder, has a mortality greater than 40%[1] and often is seen in the critical care unit as a complication of other serious health problems.

Diabetes insipidus (DI) and syndrome of inappropriate antidiuretic hormone (SIADH) are two pituitary disorders that disrupt the body's regulation of plasma osmotic pressure and circulating blood volume. Each disease rarely is seen alone, but rather develops as a result of a precipitating illness.

Thyroid crisis, also called *thyrotoxic crisis* or *thyrotoxic storm,* is an uncommon emergency that carries a high mortality. The sudden rise in the body's metabolic processes leads to tachydysrhythmias and hyperthermia. This extreme form of hyperthyroidism jeopardizes vital homeostasis.

THE PANCREAS

Description

The pancreas generally is triangular in shape and is found retroperitoneal, in a horizontal position. The base end of the organ lies in the C-shaped curvature of the duodenum, and the apex extends behind and below the stomach toward the spleen. Its size is approximately 15 cm (6 inches) long and 4 cm (1½ to 2 inches) wide. Specialized exocrine cells within the pancreas secrete digestive enzymes into a 3-mm duct that transverses the pancreas and empties into the duodenum. Fig. 41-2 shows the pancreatic duct, known also as the *duct of Wirsung,* which forms the passageway for pancreatic juice during intestinal digestion.

Function

The endocrine functions of the pancreas are accomplished by many clusters of cells that appear to form tiny islands among the exocrine cells. These islets of Langerhans (named after Paul Langerhans, the German pathologist who identified them in 1869) are composed of four distinct cell types. The cells are known as *A, B, D,* and *F cells* (see Fig. 41-2). *A cells* secrete glucagon, *B cells* secrete insulin, and *D cells* secrete somatostatin. *F cells* are the most recently identified cells and secrete pancreatic polypeptide hormone.[2]

Glucagon, insulin, somatostatin, and polypeptide hormones are released into the surrounding capillaries to empty into the portal vein, where they are distributed to target cells in the liver. They then go into general circulation to reach other target cells.

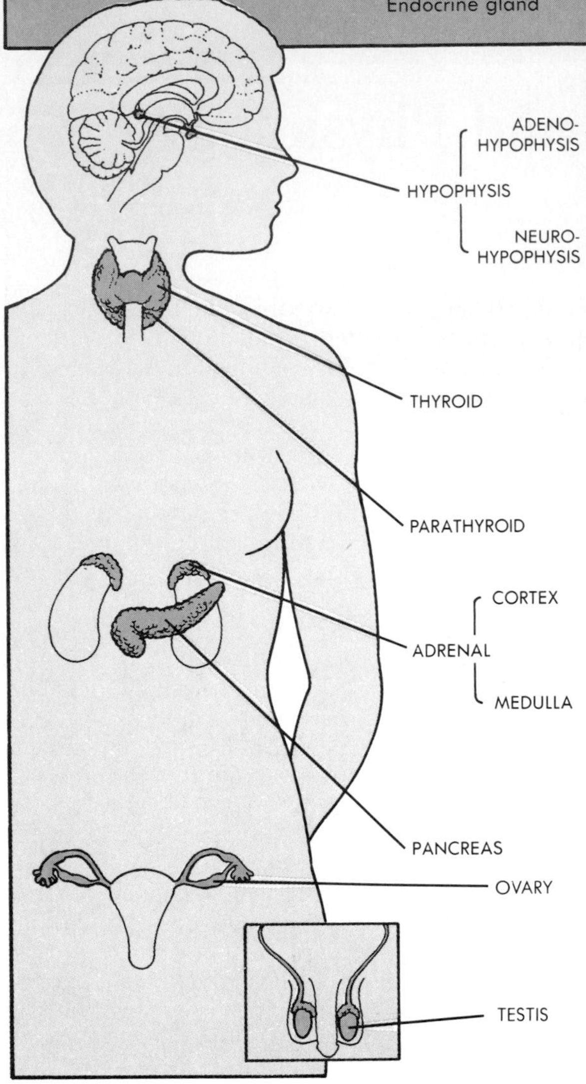

Endocrine gland	Hormone	Target cell/organ	Action
HYPOPHYSIS – ADENOHYPOPHYSIS	Corticotropin hormone	Adrenal cortex	Stimulates adrenal cortex functioning
	Somatotropin hormone	All body cells	Promotes general body growth
	Thyrotropic hormone	Thyroid	Controls thyroid gland hormones
	Gonadotropic hormones	Gonads	Stimulate primary and secondary sex characteristics
	Prolactin	Mammary glands	Breast development and lactation
HYPOPHYSIS – NEUROHYPOPHYSIS	Oxytocin	Breasts and uterus	Stimulates milk ejection and uterine contraction
	Antidiuretic hormone (arginine vasopressin)	Kidney tubules, collecting ducts	Controls permeability to water
		Arterial wall smooth muscle	Vasoconstriction
THYROID	Thyroxine	All body cells	Stimulates metabolism and increased oxygen use
	Triiodothyronine	All body cells	
	Thyrocalcitonin	Bone cells	Stimulates use of calcium and phosphorus
PARATHYROID	Parathormone	Bones, kidneys, gastrointestinal tract	Stimulates use of calcium and phosphorus
	Calcitonin	Bone cells	
ADRENAL – CORTEX	Glucocorticoids	All body cells	Increase gluconeogenesis
	Mineralcorticoids	Renal tubules	Retain sodium, excrete potassium
	Androgens	Facial, pectoral hair, vocal cords	Stimulate secondary sex traits
ADRENAL – MEDULLA	Epinephrine	Heart muscle, smooth muscle, arterioles	Increases heart rate, muscle contraction, vasoconstriction, glycogenolysis
	Norepinephrine	Blood vessels	Vasoconstriction
PANCREAS	Glucagon	Hepatic muscle tissue	Gluconeogenesis, glycogenolysis
	Insulin	Skeletal, muscle, cardiac cell	Promotes utilization of glucose, fat and protein anabolism
	Somatostatin	Pancreatic A and B cells	Inhibits secretion of both insulin and glucagon
	Pancreatic polypeptide	Gallbladder smooth muscle	Contraction
OVARY	Estrogen	Accessory sex organs, breasts	Stimulates secondary sex characteristics
	Progesterone	Uterus	Prepares uterus for fertilized ovum
TESTIS	Testosterone	Male organs, accessory sex organs	Primary and secondary sex characteristics

Fig. 41-1 Location of endocrine glands with hormones, target cell/organ, and hormone action.

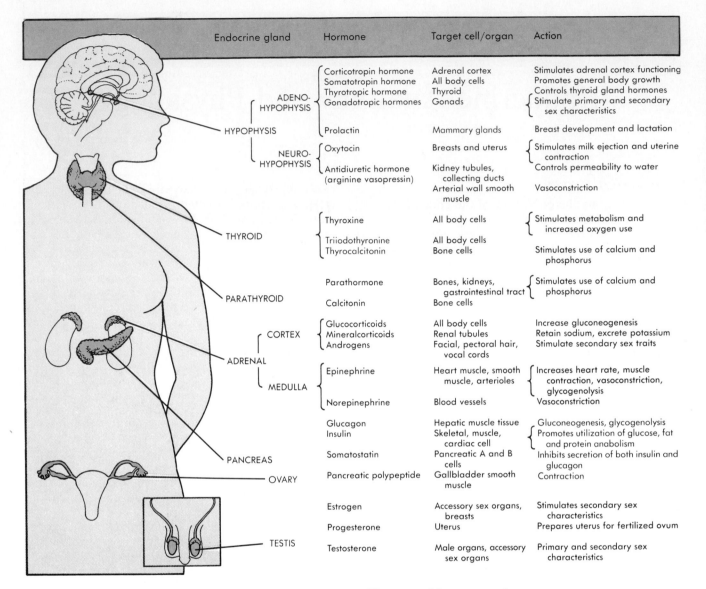

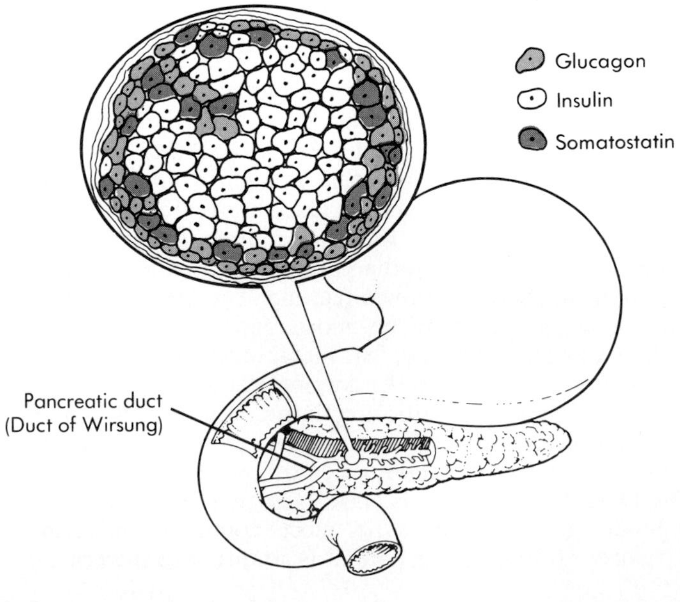

Fig. 41-2 Macroscopic and microscopic structure of the pancreas.

Table 41-1 Pancreatic endocrine cells, hormones, stimulant release factor, target tissue, and response/action

Cell	Hormone	Stimulant release factor	Target tissue	Response/action
A	Glucagon	↓ Glucose Exercise ↑ Amino acids SNS* stimulation	Hepatocyte Myocyte	↑ Glucose in blood stream ↑ Gluconeogenesis ↑ Glycogenolysis Fat mobilization Protein mobilization
B	Insulin	Glucose	Skeletal cells Muscle cells Cardiac cells	↓ Blood glucose ↓ Fat mobilization ↑ Fat storage ↓ Protein mobilization ↑ Protein synthesis ↑ Glucogenesis
D	Somatostatin	Hyperglycemia	A cells B cells	↓ Blood glucose ↓ Glycogen secretion ↓ Insulin secretion
F	Pancreatic polypeptide	Acute hypoglycemia	Gallbladder Smooth muscle	↑ Gallbladder contraction ↓ Pancreatic enzyme

*Sympathetic nervous system.

Table 41-2 Agents that release or inhibit insulin

Insulin release* (major stimulant: elevated blood glucose)	Insulin inhibition (major inhibitor: low blood glucose)
HORMONES	
Glucagon	Somatostatin
Corticotropic hormone	Norepinephrine
Thyrotropin	Epinephrine
Somatotropin	
Glucocorticoids	
Secretin	
Gastrin	
DRUGS	
Beta-adrenergic stimulators	Beta-adrenergic blocking agents
Sulfonylurea	Diazoxide
Theophylline	Phenytoin
Acetylcholine	Thiazide/sulfonamide diurectics

*NOTE: Vagal stimulation can affect insulin release also.

Hormones

◆ **Insulin.** Insulin is a potent anabolic hormone that produces hypoglycemia. It is the only hormone produced in the body that directly lowers glucose levels in the blood stream.[2] Insulin also augments the transport of potassium into the cells, decreases the mobilization of fats, and stimulates protein synthesis (Table 41-1). The major stimulant for insulin secretion is glucose (Table 41-2). When serum glucose levels are within 80 to 100 mg/dl, the serum insulin levels are between 5 to 10 μU/ml. Through the feedback mechanism of plasma glucose, rising levels—that is, 200 mg of glucose as would occur during a meal[3]—stimulate the B cells to produce 30 to 150 μU/ml.

Functions of insulin. In the presence of effective insulin, glucose is admitted to the skeletal, cardiac, and adipose cells for use as energy. Excess glucose, in the form of glycogen, is stored in the hepatic and muscle cells for use as fuel at a later time. The movement of glucose from the circulation into the intracellular compartment reduces the presence of glucose in the blood stream and helps preserve the blood's osmolality. Simultaneously, glucose is available to the cell as its main energy source.

The central nervous system is freely permeable to glucose and does not rely on insulin for the transport of glucose across the cell membrane. Brain cells store only a minimum of glycogen for energy release; these cells are unable to use the end product of gluconeogenesis for energy. Decreased insulin levels alone do not damage brain cells; however, these cells cannot survive the glucose deficiency that occurs from hypersecretion of insulin.[4]

Fat metabolism also is affected by adequate, effective insulin levels. In the presence of insulin, fat is stored in connective tissues, thereby reducing fat mobilization and fat catabolism. Protein metabolism also benefits from adequate insulin supply.

Insulin spares protein from being used as energy and permits protein synthesis. When the cells receive sufficient energy from glucose, amino acids are available for active transport into the cell, promoting the conversion of ribonucleic acid (RNA) into new protein.

Abnormal insulin levels. Insufficient or ineffective insulin levels lead to hyperglycemia, and depriving cells of their energy source. This forces the body to shift from using glucose as fuel to using fat and protein. Fats and protein are catabolized in an attempt to provide a reserve source of glucose through a process called *gluconeogenesis.* Fats are broken down to fatty acids and glycerol. The glycerol is oxidized as carbohydrate, whereas the fatty acids are converted to ketone bodies. When the ketone bodies accumulate faster than they are metabolized, ketosis results.

Protein is catabolized when the body's stores of carbohydrate and fat are depleted. As part of this process, amino acids are broken down to form ammonia and ketoacids. Nitrogen is removed from the amino groups, and the resulting ammonia is detoxified by the liver and removed by the kidneys in the form of urea. Through gluconeogenesis, the ketoacids are converted to glucose.

In a catabolic state, the body is unable to maintain the protein synthesis needed for healthy functioning and blood proteins are used for energy. Without necessary insulin to act on the cell receptor site, blood glucose levels increase. In addition, the end products of fat and protein catabolism collect in the blood stream.

◆ **Glucagon.** Glucagon, synthesized by the A cells, has the opposite effect of insulin. Glucagon counterregulates insulin levels and raises blood sugar levels. It is a potent gluconeogenic hormone. By means of gluconeogenesis it forms glucose from noncarbohydrate sources, such as fat and protein. Glucagon release is stimulated by such factors as a drop in insulin, an increase in blood amino acids, a fall in blood sugar, starvation, exercise, or stimulation of the sympathetic nervous system (Table 41-2). Glucagon is released to protect the body from the hypoglycemia that may result from these conditions.

Initially, glucagon stimulates the release of glycogen stored in the liver and muscle cells to meet short-term energy needs. Through a process called *glycogenolysis,* the glycogen stored in the liver and muscles is converted back into glucose form to be used by the cells. If the energy needs are long-term, the glucagon stimulates glucose release through the more complex process of gluconeogenesis.[5] In gluconeogenesis, fat and protein nutrients are rapidly broken down into end products that are then changed into glucose.

In the healthy body a normal blood glucose level is maintained by the insulin/glucagon ratio. When the blood glucose level is high, insulin is released and glucagon is inhibited. When blood glucose levels are diminished, glucagon rather than insulin is released (Table 41-3). The insulin/glucagon ratio is considered more important in the overall metabolism of fuel sources than is the absolute level of either hormone.[5]

◆ **Somatostatin.** Somatostatin is a protein hormone that inhibits the release of both insulin and glucagon. Somatostatin is synthesized by the pancreatic D cells, the hypothalamus, gastric mucosa, and elsewhere. The hormone decreases glucagon secretion, and in high quantities it decreases insulin release (see Table 41-1).

Hyperglycemia stimulates the activity of the D cells. It is theorized that the release of insulin causes somatostatin to keep the B cells under control. It also is believed that somatostatin allows the gradual influx of glucose into the cell after ingestion of a meal, thus preventing postprandial hyperglycemia.

Table 41-3 Insulin/glucagon ratio and its effect on carbohydrate, fat, and protein metabolism

Balanced insulin/glucagon	Decreased insulin/increased glucagon
↑ Utilization of glucose by cells	↓ Utilization of glucose by cells
↑ Movement of potassium intracellularly	↓ Movement of potassium intracellularly
↑ Carbohydrate metabolism	↑ Blood glucose
↓ Gluconeogensis	↑ Gluconeogenesis
↑ Glycogen storage	↓ Glycogen storage
↓ Glycogenolysis	↑ Glycogenolysis
↓ Lipolysis	↑ Lipolysis
↓ Fat mobilization	↑ Fat mobilization
↑ Fat storage	↓ Fat stores
↓ Protein mobilization	↑ Hepatic metabolism fats
↑ Protein synthesis	↑ Ketogenesis
	↑ Mobilization of protein
	↑ Proteolysis
	↑ Lipoprotein

◆ **Pancreatic polypeptide.** Pancreatic polypeptide is synthesized by the F cells within the islets of Langerhans. This hormone contracts the smooth muscle tissue of the gallbladder and represses pancreatic enzyme secretion.[5] Pancreatic polypeptide can be stimulated by acute hypoglycemia or by an intake that is high in protein and low in carbohydrate. Although it currently has no known metabolic function, pancreatic polypeptide is believed to play a role in nutrient homeostasis.[2]

PITUITARY GLAND AND HYPOTHALAMUS

Understanding the position of the hypothalamus in relation to the pituitary gland is necessary to appreciate the correlation that exists between these organs.

Hypothalamus

The hypothalamus lies superior to the pituitary gland. It is composed of specialized nervous tissue responsible for the integrated functioning of the nervous system and endocrine system, which is termed *neuroendocrine control.* The hypothalamus weighs approximately 4 g and forms the walls and lower portion of the third ventricle of the brain. The area composing the floor of the ventricle thickens in the center and elongates. It is from this funnel-shaped portion, called the *infundibular stalk* (or *stem*), that the pituitary gland is suspended (Fig. 41-3). The infundibular stalk contains a rich vascular supply and a network of communicating neurons that travels from the hypothalamus to the pituitary.[2] The vascular network and neural pathways transport chemical and neural signals and maintain constant communication between the nervous system and the endocrine system.

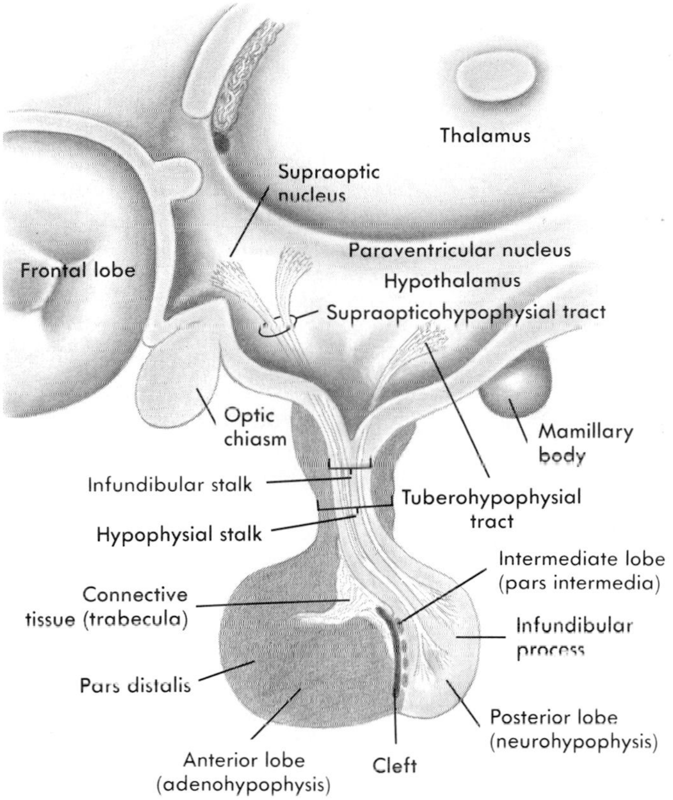

Fig. 41-3 Anatomy of the hypothalamus and the pituitary gland showing the infundibular stem (or stalk) connecting the hypothalamus to the pituitary gland. (Modified from Thompson JM and others: *Mosby's clinical nursing,* ed 3, St Louis, 1993, Mosby–Year Book.)

Pituitary Gland

◆ **Description.** The pituitary gland, also called the *hypophysis* because it is attached below the hypothalamus, is found recessed in the base of the cranial cavity in a hollow depression of the sphenoid bone known as the *sella turcica.* Secured in such a protected environment, the pituitary is one of the most inaccessible endocrine glands in humans. Yet it is because of this very location that the pituitary gland is susceptible to injury from surgical and accidental trauma of the face and head.

◆ **Function.** The pituitary gland has been known as the *master gland* because of the major influence it has over all areas of body functioning. It is now known, however, that the pituitary does not act independently. Rather, the release and inhibition of its hormones actually are controlled by the hypothalamus. The hypothalamus controls pituitary response by secreting substances termed *release-inhibiting factors.* These factors then control the release or inhibition of hormones. (See p. 682 for a discussion of thyrotropin-releasing hormone.) Virtually every function necessary to maintain the human body in a state of dynamic equilibrium is regulated in this manner. The hypophysis is composed of three parts (see Fig. 41-3): the anterior lobe, the intermediate lobe, and the posterior lobe, each with its own origin, morphology, and function.

◆ **Adenohypophysis.** The anterior lobe of the pituitary is the largest portion of the gland. It communicates with the hypothalamus by means of a vascular network. Several hormones are produced by the glandular tissue of the anterior pituitary; thus it is called the *adenohypophysis.* Although the exact number of hormones produced here is uncertain, it is undisputed that adrenocorticotropic hormone (ACTH), thyroid-stimulating hormone (TSH), follicle-stimulating hormone (FSH), luteinizing hormone (LH), growth hormone, and prolactin are manufactured here. (See p. 684 for a discussion of TSH.) Information about all the hormones, their target tissue, and action is found in Fig. 41-1.

◆ **Pars intermedia.** The intermediate lobe of the pituitary, the *pars intermedia,* is located in the central portion of the pituitary between the anterior and posterior lobes. Although the pars intermedia is present in the fetus, it gradually merges with and becomes indistinct from the posterior lobe in the adult. The functions of the pars intermedia in humans are poorly understood.

◆ **Neurohypophysis.** The posterior lobe of the pituitary is called the *neurohypophysis.* It retains its continuity with the hypothalamus by means of neural fibers running through the infundibular stalk. The neurohypophysis has no glandular properties but functions as an extension of the hypothalamus. It collects, stores, and later releases hormones that are produced in the hypothalamus.[2] After hormones are synthesized in the hypothalamus, they are transported to the posterior pituitary until the hypothalamus signals their release. Oxytocin (Pitocin) and arginine vasopressin (antidiuretic hormone) are both manufactured in the hypothalamus and stored in the neurohypophysis.

◆ **Hormones**

Oxytocin. Oxytocin stimulates smooth muscle contraction of the uterus and causes the myoepithelial cells of the breast to contract and force milk from the alveoli into the secretory ducts. Pathologic conditions caused by hypersecretion or hyposecretion of oxytocin have not been identified.[2] Insufficient amounts of oxytocin are known to result in delayed labor and delivery. Exogenous Pitocin is used clinically to induce labor, to augment contractions during the first and second stages of labor, and to manage postpartum hemorrhage.

Antidiuretic hormone. Antidiuretic hormone (ADH), known also as *arginine vasopressin* (AVP), has been identified as the single most important hormone responsible for regulating fluid balance within the body. ADH has two functions: it constricts smooth muscles within the arterial wall (pharmacologic doses may elevate blood pressure) and more important, it maintains the osmolality of the blood in a very narrow range. ADH regulates the permeability of the kidney tubule. In effect, ADH also controls the sodium levels of the extracellular fluid. Plasma osmolality is determined largely by the sodium ion concentration process in the plasma. When sodium levels rise, plasma osmolality increases. ADH is released to stimulate fluid reabsorption at the nephron to retain water and maintain sodium balance.[6]

In the presence of ADH, permeability of the kidney tubules is increased and water is reabsorbed from the renal filtrate. This process decreases water loss from the body and subsequently concentrates and reduces urine volume. Fluid conserved in this manner is returned to the circulating plasma where it dilutes the concentration (osmolality) of plasma (Fig. 41-4). The release of ADH is regulated primarily by the plasma osmotic pressure and the volume of circulating blood. Hemorrhage, sufficient to lower the blood pressure, and emesis, sufficient to reduce fluid volume, will stimulate the release of ADH. Other factors capable of influencing ADH secretion are pain, stress, malignant disease, surgical intervention, alcohol, and drugs (see Table 41-4 for additional factors that affect ADH levels).

Table 41-4 Factors affecting antidiuretic hormone levels

Antidiuretic hormone stimulation	Antidiuretic hormone restriction
Increased serum osmolality	Decreased serum osmolality
Emesis	
Hypovolemia	Hypervolemia
Hemorrhage	Water intoxication
Pain	Cold
	Congenital defect
	CO_2 inhalation
Trauma to hypothalamic-hypophyseal system	Trauma to hypothalamic-hypophyseal system
Accidental	Accidental
Surgical	Surgical
Pathologic	Pathologic
Stress	
Physical	
Emotional	
Acute infections	
Malignancies	
Nonmalignant pulmonary disorders	
Stimulated pulmonary baroreceptors	
Nocturnal sleep	
Drugs	Drugs
Nicotine	Phenytoin
Barbiturates	Chlorpromazine
Oxytocin	Reserpine
Glucocorticoids	Norepinephrine
Anesthetics	Ethanol
Acetaminophen	Narcotics
Amitriptyline	Lithium
Carbamazepine	Demeclocycline
Cyclophosphamide	Tolazamide
Chlorpropamide	
K^+ depleting diuretics	
Vincristine	
Isoproterenol	

Osmoreceptors, believed to be sodium receptors,[6] are located in the hypothalamus and are sensitive to changes in the circulating plasma osmolality. Stretch receptors located in the left atrium are sensitive to volume changes in the plasma, as may be caused by vomiting, diarrhea, or blood loss. ADH, responsible for maintaining circulating volume, is restricted when the blood volume or osmolality is low. Suppression of ADH renders the kidney tubules impermeable to water and causes an increase in the amount of water excreted by the kidneys. This restores the circulating blood volume and normal osmolality (see Fig. 41-4).

Alterations in blood tonicity and circulating blood volume also are controlled by baroreceptors located primarily in the atria, the aorta, and the carotid arteries. Information from these receptors, coupled with change reflected by the osmoreceptors, stimulates the hypothalamus to modify ADH secretion. The result is maintenance of adequate fluid balance within the extracellular and intracellular fluid compartments and normal blood pressure.

THE THYROID GLAND

Description

The thyroid gland, which is considered the largest endocrine gland, weighs from 15 to 30 g. (The size of the gland varies according to the iodine available in different parts of the world[7]). The gland, which partially encases the trachea, is wrapped around the second to fourth tracheal rings anteriorly and laterally. The gland is located at the level of the sixth and seventh cervical vertebrae, posteriorly. The bow-tie gland has two lateral lobes that are partially covered by the sternohyoid and sternothyroid muscles. The thyroid isthmus, the band of narrow thyroid tissue that connects the lateral lobes, lies directly below the cricoid cartilage (Fig. 41-5). The thyroid tissue, which is richly vascularized,[8] receives about 5 ml of blood per gram per minute. The basic functional units of the thyroid gland are spherical-shaped cells called *follicles.* Follicles are filled with a protein thyroglobulin.

Function

The functioning of the thyroid gland depends in part on the hypothalamus, adenohypophysis, dietary intake of iodine, and circulating protein bodies in the blood. The adenohypophysis, or anterior lobe of the pituitary gland, secretes thyrotropin, the thyroid-stimulating hormone (TSH) that prompts the thyroid cells to produce thyroid hormones. Through a complex process, dietary iodine is absorbed and concentrated in the thyroid follicles. The iodine is oxidized to iodide, and through active transport the amino acid tyrosine binds the iodide to the thyroglobulin and eventually yields triiodothyronine (T_3) and thyroxine (T_4). More than 99% of T_3 and T_4 circulates through the blood supply bound to the serum transporting proteins, thyroxin-binding globulin, prealbumin, and albumin.[9] The minute amount of free thyroid hormone that is not protein-bound is responsible for activating thyroid responses throughout the body.

Whereas both T_4 and T_3 are produced by the thyroid

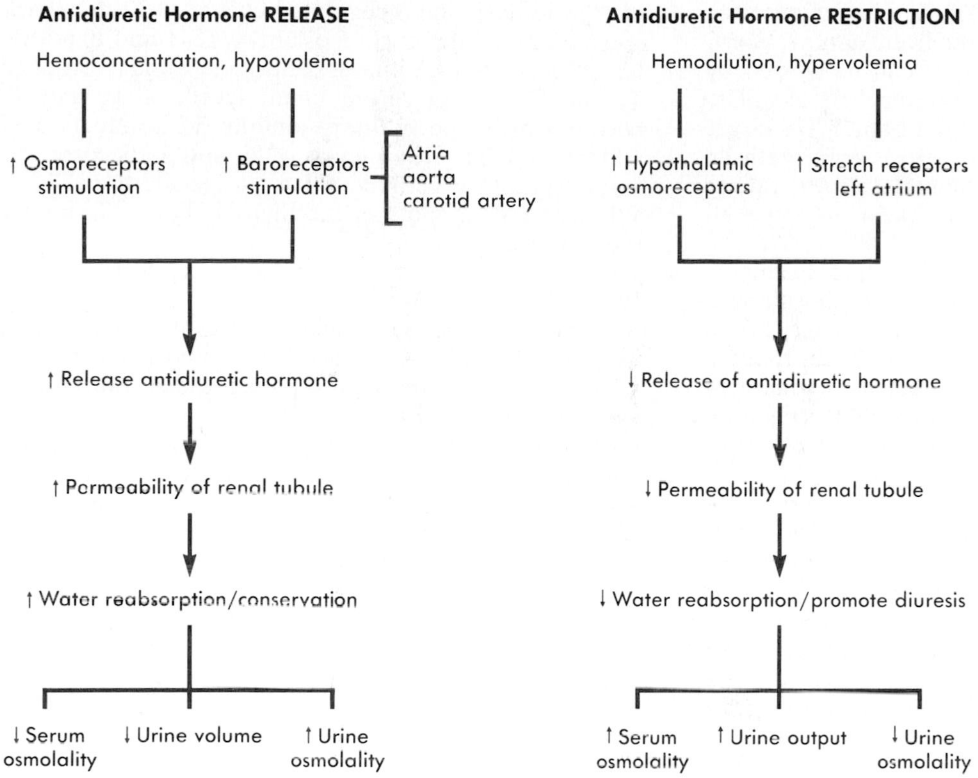

Fig. 41-4 Physiology of the release and restriction of antidiuretic hormone.

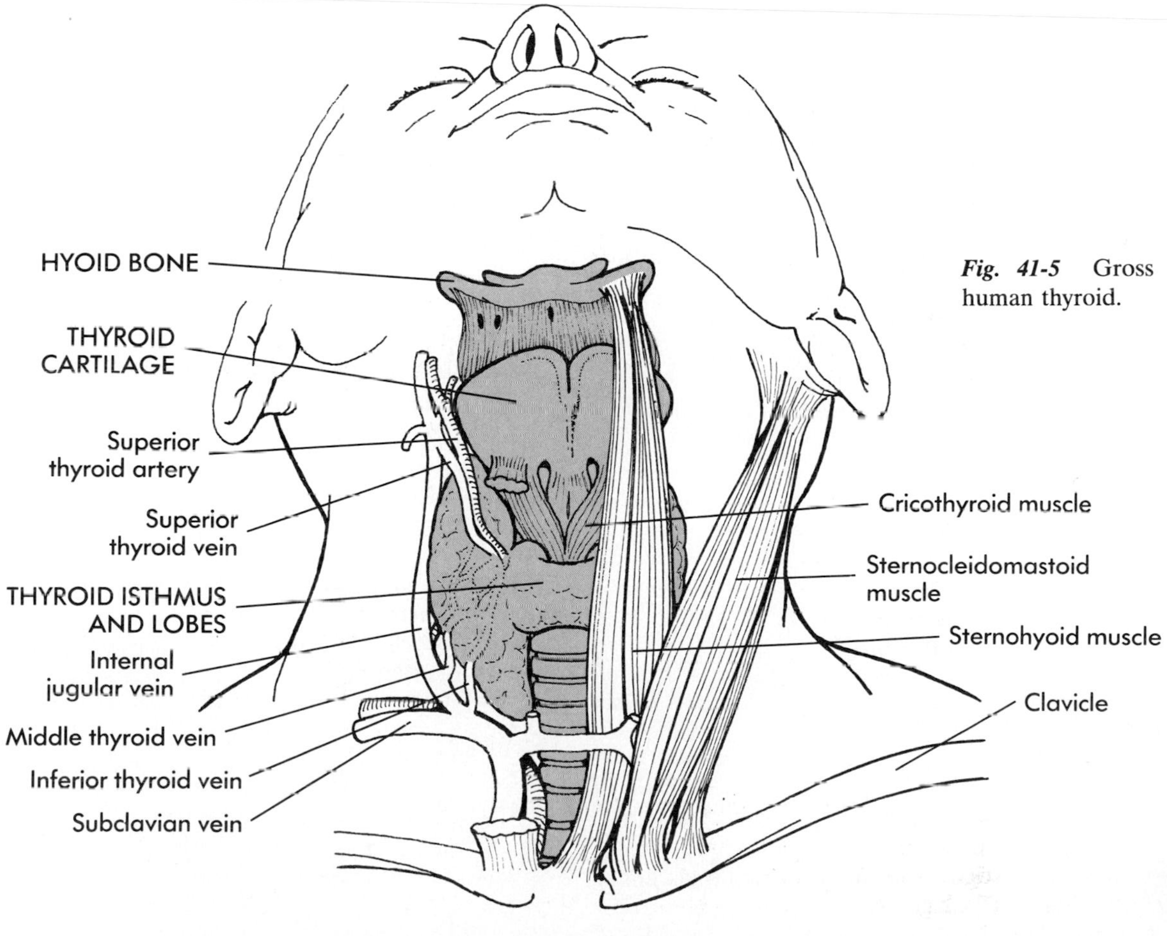

Fig. 41-5 Gross anatomy of the human thyroid.

gland, T_3 is primarily the result of the conversion of T_4 to T_3 in the peripheral tissues of the liver, kidneys, heart, and other tissues. (This conversion can be slowed by certain drugs, such as beta-adrenergic blockers, as will be seen later in the unit.) T_3 acts more rapidly on target tissues in the body than does T_4 and is more actively potent than T_4. Both thyroid hormones affect the rate at which oxygen is used in the body and therefore affect all metabolic processes in the body.

The thyroid gland also produces a third hormone, thyrocalcitronin, also called calcitonin. This hormone is produced by the parafollicular cells, or C cells, found scattered among the follicular cells. Calcitonin reduces levels of calcium in the blood stream by augmenting calcium absorption in the bone. Throughout this unit, discussion of thyroid hormone refers collectively to T_3 and T_4, not calcitonin.

The hypothalamus-pituitary-thyroid axis is responsible for the synthesis and secretion of thyroid hormone (Fig. 41-6). The hypothalamus, stimulated by neural mechanisms, secretes thyrotropin-releasing hormone (TRH). This hormone activates thyrotropin, the thyroid-stimulating hormone (TSH) in the adenohypophysis. TSH then stimulates the thyroid gland to manufacture and release the thyroid hormone. The entire production of thyroid hormone is regulated by a negative feedback mechanism at the level of pituitary TSH and hypothalamic TRH. TSH stimulates the thyroid gland to produce T_3 and T_4. When serum blood levels of T_3 and T_4 becomes high, the pituitary inhibits the production of additional TSH. When levels of T_3 and T_4 become too low, the pituitary is stimulated to secrete additional TSH. Whereas TSH stimulates the thyroid, T_3 and T_4 inhibit the pituitary.

Hormones

Thyroid hormone stimulates oxygen consumption, increases the metabolic processes in almost all cells, and activates heat production. The exact mechanism whereby these activities take place is incompletely understood.[10] Thyroxine prompts the synthesis of beta-adrenergic receptors in widespread areas of the body. These receptors trigger a sympathetic nervous system response and release epinephrine at various nerve endings. The effect is stimulation of the cardiac tissue, nervous tissue, and smooth muscle tissue, as well as increase in metabolism and thermogenesis, or the increase in body heat. Major functions of the thyroid hormones are listed in the box, p. 685.

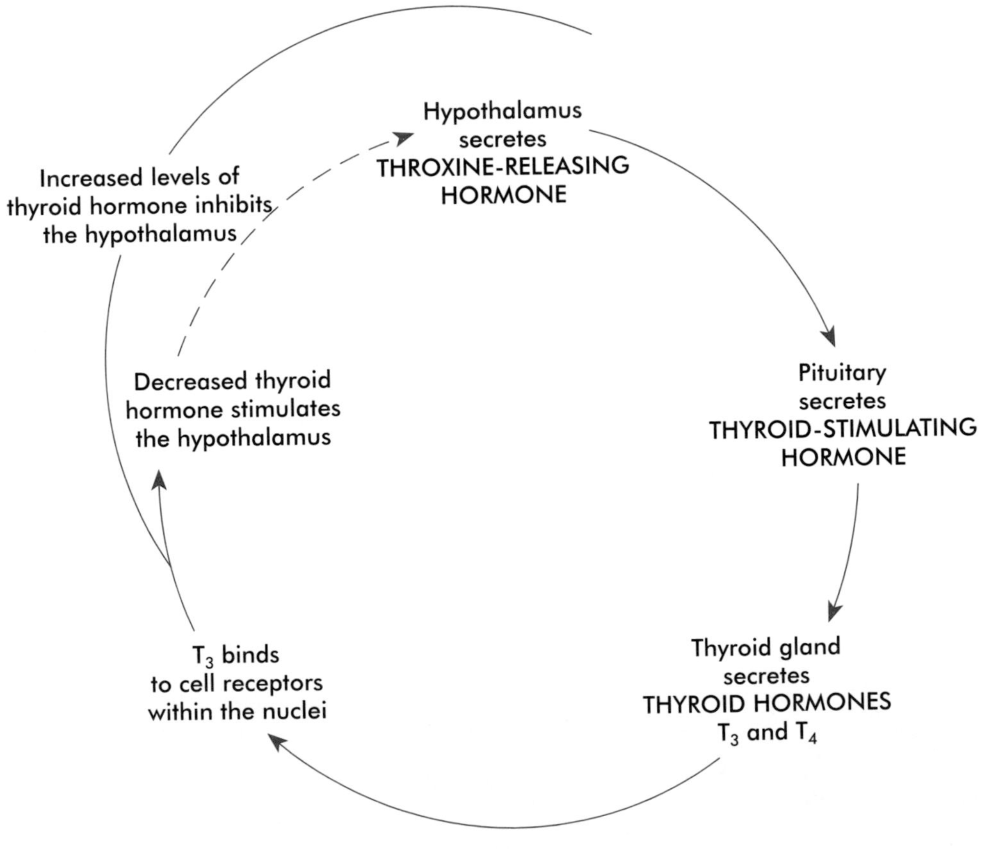

Fig. 41-6 Hypothalamus-pituitary-thyroid axis.

MAJOR FUNCTIONS OF THYROID HORMONES

- Interact with growth hormone
  - Maturation of skeletal system
  - Development of central nervous system
- Stimulate carbohydrate metabolism
  - Increase the rate of glucose absorption from the GI tract
  - Increase the rate of glucose utilization by the cells
- Accelerate the rate of fat metabolism
  - Increase cholesterol degradation in the liver
  - Decrease serum cholesterol levels
- Increase protein anabolism and catabolism
  - Mobilize protein and release amino acids into circulation
  - Increase energy from protein nutrients through gluconeogenesis
- Increase body's demand for vitamins
- Increase oxygen consumption and utilization
- Increase basal metabolic rate
- Have marked chronotropic and inotropic effects on heart
- Increase cardiac output
- Stimulate contractility and excitability of myocardium
- Increase blood volume
- Expand respiratory rate and depth necessary for normal hypoxic and hypercapnic drive
- Promote sympathetic overactivity
- Boost erythropoiesis
- Increase metabolism and clearance of various hormones and pharmacologic agents
- Stimulate bone resorption

REFERENCES

1. Kelley W, editor: *Textbook of internal medicine,* vol 2, ed 2, Philadelphia, 1992, JB Lippincott.
2. Hadley M: *Endocrinology,* ed 3, Englewood Cliffs, NJ, 1992, Prentice-Hall.
3. Rifkin H, Porte D, editors: *Ellenberg and Rifkin's diabetes mellitus: theory and practice,* ed 4, New York, 1990, Elsevier.
4. Bullock B, Rosendahl P: *Pathophysiology: adaptations and alterations in function,* ed 3, Philadelphia, 1992, JB Lippincott.
5. Slaunwhite R: *Fundamentals of endocrinology,* New York, 1988, Marcel Dekker.
6. Guyton A: *Textbook of medical physiology,* ed 8, Philadelphia, 1991, WB Saunders.
7. Kissane JM, editor: *Anderson's pathology,* vol 2, ed 9, St Louis, 1990, Mosby–Year Book.
8. Junqueira LC, Carneiro J, Kelley R: *Basic histology,* ed 7, Norwalk, Conn, 1992, Appleton & Lange.
9. Clark W, Brater DC, Johnson AR: *Goth's medical pharmacology,* ed 13, St Louis, 1992, Mosby–Year Book.
10. West JB, editor: *Best and Taylor's physiological basis of medical practice,* ed 12, Baltimore, 1991, Williams & Wilkins.

42

Endocrine Clinical Assessment and Diagnostic Procedures

CHAPTER OBJECTIVES

- Discuss the rationale involved in developing a consistent, sequential format for performing an endocrine nursing assessment.
- List the criteria for a health history that is specific in assessing for diabetic ketoacidosis and hyperglycemic hyperosmolar nonketotic coma.
- Compare and contrast at least three clinical and laboratory manifestations of diabetes insipidus and syndrome of inappropriate antidiuretic hormone.
- Identify a minimum of two clinical manifestations of thyrotoxicosis that become life-threatening in thyrotoxic crisis.
- Perform a thorough nursing assessment of a critically ill patient's endocrine system, interpret the results, and plan nursing interventions that will treat any abnormal findings.

Most of the endocrine glands are deeply encased in the human body. This protected position safeguards the glands and their link to homeostasis against injury and trauma. Although the placement of the glands provides security for the glandular functions, their inaccessibility prevents the glands from being physically appraised. Most endocrine glands cannot be assessed by palpation, percussion, or auscultation. The thyroid gland and male gonads are unusual in that the anatomic position of these endocrine glands permits palpation. An enlarged thyroid also can be auscultated for a systolic bruit or continuous venous hum.

The endocrine glands that preclude physical inspection nevertheless can be assessed by the clinician who understands the metabolic actions of the hormones involved. When percussion or palpation of the gland cannot be achieved, the nurse monitors the functioning of that gland's target tissue.

Frequently the initial focus of the hormonal disturbance is not on the gland itself, but rather on the specific cell receptor or target for the hormonal action. Posterior pituitary dysfunction, for example, is suspected when the patient has decreased urine output, clinical manifestations of hypervolemia (bounding pulse, increased blood pressure, elevated pulmonary artery or central venous pressure reading, engorged neck veins), and serum hyponatremia with hypertonic urine. An understanding that the target cell for antidiuretic hormone (ADH) is the kidney tubule and reabsorption of urine filtrate is the action of the hormone leads the clinician to suspect a compromise in ADH or posterior pituitary functioning.

Similarly, pancreatic disorders often are recognized first by noting imbalances in the B cell hormone, insulin, and its systemic effects. The cell receptor site of insulin is found on the adipose and muscle cells. The major action of insulin is to increase the uptake and utilization of glucose by the muscle and fat cells and to decrease blood glucose levels. (See Chapter 41 for a more complete discussion of the effects of insulin.) When glucose is utilized for cellular energy, insulin prevents fat and protein from being broken down for fuel. The clinician who understands the metabolic effects of insulin may suspect a dysfunctioning pancreas in a patient who is lethargic and has hot, dry skin, oliguria, and sweet-smelling breath.

In addition to obvious changes in the anatomy of the thyroid gland, the clinician assesses the hormonal effect of the glandular secretions. Thyroxine (T_4) and triiodothyronine (T_3) both affect the metabolism of almost every cell in the body. Spiking fever and tachycardia, especially tachydysrhythmia with escalating restlessness and anxiety, may be induced by increasing levels of the thyroid hormone. These changes alert the knowledgeable caregiver to look deeper for alterations in the body's metabolic processes controlled by the thyroid gland.

Collecting clues that may signal a dysfunctioning gland poses a challenge to the nurse clinician because target tissues of insulin (adipose and muscle cells), antidiuretic hormone (kidney tubule), and thyroxine (almost all body cells) are influenced by numerous other factors. Therefore the nurse starts with a pertinent data base, including history (when available) and precipitating factors. The patient in the critical care unit may not be able to provide an adequate history for the nurse's assessment data base. Changes in level of consciousness and urgent medical/nursing procedures may delay communication of the patient's personal perspective of the current problem. This initial phase of the nursing process should not be ignored, however, and sources other than the patient (family, friends, previous medical records) should be used to supply vital information.

CLINICAL ASSESSMENT

Pancreas

Insulin, which is produced by the pancreas, is responsible for glucose metabolism. The clinical assessment provides information about pancreatic functioning. Clinical manifestations of abnormal insulin levels identify the patient's response to altered glucose metabolism.

◆ **History.** A complete health history includes the patient's chief complaint and current health history. Chronic, as well as episodic, diseases are discussed (acute physiologic or psychologic stress could increase endogenous glucose). Routine treatments, such as hyperalimentation, peritoneal dialysis, and hemodialysis, are included in the health history because any one could be an exogenous source of increased glucose levels.

Also included in the data collection is the patient's past history. Has the patient ever had pancreatic surgery? Was the patient ever told that there was "too much sugar" in his or her blood or that "too much sugar" might develop later in life? What treatment was prescribed if such a condition existed?

Family history is assessed in respect to present illness. Carbohydrate metabolic imbalance commonly is influenced by hereditary factors.

Included in the medical history are questions pertaining to the patient's use of prescription or over-the-counter medications. Pharmacologic agents can alter pancreatic function by either increasing or decreasing the release of hormones. Drugs also may interfere with hormonal action at the receptor site on the target cell. Epinephrine and phenytoin are two medications that are known to decrease the effect of insulin in the body and increase serum glucose. Glucagon and glucocorticoids increase the breakdown of noncarbohydrate substances into glucose and thereby increase serum glucose levels.

In addition, information about the most recent health status of the patient is sought. An inability to balance the body's sudden physiologic changes with demands in insulin needs may develop in patients with severe infection or surgical or traumatic injury. The patient or significant other is asked about recent, unexplained changes in weight, thirst, hunger, and urination patterns, including daytime and nighttime frequency and volume. Review of the patient's activities of daily living and recent changes in activity level gives the clinician information about endurance levels, fatigue, and weakness. This information relates to glucose availability and utilization as fuel. Asking the patient or significant other about vague or obscure changes in behavior or mental status (memory loss, momentary disorientation) may reveal periods of hyperglycemia or hypoglycemia and their effect on the brain tissue.

◆ **Physical examination.** Hydration status and skin assessment provide additional information about pancreatic functioning. Normal levels of glucose in the blood stream contribute to the serum osmolality. The glucose level is a key component in the extracellular and intracellular fluid balance. Satisfactory fluid balance is easily identified by the presence of moist, shiny buccal membranes. Skin turgor that is resilient and returns to its original position in less than 3 seconds after being pinched or lifted indicates adequate skin elasticity. (Skin over the forehead, clavicle, and sternum is the most reliable for testing tissue turgor because it is less affected by aging and thus more easily assessed for changes related to fluid balance.) A well-hydrated patient has skin in the groin and axilla that is slightly moist to touch. A balanced intake and output, absence of thirst, absence of edema, stable weight, and urine specific gravity that falls within the normal range (1.005 to 1.030) all provide information that indicates the patient's hydration status is adequate for metabolic demands.

Pituitary Gland

The pituitary gland, recessed in the base of the cranium, is not accessible to physical assessment. Therefore the clinician must be aware of the systemic effects of a normally functioning neurohypophysis to identify pituitary dysfunction.

◆ **History.** When possible, the patient and/or significant other is asked about the patient's chief complaint and current health history. Does the patient have complaints of headache or fatigue? Is there an active blood loss? (Hypovolemia stimulates the presence of antidiuretic hormone.) Is the patient currently being treated for another endocrine dysfunction that potentially could interfere with the amount of ADH in the body? (Hypothyroidism and adrenal insufficiency stimulate the release of ADH regardless of serum osmolality or volume deficit.[1]) Is a head injury or neurologic disorder present that could interfere with the synthesis of ADH in the hypothalamus or its passage down to the posterior pituitary before its release? Equally important is information about pulmonary diseases or malignant diseases—tuberculosis, pneumonia, duodenal carcinoma, and especially oat cell carcinomas. Each is a disease that can cause autonomous production of ADH.

The past history may reveal information about a birth defect involving the infundibular stalk. A family history is assessed in an effort to identify familial tendencies toward ineffective ADH utilization. An inherited disorder involves kidney tubules that are insensitive to the circulating ADH.

A history of the patient's use of medications offers the clinician clues regarding potential ADH imbalance (see Table 41-4 for factors affecting ADH levels). Phenytoin, chlorpromazine, and reserpine, among other drugs, decrease the release of ADH. Barbiturates, anesthetics, vincristine, glucocorticoids, and several other drugs stimulate the release of ADH.

A psychosocial history provides an opportunity to collect data regarding any obsessional neurosis the patient may have experienced. Knowledge of compulsive activities involving insatiable water drinking is useful in determining the cause of ADH imbalance.

The patient and/or significant other is asked about the health status immediately preceding the acute care episode. Has the patient ever complained of unexplained weight loss? Has excessive urination occurred so frequently that it interferes with the patient's daily living activities and ability to sleep? Has there been an increase in thirst, and if so, is it easily satisfied?

The clinician asks the patient about any changes in mental abilities (increased or decreased fluid levels affected by circulating ADH also affect the serum sodium levels). Sodium imbalance may result from excessive sodium loss in the urine or from a disproportionate amount of extracellular fluid diluting the previously normal sodium level. Alterations in the patient's serum sodium level first may be noticed as a change in the patient's mental status inasmuch as difficulty concentrating and confusion may occur. These complaints signal changes in cerebral hydration and serum sodium levels that, unless corrected, will lead to further neurologic damage and ultimately death.

◆ **Physical examination.** Antidiuretic hormone controls the amount of fluid lost and retained within the body. The nurse uses a hydration assessment to determine the effectiveness of ADH function. A hydration assessment includes skin integrity, skin turgor, and buccal membrane moisture. Blood pressure and pulse frequently are monitored. Decreased blood pressure with an increased pulse is characteristic of hypovolemia, whereas elevated blood pressure and rapid, bounding pulse may indicate hypervolemia. Orthostatic hypotension, which occurs when extracellular fluid volume decreases, is identified by a drop in systolic blood pressure of 20 mm Hg and a drop in diastolic blood pressure of 10 mm Hg when the patient changes position from lying to standing.

Daily weight changes coincide with fluid retention and fluid loss. Sudden changes in weight could be a result of a change in fluid balance; 1 L of fluid lost or retained is equal to approximately 2 pounds, 3 ounces of weight gained or lost. To use weight as a true determinant of the body's weight changes, all extraneous variables should be eliminated and the same scale should be used at the same time each day. The patient also should wear similar clothing so as not to affect the reading.

Measuring and recording intake and output often is overlooked as a definitive tool in the critical care unit. It is a simple task that, when performed accurately and conscientiously on *all* routes of fluid intake and loss, provides information about the body's fluid balance. Precise intake and output records also are used as criteria for fluid replacement therapy. Physical characteristics of urine, such as concentration, color, and specific gravity, are significant factors in assessing the patient's fluid balance.

The patient's neurologic system frequently is evaluated in an assessment of the pituitary gland. As already mentioned, alterations in serum sodium levels adversely affect brain tissue and disrupt the patient's behavioral patterns. Muscle coordination, deep tendon reflexes, and muscle strength are included in the neurologic assessment.

Thyroid

Thyroid crisis, the focus of this presentation for critical care nurses, is a rare yet potentially lethal medical condition. It is the most extreme, severe response to overactive thyroid hormone. The thyroid hormone produces a heightened sympathetic nervous system response in the body. T_3 and T_4 increase beta-adrenergic receptors in the body, and the cardiovascular system becomes especially sensitive to catecholamines.[2] These signs occur with a variety of precipitating factors in the patient with hyperthyroidism. (Details of hyperthyroidism are presented later in the chapter.) It is important to recognize that no distinct signs or symptoms in thyroid crisis distinguish it from hyperthyroidism[3] except for the severity of the signs or symptoms. No separate laboratory values identify thyroid crisis nor differentiate it from hyperthyroidism. Therefore the responsibility rests on the clinician who is assessing the body's response to a covertly worsening condition.

To fully grasp the effect of thyroid crisis (also called *thyroid storm* or *thyrotoxic crisis*), it is necessary first to understand the effects on the body of undersecretion of thyroid hormone and oversecretion of the hormone.

Decreased secretion of thyroid hormone results in generally sluggish metabolic processes. Insufficient thyroid hormone produced during infancy and childhood results in a hypothyroid condition that may cause impaired physical growth and development and possibly mental retardation. Hypothyroidism in adults results in decreased metabolism throughout the body's systems. Fatigue, weight gain, intolerance to cold, and impaired decision making are characteristic of this disorder. Additional clinical manifestations of hypothyroidism are listed in the box, p. 689, left-hand column. Depending on etiologic factors in the dysfunction, replacement hormones are quite successful in reversing this disorder.

Increased circulating thyroid hormone results in hyperthyroidism, also known as *thyrotoxicosis.* This condition increases the breakdown of nutrients in the body and the synthesis of organic compounds within the cells. This increased metabolism requires energy to yield energy. The body responds with an effort to replenish the oxygen and energy used in a hypermetabolic state, which results in increased appetite, tachycardia, and tachypnea. The increased nutrient intake, however, is insufficient to meet accelerated needs of the body, and weight loss occurs. Most characteristic of thyrotoxicosis is the hyperthermia and heightened state of nervousness. The box mentioned above presents additional clinical manifestations of thyrotoxicosis.

Thyrotoxic crisis (thyroid crisis, thyroid storm) is a severe, life-threatening form of thyrotoxicosis. This state manifests by extremes of hypermetabolism, hyperpyrexia, and a heightened sensitivity of effector organs to adrenergic stimuli. Thyroid crisis describes a rapidly worsening state in the person with untreated or uncontrolled hyperthyroidism. Although its occurrence is relatively uncommon, it may be seen in the critical care unit in patients who are treated for superimposed medical emergencies, such as toxic systemic infections, severe cardiac myopathies, or uncontrolled diabetes. Symptoms of thyrotoxic crisis are neither unique nor do they readily identify the impending progression of thyrotoxicosis to a crisis state. As such, there is no sudden development of thyroid goiter nor revealing diagnostic tests. Because thyrotoxicosis exists before the crisis, basic assessments and laboratory data used for thyroid diseases are discussed in the next section.

CLINICAL MANIFESTATIONS OF THYROID ABNORMALITIES

ADULT HYPOTHYROIDISM

Decreased basal metabolic rate
Lethargy
Myxedema
Severe muscle cramps
Chronic anemia
Decreased bowel activity, constipation
Menstrual irregularities
Bradycardia
Bradypnea
Paresthesia
Muscle weakness
Decreased glomerular filtration
Decreased cardiac output

THYROTOXICOSIS

Increased basal metabolic rate
Fatigue, exhaustion
Diaphoresis
Intolerance to heat
Goiter
Diarrhea
Ophthalmopathy
Hyperkinesis
Increased cardiac output
Tachydysrhythmias
Frequent urination
Emotional lability
Fine tremors

SAMPLE QUESTIONS TO OBTAIN THYROID HISTORY

- Were you ever told you have a "sluggish" thyroid or "slow metabolism"?
- Have you ever had an enlarged neck from a "goiter"?
- Has anyone in your family ever been treated for a "sluggish" or fast metabolism? (Thyroid disease has a familial tendency.)
- Have you ever taken a hormone or other medication for problems with your thyroid gland?
- Do you have problems with extreme nervousness?
- Are you sensitive to heat?
- Are you always exhausted but too restless to sleep?
- Have you lost weight recently? Has your appetite increased despite the weight loss?
- Have you been aware of a high fever?
- Do you have problems with nausea, diarrhea?

◆ **History.** The history of a patient in the critical care area should be as detailed as possible. Information regarding the clinical manifestations of either hypothyroidism or hyperthyroidism must be obtained from the patient, family, or others with knowledge about the patient. Sample questions considered pertinent to thyroid disease are presented in the box, above right.

◆ **Physical examination.** The thyroid gland of normal size is not visible or apparent as a bulge in the anterior neck. Palpation of the neck to reveal a goiter or enlargement of the thyroid gland would be done before the diagnosis of thyrotoxicosis. Physical assessment by means of palpation is not necessary in the assessment of thyrotoxic storm. (For techniques used to palpate the thyroid gland, the reader is referred to a physical health assessment text). Auscultation of the thyroid is accomplished by use of the bell portion of the stethescope to identify a bruit or blowing noise from the circulation through the thyroid gland. Although the presence of a bruit indicates increased blood flow through the glandular tissue, it is not a proved method to differentiate the presence of thyrotoxic crisis from thyrotoxicosis.

Critical assessments include patient responses to increased metabolism, heightened sensitivity to adrenergic receptors, and loss of thermoregulation. Core temperatures identify the body's ability to regulate heat lost with heat generated by increased metabolism. Cardiac functioning—specifically tachydysrhythmias, premature ventricular contractions, and paroxysmal atrial tachycardia that result from the increased epinephrine effect on the myocytes—is assessed. Stroke volume and cardiac output also are monitored. Although appetite dramatically increases, nausea, vomiting, and diarrhea often thwart the body's attempt to increase food intake and replenish fuel for energy expenditure. In addition, hypermotility of the gastrointestinal tract interferes with nutrient absorption. Daily weights are taken to record changes in body mass. Hydration assessment is necessary to devise a plan to counter the effects of the hyperthermia and fluid losses from vomiting and diarrhea. Hyperglycemia may result from the increased mobilization of nutrients and insufficient insulin release. Nursing attention is given to the patient's emotional responses and sudden, unprovoked changes, for example, from laughter to hostile outbursts. Restlessness, inability to sleep, presence of tremors, and fatigue are all evaluated and documented. Interesting and important to data collection is the client's intolerance to heat. The patient who complains of profuse sweating from being too hot often follows this report with turning off room heat, opening all windows, and taking off all but minimal clothing and bed linens, even on the coldest days.

LABORATORY ASSESSMENT

Pancreas

Pertinent laboratory tests for the pancreas measure the amount of insulin produced by the pancreatic B cells and the effectiveness of insulin in transporting glucose from the blood stream into the cell. The test results reveal whether insulin can maintain a constant serum glucose level, as well as contribute to the metabolism of fats and protein. When adequate insulin is unavailable to permit glucose to be used for fuel, the body is forced to break down other noncarbohydrate sources, such as fat and protein, as alternate energy sources. The rapid, incomplete breakdown of fat and protein leaves waste products that affect the body's homeostasis. Tests to determine the osmolality, glucose, and ketone levels identify the residual effects of incomplete glucose uptake and utilization by the cells.

◆ **Insulin.** When measured by blood test, the normal value of insulin is 5 to 20 μU/ml. The amount of insulin circulating in the blood stream during a period of fasting is measured by a sensitive radioimmunoassay test. The release of insulin depends on the concentration of blood glucose; when glucose levels rise, insulin levels also rise. Conversely, when serum glucose levels are low, insulin secretion is inhibited. A fasting blood sample therefore is preferred for evaluation of serum insulin levels.

◆ **Glucose.** The normal fasting serum or plasma value of glucose, when measured by blood test, is 70 to 110 mg/dl. The fasting whole blood value is 60 to 100 mg/dl, and the nonfasting value is 85 to 125 mg/dl. Circulating blood glucose is derived from three sources: exogenous intake of glucose, release of glycogen stores, and breakdown of noncarbohydrate sources, or gluconeogenesis. A fasting blood sample is read as a simple, numeric value, but it actually measures many complex, interrelated processes. The glucose reading measures the ability of the pancreatic A cells to balance the release of glucagon with the B cell release of insulin. Circulating glucose also depends on the peripheral uptake of glucose and the functioning of the liver and its role in gluconeogenesis. Consistently elevated glucose levels signal an increase in glucagon production and an insufficient amount of effective insulin. In healthy patients a fasting serum glucose rarely exceeds 110 mg/dl of blood.

◆ **Fingerstick glucose test.** Fingerstick glucose tests involve a relatively new technique that makes frequent glucose testing rapid, economical, and convenient. This test commonly is used at the bedside for quick, accurate readings that serve as a basis for insulin coverage. The blood test also can be performed by the patient as a means of keeping track of daily glucose levels and identifying situations that cause hyperglycemia or hypoglycemia. It currently is used by patients as a means of obtaining tighter control over glucose levels and keeping the glucose as close to normal as possible with intensive insulin therapy. The test involves a reagent strip and a reflectance meter or a monitor. Numerous devices are available, each with its own specific instructions and guarantee of accuracy. Some strips can be read by comparing the color left by a drop of blood with a color chart. Strips also may be placed into a meter or monitor for an exact reading.

◆ **Glycosylated hemoglobin.** During the 120-day lifespan of erythrocytes, the hemoglobin within each cell binds to the available blood glucose through a process known as *glycosylation.* In a blood test, 4% to 7% of hemoglobin normally is glycosylated. The result is Hgb_{1A}, Hgb_{1B}, and Hgb_{1C}. Increased levels of circulating glucose cause an increase in glycosylation. Because this process is irreversible, a sample of blood provides information about the average amount of blood glucose that has been present over the previous 3 to 4 months.This test is not routinely performed as a pancreatic screening tool. It is used most frequently for patients diagnosed with diabetes mellitus. It provides information about the degree of hyperglycemia, including the actual increased values over a specific period of time. This test eliminates many variables that normally could affect the accurate interpretation of a glucose test result. Fasting state, exercise, stress, and medications do not interfere with this test result. Nor will the test outcome be influenced by patient compliance or changes in a patient's usual habits initiated only to have a fasting blood glucose value read closer to normal than it usually is.

◆ **Ketones.** In a blood test the normal results are ketones 2 to 4 mg/dl of blood; acetone 0.3 to 2 mg/dl of blood. Normally ketones are not present in the urine; thus the results of urine tests would be negative. Ketones are by-products of fat metabolism. In most cases, when the body utilizes carbohydrate as its main source of energy, fat metabolism is complete and only a trace of ketones is found in the blood. In the absence of glucose, fats are burned for energy. Lipolysis (fat breakdown) occurs so rapidly that fat metabolism is incomplete, and ketone bodies (acetone, beta-hydroxybutyric acid, and acetoacetic acid) collect in the blood (ketonemia) and are excreted in the urine (ketonuria).

Both blood and urine specimens can be tested in the laboratory or with reagent strips. Urine samples also can be tested with specially prepared tablets. Both reagent strips and tablets are compared with a color chart. These bedside urine tests are easily performed and provide immediate information regarding ketoacidosis in a person with hyperglycemia.

Ketonemia is observed by a fruity, sweet-smelling odor on the exhaled breath. This odor is the result of the body's attempt to keep the pH within the normal range. A sweet-smelling breath occurs when the lungs release carbon dioxide in an attempt to decrease the accumulated acids.

◆ **Serum osmolality.** In blood samples the normal range for serum osmolality is 285 to 300 mOsm/kg of water. Osmolality is a measurement of the number of particles in a solution (concentration of the solution) and not the size or weight of the particles. This diagnostic test is not a routine screening tool for pancreatic dysfunction. It is used commonly to identify the effects of an imbalance in carbohydrate metabolism and to assess fluid volume status.

An accumulation of ketone bodies and ketoacids results from the rapid, incomplete breakdown of fat and protein. The ketone bodies and ketoacids collect in the plasma as metabolic "debris" and, along with the increasing levels of glucose that cannot enter the cell, drastically increase the number of particles that normally circulate in the plasma. This increase in circulating particles, coupled with the fluid loss from osmotic diuresis, significantly raises the plasma osmolality.

Pituitary

No single diagnostic test identifies dysfunctioning of the posterior pituitary gland. Diagnosis usually is made through a combination of laboratory tests combined with the clinical profile of the patient.

The diagnostic tests measure the amount of antidiuretic hormone released into the blood stream. The tests include both a measurement of the ADH that is produced by the hypothalamus and tests that gauge the subsequent release of ADH by the neurohypophysis. Serum and urine osmolality tests measure the effectiveness of ADH in maintaining the correct solute concentration for the particular sample of fluid.

◆ **Serum antidiuretic hormone.** The normal result of a blood test for serum ADH is 1 to 5 pg/ml (picogram = 1 ÷ trillion), or <1.5 mg/L. The serum ADH test measures the amount of ADH present in a frozen sample of blood. The direct measurement of ADH is possible by means of a laboratory method called *radioimmunoassay*. This diagnostic procedure provides accurate results and, when available, is used in preference to water load and water deprivation tests (discussed later).

To prepare a patient for this radioimmunoassay testing, all drugs that may alter the release of ADH are withheld for a minimum of 8 hours. Medications that affect ADH levels are morphine sulfate, lithium carbonate, chlorothiazide, carbamazepine, oxytocin, and certain neoplastic and anesthetic agents (see Table 41-4 for additional drugs). Nicotine, alcohol, both positive and negative pressure ventilation, and emotional stress also can influence the ADH levels and must be considered in the interpretation of values.

The test is read by comparing serum ADH levels with the blood and urine osmolality. The presence of increased ADH in the blood stream compared with a low serum osmolality and elevated urine osmolality confirms the diagnosis of syndrome of inappropriate antidiuretic hormone (SIADH). Reduced levels of serum ADH in a patient with high serum osmolality, hypernatremia, and reduced urine concentration signal central diabetes insipidus.

◆ **Urine and blood osmolality.** Normal values are serum osmolality, 285 to 300 mOsm/kg H_2O; outermost range for urine osmolality, 50 to 1200 mOsm/kg H_2O, with the average found within 300 to 800 mOsm/kg H_2O. Osmolality measurements determine the concentration of dissolved particles in a solution. In a healthy person a change in the concentration of solutes triggers a chain of events to maintain proper dilution.

Increased serum osmolality stimulates the release of ADH, which in turn reduces the amount of water lost at the tubules. Body fluid thereby is retained to dilute the particle concentration in the blood stream. Decreased serum osmolality inhibits the release of ADH, the kidney tubules increase their permeability, and fluid is eliminated from the body in an attempt to regain normal concentration of particles in the blood stream.

The most accurate results of the body's ability to maintain a fluid balance are obtained when urine and blood samples are collected simultaneously.

◆ **Water deprivation test.** Normal values for this test are urine osmolality, >800 mOsm/kg H_2O; serum osmolality, 285 to 300 mOsm/kg H_2O. The water deprivation test is based on the premise that ADH is released to conserve urinary water when a patient is at risk of becoming dehydrated. This procedure purposely withholds all fluid while laboratory tests determine the body's response to the pending dehydration. (Sensitive radioimmunoassay serum ADH test, discussed earlier, is performed in preference to this test.)

Usually all fluids are withheld for 24 hours. Normally such a deprivation of fluids stimulates the release of ADH to conserve urine to maintain serum osmolality. In a balanced state the serum osmolality remains constant while the urine osmolality increases.

Patients with reduced levels of ADH are unable to curtail fluid losses through the urine despite increases in blood osmolality. Elevated serum osmolality with a urine osmolality that is either equal to or less than the serum concentration indicates continued loss of urinary fluid despite hemoconcentration.

To prevent serious fluid imbalances, the nurse must carefully evaluate the patient's response to this dehydration test. The patient must be weighed frequently to detect the amount of fluid lost (for every 2 pounds, 3 ounces decrease in weight, a quart of body fluid is lost). It is important that such variables as different scales, amount of clothing, and urine volume in the bladder be eliminated so that the weight recorded accurately reflects the patient's body mass. Blood pressure is taken every 1 to 2 hours to identify decreased blood volume that could indicate pending vascular collapse. Serum sodium levels also are monitored for a disproportionate rise in sodium compared with the reduced blood volume. Diabetes insipidus is suspected when reduced levels of ADH occur with increased serum osmolality and reduced urine concentration.

Water deprivation test results usually are followed up with a subcutaneous injection of aqueous Pitressin (synthetic ADH). This phase of testing provides information to differentiate the type of diabetes insipidus. Serial urine samples are collected for 2 hours, and the urine volume and osmolality are measured.

The patient with normal hypophyseal functioning responds to the exogenous ADH by reabsorbing water at the tubule and raising the urine osmolality slightly less than 5%.[4] In cases of severe central diabetes insipidus, the urine osmolality rises over 50%. This result indicates that the cell receptor sites on the renal tubules are responsive to Pitressin. Test results in which urine osmolality remains unchanged are suggestive of nephrogenic diabetes insipidus, indicating that the target tissue or cell receptor sites are no longer receptive to the ADH.

◆ **Water load test.** In urine tests, normal values of urine osmolality range from 50 to 1200 mOsm/kg H_2O, 300 to 900 mOsm/kg H_2O random specimen[5]; urine specific gravity, 1.005 to 1.030. The water load test is based on the premise that changes in the concentration of particles in the blood stream will affect the release of ADH as the body strives to maintain a homeostatic balance. This test overhydrates the patient and then provides a series of blood and urine tests to monitor the sequence of physiologic events leading to a fluid balance. (Sensitive radioimmunoassay serum ADH test, discussed on p. 691, is performed in preference to this test.)

The patient is given nothing by mouth overnight. He or she is instructed not to smoke (nicotine can stimulate ADH release) and not to take medications that alter ADH levels (see Table 41-4 for medications). The patient is asked to drink 20 ml of water per kilogram of body weight within 15 to 30 minutes. Intravenous 5% dextrose in water is given over 8 to 10 minutes if oral fluid cannot be taken.

Serial urine samples are collected for 4 to 5 hours and tested for volume, osmolality, and specific gravity. A serum osmolality also is obtained at the end of the test, and its result is compared with the entire volume of urine collected during the test.

This hypotonic fluid load test decreases the urine osmolality in a healthy subject. Patients with excessive ADH have decreased serum osmolality while maintaining either a constant or elevated urine concentration.

This test subjects patients with cardiac or renal dysfunctions to circulatory overload. Frequent assessment for the signs of cardiac decompensation, such as dyspnea, chest pain, moist breath sounds, jugular vein distention, and elevated central venous and pulmonary artery pressures, is required. The test also requires 4 to 5 hours before an accurate determination can be made.

Decreasing the patient's serum osmolality with overhydration has a dilutional effect on the serum sodium level, resulting in a mild dilutional hyponatremia. Thus the patient should be carefully observed for sodium changes, including gastrointestinal stimulation, cramps, diarrhea, apprehension, and changes in personality.

Thyroid

Thyroxine (T_4) and triiodothyronine (T_3) are found both tightly bound to plasma proteins and freely circulating in the blood stream. It is in the free state that the thyroid hormone is active. The production of T_4 and T_3 depends on a negative feedback system whereby low levels of the hormone stimulate the hypothalamus to secrete thyroid-releasing hormone (TRH). TRH then stimulates the anterior pituitary to produce thyroid-stimulating hormone (TSH).

The TSH prompts the thyroid gland to initiate the synthesis of thyroxine and triiodothyronine through a complex process of converting ingested iodine into T_4 and T_3. Thyrotoxicosis, the precursor of thyrotoxic crisis, is diagnosed in part by elevated T_4 and T_3 serum levels. Laboratory levels of TSH and TRH are measured to confirm thyrotoxicosis, as well as to identify the cause as thyroid or extrathyroid. Extrathyroid conditions implicate a source other than the thyroid gland as cause of the increased hormones. Examples of these conditions are interference with feedback system, pituitary dysfunction, and thyroid malignancy that produces hormones despite the body's needs.

The laboratory tests to determine T_3 and T_4 levels in thyrotoxicosis are not complex and require no special patient preparation. Tests most commonly performed on a thyroid panel are listed in Table 42-1. The tests, however, may be inconclusive in the critically ill patient because hormonal adaptation to the stress of the illness and common problems of protein malnutrition in critical care situations influence the thyroid hormone production.[6,7] Additional disadvantages inherent in the thyroid laboratory tests are the adjustments that need to be made for the individual variables in serum protein levels—for example, the elderly patient,[6,7] the pregnant woman, and persons with hepatitis and acute intermittent porphyria.[6,8] Concomitant use of certain drugs also must be considered. Heparin, corticosteroids, and dopamine interfere with thyroid test results. See the box, p. 694, for additional drugs that interfere with thyroid test results.[6,7,9,10]

DIAGNOSTIC PROCEDURES

Pituitary

In addition to laboratory tests, the use of radiographic examination, computerized tomography, and magnetic resonance imaging is helpful in diagnosing hypothalamic-hypophyseal disease. Although these tests may not definitively diagnose diabetes insipidus or syndrome of inappropriate antidiuretic hormone, they are useful in diagnosing the primary causes of these diseases. Cranial bone fractures that injure the hypophyseal stalk and space-occupying masses, such as tumors or blood clots that interfere with pituitary circulation, are examples of abnormalities identified and studied in diagnostic tests.

◆ **Radiologic examination.** A basic x-ray examination of the inferior skull views the sella turcica and surrounding bone formation. Bone fractures or tissue swelling at the base of the brain, which is apparent on a radiograph, suggests interference with the vascular supply and nerve impulses to the hypothalamic-pituitary system. Dysfunction may occur if the hypophysis, the infundibular stalk, or the neurohypophysis is impaired.

◆ **Computerized axial tomography.** Computerized tomography (CT) of the base of the skull (sella turcica) identifies pituitary tumors, blood clots, cysts, nodules, or other tissue masses. A skull CT scan provides more definitive results than does a radiograph and, whenever possible, is obtained in preference to a skull radiograph. The 40-minute procedure causes no discomfort except that it requires the patient to be perfectly still. A radiopaque sodium iodine solution may be given intravenously to highlight the hypothalamus, infundibular stalk, and pituitary gland. This dye may cause allergic reactions in iodine-sensitive persons, and the patient must be carefully questioned before the start of the test.

Multiple x-ray beams pass through the head from specific angles while detectors record the attenuation (absorption or scattering) of the x-ray beam. The x-rays pass through the head on a predetermined axis, producing images of minute slices or layers of brain tissue. As the x-rays pass through bone, soft tissue, and body fluid, a portion of the beam is absorbed or scattered, depending on the density of the tissue. A computer then

Table 42-1 Tests most commonly performed on a thyroid panel

Test	Normal adult value	Conditions with abnormal values: Decreased	Conditions with abnormal values: Increased	Special consideration
Serum thyroxine (T_4)	T_4, 4.5-11.5 μg/dl T_4RIA, 5-12 μg/dl	Hypothyroidism Protein malnutrition Anterior pituitary hypofunction	Hyperthyroidism Viral hepatitis Acute/chronic illness	Simple peripheral blood withdrawal Identifies amount of hormone in circulation Bound by serum protein, therefore affected by TBG Affected by pregnancy
Free thyroid index (FT_4I)	Free T_4, 0.8-2.3 ng/dl	Hypothyroidism	Hyperthyroidism	Same as above, except this measures amount of free T_4, the unbound portion of which enters the cells T_3 uptake multiplied by T_4 equals FTI
Serum triiodothyronine (T_3) (T_3RIA)	110-230 ng/dl	Hypothyroidism Malnutrition Trauma Critical illness	Thyrotoxicosis Toxic adenoma Thyroiditis	Simple peripheral blood withdrawal Measured directly by RIA Direct measurement of both bound and free T_3 Values increase in pregnancy
T_3 uptake ratio (T_3 UR) T_3 resin uptake	25%-35% uptake 0.8-1.30 ratio of laboratory result to standard control	Hypothyroidism Active hepatitis Thyroiditis	Hyperthyroidism Nephrosis Malignancy Protein malnutrition	Does not measure T_3 as name implies Indirectly measures TBG available to bind T_3 and T_4; increase in thyrotoxicosis related to increase in thyroid hormone binding[7] Affected by pregnancy Affected by diseases that alter these proteins
Serum thyroid-stimulating hormone (TSH) test	2-5.4 mU/L <3 ng/ml	Secondary hypothyroidism Anterior pituitary disorder, very low levels, 0.005 mU/L, indicate hyperthyroidism[6]	Primary hypothyroidism Cirrhosis	Identifies thyroid vs. pituitary-hypothalamus disorder
Serum thyrotropin-releasing hormone (TRH), Stimulation test, or Thyrotropin-releasing factor (TRF) test	Serum TSH rises approximately twice its normal level 30 min after IV TRH			Test confirms presence of thyrotoxicosis by measuring response of the pituitary gland's production of TSH 3-4 wk before test, thyroid medication should be discontinued 500 μg of TRH is given IV to mimic the hypothalamus Venous blood samples are taken at intervals as stated by processing laboratory; peak response occurs in 20 min and returns to normal within 2 hr

FTI, Free thyroid index; *RIA*, radioimmunoassay; *TBG*, thyroxine-binding globulin.

DRUGS THAT INFLUENCE DIAGNOSTIC THYROID LEVELS

TRIIODOTHYRONINE (T_3)

Increase	Decrease
Methadone	Anabolic steroid
Estrogens	Androgens
Progestins	Salicylates
Amiodarone	Phenytoin
	Lithium
	Reserpine
	Propranolol
	Sulfonamides
	Propylthiouracil
	Methylthiouracil

THYROXINE (T_4)

Increase	Decrease
Oral contraceptives	Phenytoin
Heparin	Steroids
Aspirin	Diphenylhydantoin
Furosemide	Chlorpromazine
Clofibrate	Lithium
Phenylbutazone	Sulfonylurea
Some nonsteroidal antiinflammatory drugs (NSAIDs)	Sulfonamides
	Reserpine
	Chlordiazepoxide
Propranolol	
Corticosteroids	
Amiodarone	

THYROID-STIMULATING HORMONE (TSH)

Increase TSH	Decrease TSH and TSH response to TRH
Metoclopramide	Glucocorticoids
Iodides	Dopamine
Lithium	Heparin
Potassium iodide	Aspirin
Morphine sulfate	Carbamazepine

THYROXINE-BINDING GLOBULIN (TBG)

Increase	Decrease
Opiates	Androgen therapy
Oral contraceptives	L-Asparaginase
Estrogens	
Clofibrate	
5-Fluorouracil (5-FU)	
Perphenazine	

calculates the degree of attenuated x-rays over very small areas. The resulting data are then projected on a viewing screen as an image of the head.

The tomogram is interpreted by a radiologist for size and shape of the sella turcica and position of the hypothalamus, infundibular stalk, and pituitary gland. Tissue density changes are noted, and a diagnostic impression is made.

◆ **Magnetic resonance imaging.** Magnetic resonance imaging (MRI) enables the radiologist to visualize internal organs, as well as examine the cellular characteristics of specific tissue. MRI uses a magnetic field rather than x-rays to produce images of internal structures of the body. The body part under examination is presented in cross-sectional slices as a high-resolution image.

The soft fluid tissue in and immediately surrounding the brain makes the brain especially responsive to MRI scanning. Although the MRI is not a definitive diagnostic test for posterior pituitary hormonal imbalance, its use identifies anatomic disruption of the gland and the surrounding area suggestive of primary causes of diabetes insipidus and SIADH.

Thyroid

◆ **Thyroid scanning.** Thyroid scanning involves the use of oral radioactive iodine. ^{123}I is the preferred isotope because of its low-energy, 13-hour output. This short half-life minimizes the patient's exposure to radioactive material. The thyroid-scanning procedure is useful in detecting the presence of ectopic thyroid tissue and thyroid carcinomas. Thyroid scans also identify the presence and amount of viable thyroid glandular tissue after irradiation treatment.

REFERENCES

1. Wilson JD and others, editors: *Harrison's principles of internal medicine,* ed 12, New York, 1991, McGraw-Hill.
2. Ganong WF: *Review of medical physiology,* ed 15, Norwalk, Conn, 1991, Appleton & Lange.
3. Kelley W, editor: *Textbook of internal medicine,* vol 2, ed 2, Philadelphia, 1992, JB Lippincott.
4. Henry J, editor: *Davidsohn's Clinical diagnosis and management by laboratory methods,* ed 18, Philadelphia, 1990, WB Saunders.
5. Horne M, Easterday Heitz U, Swearingen PL: *Fluid, electrolyte, and acid-base balance: a case study approach,* St Louis, 1991, Mosby–Year Book.
6. Sox HC, editor: *Common diagnostic tests: use and interpretation,* ed 2, Philadelphia, 1990, American College of Physicians.
7. Shoemaker W and others: *Textbook of critical care,* ed 2, Philadelphia, 1989, WB Saunders.
8. Pagana KD, Pagana TJ: *Diagnostic testing and nursing implications: a case study approach,* ed 3, St Louis, 1990, Mosby–Year Book.
9. LeFever Kee J: *Laboratory and diagnostic tests with nursing implications,* ed 3, Norwalk, Conn, 1991, Appleton & Lange.
10. Tietz N, editor: *Clinical guide to laboratory tests,* ed 2, Philadelphia, 1990, WB Saunders.

43

Endocrine Disorders and Therapeutic Management

CHAPTER OBJECTIVES

- Define the concepts of plasma hyperosmolality and osmotic diuresis; discuss why and how osmotic diuresis occurs with plasma hyperosmolality.
- Explain the pathophysiology of diabetic ketoacidosis, and list at least four clinical manifestations that identify both early and late stages of this disorder.
- List the priorities of nursing management for a patient with early clinical manifestations of diabetic ketoacidosis.
- Identify at least three factors that compose a high-risk profile for the patient with hyperglycemic hyperosmolar nonketotic coma.
- List the priorities of nursing management for a patient with either diabetes insipidus or syndrome of inappropriate antidiuretic hormone.
- Discuss the nursing interventions that are essential in the treatment of fluid volume deficit resulting from decreased secretion of antidiuretic hormone.
- Identify and describe nursing interventions that are essential in the treatment of fluid volume excess related to increased secretion of antidiuretic hormone.
- Summarize the most critical nursing considerations for the patient with thyrotoxic crisis.

DIABETIC KETOACIDOSIS

Description

Diabetic ketoacidosis (DKA) is a serious complication of diabetes mellitus. It poses a life-threatening situation to the patient with type I, insulin-dependent diabetes, although it rarely affects the patient with type II, non–insulin-dependent diabetes. Diabetic ketoacidosis is a significant community health problem with a major financial impact. Approximately 45,000 to 130,000 hospitalizations for DKA occur annually, based on a population of 10 million persons with diabetes. Of DKA episodes, 20% occur in persons with newly diagnosed diabetes, whereas the other 80% occur after the diagnosis has been made. The average age of patients with DKA is 43 years, showing that this complication occurs more in the older person with diabetes than in the adolescent.[1] Of all deaths attributed to diabetes 10% result from DKA.[2] It is estimated, however, that these deaths occur not from the ketoacidotic state alone, but rather from late complications (pneumonia, myocardial infarction, infection) resulting from DKA.[3] Available statistics show that the mortality for patients hospitalized for DKA is 9%, with DKA mortality for females higher than that for males. The death rate from DKA is 3 times higher in the nonwhite population than in the white population.[1]

Ketoacidosis may develop over several hours in a person who has had diabetes for a period of time. In an undiagnosed diabetic patient, it may take days to develop and signal an abrupt onset of the disease.

Etiology

Ketoacidosis results from an alteration in the insulin and counterregulatory hormones, glucagon, growth hormone, cortisol, and catecholamines.[1] The box on p. 696 lists the possible causes of DKA in terms of decreased insulin availability and increased presence of glucose in the blood stream. Changes in self-management of diabetes can influence this ratio, as can a decrease in insulin intake, an increase in dietary intake, or a decrease in routine exercise without adequate adjustment in insulin or diet. Life-style changes, such as growth spurts in the adolescent, require an increase in insulin intake, as do surgery, infection, and trauma. Emotional stress can increase glucose levels by releasing epinephrine or norepinephrine, or both, which triggers increased glucagon secretion. The person may be continuing a routine insulin dose that is then inadequate for the rate of glucose entry into the blood stream from gluconeogenesis and glycogenolysis triggered by the stress hormones.

Recently, DKA has been seen in patients who use the new insulin pump devices that aim to provide tighter glucose control. Improper functioning resulting in insulin leakage or pump failure[4] initially causes subtle changes in glucose levels. The patient, believing that his or her glucose level is adequately controlled by the pump, attributes the physical symptoms to extraneous health problems. Tending to trust the functioning of the pump, the patient delays testing serum glucose and urine ketones while DKA is progressively developing.

Pathophysiology

Insulin is the metabolic key to the transfer of glucose from the blood stream into the cell where it can be used immediately for energy or stored to be used at a later

ETIOLOGY OF DIABETIC KETOACIDOSIS

DECREASED EXOGENOUS INSULIN INTAKE

- Lack of knowledge, poor compliance
  - Omitting dose
  - Insufficient dose to meet glucose requirement (e.g., hyperalimentation)
- Malfunctioning insulin pump
- Pharmacologic drugs
  - Phenytoin
  - Thiazide/sulfonamide diuretics

INCREASED ENDOGENOUS GLUCOSE

- Diabetes management changes
  - Decreased exercise without decreasing food or increasing insulin
  - Increased dietary intake
- Sympathetic nervous system responses
  - Stressful events
    - Injury
    - Surgery
    - Infections
      - Respiratory tract
      - Urinary tract
      - Pancreatitis
    - Emotional trauma
- Increased glucagon
- Increased growth hormone
- Pharmacologic drugs
  - Steroid therapy
  - Epinephrine/norepinephrine

time. Without the necessary insulin, glucose remains in the blood stream, and cells are deprived of their energy source. A complex pathophysiologic chain of events follows (Fig. 43-1). The release of glucagon is stimulated when insulin is ineffective in providing the cells with glucose for energy. Glucagon increases the amount of glucose in the blood stream by breaking down stored glucose (glycogenolysis) and converting noncarbohydrate molecules into glucose (gluconeogenesis). Blood glucose levels for the patient in diabetic ketoacidosis typically range from 300 to 800 mg/dl of blood. (Blood glucose levels alone do not diagnose DKA; ketoacidosis, which is discussed later, is a major determining factor). The hyperglycemia increases the plasma osmolality, and blood becomes hyperosmolar. Cellular dehydration occurs as the hyperosmolar extracellular fluid draws the more dilute intracellular and interstitial fluid into the vascular space in an attempt to return the plasma osmolality to normal. Dehydration stimulates catecholamine production for further glycogenolysis, lipolysis, gluconeogenesis, and ketogenesis.

Excessive urination and glycosuria occur as a result of the osmotic diuresis. The excess glucose, filtered at the glomeruli, cannot be reabsorbed at the renal tubule and "spills" into the urine. The unreabsorbed solute exerts its own osmotic pull in the renal tubules, and less water is returned to circulation via the collecting ducts. As a result, large volumes of water, along with sodium, potassium, and phosphorus, are excreted in the urine.

Polydipsia occurs as the decrease in the circulating blood volume stimulates the osmoreceptors in the hypothalamus and promotes the release of angiotensin II. This initiates a strong thirst sensation intended to compensate for the loss of fluids and replenish the circulating blood volume. The fluid volume deficit also stimulates vasoconstriction as a means to preserve blood pressure. Both the vasoconstriction and the extremely elevated levels of glucose impair the delivery of oxygen to the peripheral cells, which impedes the removal of metabolic wastes.

As DKA progresses, gluconeogenesis continues to convert noncarbohydrate molecules into glucose. Ketoacidosis occurs as ketoacid end products accumulate in the blood and rapid, incomplete fatty acid metabolism releases highly acidic substances (acetoacetic acid and beta-hydroxybutyric acid) into the blood stream (ketonemia) and the urine (ketonuria).

The patient with moderate to severe DKA typically has a pH of less than 7.2, whereas in mild DKA the pH may be less than 7.36.[1] The acid ketones dissociate and yield hydrogen ions (H^+) that accumulate and cause a drop in serum pH. Normally the hydrogen ions react with bicarbonate (HCO_3^-) to produce carbonic acid (H_2CO_3). Carbonic acid dissociates to form water (H_2O) and carbon dioxide (CO_2), which are eliminated through the kidneys and the lungs, respectively. In gluconeogenesis, however, ketones accumulate in the blood stream faster than they can be metabolized. The bicarbonate and sodium loss through osmotic diuresis prevents the formation of sodium bicarbonate needed to buffer the increasing carbonic acid. The respiratory rate is altered in an attempt to compensate for the carbonic acid build-up. Breathing becomes deep and rapid (Kussmaul's respirations) to release carbonic acid in the form of carbon dioxide. Acetone is exhaled, giving the breath its characteristic "fruity" odor.

Gluconeogenesis stimulates mobilization of protein, and protein catabolism increases. Protein is broken down and converted to glucose in the liver. Continuous, uninterrupted gluconeogenesis leaves no reserve protein available for synthesis and repair of vital body tissues.

Nitrogen accumulates as protein is metabolized. Urea, added to the blood stream, increases the osmotic diuresis and accentuates the dehydration. Loss of muscle mass and reduced resistance to infection occur with impaired protein utilization. The combined states of acidosis and osmotic diuresis lead to a loss of phosphorus, further compromising peripheral tissue perfusion. Hypophosphatemia impairs the oxygen function of the hemoglobin by increasing hemoglobin's affinity for oxygen and thereby reducing delivery of oxygen to the cells.[5]

Assessment and Diagnosis

Diabetic ketoacidosis usually is preceded by patient complaints of malaise, headache, polyuria (excessive urination), polydipsia (excessive thirst), and polyphagia (excessive hunger). Nausea, vomiting, extreme fatigue, dehydration, and weight loss follow. Central nervous

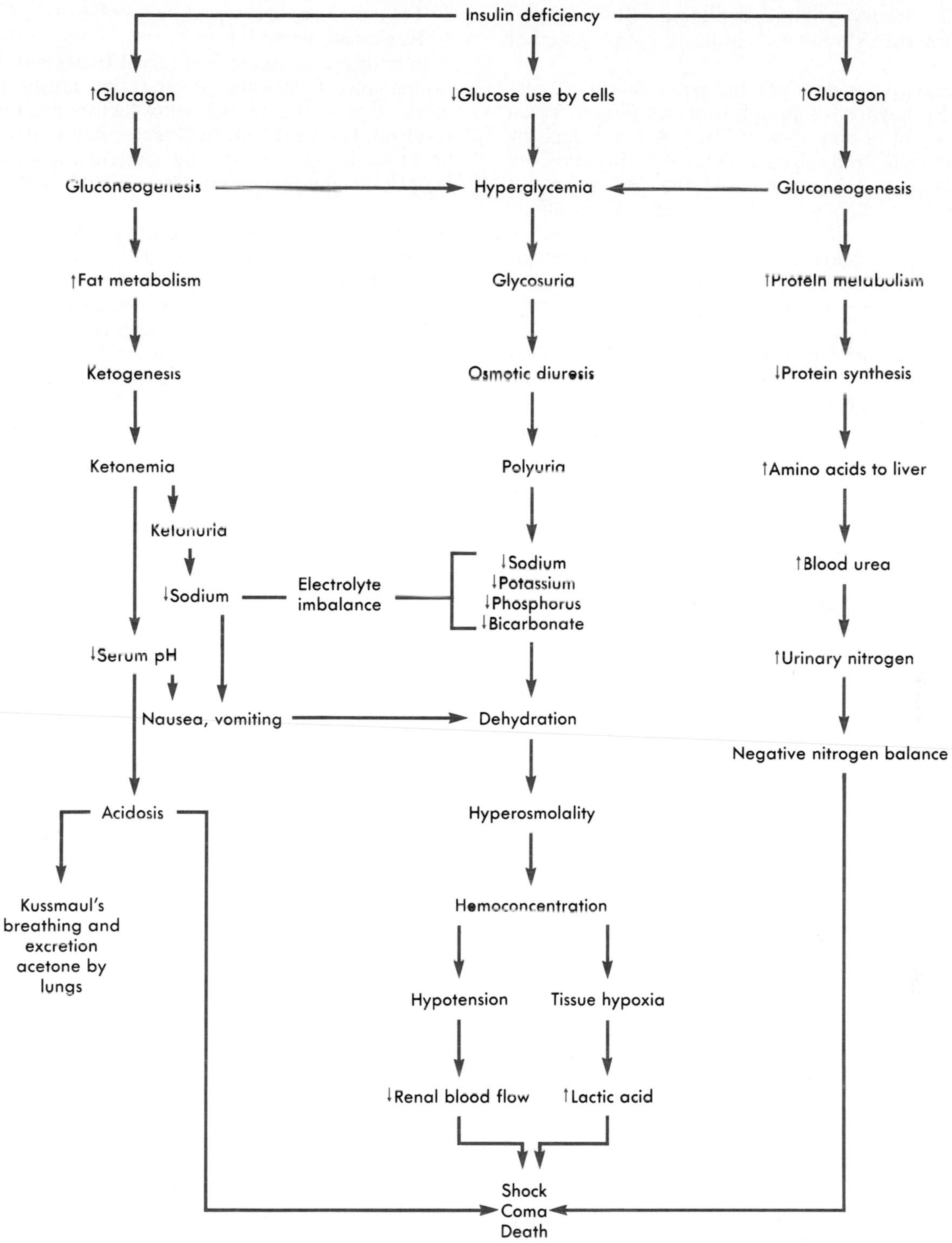

Fig. 43-1 Pathophysiology of diabetic ketoacidosis (DKA). A carbohydrate derangement affects the metabolism of both protein and fat.

system depression, with changes in the level of consciousness, can lead quickly to coma.

The patient with DKA may be stuporous or unconscious, depending on the degree of fluid-balance disturbance. The physical examination reveals evidence of dehydration, including flushed, dry skin, dry buccal membranes, and skin turgor greater than 3 seconds. Frequently, "sunken eyeballs," resulting from the lack of fluid in the interstitium of the eyeball, are observed. Tachycardia and hypotension may signal profound fluid losses. Kussmaul's air hunger continues to reveal a "fruity" odor of acetone. Normal or subnormal temperatures exist despite volume depletion. An increased temperature at this point may indicate the presence of infection.[3]

Considering the complexity and potential seriousness of DKA, the diagnosis is straightforward. With a known diabetic patient, a diagnosis of DKA is determined by heavy ketonuria and glycosuria in the presence of hyperglycemia and ketonemia. If the patient is not known to have diabetes, other causes of metabolic acidosis must be differentiated before a course of therapy is begun. Starvation, alcoholism, certain toxic chemicals, lactic acid, and uremia may result in a ketoacidotic state.[3] The treatment plan varies, depending on the cause.

Urine ketones and bedside fingerstick blood sugar determinations provide rapid confirmation of ketoacidosis in the diabetic patient. Laboratory evidence supporting the ketoacidosis includes low arterial blood pH and low plasma bicarbonate levels.[6]

Dehydration manifests by an increased serum osmolality, elevated hematocrit level, marked leukocytosis (regardless of presence of infection), increased blood urea nitrogen (BUN), and a high urine specific gravity. Extreme catabolism is seen in severe hypertriglyceridemia, ketonemia, and ketonuria.[7]

Electrolyte imbalances result from the osmotic diuresis and fluid depletion. Vomiting and polyuria cause a decrease in serum sodium and potassium levels. Hyponatremia also occurs from the shift of extracellular sodium to intracellular spaces as the potassium is depleted.

Serum potassium levels vary, depending on the phase of ketoacidosis. Potassium levels may be elevated as potassium moves from the intracellular compartment to the extracellular compartment in an exchange for hydrogen ions. Hyperkalemia is reduced quickly as potassium is lost from the body by the vomiting, diarrhea, and osmotic diuresis. Phosphorus levels also may be low, normal, or elevated despite actual serum depletion. Assessment of electrolyte levels must continue throughout the treatment phase inasmuch as both potassium and phosphorus rapidly reenter the cell when fluid and insulin therapy are provided.

Medical Management

Diagnosis of DKA is based on the combined presenting symptoms, patient history, medical history (type I diabetes mellitus), precipitating factors if known, and results of serum glucose and urine ketone testing. Additional information is obtained from laboratory serum electrolyte values, arterial blood gases, urinalysis, and a baseline electrocardiogram. Emergency medical treatment is aimed at reversing the ketoacidosis.

Once diagnosed, DKA requires aggressive medical and nursing management to prevent progressive decompensation. Treatment is needed to accomplish the following:

1. Reverse dehydration
2. Restore the insulin-glucagon ratio:
   To promote cellular use of glucose
   To reduce the counterregulatory hormone, glucagon
   To break the ketotic cycle
3. Treat and prevent circulatory collapse
4. Replenish electrolytes

In addition to vigorous medical treatment, the practitioner investigates the precipitating causes of ketoacidosis. Unless the precipitating factors are known and resolved, DKA probably will recur. After 10 to 12 hours of effective treatment, the patient's hydration and neurologic and metabolic status should improve drastically.

◆ **Hydration.** The patient with DKA is significantly dehydrated, may have lost 5% to 10% of body weight in fluids, and may have a fluid deficit of 3 to 5 L.[4] There is no consensus among medical practitioners on the use of isotonic or hypotonic solution as a replacement for lost fluid. Initially, normal physiologic saline may be given to reverse the vascular deficit, hypotension, and extracellular fluid losses. During the first hour of severe dehydration 1 L is infused. The rate, however, varies, depending on urinary output, secondary illnesses, and precipitating factors. To dilute the serum osmolality, infusions of half-strength sodium chloride may follow the initial saline replacement. Because the water deficit exceeds the sodium loss, half-strength sodium chloride can be given at a rate of 300 to 500 ml/hr until the serum osmolality returns to normal and the blood glucose levels decrease.

Once the serum glucose level is 250 to 300 mg/dl of blood, a 5% dextrose solution is infused.[4] Intravenously administered glucose is necessary to replenish glucose stores because muscle and liver glycogen reserves may have been depleted during gluconeogenesis. It also is necessary to prevent hypoglycemia, which may result from a relative drop in circulating glucose. In addition, glucose is given to prevent cerebral edema, which may result when free water is drawn across the blood-brain barrier into brain tissue (although several theories exist, the exact mechanism involved in this alteration in the blood-brain barrier is not known[8]). Intravenous glucose is maintained until the patient no longer requires intravenous fluids and is taking liquids by mouth.

◆ **Insulin administration.** Insulin is given simultaneously with intravenous fluids. A reversal of the ketoacidotic metabolic abnormalities gradually occurs as the patient becomes hydrated and receives insulin. The serum glucose level falls as large quantities of glucose are perfused through the kidneys and removed in the urine. The exogenous insulin complements the fluid therapy and promotes the entry of glucose into the cell (insulin also permits potassium and phosphorous to reenter the cell). Insulin inhibits the release of glucagon, and glucose no longer is poured into circulation as a result of gluconeogenesis and glycogenolysis. The ketoacidotic cycle gradually is broken because ketoacids no longer are produced as a by-product of incomplete fat metabolism. The serum osmolality is reduced with vigorous fluid replacement, coupled with the reduction of glucose, urea, and ketones circulating in the blood stream. Osmotic diuresis is reversed as the continuous fluids replace fluid losses, and serum glucose levels return to normal.

The traditional use of large doses of insulin has slowly given way to lower, continuous intravenous doses of insulin. A bolus of 0.3 U/kg may be given to saturate the insulin cell receptor sites and compete with any insulin resistance at the cell receptor site. Replacement of low-dose insulin, 0.1 U/kg/hr (approximately 5 to 10 U/hr), is given intravenously (or intramuscularly depending on circulatory perfusion) until acidosis is reversed.

◆ **Potassium administration.** Hypokalemia may occur as insulin promotes potassium return to the cell and acidosis is reduced. Unless the initial hypokalemia is severe, potassium may not be given for 3 to 4 hours after treatment begins or until the potassium shift stabilizes. Insulin treatment also precipitates hypophosphatemia as serum phosphate returns to the cell. Although the need to administer phosphate currently is debated, its use does seem to improve tissue oxygenation and promote the renal excretion of hydrogen ions.[3]

◆ **Bicarbonate administration.** The replacement of lost bicarbonate also is controversial. Although intravenously administered bicarbonate promotes the rapid acidotic reversal that leads to alkalosis, the sudden shift in electrolytes may cause deprivation of oxygen. Tissue hypoxia results from the reduced dissociation of oxygen from hemoglobin of cerebrospinal acidosis. It generally is agreed that bicarbonate is started for critically severe acidotic states (pH < 7)[8] and stopped when the pH level reaches 7.2.[4] An indwelling arterial line provides access to hourly sampling of blood gases.

◆ **Prevention of abdominal distention.** Some comatose patients may require gastric intubation to decompress stomach contents and to prevent vomiting and subsequent aspiration. The use of a nasogastric tube also reduces impaired ventilation that results from abdominal distention.

Nursing Management

The management of the patient with DKA demands astute assessments, critical thinking, and quick decision-making. Use of the nursing process helps to organize activities and to promote reversal of symptoms. Because the nurse simultaneously monitors several system functions, collects multiple laboratory values, and provides various interventions, an accurately maintained flow sheet is a necessity.

◆ **Hydration status.** The patient's hydration status is severely compromised in ketoacidosis. Osmotic diuresis and increased insensible loss of fluid from Kussmaul's breathing can result in loss of 10% of total body water.[3] Nausea, vomiting, and changes in level of consciousness interfere with the person's ability to ingest or retain fluids (see box, upper right).

Rapid intravenous fluid replacement requires the use of a volumetric pump when possible. Accurate intake and output measurements must be maintained to record the body's use of fluid. Hourly urine output measures renal functioning and also provides information that helps prevent overhydration or underhydration.

Skin assessment for degree of moisture indicates the body's distribution and use of fluid within body tissues. The patient with ketoacidosis has flushed, dry skin, dry buccal membranes, parched lips, and ropy saliva. The lips and tongue may adhere to the teeth because of decreased fluids. The conscious patient complains of intense thirst, but consumption of large quantities of water may be unwise if there is a concurrent problem with abdominal distention. Quickly drinking a large volume of fluid may add to the distended abdomen and stimulate vomiting. Ice chips may be used as an alternative to quench the patient's thirst, along with reassurance that the intravenous fluids will soon satisfy the thirst.

Oral care, including lip balm, helps keep lips supple and prevents cracking. Prepared sponge sticks or moist gauze pads can be used to moisten oral membranes of the unconscious patient. Swabbing the mouth moistens the tissues and displaces the bacteria that collect when saliva, which has a bacteriostatic action, is curtailed by dehydration. The conscious patient removes bacteria and provides oral comfort with frequent tooth brushing and oral rinsing.

Vital signs, especially pulse rate, hemodynamic findings, and blood pressure, are constantly monitored to assess cardiac response to the fluid replacement. Evidence that fluid replacement is effective includes normal central venous pressure (CVP), decreased heart rate, and normal pulmonary artery pressure (PAP). Further evidence of hydration includes a change from the previously weak, thready pulse to a pulse that is strong and full and a change from a previously low blood pressure to a gradual elevation of systolic blood pressure. Reduced respirations also signal a return to adequate fluid balance.

Circulatory overload from the rapid fluid volume infusion is a serious complication that can occur in the patient with a compromised cardiovascular or renal system, or both. Neck vein engorgement, dyspnea without exertion, elevated CVP and PAP, as well as moist lung sounds, signal circulatory overload. Reduction in the rate and volume of infusion, elevation of the head, administration of oxygen, and oronasopharyngeal suctioning as needed may be required to manage the increased intravascular volume.

HYDRATION ASSESSMENT FOR THE PATIENT IN DIABETIC KETOACIDOSIS (DKA) AND HYPERGLYCEMIC HYPEROSMOLAR NONKETOTIC COMA (HHNC)

Hydration status assessment includes the following:

Hourly intake
Blood pressure changes
- Orthostatic hypotension
- Pulse pressure
- Pulse rate, character, rhythm

Neck vein filling
Skin turgor
Skin moisture
Body weight
Central venous pressure
Pulmonary arterial wedge pressure
Hourly output
Complaints of thirst

Measuring hourly urine is mandatory to assess renal output and adequacy of fluid replacement. Catheterizing the alert patient remains controversial because of the risk of secondary infection. Tests for urine glucose, ketones, and specific gravity, as well as blood glucose, are performed every 30 to 60 minutes at the bedside. Serum osmolality is monitored, and blood urea nitrogen and creatinine levels are assessed for possible renal impairment related to decreased renal perfusion.

◆ **Intravenous replacement considerations.** Insulin is given intravenously to the severely dehydrated patient to ensure absorption when inadequate tissue perfusion is present. The insulin dose must be calculated to accommodate the binding that occurs, which causes insulin to be absorbed by the glass or plastic container and tubing. New inert materials currently are used in collapsible intravenous containers that minimize the drug binding. It is suggested that the institution's pharmacy department protocol be followed so that the prepared solution provides maximum absorption relative to the container and tubing. As dehydration and hypotension diminish, insulin is given intramuscularly or subcutaneously.

Throughout the insulin therapy, both patient response and laboratory data are assessed for changes relating to glucose levels. Reduction in glucose levels is fairly consistent with low-dose therapy as previously discussed. In most patients serum glucose levels decline 75 to 100 mg/dl/hr.[1] Respirations frequently are assessed for changes in rate, depth, and fruity "acetone" odor. When the blood glucose level falls to 250 to 300 mg/dl of blood, a 5% dextrose solution is infused to prevent hypoglycemia. Administration of regular insulin is not discontinued as the glucose level reaches a range of 250 to 300 mg; rather it may be decreased. Signs of hypoglycemia, such as unexpected behavioral changes, diaphoresis, and tremors (see box, upper right), may occur from a relative drop in glucose. Should hypoglycemia occur, insulin is stopped and the physician notified.

Signs of hyperglycemia, such as Kussmaul's respirations, dry skin, and fruity, acetone breath odor (see box just mentioned), also may be related to both physical and emotional stressors that the patient experiences before or during the stay in the critical care unit. Reducing these stressors and their hyperglycemic effects is a worthy challenge for the nurse.

Electrolytes fluctuate throughout the rehydration phase. Standard CCU protocols for administering electrolytes on the basis of laboratory criteria may or may not be followed. The nurse must be aware of both the obvious and the obscure signs that indicate changing electrolyte levels.

Hypokalemia can occur within the first 4 hours of the rehydration-insulin treatment. Continuous cardiac monitoring is required because potassium affects the heart's electrical condition and hyperkalemia or hypokalemia may lead to lethal cardiac dysrhythmias. Hypokalemia is depicted on the cardiac monitor by a prolonged QT interval, a flattened or depressed T wave, and depressed ST segments (see Chapter 15, Fig. 15-3, A & B). Physical signs of hypokalemia include muscle weakness, decreased gastrointestinal motility (evidenced by abdominal distention or paralytic ileus), hypotension, and a weak pulse. Respiratory arrest can occur as a result of severe hypokalemia.

CLINICAL MANIFESTATIONS OF HYPOGLYCEMIA AND HYPERGLYCEMIA

HYPOGLYCEMIA	HYPERGLYCEMIA
Restlessness	Excessive thirst
Apprehension	Excessive urination
Irritability	Hunger
Trembling	Weakness
Weakness	Listlessness
Diaphoresis	Mental fatigue
Pallor	Flushed, dry skin
Paresthesia	Itching
Headache	Headache
Hunger	Nausea
Difficulty thinking	Vomiting
Loss of coordination	Abdominal cramps
Difficulty walking	Dehydration
Difficulty talking	Weak, rapid pulse
Visual disturbances	Postural hypotension
Blurred vision	Hypotension
Double vision	Acetone breath odor
Tachycardia	Kussmaul's respirations
Shallow respirations	Rapid breathing
Hypertension	Changes in level of consciousness
Changes in level of consciousness	Stupor
Seizures	Coma
Coma	

Hyperkalemia occurs with acidosis or when potassium deficit is treated too aggressively in patients with renal insufficiency. Hyperkalemia is noted on a cardiac monitor by a large, peaked T wave, flattened P wave, and a broad, slurred QRS complex (see Chapter 15, Figs. 15-1 and 15-2). Ventricular fibrillation can follow. Additional changes related to increased potassium levels include bradycardia, increased gastrointestinal motility (with nausea and diarrhea), and oliguria. Neuromuscular signs of hyperkalemia include weakness, impaired muscle activity, and flaccid paralysis.

Serum sodium levels fall as the sodium replaces the potassium that moves out of the cells. Sodium is eliminated from the body as a result of the osmotic diuresis. In addition, the hyponatremia is compounded by the vomiting and diarrhea that occur during ketoacidosis. Clinical manifestations of hyponatremia include abdominal cramping, apprehension, postural hypotension, and unexpected behavioral changes.

Sodium chloride is infused as the initial intravenous solution. Maintenance of the saline infusion depends on clinical manifestations of sodium imbalance plus serum laboratory values.

◆ **Basic assessments.** Skin care takes on new dimensions for the patient with diabetic ketoacidosis. Dehydration, hypovolemia, and hypophosphatemia interfere with

NURSING DIAGNOSIS AND MANAGEMENT
Diabetic ketoacidosis

- ◆ Decreased Cardiac Output related to decreased preload secondary to fluid volume deficit, p. 361.
- ◆ Anxiety related to threat to biologic, psychologic, and/or social integrity, p. 763
- ◆ Knowledge Deficit: Self-Care of Diabetes Mellitus related to lack of previous exposure to information, p. 72.
- ◆ Body Image Disturbance related to functional dependence on life-sustaining technology, p. 95.
- ◆ Ineffective Individual Coping related to situational crisis and personal vulnerability, p. 762.
- ◆ Altered Health Maintenance related to lack of perceived threat to health, p. 70.
- ◆ Self-Esteem Disturbance related to feelings of guilt about physical deterioration, p. 96.
- ◆ Powerlessness related to physical deterioration despite compliance, p. 99
- ◆ Hopelessness related to perceptions of failing or deteriorating physical condition, p. 100.

oxygen delivery at the cell site and contribute to inadequate perfusion and tissue breakdown. Patients must be repositioned every hour to relieve capillary pressure and promote adequate perfusion to body tissues. The typical patient with type I diabetes is either of normal weight or underweight. Bony prominences must be assessed and circulation promoted with massage before position change. Irritation of skin from shearing force and detergents is to be avoided. Maintenance of skin integrity prevents unwanted portals of entry for microorganisms. Lung sounds are assessed every 8 hours or as needed. Encouraging the conscious patient to cough and breathe deeply every hour promotes full ventilation of the lungs and helps prevent pulmonary complications. Strict sterile technique is used to maintain all intravenous systems. All venipuncture sites are checked every 4 hours for signs of inflammation, phlebitis, or infiltration. Strict surgical asepsis is used for all invasive procedures. Careful sterile technique is used if catheterization is necessary to obtain urine samples for testing. Catheter care is given every 8 hours.

Changes in the patient's neurologic status may be insidious. Alterations in level of consciousness, pupil reaction, and motor function may be the result of fluctuating glucose levels and cerebral fluid shifts. Confusion and sudden complaints of headache are ominous signs that may signal cerebral edema. These observations require immediate action to prevent neurologic damage. Neurologic assessments performed every 4 hours or as needed, coupled with serum osmolality values, serve as an index of the patient's response to the rehydration therapy.

Throughout the treatment the precipitating causes of the patient's DKA are examined and treated. For the patient whose diabetes is newly diagnosed, teaching about the disease process and self-care is provided. Comprehensive instruction for patients and families involves various health care personnel, including the nurse, dietitian, and physician. During this instruction, emphasis is placed on reducing the anxiety associated with the critical care unit. The patient, however, must appreciate the pathophysiologic process of DKA if diabetes is not properly managed.

For patients with previously diagnosed diabetes, the knowledge level and compliance history are important in formulating a teaching plan. Learning objectives include definition of hyperglycemia, its causes, harmful effects, and symptoms. Additional objectives include a definition of ketoacidosis, its causes, symptoms, and harmful consequences. The patient and family are expected to learn the principles of diabetes management during illness. They also are expected to know the warning signs that must be brought to the attention of a health care practitioner. Education of the patient and family or other persons involved in the patient's supportive care is the goal of the teaching process.

HYPERGLYCEMIC HYPEROSMOLAR NONKETOTIC COMA

Description

Hyperglycemic hyperosmolar nonketotic coma (HHNC) is a frequently lethal complication of diabetes mellitus. The hallmarks of HHNC are extremely high levels of plasma glucose with resulting elevations in hyperosmolality and osmotic diuresis. Inability to replace fluids lost through diuresis or severe diarrhea leads to profound dehydration and changes in level of consciousness. HHNC has a 12% to 50% mortality.[9] The severity of symptoms, plus minimal or absent ketosis, distinguishes HHNC from DKA (Table 43-1).

Etiology

HHNC occurs when the pancreas produces a relatively insufficient amount of insulin for the high levels of glucose that flood the blood stream (see box, p. 703). The disorder occurs mainly, although not exclusively, in elderly obese persons with underlying conditions that require medical treatment. The patient may have type II non-insulin-dependent diabetes that is treated with diet and oral hypoglycemic agents. HHNC also can occur in persons with previously undiagnosed and therefore untreated diabetes.

The extreme hyperglycemia of HHNC can be precipitated by the stress of extensive burns, infection, or other major illness, such as myocardial infarction. The syndrome also may be precipitated by iatrogenic procedures that may increase the serum glucose levels and cause an imbalance in the insulin-glucagon ratio. Such procedures include hyperalimentation, high-calorie enteral feedings, hemodialysis, and peritoneal dialysis. Prescription medications that interfere with pancreatic insulin production may precipitate HHNC, including phenytoin, thiazide diuretics, and diazoxide. Other medications, such as sympathomimetic agents, stimulate gluconeogenesis by increasing glucose levels through the metabolism of protein and fats.

Table 43-1 General comparison of DKA and HHNC

	Diabetic ketoacidosis	Hyperglycemic hyperosmolar nonketotic coma
Cause	Insufficient exogenous insulin for glucose needs	Insufficient exogenous/endogenous insulin for glucose needs
Onset	Sudden (hours)	Slow, insidious (days, weeks)
Predisposing factors	Noncompliance to type I DM, illness, surgery, decreased activity	Elderly with recent acute illness; therapeutic procedures
Mortality	8% to 10%[1]	12% to 50%[2]
Population affected	Type I DM	Type II DM, age >65 yr
Clinical manifestations	Similarities: dry mouth, polydipsia, polyuria, polyphagia, dehydration, dry skin, hypotension, weakness, mental confusion, tachycardia, changes in level of consciousness	
	Differences: Ketoacidosis: air hunger, acetone breath odor, respirations rapid and deep, nausea, vomiting	No ketosis, no breath odor, respirations rapid and shallow, usually mild nausea and vomiting
Laboratory tests		
Serum glucose	300-800 mg/dl	600-2000 mg/dl
Serum ketones	Strongly positive	Normal or mildly elevated
Serum pH	<7.3	Normal
Serum osmolality	<350 mOsm/L	>350 mOsm/L
Serum sodium	Normal or low	Normal or elevated
Serum potassium	Low, normal, or elevated (total body K^+ is depleted)	Low, normal, or elevated
Serum bicarbonate	<15 mEq/L	Normal
Serum phosphorus	Low, normal, or elevated (may decrease after insulin therapy)	Low, normal, or elevated (may decrease after insulin therapy)
Urine glucose*	3% to 4%	4% or highest concentration
Urine acetone	Strong	Absent or mild

DM, Diabetes mellitus.
*Clinitest, 2-drop method.

Pathophysiology

The syndrome of HHNC represents a deficit of insulin and an excess of glucagon. Fig. 43-2 schematically presents the pathophysiology. Reduced insulin levels prevent the movement of glucose into the cells, thus allowing glucose to accumulate in the plasma. Glucagon release is triggered by the decreased insulin, and hepatic glucose from glycogenolysis is poured into circulation. Glucagon also stimulates the metabolism of fat and protein through gluconeogenesis in an attempt to provide cells with an energy source. Excessive glucose, along with the end products of incomplete fat and protein metabolism, collects as debris in the blood stream. As the number of particles increases in the blood, hyperosmolality increases. In an effort to decrease the serum osmolality, fluid is drawn from the intracellular compartment into the vascular bed. Profound intracellular volume depletion occurs if the patient's thirst sensation is absent or decreased, if the patient is unable to respond to thirst, or if fluids are inaccessible.

Hemoconcentration persists despite removal of large amounts of glucose in the urine (glycosuria). The glomerular filtration and elimination of glucose by the kidney tubules are ineffective in reducing serum glucose sufficiently to maintain normal glucose levels. The hyperosmolality and reduced blood volume stimulate the release of antidiuretic hormone to increase tubular reabsorption of water. ADH, however, is powerless in overcoming the osmotic pull exerted by the glucose load. Excessive fluid volume is lost at the kidney tubule with simultaneous loss of potassium, sodium, and phosphate in the urine.

Hypovolemia reduces renal circulation, and oliguria develops. Although this process conserves water and preserves the blood volume, it prevents further glucose loss, and hyperosmolality increases. Ketoacidosis is absent or very mild in HHNC despite the level of free fatty acids resulting from gluconeogenesis. The reasons for lack of ketoacidosis are unclear.[4] It is surmised that the patient may have either a glucagon resistance or sufficient insulin present to prevent the liver from converting fatty acids into ketones.[7]

Failure of the body to regain homeostatic balance further accelerates the life-threatening cycle brought about by hyperglycemia, hyperosmolality, osmotic diuresis, and profound dehydration. In an effort to restore homeostasis, the sympathetic nervous system reacts to the body's stress response. Epinephrine, a potent stimulus for gluconeogenesis, is released, and additional glucose is added to the blood stream. Unless the glycemic diuresis cycle is broken with aggressive fluid replacement, the intracellular dehydration affects fluid and oxygen transport to the brain cells. Central nervous system dysfunctioning may result and lead to coma. Hemoconcentration increases the blood viscosity, which may result in clot formation, thromboemboli, and cerebral, cardiac, and pleural infarcts.[3]

ETIOLOGY OF HYPERGLYCEMIC HYPEROSMOLAR NONKETOTIC COMA

INSUFFICIENT INSULIN
Diabetes mellitus
Pancreatic disease
Pancreatectomy
Pharmacologic
  Phenytoin
  Thiazide/sulfonamide diuretics

INCREASED ENDOGENOUS GLUCOSE
Acute stress
  Extensive burns
  Myocardial infarction
  Infection
Pharmacologic
  Glucocorticoids
  Steroids
  Sympathomimetics
  Thyroid preparations

INCREASED EXOGENOUS GLUCOSE
Hyperalimentation (total parenteral nutrition)
High-calorie enteral feedings
Hemodialysis
Peritoneal dialysis

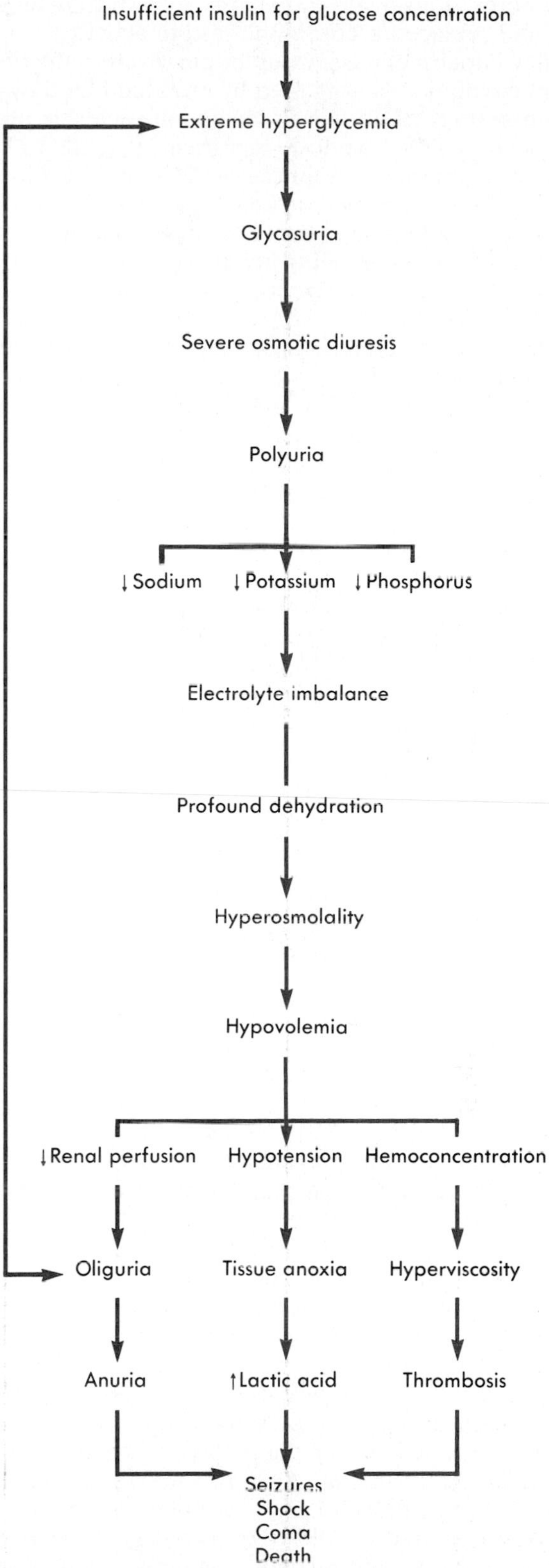

Fig. 43-2 Pathophysiology of hyperglycemic, hyperosmolar nonketotic coma (HHNC).

Assessment and Diagnosis

HHNC has a slow, subtle onset. Initially, the symptoms may be nonspecific and may be ignored or attributed to the patient's concurrent disease processes.

History reveals polyuria, polydipsia (depending on patient's thirst sensation), and advancing weakness. Medical attention may not be obtained for these nonspecific, nonacute symptoms until the patient is unable to take sufficient fluids to offset the fluid losses. Progressive dehydration follows and leads to mental confusion, convulsions, and coma.

The physical examination may reveal obtundation, with a profound fluid deficit. Signs of severe dehydration include longitudinal wrinkles in the tongue, decreased salivation, and decreased central venous pressure, with increases in pulse and respirations (Kussmaul's air hunger is not present).

Serum glucose levels are strikingly elevated, often double the levels seen in ketoacidosis (reaching 2000 mg/dl). Serum osmolality, normally 285 to 300 mOsm/kg, may reach 350 mOsm/kg, averaging 320 mOsm/kg[1]. Elevated hematocrit and depleted potassium and phosphorus levels result from the osmotic diuresis. Serum electrolyte levels vary, depending on the activity and position of the electrolyte when the laboratory test is performed.

Serial laboratory tests keep the clinician apprised of the fluctuating serum electrolyte levels and provide the basis for electrolyte replacement. Intracellular potassium usually is depleted as dehydration progresses. It quickly reenters the cells, however, when insulin is administered. Phosphate levels also are carefully monitored and replaced according to insulin activity.

Kidney impairment as a result of the severe reduction in renal circulation is suggested by elevated blood urea nitrogen and creatinine levels. Metabolic acidosis usually is absent. When acidosis is present, it tends to be mild and attributed to other factors. The mild acidosis may be a result of a starvation ketosis, a relative increase in lactic acid circulating in the reduced blood volume, or azotemia caused by impaired renal function.[3]

Medical Management

Medical management is necessary to interrupt the glycemic diuresis and to prevent vascular collapse. The underlying cause of HHNC must then be sought. The same basic principles used to treat diabetic ketoacidosis are used for the patient with hyperglycemic hyperosmolar coma: rehydration, electrolyte replacement, restoration of insulin/glucagon ratio, and prevention/treatment of circulatory collapse.

Rapid rehydration is the primary intervention. The fluid deficit may be as much as 150 ml/kg of body weight. The average 150-pound adult may lose more than 10 L of fluid a day.[1] Debate continues regarding whether isotonic or hypotonic solutions are more appropriate for treating the severe fluid deficit. Although an isotonic solution would expand the extracellular fluid and treat hypotension, it could compound the serum osmolality and exceed the body's requirement for sodium. A hypotonic solution would reduce the serum osmolality and provide free water for excretion; however, it could result in hypotonic expansion of the cells. The consensus is to use physiologic normal saline (0.9%) for the first 2 L during the first hour of treatment,[1] especially for the patient undergoing circulatory collapse.[3] Half-strength hypotonic saline (0.45%) subsequently can be used to reduce the serum osmolality. The patient may need replacement of 6 to 10 L of fluid in the first 10 hours.[6] Sodium input should not exceed that required to replace the losses. Careful monitoring for sodium and water balance is required to prevent hemolysis as hemoconcentration is reduced.[4] To prevent relative hypoglycemia, the hydrating solution is changed to 5% dextrose in water, in 0.9% saline, or in 0.45% saline when the serum glucose levels fall to 250 to 300 mg/dl.

Vigorous fluid therapy alone can reverse hyperosmolar coma.[9] Intravenously administered insulin, however, usually is given to facilitate the cellular use of glucose and to decrease the serum osmolality more rapidly.[3] Muscle, liver, and adipose cells tend to be receptive to exogenous insulin levels in the patient with HHNC, and the insulin needs are minimal; 10 to 15 U of regular insulin is given intravenously as a bolus. Maintenance doses of insulin to control hyperglycemia vary according to the practitioner. Intravenous administration of 0.1 U/kg/hr of insulin (which mimics the physiologic secretion of 5 to 10 U/hr[10]) may be given until the glucose falls between 250 and 300 mg. Another treatment method provides a one-time insulin administration of 15 U subcutaneously.[1] Once glucose levels are at 250 mg/dl, insulin treatment usually is discontinued. Aggressive treatment of the underlying causes of HHNC (severe infection, therapeutic procedures, medications) is included in the medical treatment to prevent HHNC recurrence.

Diagnostic procedures to identify and plan the treatment of HHNC are the same as those for diabetic ketoacidosis (see Table 43-1), with differences only in the frequency performed. Although arterial blood gas testing is not repeated as often in HHNC as in DKA, the serum osmolality determination is performed more frequently in HHNC than in ketoacidosis.

Nursing Management

Hyperglycemic hyperosmolar coma occurs most frequently in the patient with a precipitating stressor or illness; thus it is not unlikely for the nurse to be the first person to recognize its development. Nursing management of the patient at risk for HHNC involves prompt recognition of changes in the patient's osmolar state. A hydration assessment is outlined in the box on p. 699. The assessment provides beginning signs and symptoms of fluid imbalance that signal dehydration from the increased number of glucose molecules in the blood stream. Blood values for hematocrit, osmolality, glucose, sodium, and potassium are monitored. Urine values for osmolality and ketones also are followed.

A convenient formula used to identify the osmolality of blood on the basis of known laboratory values is the following:

$$\text{Serum osmolality} = 2\,(\text{Na}^+ + \text{K}^+) + \frac{\text{glucose mg/dl}}{18} + \frac{\text{BUN mg/dl}}{2.8}$$

Values in excess of 320 mOsm/L suggest moderate hyperosmolarity.[1] Changes in the patient's personality provide neurologic clues to the impact of fluid imbalance on the central nervous system. When unexplained behavior changes are coupled with changing laboratory values and other signs of dehydration, hyperosmolarity is to be suspected.

Once HHNC is identified, the nurse manages the alterations brought about by the fluid deficit, the increase in glucose, and the electrolyte imbalances. Because HHNC occurs most often in elderly persons, special care of this age-group is emphasized. Throughout the critical care period, the nurse collects information necessary to identify the precipitating cause of HHNC and educates the patient and family in prevention of its recurrence. Hemodynamic monitoring, including central venous pressure, pulmonary arterial wedge pressure, and pulmonary artery pressure, evaluates the degree of dehydration and the effectiveness of the hydration therapy. Because a preexisting cardiopulmonary or renal problem may exist in the elderly patient, the hemodynamic criteria must be based on the values normal for that patient's age and current medical condition. The nurse is alerted to clinical manifestations of fluid overload while vigorously rehydrating the older patient. Cardiac monitoring for sinus rhythm, CVP, and PAP continues to provide an evaluation of the patient's fluid tolerance. Symptoms of circulatory overload include elevated CVP and PAP levels, tachycardia, bounding pulse, dyspnea, tachypnea, lung crackles, and engorged neck veins. Decreasing cardiac output is signaled by hypotension and urine output less than 0.5 ml/kg/hr.

◆ **Intravenous replacement considerations.** Rigorous fluid replacement and low-dose insulin administration are best controlled with electronic volumetric pump devices when possible.

Electrolyte replacement orders are based on the patient's response to the treatment plan. Rapid fluctuations of serum potassium and phosphorus levels further compromise the patient with cardiac or renal problems. Increasing the circulating levels of insulin with therapeutic doses of intravenous insulin will promote the rapid return of potassium and phosphorus into the cell. Potassium imbalances disturb the electrocardiographic tracings (Table 43-2). Continuous cardiac monitoring provides information necessary to maintain or modify electrolyte dosages. Physical changes, such as alterations in gastrointestinal motility and neuromuscular control, also signal the effectiveness of electrolyte replacement.

◆ **Basic assessments.** Bedside serum glucose monitoring is performed every 30 to 60 minutes to determine effectiveness of treatment. Urine ketones are tested at the bedside to rule out the presence of ketoacidosis.

Alteration in the level of consciousness is directly related to osmotic diuresis and resulting intracellular dehydration. Neurologic assessments, including level of consciousness, pupillary response, motor function, and reflexes, are performed frequently to monitor the patient's response to treatment. Seizure activity may occur as a result of the hyperosmolar state, which interferes with oxygen delivery to the brain cells. Seizure precautions include nursing actions to protect the patient from injury (padded side rails, bed in low position) and to provide an open airway (oral airway, head turned to side without forcibly restraining the patient, suction equipment). Oxygen is administered via nasal cannula. Anticonvulsants, with the exception of phenytoin (which interferes with endogenous insulin [see Table 41-2]), may be ordered. Documentation of seizures includes onset, duration, and description of seizure activity.

Table 43-2 Clinical manifestations of hypokalemia and hyperkalemia

Hypokalemia	Hyperkalemia
Generalized muscle weakness	Impaired muscle activity
Fatigue	Weakness
Diminished to absent reflexes	Muscle pain/cramps
Decreased GI motility	Increased GI motility
Anorexia	Nausea
Abdominal distention	Diarrhea
Paralytic ileus	Intestinal colic
Vomiting	Oliguria
Hypotension	Dizziness
Decreased stroke volume	Bradycardia
Dysrhythmias	Ventricular fibrillation
Weak pulse	Irritability
Respiratory muscle weakness	ECG changes
Shallow respirations	Flattened P wave
Shortness of breath	Large, peaked T wave
Apathy	Broad, slurred QRS complex
Drowsiness	
Depression	
Irritability	
Tetany	
Coma	
ECG changes	
Prolonged QT interval	
Flattened, depressed T wave	
Depressed ST segments	

◆

NURSING DIAGNOSIS AND MANAGEMENT
Hyperglycemic hyperosmotic nonketotic coma

- ◆ Decreased Cardiac Output related to decreased preload secondary to fluid volume deficit, p. 361
- ◆ Anxiety related to threat to biologic, psychologic, and/or social integrity, p. 763

Interference with tissue perfusion by hypovolemia and hypophosphatemia is a serious problem for the severely compromised, dehydrated patient. Fluid replacement, range of motion, frequent positioning, and assessing skin turgor, color, temperature, and peripheral pulses are used to maintain and monitor skin integrity. Elastic support hose, elastic wraps, or antiembolism stockings may be used in an effort to prevent lower extremity venous stasis.

Continuous alertness to the clinical manifestations that identify the underlying cause of the disease is needed to prevent its recurrence. Diabetic teaching plans are necessary if the hyperglycemic coma is the result of untreated diabetes.

DIABETES INSIPIDUS/HYPOSECRETION OF ANTIDIURETIC HORMONE

Description

Diabetes insipidus (DI) occurs when there is an insufficiency or a hypofunctioning of antidiuretic hormone (ADH). ADH normally stimulates the kidney tubules to reabsorb filtered water when the body needs to increase fluid stores. ADH stimulates the tubules to increase permeability to water when particles in the blood stream increase in number (rising osmolality) or when blood pressure falls (see Table 41-4 for additional events that affect ADH). Unrestricted serum hyperosmolality develops in persons without adequately functioning ADH. An intense thirst and the passage of excessively large quantities of very dilute urine add to the characteristics of the disease.

Etiology

Diabetes insipidus is categorized into three types according to cause: central DI, nephrogenic DI, and psychogenic DI (see box, p. 706).

ETIOLOGY OF DIABETES INSIPIDUS

CENTRAL DIABETES INSIPIDUS

Primary

ADH deficiency from hypothalamic-hypophyseal malformation
- Congenital defect
- Idiopathic

Secondary

ADH deficiency from destruction to the hypothalamic-hypophyseal system
- Trauma
- Infection
- Surgery
- Primary neoplasms
- Metastatic malignancies
- Autoimmune response

NEPHROGENIC DIABETES INSIPIDUS

Inability of kidney tubules to respond to circulating ADH
- Decrease or absence of ADH receptors
- Cellular damage to nephron, especially loop of Henle
- Kidney damage, e.g., hydronephrosis, pyelonephritis, polycystic kidney
- Untoward response to drug therapy, e.g., lithium carbonate, demeclocycline

PSYCHOGENIC DIABETES INSIPIDUS

Rare form of water intoxication
- Compulsive water drinking

Central diabetes occurs when there is an interruption in the synthesis and release of ADH. It is further divided into primary and secondary categories. Primary DI occurs when structural abnormalities within the hypothalamus, infundibular stalk, and neurohypophysis prevent the release of ADH according to the body's inherent signals. Primary DI may result from an inherited familial disorder or from a neurohypophyseal system that fails to develop at birth. Primary DI also may be idiopathic or sporadic and occur without apparent cause.[11]

Secondary DI occurs as a result of trauma to or a pathologic condition of the neurohypophyseal functioning unit. Surgery or irradiation to the pituitary gland, traumatic head injury, tumors (malignant and benign), and infections, such as encephalitis, tuberculosis, and meningitis, can potentially interfere with the structure and physiology of the unit and compromise the release of ADH.

Nephrogenic diabetes insipidus (NDI) results from the inability of the kidney nephrons to respond to circulating ADH. This may result from diseased kidneys and insensitive or inadequate numbers of receptors on the nephron. Drugs can promote NDI by decreasing the responsiveness of the kidney tubules to ADH. Long-term lithium carbonate use is the most common cause of NDI.[12]

Psychogenic diabetes insipidus is a rare form of the disease that occurs with compulsive water drinking. The hypophyseal stalk is functioning adequately in psychogenic DI as are the receptor sites on the kidney nephrons. The cause of psychogenic DI is believed to be similar to obsessive neurosis inasmuch as the problem results from the consumption of abnormally large quantities of water.[13] Long-standing psychogenic DI may closely mimic nephrogenic DI; that is, the kidney tubules decrease responsiveness to ADH as a result of prolonged conditioning to hypotonic urine.

Pathophysiology

ADH is the hormone directly responsible for maintaining fluid balance within the body. The body releases ADH in an effort to maintain blood tonicity and circulating blood volume. When released into the blood stream, ADH has a twofold effect. One effect is to promote reabsorption of fluid at the distal convoluted tubule and the collecting ducts of the kidneys. The other effect is to stimulate the vascular walls to constrict.

Damage to the hypothalamus, infundibular stalk, or posterior pituitary can lead to a disruption in the normal neuroendocrine communication system and resultant secretion of ADH. When ADH is absent, inefficient, or secreted in insufficient amounts, the kidney tubules prevent the reabsorption of urinary substrate and an excessive amount of water is lost to the body. This pathologic condition is known as *diabetes insipidus.* (Fig. 43-3 is a diagram of the events postulated to occur with primary diabetes insipidus.)

A decreased amount of circulating ADH decreases the kidney tubules' reabsorption of water and leads to excessive water excretion in the urine. As free water is lost from the blood stream, the serum osmolality rises and excessive sodium concentration (hypernatremia) in the vascular space stimulate the thirst receptors. Polyuria develops as the kidneys fail to reabsorb tubular fluid and to concentrate the urine. Extremely dilute urine is excreted, and the body is depleted of the fluid necessary for hydration. Urine osmolality and specific gravity decrease. In a healthy body capable of balancing fluid losses, the rising serum osmolality triggers synthesis and release of ADH, which activates the kidney tubules to conserve water. This action returns fluid to the vascular space, thereby diluting or decreasing the osmolality. Consequently, the concentration of electrolytes, especially sodium, returns to a balanced state. In the person with the pathologic condition of decreased ADH secretion, however, this negative feedback system is interrupted, and ADH either is not released or is ineffective.

As the extracellular dehydration ensues, hypotension and hypovolemic shock can occur. The thirst mechanism is stimulated. Extreme polydipsia develops as the individual attempts to replace lost fluids. The excessive intake of water reduces the serum osmolality to a more normal level and prevents dehydration. The dramatic cycle of polydipsia and polyuria interferes with the

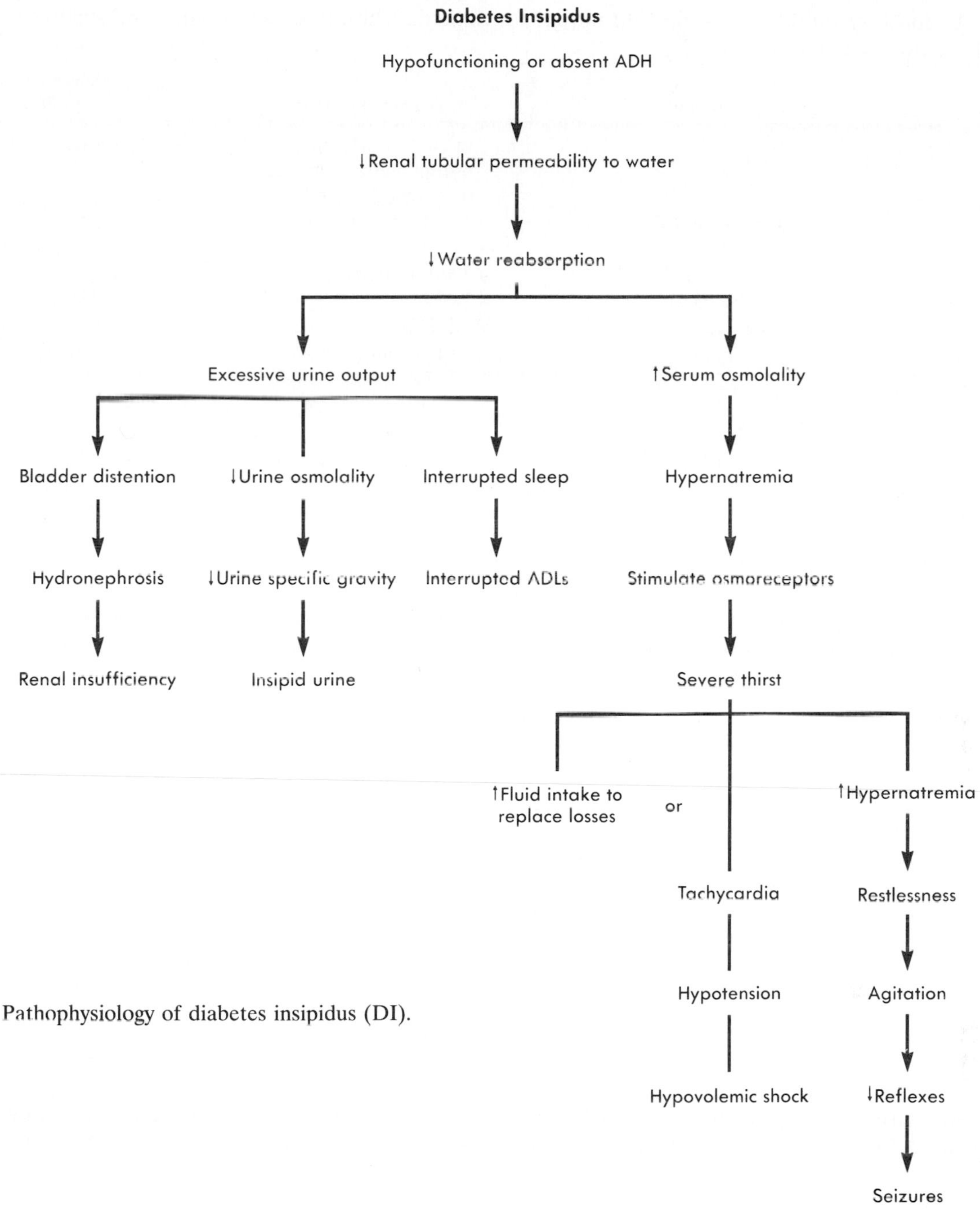

Fig. 43-3 Pathophysiology of diabetes insipidus (DI).

person's ability to work, eat, or sleep. Unless the lost fluids are replaced, severe hypernatremia, decreased cerebral perfusion, and severe dehydration disrupt the neurologic system. Seizures and loss of consciousness may lead to death.

Assessment and Diagnosis

Clinical manifestations of DI may develop gradually or may occur suddenly after head injury or other precipitating disease. Initially, urine production may exceed 300 ml/hr, accompanied by an abnormally low urine osmolality.[14] The diluted urine in DI is "insipid" or tasteless, as opposed to the sweet, honey (mellitus) taste of urine associated with diabetes mellitus. Unless the individual is able to replace the fluid loss, hypernatremia and severe dehydration result.

Diagnostic tests used to establish the presence of DI evaluate the body's innate ability to balance fluid and electrolytes. Although these tests are early markers for the disease, most are routinely performed and not specific to the endocrine system (Table 43-3). The tests performed most frequently include a comparison of serum osmolality, urine osmolality, and serum sodium values. In the well-hydrated person, the homeostatic mechanism maintains a 1:3 ratio between serum and urine concentration.[15] The serum osmolality has a nar-

Table 43-3 Laboratory values and intake and output for patients with diabetes insipidus and syndrome of inappropriate antidiuretic hormone

Value	Normal	Diabetes insipidus	Syndrome of inappropriate antidiuretic hormone
Serum ADH	1-5 pg/ml	↓ in central DI, may be normal with nephrogenic or psychogenic DI	Elevated
Serum osmolality	285-300 mOsm/kg	>300 mOsm/kg	<250 mOsm/kg
Serum sodium	135-145 mEq/L	>145 mEq/L	<120 mEq/L
Urine osmolality	300-1400 mOsm/kg	<300 mOsm/kg	Increased
Urine specific gravity	1.005-1.030	<1.005	>1.030
Urine output	1-1.5 L/24 hr	30-40 L/24 hr	Below normal
Fluid intake	1-1.5 L/24 hr	≥50 L 24 hr	Unchanged

row range between 285 and 300 mOsm/kg, whereas urine osmolality can fluctuate between 300 and 800 mOsm/kg, with extremes ranging from 50 to 1200 mOsm/kg. Severe DI could raise serum osmolality to 330 mOsm/kg while urine osmolality falls well below normal.[16]

The bedside measurement of urine output identifies polyuria. Urine specific gravity can be measured more conveniently than can urine osmolality because the procedure can take place at the bedside and does not require patient preparation. Osmolality tests, however, are preferred because they give a more accurate measurement of the renal tubules' reabsorption of water and resulting concentration or dilution of urine.[17]

In the patient with ineffective, absent, or decreased ADH, the urine osmolality is expected to be decreased while the serum osmolality is increased. The degree of serum osmolality is directly related to the degree of urine osmolality. Its measurement can provide data to support the diagnosis of DI. For a more accurate reflection of the ADH influence on water balance, the urine sample should be collected and tested simultaneously with the blood sample.

Serum sodium levels mirror the high solute concentration within the blood stream. Unconscious patients or patients unable to respond to the thirst mechanism that accompanies polyuria are at risk of rapid dehydration and hypovolemia if DI is not diagnosed and treated. For these patients a gradual rise in serum sodium level signals the fluid imbalance. Some medical clinicians suspect DI in the unconscious patient with hypoosmotic polyuria when the serum sodium level reaches 142 mEq/L before more serious problems with hemoconcentration develop.[18]

Further tests are useful in differentiating DI according to cause. In a water deprivation or dehydration test, the patient is deprived of fluids for a 24-hour period. During this time, urine and plasma osmolality measurements are taken. Adequate ADH functioning maintains the plasma osmolality within normal limits, whereas the urine osmolality increases to as high as 800 mOsm/kg. In patients with ADH deficiency, the urine is minimally concentrated after dehydration, whereas plasma osmolality rises above 300 mOsm/kg and serum sodium is greater than 145 mEq/L.

Alternate tests may include quantitative analysis of serum ADH. Absent or decreased levels of serum ADH in the presence of hyperosmolar serum and hypoosmolar urine indicate primary and secondary ADH deficiency. Normal serum ADH levels (1 to 5 pg/ml or <1.5 mg/L[17]) accompanying clinical manifestations of DI may indicate nephrogenic diabetes insipidus (NDI), in which the kidney tubule is insensitive to ADH. Normal ADH levels with elevated blood osmolality and increased urine output also may suggest pharmacologically induced DI or excessive or compulsive water drinking. The vasopressin (ADH) concentration level may be measured to differentiate the type of DI present. Exogenous ADH is given parenterally, after which urine and blood osmolality tests are recorded. Water retention and overhydration are risks with this test, which is contraindicated in patients with cardiac dysfunction.

Medical Management

Medical intervention is based on the underlying pathologic condition. When possible, treatment involves management of the primary condition that is creating the interference in ADH circulation. Fluid replacement is provided in the initial phase of the treatment to prevent circulatory collapse. Patients who are able to drink are given voluminous amounts of fluid orally to balance output. For those unable to take sufficient fluids orally, hypotonic intravenous solutions are rapidly infused and carefully monitored to restore the hemodynamic balance.

Medications have been used successfully to treat diabetes insipidus. Patients with primary and secondary DI who are unable to synthesize ADH require exogenous ADH (vasopressin) replacement therapy. One form of the hormone available for short-term substitution is aqueous, synthetic Pitressin. It is administered intramuscularly or subcutaneously or applied topically to the nasal mucosa. Onset of antidiuresis is rapid and lasts up to 8 hours. Chronic DI may be treated with a more potent substitute. Pitressin Tannate is a pituitary extract in oil. The drug is given intramuscularly, never intravenously. The onset of antidiuresis is slow, with the peak activity occurring after 48 hours. The effects of this drug last for several days. Both drugs constrict smooth muscle and can elevate systemic blood pressure. Water intoxication also can occur if the dose is higher than the therapeutic level.

Another drug for patients with mild forms of DI is a synthetic analogue of vasopressin, desmopressin acetate (DDAVP). It is administered parenterally or via the nasal mucosa (not inhaled). The drug has fewer side effects than do other vasopressin preparations. It has minimal effects on the smooth muscle tissue and does not cause hypertension.

Minute doses of pituitary extract provide greater control of the patient's fluid balance with minimal side effects. Recent trial studies have found that ultra-low doses of Pituitrin (bovine posterior pituitary extract of combined oxytocin and vasopressin) have satisfactorily regulated urine output and promoted cardiovascular stability. The dose is scrupulously measured with a syringe pump to ensure the exact amount of the hormone for the patient's hydration status.[18]

Various drugs have been found that stimulate the production and release of endogenous vasopressin for patients in whom ADH is present but in insufficient quantities. These drugs include carbamazepine (an anticonvulsive), clofibrate (a hypolipidemic), and chlorpropamide (an oral hypoglycemic agent).

Nephrogenic diabetes insipidus does not respond to hormonal replacement treatment or to administration of an anticonvulsive or hypolipidemic drug. Chlorpropamide and tolbutamide, however, have been found to be effective in increasing the responsiveness of the nephron site to circulating ADH. Trial studies have shown indomethacin, a nonsteroidal antiinflammatory, to be therapeutic in the treatment of lithium-induced polyuria and polydipsia.[12] Certain thiazide diuretics also are used in the treatment of NDI. It is not known why DI responds paradoxically to thiazide diuretics, and because of serious untoward effects, these drugs are used with extreme caution.[8]

Nursing Management

The basic nursing management of diabetes insipidus involves a continual, conscientious assessment of the patient's hydration status; DI, however, may be complicated by the primary reason for which the patient was admitted to the critical care unit. Nursing care may then include management of several dysfunctioning systems.

Critical assessment and management of the fluid status are the most important concerns for the patient with DI. Intake and output measurement, condition of buccal membranes, skin turgor, daily weights, presence of thirst, and temperature provide a basic assessment list that is vital for the patient unable to regulate fluid needs and fluid lost. A hypotonic intravenous solution (to reduce the serum hyperosmolality) may be ordered to replace loss plus 50 ml/hr to replace insensible losses.[19] Urine and blood specimens should be simultaneously collected for osmolality studies. Bedside specific gravity analysis gives immediate information regarding variations in the kidney tubules' reabsorption of water. If the patient has an indwelling urinary catheter, scrupulous asepsis is required to prevent a nosocomial infection inasmuch as the closed system is repeatedly entered. Serum sodium and potassium levels are monitored and relayed to the physician as necessary.

Meticulous skin care is necessary to preserve skin integrity and to prevent breakdown caused by dehydration. Constipation and diarrhea are common problems in the patient with DI. Constipation results from fluid loss and, depending on the patient's status, is treated with dietary fiber or stool softeners, or both. Diarrhea may accompany the abdominal cramping and intestinal hyperactivity associated with vasopressin drug therapy. Untoward effects are brought to the attention of the physician for dose modification. ADH replacement is accomplished with extreme caution in the patient with a history of cardiac disease, because vasopressin tannate may cause hypertension and overhydration. At the first signs of cardiovascular impairment, the drug is discontinued and fluid intake is restricted until urine specific gravity is less than 1.015 and polyuria resumes.

The patient who is unable to satisfy sensations of thirst or to complete any task or self-care activity without the need to urinate is confused and frightened. For patients who are able to verbalize their fears, having someone who is interested and nonjudgmental may help reduce the emotional turmoil. The nurse must recognize the patient's reluctance to engage in any activity because of the polyuria. Having a bedpan or commode constantly available will reduce anxiety for the alert patient.

Educating the patient and the family about the disease process and how it affects thirst, urination, and fluid balance will encourage patients to participate in their care and reduce the feelings of hopelessness. Patients who are discharged with the disease are taught, along with their families, the signs and symptoms of dehydration and overhydration. They are taught the procedures for correct daily weight and urine specific gravity measurements. Printed information pertaining to drug actions, side effects, dosages, and timetable is given to the patient, as well as an outline of factors that need to be reported to the physician.

NURSING DIAGNOSIS AND MANAGEMENT
Diabetes insipidus

- Fluid Volume Deficit related to decreased secretion of ADH, p. 725
- High Risk for Altered Peripheral Tissue Perfusion risk factor: high-dose vasopressor therapy (vasopressin) p. 363
- Anxiety related to threat to biologic, psychologic, and/or social integrity, p. 763
- Sensory/Perceptual Alterations related to sensory overload, sensory deprivation, and sleep pattern disturbance, p. 573

SYNDROME OF INAPPROPRIATE ANTIDIURETIC HORMONE/HYPERSECRETION OF ANTIDIURETIC HORMONE

Description

The opposite of diabetes insipidus is the syndrome of inappropriate antidiuretic hormone (SIADH). SIADH occurs when there is an increase in the release of the ADH. The excess ADH secreted in the blood stream exceeds the amount needed to maintain blood volume and serum osmolality.

Etiology

Of the numerous causes of SIADH, many are seen in patients who are critically ill (see box, p. 711). Central nervous system injury or disease interfering with the normal functioning of the hypothalamic-hypophyseal system may cause SIADH. The most common cause, however, is malignant bronchogenic oat cell carcinoma. This type of malignant cell is capable of synthesizing and releasing ADH. Other carcinomas capable of this autonomous production of ADH involve the pancreas, prostate, duodenum, and thymus. ADH levels also have been elevated in Hodgkin's disease and leukemia. In addition, ectopic endocrine production of ADH is identified in certain nonmalignant pulmonary conditions, such as tuberculosis and pneumonia. Levels of ADH also are increased by positive pressure ventilators that decrease venous return to the thorax, thus stimulating pulmonary baroreceptors to release ADH.[20]

Other causes of SIADH are neurologic disorders, such as tetanus, meningitis, and Guillain-Barré syndrome. Anesthesia, stress, pain, and such drugs as cyclophosphamide and chlorpropamide also have been implicated.

Pathophysiology

Antidiuretic hormone (vasopressin) is a powerful, complex polypeptide compound. When released into the circulation by the neurohypophysis (posterior pituitary gland), ADH has a widespread effect on the body's regulation of water and electrolyte balance. ADH activates the receptor cells in the distal tubules and collecting ducts of the nephron. The kidney tubules respond by increasing their permeability to water and by reabsorbing water intended for urinary output. ADH also activates the receptor cells located in the smooth muscles of the arterial wall to cause constriction of the vessel lumen.

Hyperosmolality (increased concentration of dissolved particles within the blood) and hypovolemia (diminished circulating blood volume) are two conditions that cause the body to release ADH. Hypotension is another causative factor that stimulates ADH release. Disease conditions such as oat cell carcinoma can result in the abnormal increase in metabolism, release of ADH, or both.

Normally, osmoreceptors in the hypothalamus and baroreceptors in the aortic arch and in the major veins signal the release of ADH from the posterior pituitary gland.[21] ADH is then circulated to its primary target cells in the nephron. The nephron stimulates the tubules to conserve water. The reabsorption of water dilutes the plasma and decreases serum osmolality. The quantity of urinary output is diminished, and the urine's concentration is increased. In the syndrome of inappropriate secretion of antidiuretic hormone (SIADH), ADH continues to be released into the blood stream despite the feedback mechanism signaling a normal serum osmolality and blood volume.

In SIADH, profound fluid and electrolyte disturbances result from the unsolicited, continuous release of the hormone into the blood stream (Fig. 43-4). Rather than providing a water balance within the body, excessive ADH stimulates the kidney tubules to retain fluid, regardless of need. Furthermore, excessive ADH alters the extracellular fluid's sodium balance. The resulting dilutional hyponatremia reduces the sodium concentration to critically low levels.[21] In the healthy adult hyponatremia inhibits the release of ADH; however, in SIADH the increased levels of circulating ADH are unrelated to the serum sodium.[23]

The hyponatremia is further aggravated as aldosterone release (normally released to retain sodium at the tubules) is suppressed. Serum hypoosmolality leads to a shift of fluid into the intracellular fluid compartment in an attempt to equalize osmotic pressure. Because minimal sodium is present in this fluid, edema usually does not result. Without ADH and aldosterone, water is retained, urine output is diminished, and further sodium is excreted in the urine. The urine has an increased osmolality from the reduction in water excretion. Urinary concentration also is increased by the continuous loss of sodium into the urine. It is believed that despite the hyponatremia, the increased release of ADH promotes sodium loss through the kidneys. It is likely that the dilute serum enters the cells in an attempt to balance the intracellular serum sodium concentration. This intracellular transport suppresses the release of aldosterone, which normally would conserve the sodium ion at the renal tubule, and sodium loss in the urine continues. Left untreated, serum hyponatremia results in neurologic changes that could ultimately lead to loss of consciousness and death.

Assessment and Diagnosis

The patient with SIADH becomes water-intoxicated. The clinical manifestations of this condition relate to the excess fluid in the extracellular compartment and the proportionate dilution of the circulating sodium. Although edema usually is not present, slight weight gain may occur from the expanded extracellular fluid volume.

Hyponatremia initially may be asymptomatic. Early clinical manifestations of dilutional hyponatremia include lethargy, anorexia, nausea, and vomiting. As the water and sodium imbalance progresses, neurologic signs of hyponatremia predominate. Inability to concentrate, mental confusion, apprehension, and seizures may progress to loss of consciousness and death.

The medical diagnosis is based on various factors. Primary disorders (oat cell carcinoma, central nervous

ETIOLOGY OF SYNDROME OF INAPPROPRIATE ANTIDIURETIC HORMONE

Malignant disease associated with autonomous production of ADH
- Bronchogenic oat cell carcinoma
- Pancreatic adenocarcinoma
- Duodenal, bladder, ureter, prostatic carcinomas
- Lymphosarcoma, Ewing's sarcoma
- Acute leukemia, Hodgkin's disease
- Cerebral neoplasm, thymoma

Central nervous system diseases that interfere with the hypothalamic-hypophyseal system and increase the production and/or release of ADH
- Head injury
- Brain abscess
- Hydrocephalus
- Pituitary adenoma
- Subdural hematoma
- Subarachnoid hemorrhage
- Cerebral atrophy
- Guillain-Barré syndrome
- Tuberculous meningitis
- Purulent meningitis
- Herpes simplex encephalitis
- Acute intermittent porphyria

Neurogenic stimuli capable of increasing ADH
- Decreased glomerular filtration rate
- Physical and/or emotional stressors
  - Pain
  - Fear
  - Trauma
  - Surgery
  - Myocardial infarction
  - Acute infection
  - Hypotension
  - Hemorrhage
  - Hypovolemia

Pulmonary diseases believed to stimulate the baroreceptors and increase ADH
- Pulmonary tuberculosis
- Viral and bacterial pneumonia
- Empyema
- Lung abscess
- Chronic obstructive lung disease
- Status asthmaticus
- Cystic fibrosis

Endocrine disturbances that hormonally influence ADH
- Myxedema
- Hypothyroidism
- Hypopituitarism
- Adrenal insufficiency—Addison's disease

Medications that mimic, increase the release of, or potentiate ADH
- Hypoglycemics
  - Insulin
  - Tolbutamide
  - Chlorpropamide
- Potassium-depleting thiazide diuretics
- Tricyclic antidepressants
  - Imipramine
  - Amitriptyline
- Phenothiazine
  - Fluphenazine
  - Thioridazine
- Thioxanthenes
  - Thiothixene
  - Chlorprothixene
- Chemotherapeutic agents
  - Vincristine
  - Cyclophosphamide
- Narcotics
- Carbamazepine
- Clofibrate
- Acetaminophen
- Nicotine
- Oxytocin
- Vasopressin
- Anesthetics

system disturbance), clinical manifestations, and laboratory tests provide data to verify the presence of SIADH. Laboratory values provide the clinical hallmarks of SIADH: hyponatremia, serum hypoosmolality, and a urine osmolality greater than would be expected of the hypotonic blood (see Table 43-3 for typical laboratory results for patient with SIADH). The patient with SIADH characteristically displays a serum hypoosmolality less than 250 mOsm/kg, with sodium levels less than 120 mEq/L. Urine osmolality that is equal to or that exceeds serum osmolality—with urinary sodium greater than 20 mEq/L in a patient with normal renal, pituitary, thyroid, and adrenal functions—indicates the inappropriate excretion of a concentrated urine in the presence of very dilute serum.[23]

To confirm the diagnosis, a water-load test may be performed. After a period of fasting, a dehydrated patient is overhydrated with water. The urine output and serum osmolality are carefully monitored to discover a decline in serum osmolality resulting from peak moments of overhydration. Patients with SIADH show a decrease in serum osmolality regardless of the fasting state and an inability to secrete dilute urine despite the hydration resulting from the water load.[17]

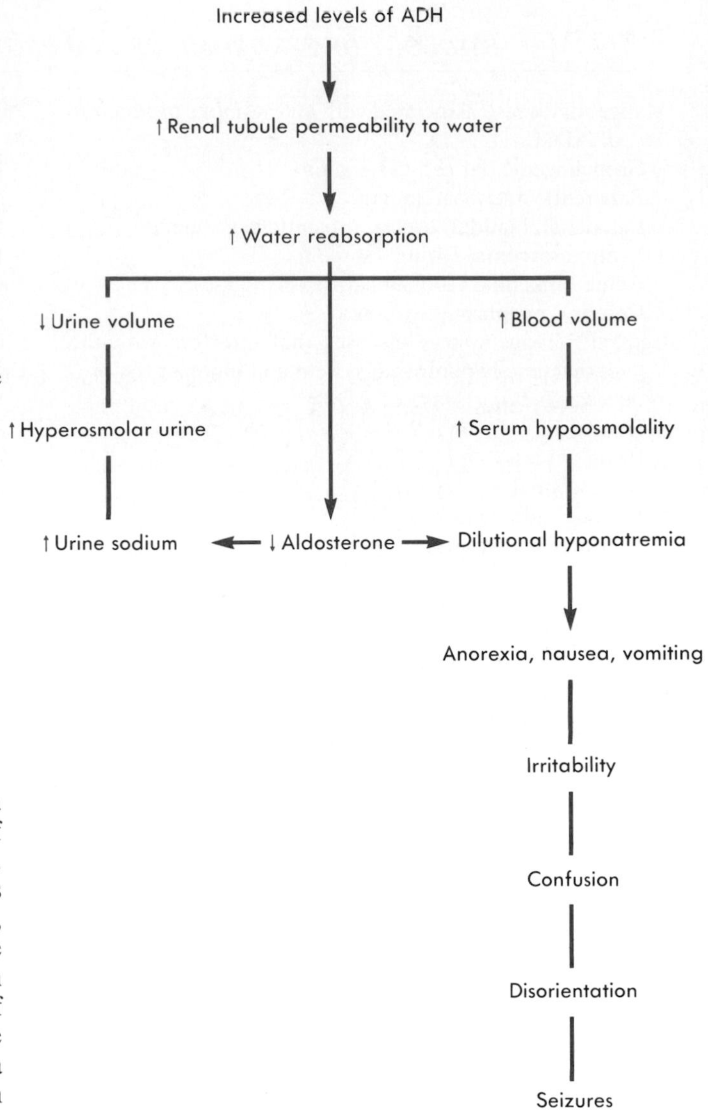

Fig. 43-4 Pathophysiology of syndrome of inappropriate antidiuretic hormone (SIADH).

Medical Management

In the critical care unit, SIADH often occurs as a secondary disease. Ideally, recognition and treatment of the primary disease will reduce the production of ADH. If the patient is receiving any of the chemical agents suspected of causing the disease, discontinuing the drug, if possible, may return ADH levels to normal. The medical therapy that is the most successful (along with treatment of the primary disease) is simple reduction of fluid intake.[4] Although fluid restrictions are to be calculated on the basis of individual needs and losses, a general criterion is to restrict fluids to 500 ml less than average daily output.[8] Patients with severe hyponatremia (<115 mEq/L) or those with seizures receive infusions with 3% to 5% hypertonic saline[24] for rapid but temporary correction of the hemodilution caused by the retention of fluid at the tubules and severe sodium loss. Furosemide is added to further increase the diuresis and to prevent risk of pulmonary edema related to the hypertonic saline solution. Hypertonic saline solution is administered very slowly and with extreme caution (0.1 mg/kg/min) until the patient's serum sodium level is increased to 125 mEq/L.[24] Treatment with a hypertonic solution is temporary inasmuch as the sodium is continuously removed from the body through the urine.

Narcotic agonists, such as oxilorphan and butorphanol, reduce the secretion of ADH in many patients with SIADH. The drugs, however, do not seem to be effective in patients with SIADH caused by lung malignancies. Patients with lung malignancies are treated with demeclocycline hydrochloride, an antibacterial tetracycline, and lithium carbonate, an alkali metal salt primarily used to alter psychogenic behavior. These drugs inhibit the tubule response to ADH and decrease the water reabsorption at the tubules.[6]

Nursing Management

Thorough, astute nursing assessments are required for care of the patient with SIADH while an attempt is made to correct the fluid and sodium imbalance: the systemic effects of hyponatremia occur rapidly and can be lethal. Evaluation of the patient's neurologic status, especially level of consciousness, occurs every 1 to 2 hours. Frequent assessment of the patient's hydration status is accomplished with serial measurements of urine output, blood and urine sodium levels, urine specific gravity, and urine and blood osmolality. Elimination patterns are assessed because constipation may occur when fluids are restricted.

Seizure precautions for the patient with SIADH are provided regardless of the degree of hyponatremia. Serum sodium levels may fluctuate rapidly, and neurologic impairment may occur with no apparent warning. The patient's altered neurologic response also may be

> ◆
>
> *NURSING DIAGNOSIS AND MANAGEMENT*
>
> **Syndrome of inappropriate antidiuretic hormone(SIADH)**
>
> ◆ Fluid Volume Excess related to increased secretion of ADH secondary to SIADH, p. 725

influenced by the acuity of the primary disease (i.e., central nervous system disease) and not solely by the result of low sodium levels. Seizure precautions include nursing actions to protect the patient from injury (padded side rails, bed in low position when patient is unattended) and to provide an open airway (oral airway, head turned to side without forcibly restraining the patient, suction apparatus). Oxygen is administered as needed.

Accurate intake and output measurement is required to calculate fluid replacement for the patient with excessive ADH. All fluids are restricted as ordered and provide only a sufficient intake to equal urine output. Frequent mouth care through moistening the buccal membrane may give comfort during the period of fluid restriction. Weights may be taken every 12 hours to gauge fluid retention or loss. Weight gain could signify continual fluid retention, whereas weight loss could indicate loss of body fluid.

Hemodynamic monitoring, including blood pressure, CVP, and pulmonary arterial wedge pressure (PAWP), are all expected to be within the normal range for the patient. Elevations in blood pressure, CVP, or PAWP may indicate cardiac overload complications from the prescribed hypertonic saline treatment.

Hypertonic saline is infused very cautiously. A volumetric pump is used to deliver 0.1 mg/kg/min,[24] or it is set to deliver a flow rate determined by the serum sodium levels. The saline infusion usually is discontinued when the patient's serum sodium levels reach 125 mEq/L. Hypertonic expansion of the vascular space is a complication of rapid infusion of hypertonic saline that must be avoided. Hypertonic expansion occurs when the hypertonic solution is infused so rapidly that it creates an immediate hyperosmolality of the blood stream. Fluid is drawn from the more diluted intracellular spaces to the blood stream in an effort to equalize the concentration of particles. The isosmotic conditions or equality of the compartments is not achieved as additional hypertonic solution continues to be rapidly infused. The hypertonic solution is discontinued if signs or symptoms occur, such as bounding pulse, increased thirst (to replace depleted intracellular fluid) and hand vein emptying longer than 5 seconds when the hand is elevated, accompanied by increased serum sodium levels.

Clinical manifestations of congestive heart failure and pulmonary edema, such as elevated blood pressure, PAWP, and CVP, also are causes to discontinue the hypertonic saline infusion. Apprehension, abrupt position changes to an upright position to breathe, dyspnea, moist cough, and increased respiratory and pulse rates also indicate the inability of the cardiopulmonary system to accommodate the increased fluid load.

An alteration in bowel elimination resulting in constipation may occur from decreased fluid intake and inactivity. Cathartics or low-volume hypertonic enemas may be given to stimulate peristalsis. Tap water or hypotonic enemas should *not* be given because the water in the enema solution may be absorbed through the bowel and potentiate water intoxication.

Rapidly occurring changes in the patient's neurologic status may frighten visiting family members. Sensitivity to the family's unspoken fears can be shown by words that express empathy and by providing time for the patient and family to communicate their feelings. The nurse should discuss with them the course of the disease and its effect on water balance. The nurse also should explain the fluid restrictions and the family's role in treating SIADH. Teaching the patient and the family to measure intake and output will encourage independence and instill a sense of usefulness.

THYROTOXIC CRISIS

Description

To describe thyrotoxic crisis it is first necessary to describe thyrotoxicosis. Thyrotoxicosis, also called *hyperthyroidism,* occurs when the thyroid gland produces thyroid hormone in excess of the body's need. Hyperthyroid conditions also may result from ingestion of excessive exogenous thyroid replacement drugs. Although rare, excess thyroid hormone may be produced by a neoplasm of ectopic thyroid tissue. Conditions associated with thyrotoxicosis are presented in the first box on p. 715.

Thyrotoxic crisis is a critical stage of hyperthyroidism. It is an uncommon, life-threatening condition that occurs when the overactive thyroid has not been diagnosed or adequately treated. Thyrotoxic crisis often is precipitated by a major stressor, such as an acute infection or a severe trauma. See the second box on p. 715 for conditions known to precipitate thyrotoxic crisis.

The signs and symptoms of thyrotoxicosis are exaggerated in the crisis stage, and unless emergency treatment is provided, death occurs from heart failure.

Etiology

Excessive circulating thyroid hormone causes cellular dysfunction in the body regardless of etiologic factors in the hypersecretion. Increased thyroid hormone causes increased metabolic activity and stimulates the beta-adrenergic receptors, which results in a heightened sympathetic nervous system response. In addition to the effects of the hypermetabolism, the increased number of epinephrine-binding sites hyperactivates cardiac tissue, nervous tissue, smooth muscle tissue metabolism, and heat production.

Pathophysiology

Thyroid hormone increases cellular oxygen consumption in almost all metabolically active cells. It is generally believed that thyroid hormones increase the rate of

RESEARCH ABSTRACT

An evaluation of interventions for meeting the information needs of families of critically ill patients.

Henneman EA, McKenzie JB, Dewa CS: *Am J Crit Care* 85 1(3):85, 1992.

PURPOSE

The purpose of this study was to evaluate the effectiveness of two methods of meeting the information needs of the families of critically ill patients: an open visiting hour policy and a family information booklet.

DESIGN

One-way between-subjects design

SAMPLE

The convenience sample consisted of 147 English-speaking, age 18 years or older, family members or significant others of patients admitted to the 12-bed medical intensive care unit (MICU) of a large West Coast medical center. The sample comprised three groups: those for whom needs were met during a restricted visiting hour period (group 1, $n = 48$); those after implementation of an open visiting hour policy (group 2, $n = 50$); and those after implementation of a family information booklet and open visiting hour policy (group 3, $n = 49$). The majority (76%) of respondents reported that they were related to the patient (spouse, child, sibling). The patient's admission to the MICU was the first critical care unit experience in 86% of the cases.

INSTRUMENTS

An instrument developed by the principal investigator consisted of three sections: a satisfaction scale addressing family members' satisfaction with having their information needs met; a knowledge evaluation tool that evaluated the family member's ability to recall certain information, such as physician and social worker name; and demographic data. Content validity of the tool was established by a panel of experts, and pilot testing of the tool demonstrated a Cronbach alpha reliability of 0.97.

PROCEDURE

Questionnaires were distributed to the family members between 24 and 48 hours after the patient's admission to the unit. Subjects were asked to complete the questionnaires within 24 hours and return them to the drop-off area in the waiting room. After the initial data collection period, an open visiting hour policy was instituted in the MICU. Four months after the open-door visiting hour policy was implemented, the questionnaires were distributed to a second set of families in the previously described manner. Six months later a family information booklet was designed and instituted, with the questionnaires distributed to a new group of families 2 months after the implementation of the booklet.

RESULTS

Significant increases ($p < .05$) in family satisfaction were reported by group 2 when compared with group 1; there was a significant ($p < .05$) increase in family member's knowledge in group 2 as compared with group 1. There were no significant differences in family satisfaction between groups 2 and 3; however, group 3 reported significantly ($p < .05$) greater knowledge of details when compared with group 2. Group 3 reported significantly ($p < .05$) greater satisfaction and knowledge than did group 1.

DISCUSSION/IMPLICATIONS

The findings of this study demonstrate that the open visiting policy and information booklet were associated with meeting the information needs of families of critically ill patients. Implementation of an open visiting policy by itself increased family satisfaction and knowledge. From this finding, it appears that even if a critical care unit does not have an information booklet, it is important to consider an open visiting hour policy. The ability to visualize the environment and spend more time in the unit will facilitate meeting important needs of family members. Even though the information booklet did not appear to increase satisfaction, it was effective in assisting family members to recall discrete pieces of information and therefore (in combination with open visiting hours) was considered to be the most effective method of meeting family needs. Recommendations for future research include replicating the study in different settings, examining the effect of staff orientation and education regarding meeting family needs, and refinement of the instrument developed specifically for this study.

sodium and potassium movement through permeable membranes by stimulation of the sodium pump. It is likely, therefore, that increased thyroid hormone levels increase the sodium-potassium–linked pumping and accelerate metabolism and heat production even more.[27] Much energy in the form of heat is lost, however, rather than utilized by the cell. Cellular oxygen demands are increased in the patient with a hyperthyroid condition, and the cardiac response is to pump more blood more rapidly to deliver oxygen and to expel carbon dioxide. The oxygen demands in the hypermetabolic state are so great, however, that the cardiac system cannot compensate adequately. Fatigue and tachydysrhythmias ensue, along with a critically high fever. Increased metabolic

CONDITIONS ASSOCIATED WITH THYROTOXICOSIS

GLANDULAR DYSFUNCTION

Grave's disease (Basedow's disease, diffuse toxic goiter)
Toxic nodular goiter
Plummer's disease (toxic multinodular adenoma)
Giant cell thyroiditis (subacute thyroiditis)
Radiation-induced thyroiditis

DRUG THERAPY

Hormonal therapy
- Iatrogenic thyroid replacement
- Thyrotoxicosis factitia (purposeful ingestion of unphysiologic doses to produce weight loss)
- Accidental ingestion of thyroid (foods or medications)

Antidysrhythmic drug
- Amiodarone (may cause thyroid dysfunction[25])
- Propranolol

TUMORS

The following cause hyperthyroidism only rarely:
- Metastatic thyroid carcinoma
- Hypophyseal tumors (increasing TSH)
- Hypothalamus tumors (increasing TRH)
- Trophoblastic tumors (malignancies with circulating thyroid stimulants), such as hydatidiform mole, testicular tumors, and choriocarcinoma[26]

CONDITIONS PRECIPITATING THYROTOXIC CRISIS

- ◆ Systemic infections
- ◆ Diabetes out of control
- ◆ Trauma
- ◆ Myocardial infarction
- ◆ Thyroid medication overdose
- ◆ Thyroid ablations (surgical or radioiodine)
- ◆ Surgery
- ◆ Parturition in patient with poorly controlled hyperthyroidism

rate requires increased oxygen and sufficient energy sources. In hyperthyroidism the patient's appetite increases to meet metabolic demands. Generally the patient is unable to take in enough food to meet the demands and prevent mobilization of carbohydrates, fats, and protein for energy sources. As a result of rapidly broken-down nutrients, nitrogen[28] and uric acid excretion are increased, and metabolic acidosis is a potential problem.[29] Intestinal peristalsis increases, often resulting in diarrhea, nausea, and vomiting. These all lead to dehydration and compound the problem of malnutrition and weight loss. Excess metabolism generates heat, and the body temperature may rise as high as 41° C (106° F). Inefficient use of oxygen also affects the muscular system. Muscular contraction and relaxation require 40% more oxygen in the patient with a hyperthyroid condition than in the healthy person.[28] Muscular weakness occurs and is compounded by the excessive protein breakdown.[30]

Hypersensitivity to the increased adrenergic-binding sites potentiates the cardiovascular and nervous system response to the hypermetabolic state. Tachydysrhythmias often progress to pulmonary edema and congestive heart failure. Increased beta-adrenergic activity manifests in emotional lability, fine muscular tremors, and delirium.

Assessment and Diagnosis

Thyrotoxic crisis is a potentially lethal complication of thyrotoxicosis. It is insidious in nature with an almost paradoxically abrupt presentation of symptoms. Thyrotoxic crisis lacks a "textbook" profile that signals its presence. The presenting symptoms and severity of the disease differ from one patient to another and change during the course of the disease, posing a profound threat to the patient's survival. Metabolic pathways are accelerated, thermoregulation is impaired, and hyperactivity of the nervous and cardiovascular system can lead to cardiac collapse and death.

Of the patients diagnosed with thyrotoxicosis 15% are older than 65 years of age, yet diagnosis of a thyroid disorder in elderly persons may present more difficulties than in any other age-group. The aging process and changes in serum protein levels reduce circulating thyroid levels up to 20%. This level can be further reduced to 50%[31] during hospitalization, when the patient is adapting to a major illness and the effects of medications. In addition, symptoms associated with thyrotoxicosis, such as hyperkinesia, often are absent in elderly persons.[31] When these symptoms are present, they frequently are attributed to senescence.

Clinical manifestations of thyrotoxicosis are exaggerated in thyrotoxic crisis. An important exception, however, is that the laboratory values of patients with thyrotoxic crisis will not show any sudden changes as a result of thyrotoxicosis. Serum triiodothyronine (T_3) and thyroxine (T_4) remain at their elevated thyrotoxic levels.[9] No diagnostic test is available to differentiate thyrotoxic crisis from its predecessor, thyrotoxicosis.[8]

Clinical manifestations of thyroid storm are exaggerated signs and symptoms of thyrotoxicosis. The clinical manifestations are listed in the box on p. 716.

Medical Management

The medical management of thyrotoxicosis is of an acute, emergency nature. Various abnormal processes are occurring in the body that, if left untreated, could quickly lead to coma and death from cardiac failure. Production of thyroid hormone and conversion of T_4 to more active, potent T_3 needs to be reduced.

The body's heightened sensitivity to the increased adrenergic and catecholamine receptors must be suppressed. Cardiac irregularities need to be controlled and

CLINICAL MANIFESTATIONS OF THYROTOXIC CRISIS

CARDIOVASCULAR

Prompted by increased number and affinity of beta-adrenergic receptors in the heart:

Tachycardia
Systolic murmur
Increased stroke volume
Increased cardiac output
Increased systolic blood pressure
Decreased diastolic blood pressure
Extra systoles
Paroxysmal atrial tachycardia
Premature ventricular contraction
Palpitations
Chest pain
Increased cardiac contractility
Congestive heart failure
Pulmonary edema
Cardiogenic shock

CENTRAL NERVOUS SYSTEM

Resulting from an increased catecholamine response:

Hyperkinesis
Nervousness
Muscle weakness
Confusion
Convulsions
Heat intolerance
Fine tremor
Emotional lability
Frank psychosis
Apathy
Stupor
Diaphoresis

GASTROINTESTINAL

Nausea
Vomiting
Diarrhea
Liver enlargement
Abdominal pain
Weight loss
Increased appetite

INTEGUMENTARY

Pruritus
Hyperpigmentation of skin
Fine, straight hair
Alopecia

CLINICAL MANIFESTATIONS OF THYROTOXIC CRISIS—cont'd

THERMOREGULATORY

Hyperthermia
Heat dissipation
Diaphoresis

SERUM/URINE

Hypercalcemia
Hyperglycemia
Hypoalbuminemia
Hypoprothrombinemia
Hypocholesterolemia
Creatinuria

progression of heart failure halted. Pyrexia must be treated with hypothermia measures such as cooling blanket and acetaminophen (aspirin is to be avoided because it is believed to free the thyroid hormone from its protein state, thus rendering it more active).[32] Vigorous fluid replacement needs to be instituted to treat or prevent dehydration. Antibiotic therapy may be warranted in the presence of systemic infection. Other existing pathologic conditions need to be treated appropriately. Table 43-4 lists the most commonly used medications and their nursing implications for the patient in thyrotoxic crisis. Pharmacologic treatment consists of blocking the synthesis and release of thyroid hormone into circulation, inhibiting the conversion of T_4 to T_3 and decreasing the body's sensitivity to the sympathetic adrenergic receptors.

Blocking the synthesis of thyroid hormone is accomplished by administration of antithyroid thioamide drugs. These drugs include propylthiouracil (PTU) and methimazole (Tapazole). Neither drug is available in parenteral form and must be given by mouth or via a nasogastric tube. Propylthiouracil is especially therapeutic because it also blocks the conversion of T_4 to T_3. Methimazole has a slower action rate but it is more potent than propylthiouracil. The anti-thyroid drugs do not block the release of previously synthesized thyroid hormone; therefore in a crisis state they are given with iodide preparations.

Drugs that reduce thyroid hormone release into circulation are the iodides and a similarly acting glucocorticoid, dexamethasone. The iodide preparations are rapid-acting with a short duration. They are given 1 hour after the administration of the antithyroid drugs to prevent the iodide from being utilized for thyroid hormone and possibly worsening the clinical state. The iodides maintain and increase the levels of protein-bound thyroid hormone, thereby decreasing the levels of free, active thyroid. The iodide most frequently used for thyrotoxic crisis is sodium iodide. Potassium iodide, saturated solution of potassium iodide, or strong iodide solution also may be used. Patients who cannot take iodides because of allergies may be given lithium carbonate, which inhibits release of the thyroid hormone.[33]

A powerful glucocorticoid, dexamethasone suppresses the release of thyroid hormone.[29] Beta-adrenergic blocking agents are used to decrease the catecholamine effects of excessive thyroid hormone. Propranolol, used in thyrotoxic crisis, has no effect on the thyroid hormone[34] but effectively reduces the exaggerated myocardial stimulation, reduces myocardial contraction force, and slows the atrioventricular (AV) conduction rate. Doses vary from patient to patient, but typically higher doses are required to affect the number of receptor sites active in the crisis. Esmolol, a short-acting beta blocker, specifically used for short-term, rapid control of atrial fibrillation, also can be used. Currently clinicians disagree on the use of beta blockers for patients with overt heart failure. Drugs that can be used when beta-adrenergic blocking agents are contraindicated[33] include reserpine and guanethidine. These drugs, used infrequently because of the numerous side effects, deplete or inhibit norepinephrine release at the adrenergic nerve endings.

Calcium channel blockers such as verapamil also are effective in controlling heart rate in patients for whom beta blockers are contraindicated.

Medical management is concurrently directed at reducing critical multiple organ dysfunction syndrome that results from the hypermetabolic effects of thyrotoxic crisis. Reduction in body temperature by use of a cooling blanket and antipyretic agents (acetaminophen is used rather than aspirin products as the latter binds to thyroid-binding globulin and displaces thyroid hormone into a free, active state). Intravenous infusion of dantrolene, used to prevent or treat malignant hyperthermia, has been used successfully in the management of pyrexia from thyrotoxic crisis.[29] Dantrolene appears to block the calcium release in select myocytes and inhibits the intense catabolism in these muscle cells. Preventing rapid breakdown of metabolites within the cells prevents the production of heat, which is believed to stimulate the critical rise in body temperature.[35]

Dehydration and metabolic acidosis are treated with large volumes of glucose and sodium solutions to replace circulating fluid and sodium and to provide calories used by the hypermetabolism. Sodium bicarbonate replacement may be ordered to reverse the metabolic acidosis. Its use is controversial, however, because it can cause further tissue hypoxia (see p. 699 for discussion of sodium bicarbonate in the treatment of diabetic ketoacidosis).

To reduce the patient's work of breathing, 100% oxygen is given. Oxygen titration is based on pulse oximeter readings or on arterial blood gas values obtained to determine the metabolic acidosis.

Medication doses usually are increased to achieve the desired effect and to compensate for the rapid metabolism and clearance of the chemicals from the body during the thyrotoxic crisis.[30] Digitalis and diuretics may be required to treat symptoms of congestive heart failure, with doses possibly increased to achieve the desired effect.

Nursing Management

Nursing management for the thyrotoxic patient is important not only to preserve homeostasis within the hyperfunctioning body, but to prevent or diagnose the beginning stages of thyrotoxic crisis. The patient with a hyperactive thyroid complains of increased body temperature, anxiety, restlessness, tremulousness, increased appetite, palpitations, sweating, and intolerance to heat. Also present are dysrhythmias and tachypnea. Uncomplicated hyperactive thyroid, however, usually is diagnosed and managed on an outpatient basis, without the need for hospitalization.[36] It is the patient who is hospitalized for a major illness—the person with either undiagnosed or previously controlled thyrotoxicosis—who is at greatest risk for experiencing the complication of thyrotoxic crisis. Thyrotoxic crisis may be precipitated by increased physical stress on the body in the form of a major illness and hospitalization. Currently no diagnostic tests specific for thyrotoxic crisis are available. Standard laboratory tests are inconclusive. The results of thyroid function tests, such as those that measure T_4 and T_3, show understandably elevated levels caused by thyrotoxicosis, but they do not reflect the gross increases one would expect with the extreme hypermetabolic state seen in a crisis condition.[9] The condition, therefore, is identified by a combination of past medical history and current clinical manifestations. The nursing history is of great importance for this patient.

Nursing management includes constant vigilance over hypermetabolic effects on the body's temperature, cardiac functioning, and nervous system responses. Hydration must be preserved, hyperglycemia treated if present, metabolic acidosis prevented and/or treated, and weight loss curtailed.

◆ **Hyperthermia.** In thyrotoxic crisis the patient has hyperthermia related to a hypermetabolic state as evidenced by critically high body temperature—often above 105° F—diaphoresis; hot, flushed skin; intolerance to heat; tachycardia; and tachypnea. Temperature is to be assessed every 15 minutes and frequency gradually tapered after the temperature reaches safe levels and stabilizes. Core temperature is identified most accurately with an invasive pulmonary arterial line. (The arterial line also is least disruptive to the patient, who is in an agitated, restless state.) If an arterial line is not used to monitor temperature, the second choice to determine accurate core body temperature is to use a tympanic membrane core temperature sensor. The tympanic sensor provides a more accurate reading of body temperature than do other noninvasive methods, including the rectal thermometer probe attached to a hypothermia cooling blanket. Its accuracy is determined by the fact that the eardrum (against which the sensor is held) shares the blood supply and is in proximity to the hypothalamus, the body's "thermostat." A reading is available in 2.3 seconds. [37]

Nursing measures to provide comfort while the patient is intolerant to heat include a room with a cool environment and a fan to circulate air, lightweight bed coverings, and comfortable, nonrestrictive bed clothes. A tepid sponge bath helps to reduce heat by evaporation, and ice application to the groin and axilla increases heat loss at major blood vessels through conduction.

Changes in cardiac functioning relate to the high metabolic activity and adrenergic response. The result-

Table 43-4 Medications and nursing implications for thyrotoxic crisis[6,8,33,34]

Drug	Dosage/frequency	Route	Action	Nursing implications	Side effects
Propylthiouracil	Loading dose: 800-1200 mg Maintenance: 100-400 mg q 4-6 hr	PO or gavage	Blocks synthesis of thyroid hormone Blocks conversion of T_4 to T_3	Monitor thyrotoxic response, i.e., heart rate, nervousness, fever, diarrhea, diaphoresis Observe for sudden conversion to hypothyroidism: headache, sluggish responses Assess for skin rash Administer with meals to reduce GI effects	Rash, nausea, vomiting Agranulocytosis Skin hyperpigmentation Prothrombin deficiency
Methimazole	10-20 mg q 6-8 hr	PO or gavage	Blocks synthesis of thyroid hormone	More toxic than propylthiouracil Presence of rash may be reason to discontinue drug Monitor signs listed for propylthiouracil	Rash Agranulocytosis
Sodium iodide	1 g/L q 12 hr	IV		Give iodide 1 hr after propylthiouracil or methimazole	
Potassium iodide	2-5 gtt q 8 hr	PO		Discontinue if rash appears	Toxic iodinism/poisoning: edema Mucosal hemorrhage/stomatitis Metallic taste Skin lesions Severe GI upset
Saturated solution of potassium iodide (SSKI)	10 gtt q 8 hr	PO	Suppresses release of thyroid hormone	Protect with covered container	
Strong iodine solution—Lugol's solution	6 gtt q 8 hr	PO		Give through a straw to prevent teeth discoloration Mix with juice or milk to lessen GI upset	
Dexamethasone	2 mg q 6 hr, variable	IV	Suppresses thyroid hormone release Blocks conversion of T_4 to T_3	Monitor intake and output; monitor serum glucose levels	Hypertension, nausea, vomiting, anorexia Increased susceptibility to infection

Propranolol hydrochloride	1-3 mg q 1-4 hr 40-80 mg q 4-6 hr	IV PO	Beta-adrenergic blocking agent Decreases conversion of T_4 to T_3	Monitor cardiac activity CVP, PCWP Be alert for bradycardia, hypotension Hold if heart rate <50 beats/min Have atropine available	Bradycardia Congestive heart failure Edema Hypotension GI upset Fatigue Weakness
Reserpine	1.0-2.5 mg q 24 hr	PO	Depletes storage of catecholamine in sympathetic nerve endings	Monitor BP, heart rate changes in hyperthyroid conditions	Bradycardia Drowsiness GI bleeding Diarrhea
Guanethidine sulfate	50-150 mg q 24 hr	PO	Inhibits norepinephrine release in response to sympathetic nerve stimulation	Monitor BP for orthostatic hypotension Measure and record intake and output Monitor diarrhea	Drowsiness Edema Fatigue Orthostatic hypotension GI upset
Esmolol hydrochloride	500 μg/kg/min for first minute, then 50 μg/kg/min for 4 min	IV	Beta-adrenergic blocker	Monitor for bradycardia, orthostatic hypotension, dysrhythmia Measure and record intake and output	Edema Hypotension Diarrhea Dizziness Diaphoresis

NURSING DIAGNOSIS AND MANAGEMENT
Thyrotoxic crisis

- ◆ Altered Nutrition: Less Than Body Protein-Calorie Requirements related to lack of exogenous nutrients and increased metabolic demand, p. 673
- ◆ Decreased Cardiac Output related to ventricular tachycardia, p. 362
- ◆ Fluid Volume Deficit related to diarrhea, wound drainage, p. 640
- ◆ Activity Intolerance related to knowledge deficit of energy/saving techniques secondary to hypermetabolic state, p. 365
- ◆ Anxiety related to threat to biologic, psychologic, and/or social integrity, p. 763
- ◆ Sensory/Perceptual Alterations related to sensory overload, sensory deprivation, and sleep pattern disturbance, p. 573

ing tachydysrhythmia and heart failure, coupled with the hyperthermia, eventually cause death.[28]

Cardiovascular assessment includes rate, rhythm, irregularities, blood pressure changes, pulse pressure variances, decrease in quality of peripheral pulses, and patient reports of chest pain and palpitations. Hemodynamic monitoring includes atrial blood pressure, CVP, PCWP, and cardiac output readings. High-output cardiac failure may occur with the demands of the hypermetabolic activity within the body, far exceeding the ability of the myocardium to pump oxygenated blood to meet those demands. Heart failure ensues as the catecholamine-driven receptors produce abnormal conduction patterns and weakening rapid contractions. The rapid heart rate allows little time for the coronary arteries to fill and supply oxygen to the cardiac tissue. Atrial fibrillation with rapid ventricular response can potentially lead to premature ventricular contractions and ventricular fibrillation.

Nursing management includes the administration of the prescribed beta-adrenergic blocking agents to decrease the catecholamine effects of the thyroid hormone. Reduction in heart rate, decreased cardiac irritability, and decreased contractile force of the myocardium should result. Administration of cardiac glycosides also may be warranted to increase the strength of the myocardial contraction while increasing stroke volume. An increase in the refractory period prolongs atrioventricular conduction, allowing the heart a longer diastole for rest and an increased time to fill coronary arteries to supply oxygen to the myocardium. Bradycardia and hypotension are to be closely monitored as potential untoward effects of the aforementioned drugs, which are given either alone or in combination.

Hyperthermia, tachypnea, diaphoresis, vomiting, and diarrhea predispose the patient to a fluid volume deficit. Fluids and electrolytes are as vigorously replaced as the decompensated cardiovascular system can manage. Glucose solutions are given to replace glycogen stores. Insulin may be administered to treat the hyperglycemia that results from mobilization of nutrients and high doses of glucocorticoids. Fingerstick glucose tests may be performed to identify the level of glucose in the blood stream and to use as a reference point for insulin dose. Hyponatremia from active loss, which is monitored by means of laboratory serum values is prevented and/or treated with appropriate sodium concentrations of intravenous fluids.

Nursing attention is focused on CVP, PAP, breath sounds, neck vein engorgement, and hourly urine output. A serious complication is circulatory overload. It is signaled by increased CVP, increased pulmonary atrial pressure, moist lung sounds, neck vein engorgement, and dyspnea without exertion. Reduction in fluid volume infusion, elevation of the head of the bed, and administration of diuretics and oxygen may be needed to support the patient's breathing and to alleviate the increased fluid load. Additional nursing measures focus on hourly hydration assessments. Intake and output measurements include estimating diaphoretic fluid loss through the number of gown and linen changes, checking buccal membranes for moisture, and recording daily weights. (See hydration assessment, p. 699, for additional information).

The patient in thyrotoxic crisis is agitated, anxious, and unable to rest and thus requires intensive care that is quiet, restful, and calm. Gradually the antithyroid medications and beta-adrenergic blocking drugs will decrease the neurologic symptoms related to the catecholamine sensitivity. Medications given for sedation include phenobarbital, which also will reduce T_4 levels in the blood stream.[34] The patient needs to be told that his or her extreme agitation is the result of the disease process and that the medications will help to control the nonstop fidgeting and tremors. (See the nursing diagnosis of anxiety related to a threat to biologic, psychologic, and/or social integrity on p. 763. Of special value to the nurse caring for the patient in thyrotoxic crisis are the nursing measures and the explanations presented in this care plan.) Frequent reassurance and clear, simple explanations regarding the patient's condition help decrease the fear brought on by the strange surroundings.

Sleep deprivation as a result of the intense neuroexcitation is another challenge for the critical care nurse. The patient needs uninterrupted blocks of time to rest even if he or she is unable to sleep during that time. The primary nurse is responsible for encouraging all members of the medical, nursing, and paramedical staff to respect these rest periods. Family and other visitors are to adhere to the treatment plan as well. The complete nursing management plans for sleep-pattern disturbance are provided on pp. 142 and 143.

The goal of intense medical and nursing management of thyrotoxic crisis is to reduce thyroid hormone levels within 24 to 48 hours. During this time the life-threatening symptoms of hyperpyrexia, cardiac excitation, and nervous system dysfunction are brought under control.

REFERENCES

1. Rifkin H, Porte D, editors: *Ellenberg and Rifkin's diabetes mellitus: theory and practice,* ed 4, New York, 1990, Elsevier.
2. Kelley W, editor: *Textbook of internal medicine,* vol 2, ed 2, Philadelphia, 1992, JB Lippincott.
3. Wilson JD and others, editors: *Harrison's principles of internal medicine,* ed 12, New York, 1991, McGraw-Hill.
4. Schroeder S, Krupp M, Tierney L: *Current medical diagnosis and treatment,* Norwalk, Conn, 1988, Appleton & Lange.
5. Tepperman J, Tepperman H: *Metabolic and endocrine physiology,* ed 5, Chicago, 1987, Mosby–Year Book.
6. Burch W: *Endocrinology,* ed 2, Baltimore, 1988, Williams & Wilkins.
7. Powers M: *Handbook of diabetes nutritional management,* Rockville, Md, 1987, Aspen.
8. Becker K: Principles and practices of endocrinology and metabolism, Philadelphia, 1992, JB Lippincott.
9. Reference deleted in proofs.
10. Torre M, Slavin M: Developing a protocol for continuous insulin infusion, *Hosp Pharm Hotline* 2(10), 1989.
11. Bullock B, Rosendahl P: *Pathophysiology: adaptations and alterations in function,* ed 3, Philadelphia, 1992, JB Lippincott.
12. Grindlinger G, Boylan M: Amelioration by indomethacin of lithium-induced polyuria, *Crit Care Med* 15(5):538, 1987.
13. Nerozzi D, Goodwin F, Costa E, editors: *Neuropsychiatric disorders,* New York, 1987, Raven Press.
14. Lubin M and others, editors: *Medical management of the surgical patient,* Boston, 1988, Butterworth.
15. Henry J, editor: *Todd, Sanford, Davidsohn's clinical diagnosis and management by laboratory methods,* ed 17, Philadelphia, 1984, WB Saunders.
16. Hadley M: *Endocrinology,* ed 2, Englewood Cliffs, NJ, 1988, Prentice Hall.
17. Fischbach F: *A manual of laboratory diagnostic tests,* ed 4, Philadelphia, 1992, JB Lippincott.
18. Chanson P and others: Ultra-low doses of vasopressin in the management of diabetes insipidus, *Crit Care Med* 15(1):44, 1987.
19. Staller A: Systemic effects of severe head trauma, *Crit Care Nurs Q* 10(1):58, 1987.
20. Hemmer M and others: Urinary ADH excretion during mechanical ventilation and weaning in man, *Anesthesiology* 52(5):395, 1980.
21. Guyton AC: *Textbook of medical physiology,* ed 8, Philadelphia, 1991, WB Saunders.
22. Methany NM: *Fluid and electrolyte balance: nursing considerations,* ed 2, Philadelphia, 1992, JB Lippincott.
23. Reference deleted in proofs.
24. Vokes T, Robertson G: Disorders of antidiuretic hormone, *Endocrinol Metab Clin North Am* 17(2):281, 1988.
25. Sox HC, editor: *Common diagnostic tests: use and interpretation,* ed 2, Philadelphia, 1990, American College of Physicians.
26. Kissane JM, editor: *Anderson's pathology,* vol 2, ed 9, St Louis, 1990, Mosby–Year Book.
27. Ganong WF: *Review of medical physiology,* ed 15, Norwalk, Conn, 1991, Appleton & Lange.
28. Ritchie AC: *Boyd's textbook of pathology,* vol 2, ed 9, Philadelphia, 1990, Lea & Febiger.
29. Bennett MH, Wainwright AP: Acute thyroid crisis on induction of anesthesia, Anesthesia 44:28, 1989.
30. West JB, editor: *Best and Taylor's physiological basis of medical practice,* ed 12, Baltimore, 1991, Williams & Wilkins.
31. Berman R, Haxby J, Pomerantz R: Physiology of aging. I. Normal changes, *Patient Care,* Jan 15, 1988.
32. Clark W, Brater DC, Johnson AR: *Goth's medical pharmacology,* ed 13, St Louis, 1992, Mosby–Year Book.
33. Shoemaker W and others: *Textbook of critical care,* ed 2, Philadelphia, 1989, WB Saunders.
34. DeGroot L, editor: *Endocrinology,* vol 1, ed 2, Philadelphia, 1989, WB Saunders.
35. Malseed RT: *Pharmacology,* ed 3, Philadelphia, 1990, JB Lippincott.
36. Isley WL: Thyroid disorders, *Crit Care Nurs Q* 13(3):39, 1990.
37. Erickson R, DiBenedetto L: Accuracy of core temperature measurement with the IVAC Core Check™; tympanic thermometer system (unpublished research), *White Paper on Clinical Issues,* Oct 31, 1991, San Diego, IVAC Corp.

44

Endocrine Nursing Diagnosis and Management

This chapter is designed to supplement the preceding chapters in the *Endocrine Alterations* unit by integrating theoretic content into clinically applicable case studies and nursing management plans.

The case study is designed to illustrate clinical problem solving and patient care management occurring in actual patients. The case, reviewed retrospectively, demonstrates how medical and nursing diagnoses may be effectively used in critical care. The case study also demonstrates revisions to the plan of care and the nursing and medical management outcomes that are apt to occur during the course of a complicated hospitalization as the patient responds physiologically to treatment. Often in a short case anecdote, such as presented in this chapter, the clinical answer may appear to be obvious from the day of admission. In practice, however, critical care patient management is sometimes investigative and the "correct" diagnosis for an individual patient may not become apparent until midway in the hospitalization. Or a patient with an apparently straightforward diagnosis may develop an unexpected complication, and the plan of care and potential outcomes will then require revision. Many of the case studies demonstrate this principle.

The nursing management plans, which—unlike the case study—are not patient-specific, provide a basis nurses can use to individualize care for their patients. In the previous *Endocrine Alterations* chapters, each medical diagnosis is assigned a Nursing Diagnosis and Management box. Using this box as a page guide, the reader can access relevant nursing management plans for each medical diagnosis. For example, nursing management of *hyperglycemic hyperosmotic nonketotic coma*, described on pp. 704-705, may involve several nursing diagnoses and management plans outlined in this chapter and in other Nursing Diagnosis and Management chapters. Specific examples are (1) *Decreased Cardiac Output related to decreased preload secondary to fluid volume deficit*, on p. 361 and (2) *Anxiety related to threat to biologic, psychologic, and/or social integrity*, on p. 763. These examples highlight the interrelationship of the various physiologic systems in the body and the fact that pathology often has a multisystem impact in the critically ill.

Use of the case study and management plans can enhance the understanding and application of the *Endocrine* content in clinical practice.

ENDOCRINE CASE STUDY

CLINICAL HISTORY

Ms. B is a 57-year-old woman who has been treated for type I diabetes mellitus for 30 years. Family members report Ms. B is careful about her diet, checks her blood glucose frequently, and gives herself insulin every day.

CURRENT PROBLEMS

Ms. B has been complaining of flu-like symptoms with nausea, vomiting, and diarrhea for the past 3 days. Her family says that she seemed confused the previous evening and could not recognize her children. This morning the family had difficulty waking her.

Assessment findings included the following: Ht, 64 in (5 ft, 4 in); wt., 47 kg (103 lbs); mentation, obtunded; T, 97.2° F; P, 140; R, 40; BP, 80/60; fingerstick glucose, >400. (See Table 44-1 for other laboratory values.) Cardiac S_1 and S_2, WNL; no S_3 or S_4 or murmurs. Kussmaul's respirations; sweet breath odor. Skin was flushed, dry and warm; skin turgor >3 seconds at clavicle. Buccal membranes were dry, lips parched, and tongue furrowed. Bowel sounds were hyperactive; abdomen was soft and tender to touch with guarding behavior. Extremities were without cyanosis or edema. Pedal pulses were equal. Ms. B was incontinent of a small amount of dark urine and approximately 50 ml diarrheal stool.

ENDOCRINE CASE STUDY—cont'd

MEDICAL DIAGNOSES

DKA (diabetic ketoacidosis) precipitated by gastroenteritis
Severe dehydration secondary to hyperosmolar status

NURSING DIAGNOSIS

◆ Fluid Volume Deficit related to diarrhea and osmotic diuresis

◆ PLAN OF CARE

1. Reverse dehydration.
2. Restore insulin-glucagon ratio.
3. Treat and prevent circulatory collapse.
4. Replenish electrolytes.
5. Identify precipitating cause to prevent DKA from recurring.

MEDICAL AND NURSING MANAGEMENT AND PATIENT OUTCOME

Ms. B began receiving an intravenous infusion of 1000 ml 0.9% sodium chloride with 30 mEq potassium chloride per hour. A bolus of 14 units of human regular insulin was started intravenously (0.3 U/kg), and regular insulin was to be added to the primary container to deliver 5 U of human regular insulin per hour (0.1 U/kg). Ms. B was placed on NPO status and was given oxygen at 2 L/min per nasal cannula. Cardiac monitoring was initiated and revealed tachycardia. An indwelling catheter was inserted into the urinary bladder, and 600 ml of dark, concentrated urine was obtained. The intravenous solution was monitored by an electronic infusion pump to assure accuracy. As a precaution, containers of 5% dextrose and 50% dextrose intravenous solutions were available for immediate use should Ms. B's serum glucose level fall too rapidly and signs of hypoglycemia manifest. Ms. B required increased stimulation to evoke a response and was placed on her side in a low-Fowler's position. Bedside fingerstick glucose tests were done every 30 minutes for the first 2 hours. Vital signs were taken every 15 minutes, at which time Ms. B's position in bed was slightly realigned to reduce pressure on the compromised skin tissues. (See Table 44-1 for other laboratory values.)

Kussmaul's respirations and fruity breath odor were assessed. Vital signs, especially BP, pulse characteristics, and hemodynamic findings, were monitored to assess for cardiac response to the rapid fluid replacement. Urine output was monitored hourly. Ms. B was assessed for circulatory overload, which could occur from such rapid rehydration; she was monitored for neck vein engorgement, sudden unexplained dyspnea, elevated central venous pressure and/or elevated pulmonary artery pressures, and moist lung sounds. Hydration assessment included temperature, skin moisture, and skin turgor.

Ms. B's oral assessment and care included moist gauze pads to keep the oral membranes moistened and to prevent buildup of bacteria in the mouth. Her neurologic status was monitored and documented every 15 minutes for the first hour to determine the effects of the hyponatremia (because of osmotic diuresis) on the central nervous system. Nurses continually evaluated the extent of Ms. B's impaired thinking. Short words and sentences were used to give simple directions and provide reorientation to her immediate hospital surroundings.

During the first two hours Ms. B showed dramatic improvement. The vigorous fluid replacement reversed the hypovolemia and diluted the relative blood osmolality. The continuous low-dose insulin therapy was used to transfer glucose from the blood stream to the cell receptor site, which reduced the need for fats to be broken down for energy. Respirations became easier as there was less carbonic acid in the blood stream to be blown off in the form of CO_2. In addition, a decrease in Kussmaul's respirations contributed to conservation of body fluid because less water was lost with each exhalation. Ms. B became more responsive and aware of her surroundings. Her level of consciousness was upgraded to lethargic. (See Table 44-1 for other laboratory values.)

She was no longer incontinent of stool, and bowel sounds returned to normal. Urine became more dilute. Serum sodium increased to 134 mEq/L, and blood pressure was 102/65. The intravenous solution was changed to 0.45% NaCl, and the flow rate was reduced to 500 ml/hour. (1500 ml of NaCl had been absorbed at that time). The bicarbonate ion was reversing itself, and subsequently a rise in pH occurred as a result of adequate fluid and insulin therapy. Bicarbonate therapy was not required. Blood glucose levels were decreasing gradually because of the low-dose insulin replacement and because no signs of hypoglycemia were present. As the patient's level of consciousness improved and she had no difficulty swallowing, Ms. B was able to rinse her mouth for comfort. As the nausea subsided, the NPO order was changed and Ms. B took sips of water, which gradually supplemented the IV replacement fluids.

At 11 AM the fingerstick glucose level was 272 mg. According to the prescribed orders the IV solution was changed from .45% NaCl to 5% Dextrose in .45% NaCl. The 30 mEq of KCl was added to the IV container, along with insulin to provide 5 U/hr. This change was made to prevent the glucose level from rapidly decreasing and precipitating hypoglycemia. The rate was set at 250 ml per hour. (See Table 44-1 for other laboratory values.)

At 12:30 PM Ms. B was alert and freely taking fluids by mouth. The serum glucose laboratory value was 226 mg/dl. At this time the IV insulin was no longer needed. BP was 129/70 and indicated that subcutaneous insulin could be absorbed and distributed throughout the body. Human regular insulin, 5 U, was given subcutaneously. Ms. B was

Continued.

ENDOCRINE CASE STUDY—cont'd

moving around in bed and asking if she could get up to go to the bathroom. (See Table 44-1 for other laboratory values.)

The remainder of Ms. B's clinical stay was uneventful. Once she was adequately hydrated and the blood osmolality returned to normal, the serum glucose levels returned to their pre-DKA status and were adequately controlled with subcutaneous injections of insulin. The blood pH continued a gradual rise to normal levels through fluid and insulin correction and without bicarbonate therapy. Potassium levels stayed within the normal range. Ms. B received discharge teaching to prevent this situation from recurring should she develop influenza or gastroenteritis again. It was recommended that she receive the influenza virus vaccine each season to minimize the course of the disease whenever she was exposed to the virus. Family members were included in the sessions, which included discussion of management of insulin doses when nausea is present and food cannot be consumed. In addition, the teaching plan for Ms. B and her family members included review of physical and emotional changes indicative of fluctuating glucose levels. Nursing instructions emphasized changes that must be brought to the attention of the health care practitioner, as well as steps that should be taken to avoid serious hyperglycemic or hypoglycemic complications.

Table 44-1 Mrs. B's laboratory data

	8 AM	9 AM	10 AM	11 AM	11:30 AM	12:30 PM	1:30 PM
Mentation	obtunded	obtunded	lethargic	lethargic	alert	alert	alert
Temperature (°F)	97.2	97.2	97.3	97.6	97.8	97.9	98.3
Pulse (/min)	140	140	138	128	123	120	113
Respiration (/min)	40	39	35	34	33	31	31
BP (mm Hg)	80/60	92/62	102/65	120/68	126/70	129/70	133/71
Urine ketones	4+	4+	4+	4+	3+	3+	2+
Plasma glucose (mg/dl)	460	350	290	272	250	226	200
Sodium (mEq/L)	129	133	134	135	136	136	138
Potassium (mEq/L)	4.5	4.3	4.1	3.9	3.9	3.8	3.7
Chloride (mEq/L)	96	98	99	99	100	100	101
Bicarbonate (mEq/L)	7.5	9.0	10.4	11.8	12.5	13.2	15
BUN (mEq/L)	34	32	31	30	29	29	28
Plasma ketones	4+	4+	4+	4+	4+	4+	4+
Po_2 (mm Hg)	100	100	100	100	100	100	100
Pco_2 (mm Hg)	20	19.3	18.9	18.5	18.4	18.3	18.1
pH	7.19	7.23	7.26	7.29	7.3	7.31	7.33
Hgb (gm/dl)	20	19.3	18.9	18.5	18.4	18.3	18.1
Hct (%/cu ml)	55.9	54.3	53.4	52.5	52.3	52.1	51.5
WBC (thousand/cu ml)	10.4	10.4	10.4	10.4	10.4	10.4	10.4

FLUID VOLUME EXCESS RELATED TO INCREASED SECRETION OF ADH

DEFINING CHARACTERISTICS

- Weight gain *without* edema
- Hyponatremia (dilutional)
- Decreased urinary output
- Urinary osmolality above normal, exceeding plasma osmolality
- Urinary specific gravity >1.030
- Evidence of water intoxication:
  Fatigue
  Headache
  Abdominal cramps
  Altered level of consciousness
  Diarrhea
  Seizures

OUTCOME CRITERIA

- Weight returns to baseline.
- Serum sodium is 135-145 mEq/L.
- Urinary output is >30 ml/hr.
- Urinary osmolality is 200-800 mOsm/kg.
- Urinary specific gravity is 1.005-1.030.
- Patient has no evidence of water intoxication.

NURSING INTERVENTIONS AND *RATIONALE*

1. Continue to monitor the assessment parameters listed under "Defining Characteristics." In addition, monitor patient closely for evidence of cardiac decompensation caused by excessive preload (i.e., elevated pulmonary artery diastolic pressure [PADP] or pulmonary capillary wedge pressure [PCWP], tachycardia, lung congestion).
2. Anticipate administration of demeclocycline, lithium carbonate, furosemide, and/or narcotic agonists.
3. With physician's collaboration, administer intravenous hypertonic sodium chloride ***to temporarily correct hyponatremia.***
4. Weigh patient daily at same time in same clothing, preferably with same scale.
5. Maintain fluid restriction.
6. Monitor hydration status.
7. Initiate seizure precautions ***because severe sodium deficit can result in seizures.***

FLUID VOLUME DEFICIT RELATED TO DECREASED SECRETION OF ADH

DEFINING CHARACTERISTICS

- Polyuria (15 L per day)
- Serum sodium 145 mEq/L (particularly in patients who are not drinking to replace losses)
- Intense thirst
- Polydipsia (alert patients)
- Urinary specific gravity <1.005
- Urinary osmolality <300 mOsm/kg
- Plasma osmolality >300 mOsm/kg

OUTCOME CRITERIA

- Urinary volume, specific gravity, and osmolality are normal.
- Thirst is reduced.
- Plasma osmolality and serum sodium level are normal.

NURSING INTERVENTIONS AND *RATIONALE*

1. Continue to monitor the assessment parameters listed under "Defining Characteristics." Additionally, monitor for signs of critical volume deficits, i.e., hypotension, fall in pulmonary artery pressures, tachycardia.
2. With physician's collaboration, administer intravenous electrolyte replacement solutions ***because critical electrolyte loss occurs along with water loss.*** Replace losses milliliter for milliliter plus 50 ml/hr for insensible losses. Avoid replacement of losses with intravenous dextrose solutions ***because of the risk of water intoxication.***
3. If patient is alert, encourage the patient to satisfy partially his or her replacement needs by drinking according to thirst. Caution should be observed regarding the patient's excessive ingestion of water (typically, the patient will crave iced water) ***because of the risk of water intoxication.***
4. With physician's collaboration, administer vasopressin intravenously, intramuscularly, or per the nasal route.
5. For patients after hypophysectomy, teach the administration of vasopressin and its reportable side and toxic effects, the monitoring of intake and output measurement, and the documentation of daily weights.

X

MULTISYSTEM ALTERATIONS

45

Trauma

CHAPTER OBJECTIVES

- Compare and contrast injuries associated with blunt and penetrating trauma.
- Discuss priorities in each phase of trauma care.
- Discuss mechanism of injury, pathophysiology, assessment findings, medical management, and nursing management of traumatic injuries to the following sites: (1) head, (2) spinal cord, (3) maxillofacial region, (4) heart, (5) lungs, (6) abdomen, (7) pelvis, and (8) lower extremities.
- Use assessment findings to identify complications and sequelae of traumatic injuries.

Trauma is a "neglected disease" of our society. In the United States, 16 traumatic deaths occur every hour, 384 deaths each day, and 150,000 deaths annually.[1] Trauma is the leading cause of death in persons 44 years of age and younger[2] and is one of America's most expensive health problems. Traumatic injuries account for one of the most expensive health care problems, costing $75 billion to $100 billion annually in direct and indirect costs.[3]

Over the past few decades major advances have been made in the management of patients with traumatic injuries, and significant improvements have been made in their care in both prehospital and emergency department settings. These improvements have affected critical care in that patients with complex, multisystem trauma are admitted to critical care units. These patients require complex nursing care. This chapter reviews nursing management of patients with traumatic injuries, particularly in the critical care setting.

MECHANISMS OF INJURY

Trauma occurs when an external force of energy impacts the body and causes structural or physiologic alterations, or "injuries." External forces can be radiation, electrical, thermal, chemical, or mechanical forms of energy. This chapter focuses on trauma from mechanical energy. Mechanical energy can produce either blunt or penetrating traumatic injuries. Knowledge of the mechanism of injury helps health care providers anticipate and predict potential internal injuries.

Blunt Trauma

Blunt trauma most often is seen with motor vehicle accidents (MVAs), contact sports, crush injuries, or falls. Injuries occur because of the forces sustained during a rapid change in velocity (deceleration). To estimate the amount of force a person would sustain in an MVA, multiply the person's weight by miles per hour of speed.[4] A 130-pound woman traveling at 60 miles per hour who hits a brick wall, for example, would sustain 7800 pounds of force within milliseconds. As the body stops suddenly, tissues and organs continue to move forward. This sudden change in velocity causes injuries that result in lacerations or crush injuries of internal body structures.

Penetrating Trauma

Penetrating injuries occur with stabbings, use of firearms, or impalement of foreign objects, which penetrate the skin, with resultant damage to internal structures. Damage is created along the path of penetration. Penetrating injuries can be misleading inasmuch as the outside of the wound does not determine the extent of internal injury. High-velocity bullets can create internal cavities up to 10 times the diameter of the bullet.[5]

Several factors determine the extent of damage sustained as a result of penetrating trauma. Different weapons cause different types of injuries. The severity of a gunshot wound depends on the type of gun, type of ammunition used, and the distance and angle from which the gun was fired. Pellets from a shotgun blast expand on impact and cause multiple injuries to internal structures. Handgun bullets, on the other hand, usually damage what is directly in the bullet's path. Once inside the body, the bullet can ricochet off bone and create further damage along its pathway. With penetrating stab wounds, factors that determine the extent of injury include type and length of object used, as well as the angle of insertion.

PHASES OF TRAUMA CARE

Care of trauma victims during wartime enhanced principles of triage and rapid transport of the injured to medical facilities.[6] The military experience has demonstrated that more lives can be saved by decreasing the time from injury to definitive care. It also has enhanced incentives and models for improvements in civilian trauma care, such as emergency medical service (EMS) systems and trauma care centers. The goal with critically injured patients is to minimize the time from initial insult to definitive care and to optimize prehospital care so that the patient arrives at the hospital alive.[7]

Statistics demonstrate that deaths as a result of

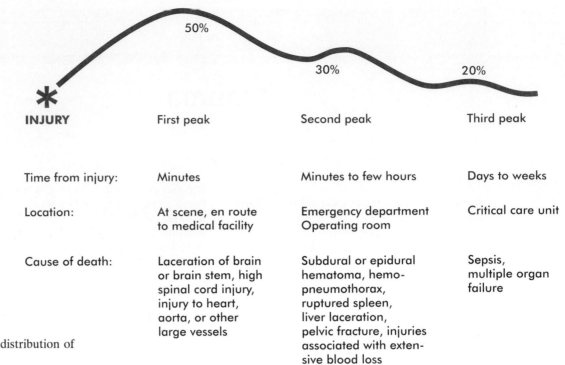

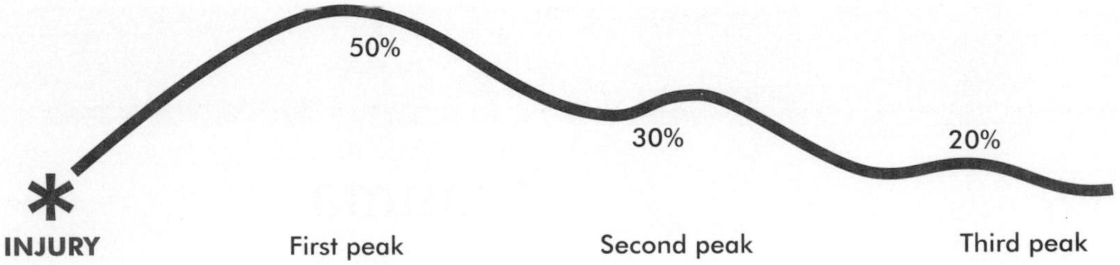

	First peak	Second peak	Third peak
Time from injury:	Minutes	Minutes to few hours	Days to weeks
Location:	At scene, en route to medical facility	Emergency department Operating room	Critical care unit
Cause of death:	Laceration of brain or brain stem, high spinal cord injury, injury to heart, aorta, or other large vessels	Subdural or epidural hematoma, hemo-pneumothorax, ruptured spleen, liver laceration, pelvic fracture, injuries associated with extensive blood loss	Sepsis, multiple organ failure

Fig. 45-1 Trimodal distribution of trauma deaths.

trauma occur in a trimodal distribution[3] (Fig. 45-1). The first peak includes victims who die before medical attention can be provided. The second peak occurs within a few hours after injury. It is this peak that commonly is referred to as the *golden hour* for those critically injured. The golden hour is a 60-minute time frame that incorporates activation of the EMS system, stabilization in the prehospital setting, transportation to a medical facility, rapid resuscitation on arrival in the emergency department, and the provision of definitive care. Chance of survival increases if all these measures can be completed within the first hour after injury.[3] The third death peak occurs days to weeks after injury as a result of complications, including infection or multiple organ dysfunction syndrome. It is a nursing challenge to influence the quality of care the trauma patient receives in an attempt to "beat" the trimodal distribution of trauma deaths.

Nursing management of the patient with traumatic injuries begins the moment a call for help is received and continues until the patient's death or return to the community.[8] Care of the trauma patient is seen as a continuum that includes six phases: prehospital, hospital resuscitation, definitive care and operative phase, critical care, intermediate care, and rehabilitation.

Prehospital Resuscitation

The goal of prehospital care is immediate stabilization and transportation. Stabilization is accomplished through assessments and interventions related to airway, breathing, and circulation (ABCs). Once stabilized at the scene, the patient is transported to an appropriate medical facility by ground or air transport.

Emergency Department Resuscitation

The American College of Surgeons developed guidelines (Advanced Trauma Life Support [ATLS]) for rapid assessment, resuscitation, and definitive care for trauma patients in the emergency department.[3] A similar nursing model (Trauma Nurse Core Course [TNCC]) was developed by the Emergency Nurses' Association.[9] Both programs emphasize the need for a systematic approach to care of the trauma patient in the emergency department: primary survey, secondary survey to be conducted simultaneously with resuscitation, and definitive management.

◆ **Primary survey.** On arrival of the trauma patient in the emergency department, the primary survey is initiated. During this assessment, life-threatening injuries are discovered and treated. The five steps in the primary survey comprise the ABCs, plus D and E—*D,* disability (mini-neurologic examination) and *E,* exposure (removal of clothes) (Table 45-1).

Airway. Airway is assessed for ineffective airway clearance and airway obstruction. The trauma patient is at high risk for ineffective airway clearance, especially in the presence of altered consciousness, drugs and alcohol, and thoracic injuries.[3] Airway obstruction can be caused by foreign bodies, blood clots, or broken teeth. Airway assessment must incorporate cervical spine immobilization by either manual cervical immobilization or placement of a rigid cervical collar, with the head, neck, and body strapped to a spine board or stretcher. The cervical spine must be immobilized in all trauma patients until a cervical spinal cord injury has been definitively ruled out. If the airway is obstructed, foreign bodies are removed. In the presence of ineffective airway clearance,

Table 45-1 Primary survey of the trauma patient

Survey component	Nursing diagnosis	Nursing assessment/care
Airway	Airway clearance: Ineffective related to obstruction or actual injury	Look, listen, and feel Immobilize C-spine Position victim/patient: Supine Sitting Log roll Clear airway: Jaw thrust Chin lift Finger sweep Suctioning Airway devices: Oropharyngeal Nasopharyngeal Endotracheal tube Cricothyrotomy
Breathing	Breathing pattern: Ineffective related to actual injury Gas exchange: Impaired related to actual injury or disrupted tissue perfusion	Assess for: Spontaneous breathing Respiratory rate, depth, and symmetry Chest wall integrity Administer high-flow oxygen Absent breathing: Intubate Positive-pressure ventilation Breathing but ineffective: Assess and treat life-threatening conditions, e.g., tension pneumothorax, flail chest
Circulation	Cardiac output, alteration in: Decreased related to actual injury Tissue perfusion, alteration in: Related to actual injury or shock Fluid volume deficit: Related to actual loss of circulating volume	Assess pulse: Quality Rate No pulse: Initiate BCLS Initiate ACLS Pulse but ineffective: Assess and treat life-threatening conditions, e.g., uncontrolled bleeding, shock Two large-bore (14- or 16-gauge) IVs Fluid replacement ECG monitoring
Disability	Injury potential for: Trauma, spinal cord, and brain related to actual injury	Brief neurologic examination Eye opening Verbal response Motor response Pupils AVPU Glasgow coma scale
Exposure	N/A	To visualize the entire body for inspection, all clothing must be removed

From Beaver BM: *Nurs Clin North Am* 25(1):13, 1990.

the airway is secured through intubation or cricothyrotomy.

Breathing. The patient is assessed for ineffective breathing patterns and impaired gas exchange. It is crucial to remember that an open, clear airway does not ensure adequate gas exchange. Assessment should include chest wall integrity, respiratory rate, depth, and symmetry. Supplemental oxygen is used in all trauma patients. Decreased breath sounds or alteration in chest wall integrity require chest tube placement. Mechanical ventilation is used for patients with a loss of consciousness or ineffective breathing patterns, or both.

Circulation. After effective airway clearance, breathing patterns, and gas exchange have been ensured, the nurse assesses for alteration in cardiac output, alteration in tissue perfusion, and fluid volume deficit. External exsanguination is identified and controlled. Rapid assessment of the circulatory status includes assessment of level of consciousness, skin color, and pulse. Level of consciousness provides data on cerebral perfusion. Assessment of skin color can provide information about the patient's circulatory volume. Ominous signs of hypovolemia include ashen, gray, or white skin. Systemic blood pressure can be rapidly evaluated by use of the 60-70-80 method.[9] If a carotid pulse is palpable, the minimal systolic pressure is estimated to be 60 mm Hg. A palpable femoral pulse can represent a systolic pressure of 70 mm Hg, and a palpable radial pulse can represent a systolic pressure of 80 mm Hg. If a pulse is not present, advanced cardiac life support (ACLS) protocols are instituted (see Appendix B). Cardiac monitoring is initiated to assess for rhythm disturbances. Life-threatening dysrhythmias are treated according to ACLS protocols. Military antishock trousers (MAST) or a pneumatic antishock garment (PASG) may be used to raise the systolic blood pressure. Both devices encompass the lower extremities and the abdomen. When inflated, these garments increase systolic blood pressure by increasing peripheral vascular resistance and myocardial afterload. Use of these garments, however, is controversial.

Disability. Once airway, breathing, and circulation have been effectively managed, the nurse begins the fourth step of the primary survey: disability (D). During this step the nurse assesses the potential for injury by completing a brief neurologic assessment to establish the patient's level of consciousness, and pupillary size and reaction. The AVPU method describes the patient's level of consciousness: *A, a*lert; *V,* responds to *v*erbal stimuli; *P,* responds to *p*ainful stimuli; and *U, u*nresponsive. A more detailed neurologic assessment is made during the secondary survey, discussed later.

Exposure. The final step in the primary survey is *E, e*xposure. All clothing is removed to facilitate a thorough examination of all body surfaces for the presence of injury.

◆ **Resuscitation phase.** After the primary survey the resuscitation phase begins. Hypovolemic shock is the most common type of shock that occurs in trauma patients.[3] Hemorrhage must be identified and treated rapidly. Vigorous intravenous (IV) fluid replacement is initiated. Large-bore peripheral IV catheters (14 to 16 gauge) or a central venous catheter should be inserted. Restoration of volume is accomplished through administration of crystalloid (lactated Ringer's solution or 0.9% saline solution), colloid (plasma or albumin), and/or blood products. During the initiation of IV lines, blood samples should be drawn (see first box in next column). High-flow fluid warmers may be used to deliver warmed IV solutions at rates up to 1000 ml/min (Model H-500 Fluid Warmer, Level I Technologies, Inc., Marshfield, Mass.). Transfusion of autologus salvaged blood (autotransfusion) also may be used to replace intravascular volume and to provide oxygen-carrying capacity.

Gastric and urinary catheters are placed, unless contraindicated. Adequate resuscitation is assessed by monitoring for improvement in vital signs, arterial blood gas levels, and urinary output.

◆ **Secondary survey.** After resuscitative measures, a rapid but thorough head-to-toe assessment of all systems is made. The history is one of the most important aspects of the secondary survey. The prehospital providers (paramedics, emergency medical technicians [EMTs]) usually can provide most of the vital information pertaining to the accident. Specific information that should be elicited pertaining to the mechanism of injury is summarized in the second box below. This information can help predict internal injuries and facilitate rapid intervention. The patient's pertinent past history can be

SERUM SAMPLES FOR LABORATORY STUDIES TO OBTAIN WITH IV PLACEMENT

Complete blood cell (CBC) count with differential
Electrolyte profile: sodium, potassium, chloride, carbon dioxide, glucose, urea, nitrogen, and creatinine
Coagulation parameters: prothrombin time (PT); partial thromboplastin time (PTT)
Type and screen (ABO compatibility)
Amylase
Ethanol
Liver function study (alanine aminotransferase—formerly SGPT)
Arterial blood gas (ABG)

HISTORY OF MECHANISM OF INJURY

PENETRATING TRAUMA

- Weapon used (handgun, shotgun, rifle, knife)
- Caliber of weapon
- Number of shots fired
- Gender of assailant
- Position of victim and assailant when injury occurred

BLUNT TRAUMA

- Length of fall
- MVA extrication time
- Ejection
- Location in automobile (passenger, driver; front seat, back seat)
- Restraint status (lapbelt, shoulder harness, or combination; unrestrained)
- Speed of automobile(s)
- Occupants (number and morbidity status)

assessed by use of the mnemonic AMPLE: *a*llergies, *m*edications, *p*ast medical illnesses, *l*ast meal, and *e*vents immediately preceding the incident/environment related to the injury.

During the secondary survey, the nurse ensures the completion of an electrocardiogram (ECG) and radiographic studies (chest, cervical spine, thorax, and pelvis). Throughout this survey the nurse continuously monitors the patient's vital signs and response to medical therapies. Emotional support to the patient and family also is imperative.

Definitive Care/Operative Phase

Once the secondary survey has been completed, specific injuries usually have been diagnosed. Definitive care related to specific injuries is described throughout this chapter. Trauma, often referred to as a *surgical disease* because of the nature and extent of the injuries, usually requires operative management of injuries. After surgery, depending on the patient's status, a transfer to the critical care unit may be indicated.

Critical Care Phase

Critically ill trauma patients are admitted into the critical care unit (CCU) as a direct transfer from the emergency department (ED) or operating room (OR). If surgery is required, the trauma patient should be directly admitted to the CCU from the OR.[2,10]

Information the CCU nurse should obtain from the ED or OR nurse, or both, is summarized in the box below. This information should be obtained before patient admission to the CCU to ensure availability of needed personnel, equipment, and supplies. This information also helps the CCU nurse to assess the impact of trauma resuscitation on the patient's CCU presentation and course. The box below summarizes the prehospital, ED, and OR resuscitative measures that can affect the trauma patient's care in the CCU.[11] Knowledge of these resuscitative measures helps the CCU nurse to identify and quantify ischemic damage that the patient experienced before admission to the CCU. The nurse can then modify nursing care in anticipation of hypoxic complications.

On the patient's arrival to the CCU, the nurse, using the primary and secondary surveys, and resuscitative measures in accordance with ATLS and TNCC guidelines, assesses the trauma patient's status. Priority nursing care during the critical care phase includes ongoing physical assessments and monitoring the patient's response to medical therapies. The CCU nurse constantly is aware that the third peak of the trimodal distribution of trauma deaths occurs in the CCU setting as a result of complications, including acute respiratory distress syndrome (ARDS), sepsis, prolonged shock states, and multiple organ dysfunction syndrome. Ongoing nursing assessments are imperative for early detection of complications.

One of the most important nursing roles is assessment of the balance between oxygen delivery and oxygen demand. Oxygen delivery must be optimized to prevent further system damage.[11] Assessment of circulatory status includes the use of noninvasive and invasive techniques as described in Chapter 14.

Tissue hypoxemia, which is a threat to the trauma patient, results from a variety of factors. The box on p. 734 lists these factors, as summarized by Von

NURSING REPORT FROM REFERRING AREA

- Name
- Age
- Mechanism of injury/injuries sustained
- Allergies
- Surgical procedures performed
- Established airway/mechanical ventilation settings
- Vital signs
- IV access
- Fluid intake (colloid and crystalloid)
- Fluid loss (urine output, chest tube drainage, estimated intraoperative blood loss)
- Invasive hemodynamic values (if in place)
- Medications administered
- Past medical/surgical history
- Family members present, assessment of coping, assessment of knowledge of nature of injuries and treatment plan

From Johnson KL: Critical care of the trauma patient. In Neff JA, Kidd PS, editors: *Trauma nursing: the art and science,* St Louis, 1992, Mosby–Year Book.

ASPECTS OF TRAUMA RESUSCITATION THAT IMPACT ON THE PATIENT'S CCU PRESENTATION AND CCU COURSE

- Prolonged extrication time (gives an indication of the length of time the patient may have been hypotensive before medical care)
- Period of respiratory or cardiac arrest with a total loss of tissue perfusion
- Length of time the patient was hypotensive or hypovolemic
- Length of time the patient was hypothermic
- Blood loss and/or massive fluid resuscitation resulting in a low hematocrit
- Time on the backboard, which potentiates the risk of sacral and occipital breakdown
- Number of units of blood received (gives an indication of the potential for development of adult respiratory distress syndrome [ARDS])

Modified from Johnson KL: Critical care of the trauma patient. In Neff JA, Kidd PS, editors: *Trauma nursing: the art and science,* St Louis, 1993, Mosby–Year Book.

FACTORS THAT CONTRIBUTE TO TISSUE HYPOXIA IN THE TRAUMA PATIENT

- Shifts to the left of the oxyhemoglobin dissociation curve (can be secondary to infusion of large volumes of banked blood, hypocarbia or alkalosis, or hypothermia)
- Reduced hemoglobin (secondary to hemorrhage)
- Reduced cardiac output (in the presence of cardiovascular insults)
- Impaired cellular oxygen consumption (associated with metabolic alterations of sepsis)
- Increased metabolic demands (associated with the stress response to injury)

From Johnson KL: Critical care of the trauma patient. In Neff JA, Kidd PS, editors: *Trauma nursing: the art and science,* St Louis, 1993, Mosby–Year Book.

Reuden.[12] Prevention and treatment of hypoxemia depend on accurate assessment of the adequacy of pulmonary gas exchange, oxygen transport, and cellular oxygen utilization. Nursing interventions must promote adequate tissue oxygenation.

Frequent and thorough nursing assessments of all body systems are important because these assessments are the cornerstone to the management of the critically ill trauma patient. The nurse can detect subtle changes and facilitate the implementation of timely therapeutic interventions to prevent complications frequently associated with trauma. The nurse must be knowledgeable about specific organ injuries, as well as their associated sequelae.

◆ Specific Trauma Injuries

HEAD INJURIES

At least 2 million persons incur head injuries each year in the United States, and more than 400,000 patients with head injuries are admitted to hospitals, approximately half of whom were involved in motor vehicle accidents (MVAs).[13] Head injuries account for 25% of all trauma deaths, and 50% to 60% of all deaths as a result of motor vehicle trauma.[13]

Mechanism of Injury

Head injuries occur when mechanical forces are transmitted to brain tissue. Mechanisms of injury include penetrating or blunt trauma to the head. Penetrating trauma can result from the penetration of a foreign object (e.g., bullet) that causes direct damage to cerebral tissue. Blunt trauma can be the result of deceleration, acceleration, or rotational forces. Deceleration causes the brain to crash against the skull after it has hit something (e.g., the dashboard of a car). Acceleration injuries occur when the brain has been hit by something (e.g., a baseball bat). In many instances, head injury can be caused by both acceleration and deceleration. Acceleration injuries occur when the skull is hit by a force that causes the brain to move forward to the point of impact, and then as the brain reverses direction and hits the other side of the skull, deceleration injuries occur.

Pathophysiology

Review of the pathophysiology of head injury can be divided into two categories: primary injury (that which occurs on impact); and secondary injury (that which occurs as a result of the original trauma).

◆ **Primary injury.** The primary injury occurs at the time of impact as a result of the dynamic forces of acceleration-deceleration or rotation. Primary injuries include contusion, laceration, shearing injuries, or hemorrhage. Primary injury may be mild, with little or no neurologic damage, or severe, with major tissue damage.

◆ **Secondary injury.** Secondary injury can be caused by further physiologic events that occur after the primary injury. Secondary injury can be caused by hypoxia, hypercapnia, hypotension, cerebral edema, or sustained hypertension. Beyond causing injury to tissue, each of these factors also contributes to significant increases in intracranial pressure (ICP).

Hypoxia produces secondary injury through two mechanisms. Tissue ischemia occurs in the area inadequately oxygenated, and the cells of the ischemic area become edematous. Extreme vasodilation of the cerebral vasculature occurs in an attempt to supply oxygen to the cerebral tissue. This increase in blood volume increases intracranial volume and ICP.

Hypercapnia is a powerful vasodilator. Most often caused by hypoventilation in an unconscious patient, hypercapnia results in cerebral vasodilation and increased cerebral blood volume and ICP.

Significant hypotension causes inadequate perfusion to neural tissue. It is important to note that hypotension rarely is associated with head injury. If a trauma patient is unconscious and hypotensive, an aggressive assessment of the chest, abdomen, and pelvis should be performed to rule out internal injuries.

Cerebral edema occurs as a result of the changes in the cellular environment caused by contusion, loss of autoregulation, and increased permeability of the blood-brain barrier. Cerebral edema can be focal as it localizes around the area of contusion (just as tissue edema occurs in other parts of the body in response to injury) or diffuse as a result of hypotension or hypoxia. The extent of cerebral edema can be minimized by controlling the other aspects of secondary injury, such as oxygenation, ventilation, and blood pressure.

Initial hypertension in the patient with severe head injury is common. As a result of the loss of autoregulation, increased blood pressure results in increased intracranial blood volume and ICP. Every effort should be made to control hypertension to prevent the secondary injury caused by increased ICP.

The effects of increases in intracranial pressure may be varied. As pressure increases inside the enclosed vault of the skull, cerebral perfusion decreases, which leads to further compromise of the intracranial contents. The effects of increasing pressure and decreasing perfusion precipitate a downward spiral of events. (For a more detailed discussion of intracranial pressure, see Chapter 29.)

RESEARCH ABSTRACT

Cerebrovascular response of patients with closed head injuries to a standardized endotracheal tube suctioning and manual hyperventilation procedure.

Crosby LJ, Parsons LC: *J Neurosci Nurs* 24 (1):40, 1992.

PURPOSE

The purpose of this study was twofold: to assess the cerebrovascular response of patients with closed head injuries to a standardized endotracheal tube suctioning/manual hyperventilation (ETTS/MH) procedure; and to determine if a 5-minute rest period after the ETTS/MH procedure was sufficient in length to allow cerebrovascular parameters to return to preintervention levels.

DESIGN

Quasi-experimental repeated measures design

SAMPLE

The nonrandom sample consisted of 49 subjects (39 males, 10 females) with a mean age of 30 years, admitted to the trauma center of a university medical center, with the diagnoses of brain contusion, subdural hematoma, intracerebral hemorrhage, and cerebral edema. Subjects were required to have an endotracheal tube in place and to be receiving mechanical ventilation with a baseline arterial oxygen pressure (Pao_2) of 70 mm Hg or greater, an arterial carbon dioxide pressure ($Paco_2$) between 28 and 32 mm Hg, a forced inspiratory oxygen concentration (FIo_2) no greater than 40%, a positive end-expiratory pressure (PEEP) less than 15 cm H_2O, and a direct mean arterial blood pressure (MABP) of greater than 50 mm Hg as measured by an arterial catheter. In addition, subarachnoid pressure bolts were in place to monitor intracranial pressure (ICP); ECG and core body temperature also were monitored (ranging between 35° and 38° C).

INSTRUMENTS

All data were recorded by a Hewlett-Packard Patient Monitoring System (H-P PMS) in digital format, stored in a Hewlett-Packard Minicomputer, and retrieved on command through paper printouts. The MABP was measured by means of an arterial catheter placed in a radial or pedal artery and connected to a Bently transducer. The ICP was measured through a Richmond subarachnoid bolt connected to either a Gould P-50 mini-pressure transducer or a Bently 800 pressure transducer. Cerebral perfusion pressure (CPP) was calculated by the H-P Minicomputer; the end-tidal carbon dioxide pressure ($Petco_2$) was measured by use of an H-P 4721A Capnometer attached to the endotracheal tube.

PROCEDURE

A research assistant, who collected data within 72 hours of the patients' head injury, used a programmed, menu-driven minicomputer at the patient's bedside with a hand-held computer keyboard. Subjects were allowed to rest undisturbed for 5 minutes before the research protocol. After the baseline data were collected, the research assistant informed the researcher when the next step in the protocol should be initiated or terminated. The researcher attached an Ohio-Onmeda soft anesthesia bag continuously filled with 100% oxygen. A two-handed method was used to administer manual hyperventilation (MH) at a rate twice the controlled ventilator rate. The first MH was maintained for 30 seconds, followed by the introduction of a 14-French Travenol plastic suction catheter, with a continuous suction pressure of between 120 and 160 mm Hg, applied for 15 seconds while the catheter was removed. The procedure lasted until three suctioning passes and four MH episodes were extended to 60 seconds (third and fourth MH episodes). On completion of the procedure the ventilator was reattached to the endotracheal tube and the 5-minute rest period was initiated. Data were collected at baseline, at the end of each 15-second time interval during the ETTS/MH procedure, and at the end of each recovery period for 5 minutes.

RESULTS

Findings indicated that those patients whose baseline mean ICP (MICP) was most elevated demonstrated significantly lower ($p < .05$) MABP, CPP, and heart rate (HR) in response to the ETTS/MH procedure when compared with those subjects with a lower baseline mean ICP. In both groups 60 seconds were required after the second and third suctioning catheter pass to reverse a stepwise increase in MICP. At least 2 full minutes of recovery time after completion of the procedure was required to allow all physiologic variables to return to baseline.

DISCUSSION/IMPLICATIONS

Findings from this study indicate that it is possible to control the stepwise increase in ICP associated with ETTS by extending the MH to 60 seconds between suction passes. Two full minutes of undisturbed rest after the procedure are necessary to return MABP, ICP, HR, CPP, and $Petco_2$ to baseline. It is important for nurses who manage head injuries to organize care with staggered interventions so that the patient's physiologic status is not compromised. Recommendations for future research include replication of this study with a larger sample; examination of the relationship of other physiologic variables with ETTS/MH techniques; inclusion of patients with a greater variability of resting MICP; and control of variables such as medications.

Classification

Injuries of the brain are described by the functional changes or losses that occur. Some of the major functional abnormalities seen in head injury are described here.

◆ **Skull fractures.** Skull fractures are common, but they do not by themselves cause neurologic deficits. Skull fractures can be classified as open (dura is torn) or closed (dura is not torn), or they can be classified as those of the vault or those of the base. Common vault fractures occur in the parietal and temporal regions. Basilar skull fractures usually are not visible on conventional skull films. Assessment findings may include cerebral spinal fluid otorrhea or rhinorrhea, Battle's sign (ecchymosis overlying the mastoid process), or "raccoon eyes" (subconjunctival and periorbital ecchymosis).

All patients with skull fractures are hospitalized for observation.[3] Open skull fractures require surgical intervention to remove bony fragments and to close the dura. The major complications of basilar skull fractures are cranial nerve injury and leakage of cerebrospinal fluid (CSF). CSF leakage may result in a fistula, which increases the possibility of bacterial contamination and resultant meningitis. Because fistula formation may be delayed, patients with a basilar skull fracture are admitted to the hospital for observation and possible surgical intervention.

◆ **Concussion.** A concussion is a brain injury accompanied by a brief loss of neurologic function, especially loss of consciousness.[3] If loss of consciousness occurs, it may last for seconds to an hour. The neurologic dysfunctions present as confusion, disorientation, and sometimes a period of posttraumatic amnesia. Other clinical manifestations that occur after concussion are headache, dizziness, irritability, inability to concentrate, impaired memory, and fatigue. The work-up for concussion probably is responsible for more emergency department visits, x-ray films, and admissions to the hospital than any other type of brain injury; despite its prevalence, however, ongoing debate continues as to the nature of the injury and its long-term sequelae.[14] The diagnosis of concussion is based on the loss of consciousness inasmuch as the brain remains structurally intact despite functional impairment. Patients with a history of 5 or more minutes of loss of consciousness usually are admitted to the hospital for a 24-hour observation period.[3]

◆ **Contusion.** Contusion, or bruising of the brain, usually is related to acceleration-deceleration injuries, which result in hemorrhage into the superficial parenchyma, often the frontal and temporal lobes. Frontal or temporal contusions can be seen in a coup-contrecoup mechanism of injury (Fig. 45-2). Coup injury affects the cerebral tissue directly under the point of impact. Contrecoup injury occurs in a line directly opposite the point of impact.

The clinical manifestations of contusion are related to the location of the contusion, the degree of contusion, and the presence of associated lesions. Contusions can be small, in which localized areas of dysfunction result in a focal neurologic deficit. Larger contusions can evolve over 2 to 3 days after injury as a result of edema and further hemorrhaging. A large contusion can produce a mass effect that can cause a significant increase in ICP.

Contusions of the tips of the temporal lobe are a common occurrence and are of particular concern. Because the inner aspects of the temporal lobe surround the opening in the tentorium where the midbrain enters the cerebrum, edema in this area can cause rapid deterioration of the patient's condition and can lead to herniation. Because of the location, this deterioration can occur with little or no warning at a deceptively low ICP.

Diagnosis of contusion is made by computed tomography (CT) scan. If the CT scan indicates contusion, especially in the temporal area, the nurse must pay particular attention to neurologic assessments and look for subtle changes in pupillary signs or vital signs, irrespective of a stable ICP.

Medical management of cerebral contusions may consist of medical or surgical therapies. Because a

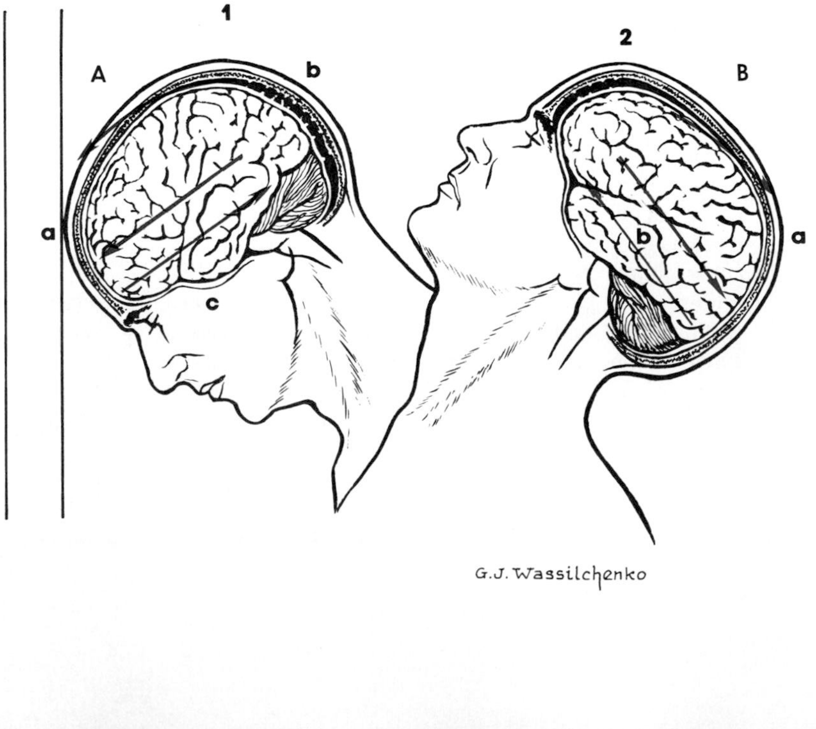

Fig. 45-2 Coup and contrecoup head injury after blunt trauma. **A,** Coup injury: impact against object. *a,* Site of impact and direct trauma to brain. *b,* Shearing of subdural veins. *c,* Trauma to base of brain. **B,** Contrecoup injury: impact within skull. *a,* Site of impact from brain hitting opposite side of skull. *b,* Shearing forces throughout brain. These injuries occur in one continuous motion—the head strikes the wall (coup), then rebounds (contrecoup).

contusion can progress over 3 to 5 days after injury, secondary injury may occur. If contusions are small, focal, or multiple, they are treated medically with serial neurologic assessments and possibly ICP monitoring. Increased ICP usually is managed medically as described in Chapter 29. Larger contusions that produce considerable mass effect require surgical intervention to prevent the increased edema and intracranial pressure as the contusion matures.[3] Outcome of cerebral contusion varies, depending on the location and the degree of contusion. These injuries often are complicated by posttraumatic epilepsy.[15]

◆ **Hematomas.** Hematomas resulting from head injury form a mass lesion and lead to increased ICP. Three types of hematomas are discussed here (Fig. 45-3). The first two hematomas, epidural and subdural, are extraparenchymal (outside of brain tissue) and produce injury by pressure effect and displacement of intracranial contents. The third type of hematoma, intracerebral, directly damages neural tissue and can produce further injury as a result of pressure and displacement of intracranial contents.

Epidural hematoma. Epidural hematoma (EDH), which is a collection of blood between the inner table of the skull and the outermost layer of the dura, most frequently is associated with skull fractures and middle meningeal artery laceration. A blow to the head that causes a linear skull fracture on the lateral surface of the head may tear the middle meningeal artery. As the artery bleeds, it pulls the dura away from the skull, creating a pouch that expands into the intracranial space.

The incidence of EDH is relatively low. This type of injury accounts for 1% to 3% of all head trauma but makes up at least 8% of severely injured patients.[15] EDH can occur as a result of low-impact injuries (such as falls) or high-impact injuries (such as motor vehicle accidents). EDH occurs from trauma to the skull and meninges rather than the acceleration-deceleration forces seen in other head trauma.

The classic clinical manifestations of EDH include brief loss of consciousness followed by a period of lucidity that may last up to 12 hours. This lucid period is followed by a progressive deterioration in level of consciousness, dilation of the pupil on the same side of the hematoma (ipsilateral), and onset of abnormal flexion (decorticate) or abnormal extension (decerebrate). Diagnosis of EDH is based on clinical symptoms and evidence of a collection of epidural blood identified on CT scan. Treatment of EDH involves surgical intervention to remove the blood and to cauterize the bleeding vessels. With early surgical intervention the prognosis is excellent.[3] Outcome varies from excellent, with no neurologic sequelae, to a persistent vegetative state or death. Outcome can depend on the timing of surgical intervention.

Subdural hematoma. Subdural hematoma (SDH), which is the accumulation of blood between the dura and underlying arachnoid membrane, most often is related to a rupture in the bridging veins between the brain and the dura. Acceleration/deceleration and rotational forces are the major causes of SDH, which often is associated with cerebral contusions and intracerebral hemorrhage.

The three types of SDH are based on the time frame from injury to clinical symptoms: acute, subacute, and chronic. Table 45-2 summarizes the time interval and presentation for each type of SDH.[16] Acute SDHs are those hematomas that are clinically symptomatic in the first 48 hours after injury. The clinical presentation of acute SDH is determined by the severity of injury to the underlying brain at the time of impact and the rapidity of accumulation of blood in the subdural space.[14] In

Table 45-2 Classification of subdural hematomas

Type	Time interval	Symptoms
Acute	Within 48 hr	Headache, drowsiness, agitation, confusion, deterioration in LOC, fixed and ipsilateral pupil dilation, contralateral hemiparesis **or** Profound coma
Subacute	2 days to 2 wk	Similar to acute SDH except that symptoms appear more slowly
Chronic	2 wk to months	Progressive lethargy, absent-mindedness, headache, vomiting, seizures, ipsilateral pupil dilation, or contralateral hemiparesis

LOC, level of consciousness.

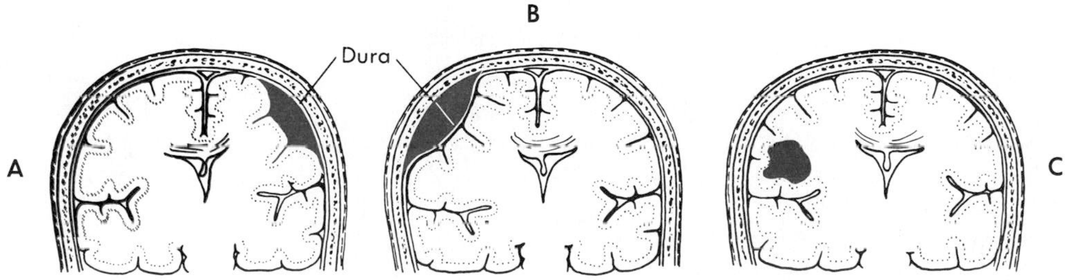

Fig. 45-3 Types of cerebral hematomas. **A,** Epidural hematoma. **B,** Subdural hematoma. **C,** Intracerebral hematoma.

other situations the patient has a lucid period before deterioration. Careful observation for deterioration in level of consciousness or lateralizing signs, such as inequality of pupils or motor movements, is essential. Surgical intervention may require craniectomy, craniotomy, or burr hole evacuation. SDH results in a mortality of 22%, which rises to 50% with injuries to other body systems.[14]

Subacute SDHs are hematomas that develop symptomatically 2 days to 2 weeks after trauma. In subacute hematomas the expansion of the hematoma occurs at a rate slower than that in acute SDH; therefore it takes longer for symptoms to become obvious. Clinical deterioration with subacute SDH usually is slower than that with acute SDH, but treatment by surgical intervention, when appropriate, is the same.

Chronic subdural hematoma is the term used when symptoms appear 2 weeks or more after injury. Most patients with chronic SDH usually are elderly or in late middle age. Many have a history of alcoholism, and some are on a regimen of anticoagulation therapy.

The pathophysiology of chronic SDH is slightly different from that of acute SDH. The initial hemorrhage is not sufficient to produce clinical signs of increasing pressure. Within 2 weeks, a vascular membrane encases the clot and the hematoma slowly enlarges. Once the hematoma becomes large enough to exert pressure on cerebral contents, symptoms appear.

Clinical manifestations of chronic SDH are insidious. The patient can report a variety of symptoms, such as lethargy, absent-mindedness, headache, vomiting, stiff neck, and photophobia, and show signs of transient ischemic attack, seizures, pupillary changes, or hemiparesis. Because history of trauma often is not significant enough to be recalled, chronic SDH seldom is seen as an initial diagnosis. CT scan evaluation can confirm the diagnosis of chronic SDH.

If surgical intervention is required, evacuation of the chronic SDH may occur by craniotomy, burr holes, or catheter drainage. Burr hole placement or catheter drainage involves drilling a hole in the skull over the site of the chronic SDH and draining the fluid. Drains or catheters are left in place for at least 24 hours to facilitate total drainage. Outcome after chronic SDH evacuation is variable. Return of neurologic status often depends on the degree of neurologic dysfunction before removal. Because this condition is most common in the elderly or debilitated patient, recovery is a slow process. Recurrence of chronic SDH is not infrequent.

Intracerebral hematoma. Intracerebral hematoma (ICH) results when there is bleeding within cerebral tissue. Traumatic causes of ICH include depressed skull fractures, penetrating injuries (bullet, knife), or sudden acceleration/deceleration motion. The ICH acts as a rapidly expanding lesion, and the mortality is high[16]; however, late ICH into the necrotic center of a contused area also is possible. Sudden clinical deterioration of a patient 6 to 10 days after trauma may be the result of ICH.

Medical management of ICH may include surgical or nonsurgical management. Generally it is believed that hemorrhages that do not cause significant ICP problems should be treated nonsurgically. Over time, the hemorrhage may be reabsorbed. If significant problems with ICP occur as a result of the ICH producing a mass effect, surgical removal is necessary. Outcome from ICH depends greatly on the location of the hemorrhage. Size, mass effect, and displacement of other intracranial structures also affect the outcome. ICH results in a mortality between 25% and 72%.[14]

◆ **Missile injuries.** Missile injuries are caused by objects that penetrate the skull to produce a significant focal damage but little acceleration/deceleration or rotational injury. The injury may be depressed, penetrating, or perforating (Fig. 45-4). Depressed injuries are caused by fractures of the skull, with penetration of bone into cerebral tissue. Penetrating injury is caused by a missile that enters the cranial cavity but does not exit. A low-velocity penetrating injury (knife) may involve only focal damage and no loss of consciousness. A high-velocity missile (bullet) can produce shock waves that are transmitted throughout the brain, in addition to injury caused by the bullet. Perforating injuries are missile injuries that enter and then exit the brain. Perforating injuries have much less ricochet effect but are still responsible for significant injury.

Risk of infection and cerebral abscess is a concern in missile injuries. If fragments of the missile are embedded

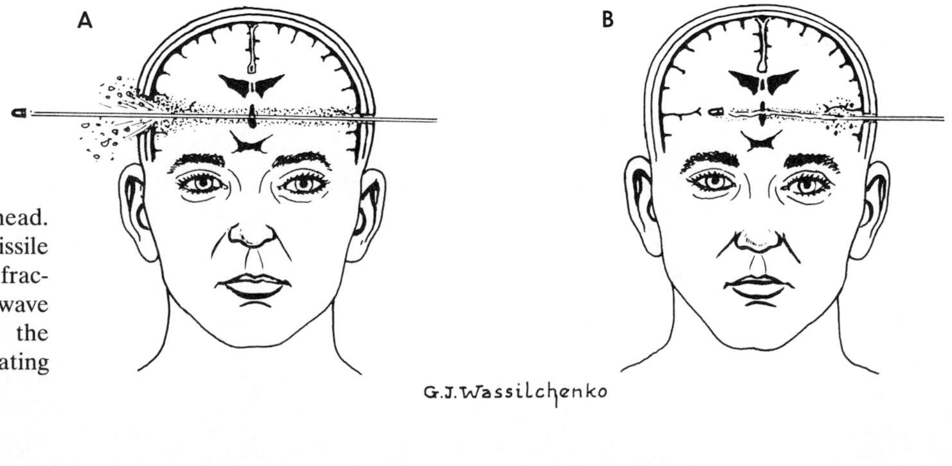

Fig. 45-4 Bullet wounds of the head. Bullet wound or other penetrating missile will cause an open (compound) skull fracture and damage to brain tissue. Shock wave effects are transmitted throughout the brain. **A,** Perforating injury. **B,** Penetrating injury.

within the brain, careful consideration of the location and risk of increasing neurologic deficit is weighed against the risk of abscess or infection. The outcome after missile injury is based on the degree of penetration and the location of the injury, as well as the velocity of the missile.

◆ **Diffuse axonal injury.** Diffuse axonal injury (DAI) covers a wide range of brain dysfunction caused by acceleration/deceleration and rotational forces. This diagnosis usually is reserved for severe dysfunction. Cerebral concussion is the least severe form of diffuse axonal injury. DAI describes prolonged coma from the time of injury that is not the result of mass lesions or ischemia.

The pathophysiology of DAI is related to the stretching and tearing of axons as a result of movement of the brain inside the cranium at the time of impact. The stretching and tearing of axons result in microscopic lesions throughout the brain, but especially deep within cerebral tissue and the base of the cerebrum. Disruption of axonal transmission of impulses results in loss of consciousness. Unless surrounding tissue areas are significantly injured, causing small hemorrhages, DAI is not visible on CT scan. The patient remains in a deep coma, often with decerebrate or decorticate posturing and autonomic dysfunction, including hyperthermia, hypertension, and diaphoresis.

Treatment of DAI includes support of vital functions and maintenance of ICP within normal limits. The outcome after severe DAI is poor because of the extensive dysfunction of cerebral pathways. DAI occurs in 44% of all coma-producing head injuries, with an overall mortality of 33%, but in its most severe form, mortality can be 50%.[3]

Assessment

Rapid assessment and triage of patients with head injury are critical to a favorable prognosis. To assist with the initial assessment, head injuries are divided into three descriptive categories on the basis of the patient's Glascow Coma Scale (GCS) and length of the unconscious state.

◆ Degree of injury

Mild injury. Mild head injury is described as a GCS score of 13 to 15, with a loss of consciousness that lasts up to 15 minutes. Patients with mild injury often are seen in the emergency department and discharged home with a family member who is instructed to evaluate the patient routinely and to bring the patient back to the hospital if any further neurologic symptoms appear.

Moderate injury. Moderate head injury is described as a GCS score of 9 to 12, with a loss of consciousness for up to 6 hours. Patients with this type of head injury usually are hospitalized. They are at high risk for deterioration from increasing cerebral edema and ICP, and therefore serial clinical assessments are an important function of the nurse. Hemodynamic and ICP monitoring and ventilatory support often are not required in this group unless other systemic injuries make them necessary. A CT scan usually is performed on admission. Repeat CT scans are indicated if the patient's neurologic status deteriorates.

Severe injury. Severe head injury is described as a GCS score of 3 to 8, with loss of consciousness for longer than 6 hours. Patients with severe head injury often receive ventilatory support along with ICP and hemodynamic monitoring. A CT scan is performed to rule out any mass lesions that can be surgically removed. Patients are placed in a critical care setting for continual assessment, monitoring, and management.

◆ **Nursing assessment.** As in all traumatic injuries, the evaluation of the ABCs (airway, breathing, and circulation) should be the first step in the assessment of the head-injured patient in the critical care unit. These assessments are particularly important in head injury because of secondary injury that can occur as a result of hypoxia, hypoventilation, and hypoperfusion. A patient with severe head injury who is breathing spontaneously may require prophylactic endotracheal or nasotracheal intubation with mechanical ventilatory support to reduce the risk of hypoxia and hypercapnia. After stabilization of the ABCs is ensured, a neurologic assessment is performed.

Level of consciousness, motor movements, pupillary response, respiratory function, and vital signs are all part of a complete neurologic assessment in the patient with severe head injury. Level of consciousness can be elicited to assess wakefulness. Consciousness should be assessed by obtaining the patient's response to verbal and painful stimuli. Determination of orientation to person, place, and time assesses mental alertness. Pupils should be assessed for size, shape, equality, and reactivity. Asymmetry should be reported immediately. Pupils should be assessed for constriction to a light source (parasympathetic innervation) or dilation (sympathetic innervation). Because parasympathetic fibers are present in the brainstem, pupils slow to react to light may indicate a brainstem injury. A "blown" pupil can be caused by compression of the third ocular nerve or transtentorial herniation. Bilateral fixed pupils can indicate midbrain involvement.

Neurologic assessments should be ongoing throughout the patient's critical care stay as part of the initial shift assessment and as part of ongoing assessments to detect subtle deteriorations. Serial assessments should include monitoring of hemodynamic status and ICP monitoring. The use of muscle relaxants and sedation for ICP control may mask neurologic signs in the patient with severe head injury. In these situations, observations for changes in pupils and vital signs become extremely important.

◆ **Diagnostic procedures.** The advent of CT scanning has greatly improved the diagnosis and management of patients with head trauma. The CT scan is a rapid, noninvasive procedure that can provide invaluable information about the presence of mass lesions and cerebral edema. With any deterioration in neurologic status, the critical care nurse should anticipate the need to transport the patient for CT scanning. A nurse should always remain with a head-injured patient during the CT scan to provide continued observation and monitoring during transport and scanning. Transporting the patient, movement from the bed to the CT table, and positioning the head flat during the CT scan are all stressful events and could cause severe increases in ICP. Continuous monitoring allows for rapid intervention.

Electrophysiology studies can aid in ongoing assessments of neurologic function. Evoked potentials and electroencephalograph (EEG) are becoming widely used in the diagnosis of head injuries. These studies are discussed in detail in Chapter 27.

Medical Management

◆ **Surgical management.** If a lesion, identified by CT scan, is causing a shift of intracranial contents or increasing ICP, surgical intervention is necessary. A craniotomy is performed to remove the EDH, SDH, or large ICH. Occasionally, if an area of contusion is large, hemorrhagic, and associated with an elevated ICP, a craniotomy for removal of the contused area may be performed to relieve pressure and prevent herniation.

◆ **Nonsurgical management.** Nonsurgical management includes management of ICP, maintenance of vital sign parameters, and treatment of any complications, such as pneumonia or infection. Medical management can include drainage of CSF through a ventricular catheter, use of diuretics, and/or administration of high-dose barbiturate therapy. For review of these treatments for increased ICP and complications, see Chapter 29.

Nursing Management

Priority nursing goals include stabilization of vital signs, prevention of further injury, and reduction of increased ICP. Ongoing nursing assessments are the cornerstone to the care of patients with head injuries. Such assessments are the primary mechanism for determining secondary brain injury from cerebral edema and increased ICP. In addition to astute neurologic assessments, it is critical to monitor ventilatory support, fluid and electrolyte balance, and nutrition. For a more extensive discussion of nursing management of intracranial pressure, see Chapter 29.

NURSING DIAGNOSIS AND MANAGEMENT
Cerebral trauma

- ◆ Altered Cerebral Tissue Perfusion related to increased intracranial pressure secondary to brain trauma, hemorrhage, edema, infection, tumor, stroke, hydrocephalus, p. 560
- ◆ High Risk for Aspiration risk factors: impaired laryngeal sensation or reflex; impaired pharyngeal peristalsis or tongue function; impaired laryngeal closure or elevation; increased gastric volume; decreased lower esophageal sphincter pressure, p. 472
- ◆ Ineffective Airway Clearance related to impaired cough secondary to artificial airway, p. 466
- ◆ Inability to Sustain Spontaneous Ventilation related to respiratory muscle fatigue secondary to mechanical ventilation, p. 468
- ◆ Impaired Gas Exchange related to ventilation-perfusion mismatching secondary to stasis of secretions, p. 470
- ◆ Altered Nutrition: Less Than Body Protein-Calorie Requirements related to lack of exogenous nutrients and increased metabolic demand, p. 673
- ◆ High Risk for Infection risk factors: invasive monitoring devices, p. 366
- ◆ Sensory/Perceptual Alterations related to sensory overload, sensory deprivation, sleep pattern disturbance, p. 573
- ◆ Body Image Disturbance related to actual change in body structure, function, or appearance, p. 94
- ◆ Altered Role Performance related to physical incapacity to resume usual or valued role, p. 97

SPINAL CORD INJURIES

According to the National Head and Spinal Cord Injury Survey, approximately 10,000 persons annually in the United States sustain a permanent spinal cord injury.[17] Of those who survive, about half have quadriplegia and half, paraplegia.[18]

Spinal cord injury (SCI) occurs mostly in males. Most victims are between the ages of 15 and 30 years, and sustain SCI as a result of vehicular accidents, assaults, falls, and sports-related injuries.[17]

Mechanism of Injury

The type of injury sustained depends on the mechanism of injury. Mechanisms of injury can include hyperflexion, hyperextension, rotation, axial loading (vertical compression), and missile or penetrating injuries.

◆ **Hyperflexion.** Hyperflexion injury most often is seen in the cervical area, especially at the level of C5-6 because this is the most mobile portion of the cervical spine. This type of injury most frequently is caused by sudden deceleration motion, as in head-on collisions. Injury occurs from compression of the cord as a result of fracture fragments or dislocation of the vertebral bodies. Instability of the spinal column occurs because of the rupture or tearing of the posterior muscles and ligaments.

◆ **Hyperextension.** Hyperextension injuries involve backward and downward motion of the head. With this injury, often seen in rear-end collisions or diving accidents, the spinal cord itself is stretched and distorted. Neurologic deficits associated with this injury often are caused by contusion and ischemia of the cord without significant bony involvement. A mild form of hyperextension is the *whiplash* injury.

◆ **Rotation.** Rotation injuries often occur in conjunction with a flexion or extension injury. Severe rotation of the neck or body results in tearing of the posterior ligaments and displacement (rotation) of the spinal column.

◆ **Axial loading.** Axial loading, or vertical compression injuries, occur from vertical force along the spinal cord. This most commonly is seen in a fall from a height in which the person lands on the feet or buttocks.

Compression injuries cause burst fractures of the vertebral body that often send bony fragments into the spinal canal or directly into the spinal cord (Fig. 45-5).

◆ **Penetrating injuries.** Penetrating injury to the spinal cord can be caused by a bullet, knife, or any other object that penetrates the cord. These types of injury cause permanent damage by anatomically transecting the spinal cord.

Pathophysiology

Spinal cord injuries are the result of a mechanical force that disrupts neurologic tissue or its vascular supply, or both. Much like the pathophysiology of head injuries, a primary injury causes a chain of secondary events in response to the injury. Spinal cord damage appears to be the result of these secondary events, which include hemorrhage, vascular damage, structural changes, and subsequent biochemical alterations.[19]

Vascular damage and hemorrhage occur as perfusion to the damaged area drops significantly. Decreased perfusion results in decreased oxygenation, ischemia, and necrosis of the spinal cord. The spinal cord becomes edematous, causing small hemorrhagic areas in the gray and white matter. Structural changes of the white and gray matter cause an opening of the tight vascular endothelial junction. This leads to an electrophysiologic alteration in neuronal conduction. Biochemical reactions to trauma result in vasoconstriction and a partial derangement in metabolism, with the release of vasoactive mediators (norepinephrine, serotonin, and histamines). These mediators generate free radicals that disrupt neuronal membranes and lead to ischemic hypoxia and rapid tissue destruction.[20] Because of the damage produced by these secondary events, neuronal conduction can no longer occur. Current medical and nursing management of the patient with a SCI is directed toward arresting or reversing these secondary events.

◆ **Functional injury of the spinal cord.** Functional injury of the spinal cord refers to the degree of disruption of normal spinal cord function. SCIs are first classified as complete or incomplete and then further divided into functional injuries (see box below).

Complete injury. Complete SCI results in a total loss of sensory and motor function below the level of injury. Regardless of the mechanism of injury, the result is a complete dissection of the spinal cord and its neurochemical pathways, resulting in one of two conditions: quadriplegia or paraplegia.

QUADRIPLEGIA. Injuries in the cervical spine region result in quadriplegia. Residual muscle function depends on the specific cervical segments involved. Cervical injuries that occur above C6 result in complete quadriplegia whereas injuries below C6 produce incomplete quadriplegia with some potential for independence in activities of daily living.[17]

PARAPLEGIA. A complete injury in the thoracolumbar region results in paraplegia. Thoracic L1 and L2 injuries produce paraplegia with variable innervation to intercostal and abdominal muscles.

Incomplete injury. Incomplete SCI results in a mixed loss of voluntary motor activity and sensation below the level of the lesion. Incomplete SCI exists if any function remains below the level of injury. Incomplete injuries can result in one of a variety of syndromes, which are classified according to the degree of motor and sensory loss below the level of injury. Some of the more common syndromes are described here.

BROWN-SÉQUARD SYNDROME. This syndrome is associated with a physiologic transverse hemisection of the cord. Injury to one side of the spinal cord produces loss of voluntary motor control on the same side of the injury, with accompanying loss of pain and temperature on the opposite side. Functionally, the side of the body with the

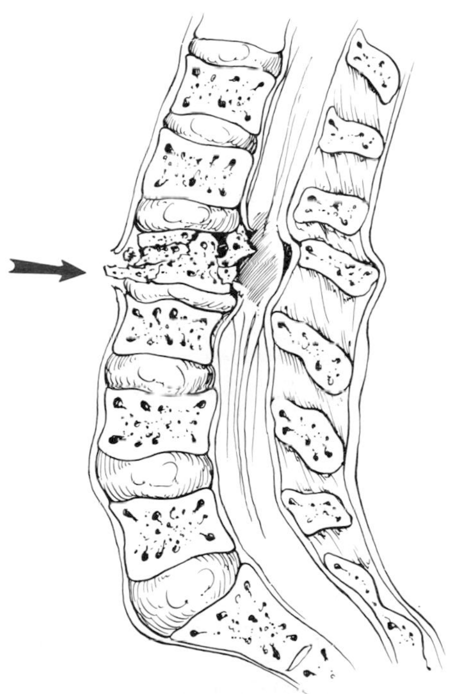

Fig. 45-5 Spinal cord compression burst injuries. Compression injuries cause burst fractures of the vertebral body that often send bony fragments into the spinal canal or directly into the spinal cord. (From Long BC, Phipps WJ, Cassmeyer VL: *Medical-surgical nursing: a nursing process approach,* ed 3, St Louis, 1992, Mosby–Year Book.)

CLASSIFICATION OF SPINAL CORD INJURIES

COMPLETE INJURY

Quadriplegia
Paraplegia

INCOMPLETE INJURY

Brown-Séquard syndrome
Central cord syndrome
Anterior cord syndrome
Posterior cord syndrome

best motor control has little or no sensation whereas the side of the body with sensation has little or no motor control.

CENTRAL CORD SYNDROME. Central cord syndrome is associated with cervical hyperextension/flexion injury. This injury produces a motor and sensory deficit more pronounced in the upper extremities than in the lower extremities. Varying degrees of bowel and bladder dysfunction may be present. This syndrome can result from contusion, compression, or hemorrhage of the gray matter of the cord.

ANTERIOR CORD SYNDROME. This syndrome is associated with injury to the anterior gray horn cells (motor), the spinothalamic tracts (pain), and the corticospinal tracts (temperature). The result is a loss of motor function, as well as loss of the sensations of pain and temperature below the level of injury. However, below the level of injury, sensations of touch, position sense, pressure, and vibrations remain intact. Anterior cord syndrome most often is caused by flexion injuries or acute herniation of an intervertebral disk.

POSTERIOR CORD SYNDROME. This syndrome is associated with cervical hyperextension. Injury results in the loss of light touch and proprioception below the level of injury. Motor function and sensation of pain and temperature remain intact.

Spinal shock. Spinal shock is a condition that occurs immediately after traumatic injury to the spinal cord. Spinal shock is the complete loss of all normal reflex activity below the level of injury, including loss of motor, sensory, reflex, and autonomic function.[19] Flaccid paralysis below the level of injury occurs in addition to bowel and bladder retention. The duration of this shock state can last several weeks after injury. The intensity of this shock is influenced by the level of injury. Spinal shock ends when spastic paralysis replaces flaccid paralysis.

Neurogenic shock. Neurogenic shock is a second shock state that can occur after an SCI above the T6 level. Injuries above this level disrupt sympathetic nervous system fibers. The parasympathetic pathway becomes predominant in spinal shock. Predominant parasympathetic innervation results in vasodilation and decreased heart rate. Vasodilation results in decreased blood pressure as a result of decreased venous return. All these events produce the classic signs of neurogenic shock: hypotension, hypothermia, and bradycardia.

Assessment

Assessment of the patient with a known or suspected SCI must include stabilization of the spinal cord. *All* trauma patients should be protected from further spinal cord damage until presence of spinal cord injury is ruled out. The cervical spinal column must remain stabilized through the use of a cervical collar, backboard, or tape to prevent motion of the spine. Movement of the patient, especially with turning, requires the use of the log-roll technique. One person maintains the patient's head and neck alignment while others assist with turning. The patient is turned in straight alignment.

◆ **Airway.** Assessment of ABCs is essential to ensure optimal oxygenation and perfusion to all vital organs, including the spinal cord, inasmuch as recovery of spinal cord tissue depends partly on adequate oxygen and blood supply.[17] Complete cardiovascular and respiratory assessments are essential to the patient's survival and prognosis. The primary assessment begins with an evaluation of airway clearance. In an unresponsive person an oral airway should be inserted while the patient's neck is maintained in a neutral position. The patient should undergo intubation before severe hypoxia can occur, which could further damage the spinal cord. Blind nasotracheal intubation generally is agreed to be the preferred route for establishing an artificial airway in the patient with an SCI.[21] Oral endotracheal intubation is contraindicated because of the degree of cervical spine manipulation required. The airway is further protected from aspiration by a nasogastric tube.

◆ **Breathing.** Assessment of breathing patterns and gas exchange is made after an airway has been secured. The level of injury dictates the degree of altered breathing patterns and gas exchange. Because complete injuries above the C3 level result in paralysis of the diaphragm,[22] these patients require ventilatory assistance. Kocan[22] described the effects of SCI on the respiratory process (Table 45-3), which affects almost all patients with SCI.

◆ **Circulation.** Assessment of cardiac output and tissue perfusion is imperative not only to detect life-threatening injuries, but to promote recovery of the injured spinal cord tissue, which depends in part on adequate perfusion of oxygenated blood.[17] The patient with SCI is at high risk for developing alterations in cardiac output and tissue perfusion because the cardiovascular system is subjected to a variety of serious and potential physiologic alterations, including dysrhythmias, cardiac arrest, orthostatic hypotension, emboli, and thrombophlebitis.[17]

In spinal shock, the cardiovascular regulatory mech-

Table 45-3 Effects of spinal cord injury on ventilatory function

Injury level	Respiratory function	Comments
Complete, above C3	Paralysis of diaphragm	Unable to sustain ventilation without mechanical assistance
C3 to C5	Varying degrees of diaphragm dysfunction	Generally able to be weaned from mechanical ventilation
C6 to T11	Intercostal muscles lost or impaired Abdominal muscles lost or impaired	Reduced inspiratory ability Paradoxic breathing patterns Diminished chest mobility Ineffective cough
Below T12	Ventilation not affected	

anisms are lost. Patients with SCI above T5 may have profound spinal shock as a result of interruption of the sympathetic nervous system and loss of vasoconstrictor response below the level of the injury.[17]

The patient with SCI should be assessed for adequate tissue perfusion by means of both invasive and noninvasive hemodynamic monitoring techniques. Cardiac monitoring is required to detect bradycardia and other dysrhythmias that occur in response to reflex vagus activity mediated by the dominant parasympathetic nervous system, as well as changes in cardiac rhythm as a result of hypothermia or hypoxia.

The critical care nurse should assess for autonomic dysreflexia as spastic movements replace flaccidity. Signs of autonomic dysreflexia include acute onset of cephalgia, hypertension, bradycardia, diaphoresis, and flushing above the level of injury. Immediate medical intervention is required to prevent cerebral hemorrhage, seizures, and acute pulmonary edema. Frequent causes of autonomic dysreflexia include a distended bowel or bladder. Patency of urinary catheters should be routinely assessed. Routine nursing assessments should include bowel elimination to aid in early detection of fecal impaction.

◆ **Neurologic.** The initial neurologic assessment may not be an accurate indication of eventual motor and sensory loss because of spinal shock.[17] It focuses on the rapid and accurate identification of present, absent, or impaired functioning of the motor, sensory, and reflex systems that coordinate and regulate vital functions. A detailed motor and sensory examination includes the assessment of all 32 spinal nerves for evidence of dysfunction. Carefully mapped pathways for the sensory portion of the spinal nerves, termed *dermatomes,* can assist in localizing the functional level of injury. Initial findings must be performed correctly and thoroughly documented in detail so that subsequent serial assessments can rapidly identify deterioration. A complete spinal cord assessment should be documented at least every 4 hours during the critical care phase.[19]

◆ **Diagnostic procedures.** Diagnostic radiographic evaluations can identify the severity of damage to the spinal cord. Initial evaluation includes anteroposterior and lateral views for all areas of the spinal cord. Films of all seven cervical vertebrae and the top of T1 must be obtained to rule out cervicothoracic junction injury.[23] Flexion and extension views can identify subtle ligamentous injuries. CT scan, tomograms, myelography, and MRI also may be used in the diagnostic process. For a more detailed discussion of these procedures, see Chapter 27.

Medical Management

After assessment and diagnosis of the SCI, medical management begins. The primary treatment goal is to preserve remaining neurologic function. Medical interventions are divided into pharmacologic, surgical, and nonsurgical interventions.

◆ **Pharmacologic management.** The use of high-dose methylprednisolone has been incorporated into the care of the patient with acute SCI. Although research has demonstrated that steroids have a beneficial effect on injured spinal cords, the mechanism for action is less clearly understood. Proposed mechanisms of action include (1) facilitation of spinal cord impulse generation, (2) enhancement of spinal cord blood flow, and (3) decreased free radical action on the neuronal membrane.[20] Key points of administration of IV methylprednisolone[20] are summarized in the box below.

◆ **Surgical management.** Surgical intervention provides spinal column stability in the presence of an unstable injury. Unstable injuries include disrupted ligaments and tendons, as well as a vertebral column that cannot maintain normal alignment. Identification and immobilization of unstable injuries are particularly important for the patient with incomplete neurologic deficit. Without adequate stabilization, movement and dislocation of the vertebral column could cause a complete neurologic deficit. A variety of surgical procedures may be performed to achieve decompression and stabilization.

Laminectomy. This procedure is the removal of the lamina of the vertebral ring to allow decompression and removal of bony fragments or disk material from the spinal canal.

Spinal fusion. This procedure entails the surgical fusion of two to six vertebral elements to provide stability and to prevent motion. Fusion is accomplished through the use of bone parts or bone chips taken from the iliac crest or by use of wire or acrylic glue.

Rodding. This procedure stabilizes and realigns larger segments of the spinal column by means of a variety of rodding procedures, such as Harrington rods. The rods are attached by screws and glue to the posterior elements of the spinal column. These types of procedures most often are performed to stabilize the thoracolumbar area.

◆ **Nonsurgical management.** If the injury to the spinal cord is stable, nonsurgical management is the treatment of choice. Nonsurgical management for cervical and thoracolumbar injuries is discussed separately.

Cervical injury. Management of cervical injuries involves the immobilization of the fracture site and realignment of any dislocation. This is accomplished through skeletal traction that involves the use of two-point tongs inserted into the skull through shallow

ADMINISTRATION OF IV METHYLPREDNISOLONE FOR SPINAL CORD INJURY

1. Concentration of methylprednisolone should be 50 mg/ml.
2. A loading dose should be administered within 8 hours after injury and infused over 15 minutes.
3. The time between loading dose and infusion doses should not exceed 45 minutes.
4. The infusion dose is administered over 23 hours.

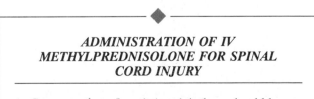

burr holes and connected to traction weights. Several types of cervical tongs are used. Gardner-Wells and Crutchfield tongs are the most common. These tongs can be applied at the bedside with the use of a local anesthetic.

After the procedure, the patient can be immobilized on a kinetic therapy or regular bed. The kinetic therapy bed is the most popular method of cervical immobilization because it maintains spinal column alignment while providing constant turning motion to reduce pulmonary and skin breakdown. Use of cervical skeletal traction on a regular bed makes it difficult to provide adequate care to the pulmonary system and skin because of the extensive degree of immobility.

After adequate realignment of the spinal column has occurred through skeletal traction, a halo traction brace often is applied. The halo vest consists of a metal ring secured to the skull with two occipital and two temporal screws. Steel bars anchor the screws to the vest to provide cervical immobilization (Fig. 45-6). The halo traction brace immobilizes the cervical spine, which allows the patient to ambulate and participate in self-care.

Thoracolumbar injury. Nonsurgical management of the patient with a thoracolumbar injury also involves immobilization. Skeletal traction may be used in high thoracic injury. For the most part, misalignment of the spinal canal does not occur in stable injuries of the thoracolumbar spine. Immobilization to allow fractures to heal is accomplished by bed rest (with bed flat) and the use of a plastic or fiberglass jacket, a body cast, or a brace.

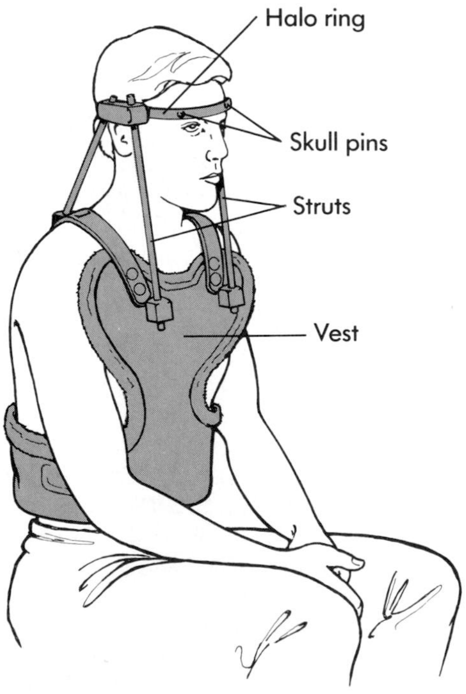

Fig. 45-6 Halo vest. The halo traction brace immobilizes the cervical spine, which allows the patient to ambulate and participate in self-care.

Nursing Management

The goal during the critical care phase is to prevent life-threatening complications while maximizing the functioning of all organ systems. Nursing interventions are aimed at preventing secondary damage to the spinal cord and managing the cardiovascular and respiratory complications of the neurologic deficit.[19] Because almost all body systems are affected by SCI, nursing management also should include interventions that optimize nutrition, elimination, skin integrity, and mobility. Prevention of complications that can delay the patient's rehabilitation is one of the goals of critical care.[19] In addition, patients with SCI have complex psychosocial needs that require a great deal of emotional support from the critical care nurse. Numerous nursing diagnoses apply to the provision of quality care for the SCI patient in the critical care unit.

◆ **Cardiovascular.** The risk for cardiovascular instability is especially profound in patients with SCI at the C3 to C5 levels, although cardiovascular alterations can occur with most injuries above T6.[24] Patients with SCI usually can tolerate a systolic blood pressure of 90 mm Hg.[17] Alteration in tissue perfusion secondary to hypotension may require the administration of IV fluids. Astute

NURSING DIAGNOSIS AND MANAGEMENT
Spinal cord injury

- Decreased Cardiac Output related to vasodilation and bradycardia secondary to sympathetic blockade of neurogenic (spinal) shock after spinal cord injury above T6 level, p. 363
- Dysreflexia related to excessive autonomic response to certain noxious stimuli (e.g., distended bladder, distended bowel, skin irritation) occurring in patients with cervical or high thorarcic (T6 or above) spinal cord injury, p. 563
- Ineffective Airway Clearance related to neuromuscular dysfunction and impaired cough secondary to quadriplegia, paraplegia, Guillain-Barré syndrome myasthenia gravis, and others, p. 467
- Impaired Gas Exchange related to alveolar hypoventilation secondary to paralysis of respiratory muscles, p. 471
- Impaired Gas Exchange related to ventilation/perfusion mismatch secondary to excessive secretions, p. 470
- High Risk for Aspiration risk factors: impaired laryngeal sensation or reflex; impaired laryngeal closure or elevation; increased gastric volume; decreased lower esophageal sphincter pressure, p. 472
- Body Image Disturbance related to actual change in body structure, function, or appearance, p. 94
- Self-Esteem Disturbance related to feelings of guilt about physical deterioration, p. 96
- Ineffective Individual Coping related to situational crisis and personal vulnerability, p. 762
- Hopelessness related to perceptions of failing or deteriorating physical condition, p. 100

assessment of fluid volume is required, however, because pulmonary edema is a threat to SCI patients. Pulmonary artery catheterization may be required to assess for this complication. Optimal ventricular function and improved perfusion usually are seen with a pulmonary artery wedge pressure of 12 to 15 mm Hg.[25] Once fluid volume status has been optimized, inotropic or vasopressor support, or both, may be implemented.

Because of the SCI patient's dependence on the environment for temperature control (poikilothermy), judicious use of heat or cold for therapeutic or comfort measures is required. Profound changes in body temperature should be avoided. Hypothermia can produce bradydysrhythmias and sinus arrest. Symptomatic bradydysrhythmias can be treated with inotropic drugs (isoproterenol), temporary transvenous or transcutaneous pacing, or propantheline.[24]

Assessment of autonomic dysreflexia requires immediate intervention, including (1) elevation of the head of bed to lower blood pressure and to reduce cerebral perfusion pressure, (2) frequent monitoring of vital signs, and (3) identification and removal of the noxious stimuli.[17]

◆ **Pulmonary.** Pulmonary complications are the most common cause of mortality in SCI patients.[17] Initial and ongoing nursing assessments of respiratory status are imperative for identifying actual or potential impairment in ventilation. These include observation of respiratory rate and rhythm, observation of symmetry of chest expansion and use of accessory muscle, inspection of quantity and character of secretions, and auscultation of breath sounds. Judicious use of serial arterial blood gas (ABG) values provides information on the adequacy of gas exchange.

Ineffective Airway Clearance is a particular problem for the SCI patient as a result of hypoventilation (paralysis of respiratory muscles), increased bronchial secretions, and atelectasis secondary to decreased cough. Frequent suctioning for airway clearance is required. Bradycardia exacerbated by hypoxia is likely to develop in patients with cervical SCI. Use of hyperventilation breaths with 100% oxygen before suctioning may help. Chest percussion and drainage facilitate removal of secretions. Kinetic therapy beds, which can rotate up to 60 degrees on each side, can provide continual postural drainage and mobilization of secretions.

Impaired Gas Exchange can occur in the SCI patient as a result of hypoventilation (paralysis of respiratory muscles), increased bronchial secretions that interfere with adequate gas diffusion, shunting secondary to atelectasis and associated pulmonary injuries, and pulmonary complications (pulmonary embolism). Nursing interventions should be directed at improving and maintaining adequate gas exchange. Deep vein thrombosis (DVT) prophylaxis should include passive range-of-motion exercises, sequential compression stockings, and kinetic therapy. Because of the loss of sensation, assessment of Homans' sign is not applicable to the SCI patient. Serial calf measurements can help detect DVT.

Depending on the level of SCI, the patient's breathing patterns may be ineffective. Spontaneous tidal volumes less than 1000 ml may indicate the need for mechanical ventilation.[22] Approximately 20% to 30% of patients with SCI require mechanical ventilatory support, although patients with lesions at the C4 level or lower generally are able to be weaned from the ventilator.[26] Weaning can be a complex process, however, because of physical requirements of the diaphragm and the psychologic effects of the fear of the inability to breathe. Weaning usually can be accomplished by slowly increasing the length of time the patient spends off the ventilator. The patient is taken off the ventilator, and a T-piece is used for a period of time. Then the patient is placed back on the ventilator for "rest" in the assist control mode, rather than the intermittent mandatory ventilation mode.[22] Setbacks are common. If reintubation is required, neuromuscular blocking agents may be used. The critical care nurse must be aware that suxamethonium (succinylcholine) never should be administered to an SCI patient any time after 72 hours after injury. Use of this depolarizing agent can produce hyperkalemic arrest. Weaning requires a well-coordinated approach planned by the nurse, physician, respiratory therapist, and patient.

The SCI patient is at high risk for aspiration. With injuries at T6 or above, a depressed cough reflex will inhibit coughing of aspirated material. Decreased gastric motility can result in retention of gastric secretions or tube feeding residuals. If possible, the head of the patient's bed should be elevated. Enteral tube feedings administered via the small intestine can help reduce the risk of aspiration as a result of delayed gastric emptying.

◆ **Maximizing mobility and skin integrity.** Nursing management of the SCI patient with impaired mobility should focus on four areas: (1) maintaining correct spinal alignment, (2) assessing for improvement or deterioration in condition, (3) facilitating progressive mobility, and (4) preventing complications of decreased mobility.[26] Once unstable fractures have been stabilized by medical intervention, nursing care can enhance spinal stability by the use of specific immobilization beds and by ensuring proper spinal alignment. Range-of-motion exercises should be initiated as soon as the spine has been stabilized. Nursing care of the patient in a halo vest includes inspection of pins and traction for security, correct positioning and turning (traction bars or the halo ring should never be used to lift or reposition the patient), placement of wrenches on the front of the vest in case of cardiac arrest, and maintenance of skin integrity inside the halo vest.

Interventions to maintain skin integrity should be started on admission to the critical care unit. Thorough skin assessments, regular turning, repositioning, meticulous skin care, and special mattresses can aid in preventing decubitus ulcers. Decubitus ulcers can cause extensive necrosis and sepsis, which will interfere or even prevent the patient's recovery and rehabilitation.[17]

◆ **Elimination.** Initially after SCI, bowel and bladder tone are flaccid. Urinary retention occurs, and insertion of an indwelling urinary catheter is required. This prevents bladder stretching and overdistention, which could permanently injure the muscular wall of the bladder and prevent the return of spastic bladder control. A bowel program to prevent fecal impaction and encourage normal, regular bowel function should be instituted.

◆ **Maximizing psychosocial adaptation.** Nursing management of the patient with SCI must include the provision of dedicated emotional support. In the critical care unit, the patient and family experience anxiety, grief, denial, anger, frustration, and hopelessness because long-term neurologic deficits remain unknown. Nursing interventions should include the promotion of coping mechanisms, support systems, and adaptive skills. Simple, accurate, and consistent information can alleviate fear and anxiety. The patient's anger may be expressed by demanding behavior, for which realistic limit setting and establishment of contracts may be helpful. Feelings of powerlessness may be reduced by including the patient and family in care and decision-making. Further psychosocial support can be given by social workers, occupational therapists, psychiatric clinical nurse specialists, and pastors.

MAXILLOFACIAL INJURIES

Trauma to the face results in complex physiologic and psychologic sequelae. Vital functions that depend on facial integrity include mastication, deglutination, perception of the environment (vision, hearing, speech, olfaction), and respiration. The face also represents a direct link to self and to expression by playing a major role in personal identity, appearance, and communication. Consequently, maxillofacial trauma has the potential to produce long-term sequelae, with emotional, sensory, and disfigurement implications. Facial injuries are common because of the exposed position of the head.

Mechanism of Injury

Maxillofacial injury results from blunt or penetrating trauma. Blunt trauma may occur from motor vehicle accidents (MVAs), industrial or athletic accidents, violent blows to the head, or falls. Penetrating maxillofacial trauma is less common, but causes include bullets or stabbings. High-velocity forces (caused by MVAs or firearms) to the maxillofacial region tend to be multiple and often are more life threatening than are injuries caused by low-velocity forces (falls, fists). Associated injuries may include concussion, skull fracture, rhinorrhea, spinal cord injury, and fractures of other bones.

Pathophysiology

The facial skeleton serves as an energy-absorbing shield to protect the brain, spinal cord, eyes, and pharynx. Nasal bones, the zygoma, and the mandibular condyle are the most susceptible to fracture.[27] Bullet wounds can be life threatening because of hemorrhage and airway obstruction. Maxillofacial trauma can result in soft tissue injury ranging from abrasions to destruction of most of the face, as well as maxillofacial skeletal fractures. This section is limited to the discussion of maxillofacial skeletal injuries.

◆ **Maxillofacial skeletal injuries.** Fractures of the maxilla are diagnosed according to Le Fort's classification. Le Fort's fractures are classified into three broad categories that depend on the level of the fracture (Fig. 45-7). The most common, Le Fort I, consists of horizontal fractures in which the entire maxillary arch moves separately from the upper facial skeleton. Le Fort II fractures are an extension of Le Fort I and involve the orbit, ethmoid, and nasal bones. Le Fort III fractures are associated with craniofacial disruption. Cerebrospinal fluid frequently leaks with these fractures.

Assessment

Assessment of the ABCs is once again critical. Patients with maxillofacial trauma are especially prone to Ineffective Airway Clearance, Fluid Volume Deficit related to hemorrhage, and High Risk for Injury. Life-threatening complications associated with maxillofacial trauma include airway obstruction, aspiration, and hemorrhage.[27]

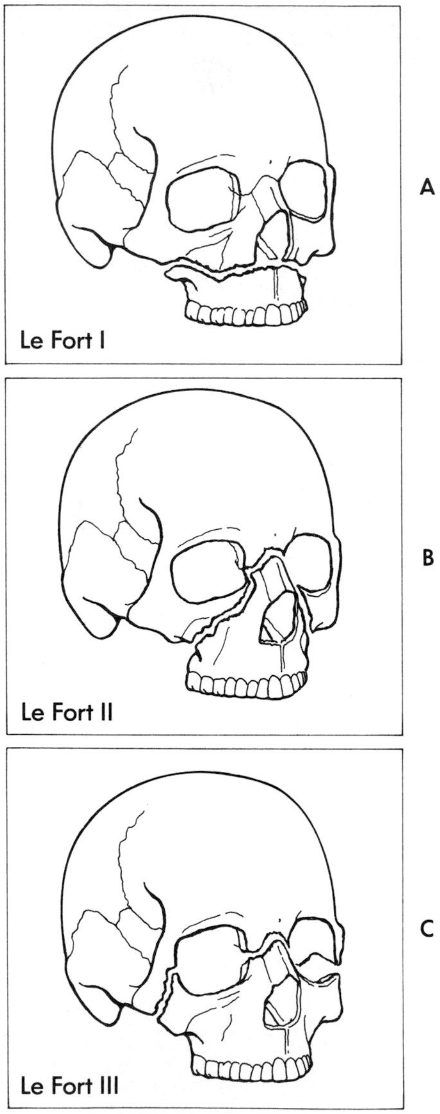

Fig. 45-7 Fractures of the maxilla are diagnosed according to Le Fort's classification, which consists of three broad categories based on the level of the fracture. **A,** Le Fort I; **B,** Le Fort II; **C,** Le Fort III.

◆ **Airway clearance.** Patients with maxillofacial trauma are at high risk for ineffective airway clearance. Edema, hemorrhage, foreign objects, vomit, broken teeth, or bone fragments can obstruct the airway. The mouth and oral pharynx should be inspected. An artificial airway may be required. An oral endotracheal tube is used unless there is a laryngeal fracture. Nasal intubation is contraindicated in the presence of facial fractures because of the risk of passing the tube into the cranium. If endotracheal intubation is unsuccessful, a cricothyrotomy may be indicated. Midface fractures may require a tracheostomy because the mouth is wired shut and massive edema can obstruct the nose. The airway must be further protected from aspiration by an orogastric tube. Nasogastric tubes are contraindicated in the presence of facial fractures because of the risk of passing the tube into the cranium.

◆ **Fluid volume deficit.** Patients with maxillofacial trauma are at high risk for fluid volume deficit related to massive hemorrhage as a result of bleeding from the ethmoid or maxillary sinuses. Effective tamponade can occur with digital pressure, manual fracture reduction, or nasal packing. Intravenously administered fluids are given to correct the fluid volume deficit.

◆ **High risk for injury.** Maxillofacial trauma frequently is associated with cervical spinal cord injury. An altered level of consciousness in the presence of maxillofacial fractures strongly suggests neurotrauma. Fractures involving the cranium and dura mater may enable oral bacterial flora to enter CSF, placing the patient at risk for meningitis. Nasal and auditory canals should be inspected for discharge. The *ring test* should be performed to determine if the drainage is CSF. This can be done by placing the drainage on a paper towel. If a double ring is formed when the fluid dries, the fluid is considered to be CSF. The drainage also can be tested for glucose inasmuch as CSF has a high glucose content.

◆ **Diagnostic procedures.** Special radiographic views are required for accurate diagnosis of maxillofacial fractures. Full maxillofacial fracture radiographic views include posteroanterior, lateral, lateral oblique, panorex, and tomograms.

Medical Management

Le Fort fractures require reduction by use of direct wiring or fixation devices. Some fractures can be reduced and immobilized immediately by the application of arch bars or intramaxillary fixation (wire) with the use of local anesthesia. Facial fractures (except mandibular fractures) can be repaired surgically up to 10 days after injury.[28]

Nursing Management

Nursing interventions are directed toward the nursing diagnoses for the patient with maxillofacial trauma. Nursing management of the patient with jaw wires requires interventions aimed at protecting the airway by reducing the risk of emesis and aspiration. Proper orogastric tube functioning should be ensured. Antiemetics may be administered. Unless contraindicated, the head of the bed should be elevated 30 degrees. If vomiting occurs, the patient should be placed in a side or forward position and oral/nasal suctioning should be used. Wire cutters must be available at the bedside in case the vomit cannot clear the wires and occludes the airway. Although this seldom is necessary, the principle in cutting the wires is to cut the vertical attachments, not the horizontal ones.[29]

NURSING DIAGNOSIS AND MANAGEMENT
Maxillofacial trauma

- ◆ High Risk for Aspiration risk factors: impaired pharyngeal peristalsis or tongue function; impaired laryngeal sensation or reflex; impaired laryngeal closure or elevation, p. 472
- ◆ Fluid Volume Deficit related to active blood loss, p. 639
- ◆ Altered Nutrition: Less Than Body Protein-Calorie Requirements related to lack of exogenous nutrients and increased metabolic demands secondary to maxillofacial trauma and wired jaws, p. 673
- ◆ Acute Pain related to transmission and perception of cutaneous, visceral, muscular, or ischemic impulses secondary to maxillofacial trauma, p. 566

THORACIC INJURIES

Thoracic injuries involve trauma to the chest wall, lungs, heart, great vessels, and esophagus. Injuries resulting from thoracic trauma account for 25% of all trauma deaths in the United States.[30] Most deaths caused by pulmonary trauma occur after the patient reaches the hospital. Thoracic trauma most commonly is the result of a violent crime or MVA.

Mechanism of Injury

◆ **Blunt thoracic trauma.** Blunt trauma to the chest most frequently is caused by MVAs or falls. The underlying mechanism of injury tends to be a combination of acceleration/deceleration injury and direct transfer mechanics, such as a crush injury. Varying mechanisms of blunt trauma are associated with specific injury patterns. After head-on collisions, drivers have a higher frequency of injury than do back-seat passengers because the driver comes in contact with the steering assembly. Severe thoracic injuries frequently are seen in patients who are unrestrained. Falls from greater than 20 feet are associated with thoracic injury.

◆ **Penetrating thoracic injuries.** The penetrating object determines the damage sustained from penetrating thoracic trauma. Low-velocity weapons (.22-caliber gun, knife) usually damage only what is in the weapon's direct path. Of particular concern, however, are stab wounds that involve the anterior chest wall between the midclavicular lines, Louis's angle, and the epigastric region inasmuch as these wounds are likely to have entered the mediastinum, heart, and/or the great vessels.[31] High-velocity weapons (rifle, shotgun, or .38 caliber) produce more serious injuries. These weapons are associated with massive energy transfer and tissue destruction. Pellets from a shotgun blast cause further damage by expanding and causing multiple injuries.

Specific Thoracic Traumatic Injuries

◆ Chest wall injuries

Rib fractures. Interruption of a single rib is the most minor and the most common chest wall injury associated with blunt thoracic trauma.[30] Fractures of certain ribs or multiple ribs can be more serious. Fractures of certain ribs are associated with more underlying life-threatening injuries. Fractures of the first and second ribs are associated with intrathoracic vascular injuries (brachial plexus, great vessels). Fractures of the seventh through tenth ribs are associated with liver or spleen injuries. The pain of rib fractures can be aggravated by movement associated with respiratory excursion. As a result, the patient often splints, takes shallow breaths, and refuses to cough, which can result in atelectasis and pneumonia.

Localized pain that increases with respiration or that is elicited by rib compression may indicate rib fractures. Definitive diagnosis can be made with a chest film. Nursing diagnoses may include Pain, Ineffective Airway Clearance, Ineffective Breathing Pattern, and Impaired Gas Exchange. Interventions should include aggressive pulmonary physiotherapy and pain control to improve chest expansion efforts and gas exchange. Intercostal nerve blocks and thoracic epidural analgesia may be used to assist with pain control. External splints are not recommended because they further limit chest wall expansion and may add to atelectasis.[32] The patient's preexisting pulmonary status may dictate the course of recovery. The major concern with rib fractures is the associated underlying injuries.

Flail chest. Flail chest, caused by blunt trauma, disrupts the continuity of chest wall structures. A flail chest occurs when three or more ribs are fractured in two or more places and are no longer attached to the thoracic cage. This results in a free-floating segment of the chest wall. This segment moves independently from the rest of the thorax and results in paradoxic chest wall movement during the respiratory cycle (Fig. 45-8). During inspiration the intact portion of the chest wall expands while the injured part is sucked in. During expiration the chest wall moves in and the flail segment moves out. Hemorrhage and edema initially occur at the site of injury, followed by an accumulation of interstitial fluid and a decrease in alveolar membrane diffusion, which leads to increased pulmonary vascular resistance, decreased pulmonary blood flow, and hypoxemia.[33]

Inspection of the chest reveals paradoxic movement. Palpation of the chest may indicate crepitus and tenderness near fractured ribs. The patient may be cyanotic and, if conscious, complain of shortness of breath. As a result of splinting the flail segment may not always be evident initially in the conscious patient. Nursing diagnoses for the patient with a flail chest include Decreased Cardiac Output, Impaired Gas Exchange, and Pain. Interventions should focus on ensuring adequate ventilation and adequate pain control, administration of oxygen, and accurate assessments of fluid balance. A pulmonary contusion beneath the flail can cause capillary leakage of fluid. This, in combination with fluid volume excess, can precipitate ARDS. Diuretics also may be used to limit interstitial fluid accumulation. Steroids may be given to reduce pulmonary capillary membrane permeability. Progressive respiratory failure is treated with intubation and mechanical ventilatory support. The patient with a flail chest also should be observed for dysrhythmias. This is especially important with anterior flail chest because of the possibility of underlying cardiac damage.[33]

Ruptured diaphragm. Diaphragmatic rupture is a frequently missed diagnosis in trauma patients because of the subtle and nonspecific symptoms this injury produces. The mechanism of injury appears to be a rapid rise in intraabdominal pressure as a result of compression force applied to the lower part of the chest or upper region of the abdomen. This injury can occur when a person is thrown forward over the tip of the steering wheel in a high-speed deceleration accident. The force can cause the diaphragm, which offers little resistance, to rupture or tear. Abdominal viscera then can gradually enter the thoracic cavity, moving from the positive pressure of the abdomen to the negative pressure in the thorax. The stomach and colon are the most commonly herniated viscera.[34] Diaphragmatic rupture can be life-threatening. Massive herniation of abdominal contents into the thoracic cavity can compress the lungs and mediastinum, which then hampers venous return and leads to decreased cardiac output. In addition, herniated bowel can become strangulated and perforate.

Diaphragmatic herniation may produce significant compromise and changes in respiratory effort. Auscultation of bowel sounds in the chest or unilateral breath sounds may indicate a ruptured diaphragm. The patient may complain of shoulder pain, shortness of breath, or abdominal tenderness. The chest film findings may be normal in 25% to 30% of cases.[34] An abnormal finding often reveals the tip of a nasogastric tube above the diaphragm, a unilaterally elevated hemidiaphragm, a hollow or solid mass above the diaphragm, and a shift of the mediastinum away from the affected side. Treatment of a ruptured diaphragm includes its immediate repair.

◆ Pulmonary injuries

Pulmonary contusion. Pulmonary contusion frequently is associated with blunt deceleration/acceleration injuries. These forces can produce bruises, tears, or lacerations under the area of blunt trauma. The pathophysiology of pulmonary contusions begins with initial hemorrhage and interstitial and alveolar edema at the contusion site, which then spreads to surrounding areas and results in general inflammation.[35] Damaged or closed alveolar capillaries result in increased pulmonary vascular resistance, reduced lung compliance, reduced pulmonary blood flow, and ventilation/perfusion imbalance.[36] Pulmonary contusion can interfere with oxygen-

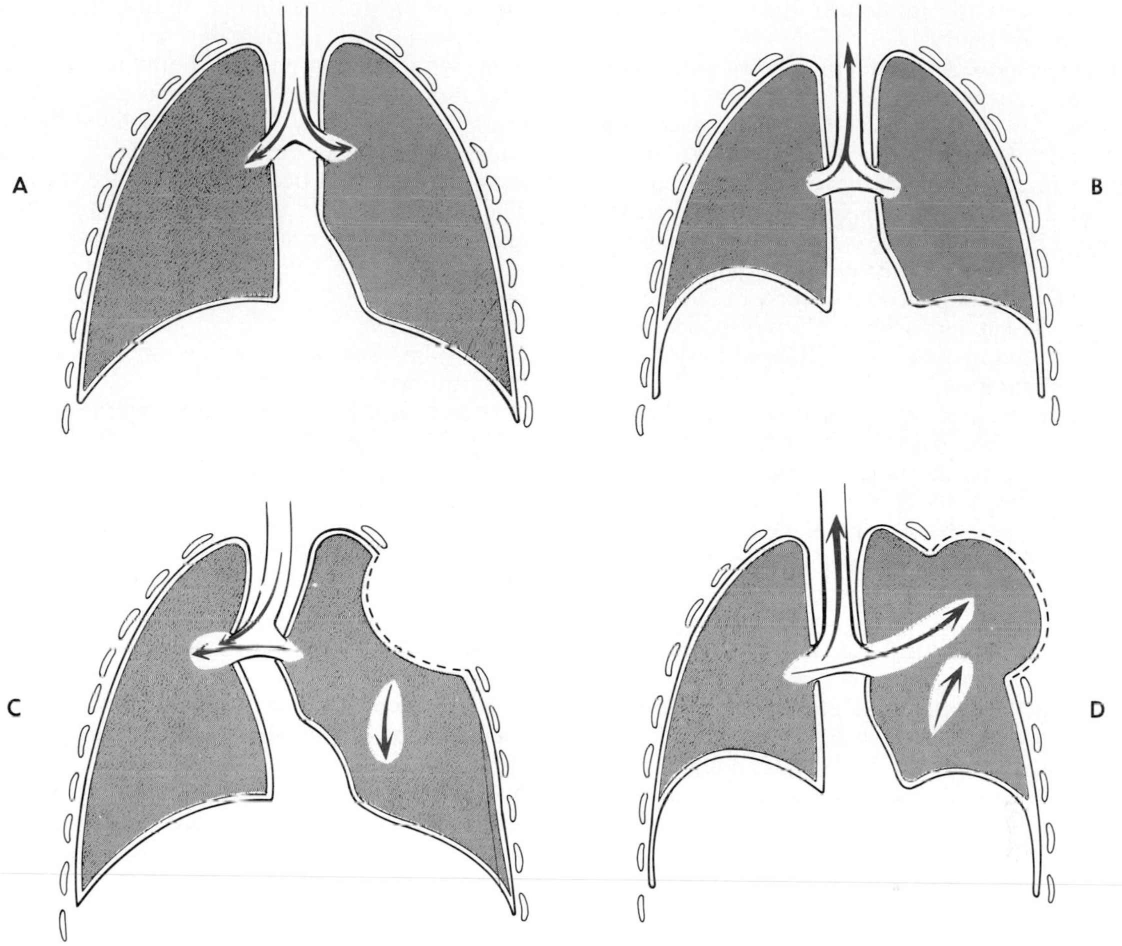

Fig. 45-8 Flail chest. **A,** Normal inspiration. **B,** Normal expiration. **C,** Inspiration: area of lung underlying unstable chest wall sucks in on inspiration. **D,** Same area balloons out on expiration. Note movement of mediastinum toward opposite lung on inspiration. (From Long BC, Phipps WJ, Cassmeyer VL: *Medical-surgical nursing: a nursing process approach,* ed 3, St Louis, 1992, Mosby–Year Book.)

ation (saturation of hemoglobin in pulmonary blood) and ventilation (removal of carbon dioxide from pulmonary blood).

Clinical manifestations of pulmonary contusion may take up to 24 to 48 hours to develop.[33] Inspections of the chest wall may reveal ecchymosis at the site of impact. Moist rales may be noted in the contused lung. A cough may be present with blood-tinged sputum. Abnormal lung function can be detected by systemic arterial hypoxemia. A chest film, within 6 hours after injury, may reveal patchy areas of density that reflect intraalveolar hemorrhage.[35] Small pulmonary parenchymal tears and lacerations can be detected by CT scan.

Nursing diagnoses for the patient with pulmonary contusions may include Impaired Gas Exchange, High Risk for Infection, Pain, Decreased Tissue Perfusion, and Ineffective Airway Clearance. Interventions generally are supportive and directed at improving ventilation and oxygenation. Patients with severe contusions may continue to show decompensation despite aggressive nursing care. Respiratory acidosis, increases in peak airway pressures, and increased work of breathing may require endotracheal intubation and mechanical ventilation with positive end-expiratory pressure (PEEP). When high levels of PEEP are required for the contused lung, synchronous independent lung ventilation (SILV) can be instituted. Aggressive removal of airway secretions is important to avoid infection and to improve ventilation. Patients with unilateral contusions should be placed with the injured side up and uninjured side down to enhance ventilation and perfusion. Because pulmonary injury can produce pulmonary interstitial edema, aggressive IV fluid administration should be avoided to prevent ARDS. A central venous pressure (CVP) of 4 mm Hg with a pulmonary arterial wedge pressure (PAWP) of 10 mm Hg or less is recommended to prevent fluid sequestration.[35] Diuretics also may be used to achieve this goal. Adequate pain control should be accomplished by administration of narcotics or intercostal nerve blocks. Complications that result from pulmonary contusions include pneumonia, ARDS, lung abscesses, empyema, and pulmonary embolism. Preinjury pulmonary status greatly influences the mortality and morbidity from this injury.

Tension pneumothorax. A tension pneumothorax usually is caused by an injury that perforates the chest wall or pleural space. Air flows into the pleural space with inspiration and becomes trapped. As pressure in the pleural space increases, the lung on the injured side collapses and causes the mediastinum to shift to the opposite side (Fig. 45-9). As pressure continues to build, the shift exerts pressure on the heart and thoracic aorta, which results in decreased venous return and decreased cardiac output. Tissue perfusion with oxygenated blood is further hampered because the collapsed lung cannot participate in ventilation.

Clinical manifestations of a pneumothorax include dyspnea or sudden chest pain extending to the shoulders. Tracheal deviation will be noted as the trachea shifts away from the injured side. On the injured side, breath sounds can be decreased or absent. Neck vein distention, cyanosis, and respiratory distress also may be present. Percussion of the chest reveals a hyperresonant sound caused by the trapped air. Diagnosis of tension pneumothorax is made by clinical assessment. There is no time for a chest film inasmuch as this potentially lethal condition must be treated immediately. A large-bore (14 gauge) needle or chest tube is inserted into the affected lung. This procedure allows immediate release of air from the pleural space. A hissing sound should be heard as the tension pneumothorax is converted to a simple pneumothorax. Nursing diagnoses for a patient with a tension pneumothorax include Decreased Cardiac Output and Impaired Gas Exchange.

Open pneumothorax. An open pneumothorax, or "sucking chest wound," usually is caused by penetrating trauma. Open communication between the atmosphere and intrathoracic pressure results in immediate lung deflation. Air moves in and out of the hole in the chest, producing a sucking sound heard on inspiration.

An open pneumothorax produces the same symptoms as a tension pneumothorax. In addition, subcutaneous emphysema may be palpated around the wound. Patients with an open pneumothorax have some degree of alteration in cardiac output and gas exchange unless treated immediately. The wound must be occluded at once. A dressing of petrolatum (Vaseline) gauze, plastic wrap, or any other occlusive substance must be applied. The dressing should be applied at the end of expiration and with only three sides taped to the skin surface. This allows the fourth side to act as a valve so that the open pneumothorax does not become a tension pneumothorax. Definitive management includes placement of a chest tube. Surgical intervention may be required to close the wound.

Hemothorax. Blunt or penetrating thoracic trauma can cause bleeding into the pleural space to produce a hemothorax (Fig. 45-10). A massive hemothorax can cause a blood loss of more than 1500 ml.[37] The source of bleeding may be the intercostal or internal mammary arteries, lungs, heart, or great vessels. Increasing intrapleural pressure results in a decrease in vital capacity. Increasing vascular blood loss into the pleural space causes decreased venous return and decreased cardiac output.

Assessment findings for patients with a hemothorax include hypovolemic shock and decreased breath sounds in the injured lung. With hemothorax, the neck veins are collapsed and the trachea is at midline.[5] Massive hemothorax can be diagnosed on the basis of clinical manifestations of hypotension associated with the absence of breath sounds and/or dullness to percussion on one side of the chest.[3] Nursing diagnoses for a patient with a hemothorax include Fluid Volume Deficit, with resulting Decreased Cardiac Output, and Impaired Gas Exchange. This life-threatening condition should be treated immediately. Resuscitation with IV fluids should be initiated to treat the hypovolemic shock. A chest tube is placed on the affected side to allow drainage of blood. An autotransfusion device can be attached to the chest

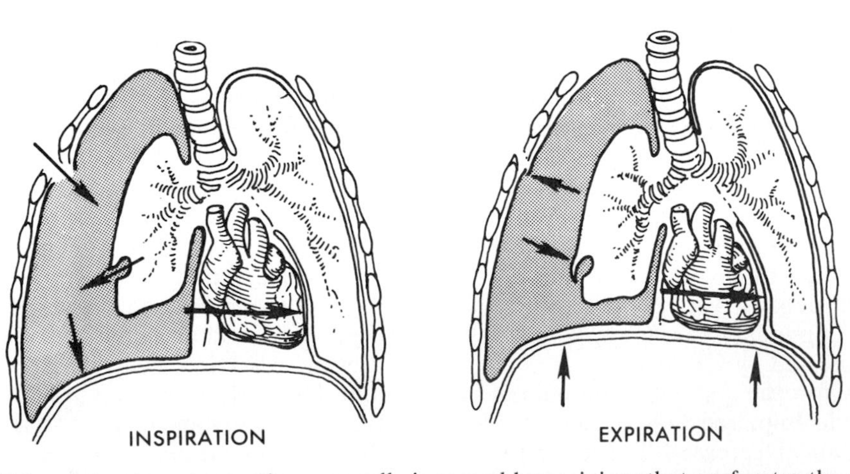

Fig. 45-9 A tension pneumothorax usually is caused by an injury that perforates the chest wall or pleural space. Air flows into the pleural space with inspiration and becomes trapped. As pressure in the pleural space increases, the lung on the injured side collapses and causes the mediastinum to shift to the opposite side. (From Rosen P and others: *Emergency medicine: concepts and clinical practice,* ed 3, St Louis, 1992, Mosby–Year Book.)

tube collection chamber. When drainage exceeds 1 L or greater than 150 ml/hr for 3 hours, a thoracotomy is indicated.[30]

◆ Cardiac injuries

Penetrating cardiac injuries. Penetrating cardiac trauma can occur from mechanical injuries as a result of bullets, knives, or impalements. The chest wall offers little protection to the heart from penetrating trauma. The most common site of injury is the right ventricle because of its anterior position. Mortality from penetrating trauma to the heart is high. Prehospital mortality for penetrating cardiac injuries is 75%, and most deaths occur within 4 or 5 minutes after injury as a result of exsanguination or tamponade.[38]

CARDIAC TAMPONADE. Cardiac tamponade is the progressive accumulation of blood in the pericardial sac (Fig. 45-11). With cardiac tamponade a progressive accumulation of blood, 120 to 150 ml, increases the intracardial pressure and compresses the atria and ventricles. Increased intracardial pressures lead to decreased venous return and decreased filling pressure, which lead to decreased cardiac output, myocardial hypoxia, cardiac failure, and cardiogenic shock.

Classic assessment findings associated with cardiac tamponade are termed *Beck's triad:* presence of elevated central venous pressure with neck vein distention, muffled heart sounds, and pulsus paradoxus. An ECG may reveal tachycardia with altered QRS complexes. The major nursing diagnosis for this injury is Decreased Cardiac Output. Immediate treatment is required to remove the accumulation of fluid in the pericardial sac. Pericardiocentesis involves the aspiration of fluid from the pericardium by use of a large-bore needle. The inherent risk in this procedure is potential laceration of the coronary artery. Other approaches include surgical procedures, such as thoracotomy or median sternotomy. The goal of these procedures is to locate and control the source of bleeding and to decompress or remove the pericardium completely.[39]

Blunt cardiac injuries. The most common causes of blunt cardiac trauma include high-speed MVAs, direct blows to the chest, and falls. The heart, because of its mobility and its location between the sternum and thoracic vertebrae, is susceptible to blunt traumatic injury. Sudden acceleration (as from contact with the steering wheel) can cause the heart to be thrown against the sternum (Fig. 45-12). Sudden deceleration can cause the heart to be thrown against the thoracic vertebrae by a direct blow to the chest (baseball, animal kick, fall). Myocardial contusion is one of the most common injuries sustained as a result of blunt cardiac trauma.

MYOCARDIAL CONTUSION. Myocardial cell injury results from the contusion. Histiologically the contused myocardium is similar to an infarcted myocardium. In a contused myocardium, however, a well-demarcated zone exists between normal and contused myocardium.[40] If the contusion is large enough and has resulted in a large area of myonecrosis, the patient may experience the same complications as those of an acute myocardial infarction. The right ventricle most often is affected because of its proximity to the sternum.

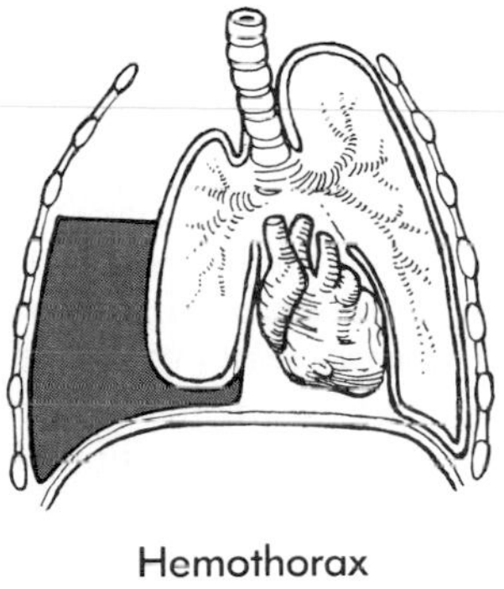

Fig. 45-10 Blunt or penetrating thoracic trauma can cause bleeding into the pleural space to form a hemothorax.

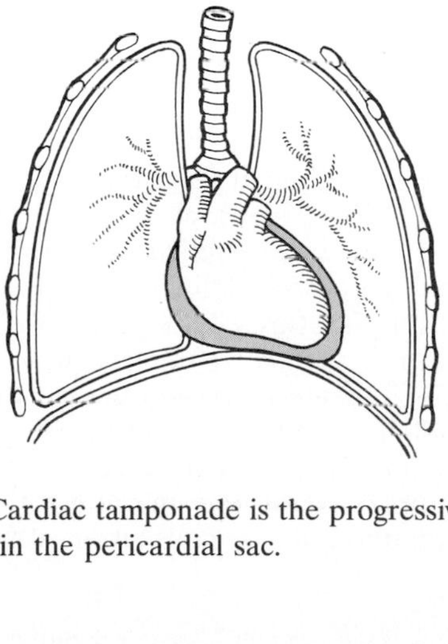

Fig. 45-11 Cardiac tamponade is the progressive accumulation of blood in the pericardial sac.

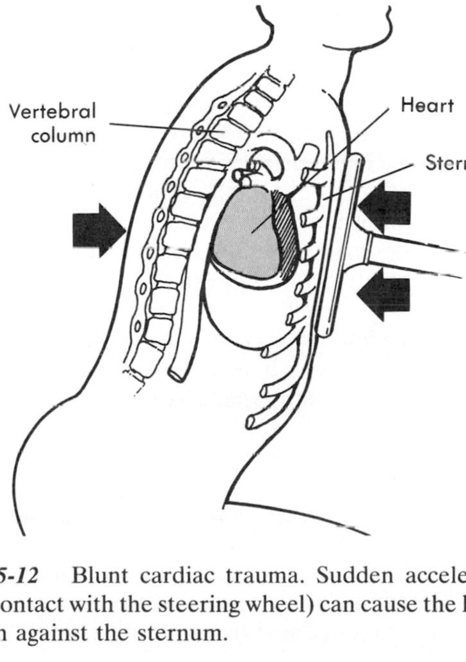

Fig. 45-12 Blunt cardiac trauma. Sudden acceleration (as from contact with the steering wheel) can cause the heart to be thrown against the sternum.

Diagnosis of myocardial contusion continues to be an area of controversy. Assessment findings associated with myocardial contusion depend on the extent and location of myocardial injury. The patient may be symptom-free or complain of dyspnea and precordial pain that is similar to that of angina, except that it typically is not relieved by nitroglycerine. If the contusion is large enough to affect cardiac output, hypotension may be present. ECG changes, which may take up to 72 hours to occur, include ST segment elevation, T wave inversion, development of new Q waves, dysrhythmias, and conduction defects. The most common rhythm changes seen with myocardial contusion are premature ventricular or atrial dysrhythmias.[39] Creatine phosphokinase–myocardial band (CPK-MB) serum assays, a routine procedure in the diagnosis of a myocardial infarction, are used in the diagnosis of myocardial contusion; they do, however, present some limitations. CPK-MB values can be elevated in the patient with multiple trauma from crush injuries and injuries to the skeletal muscle, lung, pancreas, liver, and gastrointestinal tissues. The levels of CPK-MB considered suggestive of myocardial necrosis from contusion vary from 2% to 10%.[40] These isoenzyme levels should be obtained on the patient's admission to the emergency department and every 6 to 8 hours for 24 hours to assess the degree of myocardial damage.[40] Studies have revealed, however, that the CPK-MB levels fail to detect one third to one half of all patients who subsequently are found to have evidence of myocardial damage on an echocardiogram (ECHO).[38] Therefore the use of the two-dimensional ECHO has become a more accepted method to accurately diagnose myocardial contusions.

Medical management is aimed at preventing and treating complications. This may include administration of antidysrhythmic medications, treatment of congestive heart failure, insertion of pacemakers to control heart block, or the use of intraaortic balloon pump for severe cardiac failure.[38]

Nursing diagnoses for the patient with a myocardial contusion include Decreased Cardiac Output, Altered Coronary Tissue Perfusion, and alteration in comfort: Pain. Nursing interventions should be aimed at maintaining adequate cardiac output and coronary tissue perfusion and promoting comfort. Ongoing assessments are imperative inasmuch as clinical manifestations usually appear hours after the injury. The patient's ECG rhythm and isoenzyme levels should be monitored for abnormalities. Assessment of fluid and electrolyte balance is imperative to ensure adequate cardiac output and myocardial conduction. Measures to maintain myocardial oxygenation include bed rest, administration of analgesics, maintenance of a hemoglobin level of 12 to 13 g/dl, and maintenance of adequate vascular volume.

ABDOMINAL INJURIES

Abdominal injury accounts for 10% of trauma fatalities in the United States.[41] Most persons who are injured and suffer abdominal trauma are younger than 50 years of age.[42] Abdominal injuries frequently are associated with multisystem trauma. Injuries to the abdomen are the result of blunt or penetrating trauma. Two major life-threatening conditions that occur after abdominal trauma are hemorrhage and hollow viscus perforation with its associated peritonitis.

Mechanism of Injury

◆ **Blunt trauma.** Blunt abdominal injuries are common. They result most frequently from MVAs, falls, and assaults. The spleen is the most commonly injured organ in blunt trauma and ranks second to the liver as the source of life-threatening abdominal injury.[43] In MVAs, abdominal injury is more likely to occur when a vehicle is struck from the side. In the passenger position of the front seat, hepatic injury is likely when the point of impact is on the same side as the passenger. A driver is likely to sustain injury to the spleen when the impact is on the driver's side. Seat belts, which substantially reduce morbidity and mortality, also are associated with causing bladder and bowel rupture.[41] Pedestrians hit by motor vehicles are at risk for serious abdominal injuries. Blunt trauma to the thorax can produce injuries to the liver, spleen, and diaphragm. In spinal cord injury, large abdominal arteries and veins can be injured. Deceleration and direct forces can produce retroperitoneal hematomas. Blunt abdominal injuries often are hidden and are more likely to be fatal than are penetrating abdominal injuries.

◆ **Penetrating trauma.** Penetrating abdominal trauma generally is caused by knives or bullets. The danger of penetrating abdominal trauma is that the outside appearance of the wound does not determine the extent of internal injury. The most commonly injured organs from knife wounds are liver, spleen, diaphragm, and colon.[44] Gunshot wounds to the abdomen usually are more serious than are stab wounds. A bullet destroys tissue along its path. Once inside the abdomen, a bullet can travel in erratic paths and ricochet off bone. Death from penetrating injuries depends on the injury to major vascular structures and resultant intraabdominal hemorrhage.

Assessment

The initial assessment of the trauma patient, whether in the emergency department or the critical care unit, should follow the primary and secondary survey techniques as outlined by ATLS and TNCC guidelines. Specific assessment findings associated with abdominal trauma are reviewed here.

◆ **Physical assessment.** The location of entry and exit sites associated with penetrating trauma should be assessed and documented. Inspection of the patient's abdomen may reveal purplish discoloration of the flanks or umbilicus (Cullen's sign), which is indicative of blood in the abdominal wall. Ecchymosis in the flank area (Grey Turner's sign) may indicate retroperitoneal bleeding or a possible fracture of the pancreas. A hematoma in the flank area is suggestive of renal injury. A distended abdomen may indicate the accumulation of blood, fluid, or gas secondary to a perforated organ or ruptured blood vessel. Serial measurement of abdominal girths can be helpful. The increase of abdominal girth by 1 inch can indicate intraabdominal accumulation of 500 to 1000 ml of blood.[45] Auscultation of the abdomen may reveal friction rubs over the liver or spleen and may indicate rupture. The abdomen should be assessed for rebound tenderness and rigidity. Presence of these assessment findings indicates peritoneal inflammation. Referred pain to the left shoulder (Kehr's sign) may indicate a ruptured spleen or irritation of the diaphragm from bile or other material in the peritoneum. Subcutaneous emphysema palpated on the abdomen suggests free air as a result of a ruptured bowel.

◆ **Diagnostic procedures.** Insertion of a nasogastric tube and urinary catheter serves as a useful diagnostic and therapeutic aid. A nasogastric tube can decompress the stomach, and the contents can be checked for blood. Urine obtained from the urinary catheter can be tested for the presence of blood.

Serial laboratory test results may be nonspecific for the patient with abdominal trauma. A serum amylase determination can detect pancreatic injuries. Initial leukocytosis can suggest splenic or hepatic injury. Because of hemoconcentration, hemoglobin and hematocrit results may not reflect actual values. Serial values are more valuable in diagnosing abdominal injuries.

Diagnostic peritoneal lavage (DPL) can exclude or confirm the presence of intraabdominal injury with a high accuracy rate. After the patient's bladder has been emptied, a small incision is made in the abdomen through the skin and into the peritoneum. A small catheter is inserted (Fig. 45-13). If frank blood is encountered, intraabdominal injury is obvious and the patient is taken immediately to the OR. If gross blood is not initially encountered, a liter of fluid (lactated Ringer's or 0.9% normal saline) is infused through the catheter into the abdomen. The IV bag is then placed in a dependent position and allowed to drain. The drainage fluid is sent to the laboratory for analysis. Positive DPL results signal intraabdominal trauma and usually necessitate surgical intervention (see box on right).

Abdominal CT scanning can detect retroperitoneal hemorrhage, can localize specific site(s) of abdominal injury, and can determine the relative severity of intraperitoneal or retroperitoneal hemorrhage.[46]

Specific Organ Injuries

Physical assessment findings, DPL, and CT scanning aid in making a diagnosis of specific abdominal organ injury. The medical and nursing management vary according to specific organ injuries. Liver, spleen, bowel, and pancreatic injuries, which are seen more commonly, are discussed here.

◆ **Liver injuries.** The liver is the primary organ injured in penetrating trauma and the second most commonly injured organ in blunt trauma. Detection of liver injury, as with all intraabdominal injury, is accomplished through the use of physical assessment and DPL or CT scan. The severity of liver injuries is graded to provide a mechanism for determining the amount of trauma sustained by that organ, the care needed, and possible outcomes (Table 45-4). Surgical intervention usually can correct the defect. Resection of the devitalized tissue is required for massive injuries. Hemorrhage is common

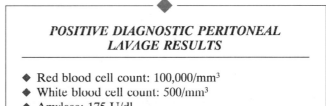

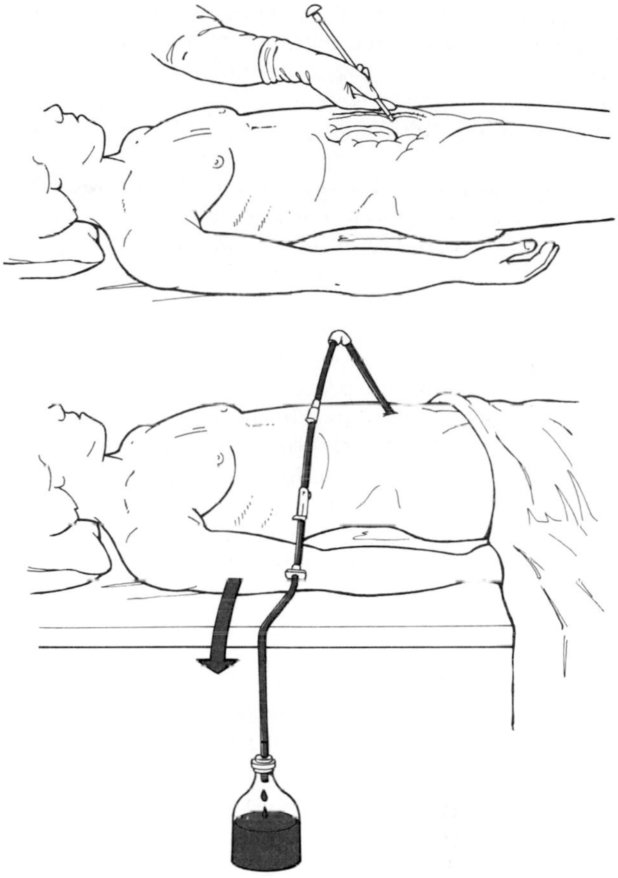

Fig. 45-13 Diagnostic peritoneal lavage (DPL) can exclude or confirm the presence of intraabdominal injury with a high accuracy rate.

POSITIVE DIAGNOSTIC PERITONEAL LAVAGE RESULTS

- ◆ Red blood cell count: 100,000/mm³
- ◆ White blood cell count: 500/mm³
- ◆ Amylase: 175 U/dl
- ◆ Presence of blood, stool, bile, bacteria

with liver injuries, and ligation of the hepatic arteries or veins may be required to control hemorrhage. Drains are placed intraoperatively to drain areas of blood and to prevent hematomas. Care of the patient with severe liver injuries can be challenging for the critical care nurse. Lack of hemodynamic stability can result from hemorrhage and hypovolemic shock, leading to fluid volume deficit, decreased cardiac output, and decreased tissue perfusion. Combinations of crystalloid and colloid IV solutions may be used to correct hypovolemia. Fresh frozen plasma, platelets, and cryoprecipitate may be administered to correct coagulopathies. A crucial nursing responsibility is to monitor the patient's response to medical therapies. Continued hemodynamic instability (hypotension, decreased cardiac output) in spite of aggressive medical intervention may indicate continued hemorrhage, in which case an exploratory laparotomy may be required to determine and correct the source of bleeding.

◆ **Spleen injuries.** The spleen is the organ most commonly injured by blunt abdominal trauma and is second to the liver as a source of life-threatening hemorrhage. Spleen injuries, like liver injuries, are graded for determining the amount of trauma sustained, the care needed, and possible outcomes (Table 45-5). The treatment of an injured spleen is controversial because of the spleen's importance in preventing infection. Hemodynamically stable patients may be monitored in the critical care unit by means of serial hematocrit values and vital signs. Progressive deterioration may indicate the need for operative management. Patients who present with hemodynamic instability require operative intervention with splenectomy, partial splenectomy, or splenorraphy. Patients who have had a splenectomy are at risk for the development of overwhelming postsplenectomy sepsis with streptococcal pneumonia. These patients require polyvalent pneumococcal vaccine (Pneumovax) to help promote immunity against most pneumococcal bacteria. Patients with isolated spleen injuries that require surgical intervention rarely are admitted to the critical care unit. Complications after splenic trauma include wound infection, sepsis, subdiaphragmatic abscess, and fistulas of the colon, pancreas, and stomach.

◆ **Intestinal injuries.** Intestinal injuries can result from blunt or penetrating trauma. Regardless of mechanism of injury, intestinal contents (bile, stool, enzymes, bacteria) leak into the peritoneum and cause peritonitis. Surgical resection and repair are required. The patient's postoperative course is dictated by the amount of spillage of intestinal contents. The patient should be observed for signs of sepsis and abscess or fistula formation.

◆ **Pancreatic injuries.** Pancreatic injury rarely occurs alone. Death is related directly to the number of associated injuries. Penetrating wounds that cause injury to the pancreas require immediate surgical intervention. The diagnosis of pancreatic injury as a result of blunt trauma is difficult. Elevated serum amylase levels may not occur for 24 hours or more after injury. Diagnostic CT findings of pancreatic edema and fluid may not develop for 24 to 48 hours after injury. Surgical intervention is required if there is any question of pancreatic injury. Postoperatively the patient must be assessed for complications of pancreatitis, pancreatic fistulas and pseudocysts, intraabdominal abscesses, and pancreatic insufficiency. Serial glucose and amylase levels should be monitored. Meticulous skin care around drainage tube insertion sites is necessary to prevent breakdown from pancreatic enzymes. Displacement of intraoperatively placed drainage tubes should be brought to the physician's attention immediately.

Table 45-4 Classification of liver injuries

Grade I	Laceration, capsular tear, minimal parenchymal damage
Grade II	Laceration, linear parenchymal tear
Grade III	Laceration, stellate fracture, moderate parenchymal tear commonly affecting posterior segment of right lobe of liver
Grade IV	Laceration, fragmented fracture, extensive parenchymal tear with involvement of hepatic fracture
Grade V	Laceration, extensive burst fracture with parenchymal tear extending into retrohepatic vasculature

From Semonin-Holleran R: *Crit Care Nurse* 8(3):52, 1988. Copyright 1988 by Cahners Publishing Co.

Table 45-5 Classification of spleen injuries

Grade I	Laceration, linear laceration along transverse axis corresponding to costal contour
Grade II	Laceration, stellate in configuration, occurring on posterolateral surface of the spleen
Grade III	Laceration, disruption of splenic parenchyma into several fragments

From Semonin-Holleran R: *Crit Care Nurse* 8(3):52, 1988. Copyright 1988 by Cahners Publishing Co.

GENITOURINARY INJURIES

Trauma to the genitourinary (GU) tract seldom occurs as an isolated injury. An associated GU injury should be suspected in any patient with trauma to the chest, flank, abdomen, pelvis, perineum, and genitalia.[47]

Mechanism of Injury

GU injuries, like all other traumatic injuries, can result from blunt or penetrating trauma. Blunt GU trauma can be caused by deceleration injuries, and penetrating injuries can occur with stabbings or gunshot wounds to the abdomen or back.

Assessment

Evaluation of GU trauma begins after the primary survey has been conducted and immediate life-threatening conditions have been effectively managed. The conscious patient may complain of flank pain or colic pain. Rebound tenderness can be elicited if intraperitoneal extravasation of urine has occurred. Inspection may reveal abdominal contusions, developing hematomas, and blood at the urethral meatus. Bluish discoloration of the flanks may indicate retroperitoneal bleeding, whereas perineal discoloration may indicate a pelvic fracture and possible bladder or urethral injury.[47] Auscultation of an abdominal bruit can signify renal vascular injury. Results of serum laboratory tests are nonspecific for GU trauma, although blood urea nitrogen (BUN) and creatinine levels should be obtained initially and monitored intermittently for trends.

Hematuria is the most common finding associated with GU trauma. The degree of hematuria, however, is not indicative of the severity of the injury.[48] The presence of hematuria necessitates further investigation to determine the extent and exact site of injury.

Specific Genitourinary Injuries

◆ **Renal trauma.** Blunt renal trauma produces 80% of all renal injuries.[47] Blunt trauma to the flank causes the twelfth rib to compress the kidney against the lumbar spine, resulting in a contusion or laceration of the kidney. Of all renal trauma 80% to 90% involves contusions or minor lacerations without urinary extravasation.[48] Intravenous pyelography (IVP) is used in the diagnosis of renal trauma because it can outline the collection system and establish the presence and function of both kidneys. Abdominal CT scan can define parenchymal lacerations, urinary extravasation, and perirenal hematoma. The major advantage of the CT scan is its ability to distinguish between superficial lacerations and major injuries. The use of renal angiography is indicated if the IVP fails to fully define the extent of injury, if the entire kidney cannot be visualized, or if CT scanning is not available.

Conditions that require surgical intervention for renal trauma include expanding hematoma, pulsatile hematoma, penetrating trauma with urinary extravasation, vascular injury, and evidence of continued hemorrhage after the patient has received 3 units of blood.[47] Postoperative complications include infection, hemorrhage, acute tubular necrosis, and hypertension.

◆ **Ureteral trauma.** Injury to the ureters is the least common result of trauma to the GU tract because the ureters are protected anteriorly by the abdominal contents and musculature and posteriorly by the psoas muscle. The patient with ureteral trauma may complain of flank pain, and hematuria may be a presenting symptom. As in renal trauma, the degree of hematuria is not indicative of the severity of injury. A "missed" ureteral injury can result in intraperitoneal extravasation and produce peritoneal signs. Ureteral injuries are surgically repaired.

◆ **Bladder trauma.** Most bladder injuries are the result of blunt trauma. The type of injury that occurs depends not only on the location and strength of the blunt force, but also on the volume of urine in the bladder at the time of injury.[48] Trauma to the bladder may result in a contusion or rupture. Urinary extravasation is the hallmark sign of a ruptured bladder. Definitive diagnosis of bladder rupture is made by means of cystographic examination.

Nursing Management

Nursing diagnoses that can be applicable in caring for a patient with GU trauma include Altered Tissue Perfusion, Pain, High Risk for Infection, and High Risk for Fluid Volume Deficit.

After the patient is admitted to the critical care unit, the nurse makes an assessment according to ATLS and TNCC guidelines. Once the patient's condition has stabilized, nursing management of postoperative renal trauma is similar to that for GU surgery. The primary nursing interventions include assessment for hemorrhage, maintenance of fluid and electrolyte balance, and maintenance of patency of drains and tubes. Measurement of urinary output should include drainage from the urinary catheter and the nephrostomy or suprapubic tubes. Drainage from these areas should be recorded separately. Urine output should be measured hourly until bloody drainage and clots have cleared.[49] Renal function should be assessed by monitoring serum BUN and creatinine levels.

PELVIC FRACTURES

The pelvis is a ring-shaped structure composed of the hip bones, sacrum, and coccyx. Because the pelvis protects the lower urinary tract and major blood vessels and nerves of the lower extremities, pelvic trauma can result in life-threatening urologic and neurologic dysfunction and in hemorrhage.[50]

Mechanism of Injury

Blunt trauma to the pelvis can be caused by MVAs, falls, or a crushing accident. Most pelvic injuries involve fractures, with or without damage to underlying tissues. Pelvic injuries frequently are associated with motorcycle accidents and accidents that involve pedestrians and vehicles. Any patient who has been projected from a vehicle should be suspected of having a pelvic fracture.

Assessment

Signs of pelvic fracture include perineal ecchymosis (testicular or labial) indicating extravasation of urine or blood, pain on palpation or "rocking" of the iliac crests, lower limb paresis or hypesthesia, hematuria, and shortening of a lower extremity.

An anteroposterior x-ray film of the pelvis permits classification of a fracture as stable or unstable. Stable fractures usually are breaks in the pelvic ring, sacrum, or coccyx, with no displacement. Unstable fractures are breaks that occur in more than one place or in the acetabulum.

Classification of Pelvic Fractures

◆ **Minor.** Minor pelvic fractures include breaks of individual bones without a break in continuity of the pelvic ring, or a single break in the pelvic ring.[51]

◆ **Major.** Major pelvic fractures involve double breaks in the pelvic ring. These fractures commonly are seen in patients in the critical care unit with multiple trauma. The condition of patients with posterior pelvic fractures is very unstable. The nearby iliac arteries frequently are damaged and can cause massive internal bleeding.

◆ **Straddle fracture.** The four-ramus, or "straddle," fracture consists of bilateral fractures of the superior and inferior pubic rami. With this fracture comes a high incidence of associated injuries, especially lower urinary tract injuries.

◆ **Malgaigne's hemipelvis fracture dislocation.** This fracture includes a variety of fracture patterns that have three separate injury components[51] (see box, p. 756). These fractures always are unstable and the result of severe trauma.

MALGAIGNE'S PELVIC FRACTURES

Fracture patterns are characterized by three separate injury components:

1. Double vertical breaks in the pelvic ring
2. Anterior break, including fractures of pubic bone, ischial rami, and/or disruption of the pubic symphysis
3. Posterior break, posterior to hip joint; may involve fractures of ilium, or sacrum, and/or disruption of the sacroiliac joint

◆ **Open fractures.** Open pelvic fractures involve an open wound with direct communication between the pelvic fractures and the buttocks, perineum, groin, pubis, or lower flank. The open wound allows contamination.

Medical Management

The priority of the medical management of pelvic fractures is to prevent or to control life-threatening hemorrhage. The use of the pneumatic antishock garment (PASG) has been advocated for control of pelvic fracture hemorrhage in the prehospital and emergency department settings.[52] Hemorrhage also may be controlled by placement of an external fixator device or use of therapeutic angiography for embolization of the lacerated vessel.

Almost every patient with a massive open pelvic fracture requires an exploratory laparotomy to treat intraabdominal injuries. A diverting colostomy is performed to prevent ongoing contamination of the pelvic wound from feces.[53] If there are no obvious intraabdominal injuries, the pelvis is stabilized.

Definitive management of pelvic fracture may include placement of internal or external fixation devices. External fixation allows pelvic stabilization until the patient can tolerate surgical open reduction and internal fixation. Using fluoroscopy, the physician inserts two or three pins percutaneously into each iliac crest. The pins are then attached to a rigid metal frame. Patients with fractures of the symphysis pubis, sacroiliac joints, iliac wings, or acetabulum usually undergo open reduction with internal fixation (ORIF).[50] ORIF occurs after bleeding has been controlled, and adequate hemodynamic stability has been achieved. In this procedure the surgeon reduces the fractures with contoured plates and screws. Six to seven units of blood may be required intraoperatively.[54]

Nursing Management

Initial assessment of the patient with a pelvic fracture in the critical care unit proceeds according to ATLS and TNCC guidelines. Nursing diagnoses include Altered Tissue Perfusion, Pain, High Risk for Infection, and High Risk for Injury.

Massive blood loss contributes to alteration in tissue perfusion. On the patient's admission to the critical care unit, hemodynamic instability, with abnormal coagulation factors, may be present. Interventions should include intravenously administered crystalloid and colloid fluids. Accurate assessment of fluid balance and tissue perfusion may require pulmonary artery catheter placement. The nurse should ensure that an appropriate amount of blood remains cross-matched and available if needed. Adequate oxygenation should be assessed by means of pulse oximetry and systemic mixed venous oxygen saturation and by monitoring serial hematocrit and hemoglobin levels.

Pelvic fractures can be extremely painful. Nursing interventions should include measures to ensure adequate pain control. The patient with pelvic fractures is at high risk for infection because of associated injuries and external fixation. Contamination of the pelvic cavity can occur with associated intestinal or GU injuries, or both. Nursing care of external fixation insertion sites should be directed at preventing infection. Most institutions have protocols for pin care that require strict compliance.

High risk for injury is secondary to neurovascular compromise, development of compartment syndrome, fat embolism syndrome, and wound infection. These syndromes are discussed in further detail later in this chapter. Routine nursing assessments should include neurovascular assessments of the lower extremities. Neurovascular complications are most common with posterior fractures and in any patient who has been treated with PASG. Neurologic injury as a result of pelvic fracture usually is temporary and lasts less than 3 weeks.[50] Open pelvic fractures may necessitate repeated wound débridement in the OR. Aggressive nutrition, fluid, and appropriate antibiotic therapies are imperative. Patients with open pelvic fractures usually have a prolonged critical care course, with varying degrees of multiple organ dysfunction syndrome.[53]

LOWER EXTREMITY ORTHOPEDIC INJURIES

The patient with only orthopedic injuries rarely is admitted to a critical care unit. However, the critical care nurse often encounters a multiple trauma patient who also has sustained lower extremity orthopedic trauma. The critical care nurse must be knowledgeable about orthopedic trauma, mechanism of injury, medical management, and nursing care.

Classification of Fractures

Orthopedic injury frequently occurs as a result of an MVA or a fall. A fracture is caused when a force exceeds the elasticity of the bone.

The classification of fractures is broad and depends on whether there is communication between the bone and outside the body. A closed or simple fracture does not expose the bone to the external environment. An open or compound fracture exposes bone to the external environment. The fracture can be complete, in which at least two pieces of bone are completely separated. A *greenstick* fracture occurs if bone is still hinged on one side. A comminuted fracture is one in which there are three or more fragments of bone. Comminuted fractures often occur as a result of crushing forces that cause the bone to collapse on itself.

Mechanism of Injury

In an MVA the knees of an unrestrained front-seat passenger can impact the dashboard with approximately 4500 pounds of force.[55] The force of this impact can result in posterior fracture-dislocation of the hip, fracture of the femoral shaft, or patellar injury. Lateral collisions can cause injury to the trochanter and head of the femur. Rotational injuries can occur when the vehicle spins.

Assessment

A fracture site should be assessed for pain and tenderness, loss of function, deformity, discoloration, altered position, abnormal mobility, crepitus (caused by bone fragments), and neurovascular dysfunction.[55]

Medical Management

Orthopedic injuries can be treated with or without surgical fixation. Nonsurgical fixation can be accomplished by aligning the bone fragments in as nearly an anatomic position as possible, then immobilizing the area. Immobilization can be performed internally by use of rods, plates, screws, or wires (Fig. 45-14) or externally by the application of an external device (Fig. 45-15). External devices, however, increasingly are being viewed as a temporary method of fracture stabilization in the patient with multiple traumatic injuries.[56]

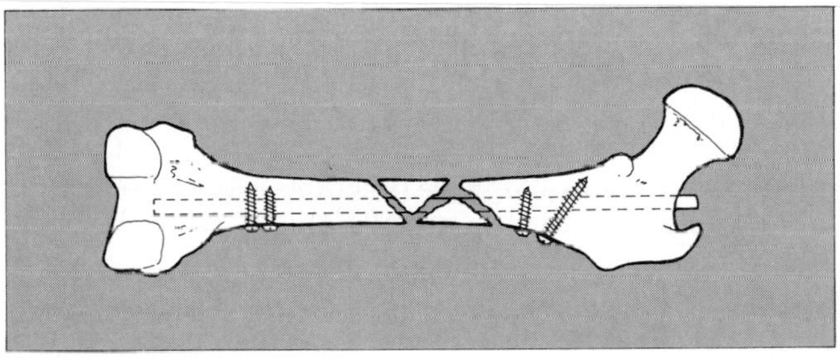

Fig. 45-14 Interlocking nails can be used for internal fracture fixation.

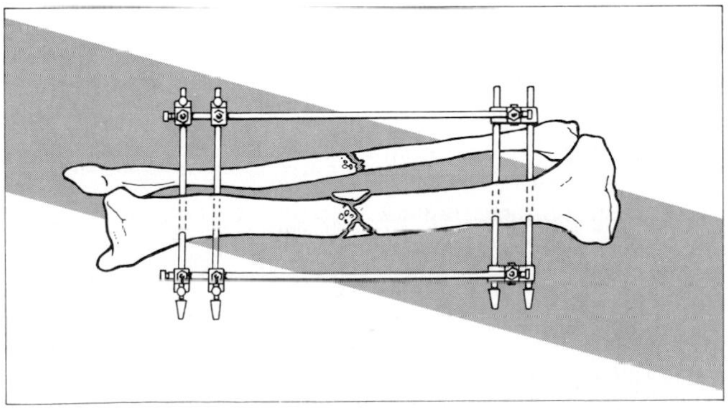

Fig. 45-15 External fracture fixation promotes stabilization of the fracture as a temporary measure.

Nursing Management

Nursing management of the patient with orthopedic injuries depends on the method of fracture reduction. Nursing diagnoses include Impaired Physical Mobility, Impaired Skin Integrity, Altered Tissue Perfusion, and Pain.

Nursing interventions should focus on assisting the patient to attain the highest level of mobility possible while injuries are healing. Proper position of splints should be ensured. Depending on other system injuries, the patient should be encouraged to ambulate as soon as possible to prevent complications associated with immobility. If the patient is unable to get out of bed, a trapeze can be added to the bed frame to assist with mobility in bed.

The patient with orthopedic injuries can have impaired skin integrity as a result of compound fractures. Meticulous wound care is required. Because of their susceptibility to pressure ulcer development, all patients with orthopedic trauma are at high risk for impaired skin integrity. A patient in traction cannot be completely turned off his or her back. Skin breakdown caused by the pressure of casts and splints can occur, for example, on the heels of a patient with fractures of the lower extremities and hips. Pillows placed under the legs can free the heels of such pressure. Turning the patient on a regular schedule is imperative.

Neurovascular assessments of extremities are critical. Irreversible neurovascular injury can occur in as little as 6 hours as a result of compression of casts or immobilization devices.[55] Assessments should be completed on both extremities, and the two sides should be compared. Assessments of tissue perfusion include capillary refill, presence of edema and pain, palpation of temperature and pulses, and evaluation of sense of touch and mobility. Capillary refill in the toes should occur within 2 seconds, and pulses should be present by palpation or Doppler examination.[56] The patient with lower extremity fractures is particularly at risk for alteration in tissue perfusion secondary to compartment syndrome. Frequent neurovascular assessments lead to early diagnoses and management of this limb-threatening condition. Orthopedic injuries can produce severe pain. Nursing interventions should ensure adequate pain control.

◆ Complications of Trauma

In the trimodal distribution of trauma deaths, the third peak of death often occurs in the critical care unit as a result of complications days to weeks after the initial injury. Ongoing nursing assessments are imperative for early detection of complications frequently associated with traumatic injuries.

INFECTION

Infection remains a major source of mortality and morbidity in critical care units. Of trauma patients who survive longer than 3 days, infection is a frequent cause of death.[57] The trauma patient is at high risk for infection because of contaminated wounds, invasive therapeutic and diagnostic catheters, intubation and mechanical ventilation, host susceptibility, and the critical care environment. Nursing management must include interventions to decrease and eliminate the trauma patient's risk of infection.

The patient with multiple trauma is at high risk for infection because of host susceptibility (including preexisting medical conditions) and the adverse effect of trauma on the immune system. Hypovolemic shock and surgery, commonly seen in the patient with multiple traumatic injuries, affect the body's inflammatory response to opportunistic bacteria. These conditions have been shown to diminish the inflammatory response for up to 24 hours, allowing opportunities for organisms to proliferate.[57] Corticosteroids, released as a stress response to trauma, further suppress the inflammatory reaction and depress humoral and cell-mediated immunity. The physiologic and psychologic stress produced by trauma increases metabolic rate and oxygen consumption. As a result of shock, the compromised cardiovascular system cannot meet all these cellular demands. The patient who has had a splenectomy for splenic trauma is further compromised by a loss of T cells.

Wound contamination poses an infective risk to the trauma patient, especially with injuries resulting from deep or penetrating trauma. Exogenous bacteria (from the external environment) can enter through open wounds. Exogenous bacteria can be introduced by dirt, grass, and debris inoculated into the wound at the time of injury, or they can be introduced by personnel during wound care. Endogenous bacteria (from the internal environment) can be released as a result of gastrointestinal or genitourinary perforation, which spills bacteria into the internal environment. Meticulous wound care is essential. The goals of wound care include minimizing infective risks, removal of dead and devitalized tissue, allowing for wound drainage, and promoting wound epithelialization and contraction. Wound healing also is accomplished through interventions that promote tissue perfusion of well-oxygenated blood and that ensure adequate nutritional support for wound healing.

SEPSIS

The patient with multiple injuries is especially at risk for overwhelming infections and sepsis. The source of sepsis in the trauma patient can be invasive therapeutic and diagnostic catheters or wound contamination with exogenous or endogenous bacteria. The source of the septic nidus must be promptly evaluated. Gram's stain and cultures of blood, urine, sputum, invasive catheters, and wounds should be obtained.

Overwhelming infection can culminate through a cascade of events into septic shock. Decreased tissue perfusion can lead to cellular death. Bacterial endotoxins released from bacteria initiate myriad events that produce cellular and humoral immune defects and an impairment of cellular oxygen utilization. (See Chapter 46 for a further discussion of septic shock.)

PULMONARY COMPLICATIONS

Respiratory Failure

Trauma to the pulmonary system is likely to result in complications through respiratory failure. This is particularly true if the patient was involved in a high-speed MVA, suffered major blunt trauma, experienced a mean arterial pressure of less than 60 mm Hg for a period of time, had 20% or more of blood volume replaced, or experienced a decrease in level of consciousness.[58] Respiratory insufficiency is one of the most common complications after multiple trauma.

Etiologic factors in posttraumatic respiratory failure[59] are listed in the box below. Posttraumatic respiratory failure often leads to the development of adult respiratory distress syndrome (ARDS). An in-depth discussion of the pathophysiology and management of ARDS is reviewed in Chapter 22. Trauma patients are especially at risk for the development of ARDS because of sepsis, multiple emergency transfusions, and pulmonary contusions. The presence of more than one of these conditions significantly increases the risk for ARDS. Sepsis most frequently is the cause of posttraumatic respiratory failure.[59]

Fat Embolism Syndrome

Fat embolism syndrome (FES) can occur as a complication of orthopedic trauma. The syndrome is characterized by pulmonary system dysfunction. FES appears to develop as a result of fat droplets that leak from fractured bone and embolize to the lungs. The droplets are broken down into free fatty acids that are toxic to the pulmonary microvascular membranes. Damage of these membranes results in edema, inactivation of surfactant, and atelectasis. Fat droplets further activate a coagulation cascade that results in thrombocytopenia. The lung becomes highly edematous and hemorrhagic. The clinical presentation is almost indistinguishable from ARDS. High pulmonary pressures can lead to increased left atrial pressures and decreased cardiac output, which further accentuates lung dysfunction. Early stabilization of unstable extremity fractures may limit the seeding of fat droplets into the pulmonary system. It has been demonstrated that early fixation of long bone fractures significantly decreases the incidence of fat embolism syndrome and death from pulmonary insufficiency.[56]

ETIOLOGIC FACTORS IN POSTTRAUMATIC RESPIRATORY FAILURE

- Pneumonia
    - Aspiration
    - Bacterial
    - Viral
- Blunt thoracic trauma
- Fat or amniotic fluid embolism
- Shock
    - Hypovolemic
    - Septic
    - Cardiogenic
- Pulmonary embolism
- Pancreatitis
- Near-drowning

GASTROINTESTINAL COMPLICATIONS

Hemorrhage

Life-threatening gastrointestinal (GI) bleeding as a result of stress ulcerations is infrequent but associated with high mortality. The patient with multiple traumatic injuries is particularly at risk for developing this complication. Risk factors associated with the development of stress ulcerations include sepsis, multiple trauma, hepatic failure, ARDS, renal failure, and major surgical procedures.[60] The pathophysiology of stress ulceration is thought to be caused by a variety of factors, including mucosal barrier breakdown, decreased mucosal blood flow, increased intraluminal acid, decreased epithelial regeneration, and lowered intramural pH. Prevention of stress ulcer development is imperative. A gastric pH greater than 3.5 should be attained through the use of histamine-2 blockers, antacids, and sucralfate.

Acalculous Cholecystitis

Prolonged critical illness predisposes the patient to bile stasis, biliary sludge development, and eventual cystic duct obstruction. Acalculous cholecystitis is inflammation of the gallbladder without evidence of gallstones. Several risk factors for acalculous cholecystitis are present in the patient with traumatic injuries: volume depletion, prolonged GI rest, morphine administration, ventilatory support, multiple transfusions, and infected wounds.[59] Diagnosis is difficult because the manifestations are similar to other posttraumatic complications. The patient's only symptoms may be unexplained leukocytosis and fever. Right upper quadrant pain is difficult to elicit from an unconscious patient, and diagnosis often is prompted by a high index of suspicion. Surgical intervention (cholecystectomy or cholecystostomy) usually is required.

RENAL COMPLICATIONS

Renal Failure

Assessment and ongoing monitoring of renal function are critical to the survival of the trauma patient. Prolonged hypoperfusion or hypoxia, or both, is the most common cause of renal failure in the patient with multiple traumatic injuries.

Prevention of renal failure is the best treatment and begins with ensuring adequate renal perfusion. Serial assessments of BUN and creatinine levels commonly are used to evaluate renal function. Urine output as a measurement to determine renal function can be misleading because posttraumatic renal insufficiency can manifest as nonoliguric renal failure. Despite an adequate urine volume, the kidneys have failed to remove metabolic wastes. Patients with nonoliguric renal failure, however, have a better chance of survival than do patients with oliguric renal failure.[61] Progressive renal failure requires prompt diagnosis and treatment. Etiologic factors in renal failure should be assessed in terms of prerenal, renal, or postrenal causes.

Myoglobinuria

Patients with a crush injury are susceptible to the development of myoglobinuria, with subsequent secondary renal failure. Crush injuries can result in arterial trauma. Loss of arterial blood flow, particularly to the extremities, results in the loss of oxygen transport to distal tissues and ischemia. This initiates a cascade of events that leads to the necrosis of skeletal muscle cells. As cells die, intracellular contents—particularly potassium and myoglobin—are released. Myoglobin, which is the muscular pigment, is a large molecule. As it circulates in the cardiovascular system, it causes acute renal tubular blockade and subsequent renal failure. Myoglobinuria frequently develops within 6 hours after injury. Signs of myoglobinuria include dark red or burgundy urine and decreasing urine output. Definitive diagnosis is made through serial testing of the urine for myoglobin.

Recognition of patients at risk for the development of myoglobinuria is imperative to its prevention. Such prevention includes early external immobilization of fractures and early serial urine testing for myoglobin.

Once the condition is diagnosed, treatment is aimed at the prevention of subsequent renal failure. Intravenously administered fluids are increased to keep the kidneys perfused. Metabolic acidosis predisposes myoglobin to crystallize and precipitate in the renal tubules. Crystallization in the renal tubules can be prevented by the administration of continuous sodium bicarbonate and mannitol solutions. Serial urine myoglobin testing should continue until three consecutive testings produce negative results.

VASCULAR COMPLICATIONS

Compartment Syndrome

Compartment syndrome is a condition in which increased pressure within a limited space compromises circulation, resulting in ischemia and necrosis of tissues within that space. Among those at high risk for the development of compartment syndrome are patients with lower extremity trauma, including fractures, penetrating trauma, vascular ruptures, massive tissue injuries, or venous obstruction. Compartment syndrome is thought to be caused by the accumulation of interstitial fluid in a closed compartment. As fluid accumulates in a closed space, decreased tissue perfusion occurs as arteries and veins become obstructed.

Clinical manifestations of compartment syndrome include obvious swelling and tightness of an extremity, paresis, and pain of the affected extremity. Elevated intracompartmental pressures confirm the diagnosis. The treatment can consist of simple interventions, such as removing an occlusive dressing, to more complex interventions, including a fasciotomy (see Chapter 48). Meticulous wound care after fasciotomy is imperative to prevent wound infection.

MISSED INJURY

Nursing assessment of the multiply injured patient in the critical care unit may reveal missed diseases or missed injuries. Missed "diseases" may include preexisting undiagnosed medical illnesses, such as endocrine disorders (diabetes, hypothyroidism), myocardial infarction, hypertension, respiratory insufficiency, renal insufficiency, or malnutrition.

Occasionally injuries may not be diagnosed in the

precritical care phases. Injuries can be subtle or masked, preventing accurate diagnosis. In the critical care unit, a missed injury may be suspected if the patient fails to show appropriate response to medical or surgical intervention. Change in the character of drainage from wounds or catheters may represent biliary or duodenal injuries. Hypotension and a falling hematocrit level despite aggressive fluid administration may indicate an expanding hematoma. Pelvic or peritoneal abscesses may develop in patients with missed rectal injuries.[59] The critical care nurse should be alert to the possibility of a missed injury, especially when the patient does not appear to be responding appropriately to interventions. The physician should be notified immediately because potential complications of infection and hemorrhage can be life-threatening.

MULTIPLE ORGAN DYSFUNCTION SYNDROME

Multiple organ dysfunction syndrome (MODS) represents the culmination of progressive organ system dysfunction. The patient with multiple injuries is particularly at risk for MODS because it can develop as a result of multiple system/organ trauma, major/emergency surgery, intraabdominal sepsis, ARDS, and renal failure. MODS is described at length in Chapter 47. Prevention of MODS depends on an aggressive approach to eliminate the "domino effect" in the patient with multiple traumatic injuries.

TRAUMA CRITICAL CARE CASE STUDY

CLINICAL HISTORY

Mr. J is a 32-year-old man who was driving home from a Super Bowl party. He hit a patch of ice and lost control of his car, hitting a guard rail and a tree. He was not wearing a seat belt. The emergency medical technicians at the scene reported a prolonged extrication time of 45 minutes.

CURRENT PROBLEMS

On arrival to the ED Mr. J's vital signs were BP, 88/56 mm Hg; HR, 130/min; respirations, 24/min; temperature, 94° F. His respirations were shallow and his airway patent, but he had diminished breath sounds on the left side. Subcutaneous air was present from the left nipple line to the left upper abdominal quadrant. A chest tube was inserted, and after placement, breath sounds were audible bilaterally. He was placed on 40% O_2 by face mask. His skin was cold and clammy. Two peripheral 16-gauge IV infusions were initiated, and with use of a fluid warmer, he was given lactated Ringer's solution (LR) at a wide-open rate. The neurologic examination showed PERLA at 5 mm, and Mr. J was combative and disoriented to place and time. He had an obvious open fracture of his left lower extremity. His ABG values revealed a metabolic acidosis. Other pertinent laboratory values included Hct, 28%; Hgb, 10 g/dl; ETOH level, 0.13; and normal urinalysis result. A Foley catheter was inserted, which yielded 100 ml clear yellow urine. A DPL was performed, and findings were positive. X-ray films revealed fractures of the fifth to tenth left ribs, comminuted fracture of the left tibia, and normal cervical spinal alignment. A head CT scan showed negative findings.

After 3 L of LR and 2 units of blood, Mr. J remained hypotensive and was taken to the OR. During surgery the exploratory laparotomy revealed a ruptured spleen. A splenectomy and placement of an external fixation device were performed in the OR. Intraoperatively, Mr. J required 15 L of fluid (10 L crystalloid, 5 L colloid) to maintain MAP >70 mm Hg. He remained hypothermic and was then transported to the trauma ICU.

MEDICAL DIAGNOSES

Ruptured spleen, SP splenectomy
Tension pneumothorax, SP chest tube placement
Fracture of fifth through tenth ribs on left side
Comminuted fracture of left tibia

NURSING DIAGNOSES

- ◆ Fluid Volume Deficit related to active blood loss (intraoperative)
- ◆ Ineffective Breathing Pattern related to abdominal or thoracic pain
- ◆ Hypothermia related to exposure to cold environment, trauma
- ◆ High Risk for Infection risk factors: altered integumentary system, invasive surgical procedures, presence of invasive lines, immobility, traumatic injuries and stress
- ◆ Acute Pain related to transmission and perception of cutaneous, visceral, muscular, or ischemic impulses secondary to chest tube, splenectomy incision, rib fractures, and tibia fracture

◆ PLAN OF CARE

1. Admit to trauma ICU.
2. Continue to monitor fluid status and oxygenation by insertion of an oximetrix pulmonary artery catheter.
3. Monitor serial Hct level, ABG values, and coagulation factors.
4. Maintain MAP >70 mm Hg.
5. Continue with mechanical ventilation, and monitor pneumothorax.
6. Treat hypothermia with warmed blankets and warmed IV fluids.
7. Monitor urine output.
8. Obtain clear thoracic and lumbar spinal films.

TRAUMA CRITICAL CARE CASE STUDY—cont'd

MEDICAL AND NURSING MANAGEMENT AND PATIENT OUTCOME (12 HOURS AFTER ICU ADMISSION)

Neuro: EMV 11T, PERLA at 3 mm

Resp: Remains intubated with FIO_2 50%, VT 1000 ml, PEEP 5, pressure support 10 on IMV 12. Respirations 20/min, equal breath sounds with scattered rhonchi. Requires suctioning q 1 to 2 hours for thin white secretions. ABGs: pH, 7.30; PCO_2, 45; PaO_2, 90; SaO_2, 92%; HCO_3^-, 20. Chest x-ray film reveals diffuse alveolar infiltrates.

CV: BP, 110/60 mm Hg; HR, 110 ST; temp, 98° F. Skin warm and dry. Capillary refill < 2 seconds. Hemodynamics: PAP, 35/22 mm Hg; PAWP, 18 mm Hg; CVP, 15 mm Hg; CO, 6 L/min; CI, 4 L/min/m²; SVR, 800 dyn/sec/cm^{-5}; SvO_2, 68%. Laboratory values: Hct, 30%; Hgb, 10 g/dl; PT, 16/12 sec; PTT, 45/28 sec. Palpable pedal pulse on the right, and left pedal pulse is positive by Doppler examination. Intake: 5000 ml crystalloid, 1000 ml colloid.

Integument: Chest tube dressing is clean and dry. Left leg is in external fixator traction; insertion sites are clean and dry. Left leg is edematous, but color, motion, and sensitivity are intact. A red, nonblanching area is noted on Mr. J's coccyx.

GI: Nasogastric tube is intact and drained 100 ml bilious fluid; guaiac finding is negative, with pH 5.5. No bowel sounds. Full-strength Traumacal at 25 ml/hr infusing via nasoenteric feeding tube.

GU: Urinary catheter in place, draining light cola-colored urine. Urine output, 30 ml/hr—heme positive; pH, 3.5; sugar/acetone, negative; protein, positive.

Lab: Ionized calcium, 1.9 mg/dl, potassium, 3.2 mEq/L.

Pain: Complains of left rib pain and left leg pain. States MSO_4 helps alleviate pain "a little."

Medications: Unasyn 3 g IV q 8 hr, gentamicin 100 mg IV q 8 hr, cimetidine 300 mg IV q 6 hr, MSO_4 4 mg IV q 1 hr prn for pain.

MEDICAL DIAGNOSES

Coagulopathy
R/O myoglobinuria

NURSING DIAGNOSES

- ◆ Ineffective Breathing Pattern related to thoracic pain
- ◆ Acute Pain related to transmission and perception of cutaneous, visceral, muscular, or ischemic impulses secondary to rib fractures and tibia fracture

◆ REVISED PLAN OF CARE

1. Decrease FIO_2 to 40%, begin slow IMV, wean within next 12 hours if ABG values are acceptable.
2. Give 2 units FFP to correct coagulation.
3. R/O myoglobinuria: send urine for myoglobin determination q 6 hr; maintain IV fluids at 150 ml/hr; and add 2 ampules $NaHCO_3^-$ to each liter IV fluid to alkalinize the urine.
4. Administer 1 g calcium gluconate.
5. Apply polyurethane dressing to coccyx. Turn patient q 2 hr.
6. Increase tube feedings to 50 ml/hr.
7. Increase MSO_4 to 8 mg IV q 1 hr.

MEDICAL AND NURSING MANAGEMENT AND PATIENT OUTCOME

Mr. J was successfully weaned from the ventilator 36 hours after injury. At 48 hours postinjury, he was on a 40% face mask. Respirations were 28/min and shallow, with scattered coarse rhonchi bilaterally. He was unable to participate in coughing and deep breathing exercises because of rib pain. Nasotracheal suctioning q 1 hr was performed to remove thick, yellow secretions. ABG values were as follows: pH, 7.50; PCO_2, 30; PO_2, 70; SaO_2, 80%; HCO_3^-, 30. Chest film revealed left lower lobe pneumonia. Mr. J underwent reintubation with an oral endotracheal tube, and breathing was assisted with mechanical ventilation. Epidural PCA was inserted to assist with pain management. Urine myoglobin finding was negative after 24 hours; at 48 hours, urine output was 50 to 100 ml/hr of clear yellow urine. Nasoenteric tube feedings were increased to 75 ml/hr. Electrolyte levels were all within normal limits, and coagulopathy was corrected. Polyurethane dressing to sacral area was intact. No further redness or blanching was present. On ICU day 5, Mr. J was successfully extubated and his polyurethane dressing was removed.

MEDICAL AND NURSING MANAGEMENT AND PATIENT OUTCOME

On day 7, Mr. J was transferred from the ICU to the floor. He was fully able to participate in aggressive pulmonary physiotherapy. His left rib pain and leg pain were well controlled with the epidural PCA morphine. His pneumothorax resolved. His Hct level remained stable at 30%, with Hgb 11 g/dl. His splenectomy incision was healing by primary intention, with minimal redness, and the staples were intact. Kidney function was normal, and urine output was 500 to 1000 ml per shift. His sacral lesion was well healed. He was fully able to participate in self-care activities except for an inability to bear weight on his left leg. The external fixator device was intact. Physical therapy began after transfer to the floor. Mr. J tolerated a full liquid diet. He made arrangements to live with his parents for a few weeks after discharge.

INEFFECTIVE INDIVIDUAL COPING RELATED TO SITUATIONAL CRISIS AND PERSONAL VULNERABILITY

DEFINING CHARACTERISTICS

- Verbalization of inability to cope. *Sample statements:* "I can't take this anymore." "I don't know how to deal with this."
- Ineffective problem solving (problem lumping). *Example:* "I have to eliminate salt from my diet. They tell me I can no longer mow the lawn. This hospitalization is costing a mint. What about my kids' future? Who's going to change the oil in the car? This is an incredible amount of time away from work."
- Ineffective use of coping mechanisms.
  - Projection: blames others for illness or pain.
  - Displacement: directs anger and/or aggression toward family. *Examples:* "Get out of here. Leave me alone." Curses, shouts, or demands attention; strikes out or throws objects.
  - Denial of severity of illness and need for treatment.
- Noncompliance. *Examples:* activity restriction; refusal to allow treatment or to take medications (see Chapter 9, "Sexuality Alterations," for interventions with patients using adaptive denial vs. patients using maladaptive denial or no denial).
- Suicidal thoughts (verbalizes desire to end life).
- Self-directed aggression. *Examples:* disconnects or attempts to disconnect life-sustaining equipment; deliberately tries to harm self.
- Failure to progress from dependent to more independent state (refusal or resistance to care for self).

OUTCOME CRITERIA

- Patient verbalizes beginning ability to cope with illness, pain, and hospitalization. *Sample statements:* "I'm trying to do the best I can." "I want to help myself get better."
- Patient demonstrates effective problem solving (lists and prioritizes problems from most to least urgent).
- Patient uses effective behavioral strategies to manage the stress of illness and care.
- Patient demonstrates interest or involvement in illness or environment. *Examples:* patient does the following:
  - Requests medications when anticipating pain.
  - Questions course of treatment, progress, and prognosis.
  - Asks for clarification of environmental stimuli and events.
  - Seeks out supportive individuals in his or her environment.
  - Uses coping mechanisms and strategies more effectively to manage situational crisis.
  - Demonstrates significant reduction in impulsive, angry, or aggressive outbursts (projection, shouting, cursing) directed toward family.
  - Verbalizes futuristic plans, with cessation of self-directed aggressive acts and suicidal thoughts.
  - Willingly complies with treatment regimen.
  - Begins to participate in self-care.

NURSING INTERVENTIONS AND *RATIONALE*

1. Continue to monitor the assessment parameters listed under "Defining Characteristics."
2. Actively listen and respond to patient's verbal and behavioral expressions. ***Active listening signifies unconditional respect and acceptance for the patient as a worthwhile individual. It builds trust and rapport, guides the nurse toward problem areas, encourages the patient to express concerns, and promotes compliance.***
3. Offer effective coping strategies to help the patient better tolerate the stressors related to his or her illness and care. Give permission to vent feelings in a safe setting. *Sample statements:* "I don't blame you for feeling angry or frustrated." "Others who are ill like you have expressed similar feelings." "I will listen to anything you want to share with me." "We don't have to talk; I'd like to sit here with you." "It's perfectly OK to cry." ***Individuals who are provided with opportunities to express their feelings will be better able to release pent-up emotions and derive a greater sense of relief and comfort. Thus they are less likely to resort to overly impulsive, aggressive acts, which may harm self or others.***
4. Inform the family of the patient's need to displace anger occasionally but that you will be working with the patient to help him or her release his or her feelings in a more constructive, effective way. ***Family members who are well-informed are better equipped to cope with their loved one's emotional anguish and outbursts. They are less likely to waste energy on feelings of guilt, fear, anger, or despair and can use their strength to help the patient in more constructive ways. The knowledge that their loved one is being cared for emotionally, as well as physically, will offer family members a greater sense of comfort and understanding. They will feel nurtured and respected by the nurse's attempt to include them in the process.***
5. With the patient, list and number problems from most to least urgent. Assist him or her in finding immediate solutions for most urgent problems; postpone those that can wait; delegate some to family members; and help him or her acknowledge problems that are beyond his or her control. ***Listing and numbering problems in an organized fashion help break them down into more manageable "pieces" so that the patient is better able to identify solutions for those that are solvable and to suppress those that are less relevant or not amenable to interventions.***
6. Identify individuals in the patient's environment who best help him or her to cope, as well as those who do not. Validate your observations with the patient. *Sample statements:* "I notice you seemed more relaxed during your daughter's visit." "After the clergy left, you were able to sleep a bit longer than usual; would you like to see him more often?" "Your grandson was a bit upset today; I'll be glad to talk to him if you like." ***Supportive persons can invoke***

INEFFECTIVE INDIVIDUAL COPING RELATED TO SITUATIONAL CRISIS AND PERSONAL VULNERABILITY—cont'd

a calming effect on the patient's physiological and psychological states. Conversely, well-meaning but non-supportive individuals can have a deleterious effect on the patient's ability to cope and must be carefully screened and counseled by the nurse.

7. Teach the patient effective cognitive strategies to help him or her better manage the stress of critical illness and care. Help him or her construct pleasant thoughts, situations, or images that can simultaneously inhibit unpleasant realities. *Examples:* a day at the beach, a walk in the park, drinking a glass of wine, or being with a loved one. ***Pleasant thoughts or images constructed during critical illness and care tend to inhibit or reduce the intensity of the unpleasant, stressful effects of the experience.***
8. Assist the patient in using coping mechanisms more effectively so he or she can better manage his or her situational crisis:
   - Suppression of problems beyond his or her control.
   - Compensation for illness and its effects; focusing on his or her strengths, interests, family, and spiritual beliefs.
   - Adaptive displacement of anger, fear, or frustration through healthy, verbal expressions to staff.

   Effective use of coping mechanisms helps to assuage the patient's painful feelings in a safe setting. Thus the patient is strengthened and need not resort to the use of more ineffective defenses to eliminate anxiety.
9. Initiate a suicidal assessment if the patient verbalizes the desire to die, states that life is not worth living, or exhibits self-directed aggression. *Sample statement:* "We know this is a bad time for you. You're saying repeatedly that you want to die. Are you planning to harm yourself?" If the response is yes, remain with the patient, alert staff members, and provide for psychiatric consultation as soon as possible. Continue to express concern to the patient and protect him or her from harm. ***Suicidal thoughts as a result of ineffective coping or exhaustion of coping devices are not an uncommon occurrence in critically ill patients. If the mood state is distressing enough, a patient may seek relief by attempting a self-destructive act. Although the patient may not imminently have the energy to succeed in his or her attempt, voicing specific plans signifies a depressed mood state and a depletion of coping strategies. Thus immediate intervention is needed, since the attempt may be successful when the patient's energy is restored.***
10. Encourage the patient to participate in self-care activities and treatment regimen in accordance with his or her level of progress. Offer praise for his or her efforts toward self-care. ***Patients who take an active role in their own treatment and progress are less apt to feel like helpless or powerless victims. This greater sense of control over their illness and environment will guide them more swiftly toward becoming as independent as possible.***

ANXIETY RELATED TO THREAT TO BIOLOGIC, PSYCHOLOGIC, AND/OR SOCIAL INTEGRITY

DEFINING CHARACTERISTICS

Subjective

- ◆ Verbalizes increased muscle tension.
- ◆ Expresses frequent sensation of tingling in hands and feet.
- ◆ Relates continuous feeling of apprehension.
- ◆ Expresses preoccupation with a sense of impending doom.
- ◆ States has difficulty falling asleep.
- ◆ Repeatedly expresses concerns about changes in health status and outcome of illness.

Objective

- ◆ Psychomotor agitation (fidgeting, jitteriness, restlessness).
- ◆ Tightened, wrinkled brow.
- ◆ Strained (worried) facial expression.
- ◆ Hypervigilance (scans environment).
- ◆ Startles easily.
- ◆ Distractibility.
- ◆ Sweaty palms.
- ◆ Fragmented sleep patterns.
- ◆ Tachycardia.
- ◆ Tachypnea.

Continued.

ANXIETY RELATED TO THREAT TO BIOLOGIC, PSYCHOLOGIC, AND/OR SOCIAL INTEGRITY —cont'd

OUTCOME CRITERIA

- Patient effectively uses learned relaxation strategies.
- Patient demonstrates significant decrease in psychomotor agitation.
- Patient verbalizes reduction in tingling sensations in hands and feet.
- Patient is able to focus on the tasks at hand.
- Patient expresses positive, futuristic plans to family and staff.
- Patient's heart rate and rhythm remain within limits commensurate with physiologic status.

NURSING INTERVENTIONS AND *RATIONALE*

1. Continue to monitor the assessment parameters listed under "Defining Characteristics."
2. Instruct the patient in the following simple, effective relaxation strategies:
   - If not contraindicated cardiovascularly, tense and relax all muscles progressively from toes to head.
   - Perform slow, deep-breathing exercises.
   - Focus on a single object or person in the environment.
   - Listen to soothing music or relaxation tapes with eyes closed.

Progressive toe-to-head relaxation releases the muscular tension that may be a stress-related effect resulting from the threat or change in the patient's health status and outcome of illness. Deep-breathing exercises provide slow, rhythmic, controlled breathing patterns that relax the patient and distract him or her from the effects of his or her illness and hospitalization. Focusing on a single object or person helps the patient dismiss the myriad of disorienting stimuli from his or her visual-perceptual field, which can have a dizzying, distorted effect. A clear sensorium allows him or her to feel more in control of his or her environment. (See "Sensory-Perceptual Alterations," p. 573.) ***Music or words expressed in soft, low tones tend to produce soothing, relaxing effects that counteract or inhibit escalating anxiety and provide respites from the patient's situational crisis. Closed eyes eliminate distracting, visual stimuli and promote a more restful environment.***

3. Actively listen to and accept the patient's concerns regarding the threats from his or her illness, outcome and hospitalization. ***Active listening and unconditional acceptance validate the patient as a worthwhile individual and assure him or her that his or her concerns, no matter how great, will be addressed. Knowledge that he or she has an avenue for ventilation will assuage anxiety.***
4. Help the patient distinguish between realistic concerns and exaggerated fears through clear, simple explanations. *Sample statements:* "Your lab results show that you're doing OK right now." "The shortness of breath you're experiencing is not unusual." "The pain you described is expected and this medication will relieve it." ***A patient who is informed about his or her progress and is reassured about expected symptoms and management of care will be better equipped to maintain a more realistic perspective of his or her illness and its outcome. Thus anxiety emanating from imagined or exaggerated fears will likely be assuaged or averted.***
5. Provide simple clarification of environmental events and stimuli that are not related to the patient's illness and care. *Sample statements:* "That loud noise is coming from a machine that is helping another patient." "The visitor behind the curtain is crying because she's had an upsetting day." "That gurney is here to bring another patient to x-ray." ***Clarification of events and stimuli that are unrelated to the patient helps to disengage him or her from the extant anxiety-provoking situations surrounding him or her, thus avoiding further anxiety and apprehension.***
6. Assist the patient in focusing on building on prior coping strategies to deal with the effects of his or her illness and care. *Sample statements:* "What methods have helped you get through difficult times in the past?" "How can we help you use those methods now?" (See Ineffective Individual Coping care plan, p. 762, for interventions that assist patients to use coping strategies effectively.) ***Use of previously successful coping strategies in conjunction with newly learned techniques arms the patient with an arsenal of weapons against anxiety, providing him or her with greater control over his or her situational crisis and decreased feelings of doom and despair.***
7. Give the patient permission to deny or suppress the effects of his or her illness and hospitalization with which he or she cannot cope or control. *Sample statements:* "It's perfectly OK to ignore things you can't handle right now." "How can we help ease your mind during this time?" "What are some things or tasks that may help distract you?" ***Adaptive denial can be helpful in reducing feelings of anxiety in patients with life-threatening illness.*** Bigus* reports that in studies of two groups of patients with myocardial infarction, the group that used adaptive denial demonstrated significantly fewer symptoms of state anxiety than those patients who failed to use it. (See Chapter 9, "Sexuality Alterations," for interventions with patients using adaptive denial vs. patients using maladaptive denial or no denial.)

*From Bigus KM: *West J Nurs Res* 3:150, 1981.

REFERENCES

1. Sheehy BS, Marvin JA, Jimmerson CL: *Manual of clinical trauma care: the first hour,* St Louis, 1989, Mosby–Year Book.
2. Boggs RL: Multiple system trauma: nursing implications, *J Adv Med Surg Nurs* 2(1):1, 1989.
3. American College of Surgeons, Committee on Trauma: *Advanced trauma life support instructor manual,* Chicago, 1989, The College.
4. Robertson L: Motor vehicles, *Pediatr Clin North Am* 32:87, 1985.
5. Martin K: Reducing complications of thoracic gunshot wounds, *Dimens Crit Care Nurs* 8(5):280, 1989.
6. Trimble P, Wallack D: Trauma nursing: past, present and future, *MMJ* 37(7):547, 1988.
7. Chabot DR: Recent advances in trauma resuscitation, *Emerg Care Q* 5(2):1, 1989.
8. Cordon V: *Trauma reference manual,* Baltimore, 1985, Brady Communications.
9. Emergency Nurses' Association: *Trauma nursing core course instructor manual,* Chicago, 1987, Award Printing Corp.
10. Meyer AA, Trunkey DD: Critical care as an integral part of trauma care, *Crit Care Clin North Am* 2(4):673, 1986.
11. Whitehorne M, Cacciola R, Quinn ME: Multiple trauma: survival after the golden hour, *J Adv Med Surg Nurs* 2(1):27, 1989.
12. Von Reuden KT: Cardiopulmonary assessment of the critically ill trauma patient, *Crit Care Nurs Clin North Am* 1(1):33, 1989.
13. Gennarelli TA: Triage of head injured patients. In Trunkey DD, Lewis FR, editors: *Current therapy of trauma,* ed 3, Philadelphia, 1991, BC Decker.
14. Stand PE: Diagnostic and therapeutic concerns in head injured patient, *J Am Acad Phys Assist* 1(2):112, 1988.
15. Gress DR: Treatment of head and spine trauma, *Emerg Care Q* 5(2):15, 1989.
16. Ammons AM: Cerebral injuries and intracranial hemorrhages as a result of trauma, *Nurs Clin North Am* 25(1):23, 1990.
17. Hughes MC: Critical care nursing for the patient with a spinal cord injury, *Crit Care Nurs Clin North Am* 2(1):33, 1990.
18. Hickey JV: *The clinical practice of neurological and neurosurgical nursing,* ed 3, Philadelphia, 1992, JB Lippincott.
19. Walleck CA: Neurologic considerations in the critical care phase, *Crit Care Nurs Clin North Am* 2(3):357, 1990.
20. Hilton G, Frei J: High-dose methylprednisolone in the treatment of spinal cord injuries, *Heart Lung* 20(6):675, 1991.
21. Kidd PS: Emergency department management of spinal cord injury, *Crit Care Nurs Clin North Am* 2(3):349, 1990.
22. Kocan MJ: Pulmonary considerations in the critical care phase, *Crit Care Nurs Clin North Am* 2(3):369, 1990.
23. Richmond TS: Spinal cord injury, *Nurs Clin North Am* 25(1):57, 1990.
24. Schwenker D: Cardiovascular considerations in the acute care phase, *Crit Care Nurs Clin North Am* 2(3):363, 1990.
25. Gilbert J: Critical care management of the patient with acute spinal cord injury, *Crit Care Nurs Clin North Am* 3:549, 1987.
26. Metcalf JA: Acute phase management of persons with spinal cord injury: a nursing diagnosis perspective, *Nurs Clin North Am* 21:589, 1986.
27. Barot LR: Maxillofacial trauma, *Top Emerg Med* 13(4):17, 1991.
28. Walton RL, Bunkis J, Borah GL: *Maxillofacial trauma*. In Trunkey DD, Lewis FR, editors: *Current therapy of trauma,* ed 3, Philadelphia, 1991, BC Decker.
29. Lower J: Maxillofacial trauma, *Nurs Clin North Am* 21(4):511, 1986.
30. Hammond SG: Chest injuries in the trauma patient, *Nurs Clin North Am* 25(1):35, 1990.
31. Ross SE, Cernaianu AC: Epidemiology of thoracic injuries: mechanisms of injury and pathophysiology, *Top Emerg Med* 12(1):1, 1990.
32. Roberts R and others: Chest trauma: emergency diagnosis and management of airway problems in intrathoracic injuries, *Top Emerg Med* 9(3):53, 1987.
33. Gough JE, Allison EJ, Raju VP: Flail chest: management and implications for emergency nurses, *J Emerg Nurs* 13(6):330, 1987.
34. Andrew L: Difficult diagnoses in blunt thoraco-abdominal trauma, *J Emerg Nurs* 15(5):399, 1989.
35. Ruth-Sahd L: Pulmonary contusion: the hidden danger in blunt chest trauma, *Crit Care Nurs* 11(6):46, 1990.
36. Rosen JE, Deluca SA: Pulmonary contusion, *Am Fam Phys,* p. 219, Nov 1988.
37. Hefti D: Chest trauma, *RN,* 54: 28, 1991.
38. Feliciano DV, Mattox KL: The heart. In Trunkey DD, Lewis FR, editors: *Current therapy of trauma,* ed 3, Philadelphia, 1991, BC Decker.
39. Turner JA: Cardiovascular trauma, *Nurs Clin North Am* 25(1):119, 1990.
40. Bartlett R: Myocardial contusion, *Dimens Crit Care Nurs* 10(3):133, 1991.
41. Merrill CR, Sparger G: Current thoughts on blunt abdominal trauma, *Top Emerg Med* 12(2):21, 1990.
42. Semonin-Holleran R: Critical nursing care for abdominal trauma, *Crit Care Nurs* 8(3):48, 1988.
43. Carrico CJ: The spleen. In Trunkey DD, Lewis FR, editors: *Current therapy of trauma,* ed 3, Philadelphia, 1991, BC Decker.
44. Wagner MM: The patient with abdominal injuries, *Nurs Clin North Am* 25(1):45, 1990.
45. Shoemaker W, Ayers S, Grenvick A: *Textbook of critical care,* ed 2, Philadelphia, 1988, WB Saunders.
46. Bresler MJ: Computerized tomography v. peritoneal lavage in blunt abdominal trauma, *Top Emerg Med* 10(1):59, 1988.
47. Kidd PS: Genitourinary trauma patients, *Top Emerg Med* 9(3):71, 1987.
48. Frevele G: Urinary tract injuries due to blunt abdominal trauma, *Phys Assist,* 13(2): 123, 1989.
49. Smith MF: Renal trauma, *Crit Care Nurs Clin North Am* 2(1):67, 1990.
50. Ruhl JM: Pelvic trauma, *RN,* p. 50, July 1991.
51. Maher AB: Early assessment and management of musculoskeletal injuries, *Nurs Clin North Am* 21(4):717, 1986.
52. Phillips TF: Pelvic fractures and perineal lacerations. In Trunkey DD, Lewis FR, editors: *Current therapy of trauma,* ed 3, Philadelphia, 1991, BC Decker.
53. Rhodes M, Smith S: Open pelvic fractures, *Emerg Care Q* 4(2):48, 1988.
54. Johnson L: Operative management of unstable pelvic fractures, *Orthop Nurs* 8(4):21, 1989.
55. Herron DG, Nance J: Emergency department management of patients with orthopedic fractures resulting from motor vehicle accidents, *Nurs Clin North Am* 25(1):71, 1990.
56. Respet P: Management of lower extremity injury: the first hour, *Emerg Care Q* 4(2):40, 1988.
57. Martin MT: Wound management and infection control after trauma: implications for the intensive care setting, *Crit Care Nurs Q* 11(2):43, 1988.
58. Thompson J, Dains J: Indices of injury: development and status, *Nurs Clin North Am* 12:655, 1986.
59. Langdale L, Schecter WP: Critical care complications in the trauma patient, *Crit Care Clin North Am* 2(4):839, 1986.
60. Konopad E, Noseworthy T: Stress ulceration: a serious complication in critically ill patients, *Heart Lung* 17(4):339, 1988.
61. Littleton M: Complications of multiple trauma, *Crit Care Nurs Clin North Am* 1(1):75, 1989.

46

Shock

CHAPTER OBJECTIVES

- Describe the generalized shock response.
- List the causes and etiologic factors of hypovolemic, cardiogenic, anaphylactic, neurogenic, and septic shock.
- Explain the pathophysiology of hypovolemic, cardiogenic, anaphylactic, neurogenic, and septic shock.
- Identify the clinical manifestations of hypovolemic, cardiogenic, anaphylactic, neurogenic, and septic shock.
- Outline the important aspects of the medical management of hypovolemic, cardiogenic, anaphylactic, neurogenic, and septic shock.
- Summarize the nursing management of the patient with hypovolemic, cardiogenic, anaphylactic, neurogenic, and septic shock.

Shock is an acute, widespread process of impaired tissue perfusion that results in cellular, metabolic, and hemodynamic derangements. Impaired tissue perfusion occurs when an imbalance develops between cellular oxygen supply and cellular oxygen demand. This imbalance can occur for a variety of reasons and eventually results in cellular dysfunction and death. This chapter presents an overview of the general shock response, or shock syndrome, followed by a discussion of the different shock states.

SHOCK SYNDROME

Description

Shock is a complex pathophysiologic process that often results in multiple organ dysfunction syndrome and death. All types of shock eventually result in impaired tissue perfusion and the development of acute circulatory failure or shock syndrome. Shock syndrome is a generalized systemic response to inadequate tissue perfusion.[1,2] It consists of four different stages: initial, compensatory, progressive, and refractory.[3] Progression through each stage varies with the patient's prior condition, duration of initiating event, response to therapy, and correction of underlying cause.[4]

Etiology

Shock can be classified as hypovolemic, cardiogenic, or distributive, depending on the pathophysiologic cause. *Hypovolemic shock* results from a loss of circulating or intravascular volume. *Cardiogenic shock* results from the impaired ability of the heart to pump. *Distributive shock* results from maldistribution of circulating blood volume and can be further classified as septic, anaphylactic, and neurogenic. *Septic shock* is the result of microorganisms entering the body. *Anaphylactic shock* is the result of a severe antibody-antigen reaction. *Neurogenic shock* is the result of the loss of sympathetic tone.[5,6]

Pathophysiology

During the *initial stage,* cardiac output (CO) is decreased and tissue perfusion is impaired. As the blood supply to the cells decreases, the cells switch from aerobic to anaerobic metabolism as a source of energy. Anaerobic metabolism produces small amounts of energy but large amounts of lactic acid. Lactic acidemia quickly develops and causes more cellular damage.[3,7]

During the *compensatory stage,* an attempt is made by the body's homeostatic mechanisms to improve tissue perfusion. The compensatory mechanisms are mediated by the sympathetic nervous system (SNS) and consist of neural, hormonal, and chemical responses. Neural compensation includes an increase in heart rate (HR) and contractility, arterial and venous vasoconstriction, and shunting of blood to the vital organs. Hormonal compensation includes activation of the renin response and stimulation of the anterior pituitary and adrenal medulla. Activation of the renin response results in the production of angiotensin II, which causes vasoconstriction and the release of aldosterone and antidiuretic hormone (ADH), leading to sodium and water retention. Stimulation of the anterior pituitary results in the secretion of adrenocorticotropic hormone (ACTH), which in turn stimulates the adrenal cortex to produce glucocorticoids, causing a rise in blood glucose levels. Stimulation of the adrenal medulla causes the release of epinephrine and norepinephrine, which further enhance the compensatory mechanisms. Chemical compensation includes hyperventilation to neutralize lactic acidosis.[3,4,7]

During the *progressive stage,* the compensatory mechanisms start to fail and the shock cycle is perpetuated. At the cellular level, the small amount of energy created by anaerobic metabolism is not enough to keep the cell functional, and irreversible damage begins to occur. The sodium-potassium pump in the cell membrane fails, causing the cell and its organelles to swell. Cellular energy production comes to a complete halt as the mitochondria swell and rupture. At this point the problem becomes one of oxygen utilization instead of oxygen delivery. Even if the cell were to receive more oxygen, it would be unable to use it because of damage to the mitochondria. The cell's digestive organelles swell, resulting in leakage of destructive enzymes into the cell. Autodigestion occurs with ensuing cell death.[7]

Every system in the body is affected by this process (see box below). Cardiac dysfunction develops as a result of myocardial hypoperfusion, lactic acidosis, and the release of myocardial depressant factor (MDF). MDF is a substance that is released from the pancreas as it becomes ischemic. Ventricular failure eventually occurs, further perpetuating the entire process.[3,7] Central nervous system (CNS) dysfunction develops as a result of cerebral hypoperfusion, leading to failure of the SNS, cardiac and respiratory depression, and thermoregulatory failure. SNS failure in turn results in vasodilation, pooling of blood in the capillaries, increased capillary membrane permeability, and the formation of microemboli.[7] Hematologic dysfunction occurs as a result of hypotension, hypoxemia, acidosis, and stasis of capillary blood flow. Disseminated intravascular coagulation (DIC) eventually develops.[3,4,8] Pulmonary dysfunction occurs as a result of increased pulmonary capillary membrane permeability, pulmonary microemboli, and pulmonary vasoconstriction. Ventilatory failure and adult respiratory distress syndrome (ARDS) eventually develop.[3,4,9] Renal dysfunction develops as a result of renal vasoconstriction and renal hypoperfusion, leading to acute tubular necrosis (ATN).[3,4,10] Gastrointestinal dysfunction occurs as a result of splanchnic vasoconstriction and splanchnic hypoperfusion, leading to failure of the gut organs. Failure of the gut organs results in the release of gram-negative bacteria into the system, which further perpetuates the entire shock syndrome.[3,11]

During the *refractory stage,* shock becomes unresponsive to therapy and is considered irreversible. As the individual organ systems die, multiple organ dysfunction syndrome (MODS), defined as failure of two or more body systems, occurs (see Chapter 47). Death is the final outcome.[3] Regardless of etiologic factors, death occurs from impaired tissue perfusion because of the failure of the circulation to meet the oxygen needs of the cell.[1,2]

CONSEQUENCES OF SHOCK

- Cardiovascular
  - Ventricular failure
- Neurologic
  - Sympathetic nervous system dysfunction
  - Cardiac and respiratory depression
  - Thermoregulatory failure
  - Coma
- Pulmonary
  - Acute respiratory failure
  - Adult respiratory distress syndrome (ARDS)
- Renal
  - Acute tubular necrosis (ATN)
- Hematologic
  - Disseminated intravascular coagulation (DIC)
- Gastrointestinal
  - Gastrointestinal tract failure
  - Hepatic failure
  - Pancreatic failure

Assessment and Diagnosis

Clinical manifestations differ according to etiologic factors and the stage of the shock. They are related to both the cause of the shock and to the patient's general response to shock.[12] (See sections on *individual shock states* for a discussion of clinical assessment and diagnosis of the patient in shock.)

Medical Management

The major focus of the treatment of shock is the improvement and preservation of tissue perfusion. Adequate tissue perfusion depends on an adequate supply of oxygen being transported to the tissues and the cell's ability to use it. Oxygen transport is influenced by pulmonary gas exchange, cardiac output, and hemoglobin level. Oxygen utilization is influenced by the internal metabolic environment. Management of the patient in shock focuses on supporting oxygen transport and oxygen utilization.[1,2]

Adequate pulmonary gas exchange is critical to oxygen transport. Establishing and maintaining an adequate airway are the first steps in ensuring adequate oxygenation. Once the airway is patent, emphasis is placed on improving ventilation and oxygenation. Therapies include administration of supplemental oxygen, mechanical ventilation, and chest physiotherapy.[13]

An adequate CO and hemoglobin level are crucial to oxygen transport. CO depends on HR, preload, afterload, and contractility. A variety of fluids and drugs are used to manipulate these parameters. The types of fluids used include both crystalloids and colloids. The categories of drugs used include vasoconstrictors, vasodilators, positive inotropes, and antidysrhythmic agents.

Fluid administration can be accomplished by use of either a crystalloid or colloid solution, or both, and is indicated for decreased preload related to intravascular volume depletion. Crystalloids are balanced electrolyte solutions that may be hypotonic, isotonic, or hypertonic. Examples of crystalloid solutions are normal saline, lactated Ringer's solution, and 5% dextrose in water. Colloids are protein or starch-containing solutions. Examples of colloid solutions are blood and blood components and pharmaceutic plasma expanders, such as hetastarch, dextran, and mannitol. The choice of fluid depends on the situation. Advantages of colloids include faster restoration of intravascular volume and use of smaller amounts. Colloids stay in the intravascular space as opposed to crystalloids, which readily leak into the extravascular space. Disadvantages include expense, allergic reactions, and difficulties in typing and crossmatching blood. Colloids also can leak out of damaged capillaries and cause a variety of additional problems, particularly in the lungs.[13-17] Blood should be used to augment oxygen transport if the patient's hemoglobin level is low.[1]

Vasoconstrictor agents are used to increase afterload by increasing the systemic vascular resistance (SVR) and improving the patient's blood pressure level. *Vasodilator agents* are used to decrease preload or afterload, or both, by decreasing venous return and SVR. *Positive inotropic agents* are used to increase contractility. *Antidysrhythmic agents* are used to influence heart rate. Table 46-1 provides examples of each of these agents.[13,15,18]

An optimal metabolic environment is very important to oxygen utilization. Once the oxygen is delivered to the cells, they have to be able to use it. The major metabolic derangement seen in shock is lactic acidosis. Interventions to correct lactic acidosis include correcting the cause, reestablishing perfusion, inducing hyperventilation, and in severe cases, administering sodium bicarbonate.[19] The patient also should be started on a nutritional support therapy. The type of nutritional supplementation initiated varies according to the cause of shock and should be tailored to the individual patient's need, as indicated by the underlying condition and laboratory data. The enteral route generally is preferred over the parenteral.[20]

Nursing Management

The nursing management of a patient in shock is a complex and challenging responsibility. It requires an in-depth understanding of the pathophysiology of the disease and the anticipated effects of each intervention, as well as a solid understanding of the nursing process.[21] (See the *individual shock states* for a discussion of specific interventions for the patient in shock.)

The psychosocial needs of the patient and family dealing with shock are extremely important. These needs, which differ with each patient and family, are based on situational, familial, and patient-centered variables. Nursing interventions for psychosocial problems include providing information on patient status, explaining procedures and routines, supporting the family, encouraging the expression of feelings, facilitating problem-solving and decision-making, involving the family in the patient's care, and establishing contacts with necessary resources.[22]

HYPOVOLEMIC SHOCK

Description

Hypovolemic shock occurs from inadequate fluid volume in the intravascular space. The lack of adequate circulating volume leads to decreased tissue perfusion and initiation of the general shock response. Hypovolemic shock is the most commonly occurring form of shock.[3,23,24]

Etiology

Hypovolemic shock can result from either absolute or relative hypovolemia. Absolute hypovolemia occurs when there is an external loss of fluid from the body. This includes external losses of whole blood, plasma, or any other body fluid. Relative hypovolemia occurs when there is an internal shifting of fluid from the intravascular space to the extravascular space. This can be the result of a loss in intravascular integrity, increased capillary membrane permeability, or decreased colloidal osmotic pressure[3,23,24] (see box, p. 769).

Pathophysiology

Hypovolemia results in a loss of circulating fluid volume. A decrease in circulating volume leads to a decrease in venous return, which in turn results in a decrease in end-diastolic volume or preload. Preload is a major determinant of stroke volume (SV) and CO. A decrease in preload results in a decrease in SV and CO. The decrease in CO leads to inadequate cellular oxygen supply and impaired tissue perfusion[3,23,24] (Fig. 46-1).

Assessment and Diagnosis

The clinical manifestations of hypovolemic shock vary, depending on the severity of fluid loss and the patient's ability to compensate for it. The *first, or initial, stage* occurs with a fluid volume loss up to 15% or an actual volume loss up to 750 ml. Compensatory mechanisms maintain CO, and the patient appears symptom-free.[6,14,23]

The *second, or compensatory, stage* occurs with a fluid volume loss of 15% to 30% or an actual volume loss of 750 to 1500 ml.[14] CO falls, resulting in the initiation of a variety of compensatory responses. The HR increases in response to increased SNS stimulation. The pulse pressure (PP) narrows as the diastolic blood pressure increases because of vasoconstriction. Respiratory rate (RR) and depth increase in an attempt to improve oxygenation. Arterial blood gas (ABG) specimens drawn during this phase reveal respiratory alkalosis and hypoxemia, as evidenced by a low $Paco_2$ and a low Pao_2, respectively. Urine output (UO) starts to decline as re-

Table 46-1 Examples of the different agents used in the treatment of shock

Vasoconstrictors	Vasodilators	Inotropes	Antidysrhythmics
Epinephrine (Adrenalin) Norepinephrine (Levophed) Alpha-range dopamine (Intropin) Metaraminol (Aramine) Phenylephrine (Neo-Synephrine) Ephedrine	Nitroprusside (Nipride, Nitropress) Nitroglycerine (Nitrol, Tridil) Hydralazine (Apresoline) Labetalol (Normodyne, Trandate)	Beta-range dopamine (Intropin) Dobutamine (Dobutrex) Amrinone (Inocor) Epinephrine (Adrenalin) Isuproterenol (Isuprel) Norepinephrine (Levephed) Digoxin (Lanoxin)	Lidocaine (Xylocaine) Bretylium (Bretylol) Procainamide (Pronestyl) Labetalol (Normodyne, Trandate) Verapamil (Calan, Isoptin) Esmolol (Brevibloc)

nal perfusion decreases. Urine sodium decreases while urine osmolarity and specific gravity increase as the kidneys start to conserve sodium and water. The patient's skin becomes pale and cool, with delayed capillary refill because of peripheral vasoconstriction. Jugular veins appear flat as a result of decreased venous return. Decreased cerebral perfusion causes a change in level of consciousness (LOC). The patient may appear disoriented, confused, restless, anxious, or irritable.[12,14,23,24]

The *third, or progressive, stage* occurs with a fluid volume loss of 30% to 40% or an actual volume loss of 1500 to 2000 ml.[14] The compensatory mechanisms become overwhelmed, and impaired tissue perfusion develops. The HR continues to increase, and dysrhythmias develop as myocardial ischemia ensues. Respiratory distress occurs as the pulmonary system deteriorates. ABG values during this phase reveal respiratory and metabolic acidosis and hypoxemia, as evidenced by a high $Paco_2$, low bicarbonate (HCO_3^-), and low Pao_2, respectively. Decreased renal perfusion results in the development of oliguria. Blood urea nitrogen (BUN) and serum creatinine levels start to rise as the kidneys begin to fail. The patient's skin becomes ashen, cold, and clammy, with marked delayed capillary refill. The patient appears lethargic as cerebral perfusion decreases and LOC continues to deteriorate.[12,14,23,24]

The *fourth, or refractory, stage* occurs with a fluid volume loss of greater than 40% or an actual volume loss of more than 2000 ml.[14] The compensatory mechanisms completely deteriorate, and organ failure occurs. Severe tachycardia and hypotension ensue. Peripheral pulses are absent, and because of marked peripheral vasoconstriction, capillary refill does not occur. The skin appears cyanotic, mottled, and extremely diaphoretic. The patient becomes unresponsive, and a variety of clinical manifestations associated with failure of the different body systems develop.[14,23,24]

Assessment of the hemodynamic parameters of a patient in hypovolemic shock reveals a decreased CO and cardiac index (CI). Loss of circulation volume leads to a decrease in venous return to the heart, which results in a decrease in the preload of the right and left ventricles. This is evidenced by a decline in the right atrial pressure (RAP) and pulmonary capillary wedge pressure (PCWP). Vasoconstriction of the arterial system results in an increase in the afterload of the heart as evidenced by an increase in the systemic vascular resistance (SVR).[12,23,25]

Medical Management

Treatment of the patient in hypovolemic shock requires an aggressive approach. The major goals of therapy are to correct the cause of the hypovolemia and to restore tissue perfusion. This approach includes

---

ETIOLOGIC FACTORS IN HYPOVOLEMIC SHOCK

ABSOLUTE

Loss of whole blood
- Trauma
- Surgery
- Gastrointestinal bleeding

Loss of plasma
- Thermal injuries
- Large lesions

Loss of other body fluids
- Severe vomiting
- Severe diarrhea
- Massive diuresis

RELATIVE

Loss of intravascular integrity
- Ruptured spleen
- Long bone or pelvic fractures
- Hemorrhagic pancreatitis
- Hemothorax or hemoperitoneum
- Arterial dissection

Increased capillary membrane permeability
- Sepsis
- Anaphylaxis
- Thermal injuries

Decreased colloidal osmotic pressure
- Severe sodium depletion
- Hypopituitarism
- Cirrhosis
- Intestinal obstruction

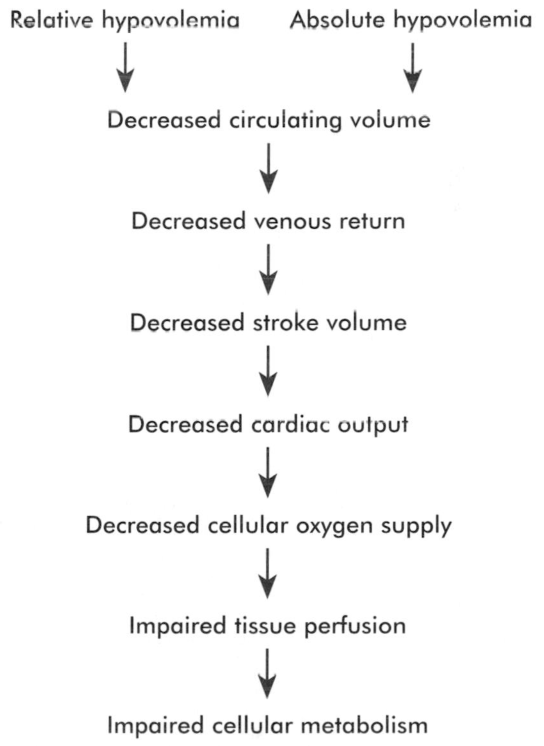

Fig. 46-1 The pathophysiology of hypovolemic shock.

identifying and stopping the source of fluid loss and vigorously administering fluid to replace circulating volume. Fluid administration can be accomplished with use of either a crystalloid or a colloid solution, or a combination of both. The type of solution used usually depends on the type of fluid lost.[13-17,23,24]

Two other therapies available for assisting with resuscitation of the patient in hypovolemic shock are autotransfusion and the pneumatic antishock garment (PASG). Autotransfusion is the collection and administration of the patient's own blood. It has been particularly useful in managing the patient with hypovolemic shock caused by chest trauma and hemorrhage.[26] PASG, also known as *military antishock trousers (MAST)*, is a one-piece suit with three individually controlled compartments: one for the abdomen and one for each leg. When inflated, the PASG acts as a vasoconstrictor to improve blood pressure and augments venous return to improve preload.[27]

Nursing Management

Prevention of hypovolemic shock is one of the primary responsibilities of the nurse in the critical care area. This includes the identification of patients at risk and constant assessment of the patient's fluid balance. Accurate monitoring of intake and output and daily weights are essential components of preventive nursing care. Early identification and treatment result in decreased mortality.[28]

The patient with hypovolemic shock may have any number of nursing diagnoses, depending on the progression of the process. Nursing interventions include minimizing fluid loss, enhancing volume replacement, and monitoring the patient's response to care. Measures to minimize fluid loss include limiting blood sampling, observing lines for accidental disconnection, and applying direct pressure to bleeding sites. Measures to enhance volume replacement include insertion of large-diameter peripheral intravenous catheters, rapid administration of prescribed fluids, and positioning the patient with the legs elevated, trunk flat, and head and shoulders above the chest. In addition, monitoring the patient for clinical manifestations of fluid overload is critical to preventing further problems.[23,28]

NURSING DIAGNOSIS AND MANAGEMENT
Hypovolemic shock

- ◆ Fluid Volume Deficit related to active blood loss, p. 639
- ◆ High Risk for Altered Peripheral Tissue Perfusion risk factor: high-dose vasopressor therapy, p. 363
- ◆ High Risk for Infection risk factor: invasive monitoring devices, p. 366
- ◆ High Risk for Aspiration risk factors: impaired laryngeal sensation or reflex; impaired laryngeal closure or elevation, p. 472
- ◆ Ineffective Airway Clearance related to impaired cough secondary to artificial airway, p. 466
- ◆ Sleep Pattern Disturbance related to fragmented sleep and/or circadian desynchronization, pp. 142 and 143
- ◆ Sensory/Perceptual Alterations related to sensory overload, sensory deprivation, sleep pattern disturbance, p. 573
- ◆ Anxiety related to threat to biologic, psychologic, and/or social integrity, p. 763

CARDIOGENIC SHOCK

Description

Cardiogenic shock is the result of failure of the heart to pump blood forward effectively. It can occur with dysfunction of either the right or the left ventricle, or both. The lack of adequate pumping function leads to decreased tissue perfusion and initiation of the general shock response.[5,29,30] It occurs in approximately 15% of the patients with an acute myocardial infarction (MI), and the mortality rate is 75% to 95%.[6]

Etiology

Cardiogenic shock can result from primary ventricular ischemia, structural problems, and dysrhythmias.[31] The most common cause is acute MI resulting in the loss of 40% or more of the functional myocardium. The damage to the myocardium may occur after one massive MI, or it may be cumulative as a result of several smaller MIs.[5,29,31]

ETIOLOGIC FACTORS IN CARDIOGENIC SHOCK

- Primary ventricular ischemia
  - Acute myocardial infarction
  - Cardiopulmonary arrest
  - Open heart surgery
- Structural problems
  - Septal rupture
  - Papillary muscle rupture
  - Free wall rupture
  - Ventricular aneurysm
  - Cardiomyopathies
    - Congestive
    - Hypertrophic
    - Restrictive
  - Intracardiac tumor
  - Pulmonary embolus
  - Atrial thrombus
  - Valvular dysfunction
  - Acute myocarditis
  - Cardiac tamponade
  - Myocardial contusion
- Dysrhythmias
  - Bradydysrhythmias
  - Tachydysrhythmias

Structural problems of the cardiopulmonary system and dysrhythmias also may cause cardiogenic shock if they disrupt the forward motion of the blood through the heart[3,30-33] (see box, p. 770, right-hand column).

Pathophysiology

Cardiogenic shock results from the impaired ability of the ventricle to pump blood forward. This leads to a decrease in SV and an increase in the blood left in the ventricle at the end of systole. The decrease in SV results in a decrease in CO, which leads to decreased cellular oxygen supply and impaired tissue perfusion. When the underlying problem involves the left ventricle, the increase in end-systolic volume results in the back-up of blood into the pulmonary system and the subsequent development of pulmonary edema. Pulmonary edema causes impaired gas exchange and decreased oxygenation of the arterial blood, which further impairs tissue perfusion (Fig. 46-2). Death may result from cardiopulmonary collapse.[5,29-32]

Assessment and Diagnosis

A variety of clinical manifestations occur in the patient in cardiogenic shock, depending on etiologic factors in pump failure, the patient's underlying medical status, and the severity of the shock state. Some of these are caused by failure of the heart as a pump, whereas many relate to the overall shock response (see box).

Initially the clinical manifestations are related to the decline in cardiac output. These signs and symptoms include systolic blood pressure less than 90 mm Hg; decreased sensorium; cool, pale, moist skin; and UO less than 30 ml/hr. The patient also may complain of chest pain. Once the compensatory mechanisms are activated, tachycardia develops to compensate for the fall in CO. A weak, thready pulse develops, and heart

CLINICAL MANIFESTATIONS OF CARDIOGENIC SHOCK

Systolic blood pressure <90 mm Hg
Heart rate >100 beats/min
Weak, thready pulse
Diminished heart sounds
Change in sensorium
Cool, pale, moist skin
Urine output <30 ml/hr
Chest pain
Dysrhythmias
Rapid, shallow breathing
Rales and rhonchi
Decreased cardiac output
Cardiac index <1.8 L/m/m^2
Increased pulmonary capillary wedge pressure
Increased right atrial pressure
Increased systemic vascular resistance

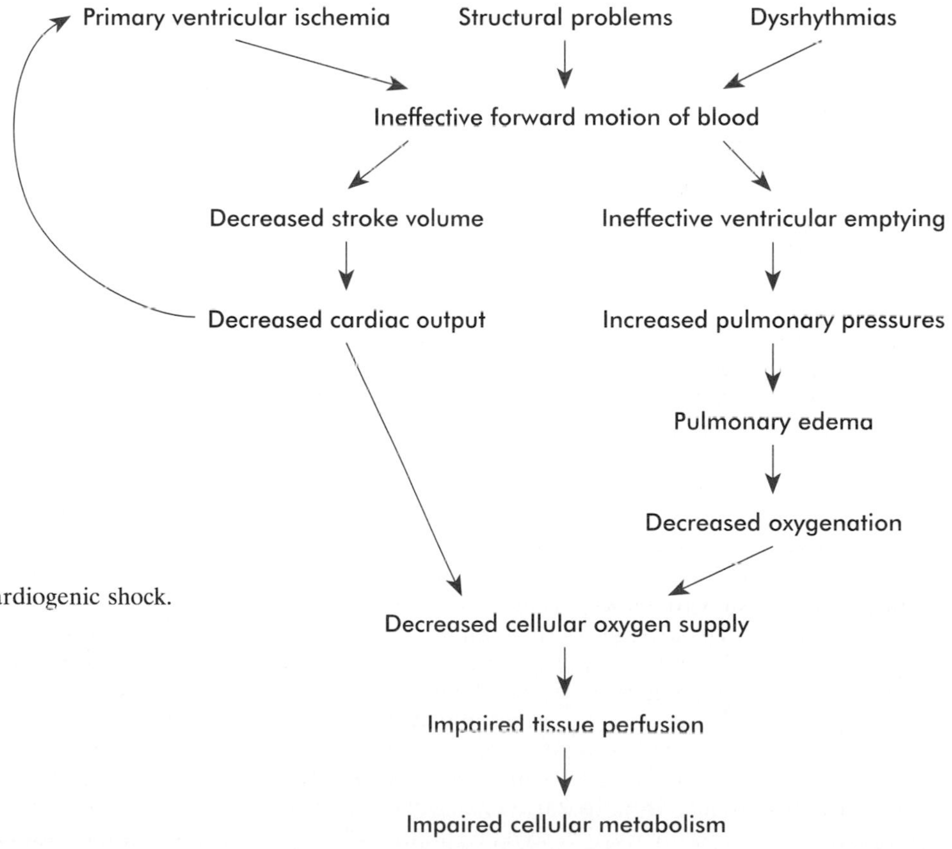

Fig. 46-2 The pathophysiology of cardiogenic shock.

sounds may reveal a diminished S_1 and S_2 as a result of the decrease in contractility. Respiratory rate increases to improve oxygenation. ABG values at this time indicate respiratory alkalosis as evidenced by a decrease in $Paco_2$. Urinalysis findings demonstrate a decrease in urine sodium and an increase in urine osmolarity and specific gravity as the kidneys start to conserve sodium and water. The patient also may experience a variety of dysrhythmias, depending on the underlying problem.[12,29-31]

In the patient with left ventricular failure a variety of additional clinical manifestations may be seen. Auscultation of the lungs may disclose rales and rhonchi, indicating the development of pulmonary edema. Hypoxemia occurs as evidenced by a fall in Pao_2 as measured by ABG values. Heart sounds may reveal an S_3 and S_4. If right-sided failure occurs, jugular venous distention may become evident.[29-31]

Once the compensatory mechanisms become overwhelmed and impaired tissue perfusion develops, a variety of other clinical manifestations appear. Myocardial ischemia progresses as evidenced by continued increases in HR, dysrhythmias, and chest pain. The pulmonary system starts to deteriorate, which leads to respiratory distress. ABG values during this phase reveal respiratory and metabolic acidosis and hypoxemia as indicated by a high $Paco_2$, low HCO_3^-, and low Pao_2, respectively. Renal failure occurs as exhibited by the development of anuria and increases in BUN and serum creatinine levels. Cerebral hypoperfusion manifests as decreasing LOC.[29]

Assessment of the hemodynamic parameters of a patient in cardiogenic shock reveals a decreased CO and a CI less than 1.8 L/min/m^2.[29] Inadequate pumping action leads to a decrease in stroke volume (SV), which results in an increase in the left ventricular end-diastolic pressure (LVEDP). This is reflected in an increase in the PCWP. Compensatory vasoconstriction results in an increase in the afterload of the heart as evidenced by an increase in the SVR. If right ventricular failure is present, the RAP also will be increased.[12,30]

Medical Management

Treatment of the patient in cardiogenic shock requires an aggressive approach. The major goals of therapy are to treat the underlying cause, to enhance the effectiveness of the pump, and to improve tissue perfusion. This approach includes identifying the etiologic factors of pump failure and administering pharmacologic agents to enhance cardiac output. Inotropic agents are used to increase contractility, whereas vasodilating agents and diuretics are used for afterload and preload reduction, respectively. Antidysrhythmic agents should be used to suppress or control dysrhythmias that can affect cardiac output.[13,29,30,32]

Once the cause of pump failure has been identified, measures should be taken to correct the problem if possible. If the problem is related to an acute MI, measures should be instituted to increase myocardial oxygen supply and decrease myocardial oxygen demand. Therapies to increase myocardial oxygen supply include supplemental oxygen, intubation and mechanical ventilation, and coronary artery vasodilator agents, such as nitroglycerine. Therapies to decrease myocardial demand include activity restrictions and pain medications and sedatives. If these measures fail, coronary angioplasty or coronary artery bypass surgery may be used to help improve myocardial oxygen supply.[13,32]

Two other therapies available to improve the effectiveness of the pumping action of the heart are the intraaortic balloon pump (IABP) and the ventricular assist device (VAD). The IABP is a temporary measure to decrease myocardial workload by improving myocardial supply and decreasing myocardial demand. It achieves this goal by improving coronary artery perfusion and reducing left ventricular afterload.[34] The VAD is a temporary external pump that takes the place of the patient's ventricle, allowing it to heal.[13]

Nursing Management

Prevention of cardiogenic shock is one of the primary responsibilities of the nurse in the critical care area. Preventive measures include the identification of patients at risk and constant assessment of the patient's cardiopulmonary status. Limiting myocardial oxygen consumption and enhancing myocardial oxygen supply are essential components of preventive nursing care. Measures to limit myocardial oxygen consumption in-

NURSING DIAGNOSIS AND MANAGEMENT

Cardiogenic shock

- ◆ Decreased Cardiac Output related to relative excess of preload and afterload secondary to impaired ventricular contractility, p. 358
- ◆ High Risk for Altered Peripheral Tissue Perfusion risk factor: high-dose vasopressor therapy, p. 363
- ◆ Activity Intolerance related to postural hypotension secondary to prolonged immobility, narcotics, vasodilator therapy, p. 365
- ◆ High Risk for Infection risk factor: invasive monitoring devices, p. 366
- ◆ High Risk for Aspiration risk factors: impaired laryngeal sensation or reflex; impaired laryngeal closure or elevation, p. 472
- ◆ Ineffective Airway Clearance related to impaired cough secondary to artificial airway, p. 466
- ◆ Sleep Pattern Disturbance related to circadian desynchronization, p. 143
- ◆ Sensory/Perceptual Alterations related to sensory overload, sensory deprivation, sleep pattern disturbance, p. 573
- ◆ Body Image Disturbance related to functional dependence on life-sustaining technology, p. 95
- ◆ Anxiety related to threat to biologic, psychologic, and/or social integrity, p. 763

clude administering pain medications and sedatives, positioning the patient for comfort, limiting activities, offering support to reduce anxiety, providing a calm and quiet environment, and providing patient teaching. Measures to enhance oxygen myocardial supply include administering supplemental oxygen, monitoring the patient's respiratory status, and administering prescribed medications.[28]

The patient with cardiogenic shock may have any number of nursing diagnoses depending on the progression of the process. Nursing interventions include administering prescribed medications, monitoring the patient's response to the medications, restricting fluids as ordered, protecting the patient, facilitating lung expansion, and preventing skin breakdown.[29,30] Patients who require IABP therapy need to be observed frequently for complications. Complications include emboli formation, infection, rupture of the aorta, thrombocytopenia, improper balloon placement, bleeding, improper timing of the balloon, balloon rupture, and circulatory compromise of the cannulated extremity.[34]

ANAPHYLACTIC SHOCK

Description

Anaphylactic shock, a type of distributive shock, is the result of an immediate hypersensitivity reaction. It is a life-threatening event that requires prompt intervention. The severe antibody-antigen response leads to decreased tissue perfusion and initiation of the general shock response.[5,35-37]

Etiology

Anaphylactic shock is caused by an antibody-antigen response. Almost any substance can cause a hypersensitivity reaction. These substances, known as *antigens,* can be introduced by injection or ingestion or through the skin or respiratory tract. A number of antigens have been identified that can cause a reaction in a hypersensitive person. This list includes foods, food additives, diagnostic agents, biologic agents, environmental agents, drugs, and venoms[5,36,37] (see box on right).

Anaphylactic reactions can be either IgE-mediated or non–IgE-mediated responses. IgE is an antibody that is formed as part of the immune response. The first time an antigen enters the body, an antibody IgE, specific for the antigen, is formed. The antigen-specific IgE antibody is then stored by attachment to mast cells and basophils. This initial contact with the antigen is known as a *primary immune response.* The next time the antigen enters the body, the preformed IgE antibody reacts with it and a secondary immune response occurs. This reaction triggers the release of biochemical mediators from the mast cells and basophils and initiates the cascade of events that precipitate anaphylactic shock.[5,35-37]

Some anaphylactic reactions are non–IgE-mediated responses in that they occur in the absence of activation of IgE antibodies. These responses occur as a result of direct activation of the mast cells to release biochemical mediators. Direct activation of mast cells can be triggered by humoral mediators, such as the complement system and the coagulation-fibrinolytic system. In addition, biochemical mediators can be released as a direct or indirect response to many drugs. This type of reaction is known as *anaphylactoid reaction.* Anaphylactoid reactions are produced in persons not previously sensitized and can occur with the first exposure to an antigen.[37]

ETIOLOGIC FACTORS IN ANAPHYLACTIC SHOCK

- Foods
  - Eggs and milk
  - Fish and shellfish
  - Nuts and seeds
  - Legumes and cereals
  - Citrus fruits
  - Chocolate
  - Strawberries
  - Tomatoes
  - Other
- Food additives
  - Food coloring
  - Preservatives
- Diagnostic agents
  - Iodinated contrast dye
  - Sulfobromophthalein (Bromsulphalein) (BSP)
  - Dehydrocholic acid (Decholin)
  - Iopanoic acid (Telepaque)
- Biologic agents
  - Blood and blood components
  - Insulin and other hormones
  - Gamma globulin
  - Seminal plasma
  - Enzymes
  - Vaccines and antitoxins
- Environmental agents
  - Pollens, molds, and spores
  - Sunlight
  - Animal hair
- Drugs
  - Antibiotics
  - Aspirin
  - Narcotics
  - Dextran
  - Vitamins
  - Local anesthetic agents
  - Muscle relaxants
  - Barbiturates
  - Other
- Venoms
  - Bees and wasps
  - Snakes
  - Jellyfish
  - Spiders
  - Deer flies
  - Fire ants

Pathophysiology

The antibody-antigen response (immunologic stimulation) or the direct triggering (nonimmunologic activation) of the mast cells results in the release of biochemical mediators. These mediators include histamine, eosinophilic chemotactic factor of anaphylaxis (ECF-A), neutrophilic chemotactic factor of anaphylaxis (NCF-A), proteinases, heparin, serotonin, leukotrienes (formerly known as *slow-reacting substance of anaphylaxis*), prostaglandins, and platelet-activating factor.

The release of histamine causes vasodilation, increased capillary permeability, bronchoconstriction, coronary vasoconstriction, cutaneous reactions, and constriction of the smooth muscle in the intestinal wall, bladder, and uterus. Leukotrienes, which are more than 1000 times as potent as histamine, result in further constriction of the small bronchial airways and coronary arteries. Coronary vasoconstriction causes severe myocardial depression. Prostaglandins produce inflammation, excessive mucus secretion, bronchoconstriction, peripheral vasodilation, and increased capillary permeability. Leukotrienes, prostaglandins, and other biochemical mediators join to stimulate nerve endings, causing itching and pain. ECF-A promotes chemotaxis of eosinophils, thus facilitating the movement of eosinophils into the area. During allergic reactions, eosinophils phagocytose the antibody-antigen complex and other inflammatory debris and release enzymes that inhibit vasoactive mediators, such as histamine and leukotrienes. In addition, secondary mediators are produced that either enhance or inhibit the already released biochemical mediators. Bradykinin, a secondary mediator, increases capillary permeability, facilitates vasodilation, and contracts smooth muscles.

Peripheral vasodilation results in decreased venous return. Increased capillary membrane permeability results in the loss of intravascular volume and the development of relative hypovolemia. Decreased venous return results in decreased end-diastolic volume and SV. The decline in SV leads to a fall in CO and impaired tissue perfusion. Death may result from airway obstruction or cardiovascular collapse, or both [5,35,36] (Fig. 46-3).

Assessment and Diagnosis

Anaphylactic shock is a severe systemic reaction that can affect any number of organ systems. A variety of clinical manifestations occur in the patient in anaphylactic shock, depending on the extent of multisystem involvement. The symptoms usually start to appear within 20 minutes of exposure to the antigen. The

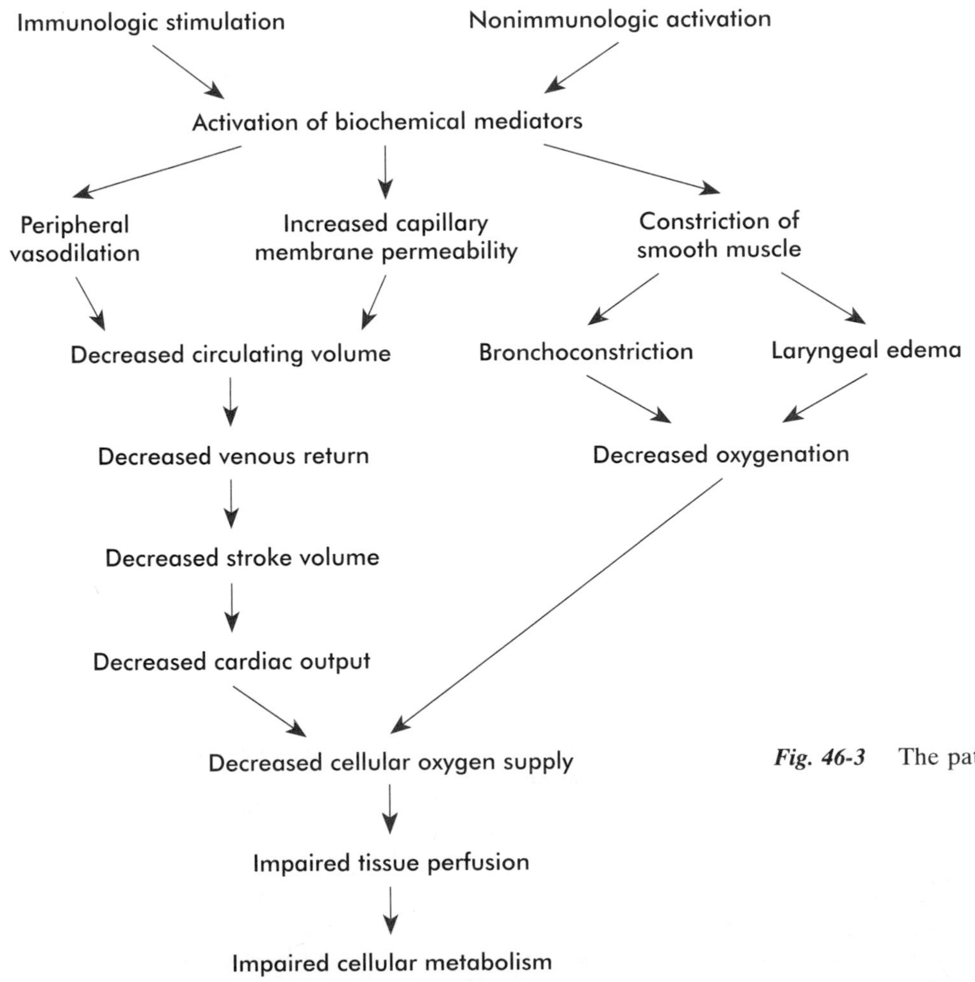

Fig. 46-3 The pathophysiology of anaphylactic shock.

severity of the reaction is directly related to the timing of the onset of clinical manifestations. The earlier they appear, the more severe the reaction[12] (see box below).

The cutaneous effects usually appear first, including pruritus, generalized erythema, urticaria, and angioedema. Angioedema develops as a result of fluid leaking into the interstitial space and is commonly seen on the face and in the oral cavity and lower pharynx. The patient may appear restless, uneasy, apprehensive, and anxious and complain of being warm. The effects on the respiratory system include the development of laryngeal edema, bronchoconstriction, and mucus plugs. Clinical manifestations of laryngeal edema include inspiratory stridor, hoarseness, a sensation of fullness or a lump in the throat, and dysphagia. Bronchoconstriction causes dyspnea, wheezing, and chest tightness.[12,35-37] In addition, gastrointestinal and genitourinary manifestations may develop as a result of smooth muscle contraction. These include vomiting, diarrhea, cramping, abdominal pain, urinary incontinence, and vaginal bleeding.[36]

As the anaphylactic reaction progresses, hypotension and reflex tachycardia develop. This occurs in response to the massive vasodilation and the loss of circulating volume. Jugular veins appear flat as right ventricular end-diastolic volume is decreased. The eventual outcome is circulatory failure and shock.[12,35-37] Pulmonary edema also may result from fluid leaking into the lungs, as evidenced by the development of rales and rhonchi.[36] The patient's level of consciousness may deteriorate to unresponsiveness.[12]

Assessment of the hemodynamic parameters of a patient in anaphylactic shock reveals a decreased CO and CI. Venous vasodilation and massive volume loss lead to a decrease in preload, which results in a decline in the RAP and PCWP. Vasodilation of the arterial system results in a decrease in the afterload of the heart, as evidenced by a decrease in the SVR.[12]

CLINICAL MANIFESTATIONS OF ANAPHYLACTIC SHOCK

- Cardiovascular
  - Hypotension
  - Tachycardia
- Respiratory
  - Lump in throat
  - Dysphagia
  - Hoarseness
  - Stridor
  - Wheezing
  - Rales and rhonchi
- Cutaneous
  - Pruritus
  - Erythema
  - Urticaria
  - Angioedema
- Neurologic
  - Restlessness
  - Uneasiness
  - Apprehension
  - Anxiety
  - Decreased level of consciousness
- Gastrointestinal
  - Nausea
  - Vomiting
  - Diarrhea
- Genitourinary
  - Incontinence
  - Vaginal bleeding
- Subjective complaints
  - Being warm
  - Dyspnea
  - Abdominal cramping and pain
  - Itching
- Hemodynamic parameters
  - Decreased CO
  - Decreased CI
  - Decreased RAP
  - Decreased PCWP
  - Decreased SVR

CO, Cardiac output; *CI,* cardiac index; *RAP,* right atrial pressure; *PCWP,* pulmonary capillary wedge pressure; *SVR,* systemic vascular resistance.

Medical Management

Treatment of anaphylactic shock requires an immediate and a direct approach. The goals of therapy are to remove the offending antigen, reverse the effects of the biochemical mediators, and promote adequate tissue perfusion. When the hypersensitivity reaction occurs as a result of administration of medications, dye, blood, or blood products, the infusion should be immediately discontinued. Many times it is not possible to remove the antigen because it is unknown or has already entered the patient's system.

Reversal of the effects of the biochemical mediators involves the preservation and support of the patient's airway, ventilation, and circulation. This is accomplished through intubation, oxygen therapy, mechanical ventilation, and administration of drugs and fluids. Epinephrine is given to promote bronchodilation and vasoconstriction and to inhibit further release of biochemical mediators. It usually is administered intravenously or via endotracheal tube. The dose is 0.1 to 0.5 mg of a 1:10,000 solution, which is repeated in 10-minute intervals (not to exceed 0.5 mg in 10 minutes) until the desired effect is achieved or until significant side effects occur. Aminophylline also may be administered in cases of severe bronchospasm. Diphenhydramine (Benadryl) is used to block the histamine response. Corticosteroids, such as methylprednisolone (Solu-Medrol), may be given with the goal of preventing a delayed reaction and stabilizing capillary membranes. Fluid replacement is accomplished by use of either a crystalloid or colloid solution. In addition, positive inotropic agents and vasoconstrictor agents may be necessary to reverse the effects of myocardial depression and vasodilation.[13,35-37]

NURSING DIAGNOSIS AND MANAGEMENT
Anaphylactic shock

- Decreased Cardiac Output related to decreased preload secondary to fluid volume deficit, p. 361
- Impaired Gas Exchange related to ventilation/perfusion mismatch secondary to *(specify)*, p. 470
- High Risk for Infection risk factor: invasive monitoring device, p. 366
- High Risk for Aspiration risk factor: impaired laryngeal sensation or reflex; impaired laryngeal closure or elevation, p. 472
- Ineffective Airway Clearance related to impaired cough secondary to artificial airway, p. 466
- Anxiety related to threat to biologic, psychologic, and/or social integrity, p. 763

Nursing Management

Prevention of anaphylactic shock is one of the primary responsibilities of the nurse in the critical care area. This includes the identification of patients at risk and cautious assessment of the patient's response to the administration of drugs, blood, and blood products. A complete and accurate history of the patient's allergies is an essential component of preventive nursing care. In addition to a list of the allergies, a detailed description of the type of response for each one should be obtained.[28]

The patient with anaphylactic shock may have any number of nursing diagnoses, depending on the progression of the process. Nursing interventions include facilitating ventilation, enhancing volume replacement, promoting comfort, and monitoring the patient's response to care. Measures to facilitate ventilation include positioning the patient to assist with breathing and instructing the patient to breathe slowly and deeply. Measures to enhance volume replacement include inserting large-diameter peripheral intravenous catheters, rapidly administering prescribed fluids, and positioning the patient with the legs elevated, trunk flat, and head and shoulders above the chest. Measures to promote comfort include administering medications to relieve itching, applying warm soaks to skin, and, if necessary, covering the patient's hands to discourage scratching. In addition, observing the patient for clinical manifestations of a delayed reaction is critical to preventing further problems.[36]

NEUROGENIC SHOCK

Description

Neurogenic shock, a type of distributive shock, is the result of the loss or suppression of sympathetic tone. Its onset is within minutes, and it may last for days, weeks, or months depending on the cause.[38] The lack of sympathetic tone leads to decreased tissue perfusion and initiation of the general shock response. Neurogenic shock is the rarest form of shock.[5]

Etiology

Neurogenic shock can be caused by anything that disrupts the SNS. The problem can occur as the result of interrupted impulse transmission or blockage of sympathetic outflow from the vasomotor center in the brain.[5] The most common cause is a spinal cord injury above the level of T6.[38] Other causes include spinal anesthesia, drugs, emotional stress, pain, and CNS dysfunction.[5]

Pathophysiology

Loss of sympathetic tone results in massive peripheral vasodilation, inhibition of the baroreceptor response, and impaired thermoregulation. Arterial vasodilation leads to a decrease in SVR and a fall in blood pressure. Venous vasodilation leads to decreased venous return because of pooling of blood in the venous circuit. A decreased venous return results in a decrease in end-diastolic volume or preload. A decrease in preload results in a decrease in SV and CO, and relative hypovolemia develops. The fall in blood pressure and cardiac output leads to inadequate or impaired tissue perfusion.[1,38,39] Inhibition of the baroreceptor response results in loss of compensatory reflex tachycardia. The HR does not increase to compensate for the fall in CO, which further compromises tissue perfusion. Impaired thermoregulation occurs because of loss of vasomotor tone in the cutaneous blood vessels that dilate and constrict to maintain body temperature. The patient becomes dependent on the environment for temperature regulation, that is, poikilothermic[38] (Fig. 46-4).

Assessment and Diagnosis

The patient in neurogenic shock usually presents with hypotension, bradycardia, hypothermia, and warm, dry skin. The decreased blood pressure is the result of massive peripheral vasodilation. The decreased heart rate is the result of inhibition of the baroreceptor response and unopposed parasympathetic control of the heart. Hypothermia occurs from uncontrolled heat loss peripherally. The warm, dry skin occurs as a consequence of pooling of blood in the extremities and loss of vasomotor control in surface vessels of the skin that control heat loss.[38,40,41]

Assessment of the hemodynamic parameters of a patient in neurogenic shock reveals a decreased CO and CI. Venous vasodilation leads to a decrease in preload, which results in a decline in the RAP and PCWP. Vasodilation of the arterial system causes a decrease in the afterload of the heart as evidenced by a decrease in the SVR.

Medical Management

Treatment of neurogenic shock requires a careful approach. The goals of therapy are to treat or remove the cause, to prevent cardiovascular instability, and to promote optimal tissue perfusion. Cardiovascular instability can occur from hypovolemia, hypothermia, hyp-

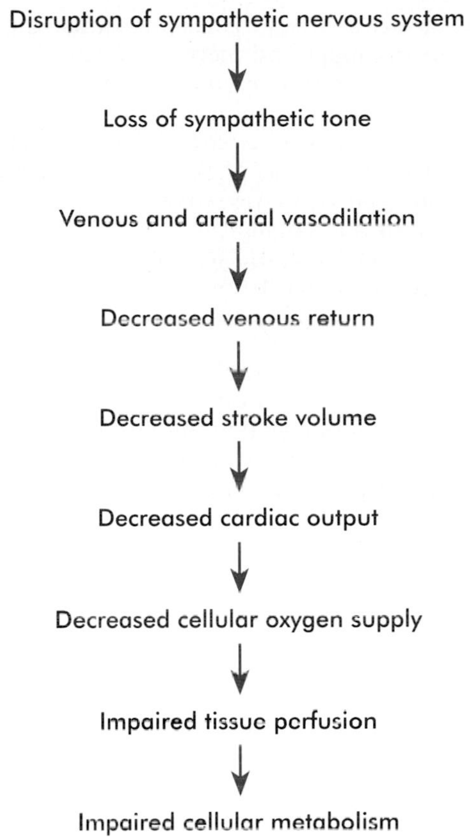

Fig. 46-4 The pathophysiology of neurogenic shock.

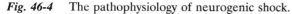

NURSING DIAGNOSIS AND MANAGEMENT
Neurogenic shock

- ◆ Decreased Cardiac Output related to vasodilation and bradycardia secondary to sympathetic blockade of neurogenic (spinal) shock after spinal cord injury above T6 level, p. 363
- ◆ High Risk for Altered Peripheral Tissue Perfusion risk factor: high-dose vasopressor therapy, p. 363
- ◆ High Risk for Infection risk factor: invasive monitoring devices, p. 366
- ◆ High Risk for Aspiration risk factors: impaired laryngeal sensation or reflex; impaired laryngeal closure or elevation, p. 472
- ◆ Ineffective Airway Clearance related to impaired cough secondary to artificial airway, p. 466
- ◆ Sleep Pattern Disturbance related to fragmented sleep and/or circadian desynchronization, pp. 142 and 143
- ◆ Sensory/Perceptual Alterations related to sensory overload, sensory deprivation, sleep pattern disturbance, p. 573
- ◆ Anxiety related to threat to biologic, psychologic, and/or social integrity, p. 763

oxia, and dysrhythmias. Specific treatments are aimed at preventing or correcting these problems as they occur.

Hypovolemia is treated with careful fluid resuscitation. The minimal amount of fluid is administered to ensure adequate tissue perfusion. Volume replacement is initiated for systolic blood pressure lower than 90 mm Hg, urine output less than 30 ml/hr, or changes in mental status that indicate decreased cerebral tissue perfusion. The patient is carefully observed for evidence of fluid overload. Vasopressors may be used as necessary to maintain blood pressure and organ perfusion.[38,40] Hypothermia is treated with warming measures and environmental temperature regulation. The goal is to maintain normothermia and avoid large swings in the patient's body temperature. The treatment of hypoxia varies with the underlying cause. Chest wall paralysis, retained secretions, pulmonary edema, and suctioning contribute to the development of hypoxia. Management of this problem may include ventilatory support, vigorous pulmonary hygiene, supplemental oxygen, and hyperoxygenation during suctioning. Continuous pulse oximetry monitoring also may be helpful in recognizing hypoxia early, before complications arise.[38,41] The major dysrhythmia seen in neurogenic shock is bradycardia, which should be treated with atropine. If necessary, isoproterenol (Isuprel), transvenous pacing, or noninvasive pacing may be initiated.

Nursing Management

Prevention of neurogenic shock is one of the primary responsibilities of the nurse in the critical care area. This includes the identification of patients at risk and constant assessment of the neurologic status. Vigilant immobilization of spinal cord injuries and slight elevation of the head of bed of the patient after spinal anesthesia are essential components of preventive nursing care. Early identification allows for early treatment and decreased mortality.[28,38,39]

The patient with neurogenic shock may have any number of nursing diagnoses, depending on the progression of the process. Nursing interventions are directed toward treating hypovolemia, maintaining normothermia, preventing hypoxia, and monitoring dysrhythmias.[38] Venous pooling in the lower extremities promotes the formation of deep vein thrombosis (DVT). All patients should receive DVT prophylaxis. This includes monitoring of calf and thigh measurements, passive range of motion, application of antiembolic stockings or sequential pneumatic stockings, or both, and administration of prescribed heparin therapy.[40,41]

SEPTIC SHOCK

Description

Septic shock, a form of distributive shock, is the result of microorganisms invading the body. The primary mechanism of this type of shock is the maldistribution of blood flow to the tissues, with some areas being overperfused and others being underperfused.[6,42] The incidence of sepsis is estimated at 70,000 to 300,000 cases annually in the United States, with 40% of these cases progressing into septic shock.[43] The mortality rate for septic shock is estimated between 40% and 95%, depending on the timeliness of identification and treatment.[44]

Sepsis is the systemic state generated by the presence of invading microorganisms and their toxins in the blood or tissues. Septic shock, which results from the body's response to the invaders, is activated by the neurologic and endocrine systems, tissue damage, and a wide variety of immune mediators. Subsequently, cellular and metabolic derangements develop that produce impairment of organ and tissue perfusion. Multiple organ dysfunction syndrome and death ensue if this process is allowed to progress.[45]

A variety of terms may be used to describe the condition the patient with an infection experiences. These include *bacteremia, sepsis,* and *septic shock.* Bacteremia simply means the presence of viable bacteria in the blood. Sepsis describes the systemic response to infection that manifests in two or more of the following conditions: temperature $>38°$ C or $<36°$ C; heart rate >90 beats/min; respiratory rate >20 breaths/min or $Paco_2$ <32 mm Hg; and white blood cell (WBC) count $>12{,}000$ cells/mm^3, <4000 cells/mm^3, or $>10\%$ bands. Septic shock is sepsis with hypotension, despite fluid resuscitation, along with the presence of perfusion abnormalities, such as altered cerebral function, acidosis, or oliguria.[46]

Etiology

Sepsis and septic shock are caused by a wide variety of microorganisms (see box below). The source of these microorganisms is varied. Exogenous sources include the hospital environment and members of the health care team. Endogenous sources include the patient's skin, gastrointestinal tract, respiratory tract, and genitourinary tract. Gram-negative bacteria are responsible for approximately two thirds of the cases of septic shock. Another one fourth of the cases are the result of a combination of microorganisms.[5,45,47-50]

Sepsis and septic shock are associated with a wide variety of intrinsic and extrinsic precipitating factors (see box below). All these factors interfere directly or indirectly with the body's anatomic and physiologic defense mechanisms. Several of the intrinsic factors are not modifiable or are very difficult to control. Several of the extrinsic factors may be required for diagnosis and management. Therefore it becomes apparent that all critically ill patients are at risk for the development of septic shock.[45,47,49-51]

Pathophysiology

Septic shock is a complex systemic response that is initiated on the entry of a microorganism into the body and the release of endotoxins or exotoxins. Endotoxins are liberated from the cell walls of gram-negative bacteria when they are destroyed by the body's immune system. Exotoxins are released from gram-positive bacteria and other microorganisms while they are alive in the body.[5,51,52] Toxic shock syndrome is an example of gram-positive, or endotoxic, shock[53,54] (see box, p. 779).

Once a microorganism invades the body and releases the toxin, a variety of mechanisms occur, including activation of the immune mediators, damage to the endothelium, and activation of the CNS and the endocrine system. Consequently, a variety of physiologic and pathophysiologic events occur that affect capillary mem-

CAUSATIVE MICROORGANISMS IN SEPTIC SHOCK

- Gram-negative bacteria
  - *Escherichia coli*
  - *Klebsiella pneumoniae*
  - *Enterobacter* organisms
  - *Pseudomonas aeruginosa*
  - Enterococcus
  - *Serratia marcescens*
  - *Bacteroides* organisms
  - *Proteus* organisms
  - *Haemophilus influenzae*
- Gram-positive bacteria
  - *Staphylococcus aureus*
  - *Staphylococcus epidermidis*
  - *Streptococcus pneumoniae*
  - *Clostridium* organisms
- Viruses
- Fungi
- Rickettsiae
- Spirochaeta
- Protozoa
- Parasites

PRECIPITATING FACTORS ASSOCIATED WITH SEPTIC SHOCK

INTRINSIC FACTORS

Extremes of age
Coexisting diseases
  Malignancies
  Burns
  Acquired immunodeficiency syndrome (AIDS)
  Diabetes
  Substance abuse
  Dysfunction of one or more of the major body systems
Malnutrition

EXTRINSIC FACTORS

Invasive devices
Drug therapy
Fluid therapy
Surgical and traumatic wounds
Surgical and invasive diagnostic procedures
Immunosuppressive therapy

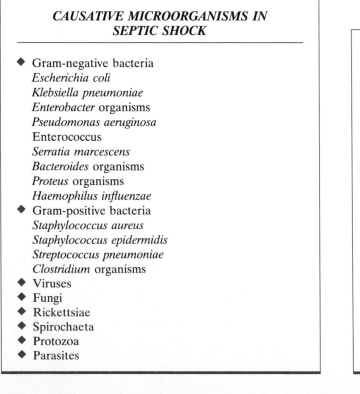

brane permeability, clotting, the distribution of blood flow to the tissues and organs, and the metabolic state of the body. Subsequently a systemic imbalance between cellular oxygen supply and demand develops that results in cellular hypoxia, damage, and death[5,44,45,48,52] (Fig. 46-5).

The septic process is initiated by the activation of immune mediators that are part of the inflammatory process and are released in response to invading microorganisms. These humoral, cellular, and biochemical mediators initiate a chain of complex interactions that are controlled by numerous feedback mechanisms.

TOXIC SHOCK SYNDROME

Toxic shock syndrome (TSS) is a form of septic shock that was first identified in 1978. TSS is a potentially lethal syndrome that is caused by a toxin-producing strain of the gram-positive bacteria *Staphylococcus aureus.* Although often associated with menstruating females who use tampons, it has been reported in males, children, and nonmenstruating females.

The syndrome starts with bacterial colonization or infection of a site. The bacteria release a toxin that is absorbed into the blood stream and circulated to the rest of the body. Once into the blood stream the septic cascade is initiated and septic shock develops.

A few features distinguish TSS. Initially the patient may have flulike symptoms, such as high fever, headache, vomiting, diarrhea, hyperactive bowel sounds, abdominal pain, arthralgia, myalgia, and malaise. The mucous membranes become hyperemic, and pharyngitis, conjunctivitis, vaginitis, and strawberry tongue may develop. In addition, a diffuse erythematous macular rash develops, which progresses to desquamation of the skin in 7 to 10 days. Blood cultures may be negative for bacteremia.

The circulating toxins can also affect the renal, hepatic, hemopoietic, and neurologic systems. Dysfunction of these systems may manifest as elevated levels of blood urea nitrogen (BUN), creatinine, lactic dehydrogenase (LDH), aspartate aminotransferase (formerly SGOT), bilirubin, and alkaline phosphatase, as well as a decline in platelets. The patient may appear disoriented, confused, and agitated.

Treatment of TSS is essentially the same as the treatment of septic shock. Definitive measures are aimed at identifying the cause of the infection. Supportive measures include administering fluid, antibiotics, and vasoactive agents, treating the fever, and protecting the patient. Generally the acute phase lasts from 2 to 5 days.

Modified from Sommers MS: *Dimens Crit Care Nurs* 4:215, 1985; and Broscious SK: *Crit Care Nurse* 11(4):28, 1991.

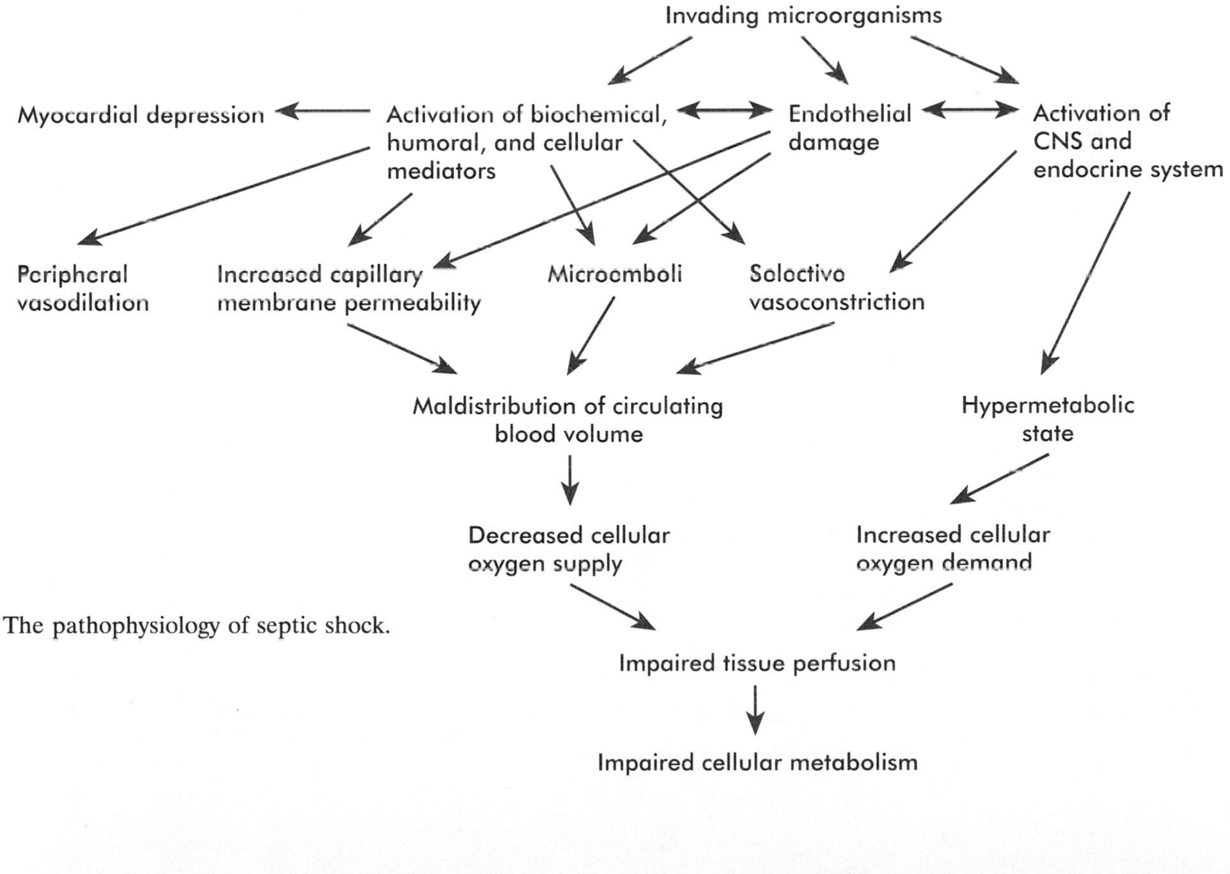

Fig. 46-5 The pathophysiology of septic shock.

Eventually the immune system is overwhelmed, the feedback mechanisms fail, and a process that was designed to protect the body actually harms the body.[5,48]

The humoral mediators involved in septic shock are the complement system, the coagulation-fibrinolytic system, and the kallikrein-kinin system. Stimulation of these systems results in activation of cellular mediators, the formation of biochemical mediators, endothelial cell damage, peripheral vasodilation, increased capillary membrane permeability, initiation of coagulation and fibrinolysis, myocardial depression, and activation of the Hageman factor (Factor XII), which potentiates the effects of the humoral mediators.

The cellular mediators involved in septic shock include polymorphonuclear (PMN) granulocytes, macrophages, lymphocytes, and platelets. Stimulation of these cells leads to the formation of biochemical mediators, the stimulation of the complement and the coagulation systems, the destruction of the invading microorganisms, the activation of T and B cells, and the formation of microemboli. The biochemical mediators involved in septic shock include oxygen-free radicals, leukotrienes, prostaglandins, interleukins 1 and 2, serotonin, tumor necrosis factor, histamine, proteinases, and platelet activating factor. Stimulation of these substances results in enhancement of the cellular and humoral mediators, peripheral vasodilation, the formation of microemboli, vasoconstriction of the renal, pulmonary, and splanchnic beds, myocardial depression, endothelial cell damage, increased capillary membrane permeability, fever, and increased metabolism.[48,55,56]

The septic cascade also is initiated by damage to the endothelial cells caused by the toxins released from invading microorganisms. Endothelial cell damage results in activation of the immune mediators, increased capillary membrane permeability, and the formation of microemboli. This leads to disruption of blood flow to the tissues, more endothelial cell damage, and further propagation of the septic process.[48]

Activation of the CNS and the endocrine system also occurs as part of the primary response to invading microorganisms. This leads to stimulation of the SNS and the release of ACTH. These events trigger the release of epinephrine, norepinephrine, glucocorticoids, aldosterone, glucagon, and renin. This results in the development of a hypermetabolic state and further contributes to the vasoconstriction of the renal, pulmonary, and splanchnic beds. Activation of the CNS also causes the release of endogenous opiates that are believed to cause vasodilation and to decrease myocardial contractility.[10,16]

Once the initial sequence of events is triggered, a series of pathophysiologic responses occur that eventually culminate in the maldistribution of circulating blood volume. These responses include massive peripheral vasodilation, microemboli formation, selective vasoconstriction, and increased capillary membrane permeability.[5,48] The maldistribution of circulating blood volume eventually results in decreased cellular oxygen supply.[42,52]

Massive peripheral vasodilation occurs in response to the release of biochemical mediators, activation of the kallikrein-kinin system, and the release of endogenous opiates. This response results in the development of relative hypovolemia and decreased tissue perfusion.[5,48,55] Microemboli formation occurs as a result of activation of the coagulation system, platelet and PMN aggregation, the release of biochemical mediators, and damage to the endothelial cells. This response leads to decreased tissue perfusion and further endothelial cell damage.[48] Selective vasoconstriction occurs as the result of stimulation of the SNS, as well as the release of renin and certain biochemical mediators. This response results in decreased tissue perfusion of the kidneys, lungs, and gastrointestinal organs, with eventual system dysfunction.[48] Increased capillary membrane permeability occurs in response to activation of the complement system and the release of biochemical mediators. It promotes fluid loss from the intravascular space (third-spacing) and potentiates the relative hypovolemic effect induced by the massive peripheral vasodilation. The formation of microemboli also is exacerbated because of the increased viscosity of the blood left in the intravascular space.[5,48]

The maldistribution of circulating blood volume decreases the amount of oxygen delivered to the cells. This situation leads to a number of cellular derangements that ultimately result in cellular death. The hypermetabolic state created by activation of the CNS and the endocrine system further enhances the situation by increasing the oxygen demands of the cells.

A number of metabolic derangements occur as a result of CNS and endocrine system activation. A hypermetabolic state develops that increases cellular oxygen demand and contributes to cellular hypoxia. Lactic acid is produced as a result of anaerobic metabolism. Glucocorticoids, ACTH, epinephrine, and glucagon are all catabolic hormones that are released as part of this response. These hormones favor the use of fats and proteins over glucose for energy production.

The hypermetabolic state also increases the cellular metabolic needs. Increased glucose requirements in conjunction with the high level of catabolic hormones result in the limited ability of the cells to use glucose as a substrate for energy production. This causes glucose intolerance, hyperglycemia, relative insulin resistance, and the use of fat for energy (lipolysis). The relative insulin resistance causes the body to produce more insulin, which inhibits the use of fat as an energy substrate. This promotes the use of protein as an energy substrate and catabolism of protein stores in the visceral organs and skeletal muscles.[48,52,55]

Assessment and Diagnosis

Clinical presentation and laboratory assessment of septic shock vary according to whether the patient is in the early or late stage of the process. The early stage of septic shock is known as the *hyperdynamic,* or *warm, phase.* The late stage is known as the *hypodynamic,* or *cold, phase* of septic shock. The hyperdynamic phase is characterized by compensatory responses, whereas the hypodynamic phase is typified by decompensatory responses (Table 46-2). Transition from one phase to another can take hours or days.[12,48,55]

◆ **Hyperdynamic phase.** During the hyperdynamic phase of septic shock, massive vasodilation occurs in both the venous and arterial beds. Dilation of the venous system leads to a decrease in venous return to the heart, which results in a decrease in the preload of the right and left ventricles. This is evidenced by a decline in the RAP and PCWP. Dilation of the arterial system results in a decrease in the afterload of the heart as evidenced by a decrease in the SVR. The patient's blood pressure falls in response to the reduction in preload and afterload. The patient's skin becomes pink, warm, and flushed as a result of the massive vasodilation.

The HR rises to compensate for the hypotension and in response to increased metabolic, SNS, and adrenal gland stimulation. This results in a normal to high CO and CI. The PP widens as the diastolic blood pressure decreases because of the vasodilation, and the systolic blood pressure increases because of the elevated CO. A full, bounding pulse develops. Myocardial contractility is decreased, as evidenced by a decline in the left ventricular stroke work index (LVSWI), an effect of myocardial depression. In the lungs a ventilation/perfusion mismatch develops as a result of pulmonary vasoconstriction and the formation of pulmonary microemboli. Hypoxemia occurs, and the RR increases to compensate for the lack of oxygen. Rales develop as increased pulmonary capillary membrane permeability leads to pulmonary interstitial edema.

Level of consciousness starts to change as a result of decreased cerebral perfusion, immune mediator activation, hyperthermia, and lactic acidosis. The patient may appear disoriented, confused, combative, or lethargic. Urine output declines because of decreased perfusion of the kidneys. The patient's temperature is elevated in response to pyrogens released from the invading microorganisms, immune mediator activation, and increased metabolic activity.[12,48,52,55]

Arterial blood gas values during this phase reveal respiratory alkalosis, hypoxemia, and metabolic acidosis. This is demonstrated by a low Pao_2, low $Paco_2$, and low HCO_3^- respectively. The respiratory alkalosis is caused by the patient's increased RR. The metabolic acidosis is the result of lack of oxygen to the cells and the development of lactic acidemia. The mixed venous oxygen saturation (Svo_2) is increased because of maldistribution of the circulating blood volume and impaired cellular metabolism.[48]

The white blood cell (WBC) count is elevated as part of the immune response to the invading microorganisms. In addition, the WBC differential reveals an increase in immature neutrophils (shift to the left). This occurs because the body has to mobilize increasing numbers of WBCs to fight the infection.[48] Hematologic alterations that may occur during this phase include prolongation of the prothrombin time (PT) and partial thromboplastin time (PTT), decreased platelet count, decreased fibrinogen level, decreased clotting factors, and increased fibrin degradation product (FDP). These processes

Table 46-2 Clinical manifestations, hemodynamic parameters, and laboratory values of septic shock

	Hyperdynamic phase	Hypodynamic phase
Clinical manifestations	Increased HR	Increased HR
	Decreased BP	Decreased BP
	Wide PP	Narrow PP
	Full bounding pulse	Weak thready pulse
	Pink, warm, flushed skin	Pale, cool, clammy skin
	Increased RR	Decreased RR
	Rales	Rales, rhonchi, and wheezes
	Change in LOC	Coma
	Decreased UO	Anuria
	Increased temperature	Increased/decreased temperature
Hemodynamic parameters	Increased CO and CI	Decreased CO and CI
	Decreased SVR	Increased SVR
	Decreased RAP	Increased RAP
	Decreased PCWP	Increased PCWP
	Decreased LVSWI	Decreased LVSWI
Laboratory values	Decreased Pao_2	Decreased Pao_2
	Decreased $Paco_2$	Increased $Paco_2$
	Decreased HCO_3^-	Decreased HCO_3^-
	Increased Svo_2	Decreased Svo_2
	Increased PT and PTT	Increased lactate level
	Decreased platelet count	Increased anion gap
	Decreased fibrinogen level	Increased BUN and Cr
	Decreased clotting factors	Electrolyte imbalances
		Increased AST, ALT, and LDH
		Increased serum amylase and lipase
	Increased serum glucose	Decreased serum glucose

LVSWI, Left ventricular stroke work index; *Svo_2*, mixed venous oxygen saturation; *Cr*, creatinine; *LDH*, lactic dehydrogenase; *AST*, aspartate aminotransferase (formerly SGOT); *ALT*, alanine aminotransferase (formerly SPGT).

reflect coagulation abnormalities caused by accelerated clotting and fibrinolysis, which indicate the onset of DIC. Increased serum glucose also occurs as part of the hypermetabolic response and the development of insulin resistance.[48,55]

◆ **Hypodynamic phase.** As the septic process progresses into the hypodynamic phase, the CO and CI decrease and profound hypotension occurs. These factors result from ventricular failure caused by myocardial ischemia, lactic acidosis, myocardial depressant factor, and a rising afterload. The RAP and PCWP increase as a result of right and left ventricular dysfunction. Vasoconstriction occurs, as evidenced by an increased SVR, to compensate for the falling BP. The patient's skin becomes pale, cold, and clammy.

The HR rises further in an attempt to compensate for the declining CO and hypotension. A variety of dysrhythmias may occur as a result of myocardial ischemia, lactic acidosis, and circulating catecholamines. The dysrhythmias exacerbate the reduction in CO. The PP narrows as the CO declines. The patient's pulse becomes weak and thready.

As the pulmonary system continues to deteriorate and ARDS develops, the patient exhibits rapid, shallow respirations and severe shortness of breath. The RR remains high until fatigue occurs and ventilatory failure develops, which causes the RR to decline. In addition, more adventitious breath sounds become apparent by increasing amounts of rales, rhonchi, and wheezes.[12,48,52,55]

The patient's LOC continues to deteriorate as the blood pressure and cerebral perfusion fall. The patient usually becomes extremely difficult to arouse. Anuria occurs as kidney function fails because of poor renal perfusion. The patient's temperature may remain elevated, or it may decline as an effect of decreased metabolic activity and thermoregulatory failure.[12,48]

ABG values during this phase of septic shock reveal a severe hypoxemia with metabolic and respiratory acidosis, which are reflected in a low PaO_2, high $PaCO_2$, and low HCO_3^-, respectively. The respiratory acidosis is caused by the decline in the patient's RR. The lactate level is elevated at this point as a result of increased anaerobic metabolism and liver failure. The patient's anion gap increases, reflecting overproduction and accumulation of lactate. The SvO_2 is decreased in response to the decreased CO and severe hypoxemia.[48]

As multiple organ dysfunction syndrome develops, a variety of laboratory data abnormalities become apparent. As the immune system fails, the WBC count declines. The blood urea nitrogen (BUN) and serum creatinine (Cr) are elevated, and an assortment of electrolyte imbalances occur as the kidneys fail. Hepatic dysfunction results in elevated levels of aspartate aminotransferase (formerly SGOT), alanine aminotransferase (formerly SGPT), and lactic dehydrogenase (LDH). Failure of the pancreas leads to elevated serum amylase and serum lipase values.[48] As the body's supplies of glucose, fats, and proteins are exhausted, the serum glucose falls.[48,52,55]

Medical Management

Treatment of the patient in septic shock requires a multifaceted approach. The goals of treatment are to control the infection, reverse the pathophysiologic responses, and promote metabolic support. This approach includes identifying and treating the infection, supporting the cardiovascular system and enhancing tissue perfusion, and initiating nutritional therapy. In addition, dysfunction of the individual organ systems must be prevented or treated.

One of the first measures that must be taken in the treatment of septic shock is finding and eradicating the cause of the infection. Blood, urine, sputum, and wound cultures should be obtained to find the location of the infection. Antibiotic therapy should be initiated as soon as possible. If the microorganism is unknown, a broad-spectrum antibiotic should be administered. Once the microorganism is identified, an antibiotic more specific to the microorganism should be started. Administration of antibiotics can be particularly hazardous in gram-negative shock because more endotoxin is released from the cell walls when the microorganisms die.[49,51] This further aggravates the entire septic process. Surgical intervention to débride infected or necrotic tissue or to drain abscesses also may be necessary to facilitate removal of the septic source.[13,51]

Another important measure in the treatment of septic shock is supporting the cardiovascular system and enhancing tissue perfusion. Specific interventions are aimed at increasing cellular oxygen supply and decreasing cellular oxygen demand. These treatments include administration of fluids, vasoactive agents, and positive inotropic agents, as well as ventilatory support, temperature control, and reversal of acidosis.

Aggressive fluid administration to augment intravascular volume and increase preload is very important during the hyperdynamic phase of septic shock. Crystalloids or colloids may be used depending on the patient's condition. No one fluid has been proved better than others. The amount of fluid that is administered may vary, but generally the goal is to restore the patient's filling pressures to the low normal range. During the hypodynamic phase, fluid administration is very limited because of the potential for fluid overload and congestive heart failure.[15,48,51,52]

The administration of vasoconstrictor agents is indicated during the hyperdynamic phase of septic shock to reverse the massive peripheral vasodilation. These agents help increase the SVR and augment the patient's blood pressure. During the hypodynamic phase, peripheral vasoconstriction is the problem and the administration of vasodilator agents is indicated. These agents help decrease the SVR and optimize the patient's CO. All these medications are titrated to the patient's response.[15,18,52,57] Myocardial depression occurs during both phases of septic shock and necessitates the administration of positive inotropic agents to increase contractility. These agents are administered in addition to the vasoactive agents, and all but digitalis are titrated to the patient's response.[15,18,52,57,58]

To optimize oxygenation and ventilation, intubation and mechanical ventilation are required. Ventilator settings should be adjusted to provide the patient with a Pa_{O_2} greater than 70 mm Hg and a pH within the normal range.[51] Temperature control also is necessary to decrease the metabolic demands created by hyperthermia. Antipyretic agents and cooling measures often are used. Reversal of lactic acidosis may be obligatory if associated complications develop. The role of sodium bicarbonate in the treatment of acidosis is controversial and usually reserved for severe cases that are refractory to other treatments, because of some associated risks. These risks include rebound increase in lactic acid production, development of hyperosmolar state, and fluid overload resulting from excessive sodium, shifting of the oxyhemoglobin curve to the left, and rapid cellular electrolyte shifts.[48]

The initiation of nutritional therapy is of utmost importance in the management of the patient in septic shock. The goal of nutritional support is to improve the patient's overall nutritional status, enhance the immune system, and promote wound healing. The ideal nutritional supplement for the patient in septic shock should be high in protein because of the metabolic derangements that develop in the hypermetabolic state. The amount of protein calories given depends on the patient's nitrogen balance. In early sepsis the mix of nonprotein calories may be divided evenly between carbohydrates and fats. In the later stages of septic shock, significant alterations in fat metabolism occur and the lipid content should be limited to 10% to 15% of the total nonprotein calories. The lipid emulsion should contain medium-chain triglycerides inasmuch as these are easier to metabolize than are long-chain triglycerides.[20,48]

Two experimental therapies that have been tested in humans are high-dose corticosteroids and naloxone (Narcan). High-dose corticosteroids are believed to antagonize the effects of several of the immune mediators. Extensive testing has failed to prove that this is true, and the use of corticosteroids in septic shock is controversial.[51,52,56] Naloxone is another therapy that has been tested a number of times with mixed results. Naloxone, an endorphin antagonist, is thought to reverse the hypotension caused by endogenous opiates.[51,52,59]

More promising studies are now being conducted with drugs that are believed to block or alter the effects of the immune mediators. These include pulmonary vasodilating prostaglandins, free radical scavengers, cyclooxygenase inhibitors, and anticomplement antibodies. Although these therapies have demonstrated positive results in animals, their efficacy in humans needs to be more extensively tested.[51,56] One other emerging therapy is the use of monoclonal antibodies. These antibodies work directly against gram-negative microorganisms by binding with the endotoxin and blocking activation of the immune mediators. Monoclonal antibody therapy has been approved for use in selected human cases. Conclusions have not been made yet as to its effectiveness.[60]

NURSING DIAGNOSIS AND MANAGEMENT
Septic shock

- Decreased Cardiac Output related to decreased preload secondary to septicemia, p. 362
- Impaired Gas Exchange related to ventilation/perfusion mismatching secondary to *(specify)*, p. 470
- High Risk for Altered Peripheral Tissue Perfusion risk factor: high-dose vasopressor therapy, p. 363
- Altered Nutrition: Less Than Body Protein-Calorie Requirements related to increased metabolic demands and/or lack of exogenous nutrients, p. 673
- High Risk for Infection risk factor: invasive monitoring devices, p. 366
- High Risk for Aspiration risk factors: impaired laryngeal sensation or reflex; impaired laryngeal closure or elevation, p. 472
- Ineffective Airway Clearance related to impaired cough secondary to artificial airway, p. 466
- Sleep Pattern Disturbance related to fragmented sleep and/or circadian desynchronization, pp. 142 and 143
- Sensory/Perceptual Alterations related to sensory overload, sensory deprivation, sleep pattern disturbance, p. 573
- Anxiety related to threat to biologic, psychologic, and/or social integrity, p. 763

Nursing Management

Prevention of septic shock is one of the primary responsibilities of the nurse in the critical care area. This includes the identification of patients at risk and reduction of their exposure to invading microorganisms. Hand washing, aseptic technique, and an understanding of how microorganisms can invade the body are essential components of preventive nursing care. Early identification allows for early treatment and decreased mortality.[28,47]

Assessment of a patient with septic shock includes monitoring for changes in the clinical manifestations, hemodynamic parameters, and laboratory values described earlier. Continual observation to detect subtle changes that indicate the progression of the septic process also is very important.[28,55]

The patient with septic shock may have any number of nursing diagnoses depending on the progression of the process. Nursing interventions include administering prescribed medications, monitoring the patient's response to the medications, implementing measures to prevent the development of concomitant infections and skin breakdown, and monitoring for effects and complications of nutritional therapy.[28,55]

SHOCK CASE STUDY

CLINICAL HISTORY

Mr. G is a 79-year-old well-nourished man. He has a history of coronary artery disease (CAD) with angina that is well controlled pharmacologically and mild chronic obstructive pulmonary disease (COPD) associated with smoking one pack a day for 32 years. He reported quitting about 5 years ago. Mr. G underwent a transurethral prostatectomy (TURP) 3 days ago to remove a benign prostate tumor. After surgery he was transferred to the telemetry unit because of numerous atrial and ventricular dysrhythmias in the post anesthesia care unit. His postoperative care has been progressing smoothly without any unusual problems except for the persistent dysrhythmias.

CURRENT PROBLEMS

This morning Mr G's vital signs were as follows: blood pressure (BP), 156/78 mm Hg; heart rate (HR), 110/min (sinus tachycardia with occasional premature atrial contractions and premature ventricular contractions); respiratory rate (RR), 26/min; temperature (T), 101.5° F. Mr. G was alert and oriented to person and place but not time. His breath sounds were clear but diminished in both bases. Mr. G's urinary drainage catheter remained patent, draining cloudy yellow urine at 40 to 50 ml/hr. This morning's complete blood count (CBC) indicated a white blood cell (WBC) count of 18,000 cells/mm^3; results of a Gram's stain of the urine showed numerous gram-negative rods.

MEDICAL DIAGNOSIS

Sepsis

NURSING DIAGNOSES

- ◆ High Risk for Decreased Cardiac Output risk factors: peripheral vasodilation, increased capillary membrane permeability, selective vasoconstriction, microemboli
- ◆ High Risk for Altered Tissue Perfusion (Cerebral, Cardiopulmonary, Renal, Gastrointestinal, Peripheral) risk factors: peripheral vasodilation, increased capillary membrane permeability, selective vasoconstriction, microemboli
- ◆ High Risk for Impaired Gas Exchange risk factors: peripheral vasodilation, increased capillary membrane permeability, selective vasoconstriction, microemboli
- ◆ High Risk for Infection risk factor: invasive monitoring devices

◆ PLAN OF CARE

1. Continue to monitor the patient for an increase in dysrhythmias or a decrease in cardiac output, or both.
2. Monitor the patient for a decrease in cerebral, cardiopulmonary, renal, gastrointestinal, and peripheral tissue perfusion.
3. Monitor the patient for impaired gas exchange.
4. Monitor for any further sources of infection, prevent the spread of the existing infection, and maintain body substance isolation.

MEDICAL AND NURSING MANAGEMENT AND PATIENT OUTCOME

Antibiotic therapy was reinstituted, and intravenous fluids were increased to 100 ml/hr. Oxygen therapy was begun at 2 L/min via nasal cannula. Eight hours later Mr. G's condition started to deteriorate. He became confused and combative. His skin appeared flushed and pink and was warm to touch. Mr. G's vital signs were: BP, 80/50 mm Hg; HR, 130 (sinus tachycardia with frequent premature ventricular contractions); RR, 30/min (shallow); T, 102.3° F. His ABG values on a 4 L/min nasal cannula were: Po_2, 70 mm Hg; $Paco_2$, 32 mm Hg; pH, 7.49; HCO_3^-, 22 mEq/L; O_2 saturation, 93%. His urine output was 20 to 30 ml/hr, with rising levels of blood urea nitrogen (BUN) and creatinine (Cr). Mr. G was moved to the critical care unit. A pulmonary artery (PA) catheter was inserted, and Mr. G's hemodynamic values were: right atrial pressure (RAP), 5 mm Hg; pulmonary capillary wedge pressure (PCWP), 6 mm Hg; cardiac output (CO), 10.5 L/min; cardiac index (CI), 7 L/min/m^2; and systemic vascular resistance (SVR), 444.

MEDICAL DIAGNOSIS

Hyperdynamic septic shock

NURSING DIAGNOSES

- ◆ Altered Tissue Perfusion related to maldistribution of circulating volume
- ◆ Anxiety related to threat to biologic, psychologic, and/or social integrity

◆ REVISED PLAN OF CARE

1. Promote tissue perfusion by administering fluids (crystalloids and colloids) and vasoconstrictor agents as ordered.
2. Decrease anxiety by providing orientation and education to environment and illness, supporting existing coping mechanisms, speaking slowly and calmly, removing excess stimulation, and promoting presence of comforting significant other.

SHOCK CASE STUDY—cont'd

MEDICAL AND NURSING MANAGEMENT AND PATIENT OUTCOME

Mr. G was given a 500 ml bolus of lactated Ringer's solution, and a dopamine drip was begun at 5 μg/kg/min to maintain his systolic BP greater than 90 mm Hg. He was also placed on a 70% nonrebreather face mask. Over the next 24 hours Mr. G's condition continued to deteriorate. He was unresponsive to verbal and tactile stimuli, his pulse was weak and thready, and his skin was pale, cool, and clammy. Mr. G's vital signs were: BP, 95/65 mm Hg (on a regimen of 12 μg/kg/min of dopamine); HR, 145/min (sinus tachycardia with frequent premature ventricular contractions); RR, 35/min (shallow); T, 102.5° F. His ABG values on a 70% nonrebreather mask were: Po_2, 50 mm Hg; $Paco_2$, 50 mm Hg; pH, 7.20; HCO_3^-,17 mEq/L; O_2 saturation, 83%. His urine output was between 5 and 10 ml/hr. Mr. G's hemodynamic parameters were: RAP, 15 mm Hg; PCWP, 18 mm Hg; CO, 3.02 L/min; CI, 2 L/min/m²; and SVR, 1600 dynes/sec/cm^{-5}.

MEDICAL DIAGNOSIS

Hypodynamic septic shock

NURSING DIAGNOSES

- ◆ Impaired Gas Exchange related to ventilation/perfusion mismatch
- ◆ Decreased Cardiac Output related to decreased preload secondary to septicemia
- ◆ Altered Nutrition: Less Than Body Requirements related to increased metabolic demands and/or lack of exogenous nutrients

◆ REVISED PLAN OF CARE

1. Support oxygenation by ensuring supplemental oxygen administration, preventing desaturation during procedures, encouraging deep breathing, facilitating frequent position changes, and providing chest physical therapy and nasotracheal suctioning if necessary.
2. Increase cardiac output by administering inotropic agents, weaning patient from vasoconstrictor agents, and administering vasodilator agents as ordered.
3. Promote optimal nutrition by administering enteral feedings as ordered and monitoring for complications.

MEDICAL AND NURSING MANAGEMENT AND PATIENT OUTCOME

Oral intubation and mechanical ventilation with an FIo_2 of 50% were used to maintain an oxygen saturation of 93%. A dobutamine drip at 5 μg/kg/min was begun while the dopamine drip was decreased slowly to 3 μg/kg/min. Enteral feedings were started at 40 ml/hr.

After 36 hours Mr. G was more responsive and following simple commands. His skin was pale and warm. His vital signs and hemodynamic parameters were: BP, 122/60 mm Hg; HR, 95/min (sinus rhythm with occasional premature atrial contractions and premature ventricular contractions); T, 99.5° F; RAP, 8 mm Hg; PCWP, 12 mm Hg; CO, 5.0 L/min (on 2.5 μg/kg/min of dobutamine); CI, 3.3 L/min/m²; and SVR, 1168 dynes/sec/cm^{-5}. Ventilation continued at a rate of 6, breathing 6 to 10 on his own. ABG values on a 50% were: Po_2, 90 mm Hg; $Paco_2$, 42 mm Hg; pH, 7.38; HCO_3^-, 21 mEq/L; O_2 saturation, 97%. Urine output was between 35 and 50 ml/hr (on 3 μg/kg/min of dopamine). Mr. G was tolerating the enteral feedings but required supplemental insulin administration to maintain a blood glucose level less than 180 mg/dl.

The remainder of Mr. G's stay in the critical care unit was uneventful. Weaning from all medication drips and mechanical ventilation was accomplished. Mr. G was transferred back to the telemetry unit for monitoring and further medical evaluation of his dysrhythmias.

REFERENCES

1. Barone JE, Snyder AB: Treatment strategies in shock: use of oxygen transport measurement, *Heart Lung* 20:81, 1991.
2. Shoemaker WC: Pathophysiology, monitoring, outcome prediction, and therapy of shock states, *Crit Care Clin* 3:307, 1987.
3. Rice V: Shock, a clinical syndrome: an update. II. The stages of shock, *Crit Care Nurse* 11(5):74, 1991.
4. Perry AG: Shock complications: recognition and management, *Crit Care Nurs Q* 11(1):1, 1988.
5. Rice V: Shock, a clinical syndrome: an update. I. An overview of shock, *Crit Care Nurse* 11(4):20, 1991.
6. Houston MC: Pathophysiology of shock, *Crit Care Nurs Clin North Am* 2:143, 1990.
7. Klein DG: Physiologic response to traumatic shock, *AACN Clin Issues Crit Care Nurs* 1:505, 1990.
8. Bell TN: Disseminated intravascular coagulation and shock: multisystem crisis in the critically ill, *Crit Care Nurs Clin North Am* 2:225, 1990.
9. Vaughan P, Brooks C: Adult respiratory distress syndrome: a complication of shock, *Crit Care Nurs Clin North Am* 2:235, 1990.
10. Lancaster LE: Renal response to shock, *Crit Care Nurs Clin North Am* 2:221, 1990.
11. Collins AS: Gastrointestinal complications in shock, *Crit Care Nurs Clin North Am* 2:269, 1990.
12. Summers G: The clinical and hemodynamic presentation of the shock patient, *Crit Care Nurs Clin North Am* 2:161, 1990.
13. Rice V: Shock, a clinical syndrome: an update. III. Therapeutic management, *Crit Care Nurse* 11(6):34, 1991.
14. Sommers MS: Fluid resuscitation following multiple trauma, *Crit Care Nurse* 10(10):74, 1990.
15. Hancock BG, Eberhard NK: The pharmacologic management of shock, *Crit Care Nurs Q* 11(1):19, 1988.
16. Kuhn MM: Colloids vs crystalloids, *Crit Care Nurse* 11(5):37, 1991.
17. Crisp CB: Fluid resuscitation in the traumatized patient: a review of crystalloid and colloid therapy, *Emerg Care Q* 3(4):57, 1988.
18. Burns KM: Vasoactive drug therapy in shock, *Crit Care Nurs Clin North Am* 2:167, 1990.
19. Lorenz A: Lactic acidosis: a nursing challenge, *Crit Care Nurse* 9(4):64, 1989.
20. Kuhn MM: Nutritional support for the shock patient, *Crit Care Nurs Clin North Am* 2:201, 1990.
21. Lancaster LE, Rice V: Nursing care planning: overview and application to the patient in shock, *Crit Care Nurs Clin North Am* 2:279, 1990.
22. Jillings CR: Shock: psychosocial needs of the patient and family, *Crit Care Nurs Clin North Am* 2:325, 1990.
23. Meyers KA, Hickey MK: Nursing management of hypovolemic shock, *Crit Care Nurs Q* 11(1):57, 1988.
24. Conn AT: Hypovolemic shock, *Emerg Care Q* 1(2):37, 1985.
25. Halfman-Franey M: Current trends in hemodynamic monitoring of patients in shock, *Crit Care Nurs Q* 11(1):9, 1988.
26. Blansfield J: Emergency autotransfusion in hypovolemia, *Crit Care Nurs Clin North Am* 2:195, 1990.
27. Frame SB, McSwain NE: Pneumatic antishock garments: where they stand today, *Emerg Care Q* 3(4):65, 1988.
28. Rice V: Shock, a clinical syndrome: an update. IV. Nursing care of the shock patient, *Crit Care Nurse* 11(7):28, 1991.
29. Roberts SL: Cardiogenic shock: decreased coronary artery tissue perfusion, *Dimens Crit Care Nurs* 7:196, 1988.
30. Jeffries PR, Whelan SK: Cardiogenic shock: current management, *Crit Care Nurs Q* 11(1):48, 1988.
31. Olsen J, Larson EB: Cardiogenic shock, *Emerg Care Q* 1(2):19, 1985.
32. Thompson JA and others: Cardiogenic shock: causes, diagnosis, and management, *J Crit Illness* 2(10):22, 1987.
33. Daily EK: Use of hemodynamics to differentiate pathophysiologic causes of cardiogenic shock, *Crit Care Nurs Clin North Am* 1:589, 1989.
34. Schott KE: Intra-aortic balloon counterpulsation as a therapy for shock, *Crit Care Nurs Clin North Am* 2:187, 1990.
35. Iseke R: Anaphylactic shock, *Emerg Care Q* 1(2):29, 1985.
36. Dickerson M: Anaphylaxis and anaphylactic shock, *Crit Care Nurs Q* 11(1):68, 1988.
37. Soto-Aguilar MC, deShazo RD, Waring NP: Anaphylaxis, *Postgrad Med* 82(5):154, 1987.
38. Schwenker D: Cardiovascular considerations in the critical care phase, *Crit Care Nurs Clin North Am* 2:363, 1990.
39. Foo D: Spinal cord injury and spinal shock, *Emerg Care Q* 1(2):77, 1985.
40. Richmond TS: A critical care challenge: the patient with a cervical spinal cord injury, *Focus Crit Care* 12(2):23, 1985.
41. Reed MA: Nursing consideration in acute spinal cord injury, *Crit Care Clin* 3:679, 1989.
42. Vincent JL, Van Der Linden P: Septic shock: particular type of acute circulatory failure, *Crit Care Med* 18:S70, 1990.
43. Bone RC and others: Sepsis syndrome: a valid clinical entity, *Crit Care Med* 17:389, 1989.
44. Iverson RL: Septic shock: a clinical perspective, *Crit Care Clin* 4:215, 1988.
45. Rice V: Septic shock: nursing implications of current medical research, NITA 10:326, 1987.
46. ACCP/SCCM Consensus Conference Committee: Definitions for sepsis and organ failure and guidelines for the use of innovative therapies in sepsis, *Crit Care Med* 20:864, 1992.
47. Hoyt NJ: Preventing septic shock: infection control in the intensive care unit, *Crit Care Nurs Clin North Am* 2:287, 1990.
48. Huddleston VB: *Multisystem organ failure: a pathophysiologic approach,* St. Louis, 1992, Mosby–Year Book.
49. Roach AC: Antibiotic therapy in septic shock, *Crit Care Nurs Clin North Am* 2:179, 1990.
50. Segreti J: Nosocomial infections and secondary infections in sepsis, *Crit Care Clin* 5:177, 1989.
51. Luce JM: Pathogenesis and management of septic shock, *Chest* 91:883, 1987.
52. Rackow EC, Astiz ME: Pathophysiology and treatment of septic shock, *JAMA* 266:548, 1991.
53. Sommers MS: Preventing complications for the toxic shock syndrome patient, *Dimens Crit Care Nurs* 4:215, 1985.
54. Broscious SK: Toxic shock syndrome and its potential complications, *Crit Care Nurse* 11(4): 28, 1991.
55. Littletone MT: Pathophysiology and assessment of sepsis and septic shock, *Crit Care Nurs Q* 11(1):30, 1988.
56. Stroud M, Swindell B, Bernard GR: Cellular and humoral mediators of sepsis syndrome, *Crit Care Nurs Clin North Am* 2:151, 1990.
57. Boyd JL, Stanford GC, Chernow B: The pharmacotherapy of septic shock, *Crit Care Clin* 5:133, 1989.
58. Schremmer B, Dhainaut JF: Heart failure in septic shock: effects of inotropic support, *Crit Care Med* 18:S49, 1990.
59. Schumann LL, Remington MA: The use of naloxone in treating endotoxic shock, *Crit Care Nurse* 10(2):63, 1990.
60. Klein DM, Witek-Janusek L: Advances in immunotherapy of sepsis, *Dimens Crit Care Nurs* 11:75, 1992.

47

Systemic Inflammatory Response Syndrome and Multiple Organ Dysfunction Syndrome

CHAPTER OBJECTIVES

- Define the concept of inflammation.
- Differentiate between the local and systemic inflammatory responses.
- Identify the actions of select inflammatory mediators in the pathogenesis of systemic inflammatory response syndrome (SIRS) and multiple organ dysfunction syndrome (MODS).
- Identify the clinical manifestations of organ dysfunction during MODS.
- Identify appropriate nursing diagnoses for patients with MODS.

Advanced cardiopulmonary life support techniques and technology have allowed the survival of critically ill or injured patients who previously would have died of an initial insult, such as trauma, infection, shock, or other acute processes. Initial survival, however, may be followed by the development of two newly named clinical syndromes of systemic inflammation and organ dysfunction that may result in death or profound disability.[1-4]

In 1992 the American College of Chest Physicians and the Society of Critical Care Medicine proposed a new conceptual framework to describe the interrelationships among the systemic inflammatory response, sepsis, bacteremia, and infection (Fig. 47-1) and multiple organ dysfunction[5,6] (Fig. 47-2). New terminology was developed to describe the clinical manifestations associated with systemic inflammation (systemic inflammatory response syndrome), its relationship to sepsis, and organ dysfunction (multiple organ dysfunction syndrome). New definitions and guidelines were proposed to standardize terminology used in diagnosis, intervention, and research protocols.

During the previous two decades, terms such as *multiple systems organ failure, multiple organ failure syndrome,* and *progressive/sequential organ failure* have

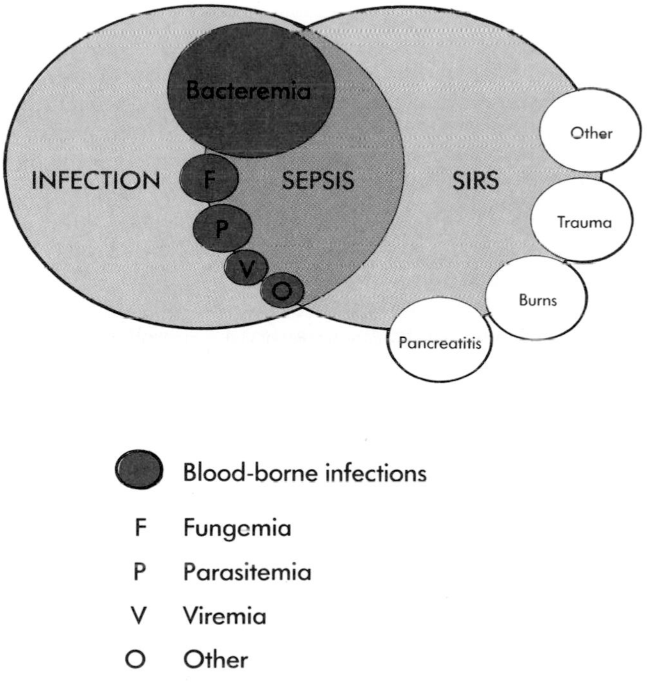

Fig. 47-1 Interrelationships among systemic inflammatory response syndrome (SIRS), sepsis, and infection. (From American College of Chest Physicians/Society of Critical Care Medicine consensus conference committee: *Crit Care Med* 20(6):865, 1992.)

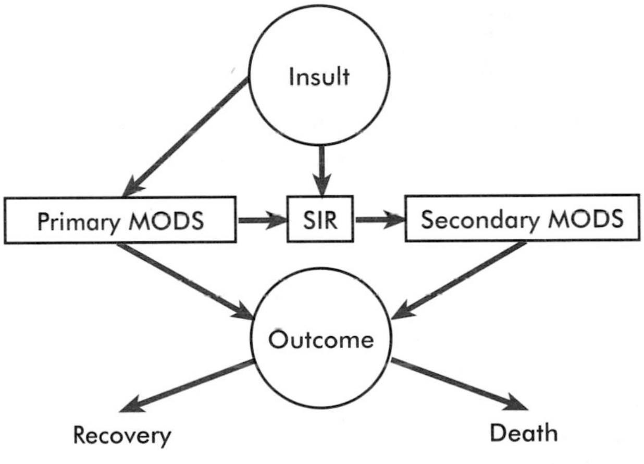

Fig. 47-2 Different causes and results of primary and secondary multiple organ dysfunction syndrome (MODS). SIR, systemic inflammatory response. (From American College of Chest Physicians/Society of Critical Care Medicine consensus conference committee: *Crit Care Med* 20(6):868, 1992.)

been used to describe clinical syndromes of organ failure in critically ill patients. Because these terms imply organ failure rather than the dynamic process of organ dysfunction, the name of the syndrome was changed to multiple organ dysfunction syndrome (MODS).[5,6]

This chapter provides information regarding the pathogenesis of the systemic inflammatory response syndrome (SIRS) and MODS within the context of critical illness. Current clinical management, including investigational therapies, is addressed. Appropriate nursing diagnoses are formulated. In addition, references are noted to appropriate chapters that address specific organ therapies and their related nursing diagnoses and interventions.

THE INFLAMMATORY RESPONSE

Inflammation is a biochemical and cellular process that occurs in vascularized tissue in response to an insult or invasion.[7] During the inflammatory process the body creates a lethal microenvironment to localize the injury and kill microorganisms. Normally the inflammatory process is contained within a restricted environment. If the response is not contained, a systemic widespread response occurs that is deleterious to organ function.[7-9] A complex system of checks and balances normally exists in the host to localize the inflammatory response.

The Local Inflammatory Response

The acute inflammatory response is a self-limiting (generally 8 to 10 days), nonspecific response that usually occurs in an identical manner regardless of the cause. The response generally starts within seconds of the insult. Mediators, the essential facilitators of the local inflammatory response, are housed in the circulation. Mediators affect the vascular bed by enhancing the movement of plasma and blood cells from the circulation into the tissue around the injury. Complex interrelationships exist among the mediators of the vascular response, including leukocytes; plasma protein cascades (complement, coagulation, kinin); platelets; and other inflammatory biochemicals, including arachidonic acid (AA) metabolites, such as prostaglandins; and monokines, such as interleukins, and tumor necrosis factor (TNF).[7]

◆ **The vascular response.** Cell injury or death initiates the acute inflammatory response. Injury may be caused by a multitude of factors, such as trauma, hypoxia, and microorganisms. The local vascular effects of inflammation start immediately and achieve a state of local increased vascular permeability that lasts through acute inflammation. Several mechanisms are operable. Arterioles near the injury constrict briefly, then dilate to increase blood flow to the injured area and allow the exudation of plasma and cells into the tissues. Exudation causes interstitial edema and slows the microcirculation, making it more viscous. Concurrently biochemical mediators, such as bradykinin, stimulate capillary and venule endothelial cells to retract, creating spaces at junctions between cells. Endothelial retraction allows leukocytes to squeeze out of the cell. The net effect is the movement of blood cells and plasma proteins into the inflamed tissue.[7]

◆ **Neutrophil function during local inflammation.** Neutrophils engage in four functions related to inflammation: margination, diapedesis, chemotaxis, and phagocytosis. Many neutrophils normally adhere to the inside of blood vessel walls until needed (margination). On activation, neutrophils move to the area of injury by squeezing through the pores of blood vessels (diapedesis), are attracted to microbial organisms or debris by chemical substances (chemotaxis), phagocytose bacteria or cellular debris, and then die. Monocytes and macrophages perform similar functions in a later stage of the inflammatory process.[7]

◆ **Plasma protein systems.** Three major plasma protein systems—the complement, coagulation, and kinin/kallikrein systems—participate in the acute inflammatory response. The complement system, a complex cascade of more than 20 serum proteins, is involved in inflammatory and immune processes that destroy bacteria and contribute to vascular changes. Eleven principal proteins known as *complements,* C1 to C9, have been identified. Activation of the complement cascade occurs through the classic pathway in response to an antigen/antibody complex or through an alternate pathway by exposure to polysaccharide from bacterial cell walls. The terminal pathway for both the classic and alternate pathways results in lysis of the target cell. The effects of complement during inflammation are outlined in the box below.[7]

The kinin/kallikrein system controls vascular tone and permeability and is activated by stimulation of the plasma kinin cascade. Hageman factor (Factor XIII) of the coagulation cascade is also directly involved in kinin activation. Kinins are biochemicals that are controlled by kinases, enzymes present in the plasma and tissues. The end result of kinin activation is the production of bradykinin. Bradykinin has profound effects, including vasodilation at low doses, pain production, extravascular smooth muscle contraction, increased vascular permeability, and leukocyte chemotaxis. As previously noted, bradykinin facilitates endothelial retraction and increased vascular permeability, processes involved in acute inflammation.[7]

The coagulation system traps bacteria in injured tissue and works with platelets to control excessive bleeding.

ACTIONS OF COMPLEMENT DURING INFLAMMATION

Opsonization/phagocytosis
Lysis of invading cell membranes
Agglutination
Neutralization of viruses
Chemotaxis
Activation of mast cells
Inflammatory effects:
- Increased hyperemia
- Increased capillary leakage
- Increased protein coagulation in tissues

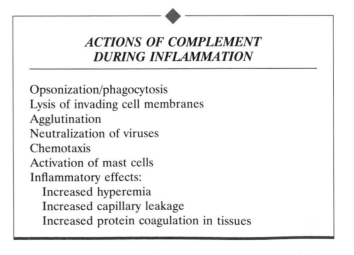

The human body normally maintains a balance between (1) clot formation (thrombosis), which is needed to minimize blood loss and to repair wounds, and (2) clot lysis (fibrinolysis), which maintains the patency of blood vessels.[10,11] The coagulation system is a plasma protein system that, like the complement cascade, can be activated through two pathways. The intrinsic pathway is activated when the Hageman factor contacts damaged vessel endothelial cells. The extrinsic pathway is activated by damaged tissue. Both pathways converge at Factor X and proceed to fibrin polymerization and clot formation. Thirteen plasma proteins (Factors I to XIII), produced primarily in the liver, participate in the coagulation cascade. The fibrinolytic system lyses fibrin clots through the actions of proteolytic and lysosomal enzymes. Plasmin splits fibrin and fibrinogen into fibrin degradation products; consequently the clots dissolves. It is this delicate balance between thrombin and plasmin in the circulation that maintains normal coagulation and lysis during the inflammatory process. The end result of these complex interactions is a lesion that is ready to heal.[7,10,11]

Normally complex systems work together to limit and localize the inflammatory response. Antiproteases, circulating albumin, vitamins C and E, red blood cells, and phagocytic cells limit the inflammatory response by three mechanisms: (1) inhibiting proteolytic enzyme activity, (2) scavenging toxic oxygen metabolites, and (3) removing the stimulus by phagocytosis.[8,9] These processes generally act together to limit and confine the potentially destructive effects of inflammatory mediators on the host. Mediator pathways are controlled by circulating activators, inhibitors, and inactivators. Feedback mechanisms exist to moderate sequential biochemical reactions involved in the production of mediators.[12]

The Systemic Inflammatory Response

The systemic inflammatory response, a continuous process, is an abnormal host response characterized by generalized inflammation in organs remote from the patient's initial insult. Systemic inflammatory response syndrome (SIRS), a newly named clinical syndrome, pertains to the widespread inflammation or clinical responses to inflammation occurring in patients with a variety of insults. Clinical conditions and manifestations associated with SIRS are listed in the box on the right. These insults produce similar or identical systemic inflammatory responses even in the absence of infection. SIRS occurs when two or more of four clinical manifestations are present in the patient at high risk. Manifestations of SIRS must represent an acute alteration from the patient's normal baseline and must not be related to other causes (e.g., neutropenia from chemotherapy or leukopenia). When SIRS is the result of infection, the term *sepsis* is used. Organ dysfunction or failure, such as acute lung injury, acute renal failure, and MODS, are complications of SIRS.[5,6]

When the inflammatory response is not contained, several consequences may occur that lead to organ dysfunction, including (1) intense, uncontrolled activation of inflammatory cells, such as neutrophils, macrophages, and lymphocytes; (2) direct damage of vascular endothelium, resulting in an uncontrolled, malignant intravascular response; (3) disruption of immune cell function; (4) a persistent state of hypermetabolism; and (5) maldistribution of circulatory volume to organ systems.[1,2,8,9]

It has been recognized recently that in the critically ill patient, damage to gastrointestinal vascular endothelial cells, along with mucosal atrophy and loss of gut barrier function, allows the release of bacteria or toxins from the intestinal tract into the circulation (endotoxemia), which provides a continual stimulus for inflammation (Fig. 47-3). Consequently, inflammation becomes a systemic and self-perpetuating process during critical illness that is inadequately regulated by the host.[7-9,12,13]

MULTIPLE ORGAN DYSFUNCTION SYNDROME

Multiple organ dysfunction syndrome (MODS) results from progressive physiologic failure of several interdependent organ systems. The patient's initial insult itself often is not the major threat to survival during critical illness. MODS is defined as the "presence of altered organ function in an acutely ill patient such that homeostasis cannot be maintained without intervention."[5] Complex interrelationships exist among dysfunctional organ systems; failure or dysfunction of one organ potentially amplifies dysfunction in another. Organ dysfunction may be absolute or relative and can occur over varying time periods. MODS, which can provide the final common pathway that leads to the death of many critically ill patients, is a leading cause of late mortality after trauma.[2,14] Organ failure may be a

CLINICAL CONDITIONS AND MANIFESTATIONS ASSOCIATED WITH SYSTEMIC INFLAMMATORY RESPONSE SYNDROME (SIRS)

CLINICAL CONDITIONS

Infection
Infection of vascular structures (heart and lungs)
Pancreatitis
Ischemia
Multiple trauma with massive tissue injury
Hemorrhagic shock
Immune-mediated organ injury
Exogenous administration of tumor necrosis factor or other cytokines
Aspiration of gastric contents
Massive transfusion
Host defense abnormalities

CLINICAL MANIFESTATIONS

Temperature $<38°$ C or $>36°$ C
Heart rate >90 beats/min
Respiratory rate >20 breaths/min or $Paco_2$ <32 torr
WBC $>12{,}000$ cells/mm^3 or <4000 cells/mm^3 or $>10\%$ immature (band) forms

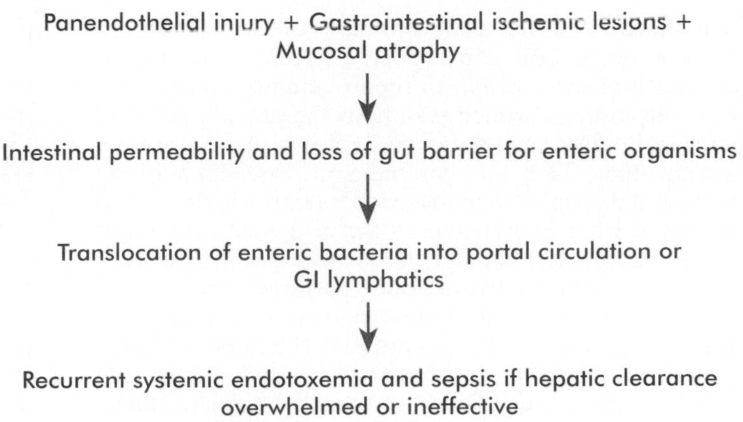

Fig. 47-3 Bacterial translocation and the development of endogenous infection.

direct consequence of the insult or can manifest latently and involve organs not directly injured or involved in the initial insult (see Fig. 47-2). Patients can experience both primary and secondary MODS. Organ dysfunction must be recognized early so that organ-specific treatment modalities can be started.[5,6] Despite modern technology and intensive medical and nursing care, the mortality rate among hospitalized patients with organ dysfunction after an acute insult remains high.[3] Patients with MODS require intensive and expert nursing care, mobilization of extensive resources, aggressive support of organ function, and appropriate physiologic monitoring of treatment responses.

Pathways for Multiple Organ Dysfunction

MODS denotes the presence of altered organ function in an acutely ill patient. As previously described, two distinct, although not mutually exclusive, pathways of organ dysfunction can develop (see Fig. 47-2). Primary MODS "directly results from a well-defined insult in which organ dysfunction occurs early and is directly attributed to the insult itself."[5] Direct insults cause localized inflammatory responses initially. Examples of primary MODS include the immediate consequences of trauma, such as pulmonary contusion, acute renal failure as a result of rhabdomyolysis, or coagulopathy caused by multiple blood transfusions. During primary MODS the abnormal and excessive host inflammatory response both at the onset and during the progression of the syndrome is less evident than in secondary MODS.[5,6]

Secondary MODS is a consequence of trauma or infection in one system that results in the systemic inflammatory response and dysfunction of organs elsewhere. Secondary MODS is not a direct response to the insult itself but is the consequence of a host response and is identified within the context of the SIRS.[5,6]

Incidence

In the past, lack of consensus regarding acceptable definitions of organ dysfunction or failure, the number of organs involved, and the duration of organ failure has hampered an accurate account of organ failure in critically ill patients. Data suggest that 7% to 15% of critically ill patients experience organ failure or dysfunction in at least two organ systems. Patient outcome is directly related to the number of organs that fail. Failure of three or more organs is associated with a 90% to 95% mortality rate.[3] The incidence of this newly defined syndrome, MODS, as such, is unknown.[5,6]

Patients at High Risk

Although various patient populations are at risk for organ dysfunction, trauma patients are particularly vulnerable because they frequently experience prolonged episodes of circulatory shock, with tissue hypoxemia, tissue injury, and infection.[4] Others at high risk include those who have experienced a shock episode associated with a ruptured aneurysm, acute pancreatitis, sepsis, burns, or surgical complications.[1,4,15] Patients older than 65 years of age are at increased risk because of their decreased organ reserve.[4]

Clinical Course and Progression of Primary MODS

As noted, primary MODS occurs in direct response to an insult. (See discussions on acute organ failure that result as direct complications from an initial insult, such as the immediate development of respiratory failure after a pulmonary contusion.) The focus here pertains to the relationship between the systemic inflammatory response and organ dysfunction currently referred to as *secondary MODS.*[5,6]

Clinical Course and Progression of Secondary MODS

Secondary MODS occurs as a result of uncontrolled systemic inflammation, with resultant organ dysfunction in populations at high risk (such as those with infection, trauma, or shock). This syndrome develops latently after a variety of insults. The early impairment of organs normally involved in immunoregulatory function, such as the liver and gastrointestinal tract, intensifies the host response to an insult.[4,8,9,13]

Sepsis is a common initiating event in the development of secondary organ dysfunction. Severe sepsis appears to initiate a period of circulatory instability and relative physiologic shock that perpetuates an inflammatory focus and resultant organ damage (see Chapter 46). Noninfectious stimuli (inflammation, perfusion deficit, or dead tissue) also effectively initiate similar cellular consequences. Physiologic shock may create a tissue oxygen debt that sets the stage for activation of the systemic inflammatory response.[16]

At present the definitive clinical course of secondary

MODS has not been completely identified. Clinical observations suggest that organ dysfunction may occur in a progressive pattern; however, organs may fail simultaneously.* Renal dysfunction, for example, may occur concurrently with hepatic dysfunction. In secondary MODS, organ dysfunction is latent.[5,6] The lungs generally are the first major organ affected. After the initial insult and resuscitation, a state of persistent hypermetabolism develops, most likely as a metabolic consequence of sustained systemic inflammation and physiologic stress, followed closely by lung dysfunction, manifested as adult respiratory distress syndrome (ARDS).

Hypermetabolism, which may not occur immediately after insult, may last for 14 to 21 days. During this period of hypermetabolism, changes occur in cellular anabolic and catabolic function, resulting in autocatabolism. Autocatabolism manifests by a severe decrease in lean body mass, severe weight loss, anergy, and increased cardiac output and volume of oxygen consumption (VO_2). The patient experiences profound alterations in carbohydrate, protein, and fat metabolism (see Chapter 50). Concurrently, gastrointestinal, hepatic, and immunologic dysfunction also may occur, which intensifies the systemic inflammatory response. Clinical manifestations of cardiovascular instability and central nervous system dysfunction may be present. Ongoing perfusion deficits and septic foci continue to perpetuate the systemic inflammatory response. About 25% to 40% of patients die during hypermetabolism. It has been suggested that the development of renal and hepatic failure are preterminal events in MODS.[15] The sequential pattern of organ involvement in MODS is not fully discerned. Clinical manifestations may indicate multiple organ involvement. Encephalopathy, coagulopathy, gastrointestinal bleeding, cardiovascular dysfunction, and recurrent infection are characteristic.* Death may occur in 21 to 28 days after the initial insult.[15] Clinical manifestations of organ dysfunction may occur earlier after an insult in patients with decreased physiologic organ reserve than in the normal patient population.[16] Patients who survive MODS often require prolonged and expensive rehabilitation, and generalized polyneuropathy may complicate their recovery. In addition, ARDS may result in a chronic form of lung disease.[3]

Biologic and Pathophysiologic Mechanisms in SIRS and Secondary MODS

Secondary organ dysfunction results from altered regulation of the patient's acute immune and inflammatory responses. Dysregulation or failure to control the host inflammatory response leads to the excessive production of inflammatory cells and biochemical mediators that in turn cause widespread damage to vascular endothelium, as well as organ damage.[19] The critically ill patient's compromised immune state also fosters an environment conducive to organ failure.

◆ **Mediators.** The inflammatory and immune responses implicated in SIRS and secondary MODS are mediated by certain cells and biochemicals that in turn affect cellular activity. As outlined in the box below, mediators associated with SIRS and MODS can be classified as inflammatory cells, plasma protein systems, and inflammatory biochemicals. Mediators either (1) facilitate cell-to-cell interaction and function or (2) cause direct tissue damage. Biochemical mediators are preformed or generated in response to select stimuli. Preformed mediators are released without specific cell activation. Direct cellular injury, for example, elicits mediator release by exocytosis; during phagocytosis mediators leak into the extracellular spaces. In contrast, generated mediators require direct cell activation to stimulate their release. Examples of generated mediators include prostaglandins and oxygen metabolites.[12]

Complex interactions occur among the multitude of inflammatory cells and biochemicals implicated in organ dysfunction after an insult. Activation of one mediator often leads to activation of another. Plasma levels are not always indicative of cellular levels. The biologic activity of inflammatory cells, biochemical mediators, and plasma protein systems and how they work in concert to cause SIRS and MODS are not yet totally defined. However, the actions of inflammatory cells and some biochemical mediators after an insult are well defined.

Inflammatory cells. Neutrophils, macrophages, mast cells, platelets, and endothelial cells mediate the SIRS through their production of cytokines (biochemical mediators). Along with proinflammatory biochemicals released from damaged or necrotic tissue and circulating

INFLAMMATORY MEDIATORS ASSOCIATED WITH SIRS AND MODS

INFLAMMATORY CELLS

Neutrophils
Macrophages/monocytes
Mast
Endothelial

BIOCHEMICAL MEDIATORS

Interleukins
Tumor necrosis factor
Platelet activating factor
Arachidonic acid metabolites
- Prostaglandins
- Leukotrienes
- Thromboxanes

Oxygen radicals
- Superoxide radical
- Hydroxyl radical
- Hydrogen peroxide

Proteases

PLASMA PROTEIN SYSTEMS

Complement
Kinin
Coagulation

*References 1, 2, 4, 15, 17, 18.

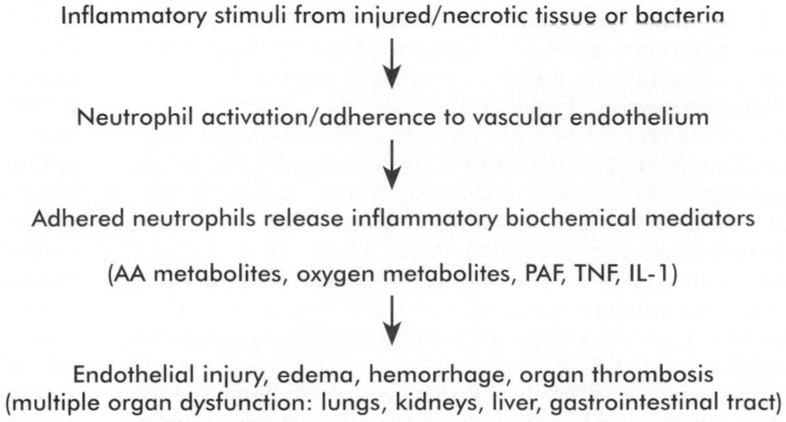

Fig. 47-4 Effects of select inflammatory mediators.

catecholamines (stress response), inflammatory cells create a hypermetabolic state, cause maldistribution of circulatory volume, and alter inflammatory and immune function.[19]

NEUTROPHILS. The activity of the neutrophil during SIRS is noteworthy. As previously defined, circulating neutrophils play a direct role in both tissue injury and defense against invading organisms. During SIRS, neutrophils release multiple preformed and generated mediators, including enzymes, arachidonic acid (AA) and oxygen metabolites, tumor necrosis factor (TNF), interleukins, and platelet-activating factor (PAF).

The neutrophil is directly implicated in systemic inflammation and organ dysfunction because it overreacts systemically and damages host cells, as well as bacteria. Neutrophils adhere to vascular endothelium throughout the microvasculature and release cytotoxic inflammatory biochemicals, including PAF, AA metabolites, and toxic oxygen metabolites.* These substances cause tissue damage, vascular injury, edema, thrombosis, and hemorrhage in multiple organ systems (Fig. 47-4). During a septic episode, neutrophilic function also is modulated by other circulating mediators, thereby intensifying the neutrophil's inflammatory response.[19] As discussed later, the pharmacologic modification of neutrophil activity is a future goal in the treatment of MODS.

MONOCYTES AND MACROPHAGES. Monocytes and macrophages normally perform three major functions relative to inflammation: (1) antigen processing and presentation, (2) bacterial phagocytosis, and (3) mediator production. Monocytes and macrophages detect, process, and present antigen to lymphocytes for initiation of the humoral and cellular components of the lymphocytic immune response. Macrophages play a significant role in organ injury by producing oxygen metabolites, initiating procoagulant activity, and releasing interleukin-1 (IL-1) and TNF. Both TNF and IL-1 then stimulate neutrophils and lymphocytes to activate the AA cascade. AA metabolites are vasoactive and cause vascular instability and altered organ blood flow.[19,20]

In the lungs, alveolar macrophages produce toxic oxygen metabolites and proteolytic enzymes that destroy alveolar epithelial cells. The role of macrophages and monocytes in organ dysfunction is most directly linked to their production of TNF and IL-1.[21-23]

MAST CELLS. Mast cells are found in all body tissues, especially those adjacent to blood vessels. As tissue-based cells, mast cells contain large amounts of preformed mediators that when released have systemic as well as local effects. Endotoxin, direct cellular injury, complement proteins (C3a and C5a), and bradykinin stimulate the release of mast cell mediators. Preformed mediators from mast cells include histamine, proteases, heparin, TNF, select AA metabolites, and PAF.[12]

LYMPHOCYTES. Lymphocytes contribute to the inflammatory response by adhering to and sequestering in the microvascular endothelium. Stimulated T and B lymphocytes produce cytokines such as IL-1 and IL-2, which in turn activate other inflammatory cells.[12]

ENDOTHELIAL CELLS. As noted, endothelial cells are common targets for leukocyte-derived mediators during the systemic inflammatory response. Widespread endothelial destruction leading to increased vascular permeability is a key element in sepsis and the systemic inflammatory response. Inflammatory mediators that cause endothelial damage include endotoxin, TNF, IL-1, and PAF. Most of these mediators also recruit and activate neutrophils and activate complement. The end result is sustained inflammation and the continued destruction of the endothelium.[19]

Endothelial cells manufacture chemotactic agents that attract neutrophils to areas of inflammation and endothelial injury. Consequently the interaction between endothelial cells and neutrophils greatly influences the magnitude of the systemic inflammatory response. Endothelial cells also produce and normally maintain a balance between endothelin (a vasoconstrictor) and endothelial-derived relaxant factor. Evidence suggests that an alteration in this delicate balance leads to vascular instability and subsequent perfusion abnormalities commonly seen in patients with sepsis. In addition, endothelial cells produce procoagulants, such as PAF and plasminogen-activating inhibitors; angiotensin II; and prostacyclin (AA metabolite), substances implicated in the inflammatory response.[19]

*References 1, 4, 8, 9, 12, 15.

Biochemical mediators. Multiple biochemical inflammatory mediators play a role in the host inflammatory response and organ injury, including TNF, interleukins, PAF, AA metabolites, and oxygen metabolites.

TOXIC OXYGEN METABOLITES. Toxic oxygen metabolites (oxidants), including the superoxide ion (O_2^-), hydrogen peroxide (H_2O_2), and the hydroxyl radical (OH), may be produced in excessive amounts during critical illness and have been implicated in organ dysfunction.

Oxidants normally are produced during the sequential single electron reduction of oxygen to water. Metal ions, including iron and copper, are needed for the production of OH, the most destructive oxidant. Normally cellular antioxidant enzymes neutralize the effects of oxidants so that cellular integrity is maintained. Cell injury occurs, however, when the production of oxygen metabolites exceeds antioxidant cellular mechanisms. Oxygen metabolites cause lipid peroxidation and damage to the cell membrane, activate the complement and coagulation cascades, and cause deoxyribonucleic acid (DNA) damage.[24]

Neutrophils produce toxic oxygen metabolites that together with proteases cause tissue injury. Toxic oxygen metabolites, for example, cause lung injury in ARDS. In addition, oxygen metabolites can cause organ injury after reperfusion in the small intestines, liver, lungs, muscles, heart, brain, stomach, and skin. Reperfusion of ischemic tissues generates the production of highly toxic oxygen metabolites that in the presence of certain metals cause organ damage.[24] Reperfusion injury occurs after the reestablishment of blood supply to an organ after an ischemic event. Antioxidant drug therapy in the future may be effective in preventing organ dysfunction.[20]

TUMOR NECROSIS FACTOR. TNF, also known as *cachectin,* is an inflammatory biochemical secreted by monocytes and macrophages, particularly in the lung and liver in response to endotoxin or noninfectious agents. TNF is not stored in body cells but probably is produced in varying amounts in response to various stressors. TNF receptors have been found on endothelial cells, adipocytes, and monocytes, and in fibroblasts. Low levels of TNF mediate the normal host response to an antigen, whereas high circulatory levels of TNF have been detected in patients with multiple organ failure. TNF, which is released by cells in 30 to 60 minutes and peaks in 1 to 2 hours after exposure to endotoxin, is primarily responsible for the pathophysiologic changes that cause organ damage in sepsis and gram-negative shock. The destructive effects of TNF are exacerbated by AA metabolites from the cyclooxygenase pathways, including prostaglandins PGE_1 and PGE_2.[19,21-23]

The biologic effects of TNF are numerous and are outlined in the box on the right. Responses to TNF, which parallel the clinical manifestations of sepsis and shock, include fever, hypotension, decreased organ perfusion, and increased capillary permeability. TNF may precipitate organ injury after trauma and infection by causing generalized endothelial injury, fibrin deposition, and a procoagulant state. TNF causes disseminated intravascular coagulopathy (DIC); interstitial pneumonitis; acute renal tubular necrosis; and necrosis of the gastrointestinal tract, liver, and adrenal glands. Metabolically, TNF causes hyperglycemia that progresses to hypoglycemia and hypertriglyceridemia. Recent evidence suggests that the stress hormones significantly influence the biologic response to TNF.[19,21-23]

INTERLEUKINS. The interleukins are a class of cytokines (biochemical mediators). At this time there are 12 known interleukins. Interleukin-1 (IL-1) has two known forms. Although structurally different, they produce similar biologic responses. As depicted in the box below, the effects of IL-1 in the host inflammatory response parallel those of TNF and are synergistic with TNF activity. Both IL-1 and TNF have profound systemic effects on host function. Endotoxin stimulates the production of IL-1 from macrophages and endothelial cells. IL-1 plays a major role in the systemic inflammatory response, particularly in mediating the vascular

SELECT EFFECTS OF TUMOR NECROSIS FACTOR AND INTERLEUKIN-1

VASCULAR

Endothelial permeability
Increased procoagulant activity
Local vasodilation
Release of platelet activating factor (PAF)
Release of endothelial cytokines
Disseminated intravascular coagulation (DIC)
Leukocyte adherence

HEMATOLOGIC

Chemotaxis
Release of leukocyte AA metabolites
Initial neutropenia
Stimulation of polymorphonuclear leukocytes

HEPATIC

Increased triglycerides caused by suppression of lipoprotein lipase
Decreased synthesis of plasma proteins: albumin and transferrin
Increased synthesis of acute phase proteins
Production of complement components
Synthesis of clotting factors

CENTRAL NERVOUS SYSTEM

Prostaglandin release in the brain
Fever
Headache
Anorexia

CARDIOVASCULAR SYSTEM

Tachycardia
Increased cardiac output
Decreased systemic vascular resistance
Hypotension

Modified from Zimmerman JJ, Ringer TV: *Crit Care Clin* 8:163, 1992.

congestion, capillary leakage, and altered coagulation associated with sepsis. Like TNF, IL-1 has profound vascular endothelial effects, including stimulation of (1) the production of two vasodilators, PGI_2 and PGE_2 (AA metabolites) and (2) leukocyte adherence to the endothelium.[19]

IL-1 fosters a procoagulant state by stimulating the production of procoagulants such as PAF and plasmin-activation inhibitor by endothelial cells. IL-1 increases the production of acute phase reactant proteins, increases catabolism of muscle tissue, and causes neutrophilia. Neutrophilia occurs as a result of the release of neutrophils from the bone marrow. The cardiovascular and inflammatory manifestations of IL-1 most commonly include hypotension, fever, tachycardia, diarrhea, acute lung injury, leukopenia, platelet aggregation, and intravascular coagulation.[19,22]

PLATELET ACTIVATING FACTOR. PAF is a lipid that attaches to cell membrane phospholipids and is released from inflammatory and immune cells in response to a multitude of factors or stimuli that also initiate AA metabolism. PAF is released by platelets, mast cells, monocytes, macrophages, neutrophils, and endothelial cells. PAF has widespread effects on the heart, vascular system, coagulation, platelets, and the lungs. Effects of PAF include platelet aggregation, with resultant microvascular stasis and ischemia in the microvascular bed; platelet release of serotonin, which increases vascular permeability; and increased vasoconstriction from increased production of thromboxane A_2, an AA metabolite.

ARACHIDONIC ACID METABOLITES. AA is a highly metabolic fatty acid that is a precursor of many biologically active substances known as *eicosanoids.* AA metabolites (eicosanoids) play a primary role in the pathogenesis of SIRS and MODS. Activation of the AA cascade by numerous stimuli, including hypoxia, ischemia, endotoxin, catecholamines, and tissue injury, produces metabolites from both the cyclooxygenase and lipooxygenase pathways. AA metabolites produced via the cyclooxygenase pathway are termed *prostaglandins* (PG) and thromboxanes (Tx), whereas those from the lipooxygenase pathway are called *leukotrienes* (LT). AA metabolites have profound effects on vasculature and cause vascular instability and maldistribution of blood flow. Eicosanoids, such as PGH_2 and PGF_2; TxA_2 and TxB_2; and LTD_4, LTC_4, and LTE_4 are vasoconstrictors. In contrast, some eicosanoids have vasodilatory properties. All leukotrienes and TxA_2 enhance capillary membrane permeability and increase vascular leakage. TxA_2, PGH_2, and PGF_2 are potent platelet aggregators.[25-28]

AA metabolites also affect leukocytes. LTB_4 stimulates leukocyte chemotaxis and adherence to vascular endothelium, with subsequent tissue injury. TxA_2 causes neutrophil aggregation, vasoconstriction, and pulmonary bronchoconstriction, processes implicated in ARDS. In summary, eicosanoids play a role in organ failure by altering vascular reactivity and permeability and by fostering the accumulation and activation of inflammatory cells.[22-28]

PROTEASES. Proteases are proteolytic (protein-digesting) enzymes released from inflammatory cells upon activation. Because most tissue is made of protein, proteases can cause significant parenchymal damage. Neutrophils in the lung, for example, produce proteases that destroy lung tissue. In the gastrointestinal tract protease-induced mucosal injuries are associated with acute ulcerative colitis, colitis associated with antibiotic treatment, and acute ischemic enteropathy.[13]

COMPLEMENT. Complement is directly implicated in systemic inflammation and organ dysfunction. As previously described, complement activation occurs in response to various stimuli, including endotoxin and TNF. Circulating complement concentrations are greatly increased in patients with sepsis. Recent evidence suggests that ARDS patients may have a functional deficiency in a C5a inhibitor called *chemotactic factor inactivator.*[20]

Organ-Specific Manifestations of Secondary MODS

Secondary MODS is a systemic disease with organ-specific manifestations. As noted, organ dysfunction or failure results from (1) the adherence of neutrophils to vascular endothelial surfaces and the release of toxic mediators, (2) direct effects of mediators on organ parenchymal endothelial cells, (3) metabolic abnormalities, and (4) poor oxygen delivery and consumption by individual organs. Organ dysfunction is influenced by numerous factors, including (1) organ host defense function, (2) response time to the injury, (3) metabolic requirements, (4) organ vasculature response to vasoactive drugs, and (5) organ sensitivity to damage and physiologic reserve. Discussion of the responses of the gastrointestinal, hepatobiliary, cardiovascular, pulmonary, renal, and coagulation systems in organ dysfunction follow. Clinical manifestations of organ dysfunction are outlined in the box on p. 795.

◆ **Gastrointestinal dysfunction.** The gastrointestinal tract plays an important role in secondary MODS. Early dysfunction of gastrointestinal organs that also have immunoregulatory function amplifies the systemic inflammatory response during critical illness. The gut is a common target organ during SIRS and MODS. As mentioned, gut damage is hypothesized to lead to bacterial translocation and endogenous endotoxemia.[4,9,13,29]

Three specific mechanisms link the gastrointestinal tract and latent organ dysfunction (see Fig. 47-3). First, hypoperfusion or shocklike states, or both, disrupt the normal mucosa barrier of the gastrointestinal tract. The gastrointestinal tract is extremely vulnerable to oxygen metabolite–induced reperfusion injury. Endothelial injury and gastrointestinal lesions occur in response to mediator-induced tissue damage. In addition, ischemic events and the absence of feedings can disrupt the normal metabolism of the gastric/intestinal lumen and the normal protective function of the gut barrier.[13] The low glycogen reserve of the gastric mucosa may require enteral feedings to maintain normal metabolism. Atrophy of the intestinal villi and ulceration may occur when patients do not receive enteral feedings.[13] Clinical

CLINICAL MANIFESTATIONS OF ORGAN DYSFUNCTION

GASTROINTESTINAL

Abdominal distention
Intolerance to enteral feedings
Paralytic illeus
Upper/lower GI bleeding
Diarrhea
Ischemic colitis
Mucosal ulceration
Decreased bowel sounds
Bacterial overgrowth in stool

LIVER

Jaundice
Increased serum bilirubin (hyperbilirubinemia)
Increased liver enzymes (AST, ALT, LDH, alkaline phosphatase)
Increased serum ammonia
Decreased serum albumin
Decreased serum transferrin

GALLBLADDER

Right upper quadrant tenderness/pain
Abdominal distention
Unexplained fever
Decreased bowel sounds

METABOLIC/NUTRITIONAL

Decreased lean body mass
Muscle wasting
Severe weight loss
Negative nitrogen balance
Hyperglycemia
Hypertriglyceridemia
Increased serum lactate
Decreased serum albumin, serum transferrin, prealbumin
Decreased retinol-binding protein

IMMUNE

Infection
Decreased lymphocyte count
Anergy

PULMONARY

Tachypnea
ARDS pattern of respiratory failure (dyspnea, patchy infiltrates, refractory hypoxemia, respiratory acidosis, abnormal O_2 indexes)
Pulmonary hypertension

RENAL

Increased serum creatinine, BUN levels
Oliguria, anuria, or polyuria consistent with prerenal azotemia or acute tubular necrosis
Urinary indexes consistent with prerenal azotemia or acute tubular necrosis

CARDIOVASCULAR

Hyperdynamic

Decreased pulmonary capillary wedge pressure
Decreased systemic vascular resistance
Decreased right atrial pressure
Decreased left ventricular stroke work index
Increased oxygen consumption
Increased cardiac output, cardiac index, heart rate

Hypodynamic

Increased systemic vascular resistance
Increased right atrial pressure
Increased left ventricular stroke work index
Decreased oxygen delivery and consumption
Decreased cardiac output and cardiac index

CENTRAL NERVOUS SYSTEM

Lethargy
Altered level of consciousness
Fever
Hepatic encephalopathy

COAGULATION/HEMATOLOGIC

Thrombocytopenia
DIC pattern

manifestations of altered gastrointestinal function may include abdominal distention, intolerance to enteral feedings, paralytic illeus, gastrointestinal bleeding, diarrhea, and ischemic colitis.[13,29]

Second, the translocation of normal flora bacteria of the gut into the systemic circulation initiates and perpetuates an inflammatory focus. The gastrointestinal tract harbors organisms that, when translocated from the gut into the portal circulation and inadequately cleared by the liver, present an inflammatory focus in a critically ill patient. Hepatic macrophages respond to an increase in enteric organisms by producing tissue-damaging amounts of TNF. The effects of TNF have been discussed previously. Variables associated with bacterial translocation include paralytic ileus, antibiotics, antacids, and histamine blockers.[13]

The third mechanism linking the gastrointestinal tract and organ dysfunction is colonization. The oropharynx of critically ill patients becomes colonized with potentially pathogenic organisms from the gastrointestinal tract. Pulmonary aspiration of colonized sputum presents the critically ill patient with an inflammatory focus. Antacids, histamine blockers, and antibiotics increase colonization of the upper gastrointestinal tract.[13,29]

◆ **Hepatobiliary dysfunction.** The liver plays a vital role in host homeostasis related to the acute inflammatory response. Consequently, hepatic dysfunction after a critical insult may be a primary threat to survival. The liver normally controls the inflammatory response by several mechanisms. Kupffer's cells, which are hepatic macrophages, detoxify substances that might normally induce systemic inflammation, as well as vasoactive substances that cause hemodynamic instability. Failure to detoxify gram-negative bacteria translocated from the intestinal tract causes endotoxemia and perpetuates the systemic inflammatory response and may lead to organ dysfunction. In addition, the liver produces proteins and antiproteases to control the inflammatory response; however, hepatic dysfunction limits this response.[8,9]

The splanchnic organs, including the liver, pancreas, and gallbladder, are extremely susceptible to ischemic injury. Ischemic hepatitis occurs after a prolonged period of physiologic shock and is associated with centrilobular hepatocellular necrosis. Histologic data suggest that the degree of hepatic damage is related directly to severity and duration of the shock episode. Terms such as *shock liver* and *posttraumatic hepatic insufficiency* have been used to describe ischemic hepatitis. Both anoxic and reperfusion injury damage hepatocytes and the vascular endothelium.[30]

Patients at high risk for ischemic hepatitis after a hypotensive event include those with a history of cardiac failure or cardiac dysrhythmias, or both. Clinical manifestations of hepatic insufficiency are evident 1 to 2 days after the insult. Jaundice and transient elevations in serum transaminase and bilirubin levels occur. Changes in the serum bilirubin may lag behind changes in transaminase levels. Indirect bilirubin values may increase 3 to 10 times normal. Significantly higher bilirubin values occur, however, if the patient has experienced severe hemolysis. Hyperbilirubinemia results from hepatocyte anoxic injury and an increased production of bilirubin from the hemoglobin catabolism. Ischemic hepatitis may either resolve spontaneously or progress to hepatic failure and hepatic encephalopathy. Although ischemic hepatitis is not a life-threatening complication, it can contribute to patient morbidity and mortality as a component of multiple organ dysfunction.[30]

Acalculous cholecystitis, a component of MODS, appears 3 to 4 weeks after the initial insult. Its pathogenesis is unclear but may be related to various factors, including ischemic reperfusion injury, narcotics, and cystic duct obstruction as a result of hyperviscous bile. Mediator-induced gallbladder dysfunction associated with acalculous cholecystitis may be related to the release of TxA_2 and leukotrienes (vasoactive substances) into the microcirculation in response to a damaged endothelium, aggregated platelets, and neutrophils. Clinical manifestations of acalculous cholecystitis may mimic acute cholecystitis with gallstones. Patients may demonstrate vague symptoms, however, including right upper quadrant pain and tenderness. Critical to the detection of acalculous cholecystitis is the recognition of abdominal distention, unexplained fever, loss of bowel sounds, and a sudden deterioration in the patient's condition. Data suggest that 50% of patients with acalculous cholecystitis have gallbladder gangrene and 10% have gallbladder perforation. Consequently, surgical removal of the gallbladder may be performed. A high mortality rate is associated with acalculous cholecystitis because of the seriousness of the underlying disease process.[31]

◆ **Pulmonary system failure.** The lungs are a frequent target organ for mediator-induced injury. Acute lung injury most frequently manifests as acute respiratory distress syndrome (ARDS). This clinical syndrome, described in Chapter 22, is addressed here only briefly. Although MODS does not develop in all patients with ARDS, acute respiratory failure as a result of ARDS generally occurs in those with organ dysfunction. ARDS patients who experience persistent inflammation with sepsis concurrently with respiratory failure are at greatest risk for multiple organ dysfunction.[1]

Clinical manifestations of mediator-induced pulmonary injury are consistent with ARDS. Damage to the pulmonary vascular endothelium and the alveolar epithelium from a multitude of mediators results in surfactant deficiency, pulmonary hypertension, increased lung water (noncardiogenic pulmonary edema) because of increased pulmonary capillary permeability and hypoxemia. Pulmonary hypertension and hypoxic pulmonary vasoconstriction may be the result of loss of the vascular bed during the proliferative phase of ARDS. Pulmonary function is acutely disrupted, resulting in altered airway mechanics and bronchoconstriction. The patient demonstrates a low-grade fever, tachycardia, dyspnea, and mental confusion. Diagnostic studies show patchy infiltrates on chest film, thrombocytopenia, and consumptive coagulopathy. Dyspnea worsens, and intubation and mechanical ventilation are required. Mediators associated with acute lung injury include AA metabolites, toxic oxygen metabolites, proteases, TNF, and interleukins[1,3] (discussed in conjunction with ARDS in Chapter 22).

◆ **Renal dysfunction.** Acute renal failure is a frequent manifestation of both primary and secondary MODS. As discussed in Chapter 34, acute renal failure can result from renal hypoperfusion (prerenal cause) or from direct damage to renal tubular cells (intrarenal cause). The kidney is highly vulnerable to reperfusion injury. Renal ischemic-reperfusion injury may be a major cause of renal failure in MODS. Patients may demonstrate oliguria secondary to decreased renal perfusion and relative hypovolemia. The condition may become refractory to diuretics, fluid challenges, and dopamine. Prerenal oliguria may progress to acute renal failure and require hemodialysis or other renal therapies. The frequent use of nephrotoxic drugs during critical illness also intensifies the risk of renal failure[32] (see Chapter 34).

◆ **Cardiovascular dysfunction.** The initial cardiovascular response associated with systemic inflammation is characterized by a period of cardiac excitation and altered vascular resistance during hypermetabolism. This response parallels the hyperdynamic response seen in septic patients and is characterized by decreased right atrial pressure and systemic vascular resistance (SVR), as well as increased venous capacitance, VO_2, cardiac output (CO), and heart rate (HR). During this hyperdynamic phase, the patient has increased volume requirements. The inability to increase CO as response to a low SVR, which may indicate myocardial failure or inadequate fluid resuscitation, is associated with increased mortality. VO_2 may be twice normal and may be flow-dependent. Mediators implicated in the hyperdynamic response include bradykinin, vasodilator prostaglandins, PAF, endogenous opioids, and β-adrenergic stimulators.[4,33-35]

As organ failure progresses and mediator effects become more deleterious, cardiac failure develops. Recent evidence suggests that cardiac dysfunction is characterized by ventricular dilation, decreased diastolic compliance, and decreased systolic contractile function. Cardiovascular function becomes vasopressor-dependent. Cardiac failure may be caused by immune mediators, TNF, acidosis, or myocardial depressant factor (MDF), a substance thought to be secreted by the pancreas. TNF has a myocardial-depressant effect and is associated with myocardial depression during septic shock.[36] Myocardial depression is exacerbated by myocardial hypoperfusion from a low CO state and persistent lactic acidosis. Late cardiovascular responses include decreased CO and an increased SVR and VO_2. Cardiogenic shock and biventricular failure occur and lead to death.

◆ **Coagulation system dysfunction.** Failure of the coagulation system may manifest as disseminated intravascular coagulation (DIC). DIC results in simultaneous microvascular clotting and hemorrhage in organ systems because of the depletion of clotting factors and excessive fibrinolysis. As depicted in Fig. 47-5, cell injury and damage to the endothelium initiate the intrinsic or extrinsic coagulation pathways. The endothelium is closely involved in DIC. Several relationships have been proposed. Endotoxins may roughen and expose the endothelial lining of blood vessels and consequently stimulate clotting. Low flow states during hypotensive episodes may damage vessel endothelium and release tissue thromboplastin, with subsequent activation of the extrinsic pathway. A variety of clinical conditions, such as trauma, burns, and radiographic procedures, also can cause damage to the local endothelium and activation of the intrinsic coagulation pathway.[10,11]

DIC is a complex consumptive coagulopathy that occurs in patients with a variety of disorders, including sepsis, tissue injury, and shock, and is an overstimulation of the normal coagulation process. Thrombosis and fibrinolysis are magnified to life-threatening proportions. The initial alteration in DIC is a generalized state of systemic hypercoagulation that produces organ ischemia. All organs, particularly the skin, lungs, and kidneys, are involved.[10,11] The thrombotic clinical manifestations of DIC are presented in the box on the right.

Hemorrhage is the second pathophysiologic alteration in DIC. The lysis of clots (fibrinolysis) normally is initiated by the coagulation cascade. The intensity of the thrombosis in DIC enhances an equally intense lysis; however, clot lyse cannot effectively maintain blood vessel patency. As depicted in Fig. 47-5, the production of fibrin split products exerts further anticoagulant effects and hemorrhage ensues. Clotting factors, platelets, fibrinogen, and thrombin are consumed in large quantities during the thrombosis. Consequently coagulation substances are depleted. The hemorrhagic signs and symptoms of DIC are presented in the box below.

The abnormal clotting studies in patients with DIC may indicate thrombocytopenia, prolonged clotting times, depressed levels of clotting factors, particularly Factor VII, and fibrinogen/fibrin and high levels of breakdown products of fibrinogen and fibrin (fibrin degradation products, D-dimer). Medical management of DIC includes immediate treatment of the underlying cause; transfusion of blood products, such as red blood cells, platelets, and fresh frozen plasma, to correct the clotting factor deficiencies; and cryoprecipitate to treat hypofibrinogenemia. The use of heparin therapy in DIC remains controversial. Heparin must be used with caution; however, it is contraindicated in patients with bleeding in critical areas such as the cranium. Antifibrinolytic agents may be used concurrently with heparin

CLINICAL MANIFESTATIONS OF DISSEMINATED INTRAVASCULAR COAGULATION

THROMBOTIC CLINICAL MANIFESTATIONS

Skin involvement
Red, indurated areas along vessel wall
Purpura fulminans (diffuse skin infarction)
Acral cyanosis
Necrosis of fingers, toes, nose, and genitalia
Cool, pale extremities with mottling, cyanosis, or edema
Renal involvement
  Renal failure
Cerebral infarcts or hemorrhage
Focal neurologic deficits, e.g., hemiplegia or loss of vision
Nonspecific changes, e.g., altered LOC, confusion, headache, or seizures
Bowel infarction
Melena, hematemesis, abdominal distention, or absent or hyperactive bowel sounds
Thrombophlebitis
Pulmonary embolism

HEMORRHAGIC CLINICAL MANIFESTATIONS

Spontaneous hemorrhage into body cavities and skin surfaces
Classic symptom of oozing or bleeding from invasive-line insertion sites or from body orifices
Bleeding from body orifices such as the rectum, vagina, urethra, nose, and ears, as well as from the lung and GI tract
Petechiae, purpura, or ecchymosis
Gingival, nasal, or scleral hemorrhage on physical examination
Hemorrhaging into all body cavities, including the abdomen, retroperitoneal space, cranium, and thorax

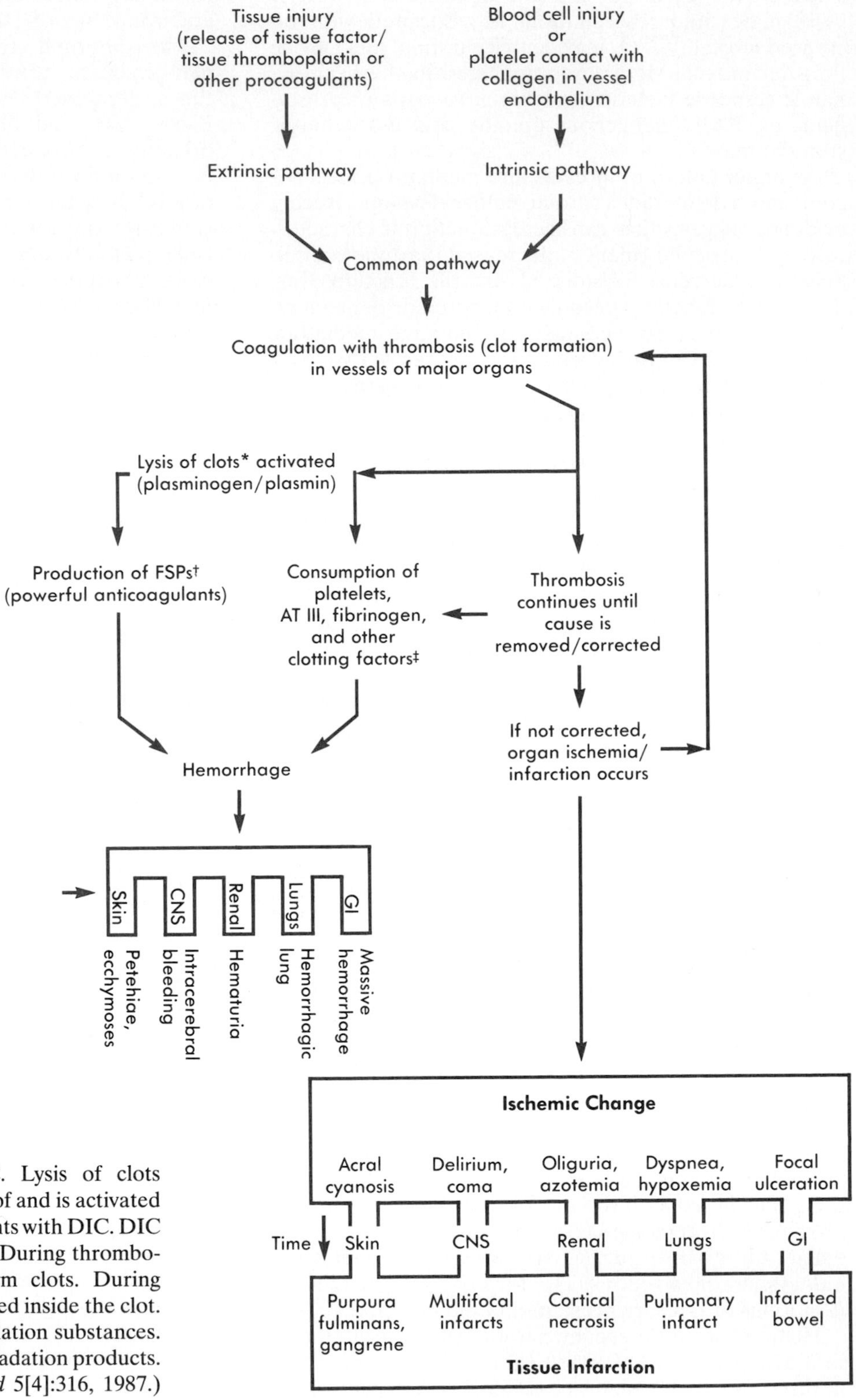

Fig. 47-5 Pathophysiology of DIC. Lysis of clots (fibrinolysis) is a natural consequence of and is activated by coagulation. It is intensified in patients with DIC. DIC is termed a *consumptive coagulopathy.* During thrombosis, clotting factors are used to form clots. During fibrinolysis, clotting factors are destroyed inside the clot. The end result is a depletion of coagulation substances. *FSP,* Fibrin split products or fibrin degradation products. (Modified from Carr M: *J Emerg Med* 5[4]:316, 1987.)

therapy but generally are contraindicated because of the risk of thrombotic complications. Strict adherence to bleeding precautions is essential to minimize tissue and vascular trauma.[10,11]

Nursing Assessment of Patients at High Risk

The nurse caring for patients at high risk for MODS engages in a multitude of assessment strategies to detect early organ manifestations of this syndrome. Initial identification of patients at high risk for primary and secondary MODS involves an awareness of the complications related to the patient's initial insult. Because the SIRS is related directly to the development of secondary MODS, patients at risk for systemic inflammation (pancreatitis, burns, multitrauma and tissue injury, ischemia, hemorrhagic shock, or immune-mediated organ injury) should be continuously assessed for organ dysfunction. Patients who continue to experience sites of inflammation, septic foci, and inadequate tissue perfusion may be at even higher risk.

◆

NURSING DIAGNOSIS AND MANAGEMENT

Multiple organ dysfunction syndrome (MODS) and disseminated intravascular coagulation (DIC)

- ◆ High Risk for Infection risk factors: invasive monitoring devices, p. 366
- ◆ High Risk for Infection risk factors: malnutrition and immunodeficiencies, p. 674
- ◆ High Risk for Aspiration risk factors: impaired laryngeal sensation or reflex; impaired laryngeal closure or elevation; increased gastric volume; decreased lower esophageal sphincter pressure, p. 472
- ◆ Acute Pain related to transmission and perception of cutaneous, visceral, muscular, and ischemic impulses secondary to multiple invasive procedures, tissue trauma, exposure to noxious stimuli, p. 566.
- ◆ Fluid Volume Deficit related to active blood loss (DIC), p. 639
- ◆ Decreased Cardiac Output related to relative excess of preload and afterload secondary to impaired ventricular contractility, p. 358
- ◆ Impaired Gas Exchange related to ventilation-perfusion mismatch secondary to damage to pulmonary vascular endothelium and alveolar epithelium, p. 470
- ◆ Impaired Gas Exchange related to alveolar hyperventilation secondary to hypoxemia, hypercatabolism, p. 471
- ◆ Ineffective Airway Clearance related to excessive secretions or abnormal viscosity of mucus, p. 464
- ◆ Ineffective Airway Clearance related to impaired cough secondary to artificial airway, p. 466
- ◆ Altered Nutrition: Less Than Body Protein-Calorie Requirements related to lack of exogenous nutrients and increased metabolic demand, p. 673
- ◆ Sensory/Perceptual Alterations related to sensory overload, sleep pattern disturbance, p. 573
- ◆ High Risk for Altered Tissue Perfusion risk factor: high-dose vasopressor therapy, p. 363

Management of MODS Patients at High Risk

The patient at high risk for MODS requires interdisciplinary collaboration in clinical management, which involves prevention and treatment of infection, maintenance of tissue oxygenation, nutritional/metabolic support, and support for individual organs.[1,2,4,17,37] Currently the use of investigational therapies frequently is part of the patient's clinical management.

◆ **Prevention, detection, and treatment of infection.** Elimination of the source of inflammation or infection can reduce mortality. Therefore surgical procedures such as early fracture stabilization, removal of infected organs or tissue, and burn excision may be helpful in limiting the inflammatory response. Appropriate antibiotics are needed if the focus cannot be removed surgically; however, antibiotics may contribute to the systemic inflammation by breaking down microbes and releasing endotoxin, an inflammatory mediator.[38] Although steroids have been used in the past to suppress malignant inflammation, their use does not significantly decrease mortality in this patient population.[38]

Patients should be assessed closely for infection. Subtle expressions of infection warrant investigation. High Risk for Infection is a highly relevant nursing diagnosis during this time period. Nursing care includes strict adherence to standards of practice to prevent infection as they relate to infection control in the use of invasive procedures such as hemodynamic monitoring, urinary catheters, endotracheal tubes, intracranial pressure monitoring, total parenteral nutrition, and wound care.

Despite compliance with meticulous infection control practices, critically ill patients may "infect" themselves. As previously noted, bacterial contamination of the highly vulnerable respiratory tract and pneumonia can result from the colonization of gastrointestinal tract bacteria. Recently several new approaches to infection control have been proposed, including selective decontamination of the gastrointestinal tract with enteral antibiotics to prevent nosocomial infections, topical antibiotics in the oral pharynx to prevent colonization, monoclonal antibodies against endotoxin, and passive antibody protection.[15,21] Data suggest that gut decontamination and prevention of oral pharyngeal colonization reduce the incidence of infection; however, the death rate from multiple organ dysfunction has not significantly been affected.[29]

Several approaches to infection and inflammation control currently are being investigated, including immunotherapy. Immunotherapy is antibody therapy that lessens the systemic inflammatory response to microbes (antiinflammatory immunotherapy) and is based on the principle that antibodies directed against endotoxin can prevent the endotoxin from stimulating the systemic inflammatory response.[38]

◆ **Maintenance of tissue oxygenation.** Hypoperfusion and resultant organ hypoxemia frequently occur and subject essential organs to failure. (The role of the cardiovascular system in oxygen transport, delivery, and consumption is discussed in Chapter 13.) Failure to maintain adequate oxygenation to vital organs results in organ dysfunction or failure. Despite adequate oxygen delivery, VO_2 may not meet the needs of the body during MODS. Normally under steady state conditions, VO_2 is relatively constant and independent of oxygen delivery unless delivery becomes severely impaired.[40] Patients with inflammatory responses such as ARDS and sepsis, however, may have an abnormality in which tissue VO_2 becomes dependent on the amount of oxygen delivered. Patients are unable to use oxygen appropriately despite normal delivery.[33,34,39,40] Possible causes of this flow-dependent VO_2 include abnormal mitochondrial function, redistribution of blood flow to organs, decreased SVR (secondary to prostaglandins), maldistribution of blood flow, microembolization, and capillary obstruction.[37,40]

Currently, information about organ blood flow and oxygen delivery generally is not available at the bedside of most MODS patients; therefore, nurses must rely on systemic measures of oxygenation, including pulse oximetry and data concerning mixed venous oxygen saturation (SvO_2). Interventions that decrease oxygen demand and increase oxygen delivery are essential. Decreasing oxygen demand may be accomplished by sedation, mechanical ventilation, temperature control, and rest. Oxygen delivery may be increased by maintenance of a normal hematocrit and Pao_2, by positive end-expiratory pressure, by increasing preload or myocardial contractility to enhance cardiac output, or by reducing afterload to increase cardiac output. Recent evidence suggests that the maintenance of supranormal oxygen levels significantly decreases the incidence of organ failure in trauma patients.[14]

◆ **Nutritional/metabolic support.** Hypermetabolism in MODS results in profound weight loss, cachexia, and loss of organ function. Nutritional support may not alter the course of organ dysfunction but prevents generalized nutritional deficiencies. The enteral route is preferable to parenteral support.[15] The advantages and disadvantages of both enteral and parenteral nutrition are discussed in Chapter 50.

Recent guidelines have been proposed regarding nutritional support during MODS. Patients should receive 25 to 30 kcal/kg/day with 3 to 5 g/kg/day as glucose. The respiratory quotient should be monitored and maintained under 0.9. Fat emulsions should be limited to 0.5 to 1 g/kg/day to prevent iatrogenic immunosuppression associated with lipids and fat overload syndromes. Plasma transferrin and prealbumin levels should be used to monitor hepatic protein synthesis.[15]

Experimental Pharmacologic Approaches in SIRS and MODS

Organ-specific interventions have not been effective in improving survival rates in patients with multiple organ involvement. Although organ-specific therapies such as mechanical ventilation and hemodialysis are needed for immediate survival, future medical treatment must be aimed at targeting and controlling the destructive activity of mediators that cause cell and organ death. Studies with animal models continue to provide information regarding the efficacy of agents and drugs in preventing organ dysfunction. Several experimental drugs and agents currently are undergoing clinical trials in human beings. As previously described, endothelial cells are common targets for inflammatory mediators; consequently endothelial cell protection is a primary goal in pharmacologic management. Endothelial cell protection against the effects of inflammatory cells and mediators may include therapeutic agents that act as neutrophil inhibitors, WBC adherence inhibitors, antioxidants, eicosanoid modulators, PAF inhibitors, and monoclonal antibodies aimed at cytokines and cell surface receptors. Monoclonal antibodies are antibodies that have specific antigens as targets and a constant binding affinity.[20]

Drugs that can act as inhibitors of neutrophil function hold great promise in the treatment of MODS. As noted, mediators such as endotoxin, TNF, IL-1, and PAF cause endothelial damage. These inflammatory mediators all recruit and activate neutrophils. Subsequently activated neutrophils release destructive mediators. TNF also activates complement, a process that ultimately affects neutrophils. Proinflammatory effects also are mediated through the lipooxygenase and cyclooxygenase pathways. Drugs that inhibit neutrophil function may be beneficial in the systemic inflammatory response and are listed in the box, p. 801. At this time limited information is available regarding the effects of these drugs with SIRS and MODS patients. As immunomodulators, these drugs moderate neutrophil-induced injury in endothelial cells. It has been suggested that pentoxifylline has pronounced effects on neutrophils preexposed to cytokines. Specifically, pentoxifylline (1) reduces the adhesiveness of activated neutrophils to the endothelium, (2) reduces the release of toxic oxygen metabolites and lysosomal enzymes, and (3) inhibits neutrophil activation by endotoxin, TNF, and IL-1. Current data regarding the effectiveness of pentoxifylline in human beings with sepsis or systemic inflammation are limited. Adenosine, another potential neutrophil inhibitor, reduces granulocyte adherence, inhibits superoxide ion formation, limits the effects of reperfusion injury, and protects endothelial cells.[20]

Naturally occurring substances, including some interleukins, inhibit the adherence of neutrophils to the endothelium. In the future, monoclonal antibodies may be available to decrease the adhesion of neutrophils to the endothelium. Antioxidants, drugs that scavenge superoxide or hydrogen peroxide radicals, or xanthine oxidase (an enzyme that facilitates the production of oxygen radicals); oxygen radical scavengers, drugs that bind free oxygen radicals; and protease inhibitors may be effective in the treatment of systemic inflammation and sepsis. Combinations of drugs may be needed to suppress the systemic inflammatory response to prevent organ dysfunction.[20]

Eicosanoid modulation involves the use of pharmacologic agents to negate the destructive effects of AA metabolites. Agents that may inhibit the release or destructive activity of AA metabolites are listed in the box on right. The effectiveness of these agents in modulating the response to sepsis is under investigation. In contrast to AA metabolites that have damaging effects, the administration of PGI_1 may be effective in limiting the systemic inflammatory response because of its local vasodilatory effects and antiplatelet properties.[26]

Other therapies currently under investigation include the modulation of macrophage function with n-3 polyunsaturated fatty acids, and stimulation of lymphocyte function with arginine and n-3 polyunsaturated fatty acids.[15] Antiendorphin therapy has been used in patients with sepsis. No scientific evidence exists that endorphin neutralization with naloxone benefits patients with sepsis or multiple organ involvement. In some patients, however, naloxone has pressor effects.[41] Other investigational therapies that have not demonstrated significant effects in limiting systemic inflammation and organ dysfunction include antihistamines and glucocorticoids.[8]

EXPERIMENTAL PHARMACOLOGIC APPROACHES IN SIRS AND MODS

- Neutrophil inhibitors (pentoxifylline, adenosine, aminophylline, terbutaline, dibutyl-cAMP, caffeine, forskolin)
- WBC adherence inhibitors
- Antioxidants/oxygen radical scavengers
- Arachidonic acid metabolite modulators
  - Monoconal antibodies to phospholipase A_2
  - Cyclooxygenase inhibitors (ibuprofen, indomethacin)
  - Thromboxane synthetase inhibitors
  - Thromboxane receptor blockers
  - Lipooxygenase inhibitors
  - Leukotrienes antagonists
- PAF inhibitors
- Monoconal antibodies to decrease adhesion of neutrophils to the endothelium
- Protease inhibitors
- Modulation of macrophage function (n-3 polyunsaturated fatty acids)
- Stimulation of lymphocyte function (arginine, n-3 polyunsaturated fatty acids)
- Antiendorphin therapy
- Antihistamines
- Glucocorticoids

MULTIPLE ORGAN DYSFUNCTION SYNDROME CASE STUDY

CLINICAL HISTORY

Mr. H is a 38-year-old white, well-nourished, construction worker who sustained abdominal injuries and a liver laceration that required surgical intervention (exploratory laparotomy, repair of liver laceration, splenectomy) after volume resuscitation in the field and emergency room. His previous medical history reveals no chronic health problems. He is, however, a 20 pack/year smoker.

CURRENT PROBLEMS

During the immediate postoperative period (days 1 and 2), extubation occurred. Mr. H was lethargic but oriented and hemodynamically stable, with mild volume depletion (as evidenced by measured and derived hemodynamic data from the pulmonary artery catheter). He required low-flow nasal oxygen (2 L/min) to maintain a PaO_2 of 75 mm Hg and an O_2 saturation above 95% (assessed continuously via pulse oximetry). Despite his relatively stable hemodynamic profile, he was tachycardic (sinus) and mildly tachypneic (RR, 26 breaths/min), with diminished breath sounds at both bases. He comprehended and was able to use patient-controlled analgesia (PCA) but frequently awakened anxious and in pain. Urine output was low but adequate for intravenous intake; skin and extremities were cool to the touch, and core temperature (CT) was 37° C. Mr. H's abdomen was distended, with absent bowel sounds. A nasogastric tube was draining small amounts of dark green drainage. His surgical wound was well approximated, with no redness or drainage. Laboratory data revealed normochromic normocytic anemia (hemoglobin, 9.8 g/dl; hematocrit, 25%), leukocytosis (WBC, 13,000 cells/mm^3), and an elevated serum lactate level. Arterial blood gas (ABG) values indicated a primary respiratory alkalosis and metabolic acidosis. Serum potassium levels were high; consequently all potassium was removed from intravenous fluids.

MEDICAL DIAGNOSES

Abdominal trauma, exploratory laparotomy with repair of liver lacerations

Systemic inflammatory response syndrome: multiple trauma

NURSING DIAGNOSES

- ◆ High Risk for Altered Tissue Perfusion: Cardiopulmonary, Renal, Gastrointestinal risk factors: systemic inflammation, volume depletion
- ◆ High Risk for Impaired Gas Exchange risk factors: alveolar hypoventilation and ventilation/perfusion mismatch
- ◆ High Risk for Ineffective Airway Clearance risk factors: abdominal or thoracic pain
- ◆ High Risk for Infection risk factors: invasive monitoring, impaired skin integrity, depressed immune response after trauma, altered skin barrier
- ◆ Acute Pain related to transmission and perception of cutaneous, visceral, muscular, or ischemic impulses secondary to surgical incision
- ◆ Fluid Volume Deficit related to active blood loss
- ◆ Anxiety related to threat to biologic, psychologic, and/or social integrity

◆ PLAN OF CARE

1. Minimize proinflammatory stimuli, such as perfusion deficits, hypoxia, hypotension, and bacteria, that further activate the systemic inflammatory response.
2. Maintain optimal pulmonary function by aggressive use of incentive spirometry, turning, and effective pain control.
3. Optimize tissue perfusion and oxygen transport and delivery to organ systems.
4. Monitor closely for clinical manifestations of SIRS and progression to organ dysfunction.

MEDICAL AND NURSING MANAGEMENT AND PATIENT OUTCOME

Despite his relatively stable clinical status during the first 2 postoperative days, on day 3 Mr. H was becoming progressively more tachycardic, tachypneic, and anxious. He required 100% oxygen via face mask. Chest film results demonstrated widespread alveolar opacification consistent with adult respiratory distress syndrome (ARDS). ABG values revealed refractory hypoxemia, with high anion gap primary metabolic acidosis and respiratory acidosis. Consequently, oral intubation and volume-cycled mechanical ventilation were used. Positive end-expiratory pressure (PEEP) at 10 cm H_2O was added incrementally to maximize oxygenation without compromising cardiac output and oxygen delivery. Measures of static and dynamic lung compliance were consistent with decreasing lung compliance; oxygen indexes and derived shunt calculations demonstrated severe ventilation/perfusion mismatch. Hemodynamic data continued to show a hyperdynamic cardiovascular profile. ABG values remained unchanged. Energy expenditure as measured with use of a metabolic cart demonstrated hypermetabolism, with increased oxygen consumption and carbon dioxide production. Enteral nutrition via a small-bore jejunal feeding tubing was attempted without success; consequently, total parenteral nutrition (TPN) was started at 25 to 30 kcal/kg/day via a newly placed internal jugular catheter. Appropriate fat supplementation also was provided.

MULTIPLE ORGAN DYSFUNCTION SYNDROME CASE STUDY—cont'd

MEDICAL DIAGNOSIS

Acute respiratory failure secondary to adult respiratory distress syndrome

NURSING DIAGNOSES

- High Risk for Infection risk factors: invasive monitoring, altered immune responses after trauma, hypermetabolism
- Altered Tissue Perfusion: Cardiopulmonary, Renal, Gastrointestinal related to systemic inflammation, hypoxemia
- Impaired Gas Exchange related to ventilation/perfusion mismatch secondary to mediator-induced pulmonary injury
- Ineffective Airway Clearance related to impaired cough secondary to artificial airway
- Altered nutrition: Less than Body Protein-Calorie Requirements related to lack of exogenous nutrients and increased metabolic demand

MEDICAL AND NURSING MANAGEMENT AND PATIENT OUTCOME

On days 6 and 7 Mr. H remained intubated and required 100% O_2 to maintain a Pao_2 of 70 mm Hg. CT was 38.4° C and WBC, 18,000/mm^3 with a shift to the left. However, blood, urine, and wound cultures were negative. Despite the aggressive administration of diuretics (furosemide and mannitol), Mr. H was oliguric and azotemic, with renal indexes consistent with acute tubular necrosis. Serum creatinine and BUN levels were approaching the need for hemodialysis. His level of consciousness was difficult to evaluate because paralytic agents and narcotics had been used to facilitate effective mechanical ventilation. Since admission, Mr. H had lost 8 pounds. His condition was highly catabolic, hyperglycemic, and in a negative nitrogen balance. Visceral protein (serum albumin, transferrin, prealbumin) levels were low despite nutritional and metabolic support. Hepatic function was altered as evidenced by elevated serum bilirubin, AST, ALT, and LDH levels; clinical jaundice was evident. Mr. H's abdomen was distended and bowel sounds were absent. He was unresponsive to all noxious stimuli and no longer required paralytics or narcotics for effective ventilation. Cardiovascular function was dependent on vasoactive drugs (dopamine at 10 µg/kg/min) to maintain a subnormal cardiac output. Mr. H's family was notified of his grave prognosis. They were angry and grief stricken.

MEDICAL DIAGNOSIS

Multiple organ dysfunction syndrome; acute respiratory, renal, and hepatic failure

NURSING DIAGNOSES

- Anticipatory Grieving related to unexpected impending loss of family member
- Altered Tissue Perfusion: Cardiopulmonary, Renal, Gastrointestinal related to systemic inflammation, hypoxemia
- Impaired Gas Exchange related to ventilation/perfusion mismatch secondary to mediator-induced pulmonary injury
- Ineffective Airway Clearance related to impaired cough secondary to artificial airway
- Altered nutrition: Less than Body Protein-Calorie Requirements related to lack of exogenous nutrients and increased metabolic demand

REFERENCES

1. Cerra FB: The multiple organ failure syndrome, *Hosp Pract* 1:69, Aug 15, 1990.
2. DeCamp MM, Demling RH: Posttraumatic multisystem organ failure, *JAMA* 260:530, 1988.
3. Knaus WA, Wagner DP: Multiple systems organ failure: epidemiology and prognosis, *Crit Care Clin* 5:221, 1989.
4. Matuschak GM: Multiple systems organ failure: clinical expression, pathogenesis, and therapy. In Hall JB, Schmidt GA, Wood LD, editors: *Principles of critical care,* New York, 1992, McGraw-Hill.
5. American College of Chest Physicians/Society of Critical Care Medicine consensus conference: Definitions for sepsis and organ failure and guidelines for the use of innovative therapies in sepsis, *Crit Care Med* 20:864, 1992.
6. Bone RC, Sprung CL, Sibbald WJ: Definitions for sepsis and organ failure, *Crit Care Med* 20:724, 1992.
7. Rote NS: Inflammation. In McCance KL, Huether SE, editors: *Pathophysiology: the biologic basis for disease in adults and children,* St Louis, 1990, Mosby–Year Book.
8. Pinsky MR: Multiple systems organ failure: malignant intravascular inflammation, *Crit Care Clin* 5:195, 1989.
9. Pinsky MR, Matuschak GM: Multiple systems organ failure: failure of host defense homeostasis, *Crit Care Clin* 5:199, 1989.
10. Bell TN: Disseminated intravascular coagulation and shock, *Crit Care Nurs Clin* 2:255, 1990.
11. Guyton AC: *Textbook of medical physiology,* ed 8, Philadelphia, 1991, WB Saunders.
12. Yurt RW, Lowry SF: Role of the macrophage and endogenous mediators in multiple organ failure. In Deitch EA, editor: *Multiple organ failure pathophysiology and basic concepts of therapy,* New York, 1990, Thieme Medical.
13. Deitch EA: Gut failure: its role in the multiple organ failure syndrome. In Deitch EA, editor: *Multiple organ failure pathophysiology and basic concepts of therapy,* New York, 1990, Thieme Medical.
14. Bishop M and others: Prospective trial of supranormal values in severely traumatized patients, *Crit Care Med* 20:S93, 1992 (abstract).
15. Cerra FB: The syndrome of hypermetabolism and multiple systems organ failure. In Hall JB, Schmidt GA, Wood LD, editors: *Principles of critical care,* New York, 1992, McGraw-Hill.
16. Waxman K: Postoperative multiple organ failure, *Crit Care Clin* 3:429, 1987.
17. Cerra FB: Hypermetabolism–organ failure syndrome: a metabolic response to injury, *Crit Care Clin* 5:289, 1989.
18. Cerra FB: Nutritional pharmacology: its role in the hypermetabolism–organ failure syndrome, *Crit Care Med* 18:S154, 1990.
19. Zimmerman JJ, Ringer TV: Inflammatory host responses in sepsis, *Crit Care Clin* 8:163, 1992.
20. Bone RC: Inhibitors of complement and neutrophils: a critical evaluation of their role in the treatment of sepsis, *Crit Care Med* 20:891, 1992.
21. Beutler B: Cachectin in tissue injury, shock, and related states, *Crit Care Clin* 5:353, 1989.
22. Damas P and others: Tumor necrosis factor and interleukin-1 serum levels during severe sepsis in human, *Crit Care Med* 17:975, 1989.
23. Demets JM and others: Plasma tumor necrosis factor and mortality in critically ill septic patients, *Crit Care Med* 17:489, 1989.
24. Nahum A, Sznajder JI: Role of free radicals in critical illness. In Hall JB, Schmidt GA, Wood LD, editors: *Principles of critical care,* New York, 1992, McGraw-Hill.
25. Bernard GR: Cyclooxygenase inhibition, *Crit Care Report* 1:193, 1990.
26. Bone RC: Phospholipids and their inhibitors: a critical evaluation of their role in the treatment of sepsis, *Crit Care Med* 20:884, 1992.
27. Petrak RA, Balk RA, Bone RC: Prostaglandins, cyclo-oxygenase inhibitors, and thromboxane synthetase inhibitors in the pathogenesis of multiple systems organ failure, *Crit Care Clin* 5:303, 1989.
28. Sprague RS and others: Proposed role of leukotrienes in the pathophysiology of multiple systems organ failure, *Crit Care Clin* 4:315, 1989.
29. van Saene HK, Stoutenbeek CC, Stoller JK: Selective decontamination of the digestive tract in the intensive care unit: current status and future prospects, *Crit Care Med* 20:691, 1992.
30. Vickers SM, Bailey RW, Bulkley GB: Ischemic hepatitis. In Marston A and others, editors: *Splanchnic ischemia and multiple organ failure,* St Louis, 1989, Mosby–Year Book.
31. Haglund UH, Arvidsson D: Acute acalculous cholecystitis. In Marston A and others, editors: *Splanchnic ischemia and multiple organ failure,* St Louis, 1989, Mosby–Year Book.
32. Gamelli RL, Silver GM: Acute renal failure. In Deitch EA, editor: *Multiple organ failure pathophysiology and basic concepts of therapy,* New York, 1990, Thieme Medical.
33. Berstern A, Sibbald WJ: Circulatory disturbances in multiple systems organ failure, *Crit Care Clin* 5:233, 1989.
34. Shoemaker WC, Kram HB, Appel PL: Therapy of shock based on pathophysiology, monitoring, and outcome prediction, *Crit Care Med* 18:S19, 1990.
35. Vincent JL, De Backer D: Initial management of circulatory shock as prevention of MSOF, *Crit Care Clin* 5:369, 1989.
36. Kumar A and others: Tumor necrosis factor produces depression of myocardial cell contraction in vitro, *Crit Care Med* 20:S52, 1992 (abstract).
37. Macho JR, Luce JM: Rational approach to the management of multiple systems organ failure, *Crit Care Clin* 5:379, 1989.
38. Sheagren JN: Mechanism-oriented therapy for multiple systems organ failure, *Crit Care Clin* 5:393, 1989.
39. Edwards JD: Use of survivors' cardiopulmonary values as therapeutic goals in septic shock, *Crit Care Med* 17(11):1098, 1989.
40. Feustel PJ and others: Oxygen delivery and consumption in head-injured and multiple trauma patients, *J Trauma* 30:30, 1990.
41. Hacksaw KV, Parker GA, Roberts JW: Naloxone in septic shock, *Crit Care Med* 18:47, 1990.

48

Burns

CHAPTER OBJECTIVES

- Differentiate full-thickness and partial-thickness burn injuries using the recommended classification criteria.
- List the American Burn Association's criteria for determining burn injuries that should be referred to a regional burn center.
- Describe emergency management of thermal, chemical, electrical, and inhalation injury.
- Develop nursing diagnoses and management approaches for the patient with burn injuries in the resuscitation, acute, and rehabilitation phases.
- Identify medical and nursing management approaches to burn wound closure.
- State common stressors in the specialty practice of burn nursing.

Some authorities estimate that 75% of all burn injuries could be prevented with reasonable caution and adherence to safety measures. The nurse can play an active role in preventing fires and burns by promoting legislation and teaching safety practices. Many programs and organizations are dedicated to the prevention of burn injury; yet 2 million Americans each year require medical attention for burns.[1] Each year, in the United States, more than 500,000 persons visit an emergency department because of burn injury. Approximately 70,000 to 100,000 are hospitalized, of whom 10,000 to 12,000 will die. Approximately 21,000 patients with burns are admitted directly or by referral to a facility with special resources dedicated to burn care.[2]

To provide comprehensive, holistic care for burn patients, close collaboration is required among members of the multidisciplinary team. This *burn team* comprises nurses, physicians, physical therapists, occupational therapists, recreational therapists, nutritionists, psychologists, social workers, family, and spiritual support staff members. The burn patient is characterized as the universal trauma model.[3] The patient's response to a major burn injury is dramatic and involves multisystem alteration. Knowledge of local and systemic changes associated with patient needs is essential, which places extraordinary demands on the nurse in burn practice who must be both a specialist and a broadly based generalist.

The purpose of this chapter is to provide a basic understanding of the complexities of burn care and the patient's response to burn injury.

ANATOMY AND FUNCTIONS OF THE SKIN

The skin is the largest organ of the human body, ranging from 0.2 m^2 in the newborn to more than 2 m^2 in the adult.[4] The integumentary system consists of two major layers: the epidermis and the dermis (Fig. 48-1).

The outermost layer of epidermis varies from 0.07 to 0.12 mm in thickness, with the deepest layer found on the soles of the feet and palms of the hand. The epidermis is composed of dead, cornified cells that act as a tough protective barrier against the environment. From the surface inward the five layers are stratum corneum, stratum lucidum, stratum granulosum, stratum spinosum, and stratum basale. The second, thicker layer, the dermis, ranges from 1 to 2 mm in thickness and lies below the epidermis. The dermis is composed of two layers: the papillary layer next to the stratum basale and the reticular layer. This layer, composed primarily of connective tissue and collagenous fiber bundles, provides nutritional support to the epidermis. The dermis contains the blood vessels, sweat and sebaceous glands, hair follicles, nerves to the skin and capillaries that nourish the avascular epidermis, and sensory fibers for pain, touch, and temperature. Mast cells in the connective tissue perform the functions of secretion, phagocytosis, and production of fibroblasts. Beneath the dermis is the hypodermis, which contains the fat, smooth muscle, and areolar tissue. The hypodermis acts as a heat insulator, shock absorber, and nutritional depot.

The skin provides functions crucial to human survival. These functions include maintenance of body temperature; barrier to evaporative water loss; metabolic activity (vitamin D production); protection against the environment through sensations of touch, pressure, and pain; overall cosmetic appearance; and other functions that remain unknown.

PATHOPHYSIOLOGY AND ETIOLOGY OF BURN INJURY

A burn is an injury resulting in tissue loss or damage. Injury to tissue can be caused by exposure to thermal, electrical, chemical, and/or radiation sources. Injury to the tissue is determined by the temperature or causticity of the burning agent and duration of tissue contact with the source.

At the cellular level the burning agent produces a dilation of the capillaries and small vessels, thus increasing the capillary permeability. Plasma seeps out into the surrounding tissue, producing blisters and edema. The type, duration, and intensity of the burn affect the amount and extent of fluid loss. This progressive fluid

Fig. 48-1 Anatomy of the skin. (From Dains JE: Integumentary system. In Thompson JM and others: *Mosby's clinical nursing,* ed 3, St Louis, 1993, Mosby–Year Book.)

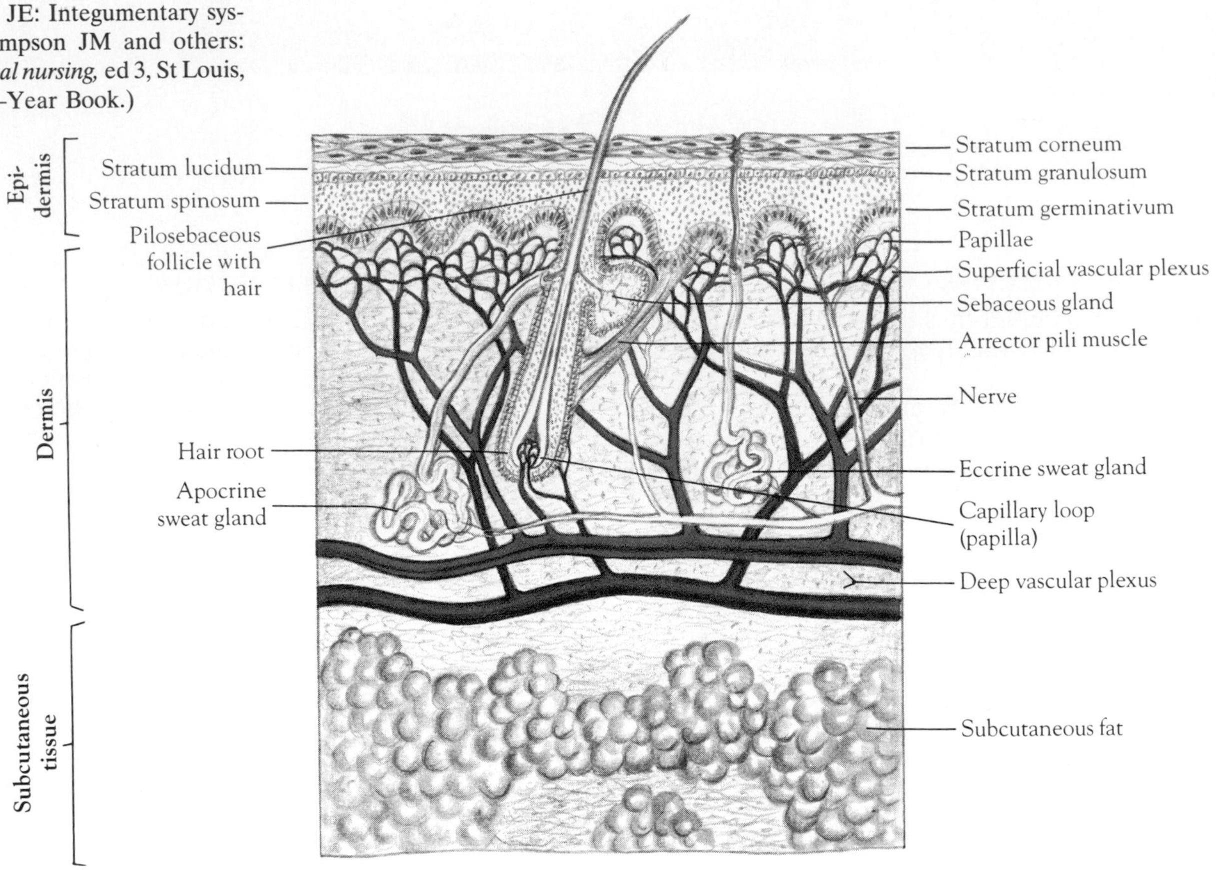

loss in major burns results in significant intravascular fluid volume deficit. The pathophysiologic response to injury is twofold. Early postinjury organ hypoperfusion develops as a result of low cardiac output, as well as increased peripheral vascular resistance because of the normal neurohormonal response to trauma. With adequate volume repletion, hemodynamic functions improve, and as plasma volume increases, cardiac output rises, which results in a hypermetabolic response and overall increase in organ perfusion.

The clinical course of a burn injury comprises three phases: the resuscitative phase, acute care phase, and the rehabilitative phase. The resuscitative phase begins with the initial hemodynamic response to injury and lasts until capillary integrity is restored and the repletion of plasma volume by fluid replacement occurs. The acute phase begins with the onset of diuresis of fluid mobilized from the interstitial space and ends with the closure of the burn wound. The rehabilitative phase often commences on the patient's admission, and correction of functional deficits and scar management are major considerations. The rehabilitative phase may last from months to years depending on the severity of injury.

CLASSIFICATION OF BURN INJURIES

Burns are classified primarily according to the size and depth of the injury. The type and location of the burn, as well as the patient's age and medical history, however, are significant considerations. Recognition of the magnitude of burn injury, which is based on the depth, size, and prior health of the host, is of crucial importance in the overall care plan.[4] Decisions concerning complete patient management are based on this assessment. Age and burn size are the cardinal determinants of survival.[5,6]

Size of Injury

Several different methods can be used to estimate the size of the burn area. A quick and easy method is the *rule of nines,* which often is used in the prehospital setting for initial triage of the burn patient (Fig. 48-2). With this method the adult body is divided into surface areas of 9%. This method is modified in infants and very small children. The head and the anterior and the posterior surfaces of the trunk are each 18%, each arm is 9%, each leg is 14%, and the perineum is 1%.

In the hospital setting the Lund and Browder method (Fig. 48-3) is the most accurate and accepted method for determining the percentage of burn. Surface area measurements are assigned to each body part in terms of the age of the patient. Therefore this method is highly recommended for use with children younger than 10 years of age because it corrects for smaller surface areas of the lower extremities. It also is used for adult burn victims because it provides additional accuracy.

Small and scattered areas of burns can be calculated with use of the principle that the palmar surface of the victim's hand represents 1% of the total body surface area (TBSA).

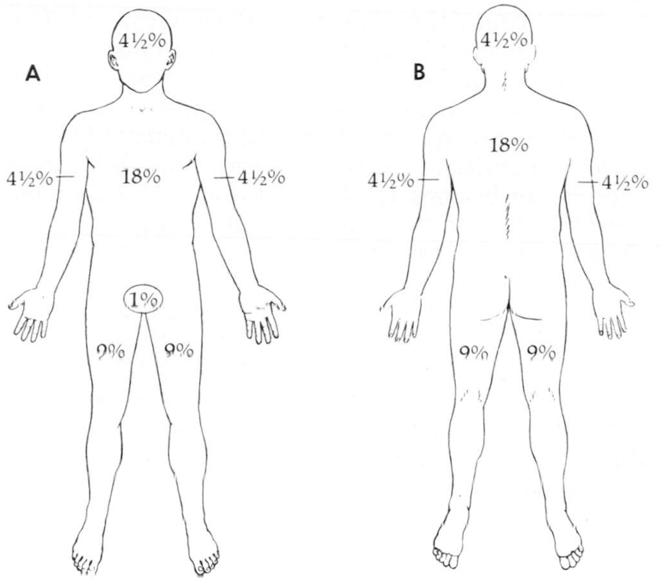

Fig. 48-2 Estimation of adult burn injury: rule of nines. **A,** Anterior view. **B,** Posterior view. (From Dains JE: Integumentary system. In Thompson JM and others: *Mosby's clinical nursing,* ed 3, St Louis, 1993, Mosby–Year Book.)

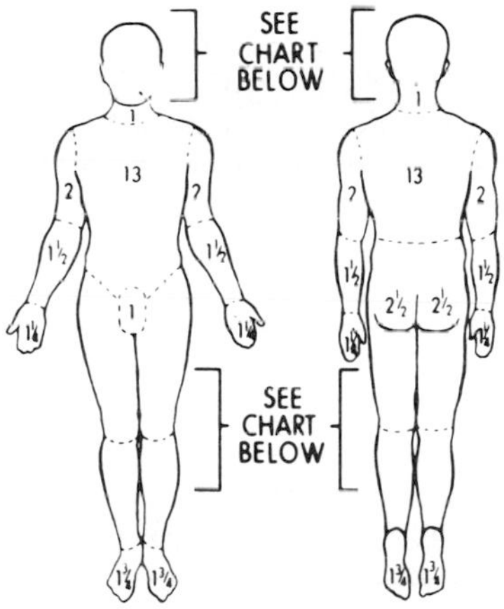

AGE: ____________
SEX: ____________
WEIGHT: ____________
HEIGHT: ____________

COLOR CODE

RED - Full
BLUE - Partial
GREEN - Available donor sites

Fig. 48-3 Lund and Browder's burn estimate diagram. (From Jacoby FG: *Nursing care of the patient with burns,* St Louis, 1976, Mosby–Year Book.)

AREA	Inf.	1-4	5-9	10-14	15	Adult	Part.	Full	Total	Donor areas
HEAD	19	17	13	11	9	7				
NECK	2	2	2	2	2	2				
ANT. TRUNK	13	13	13	13	13	13				
POST. TRUNK	13	13	13	13	13	13				
R. BUTTOCK	2½	2½	2½	2½	2½	2½				
L. BUTTOCK	2½	2½	2½	2½	2½	2½				
GENITALIA	1	1	1	1	1	1				
R.U. ARM	4	4	4	4	4	4				
L.U. ARM	4	4	4	4	4	4				
R.L. ARM	3	3	3	3	3	3				
L.L. ARM	3	3	3	3	3	3				
R. HAND	2½	2½	2½	2½	2½	2½				
L. HAND	2½	2½	2½	2½	2½	2½				
R. THIGH	5½	6½	8	8½	9	9½				
L. THIGH	5½	6½	8	8½	9	9½				
R. LEG	5	5	5½	6	6½	7				
L. LEG	5	5	5½	6	6½	7				
R. FOOT	3½	3½	3½	3½	3½	3½				
L. FOOT	3½	3½	3½	3½	3½	3½				
						TOTAL				

Berkow's method also is used to estimate burn size for infants and children because it accounts for the proportionate growth. (This method requires special charts provided by the National Burn Institute, which are not always available in local hospitals but may be at hand in a designated burn center.)

Depth of Injury

Traditionally, burn depth has been classified in degrees of injury based on the amount of injured epidermis or dermis, or both—that is, first-, second-, or third-degree burns. These terms, however, are not descriptive of the burn surface.

Currently, burns are classified as *partial thickness* and *full thickness.* This description is based on the surface appearance of the wound. Partial thickness includes first and second degree. Full thickness includes third degree. Partial-thickness burns are further classified as *superficial, moderate,* and *deep dermal partial-thickness.* Wound assessment involves recognition of the depth of injury and size of burn.

A *superficial partial-thickness burn (first degree)* involves only the first two or three of the five layers of the epidermis. Superficial partial-thickness wounds are characterized by erythema and mild discomfort. Pain, the chief symptom, usually resolves in 48 to 72 hours. Common examples of these burn injuries are sunburns and minor steam burns that occur while the person is cooking. Generally these wounds heal in 2 to 7 days and usually do not require medical intervention aside from pain relief and oral fluids.

A *moderate partial-thickness burn (second degree)* involves the upper third of the dermis. These burns usually are caused by brief contact with flames, hot liquid, or exposure to dilute chemicals. Superficial second-degree burns are characterized by light- to bright-red or mottled appearance. These wounds may appear wet and weeping, may contain bullae, and are extremely painful and sensitive to air currents. The microvessels that perfuse this area are injured, and permeability is increased, resulting in the leakage of large amounts of plasma into the interstitium. This fluid, in turn, lifts off the thin damaged epidermis, causing blister formation. Despite the loss of the entire basal layer of the epidermis, a burn of this depth will heal in 7 to 21 days. Minimal scarring can be expected to occur. Moderately deep partial-thickness wounds frequently take 4 to 6 weeks to heal.

A *deep dermal partial-thickness burn* (second degree) involves the entire epidermal layer and part of the dermis. These burns often result from contact with hot liquids, solids, and intense radiant energy. A deep dermal partial-thickness burn generally is not characterized by blister formation. Only a modest plasma surface leakage occurs because of severe impairment in blood supply. The wound surface usually is red, with white areas in deeper parts, and blanching will follow capillary refill. The appearance of the deep dermal wound changes over time. Dermal necrosis, along with surface coagulated protein, turns the wound white to yellow. These wounds have a prolonged healing time. They can heal spontaneously as the epidermal elements germinate and migrate until the epidermal surface is restored. This process of healing by epithelialization can take up to 6 weeks. Left untreated, these wounds can heal primarily with unstable epithelium, late hypertrophic scarring, and marked contracture formation. The treatment of choice is surgical excision and skin grafting. Partial-thickness injuries can become full-thickness injuries if they become infected, if blood supply is diminished, or if further trauma occurs to the site.

A *full-thickness burn (third degree)* involves destruction of all the layers of the skin down to and including the subcutaneous tissue. The subcutaneous tissue is composed of adipose tissue, includes the hair follicles and sweat glands, and is poorly vascularized. A full-thickness burn appears pale white or charred, red or brown, and leathery. At first a full-thickness burn may resemble a partial-thickness burn. The surface of the burn may be dry, and if the skin is broken, fat may be exposed. Full-thickness burns usually are painless and insensitive to palpation. All epithelial elements are destroyed; therefore the wound will not heal by reepithelialization. Wound closure of small full-thickness burns (less than a 4-cm area) can be achieved with healing by contraction. All other full-thickness wounds require skin grafting for closure. Extensive full-thickness wounds leave the patient extremely susceptible to infections, fluid and electrolyte imbalances, alterations in thermoregulation, and metabolic disturbances.

The exact depth of many burn wounds cannot be clearly defined on the first inspection. A major difficulty is distinguishing deep-dermal from full-thickness injury. Burn wounds may evolve over time and require frequent reassessment. Special consideration must always be given to the very young and elderly patient because of the thin dermal layer. Burn injuries in these age-groups may be more severe than they initially appear.

At the same time wound assessment for depth occurs, the total percentage, or total body surface area (TBSA), of the burn should be calculated by means of either the rule of nines or the Lund and Browder chart. This calculation provides the basis for determining the amount of fluid that will be required for treatment.

Zones of Injury

Thermal burns are additionally classified into three concentric zones of injury—the central zone being most severe and the peripheral zone being least damaged. The outermost zone is termed the *zone of hyperemia* and is analogous to a first-degree burn. Next to the zone of hyperemia is the zone of stasis, in which tissue perfusion is compromised. The innermost zone is the *zone of coagulation.* This zone had most direct contact with the heat source. Cellular death occurs in this zone.[7]

Types of Injury

◆ **Thermal burns.** The most common burns are thermal burns caused by steam, scalds, contact, and fire injuries. The most common age-groups involved are toddlers (2 to 4 years), for whom scalds are the most common cause, and young adults (17 to 25 years), usually male, for whom the most common cause is flammable liquid. Structural fires account for fewer than 5% of hospital admissions but are responsible for more than 45% of burn-related deaths.[4]

◆ **Electrical burns.** Electrical and lightning injuries result in 1000 deaths per year in the United States. The incidence of electrical burn injury is 17 times greater in males. Electrical burns can be caused by low-voltage (alternating) current or high-voltage (alternating or direct) current. Common situations that may increase the risk for electrical injuries include occupational exposure and accidents involving household current. Lightning causes death in approximately 25% of those injured, and permanent sequelae in about 75%.[8]

◆ **Chemical burns.** Chemical burns are caused by acids and alkalies. Alkalies frequently result in more severe injuries than do acid burns. Acids and alkali agents are found in household substances, such as drain cleaner, and occupational substances, such as liquid concrete. The concentration of the chemical agent and the duration of exposure are the key factors that determine the extent and depth of damage. Time should not be wasted in looking for specific neutralizing agents because the injury is related directly to the concentration of the chemical and the duration of the exposure; also, the heat of neutralization can extend the injury.[9] Tar and asphalt burns are serious and rather common injuries. Approximately 70% of these burns occur to the hands.

◆ **Radiation.** Burns associated with radiation exposure are uncommon injuries. Radiation burns usually are localized and indicate high radiation doses to the affected area. Radiation burns may appear identical to thermal burns. The major difference is the time between exposure and clinical manifestation—days to weeks depending on the level of the dose. Radiation injury can occur with exposure to industrial equipment, such as accelerators and cyclotrons, and equipment used for medical treatment.

Location of Injury

Location of injury can be a determinant factor in differentiating a minor burn from a major burn. According to triage criteria (see box on right), burns on the face, hands, feet, and perineum are considered major burns. These involve functional areas of the body and often require specialized intervention. Injuries to these areas can result in significant long-term morbidity, both from impaired function and altered appearance.

Patient Age and History

Age and history are significant determinants of survival. Patients considered most at risk are younger than 2 years of age and older than 65 years. History of inhalation injury, electrical burns, and all burns complicated by trauma and fractures significantly increase mortality and are considered major burns. Obtaining a past medical history is important, particularly relating to cardiac, pulmonary, and renal disorders, as well as diabetes and central nervous system disorders.

INITIAL EMERGENCY BURN MANAGEMENT

The goals of acute care of the patient with thermal injuries are to save life, minimize disability, and prepare the patient for definitive care. The burn injury may involve multiple organ systems, and the approach to the injured patient must be expeditious and methodic in identifying problems and establishing priorities of care.[10]

The resuscitation phase begins immediately after the burn insult has occurred; therefore the nurse is concerned with patient management at the scene until admission to an appropriate medical facility and preparation for care of the burn injury can occur. As with any major trauma, the first hour is crucial but the first 24 to 36 hours also are vitally important in burn patient management. This time interval has a major impact on the patient's survival and ultimate rehabilitation.

Obtaining a history of the nature of the injury is extremely valuable in management. Water heater, propane gas, grain elevator, and other types of explosions frequently throw the patient some distance and may result in concomitant orthopedic, neurologic, and/or internal trauma. It is valuable to know the specific agents involved if the burns are chemical. It also helps to know what was burned or inhaled and how long the patient was exposed to superheated air.

TRIAGE CRITERIA FOR BURN PATIENTS

Minor burn injury: can be treated initially on outpatient basis

1. Second-degree burn
   a. Less than 15% of body surface in adult
   b. Less than 10% of body surface in child
2. Third-degree burn
   a. Less than 2% of body surface

Moderate uncomplicated burn injury: usually requires hospitalization (general hospital) with experience in burn care or specialized burn treatment facility)

1. Second-degree burn
   a. 15%-20% of body surface in adult
   b. 10%-20% of body surface in child
2. Third-degree burn
   a. 2%-10% of body surface

Major burn injury: requires hospitalization in a specialized burn treatment facility

1. Second-degree burn
   a. More than 25% of body surface in adult
   b. More than 20% of body surface in child
2. Third-degree burn
   a. More than 10% of body surface
3. Smaller burns with complicating features
   a. Extremes of age: less than 5 or more than 60
   b. Burns of hands, face, perineum, feet
   c. Chronic alcoholism or drug addiction
   d. Inhalation injury
   e. Significant preexisting disease, e.g., diabetes mellitus
   f. Associated trauma
   g. Unreliable home environment for small children
   h. Child abuse

From Shires GT, *Principles of trauma care,* New York, 1985, McGraw-Hill, p 175.

Airway Management

The first priority of emergency burn care is to secure and protect the airway. For patients with facial burns or exposure to an enclosed space fire, or both, a high index of suspicion exists for inhalation injury. Carbon monoxide poisoning or intoxication is associated with high mortality at the scene. Carboxyhemoglobin levels are obtained, and oxygen therapy is continued until levels are no longer toxic. All patients with major burns or suspected inhalation injury are initially administered 100% oxygen.[10] The nurse should continue to observe the patient for clinical manifestations of impaired oxygenation, such as tachypnea, agitation, anxiety, and upper airway obstruction—for example, hoarseness, stridor, and wheezing. Endotracheal intubation may be necessary. Immobilization of the cervical spine should be maintained until full evaluation is completed in a patient with prior history. Cross-table lateral films, however, may not be possible to obtain before intubation. A detailed patient history is important, including the mechanism of injury, age, location and size of burn, type and amount of fluid already administered, known allergies, status of tetanus immunization, and significant past medical history. All rings, watches, and jewelry should be removed from injured limbs to avoid a tourniquet effect when edema occurs as a result of fluid shifts and fluid resuscitation.

Circulatory Management

At this point the extent and depth of the burn are assessed. The extent or TBSA of the burn is calculated by means of one of the formulas for estimation of fluid resuscitation requirements (Table 48-1). The Parkland formula is the most widely used. Depth is assessed according to the percentage of partial- and full-thickness wounds present. Burn shock is the result of the loss of fluid from the vascular compartment into the area of injury. Therefore the larger the percentage of burn, the greater the potential for development of shock. Lactated Ringer's solution is infused via large-bore cannula in a peripheral vein. Lactated Ringer's solution, an isotonic crystalloid, is the most popular resuscitation fluid. Lactated Ringer's solution given in large amounts can restore cardiac output toward normal in most patients. It is preferred to normal saline because it most closely matches extracellular fluid. Because isotonic salt solutions generate no difference in osmotic pressure between plasma and interstitial space, the entire extracellular space must be expanded to replace intravascular losses. The Parkland formula is as follows:

4 ml lactated Ringer's solution per body weight in kg/% BSA burn = the 24-hour fluid requirement.

In the first 8 hours after injury, half the calculated amount is administered to the patient; 25% is given in the second 8 hours and 25% in the third 8 hours. It is important to remember that calculated fluid requirements are guidelines. The quantity of crystalloid needed depends on the patient's response to treatment and is determined by monitoring the volume of urine output. Meticulous attention to detail is taken to ensure that patients are neither underresuscitated nor overresuscitated. Underresuscitation may result in inadequate organ perfusion and potential for wound conversion from partial- to full-thickness. Overresuscitation may lead to severe pulmonary edema, excessive wound edema causing a decrease in perfusion of unburned tissue in the distal portions of the extremities, or edema impeding perfusion of the zone of stasis, causing wound conversion.

Table 48-1 Formulas for fluid replacement resuscitation

	First 24 hours			Second 24 hours		
Formulas	**Electrolyte**	**Colloid**	**Glucose in water**	**Electrolyte**	**Colloid**	**Glucose in water**
ABA consensus	Lactated Ringer's solution, 2-4 ml/kg/% BSA to maintain urinary output at 30-50 ml/hr					
Brooke	Lactated Ringer's solution, 1.5 ml/kg/% burn	0.5 ml/kg/% burn	2000 ml	One half to three quarters of first 24-hr requirement	One half to three quarters of first 24-hr requirement	2000 ml
Parkland	Lactated Ringer's solution, 4 ml/kg/% burn				20%-60% of calculated plasma volume	
Hypertonic sodium solution	Volume to maintain urinary output at 30 ml/hr (fluid contains 250 mEq sodium/L)			One third of salt solution orally, up to 3500 ml limit		

Modified from Hudak C, Gallo B, Lohr T: *Critical care nursing: a holistic approach*, ed 4, Philadelphia, 1986, JB Lippincott.

Renal Management

If fluid resuscitation is inadequate, acute renal failure may occur. A Foley catheter is placed to monitor renal perfusion and effectiveness of fluid resuscitation. The nurse should measure urine output hourly. For thermal injuries, adequate urine output is 30 to 50 ml/hr.[1]

Gastrointestinal Management

Patients with burns of more than 20% BSA are prone to gastric dilation as a result of paralytic ileus. Nasogastric tubes are placed in these patients to prevent abdominal distention, emesis, and potential aspiration. This decrease in gastrointestinal function is caused by a combination of the effect of hypovolemia and the neurologic and endocrine response to injury. Gastrointestinal activity usually returns in 24 to 48 hours.

Pain Management

Pain is assessed frequently. Morphine is indicated for pain management; however, narcotics should be administered intravenously only in small doses. Changes in fluid volume and fluid shifts make the absorption of any drug given intramuscularly or subcutaneously unpredictable.

Extremity Pulse Assessment

In cases of circumferential extremity burns, arterial blood flow must be assessed frequently. Edema that develops beneath the eschar initially obstructs venous return. If this is not corrected, arterial flow will be reduced to a level resulting in ischemia, necrosis, and eventually gangrene. Early signs include numbness and pain in the extremity. When venous return is interrupted, an *escharotomy,* or surgical incision into burned tissue to relieve pressure, is indicated. The nurse assesses blood flow with an ultrasonic Doppler device.

Laboratory Assessment

Initial laboratory studies are performed: hematocrit, electrolytes, blood urea nitrogen, urinalysis, and chest roentgenogram. Special situations warrant arterial blood gas, carboxyhemoglobin, and alcohol and drug screens. An electrocardiogram (ECG) is obtained for all patients with electrical burns or preexisting cardiac problems.

Wound Care

Once the wounds have been assessed, during emergency care, topical antimicrobial therapy is not a priority. The wounds should be covered with clean, dry dressings or sheets. Every attempt should be made to keep the patient warm because of the high risk for hypothermia.

Burn Center Referral

After initial treatment and stabilization at an emergency department, referral to a burn center should be considered. By definition a burn center must be capable of delivering all therapy required, including rehabilitation, and must perform training of personnel and burn research.[4] Patients meeting the criteria for referral require the expertise of a multidisciplinary team. The United States and Canada are divided into 12 regions, each with one or more tertiary burn care centers.[11] Referring hospitals should always contact the burn center in their region.

SPECIAL MANAGEMENT CONSIDERATIONS

Inhalation Injury

Inhalation injury can occur either in the presence or the absence of cutaneous injury. Inhalation injuries are highly associated with burns sustained in a closed space. Smoke inhalation accounts for 20% to 30% of burn center admissions and 60% to 70% of burn center fatalities.[10] Inhalation injury appears in three basic forms, alone or in combination: carbon monoxide poisoning, direct heat injury, and chemical damage. In the strict sense, carbon monoxide poisoning is not an injury but an intoxication.[10] There are three distinguishable types of inhalation injury: carbon monoxide poisoning, upper airway injury, and lower airway injury. Immediate measures to save the life of the burn patient include management of the airway. The burn patient may present few, if any, signs of airway distress; however, thermal injury to the airway should be anticipated if there are facial burns, singed eyebrows and nasal hair, carbon deposits in the oropharynx, or carbonaceous sputum or if the history suggests confinement in a burning environment. Any of these findings indicate acute inhalation injury and require immediate and definitive care. To prevent the necessity of tracheostomy or cricothyrotomy, the use of early intubation and respiratory support should be considered before tracheal edema occurs.

◆ **Carbon monoxide poisoning.** Persons found dead at the scene of a fire often have little or no cutaneous thermal injury but have died of carbon monoxide poisoning. Carbon monoxide is a colorless, odorless, and tasteless gas. It binds with hemoglobin at the expense of hemoglobin's oxygen-carrying capacity, and the affinity of hemoglobin molecules for carbon monoxide is approximately 200 times that for oxygen. Carboxyhemoglobin binds poorly with oxygen, reducing the oxygen-carrying capacity of blood and causing hypoxia. The major clinical manifestations of severe carbon monoxide poisoning are related to the central nervous system and the heart. Measurement of arterial oxygen tension is of no value, because oxygen tension may be quite high in the presence of a dangerously low oxygen content of carbon monoxide–saturated hemoglobin. The most reliable treatment of carbon monoxide poisoning consists of 100% oxygen administration by a tight-fitting mask or endotracheal tube if the patient is unresponsive. Carboxyhemoglobin levels of 40% to 60% frequently produce unresponsiveness or obtundation; 15% to 40% may manifest central nervous system dysfunction of varying degrees; and less than 15% levels often are found in cigarette smokers and rarely are symptomatic.[10]

◆ **Upper airway injury.** Burns of the upper respiratory tract include those involving the pharynx, larynx, glottis, trachea, and larger bronchi. Injuries are caused either by direct heat or by chemical inflammation and necrosis.

The resuscitation phase is from immediately after injury to the onset of spontaneous diuresis, the hallmark

Except for rare events, respiratory injury is confined to the upper airway. The heat exchange capability is so efficient that most heat absorption and damage occur in the pharynx and larynx above the true vocal cords.

Heat damage often is severe enough to cause upper airway destruction, which also may cause destruction at any time during the resuscitation. Caution is taken for patients with severe hypovolemia, because supraglottic edema may be delayed until fluid resuscitation is underway. Patients should be monitored for hoarseness, stridor, audible air-flow turbulence, and the production of carbonaceous sputum.

◆ **Lower airway injury.** Heated air rarely causes lower airway injury. If it does, it usually is associated with death at the scene. Lower airway injuries also may be caused by chemical damage to mucosal surfaces. Tracheobronchitis with severe spasm and wheezing may occur in the first minutes to hours after injury. The most accurate method of documenting lower airway injury is the xenon-ventilation perfusion lung scan. Prolonged retention or asymmetry of washout of the radioisotope indicates pulmonary parenchymal injury on the side of the retained emissions.[12] Treatment is largely symptomatic. The fiberoptic bronchoscope is used both in the diagnosis and in the management of inhalation injury associated with complications. The burn surgeon diagnoses inhalation injury by bronchoscopic examination. The onset of symptoms is so unpredictable with possible smoke inhalation that patients at risk must be closely observed for at least 24 to 48 hours.

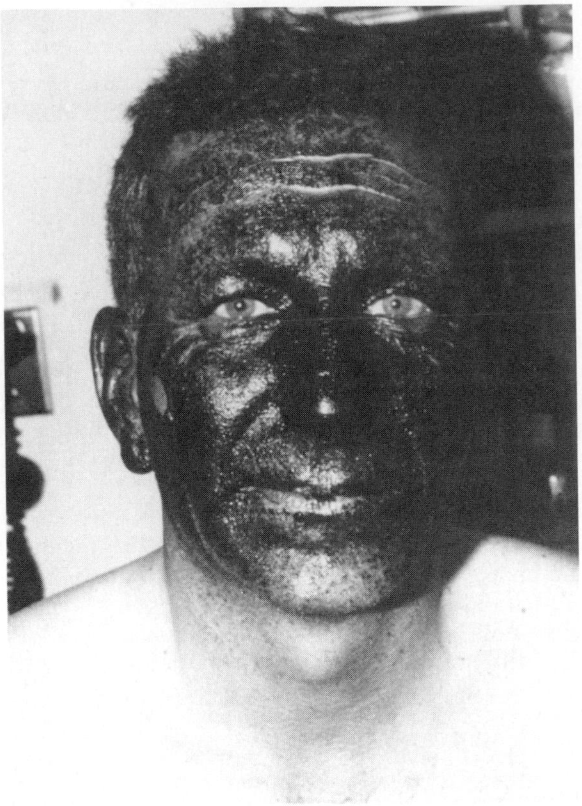

Fig. 48-4 Tar burn to the face.

Nonthermal Burns

◆ **Chemical burns.** In the past, the irrigation of acid, alkali, and organic compound burns with neutralizing solutions was recommended to limit the extent and depth of chemical burns. Neutralizing agents, however, may cause reactions that are exothermic—that is, produce heat—thereby increasing the extent and depth of the burn. It also is possible that the neutralizing agent is not immediately known nor available. Therefore the use of large amounts of water to flush the area is recommended. Alkali burns of the eyes require continuous irrigation for many hours after the injury. Once the chemical agent has been diluted, more individualized treatment can be initiated to reduce systemic absorption of the toxin.

Phenol burns are first diluted, and then the skin is wiped quickly with polyethylene glycol or vegetable oil to decrease the severity of the burn. Areas exposed to hydrofluoric acid should also be copiously irrigated with water; the burned area then can be treated with 2.5% calcium gluconate gel. The patient may need calcium gluconate replacements because the fluoride ion will precipitate serum calcium, causing hypocalcemia. White phosphorous can ignite if kept dry; therefore wounds must be covered with moist dressings.[9]

After a tar or asphalt injury, the removal of tar and asphalt is best accomplished with the use of bacitracin or Neosporin ointment. The tar should not be peeled off because of potential damage to the involved hair and skin (Fig. 48-4). According to Hill, Achauer, and Martinez,[13] there is no real advantage to early tar removal; it may result only in greater pain and discomfort. Thus patients usually find delayed removal acceptable. Daily wound care, consisting of débridement of loose skin and tar, followed by application of an antibiotic-containing emollient, is preferable. All chemical wounds are treated with appropriate topical therapy once the chemical has been diluted, neutralized, or removed.

◆ **Electrical burns.** In electrical burns, the type and voltage of the circuit, resistance, pathway of transmission through the body, and duration of contact should be considered in determining the amount of damage sustained. Frequently in these situations the rescuer also may be injured if he or she becomes part of the electrical circuit. The rescuer must disconnect the electrical source to break the circuit or must know how not to become part of the circuit. The use of appropriately insulated equipment that diverts the circuit elsewhere is essential. Extreme caution should be used in the rescue of victims.

Electricity always travels toward the ground. It travels most quickly through the circulatory system, then through nerves, muscles, the integumentary system, and finally bone. Electrical burns frequently are much more serious than their surface appearance suggests. As the electrical current passes through the body, it damages the inner tissues and may leave little evidence of a burn on the skin surface (Fig. 48-5).

A

B

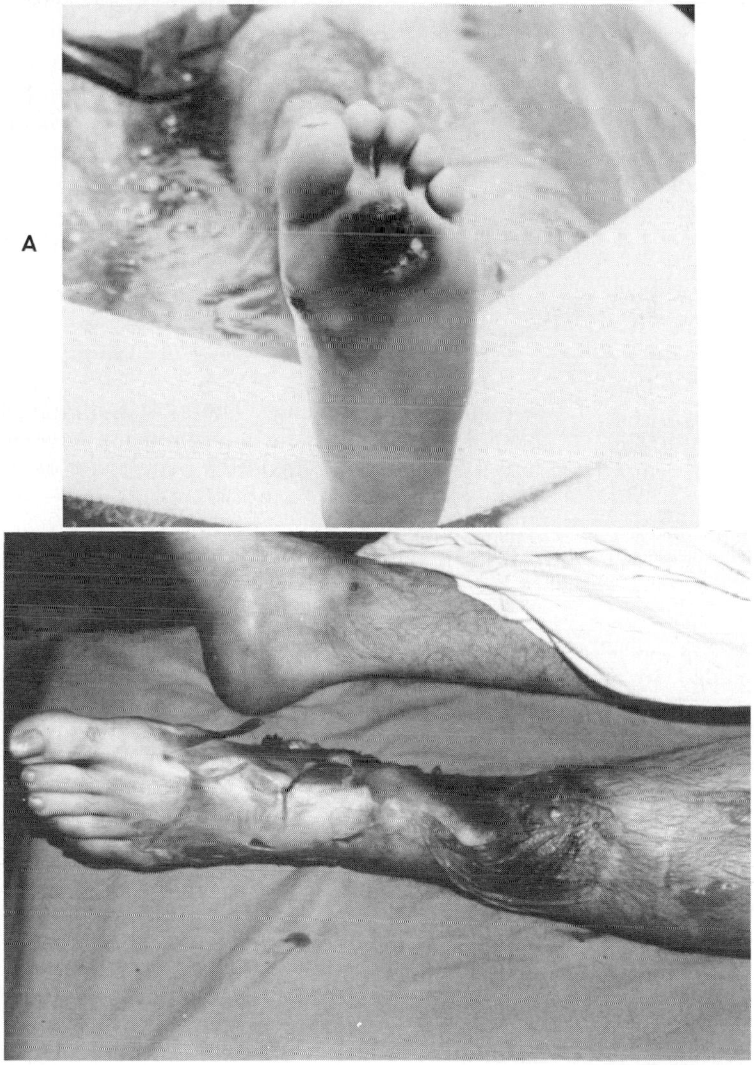

Fig. 48-5 **A,** Exit site of electrical burn on sole of foot. **B,** Same leg several days later, illustrating extension of tissue damage after the injury.

The electrical burn process can result in a profound alteration in acid-base balance and the production of myoglobinuria, which poses a serious threat to renal functioning. Fluid resuscitation does not correlate with the Parkland formula, and the fluid is adjusted according to the patient's urine output. If hemochromogen is present in the urine, a urine output of 100 to 150 ml/hr is established until the urine clears of all gross pigment. Myoglobin is a normal constituent of muscle; with extensive muscle destruction it is released into the circulatory system and filtered by the kidney. It can be highly toxic and can lead to intrinsic renal failure.

The immediate management of an electrical burn includes placement of a large-bore intravenous (IV) line and a Foley catheter to monitor kidney function. In the presence of hemoglobinuria, one must assume that myoglobinuria and acidosis are present. Sodium bicarbonate may be administered to bring the pH into normal range, to correct a documented acidosis, and/or to alkalize urine to promote myoglobin excretion. Mannitol also may be administered intravenously until the qualitative myoglobinuria disappears. A baseline ECG and cardiac enzyme levels are obtained while the patient is in the emergency department. Purdue and Hunt[14] established the following criteria for cardiac monitoring of patients:

- ◆ A history of loss of consciousness or cardiac arrest
- ◆ Documentation of cardiac dysrhythmia at the scene of the accident or in the emergency department
- ◆ Abnormal ECG findings on admission
- ◆ Large BSA burns
- ◆ Very young or elderly persons

Other patients may be admitted to unmonitored settings and observed closely. Cardiac dysrhythmias must be treated promptly, and a protocol to rule out myocardial infarction should be followed.

◆ Burn Nursing Diagnosis and Management

Management of the patient with burn injuries can be divided into three phases: resuscitation, acute care, and rehabilitation. Each phase is unique and has its own set of actual and potential problems.

that demonstrates the capillaries have regained their integrity. The major focus of the acute phase that follows is wound healing, wound closure, and prevention of infection and other complications. The rehabilitation phase overlaps the acute phase and may continue for up to 2 years after the burn injury. The rehabilitation phase focuses on support for adequate wound healing and prevention of scarring and contractures.

RESUSCITATION PHASE

The resuscitation phase, or shock phase, of burn injury is characterized by cardiopulmonary instability, life-threatening airway and breathing problems, and hypovolemia. Every organ is involved in the physiologic response that occurs with thermal injury. The magnitude of this pathophysiologic response is proportional to the extent of cutaneous injury, which is maximal when approximately 60% of the total BSA is burned.[3]

After thermal injury, a marked increase in capillary hydrostatic pressure occurs in the injured tissue early in the postinjury phase. Later, an increase in capillary permeability occurs, which returns toward normal during the latter half of the first 24 hours. A marked increase in peripheral vascular resistance, accompanied by a decrease in cardiac output, is one of the earliest manifestations of the systemic effects of thermal injury. Organ hypoperfusion develops as a result of low cardiac output and increased peripheral vascular resistance caused by the normal neurohormonal response to trauma. With adequate volume repletion, hemodynamic functions improve, and as plasma volume increases, cardiac output rises, resulting in a hyperdynamic state and overall increase in organ perfusion.

These initial changes appear to be unrelated to hypovolemia and have been attributed to neurogenic and humoral effects.[4] These alterations result in the formation of edema within the wound. This progressive loss of fluid may result in significant intravascular fluid volume deficit. With adequate volume repletion, hemodynamic performance improves, and as plasma volume increases during the second 24 hours, cardiac output increases to supernormal levels, characteristic of the hypermetabolic response to injury.

The goal of the shock phase is to maintain vital organ function and perfusion. Emergent interventions for inhalation injury, airway management, and hypovolemia are concurrently addressed.

Oxygenation Alterations

Forty to fifty years ago, burn shock accounted for most burn deaths, followed in more recent years by burn wound sepsis. Currently, inhalation injuries have emerged as the most frequent cause of death in burn patients. Three separate oxygenation complications are associated with smoke inhalation during the resuscitation phase: *carbon monoxide poisoning, upper airway obstruction,* and *chemical pneumonitis.* Early diagnosis of inhalation injuries is vital to minimize complications and to decrease the mortality rate.

The assessment of a patient for inhalation injury should include the following parameters: physical assessment, arterial blood gas analysis, carboxyhemoglobin levels, chest radiography, flexible fiberoptic bronchoscopy, xenon-133 lung scan, and pulmonary function tests.[15] Nursing actions include the following:

- ◆ Assess breath sounds, as well as the rate and quality of respirations, and document.
- ◆ Administer oxygen as prescribed.
- ◆ Monitor carboxyhemoglobin levels.
- ◆ Assess and document pulmonary secretions.
- ◆ Provide suction as needed.
- ◆ Observe for signs of airway obstruction, e.g., stridor, wheezing, hoarseness, crackles.
- ◆ Prepare for endotracheal intubation and mechanical ventilation.

◆ **Impaired gas exchange.** The most common pulmonary burn complication is carbon monoxide poisoning. Inhalation of carbon monoxide, a by-product of the incomplete combustion of carbon, results in its bonding to available hemoglobin, producing carboxyhemoglobin (HbCO), which effectively decreases oxygen saturation of hemoglobin.

Symptoms associated with carbon monoxide poisoning include headache, dizziness, nausea, vomiting, dyspnea, and confusion. In severe cases carbon monoxide poisoning may lead to myocardial ischemia and central nervous system complications caused by lowered oxygen tension and the already compromised circulatory system. The shortage of oxygen at the tissue level is worsened by a leftward shift of the oxyhemoglobin dissociation curve, reflecting a heightened affinity of carbon monoxide for the hemoglobin molecule. Early signs of carbon monoxide poisoning may include tachycardia, tachypnea, confusion, and lightheadedness. As the level of carbon monoxide rises, the patient will demonstrate cherry red skin and membranes and a decreased level of responsiveness, which may progress to unresponsiveness and respiratory failure.

The treatment of choice is high-flow oxygen administered at 100% through a nonrebreathing mask or through endotracheal intubation. The half-life of carbon monoxide in the body is 4 hours at room air (21% oxygen), 2 hours at 40% oxygen, and 60 to 80 minutes at 100% oxygen. The half-life of carbon monoxide is 30 minutes in a hyperbaric oxygen chamber at 3 times atmospheric pressure. Currently the use of hyperbaric oxygen is not recommended for most burn patients.

Chemical pneumonitis is caused by inhalation of the by-products of combustion of such substances as are present in burning cotton, aldehydes, oxides of sulfur, and nitrogen. Burning polyvinylchloride yields at least 75 potentially toxic compounds, including hydrochloric acid and carbon monoxide. Within 2 to 3 days after a burn, adult respiratory distress syndrome (ARDS) frequently develops in patients with chemical pneumonitis, with the chief manifestation being hypoxemia refractory to oxygen therapy. Early signs include increased pH, decreased partial pressure of carbon dioxide (Pco_2), and increased respiratory rate. Ventilatory support with the use of positive end-expiratory pressure (PEEP) is the treatment of choice. (See Chapter 20 for a discussion of ARDS.)

◆ **Ineffective airway clearance.** Laryngeal swelling and upper airway obstruction generally occur 4 to 6 hours after the burn injury. Endotracheal intubation should be accomplished early because this simple procedure can become extremely difficult in the presence of laryngeal edema. Generally, however, time to intervene is available after obtaining the history and transporting the patient to the primary hospital. Edema may continue to develop for 72 hours after the burn incident. An oral airway may adequately maintain airway patency but frequently is contraindicated in the awake patient. The patient who has not initially undergone intubation should be carefully monitored during this critical period.

The prediction of an upper airway obstruction is based on consideration of the following variables: extent of injury to the face and neck, the presence of blisters on or redness of the posterior pharynx, signs of singed nasal hair, increased carboxyhemoglobin levels, increased rate and decreased depth of breathing, hoarseness (which indicates a significant decrease in the diameter of the airway), increased amount of sputum, and the circumstances of the burn event (i.e., whether it occurred in an enclosed space and/or if it involved superheated gases or steam). Only steam has a heat-carrying capacity many times that of dry air and is capable of overwhelming the extremely efficient heat-dissipating capabilities of the upper airway.

Extubation should occur only if these patients can meet extubation criteria: awake level of consciousness, intact cough and gag reflexes, inspiratory effort greater than −25, vital capacity of 10 cc/kg, and decreased volume and tenacity of the sputum.[15]

Laryngospasm is another complication that, although not frequently seen, should be addressed. It generally is brought on by airway irritation secondary to inhalation of noxious agents.

◆ **Ineffective breathing pattern.** Circumferential full-thickness burns to the chest wall can lead to restriction of chest wall expansion and decreased compliance. Decreased compliance requires higher ventilatory pressures to provide the patient with oxygen. In the patient who has not undergone intubation, clinical manifestations include rapid, shallow respirations; poor chest wall excursion; and severe agitation.

Escharotomies should immediately be performed to increase compliance, leading to improved ventilation. Eschartomies are incisions made to relax the pressure and tension of the edema that is being exerted against the venous and arterial systems and, in this case, the chest wall. Only the dead eschar is incised. These incisions generally are made down the lateral sides of the chest. The wound spreads spontaneously as the edema continues to form. Electrocautery or a scalpel can be used to perform the escharotomies.

Fluid Resuscitation

As mentioned, current resuscitation protocols emphasize fluid delivery rates based on the extent of burn and the patient's weight. Therefore a weight measured in kilograms should be obtained on the patient's admission. The extent of the burn should be calculated by use of one of the methods previously described. Although several formulas exist, the Parkland formula remains the one most commonly used by burn centers around the country (see Table 48-1). Adequate tissue perfusion is ensured by achieving urine outputs of 30 to 40 ml/hr in adults.

Ideally, the capillary leak seals approximately 24 hours after the injury; therefore it is possible to give colloid without leakage of protein into the interstitium. Colloid deficits are replaced in the next 24 hours with salt-free albumin or fresh frozen plasma, at 0.3 to 0.5 ml/kg/% BSA burn. In addition, 5% dextrose solution is given to replace evaporative losses and the amount adjusted according to the patient's serum sodium level.

◆ **Fluid volume Deficit.** Tissue damage that occurs after the burn insult is complicated by the physiologic effects of the burn. Coagulation factors are affected, protein is denatured, and cellular content is ionized. These factors, coupled with the dilation of capillaries and small vessels, lead to increased capillary permeability and fluid shifts. The lymphatic system, which normally would carry away the increased interstitial fluid, may be damaged or overloaded and unable to function to its normal capacity.

In addition to the protein and electrolyte shift, there is an increased insensible water loss. In the healthy adult this loss is estimated at 35 to 50 ml/hr. The burn patient's insensible loss may be as much as 300 to 3000 ml. This increase may be related to temperature elevation, tracheostomy, and the size of the burn.

Burn shock is proportional to the extent and depth of injury. The loss of plasma begins almost immediately after the injury and reaches its peak within the first 48 hours. Fluid volume deficit must be addressed during the first 24 to 36 hours of the resuscitation phase.

NURSING DIAGNOSIS AND MANAGEMENT

Burn injury

- ◆ Impaired Gas Exchange related to ventilation/perfusion mismatch secondary to inhalation injury, p. 470
- ◆ Ineffective Airway Clearance related to excessive secretions or abnormal viscosity of mucus, p. 464
- ◆ Fluid Volume Deficit related to active plasma loss and fluid shift into interstitium secondary to burns, p. 640
- ◆ High Risk for Infection risk factors: invasive lines, immunodeficiencies, pp. 366 and 866
- ◆ Sensory/Perceptual Alterations related to sensory overload, sensory deprivation, sleep pattern disturbance, p. 573
- ◆ Body Image Disturbance related to actual change in body structure, function, or appearance, p. 94
- ◆ Powerlessness related to physical deterioration despite compliance, p. 99

Several formulas are used to guide fluid resuscitation, each with its advantages and disadvantages (see Table 48-1). They differ primarily in terms of administration, volume, and sodium content. Lactated Ringer's solution is the crystalloid solution of choice because of its physiologic similarity to the composition of extracellular fluid. In addition, it is an excellent volume expander because of its large molecules. Whichever fluid resuscitation formula is used, it is only a guideline. The actual amount of fluid given to any patient should be based on that individual's response.

Desired clinical responses to fluid resuscitation include a urinary output of 30 to 50 ml/hr, pulse rate below 120/min, blood pressure in normal to high ranges, central venous pressure less than 12 cm H_2O or a pulmonary capillary wedge pressure below 18 torr, clear lung sounds, clear sensorium, and the absence of intestinal events, such as nausea and paralytic ileus. Heart rate, blood pressure, and central venous pressure values are not always accurate or reliable predictors of successful fluid resuscitation.

Potassium and sodium, the two electrolytes of concern during the resuscitation period, should be monitored carefully until the wounds are healed. *Hyperkalemia* can occur during this phase because of the release of potassium from damaged cells, metabolic acidosis, and/or impaired renal function secondary to hemoglobinuria, myoglobinuria, or decreased renal perfusion; the patient should be assessed for its clinical manifestations. Treatment should include correction of acidosis. During the resuscitation phase, however, it is not recommended to use cation-exchange resins or intravenously administered insulin and hypertonic dextrose to transport potassium back into the cell.

Hypokalemia also can occur during the resuscitation phase because of the massive loss of fluids and electrolytes through the burn wounds or because of hemodilution. During the acute phase it may be related to hemodilution, inadequate replacement, loss associated with diuresis, diarrhea, vomiting, nasogastric drainage, long hydrotherapy sessions, and/or the shift of potassium from the intravascular space to the cell after the acidosis has been corrected. Nursing interventions include treating nausea and vomiting, limiting hydrotherapy sessions, preventing fluid volume excess, and monitoring potassium replacement.

Hyponatremia is not uncommon during the resuscitation phase because of the loss of sodium through the burn wound, the shift into interstitial space, vomiting, nasogastric drainage, diarrhea, and/or the use of hypotonic salt solutions during the early phase of resuscitation. During this phase it may be necessary to monitor serum sodium levels every 2 to 4 hours. Hyponatremia also may occur during the acute phase because of hemodilution, loss through the wound, lengthy hydrotherapy sessions, and excessive diuresis resulting from the fluid shift back into the intravascular space. Interventions should be followed for treating nausea and vomiting, hydrotherapy sessions should be limited, and consideration should be given to the intravenous replacement of sodium. During diuresis, which occurs during the acute phase, restricting free water intake usually is the only required intervention to increase the serum sodium.

High Risk for Infection

Preventing infection in the burn patient is a true challenge and involves complex decision making. There are both advantages and disadvantages to invasive and noninvasive physiologic monitoring. Monitoring of a major burn victim is multisystem and complex in nature.

There has been considerable discussion in recent years about the type of isolation precautions to use with burn patients. Studies[16,17] suggest that hand washing and the use of gowns, gloves, and masks alone are effective in controlling contamination and infection in the adult patient with burns. Significant contributors to infection are autocontamination from exogenous sources. Cross-contamination by direct contact is the most significant source of infection and subsequent cause of sepsis.[18]

Proper hand-washing technique cannot be overemphasized. Nurses should wash their hands and change gloves when moving from area to area on the same patient. For example, after changing the chest dressing, which may be contaminated with sputum from the tracheostomy, hands should be washed and gloves changed before the nurse moves to the legs. Gowns, gloves, and masks should be changed and hands washed before caring for a different patient.

Whichever precautions are used, it is vital that everyone coming in contact with the patient (including the family and visitors) be knowledgeable about the standard for infection control and that it be strictly followed by all. Precautions should have sound rationale and must not increase the workload or the frustration of the burn team. Otherwise, compliance and consistent application of the standard will not occur, thus increasing the risk of infection and sepsis for the burn patient.

Tissue Perfusion

◆ **Altered renal tissue perfusion.** Urinalysis to determine the myoglobin level should be performed early in burn care. Myoglobinuria can be detected grossly by a dark, port wine color of the urine. Myoglobin is extremely toxic to the kidneys and can cause massive tubular destruction. It is best treated with rapid fluid administration and forced diuresis with mannitol, an osmotic diuretic. The goal is an hourly urinary output that is at least double the general recommendations to flush the tubules. All other diuretics should be avoided because they will deplete the already compromised intravascular volume.

Maintaining and monitoring the renal system are vital in burn patient management. Impairment of the renal system may be related to hemoglobinuria, myoglobinuria, hypoperfusion, and hypovolemia. Urinary output should be monitored every hour for the first 48 to 72 hours, and specific gravity values should be used to determine adequacy of hydration status and renal compe-

---

*See also High Risk for Infection risk factors: invasive monitoring devices, p. 366.

tency. Urinary glucose is monitored, as are urinary sodium, creatinine, and blood urea nitrogen (BUN) levels. Use of a Foley catheter is appropriate for the first 48 to 72 hours. Because of the tremendous risk of infection related to indwelling catheters, they should be removed as soon as possible. Leaving the catheter in place may be necessary if perineal burns are involved. Oliguria usually is related to inadequate fluid resuscitation but may be associated with acute renal failure. Other signs of renal failure include increasing creatinine, BUN, phosphorus, and potassium levels; weight gain; edema; elevated blood pressure; lethargy; and confusion.

The presence of glucose in the urine causes osmotic diuresis, which does not necessarily reflect the patient's volume status and may, in fact, suggest the need for additional fluid to make up for the compensatory mechanism.

◆ **Altered cerebral tissue perfusion.** The patient's neurologic status should be assessed frequently during the first few days. Changes may be related to an associated head injury that occurred with the burn, hypoperfusion related to hypovolemia, hypoxemia associated with inadequate ventilation, carbon monoxide poisoning, and/or electrolyte imbalances. Patients with electrical burns or major thermal burns may have peripheral neurologic injuries, which may not become evident for several days after the injury. The neurologic assessment should include use of the *Glasgow Coma Scale,* detailed in Chapter 26. It is not unusual for the patient to be agitated, restless, and extremely anxious during the emergent phase of burn injury as a result of hypovolemia or the fear of disfigurement or even death. The possibility of neurologic involvement, however, should not be overlooked.

◆ **Altered peripheral tissue perfusion.** Altered peripheral tissue perfusion results from third spacing of fluid during the emergent phase, which restricts blood flow to extremities. As hypovolemia ensues, vasoconstriction increases and can be potentiated by the loss of body temperature. Peripheral tissue perfusion should be monitored carefully in all burn patients. The blood pressure, pulse, and respirations should be monitored in all burn patients. The patient's blood pressure pulse, and respirations should be monitored as previously discussed. Burned and unburned areas should be carefully assessed for warmth, color, and peripheral pulses. Capillary refill time should be less than 3 seconds. Any clinical manifestations of diminished systemic tissue perfusion should be reported immediately. Nursing actions should be taken to minimize any compromise of peripheral circulation. Fluid resuscitation must be maintained and monitored to enhance peripheral circulation. Care should be taken not to position the patient in a way that compromises blood flow, such as crossing legs, pillows under knees, or dependent positioning. If possible, limbs should be elevated to decrease the peripheral edema by enhancing venous return.

Monitoring the peripheral circulation is vital in the burn patient with circumferential full-thickness burns of the extremities. The resulting edema may severely compromise the venous system and then the arterial system. Neurovascular integrity of extremities with circumferential burns should be assessed every hour for the first 24 to 48 hours using the "six p's": *pulselessness, pallor, pain, paresthesia, paralysis,* and *poikilothermy.* The use of a Doppler flowmeter may be necessary. Loss of pulses may be a late sign. If any other changes are noted, the physician should be notified immediately. Numbness and paresthesias can occur in 30 minutes. Irreversible nerve ischemia resulting in a loss of function may begin after 12 to 24 hours.[19]

A most unfortunate scenario results when the patient's reports of ischemic pain and paresthesia in a circumferentially burned extremity go unheeded and neurovascular compromise is allowed to persist. Sensory nerve fibers become damaged and altered sensations cease, which may be misinterpreted as improvement in neurovascular status. Permanent disability and quite possibly loss of limb are eventual outcomes.

Extremities should be elevated and put through passive range-of-motion exercises to reduce edema. This, however, may not be sufficient intervention to improve circulation. An escharotomy, which is an incision into the full thickness of the eschar, may become necessary to allow the underlying tissue to expand. In deeper wounds it may be necessary to perform a fasciotomy, which involves incision of the fascia. These procedures can be performed at the bedside with use of either a scalpel or electrocautery.

◆ **Altered gastrointestinal tissue perfusion.** Paralytic ileus is a common gastrointestinal (GI) complication during resuscitation or when sepsis develops. The abdomen and the bowel sounds should be assessed every 2 hours during the initial phase and every 4 hours thereafter. If clinical manifestations of a paralytic ileus occur, all oral intake should be withheld and a nasogastric tube inserted, using low to medium suction.

A paralytic ileus can be related to hypokalemia, the sympathetic response to severe trauma, and/or decreased tissue perfusion related to hypovolemia. A stress ulcer (Curling's) may develop as a result of decreased tissue perfusion to the GI tract, a change in the quantity or quality of mucus (which has a pH of 1), and/or an increase in gastric acid secretion resulting from the stress response. Gastric acid should be maintained above pH 5 through the administration of antacids, cimetidine, or ranitidine to prevent the development of these ulcers. The patient should be carefully monitored for GI bleeding. All stools and gastric content should be tested for occult blood. The patient should be observed for epigastric discomfort or fullness, decreased blood pressure, or increased pulse.

Invasive Monitoring

The decision to use invasive techniques requires careful consideration of the potential risk factors and how the data collected will actually influence the course of treatment. Invasive monitoring certainly should be considered if treatment seems ineffective or if complicating factors occur such as severe respiratory involvement, major life-threatening injuries, head injuries, pneumothorax, or preexisting medical conditions such as chronic obstructive pulmonary disease (COPD), congestive heart failure, and renal failure.[19]

During the past 10 years invasive cardiovascular monitoring has become commonplace. This procedure includes direct measurement of central venous pressure, pulmonary artery pressure, arterial pressure, core temperature, cardiac output, systemic vascular resistance, and pulmonary vascular resistance. The use of *arterial lines* is considered if data about serial and frequent arterial blood gas values are required for respiratory management or if vasoactive drugs are being titrated. *Central venous catheters* often are required for fluid resuscitation in the early stages to deliver the massive amount of fluids required. The physician placing these catheters should consider where the burns are located and the purpose of the catheter. It is preferable not to insert these catheters through burns. It may be appropriate to use a multilumen catheter that can serve for fluid resuscitation and maintenance, antibiotic therapy, and vasoactive drugs. The risks involved include the increased chance of infection, potential for pneumothorax, and difficulty with the procedure if hypovolemia is present.

Pulmonary artery catheters should be placed only when necessary for optimal care. They may be absolutely essential to the survival of the septic patient despite the risks involved. Pulmonary artery catheters can provide data about pulmonary artery wedge pressure, cardiac output, systemic and pulmonary vascular resistance, core temperature, and oxygen saturation, all of which are discussed at length in other chapters.

These catheters require meticulous care. Strict guidelines should be established and monitored. It is highly recommended that these catheters be changed over a guidewire every 3 days and the site rotated every 6 days. All catheters should be inserted under sterile conditions, and the dressings should be changed under the same conditions.

Hypothermia

The patient with extensive burn injury is at high risk for hypothermia. Hypothermia is especially problematic during initial treatment, hydrotherapy, and immediately after surgery. Heat is lost through open burn wounds by means of evaporation and radiation. The patient's core temperature should be maintained at 99.6° to 101° F. Thermoregulation is a nursing challenge. Heat shields/lamps, hypothermia blankets, and fluid warmers can be individually or simultaneously used to maintain body temperature.

Laboratory Assessment

Laboratory assessment is another important aspect of burn care. Because of the invasive nature of drawing blood, it should be done only if absolutely indicated. Consideration should be given to the age of the patient, the size of the burn, the time since injury, and any underlying disease process.

White blood cell (WBC) counts usually are monitored for elevation as a sign of sepsis. It is not unusual, however, for the WBC count to fall below 5000/mm^3 within the 48 hours after injury. It may drop even lower—1500 to 2000 mm^3—with the use of silver sulfadiazine. If the WBC count stays in this range for more than 12 hours, the use of a different topical agent is recommended. The WBC count generally will become normal again. At this point the use of silver sulfadiazine can be tested again by applying it to a small area. If the WBC count does not drop again within 12 hours, its use can be resumed. In practice, discontinuation of silver sulfadiazine is not common but should be considered if the WBC count continues to fall.[19]

ACUTE CARE PHASE

The acute care phase of burn management begins after resuscitation and lasts until complete wound closure is achieved. The early postresuscitation phase is a period of transition from the shock phase to the hypermetabolic phase. Major cardiopulmonary and wound changes occur that substantially alter the manner of patient care from that during resuscitation. In general, cardiopulmonary stability is optimal during this period because wound inflammation and infection have not developed. Hypermetabolic changes, however, may become complicated with the onset of wound infection and sepsis. Early wound excision and skin grafting procedures, local wound care, nutritional support, and infection control characterize this phase.

Twenty-five years ago, patients with extensive burn injuries had little chance of survival. Many of those who survived the resuscitation phase of care died of infection early in the acute care phase. Today, with advances in fluid resuscitation, surgical techniques, and early diagnosis of infection, the prognosis for these patients is markedly improved. Critical care nurses play a major role in the healing process. Nurses, as skilled clinicians of the burn team, provide daily wound assessment, hydrotherapy, débridement, preoperative and postoperative management, and pain management. Appropriate treatment results in critical differences in patient care and outcomes. Immediately after injury, the body responds by initiating a series of physiologic changes to restore skin integrity. These physiologic changes include the inflammatory phase, the proliferative phase, and the maturation phase.

◆ **The inflammatory phase.** The inflammatory phase begins immediately after injury. This period is characterized by vascular changes and cellular activity. Cooper[20] explains that changes in the severed vessels occur in an attempt to wall the wound off from the external environment. Platelets, activated as a result of vessel wall injury, aggregate; blood coagulation is initiated; and in larger vessels, smooth muscle tissue contraction occurs, resulting in reduction in the diameter of the vessel lumen. These brief but important compensatory mechanisms serve to protect the entire organism from excessive blood loss and increased exposure to bacterial contamination.[20] As vasodilation occurs, there is an increase in vascular permeability and increased blood supply to the wound site. As extravascular volume increases, signs of erythema, edema, and tenderness become apparent. Granulocytes invade the wound within 24 hours and initiate the phagocytosis of necrotic tissue and bacteria. Fibroblasts migrate to the wound and multiply, producing a bed of collagen. This phase of healing lasts from the moment of injury to day 3 or 4 after the traumatic event.

◆ **The proliferative phase.** This phase of healing occurs approximately 4 to 20 days after injury. The key cell in this phase of healing, the fibroblast, rapidly synthesizes collagen. Collagen synthesis provides the needed strength for a healing wound. Epithelial cells migrate across the wound bed. Once these cells contact each other, the wound is covered. This process is known as *epithelialization.* Myofibroblasts also play a role in healing by pulling down the wound edge toward the center in an effort to close the wound; this process is known as *wound contraction.*

◆ **The maturation phase.** This phase of healing occurs from approximately 20 days after injury to longer than 1 year after injury. During this period the wound develops tensile strength as collagen deposits form scar tissue. Regardless of how well collagen realigns itself, the tissue of the wound will never regain the degree of strength or intactness inherent in uninjured tissue. Over time, scar tissue matures and becomes smaller and less bulky, and pigmentation returns.

Impaired Tissue Integrity

Management of the burn wound is the top priority after the resuscitation phase. Expedient closure of the wounds will decrease the potential for multiple complications such as fluid and electrolyte imbalances, loss of proteins and nitrogen, and infection. The major goal of burn wound care is to close the wound. Several objectives must be met for optimal wound closure: to control infection through meticulous cleansing and débridement, to promote reepithelization, and to prepare the wound for grafting. Other goals are to reduce scarring and contracture formation and to provide patient comfort with appropriate psychologic support and pharmacologic intervention.

◆ **Wound cleansing.** A variety of equally appropriate methods can be used to cleanse burn wounds, for example, sterile normal saline at the bedside or tap water in a hydrotherapy room. Generally a mild antimicrobial cleansing agent is used, such as chlorhexidine (Hibiclens) and dilute povidone-iodine. Wounds should be gently rinsed and patted dry before application of topical agents. Hydrotherapy facilitates the removal of debris and loose eschar. Daily cleansing and inspection of the wound and remaining skin integrity are performed for assessment of healing and local infection. Generally this therapy is performed once or twice daily and should last no longer than 20 or 30 minutes per session. Pain management and measures to reduce hypothermia are employed. Patients should receive adequate premedication with analgesics, narcotics, and/or sedatives. Morphine sulfate, the drug of choice, is administered subcutaneously or titrated intravenously in small doses. The patient's vital signs should be carefully monitored during this time, especially body temperature and blood pressure. Mechanical débridement with scissors and forceps can be performed during these treatments. Total immersion is not as popular as it once was. Currently, spray tables and specially designed upright and chair showers are being used. The force of the spray assists in the removal of topical agents and débridement.

◆ **Wound débridement.** Débridement has two major aims: (1) removal of tissue contaminated by foreign bodies and bacteria, thus protecting patients from invasive infection; and (2) removal of devitalized tissue. There are three types of débridement:

- ◆ Mechanical
- ◆ Enzymatic
- ◆ Surgical

Eschar is the nonviable tissue that forms after the burn injury. This tissue has no blood supply. Therefore polymorphonuclear leukocytes, antibodies, and systemic antibodies cannot reach these areas. Eschar provides an excellent medium for bacterial growth; thus it is vital that the burn wounds be cleansed daily and loose eschar débrided as necessary.

Mechanical débridement involves the use of scissors and forceps to lift gently and to trim loose, necrotic tissue. This procedure is performed by experienced professional nurses and physicians. Sterile gauze also may be used in the form of a wet-to-dry or wet-to-wet dressing to further débride the wound bed. Enzymatic débridement involves the topical application of proteolytic substances to the wound bed. These agents are useful in softening eschar and dissolving devitalized tissue. They promote the separation of eschar, which can lead to earlier wound closure. Surgical débridement employs the use of two techniques: tangential excision and fascial excision. Tangential excision involves sequentially excising the eschar down to bleeding, viable tissue and then placing a split-thickness skin graft over the wound. Fascial excision is used when the wounds are particularly deep and the fat does not appear viable. Split-thickness skin grafts are harvested at approximately twelve thousandths of an inch in thickness by means of a dermatome.[21] Improved survival has not been clearly established with early excision and grafting; however, hospital stay in patients with burns of 20% total BSA has been reduced.[22] Surgical intervention with split-thickness skin grafts often yields a better cosmetic result than does the natural healing process with deep-partial and full-thickness injuries.

This surgical débridement technique may begin as early as 3 to 5 days after the burn insult when hemodynamic stability has been achieved. It involves excision of full-thickness tissue down to freely bleeding and viable tissue. The area that has been excised is immediately grafted with autografts or temporary biologic or synthetic dressings. This procedure is not without risk because the blood loss can be significant (up to 200 ml/% of burn tissue removed). Therefore the procedures may be staged. Use of this method may require many surgical procedures spaced several days apart. Generally the wound can be covered and grafted much sooner by means of this method, thereby decreasing the potential for wound infections or sepsis.

After cleansing and mechanical or enzymatic débridement has been performed, burn wounds are managed in one of three methods. The *open method* involves leaving the burn open with only a topical agent applied. Advantages to this method are (1) the wound can be easily assessed, (2) there are no dressings that would limit range of motion, and (3) the risk of diminishing circulation is decreased. There are, however, several disadvantages to the open method, including the need for strict isolation techniques. In addition, patients may experience more discomfort with this method because of exposure of the wound to air currents and environmental temperatures.

The *semiopen method* consists of covering the wound with topical antimicrobial agents and then applying a thin layer of gauze and netting material to keep the antimicrobial agent in place.

The *closed method* of management generally consists of the application of topical agents covered with gauze or a nonadherent dressing (e.g., Adaptic, Xerform) followed by a woven gauze dressing (e.g., Kerlix) to secure it in place. Advantages to this method include (1) greater ease for patient mobility and (2) the decreased likelihood that the agent will be wiped off with movement. Disadvantages of this method include (1) the amount of nursing time required to change these dressings, (2) the inability to assess the wound directly, and (3) the increased risk of impaired peripheral circulation.

Topical Antibiotic Therapy

Burn injuries destroy the function of the skin's protective mechanism, including that of the sebaceous glands. Sebaceous glands normally secrete sebum, which contains fatty acids, including oleic acid. In addition to lubricating the skin, sebum is believed to help destroy some microorganisms, such as streptococci, and some strains of staphylococci. In addition, serum is lost from damaged capillaries, providing a rich nutritional medium for bacterial colonization. Topical antibiotic agents are used to control this colonization.

Effective antibacterial agents should control colonization so that specimens for wound biopsy reflect fewer than 10^{-4} microorganisms per gram of tissue. More microorganisms than this number make control of wound sepsis with topical antibiotics questionable. Consideration must then be given to parenteral therapy. Topical antibiotics selected should meet the following criteria: side effects should be minimal; resistant strains should not develop with use; application should be easy and rapid; and use should be relatively economical. Currently the most commonly used topical antibiotics are silver sulfadiazine (Silvadene), bacitracin ointment, 0.5% silver nitrate solution, and mafenide acetate (Sulfamylon).

Silver sulfadiazine is a broad-spectrum antimicrobial agent that has bactericidal action against many gram-negative and gram-positive bacteria. It does not penetrate eschar as readily as does mafenide acetate. Its application, however, is much more comfortable for the patient. A frequent side effect of silver sulfadiazine is leukopenia, which may develop 24 to 72 hours after application. Silver sulfadiazine is indicated for use in partial- and full-thickness wounds. Bacitracin ointment is a topical agent applied to superficial burns and facial burns; 0.5% silver nitrate is indicated for use with patients who are sensitive to sulfa drugs. It is applied two or three times daily in the form of saturated dressings. This agent does not penetrate eschar and may cause severe electrolyte imbalances. Silver nitrate possesses a broad-spectrum antimicrobial property. It ideally is used early in the postburn course before establishment of a heavy population of bacterial organisms. Mafenide acetate penetrates through burn eschar and is bacteriostatic against many gram-negative and gram-positive organisms. Its application generally is uncomfortable for the patient. It routinely is used for coverage of wounds involving anatomic areas that contain cartilage. Metabolic acidosis that results from use of mafenide acetate is not uncommon. The patient should be observed closely for hyperventilation.

Research is being conducted to determine the effectiveness of parenteral antibiotics for use as topical agents. Antibiotics being studied are aminoglycosides, cephalosporins, penicillin, colistin (Coly-Mycin), and amphotericin B (Fungizone). In one study[18] these antibiotics were applied with wet dressing, spray, or immersion; toxicity from topical solutions of parenteral antibiotics did not occur. Peaks or troughs, or both, of the aminoglycosides did not approach the low therapeutic ranges of the drugs. It is believed that much of the bolus of the topical antibiotic solution is sequestered in the burn wound eschar and an indeterminate amount is evaporated. The strength and amount of the solution required to control microorganisms within the acceptable range apparently are small enough for this to be an economically sound approach.[18]

Factors Affecting Healing of the Burn Wound

For a short period of time after injury the burn wound is sterile. If topical antimicrobial therapy is not initiated in a timely fashion, however, bacteria will contaminate the surface of the wound within 48 hours. The sources of contamination are many and include the patient's endogenous flora found on the skin, the upper respiratory tract, and the gastrointestinal tract. Exogenous flora found in the patient care setting include bacteria carried by staff members and the environment. Patient-specific factors, as distinct from local wound factors, that predispose infection include age, diabetes, steroid therapy, extreme obesity, severe malnutrition, and infections in remote sites. Because both wound healing and clinical infection are inflammatory responses, it is essential to differentiate between normal wound inflammation in the presence of colonization of microorganisms and that of invading organisms.[23] In diagnosing infection, the importance of microbiologic results must be evaluated in conjunction with clinical findings such as excessive erythema, edema, pain, and purulence. Generally, clinical findings in conjunction with burn wound biopsy results are the hallmark determinants of wound sepsis.

Autograft

An autograft is a skin graft harvested from a healthy, uninjured donor site and placed over a clean excised burn wound on the same individual to provide permanent coverage of the wound. Autografts are the only grafts that provide permanent wound coverage. Preferred sites for obtaining these grafts are thighs, back, and abdomen. Grafts, however, can be harvested from almost anywhere on the body. Surgical excision is performed to mechanically remove necrotic tissue from the burn wound. As previously discussed, excision is performed tangentially or fascially. Sheets of the patient's epidermis and a partial layer of the dermis are harvested with use of a dermatome. These grafts are referred to as *split-thickness* and can be applied to the wound bed as a sheet or in meshed form (Fig. 48-6). The split-thickness skin graft can be meshed 1½:1 in a mesher and then placed on the wound. This meshing maneuver prevents serum accumulation under the graft and permits coverage of a larger surface area than its original surface. If enough donor site skin is available, however, sheet grafts are used because of frequently improved cosmetic result.[21] Grafts that are placed on the face, neck, lower portions of the arms, and hands generally are sheet grafts. Grafts that are meshed can cover more area but may not produce the cosmetic appearance desired and therefore usually are placed on areas generally covered by clothing.

Autografting usually is performed in the operating room. The grafts can be secured with sutures, fibrin glue, or staples. Fine mesh gauze impregnated with an emollient is placed over the graft, covered with a heavy gauze dressing, and secured to the patient with or without a splint, depending on the anatomic area of the graft.[21] Great care should be taken not to disturb the graft. The dressings are removed by trained nursing professionals, routinely on postoperative day 3 for assessment. Secure graft adherence should occur in 48 to 72 hours. Autograft sites are assessed for adherence, presence of infection, and closure of interstices. Nursing management during the postoperative period includes proper positioning, splinting, and pain management.

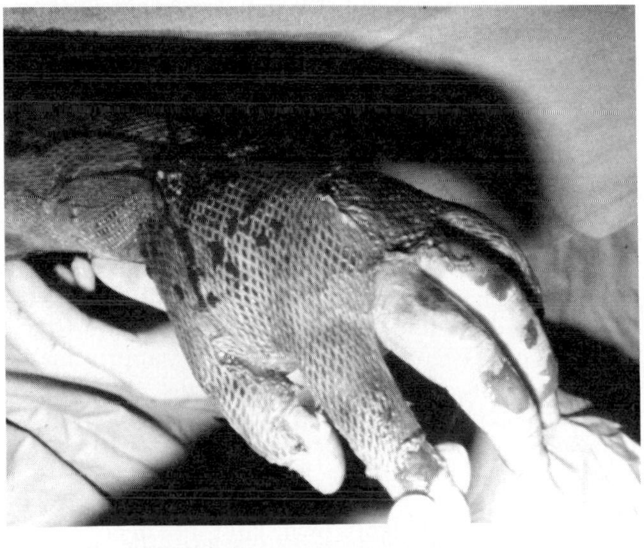

Fig. 48-6 Meshed autograft.

Care of the donor site is equally important because it represents a wound similar to that of a partial-thickness injury. Because donor sites often are selected for cosmetic reasons frequently they are limited as a result the extent of the burn injury. Donor sites can be covered with many different types of dressings. The most effective dressing is yet to be defined. Three popular donor site dressings are Biobrane, Op-Site, and DuoDerm.[21] Biobrane, which is semipermeable, is composed of a silicone rubber bonded to a fine-knit, flexible nylon fabric. Op-Site is a semipermeable polyurethane film, whereas DuoDerm is an occlusive impermeable dressing. The latter two dressings result in expedient healing with less pain. The DuoDerm dressing had been reported to heal with an average healing time of 7.4 days compared with 9 days for fine mesh gauze.[24]

Burn Wound Closure

The primary goal of burn wound management is closing the wound during the acute phase. Many methods are available to achieve this goal. Creative attempts have been initiated to establish a skin substitute that permanently closes the wound in a cosmetically acceptable fashion. Temporary skin substitutes may be used but to date do not provide permanent wound closure. These materials temporarily restore the protective barrier that the skin provides naturally. Skin substitutes can be used until the patient's own skin is available for harvesting.

Skin substitutes may be biologic or synthetic. Biologic substitutes include homograft (allograft) and heterograft (xenograft skin) techniques.

◆ Biologic skin substitutes

Homograft (allograft). Homograft skin can be obtained from live or deceased donors (cadaver skin). The homograft is harvested from cadaver skin and with advances in cryopreservation can be frozen and stored in a tissue bank. It is possible to transmit disease through the application of a homograft; therefore tissue banks must adhere to strict guidelines. Before application, homograft skin is tested for a variety of transmissible diseases, including HIV and hepatitis B surface antigens. Homograft skin can be used as a biologic dressing for débridement applied at the bedside or a temporary wound coverage on excised burn wounds. The patient's wound readily accepts the homograft. Vascular ingrowth occurs, and the homograft seals the wound and protects it from bacterial invasion; however, it is rejected approximately 2 weeks after its application. Allografts should be handled and applied very carefully. They should be placed with the shiny surface down and should be wrinkle-free. They should neither overlap each other nor lap over infected areas or uninjured areas. The grafts can be dressed with a nonadherent agent that usually is not changed for 24 to 48 hours (Fig. 48-7).

Disadvantages include the homograft's antigenicity, lack of accessibility, difficulties with storage and quality

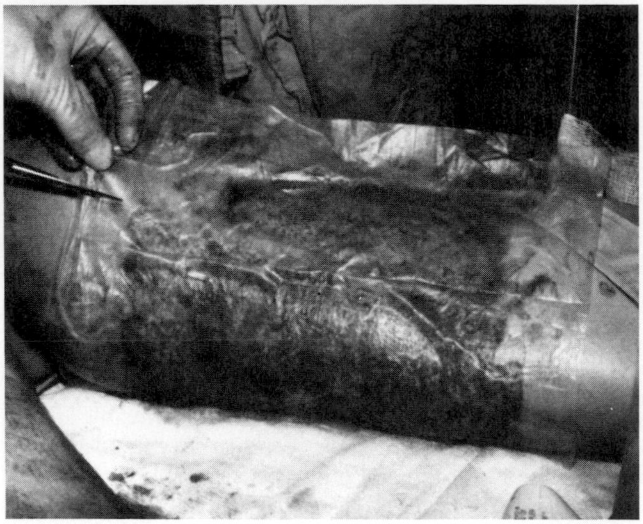

Fig. 48-7 Biosynthetic skin substitute.

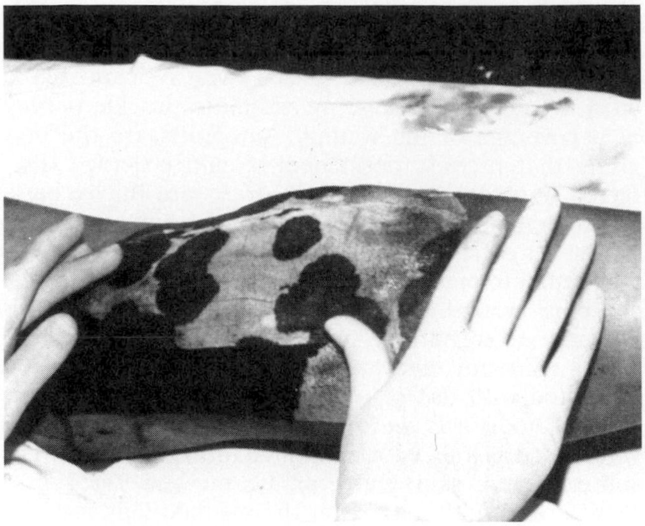

Fig. 48-8 Xenograft (pigskin).

control, expense of procurement, and possibility of disease transmission from the donor. The microbiologic cleanliness of the cadaver skin is of extreme concern because of the burn patient's debilitated immunologic condition. Allografts are harvested during the first 4 hours after death. They generally are taken from the abdomen, thighs, and back. Partial-thickness grafts are obtained, leaving the graft sites looking as if they were sunburned. These areas generally do not interfere with the presentation or appearance of the donor's body at the funeral. Allografts usually are available only in centers in which the rigorous processing procedure can be achieved. These centers usually have skin and tissue bank facilities. Procurement of the allograft is much the same as for any other donated organ. The public, however, is not nearly as well educated about this organ as it is about eyes, kidneys, and hearts.

Xenograft. The xenograft, or heterograft, is a graft transferred between two different species to provide temporary wound coverage. The most common and widely accepted xenograft is pigskin (porcine). Pigskin is available in frozen and shelf forms, with each type having a much longer storage life than does allograft. Depending on how the pigskin was prepared, it can have a shelf life of 1 month to 1 year. The pigskin is packaged in a variety of ways and in various sizes. It can be treated with silver sulfadiazine and can be meshed or nonmeshed. Pigskin can be used for temporary coverage of full- and partial-thickness wounds, burn wounds, and donor sites. It meets many of the ideal skin substitute properties mentioned previously. It has two disadvantages, however; it is antigenic, and it has the potential for digestion by the wound collagenase, possibly leading to infection.

Pigskin is applied in the same manner as allograft (Fig. 48-8). If the pigskin is frozen, it is thawed in a warm saline-solution bath. If it has been treated with silver sulfadiazine, it is thawed in water. The pigskin is placed on the wound with the dermal side down (the dermal side faces the center of the roll) and may be distinguished by its tendency to curl toward the dermal surface when held up at one end. Shelf-stored pigskin may be applied with either side to the wound. Once the pigskin is in place, it may be dressed with antibacterial-impregnated dressings or other forms of dressings. Pigskin usually is removed in 3 to 4 days. If sloughing or purulent drainage occurs, the xenograft should be removed.

◆ **Synthetic skin.** The lack of available donor sites for major burn injury often delays wound closure. In an effort to minimize infection and promote healing, many attempts have been made to develop skin substitutes that will seal the wound in a cosmetically acceptable fashion. This goal has yet to be achieved. A technique that involves the growth and subsequent graft placement of cultured epithelial autografts has become an important adjunct to treatment of burn wounds. Burke and others[25] created a synthetic dermis that has been used on full-thickness wounds but still requires a split-thickness skin graft to complete closure. Beginning with O'Connor and others[26] several researchers have used autologous epithelium grown in culture. Biopsy specimens obtained from areas of unburned skin are minced and trypsin crystallized to reduce the epithelial layers to single cells. This mixture of single cells is placed in a flask that contains growth medium. During the primary culture, which takes from 8 to 10 days, the surface area will expand to 50 to 70 times the size of the initial biopsy specimens. The cells are again separated into single cells and replated in culture medium. Between days 10 and 12, those cells become confluent and are approximately three to eight cell layers thick in the flask. These confluent sheets of cultured epithelial cells are attached to a gauze backing and placed on the wound. Epidermal cells also can be grown from cadaver skin.[27] The advantage of using allogeneic cells is that they are readily available and the patient's own skin is not needed. They differentiate into sheets composed of stratified cells 10 to 15 cells layers in thickness. The combination of epidermal cultures with a dermal substitute may be required. To date, successful wound coverage has been reported with autologous grafts alone without the need for a dermis.[28] The exact role of skin substitutes is not yet clearly defined. The role of the nurse caring for the burn patient undoubtedly involves gaining knowledge and awareness of current research trends.

Synthetic skin dressings. The use of synthetic skin substitute has gained popularity throughout the United States during the past 5 to 10 years. Synthetic skin dressings include a deluge of products currently available on the market, and they are composed of a variety of materials. These products can be characterized as nonsynthetic gauze (Scarlet Red, Xeroform), synthetic and semisynthetic polymers (Op-Site and Biobrane), and synthetic and semisynthetic hydrocolloid polymers (DuoDerm).

Each dressing has specific indications for use. Skin barrier substitutes must possess several properties to accomplish their desired effect as a temporary wound covering to protect the granulating tissue and/or to preserve a clean, viable wound surface for future autografting[29] (see box below). The most important property of these materials is adherence so that the skin substitute can simulate the function of the skin. Adherence must be uniform to prevent fluid accumulation beneath its surface, which could lead to bacterial proliferation. For application of skin substitutes, the wound must be clean and ideally have a bacterial count of less than 10^5 organisms per gram of tissue. The burn wound must be free from eschar, and hemostasis must be present. Both eschar and blood provide an excellent medium for bacterial proliferation, and the presence of blood may interfere with adherence. The surfaces should be cleaned and rinsed with saline solution, and the skin substitutes should be applied according to established procedures by means of sterile techniques.[18]

Scarlet Red and Xeroform. Scarlet Red, which is a fine mesh gauze impregnated with a blend of lanolin, olive oil, and petroleum, is used primarily over the donor sites.

IDEAL PROPERTIES OF SKIN SUBSTITUTES

- Adherence
- Minimal discomfort or pain
- Easy application and removal
- Intact bacterial barrier
- Shelf storage capability
- Inexpensive in relation to alternatives
- Nonantigenic
- Similar to normal skin in transport of water vapor
- Nontoxic
- Elastic
- Hemostatic
- Decreased protein and electrolyte loss
- Enhanced natural healing processes

It possesses many of the ideal skin substitute properties; however, it has several serious disadvantages. It causes red stains on clothing and linen and can cause discomfort related to the way the material dries, hardens, stretches, and pulls underlying skin.

Xeroform is a fine mesh gauze that contains 3% bismuth tribromphenate in a petrolatum blend. It, too, generally is used on donor sites. Xeroform has no major disadvantages and possesses many of the ideal properties. Application is easy, and it does not have the disadvantages of Scarlet Red. As the donor site heals, the edges of the Scarlet Red and Xeroform loosen and may be trimmed. These dressings should not be removed forcibly, because this would interfere with the reepithelialization process.

The disadvantages of using gauze on burn sites include delayed healing times and increased pain.

◆ **Biosynthetic dressing.** Biobrane is a semipermeable biosynthetic temporary wound dressing. It is composed of a nylon and Silastic membrane combined with a collagen derivative. It also can be used on several types of wounds, including partial- and full-thickness burns and wounds, granulating wounds, and donor sites and over split-thickness grafts.

Biobrane has many of the properties of an ideal skin substitute. It has two advantages that other skin substitutes do not share. Biosynthetic skin has elasticity in all directions and conforms well to surfaces that are difficult to dress, such as breast, joints, and axilla. Also, because of its porosity, it allows the passage of some topical antibiotics, such as silver sulfadiazine, to penetrate its membrane, reducing the bacterial count of the burn wound. Biosynthetic skin may be applied after daily cleaning at the bedside or in the operating room. It is applied with the dull or nylon mesh side facing the wound. It can be held in place with sutures, staples, Steri-Strips, or stent. If fluid accumulates under the biosynthetic skin, it may be slit and the fluid expressed. If a large amount of fluid accumulates, the biosynthetic skin should be removed and replaced. Biosynthetic skin initially adheres to the wound fibrin, which binds to the collagen and nylon backing of the material. Later the cells migrate into the nylon mesh and further bind to the wound.

Polyurethane film. Polyurethane film is a semiocclusive dressing that is impermeable to bacteria and liquid. Polyurethane film is used primarily in the coverage of donor sites, but some practitioners report using it over some partial-thickness burn wounds. Polyurethane film dressings possess many of the properties of an ideal skin substitute. Fluid collects under the dressing in large quantities. When fluid collects, it often leaks and decreases the adherence of the dressing. The fluid can be removed with a needle and syringe; however, the needle puncture must be patched with a small piece of polyurethane film. The wound exudate trapped under the dressing may provide a physiologic milieu that enhances healing.

Polyurethane film has an adhesive side that is designed to adhere to normal skin adjacent to the wound. It generally takes two persons to apply large pieces of polyurethane film because of its tendency to wrinkle and stick to itself. The dressing may be further secured with an elastic wrap or netting material.

Hydrocolloid dressings. DuoDerm is an oxygen-impermeable, occlusive, hydrocolloid dressing. It is composed of an outer layer of polyurethane foam and an inner layer of hydrocolloid polymer complex. Hydrocolloid dressings are indicated for use on donor sites and partial-thickness wounds. The dressing does not adhere to the wound bed; therefore it does not damage new epithelium and decreases pain. Numerous studies have reported that occlusive dressings provide an optimal environment for reepithelialization.[23,24] Historically, bacterial proliferation has been feared with the use of occlusive dressings. To date clinical investigations have revealed colonization but not clinical infection.

Dressings are applied to donor sites in the operating room after cleansing of partial-thickness wounds at the bedside. The adhesive side is applied to the wound bed. Disadvantages with the use of hydrocolloid dressings include large amounts of exudate, odor, and an inability to visualize the wound bed. Advantages include rapid healing times and decreased pain, and because the dressing is self-adhesive, staples are not required.

◆ **Closed burn wound care.** Two to six weeks after wound closure, a problem with the formation of tiny water blisters frequently occurs. These blisters usually open and heal without incident in 3 to 5 days. These areas should be kept clean with mild soap and should be covered with a bland ointment. For 6 to 8 weeks, a mild, nonalcohol-based skin cream should be applied every 4 hours to these areas to lubricate the skin until natural lubrication occurs. Pruritus is common in the maturing burn wound. Patients can be relieved of this discomfort by the administration of an antipruritic agent, such as diphenhydramine hydrochloride or hydroxyzine, and by the application of moisturizing creams.

Another concern in burn wound healing is the prevention or reduction of hypertrophic scarring. Its prevention or reduction depends on the timely application of uniform pressure. Hypertrophic scarring can be controlled with the use of tubular support bandages applied within 5 to 7 days after the graft. Bandages are available in a variety of sizes and have the advantage of applying pressure to selected body areas while allowing the remaining burned area to heal sufficiently. They are also readily available for immediate use during the wait for the commercial manufacture of the customized elastic pressure garment for long-term use, which can take up to 3 or 4 weeks.

Tubular support bandages apply a tension in the medium range of 10 to 20 mm Hg. Tensions lower than this do not exert adequate pressure to control scarring, and higher tensions tend to cause edema in the distal parts of the extremities and may be too abrasive to newly grafted skin. Tension can be elevated if needed by placing silicone foam under the tubular support bandages over areas such as the axilla and knees.[30]

Custom-made elastic pressure garments generally are worn for 6 months to 1 year after grafting. It is important to assess the patient for pressure points during this time as weight is gained and as children grow (Fig. 48-9). It also is necessary to assess the garment for elasticity; with many washings over time this property may be decreased.

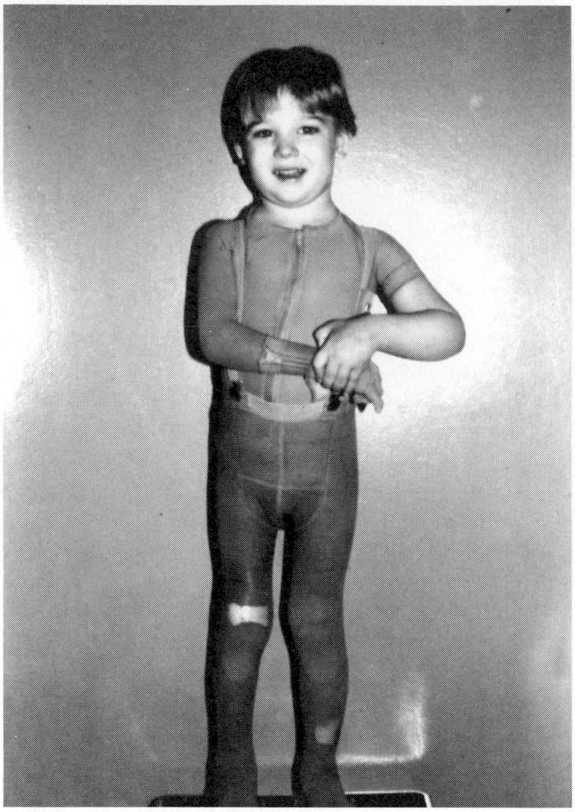

Fig. 48-9 Custom-made elastic pressure garment.

Adjunct Therapy in Burn Wound Healing

For patients with extensive posterior burns or large graft sites and those immobilized for long periods of time, providing adjunct support should be considered. Support may be the use of fluidized air therapy or controlled air suspension. Each has its advantages and disadvantages.[31]

To allow better wound healing, it is useful to reduce skin pressure as much as possible, because skin pressure is significantly less than capillary pressure. Fluidized air therapy reduces this pressure, reduces shearing force, and reduces moisture to the posterior surface through flotation and the circulation of dry air. Because of these advantages, conversion of wounds from partial thickness to full thickness is reduced, wound infections are reduced, healing time is improved, and patient comfort is enhanced.[32]

Three areas of concern must be addressed if fluidized air therapy is used. The most significant complication is dehydration, which is related to evaporation as the dry air circulates around the patient. Evaporation can increase insensible fluid loss by twice the normal amount. In the burn patient a significant loss of fluid related to the loss of skin integrity already has occurred. This complication must be carefully considered in the use of this therapy and appropriate steps taken to maintain the patient's fluid and electrolyte balance. This risk factor can be reduced by the use of a latex sheet, which decreases the dry air circulating around intact body surface areas. Contracture of the shoulders also can occur. This usually is an anterior rotation that can be avoided by the use of a foam wedge under the shoulders several times a day. Because the use of the foam decreases the advantages of the therapy, it should not be used for several hours at a time. The last concern with this therapy is that patients occasionally become confused and disoriented when they are suspended in this "weightless" state. This concern generally can be compensated by stopping or freezing the flotation of the bed. One of the significant issues involved in burn care and wound management is development of an explicit protocol and adequate education of staff members. Constant review of outcomes within the burn unit is mandatory. What works well in one unit may not in another for a multitude of reasons.

Acute Pain

Pain is an individualized and subjective phenomenon. It comprises both physiologic and psychologic aspects. Pain after burn injury is significant. Physiologic changes associated with pain include the damage or exposure of the nerve endings within a partial-thickness burn, donor sites, range of motion of the affected limbs, tightening scar tissue, and/or extensive and frequent treatments in tubs and débridement. Other pain-producing interventions include arterial punctures, chest physical therapy, injections, and use of nasogastric tubes, suction, and pressure garments. Loss of control, forced dependence, loneliness, and separation from home and family can all contribute to anxiety, which heightens the patient's perception of the pain. The patient's fears abound in thoughts of disfigurement and loss of love, function, and job. The psychologic experience or subjective component may be related to past experiences, anxiety, and altered coping mechanisms. Attention to the psychologic component of the patient's pain may lead to very useful strategies in decreasing perceived pain. If possible, how the patient has responded in the past to pain and which interventions, if any, were successful in relieving pain should be determined.

Patients with partial-thickness burns experience a great deal of discomfort. The slightest air current to the surface of the burn may stimulate pain. Covering wounds with topical agents, dressings, and linen will significantly decrease the pain.

Use of narcotics for management of pain in burn patients is controversial. Pharmacokinetics of drugs such as aminoglycosides, digitalis, phenytoin, and meperidine are altered in the burn patient. Perry and Inturrisis studied the pharmacokinetics of morphine in eight patients with burns less than 40% of BSA and at least 2 weeks old. Their findings in this limited sample showed that burn patients could eliminate morphine normally and could receive effective pain relief when plasma concentration was sufficient. However, the effects on the respiratory system, fear of iatrogenic addiction, the pharmacokinetics of patients immediately after burn injury, and the influence of the size of the burn are causes of concern.

Narcotics and other sedatives should be administered intravenously. Intramuscular injections should not be used until hemodynamic stability and adequate tissue perfusion have been achieved.

Nonpharmacologic techniques, such as imagery, hypnosis, distraction, and methods adapted from some of the popular childbirth techniques, can be effective in reducing anxiety and the pain experience. Giving the patient some management control also can reduce the anxiety and the pain experience. The perception of pain often is increased in the patient who is anxious and lacks control of the situation. A study[34] was performed to determine if interrupted débridement would decrease the pain experienced during daily tub treatments. Patients could suspend débridement for 15 seconds each minute. It was predicted that this increased sense of control would decrease anxiety and thereby diminish the pain experience. It was found that having a choice in the method of débridement did make a difference in the patient's pain experience. It also was found that during continuous débridement, nurses were not conscious of the patient's continuous pain; during continuous débridement procedures there was no correlation between the patient's and nurse's ratings of distress and pain. During the interrupted procedures high positive correlations were found between the ratings by nurses and patients. In the continuous procedures, nurses consistently underestimated the pain, anxiety, and distress of the patient, perhaps because of their intense concentration on the physical task at hand. Nurses involved in the interrupted procedures, however, were much more aware of patients' pain and their reaction.[35]

Altered Nutrition: Less Than Body Requirements

The basic metabolic rate of a burn patient may be elevated 40% to 100% above the normal rate, depending on the amount of BSA involved. The metabolic rate is influenced by the amount of protein and albumin lost through the wounds, the catabolic response associated with stress and other associated injuries, fluid loss, fever, infection, immobility, gender, and the height and weight of the patient before the injury.[36] The goal in nutritional management of the burn patient is to provide adequate calories to prevent starvation and to enhance wound healing. To achieve this goal, nutritional support is imperative and the reduction of energy demand also is vital. Every effort should be made to reduce the release of catecholamines, which increase metabolic rate (see Chapter 50). Release of catecholamine stores is stimulated by pain, fear, anxiety, and cold. Appropriate interventions for each of these stimuli should be performed.

The use of enteral and oral routes is preferred in the management of burn patients. Caloric requirements should be calculated on the basis of the size of the burn; the age, height, and weight of the patient; and the stress factors. Protein and caloric requirements of each patient are highly individualized and should be assessed on a daily basis. The daily protein requirement for the burn patient is elevated in light of a negative nitrogen balance. The daily protein requirement may increase to 2 to 4 times the normal 0.8 g/kg of body weight. Carbohydrates and fat are used for energy and to spare proteins required for wound healing. Daily caloric intake can be 2 to 20 times higher than normal. Vitamins and minerals generally are given in doses higher than normal. Serum iron, zinc, calcium, phosphate, and potassium values should all be monitored and supplements given as indicated.

REHABILITATION PHASE

This rehabilitation phase is one of recuperation and healing, both physically and emotionally. The patient is not acutely ill but may or may not be ready for discharge. This phase can last several years. The patient may require extensive reconstructive surgery. Psychologically, the patient focuses on attaining specific personal goals related to achieving as much preburn function as possible.[33] Minor and major accomplishments should be praised. This phase is characterized by scar management techniques and by physical and occupational therapy. The burn team and the patient prepare the patient for the transition to the outside world. The use of group therapy is a valuable tool used at many burn centers. Patients, family members, and health care providers express ideas and feelings. Many times the burn patients establish priorities and make realistic decisions about their lives. Staff intervention during this phase is primarily one of support.

Impaired Physical Mobility

Tremendous advances have been made in the physical care of the burn patient over the past 10 to 15 years. The survival rate of patients with full-thickness burns greater than 40% of total BSA has increased significantly. Currently, survival of patients with burns greater than 90% is not impossible. As patients with larger and deeper burns survive, the challenge to maintain their optimal mobility and cosmetic appearance has met with increased success. It is imperative that rehabilitation needs are addressed early in burn care. Nursing prescriptions for range-of-motion exercises, positioning, splinting, ambulation, and activities of daily living are initiated within the first 48 hours of hospitalization.

Contracture may develop after a burn injury because of a variety of factors: the extent, depth, location, and configuration of the burn; the position of comfort the patient most frequently assumes; the relative underlying muscle strength; and the patient's motivation and compliance. Positioning the affected body parts in *antideformity positions* is vital. Frequent change of position also is important and may need to be performed as frequently as every hour. Burn patients are at greater risk for the development of pressure sores than the general hospital population, as well as the possible conversion of their partial-thickness burns to full-thickness burns.

Splints can be used to prevent and/or correct contracture or to immobilize joints after grafting (Fig. 48-10). If splints are used, they should be checked daily for proper fit and effectiveness. Splints used to immobilize body parts after grafting should be left on at all times except to assess the graft site for pressure points every shift. Splints to correct severe contracture may be off for 2 hours per shift to allow burn care and range-of-motion exercises. Mild contracture may be in splints for 4 hours and out for 4 hours to promote exercise and mobility.[36]

Active exercise should be encouraged and is preferred, although active-assisted or gentle-passive exercise also may be an important part of the rehabilitation program. Active exercise maintains muscle mass, aids in restoring protein structures within the muscle tissue, aids in venous and lymphatic return, and reduces the risk of pulmonary embolus and deep vein thrombosis. Patient tolerance should be carefully evaluated. The number of repetitions should be proportional to the degree of anticipated contracture and the patient's tolerance. Anticipation of the patient's pain also should be carefully considered. Before range-of-motion exercises and activities of daily living are performed, the need for pain medication should be assessed.

Outpatient Burn Care

Outpatient burn care should be considered for minor burns. It is cost effective and removes the potential for a wound infection from endemic, drug-resistant microorganisms within the hospital environment. The hospital environment also changes many of the self-care routines, such as diet, family contact, hygiene, and coping mechanisms. Patients considered for outpatient burn care, however, should be well screened. Nursing evaluation of the patient or family, or both, includes consideration of motivation, willingness to participate in care, ability to

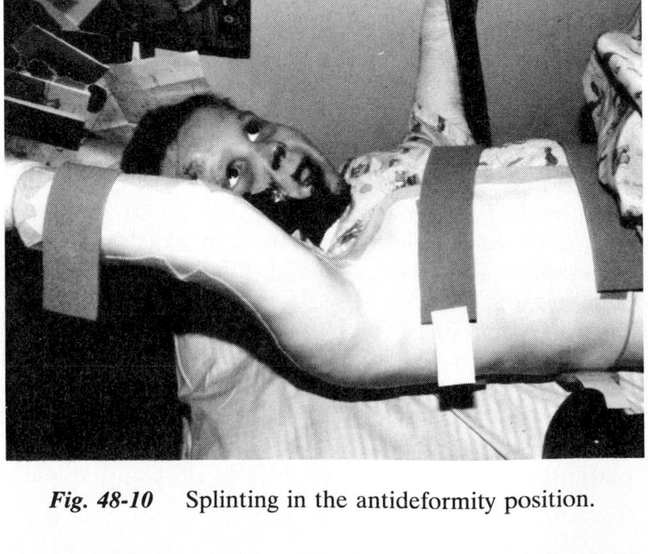

Fig. 48-10 Splinting in the antideformity position.

understand and perform the necessary procedures, potential aversions to wound care or dressing changes, and reliability of transportation. Medical considerations include hemodynamic stabilization, nutritional status, fluid and electrolyte balance, adequate pain control, and ruling out any complications.

In general, small burns should be washed daily with a mild soap and water, and a bland ointment and/or synthetic antimicrobial agent can be applied and held in place with dressings. Initially these wounds should be followed daily and then on a weekly basis until the wound begins to reepithelialize. Generally, if epithelialization of these wounds has not occurred in 2 to 3 weeks, use of primary excision and grafting should be considered.

To check for evidence of scarring, partial-thickness injuries should be followed until the epithelialization has occurred. If scarring occurs, compression dressings should be fitted and worn until the wound becomes quiescent, which requires 12 to 18 months.

STRESSORS OF BURN NURSING

Burn units are fascinating environments in which to work. They offer the fast-paced, high-technology atmosphere of any critical care setting, the complexity of advanced nursing management, and the dynamics of an interdisciplinary, collaborative model of practice. All these elements combined, however, contribute to a potentially stressful work environment for the nurse. The physical environment can be a difficult one in which to work for a variety of reasons. The amount of equipment necessary to maintain the patient can be overwhelming and can limit the work space dramatically. The temperature of the room generally is kept at approximately 85° F and can get much warmer, depending on the amount of equipment in the room. Odors vary and can be very unpleasant. Noise levels within a unit also are distressing. These variables exact a physical toll on nursing staff members.

In addition, there are patient care complexities unique to burn nursing. The daily tub treatments and dressing changes are extremely stressful for both the nurse and the patient. The nursing management of patients' pain is a complex issue in burn care and is one that contributes significantly to the stress level of nurses who specialize in burn injuries. The psychodynamics associated with the patient's burn injury experience are just that—*dynamic*—and require constant, high-level nursing assessment and intervention.

The decision to specialize in burn nursing is a meaningful one, an important one; this decision, however, also must be an informed one. For an excellent discussion of the nature of stress in critical care nursing and specific stress management strategies, see Chapter 6. Self-care and care of other nurses are just as important issues as the care of the patient and his or her significant other.

REFERENCES

1. Nebraska Burn Institute: *Advanced burn life support (ABLS) course* (first rev), Lincoln, 1990, Nebraska Burn Institute.
2. American Burn Association: Hospital and prehospital resources for optimal care of patients with burn injury: guidelines for development and operation of burn centers, *J Burn Care Rehabil* 11:97, 1990.
3. Pruitt BA Jr: The universal trauma model, *Bull Am Coll Surg* 70:2, 1985.
4. Demling RH, LaLonde C: *Burn trauma,* ed 9, New York, 1989, Thieme Medical Publishers.
5. Feller I, Crane KL, Flanders S: Baseline data on the mortality of burn patients, *QRB* 5.4, 1979.
6. Feller I, Jones CA: The National Burn Information Exchange, *Surg Clin North Am* 67:167, 1987.
7. Moncrief JA: The body's response to heat. In Artz CP, Moncrief JA, Pruitt BA Jr, editors: *Burns: a team approach,* Philadelphia, 1979, WB Saunders.
8. Finkelstein JL and others: Management of electrical injuries, *Inf Surg,* p 43, Oct 1990.
9. Madden MR and others: The acute management and surgical treatment of the burned patient. I. *Surg Rounds,* June 1990.
10. Madden MR, Finkelstein JL, Goodwin CW Jr: Respiratory care of the burn patient, *Clin Plast Surg* 13(1):29, 1986.
11. Pruitt BA Jr, Mason AD Jr, Goodwin CW Jr: Epidemiology of burn injury and demography of burn care facilities, *Probl Gen Surg* 7:235, 1990.
12. Agee RN and others: Use of 133-xenon in early diagnosis of inhalation injury, *J Trauma* 16:218, 1976.
13. Hill ME, Achauer BM, Martinez S: Tar and asphalt burns, *J Burn Care Rehabil* 5:271, 1984.
14. Perdue GF, Hunt HL: Electrocardiographic monitoring after electrical injury: necessity or luxury, *J Trauma* 26:166, 1986.
15. Desai MH: Inhalation injuries in burn victims, *Crit Care Q* 7:1, 1984.
16. Jacoby F: Care of the massive burn wound, *Crit Care* 7:44, 1984.
17. Kealey CP and others: Cytomegalovirus infection in burn patients, *J Burn Care Rehabil* 8(6):543, 1987.
18. Mangus DJ and others: Quantitative evaluation and laboratory studies of topical antibiotic therapy in burns, *J Burn Care Rehabil* 6:39, 1985.
19. Moore S, Marvin JA: Monitoring the burn patient. In Boseick JA, editor: *The art and science of burn care,* Rockville, Mass, 1987, Aspen.
20. Cooper D: Optimizing wound healing. A practice within nursing domain, *Nurs Clin North Am* 25(1):165, 1990.
21. Madden MR and others: The acute management and surgical treatment of the burned patient. II. *Surg Rounds,* July 1990.
22. Curreri PA and others: Burn injury: analysis of survival and hospitalization time for 937 patients, *Am Surg* 192:472, 1980.
23. Hutchinson JJ, McGuckin M: Occlusive dressing: a microbiologic and clinical review, *Am J Infect Control* 18(4):257, 1990.
24. Madden MR and others: Comparison of an occlusive and semiocclusive dressing and the effect of the wound exudate upon keratinocyte proliferation, *J Trauma* 29(7):924, 1989.
25. Burke JF and others: Successful use of a physiologically acceptable artificial skin, *Ann Surg* 194:413, 1981.
26. O'Conner NG and others: Grafting of burns with cultured epithelium prepared from autologous epidermal cells, *Lancet* 1:75, 1981.
27. Madden MR and others: Grafting of cultured allogeneic epidermis on second- and third-degree burn wounds on 26 patients, *J Trauma* 26(11):955, 1986.

28. Compton CC and others: Skin regenerated from cultured epithelial autografts from six days to five years after grafting: a light electron microscope and immunohistochemical study, *Lab Invest* 60(5):600, 1989.
29. Nowicki CR, Springer CK: Temporary skin substitutes for burn patients: a nursing perspective, *J Burn Care Rehabil* 9:209, 1988.
30. Judge JC, May R, Declement FA: Control of hypertrophic scarring in burn patients using tubular support bandages, *J Burn Care Rehabil* 5:221, 1984.
31. Peltier GL, Poppe SR, Twomey JA: Controlled air suspension: an advantage in burn care, *J Burn Care Rehabil* 8:558, 1987.
32. Scheulen JJ, Munster AM: Clinitron air-fluidized support: an adjunct to burn care, *J Burn Care Rehabil* 4:271, 1983.
33. Watkins PN, Cook EL, May SR: A method for facilitating psychological recovery of burn victims, *J Burn Care Rehabil* 9:376, 1986.
34. Powers PS and others: Interrupted debridement, *J Burn Care Rehabil* 5:398, 1985.
35. Schane J, Goede M, Silverstein P: Comparison of energy expenditure measurement techniques in severely burned patients, *J Burn Care Rehabil* 8:366, 1987.
36. Nadel E, Kozerefski PM: Rehabilitation of the critically iil burn patient, *Crit Care Q* 7:19, 1984.

49

Transplantation

CHAPTER OBJECTIVES

- Discuss the specialized cells of the immune system as they relate to organ transplantation.
- Explain the mode of action of the major immunosuppressive drugs used to prevent organ rejection.
- Describe the selection criteria, surgical procedures, major postoperative complications, and long-term outcomes for recipients of heart transplant, heart-lung transplant, single-lung transplant, liver transplant, kidney transplant, and pancreas transplant.

Major advances in transplantation have been achieved since the first cadaver organ transplants in the 1960s. Today transplantation has become an accepted form of therapy for end-stage organ failure. The field of transplantation is highly specialized and requires expert teams of surgeons, immunologists, and medical and nurse specialists to achieve successful outcomes.

Many problems are yet to be solved in the field of transplantation. Organs are a scarce commodity, and a lack of available organs restricts the availability of transplantation for many individuals. Safe and efficacious control of the immune system remains elusive. Rejection and infection as a result of immunosuppression persist as the major causes of death in recipients. Chronic rejection is still not well understood. This type of rejection results in eventual graft failure and limits long-term survival in many types of organ recipients.

This chapter overviews the specialized areas of solid organ transplantation, the immune system, and current therapies to prevent rejection.

IMMUNOLOGY OF TRANSPLANT REJECTION

Organ transplantation has become a commonly practiced procedure for end-stage cardiac, pulmonary, hepatic, renal, and pancreatic disease. Major advances have been made in organ procurement and preservation, surgical techniques, and identifying and treating rejection. The ultimate long-term success of any organ transplant depends on the immune system's tolerance of the transplanted graft. Virtually every body cell carries distinctive molecules that enable the immune system to distinguish self from non-self. When non-self is recognized, a normally functioning immune system is designed to eliminate the foreign invader. Tolerance of the transplanted organ can be achieved only by suppressing or regulating this normal immune response to the foreign organ.

To understand the principles of immunosuppressive therapy, it is important to have some understanding of the cells of the immune system, the immune response, and the process of organ rejection.

Immune Mechanism

Whenever the body is confronted with any substance that is non-self, a primary immune response is elicited. There are three phases to each *primary* immune response: (1) recognition of the substance as non-self, (2) proliferation of immunocompetent cells, and (3) the effector phase or action against the foreign substance.[1] During this primary response, immunologic memory is established and any subsequent encounter with the same substance will provide a more rapid and intense immune response. Subsequent encounters are termed *secondary immune responses.*

An antigen is a substance that is capable of eliciting an immune response. Each cell has antigens on its surface that are genetically predetermined by a series of linked genes known as the *major histocompatibility complex* (MHC).[2] If tissue from one person is transplanted into a genetically different person, the antigens on the transplanted tissue cells are immediately recognized as non-self and rejection occurs. MHC determines the antigens to which the immune system should respond. The human MHC is called *human leukocyte antigen* (HLA) because these markers were first discovered on lymphocytes. The HLA gene complex is located on chromosome number 6. Each chromosome contains four loci: HLA-A, -B, -C, and -D. More than 150 antigens have been recognized in the HLA system: 23 on the A locus, 52 on the B locus, 11 on the C locus, and 61 on the D locus.[2] Because a potential for millions of different arrangements of these antigens exists, the chances of finding a donor organ with the same histocompatibility genes as a recipient are virtually impossible unless donor and recipient are identical twins.

HLA antigens are divided into three classes of antigens. Class I antigens are present on almost all body cells and are thus the markers of self. The class II antigens are present on B lymphocytes, macrophages, and other cells responsible for presenting foreign antigen to the immune system and inducing the immune response. Class III antigens include some red blood cell antigens and complement.

Cells of the Immune System

The immune system houses a vast number of cells responsible for general defense and very specific immune responses. Only a few cells of each specificity are stored. When a specific antigen appears, those few cells are stimulated to multiply and mount a response to the foreign antigen. Immune cells are originally produced in the bone marrow as stem cells. Their descendants become either lymphocytes or phagocytes (Fig. 49-1).

There are two major classes of lymphocytes: B cells and T cells. B cells remain in the bone marrow to complete their maturation. The T cells migrate to the thymus gland where they mature. In the thymus, T cells acquire the ability to distinguish self from non-self. Once mature, some B and T cells will be housed in the lymph nodes while others circulate in the blood and lymph system.

Humoral immunity is mediated by B cells. They are responsible for the production of antibody or immunoglobulin. When a B cell encounters an antigen to which it is specifically coded to respond, the B cell enlarges, divides, and differentiates into a plasma cell. It is the plasma cell that actually produces and secretes antigen-specific antibody (Fig. 49-2). Once exposed to an antigen, the immune system retains a memory of that antigen. Subsequent exposure stimulates the B cell memory cells, resulting in a rapid mobilization of antibody-secreting cells. Antibodies work in several ways, but their primary purpose is to mark an antigen for destruction by the immune system. Other antibodies are capable of neutralizing toxins produced by bacteria or can trigger the release of serum proteins known as *complement.*

Cell-mediated immunity is determined by T cells that are specifically sensitized. Approximately 65% to 80% of all lymphocytes are T cells, of which there are three basic types.

Cytotoxic T cells are cells capable of killing invading cells. Their primary role is to rid the body of cells that have become infected, transformed by cancer, or are non-self, as in the case of transplanted tissue. They also are called *T8* or *CD8 lymphocytes,* referring to a marker that distinguishes cytotoxic T cells from other T cells. Cytotoxic T cells are activated by macrophages that present the foreign antigen to immature cytotoxic T cells. With the assistance of the helper T cell and its release of chemical mediators, the cytotoxic T cell matures and kills foreign cells that carry that specific antigen (Fig. 49-3).

Helper T cells up-regulate the immune response by stimulating B cells to differentiate into plasma cells and begin antibody production, by activating cytotoxic T cells, and by stimulating natural killer cells and macrophages. Helper T cells are identified by their T4 or CD4 marker. Fig. 49-4 illustrates the process responsible for activating helper T cells. Macrophages are responsible for presenting processed antigen to the immature helper T cells. With the assistance of chemical mediators released by the macrophage, the helper T cell matures and begins to activate other cells of the immune system previously described.

A third type of T cell is the suppressor T cell. These cells suppress or down-regulate the immune response. They play an important role in keeping the immune response controlled and in turning off the response once the antigenic threat is no longer present.

Natural killer cells represent another type of lymphocyte. These cells are not targeted for any specific antigen but will attack and destroy any cell that is identified as non-self. Natural killer cells contain granules filled with

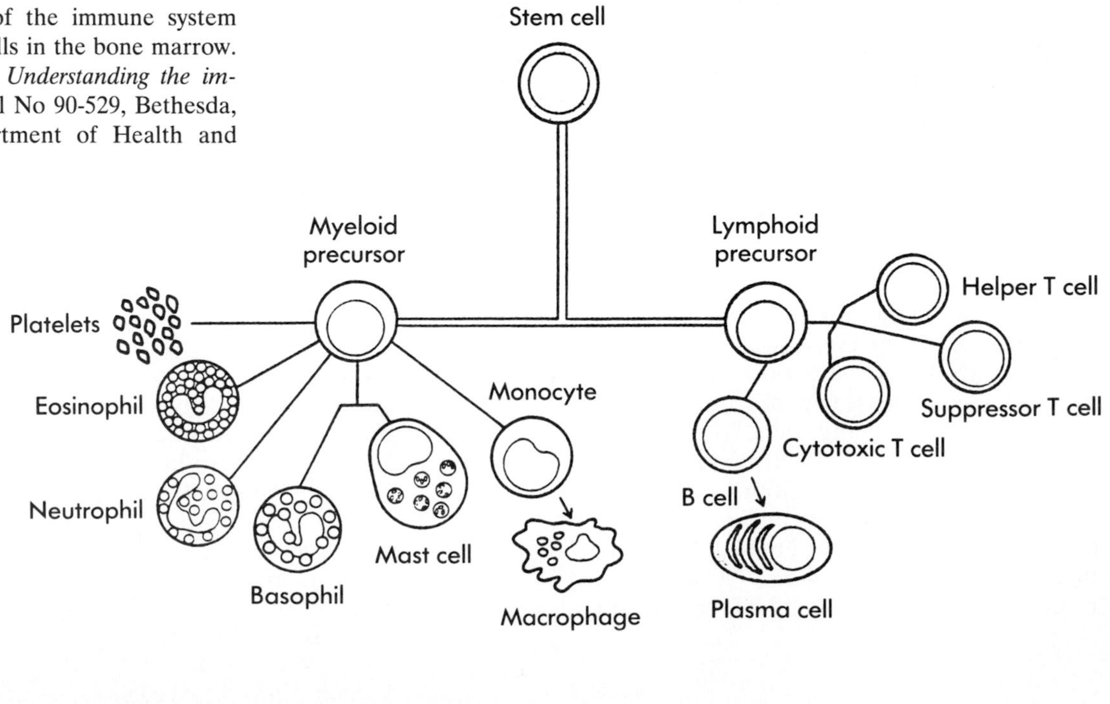

Fig. 49-1 All cells of the immune system originate from stem cells in the bone marrow. (From Schindler LW: *Understanding the immune system,* NIH Publ No 90-529, Bethesda, Md, 1990, US Department of Health and Human Services, p 5.)

potent chemicals that are released when the natural killer cell binds to the targeted non-self cell. These chemicals are capable of lysing the cell membrane and causing the cell's death.

Phagocytes are a major category of immune cells capable of destroying alien cells. Critical phagocytes include monocytes, macrophages, neutrophils, eosinophils, and basophils. Table 49-1 outlines the primary function of these cells. Macrophages are vitally important to the immune response because of their role in "presenting" the antigen to the helper and cytotoxic T cells. This presentation alerts the T cells to the presence of antigen. Macrophages also produce chemical regulators that stimulate the maturation of helper and cytotoxic T cells.

As just described, chemical substances are released by macrophages, helper T cells, and cytotoxic T cells, which allows these immune cells to communicate with each other. These substances provide a network of soluble, low–molecular-weight peptides called *cytokines,* or more specifically, *interleukins.*[3] Interleukins are capable of activating or suppressing the proliferation of lymphocyte subsets. Several different types of interleukins with specific functions have been identified, but researchers are just beginning to understand the role that interleukins play in modulating the immune response.

An important system in the immune response is complement. Complement consists of a series of 25 proteins, which, when activated, develop into a powerful enzyme capable of lysing alien cell walls. Complement is triggered by the presence of antibody bound to an alien cell or antigen (antigen-antibody complex). Complement also stimulates basophils, attracts neutrophils, and coats alien cells to make them more attractive to phagocytes. The latter action is referred to as *opsonization.*

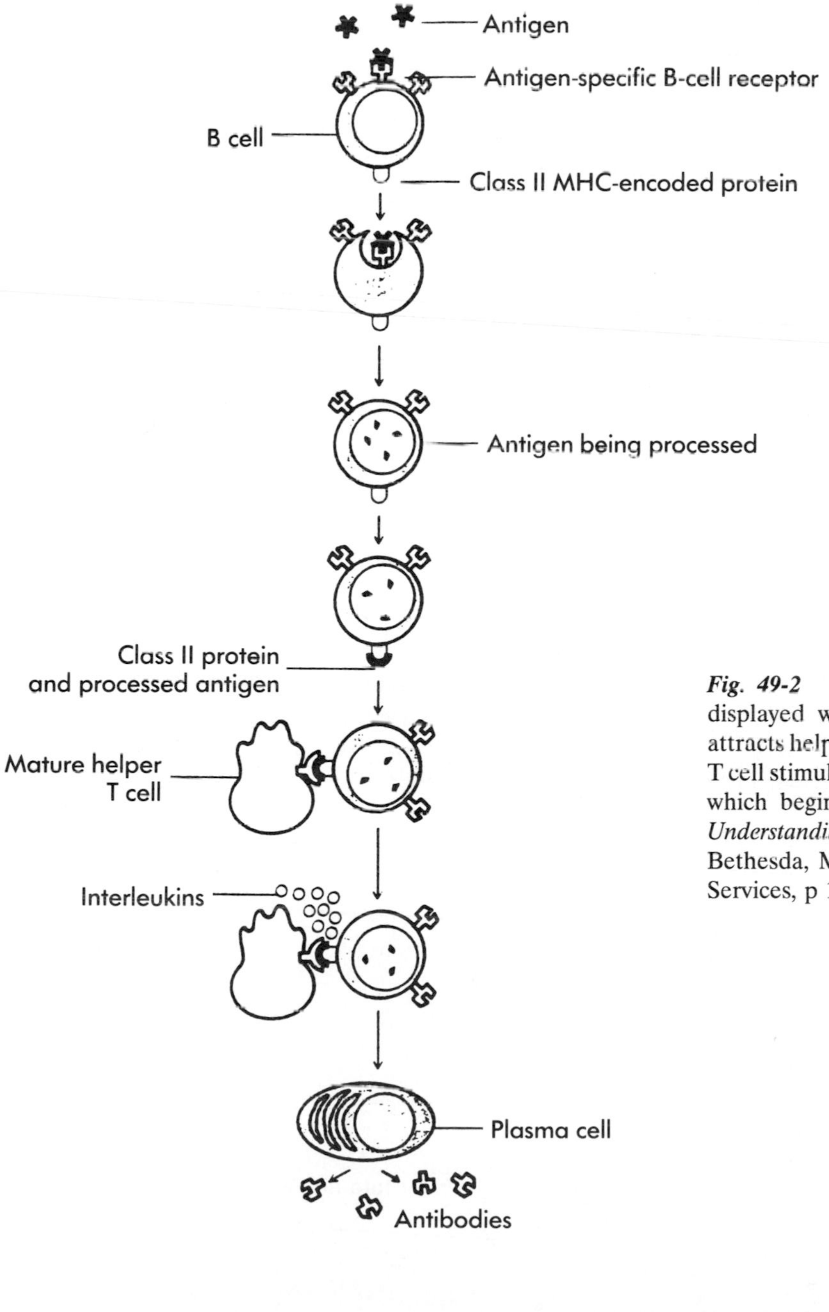

Fig. 49-2 Foreign antigen is processed by the B cell and displayed with its MHC class II antigen (protein), which attracts helper T cells. The release of interleukins by the helper T cell stimulates differentiation of the B cell into a plasma cell, which begins to produce antibody. (From Schindler LW: *Understanding the immune system,* NIH Publ No 90-529, Bethesda, Md, 1990, US Department of Health and Human Services, p 16.)

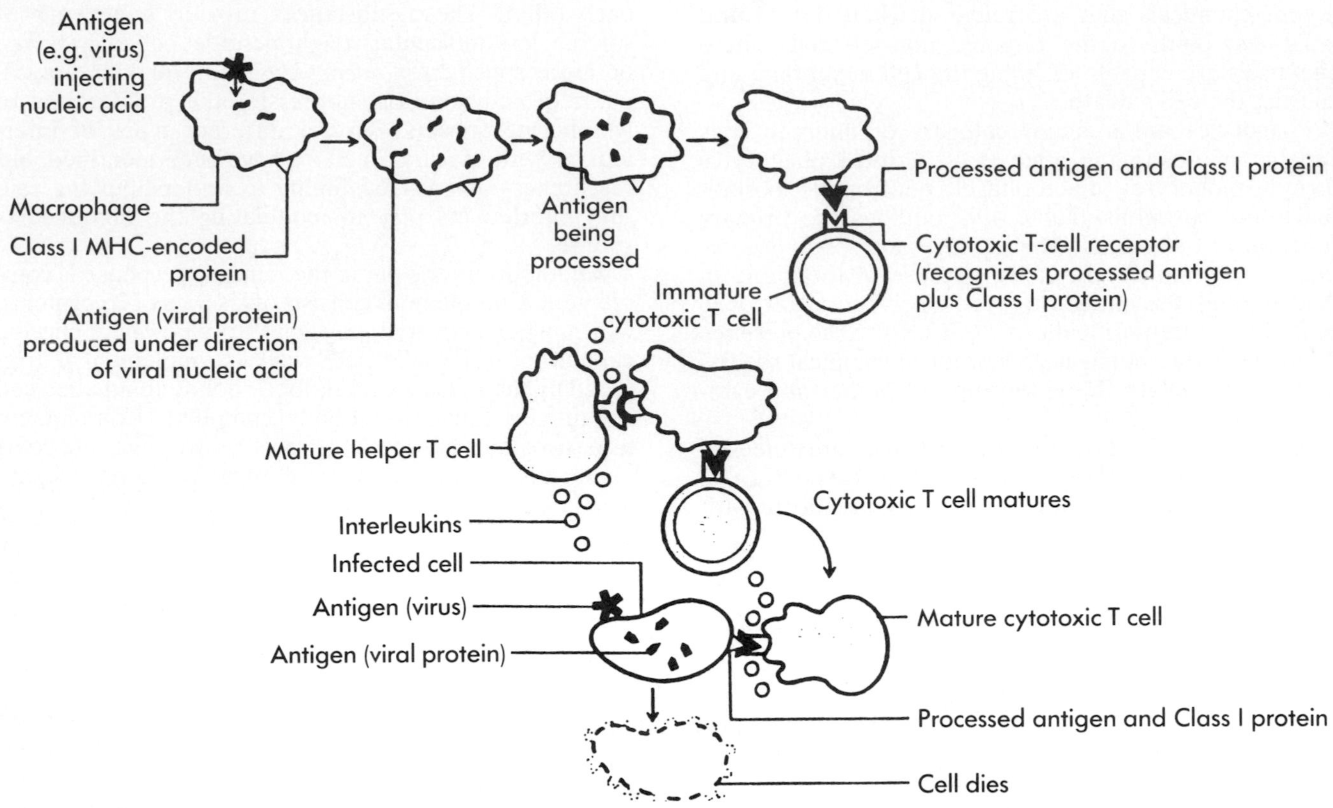

Fig. 49-3 The macrophage presents MCH class I antigen (protein) and processed antigen from the foreign organism to the cytotoxic and helper T cell. Aided by the helper T cell, the cytotoxic T cell matures and kills the foreign cell. (From Schindler LW: *Understanding the immune system,* NIH Publ No 90-529, Bethesda, Md, 1990, US Department of Health and Human Services, p 17.)

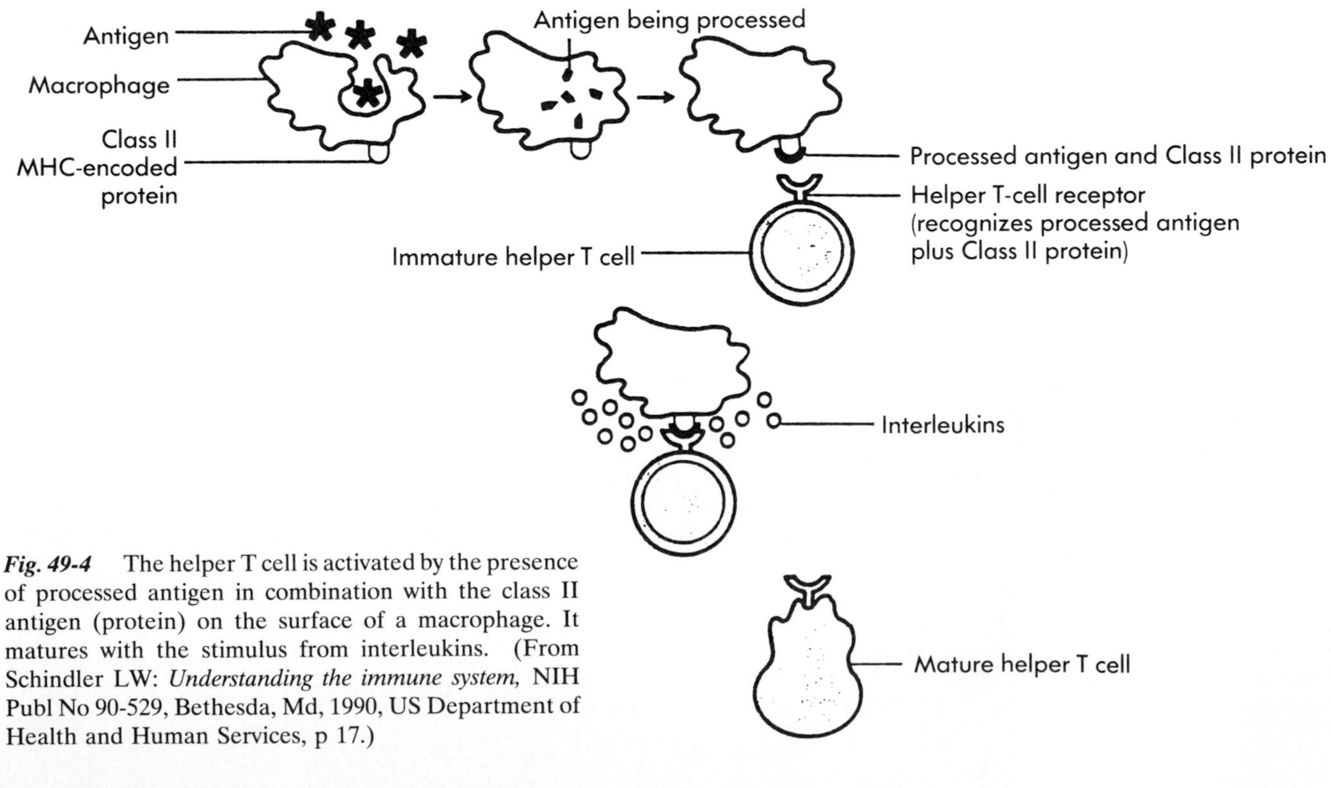

Fig. 49-4 The helper T cell is activated by the presence of processed antigen in combination with the class II antigen (protein) on the surface of a macrophage. It matures with the stimulus from interleukins. (From Schindler LW: *Understanding the immune system,* NIH Publ No 90-529, Bethesda, Md, 1990, US Department of Health and Human Services, p 17.)

Table 49-1 Phagocytes and their functions

Phagocyte	Function
Monocytes	Migrate from blood tissues to become macrophages
Macrophages	Scavenger cells in tissues Present antigen to T cells Secrete enzymes, complement proteins, and immune regulatory factors (cytokines) Activated by lymphokines
Neutrophils	Contain granules capable of destroying alien organisms Key role in inflammatory reactions
Eosinophils	Contain granules capable of destroying alien organisms Weaker phagocyte
Basophils	Contain granules capable of destroying alien organisms Key role in allergic reaction

Graft Rejection

Rejection of any transplanted organ occurs when the transplanted tissue is recognized as non-self by the immune system. Cellular-mediated rejection occurs when HLA class II antigens, displayed on donor cells, activate helper T cells that promote the expansion of cytotoxic T cells and recruitment of macrophages into the transplanted tissue. Natural killer cells also begin to attack any cell with foreign HLA class I antigens. As a result, the transplanted organ becomes infiltrated with these cells, which proceed to destroy the foreign graft tissue.

At the same time, antibody-mediated or humoral-mediated rejection occurs as antigen-antibody complexes form. These complexes also are present in the transplanted organ and release complement that is capable of cell destruction. Complement plays a role in recruiting basophils and tissue-destroying neutrophils to the site. Antibody also coats the foreign cells, making them more attractive to macrophages.

Graft rejection can occur at different time intervals and has different injury patterns. There are three different types of rejection patterns: hyperacute rejection, acute rejection, and chronic rejection. Hyperacute rejection occurs within hours after transplantation and results in immediate graft failure. The primary mechanism triggering this response is activation of humoral-mediated rejection. Such an immediate response by the immune system is caused by the presence of preformed reactive antibodies resulting from previous exposure to antigens. Presensitization can be the result of previous blood transfusions, multiple pregnancies, or previous organ transplants.[4] Transplanting an organ from a donor with an incompatible blood type can have the same effect. Hyperacute rejection is prevented by testing for the presence of preformed antibodies in the recipient and by selecting donors with compatible blood types. Acute rejection occurs weeks to months after transplantation. Class I or II antigens on the cells of the transplanted graft activate cellular-mediated rejection. Chronic rejection occurs at varying times after transplantation and progresses for years until ultimate deterioration of the transplanted organ. Chronic rejection is the result of both humoral- and cellular-mediated immune responses. Chronic inflammation results in diffuse scarring of tissue and stenosis of the vasculature of the organ. Lack of blood supply leads to ischemia and necrosis of tissue. Chronic lung rejection results in small airway destruction, and chronic liver rejection causes diminution of bile ducts.

Immunosuppressive Therapy

Immunosuppressive protocols vary among institutions and with specific organ transplants. The primary goal of all protocols is to suppress the activity of helper and cytotoxic T cells. Therapy ideally interferes with the secretion of interleukins, which stimulate the immune response. The five most common agents used for immunosuppression include cyclosporine, corticosteroids, azathioprine, orthoclone T3 (OKT3), and antithymocyte preparations. Table 49-2 summarizes the adverse effects of these drugs. Absolute care must be taken to monitor the effectiveness of drug therapy and to minimize unnecessarily high doses of these agents, which could predispose patients to greater risks for infection or malignancy.

◆ **Cyclosporine.** Graft survival has improved dramatically since the introduction of cyclosporine. Its primary action seems to be inhibition of cytotoxic T cell generation.[5] It also interferes with the secretion of interleukins by helper T cells and the ability for cytotoxic T cells to respond to interleukins. Interleukin secretion by macrophages also is impaired. Because cyclosporine is specifically targeted for T cells, the patient's immune system is not totally impaired and some ability to protect the body from infection is preserved. T cells play a major role in providing protection from viral infections; thus cyclosporine's interference with T cell function prevents full immunologic competence against viral infection.[6]

◆ **Corticosteroids.** Corticosteroids (IV methylprednisolone [Solu-Medrol] and oral prednisone) have complex and diverse effects on the immune system. They are used both for maintenance therapy and to treat acute rejection. The antiinflammatory actions of steroids provide important protection of the transplanted organ from permanent damage from the rejection process. As a maintenance therapy, steroids impair the sensitivity of T cells to antigen, decrease the proliferation of sensitized T cells, and impair the production of interleukins.[7] Steroids also decrease macrophage mobility. Chronic steroid therapy is associated with numerous adverse effects and predisposes the patient to an increased risk of infection (see Table 49-2). A primary goal of therapy is to titrate the drug dose to as minimal a level as possible.

◆ **Azathioprine.** Azathioprine (Imuran) is an antimetabolite that interferes with the purine synthesis necessary for the production of antibodies. Purine synthesis also is

Table 49-2 Major adverse side effects of immunosuppressive agents and clinical manifestations

Drug	Adverse effects	Clinical manifestations
Cyclosporine	Nephrotoxicity	Elevated BUN and creatinine Decreased urine output Weight gain, edema
	Hypertension	Elevated blood pressure
	Hepatotoxicity	Elevated bilirubin level Elevated alkaline phosphatase, aspartate aminotransferase (AST), and alanine aminotransferase (ALT) levels Jaundice
	Hypertrichosis	Excessive hair growth all over body
	Tremors, seizures	Fine motor tremors, especially hands Associated paresthesias Seizure activity
	Increased risk of malignancy when associated with high doses of multiple agents	Dependent on type and location of malignancy
	Gingival hyperplasia	Growth of gums over teeth Bleeding of gums
Corticosteroids	Aseptic necrosis of bone, osteoporosis	Pain in weight-bearing joints Pathologic fractures
	Hyperglycemia, steroid-induced diabetes mellitus	Elevated serum glucose Polydipsia, polyuria
	Salt and water retention	Weight gain/fluctuations associated with edema
	Hypertension	Elevated blood pressure
	Skin alterations	
	Acne	Rash or pimples on face and/or trunk
	Sun sensitivity	Susceptibility to sunburn
	Hirsutism	Excessive hair growth on face, trunk, extremities
	Growth retardation in children	Failure to reach normal height for age
	Gastritis/gastrointestinal ulcerations	Abdominal pain, dysphagia Hematemesis, guaiac-positive stools
	Cataracts	Visual acuity problems

necessary for the synthesis of nucleic acids in rapidly proliferating cells, such as the cells of the immune system. Azathioprine is used as a maintenance drug to prevent the activation and rapid proliferation of T cells responding to an antigen. A common adverse effect is the suppression of other rapidly proliferating cells, resulting in leukopenia, thrombocytopenia, and anemia. The dose of the drug is adjusted to keep the white blood cell count between 3000 and 5000 cells/mm^3, thus protecting the patient from an increased risk of infection. The actual minimum acceptable white blood cell count varies with institutional preferences and type of organ transplant.

◆ **Orthoclone.** Orthoclone (OKT3) was one of the first drugs introduced to target distinct subpopulations of T cells. The drug is a monoclonal antibody produced in mice to specifically target cells with the T3 surface antigen found on mature T cells. OKT3 removes these cells from circulation by forming antibody-antigen complexes. OKT3 also interferes with T cell recognition of foreign antigen, which renders the T cells incapable of responding.[8] The drug is used as induction therapy by some centers to eliminate T cell response for the first 2 weeks after transplantation. Other centers use it to treat and reverse a severe rejection episode. Because it is an animal protein, antibodies against the drug develop in some patients. For that reason it cannot be used repeatedly in those patients with sensitivity. Its adverse effects seem to be caused by the massive destruction of T cells, resulting in fever, general malaise, and rigors.[6] Reactions usually subside with subsequent doses. As the T cell population declines, the severity of the reaction diminishes. OKT3 usually is administered for 14 days and then stopped.

◆ **Antithymocyte preparations.** Antithymocyte preparations are made by injecting human thymocytes into an animal, usually a horse, rabbit, or goat. The animal produces antibody in response to the foreign human antigen. Antibody to human thymocytes can then be extracted from the serum of the animal. The same process can be used to obtain antilymphocyte preparations. Antibody preparations are made with serum or

Table 49-2 Major adverse side effects of immunosuppressive agents and clinical manifestations—cont'd

Drug	Adverse effects	Clinical manifestations
Azathioprine	Bone marrow depression	Leukopenia, thrombocytopenia, anemia
	Hepatotoxicity	Elevated bilirubin level Elevated alkaline phosphatase, AST, and ALT Jaundice
	Increased risk of malignancy when associated with high doses of multiple agents	Dependent on type and location of malignancy
	Sun sensitivity of skin	Susceptibility to sunburn Skin malignancies
Orthoclone (OKT3)	Pyrexia, malaise	Fever, chills, flulike symptoms Headache, diarrhea
	Respiratory distress associated with initial doses and fluid overload	Chest tightness, dyspnea, wheezing
	Increased risk of malignancy when associated with high doses of multiple agents	Dependent on type and location of malignancy
Antithymocyte preparations	Anaphylactic reactions	Hypotension, dyspnea, wheezing, fever, chills
	Serum sickness associated with antibody formation to foreign protein	Fever, joint pain
	Bone marrow depression associated with prolonged use in conjunction with azathioprine	Leukopenia Thrombocytopenia Anemia
	Local inflammatory reactions associated with IM administration	Pain, redness, extreme muscle soreness, swelling
	Increased risk of malignancy when associated with high doses of multiple agents	Dependent on type and location of malignancy
FK506	Nephrotoxicity associated with high doses	Elevated BUN and creatinine levels Decreased urine output
	Hyperkalemia	Elevated potassium levels
	Insomnia	Sleep disturbances
	Malaise	Headaches, nausea, and vomiting associated with IV administration

globulin. If globulin is produced, globulin molecules are extracted from the animal serum.[6] Many centers make their own preparations. Only two preparations are commercially available in the United States, and they are made from horse serum. Depending on the protocol of the institution and the type of organ transplant, antithymocyte or antilymphocyte preparations may be given as part of induction therapy or may be used only to treat rejection. The duration of therapy is typically around 7 days but may be shorter or longer, depending on institutional preference. Administration of the drug depletes circulating T cells and reduces the proliferative function of the T cells. As with OKT3, patients are subject to reactions from the release of pyrogens during the massive T cell lysis, as well as to the foreign animal protein contained in the preparation. OKT3, antilymphocyte, and antithymocyte preparations are referred to as *cytolytic drugs*. Use of cytolytic drugs has been associated with an increased incidence of malignancy. This increased incidence is most likely caused by the suppression of cytotoxic T cells, which play an important role in identifying and eliminating cancer cells. For that reason, many centers use these drugs only to reverse rejections that are unresponsive to conventional treatment with increased corticosteroid.

◆ **FK506.** FK506 is a relatively new immunosuppressant first released for human clinical trials in February 1989 for use in liver transplant patients at the University of Pittsburgh.[9] Since that time, trials have begun with recipients of heart and kidney transplants. The immunologic action of FK506 is mediated through the inhibition of a specific type of interleukin release (interleukin-2).[10] FK506 has been shown to have fewer side effects than cyclosporine and is used in place of cyclosporine in the immunosuppressive regimen. If cyclosporine has been used in a patient, the recommendation is that before the first dose of FK506 is administered, cyclosporine be discontinued for a minimum of 24 hours to prevent synergistic side effects. These effects include hypertensive episodes and body rash.[11]

Initially, intravenously administered FK506 is given during the perioperative period and then every 12 hours.

RESEARCH ABSTRACT

Infection control practice in cardiac transplant recipients.

Lange SS and others: *Heart Lung* 21(2):101, 1992.

PURPOSE

The purpose of this study was to identify the infection control methods used in transplant centers nationwide.

DESIGN

Descriptive survey design

SAMPLE

The sample consisted of 68 heart transplant programs identified by the North American Transplant Coordinators Organization. Only 30.2% of the transplant centers performed more than 20 transplants annually, and fewer than one fifth of the centers had been performing transplants more than 5 years. There was a mean 1-year survival rate of 85%, with a 74% 5-year mean survival rate. Average CCU stay was 6.7 days, with an average of 19.2 hospital days; 76.6% accepted diabetic patients for transplantation. The median age of the transplant recipients was 63 years.

INSTRUMENTS

A 156-item questionnaire developed by the investigators requested information regarding isolation procedures, dressings, invasive lines, medications, staffing, education, dress codes, unit design, visitation, length of stay, survival rates, and demographics. Content validity of the instrument was established by a panel of six experts on transplantation; reliability was not established.

PROCEDURE

A cover letter and questionnaire were sent to the heart transplant coordinators of 120 heart transplant centers on the mailing list of the North American Transplant Coordinators Organization. Participants were asked to complete the questionnaires and return within 6 weeks. At the end of 6 weeks, follow-up telephone calls were made to the institutions that had not responded. There was an overall 61.8% return rate of the questionnaires.

RESULTS

Data were divided into two groups: group I consisted of those using maximal precautions (four to eight infection control measures), and group II used minimal precautions (one to three infection control measures). Group I accounted for 51.6% of the sample; group II consisted of 48.4%. Programs that had been in existence longer used significantly fewer infection control measures ($p < .0002$). There was no significant relationship between the number of infection control measures and survival rates. All the centers reported use of triple-drug therapy (corticosteroids, cyclosporine, and azathioprine). Scrubs were worn by 92% of respondents, with most donned at work. Of the transplant recipients, 86.6% were placed into a general medical-surgical critical care unit on admission, with 64% admitted to a private room with limited access immediately after surgery. Fewer than 22% reported an "open" visitation policy. There was a 1:1 nurse-to-patient ratio for the first 24 hours after surgery in 64.2% of the centers. Most centers (83.3%) required that staff members receive instruction in the care of transplant recipients.

DISCUSSION/IMPLICATIONS

This survey contributed to the existing body of knowledge regarding infection control measures used with heart transplant recipients inasmuch as it is representative of nationwide centers (response rate was 61.8%). The results of this study indicate that more than 50% of heart transplant centers use maximal infection control precautions in caring for recipients. There appeared to be no relationship between survival rates and the number of infection control practices implemented in this sample. This finding has fiscal implications in that fewer isolation restrictions would lower the unit costs and decrease staffing needs. To clearly describe the impact of infection control measures, however, other areas of research need to be undertaken. Future studies might include examining the relationship of the number of infection control measures with nosocomial infection rate, length of stay, or other outcome indicators. An additional focus of study might be the further refinement of the instrument developed by the investigators for this study.

The dose is adjusted according to the patient's liver chemistry findings, blood levels, and the degree to which the drug is tolerated. On the basis of these factors, dosing schedules can be varied, and some patients may not require the drug on a 12-hour regimen or even on a daily basis. Conversion to oral administration occurs when patients are able to tolerate oral intake.

Side effects are encountered most frequently with intravenous administration. These untoward effects include headaches, nausea, and vomiting.[11] Hyperkalemia associated with low aldosterone and renin levels has occurred and may require treatment with potassium-restricted diets. FK506 does not appear to be as nephrotoxic as cyclosporine, nor does it cause hypertension.

◆ **Risk of infection.** A major adverse effect of all immunosuppressive drugs is an increased risk for infection. Patients on a multiple drug regimen that is administered at high doses are at greatest risk. Few patients complete their first year of immunosuppressive therapy without an episode of infection. It is important for the clinician to be astute and look for subtle signs of infection. Infections can be treated successfully if clinicians are vigilant, if patients are taught to recognize signs of possible infection, and if aggressive treatment is started early. The nursing management plan at the end of this chapter outlines important interventions.

HEART TRANSPLANTATION

Laboratory research and development of tissue and organ transplantation were initiated in 1904 when Guthrie and Carrel began their investigations of whole organ transplant at the University of Chicago. Initial studies of heart rejection were described as early as 1914 by Frank C. Mann at the Mayo Clinic. It was not until the mid 1940s that Russian researchers Demikhov and Sinitsyn successfully transplanted heart-lung blocks in dogs. In addition, heterotopic heart transplantation was achieved, again in a dog, with survival to 32 days. Early years of research focused on heterotopic (transplanting a heart as an augmentation to the native heart) transplant because of the unavailability of cardiopulmonary bypass. The first heart preservation techniques evolved in the mid-1950s, coinciding with the advent of the cardiopulmonary bypass. These developments opened the door for investigations of orthotopic (replacement of the heart in the native position) transplantation in animals. In 1960 Lower and Shumway first reported the surgical technique of orthotopic transplantation in dogs, with a maximum survival of 2 weeks without immunosuppression. The validity of using the electrocardiogram to detect rejection subsequently was reported by Lower, Dong, and Shumway. Recognition of rejection resulted in longer survival.[12]

The first human heart transplant was performed at the University of Capetown in 1967 by Dr. Christiaan Barnard, with the patient surviving 18 days. In 1968 American heart transplant pioneer Norman Shumway performed the first transplant in the United States at Stanford University. Heart transplant procedures dramatically grew in number for the first few years and then rapidly declined because of poor results. It was not until 1972-1974 that improvements were seen and interest regenerated. The development of the endomyocardial biopsy in 1972 was a major milestone in the detection of allograft rejection. In addition, the introduction of T cell–specific agents, such as rabbit antithymocyte globulin, and the ability of laboratories to measure specific T cells (rosette counts) contributed to an increase in 1-year survival by approximately 20%. In 1981 cyclosporine was introduced in the clinical setting, which marked another significant advancement in transplantation science. Again, survival increased dramatically by about 20% at 1 year with the use of cyclosporine. Once again the number of transplant procedures grew rapidly.[12]

Indications and Selection

General candidate criteria for heart transplantation is a life expectancy of only 6 to 12 months because of end-stage cardiac disease.[13] Common causes of such conditions are cardiomyopathy of various origins (idiopathic, viral, valvular) and coronary artery disease.[13,14] Other less common etiologic factors include severe heart failure resulting from chemotherapy, radiation treatment, myocardial tumor, and complex congenital defects. Many centers grade the severity of heart failure by the New York Heart Association (NYHA) functional classification (Table 49-3), which is based on the amount of exertion required to cause symptoms. Although most patients fall into the category of NYHA class IV, the condition of some is graded class III because of recent recompensation.[13,14]

In addition to satisfying medical criteria, patients generally are evaluated for the presence of familial or social support, absence of chemical dependence, and commitment to adhering to a strict, lifelong medical regimen and follow-up.

Specific contraindications to cardiac transplantation are listed in the box below. The age range in heart transplantation is from the neonatal period to approximately 65 years; upper age limits vary among transplant

Table 49-3 New York Heart Association functional classification of heart disease

Class	Physical manifestation
I	No limitation of physical activity. No dyspnea, fatigue, or palpitation with ordinary physical activity.
II	Slight limitation of physical activity. These patients have fatigue, palpitations, and dyspnea with ordinary physical activity but are comfortable at rest.
III	Marked limitation of activity. Less than ordinary physical activity results in symptoms, but patients are comfortable at rest.
IV	Symptoms are present at rest, and any physical exertion exacerbates the symptoms.

CONTRAINDICATIONS TO HEART TRANSPLANTATION

- Advanced Age
- Significant systemic or multisystem disease
- Fixed severe pulmonary hypertension
- Active infection
- Recent pulmonary infarction
- Cachexia or obesity
- Psychiatric illness
- Drug or alcohol abuse

institutions. Preexisting malignancy has been an absolute contraindication because of the potential for recurring cancer or development of second cancers as a result of therapeutic immunosuppression. Some centers, however, consider cured, nonmetastatic malignancies as a relative contraindication.[15,16] Severe liver and kidney dysfunctions that are not reversible by the increase in cardiac output are contraindications for transplantation.[13,14] Diabetes mellitus (DM) was once an absolute contraindication because steroid administration can cause exacerbation of the condition. With good medical management, however, the hyperglycemia can be controlled.

It also was believed that diabetic persons would incur an increased risk for infectious complications. Currently, however, DM is considered a relative contraindication if the hyperglycemia is adequately treated, because it has been demonstrated that the early survival rates of patients with DM are equal to those without DM.[17-19] If patients have active infections, transplantation is delayed until the infection is cleared. Recent pulmonary infarctions increase the risk for postoperative infection and complicate oxygenation and ventilation. Thus a recent history of infarction often precludes transplantation.

The active waiting list is prioritized by acuity, length of time on the list, ABO blood group, and weight. Distribution of organs is regulated by a regional, state, and national network organized and managed by the federal government. Acuity is determined by a patient's need for inotropic support or mechanical assist devices. Patients requiring this degree of assistance are listed as *status one.* All other heart transplant candidates are listed as *status two.*

Surgical Procedure

The standard surgical procedure has changed little since its development by Lower and Shumway.[20] A standard median sternotomy is used, the great vessels are cannulated, and cardiopulmonary bypass (CPB) is instituted after anticoagulation with standard hypothermic technique. Continuous topical cold saline solution at 4° C is used to protect the myocardium from ischemia. The donor heart is prepared by interconnecting the pulmonary veins to form a single left atrial cuff and trimming the aorta and pulmonary artery to fit the recipient's anatomy. All of the recipient's heart is removed except the posterior walls of the atria that contain the orifices of the pulmonary veins and vena cava, which minimizes the need for multiple anastomoses. Three major anastomoses are performed between the donor heart and recipient's native atrial remnant. These include the anastomoses and connection of the atria, the aorta, and the pulmonary artery, in that order[20] (Fig. 49-5). Atrial and ventricular epicardial pacing wires are placed before sternal closure in the event pacing is needed in the postoperative period.

The native atrial remnant remains innervated by the parasympathetic and sympathetic nerve fibers from the autonomic nervous system (ANS). The donor heart, however, is now denervated, resulting in a faster resting heart rate of 90 to 100 beats/min. The rate of the transplanted heart is the normal intrinsic rate generated by the donor sinoatrial (SA) node located in the right atria. Even though the donor SA node paces the heart,

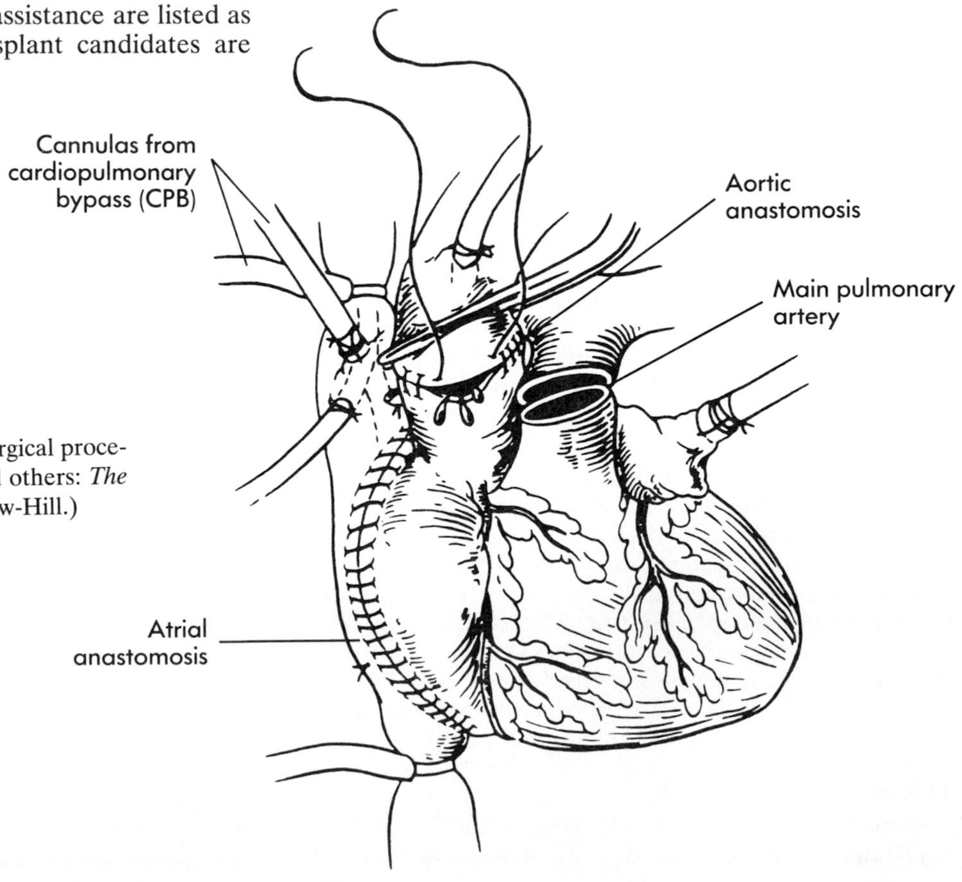

Fig. 49-5 Heart transplantation: surgical procedure. (Modified from Hurst JW and others: *The heart,* ed 7, New York, 1990, McGraw-Hill.)

the remnant native atria will have a separate rate of conduction influenced by the ANS. Manipulation of the atria during surgery and edema around the suture line can cause conduction disturbances that may result in postoperative bradycardia.

Postoperative Medical and Nursing Management

Immediate postoperative management of the transplant recipient is similar to that of patients undergoing other heart surgery procedures. The transplant recipient's most common nursing diagnosis in the postoperative period is Decreased Cardiac Output (CO). Possible causes for a decrease in CO are dysrhythmia, hypothermia, myocardial depression, tamponade, and rejection. Variables that influence myocardial performance are prolonged ischemic times (time from excision of heart from the donor to removal of aortic cross clamp after the implant to the recipient), reperfusion injury, and hypothermia. Dysrhythmia may occur as a result of myocardial irritation, local ischemia, edema around the atrial suture line, and disruption of the SA nodal blood supply.[21] An electrocardiogram abnormality unique to the transplanted heart is the presence of a second P wave, generated by the native SA node left in the atrial cuff. Because this impulse does not cross the suture line, it is capable of conducting only through the remnant of the native recipient atria.

Isoproterenol, a powerful beta-adrenergic antagonist, is the agent most used in the postoperative period for inotropic and chronotropic support. Its chronotropic and vasodilator properties effectively sustain heart rate, increase CO, and decrease pulmonary vascular resistance (PVR). PVR may be increased as a result of preexisting left ventricular failure and may be a cause of transient right ventricular dysfunction in the newly transplanted heart. Dopamine is the most frequently used drug for inotropic support in the postoperative period. Usually, within 48 hours the inotropic support drugs can be gradually discontinued, and the need for isoproterenol decreases as the heart begins to maintain its normal intrinsic rate of 100 beats/min. Temporary pacing is required only occasionally, and fewer than 10% of transplant patients will require a permanent pacemaker implant.[21]

Cardiac tamponade generally does not occur with greater frequency in transplantation than in other cardiac surgeries, but it may do so insidiously as a result of an enlarged pericardial sac from long-standing cardiomyopathy.[22] Patients who have had chronic right ventricular failure, subsequent liver enlargement, and abnormal coagulation studies may benefit from preoperative administration of fresh plasma or fresh frozen plasma (FFP). Plasma contains most clotting factors and is indicated for liver dysfunction. Administration of plasma may decrease the risk of bleeding and tamponade.[23]

Rejection is the most common etiologic factor in low CO for the first 3 months after transplantation.[22] Hyperacute rejection occurs only in the immediate postoperative period. It is a rare complication that requires retransplantation for survival. Acute rejection occurs most frequently in the first 3 to 6 months after transplantation. It is graded according to the institution's numerical scale: mild, moderate, or severe. Diagnosis of rejection is determined by endomyocardial biopsy. Biopsy specimens are obtained by inserting a bioptome percutaneously through the right internal jugular vein, advancing through the right atrium to the right ventricle with the aid of fluoroscopy. Four to five samples of myocardial tissue are obtained from the interventricular septum. The samples are microscopically evaluated for interstitial and perivascular infiltration. Surveillance for rejection is performed on a weekly basis for the first 4 to 6 weeks. Surveillance frequency gradually is decreased relative to the patient's rejection history. A major but rare complication of biopsy is ventricular perforation, resulting in cardiac tamponade. This emergency situation requires open heart surgical repair. Pneumothorax may result from the perforation of the visceral pleura during cannulation of the jugular vein. Clinical manifestations are a sudden onset of sharp pain in the affected side and dyspnea. Transplant patients require biopsy monitoring for the rest of their lives.

Treatment of the initial and second rejection episodes requires intravenously administered methylprednisolone (Solu-Medrol). Recurrent rejection is treated with various pharmacologic agents, depending on the institution. OKT3, a monoclonal antibody, frequently is used for recurrent rejection. It also is used as an induction immunosuppressive agent for the first 10 to 14 days after surgery. If OKT3 is being used for a second time, the patient must be tested for the presence of antibodies. Antibodies may contraindicate use of OKT3. Other agents used for recurrent rejection are polyclonal antibodies, such as antilymphocyte globulin (ALG) or antithymocyte globulin (ATG). Salvage therapy for

NURSING DIAGNOSIS AND MANAGEMENT

Heart transplantation

- High Risk for Decreased Cardiac Output risk factors: dysrhythmias, impaired ventricular contractility, open heart surgery, pp. 359, 360, 358, 362
- High Risk for Infection risk factor: immunosuppressive drugs required to prevent rejection of transplanted organ, p. 866
- Body Image Disturbance related to actual change in body structure, function, or appearance, p. 94
- Anxiety related to threat to biologic, psychologic, and/or social integrity secondary to immunologic rejection of the transplanted heart, p. 763
- Knowledge Deficit: Posttransplant Self-care Regimen, specifically immunosuppressive drugs, cardiac drugs, diuretics, and clinical manifestations of infection related to lack of previous exposure to information, p. 72
- Sensory/Perceptual Alterations related to sensory overload, sensory deprivation, sleep pattern disturbance, p. 573

persistent rejection that has not responded to conventional immunosuppression, multiple steroid boluses, or anti–T cell antibodies consists of total lymphoid irradiation (TLI). Low-dose ionizing radiation is used to treat the lymphoid tissue. Areas exposed to radiation are the axilla, sternum, clavicle, paraaorta, ilium, the inguinofemoral lymph nodes, and the spleen.[24]

Infection surveillance is a high priority for the immunocompromised person. It is well known that immunosuppression predisposes the patient to infection by a multitude of opportunistic pathogens, which cannot easily be prevented with infection control. Development of infection is encountered most frequently in the early postoperative period when immunosuppression is maximized. Infection is the leading cause of death during this period (up to 2 years after surgery).[20,25] Great care must be taken to use aseptic technique for all line and dressing changes. Centers differ widely in protective practices regarding the transplant recipient. Some use reverse isolation, whereas others room transplant recipients with other patients and simply employ universal precautions.

Any development of fever is aggressively pursued by systematic blood, wound, and respiratory tract cultures, chest x-ray films, and observation. Because steroids are known to suppress the body's inflammatory reaction, a temperature generally is considered significant at 38° C. Nurses should be suspicious of any new productive cough, dry cough, change in type of secretions, or change in chest roentgenogram findings. (see p. 866).

A particular threat to transplant recipients is cytomegalovirus (CMV). CMV is a herpesvirus that can produce latent infection that persists throughout life; approximately 50% of the population is infected. The virus can be transmitted through organ and blood product donation; thus the transplantation from a CMV-seropositive donor to a CMV-negative recipient poses a risk to the recipient. An antiviral agent, ganciclovir, can inhibit viral replication and ameliorate symptoms and thus is used in the prophylaxis and treatment of CMV infections.[26,27]

Long-Term Considerations

Chronic immunosuppression results in significant morbidity. Steroid administration can result in osteoporosis, avascular necrosis of joints, fragile skin, and obesity. Cyclosporine can induce renal insufficiency, excessive hair growth, gingival hyperplasia, tremor, and hypertension that requires pharmacologic control. Azathioprine can be hepatotoxic. Concomitant use of these immunosuppressants also leaves patients more susceptible to malignancies and late infections (see Table 49-2).

Accelerated graft atherosclerosis (AGAS), or coronary artery disease in the transplanted heart, is a major cause of late morbidity and mortality.[28] AGAS is a diffuse and rapidly progressive type of coronary artery disease that causes concentric narrowing of the coronary arteries. Because the lesions are not discrete, they are not amenable to angioplasty or bypass grafting.[28] The etiology of AGAS remains unclear, but chronic rejection likely plays a role.[29] Patients with denervated hearts usually cannot feel anginal pain; however, recent literature reports evidence of reinervation and subsequent chest pain.[30] More often, their symptoms are ischemic injury, heart failure, or sudden death. The disease is recognized initially by angiographic screening and, later in the course of the disease, by the presence of silent infarctions on electrocardiogram. Many patients may have the disease and demonstrate no clinical sequelae.[28] The only therapy for advanced AGAS is retransplantation.

In general, heart transplant recipients report being highly satisfied with their quality of life.[31,32] Fewer than 35% return to full-time employment, but many who are able to work cannot find suitable employment because of employers' concerns about liability, lack of health insurance, and the need to qualify for medical disability.[33,34]

In 1990 there were 1988 cardiac transplants performed in the United States. In the same year 1796 persons were registered on waiting lists.[35] The number of cardiac transplants performed is greatly influenced by the limited donor pool. Current 1-year survival for heart transplant recipients, as reported by the United Network for Organ Sharing,[35] is 83% (±1.0%), which parallels results compiled by the International Society for Heart and Lung Transplantation.

HEART AND LUNG TRANSPLANTATION

Heart and lung transplantation research has been built on the foundation established by heart transplantation through years of laboratory investigation. The first attempts at heart-lung transplantation in humans were in 1968 by Cooly and his associates, with a 14-hour survival; in 1969 by Lellehei, which produced a survival of several days; and in 1971 by Barnard, whose patient survived for 23 days. Interest in the procedure gained momentum with the introduction of cyclosporine because it permitted the delay of high-dose steroid therapy (its use impaired bronchial healing and favored early postoperative infections). In 1981 at Stanford University, Bruce Rietz performed the first heart-lung transplant resulting in long-term survival; the patient lived for more than 5 years.

Heart and lung transplantation, now in its third decade, currently is the therapy of choice for some cardiac and cardiopulmonary diseases. Research and laboratory investigations continue in the development of new immunosuppressants, preservation solutions, and techniques. Recent advances have led to single-lung and double-lung transplantation, lobar lung transplantation, and single-lung transplantation with cardiac repair.

Indications and Selection

Heart-lung transplantation (HLT) is an established treatment for selected patients with irreversible, progressively disabling end-stage cardiopulmonary and pulmonary disease.[36-38] Transplantation usually is offered to patients as an option when life expectancy is limited to 15 to 24 months.[36,37] Patients are evaluated and listed earlier than are heart transplant recipients because of the paucity of heart-lung donors and the inevitable long wait to transplantation.

Specific etiologic factors in pulmonary disease can be

grouped according to the type of lung abnormality. Categories are pulmonary vascular disease, obstructive lung disease, and restrictive lung disease[36,37] (see box below). Optional lung transplantation, such as single-lung transplantation, is discussed in a later section.

HLT is the operation of choice for patients whose pulmonary disease process has irreversibly disabled the heart. HLT is considered the preferential procedure because transplantation of the entire heart-lung block eliminates having to separate the pulmonary artery and veins, avoiding subsequent reanastomoses, and thus decreasing bleeding complications. However, in the case of disease processes in which the heart is judged to be only temporarily dysfunctional and can be expected to regain adequate function after the transplantation of a healthy lung or lungs, the native heart may be left in place[37,39] and a single-lung or double-lung transplant performed. Another option is to transplant the heart-lung block into such an individual and then donate the native heart to another recipient, which is referred to as the *domino procedure.*

The evaluation of HLT candidates is similar to that for heart transplant recipients with respect to patient commitment to compliance with a strict lifelong medical regimen. Contraindications to HLT are listed in the box in the right-hand column. Systemic disease, active extrapulmonary infection, and other organ disease are absolute contraindications. Cachexia and obesity are obstacles that can be eliminated by nutritional support and weight reduction. Truncal obesity is especially undesirable because it significantly decreases diaphragmatic excursion, hinders postoperative mobilization, and may complicate recovery.[36] Preoperative use of corticosteroids has been implicated as a cause of tracheal and bronchial dehiscence in the early postoperative period.[36,37] Prior cardiothoracic surgery is a relative contraindication because of the risk of bleeding associated with the presence of pleural adhesions.[36] Removal of the native lung may precipitate pleural bleeding in the posterior pleural space, which can be particularly difficult to control because of location.[40]

HEART-LUNG TRANSPLANTATION INDICATIONS

- Pulmonary vascular disease
  - Primary pulmonary hypertension
  - Eisenmenger's syndrome
  - Cardiomyopathy with pulmonary hypertension
- Obstructive lung disease
  - Emphysema—idiopathic
  - Emphysema—$alpha_1$-antitrypsin deficiency
  - Cystic fibrosis
  - Bronchiectasis
  - Posttransplant obliterative bronchiolitis
- Restrictive lung disease
  - Idiopathic pulmonary fibrosis
  - Sarcoidosis
  - Lymphangiomyomatosis

Surgical Procedure

Success of HLT depends in part on selection and procurement of suitable donor organs. The lungs are particularly difficult to procure because they are vulnerable to complications related to brain death. Prolonged mechanical ventilation is required, which increases the risk of infection. Any infection precludes donation. Neurogenic pulmonary edema also may damage the lungs, making their donation impossible. Lungs have a limited ischemic time of about 4 hours, which limits the geographic area for donor procurement.[40] Lung preservation has improved, and distant procurement with 2 to 3 hours transport time has increased the donor pool.[41]

Before the removal of the heart-lung block, prostaglandin E_1 (PGE_1) is administered gradually until a systemic effect is achieved. PGE_1 is used to ensure complete pulmonary vasodilation for uniform cooling and distribution of pulmonoplegia.[41,42]

The operative procedure for the recipient is through a median sternotomy or a bilateral thoracosternotomy (clam shell) incision. The patient is heparinized and placed on cardiopulmonary bypass, and the heart is excised.[43] Care is used to ensure the preservation of the recipient's phrenic, vagus, and laryngeal nerves. The bronchus is divided, and the lungs are removed separately to decrease the risk of nerve damage. The donor heart and lungs are implanted as a block. The heart is put into the orthotopic position and anastomosed to the native aorta and remnant recipient aorta. The tracheal anastomosis is performed just above the level of the carina[42] (Fig. 49-6).

Postoperative Medical and Nursing Management

Immediate postoperative care of the HLT recipient is similar to that used for the heart transplant recipient. The most common complication is bleeding. Patients who have been cyanotic often have large bronchial vessels that cross behind the trachea, which tend to be a source of bleeding. Control of bleeding at this site is difficult because of the location. Patients who have had previous thoracic surgery require more surgical

ABSOLUTE AND RELATIVE CONTRAINDICATIONS TO HEART-LUNG TRANSPLANTATION

ABSOLUTE CONTRAINDICATIONS

- Significant systemic or multisystem disease
- Active extrapulmonary infection
- Cachexia or obesity
- Current cigarette smoking
- Psychiatric illness
- Drug or alcohol abuse

RELATIVE CONTRAINDICATIONS

- Corticosteroid therapy
- Previous cardiothoracic surgery

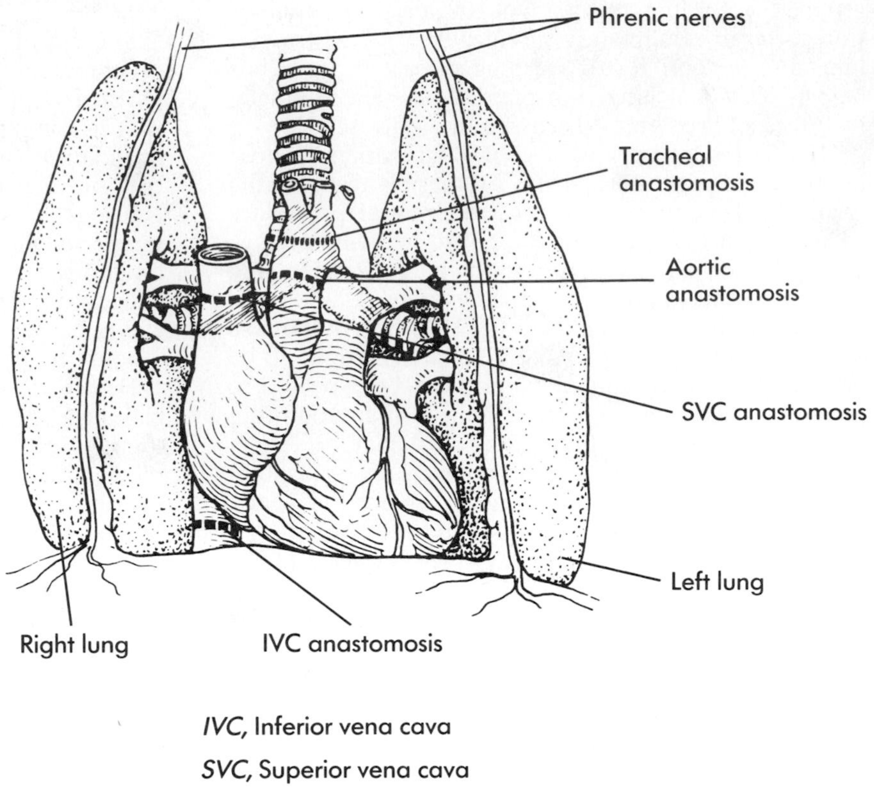

Fig. 49-6 Heart-lung transplantation: surgical procedure. (Modified from Reitz BA and others: Heart and lung transplantation, *J Thorac and Cardiovasc Surg* 80(3):360, 1980.)

NURSING DIAGNOSIS AND MANAGEMENT
Heart-lung transplantation

- Ineffective Airway Clearance related to impaired cough secondary to artificial airway, p. 466
- Ineffective Airway Clearance related to excessive secretions or abnormal viscosity of mucus, p. 464
- High Risk for Impaired Gas Exchange risk factor: ventilation-perfusion mismatch secondary to rejection of transplanted lungs, p. 470
- High Risk for Decreased Cardiac Output risk factors: dysrhythmias, impaired ventricular contractility, open heart surgery, pp. 359, 360, 358, 362
- High Risk for Infection risk factors: immunosuppressive drugs required to prevent rejection of transplanted organ, p. 866
- Body Image Disturbance related to actual change in body structure or appearance, p. 94
- Anxiety related to threat to biologic, psychologic, and/or social integrity secondary to immunologic rejection of the transplanted heart and lungs, p. 763
- Knowledge Deficit: Posttransplant Self-care Regimen, specifically immunosuppressive drugs, cardiopulmonary drugs, diuretics, and clinical manifestations of infection related to lack of previous exposure to information, p. 72
- High Risk for Powerlessness risk factor: physical deterioration despite compliance, p. 99
- Sensory/Perceptual Alterations related to sensory overload, sensory deprivation, and sleep pattern disturbance, p. 573

dissection because of scarring and therefore achieve hemostasis with more difficulty. Careful monitoring of bleeding and maintenance of the patency and function of mediastinal and pleural chest tubes are essential. Bleeding of greater than 100 to 200 ml/hr for more than 3 hours with normal coagulation studies is cause for concern. If bleeding of this nature persists, reexploration of the chest usually is indicated. The transplanted lung is susceptible to fluid overload because of the disruption of pulmonary lymphatics and the increase in extravascular lung water that is common after lung transplantation.[37] Replacement of blood loss with crystalloid or colloid therapy must be used carefully to minimize the risk of fluid overload of the transplanted lungs and the development of adult respiratory distress syndrome (ARDS).

Patients are maintained on mechanical ventilation to support oxygenation for 24 to 48 hours. At least 5 mm Hg of positive end-expiratory pressure is used routinely to prevent atelectasis. Endotracheal tube placement is monitored by auscultation and chest x-ray evaluation. It should be well secured and movement minimized to protect the tracheal anastomosis. In addition, suctioning should be gentle, and, to avoid disruption of the suture line, the suction catheter should not be advanced beyond the end of the tube. Small amounts of bloody secretions can be expected with suctioning, but overt hemoptysis can be a sign of dehiscence, which requires immediate attention. Patients are weaned from ventilatory support as soon as possible. The longer the period of intubation, the higher the risk of pneumonia.[37] After extubation, patients are encouraged to cough, deep-breathe, and ambulate in the room.

Pharmacologic support is similar to that used for heart transplantation. Isoproterenol is given to augment heart rate, and dopamine is used for inotropic support and renal vasodilation. Additional inotropic support is achieved with epinephrine if necessary. PGE_1 is administered primarily for pulmonary vasodilation, and sodium nitroprusside is given for its systemic vasodilatory properties. Initial immunosuppression usually does not include the use of methylprednisone. A single dose of methylprednisone usually is given in the operating room, and maintenance dosing begins within the first 2 weeks. The use of methylprednisone in the immediate postoperative period varies with institution. Daily steroid use is avoided for the first 2 to 3 weeks because of the deleterious effects on wound healing, especially the tracheal anastomosis.

Surveillance for infection and rejection in the HLT recipient is accomplished by bronchoscopy. This is performed initially at weekly or biweekly intervals to monitor the tracheal anastomosis for evidence of healing, to obtain bronchoalveolar lavage washings for appropriate cultures, and to take biopsy specimens for the diagnosis of rejection. Bronchoscopic examination provides visual evidence of tracheal anastomosis healing which determines when maintenance corticosteroids should be introduced to the immunosuppressive regimen.[37]

As in the heart transplant recipient, presence of fever is an indication for aggressive evaluation. Serial chest roentgenograms are used to monitor for infiltrates. It is difficult, however, to distinguish infection from rejection by means of chest roentgenograms. Radiographic changes are used with other clinical evidence, including Pao_2, O_2 saturation, presence or absence of fever, and culture reports to determine the course of action. Documented infections are treated with appropriate antibiotics.

Rejection, which can be definitively diagnosed only by biopsy, is treated either by augmentation of immunosuppression or by pulses of intravenously administered corticosteroid. Augmentation may be in the form of increasing the cyclosporine dose to achieve a higher cyclosporine level and/or increasing the azathioprine to lower the white blood cell (WBC) count and/or increasing the maintenance prednisone dose slightly. Pulsing is the method of administering large doses of corticosteroids over a relatively short period of time. A common pulse of steroid is 1 g of Solu-Medrol every day for 3 consecutive days. Quick resolution of radiographic changes after steroid pulses provides a retrospective confirmation of the diagnosis of rejection. Procedural complications after bronchoscopic examination are a transient fever, fall in Pao_2, infection, and pneumothorax. Chest x-ray examination should follow each bronchoscopy to rule out pneumothorax.

Pulmonary function testing is a noninvasive method of assessing lung function and the presence of rejection. Lung denervation does not adversely affect the control of ventilation during exercise inasmuch as nervation is not necessary for the overall function of the respiratory system.[44] Pulmonary function testing employs a wide range of parameters used to measure the function of the lung at rest and with exercise. The functions are measured in percentages based on weight, gender, and age. The focus is usually on forced expiratory volume in 1 second (FEV_1), forced vital capacity (FVC), forced expiratory flow rate between 25% and 75% of FVC (FEF 25% to 75%), and the measurement of arterial blood gases. These functions are sensitive to slight changes in oxygenation and ventilation caused by infection or rejection. Acute changes in pulmonary function test (PFT) results and in Pao_2 are indications for transbronchial biopsy.[40]

Heart rejection occurs less often in the HLT recipient. Thus endomyocardial biopsy is performed less often[45]; when required, the procedure is similar to that in the heart transplant recipient.

Long-Term Considerations

Chronic immunosuppression in the HLT patient carries the same consequences as it does in the heart transplant recipient. Accelerated graft atherosclerosis can be a late complication in HLT patients and follows a course similar to that in the heart recipient. A major long-term complication in the pulmonary transplant patient is obliterative bronchiolitis (OB). Obliterative bronchiolitis is an inflammatory disorder of the small airways, which leads to obstruction and destruction of pulmonary bronchioles.[46] Features of obliterative bronchiolitis are listed in the box below. Obliterative bronchiolitis may represent a manifestation of chronic pulmonary allograft rejection.[47] The only treatment for end-stage obliterative bronchiolitis is retransplantation. Retransplantation in the HLT group carries a high risk for complications related to infection, delayed healing as a result of steroids, renal insufficiency related to chronic cyclosporine use, and bleeding from scarring from the previous surgery.

Heart-lung transplantation has increased annually for 10 years. In 1990 52 HLTs were performed in the United States. The number of patients listed as candidates in the same year were cited as 226.[35] National 1-year survival for HLT was 57%,[35] which closely parallels international survival rates. The limited donor pool remains the major factor limiting the number of HLTs performed.

FEATURES OF OBLITERATIVE BRONCHIOLITIS

- Rapid rate of development; several months to 1 to 2 years
- Bronchitic symptoms followed by early development of dyspnea
- Distinct infiltrative component on chest film
- Severe obstructive and restrictive disease
- Decreased total lung capacity
- Largely irreversible with bronchodilator

SINGLE-LUNG TRANSPLANTATION

Single-lung transplantation (SLT) is an alternative to HLT in a select group of patients. Transplant teams have explored, modified, and successfully pursued the development of pulmonary transplantation. Indications for single-lung transplantation are similar to those listed for HLT with some exceptions. Pulmonary diseases that typically are associated with chronic lung infections, such as cystic fibrosis and bronchiectasis, require transplantation of both lungs because of the risk of cross contamination. In addition, severe cardiac disease mandates heart replacement.[36] Thorough evaluation of cardiac function is essential to the success of SLT. Contraindications to SLT parallel those for HLT (see box, p. 841). Advantages to SLT are better use of donor resources, decreased operative risks, and decreased short- and long-term complications (see box on right).

Surgical Procedure

Considerations in choosing lung transplantation include the specific disease process, the need for cardiac repair, and donor availability. Transplantation contralateral to a previous thoracotomy is preferable to avoid adhesions that require further surgical dissection.[36] The left lung is preferred because it is easier to expose and has a longer left main bronchus. The longer bronchus gives the surgeon more flexibility in trimming the suture site as needed for anastomosis.[48] If there is a significant disproportion of ventilation and perfusion to one side, then transplantation of the worse side may be the preferred option.[37]

Use of cardiopulmonary bypass (CPB) depends on the disease process. Patients with pulmonary hypertension usually require CPB, whereas patients with pulmonary fibrosis or emphysema do not.[48] Surgical intervention first requires the removal of the diseased lung. The pulmonary artery is then divided and the pulmonary vein mobilized. Donor and recipient arteries are trimmed to suitable lengths, and an end-to-end anastomosis is performed. Bronchial anastomosis is performed with a running suture. After the atrial clamp is slowly removed, the patient is assessed for bleeding[37,48] (Fig. 49-7). In some transplant centers the omentum is brought through the diaphragm from the abdomen and is wrapped around the bronchus for added stability of the anastomosis and increased vascular supply. Disadvantages of this maneuver include a larger incision and involvement of the abdominal cavity.[37]

◆ **Double-lung transplant.** A double-lung transplant may be performed for clinical conditions, such as cystic fibrosis, pulmonary fibrosis or bronchiectasis. In these situations the native heart remains healthy but the lungs are diseased. The surgical technique involves removal of the heart-lung block from the donor. The heart is transplanted into one recipient (see Fig. 49-5). The lungs are transplanted into another recipient (Fig. 49-8). The surgical anastomosis sites are the back wall of the atria (the back wall of the left atrium contains the four pulmonary vein orifices), the trachea, and the main pulmonary artery.

ADVANTAGES OF SINGLE-LUNG TRANSPLANTATION

- ◆ One lung donor provides organs for two lung recipients
- ◆ Increased donor availability
- ◆ Decreased recipient waiting time
- ◆ Decreased need for intraoperative cardiopulmonary bypass
- ◆ Potential shorter recovery and hospital stay
- ◆ Preservation of native heart
- ◆ Heart rejection avoided
- ◆ Accelerated graft atherosclerosis not as prevalent

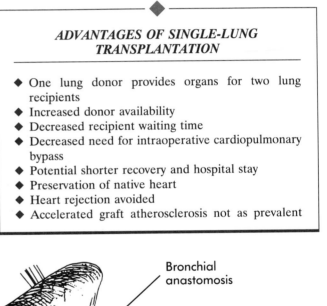

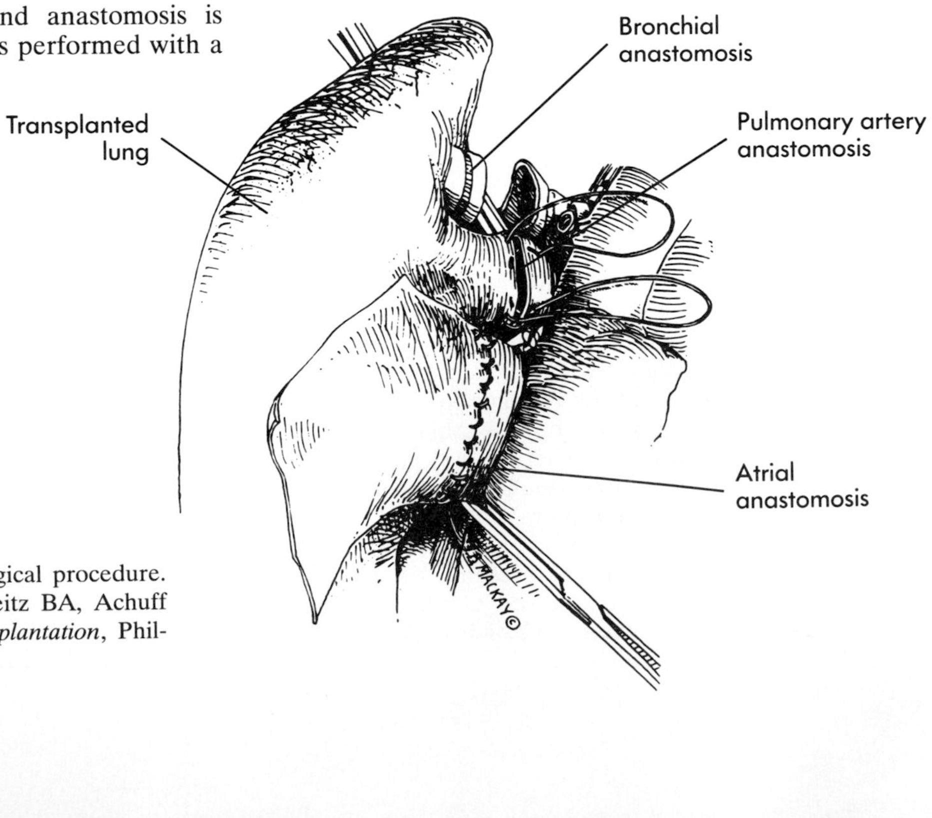

Fig. 49-7 Single-lung transplant: surgical procedure. (Modified from Baumgartner WA, Reitz BA, Achuff SC, editors: *Heart and heart-lung transplantation*, Philadelphia, 1990, WB Saunders.)

Postoperative Medical and Nursing Management

Postoperative care of the single-lung transplant recipient is similar to that of HLT patients, as mentioned in the previous discussion. SLT patients generally require mechanical ventilation of shorter duration. Less bleeding can be anticipated because of the brevity of the surgical procedure. A single pleural chest tube usually is sufficient for drainage. A pulmonary artery catheter may be used to measure right ventricular response when significant ventilation/perfusion (V/Q) mismatch occurs. In the event of elevated pulmonary artery pressures, pharmacologic vasodilation or afterload reduction can be instituted. The patients with pulmonary hypertension potentially may have a greater V/Q mismatch, resulting in larger A-ao_2 gradients. These patients, however, are not functionally impaired, and oxygenation can occur as effectively as in patients with parenchymal disease.[48]

Immunosuppression for SLT recipients is essentially the same as that for HLT patients. Initiation of steroids depends on institutional preference and healing of the bronchial anastomosis.

Surveillance of rejection and infection is similar to that in HLT. Pulmonary function testing is not initiated until the second or third week postoperatively to allow for surgical recovery. Decreased lung function because of fluid shifts, microatelectasis, and splinting from incisional pain would interfere with accurate testing. Unlike HLT, in unilateral lung transplantation the transplanted lung functions in parallel with the native lung, which can be expected to retain any pathology.[49] The patient must be measured by a comparison with his or her own baseline and not with normal standards. This concept also can be applied to the immediate postoperative period of intubation during the evaluation of arterial blood gases. Oxygenation and ventilation occur in both the diseased and transplanted lung, and parameters for evaluation need to be adjusted accordingly. Clinically, SLT recipients function as well as other patients with only one lung. With physical exertion, some patients may complain of shortness of breath. A combination of chest roentgenogram, bronchoscopic examination, and pulmonary function testing is used in the detection and diagnosis of rejection and infection.

Long-term outcome for SLT parallels that of HLT. One-year survival for patients with SLT is quoted from 48%[35] as a national figure to 68%[48] at some institutions.

NURSING DIAGNOSIS AND MANAGEMENT
Single-lung transplantation

- ◆ Ineffective Airway Clearance related to impaired cough, secondary to artificial airway, p. 466
- ◆ Ineffective Airway Clearance related to excessive secretions or abnormal viscosity of mucus, p. 464
- ◆ High Risk for Impaired Gas Exchange risk factor: ventilation/perfusion mismatch secondary to rejection of transplanted lungs, p. 470
- ◆ High Risk for Infection risk factors: immunosuppressive drugs required to prevent rejection of transplanted organ, p. 866
- ◆ Body Image Disturbance related to actual change in body structure or appearance, p. 94
- ◆ Anxiety related to threat to biologic, psychologic, and/or social integrity secondary to immunologic rejection of the transplanted heart and lungs, p. 763
- ◆ Knowledge Deficit: Posttransplant Self-care Regimen, specifically immunosuppressive drugs, cardiopulmonary drugs, diuretics, and clinical manifestations of infection related to lack of previous exposure to information, p. 72
- ◆ Sensory/Perceptual Alterations related to sensory overload, sensory deprivation, and sleep pattern disturbance, p. 573

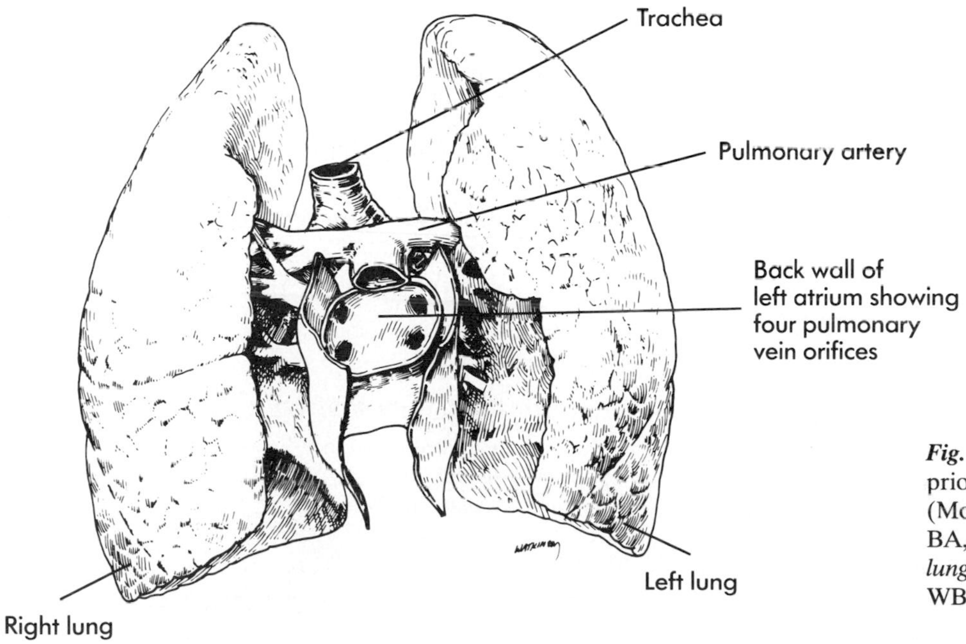

Fig. 49-8 Double-lung transplant graft prior to implantation into a recipient. (Modified from Baumgartner WA, Reitz BA, Achuff SC, editors: *Heart and heart-lung transplantation*, Philadelphia, 1990, WB Saunders.)

International statistics compare equally. Lung transplantation is a relatively new procedure. Thus data are limited, but the numbers of transplants are increasing on an annual basis. In 1990, 309 SLT candidates were listed with the United Network for Organ Sharing and 265 patients received transplants.

LIVER TRANSPLANTATION

Liver transplantation was first attempted in canine models in the 1950s. The outcomes were unsuccessful because of technical complications, infection, and graft failure.[50,51] The effort to improve surgical technique continued, and successful liver transplantation in dogs was achieved several years later by both Moore and others[52,53] and Starzl and others.[54] In 1963 Starzl and colleagues performed the first human liver transplant operation.[55] Although the patient died intraoperatively, this attempt pioneered the possibility of liver transplantation in human beings.

The first successful human liver transplant was performed in 1967, also by Starzl and co-workers,[56] in a patient with malignant hepatoma. The success of this procedure was largely because of refinements in both surgical technique and immunosuppressive therapy. The patient survived 1 year before succumbing to recurrent disease.

Despite this monumental achievement, complications after liver transplantation were numerous and resulted in an associated mortality rate of approximately 70%.[57] Advances in surgical technique, anesthesia, and intraoperative management contributed to improved patient survival in the immediate postsurgical phase, but the complexity of the immune system and limited availability of immunosuppressive agents resulted in life-threatening infection and rejection. Attempts at human liver transplantation decreased over the next decade as a result of poor patient outcomes.

During this moratorium, important advances were achieved in the area of immunobiology. Cyclosporine, a powerful antirejection agent, was developed in the late 1970s and became widely available in the early 1980s. The addition of cyclosporine to the agents already in use dramatically improved the survival statistics of all solid organ transplants.[58-62] Better survival statistics prompted the National Institutes of Health (NIH) to declare liver transplantation to be no longer experimental, but rather an accepted therapeutic modality for some patients with end-stage liver disease.[63] This position statement issued by the NIH resulted in an increase in the number of liver transplant centers worldwide, and an estimated 3000 liver transplants had been performed by 1988.[64]

Indications and Selection

Many persons in the United States would benefit from liver transplantation. The Centers for Disease Control (CDC) reported more than 26,000 deaths related to end-stage liver disease in 1990.[65] Liver transplantation should be considered for any patient who suffers from irreversible acute or chronic liver disease that is likely to progress to end-stage and for whom other medical or surgical treatment options are not beneficial. In addition, the patient should have no absolute contraindications for liver transplantation. Diseases of the liver may be divided into four categories: advanced chronic liver disease, acute fulminant hepatic failure, unresectable hepatic malignancies, and inborn errors of metabolism. Specific diseases that fall into these categories are listed in the box below. Candidate selection continues to be an important aspect of transplantation.

In general, liver transplantation should not be offered to those persons who (1) would not survive major surgery, (2) would not survive the side effects of lifelong immunosuppression, or (3) have a disease that is likely to recur quickly and fatally after transplantation. This last category may include those with certain hepatic or biliary malignancies or extremely active states of hepatitis B virus (HBV), all of which have been shown to recur after transplantation.[66-70] The decision to offer transplantation must be based on thorough case-by-case evaluation. Criteria, which may vary slightly among institutions, will continue to be modified as advances in technical ability, immunosuppression, and perioperative management continue. Relative and absolute contraindications to liver transplantation are listed in the box on p. 847, left-hand column.

INDICATIONS FOR LIVER TRANSPLANTATION

ADVANCED CHRONIC LIVER DISEASE

- Cholestatic syndromes
  - Primary biliary cirrhosis
  - Sclerosing cholangitis
  - Biliary atresia
  - Others
- Hepatocellular diseases
  - Chronic viral hepatitis
  - Chronic drug-induced hepatitis
  - Alcoholic liver disease
- Autoimmune liver disease
- Vascular diseases of the liver

ACUTE HEPATIC FAILURE

- Viral hepatitis
- Drug-induced hepatitis
- Metabolic liver disease

HEPATIC MALIGNANCIES

- Hepatocellular carcinoma
- Cholangiocarcinoma

METABOLIC LIVER DISEASE

- $Alpha_1$-antitrypsin deficiency
- Wilson's disease
- Hemoachromatosis
- Tyrosinemia
- Others

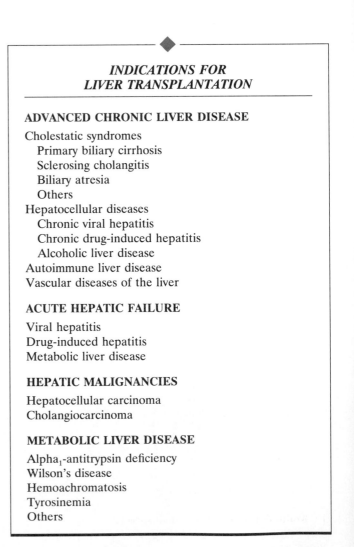

◆ **Recipient evaluation.** Patients being considered for liver transplantation must undergo a comprehensive multidisciplinary evaluation that includes a thorough psychosocial assessment. The goal of the evaluation is several-fold: (1) to determine the medical need for liver transplantation, (2) to identify any absolute or relative medical or psychologic contraindications to transplantation, and (3) to identify any medical and/or psychosocial issues that require intervention before transplantation. The evaluation may be completed on an inpatient or outpatient basis. The patient undergoes a multitude of tests and consultations to accomplish the goals of the evaluation (see box in right-hand column). In addition, the patient and family receive education regarding transplant surgery, postoperative management, and long-term follow-up. One of several outcomes is possible at the conclusion of the evaluation: (1) the patient is not a candidate for transplant; (2) the patient is a candidate for transplant; or (3) the patient may be a candidate sometime in the future if certain criteria are met. This last category might include patients who have psychosocial issues that need attention, such as alcohol rehabilitation or treatment for depression.

◆ **Pretransplantation phase.** After candidacy has been determined and the patient is essentially ready for transplant, his or her name is entered into the national computer system operated by the United Network for Organ Sharing (UNOS) in Richmond, Virginia. The patient then begins what may be the most difficult phase of transplantation—the waiting period. It is not possible to anticipate when an appropriate organ may become available; thus patients may feel as though their lives are temporarily "on hold." Knowing that another person must die so that he or she may live may cause feelings of guilt as the patient hopes for a donor to become available. In addition, the candidate with end-stage liver disease knows that the only alternative to transplant is death. It is therefore important for the patient and family to receive ongoing psychosocial assessment and to attend pretransplant support groups, which are available at many transplant centers.

The patient is followed up at regular intervals in the outpatient clinic where a thorough assessment is performed to monitor disease status. The numerous sequelae associated with end-stage liver disease may result in intermittent hospitalizations during the waiting period (Table 49-4). An increasing frequency of these complications indicates advancement of disease status. Pretransplant morbidity has been shown to adversely affect posttransplant rehabilitation.[71] It is therefore important to treat as many health problems as possible, so that the patient will be at his or her maximum level of wellness at the time of transplantation.

ABSOLUTE AND RELATIVE CONTRAINDICATIONS FOR LIVER TRANSPLANTATION

ABSOLUTE CONTRAINDICATIONS

Active drug or ethanol abuse
Extrahepatobiliary sepsis
Extrahepatobiliary malignancy, primary or metastatic
Metastatic hepatic malignancy
Serologic markers indicative of actively replicating HBV
Advanced cardiopulmonary disease
Presence of HIV antibody with decreased CD4 lymphocytes

RELATIVE CONTRAINDICATIONS

Age >60 years
Presence of hepatitis B surface antigen
Presence of HIV antibody
Portal vein or superior mesenteric vein thrombosis
Advanced renal disease
Primary hepatic malignancy
Multiple previous abdominal surgeries

METHODS USED TO EVALUATE CANDIDATES FOR LIVER TRANSPLANTATION

ASSESSMENT OF LIVER FUNCTION

Liver biopsy
Serologic indexes of disease status:
- Hepatitis screen
- Serum transaminases—indicators of hepatocellular damage
  - AST, ALT
- Serum phosphatases—indicators of bile duct damage
  - Alkaline phosphatase, gamma glutamyltransferase (GGT)
- Serum bilirubin level
- Indicators of protein synthesis
  - Albumin, PT, PTT, clotting factors

RADIOLOGIC STUDIES

Assessment of liver and portal circulation

CT scan for liver and spleen volume
Doppler ultrasound of liver, vessels, and bile ducts
Others as needed

ASSESSMENT OF OTHER SYSTEMS

Cardiovascular: baseline 12-lead ECG, thallium stress test or multiple gated acquisition (MUGA) scan
Pulmonary: ABGs, PFTs, chest film
Renal: creatinine clearance, BUN
Psychosocial evaluation
Dental: correction of abnormalities, extraction as necessary
Obstetric/gynecologic examination as indicated
Blood bank: type and antibody screen
Anesthesia consultation

Table 49-4 Sequelae associated with end-stage liver disease

Complication	Management
Massive ascites	Diuretics, paracentesis
Hepatic encephalopathy	Laxatives, antibiotics, enemas
Gastrointestinal hemorrhage	Propranolol, sclerotherapy, portosystemic shunt surgery
Hepatorenal syndrome	No real treatment except transplant
Infection: Spontaneous bacterial peritonitis, cholangitis	Antibiotics

Blood type and body size are the two criteria necessary for matching a donor liver to a recipient. Human lymphocyte antigen (HLA) tissue typing is not used in the matching of donor livers because this has not been shown to significantly affect patient outcomes, nor is it feasible because of the relative shortage of donor livers. The transplant center is notified by UNOS by the regional Organ Procurement Organization (OPO) of an available donor. If the center accepts the donor organ, the recipient is contacted by the transplant team.

Surgical Procedure

Liver transplant surgery is a lengthy and technically difficult operation, often lasting between 8 and 10 hours. The procedure involves the combined efforts of surgeons, anesthesiologists, nurses, perfusionists, and blood

LEGAL REVIEW: Organ transplantation

Among the most rapid developments in medical technology has been the evolution of organ transplantation, which raises many legal issues. Of major import are the issues of supply and demand, rationing and allocation, cost and reimbursement, locating organ donors, organs from live donors, and confidentiality and access to donor-donee data.

Critical care nurses are involved in the process of organ procurement for donation and transplantation, as well as the care of the organ donee—that is, the recipient. Federal and state statutes and regulations govern this area of health care delivery.

Federal law has established a national system of organ donation and procurement for the purpose of maximizing supply to meet increasing demand but simultaneously prohibiting the sale of organs. It is unlawful for any person to knowingly acquire, receive, or otherwise transfer any human organ for valuable consideration for use in human transplantation if the transfer affects interstate commerce. Violations of this law can result in substantial fines and incarceration.

Because there is a paucity of available organs for donation, a need exists for rationing and allocation. The purpose and intent of the Uniform Anatomical Gift Act (UAGA) are to establish the legal framework for cadaveric organ donation and to locate donors for organ transplantation; each state has adopted a variation of this uniform statute. Generally, the law provides that any adult of sound mind may donate any part or all of his or her body. In most states this individual decision cannot be overruled by a family member after death. In some states, however, family members can reverse this bequest. State law also specifies who may donate, who may receive the anatomic gift, and how the gift is made. In addition, state law includes restrictions. The physician who certifies or determines the time of death, for example, may not participate in the removal or transplantation of organs.

To increase the availability of organs, state and federal laws and regulations have been passed that require hospitals to ask patients or their family members about organ donation. At the federal level, hospitals receiving Medicare or Medicaid funding must establish written protocols for the identification of potential donors. Under state law hospitals establish policies addressing the request for organ donations. These policies should specify clearly the nurse's duties and responsibilities in organ procurement.

The major legal problem surrounding live donors arises when the potential donor is a minor or is incompetent. The courts have reached various decisions in these cases. In some jurisdictions the courts have adopted the substituted judgment rule. In others, the courts have rejected this doctrine and have adopted in its place the rule that the guardian must act, if at all, in the best interests of the guardian's ward, who is the potential donor.

Other legal issues have arisen, for example, questions about the right of access of a person in need of an organ to a hospital's records of the identities of potential donors. In the Iowa case cited in the footnote, the court held that the records of potential donors were confidential.

See Bouressa Fr G, O'Mara RJ: Ethical dilemmas in organ procurement and donation, *Crit Care Nurs Q* 10(2):37, 1987; *Guardianship of Pescinski,* 226 NW2d 180 (Wis 1975); *Head v Colloton,* 331 NW2d 870 (Iowa 1983); National Organ Transplant Act (NOTA), PL 98-507 (1984); 42 USCA Sec 274(e) (1986); O'Connell DA: Ethical implications of organ transplantation. *Crit Care Nurs Q,* 1990, 13(4):1, 1991; Smith SL: *AACN tissue and organ transplantation: implications for professional nursing practice,* St Louis, 1990, Mosby–Year Book; *Strunk v Strunk,* 445 SW2d 145 (Ky App 1969); Uniform Anatomical Gift Act (UAGA), 8A Uniform Law Acts [ULA] (1983).

bank, laboratory, and radiology personnel, to name a few. The surgical component of transplantation can be divided into three phases: (1) donor hepatectomy, (2) recipient hepatectomy, and (3) graft insertion and reperfusion.

◆ **Donor hepatectomy.** Recovery of a donor liver usually occurs in conjunction with the recovery of other organs, such as the heart, kidneys, and pancreas. Because each of these organs may be intended for recipients at different transplant centers, recovery requires the coordination of several recipient teams. At the time of recovery, the donor liver is visually inspected in situ by the receiving transplant surgeon. Abnormalities such as tumor, anomalies, contamination, or donor instability may preclude donation at this time.

A midline incision is made that extends from the sternal notch to the pubis. The liver is dissected free from the restraining ligaments that keep it secured to the diaphragm and abdominal wall. The aorta is isolated and cross-clamped. The bile duct is transected proximal to the ampulla of Vater, and the gallbladder is flushed free of bile. The liver is then flushed, first with a saline solution to clear blood, followed by cold heparinized perservative solution. The vessels of the liver are then divided, beginning with the suprahepatic vena cava, which is transected at the level of the right atrium. The infrahepatic vena cava is then transected above the level of the renal veins, thereby retaining them for renal transplantation. The portal vein is divided just proximal to the confluence of the splenic and superior mesenteric vein. The hepatic artery is resected with a generous patch of aorta, if possible. The entire organ and vessels are then removed from the donor. Other structures, such as portions of the distal aorta, iliac arteries, and iliac veins, also are procured. These extra tissues may be needed for grafting during the transplantation procedure. All recovered tissue is packed in iced preservative solution and transported to the recipient center.

Until recently, Euro-Collins solution was the only commercially available solution for organ preservation. This solution allowed only a cold ischemic time of approximately 10 to 12 hours for donor livers. This narrow margin of time created logistic problems because it was necessary for recipients to be admitted immediately for surgery, regardless of the time of day or night. In addition, organs that were preserved for the longer amount of time were associated with postoperative complications, such as delayed graft function.[72] The University of Wisconsin developed a solution that has been shown to lengthen cold ischemic time to 30 hours in canine livers.[73] Longer preservation time makes donor retrieval possible in centers distant from the receiving hospital, and it also allows the delay of surgery until the day shift when the hospital is better staffed to manage the complex operation.

◆ **Recipient hepatectomy.** The recipient is taken to the operating room for anesthesia induction and the insertion of large-bore intravenous catheters that allow high-volume fluid infusion and a pulmonary artery catheter for hemodynamic monitoring. Other devices, such as an arterial line, a nasogastric tube, and a urinary drainage catheter, also are inserted. The patient is positioned on the operating room table in such a way as to minimize pressure that might cause ischemia and subsequent injury to tissue and peripheral nerves.

Chronic liver disease has associated sequelae that can make the recipient hepatectomy one of the most difficult aspects of the transplantation procedure. The patient most likely has some degree of portal hypertension as a result of cirrhosis, which causes the development of massive collateral circulation around the liver. The dissection of these collateral vessels combined with the severe coagulopathy, which accompanies liver disease, greatly increases the risk of intraoperative hemorrhage, and the infusion of many units of packed red blood cells, fresh frozen plasma, platelets, and cryoprecipitate often is necessary.

A large subcostal transverse incision is made, which extends upward at the midline to the xiphoid process. The surgeon then begins the cumbersome task of dissecting down to the liver. This entails lysing adhesions that may have developed in the course of cirrhosis, as well as cauterizing numerous vessels. All surrounding structures are isolated and identified.

During this time another surgeon is preparing the donor liver for implantation. While still immersed in preservative solution, the organ is trimmed of fat and extra tissue and the gallbladder is removed. Any vascular anomalies that necessitate the use of grafts are corrected by use of the additional vessels obtained during procurement.

To remove the recipient's diseased liver, the vena cava must be crossed-clamped in two places: just below the diaphragm and just above the level of the renal veins. This interrupts the flow of blood through the vena cava and subsequently to the right atrium. To minimize the consequences of interrupting venous return, the patient is placed on venovenous bypass before the hepatectomy. Large-bore cannulas are placed in the patient's portal vein, left external iliac vein, and left axillary vein. A centrifugal pump cycles blood out via the iliac and portal vein cannulas and returns this blood into the central circulation via the axillary vein cannula (Fig. 49-9). Bypass accomplishes several goals: (1) it maintains venous return and therefore cardiac output; (2) it prevents engorgment of the intestinal vessels, which occurs with cross-clamping of the vena cava; and (3) it decreases the amount of blood in the surgical field. After the patient is placed on venovenous bypass, the portal vessels and bile duct are transected and the organ is removed. This begins what is known as the *anhepatic phase.*

◆ **Graft insertion and reperfusion.** The donor liver, or graft, is placed in the hepatic fossa. Anastamosis begins with the suprahepatic inferior vena cava, followed by the infrahepatic vena cava, by means of an end-to-end technique between the donor and recipient structures. The donor and recipient portal veins also are anastamosed in this manner, and venovenous bypass is discontinued after this step is completed. The liver is reperfused with blood, and any leakages of the venous anastamoses are identified and corrected. The hepatic artery is then anastamosed, also by means of the end-to-end method. At this point the patient is actively

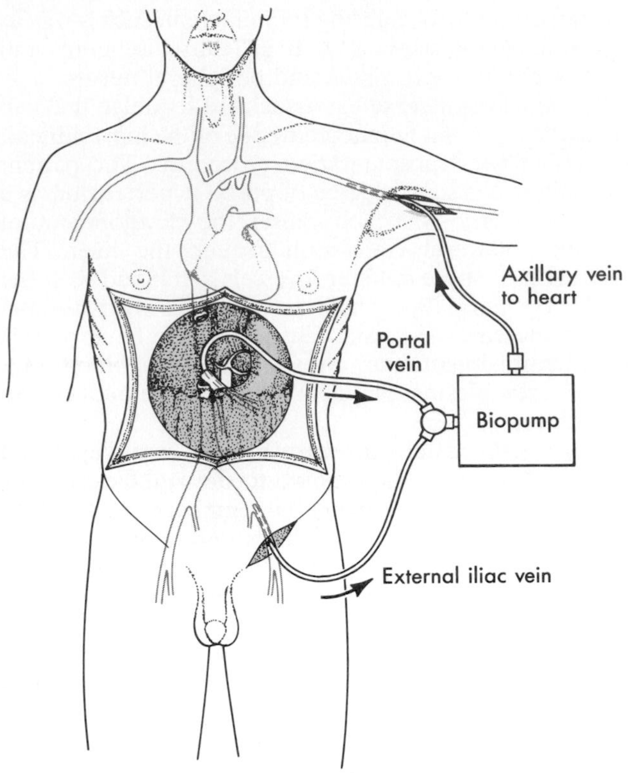

Fig. 49-9 Venovenous bypass for liver transplant surgery. (From Smith SL: *AACN tissue and organ transplantation: implications for professional nursing practice*, St Louis, 1990, Mosby–Year Book.)

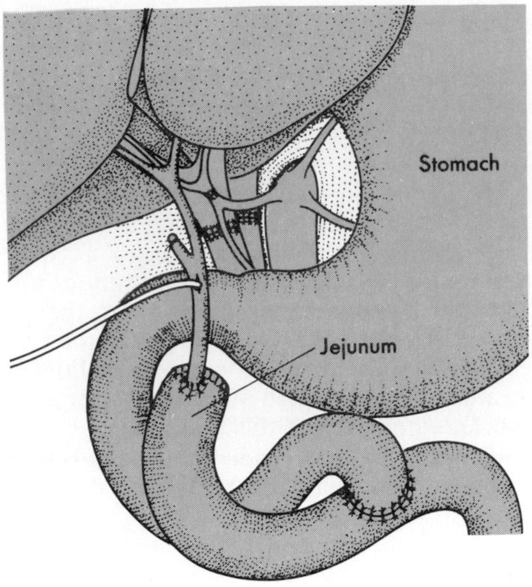

Fig. 49-10 Choledochojejunostomy for biliary drainage. (From Smith SL: *AACN tissue and organ transplantation: implications for professional nursing practice*, St Louis, 1990, Mosby–Year Book.)

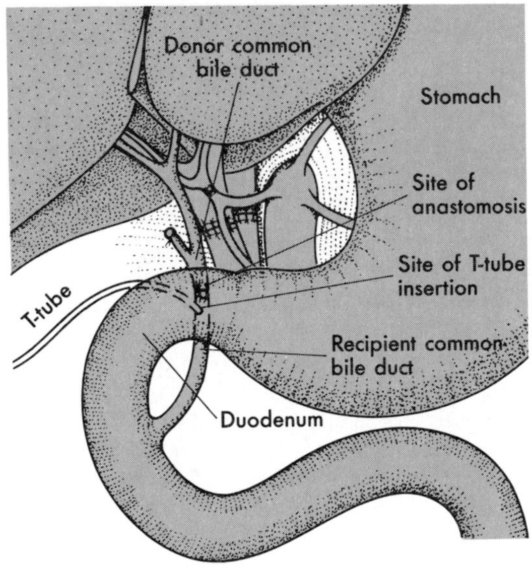

Fig. 49-11 Choledochocholedochostomy for biliary drainage. (From Smith SL: *AACN tissue and organ transplantation: implications for professional nursing practice*, St Louis, 1990, Mosby–Year Book.)

rewarmed with warm irrigants and intravenous fluids. Clotting studies are obtained to determine synthetic ability of the graft. Once the patient has been rewarmed and proper hemostasis is achieved, the biliary anastamosis begins.

There are two standard procedures for the biliary anastomosis; the technique used depends on the recipient's liver disease. For patients who had primary disease of the large bile ducts of the liver, such as sclerosing cholangitis, it is not possible to use the recipient native bile duct in transplanting the donor liver. In these cases a choledochojejunostomy is performed (Fig. 49-10). For patients with other types of liver disease, it is possible to anastomose the donor bile duct directly to the recipient bile duct as in a choledochocholedochostomy (Fig. 49-11). The latter procedure requires the placement of a T-tube stent, which not only secures the area, but also diverts bile from the anastomosis. The bile drains into an external drainage bag. This allows direct monitoring of bile production, which is an important indicator of proper graft function.

On completion of the biliary anastomosis, an intraoperative cholangiogram is performed to determine integrity of the biliary system. If the structures are intact, three surgical drains are placed in the abdominal cavity and the abdomen is sutured closed. The patient is then transported directly to the critical care unit.

Postoperative Medical and Nursing Management

The patient arrives in the critical care unit unreversed from anesthesia. Mechanical ventilation is necessary until the patient has awakened and begun effective spontaneous respirations. Postoperative hypothermia, which is caused by many factors (see first box on p. 851), delays renal excretion of anesthesia and prolongs sedating effects. Prolonged hypothermia may cause other complications, such as cardiac dysrhythmias, altered platelet func-

LIVER TRANSPLANTATION FACTORS CONTRIBUTING TO POSTOPERATIVE HYPOTHERMIA

- General anesthesia
- Low ambient temperature of operating room
- Wet surgical preparation techniques
- Muscle relaxants
- Narcotics
- Prolonged exposure of large body cavity
- Cold preservation techniques of donor organ
- Infusion of unwarmed intravenous fluids
- Use of unwarmed irrigants

NURSING DIAGNOSIS AND MANAGEMENT
Liver transplantation

- Hypothermia related to cold environment secondary to prolonged surgery and cold preservation techniques of donor organ, p. 562
- Altered Nutrition: Less than Body Protein-Calorie Requirements related to lack of exogenous nutrients and increased metabolic demands secondary to preoperative cachexia, p. 673
- High Risk for Infection risk factor: the immunosuppressive drugs required to prevent rejection of the transplanted liver, p. 866
- High Risk for Fluid Volume Deficit risk factor: active blood loss, p. 639
- Anxiety related to threat to biologic, psychologic, and/or social integrity secondary to immunologic rejection of the transplanted liver, p. 763
- Knowledge Deficit: Posttransplant Self-care Regimen, specifically immunosuppressive drugs and clinical manifestations of infection related to lack of previous exposure to information, p. 72
- Body Image Disturbance related to actual change in body function or appearance, p. 94
- Sensory/Perceptual Alterations related to sensory overload, sensory deprivation, and sleep pattern disturbance, p. 573

tion, coagulopathy, and decreased oxygen delivery to tissues. Most of the critical care nurse's efforts in this early postoperative period therefore are directed toward safely rewarming the patient. The use of warmed blankets, heating lamps, and a head cover are all important in achieving this goal. Core temperature is monitored by an indwelling pulmonary artery catheter or urinary drainage catheter. Measurements of hemodynamic function, such as arterial blood pressure, central venous pressure, pulmonary artery pressure, pulmonary capillary wedge pressure, cardiac output, and urinary output, are obtained frequently during the rewarming process. Such

LIVER TRANSPLANTATION EARLY INDICATORS OF PROPER GRAFT FUNCTION

- Adequate bile output from T tube
- Decrease in hepatocellular and biliary enzyme levels
- Increase in serum protein levels
- Timely recovery from anesthesia
- Normal or mildly elevated serum glucose level
- Adequate urine output

changes as decreased arterial blood pressure, decreased systemic vascular resistance, and decreased cardiac output are anticipated inasmuch as rising core temperature results in vasodilation. Serologic tests, such as serum bilirubin level, liver enzymes, blood glucose level, and clotting factors, are performed at regular intervals to monitor graft function. Serial blood counts, such as hemoglobin and hematocrit, as well as the character of surgical drain output, are assessed to determine the possibility of intraabdominal hemorrhage. Deficiencies in clotting components are supplemented by the infusion of fresh frozen plasma and platelets. If a T tube is present, bile output and character are assessed frequently. Early indicators of proper graft function are listed in the box above.

After the removal of the endotracheal tube, the patient begins physical therapy and mobilization. If there is no contraindication, the nasogastric tube is removed and clear liquids are begun. The diet is advanced as tolerated. The frequency of hemodynamic monitoring decreases, and the pulmonary artery catheter is replaced with a multilumen central venous catheter and the arterial catheter is removed. The urinary catheter also is removed several days after surgery. The patient begins to participate in self-care and discharge planning. Plans are made to transfer the patient to the general nursing unit.

During the post-ICU phase, laboratory data and vital signs continue to be monitored on a routine basis. Much of the nurse's effort is directed at patient education and discharge planning. Discharge booklets are helpful in the education process. It is important for the patient to learn how to self-administer medications, monitor blood pressure, care for the T tube if present, prevent infections, and identify problems that should prompt seeking medical attention. Before discharge, at some centers, a multidisciplinary conference is held to allow the patient to ask any questions about issues related to rehabilitation at home. The length of hospitalization after liver transplantation may be 20 to 30 days, or longer if complications arise.

Complications

A variety of possible complications are associated with liver transplantation. It is not possible to predict which complications individual patients may experience, but most patients have some type of complication. Although all patients are maintained on immunosuppressive therapy, rejection is always a possibility and is estimated to occur in approximately 80% of liver transplants.[74] Rejection can occur at any time after transplantation, but the risk for rejection is highest within the first 10 to 14 days after transplant. Acute rejection is suspected when an elevation in serum liver enzyme levels occurs (Table 49-5), especially when accompanied by fever. The diagnosis and severity of rejection, which are determined by percutaneous liver biopsy, can range from the mildly acute type, which requires no treatment, to chronic rejection, which requires retransplantation. Most often the severity of rejection falls between these two extremes and is treated pharmacologically.

Immunosuppressive therapy (cyclosporine, FK506, prednisone, azathioprine) places the transplant patient at an increased risk of infection, which is the leading cause of morbidity and mortality in this patient population.[75] The potential for infection is greatest in patients who have required additional immunosuppressive agents for the treatment of rejection. The patient is educated regarding infection control. Good handwashing techniques should be practiced by all persons who come in contact with the patient during the hospitalization phase. Infection is treated with pharmacotherapy specific to the invading organism. Other complications after liver transplantation are listed in the box, lower right.

Long-Term Considerations

After discharge, the patient is seen at regular intervals in the outpatient clinic. Serologic testing is performed to monitor graft function and to determine blood levels of certain immunosuppressive drugs (cyclosporine, FK506). Readmission to the hospital often is necessary to evaluate problems that may be detected during clinic follow-up. Because the possibility of readmission may create anxiety for the patient and family, they are encouraged to attend posttransplant support groups if offered by the center.

Financial concerns also are a major source of stress in this patient population. The largest group of liver transplant recipients are those who have suffered from some type of chronic liver disease. They often are disabled for some length of time before transplant and already have experienced financial stressors related to illness.

Transplant offers hope for survival, but at considerable expense. Many insurance companies, including Medicare, provide partial reimbursement for liver transplantation. The remaining costs, however, can be staggering. Liver transplant surgery has been reported to cost between $75,000 and $630,000, depending on the incidence of postoperative complications.[76-78] These figures refer to the transplant hospitalization and do not take into account the additional costs associated with long-term follow-up, lifelong pharmacologic therapy, tests, and rehospitalization.

Future of Liver Transplantation

The future of liver transplantation holds many possibilities. The most significant challenge of successful transplantation is achieving immunosuppression that is adequate at preventing rejection but does not cause increased morbidity and mortality from overwhelming infection. Clinical trials are seeking to identify possible new drugs and to define treatment protocols.[79-81] Research also has explored methods of inducing tolerance to donor antigens in the recipient during the anhepatic phase of transplantation surgery.[82] Tolerance would suppress the immunologic mechanism responsible for rejection and therefore decrease the amount of maintenance immunosuppression required by the recipient.

Attention also is being focused on ways to increase the number and availability of donor organs. Mechanisms include alternatives to whole-organ transplantation, such as surgical reduction of large livers to fit small recipients, splitting one donor liver between two recipients, and considering segmental transplantation from living donors.[83] Public education and legislature regarding donation are other issues that will affect the number of available organs. Xenografting, which is transplanting tissue from one species to another, also is being explored[84] (see box, p. 853).

Table 49-5 Enzymes used to monitor graft function after liver transplantation*

Enzyme	Normal range
Transaminases	
AST	7-40 U/L
ALT	7-35 U/L
Phosphatases	
Alkaline phosphatase	30-115 IU/L
Gamma GT (GGT)	5-55 U/L

AST, Aspartate aminotransferase—previously known as SGOT; *ALT,* alanine aminotransferase—previously known as SGPT.

*Normal reported enzyme values will vary from laboratory to laboratory, depending on the specific methods used to measure enzymes in each setting.

COMPLICATIONS AFTER LIVER TRANSPLANTATION

- Primary graft nonfunction
- Hemorrhage
- Biliary leak, obstruction, or stricture
- Hepatic artery or portal vein thrombosis
- Infection
  - Viral, bacterial, opportunistic
- Rejection
  - Acute, chronic
- Side effects of immunosuppressive therapy
- Psychosocial issues

FACTORS INFLUENCING THE FUTURE OF LIVER TRANSPLANTATION

- Better candidate selection
- Advances in organ recovery and preservation
- Advances in perioperative management
- Advances in immunobiology and immunosuppression
- Innovative use of organs
- Xenografting
- Public education regarding donation
- Timely referral of patients to transplant centers
- Cost-effective management

KIDNEY TRANSPLANTATION

In 1954 a team of surgeons led by Dr. Joseph Murray performed a successful renal transplant between identical (monozygotic) twins at Peter Bent Brigham Hospital in Boston. Although transplantation had been attempted since the beginning of the twentieth century, this landmark event marked the potential for renal transplantation as a treatment for end-stage renal disease (ESRD).[85] Improved surgical techniques and better understanding of the immune system have resulted in renal transplantation becoming the treatment of choice for many individuals rather than an experimental procedure. In 1991, 9943 renal transplants were performed in the United States.[86] Not only is transplantation the most cost-effective treatment for ESRD; it also offers successful transplant recipients an improved quality of life and increased activity levels compared with other forms of ESRD treatments.[87,88]

In the early years of renal transplantation, information was limited about the immune system and long-term effects of immunosuppressive medications. High dosages of these medications led to liver malfunction, facial disfigurement, severe osteoporosis, cancer, and fatal infections. During the 1970s, procedures such as total body irradiation, splenectomy, and depleting the lymphatic system of lymphocytes through thoracic duct drainage were used to modify the immune system of kidney transplant recipients. This, it was hoped, would permit administration of lower doses of immunosuppressive medications. The complications of these procedures, however, including severe infections, have prevented these treatments from becoming routine in transplantation today.[89] Preconditioning recipients with blood transfusions before transplantation was begun in the late 1970s. This practice has decreased in recent years because of the success of cyclosporine in prolonging graft survival.[90]

Indications and Selection

Because of the broad range of diseases that can lead to ESRD, the potential transplant recipient must undergo extensive evaluation to determine whether transplantation is a viable treatment option. The first box on p. 854 lists the laboratory tests and diagnostic studies most often performed during an evaluation. Specific findings that would contraindicate transplantation are listed in the box on p. 854, bottom of left-hand column. Because ESRD affects many of the body's systems, many patients who are evaluated have abnormal findings, which must be assessed on an individual basis. If active infection is present, the evaluation may need to be resumed when the infection is controlled. An extensive cardiac evaluation may be needed, including possible angioplasty or coronary artery bypass surgery before a patient is considered a candidate. Some individuals who are overweight are recommended for transplantation on the condition that they lose weight to decrease surgical risk. Smokers, especially those with diabetes or chronic obstructive pulmonary disease (COPD), are strongly advised to quit smoking. Patients with malignancies that have been in remission for 2 to 5 years, depending on the type of malignancy, may be considered as candidates. Persons with ESRD as a result of active vasculitis or glomerulonephritis, or both, may be considered when the disease process becomes inactive. Patients with substance abuse problems are required to have treatment, and close substance screening will be required for an appropriate amount of time to monitor compliance. Patients who are noncompliant with their medical treatment also may be given a period of time to improve their compliance before transplantation occurs. Persons with severe learning deficits, mental retardation, or other process that may alter their mental status may be considered for transplantation if there is strong, consistent support from a family member or significant other.

Once transplantation is considered as a possible treatment, the patient must either be placed on the UNOS waiting list for a cadaveric donation or receive a kidney from a living related donor. Several factors are considered in allocation of cadaveric kidneys, including blood type, degree of human lymphocyte antigen (HLA) match between the donor and recipient, the length of time the patient has been on the waiting list, and the proximity of the organ to the patient.[91] The supply of cadaveric organs does not meet the demand of the number of persons on the waiting list. To avoid this wait, a living donor may be considered. A living donor should be evaluated to rule out surgical risks and to consider any medical risk in having one kidney. The box on p. 854, right-hand column, lists the tests required in evaluation of a potential living donor. There has been some concern over whether the use of living donors is justified. If, however, there is no perceived risk to the donor and the gift of the organ is freely given, most transplant centers will use a living donor.[92]

Surgical Procedure

When the kidney is harvested, the ureter, renal vein, and renal artery are dissected. If the kidney is taken from a living donor, the organ is flushed with an iced solution to remove formed blood elements. It is then taken to the recipient's operating room for transplantation. When the kidney is taken from a cadaveric donor, the organ is flushed with a hyperosmolar, hyperkalemic, and hypo-

EVALUATION TESTING FOR KIDNEY TRANSPLANTATION

Laboratory tests
- SMA-18, CBC with differential, RPR, HBsAg and HBsAb (anti-HBS)
- HIV, HCVAB and HTLVI antibody, CMV, EBV, HSV and VZV titers, fasting lipid profile and PSA
- Platelet count, PT, PTT, HLA typing, urine for urinalysis and C&S (If patient is receiving peritoneal dialysis, then the peritoneal fluid should also be sent for C&S and AFB)

Roentgenograms
- Posteroanterior (PA) and lateral chest films
- Hand films to evaluate possible osteodystrophy
- Possible Panorex films as part of the dental work-up
- Mammogram for women over 35 years old

Renal ultrasound

12-Lead Electrocardiogram (ECG)

Thallium scan
- 45 years of age or older
- Diabetes mellitus
- Abnormal ECG findings
- History of angina or myocardial infarction

Noninvasive vascular studies
- Diabetes mellitus

Consultations
- Psychiatry, urology, transplant nephrology, social services, dental, nursing, gynecology for female patients, nutritional assessment

SMA, Sequential Multiple Analyzer; *RPR,* rapid plasma reagin; *HBsAg,* hepatitis B surface antigen; *HBsAb,* hepatitis B surface antigen antibody; *HIV,* human immunodeficiency virus; *HCVAB,* hepatitis C virus antibody; HTLVI, human T-cell leukemia virus; *CMV,* cytomegalovirus; *EBV,* Epstein-Barr virus; *HSV,* herpesvirus; *VZV,* varicella-zoster virus; *PSA*, prostatic-specific antigen; *PT,* prothrombin time; *PTT,* partial thromboplastin time; *C&S,* culture and sensitivity; *AFB,* acid-fast bacillus.

CONTRAINDICATIONS TO KIDNEY TRANSPLANTATION

- Active infections, including active HIV, tuberculosis, or systemic infections
- Active vasculitis/glomerulonephritis: lupus, Wegener's granulomatosis, Goodpasture's syndrome
- Advanced cardiopulmonary disease
- Persons at high risk for surgery, e.g., advanced chronic obstructive pulmonary disease (COPD), obesity
- Malignancy
- Active IV drug use
- Noncompliance with medical course of therapy
- Mental incompetence
- Positive T-cell lymphocytotoxic crossmatch

EVALUATION TESTING FOR LIVING KIDNEY DONORS

Laboratory test
- SMA-18, CBC with differential, RPR, HBsAg and HBsAb (anti-HBS), HTLVI antibody, HCV antibody, HIV, amylase, CMV, EBV, HSV, and VZV titers, platelet count, PT, PTT, urine for urinalysis and C&S, 24-hr urine collection for creatinine clearance, serum creatinine, and protein

Roentgenograms
- PA and lateral chest films

12-Lead electrocardiogram (ECG)

Renal scan

Renal arteriogram

Consultations
- Psychiatry, urology, transplant nephrology, social services, nursing, and gynecology for female donors

thermic preservation solution and then placed in an iced solution. Once the kidney is in this hypothermic solution, metabolism is slowed and the organ may be preserved for up to 48 hours. To decrease the potential for acute tubular necrosis (ATN), most centers attempt to transplant the organ as soon as possible.

After the patient is anesthetized, a urinary catheter is inserted and irrigated with a sterile antibiotic fluid or povidone-iodine solution.[93] A curved incision is made just above the symphysis pubis that extends to the iliac crest. The transplanted kidney is placed in the extraperitoneal site of either the right or the left iliac fossa (Fig. 49-12). The muscles and facia are divided, and the peritoneum is freed and retracted medially, exposing the iliac vessels.[93] The renal artery is anastomosed end-to-end to the external iliac artery, and the vein is sutured end-to-side to the external iliac vein. If the aortic cuff is recovered from a cadaveric donation, a Carrel patch may be used to attach the renal artery end-to-side to the external iliac artery. Examples of potential anastomoses can be seen in Fig. 49-13.

During the surgery a central venous pressure (CVP) of 8-16 mm Hg should be maintained. Systolic blood pressure at or above preoperative levels also is recommended.[93] This is necessary to ensure adequate reperfusion of the transplanted kidney.

Once revascularization is completed, the ureteral anastomosis is begun, with the most common being the ureteroneocystostomy. This involves making an incision into the dome of the bladder. After the donor ureter is tunneled through the mucosal layer of the bladder, it is sutured end-to-side into the mucosal opening[93] (Fig. 49-14). With each bladder contraction the tunnel prevents reflux by acting as a one-way valve, thus reducing the potential for bladder contamination.[93] If the recipient has had multiple bladder surgeries or has a history of infections, a ureteroureterostomy may be performed. This involves an anastomosis of the donor ureter to the native ureter.

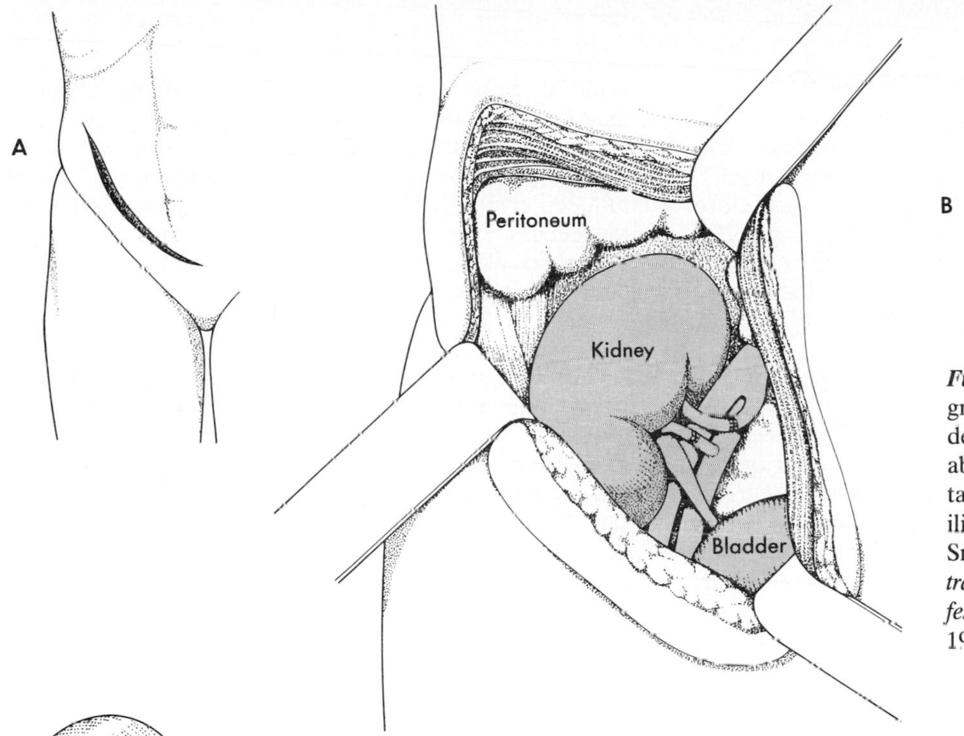

Fig. 49-12 Placement of the renal graft into iliac fossa. **A,** The incision is depicted for the right side of the abdomen, representing graft implantation in the right iliac fossa. **B,** The iliac vessels are exposed. (From Smith SL: *AACN tissue and organ transplantation: implications for professional nursing practice*, St Louis, 1990, Mosby–Year Book.)

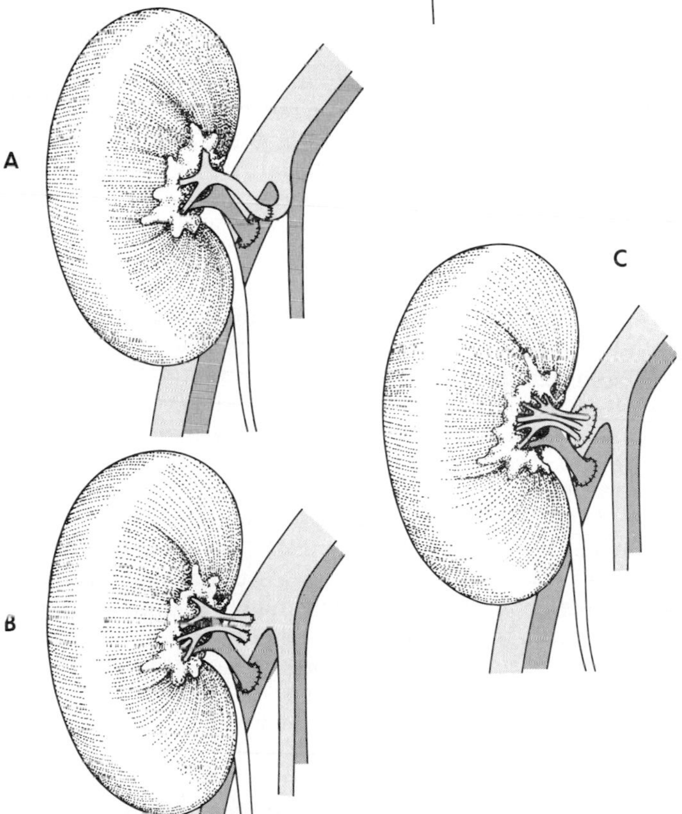

Fig. 49-13 Anastomosis of the renal artery to the iliac artery. **A,** Single renal artery to internal iliac artery and renal vein to external iliac vein. **B,** Multiple renal arteries to external iliac artery. **C,** Carrel patch containing multiple renal arteries to external iliac artery. (From Smith SL: *AACN tissue and organ transplantation: implications for professional nursing practice*, St Louis, 1990, Mosby–Year Book. Redrawn from Whelchel JD: Renal transplantation. In Grabar GB, editor: *Anesthesia for renal transplantation,* vol 14, Norwell, Mass, 1987, Cluwer Academic Publishers.)

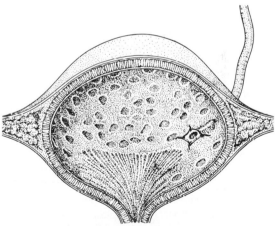

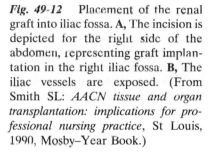

Fig. 49-14 Ureteroneocystostomy reconstruction of the urinary tract. The donor ureter is passed through a posterior bladder wall tunnel and anastomosed to the bladder mucosa. (From Smith SL: *AACN tissue and organ transplantation: implications for professional nursing practice*, St Louis, 1990, Mosby–Year Book. Redrawn from Whelchel JD: Renal transplantation. In Grabar GB, editor: *Anesthesia for renal transplantation,* vol 14, Norwell, Mass, 1987, Cluwer Academic Publishers.)

Postoperative Medical and Nursing Management

Depending on the transplant center's protocol, the recipient is transferred either to the intensive care unit (ICU) or the transplant nursing unit after surgery. Regardless of where the patient begins recovery, close monitoring is needed. A knowledge of surgical postoperative care, renal function, and immunosuppression is necessary to detect any complications. An immediate response to complications ensures graft, and possibly patient, survival.

If the graft is functioning well, the patient may become dehydrated or hypotensive as a result of diuresis. Adequate hydration and blood pressure are necessary to ensure adequate blood flow to the transplanted organ. Inadequate blood flow may cause acute tubular necrosis (ATN) and, if uncorrected, possible graft failure.[94] The amount of urine output may vary as a result of such factors as cold ischemia time or administration of diuretics. Therefore IV fluid replacement of 1 ml for each milliliter of urine may be indicated. However, a limit on total fluid given each hour is necessary to avoid complications of fluid overload.

The patient's CVP should not fall below 4 mm Hg, and the systolic blood pressure should remain above 110 mm Hg.[94] Albumin may be needed to maintain these levels in the event of extensive diuresis. Noninvasive monitoring of fluid status includes accurate recording of intake and output, daily weights, and assessment of skin turgor, sacral edema, and jugular venous distention.

Monitoring of serum electrolyte levels is required every 4 to 6 hours for the first 24 hours. Blood urea nitrogen (BUN) and serum creatinine levels are needed to monitor graft function. A steady decline of these levels is seen as graft function improves. Hypokalemia may occur if there is excessive diuresis, and hyperkalemia may occur if the graft is not functioning well. Both require assessment of frequent potassium levels, and cardiac monitoring sometimes is indicated. Steroid-induced hyperglycemia is a potential complication. If this occurs, an insulin drip is necessary in the immediate postoperative phase. When the patient's condition becomes stable, obtaining daily serum electrolyte levels is adequate for monitoring graft function.

Because of the surgical anastomoses that involve the renal artery and vein, there is potential for hemorrhage. Frequent serum hematocrit (Hct) measurements are obtained. Any drainage or swelling at the incision site, or a sudden drop in blood pressure or Hct level should alert the nurse to possible hemorrhage. In addition, leakage at the bladder anastomis can occur, resulting in decreased urine output or leakage of urine from the incision. In the immunosuppressed patient a urine leak can lead to life-threatening peritonitis. These complications must be surgically corrected as soon as possible.

These patients are immunocompromised to prevent rejection, which also places them at an increased risk for infections. All dressing changes are performed with use of aseptic technique, and any unnecessary intravenous line should be discontinued. Any fever or elevation in white blood cell count is a cause for concern, and blood and urine cultures should be obtained. Not only are these patients susceptible to wound and urinary tract infections; they are at risk for opportunistic infections. As the patient recovers from surgery, the importance of good hand washing and hygiene, as well as the recognition of the clinical manifestations of infection, should be stressed. See nursing management plan on p. 866 for additional information on infection control.

In addition, during their hospitalization, patients are taught the clinical manifestations of rejection (see box below), record keeping of laboratory values and vital signs, and the importance of compliance with the posttransplant regimen. Many centers place recipients on a self-medication program before discharge. Frequent clinic visits during the first 3 to 6 months are needed to monitor progress and to adjust medications. As the patient progresses, a schedule is established for routine laboratory tests and clinic visits to ensure long-term success of the transplant.[95]

NURSING DIAGNOSIS AND MANAGEMENT
Kidney transplantation

- High Risk for Infection risk factors: immunosuppressive drugs to prevent rejection of the transplanted kidney, p. 866
- Body Image Disturbance related to actual change in body function or appearance, p. 94
- Anxiety related to threat to biologic, psychologic, and/or social integrity secondary to immunologic rejection of the transplanted kidney, p. 763
- Knowledge Deficit: Posttransplant Self-care Regimen, specifically immunosuppressive drugs and clinical manifestations related to lack of previous exposure to information, p. 72
- High Risk for Decreased Cardiac Output risk factors: decreased preload secondary to postoperative bleeding at graft anastomoses, p. 361
- Sensory/Perceptual Alterations related to sensory overload, sensory deprivation, and sleep pattern disturbance, p. 573

KIDNEY TRANSPLANTATION CLINICAL MANIFESTATIONS OF REJECTION

- Tenderness at graft site
- Decrease in urine output
- Sudden increase in weight: 3 to 5 pounds in a 24-hour period
- Edema – usually begins in hands and feet
- Elevated temperature
- Elevated serum creatinine above the individual's baseline

Long-Term Considerations

As with any transplant patient, rejection is always a possibility. If rejection is suspected, a biopsy specimen of the kidney will determine which medication is indicated for treatment. This can be an emotionally charged time for the patient. The uncertainty of graft survival and concerns regarding the possible return to dialysis are areas that need to be discussed with patients and their significant others. Frequent outpatient monitoring after a rejection episode is necessary until graft function is determined to be stable.

The future of renal transplantation lies in the improvement of immunosuppressive medications. As cyclosporine increased the graft survival of transplanted organs in the 1980s, future medications may lead to effective immunosuppression with fewer side effects. Many organizations also are investigating methods to improve organ donation. An increase in donation, combined with improved immunosuppression, can enhance the quality of life for thousands of individuals waiting for a transplant each year.

PANCREAS TRANSPLANTATION

The devastating effects of insulin-dependent diabetes mellitus (IDDM) are well documented.[96,97] Providing the diabetic person with a functioning pancreas, thus eliminating the need for insulin and, it is hoped, reducing the complications of the disease, are the goals of pancreatic transplantation. Many years of experimentation and research led to the first human pancreas transplant in 1966 at the University of Minnesota. The patient, who had diabetic uremia, received a simultaneous renal-pancreas transplant. Unfortunately, sepsis and rejection proved fatal 2 months after the procedure.[98] During the 1960s and 1970s the progress in pancreas transplantation was slow and relatively unsuccessful. This was because of difficulties involving organ grafting, management of exocrine graft function, and immunosuppression. In the 1980s, however, with improved surgical technique and the use of medications such as cyclosporine, the success rate of this procedure has improved. Many centers now report 1-year graft survival and function of approximately 70%.[99]

Indications and Selection

Persons with diabetes who are considered for pancreas transplantation must undergo a thorough medical evaluation. Systems that are adversely affected by IDDM are examined closely. A cardiac evaluation is necessary. Extensive vascular studies are required to ensure adequate vascularization of the graft. Nerve conduction studies are needed to evaluate neuropathy. Depending on the type of surgical technique used, urologic and bladder function testing may be needed to evaluate possible difficulties with a bladder anastomosis. An endocrinologist will evaluate the patient and decide appropriate endocrine function tests. If the pancreas is to be transplanted simultaneously with another organ, the patient should complete all the evaluation procedures required for the additional organ, including the psychologic evaluation.

Because of diabetic glomerular nephropathy resulting in ESRD, many candidates for pancreas transplant often will be candidates for renal transplant. Many programs perform simultaneous renal-pancreas transplants.[100] Combined renal-pancreas transplants have a 1-year graft survival of approximately 75%. Patients who receive a kidney from one donor and subsequently receive a pancreas from another donor have a 1-year insulin-free graft survival of 55%.[100] Diabetic persons with a successful renal-pancreas transplant have a higher quality of life than do those who have received only a kidney transplant.[101] Regardless of whether the transplant program performs single pancreas or combined renal pancreas transplantations, the surgery is performed if the projected benefits outweigh the risk of the procedure.[100,102]

Surgical Procedure

Transplantation of the pancreas may involve islet cell transplantation, segmental transplantation, or whole organ transplantation. Regardless of the type of surgery performed, the native pancreas is left intact for continued exocrine function. The purpose of a pancreas transplant is to replace the endocrine function (insulin production). Islet cell transplantation involves isolation and extraction of endocrine cells from a donor, which are then inoculated into the recipient. Inoculation sites include the peritoneal cavity, liver, spleen, capsule of the kidney, testes, omentum, and cerebral ventricles.[98] The complications to this procedure include an inadequate amount of cell mass, damage of the cells, and rejection. Success with this procedure is limited, and research is continuing to improve the technique and immunosuppression involved.[103]

Segmental transplantation involves grafting the body and tail of the donor pancreas. The segmental pancreas can be recovered from either a cadaveric or a living donor, although pancreas transplantation involving a living donor remains controversial. The success rates between the two methods are comparable, although whole organ transplantation is performed more often than segmental. The advantages of whole organ transplantation include a larger mass of islet cells and adequate vessel perfusion.[104]

When the pancreas is recovered for whole organ transplantation, the superior mesenteric and splenic arteries also are procured. A 5- to 8-cm segment of the duodenum is resected, which assists in handling the organ and, depending on the surgical technique, may be used for surgical drainage. Once it is recovered, the cold ischemic time is 18 to 24 hours.[105] Initially the pancreas was placed extraperitoneally, similar to kidney grafts. Complications of delayed wound healing and infections were not uncommon as a result of exocrine drainage from the surface of the graft. More recently, these grafts are placed in the intraperitoneal space. This allows the peritoneum to absorb the exocrine drainage. The pancreas is placed in the right iliac fossa. In this placement the relationship between the donor and the recipient veins decreases the possibility of obstruction.[105] The donor arterial supply is anastomosed to the common iliac vein. If a kidney is transplanted simultaneously, the

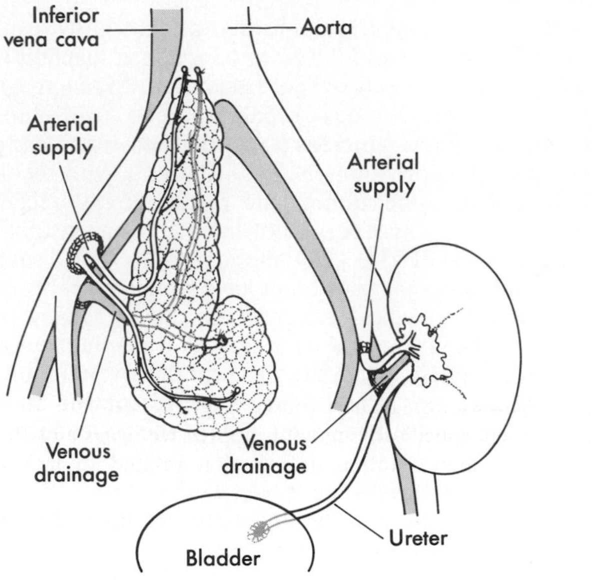

Fig. 49-15 Placement of organs during simultaneous kidney-pancreas transplant. (From Smith SL: *AACN tissue and organ transplantation: implications for professional nursing practice*, St Louis, 1990, Mosby–Year Book.)

kidney is placed in the left iliac fossa. Fig. 49-15 shows placement of both organs. Once the blood flow to the pancreas is established, provisions for elimination of the exocrine drainage must be made.

Endocrine function of the transplanted pancreas is all that is needed to eliminate the need for insulin therapy. In most cases there is adequate exocrine function (digestive enzymes) of the native pancreas, thus creating a need for elimination of the exocrine function of the transplanted graft. Management of these digestive enzymes has proved to be the surgical challenge of this procedure. Over the years the three most common techniques that have developed are ductal occlusion, enteric drainage, and urinary diversion.

Ductal occlusion involves injecting a polymer substance into the main pancreatic duct (Fig. 49-16). This injection causes hardening and occlusion of the duct. Although there are short-term complications, such as leakage and wound infection, the major concerns are the potential for long-term complications. Fibrosis resulting from the injection may involve the islet cells and ultimately cause graft failure.[104]

Anastomosing the graft to a Roux-en-Y loop of recipient jejunum is the second method of eliminating exocrine drainage (Fig. 49-17). This method of enteric drainage, pancreaticojejunostomy, is used if both endocrine and exocrine function is desired from the transplanted pancreas or if the recipient has chronic bladder dysfunction and cannot tolerate urinary diversion.[106] The reabsorption of the pancreatic enzymes creates fewer metabolic imbalances; however, the inability to monitor enzyme secretion eliminates a method of detecting graft dysfunction or rejection.[107]

The third technique, which manages exocrine drainage by urinary diversion, is termed *pancreaticoduodenocystostomy.* This technique involves anastomosing the pancreas to the recipient's bladder. A portion of the

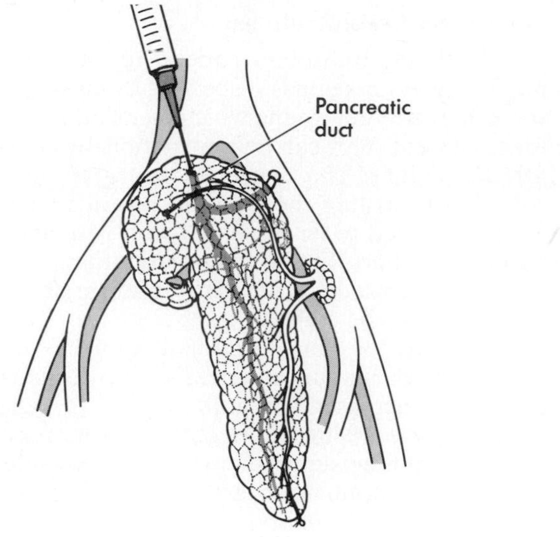

Fig. 49-16 Exocrine management by ductal injection. (From Smith SL: *AACN tissue and organ transplantation: implications for professional nursing practice*, St Louis, 1990, Mosby–Year Book.)

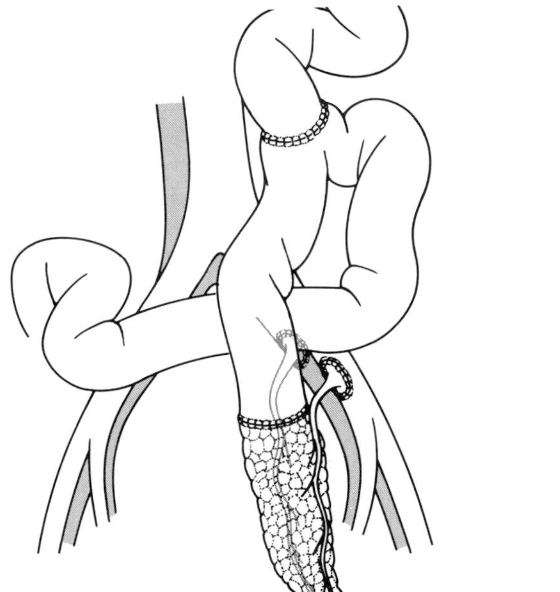

Fig. 49-17 Exocrine management by enteric drainage (Roux-en-Y jejunum). (From Smith SL: *AACN tissue and organ transplantation: implications for professional nursing practice*, St Louis, 1990, Mosby–Year Book.)

donor duodenum is recovered with the pancreas, and this is sutured into place as a conduit for drainage (Fig. 49-18). Adequate bladder function is necessary if this technique is to be successful. Complications of this procedure include ulceration and cystitis resulting from duodenal irritation by the pancreatic enzymes. If a simultaneous renal-pancreas transplant is performed, there may be leakage because of the multiple bladder anastomoses.[108] Also, there is a significant amount of sodium and bicarbonate lost in the urine. Patients who have this procedure are at high risk for hypotension and

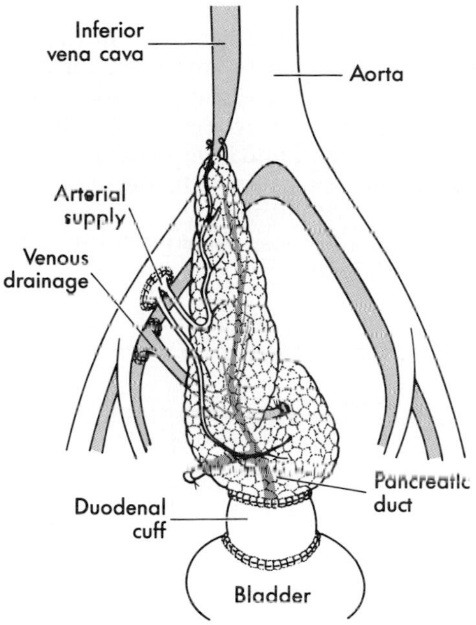

Fig. 49-18 Exocrine management by urinary diversion. (From Smith SL: *AACN tissue and organ transplantation: implications for professional nursing practice*, St Louis, 1990, Mosby–Year Book.)

metabolic acidosis. Daily oral sodium bicarbonate replacement is necessary, and intravenous hydration sometimes is needed. Despite the potential complications of this procedure, several advantages are noteworthy. The incidence of fistulas is decreased as a result of inactivation of pancreatic enzymes in the urine. Also, the urinary tract is free from bacteria, which reduces the risk of infection.[98] This is extremely important because these patients are immunosuppressed. The main advantage of this procedure is the ability to evaluate pancreatic function by monitoring urinary amylase levels. A decrease in urinary amylase has proved to be one of the earliest indicators of graft dysfunction and rejection.[107]

Postoperative Medical and Nursing Management

After surgery the patient is taken to the ICU. Although these patients have a functioning pancreas, they are at increased risk for surgical complications because of the long-term adverse effects of diabetes. Oxygenation, hemodynamics, and cardiac status are monitored closely. If a simultaneous renal transplant has been performed, fluid and electrolyte management is indicated, including fluid replacement, recording intake and output, and monitoring potassium, BUN, and serum creatinine levels. A nasogastric tube usually is in place for 24 to 48 hours after surgery. The patient also may be receiving a continuous insulin infusion to rest the graft. Frequent monitoring of blood glucose level is needed, and the infusion is discontinued as soon as possible. Because of the immunosuppressed status of these patients, good hand washing and aseptic technique are necessary with all procedures.

Because of the fragility of the pancreas and the delicate anastomosis performed in this surgery, these patients are at high risk for graft thrombosis. Activity is restricted to bed rest for up to 5 days, with no hip flexion on the side of the graft for up to 7 days. Gentle log rolling, an air mattress, and an overhead trapeze are needed to maintain skin integrity. Low molecular–weight dextran is given during this time to decrease blood viscosity. Aspirin therapy is started when oral intake is resumed.

If there has been a urinary diversion for exocrine management, the potential for metabolic acidosis exists because of the loss of bicarbonate in the urine. Intravenously administered bicarbonate replacement is given until oral replacement is possible. The increased loss of sodium in the urine predisposes this patient to dehydration and hypotension. Hematuria also may occur because of the anastomosis, and cystitis may occur. Careful urinary irrigation may be required.

Rejection in this patient population may be difficult to detect. Serum amylase levels have not proved effective in monitoring graft function, and blood glucose levels seem to become elevated only in the late phases of rejection. A decrease in urine amylase in patients with urinary diversions has proved to be the best indicator of rejection[109]. During the postoperative stay, urine amylase collections are obtained every 12 to 24 hours. If a simultaneous renal-pancreas transplant has been performed, a rise in serum creatinine level also is useful in diagnosing rejection. In these cases, because of the fragility of the pancreas, a renal biopsy specimen may be obtained to determine rejection and treatment. If the transplant is a single organ, a CT scan–directed biopsy of the pancreas may be indicated.

NURSING DIAGNOSIS AND MANAGEMENT
Pancreas transplantation

- Altered Nutrition: Less than Body Protein-Calorie Requirements related to lack of exogenous nutrients and increased metabolic demand, p. 673
- High Risk for Infection risk factor: immunosuppressive drugs required to prevent rejection of pancreas, p. 866
- Anxiety related to threat to biologic, psychologic, and/or social integrity secondary to immunologic rejection of the transplanted pancreas, p. 763
- Knowledge Deficit: Posttransplant Self-care Regimen, specifically immunosuppressive drugs and clinical manifestation of infection related to lack of previous exposure to information, p. 72
- Body Image Disturbance related to actual change in body structure or function, p. 94
- Sensory/Perceptual Alterations related to sensory overload, sensory deprivation, and sleep pattern disturbance, p. 573
- If simultaneous renal-pancreas transplant has been performed, see box on p. 856

Long-Term Considerations

As with all transplant patients, postoperative care includes educating the patient regarding compliance and record keeping. Patients may be required to check their blood glucose levels at home. Blood pressure monitoring is necessary after discharge to detect the development of hypotension. Outpatient 24-hour urine collections are obtained to monitor urinary amylase levels. At first, frequent clinic visits are needed to monitor progress and adjust medications. As the patient progresses, a schedule is established for routine laboratory tests and clinic visits to ensure long-term success of the transplant.

Although islet cell transplantation remains investigational, ongoing research continues in this area.[110] In the future this procedure may offer a nonsurgical method of transplantation. Improvements in matching single organ grafts with recipients also may improve graft survival.[109] Continued improvement of surgical technique, immunosuppressive medications, and organ donation will offer an insulin-free treatment option and may one day be the most effective form of treatment available for diabetes.

HEART TRANSPLANTATION CASE STUDY

CLINICAL HISTORY

AB is a 58-year-old man who is diagnosed with ischemic cardiomyopathy. He has been accepted as a transplant candidate and is currently waiting in the coronary care unit.

CURRENT PROBLEMS

AB is receiving 8 mcg/kg/min of dopamine hydrochloride; 12 mcg/kg/min of dobutamine; 2 mcg/kg/min of nitroglycerine; and a heparin drip of 50 units/hour. He has been intubated and mechanically ventilated for 48 hours. His nutrition is being supported with hyperalimentation. He has been anorexic for the past 3 weeks, and his weight had dropped from 78 kg to 70 kg. Current cardiac index (CI) ranges from 2.0 to 2.3 L/min/m². Serum creatinine is 1.7 mg/dl. During the ensuing 24 hours, a suitable heart is obtained.

The operation proceeded without incident. Six hours after his return to the intensive care unit, he is mechanically ventilated with an FIo_2 of 50% and a rate of 10 breaths/min. His blood pressure (BP) is 102/52 mm Hg (mean 68), heart rate (HR), 78; pulmonary artery pressure (PAP), 40/18 mm Hg (wedge 17mm Hg); central venous pressure (CVP), 15mm Hg. His most recent CI is 2.2 L/min/m². Hourly urine output for the past 2 hours averages 40 ml/hr. Peripheral pulses are present, but his legs are cool to touch from feet to knees. His temperature is 36.2° C (core). Chest tube drainage averages 25-35 ml/hr over the last 2 hours.

Hemodynamic support consists of dopamine at 3 mcg/kg/min; sodium nitroprusside at 0.5 μg/kg/min; nitroglycerin at 1 μg/kg/min; and isoproterenol is hanging (ready to infuse), but currently is turned off.

MEDICAL DIAGNOSIS

Orthotopic heart transplant

NURSING DIAGNOSES

- Decreased Cardiac Output related to relative excess of preload and afterload secondary to impaired ventricular contractility
- Hypothermia related to exposure to cold environment (decreased temperature intraoperataively and cardiopulmonary bypass)

◆ PLAN OF CARE

1. Initiate inotropic and chronotropic support with isoproterenol.
2. Monitor for improvement in CI.
3. Monitor for HR greater than 115 beats/min.
4. Consult with physician about need for standby pacemaker; obtain parameters.
5. Monitor for any new-onset dysrhythmia

MEDICAL AND NURSING MANAGEMENT AND PATIENT OUTCOME

Over the next 2 hours CI increased to 3.1 L/min/m² after initiating isoproterenol at 3 mcg/min. HR was then 100 beats/min. Urine output ranged from 50 to 60 ml/hr. The patient received his first postoperative dose of methylprednisolone (125 mg) and an IV cyclosporine dose of 50 mg, which continued bid. He was extubated 16 hours after admission and placed on 40% oxygen by mask. He was oriented and moved all extremities. He received a total of 90 mg of cyclosporine IV. His first cyclosporine level was 220 ng/ml. At 18 hours postoperatively his serum creatinine was 2.5 mg/dl with a urine output decreased to 35 ml/hr. A later 12-hour urine creatinine clearance revealed a clearance of 40 ml/hr. The patient had a very weak cough, but fairly clear lung fields. He refused clear liquids. Sodium nitroprusside and nitroglycerine were weaned off.

MEDICAL DIAGNOSIS

Orthotopic heart transplant

NURSING DIAGNOSES

- High Risk for Impaired Gas Exchange risk factor: alveolar hypoventilation secondary to debilitated state
- Altered Nutrition: Less than Body Protein-Calorie Requirements related to lack of exogenous nutrients and increased metabolic demand

◆ REVISED PLAN OF CARE

1. Consult with physician about adjusting or holding cyclosporine.
2. Monitor for clinical manifestations of fluid volume excess.
3. Monitor for elevations in potassium.
4. Monitor for changes in respiratory pattern, rate, and character and quality of chest expansion and cough.
5. Evaluate breath sounds every 2 to 4 hours.
6. Mobilize patient as soon as possible.
7. Consult with physician about possible need for respiratory therapy treatments.
8. Consult with physician about need to augment nutrition via enteral feedings if patient unable or uninterested in taking nutrition by mouth.
9. Monitor cyclosporine level.

MEDICAL AND NURSING MANAGEMENT AND PATIENT OUTCOME

The cyclosporine dose was held for 36 hours. By postoperative day 3 the patient's cyclosporine level fell to 150 ng/ml with a serum creatinine of 2.1 mg/dl. Oral cyclosporine was instituted at a dose of 25 mg bid and was to be gradually increased according to the cyclosporine level. Oral prednisone and azathioprine were begun after extubation. An inability to take in adequate nutrition led to a prescription for supplementary Ensure taken between meals. By day 3 AB was ambulating in his room with the assistance of physical therapy. His ability to clear secretions with a stronger cough maintained clear lung fields. Isoproterenol was weaned off, and he consistently maintained a HR of 90 to 100 beats/min with a CI of 3.2 L/min/m². He was transferred to the intermediate intensive care unit on 2 μg/kg/min of dopamine for renal perfusion. At that point minimal teaching had been done.

MEDICAL DIAGNOSIS

Orthotopic heart transplant

NURSING DIAGNOSES

- ◆ Knowledge Deficit: Dietary Needs, Medications, Reportable Symptoms related to lack of previous exposure to information
- ◆ Altered Nutrition related to lack of exogenous nutrients and increased metabolic demand

◆ REVISED PLAN OF CARE

1. Continue instruction and activity progression with the assistance of physical therapy.
2. Obtain a dietary consult to increase caloric intake.
3. Encourage spouse to suggest favorite foods and bring in favorite foods from home.
4. Begin teaching patient and spouse about care regimen at home, medications, and side effects to watch for.
5. Teach patient about clinical manifestations of infection.

MEDICAL AND NURSING MANAGEMENT AND PATIENT OUTCOME

AB underwent endomyocardial at day 7. The results indicated no evidence of rejection. His appetite improved, and he took in adequate nutrition without supplements. He was able to cycle on a stationary bicycle for 15 minutes with some resistance. His BP was 165/95 mm Hg. His cyclosporine level stabilized at 200 ng/ml and a dose of 40 mg bid. AB and his spouse demonstrated a knowledge of medications, side effects, and clinical manifestations of infection. The patient administered his own medications without error.

MEDICAL DIAGNOSES

Orthotopic heart transplant
Hypertension related to cyclosporine

NURSING DIAGNOSIS

- ◆ Knowledge Deficit: Instruction on Home Monitoring of Blood Pressure related to lack of previous exposure to information

◆ REVISED PLAN OF CARE

1. Consult with physician about the need for antihypertensive medication.
2. Teach patient and spouse how to take blood pressure.
3. Acquire equipment so patient can take his blood pressure at home.

MEDICAL AND NURSING MANAGEMENT AND PATIENT OUTCOME

AB was started on captopril, which controlled his blood pressure by postoperative day 9. He and his spouse demonstrated their ability to accurately measure his blood pressure. AB was discharged on postoperative day 10 with a stethoscope and sphygmomanometer, confident that he could manage his own health outside the hospital.

LIVER TRANSPLANTATION CASE STUDY

CLINICAL HISTORY

Mr. B is a 20-year-old man diagnosed with primary sclerosing cholangitis six years ago. This disease is characterized by progressive narrowing of the bile ducts, which prevents the normal outflow of bile from the liver. Cirrhosis is the result of prolonged cholestasis. Mr. B has successfully completed evaluation and is followed at regular intervals through the outpatient clinic.

CURRENT PROBLEMS

After undergoing orthotopic liver transplantation, Mr. B arrives in the intensive care unit directly from the operating room. He is mechanically ventilated at a rate of 12 breaths/min with an FIO_2 of 60%. He has a pulmonary artery catheter, which indicates a core temperature of 35.5° C. Other initial vital signs are a blood pressure (BP) of 150/95 mm Hg; pulse (P), 70; pulmonary artery pressure (PAP), 45/25 mm Hg; pulmonary capillary wedge pressure (PCWP), 16 mm Hg; central venous pressure (CVP), 12 mm Hg. His cardiac output (CO) is 5 L/min with an index of 2.2 L/min/m^2. He has an indwelling urinary catheter. Urine output during the first hour totals 160 ml. Initial arterial blood gases (ABGs) reveal a PaO_2 of 100, PCO_2, 32; pH, 7.49; O_2 saturation, 99%. Serum liver enzyme levels show marked elevations, which often occur as a result of manipulation of the graft during procurement and transplantation (harvest injury).

MEDICAL DIAGNOSIS

Orthotopic liver transplant

NURSING DIAGNOSES

- Hypothermia related to exposure to cold environment secondary to surgery
- Impaired Gas Exchange related to ventlation/perfusion mismatch secondary to mechanical overventilation

◆ PLAN OF CARE

1. Use rewarming techniques.
2. Wean mechanical ventilations.
3. Begin immunosuppressive medications.

MEDICAL AND NURSING MANAGEMENT AND PATIENT OUTCOME

Warm blankets and a head cover were applied to the patient, and a heating lamp was positioned 3 feet from the thorax. The ventilator was weaned to 8 respirations/min after satisfactory arterial blood gases were obtained with each decrease. The patient remained anesthetized. Two hours after admission, the vital signs were as follows: BP, 105/60 mm Hg; P, 108; PAP, 20/8 mm Hg; PCWP, 6 mm Hg; CVP, 4 mm Hg; CO, 7.2 L/min; CI, 3.3 L/min/m^2. The urine output for the last hour totaled 20 ml. Core temperature rose to 37° C.

MEDICAL DIAGNOSIS

Orthotopic liver transplant

NURSING DIAGNOSES

- Fluid Volume Deficit related to wide spread vasodilation
- Increased Cardiac Output related to increased heart rate and vasodilation

◆ REVISED PLAN OF CARE

1. Infuse 250 ml of 5% albumin over 1 hour.
2. Remove warming apparatus—cover patient with one sheet and blanket.

MEDICAL AND NURSING MANAGEMENT AND PATIENT OUTCOME

After the revised plan of care was instituted, Mr. B's blood pressure rose to 130/75 mm Hg and his pulse returned to 70 bpm. Other measurements were as follows: PAP, 30/12 mm Hg; PCWP, 10 mm Hg; CVP, 7 mm Hg; CO, 6 L/min. His core temperature remained at 37° C. Fifteen hours after surgery, the patient was awake and alert. Successful weaning from the ventilator allowed extubation. The patient was placed on 40% oxygen by face mask, and ABGs were monitored every 6 to 8 hours. Other vital signs remained stable.

LIVER TRANSPLANTATION CASE STUDY—cont'd

MEDICAL DIAGNOSIS

Orthotopic liver transplant

NURSING DIAGNOSIS

- ◆ Ineffective Breathing Pattern related to abdominal pain secondary to surgical incision

◆ REVISED PLAN OF CARE

1. Institute mobilization—assist patient out of bed three times daily.
2. Incorporate aspects of self-care with ADLs.
3. Facilitate vigorous deep-breathing regimen q 2 hours.
4. Assist with incentive spirometry q 2 hours.
5. Advance diet to full liquids/regular diet.

MEDICAL AND NURSING MANAGEMENT AND PATIENT OUTCOME

On the second postoperative day, the route of oxygen administration was changed to nasal cannula. The nurse auscultated bowel sounds in all four quadrants. The nasogastric (NG) tube was removed, and the patient began to sip clear liquids. Liver enzyme values were decreasing appropriately, and other laboratory values were stable. Urine output and vital signs also were stable. On the fourth postoperative day, the pulmonary artery catheter was removed, and a multilumened central venous catheter was inserted. All unnecessary peripheral intravenous lines were removed.

On the fifth postoperative day, Mr. B's temperature spiked to 39° C. His pulse was 130; BP, 110/55 mm Hg; and RR, 34/min. His central venous pressure dropped to 4 mm Hg.

MEDICAL DIAGNOSIS

Orthotopic liver transplant

NURSING DIAGNOSES

- ◆ High Risk for Infection risk factor: immunosuppressive drugs required to prevent rejection of liver
- ◆ Ineffective Breathing Pattern related to abdominal pain secondary to surgical incision

◆ REVISED PLAN OF CARE

1. Culture blood, urine, and sputum for bacterial, fungal, and viral organisms (Culture bile from T tube in appropriate patients).
2. Remove and culture indwelling IV catheters.
3. Institute measures to decrease body temperature.
4. Administer antibiotics.
5. Obtain abdominal CT scan if all cultures are negative.

MEDICAL AND NURSING MANAGEMENT AND PATIENT OUTCOME

On day 6, preliminary blood culture results revealed enterococcus. Mr. B's antibiotic regimen was tailored to combat the specific organism. His temperature decreased to 37.5° C. His pulse decreased to 76, and his blood pressure was 140/88 mm Hg. His liver enzymes continued to decrease over the next day to the following levels: AST(SGOT), 123 u/L; ALT(SGPT), 94 u/L; GGT, 174 Iu/L; and alkaline phosphatase, 145u/L. His total bilirubin was 2.5 (normal ranges from 0.1 to 1.1 mg/dl).

By the seventh postoperative day Mr. B was taking a regular diet, ambulating small distances, and performing most activities of daily living (ADLs). He began to learn how to self-administer his oral medications. One of his abdominal drains was discontinued, and the remaining two other three were draining minimal amounts of serosanguineous drainage. His urinary catheter was discontinued. On day 8 he was transferred to the floor.

Mr. B continued to learn aspects of self-care on the general nursing unit. He participated in physical and occupational therapy for muscle strengthening. He attended posttransplant support groups. On day 14, Mr. B's liver enzymes were as follows: AST(SGOT), 160 u/L; ALT(SGPT), 156 u/L; GGT, 230 Iu/L; and alkaline phosphatase, 223 u/L. He underwent a percutaneous liver biopsy under ultrasound guidance. The biopsy revealed moderate acute cellular rejection.

MEDICAL DIAGNOSES

Orthotopic liver transplant
Acute cellular rejection (moderate)

NURSING DIAGNOSES

- ◆ Anxiety related to threat of acute cellular rejection
- ◆ Knowledge Deficit: Dietary Needs, Medications, Reportable Symptoms related to lack of previous exposure to information

Continued.

LIVER TRANSPLANTATION CASE STUDY—cont'd

◆ REVISED PLAN OF CARE

1. Administer IV bolus of solumedrol 500 mg.
2. Administer oral prednisone as follows:
   80 mg/day times 2 days; then
   60 mg/day times 2 days; then
   40 mg/day times 2 days; then
   20 mg/day maintenance dose thereafter.
3. Measure blood glucose twice daily.
4. Begin teaching patient and spouse about self-care regimen, medications and side effects.

MEDICAL AND NURSING MANAGEMENT AND PATIENT OUTCOME

During the treatment Mr. B's blood glucose levels elevated in response to the extra doses of steroids. He required subcutaneous regular insulin coverage to maintain normal blood glucose levels during the steroid cycle. During the treatment Mr. B's enzymes decreased. On day 20, they reached normal levels and his blood glucose levels again were normal. By this time he had learned all aspects of self-care. By day 23, Mr. B's blood pressure trended up to 160/98 mm Hg and remained elevated. He learned that this is a common side effect of both cyclosporine and prednisone; antihypertensive medication was begun. He learned how to monitor his own blood pressure measurements. On day 26, a discharge conference was held for Mr. B. He went home the following day.

KIDNEY-PANCREAS TRANSPLANTATION CASE STUDY

CLINICAL HISTORY

Mr. G is a 36-year-old man with a 20-year history of insulin-dependent diabetes mellitus (IDDM). Complications from the diabetes include retinopathy, neuropathy, and end-stage renal disease (ESRD). He has been on continuous ambulatory peritoneal dialysis (CAPD) for 18 months. He has undergone a simultaneous kidney-pancreas transplant and arrives to the ICU in stable condition.

CURRENT PROBLEMS

On admission to the ICU, Mr. G had a serum creatinine of 14.3 mg/dl; Hct, 26%; blood glucose level, 100 mg/dl. He had a nasogastric tube connected to continuous low-pressure wall suction; 4L oxygen per nasal cannula; a right triple-lumen central line was present with the following fluids infusing: milliliter per milliliter replacement fluid of NS (did not exceed 300 ml/hr), low molecular dextran infused at 20 ml/hr, and an insulin drip. An abdominal midline dressing was dry and intact. A urinary catheter was in place and drained approximately 200 ml of slightly blood-tinged urine each hour. Mr. G was on bedrest with no hip flexion. Continuous 12-hour urine specimens were collected to monitor urinary amylase levels. His blood pressure was stable at 130/70 mm Hg; CVP remained at 7 mm Hg.

MEDICAL DIAGNOSIS

Kidney-pancreas transplant

NURSING DIAGNOSES

- ◆ High risk for Infection risk factor: immunosuppressive drugs required to prevent rejection of kidney and pancreas
- ◆ High Risk for Fluid Volume Deficit risk factors: active blood loss, osmotic diuresis
- ◆ High Risk for Impaired Gas Exchange risk factors: alveolar hypoventilation and acute pain
- ◆ Altered Nutrition: Less than Body Protein-Calorie Requirements related to lack of exogenous nutrients

◆ PLAN OF CARE

1. Maintain aseptic technique with all lines/catheters.
2. Accurately measure and record intake and output, and continuously monitor volume status.
3. Assist patient with incentive spirometer q 2 hours.
4. Administer pain medication as needed for adequate relief.

MEDICAL AND NURSING MANAGEMENT AND PATIENT OUTCOME

Over the first 5 postoperative days, Mr. G's creatinine decreased to 1.3 mg/dl. Urinary amylase levels remained at approximately 40,000 u/ml. He began to have positive bowel sounds, and his NG tube was discontinued. He tolerated liquids well. His blood glucose was stable with values between 50 and 120 mg/dl. On day 6 he was transferred to the general transplant unit. On day 11 Mr. G began to ambulate and ask questions regarding his medications. He was tolerating a low-sodium, low-fat diet without difficulty.

MEDICAL DIAGNOSIS

Kidney-pancreas transplant

NURSING DIAGNOSES

- ◆ Activity Intolerance related to postural hypotension secondary to prolonged immobility
- ◆ Knowledge Deficit: Medications, interpretation of laboratory values related to lack of previous exposure to information

◆ REVISED PLAN OF CARE

1. Assist in increasing activity as tolerated.
2. Incorporate ADLs and self-care into daily activity.
3. Begin self-medication program; teach patient regarding laboratory values.

MEDICAL AND NURSING MANAGEMENT AND PATIENT OUTCOME

By day 14, Mr. G had a stable creatinine that ranged from 1.3 to 1.5 mg/dl. Blood glucose values were stable, and he did not require any insulin. A cystoscopy revealed healing sutures, and the urinary catheter was removed. On day 15 Mr. G's white blood cell count rose slightly, and by day 18 his WBC had climbed from 7.8 to 15.7. He had orthostatic hypotension with blood pressures of 138/80, lying; 110/70 mm Hg, sitting; and 80/50 mm Hg, standing. His temperature ranged between 99° and 100.6° F. He complained of dizziness when he first stood, but otherwise he felt well. An infection was suspected. Blood, throat, urine, and CMV cultures were obtained. On postoperative day 19, Mr. G was transferred back to the ICU with a temperature of 102° F, WBC count of 7.8 to 15.7mm^3, and a blood pressure of 90/50 mm Hg supine.

MEDICAL DIAGNOSIS

Kidney-pancreas transplant

NURSING DIAGNOSES

- ◆ High Risk for Infection risk factor: immunosuppressive drugs required to prevent rejection of kidney and pancreas
- ◆ Activity Intolerance related to postural hypotension-secondary to vasodilation caused by an infectious process

◆ REVISED PLAN OF CARE

1. Use aseptic technique with all lines and catheters.
2. Administer IV and PO fluids.
3. Closely monitor blood pressure. Maintain systolic BP > 100 mm Hg.
4. Reassure patient of need for close monitoring to ensure his well-being.

MEDICAL AND NURSING MANAGEMENT AND PATIENT OUTCOME

Mr. G's blood cultures showed that he had a staphylococcus infection. After treatment with appropriate antibiotics and aggressive fluid replacement, Mr. G became afebrile and maintained a stable blood pressure range of 120-130's/70-80's mm Hg. However, over the next 48 hours his creatinine rose from 1.3 to 1.7 mg/dl despite hydration. Also, his urine amylase levels decreased from 30,210 to 12,620 u/ml. His blood sugar levels remained stable. Rejection was suspected, and a renal biopsy was obtained. The biopsy revealed acute rejection (mild).

MEDICAL DIAGNOSES

Kidney-pancreas transplant
Post-Staphylococcus infection
Acute rejection (mild)

NURSING DIAGNOSES

- ◆ High Risk for Infection risk factor: immunosuppressive drugs required to prevent rejection of kidney and pancreas
- ◆ Anxiety related to threat to biologic, psychologic, and/or social integrity
- ◆ Knowledge Deficit: Self-care Regimen related to lack of previous exposure to information

Continued

KIDNEY-PANCREAS TRANSPLANTATION CASE STUDY—cont'd

◆ REVISED PLAN OF CARE

1. Use aseptic technique with all lines and catheters.
2. Discuss patient's concerns regarding this rejection episode.
3. Continue teaching patient about self-care regimen, medications, and side-effects.

MEDICAL AND NURSING MANAGEMENT AND PATIENT OUTCOME

Mr. G was treated with IV Solu-Medrol. By the third treatment day his creatinine was 1.4 mg/dl, and his urinary amylase was 40,700 u/ml. He was transferred to the general transplant unit. He continued to improve and became very knowledgeable regarding medications, laboratory values, symptoms of rejection, physical limitations, diet, and clinic appointments. On postoperative day 25 he was discharged to home.

HIGH RISK FOR INFECTION RISK FACTOR: IMMUNOSUPPRESSIVE DRUGS REQUIRED TO PREVENT REJECTION OF TRANSPLANTED ORGAN

DEFINING CHARACTERISTICS

- ◆ Temperature >38° C or persistent temperature >37.5° C
- ◆ Leukocytosis or leukopenia
- ◆ Infiltrate on chest x-ray film
- ◆ Cough (may be nonproductive)
- ◆ Redness, pain, tenderness or drainage over wounds or IV access sites
- ◆ Positive blood, urine, or sputum cultures
- ◆ Specific manifestations related to site of infection (e.g., decreased Po_2 with lung infection)

OUTCOME CRITERIA

- ◆ Temperature is normal.
- ◆ Chest film is clear.
- ◆ No clinical signs of infection are present.
- ◆ Wounds are healing normally.
- ◆ All cultures are negative.
- ◆ Patient is knowledgeable about clinical manifestations of infection and when to seek medical care.

NURSING INTERVENTIONS AND *RATIONALE*

1. Monitor for temperature elevation >37.5° C, and report elevations to physician.
2. Obtain blood, urine, and sputum cultures for temperperature elevations >38° C ***inasmuch as elevation likely is caused by bacteremia or bladder or pulmonary infection.***
3. Auscultate breath sounds at least every 6 hours. ***Pulmonary infection is the most common type of infection, and changes in breath sounds might be an early indication.***
4. Inspect wounds at least every 8 hours for redness, swelling, and/or drainage, ***which may indicate infection.***
5. Inspect overall skin integrity and oral mucosa for signs of breakdown, ***which place the patient at risk of infection.***
6. Notify physician of any new onset cough. ***Even a nonproductive cough may indicate pulmonary infection.***
7. Monitor WBC count daily, and report leukocytosis or sudden development of leukopenia, ***which may indicate an infectious process.***
8. Protect patient from exposure to any staff or family member with contagious lesions (e.g., herpes simplex) or respiratory infections.
9. Evaluate nutritional status, and suggest augmentation of nutritional intake as necessary ***to prevent debilitation and increased susceptibility to infection.***
10. Encourage physician to remove invasive lines and catheters as soon as possible ***to decrease potential portals of entry.***
11. Teach patient the clinical manifestations of infection. ***A knowledgeable patient will seek medical attention promptly, which will result in earlier treatment and a decreased risk that an infection will become life-threatening.***

REFERENCES

1. Shumway SJ: Basic immunologic concepts involved in organ transplantation. In Baumgartner WA, Reitz BA, Achuff, SC editors: *Heart and heart-lung transplantation,* Philadelphia, 1990, WB Saunders.
2. Bartucci MR, Seller MC: The immunology of transplant rejection. In Sigardson-Poor KM, Haggerty LM, editors: *Nursing care of the transplant patient,* Philadelphia, 1990, WB Saunders.
3. Dinarello CA, Mier JW: Current concepts: lymphokines, *N Engl J Med* 317:940, 1987.
4. Colling EG, Hubbell EA: Immunologic aspects of organ transplantation. In Williams BAH, Grady KL, Sandiford-Guttenbiel DM, editors: *Organ transplantation,* New York, 1991, Springer.
5. Hess AD, Colombani PM, Esa A: Cyclosporine: immunobiologic aspects in transplantation. In Williams GM, Burdick JF, Solez K, editors: *Kidney transplant rejection: diagnosis and treatment,* New York, 1986, Marcel Dekker.
6. Crandell B: Immunosuppression. In Sigardson-Poor KM, Haggerty LM, editors: *Nursing care of the transplant recipient,* Philadelphia, 1990, WB Saunders.
7. Rana AN, Lusking A: Immunosuppression, autoimmunity and hypersensitivity, *Heart Lung* 9:651, 1980.
8. Cosimi AB and others: Treatment of acute renal allograft rejection with OKT3 monoclonal antibody, *Transplantation* 32:535, 1981.
9. Starzl TZ and others: *Clinical trials of FK506.* Paper presented at the Fourth Congress of the European Society for Organ Transplantation, Barcelona, Spain, 1989.
10. Warty V and others: FK506: a novel immunosuppressive agent, *Transplantation* 46(3):453, 1988.
11. Staschak SM, Zamberlan K: Recent development: FK506. In Sigardson-Poor KM, Haggerty LM, editors: *Nursing care of the transplant patient,* Philadelphia, 1990, WB Saunders.
12. Reitz B: The history of heart and heart-lung transplantation. In Baumgartner WA, Rietz BA, Achuff SC, editors: *Heart and heart-lung transplantation,* Philadelphia, 1990, WB Saunders.
13. Losse B: Indications and selection criteria for cardiac transplantation, *Thorac Cardiovasc Surg* 38:276, 1990.
14. Stevenson LW and others: Cardiac transplantation selection, immunosuppression, and survival, *West J Med* 149:572, 1988.
15. Dillon TA and others: Cardiac transplantation in patients with preexisting malignancies, *Transplantation* 52:82, 1991.
16. Edwards BS and others: Cardiac transplantation in patients with preexisting neoplastic diseases, *Am J Cardiol* 65:501, 1990.
17. Badellino NM and others: Cardiac transplantation in diabetic patients, *Transplant Proc* 22:2384, 1990.
18. Ladowski JS and others: Heart transplantation in diabetic recipients, *Transplantation* 49:303, 1990.
19. Rhenman MJ and others: Diabetics and heart transplantation, *J Heart Transplant* 7:356, 1988.
20. Hurst JW and others: *The heart,* ed 7, New York, 1990, McGraw-Hill.
21. Dibiase A and others: Frequency and mechanism of bradycardia in cardiac transplant recipients and need for pacemakers, *Am J Cardiol* 67:1385, 1991.
22. Whitman GR, Hicks LE: Major nursing diagnoses following cardiac transplantation, *J Cardiovasc Nurs* 2:1, 1988.
23. Masoorli ST, Piercy S: A lifesaving guide to blood products, *RN* 47:32, 1984.
24. Hunt SA and others: Total lymphoid irradiation for treatment of intractable cardiac allograft rejection, *J Heart Lung Transplant* 10:211, 1991.
25. Futterman LG: Cardiac transplantation: a comprehensive nursing perspective. II. *Heart Lung* 17:631, 1988.
26. Whitley RJ: Ganciclovir—have we established clinical value in the treatment of cytomegalovirus infections? *Ann Intern Med* 108:452, 1988.
27. *Cytomegalovirus infections in the immunocompromised transplant patient: diagnosis and treatment* (special symposium review), San Francisco, 1991, Professional Healthcare Communications.
28. Gao S and others: Accelerated coronary vascular disease in the heart transplant patient: coronary arteriographic findings, *J Am Coll Cardiol* 12:334, 1988.
29. Sharples LD and others: Risk factor analysis for the major hazards following heart transplantation, rejection, infection and coronary occlusive disease, *Transplantation* 52:244, 1991.
30. Stark RP, McGinn AL, Wilson RF: Chest pain in cardiac transplant recipients, *N Engl J Med* 324:1791, 1991.
31. Lough ME and others: Impact of symptom frequency and symptom distress on self-reported quality of life in heart transplant recipients, *Heart Lung* 16:193, 1987.
32. Packa RD: Quality of life of adults after a heart transplant, *J Cardiovasc Nurs* 13:12, 1989.
33. Evans RW and others: *The national heart transplantation study: final report,* Seattle, 1984, Battelle Human Affairs Research Centers.
34. Lough ME: Quality of life issues following heart transplantation, *Prog Cardiovasc Nurs* 1:17, 1986.
35. Cate FH, Laudicina SS: *Current statistical information about transplantation in America.* Washington, DC, 1991, Transplantation White Paper, The Annenberg Washington Program, United Network for Organ Sharing.
36. Marshall SE and others: Selection and evaluation of recipients for heart-lung and lung transplantation, *Chest* 98:1488, 1990.
37. Egan TM, Kaiser LR, Cooper JD: Lung transplantation, *Curr Probl Surg* 10:673, 1989.
38. Hutter JA: Heart-lung transplantation: better use of resources, *Am J Med* 85:4, 1988.
39. Klepetko W and others: Domino transplantation of heart-lung and heart: an approach to overcome the scarcity of donor organs, *J Heart Lung Transplant* 10:129, 1991.
40. Theodore J, Lewiston N: Lung transplantation comes of age, *N Engl J Med* 322:772, 1990.
41. Hakim M and others: Selection and procurement of combined heart and lung grafts for transplantation, *J Thorac Cardiovasc Surg* 95:474, 1988.
42. Starnes VA: Heart-lung transplantation: an overview, *Cardiol Clin* 8:159, 1990.
43. Starnes VA and others: Cystic fibrosis: target population for lung transplantation in North America in the 1990's, *J Thorac Cardiovasc Surg* 103(5):1008, 1992.
44. Theodore J: Pulmonary function in the uncomplicated human transplanted lung, *ACP* 2:301, 1987.
45. Baldwin JC: Comparison of cardiac rejection in heart and heart-lung transplantation, *J Heart Transplant* 6:352, 1987.
46. Theodore J, Starnes VA, Lewiston NJ: Obliterative bronchiolitis, *Clin Chest Med* 11:309, 1990.
47. Glanville AR and others: Obliterative bronchiolitis after heart-lung transplantation: apparent arrest by augmented immunosuppression, *Ann Intern Med* 107:300, 1987.
48. Starnes VA and others: Current trends in lung transplantation: lobar transplantation and expanded use of single lungs, *J Thorac Cardiovasc Surg,* 104:1060. 1992.
49. Marshall SE and others: Prospective analysis of serial pulmonary function studies and transbronchial biopsies in single-lung transplant recipients, *Transplant Proc* 23:1217, 1991.
50. Welch CS: A note on transplantation of the whole liver in dogs, *Transplant Bull* 2(2):54, 1955.
51. Cannon JA: Organs *Transplant Bull* 3(1):7, 1956 (communication).
52. Moore FD and others: One-stage homotransplantation of the liver following total hepatectomy in dogs, *Transplant Bull* 6:103, 1959.
53. Moore FD and others: Experimental whole organ transplantation of the liver and of the spleen, *Ann Surg* 152(3):374, 1960.

54. Starzl TE and others: Reconstructive problems in canine liver homotransplantation with special reference to the postoperative role of hepatic venous flow, *Surg Gyn Obstet* 11:733, 1960.
55. Starzl TE and others: Homotransplantation of the liver in humans, *Surg Gyn Obstet* 117(6):659, 1963.
56. Starzl TE and others: Orthotopic homotransplantation of the human liver, *Ann Surg* 168(3):392, 1968.
57. Cosimi AB: Update on liver transplantation, *Transplant Proc* 23(4):2083, 1991.
58. Kahan BD and others: Complications of cyclosporine-prednisone immunosuppression in 402 renal allograft recipients exclusively followed at a single center for from one to five years, *Transplantation* 43(2):197, 1987.
59. Griffith BP and others: Cardiac transplantation with Cyclosporin A and prednisone, *Ann Surg* 196(3):324, 1982.
60. Starzl TE and others: Evolution of liver transplantation, *Hepatology 2(5):614, 1982.*
61. Sutherland DER and others: Experience with 49 segmental pancreas transplants in 45 diabetic patients, *Transplantation* 34(6):330, 1982.
62. Hows JM, Palmar S, Gordon-Smith EC: Use of cyclosporin A in allogenic bone marrow transplantation for severe aplastic anemia, *Transplantation* 33(4):382, 1982.
63. National Institutes of Health: National Institutes of Health consensus development conference statements: Liver transplantation, *Hepatology* 4(1S):107S, 1984.
64. Van Thiel DH, Makowka L, Starzl TE: Liver transplantation: where it's been and where it's going, *Gastroenterol Clin North Am* 17(1):1, 1988.
65. Deaths from chronic liver disease—United States, 1986, *JAMA* 263(3):355, 1990.
66. O'Grady JG and others: Liver transplantation for malignant disease, *Ann Surg* 207(4):373, 1988.
67. Koneru B and others: Liver transplant for malignant tumors, *Gastroenterol Clin North Am* 17(1):177, 1988.
68. Demetrius JA and others: Recurrent hepatitis B in liver allograft recipients, *Am J Pathol* 125(1):161, 1986.
69. Demetrius AJ and others: Evolution of hepatitis B virus liver disease after hepatic replacement, *Am J Pathol* 137(3):667, 1990.
70. Van Thiel DH and others: Interferon therapy of hepatitis following liver transplantation under FK 506 or cyclosporine, *Transplant Proc* 23(6):3052, 1991.
71. Shaw BW and others: Stratifying the causes of death in liver transplant recipients: an approach to improving survival, *Arch Surg* 124:895, 1989.
72. Sanflippo F and others: The detrimental effects of delayed graft function in cadaver donor renal transplantation, *Transplantation* 1984(38):643, 1984.
73. Jamieson NV and others: Successful 24 and 30 hour preservation of the canine liver: a preliminary report, *Transplant Proc* 20(1S):945, 1988.
74. Ascher NL and others: Rejection of the liver. In Maddrey WC, editor: *Current topics in gastroenterology: transplantation of the liver,* New York, 1988, Elsevier.
75. Koneru B and others: Postoperative surgical complications, *Gastroenterol Clin North Am* 17(1):71, 1988.
76. Staschak S and others: A cost comparison of liver transplantation with FK 506 or CyA as the primary immunosuppressive agent, *Transplant Proc* 22(1S):47, 1990.
77. Millikan WJ and others: Changes in hepatic function, hemodynamics, and morphology after liver transplantation, *Ann Surg* 209(5):513, 1989.
78. Van Thiel DH and others: Liver transplantation in adults, *Gastroenterology* 90(1):211, 1986.
79. Lautenschlager I and others: Efficiency of FK 506 and CyA to prevent acute cellular rejection of pig liver allografts, *Transplant Proc* 23(4):2233, 1991.
80. Chen HF and others: The immunosuppressive effect of rampamycin on pancreaticoduodenal transplants in the rat, *Transplant Proc* 23(4):2239, 1991.
81. Merion RM and others: Early immunological benefits of gluathione-supplemented UW solution in hepatic transplantation, *Transplant Proc* 23(4):2243, 1991.
82. Madsen JC and others: Immunological unresponsiveness induced by recipient cells transfected with donor MHC genes, *Nature* 332(6160):161, 1988.
83. Thistlewaite JR and others: Innovative use of organs for liver transplantation, *Transplant Proc* 23(4):2147, 1991.
84. Morris PJ: Prospects in transplantation, *Transplant Proc* 23(4):2133, 1991.
85. Gutkind L: *Many sleepless nights,* New York, 1988, WW Norton.
86. Data Source: United Network for Organ Sharing (UNOS), 1991.
87. Eggers PW: Effect of transplantation on the medicare end-stage renal disease program, *N Engl J Med* 318(4):223, 1988.
88. Gallagher-Lepak S: Functional capacity and activity level before and after renal transplantation, *ANNA J* 18(4):378, 1991.
89. Perryman JP, Stillerman PU: Kidney transplantation. In Smith SL, editor: AACN tissue and organ transplantation: implications for professional nursing practice, St Louis, 1990, Mosby–Year Book.
90. Kahan BD and others: Clinical and experimental studies with cyclosporine in renal transplantation, *Surgery* 97(2):125, 1985.
91. McDonald JC: The national organ procurement and transplant network, *JAMA* 259(5):725, 1988.
92. Jones MB: Ethical issues involving living related donors and recipients, *ANNA J* 14(6):398, 1987.
93. Whelchel JD: Overview of renal transplantation, *Emory U J Med* 1(2):89, 1987.
94. Cunningham NH, Boteler S, Windham S: Renal transplantation, *Crit Care Nurs Clin North Am* 4(1):79, 1992.
95. Smith SL, Cunningham N: Postoperative care of the renal transplant patient, *Crit Care Nurse* 10(9):74, 1990.
96. Groer MW: Mechanisms of nutritional disequilibrium. In Groer MW, Shekleton ME, editors: *Basic pathophysiology: a holistic approach*, ed 3, St Louis, 1989, Mosby–Year Book.
97. Guthrie DW. Guthrie RA: Chronic complications. In Guthrie DW, Guthrie RA, editors: *Nursing management of diabetes mellitus*, New York, 1991, Springer.
98. Wills BG, Post CL: Pancreas transplantation. In Smith SL, editor: *AACN tissue and organ transplantation: implications for professional nursing practice,* St Louis, 1990, Mosby–Year Book.
99. Velosa GA and others: Pancreas transplantation at Mayo: patient selection, *Mayo Clin Proc* 65:475, 1990.
100. Hunsicker LG: Renal transplantation for the nephrologist: is pancreas transplantation for diabetic ESRD now accepted therapy? *Am J Kidney Dis* 15(1):93, 1990.
101. Nakache R, Tyden G, Groth C: Quality of life after combined pancreas-kidney or kidney transplantation, *Diabetes* 38(1):40, 1989.
102. Tattersall R: Is pancreas transplantation for insulin-dependent diabetics worthwhile? *N Engl J Med* 321(2):112, 1989.
103. Scharp DW and others: Insulin independence after islet transplantation into type I diabetic patient, *Diabetes* 39(4):515, 1990.
104. Sutherland DER and others: Pancreas transplantation, *Surg Clin North Am* 66(3):557, 1986.
105. Perkins JD and others: Pancreas transplantation at Mayo: operative and perioperative management, *Mayo Clin Proc* 65:483, 1990.
106. Corry RJ, Wright FH, Smith JL: Whole organ pancreas transplantation, *Transplant Proc* 20(3S):420, 1988.
107. Perkins JD and others: Pancreas transplantation at Mayo: multidisciplinary management, *Mayo Clin Proc* 65:496, 1990.
108. Trusler LA: Simultaneous kidney-pancreas transplantation, *ANNA J* 18(5):487, 1991.
109. Corry RJ: Status report on pancreas transplantation, *Transplant Proc* 23(4):2091, 1991.
110. Warnock GL and others: Studies of the isolation and transplantation of purified islets in adult humans, *Transplant Proc* 23(1):781, 1991.

50

Nutritional Alterations and Management

CHAPTER OBJECTIVES

- ◆ Describe the adverse effects of nutritional impairments on critically ill patients.
- ◆ Assess the nutritional status of critically ill patients.
- ◆ Participate with other health care team members in designing an effective nutrition support program for a patient in the critical care unit.
- ◆ Identify complications of nutrition support and nursing measures for prevention and treatment of these complications.
- ◆ Recognize nutritional alterations commonly associated with cardiovascular, pulmonary, neurologic, renal, gastrointestinal, endocrine, and hematoimmune systems.
- ◆ Assess the nutritional status of a patient with cardiovascular, pulmonary, neurologic, renal, gastrointestinal, endocrine, and/or hematoimmune system dysfunction(s).
- ◆ Evaluate the success of and make the necessary changes in the nursing management plan/nutritional teaching plan for a critically ill patient.

NUTRIENT METABOLISM

Macronutrients

The major macronutrients are carbohydrates, proteins, and fats. For proper metabolic functioning, adequate amounts of vitamins, electrolytes, minerals, and trace elements (micronutrients) also must be supplied. The process by which these nutrients are used at the cellular level is known as *metabolism.* The major purpose of nutrient metabolism is the production of energy and the preservation of lean body mass.

◆ **Carbohydrates.** Of the three macronutrients, carbohydrates provide the preferred source of energy for cellular activity. Through the process of digestion, carbohydrates are broken down into glucose, fructose, and galactose. After absorption from the intestinal tract, fructose and galactose are converted to glucose, the primary form of carbohydrate used at the cellular level.

The primary function of glucose is to produce the energy needed to maintain cellular functions, including transport of substrates across cellular membranes, secretion of specific hormones, muscular contraction, and the synthesis of new substances. Most of the energy produced from carbohydrate metabolism is used to form adenosine triphosphate (ATP), the principal form of immediately-available energy within the cytoplasm and nucleoplasm of all body cells. One gram of carbohydrate provides approximately 4 kcal of energy.

Inside the cell, glucose is either stored as glycogen or lipid or metabolized for the release of energy. All cells can store glycogen for future use; however, liver and muscle cells have the largest glycogen reserves, providing glucose sufficient to meet the body's needs for up to 6 to 12 hours. Moderate amounts of glucose can be formed from lactate, amino acids, and glycerol. This process of manufacturing glucose from nonglucose precursors is called *gluconeogenesis,* a normal body defense mechanism that preserves the source of energy in times of increased physiologic need and limited exogenous supply.[1]

◆ **Protein.** Protein has important structural and functional duties within the body. It is the structural basis of all lean body mass, such as organ mass and skeletal muscle. Proteins are important for such visceral (cellular) functions as initiation of chemical reactions (hormones and enzymes), transportation of other substances (apoproteins), preservation of immune function (antibodies), and maintenance of osmotic pressure (albumin) and blood neutrality (buffers).

Proteins constantly are synthesized, broken down into amino acids, and then resynthesized into new protein. This three-step process is called *protein turnover.* In very active tissues—such as those composing the gut, liver, and kidney—protein turnover occurs every few days. The average turnover time of all body protein has been estimated at 80 days; the rate of turnover is fastest in enzymes and hormones involved in metabolic activities. Therefore to preserve lean body mass, a constant supply of protein must be ensured.

The functional protein component that is used at the cellular level is the amino acid. Through digestion, complex proteins are broken down into dipeptides and amino acids and are transported to the liver. The liver not only metabolizes the majority of amino acids, but also regulates amino acid flow to other cells of the body. One gram of protein provides approximately 4 kcal of energy.

Specific amino acids are *essential;* that is, they cannot be produced by the body. They must be supplied by the diet. Other *nonessential* amino acids can be manufactured by the body under normal circumstances if the *essential* amino acids are in adequate supply.

Similar to carbohydrates and fat, amino acid molecules contain carbon, hydrogen, and oxygen. Amino acids, however, also contain nitrogen in the form of the amine group NH_2. It is the nonamine group that is used to produce glucose in times of need. However, if amino acids are broken down and used for making glucose (i.e., *gluconeogenesis*), proteins are not available for their usual structural and functional activities, resulting in a depletion of both lean body mass (structural protein) and visceral (cellular) proteins, amino acids that are needed for survival. It is therefore the preservation of body protein that is the basis for nutritional support of critically ill patients.

◆ **Fat (lipids).** Lipids include fatty acids, triglycerides, phospholipids, cholesterol, and cholesterol esters. Aside from their involvement in such functions as the maintenance of cell membranes and the manufacture of prostaglandins, lipids—primarily in the form of triglycerides—provide a stored source of energy. Triglycerides are more easily stored than is glycogen. They are calorically dense molecules, providing more than twice the amount of energy per gram (9 kcal) as protein and carbohydrates.

Dietary lipids—mainly triglycerides—are hydrolyzed in the intestine to form micelles, which are emulsions of chains of fatty acids, monoglycerides, and bile salts. Short-chain fatty acids are passively absorbed through the intestine and are transported to the liver via the portal vein. Long-chain fatty acids are surrounded by specific proteins to form chylomicrons. These chylomicrons are transported out of the intestine through the lymphatic system, finally entering blood circulation through the thoracic duct. A portion of the chylomicrons is taken up by the liver, but the majority are directly transported to other tissues. With the aid of the enzyme *lipoprotein lipase,* triglyceride-containing chylomicrons are broken down outside the cell and enter the cell as fatty acids and glycerol. Once inside the cell, the fatty acids are oxidized or reformed into triglycerides for storage. Insulin also facilitates the cellular uptake of triglycerides.[1]

During an overnight fast, prolonged starvation, or metabolic stress when the carbohydrate supply is low, a process called *lipolysis* causes the breakdown of intracellular triglycerides, which provides fatty acids for energy production and glycerol for gluconeogenesis. Therefore the use of fatty acids is directly related to the level of blood glucose.

The fatty acids released from adipose tissue are used by either the liver or peripheral tissue. In the liver, fatty acids are further degraded to ketones (betahydroxybutyrate, acetoacetate, and acetone). In the absence of glucose, fatty acid breakdown and ketone production are increased. Ketone bodies can be directly oxidized by skeletal muscle and used for energy. During prolonged starvation, the brain—which normally uses glucose—converts to ketones as its primary energy source. This is another body defense mechanism to ensure a supply of energy when exogenous glucose intake is curtailed.

Protein-Calorie Malnutrition

Malnutrition results from the lack of necessary nutrients in the body or improper absorption and distribution of them. Although an inadequate supply of both macronutrients and micronutrients can lead to deficiencies and decreased functioning, the lack of protein and calories further debilitates the critically ill patient—thus the use of the term *protein-calorie malnutrition.* To put it simply, an inadequate exogenous supply of calories for energy results in the breakdown of endogenous protein for gluconeogenesis, severely restricting the availability of protein and amino acids for other peripheral and visceral functions. Malnutrition can be caused by simple starvation—the inadequate intake of nutrients. It also can be the result of physiologic events that increase metabolism beyond the supply of nutrients. In the hospitalized patient, if malnutrition occurs, usually it is the result of the combined effects of starvation and hypermetabolism.

Metabolic Response to Starvation and Stress

To understand the development of malnutrition in the hospitalized patient, the nurse must understand the metabolic response to starvation and physiologic stress.[1,2] Changes in endocrine status and metabolism work together to determine the onset and extent of malnutrition. Nutritional imbalance occurs when the demand for nutrients is greater than the exogenous nutrient supply. The major difference between one who is starved and one who is starved *and* injured is that the latter experiences an increased reliance on endogenous protein breakdown to provide precursors for glucose production to meet increased energy demands. Therefore although carbohydrate and fat metabolism are also affected, the main concern is with protein metabolism and homeostasis.

During the postabsorptive state, the normal diet provides exogenous sources of carbohydrate and fat to meet the body's demand for fuel. Any carbohydrate or fat not immediately used for energy is converted and stored as triglycerides (adipose tissue). Dietary protein enters the amino acid pool and is used to replace protein that has been degraded during routine protein turnover. If necessary, 95% of endogenous protein can be reused, with the diet providing the remaining 5% for protein synthesis.

During an acute, nonstressed fast, the fuel demands of the body still must be met. Some amino acids, instead of being resynthesized into new protein or further broken down and excreted, are shuttled to the liver for gluconeogenesis. In the liver the amino acid is degraded, which means that the nitrogen-containing amine group is released, converted to urea, and then transported to the kidney for excretion. The remaining hydrogen, carbon, and oxygen radical (called the *carbon skeleton*) enters the Kreb's cycle, which eventually produces ATP.

As fasting is prolonged, the metabolic rate decreases, blood levels of insulin fall, and glucagon levels rise. Glucagon promotes the use of glycogen reserves, which become quickly exhausted. Cellular triglycerides are then mobilized as the primary source of fuel.

The triglycerides are degraded to fatty acids and glycerol. In the liver the glycerol is used to make glucose and the fatty acids are further metabolized to ketones. Once the circulating ketone level rises, the brain is able to use ketones for 70% of its energy, thereby decreasing the total body's reliance on glucose as a major energy source. As gluconeogenesis from protein precursors decreases, protein breakdown and nitrogen excretion also slow. Obligatory glucose users—such as white blood cells, the renal medulla, and 30% of brain cells—still require a small amount of amino acids, because they continue to rely on glucose as their preferred source of fuel. Although the events of an acute fast are usually short lived, the continued absence of exogenous calories means that the body will use degraded triglycerides as its primary energy source. Endogenous protein stores are "spared" from use for gluconeogenesis, and protein homeostasis is partially restored.

Of concern to those caring for critically ill patients is the combination of starvation and the physiologic stress resulting from injury, trauma, major surgery, and/or sepsis. This physiologic stress results in profound metabolic alterations that persist from the time of the stressful event until the completion of wound healing and recovery. Stress normally causes an increased metabolic rate (hypermetabolism) that necessitates a rise in oxygen consumption and energy expenditure[3] (see box below).

Hormonal changes that occur at the initiation of the stressful event begin the hypermetabolic process. With stimulation of the sympathetic nervous system, the adrenal medulla releases catecholamines (epinephrine and norepinephrine).[4] These in turn stimulate the body's metabolic response to stress. Also released in response to stress are adrenocorticotropic hormone (ACTH) and antidiuretic hormone (ADH), as well as glucocorticoids and mineralocorticoids.[4] Insulin resistance caused by the release of glucagon allows nutrient substrates, primarily amino acids, to move from peripheral tissues (e.g., skeletal muscle) to the liver for gluconeogenesis.[3]

This hypermetabolic process is the body's effort to mobilize the supply of circulating nutrient substrates, such as glucose and amino acids. Unfortunately, this mobilization occurs at the expense of body tissue and function at a time when the needs for protein synthesis (e.g., for wound healing and acute phase proteins) also are high. Hyperglycemia prevails as the effects of insulin and the release of free fatty acids are diminished by the effects of increased catecholamines, glucocorticoids, and glucagon. Again the body relies on its protein stores to provide substrates for gluconeogenesis, because glucose now becomes the major fuel source. Loss of protein results in a negative nitrogen balance and weight loss. The classic response to metabolic stress is the use of protein for fuel.

METABOLIC RESPONSES DURING STARVATION WITH STRESS

BRIEF STARVATION

- ↓ Metabolic rate
- ↓ Body temperature
- ↓ Blood insulin levels
- ↑ Catecholamine, glucagon, cortisol levels
- ↑ Glucose levels
- ↑ Blood lactate levels
- ↑ Plasma free fatty acid levels
- ↑ Urinary nitrogen excretion

PROLONGED STARVATION

- ↑ Metabolic rate ↑ or ↓ metabolic rate
- ↑ Body temperature
- ↑ or normal insulin levels
- ↑ or normal catecholamine, glucagon, cortisol levels
- ↑ or normal blood glucose levels
- ↑ Blood lactate levels
- ↑ Free fatty acid levels
- ↑ Urinary nitrogen excretion

IMPLICATIONS OF UNDERNUTRITION FOR THE SICK OR STRESSED PATIENT

Surveys of hospitalized patients have revealed that malnutrition is widespread at admission.[5,6] Critically ill patients are especially vulnerable, with more than 40% of these patients malnourished at the time of admission.[7] Other possible contributing factors include lack of communication among the nurses, physicians, and dietitians responsible for the care of these patients; frequent diagnostic testing, which causes patients to miss meals or to be too exhausted for meals; medications and other therapies that cause anorexia, nausea, or vomiting and thus interfere with food intake; or inadequate use of tube feedings or total parenteral nutrition to maintain the nutritional status of these patients.

When protein and calorie intake are inadequate for more than a few hours, existing body proteins will be broken down to meet the body's needs. Even when the individual has large fat reserves, catabolism of body proteins will occur. Unlike fat, proteins can provide the amino acids that are needed for tissue synthesis and repair and can also provide a significant source of glucose. The well-nourished individual tolerates a few days of starvation when not exposed to stress, but a patient with trauma, surgery, burns, or infection, along with inadequate nutritional intake, will have accelerated catabolism. An already undernourished patient exposed to stress (e.g., a cancer patient with anorexia and weight loss who undergoes surgery) is especially vulnerable.

Malnutrition is an ominous finding among very ill patients. Undernourished patients are more likely than are well-nourished patients to have major surgical complications. In addition, wound dehiscence, decubitus ulcers, sepsis, and pulmonary infections are more common among undernourished patients. Length of hospital stay for malnourished medical patients is longer than for those who are well-nourished.[5]

Nutrition assessment is the process of obtaining and interpreting patient data about nutritional status. It provides a basis for identifying patients who are malnourished or at risk of becoming malnourished, determining the nutritional needs of individual patients, and selecting the most appropriate methods of nutritional support for patients with or at risk of developing nutritional deficits. Nutrition support (the provision of specially formulated or delivered enteral or intravenous nutrients to prevent or treat malnutrition)[8] provides a method of coping with the nutritional problems of very ill patients both in the hospital and at home.

ASSESSING NUTRITIONAL STATUS

Nutrition assessment is a multistep process involving the collection and evaluation of pertinent information from the patient's diet and medical history, physical examination, and laboratory values. The assessment can be performed by a designated member of the health care team, such as the dietitian or the nurse, or it can be a team effort.

History

Information about dietary intake and significant variations in weight is a vital part of the history. A change of 10% or more in body weight during the past year or 5% to 6% during the past 3 months is usually considered significant. Dietary intake can be evaluated in several ways, including a diet record, a 24-hour recall, and a diet history. The diet record, a listing of the type and amount of all foods and beverages consumed for some period (usually 3 days), is useful for evaluating the patient's intake in the critical care setting if there is a question about the adequacy of intake. However, such a record reveals little about the patient's habitual intake before the illness or injury. The 24-hour recall of all food and beverage intake is easily and quickly performed, but it, too, may not reflect the patient's usual intake and thus has limited usefulness. The diet history consists of a detailed interview about the patient's usual intake, along with social, familial, cultural, economic, educational, and health-related factors that may affect intake. Although the diet history is time consuming to perform and may be too stressful for the acutely ill patient, it provides a wealth of information about food habits over a prolonged period and provides a basis for planning specific patient teaching, if changes in eating habits are desirable. Other information to include in a nutrition history is listed in Table 50-1.

Physical Examination

◆ **Anthropometric measurements.** Obtaining anthropometric or body measurements, of which height and weight are the most important, is the first step in physical evaluation. If at all possible, height and weight should be measured, rather than obtained through patient or family report. Skinfold measurements, another anthropometric parameter, provide an estimate of body fat, which is helpful in diagnosing obesity and malnutrition. The triceps skinfold (TSF) is the most commonly used.

Table 50-1 Nutrition history information

Area of concern	Significant findings	Nutrients of special concern
Inadequate intake of nutrients	Avoidance of specific food groups because of poverty or poor dentition	Protein, iron
	Alcohol abuse	Protein, vitamin B_1, niacin, folate
	Anorexia, nausea, vomiting	Most nutrients, particularly protein, electrolytes
	Confusion, coma	All nutrients
Inadequate absorption of nutrients	Previous GI surgeries:	
	Gastrectomy	Vitamin B_{12}, minerals, calories (if the patient experiences dumping syndrome)
	Ileal resection	Vitamins B_{12}, A, E; minerals; calories (in extensive small bowel resection)
	Certain medications:	
	Antacids, cimetidine (reduce upper duodenal acidity)	Minerals
	Cholestyramine (binds fat-soluble nutrients)	Vitamins A, D, E, K
	Corticosteroids	Protein
	Anticonvulsants	Calcium
Increased nutrient losses	Chronic or acute blood loss	Iron
	Severe diarrhea	Fluid, electrolytes
	Fistulas, draining abscesses, wounds	Protein, zinc
	Nephrotic syndrome	Protein, zinc
	Peritoneal dialysis or hemodialysis	Protein, zinc, water-soluble vitamins
Increased nutrient requirements	Fever*	Calories
	Surgery, trauma, burns, infection	Calories, protein, zinc, vitamin C
	Neoplasms (some types)	Calories, protein
	Physiologic demands (pregnancy, lactation, growth)	Calories, protein, iron

*Each 1° C (1.8° F) elevation in temperature increases caloric needs by approximately 13%.

It is measured at the midpoint of the upper arm, which is half the distance between the olecranon and acromion. The TSF measurement is obtained by grasping the skin and subcutaneous tissue at the back of the arm about 1 cm from the midpoint. Special calipers are then applied to the skinfold at the midpoint, and the skinfold reading is taken to the nearest millimeter. Skinfold measurements are best performed by specially trained nurses and dietitians, because the measurements tend to vary greatly when performed by inexperienced personnel.

Anthropometric measurements are sometimes compared with tables of standard values for large numbers of healthy people. Generally, measurements are considered abnormal if less than the 10th percentile or greater than the 90th. A guideline often used for evaluating body weight states that ideal weight for men is 106 pounds plus 6 pounds for every inch in height over 5 feet, and ideal weight for women is 100 pounds plus 5 pounds for every inch over 5 feet. Thus a man 6 feet 2 inches tall would be expected to weigh 190 pounds (86.4 kilograms). However, standard tables are not always reliable. For instance, an obese woman who has lost 33 pounds (15 kilograms) over the previous 4 months may be within the normal range for weight while suffering from malnutrition. Furthermore, standard tables fail to take into account variations in weight with body build. The best use of anthropometric measurements is for comparison of changes in an individual over a period of time. Good judgment must be used in interpreting anthropometric data. As an example, edema may mask significant weight loss and also may falsely elevate skinfold readings.

A thorough physical examination is an essential part of nutrition assessment. Table 50-2 lists some of the more common findings that may indicate an altered nutritional state. It is especially important for the nurse to check for signs of muscle wasting, loss of subcutaneous fat, skin or hair changes, and impairment of wound healing.

Laboratory Data

A wide range of diagnostic tests can provide information about nutritional status. Those most often used in the clinical setting are described in Table 50-3. As the table emphasizes, there are no perfect diagnostic tests for evaluation of nutrition, and care must be taken in interpreting the results of the tests.

EVALUATING NUTRITIONAL ASSESSMENT FINDINGS AND DETERMINING NUTRITIONAL NEEDS

It is rare for a patient to exhibit a lack of only one nutrient. Usually nutritional deficiencies are combined, with the patient lacking adequate amounts of protein, calories, and possibly vitamins and minerals. A common

Table 50-2 Clinical manifestations of nutritional alterations

Finding	Possible deficiency	Possible excess
HEAD AND NECK		
Hair loss	Protein, zinc, biotin	Vitamin A
Dull, dry, brittle hair; loss of hair pigment	Protein	
Conjunctival and corneal dryness	Vitamin A	
Blue sclerae	Iron	
Pale conjunctiva	Iron	
Gingivitis	Vitamin C	
Cheilosis or angular stomatitis (lesions at corners of mouth)	Vitamin B_2	
Glossitis	Niacin, folate, vitamin B_{12}, other B vitamins	
Hypogeusia (poor sense of taste), dysgeusia (bad taste)	Zinc	
SKIN AND NAILS		
Dry, scaly	Vitamin A, zinc, essential fatty acids	Vitamin A
Follicular hyperkeratosis (resembles gooseflesh)	Vitamin A	
Eczematous lesions	Zinc	
Petechiae, ecchymoses	Vitamin C, K	
Poor wound healing	Protein, zinc, vitamin C	
Koilonychia (spoon-shaped nails)	Iron	
ABDOMEN		
Hepatomegaly	Protein	Vitamin A
MUSCULOSKELETAL AND EXTREMITIES		
Muscle wasting	Calories	
Edema	Protein, vitamin B_1	
Paresthesias	Vitamins B_1, B_6, B_{12}; biotin	

form of combined nutritional deficit among hospitalized patients is protein-calorie malnutrition (PCM). Two types of PCM are *kwashiorkor* and *marasmus*. Kwashiorkor is evidenced by low levels of the serum proteins albumin, transferrin, and prealbumin; low total lymphocyte count; impaired immunity; loss of hair or hair pigment; edema; and an enlarged, fatty liver. Marasmus is recognizable by weight loss, a decrease in skinfold measurements, loss of subcutaneous fat, muscle wasting, and low levels of creatinine excretion. Because PCM weakens musculature, increases vulnerability to infection, and can prolong hospital stays, the health care team should diagnose this serious disorder as quickly as possible so that appropriate nutritional intervention can be implemented.

Nutrition assessment provides a basis for estimating nutritional needs. Methods that are frequently used in estimating the calorie and protein needs of patients can be found in Appendix C.

NUTRITION AND CARDIOVASCULAR ALTERATIONS

Diet and cardiovascular disease may interact in a variety of ways. In one situation, excessive nutrient intake—manifested by overweight or obesity and a diet rich in cholesterol and saturated fat—is a risk factor for

Table 50-3 Diagnostic tests used in nutrition assessment

Area of concern	Possible deficiency	Comments
SERUM PROTEINS		
Decrease of serum albumin, transferrin (iron transport protein), or thyroxine-binding prealbumin*	Protein	These proteins are produced in the liver, are depressed in hepatic failure, and are falsely low in fluid volume excess and elevated in volume deficit. Albumin has a long half-life (14-20 days) and is slow to change in malnutrition and repletion; transferrin has a half-life of 7-8 days, but levels increase in iron deficiency, and prevalence of iron deficiency limits usefulness in diagnosing protein deficits; prealbumin half-life is 2-3 days, and levels fall in trauma and infection.
HEMATOLOGIC VALUES		
Anemia (decreased Hct, Hgb)		Hct and Hgb are falsely low in fluid volume excess and falsely high in fluid volume deficit.
Normocytic (normal MCV, MCHC)	Protein	
Microcytic (decreased MCV, MCH, MCHC)	Iron, copper	
Macrocytic (increased MCV)	Folate, vitamin B_{12}	
Total lymphocyte count (TLC = WBC × % lymphocytes)		
TLC of <1200/mm³	Protein	TLC is decreased in severe debilitating disease.
URINARY CREATININE		
Creatinine excretion of <17 mg/kg/day (women), <23 mg/kg/day (men)	Protein (reflects lean body mass)	It is difficult to collect accurate 24-hr urine; creatinine excretion varies widely from day to day; levels decline with age as percentage of lean body mass declines.
NITROGEN BALANCE†		
Negative values	Protein, calories (during calorie deficit, protein is metabolized to provide calories)	Negative values occur when more nitrogen is excreted than is consumed (reflects inadequate intake or increased needs); positive values occur when more is consumed than lost (e.g., during nutrition repletion, growth, or pregnancy); normal healthy adults excrete exactly what they consume. Limitations: it is difficult to collect accurate 24-hr urine; retention of nitrogen does not necessarily mean that it is being used for tissue synthesis.

*Evaluation of at least one of these is a part of almost every nutritional assessment.

†Protein is 16% nitrogen. Thus nitrogen balance = [24-hr protein intake (g) × 0.16] − [24-hr urine urea nitrogen (g) + 4 g]. The 4 g is an estimate of fecal, skin, and other minor losses.

development of arteriosclerotic heart disease. Conversely, the consequences of chronic myocardial insufficiency can include malnutrition.

Nutrition Assessment in Cardiovascular Alterations

A nutrition assessment provides the nurse and other members of the health care team the information necessary to plan the patient's nutrition care and teaching. Key points of the nutrition assessment of the cardiovascular patient are summarized in Table 50-4. The major nutritional concerns relate to appropriateness of body weight and the levels of serum lipids and blood pressure.

Nutrition Intervention in Cardiovascular Alterations

◆ **Myocardial infarction.** The following guidelines will assist the nurse in providing appropriate nutritional care for the patient in the immediate post–myocardial infarction (MI) period:

1. Limit meal size for the patient with severe myocardial compromise or postprandial angina. Although a meal of typical size is less stressful than is a bed bath or shower for the patient with an uncomplicated condition, these meals increase cardiac index, stroke volume, heart rate, myocardial oxygen consumption, and whole-body oxygen consumption; thus they increase cardiac work. Five to six small meals daily are less likely than are three larger meals to increase myocardial work, promote ischemia, and cause angina.[9]
2. Monitor the effect of caffeine on the patient, if caffeine is included in the diet. Because caffeine is a stimulant, it might be expected to increase heart rate and myocardial oxygen demand. In the United States and in most industrial nations, coffee is the richest source of caffeine in the diet, with about 150 mg of caffeine per 180 ml (6 fluid oz) of coffee. In comparison, the caffeine content of the same volume of tea or cola is approximately 50 mg or 20 mg, respectively.
3. Avoid serving foods at temperature extremes. Although most patients appear to tolerate cold fluids (ice water) well, a subset of patients manifest electrocardiographic changes after drinking ice water.[10] Therefore very hot or very cold foods could trigger vagal or other neural input and cause cardiac dysrhythmias.

◆ **Hypertension.** The primary nutritional intervention for hypertensive patients is to limit sodium intake, usually to no more than 2 g/day. To achieve this level of intake, the patient usually must be helped to avoid foods high in sodium. The primary sodium source in the American diet is salt (sodium chloride) added during food processing and preparation or at the table. One teaspoon of salt provides about 2.3 g of sodium. Most salt substitutes contain potassium chloride and may be used with the physician's approval by the patient who has no renal impairment. "Lite salt" is about half sodium chloride and half potassium chloride. It too may be used if the physician agrees, but it must be used very sparingly to achieve a sodium intake of 2 g or less daily.

◆ **Heart failure.** Nutrition intervention in heart failure (HF) is designed to reduce fluid retained within the body and thus reduce the preload. Because fluid accompanies sodium, limitation of sodium is necessary to reduce fluid retention. Specific interventions include (1) limiting sodium intake, usually to 2 g/day or less and (2) limiting fluid intake as appropriate. The amount ordered is usually 1.5 to 2 L/day, to include both fluids in the diet and those given with medications and for other purposes. The nurse should remember that some foods that are normally served as solids are actually liquids at body temperature. These include gelatins (100% water), custard (75% water), sherbet and fruit ices (50% water), and ice cream (33% water).

◆ **Cardiac cachexia.** The severely malnourished cardiac patient often suffers from CHF. Therefore sodium and fluid restriction, as previously described, are appropriate. It is important to concentrate nutrients into as small a volume as possible and to serve small amounts frequently, rather than three large meals daily, which may overwhelm the patient. The patient also can be given calorie-dense foods and supplements.

Because the patient is likely to tire quickly and to suffer from anorexia, tube feeding or total parenteral nutrition (TPN) may be necessary. When tube feeding is needed, formulas with 2 or more calories/ml are preferable. (Most commonly used formulas provide 1 calorie/ml.) Formulas appropriate for the fluid-restricted patient include Magnacal (Sherwood), Isocal HCN (Mead Johnson), TwoCal HN (Ross), and Nutrisource (Sandoz). During TPN, 20% lipid emulsions with 2 calories/ml provide a concentrated energy source. (The 10% emulsions, in contrast, contain only 1.1 calorie/ml.)

The nurse must monitor the fluid status of these patients carefully when they are receiving nutrition support. Body weight must be recorded daily; a consistent gain of more than 0.11 to 0.22 kg (¼ to ½ lb) a day usually indicates fluid retention rather than gain of fat and muscle mass. The nurse also must check the patient frequently for increasing pulmonary and peripheral edema.

Nutrition Teaching in Cardiovascular Alterations

◆ **Myocardial infarction.** The patient recovering from MI must recognize the need for permanent changes in diet and life-style to reduce the risk of additional MIs. These changes include the following:

1. Weight reduction, if the patient is overweight. Gradual loss of 0.45 to 0.9 kg (1 to 2 lb) per week should be the goal. This can be achieved through moderate exercise and reduction of dietary intake – in particular, reducing intake of fried and fatty foods, because fat is the most concentrated source of calories. In addition, although there is no concrete evidence that a high-fiber diet is effective in promoting weight loss,[11,12] the patient should be encouraged to choose high-fiber foods. Foods high in fiber or "bulk" are usually low in caloric density. They also take longer to consume than more refined foods, allowing the patient to attain satiety before he or she has consumed large numbers of calories.

2. Control of cholesterol, fat, and saturated fat intake. For individuals with no elevation in serum cholesterol and LDL-cholesterol levels, a diet in which fat provides no more than 30% of the calories and saturated fat no more than 10% of the calories is recommended.[13,14] Cholesterol intake should average no more than 300 mg/day. Animal products are the major sources of saturated fat and cholesterol in the diet, with tropical oils (coconut, palm, and palm kernel, which are used frequently in processed foods, popcorn oils, and bakery items) and hydrogenated fats (margarine and shortening) providing additional amounts. To control fat, saturated fat, and cholesterol intake, meat intake is limited to approximately 6 oz/day.

The National Cholesterol Education Program has recommended intensive dietary therapy for individuals with LDL-cholesterol levels of 160 mg/dl and above and those with levels of 130 to 159 mg/dl who have definite coronary heart disease or two other risk factors (i.e., male gender, coronary heart disease before age 55 in a parent or sibling, diabetes mellitus, history of cerebrovascular or peripheral vascular disease, and >30% overweight). A two-step program (Table 50-5) has been established to reduce saturated fat and cholesterol intake, and total fat intake is limited as well, to aid in weight reduction. Initially, the patient receives counseling about the Step-One Diet (Table 50-6), which reduces the most common and obvious sources of saturated fatty acids and cholesterol in the diet and can be implemented without drastic diet or life-style changes for most patients. If, after adhering to the diet for a period of 3 months, the patient does not succeed in lowering LDL-cholesterol to the desirable level, he or she may progress to the Step-Two Diet. Although the physician or nurse often can provide education about the Step-One Diet, referral to a dietitian is valuable for patients who have difficulty in adhering to the diet or who have a disappointing response to the diet. The dietitian's help is particularly needed by patients who progress to the Step-Two Diet.

Diet teaching should emphasize that changes do

Table 50-4 Nutrition assessment of the cardiovascular patient

	Significant findings		
Area of concern	**History**	**Physical assessment**	**Laboratory data**
Overweight/obesity	Excessive kcal intake (consult dietitian regarding nutrition history) Sedentary life-style	Weight >120% of desirable Triceps skinfold measurement of >90th percentile*	
Protein-calorie malnutrition (cardiac cachexia)	Chronic cardiopulmonary disease causing the following: Decreased food intake related to angina, respiratory embarrassment, or fatigue during eating Malabsorption of nutrients caused by hypoxia of the gut Medications that impair appetite (e.g., digitalis, quinidine)	Weight <85% of desirable Triceps skinfold measurement of <10th percentile† Muscle wasting Loss of subcutaneous fat	Serum albumin <3.5 g/dl (or low serum transferrin or prealbumin level) Negative nitrogen balance Creatinine excretion <17 mg/kg/day (women) or <23 mg/kg/day (men)
Elevated serum lipid levels	Frequent or daily use of foods high in cholesterol and saturated fat, including red meat, cold cuts, bacon or sausage, butter, cream or nondairy creamer, foods containing shortening or lard or fried in those products, eggs, organ meats, cheese, ice cream Sedentary life-style Family history of hyperlipidemia Overweight or obesity	Xanthomas, or yellowish plaques deposited in the skin (uncommon)	Serum cholesterol >200 mg/dl[5] Low-density lipoprotein cholesterol >130 mg/dl[13]
Elevated blood pressure	Daily use of high-sodium foods and salt at the table Consumption of >2 oz of alcohol/day		

Modified from Moore MC: *Pocket guide to nutrition and diet therapy*, ed 2, St Louis, 1993, Mosby–Year Book.
*20 mm for men and 34 mm for women.
†6 mm for men and 14 mm for women.

not have to result in a restrictive or unpalatable diet. Patients should be encouraged to consume a diet rich in complex carbohydrates (starches and fibers), which are found primarily in breads, cereals, and fresh vegetables and fruits. Not only do carbohydrates help to replace fats in the diet, but also the "soluble fibers"—such as those in oat products and legumes (but not the cellulose found in wheat bran)—are hypocholesterolemic. Animal protein intake should be limited to no more than approximately 6 oz/day; dried beans and peas are good meat substitutes for individuals seeking to lower their fat intake. Epidemiologic studies indicate that frequent consumption of fish helps to lower the risk of coronary heart disease; therefore fish intake should be encouraged. Use of fish oil supplements, however, has not been shown to lower LDL-cholesterol levels or the risk of MI and should not be recommended. Because egg yolks are rich in both cholesterol and saturated fat, the person on the Step-One Diet should eat no more than three egg yolks a week, and the person on the Step-Two Diet should eat no more than one yolk. Egg whites, which are free of fat and cholesterol, can be used liberally. Fat intake should be limited to approximately 6 to 8 tsp/day, with the unsaturated vegetable oils being the most desirable dietary fats (Table 50-6). Moderate alcohol intake usually is allowed, but excessive intake should be discouraged—especially for obese or overweight individuals—because it is relatively high in calories.

◆ **Hypertension.** The patient must understand the rationale for the necessary dietary changes, as well as the risks associated with noncompliance. Recommended dietary changes include the following:

1. Reduce weight, if overweight or obese. Even if the patient does not achieve the ideal weight, weight loss helps to control hypertension.

Table 50-5 Dietary therapy of high blood cholesterol

	Recommended intake	
Nutrient	**Step-one diet**	**Step-two diet**
Total fat	<30% of total calories	
Saturated fatty acids	<10% of total calories	<7% of total calories
Polyunsaturated fatty acids	Up to 10% of total calories	
Monounsaturated fatty acids	10% to 15% of total calories	
Carbohydrates	50% to 60% of total calories	
Protein	10% to 20% of total calories	
Cholesterol	<300 mg/day	<200 mg/day
Total calories	To achieve and maintain desirable weight	

From National Cholesterol Education Program: *Report of the Expert Panel on Detection, Evaluation, and Treatment of High Blood Cholesterol in Adults*, NIH Publ No 89-2925, Washington DC, 1989, US Department of Health and Human Services.

2. Restrict sodium intake. Although the patient with no renal impairment may use a salt substitute with the physician's approval, many patients do not care for the taste of the substitutes. The patient and/or the person normally responsible for the patient's food preparation can be encouraged to experiment with the use of low-sodium herbs and seasonings to replace salt. The patient may be encouraged to know that the taste for sodium declines after approximately 3 months if the low-sodium regimen is followed conscientiously.

   Almost all fresh fruits and vegetables are low in sodium and can be used to provide interest in the diet. These foods are also a good source of potassium, and some evidence suggests that a high potassium intake helps to maintain a normal blood pressure, although this has not been proved.
3. Consume no more than 2 oz of alcohol daily. One ounce of alcohol is the equivalent of 2 oz of 100-proof whiskey, 8 oz of wine, or 24 oz of beer. Alcohol has a direct pressor effect.[15]

◆ **Heart failure.** Recommended dietary changes include the following:

1. Restrict sodium intake. This teaching is the same as that for the hypertensive patient.
2. Restrict fluid intake, if appropriate. The patient and family need help in learning to measure and record fluid intake, including those foods that are consumed as solids, such as ice cream, custard, and sherbet.
3. Consume a balanced, nutritious diet if cachectic or undernourished. Patients should be encouraged to avoid low-caloric foods and choose instead those with high-caloric density.

NUTRITION AND PULMONARY ALTERATIONS

Malnutrition has extremely adverse effects on respiratory function, decreasing both surfactant production and vital capacity.[16] Moreover, individuals who lose weight lose proportionately more mass from the diaphragm than total body mass, and this further impairs ventilation.[16] Early detection and treatment of nutritional deficits seem to be especially important in patients with pulmonary alterations. Patients with acute respiratory disorders find it difficult to consume adequate oral nutrients and can rapidly become malnourished. Patients with chronic disorders and long-term weight loss have proved challenging to rehabilitate nutritionally. Patients who do tolerate nutritional repletion demonstrate significant improvements in forced expiratory volume at 1 minute (FEV_1) and forced vital capacity (FVC), as well as increased sensitivity to $Paco_2$ levels.[17] Patients with undernutrition and end-stage chronic obstructive pulmonary disease (COPD), however, are unable to tolerate the increase in metabolic demand that occurs during refeeding. In addition, they are at significant risk for development of cor pulmonale and often fail to tolerate the fluid required for delivery of enteral or parenteral nutrition support. Prevention of severe nutritional deficits, rather than correction of deficits once they have occurred, is the key to nutritional management of these patients.

Nutrition Assessment in Pulmonary Alterations

Nutrition assessment is summarized in Table 50-7. The patient with respiratory compromise is especially vulnerable to the effects of fluid volume and carbohydrate excess and must be assessed continually for these complications.

Nutrition Intervention in Pulmonary Alterations

◆ **Prevent or correct undernutrition and underweight.** The nurse and dietitian can work together to encourage oral intake in the undernourished or potentially undernourished patient who is capable of eating. Small, frequent feedings are especially important, because a very full stomach can interfere with diaphragmatic movement. Mouth care needs to be provided before meals and snacks to clear the palate of the flavors of sputum and medications. Administering bronchodilators with food can help to reduce gastric irritation.

Because of anorexia, dyspnea, and debilitation, however, many patients will require tube feeding or TPN. It is especially important for the nurse to be alert to the risk of pulmonary aspiration in the patient with an artificial airway. To reduce the risk of this complication, the nurse should (1) keep the patient's head elevated at least 30 degrees during feedings, unless contraindicated, (2) discontinue feedings 30 to 60 minutes before any procedures that require lowering the head, (3) keep the cuff of the artificial airway inflated during feeding, if possible, (4) measure the patient's gastric residuals at frequent intervals and discontinue feedings if residuals

Table 50-6 Recommended diet modifications to lower blood cholesterol: the step-one diet

Food Source	Choose	Decrease
Fish, chicken, turkey, and lean meats	Fish, poultry without skin, lean cuts of beef, lamb, pork or veal, shellfish	Fatty cuts of beef, lamb, pork; spare ribs, organ meats, regular cold cuts, sausage, hot dogs, bacon, sardines, roe
Skim and low-fat milk, cheese, yogurt, and dairy substitutes	Skim or 1% fat milk (liquid, powdered, evaporated) Buttermilk	Whole milk (4% fat); regular, evaporated, condensed; cream, half and half, 2% milk, imitation milk products, most non-dairy creamers, whipped toppings
	Nonfat (0% fat) or low-fat yogurt	Whole-milk yogurt
	Low-fat cottage cheese (1% or 2% fat)	Whole-milk cottage cheese (4% fat)
	Low-fat cheeses, farmer, or pot cheeses (all of these should be labeled no more than 2-6 g fat/oz)	All natural cheeses (e.g., blue, roquefort, camembert, cheddar, swiss)
		Low-fat or "light" cream cheese, low-fat or "light" sour cream
		Cream cheeses, sour cream
	Sherbet Sorbet	Ice cream
Eggs	Egg whites (2 whites = 1 whole egg in recipes), cholesterol-free egg substitutes	Egg yolks
Fruits and vegetables	Fresh, frozen, canned, or dried fruits and vegetables	Vegetables prepared in butter, cream, or other sauces
Breads and cereals	Homemade baked goods using unsaturated oils sparingly, angel food cake, low-fat crackers, low-fat cookies	Commercially baked goods: pies, cakes, doughnuts, croissants, pastries, muffins, biscuits, high-fat crackers, high-fat cookies
	Rice, pasta	Egg noodles
	Whole-grain breads and cereals (oatmeal, whole wheat, rye, bran, multigrain, and so on)	Breads in which eggs are major ingredient
Fats and oils	Baking cocoa	Chocolate
	Unsaturated vegetable oils: corn, olive, rapeseed (canola oil), safflower, sesame, soybean, sunflower	Butter, coconut oil, palm oil, palm kernel oil, lard, bacon fat
	Margarine or shortening made from one of the unsaturated oils listed above	
	Diet margarine	
	Mayonnaise, salad dressings made with unsaturated oils listed above	Dressings made with egg yolk
	Low-fat dressings	
	Seeds and nuts	Coconut

From National Cholesterol Education Program: *Report of the Expert Panel on Detection, Evaluation, and Treatment of High Blood Cholesterol in Adults*, NIH Publ No 89-2925, Washington, DC, 1989, US Department of Health and Human Services.

Table 50-7 Nutrition assessment of the pulmonary patient

Area of concern	Significant findings		
	History	**Physical assessment**	**Laboratory data**
Protein-calorie malnutrition	Chronic lung disease: Poor intake of protein and calories because of the following: Breathing difficulty from pressure of a full stomach on the diaphragm Unpleasant taste in the mouth from chronic sputum production Gastric irritation from bronchodilator therapy Increased energy expenditure from increased work of breathing[16]	Muscle wasting Loss of subcutaneous fat Recent weight loss, or weight measurement of <90% of desirable Triceps skinfold measurement of <10th percentile*	Serum albumin <3.5 g/dl, or low transferrin or prealbumin level Total lymphocyte count $<1200/mm^3$ Creatinine excretion <17 mg/kg (women) or <23 mg/kg (men)
	Acute respiratory alterations: Inadequate intake of protein and calories because of the following: Upper airway intubation Altered state of consciousness Dyspnea Increased protein and calorie requirements caused by increased work of breathing or acute pulmonary infections Catabolism resulting from corticosteroid use	Same as for chronic disease	Same as for chronic disease
Overweight/obesity (in patients with chronic lung disease)	Decreased caloric needs resulting from decreasing metabolic rate with aging (metabolic rate declines by 2%/decade after age 30) or decreased activity to compensate for impaired respiratory function	Weight >120% of desirable Triceps skinfold measurement >90th percentile†	
Elevated respiratory quotient (RQ)‡	Use of glucose or other carbohydrate to provide 70% or more of nonprotein calories Consumption of excess calories	Tachypnea, shortness of breath	RQ ≥1 Elevated Vo_2 and Vco_2 Elevated $Paco_2$ (not always present)
Fluid volume excess	Administration of more than 35-50 ml fluid/kg/day Increased antidiuretic hormone (ADH) release resulting from stress and ventilator dependency	Dependent edema Pulmonary rales Bounding pulse Shortness of breath	Serum sodium <135 mEq/L BUN, hematocrit, and serum albumin decreased from previous values
Excess lipid intake	Administration of IV lipids		Serum triglyceride >150 mg/dl Low VA/Q§

*6 mm for men and 14 mm for women.

†20 mm for men and 34 mm for women.

‡RQ, or CO_2 produced ÷ O_2 consumed, is measured by indirect calorimetry, which is not available in all institutions. However, pulmonary function tests can provide some indication of RQ, as the "laboratory data" column demonstrates. Carbon dioxide production (and RQ) rises in the patient who is depending primarily on carbohydrate for fuel (e.g., the patient receiving TPN in whom dextrose is supplying almost all calories, rather than receiving a balance between dextrose and lipid calories) and especially in the patient who is being overfed so that adipose tissue is being accumulated.

§The defect is not usually sufficient to alter Pao_2 or $Paco_2$, except in patients with the most severe lung disease.

exceed the guidelines established for the patient (if no guidelines are set, 150 ml is often considered excessive for intermittently fed and 10% to 20% more than the hourly flow rate is considered excessive for continuously fed patients), and (5) monitor the patient for increasing abdominal distension.

◆ **Avoid excess carbohydrate administration.** The production of carbon dioxide increases when carbohydrate is relied on as the primary energy source, and this raises the respiratory quotient (see the section on assessment). This is unlikely to be significant in the patient who is eating foods. Instead, it is an iatrogenic complication of TPN, in which glucose is often the predominant calorie source, or occasionally of tube feeding in a patient with a very high carbohydrate formula.[18] Excessive carbohydrate intake can raise $Paco_2$ sufficiently to make it difficult to wean a patient from the ventilator. Patients who are not dependent on a ventilator may experience tachypnea or shortness of breath on a high carbohydrate regimen.

The nurse who notes an increasing $Paco_2$ in a patient receiving carbohydrate-based TPN should discuss with the physician the possibility of providing daily lipid infusions for the patient. A regimen with both lipids and carbohydrates providing the nonprotein calories is optimal for the patient with respiratory compromise. Table 50-8 illustrates a sample TPN prescription for a patient with acute respiratory failure.

◆ **Avoid excessive serum lipid levels.** Excessive lipid intake can impair capillary gas exchange in the lungs, although this is not usually sufficient to produce an increase in $Paco_2$ or decrease in Pao_2. However, the patient with severe respiratory alteration may be further compromised by lipid overdose. If lipid intake is maintained at no more than 2 g/kg/day, lipid excess is rarely a problem. Lipids are available as 20 g lipid per 100 ml (20% lipid emulsion) and 10 g/100 ml (10% emulsion). Serum triglyceride levels are usually maintained at less than 150 mg/dl. Higher levels may indicate inadequate clearance and a need to decrease the lipid dosage.

◆ **Prevent fluid volume excess.** Pulmonary edema and failure of the right side of the heart, which may result from fluid volume excess, further worsen the status of the patient with respiratory compromise. Strict intake records must be maintained to allow for accurate totals of fluid intake. Usually the patient requires no more than 35 to 50 ml/kg/day of fluid. For the patient receiving nutrition support, fluid intake can be reduced by using 20% lipid emulsions as a source of calories, using tube feeding formulas providing at least 2 calories/ml (the dietitian can suggest appropriate choices), and choosing oral supplements that are low in fluid. Some examples are cottonseed oil (Lipomul [Upjohn]), an oral lipid supplement providing 6 calories/ml, and powdered glucose polymers, which increase caloric intake without increasing volume. The nurse plays a valuable role in continually reassessing the patient's state of hydration and alerting other team members to changes that may dictate an increase or decrease in fluid intake.

Table 50-8 Sample TPN prescription for a patient with acute respiratory failure

PATIENT INFORMATION

Estimated nonprotein calorie need = 2200 calories/day
Estimated protein need = 90 g/day

NUTRIENT SOLUTIONS

	Nonprotein calories/L	Protein (g/L)
1. Glucose–amino acid TPN solution, each liter containing the following:		
70% glucose, 400 ml	952	0
8.5% amino acids, 600 ml	0	51
Vitamins, minerals, and electrolytes to meet patient requirements	0	0
2. 20% lipid emulsion	2000	0

NUTRITION ORDERS

Infuse 1.8 L glucose–amino acid solution (1714 nonprotein calories and 92 g amino acids) and 250 ml lipid emulsion (500 calories) daily.

Nutrition Teaching in Pulmonary Alterations

Teaching focuses on achieving or maintaining the desirable body weight and avoiding nutritional deficits.

◆ **Undernourished patients and patients at risk of undernutrition.** Undernourished patients should be encouraged to follow the previously outlined suggestions concerning nutrition intervention. Specifically, they should continue to eat frequent small meals and choose calorie-dense foods. They may need help in determining which foods are good calorie sources and in learning to increase calories by adding fat or by using nutritional supplements.

◆ **Overweight or obese patients.** Some patients with chronic lung disease become overweight or obese, rather than underweight, primarily because they restrict their activity because of their disease. The nurse can help them to reduce their weight, which often improves their activity tolerance. In addition, with the physician's agreement, the nurse may recommend a graduated exercise program designed to assist the patient in increasing the metabolic rate and the number of calories used.

NUTRITION AND NEUROLOGIC ALTERATIONS

Because neurologic disorders tend to be long-term problems, they necessitate good nutritional care to prevent nutritional deficits and promote well-being.

Nutrition Assessment in Neurologic Alterations

Nutrition-related assessment findings vary widely in the patient with neurologic alterations, depending on the type of disorder present. Some common findings are shown in Table 50-9.

Table 50-9 Nutrition assessment of the patient with neurologic alterations

	Significant findings		
Area of concern	**History**	**Physical assessment**	**Laboratory data**
DISORDERS OF PROTEIN AND CALORIE NUTRITURE			
Protein calorie malnutrition	Decreased intake because of the following: Coma or confusion Feeding/swallowing difficulties such as dribbling of food and beverages from mouth, dysphagia, weakness of muscles involved in chewing and swallowing Ileus resulting from spinal cord injury or use of pentobarbital Anorexia resulting from depression Increased needs because of the following: Hypermetabolism and catabolism after head injury Catabolism resulting from corticosteroid use Trauma and surgical wounds Loss of protein from decubitus ulcers	Muscle wasting Loss of subcutaneous fat Weight <90% of desirable Triceps skinfold measurement <10th percentile* Change in hair texture, loss of hair	Serum albumin <3.5 g/dl (or low transferrin or prealbumin values) Negative nitrogen balance Total lymphocyte count <1200/mm³ Creatinine excretion <17 mg/kg/day (women) or <23 mg/kg/day (men)
Overweight/obesity	Decreased caloric needs resulting from inactivity Reliance on soft or pureed foods, which are often more dense in calories than higher fiber foods Increased food intake resulting from depression/boredom	Weight >120% of desirable Triceps skinfold >90th percentile†	
VITAMIN AND MINERAL DEFICIENCIES			
Iron (Fe)	Poor intake of meats resulting from chewing difficulties (e.g., as occurs with myasthenia gravis) Loss of blood in trauma	Pallor, blue sclerae Koilonychia	Microcytic anemia (low Hct, Hgb, MCV, MCH, MCHC) Serum Fe <50 μg/ml
Zinc (Zn)	Poor intake of meat resulting from chewing problems Increased needs for healing decubitus ulcers, trauma, or surgical wounds	Hypogeusia, dysgeusia Diarrhea Seborrheic dermatitis Alopecia	Serum Zn <60 μg/ml
FLUID ALTERATIONS			
Fluid volume deficit	Poor intake resulting from difficulty swallowing (e.g., as occurs with cerebrovascular accident), inability to express thirst, fluid restriction in an effort to reduce intracranial edema	Poor skin turgor Decreased urinary output Dry, sticky mucous membranes	Serum sodium >145 mEq/L Serum osmolality >300 mOsm/kg Increased BUN and Hct levels Urine specific gravity >1.030

From Moore MC: *Pocket guide to nutrition and diet therapy*, St Louis, 1988, Mosby–Year Book.
HCT, Hematocrit; *Hgb*, hemoglobin; *MCV*, mean cell volume; *MCH*, mean cell hemoglobin; *MCHC*, mean cell hemoglobin concentration; *BUN*, blood urea nitrogen.
*6 mm (men) or 14 mm (women).
†20 mm (men) or 34 mm (women).

Nutrition Intervention in Neurologic Alterations

◆ **Prevention or correction of nutritional deficits**

Oral feedings. Patients with dysphagia or weakness often experience the greatest difficulty in swallowing foods that are dry or thin liquids, such as water, that are difficult to control. For these patients, the nurse and dietitian can work together to plan suitable meals and evaluate patient acceptance and tolerance. Some suggestions that may help the patient with dysphagia or weakness of the swallowing musculature include the following:

1. Serve soft, moist foods.
2. Thicken beverages with infant cereal, yogurt, or ice cream if the patient has difficulty swallowing fluids or chokes on water and other thin liquids. Alternatively, fluid can be provided by gelatin, sherbet, sorbet, fruit ices, popsicles, and ice cream. Fruit nectars may be better tolerated than juices.
3. Do not rush the patient who is eating, because this may increase the risk of pulmonary aspiration. Providing small amounts of food at frequent intervals, rather than larger amounts only at mealtimes, may help the patient feel less need to hurry. Keep suction equipment available in case aspiration does occur.
4. Place the patient in Fowler's position before feedings, if possible, to allow gravity to facilitate effective swallowing.

Tube feedings or TPN. Patients who are unconscious or unable to eat because of severe dysphagia, weakness, ileus, or other reasons will need tube feedings or TPN. Prompt initiation of nutrition support must be a priority in the patient with neurologic impairments. Needs for protein and calories are increased by infection and fever, as may occur in the patient with encephalitis and meningitis. Needs for protein, calories, zinc, and vitamin C are increased during wound healing, as occurs in the trauma patient and the patient with decubitus ulcers.

Tube feeding can be successful in some patients with neurologic impairment. Because these patients have an increased risk of certain complications, particularly pulmonary aspiration, they require especially careful nursing care. Patients of most concern are (1) those with an impaired gag reflex, such as some patients with cerebral vascular accident, (2) those with delayed gastric emptying, such as patients in the early period after spinal cord injury and patients with head injury treated with barbiturate coma, and (3) patients likely to experience seizures. To help prevent pulmonary aspiration, the patient's head should be kept elevated at 30 degrees, if possible; when elevation of the head is not possible, administering feedings with the patient in the prone or lateral positions will allow free drainage of emesis from the mouth and decrease the risk of aspiration.

Although it has been reported that formulas for enteral feeding can interfere with phenytoin absorption,[19] two investigations failed to find any effect on overall absorption of phenytoin.[20,21] Until this issue has been resolved, phenytoin levels should be monitored carefully in patients receiving enteral feedings.

Hyperglycemia is a common complication in patients receiving corticosteroids. Patients treated with these drugs should have blood glucose levels monitored regularly and may require insulin to prevent substantial loss of glucose in the urine, as well as osmotic diuresis, loss of excessive amounts of potassium, and other fluid and electrolyte disturbances.

Tube feedings may not be possible in some patients with neurologic alterations.[22] Certain patients with head injury may not tolerate tube feedings for a prolonged period because of vomiting and poor gastrointestinal motility. Another group of patients who are not good candidates for enteral feedings are those with frequent or uncontrolled seizures.

TPN is needed by most patients who fail to tolerate tube feedings or those who cannot be enterally fed for at least 5 to 7 days. Prompt use of TPN is especially important for patients with head injuries, because head injury causes marked catabolism,[23] even in patients who receive barbiturates, which should decrease metabolic demands.[23,24] Head-injured patients rapidly exhaust glycogen stores and begin to utilize body proteins to meet energy needs, a process that can quickly cause PCM. The catabolic response to head injury is partly a result of the corticosteroids often used in treatment. However, the hypermetabolism and hypercatabolism are also caused by dramatic hormonal responses to this type of injury.[23] Levels of cortisol, epinephrine, and norepinephrine increase, with levels of norepinephrine elevating as much as 7 times normal. These hormones increase the metabolic rate and caloric demands, causing mobilization of body fat and proteins to meet the increased energy needs. Furthermore, head-injured patients undergo an inflammatory response and may be febrile, creating increased needs for protein and calories. Improved survival has been observed in head-injured patients who receive adequate nutrition support early in the hospital course.[23]

◆ **Prevention of overweight and obesity.** Many stable patients with neurologic disorders are less active than their healthy counterparts and require fewer calories. Thus they may become overweight or obese if given normal amounts of calories for their age and gender. An example is the patient with spinal cord injury.[25] Within 1 or 2 months, substantial amounts of muscle atrophy and loss of body mass begin to occur as a result of denervation and disuse.[26] Consequently, body weight and caloric needs decline. Ideal body weights for paraplegics and quadriplegics are 4.5 kg and 9 kg, respectively, less than those for healthy adults of the same height. Stable, rehabilitating paraplegics need approximately 27.9 calories/kg/day, and quadriplegics need 22.7 calories/kg/day.[27] Patients with dysphagia or extreme weakness may rely on very soft, easy-to-chew foods that are usually more dense in calories than are bulky, high-fiber foods. Thus they also may gain unneeded weight that will hamper their care and impede mobility. Decreased use of high-fat foods —such as shakes, ice cream, butter, margarine, and pastries—will help to reduce calorie intake.

Nutrition Teaching in Neurologic Alterations

The primary nutrition teaching needs of the patient

and family are coping with dysphagia and preventing unwanted weight gain. The nurse can share with them the suggestions for dealing with dysphagia that are described in the section concerning nutrition interventions in neurologic alterations (p. 882). Dysphagia is frustrating and frightening for the patient and requires much understanding and patience by the family. Support and empathy on the part of the nurse can make their coping process easier. For the patient who is at risk of overweight or obesity, suggestions for reducing caloric intake are appropriate.

NUTRITION AND RENAL ALTERATIONS

Providing adequate nutritional care for the patient with renal disease can be extremely challenging. Although renal disturbances and their treatments can markedly increase needs for nutrients, necessary restrictions in intake of fluid, protein, phosphorus, and potassium make delivery of adequate calories, vitamins, and minerals difficult. Thorough nutrition assessment provides the basis for successful nutritional care in patients with renal disease.

Nutrition Assessment in Renal Alterations

Assessment is summarized in Table 50-10.

Nutrition Intervention in Renal Alterations

The goal of nutritional interventions is to administer adequate nutrients, including calories, protein, vitamins, and minerals, while avoiding excesses of fluid, protein, electrolytes, and other nutrients with potential toxicity.

◆ **Protein.** Evidence suggests that a low-protein diet retards the progression of renal damage. It is postulated that a high-protein intake increases glomerular flow and pressures, as the kidney attempts to excrete the urea and other nitrogenous products derived from the protein. The increase in glomerular pressures may hasten the death of the glomeruli.[28] Consequently, decreased protein intake (0.6 g/kg/day compared with the 0.8 g/kg/day recommended for the healthy person and the 1.7 g/kg/day actually consumed by the average American) is recommended for the undialyzed patient with renal failure. Although uremia necessitates control of protein intake, the patient with renal failure often has many problems that actually increase protein/amino acid needs: losses in dialysis, wounds, and fistulae; use of corticosteroid drugs that exert a catabolic effect; increased endogenous secretion of catecholamines, corticosteroids, glucagon, and parathyroid hormone, all of which can cause or aggravate catabolism; and catabolic conditions, such as trauma, surgery, and sepsis associated or coincident with the renal disturbances. Therefore protein needs may actually be increased. During hemodialysis and arteriovenous (A-V) hemofiltration, amino acids are freely filtered and lost but such proteins as albumin and immunoglobulin are not. Both proteins and amino acids are removed during peritoneal dialysis, creating a greater nutritional requirement for protein.[29] Protein needs are estimated at approximately 1.2 g/kg/day for patients receiving hemodialysis or hemofiltration,[30] and 1.2 to 1.5 g/kg/day for those receiving peritoneal dialysis.[29] Although these amounts are greater than the recommended daily level for healthy adults, they are lower than the amount found in the diet of most adults, and thus most patients will perceive them as restrictions.

Controversy exists regarding the type of amino acids to be provided to the patient in renal failure. Some authorities advocate using primarily essential amino acids, those which the body cannot make, with the idea that the patient will form adequate amounts of nonessential amino acids via the process of transamination (transfer of amine groups from one carbon backbone to another). Foods containing protein of high biologic value—such as eggs, milk, beef, poultry, and fish—are richer in essential amino acids than are foods with lower biologic value protein, such as grains, legumes, and vegetables. Therefore foods containing lower biologic value protein would need to be especially restricted. Specialized essential amino acid products have been developed for nutrition support. These include Amin-Aid (Kendall McGaw) and Travasorb Renal (Clintec) for enteral feedings and Aminosyn RF (Abbott), Ren-Amin (Clintec), and Nephramine (Kendall McGaw) for use in preparation in TPN. Reliance on these solutions may delay the need for dialysis. However, it is not clear that outcome is improved in patients receiving essential amino acid preparations, and many physicians now recommend the use of more balanced preparations, containing both essential and nonessential amino acids, in settings in which dialysis is available.[31] For the stressed, catabolic renal patient, provision of adequate amounts of all types of amino acids required for anabolism appears to be more important than delaying initiation of dialysis.

Some nephrologists advocate the use of ketoanalogs (carbon structures related to the amino acids, but lacking the amine group) rather than or in addition to essential amino acids. Patients can form amino acids from the ketoanalogs and circulating nitrogenous compounds. Use of ketoanalogs requires reduction of protein intake to at least 0.4 g/kg/day.[31] Because these compounds are relatively unpalatable, they may need to be given by tube.

◆ **Fluid.** Patients are usually limited to a fluid intake resulting in a gain of no more than 0.45 kg (1 pound) per day on the days between dialysis. This generally means a daily intake of 500 ml plus the volume lost in urine, diarrhea, and vomitus. With the use of continuous peritoneal dialysis, hemofiltration, or arteriovenous hemodialysis, the fluid intake can be liberalized. A liberal fluid allowance permits more adequate nutrient delivery, whether by oral, tube, or parenteral feedings. Enteral formulas providing 2 calories/ml or more—such as Nutrisource (Sandoz), TwoCal HN (Ross), Isocal HCN (Mead Johnson), and Magnacal (Sherwood)—are useful in providing a concentrated source of calories for tube-fed patients who require fluid restriction. Intravenous lipids, particularly 20% emulsions, can be used to supply concentrated calories for the TPN patient.

◆ **Calories.** It is essential that the renal patient receive an adequate number of calories to prevent catabolism of body tissues to meet energy needs. Catabolism not only

Table 50-10 Nutrition assessment of the renal patient

Area of concern	History	Physical assessment	Laboratory data
Protein-calorie malnutrition	Poor dietary intake because of the following: Dietary restrictions on protein-containing foods Anorexia caused by zinc deficiency (lost in dialysis or decreased in diet because of restrictions on meats, whole grains, legumes) Increased protein and amino acid losses from the following: Dialysis (hemodialysis losses ≈ 10-13 g/session; CAPD losses ≈ 5-15 g/day)† Tissue catabolism resulting from corticosteroid use Proteinuria (e.g., as occurs with nephrotic syndrome) Increased needs for protein and calories during peritonitis and other infections	Muscle wasting Loss of subcutaneous tissue Weight <90% of desirable Triceps skinfold <10th percentile* (Loss of weight and subcutaneous fat may be masked by edema) Loss of hair, change of hair texture	Serum albumin <3.5 g/dl or low transferrin or prealbumin levels Total lymphocyte count <1200/mm³ Negative nitrogen balance
Altered lipid metabolism	Nephrotic syndrome, with elevated cholesterol levels Excess carbohydrate (CHO) consumption from the following: Emphasis on CHO in the diet to replace some of the calories normally provided by protein Use of glucose as an osmotic agent in dialysis		Serum cholesterol >250 mg/dl Serum triglyceride >180 mg/dl
Potential fluid volume excess	Oliguria or anuria Patient knowledge deficit about or noncompliance with fluid restriction	Edema Hypertension Acute weight gain (≥1%-2% of body weight)	Hematocrit decreased from previous levels
DISORDERS OF MINERALS/ELECTROLYTES			
Phosphorus (P) excess	Oliguria or anuria	Tetany	Serum P > 4.5 mg/dl Calcium × P product (Ca in mg/dl × P in mg/dl) >70
Zinc (Zn) deficit	Poor intake because of restriction of protein-containing foods Loss in dialysis	Hypogeusia, dysgeusia Alopecia Seborrheic dermatitis Diarrhea	Serum Zn <60 μg/ml
Iron (Fe) deficit	Decreased intake because of restriction of protein-containing foods Loss of blood in dialysis tubing	Fatigue Pallor, blue sclerae Koilonychia	Hematocrit <37% (women) or <42% (men); hemoglobin <12 g/dl (women) or <14 g/dl (men); low MCV, MCH, MCHC levels
Sodium excess	Oliguria or anuria	Edema Hypertension	

From Moore, MC: *Pocket guide to nutrition and diet therapy*, St Louis, 1988, Mosby–Year Book.

CAPD, continuous ambulatory peritoneal dialysis; *MCV*, mean cell volume; *MCH*, mean cell hemoglobin; *MCHC*, mean cell hemoglobin concentration.

*6 mm for men, and 14 mm for women.

†Increased by 50%-100% in peritonitis.

Table 50-10 Nutrition assessment of the renal patient—cont'd

Area of concern	History	Physical assessment	Laboratory data
Potassium (K^+) excess	Oliguria or anuria	Weakness, flaccid muscles	Serum K^+ >5 mEq/L Elevated T wave and depressed ST segment on ECG
Aluminum (Al) excess	Use of aluminum-containing phosphate binders Al contamination of TPN constituents	Ataxia, seizures Dementia Renal osteodystrophy with bone pain and deformities	Plasma Al >100 μg/L
DISORDERS OF VITAMIN NUTRITURE			
A excess	Oliguria or anuria Daily administration of tube feedings, TPN, or oral supplement with vitamin A	Anorexia Alopecia, dry skin Hepatomegaly Fatigue, irritability	Serum retinol level of >80 μg/dl
C deficit	Loss in dialysis Decreased intake due to restriction of K^+-containing fruits and vegetables	Gingivitis Petechiae, ecchymoses	Serum ascorbate <.4 mg/dl
B_6	Failure of the diseased kidney to activate vitamin B_6 Loss in dialysis	Dermatitis Ataxia Irritability, seizures	Plasma pyridoxal phosphate <34 nmol (normal levels not well established)
Folic acid	Loss in dialysis Decreased intake resulting from restriction of meats, fruits, and vegetables	Glossitis (inflamed tongue) Pallor	Hematocrit <37% (women) or <42% (men), elevated MCV level Serum folate <6 ng/ml

reduces the mass of muscle and other functional body tissues, but also releases nitrogen that must be excreted by the kidney. Adults with renal failure need about 35 to 40 calories/kg/day, compared with the 25 to 30 calories/kg needed by healthy adults, to prevent catabolism and ensure that all protein consumed is used for anabolism rather than to meet energy needs. After renal transplantation, when the patient usually receives large doses of corticosteroids, it is especially important to ensure that adequate caloric intake continues to prevent undue catabolism.

High-carbohydrate foods, such as hard candies, sugar, honey, jelly, jellybeans, and gumdrops, are often used as a means of supplying calories to the patient with renal failure, because these foods are low in sodium and potassium, which are retained in renal failure. However, hypertriglyceridemia is found in a substantial number of patients with renal disorders. This condition is worsened by excessive intake of simple refined sugars, such as sucrose (table sugar) or glucose. To help control hypertriglyceridemia, only about 30% to 35% of the patient's calories should come from carbohydrates, with the emphasis placed on complex carbohydrates (starches and fibers). When glucose is used as the osmotic agent in peritoneal dialysis and A-V hemodialysis, approximately 70% of the glucose in the dialysate may be absorbed and this must be considered part of the patient's carbohydrate intake.[32] The glucose monohydrate used in intravenous and dialysate solutions supplies 3.4 calories/g. Thus if the patient receives 4.25% glucose (4.25 g glucose/100 ml solution) in the dialysate, he or she receives the following:

$$42.5 \text{ g/L} \times 70\% \times 3.4 \text{ calories/g} = 101 \text{ calories/L of dialysate}$$

For the tube-fed patient, enteral formulas that contain some fiber, such as Compleat (Sandoz) and Enrich (Ross), may help to control hypertriglyceridemia.

To help control hypertriglyceridemia and to provide concentrated calories in minimal fluid, fat should supply about half or more of the patient's calories. Because hypercholesterolemia is frequently found in patients with renal failure, polyunsaturated fats and oils are preferred over saturated fats, which tend to raise cholesterol levels. The necessary restriction of meat, milk, and other protein foods in the diet will help to lower cholesterol and saturated fat intake. For patients who need a caloric supplement, Lipomul (Upjohn) is a palatable oral lipid supplement providing 6 calories/ml with minimal sodium and potassium. Intravenous lipids and the long-chain fats found in most enteral formulas, except those prepared from blended foods, are primarily polyunsaturated. Some formulas are rich in medium-chain triglycerides, or fats. Although these triglycerides are saturated, they do not contribute to hypercholesterolemia and thus may be used for the renal patient.

◆ **Other nutrients.** Table 50-11 is a summary of the recommended nutrient intake for patients with renal disorders, for whom recommendations are different from those for healthy adults. The recommendations for

Table 50-11 Daily nutritional recommendations for patients with renal failure

Nutrient	Recommended dietary allowance (RDA) for healthy adults	Daily amount in renal failure
Protein or amino acids (g/kg)	0.8	0.6 (undialyzed)* 1.2+ (hemodialysis)* 1.2-1.5 (peritoneal dialysis)*
Calories/kg	25-30	35-40
Electrolytes and minerals†		
Sodium	Unspecified	87-109 mEq (2-2.5 g)‡
Potassium	Unspecified	70-80 mEq (2.7-3.1 g)
Calcium (mg)	800	1000-1500
Phosphorus (mg)	800	700-800
Magnesium (mg)	280-350	200-300
Trace minerals		
Iron (mg)	10-15	15 mg +, as needed to prevent deficiency
Zinc (mg)	12-15	15 mg +, as needed to prevent deficiency
Vitamins		
C (mg)	60	70-100
B_6 (mg)	1.6-2.0	5-10
Folic acid (μg)	180-200	1000

From Feinstein EI: *Nutr Clin Prac* 3:9, 1988; Kopple JD, Blumenkrantz MJ: *Kidney Int Suppl* 16:S295, 1983; Maschio G and others: *Kidney Int* 22:371, 1982; and *Recommended dietary allowances*, Washington, DC, 1989, National Academy of Sciences—National Research Council.

*Based on estimated dry weight.

†Dosages given are representative ranges; serum levels and physical findings help to determine actual individual intake. For instance, the presence of edema and hypertension usually necessitates a reduced sodium allowance. These are enteral recommendations, and parenteral levels may be lower.

‡Levels for continuous ambulatory peritoneal dialysis (CAPD) may be higher.

healthy adults are included to provide a basis for comparison. Certain nutrients are restricted because they are excreted by the kidney. Phosphorus is one example: its restriction appears to delay progression of renal damage.[31] Phosphorus is found primarily in meat, milk, nuts, and whole grains, so that limitation of protein intake will also help to lower phosphorus levels. The patient has no specific requirement for the fat-soluble vitamins A, E, and K, because they are not removed in appreciable amounts by dialysis and restriction prevents development of toxicity. Elevated levels of vitamin A are a common finding in dialyzed patients. On the other hand, needs for several water-soluble vitamins and trace minerals are increased in the dialysis patient because they are small enough to pass freely through the dialysis filter. If the patient is not receiving supplements of the water-soluble vitamins listed in Table 50-11 or levels of trace elements are not being monitored, the nurse should consult with the physician about the need for such measures. Similarly, if the patient is receiving vitamin A–containing TPN or tube feeding daily, the nurse can discuss with the physician, pharmacist, and dietitian the desirability of devising nutrient solutions providing only the water-soluble vitamins.

Nutrition Teaching in Renal Alterations

Although the primary nutrition teaching for such a complex dietary regimen will normally be performed by the dietitian, the nurse can reinforce and supplement the dietary instruction. In addition, an understanding of the need for a generous caloric intake may make the patient more cooperative in consuming meals and supplements or when it is apparent that tube feeding or TPN is necessary. The nurse can help the patient and family learn to recognize sources of high and low biologic value protein and to select moderate amounts of the high biologic value protein, to measure all fluid intake and maintain daily records of all fluid intake, and to control sodium and potassium intake as necessary.

NUTRITION AND GASTROINTESTINAL ALTERATIONS

Because the gastrointestinal (GI) tract is so inherently related to nutrition, it is not surprising that catastrophic occurrences in the GI tract—hemorrhage, perforation, infarct, or related organ failure—have acute and severe adverse effects on nutritional status.

Nutrition Assessment in Gastrointestinal Alterations

Assessment is summarized in Table 50-12. The area and amount of the GI tract affected determine, to a large extent, the likelihood and degree of nutritional deficits, because each portion of the bowel has a role to play in absorption (Fig. 50-1). The ileum is among the most nutritionally important areas. Fat and bile salt absorption occurs in this area, as does absorption of vitamin B_{12}. Patients with ileal disease or resection are likely to become malnourished as a result of significant loss of calories, as well as vitamins and minerals, in the feces. The ileocecal valve is especially critical in maintaining adequate nutrition. Not only does it slow entry of GI contents into the large bowel, allowing more time for

Table 50-12 Nutrition assessment of the patient with a gastrointestinal disorder

Area of concern	History	Physical assessment	Laboratory data
Protein-calorie malnutrition	Decreased oral intake caused by the following: Fear of symptoms—pain, cramping, diarrhea—associated with eating (e.g., as occurs with peptic ulcer, dumping syndrome) Alcohol abuse Nausea, vomiting, anorexia Increased losses because of the following: Maldigestion or malabsorption (e.g., as occurs with inadequate bile salt production, increased loss of bile salts in short bowel syndrome, diarrhea, inadequate absorptive area in short bowel syndrome) GI bleeding Fistula drainage Increased requirements caused by the following: Needs for healing (e.g., surgical wounds, fistulae)	Muscle wasting Loss of subcutaneous fat Weight <90% of desirable or recent weight loss Triceps skinfold measurement <10th percentile* Hair loss or change in hair texture	Serum albumin <3.5 g/dl or low transferrin level Total lymphocyte count <1200/mm³ Creatinine excretion <17 mg/kg/day (women) or <23 mg/kg/day (men) Negative nitrogen balance Fecal fat >5 g/day or >5% of intake
Potential fluid volume deficit	Losses caused by severe vomiting or diarrhea (e.g., as occurs with GI obstruction, short bowel syndrome)	Poor skin turgor Dry, sticky mucous membranes Complaint of thirst Loss of ≥0.23 kg (0.5 pounds) in 24 hr	Hct >52% (men) or >47% (women) BUN >20 mg/dl Serum sodium >145 mEq/L Serum osmolality >300 mOsm/kg Urine specific gravity >1.030
DISORDERS OF MINERAL/ELECTROLYTE NUTRITURE			
Calcium (Ca)	Increased loss because of steatorrhea (Ca forms soaps with fat in the stool and thus becomes unabsorbable)	Tingling of fingers Muscular tetany and cramps Carpopedal spasm Convulsions	Serum Ca level of <8.5 mg/dl (severe deficits only)
Magnesium (Mg)	Inadequate intake because of poor diet in alcoholism Increased losses because of the following: Diarrhea or steatorrhea Loss of small bowel fluid (e.g., as occurs with short bowel syndrome, fistulae)	Tremor Hyperactive deep reflexes Convulsions	Serum Mg <1.5 mEq/L
Iron (Fe)	Blood loss Impaired absorption because of decreased upper GI acidity with gastrectomy or use of antacids and cimetidine Inadequate intake (e.g., restriction of protein foods in hepatic failure)	Pallor, blue sclerae Fatigue Koilonychia	Hct <42% (men) or <37% (women); Hgb <14 g/dl (men) or <12 g/dl (women); low MCV, MCH, MCHC Serum Fe <60 μg/dl

Modified from Moore MC: *Pocket guide to nutrition and diet therapy, ed 2*, St Louis, 1993, Mosby–Year Book.

Hct, hematocrit; *BUN*, blood urea nitrogen; *Hgb*, hemoglobin; *MCV*, mean cell volume; *MCH*, mean cell hemoglobin; *MCHC*, mean cell hemoglobin concentration; *Ca*, calcium.

*6 mm for men and 14 mm for women.

Continued.

Table 50-12 Nutrition assessment of the patient with a gastrointestinal disorder—cont'd

Area of concern	History	Physical assessment	Laboratory data
Zinc (Zn)	Increased losses caused by the following: Diarrhea, steatorrhea Loss of small bowel fluid Diuretic use (in hepatic failure) Increased urinary losses in alcoholism Inadequate intake caused by the following: Protein restriction in hepatic failure Poor diet in alcoholism	Anorexia Hypogeusia, dysgeusia Seborrheic dermatitis	Serum Zn <60 μg/dl
Potassium (K^+)	Increased loss caused by the following: Diarrhea Diuretic use Hyperaldosteronism (in hepatic failure) GI suction	Muscle weakness, ileus Diminished reflexes	Serum K^+ <3.5 mEq/L
DISORDERS OF VITAMIN NUTRITURE			
A	Increased loss in steatorrhea (vitamin A dissolves in fatty stools) Impaired release of vitamin A from storage in the liver because of inadequate production of retinol-binding protein, the transport protein, in malnutrition or liver failure	Drying of skin and cornea Poor wound healing Follicular hyperkeratosis (resembles gooseflesh)	Serum retinol <20 μg/dl
K	Impaired absorption in steatorrhea Decreased production because of destruction of intestinal bacteria by antibiotic usage	Petechiae, ecchymoses Prolonged bleeding	Prothrombin time >12.5 sec (not accurate in liver failure)

absorption to take place in the small bowel, but it also helps prevent migration of the microorganisms from the large bowel into the small bowel. Proliferating microorganisms in the small bowel deconjugate the bile salts, impairing fat absorption. Deconjugated bile salts also irritate the intestinal mucosa and raise the osmolality level within the bowel, promoting diarrhea.[33] The ileum can absorb most of the nutrients normally absorbed in the upper half of the small bowel, but it is impossible for the duodenum and jejunum to compensate for the loss of the ileum.

Nutrition Intervention in Gastrointestinal Alterations

The GI tract is the preferred route for delivery of nutrients in GI disease, as it is in all other disease states. However, after damage or resection, enteral nutrition support may be inadequate or impossible, at least temporarily. The most common indications for parenteral and enteral feedings in GI patients are listed in the box on p. 889. Because bowel resection and hepatic failure are two of the most nutritionally challenging GI alterations, most of this discussion is devoted to them.

◆ Short bowel syndrome

Administration of fluids and electrolytes. Extensive bowel resection is associated with marked gastric hypersecretion. The increase in gastric juices, coupled with the sudden loss of absorptive area, results in the loss of several liters of fluid daily, along with potassium, magnesium, and zinc. The nurse's role in management of these patients includes (1) keeping strict intake and output records, including volume or weight of stools if they are frequent or loose, (2) continually assessing the patient's state of hydration, and (3) administering fluids

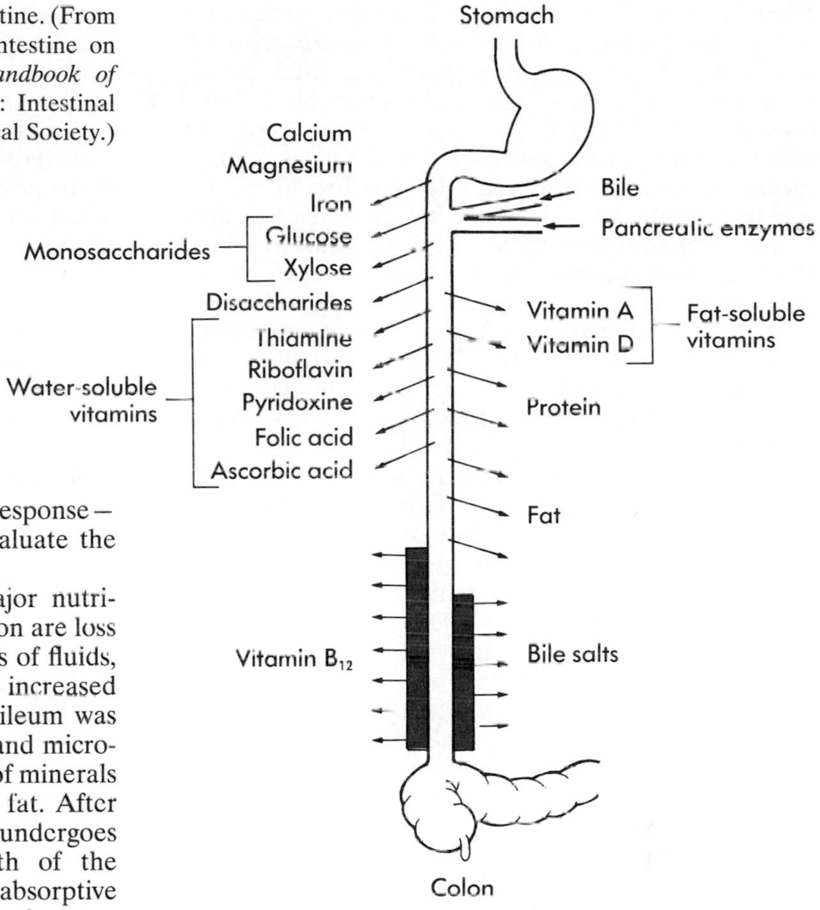

Fig. 50-1 Sites of absorption along the small intestine. (From Booth CC: Effect of location along the small intestine on absorption of nutrients. In Code CF (ed): *Handbook of physiology,* Section 6: Alimentary Canal, Vol. III: Intestinal Absorption, Bethesda, 1968, American Physiological Society.)

and electrolytes and evaluating the patient's response—including daily weight measurements—to evaluate the adequacy of fluid replacement.

Administration of nutrition support. The major nutritional problems associated with bowel resection are loss of absorptive area, with increased fecal losses of fluids, electrolytes, fat, protein, and other nutrients; increased loss of bile salts, especially if the terminal ileum was resected, with further malabsorption of fat; and micronutrient deficiencies resulting from trapping of minerals and fat-soluble vitamins within the excreted fat. After bowel resection, the remaining intestine undergoes marked hyperplasia, with increasing length of the remaining villi, which increases the available absorptive area. The result is improved absorption of water, electrolytes, and glucose.[33] Some patients with 70% to 80% resection of the small bowel can eventually be maintained on enteral feedings only, especially if the terminal ileum and ileocecal valve are retained, but patients with resection of more than 90% of the small bowel usually require permanent TPN.[34] The small bowel is estimated to be approximately 350 to 600 cm in length, depending on whether measurements are made during surgery, when the GI tract retains much of the muscle tonus, or on postmortem examination, when minimal tone is present.[33] It is difficult to estimate the amount remaining at the time of intestinal resection, and thus many patients undergo contrast radiographs when stable to determine the length of the remaining bowel. The adaptive response may take up to a year to become complete, and it does not occur without the presence of nutrients within the gut.[33]

The first priority in nutrition support of the patient with short bowel syndrome is stabilization of fluid and electrolyte balance. After that is accomplished, TPN is initiated. Small enteral feedings are begun early to stimulate adaptation of the remaining bowel. Feedings may consist of an elemental, or predigested, diet given by tube. Fat is the most difficult nutrient to absorb, and the formula will ordinarily be very low in fat or will be high in medium-chain triglycerides (MCTs), which are more readily absorbed than are the long-chain triglycerides predominating in most foods. Tube feedings should be given on a continuous basis to

INDICATIONS FOR SPECIALIZED NUTRITION SUPPORT IN GI ALTERATIONS

PARENTERAL NUTRITION

Complete obstruction of the small or large bowel
Ileus or severe hypomotility of the intestine
Short bowel syndrome (>50% small bowel resection)
High-output (>500 ml/day) enterocutaneous fistulae, where bowel rest may reduce GI secretions and promote healing
Severe diarrhea unresponsive to pharmacologic therapy

ENTERAL NUTRITION

Short bowel syndrome (50% to 90% small bowel resection), in conjunction with TPN
Low-output enterocutaneous fistulae, especially if feedings can be given distal to the fistulae
Anorexia caused by hepatic failure and the unpalatable diet required for its treatment
Stupor or coma

promote optimal absorption. Intragastric rather than transpyloric feedings are preferable to use every available centimeter of intestinal surface area. Alternatively, a low-fat, high-starch diet may be given by mouth.[35] Lactose, or milk sugar, is often tolerated poorly by patients with bowel resection, but low-fat cottage cheese or yogurt, which are relatively low in lactose, may be tolerated. MCTs can be served in juice or used in food preparation to increase caloric intake. Patients receiving oral feedings often require much encouragement to eat, because they may associate eating with worsening of diarrhea. As more and more enteral intake is tolerated, TPN is gradually tapered. Careful records must be kept of all enteral and parenteral intake to determine when TPN can be decreased or discontinued.

Administration of medications. In some patients with short bowel syndrome, in whom diarrhea is prolonged or especially severe and causes anal excoriation or copious ostomy output, antidiarrheal agents, such as diphenoxylate with atropine or codeine, may be beneficial. Anticholinergic drugs, such as glycopyrrolate, can also be used to counteract the gastric hypersecretion.

◆ **Hepatic failure.** Hepatic failure is associated with a wide spectrum of metabolic alterations. Because the diseased liver has impaired ability to deactivate hormones, levels of circulating glucagon, epinephrine, and cortisol are elevated. These hormones promote catabolism of body tissues. Glycogen stores are rapidly exhausted. Although release of lipids from their storage depots is accelerated, the liver has decreased ability to metabolize them for energy. Furthermore, as many as half of the patients with hepatic failure may have malabsorption of fat because of inadequate production of bile salts by the liver. Therefore body proteins are increasingly used for energy sources, producing rapid tissue wasting. The branched chain amino acids (BCAAs)—leucine, isoleucine, and valine—are especially well utilized for energy, and their levels in the blood decline. Conversely, levels of the aromatic amino acids (AAAs)—phenylalanine, tyrosine, and tryptophan—rise as a result of tissue catabolism and impaired ability of the liver to clear them from the blood. Although hyperammonemia is a feature of hepatic failure, it probably is not the causative agent in encephalopathy; it is postulated that AAAs cause encephalopathy. After transport across the blood-brain barrier, they can be converted to "false neurotransmitters," which compete with the normal neurotransmitters for binding sites. The net result is to impede normal neurotransmission and produce hepatic encephalopathy.[36]

Monitoring of fluid and electrolyte status. Ascites and edema result from decreased colloid osmotic pressure in the plasma, because the diseased liver produces less albumin and other plasma proteins; increased portal pressure caused by obstruction; and renal sodium retention from secondary hyperaldosteronism. To control the fluid retention, restriction of sodium (usually 500 to 1500 mg, or 20 to 65 mEq, daily) and fluid (1500 ml or less) is generally necessary, in conjunction with administration of diuretics. Patients must be weighed daily to evaluate the success of treatment. In addition, laboratory and physical status must be closely observed for potassium deficits caused by diuretic therapy and hyperaldosteronism.

Provision of a nutritious diet and evaluation of response to dietary protein. Nutrition intervention in hepatic failure is based on the metabolic alterations. Initially, protein allowances are increased to 1 to 1.5 g/kg/day, in an effort to suppress catabolism and promote liver regeneration. However, if encephalopathy occurs or appears to be impending, protein intake is reduced to 0.5 g/kg/day or less. A high-calorie diet (45 to 50 calories/kg/day, compared with approximately 25 to 30 calories for the healthy adult) is provided to help prevent catabolism and to prevent the use of dietary protein for energy needs. Moderate amounts of fat are given, unless the patient has steatorrhea, in which case it is necessary to rely heavily on carbohydrates and MCTs to meet caloric needs. Soft foods are preferred, because the patient may have esophageal varices that might be irritated by high-fiber foods. Because alcoholism is often the cause of hepatic failure and the diets of alcoholics have been shown to be low in zinc, vitamin B complex, folate, and magnesium, supplements of these nutrients are usually provided daily.[36] Anorexia, malaise, and confusion may interfere with oral intake, and the nurse may need to provide much encouragement to the patient to ensure intake of an adequate diet. Small, frequent feedings are usually better accepted by the anorexic patient than are three large meals daily. The nurse must assess the patient's neurologic status daily to evaluate tolerance of dietary protein. Increasing lethargy, confusion, or asterixis may signal a need for decreased protein intake. Anorexia—coupled with the unpalatable nature of the very low-sodium, low-protein diet required in impending coma—may result in a need for tube feedings.

Although experimental results are conflicting,[37-40] some authorities feel that administration of increased amounts of BCAAs in encephalopathy may improve electroencephalograms, arousal, and survival, as well as nutritional status. BCAA-enriched enteral formulas (Hepatic-Aid II [Kendall McGaw] and Travasorb Hepatic [Clintec]) and parenteral amino acid solutions (Hepatamine [Kendall McGaw]) are available. Diarrhea from concurrent administration of lactulose should not be confused with intolerance of the enteral formulations. Thus far, evidence is lacking that BCAA-enriched formulas are beneficial in hepatic failure without encephalopathy.

Nutrition Teaching in Gastrointestinal Alterations

Teaching usually focuses on three areas: the rationale for dietary modifications and nutrition support, components of a nutritious and balanced diet, and the need to take vitamin/mineral supplements as ordered. Both the patient with hepatic failure and the one with short bowel syndrome require high-calorie, high-protein diets during convalescence. In addition, the patient with short bowel syndrome should adhere to a low-fiber diet with generous amounts of fluids. Although fat is an excellent source of calories, fat malabsorption is a problem for both groups of patients. Even with intestinal adaptation and hyperplasia, fat absorption may never normalize in the patient with short bowel syndrome, and the patient may experience less diarrhea and discomfort if a low-fat diet is followed permanently.[35] Glucose oligosaccharides (e.g., Polycose [Ross] and Moducal [Mead Johnson])—which can be added to beverages, cereals, or soups without increasing the sweetness—and MCT oil are two caloric supplements that also can be used. Patients with steatorrhea usually need daily oral water-miscible supplements of the fat-soluble vitamins A and E to prevent deficiencies. Supplements of calcium, zinc, and magnesium may also be needed. The nurse needs to ensure that the patient understands the dosage and is capable of administering these supplements.

In addition, patients who will be discharged while still receiving tube feedings or TPN (usually those with short bowel syndrome) must be taught the mechanics of administering their feedings and maintaining their feeding tube or catheter, as well as methods of preventing and coping with problems and complications. The need for long-term nutrition support may have severe emotional and financial effects.[41] Providing emotional support and counseling are among the nurse's most important roles in assisting these patients. In an effort to encourage resumption of normal activity patterns, many patients are begun on cyclic feedings—usually administered nocturnally—as discharge is anticipated. The costs of long-term home nutrition support are high, although not nearly as high as continued hospitalization, and the social worker or financial counselor should be involved early in the patient's hospitalization in exploring routes of payment, as plans are made for discharge.

NUTRITION AND ENDOCRINE ALTERATIONS

Because of the far-reaching effects on all body systems, endocrine alterations have an impact on nutritional status in a variety of ways.

Nutrition Assessment in Endocrine Alterations

The nutrition assessment process is summarized in Table 50-13. Because of the prevalence of non–insulin-dependent diabetes mellitus (NIDDM) patients among the hospitalized population, the nutritional problems most commonly noted in patients with endocrine alterations are overweight and obesity.

Nutrition Intervention in Endocrine Alterations

◆ **Underweight and malnourished patients.** The most severely undernourished patients are usually those with pancreatitis, because of loss of pancreatic exocrine function. Pancreatic insufficiency—with inadequate release of trypsin, chymotrypsin, and pancreatic lipase and amylase—results in impaired digestion and subsequent loss of nutrients in the stool. Fat malabsorption is the most marked effect of pancreatic insufficiency. Fat lost in the stools is accompanied by calcium, zinc, and other minerals, along with the fat-soluble vitamins. Nutritional care in malabsorptive disorders is discussed more thoroughly in the section concerning nutrition in gastrointestinal alterations.

Patients with insulin-dependent diabetes mellitus (IDDM) or endocrine dysfunction caused by pancreatitis often have weight loss and malnutrition as a result of tissue catabolism, because they cannot utilize dietary carbohydrates to meet energy needs. Although patients with NIDDM are more likely to be overweight than underweight, they too may become malnourished as a result of chronic or acute infections, trauma, major surgery, or other illnesses. Delivery of nutrition support in these patients, especially control of blood glucose, can be challenging. Blood glucose should be monitored regularly, usually several times a day until the patient is stable. Regular insulin added to the solution is the most common method of managing hyperglycemia in the patient receiving TPN. The dosage required may be larger than the patient's usual subcutaneous dose, because some of the insulin adheres to glass bottles and plastic bags or administration sets. Continuous subcutaneous infusion of insulin also may be used. Hyperglycemia is also a common problem in tube-fed patients, particularly when feedings are given continuously. Twice-daily doses of intermediate-acting insulin or more frequent doses of regular insulin may be inadequate to control hyperglycemia in continuously fed patients. One solution is to administer feedings intermittently, on a "meal-type" schedule, and to administer oral hypoglycemics, regular insulin, or intermediate-acting insulin based on this schedule.[42] However, some diabetic patients require continuous feedings. For example, patients with severe gastroparesis may need transpyloric feedings because poor gastric emptying makes intragastric feedings impossible or inadequate. Transpyloric feedings must almost always be given continuously, because dumping syndrome and poor absorption often occur if feedings are given rapidly into the small bowel. For the continuously tube-fed diabetic patient, control of blood glucose may be improved either with continuous insulin infusion or by use of a formula containing fiber, if possible. Examples are Compleat (Sandoz) and Enrich (Ross). Fiber slows the absorption of the carbohydrate in the formula, producing a more delayed and sustained glycemic response.

◆ **Overweight patients.** Aggressive attempts at weight loss are rarely warranted among very ill patients, although weight loss in overweight patients with NIDDM improves glucose tolerance. Instead of suggesting a low-calorie diet, nurses should encourage patients to select foods providing fiber and starches. Diets rich in complex carbohydrates have been shown to lower insulin requirements, increase the sensitivity of the peripheral tissues to insulin, and decrease serum cholesterol levels.[43]

Nutrition support should not be neglected simply because a patient is obese, because PCM develops even among such patients. When a patient is not expected to be able to eat for at least 5 to 7 days or inadequate intake persists for that period, the nurse should consult with the physician regarding initiation of tube feedings or TPN if no steps have been taken to do so. No disease process benefits from starvation, and development or progression of nutritional deficits may contribute to complications (e.g., decubitus ulcers, pulmonary or urinary tract infections, and sepsis, which prolong hospitalization, increase the costs of care, and may even result in death[44]).

◆ **Severe vomiting or diarrhea in the insulin-dependent diabetic patient.** When insulin-dependent patients experience vomiting and diarrhea severe enough to interfere significantly with oral intake or result in excessive fluid and electrolyte losses, adequate carbohydrates and fluids must be supplied. If patients are receiving oral feedings, they may not be able to adhere to their usual diet, but they generally should consume 10 to 20 g of carbohydrates every 1 to 2 hours[45]; the physician usually provides guidelines as to the amount. Small amounts of liquids taken every 15 to 20 minutes are generally tolerated best by the patient with nausea and vomiting. Blood glucose and urine ketone levels should be monitored frequently and the physician notified of increasing hyperglycemia, ketonuria, difficulty retaining fluids, or signs of dehydration.

Nutrition Teaching in Endocrine Alterations

Most nutrition teaching in the patient with endocrine alterations focuses on understanding of the diet of the diabetic patient and on achieving the desirable body weight. The underweight or overweight patient should be helped to understand the need for weight changes. For example, weight loss in the obese diabetic individual improves glucose tolerance and may reduce or eliminate the need for insulin. In addition, it usually has beneficial effects on blood pressure and serum cholesterol levels.

Diet instruction for the diabetic patient is usually carried out by the dietitian, but the nurse should reinforce the information given.

In addition to the importance of achieving and/or

Table 50-13 Nutrition assessment of the patient with an endocrine disorder

Area of concern	History	Physical findings	Laboratory data
Underweight or protein-calorie malnutrition	Increased losses of calories in urine or feces caused by the following: Impaired glucose metabolism and glucosuria in type I diabetes mellitus Steatorrhea in pancreatitis Decreased intake because of the following: Discomfort with eating (in pancreatitis) Alcoholism (often a cause of pancreatitis)	Weight of <90% of desirable Recent weight loss Wasting of muscle and subcutaneous tissue Triceps skinfold measurement of <10th percentile*	Urine glucose >0.5% Fecal fat >5 g/24 hr or <95% of intake Serum albumin <3.5 g/dl, or low transferrin or prealbumin levels Total lymphocyte count <1200/mm^3 Creatinine excretion <17 mg/kg/day (women) or <23 mg/kg/day (men)
Overweight	NIDDM Sedentary life-style	Weight of >120% of desirable Triceps skinfold measurement of >90th percentile†	
High risk for fluid volume deficit	Diuresis (from diabetes insipidus or osmotic diuresis of HHNK or Ketoacidosis)	Poor skin turgor Dry, sticky mucous membranes Thirst Loss of >0.23 kg (0.5 pound) in 24 hr Increased urine output	Serum glucose >250 mg/dl Urine glucose >0.5% Serum sodium >145 mEq/L Increasing Hct BUN >20 mg/dl
High risk for fluid volume excess	Fluid retention caused by SIADH	Edema (peripheral and/or pulmonary) Gain of >0.23 kg (0.5 pound) in 24 hr	Serum sodium <135 mEq/L Decreasing Hct
Potential zinc deficiency	Impaired absorption in steatorrhea associated with pancreatitis Increased urinary losses in diuresis, diabetes mellitus, and alcoholism Poor intake in alcoholism	Hypogeusia, dysgeusia Alopecia Seborrheic dermatitis Impaired wound healing	Serum zinc <60 μg/ml

Modified from Moore MC: *Pocket guide to nutrition and diet therapy,* ed 2, St Louis, 1993, Mosby–Year Book.
Hct, hematocrit; *BUN*, blood urea nitrogen; *SIADH*, syndrome of inappropriate secretion of antidiuretic hormone.
*6 mm for men and 14 mm for women.
†20 mm for men, and 34 mm for women.

maintaining the desirable body weight, the diabetic patient should understand the following key concepts:

1. Both hypoglycemia and hyperglycemia can have serious consequences. The patient should be aware of the precipitating factors and symptoms associated with each condition. Precipitating factors for hypoglycemia include failing to eat scheduled meals or snacks, eating meals or snacks late, vomiting or poor food intake during acute illness, prolonged or intense physical activity without a compensatory increase in carbohydrate intake or decrease in insulin dosage, impaired gluconeogenesis with alcohol intake, and impaired mentation and self-care skills resulting from alcohol intoxication or use of controlled drugs. Clinical manifestations include hunger, irritability, headache, shakiness, sweating, and altered neurologic status, ranging from drowsiness to unconsciousness and convulsions.

   Diabetic ketoacidosis or hyperglycemic hyperosmolar nonketotic coma may result from uncontrolled hyperglycemia. Acute infectious illnesses or failure to take the prescribed dosage of insulin or oral hyperglycemia agents are common causes of severe hyperglycemia. Clinical manifestations of diabetic ketoacidosis include thirst; warm, dry skin; nausea and vomiting; "fruity"-smelling breath; pain in the abdomen; drowsiness; and polyuria. Excessive thirst, polyuria, dehydration, shallow respirations, and an altered sensorium often accompany hyperglycemic hyperosmolar nonketotic coma.

   The patient should be taught measures to prevent hypoglycemia and excessive hyperglycemia. No planned meal or snack should ever be omitted, particularly if the patient is using insulin or an oral hypoglycemic agent. Food exchanges should not be transferred from one meal to another. The planned exchanges should be eaten at regular times each day to avoid undue fluctuations in blood glucose. No foods should be added to the diet, unless hypoglycemia occurs or unless the patient is engaging in vigorous physical exertion. The best way to know whether increased food is needed during exercise is to monitor the blood glucose level. Alcohol should be consumed only if the physician is aware of the patient's alcohol use, and it is best if consumption is limited to no more than 2 oz once or twice a week.[45] In addition, the patient should be taught to monitor his or her own blood glucose level and instructed to self-monitor such whenever clinical manifestations of hypoglycemia or hyperglycemia occur.
2. Arteriosclerosis and hypertension are more common in individuals with diabetes than in the general population. Therefore control of cholesterol and saturated fat intake (see Table 50-6) and limitation of sodium intake to no more than 3 g/day are recommended.[45,46]
3. Emphasizing foods high in complex carbohydrate improves glucose tolerance and may promote gradual weight loss.
4. "Dietetic" and "diabetic" foods are unnecessary. Also, labels containing these words do not always mean that foods are unsweetened. They may be sweetened with fructose, sorbitol, or other absorbable sweeteners. The patient who wishes to use these products should read the label carefully to determine exactly what dietetic or diabetic means in this context. Some "dietetic" cookies contain more calories than does the standard version of the product. Fruits canned in water or juice (with the juice drained before serving) are available in all supermarkets and are suitable for the diabetic patient.
5. Moderate exercise has many benefits for patients with NIDDM, including increased insulin sensitivity and improved glucose tolerance, weight control, reduced blood cholesterol levels, and lowered blood pressure.[47,48] If the physician approves, the patient should be encouraged to begin an exercise program, gradually increasing the length and intensity of the exercise sessions.

NUTRITION AND HEMATOIMMUNE ALTERATIONS

Malnutrition has well-known adverse effects on hematoimmune function. Generalized PCM, for example, depresses cell-mediated immunity, secretory immunity, complement levels, and phagocyte activity. Deficiencies of single nutrients—especially iron, zinc, selenium, folic acid, and vitamins B_{12}, B_6, C, and A—also impair immunologic function.[49] In the patient with an existing hematoimmune disorder, therefore, maintenance of adequate nutrition is essential to prevent additional immunologic deficits.

Nutrition Assessment in Hematoimmune Alterations

Assessment of the patient with a hematoimmune disorder is summarized in Table 50-14. Acquired immunodeficiency syndrome (AIDS) is the hematoimmune disorder most likely to have profound nutritional consequences. Unfortunately, generalized PCM is a common sequela of AIDS. There are multiple etiologic factors for the malnutrition. AIDS itself may be associated with a poorly understood enteropathy that causes diarrhea and malabsorption.[50] Furthermore, opportunistic gastrointestinal (GI) infections caused by various fungi, viruses, bacteria, and protozoans may cause diarrhea. *Cryptosporidium,* a particularly resistant protozoan, can cause intractable, profuse, watery diarrhea lasting for months.[51,52] Calorie and protein needs are elevated in persons with AIDS, because metabolic rate and catabolism increase as a result of infection, fever, and such malignancies as lymphoma and Kaposi's sarcoma. At the same time, oral intake is frequently suppressed by emotional reactions to the personal, family, and financial stresses imposed by AIDS; oral and esophageal pain from lesions of Kaposi's sarcoma, herpes, candidiasis, and/or chemotherapy; nausea, vomiting, and anorexia associated with antibiotic therapy, chemotherapy for malignancies, or antiviral agents used in the treatment of AIDS (see box, p. 895); and impaired motor ability, confusion, and dementia caused by AIDS encephalitis or opportunistic central nervous system infections. AIDS patients often have marked weight loss, hypoalbuminemia, and low levels of zinc, selenium, and other minerals.[53-56]

Nutrition Intervention in Hematoimmune Alterations

Nutritional needs may be quite high in some patients with AIDS, particularly those with sepsis. Ideally, nutrition intervention in patients with AIDS can be achieved via the gastrointestinal tract. Enteral feedings (oral or tube) maintain the integrity of the gut mucosa, are relatively inexpensive, and are the most physiologic means of nutritional support.

◆ **Promotion of adequate oral intake.** As mentioned, a host of factors may interfere with adequate oral intake in the individual with AIDS. With thorough assessment and careful planning to meet the needs of the individual, however, it is often possible to increase oral intake significantly. If nutritional supplements must be given to improve intake, it is usually best to choose those that are lactose-free. Patients with disease of the small bowel often have lactose intolerance, which causes diarrhea when lactose (milk sugar) is ingested. Awareness of the

Table 50-14 Nutrition assessment of the patient with a hematoimmune disorder

Area of concern	History	Physical findings	Laboratory data
Protein-calorie malnutrition	Nutrient losses caused by malabsorption and diarrhea (AIDS) Increased needs caused by infection and fever Poor intake caused by the following: Anorexia (related to respiratory or other infections, emotional stress, medication side effects) Pain associated with eating (e.g., *Candida* esophagitis and endotracheal Kaposi's sarcoma in the immunosuppressed patient) Dementia or CNS infections associated with AIDS Dysphagia	Recent weight loss Weight <90% of desirable Wasting of muscle and subcutaneous tissue Triceps skinfold measurement of <10th percentile*	Serum albumin <3.5 g/dl, or low transferrin or prealbumin level Negative nitrogen balance Urinary creatinine <17 mg/kg (women) or <23 mg/kg (men)
DISORDERS OF MINERAL AND VITAMIN NUTRITURE			
Iron (Fe)	Blood loss Poor intake of meats, whole-grain or enriched breads and cereals, legumes because of the following: Anorexia Pain associated with eating	Pallor, blue sclerae Koilonychia Fatigue Tachycardia	Hct level of <37% (women) or <42% (men); Hgb level of <12 g/dl (women) or <14 g/dl (men); low MCV, MCH, MCHC
Zinc (Zn)	Impaired absorption in diarrhea Poor intake of meats, whole grains, legumes because of the following: Anorexia Pain associated with eating	Hypogeusia, dysgeusia Alopecia Seborrheic dermatitis Impaired wound healing	Serum Zn <60 μg/dl
Selenium (Se)	Impaired absorption in diarrhea Poor intake of meats, fish, poultry	Congestive cardiomyopathy Muscle weakness Pallor, fatigue, tachycardia (anemia caused by RBC fragility)	Serum Se level of <0.08 μg/ml Presence of nucleated RBC, Howell-Jolly bodies, Heinz bodies (hemolytic anemia)
Vitamin B_{12}	Small intestinal disease with malabsorption Macrobiotic or other vegetarian diet that does not include vitamin B_{12} sources	Pallor Glossitis Neuropathy Psychiatric symptoms (e.g., dementia, psychosis, depression)	Hct <37% (women) or <42% (men); Hgb, <12 g/dl (women) or <14 g/dl (men); increased MCV

Hct, hematocrit; *Hgb*, hemoglobin; *MCV*, mean cell volume; *MCH*, mean cell hemoglobin; *MCHC*, mean cell hemoglobin concentration; *RBC*, red blood cell.
*6 mm for men; 14 mm for women.

effects of drugs on nutrient intake (see box below) help the nurse to plan appropriate interventions and patient teaching to maximize oral intake.

◆ **Administration of nutrition support.** Despite dietary modifications and encouragement, some patients may find consuming an adequate diet impossible. Temporary oral or esophageal disorders—such as candidiasis, which produces painful lesions—may temporarily impair oral intake. Other individuals may have such severe diarrhea and malabsorption that they are unable to maintain their nutritional state with oral feedings alone. Nasogastric, nasoduodenal, or nasojejunal feeding tubes can be used to administer tube feedings if the patient does not have severe oral or esophageal disease. Continuous feedings (given either 24 hours a day or only nocturnally) are recommended, because these are likely to result in improved absorption in individuals with small bowel disease.[57] Gastrostomy or jejunostomy tubes are used when long-term feedings are needed or when oral and/or esophageal complications prevent nasal intubation. For patients with malabsorption, elemental formulas often are used. These contain predigested nutrients, no lactose, and little fat, thereby maximizing absorption in the patient with impaired absorptive ability.

NUTRITION-RELATED SIDE EFFECTS OF SOME MEDICATIONS USED IN TREATMENT OF PATIENTS WITH AIDS

NAUSEA AND VOMITING

Amphotericin B
Clindamycin
Dihydroxyphenoxymethylguanine (DHPG)
Ketoconazole
Nystatin
Pentamidine (IV or aerosol administration)
Zidovudine (AZT)

DIARRHEA

Acyclovir
Amphotericin B
Clindamycin
Ketoconazole
Nystatin
Pentamidine (IV administration)
Zidovudine

ALTERED TASTE SENSATION/BAD TASTE

Acyclovir
Amphotericin B
Pentamidine (IV or aerosol)
Zidovudine

SORE MOUTH AND/OR THROAT

Acyclovir
Dapsone
Pentamidine (IV or aerosol)

lactose, and little fat, thereby maximizing absorption in the patient with impaired absorptive ability.

Parenteral nutrition is reserved for patients for whom enteral feeding is not feasible or beneficial. For example, patients with inadequate absorption caused by disease involving the entire small intestine are candidates for receiving parenteral nutrition.[57] Strict asepsis should be maintained to reduce the risk of catheter-related infection. Patients with sepsis often are glucose intolerant, and therefore it is especially important to monitor their blood glucose levels frequently.

Nutrition Teaching in Hematoimmune Disorders

Nutrition teaching for the patient with AIDS should include the importance of good nutrition in maintaining strength and optimal functioning and in preventing additional deficits in immune function and wound healing. The patient should be discouraged from viewing nutrition itself as a panacea; its major role is in supportive care.

◆ **Consumption of an adequate diet.** The AIDS patient should be encouraged to consume an adequate diet of regular foods, if at all possible. High-fat foods are a good source of calories. However, their intake may need to be limited or avoided if the patient has diarrhea and malabsorption, because they tend to exacerbate the problem. Frequent small feedings are often better tolerated than are a few larger daily meals. Many individuals with disease of the small bowel exhibit lactose intolerance. Patients with lactose intolerance may be able to tolerate yogurt, chocolate milk, and aged cheeses even if they experience symptoms (bloating, abdominal cramping, and diarrhea) when they consume liquid milk. Lactase enzyme, available at many pharmacies and supermarkets, can be added to liquid milk to allow such patients to digest the lactose. Lactose-free commercial supplements also can be used to promote caloric and protein intake in patients with lactose intolerance.

A multivitamin/mineral supplement providing 100% of the recommended dietary allowances (RDAs) is suggested for patients with inadequate diets, but there is no evidence that any particular vitamin or mineral has a beneficial effect in treating AIDS or its associated complications.[57]

◆ **Food safety.** Individuals with AIDS are especially susceptible to infections caused by foodborne organisms. To prevent such infections, food should be stored, prepared, and served with scrupulous cleanliness. All individuals preparing food for the patient should be taught to avoid cross-contaminating food (e.g., using a cutting board to slice meat when it has just been used to prepare raw vegetables). All raw fruits and vegetables should be washed well, and meat should be thoroughly cooked. Consumption of raw eggs, fish or shellfish (e.g., sushi or raw oysters), and meat should be avoided, as should unpasteurized milk. Leftover food should be promptly refrigerated and then discarded if not consumed within 3 days.[58]

◆ **Food fads and medicinal uses of foods.** As with patients suffering from other chronic and serious diseases, individuals with AIDS often adhere to alternative or nontraditional treatments. A variety of diets, special foods, and supplements are used by individuals with AIDS.[59] Some of these are listed in Table 50-15. Some of the practices, such as use of megadoses of fat-soluble vitamins and minerals or use of a macrobiotic diet, can be harmful. While maintaining a nonjudgmental and accepting attitude, the nurse should discourage alternative dietary practices and encourage the patient to follow a balanced diet instead.

Table 50-15 Food fads and unproven therapies for AIDS

Therapy	Use/Comments
Vitamin and mineral supplements, including vitamins A, C, and E, and zinc and selenium, often in megadoses	To restore immune function; chronic high intakes of vitamin A, zinc, and selenium have resulted in toxicity.
Macrobiotic or strict vegetarian diet	Includes no animal products. Macrobiotic diet consists of whole grains, vegetables, fermented soy, and seaweed. These diets are inadequate in vitamin B_{12} and calcium and are likewise often deficient in calories, protein, and iron.
Yeast-free diet	To prevent opportunistic yeast infection. Eliminates yeast and sugars in diet. Prohibits yeast breads, wine, beer, cheese, peanuts, processed meats, and mushrooms. No evidence of efficacy.
Lecithin supplements	To kill HIV; no evidence of efficacy.
Dr. Berger's Immune Power Diet	To "revitalize" the immune system. Initial elimination diet for foods purported to cause allergies, followed by reintroduction diet. Foods that are singled out as common allergens include milk products, wheat, corn, soy, sugar, and eggs. Suggested menus are low in calories and calcium.
Purgatives and laxatives	To purify the system.
Garlic	To purify the system.
Herbal remedies (including pepiñillo, available in Mexico)	To stimulate immune function; no proven efficacy.

From Berger M: *Dr. Berger's immune power diet*, New York, 1985, Avon Books; Chelluri L, Jastremski MS: *Nutr Clin Prac* 4:16, 1989; Crook WG: *The yeast connection*, New York, 1986, Random House; Resler SS: *J Am Diet Assoc* 88:828, 1988; and Task Force on Nutrition Support in AIDS: *Nutrition* 5:39, 1989.

◆ **Nutrition support modalities.** Patients with AIDS should be made aware of the nutrition support options available to them.[57,60] With this information, the patient will have a basis for making an informed decision about initiating or continuing nutrition support. The patient's family or friends also may need this information to assist the health care team in making decisions about providing nonvolitional nutrition support in a patient with severe dementia.

ADMINISTERING NUTRITION SUPPORT

Enteral Nutrition Support

The enteral route is the preferred method of feeding whenever possible, because this route is generally safer, more physiologic, and much less expensive than is parenteral feeding. There are a variety of enteral feeding products, some of which are designed to meet the specialized needs of very sick patients. Some products can be consumed orally, but many of the specialized ones are so unpalatable that they are reserved solely for tube feeding. Table 50-16 provides more information about the major categories of products.

◆ **Oral supplementation.** For patients who can eat and have normal digestion and absorption but simply cannot consume enough regular foods to meet caloric and protein needs, oral supplementation may be necessary. Patients with mild to moderate anorexia, burns, or trauma sometimes fall into this category. To improve intake and tolerance of supplements, the critical care nurse should do the following:

1. Collaborate with the dietitian to choose appropriate products and allow the patient to participate in the selection process if possible. Milk shakes made with ice cream and half-and-half; powdered milk added to cereal and fluid milk; and instant breakfast are often more palatable and economic than are commercial supplements. However, intolerance of lactose (milk sugar) is common among adults, especially blacks, Orientals, native Americans, and Inuits. Furthermore, many disease processes (e.g., Crohn's disease, radiation enteritis, and severe gastroenteritis) are associated with lactose intolerance. Individuals with this problem experience abdominal cramping, bloating, and diarrhea after lactose ingestion and may require commercial lactose-free supplements.
2. Serve commercial supplements well chilled or on ice, because this improves flavor.
3. Advise patients to sip formulas slowly, consuming no more than 240 ml over 30 to 45 minutes. These products contain easily digested carbohydrates. If formulas are consumed too quickly, rapid hydrolysis of the carbohydrate in the duodenum can contribute to dumping syndrome, characterized by abdominal cramping, weakness, tachycardia, and diarrhea.
4. Record all supplement intake separately on the intake and output sheet so that it can be differentiated from intake of water and other liquids.

◆ **Enteral tube feedings.** Tube feedings are used for

patients who have at least some digestive and absorptive capability but are unwilling or unable to consume enough by mouth. Patients with profound anorexia and those experiencing severe stress that greatly increases their nutritional needs[61] (e.g., those with major burns or trauma) often benefit from tube feedings. Individuals who require elemental formulas because of impaired digestion or absorption or the specialized formulas for altered metabolic conditions (see Table 50-16) usually require tube feeding, because the unpleasant flavors of the free amino acids, peptides, or protein hydrolysates used in these formulas are very difficult to mask.

◆ **Location and type of feeding tube.** Whether temporary tubes (nasogastric or nasoduodenal/nasojejunal) or more permanent ones (gastrostomy or jejunostomy) are used depends largely on the length of time that feedings are anticipated to be needed. Usually 3 months or longer constitutes long-term feedings. However, the patient who is extremely agitated or confused or for some other reason does not tolerate nasal intubation may require a permanent tube earlier. In addition, the advent of the percutaneous gastrostomy tube, which can be inserted without a general anesthetic, has made gastrostomy increasingly popular, even in patients who do not require long-term feeding.

The site for intubation also is determined by patient need. Nasoduodenal, nasojejunal, or jejunostomy tubes are most often used when there is a high risk for pulmonary aspiration, because the pyloric sphincter is believed to provide a barrier that lessens the risk of regurgitation and aspiration.[62] One small prospective study failed to find any reduction in aspiration with

Table 50-16 Enteral formulas

Formula type	Examples of formulas	Oral or tube feeding	Nutritional problem	Clinical examples
Complete diet with intact protein and LCT*† (some contain blended foods)	Ensure and Osmolite (Ross), Sustacal and Isocal (Mead Johnson Nutritional), Meritene and Compleat (Sandoz). For fluid restriction: Magnacal (Sherwood Medical), Isocal HCN (Mead Johnson Nutritional), TwoCal HN (Ross)	Some are suited to both (e.g., Ensure), some primarily to oral (e.g., Sustacal, Meritene), and some primarily to tube feeding (e.g., Compleat, Osmolite, Isocal)	Inability to ingest food Inability to ingest enough food to meet needs	Oral or esophageal cancer Coma Anorexia resulting from chronic illness Burns or trauma
Elemental diets‡	Criticare HN (Mead Johnson Nutritional), Vital High Nitrogen (Ross), Reabilan (O'Brien), Vivonex and Vivonex T.E.N. (Norwich Eaton), Travasorb HN (Clintec Nutrition)	Tube feeding	Impaired digestion and/or absorption	Pancreatitis Inflammatory bowel disease Radiation enteritis Short bowel syndrome Malnutrition
SPECIALIZED DIETS FOR METABOLIC ALTERATIONS				
Diets high in essential amino acids, low in nonessential amino acids	Amin-Aid (Kendall McGaw), Travasorb Renal (Clintec Nutrition)	Both (especially tube)	Renal failure	Undialyzed end stage renal disease
Diets high in branched chain amino acids, low in aromatic amino acids§	Hepatic-Aid II (Kendal McGaw), Travasorb Hepatic (Clintec Nutrition)	Both (especially tube)	Hepatic failure	Impending hepatic coma
Diets high in branched chain amino acids§‖	Stresstein (Sandoz), TraumaCal (Mead Johnson Nutritional), Traum-Aid HBC (Kendall McGaw)	Both (especially tube)	Stress	Trauma and injury Sepsis

**LCT*, long-chain triglycerides or fat (used in formulas for patients with no digestive or absorptive abnormality).
†Some of these formulas contain lactose. If the patient has a lactose intolerance, the dietitian can recommend an appropriate lactose-free formula.
‡Contain "predigested" nutrients: protein in the form of amino acids and/or peptides or protein hydrolysates, fat as medium chain triglycerides (which require less emulsification by bile salts and enzymatic digestion than LCT) or minimal fat, and easily digested carbohydrates (no lactose).
§Not conclusively proven to improve patient outcome.
‖Branched-chain amino acids (leucine, isoleucine, and valine) contain a branch in their carbon chain structure. They are required for protein synthesis, but they are especially important because they serve as a valuable energy source after injury.

transpyloric tubes, in comparison with intragastric ones, however.[63] Jejunostomy tubes have the added advantage of being able to bypass an upper gastrointestinal (GI) obstruction.

◆ **Nursing management.** The nurse's role in delivery of tube feedings usually includes insertion of the tube, if a temporary tube is used; maintenance of the tube; administration of the feedings; prevention of complications associated with this form of therapy; and participation in assessment of the patient's response to tube feedings. Assessment of response is discussed later in this chapter.

Critical care nurses are usually familiar with tube insertion, and therefore this topic is not discussed in depth here. However, transpyloric passage of tubes deserves special mention. Tubes with mercury, stainless steel, or tungsten weights on the proximal end are often used when transpyloric tube placement is desired, in the belief that the weight will encourage transpyloric passage of the tube or that the weight will help the tube maintain its position once it passes into the bowel. However, unweighted tubes are just as likely as weighted ones to migrate through the pylorus.[64,65] Furthermore, weighted tubes appear to offer no advantage over unweighted ones in regard to remaining in place.[65] Because the weights sometimes cause discomfort while being inserted through the nares, unweighted tubes may be preferable. One technique that has been shown to promote transpyloric passage of tubes is the administration of metoclopramide hydrochloride before tube insertion. Administering the drug after the tube's proximal tip is already in the stomach is much less effective.[66,67]

Maintenance of the tube includes regular irrigation of the tube to maintain patency, skin care around the insertion site, and mouth care. The newer small-bore (usually 8 French) "nonreactive" tubes made of polyurethane, silicone rubber, and similar materials are much more comfortable for the patient than are the older polyethylene or polyvinylchloride tubes (usually 12 to 16 French), and patient complaints of discomfort and nasal and skin erosion have decreased with the use of the nonreactive tubes. Unfortunately, these small tubes tend to clog readily. Regular irrigation helps to prevent tube occlusion. Generally, 30 to 60 ml of irrigant every 3 to 4 hours or after each feeding is appropriate. The volume of irrigant may have to be reduced during fluid restriction. The irrigant is usually water, but other fluids, such as cranberry juice or cola beverages, are sometimes used in an effort to reduce the incidence of tube occlusion. However, cranberry juice is inferior to, and cola beverages appear no better than, water for irrigating tubes.[68] Furthermore, once a tube has occluded, cranberry juice and cola are of little use in clearing the occlusion. Polyurethane tubes clog less readily than do those made of silicone rubber, an important consideration for the nurse in selecting a feeding tube.[68]

The skin around the tube should be cleaned at least daily, and the tape around the tube replaced whenever loosened or soiled. Secure taping helps to prevent movement of the tube, which may irritate the nares or skin or result in accidental dislodgement of the tube. Dressings are used initially around gastrostomy insertion sites. The dressing should be changed daily and the skin cleansed with half-strength hydrogen peroxide. If leakage of gastric fluid occurs around a gastrostomy tube, the skin can be protected with karaya.

To prevent dryness of the mouth (a common complaint during tube feeding), the patient should be encouraged to breathe through the nose as much as possible, drink and eat as much as desired (if compatible with the patient's nutrition orders), suck sugarfree candies or chew sugarfree gum (if allowed), and perform regular mouth care. If the patient is unconscious or otherwise unable to perform mouth care, the nurse should do it or should enlist the family in performing it. Patients often report that they can "taste" the tube feedings, and frequent mouth care will clear the palate of unpleasant flavors from the formula, as well as clean the teeth, tongue, and oral mucous membranes.

Careful attention to administration of tube feedings can prevent many complications. Very clean techniques in the handling and administration of the formula can help prevent bacterial contamination and a resultant infection.[69] The schedule for delivery of feedings also is important. Tube feedings may be administered intermittently or continuously. Intermittent feedings are best suited to those patients who are disoriented and attempt to remove the feeding tube when they are alone. Bolus feedings, which are intermittent feedings delivered rapidly into the stomach or small bowel, are likely to cause distention, vomiting, and dumping syndrome with diarrhea.[70] Instead of using bolus feedings, nurses should gradually drip intermittent feedings, with each feeding lasting 20 to 30 minutes or longer, to promote optimal assimilation. Regardless of how slowly intermittent feedings are given, however, continuous feedings are usually better absorbed by patients who have compromised digestion or absorption. Even patients who might be expected to have normal GI function, such as those with burns or trauma, have been shown to absorb the feedings better, tolerate larger volumes of formula, and experience less diarrhea with continuous feedings than with intermittent ones.[71] Therefore continuous feedings are usually preferable for very sick patients.

◆ **Prevention and correction of complications.** Some of the more common and serious complications of tube feeding are pulmonary aspiration,[72,73] diarrhea, constipation, tube occlusion, and delayed gastric emptying. Delayed gastric emptying limits the amount of feeding that the patient can tolerate and thus interferes with adequate nutrition support. Nursing management of these problems is detailed in Table 50-17.

Total Parenteral Nutrition

Total parenteral nutrition (TPN) refers to the delivery of all nutrients by the intravenous route. TPN is generally not worthwhile when enteral intake is expected to be adequate within 5 to 7 days. Likely candidates for TPN include patients who are unable to ingest or absorb nutrients via the GI tract, as in short bowel syndrome; who have severe disease of the small bowel (e.g., inflammatory bowel disease, collagen-vascular diseases, intestinal pseudo-obstruction, or radiation enteritis); or who are experiencing intractable vomiting. TPN may be warranted in patients receiving high-dose chemotherapy, radiation, and bone marrow transplantation, where nutritional intake is apt to be poor for several weeks because of stomatitis, nausea, vomiting, diarrhea, and anorexia. It may also be useful in patients who can benefit from a period of bowel rest, including those with moderate to severe pancreatitis or with enterocutaneous fistulae. In both cases, enteral intake (which stimulates secretion of digestive enzymes) is likely to exacerbate the condition, whereas bowel rest may promote healing. In addition, some postoperative, trauma, or burn patients may need temporary TPN.

◆ **Routes for TPN.** TPN may be delivered through either

Table 50-17 Nursing management of enteral tube feeding complications

Complication	Contributing factor(s)	Prevention/correction
Pulmonary aspiration	Feeding tube positioned in esophagus or respiratory tract	Check tube placement before intermittent feeding and every 4-6 hr during continuous feedings; be aware that an in-rush of air can sometimes be auscultated over the right upper quadrant even when the distal tip of the tube is in the esophagus or respiratory tract[73a,b]; if there is a question about the tube position, check the pH level of fluid aspirated from the tube (usually gastric juice pH is 1.0-3.5) or perform an x-ray examination.[73b]
	Regurgitation of formula (most common in patients with inadequate gag reflex, artificial airways, or altered state of consciousness and also in those with delayed gastric emptying)	Add food coloring (usually blue, to avoid mistaking it for any body secretion) to all formula to facilitate diagnosis of aspiration. Elevate head to 30 degrees during feedings; if it is imposible to raise the head, position patient in lateral or prone position to improve drainage of vomitus from the mouth (the right lateral position is especially advantageous because it facilitates gastric emptying); if head must be in a dependent position (e.g., for postural drainage), discontinue feedings 30-60 min earlier and restart them only when the head can be raised. Keep cuff of endotracheal or tracheostomy tube inflated during feedings, if possible.[62] Measure gastric residual before each intermittent feeding and at least every 4-6 hr during continuous feedings; guidelines vary, but often a volume of >150 ml or 110%-120% of the hourly rate is considered excessive; it is difficult to aspirate GI contents via small-bore nonreactive tubes without collapsing the tube, but use of large syringes (35-60 ml) is least likely to cause tube collapse. If a patient is at risk for pulmonary aspiration and it proves impossible to measure gastric residuals with an 8-French tube, substitute a 10- or 12-French one.
Diarrhea	Medications with GI side effects (antibiotics, which can alter gut flora, are common culprits, but others include digitalis, laxatives, magnesium-containing antacids, and quinidine)	Evaluate the patient's medications to determine their potential for causing diarrhea, consulting the pharmacist if necessary.
	Hypertonic formula or medications (e.g., oral suspensions of antibiotics, potassium, or other electrolytes), which cause fluid to be drawn into the gut to dilute the hypertonic load	Consult the physician about using continuous feedings (if feedings are currently intermittent) or diluting or slowing tube feedings temporarily; dilute enteral medications well.
	Malnutrition (hypoalbuminemia impairs absorption by decreasing plasma oncotic pressure; malnutrition also results in loss of intestinal microvilli, reducing brush border enzymes needed for digestion, as well as the absorptive area)	Consult with the physician about using continuous feedings, which may facilitate absorption.

Continued.

Table 50-17 Nursing management of entcral tube feeding complications—cont'd

Complication	Contributing factor(s)	Prevention/correction
	Bacterial contamination	Use scrupulously clean technique in administering tube feedings; keep opened containers of formula refrigerated and discard them within 24 hr; discard enteral feeding containers and administration sets every 24 hr[69]; hang formula for no more than 4-8 hr unless it comes prepackaged in sterile administration sets; be especially careful with feedings given to patients being fed transpylorically or those receiving cimetidine or antacids, because these patients lack the normal antibacterial barrier of the stomach's hydrochloric acid.
	Fecal impaction with seepage of liquid stool around the impaction	Perform a digital rectal examination to rule out impaction; see guidelines for prevention of constipation (below).
Constipation	Low-residue formula, creating little fecal bulk	Consult with the physician regarding the use of fiber-containing formula (e.g., Enrich [Ross], Compleat [Sandoz]), although this is not possible if the patient requires an elemental diet; consult with the physician about adding bran or bulk-type laxatives to the patient's regimen.
	Inadequate fluid intake	Check patient's fluid intake to see that it totals 50 ml/kg/day, unless there is need for fluid restriction.
Tube occlusion	Giving medications via tube (medications may physically plug the tube or may coagulate the formula, causing it to clog the tube)	If medications must be given by tube, avoid use of crushed tablets; consult with the pharmacist to see whether medications can be dispensed as elixirs or suspensions; irrigate tube with water before and after administering any medication; never add any medication to the tube-feeding formula unless the two are known to be compatible.
	Sedimentation of formula	Irrigate tube every 4-8 hr during continuous feedings and after every intermittent feeding.
Gastric retention	Delayed gastric emptying resulting from neural impairment or serious illness (e.g., diabetic gastroparesis, trauma)	Measure gastric residual at least every 4-6 hr or before every feeding; consult with physician about use of transpyloric feedings, temporary reduction of formula volume, or metoclopramide hydrochloride to stimulate gastric emptying; encourage patient to lie in right lateral position frequently, unless contraindicated.

central or peripheral veins. Because it requires an indwelling catheter, central vein TPN carries an increased risk of sepsis, as well as potential insertion-related complications, such as pneumothorax and hemothorax.[74] Air embolism is also more likely with central vein TPN. However, central venous catheters provide very secure IV access and allow delivery of more hyperosmolar solutions than does peripheral TPN. TPN solutions containing 25% to 35% dextrose are commonly used via central veins, and this provides an inexpensive source of calories. It is increasingly common for patients requiring multiple IV therapies and frequent blood sampling to have multilumen central venous catheters and for TPN to be infused via these catheters. Infection rates in patients receiving TPN via multilumen catheters have been reported to be as much as 3 times higher than those in patients with single-lumen catheters.[75] Scrupulous aseptic technique is essential in maintaining multilumen catheters; the manipulation involved in frequent changes of IV fluid and obtaining blood specimens through these catheters increases the risk of catheter contamination. Also, patients requiring these catheters are likely to be very ill and immunocompromised.

Peripheral TPN rarely is associated with serious infectious or mechanical complications, but it does necessitate good peripheral venous access. Therefore it may not be appropriate for long-term nutrition support or for patients receiving multiple IV therapies. Furthermore, peripheral veins tolerate very hyperosmolar solutions poorly, and thus peripheral solutions are limited to about 10% dextrose. Daily use of IV lipid emulsions, which are isotonic, is necessary to provide adequate calories during peripheral TPN, unless the patient is consuming substantial amounts by mouth and the TPN is being used only as a supplement.

◆ **Nursing management.** Nursing care of the patient receiving TPN includes catheter care, administration of solutions, prevention or correction of complications, and evaluation of patient responses to IV feedings. Evaluation of patient response is discussed later in this chapter.

The indwelling central venous catheter provides an excellent nidus for infection.[76-78] The nurse has a major role in preventing this complication of TPN therapy. Catheter care includes maintaining an intact dressing at the catheter insertion site and manipulating the catheter and administration tubing with aseptic technique. Dressings for TPN catheters may consist of either gauze and tape or transparent film. Usually gauze dressings are changed three times weekly, and transparent dressings are changed every 5 to 7 days. Both types are also changed whenever they become wet, soiled, or nonadherent. These types of dressings are associated with comparable rates of catheter-related sepsis,[79,80] but the transparent dressings usually decrease nursing time spent on dressing changes and may reduce irritation of sensitive skin.[79,80] After removal of the old dressing, the skin at the insertion site is commonly cleansed with povidone iodine, which is used because it has both antibacterial and antifungal activity. Chlorhexidine hydrochloride can be substituted for povidone iodine for patients allergic to iodine.

TPN solutions usually consist of amino acids, dextrose, electrolytes, vitamins, minerals, and trace elements. Although dextrose–amino acid solutions are commonly thought of as good growth media for microorganisms, they actually suppress the growth of most organisms usually associated with catheter-related sepsis, except yeasts. However, because the many manipulations required to prepare solutions increase the possibility of contamination, TPN solutions are best used with caution. They should be prepared under laminar flow conditions in the pharmacy, with avoidance of additions on the nursing unit. Solution containers should be inspected for cracks or leaks before hanging, and solutions should be discarded within 24 hours of hanging. An in-line 0.22 μm filter, which eliminates all microorganisms but not endotoxins, may be used in administration of solutions. Use of the filter, however, should not be substituted for scrupulous aseptic technique, because there is no conclusive evidence that filters decrease sepsis rates.

In contrast to dextrose–amino acid solutions, IV lipid emulsions support the proliferation of many microorganisms. Furthermore, lipid emulsions cannot be filtered through an in-line 0.22 μm filter, because some particles in the emulsions have larger diameters than this. Lipid emulsions should be handled with strict asepsis, and they should be discarded within 12 to 24 hours of hanging. There is a trend toward mixing lipid emulsions with dextrose–amino acid TPN solutions. Although this saves nursing time, the nurse must be extremely careful in administering these solutions. TPN solutions containing lipids cannot be filtered through an in-line 0.22 μm filter, and they support the growth of most bacteria and *Candida albicans* better than do dextrose–amino acid TPN solutions.

◆ **Prevention or correction of complications.** Some of the more common and serious complications of TPN include catheter-related sepsis, air embolism, pneumothorax, central venous thrombosis, catheter occlusion, and metabolic imbalances such as hypoglycemia and hyperglycemia. These complications, along with nursing approaches to their management, are described in Table 50-18.

EVALUATING RESPONSE TO NUTRITION SUPPORT

Assessment of response to nutrition support is an ongoing process that involves anthropometric measurements, physical examination, and biochemical evaluation. Table 50-19 summarizes some of the parameters that are used most frequently. Daily weighings and the maintenance of accurate intake and output records are especially crucial for evaluating nutritional progress and state of hydration in the patient receiving nutrition support. In addition, the nurse is the health care team member who has the most constant contact with the patient; therefore he or she is uniquely qualified to evaluate bowel function, determining whether the patient has enough diarrhea to preclude advancement of enteral feedings or whether the patient is at risk of pulmonary aspiration because of slow gastric emptying. Also, the nurse should alert other team members to changes in laboratory parameters.

Table 50-18 Nursing management of TPN complications

Complication	Clinical manifestations	Prevention/correction
Catheter-related sepsis	Fever, chills, glucose intolerance, positive blood culture	Maintain an intact dressing, change if contaminated by vomitus, sputum, and so on; use aseptic technique when handling catheter, IV tubing, and TPN solutions; hang a bottle of TPN no longer than 24 hr, lipid emulsion no longer than 12-24 hr; use an in-line 0.22 μm filter with TPN to remove microorganisms; avoid drawing blood, infusing blood or blood products, piggybacking other IV solutions into medications into TPN IV tubing, or attaching manometers or transducers via the TPN infusion line, if at all possible. If catheter-related sepsis is suspected, remove catheter or assist in changing the catheter over a guidewire and administer antibiotics as ordered.
Air embolism	Dyspnea, cyanosis, apnea, tachycardia, hypotension, "millwheel" heart murmur; mortality estimated at 50% (depends on quantity of air entering)	Use Luer-Lok syringe or secure all connections well; use an in-line 0.22 μm air-eliminating filter; have patient perform Valsalva maneuver during tubing changes; if the patient is on a ventilator, change tubing quickly at end expiration; maintain occlusive dressing over catheter site for at least 24 hr after removing catheter to prevent air entry through catheter tract. If air embolism is suspected, place patient in left lateral decubitus and Trendelenburg's position (to trap air in the apex of the right ventricle, away from the outflow tract) and administer oxygen and CPR as needed; immediately notify physician, who may attempt to aspirate air from the heart.
Pneumothorax	Chest pain, dyspnea, hypoxemia, hypotension, radiographic evidence, needle aspiration of air from pleural space	Thoroughly explain catheter insertion procedure to patient, because when a patient moves or breathes erratically he or she is more likely to sustain pleural damage; perform x-ray examination after insertion or insertion attempt. If pneumothorax is suspected, assist with needle aspiration or chest tube insertion, if necessary; chest tubes are usually used for pneumothorax of >25%.
Central venous thrombosis	Edema of neck, shoulder, and arm on same side as catheter; development of collateral circulation on chest; pain in insertion site; drainage of TPN from the insertion site; positive findings on venogram	Follow measures to prevent sepsis; repeated or traumatic catheterizations are most likely to result in thrombosis. If thrombosis is suspected, remove catheter and administer anticoagulants and antibiotics as ordered.
Catheter occlusion or semiocclusion	No flow or a sluggish flow through the catheter	If infusion is stopped temporarily, flush catheter with heparinized saline. If catheter appears to be occluded, attempt to aspirate the clot; if this is ineffective, physician may order thrombolytic agent such as streptokinase or urokinase instilled in the catheter.
Hypoglycemia	Diaphoresis, shakiness, confusion, loss of consciousness	Infuse TPN within 10% of ordered rate; observe patient carefully for signs of hypoglycemia after discontinuance of TPN. If hypoglycemia is suspected, administer oral carbohydrate; if the patient is unconscious or oral intake is contraindicated, the physician may order a bolus of IV dextrose.
Hyperglycemia	Thirst, headache, lethargy, increased urinary output	Administer TPN within 10% of ordered rate; monitor blood glucose level at least daily until stable; the patient may require insulin added to the TPN if hyperglycemia is persistent; sudden appearance of hyperglycemia in a patient who was previously tolerating the same glucose load may indicate onset of sepsis.

Table 50-19 Evaluating response to nutrition support

Parameter	Frequency of measurement*	Purpose/comments
ANTHROPOMETRIC MEASUREMENTS		
Weight	Daily	Indicator of efficacy or of overfeeding; underweight patient should have steady gain, and normal weight or overweight patient should maintain current weight. Detection of overhydration: a consistent gain of >0.11-0.22 kg (0.25-0.5 lb)/day usually indicates fluid retention.
Skinfold	Weekly, if trained personnel available	Indicator of efficacy.
PHYSICAL EXAMINATION		
State of hydration	Daily	Detection of overhydration: check for edema of dependent body parts, shortness of breath, rales in lungs, fluid intake consistently >output. Detection of dehydration: look for poor skin turgor, dry mucous membranes, complaints of thirst, output >intake (measure stool volumes if liquid), >10% difference between blood pressure when lying and standing.
Bowel motility	Daily	Detect hypermotility or hypomotility: auscultate bowel sounds to be sure that peristalsis is present in patients receiving enteral feedings and to help determine when feedings can start in those not being enterally fed; evaluate stool consistency: hard, dry stools, decreased stool frequency, or <3 stools/wk may indicate constipation in the tube-fed patient, although infrequent stools are expected in the patient who is receiving nothing by mouth; loose or liquid stools, increased frequency or >3 stools/day may indicate diarrhea.
Gastric emptying (tube-fed patients)	Every 4-6 hr or as indicated	Detect gastric retention: measure gastric residual as described in the discussion of tube feeding complications.
HEMATOLOGIC AND BIOCHEMICAL MEASUREMENT		
Serum albumin, transferrin, or prealbumin level	Weekly	Indicator of efficacy: levels should be maintained or improved if protein nutriture is adequate.
Serum glucose and electrolyte levels	Daily until stable, then 2-3/wk	Indicates whether intake is adequate or excessive.
Blood urea nitrogen (BUN) level	1-2/wk	Increased level indicates inadequate fluid intake, renal impairment, or excessive protein intake.
Serum calcium, phosphorous, and magnesium levels	1-2/wk	Measure of adequacy of intake.
Serum triglyceride levels (patients receiving IV lipid emulsions)	After each increase in lipid dosage; then 2-3/wk when stable	Elevated levels indicate lipid clearance and possibly a need for reduction in lipid dosage
REE (resting energy expenditure)—measured by indirect calorimetry, not available in all institutions)	At beginning of nutrition support and as indicated	Permits very accurate determination of energy expenditures, allowing the nutrition support regimen to be planned to avoid overfeeding or underfeeding.

Modified from Moore MC: *Pocket guide to nutrition and diet therapy,* ed 2, St Louis, 1993, Mosby–Year Book.
*These are suggested frequencies only; individual patients may need more or less frequent assessment.

REFERENCES

1. Crocker KS, Gerber F, Shearer J: Metabolism of carbohydrate, protein and fat, *Nurs Clin North Am* 18(1):3, 1983.
2. Evans NJ, Sorouri BK, Feurer ID: Constraints of nutrient supply in the intensive care unit, *JPEN* 15(suppl 1):34S, 1991.
3. Forlaw L: The critically ill patient: nutritional implications, *Nurs Clin North Am* 18(1):111, 1983.
4. Long CL, Lowry SF: Hormonal regulation of protein metabolism, *JPEN* 14(6):555, 1990.
5. Messner RL and others: Effect of admission nutritional status on length of hospital stay, *Gastroenterol Nurs* 13:202, 1991.
6. Weinsier RL and others: Hospital malnutrition: a prospective evaluation of general medical patients during the course of hospitalization, *Am J Clin Nutr* 32:418, 1979.
7. Driver AG, LeBrun M: Iatrogenic malnutrition in patients receiving ventilatory support, *JAMA* 244:2195, 1980.
8. American Society for Parenteral and Enteral Nutrition: Standards for nutrition support: hospitalized patients, *Nutr Clin Prac* 3:28, 1988.
9. Bagatell CJ, Heymsfield SB: Effect of meal size on myocardial oxygen requirements: implications for postmyocardial infarction diet, *Am J Clin Nutr* 39:421, 1984.
10. Kirchoff KT and others: Electrographic response to ice water, *Heart Lung* 19:41, 1990.
11. Stevens J: Does dietary fiber affect food intake and body weight? *J Am Diet Assoc* 88:939, 1988.
12. Rock CL, Coulston AM: Weight-control approaches: a review by the California Dietetic Association, *J Am Diet Assoc* 88:44, 1988.
13. National Cholesterol Education Program: *Report of the Expert Panel on Detection, Evaluation, and Treatment of High Blood Cholesterol in Adults,* NIH Pub No 89-2925, Washington, DC, 1989, US Department of Health and Human Services.
14. *Nutrition and your health: dietary guidelines for Americans,* ed 3, Washington, DC, 1990, US Department of Agriculture and US Department of Health and Human Services.
15. National Education Programs Working Group: Report on the management of patients with hypertension and high blood cholesterol, *Ann Intern Med* 114:224, 1991.
16. Rothcopf MM and others: Nutritional support in respiratory failure, *Nutr Clin Prac* 4:166, 1989.
17. Donahue M, Rogers RM: Nutritional assessment and support in chronic obstructive pulmonary disease, *Clin Chest Med* 11:487, 1990.
18. Benotti PN, Bistrian B: Metabolic and nutritional aspects of weaning from mechanical ventilation, *Crit Care Med* 17:181, 1989.
19. Olsen KM and others: Effect of enteral feedings on oral phenytoin absorption, *Nutr Clin Prac* 4:176, 1989.
20. Nishimura LY and others: Influence of enteral feedings on phenytoin sodium absorption from capsules, *DICP* 22:130, 1988.
21. Marvel ME, Bertino JS Jr: Comparative effects of an elemental and a complex enteral feeding formulation on the absorption of phenytoin suspension, *JPEN* 15:316, 1991.
22. Chin DE, Kearns P: Nutrition in the spinal-injured patient, *Nutr Clin Prac* 6:213, 1991.
23. Ott L, Young B: Nutrition in the neurologically injured patient, *Nutr Clin Prac* 6:223, 1991.
24. Lander V and others: Enteral feeding during barbiturate coma, *Nutr Clin Prac* 2:56, 1987.
25. Rodriguez DJ and others: Obligatory negative nitrogen balance following spinal cord injury, *JPEN* 15:319, 1991.
26. Shizgal HM and others: Body composition in quadriplegic patients, *JPEN* 10:364, 1986.
27. Cox SAR and others: Energy expenditure after spinal cord injury: an evaluation of stable rehabilitating patients, *J Trauma* 25:419, 1985.
28. Ihle BU and others: The effect of protein restriction on the progression of renal insufficiency, *N Engl J Med* 321:1773, 1989.
29. Gahl GM, Hain H: Nutrition and metabolism in continuous ambulatory peritoneal dialysis, *Contrib Nephrol* 84:36, 1990.
30. Alvestrand A: Protein metabolism and nutrition in hemodialysis patients, *Contrib Nephrol* 78:102, 1990.
31. Mitch WS, Klahr S: *Nutrition and the kidney,* Boston, 1988, Little, Brown.
32. Grodstein GP and others: Glucose absorption during continuous ambulatory peritoneal dialysis, *Kidney Int* 19:564, 1981.
33. Purdum PP III, Kirby DF: Short-bowel syndrome: a review of the role of nutrition support, *JPEN* 15:93, 1991.
34. American Society for Parenteral and Enteral Nutrition Board of Directors: Guidelines for the use of enteral nutrition in the adult patient, *JPEN* 11:435, 1987.
35. Beyer PL, Frankenfield DC: Enteral nutrition in extreme short bowel, *Nutr Clin Prac* 2:60, 1987.
36. Hiyama DT, Fischer JE: Nutritional support in hepatic failure: current thought in practice, *Nutr Clin Prac* 3:96, 1988.
37. Cerra FB and others: Disease-specific amino acid infusion (F080) in hepatic encephalopathy: a prospective, randomized, double-blind, controlled trial, *JPEN* 9:288, 1985.
38. Millikan WJ Jr, Hooks MA: Nutritional support in hepatic failure: clinical controversies, *Nutr Clin Prac* 3:94, 1988.
39. Wahren JJ and others: Is intravenous administration of branched chain amino acids effective in the treatment of hepatic encephalopathy? A multicenter study, *Hepatology* 3:475, 1983.
40. McCullough AJ and others: Nutritional therapy and liver disease, *Gastroenterol Clin North Am* 18:619, 1989.
41. Gulledge AD and others: Psychosocial issues of home parenteral and enteral nutrition, *Nutr Clin Prac* 2:183, 1987.
42. Phillips ML: Enteral nutrition support in diabetes mellitus, *Nutr Clin Prac* 2:152, 1987.

43. Anderson JW and others: Dietary fiber and diabetes: a comprehensive review and practical application, *J Am Diet Assoc* 87:1189, 1987.
44. Reilly JJ and others: Economic impact of malnutrition: a model system for hospitalized patients, *JPEN* 12:371, 1988.
45. *Physician's guide to insulin-dependent (type I) diabetes: diagnosis and treatment,* Alexandria, Va, 1988, American Diabetes Association.
46. *Physician's guide to non-insulin-dependent (type II) diabetes: diagnosis and treatment,* Alexandria, Va, 1988, American Diabetes Association.
47. Diabetes mellitus and exercise, *Diabetes Care* 14(suppl 2):36, 1991.
48. Nutritional recommendations and principles for individuals with diabetes mellitus, *Diabetes Care* 14(suppl 2):20, 1991.
49. Bower RH: Nutrition and immune function, *Nutr Clin Prac* 5:189, 1990.
50. Batman PA and others: Jejunal enteropathy associated with human immunodeficiency virus infection: quantitative histology, *J Clin Pathol* 42:275, 1989.
51. Crocker KS: Gastrointestinal manifestations of acquired immunodeficiency syndrome, *Nurs Clin North Am* 24:395, 1989.
52. Cuff PA: Acquired immunodeficiency syndrome and malnutrition: role of gastrointestinal pathology, *Nutr Clin Prac* 5:43, 1990.
53. Garcia ME, Collins CL, Mansell PWA: The acquired immune deficiency syndrome, *Nutr Clin Prac* 2:108, 1987.
54. Kotler D and others: Magnitude of body-cell-mass depletion and the timing of death from wasting in AIDS, *Am J Clin Nutr* 50:444, 1989.
55. Chelluri L, Jastremski MS: Incidence of malnutrition in patients with acquired immunodeficiency syndrome, *Nutr Clin Prac* 4:16, 1989.
56. Resler SS: Nutrition care of AIDS patients, *J Am Diet Assoc* 88:828, 1988.
57. Task Force on Nutrition Support in AIDS: Guidelines for nutrition support in AIDS, *Nutrition* 5:39, 1989.
58. Keithley JK, Kohn CL: Managing nutritional problems in people with AIDS, *Oncol Nurs Forum* 17:23, 1990.
59. Dwyer JT and others: Unproven nutrition therapies for AIDS: what is the evidence? *Nutr Today* 23:25, 1988.
60. Taber J: Nutrition in HIV infection, *Am J Nurs* 89:1446, 1989.
61. Moore F and others: Enteral feeding reduces postoperative septic complications, *JPEN* 15(1):22S, 1991.
62. Treloar DM, Stechmiller J: Pulmonary aspiration in tube-fed patients with artificial airways, *Heart Lung* 13:667, 1984.
63. Strong RM and others: Equal aspiration rates from postpylorus and intragastric-placed small-bore nasoenteric feeding tubes: a randomized, prospective study, *JPEN* 16:59, 1992.
64. Levenson R and others: Do weighted nasoenteric feeding tubes facilitate duodenal intubations? *JPEN* 12:135, 1988.
65. Rees RGP and others: Spontaneous transpyloric passage and performance of fine-bore polyurethane feeding tubes: a controlled clinical trial, *JPEN* 12:469, 1988.
66. Kittinger JW, Sandler RS, Heizer WD: Efficacy of metoclopramide as an adjunct to duodenal placement of small-bore feeding tubes: a randomized, placebo-controlled, double-blind study, *JPEN* 11:33, 1987.
67. Whatley K and others: When does metoclopramide facilitate transpyloric intubation? *JPEN* 8:679, 1984.
68. Metheny N, Eisenberg P, McSweeney M: Effect of feeding tube properties and three irrigants on clogging rates, *Nurs Res* 37:165, 1988.
69. Kohn CL: The relationship between enteral formula contamination and length of enteral delivery set usage, *JPEN* 15:567, 1991.
70. Guenter PA and others: Tube feeding–related diarrhea in acutely ill patients, *JPEN* 15:277, 1991.
71. Hiebert JM and others: Comparison of continuous vs intermittent tube feedings in adult burn patients, *JPEN* 5:73, 1981.
72. Sands JA: Incidence of pulmonary aspiration in intubated patients receiving enteral nutrition through wide- and narrow-bore nasogastric feeding tubes, *Heart Lung* 20(1):75, 1991.
73. Kingston GW, Phang PT, Leathley MJ: Increased incidence of nosocomial pneumonia in mechanically ventilated patients with subclinic aspiration, *Am J Surg* 161(5):589, 1991.
73a. Hiebert SM and others: Comparison of continuous versus intermittent tube feeding in adult burn patients, *JPEN* 5:73, 1981.
73b. Kagawa Busby KS and others: Effects of diet temperature on tolerance of enteral feedings, *Nurs Res* 29:276, 1980.
74. Clark-Christoff N and others: Use of triple lumen subclavian catheters for administration of TPN, 1992.
75. Powell C, Fabri PJ, Kudsk KA: Risk of infection accompanying the use of single-lumen vs double-lumen subclavian catheters: a prospective randomized study, *JPEN* 12:127, 1988.
76. Corona ML and others: Infections related to central venous catheters, *Mayo Clin Proc* 65:979, 1990.
77. Armstrong CW and others: Clinical predictors of infection of central venous catheters used for total parenteral nutrition, *Infect Control Hosp Epidemiol* 11(2):71, 1990.
78. Horowitz HW and others: Central catheter-related infections: comparison of pulmonary artery catheters and triple lumen catheters for the delivery of hyperalimentation in a critical care setting, *JPEN* 14(6):588, 1990.
79. Kellam B, Fraze DE, Kanarek KS: Central line dressing material and neonatal skin integrity, *Nutr Clin Prac* 3:65, 1988.
80. Young GP and others: Catheter sepsis during parenteral nutrition: the safety of long-term OpSite dressings, *JPEN* 12:365, 1988.

51

Gerontologic Alterations and Management

CHAPTER OBJECTIVES

- Describe the age-associated physiologic changes that occur in the cardiovascular, respiratory, renal, gastrointestinal, hepatic, integumentary, and central nervous systems.
- State the clinical significance of age-related physiologic changes and the expected nursing considerations or interventions used in caring for the elderly critical care patient.
- Explain any modifications in the physical examination of the older critical care patient, along with age-associated changes in laboratory values.
- Relate the age-related changes in hepatic function and accompanying pharmacokinetic changes to the administration of various cardiovascular medications.

More than 50% of critical care patients are older than 65 years of age.[1] Patients who are 65 years or older also are hospitalized for longer periods in the critical care unit.[1,2] Henning and others[2] found the average length of stay in the critical care unit for an elderly person (i.e., >59.5 years of age) was 3.7 days, compared with 2.1 days for younger adults (i.e., <56.5 years of age). The survival rate for the former group was 81%, compared with 98% for the latter group.[1]

In the United States, individuals who are over 65 years of age account for 12% of the total population. It is expected that in the next decade, such individuals will account for at least 20% of the general population.[3] Individuals over the age of 85 are the fastest growing cohort of the elderly population. The overall life expectancy for a person born in 1913 is 74.9 years of age.[4] Currently the terms *senescent* and *elderly* apply to individuals aged 65 years and older. The term *young-old* is used to describe individuals 65 to 75 years of age, *old-old* refers to persons aged 75 to 84 years of age, and *oldest-old* is 85 years plus.[5]

Advancing age is accompanied by physiologic changes in the cardiovascular, respiratory, renal, gastrointestinal, hepatic, integumentary, and central nervous systems. With advancing age the incidence of disease increases, with cardiovascular and neoplastic diseases being the most common cause of death.[6,7] However, although physiologic decline and disease processes influence each other, physiologic decline occurs independently of disease. Therefore changes in physiologic function are important to consider when caring for the elderly patient.[6] The purpose of this chapter is to acquaint the critical care nurse with literature and research on the age-associated changes in physiologic function in healthy older adults and to describe implications for this population in critical care.

Aging is inevitable, independent of environmental exposures or life-style patterns. However, numerous environmental factors and life-style habits influence or accelerate the aging process. For example, exposure to environmental pollutants, excessive ultraviolet light, and radiation and repeated toxin and chemical exposure are environmental factors that can affect the aging process. In addition, two life-style variables are an individual's physical activity and nutritional status.

Most of our information on aging is derived from studies on animals and longitudinal or prospective studies on healthy elderly persons. Interestingly, many studies were conducted between 1974 and 1985, which corresponds to the establishment of the National Institute on Aging (NIA), within the National Institutes of Health.[8] Most of our knowledge of age-related cellular and subcellular changes in various organ systems has come from animal models of aging. Ethical constraints and considerations have prevented the rigorous investigation of cellular and subcellular changes in the organ systems of aging humans. In addition, because of the increased incidence of disease with aging, it becomes difficult to recruit healthy elderly subjects. Some current areas of research supported by the NIA include clinical problems of the geriatric population that are associated with increased morbidity and mortality, clinical problems of nursing home patients, control of gene expression in aging, and genetic theories of aging.[8]

AGING OF THE CARDIOVASCULAR SYSTEM

Advancing age has many effects on the cardiovascular system. With advancing age both the myocardium and the vascular system undergo a multitude of anatomic, cellular, and genetic changes that alter the function of both the myocardium and peripheral vascular system.[9]

Age-Related Morphologic Changes in the Myocardium

Myocardial collagen content increases with age.[10,11] Collagen is the principal noncontractile protein occupying the cardiac interstitium.[12] There are two types of collagen, type I and type III. The increase in myocardial stiffness in the aging heart probably results from an increase in type I collagen, which is associated with scar-tissue formation and has a higher tensile strength.[12] Type III collagen is different from type I in that it is a "softer" type and is associated with the reparative process of wound healing. Increased myocardial collagen content renders the myocardium less compliant.

The decrease in myocardial compliance can adversely affect diastolic filling (through decreased distensibility and dilation) and myocardial relaxation. Consequently, the left ventricle must develop a higher filling pressure for a given increase in ventricular volume. The functional consequence could be an increase in myocardial oxygen consumption.

Under normal physiologic conditions, an increase in myocardial oxygen demand is met with a corresponding increase in coronary artery blood flow. However, in the presence of coronary artery disease, coronary artery blood flow can be limited because of atherosclerotic-mediated narrowing of the coronary arteries. Hence the patient is at risk for developing myocardial ischemia and/or infarction. Clinical manifestations of myocardial ischemia include electrocardiographic changes and chest pain. However, the cessation of chest pain is altered in the elderly person. Muller and others[13] found that complaints of chest pain were absent in 75% of elderly patients (over the age of 85 years) who sustained a myocardial infarction. Others[14] have also reported that chest pain is less intense and of shorter duration and originates in other areas of the chest besides the substernal region.

The aging heart undergoes a modest degree of hypertrophy that is similar to pressure-overload–induced hypertrophy. Such hypertrophy entails a thickening of the left ventricular wall without appreciable changes in the size of the left ventricular chamber (dilation).[15] Progressive increases in left ventricular wall thickness have been found in normotensive men age 15 to 80 years.[15] Walsh[16] has suggested that the hypertrophy in elderly individuals may result from the increased aortic input impedance caused by age-related changes in the peripheral vasculature; the compliance of vascular smooth muscle decreases and blood pressure increases with advancing age.

Functional Changes: Myocardial Contraction and Relaxation

When measured under similar experimental conditions, the developed contractile force of isolated papillary muscle strips removed from aged and young-adult animals is the same.[17] The rate of tension rise is also similar between senescent and young-adult papillary muscles; however, the duration of contraction is prolonged in the aged animal. For example, twitch contractile recordings from adult (7-month) and aged (24-month) rats shows that the duration of the contraction in the adult muscle strip is 350 msec, as compared with 500 msec in the aged muscle strip. Peak contractile force is 7.5 (g/mm^2) in each preparation.[18]

Myocardial contractility depends on numerous factors. However, the most important determinants of myocardial contraction are the intracellular level of free calcium (Ca^{2+}) and the sensitivity of the contractile proteins for calcium.[19] Peak contractile force in the senescent myocardium is unaltered, suggesting that neither the amount of intracellular free calcium during systole nor the sensitivity of the contractile proteins for calcium is altered.

The prolonged duration of contraction is caused in part by a slowed or delayed rate of myocardial relaxation.[9,20] Myocardial relaxation depends on removal of calcium from the cell by uptake into the sarcoplasmic reticulum (SR) and extrusion of calcium across the plasma membrane (sarcolemma) by the action of the sarcolemmal sodium-calcium exchanger and sarcolemmal Ca-ATPase pump.[19]

In heart cells the decrease in intracellular calcium ion concentration at the start of diastole results primarily from uptake into the SR and, to a lesser extent, from efflux out of the cell via the sarcolemmal sodium-calcium exchanger. The age-associated decrease in the rate of relaxation may be partly the result of a reduced rate of calcium uptake (sequestration) by the SR.[21,22] Calcium uptake by the SR occurs through a Ca-ATPase pump, which is embedded in the membrane of the SR. Investigators have found a decrease in the amount of messenger RNA (mRNA) coding for the SR Ca-ATPase pump in the aging myocardium.[23] Messenger RNA is transcribed from the DNA molecule and serves as the template for protein synthesis. A decrease in mRNA or "message" for the synthesis of SR Ca-ATPase pumps results in a decreased number of SR Ca-ATPase pumps or decreased amount of Ca-ATPase enzyme protein. These findings may explain, in part, the reduced uptake of calcium by the SR during relaxation. Table 51-1 summarizes the age-associated changes in excitation-contraction coupling and the effects of inotropic agents in the myocardium.

In the elderly human myocardium, several indexes of relaxation—such as the isovolumic phase of diastole and early diastolic filling—are prolonged.[24,25] The duration of the QT interval on the ECG also increases.[26] Theoretically, impaired relaxation can affect ventricular filling and myocardial perfusion, because most of the myocardial layers are perfused during diastole. In the healthy elderly person, impaired relaxation may not cause any appreciable change in ventricular filling and therefore cardiac output (CO) or myocardial perfusion. However, in an elderly person with ischemic heart disease, the delay in the rate of relaxation could compromise perfusion of the myocardium, especially the subendocardial layer.[19]

Changes in Myocardial Gene Expression

Some of the age-related changes in myocardial function are possibly the result of altered gene expression. Genes are sequence bases of deoxyribonucleic acid (DNA) that specify the amino acid sequence of a protein molecule. Gene expression refers to the process in which certain amino acids are assembled into proteins; genes are composed of DNA, and genes carry the chemical message that informs the cells how to synthesize the new protein.[27] Sometimes there is a change in the DNA that alters the message to the cells, and a different type of protein and/or enzyme is synthesized. The change in gene expression may be an "adaptive" or "protective" response, or it may produce an undesirable change that leads to abnormal tissue growth or carcinogenesis.

In the hearts of senescent animals, there are changes in the contractile proteins—specifically myosin, the large contractile protein that contains the actin-binding site and myosin ATPase. In the adult animal myocardium and human myocardium, one form of the myosin (V1 [alpha] heavy chain) is preferentially expressed. In animal models of aging, investigators have found that a different isoform of myosin V1 heavy chain is expressed.[28,29] Isoforms (or isoenzymes) of a protein differ structurally but provide the same overall function.[19] For example, one isoform of a specific enzyme (protein) may catalyze a reaction more quickly than does another isoform. The isoform of myosin V1 heavy chain found in the aging myocardium is myosin V3 (beta) heavy chain and is associated with a low myosin ATPase activity and a reduced shortening velocity.[29]

Table 51-1 Age-related changes in the senescent animal myocardium

Age-related changes	Physiologic consequences
Increase in the duration of myocardial contraction Increase in the duration of the Ca^{++} transient, which may in part be related to a decrease in the rate of SR Ca^{++} sequestration	Decrease in the rate of relaxation (diastole is shorter)
No change in myofilament response (sensitivity) to Ca^{++}	No change in isometric force development
Decrease in myosin ATPase activity A different form of myosin (isoform) is synthesized, which hydrolyzes ATP at a slower rate	Decrease in the speed and extent of muscle shortening
Decrease in beta-adrenergic inotropic and chronotropic effects No change in beta-adrenoreceptor density or affinity Possibly changes in postreceptor events	Decreased heart rate response to exercise and stress Decreased chronotropic and inotropic responses to exogenously administered catecholamines
Decreased pharmacologic response to ouabain Decrease in the activity of the sarcolemmal Na-Ca exchanger Decrease in number of sarcolemmal Na^{+}-K^{+}-ATPase pumps	Decreased inotropic response to ouabain

From Gerstenblith G and others: *Circ Res* 44:517, 1979; Guarnieri T and others: *Am J Physiol* 239:H501, 1980; Lakatta EG and others: *J Clin Invest* 55:61, 1975; Maciel LM and others: *Circ Res* 67(1):230, 1990; Scarpace PJ: *Fed Proc* 45:51, 1986; and Spurgeon HA, Steinbach MF, Lakatta EG: *Am J Physiol* 244:H513, 1983.

Ca^{++}, calcium; ATP, adenosine triphosphate; SR, sarcoplasmic reticulum.

Hemodynamics and the Electrocardiogram

Resting (supine) heart rate decreases with age. By age 70 there is approximately a 16 beat/min decrease in the resting heart rate, as compared with the heart rate values of younger adults.[30,31] Cinelli and others[30] reported a decrease in the resting heart rate from 78.8 beats/min in young adults to 62.3 beats/min in elderly adults. Heart rate is an important determinant of CO, and the normal resting heart beats approximately 70 times a minute. At rest or with minimal activity, the elderly person probably will not experience any untoward cardiovascular effect (i.e., a decrease in CO) with a heart rate of 62 beats/min. However, if the heart rate response is attenuated during exercise, the elderly person's capacity for exercise may be limited.

Intrinsic heart rate also decreases with aging.[32] Resting heart rate is modulated by both divisions of the autonomic nervous system. In healthy resting individuals, parasympathetic (cholinergic) influences predominate, which causes a heart rate of approximately 70 beats/min.[19] In the absence of both parasympathetic and sympathetic influences, the heart rate of young adults averages about 100 beats/min and is referred to as the *intrinsic heart rate.* Jose[32] found that the intrinsic heart rate (in the presence of both sympathetic and parasympathetic blockers) in a 20-year-old person was 100 beats/min, as compared with a heart rate of 74 beats/min in a 80-year-old man. This decrease in intrinsic heart rate may in part explain the decrease in the resting (supine) heart rate that occurs with aging.

Early reports indicate that resting CO and stroke volume decrease with advancing age.[33] There are also reports that these indexes decrease in various animal models of aging.[34] More recently, Rodeheffer et al.[35] studied subjects without coronary artery disease or other types of illnesses over a 30- to 80-year period in the Baltimore Longitudinal Study of Aging. They reported no change in resting CO or cardiac index in participants.[35] Lakatta[33] suggests the differences among studies may be because of different or mixed study populations; that is, some of the subjects may have had coronary artery disease or other diseases that went undetected. As noted earlier, the incidence of all types of chronic diseases increases with aging, especially cardiovascular-related diseases. Hence it becomes very difficult to find subjects who are free of disease to participate in an aging study.

At rest, left ventricular end-diastolic volume (preload), end-systolic volume (the volume of blood remaining in the ventricle after systole), and the ejection fraction are not affected by age.[33] In addition, Kennedy and Caird[36] reported that pulmonary artery pressures are similar between young and elderly persons.

Advancing age produces changes in the ECG. The

incidence of asymptomatic cardiac dysrhythmias also increases in elderly patients.[37] R-wave and S-wave amplitude significantly decrease in persons over 49 years of age, whereas Q-T duration increases (Table 51-2).[26] The increase in the duration of the Q-T interval is reflective of the prolonged rate of relaxation.[26] There is also a downward shift in the frontal plane axis from 48.93 to 38.83 degrees between the ages of 30 and 49, suggestive of a modest degree of cardiac enlargement or hypertrophy.[26]

The most frequent dysrhythmia occurring in elderly individuals is the premature ventricular contraction (PVC). Camm and others[38] and Fleg and Kennedy[39] report that 70% to 80% of all patients over 60 years of age experience PVCs. In a healthy geriatric population (60 to 85 years of age), 24-hour ambulatory electrocardiographic recordings revealed that 80% of the 98 subjects studied experienced asymptomatic ventricular ectopic beats. The findings of this study suggest that aging per se is associated with an increase in the occurrence of PVCs.

Other common types of dysrhythmias are sinus node dysfunction (atrial fibrillation, atrial flutter, or paroxysmal supraventricular tachycardia) and atrioventricular conduction disturbances.[37-39] Because the majority of patients are asymptomatic, the use of antidysrhythmics is generally not recommended. The side effects and toxic effects of antidysrhythmics impose more of a risk, as compared with the risk of mortality or morbidity related to the dysrhythmia.[37] In contrast, in patients who are symptomatic and have malignant ventricular dysrhythmias (sustained ventricular tachycardia and/or fibrillation), pharmacologic therapy is warranted.[37]

Age-Related Changes in Baroreceptor Function

Baroreceptor-reflex function is altered with aging.[40] Baroreceptors are mechanoreceptors that respond to stretch and other changes in the blood vessel wall and are located at the bifurcation of the common carotid artery and aortic arch.[19] Impulses arising in the baroreceptor region project to the vasomotor center (nucleus of tractus solitarius) in the medulla. Abrupt changes in blood pressure caused by increases in peripheral resistance, CO, or blood volume are sensed by the baroreceptors, resulting in an increase in the impulse frequency to the vasomotor center within the medulla. This increase inhibits vasoconstrictor impulses arising from the vasoconstrictor region within the medulla.[19] The result is a decrease in heart rate and peripheral vasodilation; both of these effects return the blood pressure to within normal limits. The baroreflex can be tested by measuring the heart rate response (i.e., increase or decrease in heart rate) after the administration of either a pressor or depressor agent and by changing a person's position from lying to standing. Yin and others[41] and Elliott and others[42] found an attenuated increase in heart rate response in elderly subjects after the infusion of phenylephrine, an alpha-adrenoreceptor agonist that produces vasoconstriction and increases the blood pressure. Likewise, the baroreflex-mediated tachycardia response to depressor agents is also attenuated in elderly subjects.[41] There are several reports of an attenuation in the heart rate response of elderly subjects after changes in position (supine to standing).[43,44]

The change in baroreceptor function may explain in part the occurrence of postural or orthostatic hypotension in elderly persons. When an individual changes his or her position from supine to standing, the distribution of blood volume changes. This can result in a reduction in CO and hence blood pressure.[19] However, when a person changes position, there are simultaneous baroreceptor-mediated increases in the heart rate that serve to maintain the blood pressure by increasing the CO. The baroreceptor reflex response also mediates changes in the peripheral resistance and force of myocardial contraction, which likewise serve to offset the drop in blood pressure. It was once thought that postural hypotension occurred more frequently in elderly subjects and was an age-related phenomenon. However, recent studies have shown that the prevalence of postural hypotension is quite low in elderly persons.[45,46] The prevalence of orthostatic hypotension is greater in institutionalized elderly patients who are receiving antihypertensive medications.[44]

Left Ventricular Function in Elderly Persons at Rest and During Exercise

Several investigators using echocardiography and radionuclide scintigraphy found no change in resting left ventricular function in healthy subjects.[35] However, several indexes of relaxation, such as the isovolumic phase of diastole and early diastolic filling, are found to be prolonged and slowed in the myocardium of elderly persons.[24,25] These findings are consistent with those

Table 51-2 Age-related changes in electrocardiographic variables

ECG variable	<30 years	30-39 years	40-49 years	>49 years
R-wave amplitude (mm)	10.43	10.53	9.01	9.25
S-wave amplitude (mm)	15.21	14.21	12.22	12.42
Frontal plane axis (degrees)	48.93	48.13	36.50	38.83
P-R duration (ms)	15.89	16.23	16.04	16.25
QRS duration (ms)	7.64	7.51	7.36	8.00
Q-T duration (ms)	37.83	37.50	37.99	39.58
T-wave amplitude (ms)	5.21	4.57	4.31	4.42

Modified from Bachman S, Sparrow D, Smith LK: *Am J Cardiol* 48:513, 1981.

found in isolated cardiac muscles removed from aged animals.

It is well established that an elderly person's ability to exercise decreases.[26] However, Rodeheffer and others[35] reported that the elderly person's diminished ability to exercise is not because of the maximal CO that can be achieved during exercise. These investigators found no difference in CO response to different levels of exercise in subjects from the Baltimore Longitudinal Study on Aging.[35] During exercise, CO is increased by four mechanisms: an increased heart rate, increased inotropic state of the myocardium, decreased aortic impedance or afterload, and increased dependence on Starling's law of the heart.[35] With advancing age, exercise causes decreases in the first three mechanisms; however, there is a striking increase in the left ventricular end-diastolic volume, which suggests an increased dependence on Starling's law of the heart. This means that at the same end-diastolic volume, the older myocardium develops more force, as compared with a younger myocardium. Because the former contracts more forcefully, a greater stroke volume and CO are achieved, but at the same end-diastolic volume. In elderly subjects during exercise, CO is augmented through Starling's law of the heart, thereby compensating for the attenuated heart rate response, inotropic response, and reduced afterload response.[35]

Inotropic Response to Catecholamines and Cardiac Glycosides

The inotropic response of the elderly person's myocardium to catecholamines also decreases. This is exemplified by an attenuated force development and heart rate increase to exogenously-administered norepinephrine.[47] The age-associated decrease in inotropic effect to catecholamines does not appear to be receptor mediated, because Guarnieri and others[48] found no change in beta-receptor number or affinity in the myocardium of aged rats. Age-associated changes in postreceptor events, such as coupling of the beta-adrenoreceptor to the enzyme adenylate cyclase or changes in the amount of the second messenger cyclic adenosine monophosphate, may be responsible for the attenuated inotropic effect of beta-adrenergic agents.[47,49] Interestingly, when isolated cardiac muscles of aged animals are exposed to high concentrations of calcium, they have the ability to respond and generate as much force as do cardiac muscles of adult animals.[47] These results suggest that there is no change in the contractile machinery or myofilaments that are responsible for generating the force within cardiac muscle. There are also reports of a decrease in catecholamine content of the heart, as well as a decrease in the adrenergic nerve density, which could in part explain reports of decreased heart rates and inotropic responses to the release of endogenous catecholamines.[50,51]

The contractile response to the cardiac glycoside *ouabain* is diminished in the myocardium of the senescent animal.[52] Ouabain increases myocardial contractility by increasing the intracellular level of calcium. Ouabain inhibits the sarcolemmal Na^+-K^+-ATPase pump; this produces a rise in intracellular sodium, which in turn activates the sarcolemmal sodium-calcium exchanger.[19] Calcium is pumped into the cell in exchange for sodium, resulting in an elevated intracellular level of calcium and concomitant increase in the force of myocardial contraction. Gerstenblith and others[52] suggested that the diminished inotropic effect of ouabain is the result of changes in the activity of the sodium-calcium exchanger or ATPase receptor density, because—as noted earlier—the inotropic response of the isolated aged muscle to calcium is similar to the inotropic response in adult animals.

To date there are no reports on the inotropic effects of the cardiac glycoside *digoxin* in either the aged human or animal myocardium. Because digoxin is the most frequently-used cardiac glycoside, it may be important to examine whether the cardiac response diminishes with the use of digoxin.

The Peripheral Vascular System

The effects of aging on the peripheral vascular system are reflected in the gradual, but linear, rise in systolic blood pressure.[53,54] Diastolic blood pressure is less affected by age and generally remains the same or decreases.[54] Important determinants of systolic blood pressure include the compliance of the vasculature and the blood volume within the vascular system. Similar to the heart, the compliance of the vasculature is determined by its composition. With advancing age, the intimal layer thickens, principally because of an increase in smooth muscle cells (which have migrated from the medial layer), and the amount of connective tissue (collagen and elastic tissue) increases.[53] These changes occur in the intima of the large and distal arteries. This gradual decrease in arterial compliance or "stiffening of the arteries" is sometimes referred to as *arteriosclerosis.*

Arteriosclerotic changes are also accompanied by changes caused by *atherosclerosis,* which is the accumulation of lipoproteins and fibrinous products—such as platelets, macrophages, and leukocytes—within a vessel.[55] The consequences of arteriosclerotic and atherosclerotic processes are that the arteries become progressively less distensible and the vascular pressure-volume relationship is altered. These changes are clinically significant, because small changes in intravascular volume are accompanied by disproportionate increases in systolic blood pressure.[56] The decrease in arterial compliance and disproportionate increase in systolic blood pressure may lead to an increase in afterload and the development of concentric (pressure-induced) ventricular hypertrophy in the elderly patient.[56]

It is well recognized that increased serum lipoprotein levels are risk factors in the development and progression of atherosclerosis.[55] Lipoprotein levels increase with advancing age. However, innumerable factors can influence the serum lipoprotein level, making it very difficult to determine whether such changes contribute to the aging of the peripheral vascular system.[57,58]

Serum lipoproteins are particles that contain varying amounts of cholesterol, triglycerides, phospholipids, and apoproteins.[55] There are five principal serum lipoproteins: chylomicrons, low-density lipoproteins (LDLs), very low-density lipoproteins (VLDLs), intermediate-density lipoproteins (IDLs), and high-density lipoproteins (HDLs). The lipoprotein classification is based on the lipoprotein's size and relative concentration of cholesterol, triglycerides, and apoproteins.[55] In men, the serum total cholesterol level (all of the lipoproteins combined) increases progressively from 150 to 200 mg/dl between the ages of 20 and 50 years and remains relatively unchanged until the age of 70 years.[58] As is predicted, the age-related changes in serum LDL levels parallel the changes in the total serum cholesterol level. All lipoprotein fractions transport cholesterol; however, in healthy people, three fourths of the total cholesterol is transported within the LDL.[55] There are relatively few age-related changes in VLDL and HDL levels in men, in whom serum triglyceride levels peak at approximately age 40 and then decrease.[57,58]

In women, serum total cholesterol levels are low between the ages of 20 and 50 years.[57,58] However, between the ages 55 to 60 years, serum total cholesterol levels progressively increase, usually simultaneously with changes in the hormonal production of estrogen.[58] The increase in total serum cholesterol level is primarily the result of an increase in the LDL fraction and, to a lesser extent, the VLDL and HDL fractions, which do not change appreciably with age in women. In women, serum triglyceride levels progressively increase with age.[58]

Arterial pressure is also governed by the amount of blood volume, which in turn is regulated by plasma levels of sodium and water and the activity of the renin-angiotensin system (RAS).[59] Plasma renin activity declines with age, and aging per se has no appreciable effect on sodium and water homeostasis.[60,61] However, as noted earlier, there are age-related changes in tubular function, as well as a decrease in the glomerular filtration rate (GFR), both of which can affect overall sodium and water homeostasis. Circulating levels of sodium-regulating hormones—such as natriuretic hormone, aldosterone, and antidiuretic hormone (ADH)—are not appreciably altered by advancing age.[61,62] However, a delayed natriuretic response after sodium loading and plasma volume expansion and diminished renal response to ADH secretion have been reported in elderly people.[62]

THE RESPIRATORY SYSTEM

Many of the changes in the pulmonary system that occur with aging are reflected in tests of pulmonary function and include changes in thoracic wall expansion, respiratory muscle strength, and morphology of alveolar parenchyma and decreases in arterial oxygen tension (Pa_{O_2}) (Tables 51-3 and 51-4).[63] These changes occur progressively as age advances and should not alter the elderly person's ability to breathe effortlessly. However, such factors as repeated exposure to environmental pollutants, cigarette smoking, and frequent pulmonary infections can accelerate age-related changes, thereby making it difficult to identify the age-associated changes in pulmonary function. Interestingly, Thurlbeck[64] did not find age-related morphologic changes in the lung tissue of aging mice raised in a pollution-free and infection-free environment, suggesting the immense effect of environmental variables on pulmonary function.

Thoracic Wall and Respiratory Muscles

The chest wall (thoracic skeleton) and vertebrae undergo a small degree of osteoporosis, and at the same time the costal cartilages that connect the rib cage together become calcified and stiff. These changes may produce kyphosis and reduce chest wall compliance, respectively (Fig. 51-1).[63,65,66] The functional effect is a decrease in thoracic wall excursion. Other factors, such as an increase in abdominal girth and change in posture, will also decrease thoracic excursion. These anatomic structural changes are reflected by an in-

Table 51-3 Age-related changes in frequently performed pulmonary function tests

Pulmonary function tests	Descriptions	Standard lung volumes and capacities (ml)	Age-related changes (ml)
Total lung capacity	Vital capacity plus residual volume	6000	6000
Vital capacity	Amount of air exhaled after a maximal inspiration	5000	↓ 3750
Tidal volume (VT) (ml)	Amount of air inhaled or exhaled with each breath	500	500
Residual volume (RV) (ml)	Amount of air left in lungs after forced exhalation	1200	↑ 1800
Inspiratory reserve volume (IRV)	Amount of air that can be forcefully inhaled after inspiring a normal VT	3100	↓ 2800
Expiratory reserve volume (ERV)	Amount of air that can be forcefully exhaled after expiring a normal VT	1200	↓ 1000
Forced expiratory volume in 1 sec (FEV_1)	Volume exhaled in the first second of a single forced expiratory volume; expressed as a percent of the forced vital capacity	80%	↓ 75%

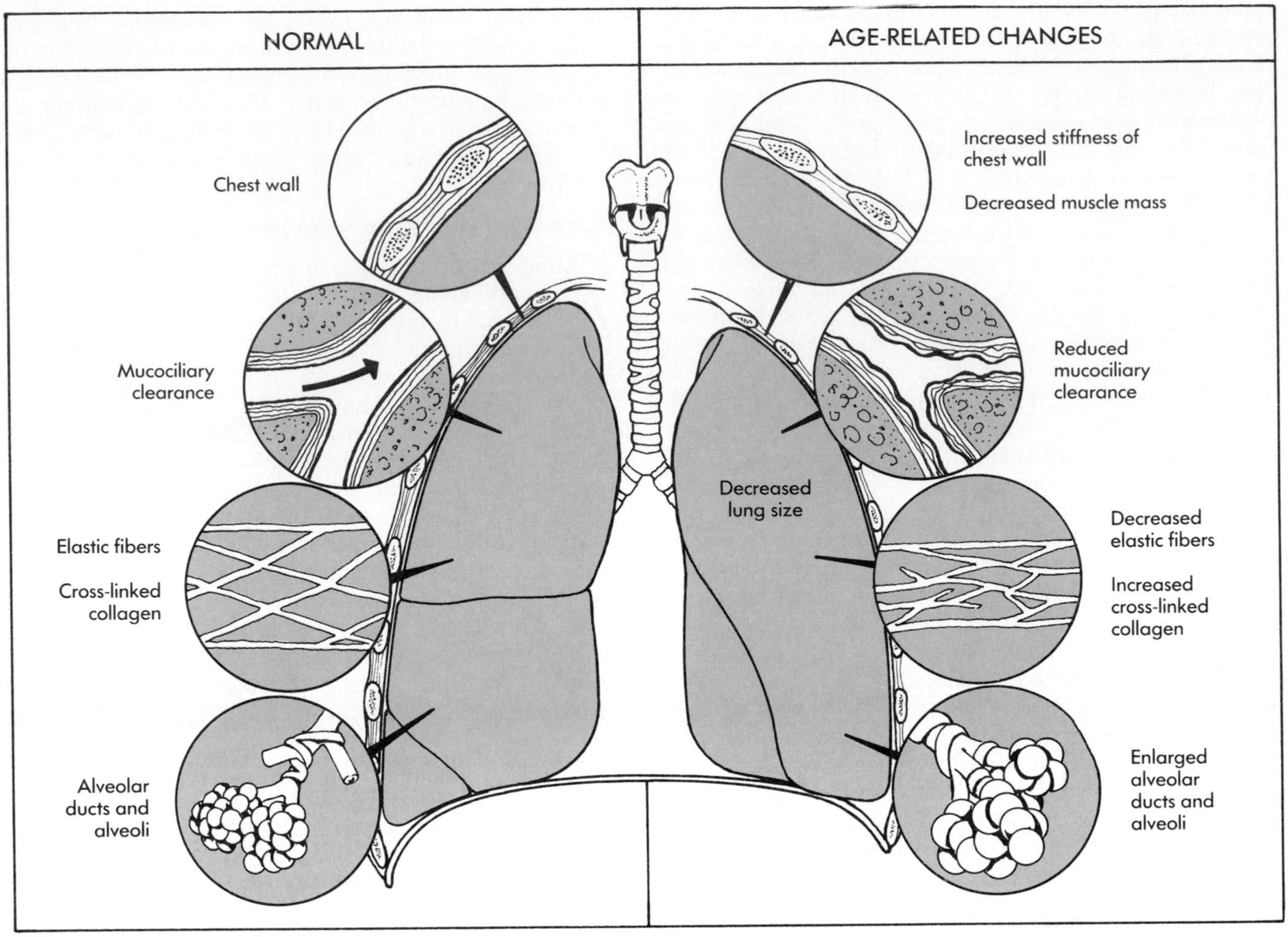

Fig. 51-1 Age-related changes in the respiratory system. With advancing age, the compliance of the chest wall and lung tissue change. There is also a reduced clearance of mucus by the cilia that line the pulmonary tree and an enlargement of the alveolar ducts and alveoli. More age-related changes in respiratory function are described in the text. (From Webster JR, Kadah H: *Geriatrics* 46:31, 1991.)

Table 51-4 Progressive changes in arterial oxygen tension (Pa_{O_2}) and carbon dioxide tension (Pa_{CO_2})

Age-groups	Pa_{O_2} (mm Hg)	Pa_{CO_2} (mm Hg)
<30 years	94	39
31-40	87	38
41-50	84	40
51-60	81	39
>60	74	40

Adapted from Sorbini CA and others: *Respiration* 25:3, 1968.

crease in residual volume and decrease in vital capacity (see Table 51-1).

There is a gradual decrease in the strength of the respiratory muscles: the diaphragm and both the external and internal intercostal muscles. The diaphragm is the most important inspiratory muscle, because its movement accounts for 75% of the change in intrathoracic volume during quiet respiration.[67] The respiratory muscles are composed of skeletal muscle fibers.[67] During aging, skeletal muscle progressively atrophies and its energy metabolism decreases, which may partially explain the declining strength of the respiratory muscles.[68,69] In addition, there is an age-associated decrease in the effectiveness of the cough reflex, which is possibly caused by a decrease in ciliary responsiveness and motion.[70] These changes underscore the importance of deep breathing and coughing for the bedridden elderly patient in the critical care unit.

As noted previously, the age-associated changes in pulmonary function do not alter the elderly person's ability to breathe effortlessly. However, the decrease in respiratory muscle strength may be a limiting factor during exercise, because the respiratory muscles—specifically the accessory inspiratory muscles (sternocleidomastoid, scalene, and trapezius)—facilitate inspiration during exercise. However, this theory is not supported by the findings of Belman and Gaesser,[71] who reported that although ventilatory muscle strength

RESEARCH ABSTRACT

Skin ulcers of elderly surgical patients in critical care units.

Marchette L, Arnell I, Redick E: *DCCN* 10(6):321, 1991.

PURPOSE

The purpose of this study was to describe the relationships among several patient characteristics—such as skin condition, nursing care, and medical care—and to compare the characteristics of those patients who developed skin ulcers with those who did not.

DESIGN

Correlational design

SAMPLE

The random sample consisted of 161 subjects (89 men and 72 women) with a mean age of 70 years who were in a critical care unit after surgery. The surgical specialties of the subjects were cardiac (30%), gastrointestinal (30%), orthopedic (19%), pulmonary (15%), and neurosurgical (5%). Subjects had been in the critical care unit for an average of 14 days. Most of the subjects (70%) were unconscious for at least 1 day; 33% of subjects had urinary incontinence, and 55% experienced fecal incontinence.

INSTRUMENTS

The investigators developed a data collection form based on literature regarding skin problems. Skin ulceration was operationally defined as any skin problem caused by pressure, shearing, friction, maceration, and/or lack of oxygen to tissues secondary to vascular insufficiency. The instrument was pilot tested and modified; content validity was established by the consensus of eight health care providers familiar with skin care problems.

PROCEDURE

Data were collected from the medical records of the 161 subjects by the principal investigator and a medical-surgical nurse (interrater reliability correlation of .96).

RESULTS

There was a significant relationship ($p < .00001$) between the incidence of redness and skin ulcers. Most of the skin ulcers were stage 1 or 2, with an average diameter of 7.5 cm. Surgical specialty was not related to whether patients had skin ulcers. Operating room (OR) time was significantly related to the incidence of skin redness ($p < .04$), skin ulcers ($p < .02$), and skin ulcer stage ($p < .0007$). There was a significant relationship between fecal incontinence and skin redness ($p < .02$) and skin ulcers ($p < .001$). The incidence of diarrhea was related to the incidence of skin redness ($p < .01$) and skin ulcers ($p < .001$), but not to the stage of skin ulcers. Steroid use was not related to skin redness but was significantly related ($p < .05$) to the incidence of skin ulcers. Subjects with skin ulcers showed significantly lower levels of protein ($p < .05$) and albumin ($p < .04$). The combination of five variables was found to predict the occurrence of skin ulcers with 74.4% accuracy: skin redness, number of days that static air mattress was used for prevention, fecal incontinence, diarrhea, preoperative albumin level, number of days that heel protectors were used, preoperative protein level, and number of days that alternating pressure pad was used.

DISCUSSION/IMPLICATIONS

Based on the findings of this study, the implications for the care of the elderly patient in surgical critical care unit are as follows: elimination of skin redness, development of a protocol for air mattress use, the rapid and aggressive treatment of incontinence, and close monitoring of serum laboratory values. It is important for critical care nurses to understand the complex relationships among the variables causing skin ulcers in the vulnerable elderly patient population. Recommendations for future research include determining the effectiveness of specific interventions on skin ulcer formation or treatment, studying the predictors of skin ulcers in elderly medical patients, and examining the relationship of other variables—such as vasopressor drugs and protein status—on the development of skin ulcers in elderly persons.

improved after elderly men and women received ventilatory muscle training, neither submaximal or maximal exercise tolerance improved.

Alveolar Parenchyma

With advancing age a diminished recoil (or increased compliance) of the lung occurs, as exemplified by a leftward shift in the pressure-volume curve.[72] The reduced recoil results from the increase in the ratio of elastin to collagen content that occurs with advancing age.[73] Collagen, elastin, and reticulin are the primary connective tissue proteins of the lung tissue (see Fig. 51-1).[74,75] They are responsible for the elasticity and performance of the airways of the lung. Whereas total lung collagen remains unaltered, the amount of elastin increases with age in the interlobular septa and pleura and possibly within the bronchi and their vessels.[74,75] These anatomic structural changes are reflected by an increase in residual volume and a decrease in forced expiratory volume.

An additional anatomic structural change is the increase in the size of the alveolar ducts, which occurs after 40 years of age.[63] The bronchial enlargement displaces inhaled air volume away from the alveoli that line the alveolar ducts (see Fig. 51-1).[63] Ventilation and the process of oxygen and carbon dioxide exchange (diffusion) depend on numerous factors, one of which is the surface area available for diffusion. A displacement of inhaled air volume away from the alveoli limits the surface area available for gas exchange. This may in part explain the progressive and linear decrease in the pulmonary diffusion capacity, which depends on both the surface area and capillary blood volume. There are reports that capillary blood volume decreases with advancing age.[76]

Pulmonary Gas Exchange

The arterial oxygen tension (PaO_2) decreases with age, such that the median PaO_2 for healthy persons over 60 years of age is 74.3 mm Hg, as compared with 94 mm Hg for younger adults.[77] In contrast, arterial carbon dioxide ($PaCO_2$) does not change with advancing age (Table 51-4).[77]

The decrease in PaO_2 may be the result of an increase in the closing volume in the dependent lung zones during resting tidal breathing in older subjects.[78,79] Consequently, dependent lung zones may be ventilated intermittently, leading to regional differences in ventilation. It is possible that alterations in blood volume and vascular resistance within the pulmonary circulation may also contribute to ventilation/perfusion (V/Q) mismatching. Other factors, such as smoking and pulmonary disease, also have an impact on the level of arterial oxygenation.

Lung Volumes and Capacities

With advancing age, total lung capacity and tidal volume do not change[65] (see Table 51-3). Residual volume (RV) increases with age, paralleling the decrease in chest wall compliance and reduced strength of the respiratory muscles (see Table 51-3).[63] The increase in RV may also add to the diminished strength of the inspiratory muscles by stretching the diaphragm and altering the tension-length relationship.

Results from studies are conflicting with regard to age-related changes in functional residual capacity (FRC), which is the volume of air in the lungs at the normal resting end-expiratory position. There are reports of no change[80] and decreases[65] in FRC in elderly persons. The balance of two opposing forces, the elastic recoil of the lung and the outward recoil of the chest wall, determine the FRC.[67] These factors change in opposite directions with age: the elastic recoil of the lung decreases, thereby increasing compliance, while the outward recoil of the chest wall decreases, thus decreasing the compliance of the chest wall. One would predict that because these factors change in opposite directions, FRC would remain unaltered. In fact, Knudson and others[80] found no change in FRC in elderly people, supporting this prediction.

Other lung volumes that decrease with age include the inspiratory reserve volume (IRV) and the expiratory reserve volume (ERV).[65] The decrease in the ERV is the result of an increase in the RV. The decrease in IRV, however, has been found only in studies reporting a corresponding increase in FRC. See Table 51-3 and Fig. 51-1 for a summary of age-related changes in pulmonary function.

The following dynamic measurements of lung volume are decreased in aging: maximal expiratory flow rate, maximal midexpiratory flow rate, forced expiratory volume in 1 second (FEV_1), and the ratio of FEV_1 to forced vital capacity.[81] Dynamic measurements of lung volume reflect changes in air flow rate; air flow rate depends on the resistance of airways and chest wall compliance. Hence the age-related decrease in the dynamic lung volume is probably caused by decreased chest wall compliance, increased likelihood of small airways closing during forced expiratory efforts (increasing airway resistance), and decreased strength of expiratory muscles.[82]

THE RENAL SYSTEM

Aging produces changes in renal structure and function, many of which begin at approximately 30 to 40 years of age.[83] One of the prominent changes is a decrease in the number and size of the nephrons, which begins in the cortical regions and progresses toward the medullary portions of the kidney.[84] The decrease in the number of nephrons corresponds to a 20% decrease in the weight of the kidney between 40 and 80 years of age.[84] Initially, this loss of nephrons does not appreciably alter renal function because of the large renal reserve: the kidney contains approximately two to three million nephrons, all of which are not required to maintain adequate fluid and acid-base homeostasis. However, with time the geriatric patient also loses this "renal reserve."[84]

Nephron loss is caused by a gradual reduction in blood flow to the glomerular capillary tuft.[85] Total renal blood flow declines after the fourth decade of life,[83] because of hyaline arteriolosclerosis.[85,86] The etiology of this vascular lesion within the glomerular tuft is unknown. By the eighth decade of life, 50% of the glomeruli are lost as a result of this arteriolar hyalinization.[84]

The glomerular filtration rate (GFR) decreases with advancing age.[83,84] The GFR is the volume of fluid traversing the glomerular membrane in a given period and is an important regulator of water and solute excretion. GFR depends on the permeability of the glomerular capillary and the surface area available for filtration, as well as the balance of pressure gradients between the glomerular capillary and Bowman's space.[59] In elderly persons, the decrease in GFR is most likely caused by the decrease in nephron number, as well as the decrease in renal blood flow.[83]

Even though the remaining nephrons adapt to the loss of nephrons by glomerular hyperfiltration and increased solute load per nephron, the reduced GFR predisposes the elderly patient to adverse drug reactions and drug-induced renal failure. Some drugs are excreted unchanged in the urine, whereas other drugs have active or nephrotoxic metabolites that are excreted in the urine. In addition, the senescent kidney is more susceptible to injury by hypotensive episodes, because of the age-related decrease in renal blood flow and reduced pressure gradient across the afferent arteriole.[87]

There are also age-related changes in tubular function. The functions that are primarily carried out in the renal tubules are sodium and water concentration and conservation and acidification of the urine.[59] These functions are governed by the amount of sodium and water delivered to the tubules and overall acid-base balance. The age-related changes in tubular function become apparent when there are extreme changes in the body fluid composition or acid-base balance. For example, with systemic acidosis the rate and amount of total acid excretion (bicarbonate, titratable acid, and ammonium) are reduced.[83,87] This predisposes the elderly patient to metabolic acidosis, volume depletion, and hyperchloremia. However, at a normal pH level, the kidney of an elderly person is able to maintain acid-base homeostasis.

There is a diminished ability of the senescent kidney to excrete a free water load, conserve water during periods of dehydration, and conserve sodium during periods of low salt intake.[83] There are also age-related changes in extrarenal mechanisms, such as the decreased activity and responsiveness of the senescent kidney to the sympathetic nervous system and renin-angiotensin-aldosterone system, which are important in integrating overall fluid homeostasis and maintaining blood pressure in response to changes in body position.[60]

THE GASTROINTESTINAL SYSTEM

Age-related gastrointestinal changes occur in the processes of swallowing, motility, and absorption.[88,89] Swallowing may be difficult for the elderly person because of incomplete mastication of food.[89] Deteriorating dentition, diminished lubrication, and ill-fitting dentures result in insufficient mastication of food within the oral cavity, thereby predisposing the elderly patient to aspiration.[88] In addition, the number and velocity of the peristaltic contractions of the elderly person's esophagus decrease and the number of nonperistaltic contractions increases.[89] These changes in esophageal motility are referred to as *presbyesophagus.* These changes may predispose the patient to erosion of the esophageal wall (recurrent esophagitis), because food will remain in the esophagus longer. In addition, bed rest and reclining in a supine position for a prolonged period can cause esophageal reflux, which also can lead to esophagitis.

The aging process produces thinning of the smooth muscle within the gastric mucosa.[90] The epithelial layer of the gastric mucosa, which contains the chief and parietal cells, undergoes a modest degree of atrophy, resulting in the hyposecretion of pepsin and acid, respectively.[91] Furthermore, mucin secretion from the mucus cells decreases, thereby altering the protective function of the gastric mucosal (bicarbonate) barrier. Because of this, the stomach wall is more susceptible to acid injury, thus increasing the incidence of gastric ulcerations.[92] Aging does not appreciably alter gastric emptying of solid foods. However, Moore and others[93] found a delay in the emptying of liquids from the stomach in elderly persons.

To our knowledge, there are no reported changes in small intestinal peristalsis or segmental movements with aging.[94] Alterations within the small intestine include a decrease in intestinal weight after the age of 50 and a flattening of jejunal villi.[94] Age produces no change in the small intestine's absorption of fats and proteins; however, decreased carbohydrate absorption has been reported.[95,96] There is essentially no change in vitamin or mineral absorption, except for a decrease in calcium absorption from the aged duodenum.[89]

THE LIVER

With advancing age, both hepatocyte number and liver weight decrease.[97] There is also a significant decrease in total liver blood flow, such that between 25 and 65 years of age there is a 50% decrease in total liver blood flow.[97-99] The liver has many complex functions, including carbohydrate storage, ketone body formation, reduction and conjugation of adrenal and gonadal steroid hormones, synthesis of plasma proteins, deamination of amino acids, storage of cholesterol, urea formation, and detoxification of toxins and drugs. However, despite changes in hepatocyte number and blood flow, liver function is not appreciably altered.[99] Several tests of liver function—such as serum bilirubin, alkaline phosphatase, and glutamic oxaloacetic transaminase levels—are not altered with advancing age.

The most important age-related change in liver function is the decrease in the liver's capacity to metabolize drugs.[100,101] Although clinical tests of liver function do not reflect this change in metabolism, it is well recognized that drug side effects and toxic effects occur more frequently in older adults than young adults.[101] This reduced drug-metabolizing capacity is caused by a reduction in the activity of the drug-metabolizing enzyme system (MEOS) and decrease in total liver blood flow.[98,102]

Changes in Pharmacokinetics and Pharmacodynamics

There are many age-related changes in drug pharmacokinetics, which is the manner in which the body absorbs, distributes, metabolizes, and excretes a drug.[102,103] The aging process alters various gastrointestinal properties, such as the gastric pH level, which can alter the ionization or solubility of a drug and hence its absorption (Table 51-5).[101,102]

Drug distribution depends on body composition, as well as the physiochemical properties of the drug. With advancing age, fat content increases and intracellular water concentration decreases, which can alter the drug disposition.[102] For example, because of the increase in the ratio of body fat content to body weight, lipophilic drugs have a greater volume of distribution per body weight in elderly persons, as compared with younger adults. Other age-related factors affecting drug disposition are listed in Table 51-5.

As noted previously, the senescent liver has a decreased ability to metabolize drugs, which also affects the clearance of some drugs. For example, there is a reduced clearance of loop diuretics in elderly patients, which reduces the peak plasma concentration of the diuretic, as well as decreases the magnitude of the diuretic response.[105] Other drugs—such as angiotensin

Table 51-5 Age-related changes in pharmacokinetics

Pharmacokinetic parameters	Definitions	Age-related changes
Absorption	Receptor-coupled or diffusional uptake of drug into tissue	Decreased absorptive surface area of small intestine Decrease in splanchnic blood flow Increase in gastric acid pH Decrease in gastrointestinal motility
Distribution	Theoretic space (tissue) or body compartment into which free form of drug distributes	Decreased lean body mass and total body water Increased total body fat Decreased serum albumin level Increased $alpha_1$-acid glycoprotein
Metabolism	Chemical change in drug that renders it active or inactive	Decreased liver mass Decrease in activity of microsomal drug-metabolizing enzyme system Decrease in total liver blood flow
Excretion	Removal of drug through an eliminating organ, which is often the kidney; some drugs are excreted in the bile or feces, in the saliva, or via the lungs	Decreased renal blood flow and GFR Decrease in distal renal tubular secretory function

From Gilman and others, editors: *Goodman and Gilman's the pharmacological basis of therapeutics*, London, 1990, Pergamon Press, and Vestal RE, Cusack BJ: Pharmacology and aging. In Schneider EL, Rowe JW, editors: *Handbook of the biology of aging*, San Diego, 1990, Academic Press.

II–converting enzyme (ACE) inhibitors—have delayed excretion, increased serum concentration, and more prolonged duration of action, because they are excreted by GFR.[106] GFR progressively decreases with aging. See Table 51-5 for age-related changes in drug pharmacokinetics and Table 51-6 for the potential side effects, nursing interventions, and/or special considerations for frequently-used pharmacologic agents in the elderly patient in the critical care unit.

There are reports of age-related changes in pharmacodynamics. Pharmacodynamics refers to the pharmacologic or physiologic response to a drug that occurs after the drug interacts with its receptor on the plasma membrane. The chronotropic and inotropic effects of beta-adrenergic agonists reportedly decrease in elderly patients.[112,113] There also are reports that age produces no change in heparin-stimulated increases in partial thromboplastin time, whereas there is a diminished effect of coumadin (less of an increase in the prothrombin time). See Schwertz and Bushmann[103] for an extensive review of the pharmacologic considerations for the elderly patient in the critical care unit.

THE CENTRAL NERVOUS SYSTEM

In some individuals, aging is associated with such changes in cognitive function as impairments in short-term memory, speed of cognitive processing, and verbal intelligence. Some elderly people also experience changes in sensorimotor function; for example, vision and hearing are less acute and gait may become slightly unsteady. It is thought that some of these changes may be related to the numerous structural and morphologic changes that occur within the brain with advancing age.[114]

The changes in neurologic function generally do not interfere with the elderly person's ability to carry out activities of daily living. However, neurologic disorders—such as Alzheimer's disease, stroke, and Parkinson's disease—account for almost 50% of the functional incapacity experienced by elderly persons.[114,115] As with other aging processes, the onset of age-associated changes in neurologic function occur at different rates and may be exaggerated by the coexistence of other neurologic disorders or nutritional alterations. In addition, some older adults may experience little or no neurologic deficit or decline in cognitive or memory function. Finally, with advanced age (over 85 years of age), it also becomes difficult to distinguish between normal and disease-associated changes in neurologic functioning.[115]

Changes in Structure and Morphology

The brain decreases approximately 20% in size between 25 and 95 years of age (Fig. 51-2).[114] The reduced brain weight may be related in part to the overall decrease in the number of neurons that occurs with advancing age. Neurons are lost from the hippocampus, amygdala, and cerebellum, and such areas of the brainstem as the locus ceruleus, the dorsal motor nucleus of the vagus, and substantia nigra.[114,116] This is in contrast to such areas as the hypothalamus, where very few neurons disappear with advancing age.[114] In addition, portions of the cerebral cortex atrophy, principally the frontal and temporal cortical association areas (the superior frontal gyrus and superior temporal gyrus, respectively).[115]

The cerebral ventricles enlarge and develop an asymmetric appearance.[117] Cerebrospinal fluid (CSF) also accumulates in the ventricles; however, total brain CSF is not increased.[117]

Accompanying the loss of neurons are changes in the

ultrastructure and intracellular structures of the neuron.[116] The neuron is composed of a cell body, dendrite, and axon. Dendrites are long, spiny processes extending out from the cell body. One of the most ubiquitous changes in the aging brain is a decrease in the number of dendrite spines. Interestingly, between middle and late old age the length of the dendritic spines increases, but then decreases after late old age (over 90 years).[114] There are also reports of large neuron shrinking and degenerative changes occurring in the cell bodies and axons of certain acetylcholine secreting neurons. These changes may affect the transmitting and processing of sensory and motor information, thereby affecting learning, memory, and other complex, integrative intellectual functions.[114]

With advancing age, lipofuscins, neuritic plaques, and neurofibrillary bodies appear within the cytoplasm of the neuron.[114] Lipofuscins, or age pigment, are granules containing a dark fluorescent pigment. They are derived from lipid-rich membranes that have been partially disintegrated and oxidized. It is still not clear whether lipofuscin accumulation is harmful to the brain.[114]

Neuritic, or senile, plaques are aggregates of the beta-amyloid protein, and they also accumulate in the brain of normal senescent persons. Neuritic plaques are found in the hippocampus, cerebral cortex, and other brain regions.[114] However, large numbers of neuritic plaques are also found in the brains of patients with Alzheimer's disease.[114] Neurofibrillary tangles, which are bundles of helically wound protein filaments, occur in the hippocampus with advancing age in healthy persons.[115] However, they are present in larger numbers in persons with such neuropathologic disorders as Alzheimer's disease. It has been suggested that neurofibrillary tangles could interfere with neuronal signaling.[114]

In the senescent brain, synaptogensis (synaptic regeneration) still occurs after partial nerve degeneration.[118] After a nerve fiber is damaged, neighboring undamaged neurons often sprout new fibers and form new connections. However, synaptogensis occurs at a slower rate in the older brain.[118]

Neurotransmitter Synthesis

Advancing age is associated with changes in neurotransmitter function. Altered neurotransmitter function can result from changes in the available precursors for neurotransmitter synthesis, changes in the neurotransmitter receptor, and changes in the activity of the enzymes that synthesize and degrade the neurotransmitter. Investigating neurotransmitter levels and turnover is complex, and results from studies have differed, depending on the medium (tissue or body fluid) and experimental technique used to quantify the neurotransmitters.[119] For example, in some studies, neurotransmitters have been quantified by measuring (1) the concentration of the neurotransmitter, (2) the breakdown or activation products and (3) the activity of the enzyme responsible for the synthesis or breakdown of the neurotransmitter. Following is a brief summary of age-related changes in these established neurotransmitters: acetylcholine (ACh), dopamine (DA), norepinephrine (NE), and serotonin (5-HT).

ACh and DA are the most frequently studied neurotransmitters. With advancing age, the effect of ACh in the CNS and the number of muscarinic receptors are both reduced.[120] DA levels in both the human and rat brain diminish with aging.[120] DA is the precursor for NE, and because of this, synthesis of NE may be affected by aging. However, there are reports of no change, and specifically no decrease, in NE. DA and ACh are also altered in two major age-related neurodegenerative disorders: Alzheimer's disease and Parkinson's disease. There are also reports of no change and decreases in 5-HT levels.[120]

These neurotransmitters have many functions within the CNS and are localized in different areas of the brain. Gottstein and Held[121] suggested that age-related changes in neurotransmitter levels may cause a "desynchronization" in neurotransmission, thereby affecting many neurologic functions.

Cerebral Metabolism and Blood Flow

Cerebral blood flow (CBF) decreases with advancing age. This decrease parallels the decrease in brain weight and is most likely caused by the reduction in neuronal number and metabolic needs of the cerebral tissue.[122]

PHYSICAL EXAMINATION AND DIAGNOSTIC PROCEDURES

The various physiologic changes that occur with aging warrant special physical examination techniques. The clinician must distinguish between changes in health caused by physiologic versus pathologic processes; therefore the nurse must ensure that the physical examination is conducted under optimal conditions. When beginning a physical examination, the clinician needs to consider the ability of the gerontologic patient to cooperate and hear, as well as his or her activity level. In addition, the patient's comfort and energy levels must be considered. Before beginning an examination, the nurse must ensure that the room's noise level and temperature and the patient's position in the bed are optimal and comfortable.[123]

Head and Neck

Normal funduoscopic findings include a diminished pupillary response to penlight, a decrease in near and peripheral vision, and loss of visual acuity to dim light. These changes result from an increase in opacity of the lens and decrease in ciliary movement.[126] It is not uncommon to find irises that are pale blue or light gray in color, stemming from a decrease in melanocyte production.[124] Around the periphery of the iris, fat deposits may also be found, which is referred to as *arcus senilis.* The eyes also may appear sunken or recessed, because of a loss of subcutaneous tissue. These clinical manifestations may also be signs of dehydration; however, in elderly persons, these are normal findings. The pupils may appear small, which can be unrelated to changes in neurologic status or medication administration. The pupil at age 60 is one third the size of a pupil at age 20.[124] Patients may complain of dry, itching eyes, which results from a decrease in lacrimal activity.[124] Less remarkable deficits are noted in gerontologic patients'

Table 51-6 Pharmacologic agents used in the critical care unit and frequent side effects experienced by the gerontologic patient

Pharmacologic agent	Drug actions	Adverse drug effects*	Nursing interventions and/or special considerations
ACE INHIBITORS			
Enalapril	Inhibits the conversion of angiotensin I to angiotensin II	Hypotension, especially in patients taking diuretics Hypokalemia	Monitor HR and BP. Monitor serum creatinine level. Monitor serum K^+ level. Excreted by the kidney so the dosage should be reduced if the GFR is reduced.
DIURETICS			
Lasix	Inhibits Na^+ and Cl^- absorption from the proximal tubule and loop of Henle	Hypokalemia Volume depletion	Reduced rate of clearance and magnitude of the diuretic response.
CARDIAC GLYCOSIDES			
Digoxin	Inhibits the sarcolemmal Na^+K^+-ATPase	Digitalis toxicity	Monitor HR and serum K^+ and serum digoxin levels. Verapamil, quinidine, and amidarone increase serum digoxin levels.
ANTIDYSRRHYTHMICS			
Procainamide	Decreases myocardial conduction velocity and excitability and prolongs myocardial refractoriness	Procainamide toxicity	Procainamide is converted to its active metabolite N-acetyl-procainamide (NAPA) in the liver. NAPA may accumulate and cause side effects, even though the procainamide plasma level is within therapeutic range.
Lidocaine	Decreases automaticity (especially in Purkinje fibers) and prolongs conduction and refractoriness	Dizziness, paresthesia, and drowsiness at lower plasma concentrations	Can be administered only parenterally.
CALCIUM CHANNEL BLOCKERS			
Verapamil	Blocks the entry of Ca^{2+} through voltage-dependent Ca^{2+} chan- nels and decreases SA automaticity and AV conduction	Constipation May alter liver function	Monitor liver function tests. Contraindicated in heart failure, sick sinus syndrome, or first-degree AV block.
Nifedipine	Same as verapamil	Headaches, tachycardia, palpitations, flushing, and ankle edema	Calcium channel blockers have a negative inotropic effect, but nifedipine produces less of a negative inotropic effect as compared with verapamil.
Diltiazem	Same as verapamil	Constipation	Monitor liver function tests. Contraindicated in heart failure, sick sinus syndrome, or first-degree AV block.

From Creasy WA and others: *J Clin pharmacol* 26:264, 1986; Gilman AG and others, editors: *Goodman and Gilman's the pharmacological basis of therapeutics*, London, 1990, Pergamon Press; Hockings N, Ajayi AA, Reid JL: *Br J Pharmacol* 21:341, 1986; Lynch RA, Horowitz LN: *Geriatrics* 46:41, 1991; Pederson KE: *Acta Med Scand* 697(suppl 1):1, 1985; Vidt GD, Borazanian RA: *Geriatrics* 46:28, 1991; Wall RT: *Clin Geriatr Med* 6:345, 1990; and Watters JM, McClaran JC: The elderly surgical patient. In Wilmore DW and others, editors: *In care of the surgical patient*, vol III, Special problems, New York, 1990, Scientific American.

*Not all side effects are listed for each drug.

BP, blood pressure; *SA*, sinus node; *AV*, atrioventricular node; *CNS*, central nervous system; *GFR*, glomerular filtration rate; *HR*, heart rate; *ACE*, angiotensin II–converting enzyme.

Table 51-6 Pharmacologic agents used in the critical care unit and frequent side effects experienced by the gerontologic patient—cont'd

Pharmacologic agent	Drug actions	Adverse drug effects*	Nursing interventions and/or special considerations
NARCOTIC ANALGESICS			
Demerol	Blocks the transmission of pain and inhibits the release of substance P; site of action is within the CNS	Respiratory depression and oversedation Tremors and muscle twitches related to effects of the metabolite normeperidine	Accumulation of normeperidine can produce CNS hyperexcitability.
Morphine	Synthetic analgesic; mechanism similar to demerol	Respiratory depression and oversedation	The volume of distribution for morphine is small; hence plasma and tissue levels are greater at a specific plasma concentration.

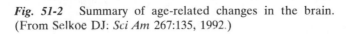

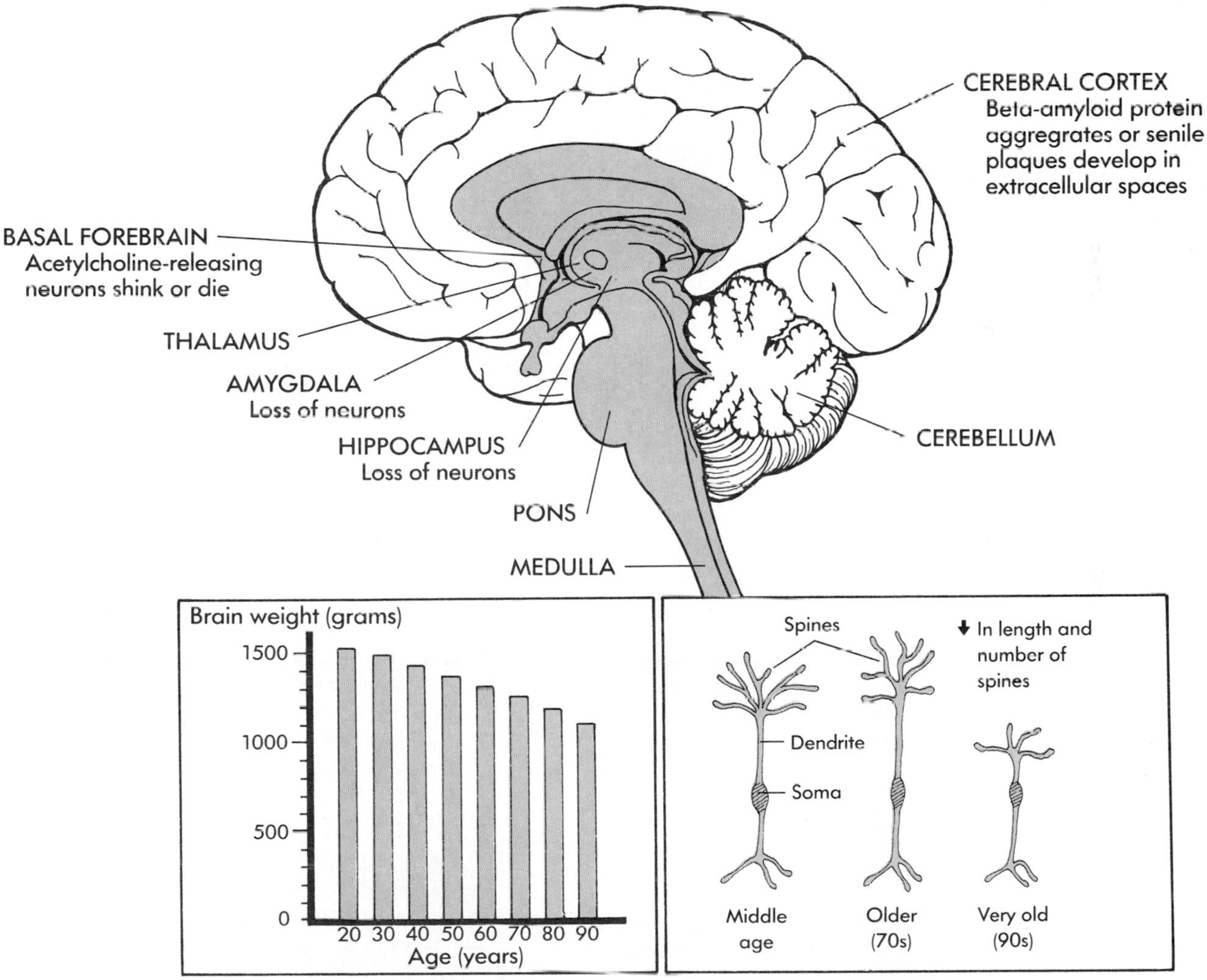

Fig. 51-2 Summary of age-related changes in the brain. (From Selkoe DJ: *Sci Am* 267:135, 1992.)

olfactory and gustatory senses.[125,126] However, they do report a lack of enjoyment at mealtime or lack of ability to taste flavor in food.[127]

Loss of dentition is not a normal process of aging. It indicates poor nutrition and/or poor oral hygiene. Elderly patients frequently experience gradual hearing loss.[128] On physical examination, the elderly person may have a reduced ability to distinguish low and high sounds and have difficulty in understanding high-pitched and rushed speech. The hearing loss is related to atrophy of the auditory nerve and the organ of Corti.[128]

Integumentary and Musculoskeletal Systems

As noted previously, the loss of elastic and connective tissue causes the skin to wrinkle; both skin wrinkles and sagging may be found over many areas of the body. The appearance and number of skin wrinkles also depends greatly on environmental agents and exposure to ultraviolet rays.[129] The nurse will also find that underlying structures, such as the veins and muscles, are more visible because of the transparency of the skin. Because of the loss of skin turgor, especially in the hands, the nurse should assess for dehydration by pinching the skin tissue over the sternum or forehead. (See Table 51-7 for age-related changes in the skin and underlying mechanisms.)

The nurse may also find multiple ecchymotic areas, because of decreased protective subcutaneous tissue layers, increased capillary fragility, and flattening of the capillary bed, which predisposes elderly persons to developing ecchymosis.[130-132] In conjunction with frequent aspirin use, these physiologic factors result in increased bleeding tendencies and the appearance of ecchymotic areas. However, areas of ecchymosis may also indicate elder abuse. The nurse should assess for discrepancies between the patient's history and physical findings. Patients at high risk for abuse are those who require maximal physical assistance in the home setting.[133] Caregiver frustration may be expressed by physical assault.

Changes that occur in the musculoskeletal system are a decrease in lean body mass; a compression of the spinal column, which results from the thinning of cartilage between vertebra; and a decrease in the mobility of skeletal joints.[133] Despite the ubiquitous finding of reduced joint mobility, no exact physiologic process gives rise to the altered mobility. It is possible that the reduced synovial fluid production that occurs with aging causes changes in function. There is also an increase in muscle rigidity, especially in the neck, shoulders, hips, and knees.[133] These may produce some changes in range of motion.

Bone demineralization afflicts both men and women as they age; however, it occurs 4 times more frequently in women than in men. Bone demineralization refers to an increase in osteoplast and osteoclast activity, which decreases calcium absorption into the bone.[134] Mineral loss (calcium and phosphorous), along with a decrease in bone mass, is referred to as *osteoporosis.*[134] Osteoporosis produces bones that are more "porous" or fragile. With extensive bone demineralization, an elderly patient may sustain multiple fractures. There is an accelerated incidence of osteoporosis in women, which occurs after the onset of menopause. A decrease in estrogen is implicated in this process, because estrogen replacement may arrest the osteoporosis process (although it will not

Table 51-7 Age-related changes in the integumentary system

Skin problems	Nursing interventions	Rationale
Delayed wound healing	Use nonrestrictive dressings. Weigh patient daily. Support nutritional needs.	↓ Vascular supply to dermis ↓ Connective tissue layer ↓ SQ tissue layer Impaired inflammatory response ↓ New connective tissue proliferation
Thermoregulation	Monitor room temperature.	↓ SQ tissue layer ↓ Number of capillary arterioles supplying skin ↓ Number of eccrine (sweat) glands
Pressure ulcers	Reposition patient every 2 hours. Use pressure-relieving devices.	↓ Flattening of capillary bed ↓ Thinning of epidermis
IV infiltrations	Monitor peripheral IV site hourly. Discontinue IV at first sign of infiltration.	↓ Connective tissue layer Vascular fragility
Diminished skin turgor	Bathe with tepid water. Avoid use of deodorant soap.	↓ Connective tissue layer ↓ Eccrine and sebaceous gland activity

CBC, complete blood cell count; *IV*, intravenous; *SQ*, subcutaneous.

reverse the process). The exact mechanism whereby estrogen affects bone mass is unknown, but recently estrogen receptors have been found on human osteoblasts.[134] Decreased intake of dietary calcium, immobility, excess glucocorticoid secretion, and smoking all contribute to the development of osteoporosis.

Respiratory and Cardiovascular Systems

Many of the physiologic changes that occur with aging and the mechanisms underlying them have been addressed previously. The physical correlates to these changes are only noted in this section. On inspection of the aging thorax, the nurse will find a greater anterior-posterior diameter and some degree of kyphosis. On initial auscultation, bibasilar crackles may be heard; however, with several deep breaths and coughing they should be cleared. Bibasilar crackles that do not clear with deep inspirations are suggestive of pathology. There is also a diminished cough reflex, which predisposes the elderly patient to aspiration. No changes are noted with palpation, but the nurse should assess for areas of tenderness, which could be the result of old fractures. With percussion there is increased resonance. Changes in tests of pulmonary function are noted in Tables 51-3 and 51-4.

There are relatively few modifications in the assessment of cardiovascular function and age-related physical findings in the elderly patient. As noted earlier, resting heart rate decreases and systolic blood pressure increases with age. Blood pressure should be taken in both arms, and both pressure determinations should be recorded. If there are large differences in these blood pressure measurements, the higher blood pressure is considered to be more reliable.

Gastrointestinal and Renal Systems

On physical examination of the nonobese elderly patient, the abdominal organs are more easily palpated because of a decrease in subcutaneous tissue. Despite a change in gastrointestinal (GI) motility, bowel sounds are normoactive. There are no remarkable physical assessment considerations with the hepatic-biliary and renal systems and no age-related change in liver function tests.

Blood urea nitrogen (BUN) and serum creatinine levels can be normal or decreased in elderly patients (see box on right). As noted earlier, the glomerular filtration rate (GFR) decreases with age. In the hospital the GFR is estimated by the creatinine clearance. Endogenous creatinine is a metabolic by-product of muscle metabolism that is excreted by the kidney and is not reabsorbed. Usually the creatinine clearance is estimated by collecting a 24-hour urine sample to measure creatinine excretion. With advancing age, muscle mass decreases, thereby reducing the renal load of serum concentration of creatinine. Therefore, in the geriatric patient, neither the creatinine excreted nor the plasma creatinine level may reflect the change in GFR. In elderly patients, the Cockroft-Gault equation often is used to assess creatinine clearance (CrCl) and GFR (ml/min), because it incorporates serum creatinine levels, body weight, age, and gender as variables.[77] The Cockroft-Gault equation is as follows:

$$\text{CrCl (ml/min)} = \frac{\begin{array}{c}(140 - \text{age}) \times \text{Weight (kg)}\\ \text{(multiply by 0.85 for women)}\end{array}}{(72 \times \text{Serum creatinine level [m/dl]})}$$

The box below also lists the effects of aging on other laboratory tests that may or may not have clinical significance.[135]

Neurologic System

Physical examination of the neurologic system begins with a review of the elderly patient's mental status. The nurse assesses the patient's level of consciousness, ability to communicate and follow commands, and short-term and long-term memory. In the critical care unit, parameters may be altered by hypoxia, electrolyte imbalances, or various medications. The practitioner may observe that the patient occasionally forgets minor details. Forgetfulness of important information—such as name, address, and marital status—is *not* part of the normal aging process. Although some elderly patients may have problems with short-term memory, long-term memory should still be intact. Elderly persons are frequently labeled "demented" or "confused." These cognitive

EFFECTS OF AGING ON VARIOUS LABORATORY VALUES

VALUES THAT DO NOT CHANGE WITH AGE

Hemoglobin/hematocrit
Platelet count
White blood cell count with differential
Serum electrolytes
Coagulation profile
Liver function tests
Thyroid function tests
↔ or ↓ Blood urea nitrogen
↔ or ↓ Creatinine

VALUES THAT CHANGE WITH AGE BUT HAVE LITTE CLINICAL SIGNIFICANCE

↓ Calcium
↑ Uric acid

VALUES THAT CHANGE WITH AGE AND HAVE CLINICAL SIGNIFICANCE

↓ Erythrocyte sedimentation rate
↓ Arterial oxygen pressure
↑ Blood glucose
↓ or ↑ Serum lipid profile
↓ Albumin

From Duthie EH, Abbasi AA: *Geriatrics* 46:41, 1991.
↓, decrease; ↑, increase; ↔ no change.

syndromes have different etiologies and are not a normal part of aging. See Foreman, Gillies, and Wagner[136] for further review of impaired cognition in the elderly patient.

The neurologic examination for the geriatric patient should always include an assessment of muscle strength, reflexes, sensation, and cranial nerves.[137] There may be some changes in fine and gross motor skills. Handgrip strength declines with age and may correlate with a decreased ability to perform fine motor activity (e.g., tying a shoelace). Age diminishes the elderly patient's vibratory sense, primarily in the lower extremities. Reflexes are slowed, which is caused by neuronal loss.[137] Neurologic deficits may ultimately alter the patient's ability to perform self-care. In addition, changes in the elderly patients' cognitive function may alter their ability to follow instructions and interpret patient-teaching instructions regarding their care in the critical care unit. Also, the critical care nurse should evaluate the patient's gait if the patient is ambulatory.

SUMMARY

The elderly patient requires more intense observation and consideration in the critical care unit, because his or her system has become less adaptable to stress and illness. Table 51-8 summarizes the major changes in the various systems, along with clinical considerations.[138] As shown in Fig. 51-3, many physiologic changes occur with advancing age and each change may render a particular system less adaptable to stress. In addition, the change in one system may affect another system in the presence of disease.

The critical care nurse must also be aware of socioeconomic factors that confront elderly patients, as well as life-style adjustments, such as the death of a spouse or friend. Changes in Medicare payment for hospitalization and medication have also placed a financial burden on such patients. To provide the best care and prevent iatrogenic complications, the critical care nurse must consider all physiologic and psychologic factors that affect the elderly patient.

THE USE OF PHYSICAL RESTRAINTS ON ELDERLY PATIENTS IN THE CRITICAL CARE UNIT

Physical restraints are commonly used in the critical care unit to reduce the risk of injury to the sick, elderly patient or to prevent the patient from prematurely removing pacemakers, Swan-Ganz catheters, and so on. Physical restraints may be used in young, as well as elderly, patients. However, Catchen[139] found that physical restraints were more frequently used in elderly patients.

Previously, the most common rationale for the use of physical restraints was the prevention of injury to self or others.[140] More recently, Kapp[141] reported that nurses most often decide to restrain patients because of potential litigation resulting from injuries associated with falls or the premature removal of facilitative treatments. Among elderly people, falls represent a primary cause of injury, disability, and death.[142] Elderly patients experience the largest percentage of these falls in institutions, and the most frequent site is at the bedside.[142]

Nurses can use restraints intermittently, depending on the patient's level of alertness, or nurses can chronically restrain the patient. Interestingly, patients who were chronically restrained fell more frequently than did those who were not, because the restraints produced more agitation and combative behavior.[140] In addition, several investigators report that patients lose their balance and steadiness and develop elimination problems when restraints are used.[140,143] Of particular interest to critical care nurses is that elderly restrained patients are predisposed to aspiration pneumonia,[144] circulatory obstruction,[145] circulatory stress,[146] dehydration,[147] and orthostatic hypotension.[148] Other potential problems include discomfort, weakening and contracture of the affected limb, pressure sores, diminished respiratory excursion, and possible death from strangulation.[140]

Interestingly, once the medical order to use physical restraints is obtained, it is seldom discontinued. Restraints may magnify the patient's fear of losing control, diminish his or her sense of dignity, and distort others' future perceptions of the patient's mental competence.

Considering these deleterious effects of physical restraints, critical care nurses must carefully consider the risks and benefits of restraints. For example, it is well recognized that premature removal of an arterial balloon pump catheter may produce excessive bleeding and cardiogenic shock. The best alternative to the use of physical restraints is continuous surveillance. However, this is not always feasible in a critical care unit, because of sudden emergencies or staffing conditions.

Protecting the patient from falls or inappropriate removal of treatments, such as catheters and intravenous tubing, can be achieved by limiting the movement of the patient's limbs or torso with the use of soft wrist/ankle restraints and a posey jacket, respectively. The nurse should observe the patient frequently and listen to his or her concerns. The call light should be within the patient's reach, and the nurse should encourage family and friends to visit frequently. In the event that physical restraints are deemed necessary, it is important to follow the institution's policy regarding the use of physical restraints. In addition, the nurse should release the restraints every hour to check color, motor skills, and sensation of torso and extremities and make an ongoing assessment about the necessity of using the restraints.

Table 51-8 Summary of age-related physiologic changes and related clinical considerations

Age-related effects	Clinical considerations
CARDIOVASCULAR SYSTEM	
↓ Inotropic and chronotropic response of myocardium to catecholamine stimulation	The increase in CO achieved during stress or exercise is achieved by an increase in diastolic filling (increased dependence on Starling's law of the heart)
↑ Myocardial collagen content	Leads to a decrease in the compliance of the ventricle (higher filling pressures are needed to maintain stroke volume)
↓ Baroreceptor sensitivity	↑ Tendency for orthostatic hypotension after prolonged bed rest, or if patient is taking antihypertensive medication or has systolic hypertension
Prolonged rate of relaxation	May predispose the elderly patient to hemodynamic derangements in the presence of tachydysrhythmias, hypertension, or ischemic heart disease
↓ Compliance of blood vessels	↑ Peripheral vascular resistance and blood pressure
RESPIRATORY SYSTEM	
↓ Strength of the respiratory muscles, recoil of lungs, chest wall compliance, and efficiency and number of cilia in airways	↑ Susceptibility to aspiration, atelectasis, and pulmonary infection Patient may require more frequent deep breathing, coughing, and position change
↓ Pa_{O_2} level	↓ Ventilatory response to hypoxia and hypercapnia ↑ Sensitivity to narcotics
RENAL SYSTEM	
↓ GFR	Careful observation of patient when administering aminoglycosides, antibiotics, and contrast dyes
↓ Ability to concentrate and conserve water	May predispose patient to development of dehydration and hypernatremia, especially if patient is fluid restricted and insensible losses are high (e.g., during mechanical ventilation or fever)
↓ Ability to excrete salt and water loads, as well as urea, ammonia, and drugs	Observe for clinical manifestations of fluid overload and drug reactions
↓ Response to an acid load	After an acid load (i.e., metabolic acidosis) the elderly patient may be in a state of uncompensated metabolic acidosis for a longer period
LIVER	
↓ Total liver blood flow	Adverse drug reactions, especially with polypharmacy
GASTROINTESTINAL SYSTEM	
Diminished ability to swallow	May predispose elderly patient to aspiration pneumonia Assess for proper fit of dentures and ability to chew Flex head forward 45 degrees
Impaired esophageal motility	Develop awareness for complaints of food or medications "sticking in throat" Assess for complaints of heartburn or epigastric discomfort Avoid prolonged supine position
Delayed emptying of liquids	Examine abdomen for distention Investigate complaints of anorexia
↓ Stool weight and transit time	Obtain thorough bowel history, and note routine use of laxatives Increase intake of dietary fiber, and assess for fecal incontinence and impaction
NEUROLOGIC SYSTEM	
↑ In cranial dead space	Elderly persons may sustain a significant amount of hemorrhage before symptoms are apparent
↓ In number of neurons and dendrites and length of dendrite spines	Delayed or impaired processing of sensory and motor information
Delay in the rate of synaptogenesis	
Changes in neurotransmitter turnover	May cause desynchronization of neurotransmission

Modified from Rebenson-Piano M: *Crit Care Q* 12:1, 1989.
GFR, glomerular filtration rate; *CO*, cardiac output; *Pa_{O_2}*, arterial oxygen.

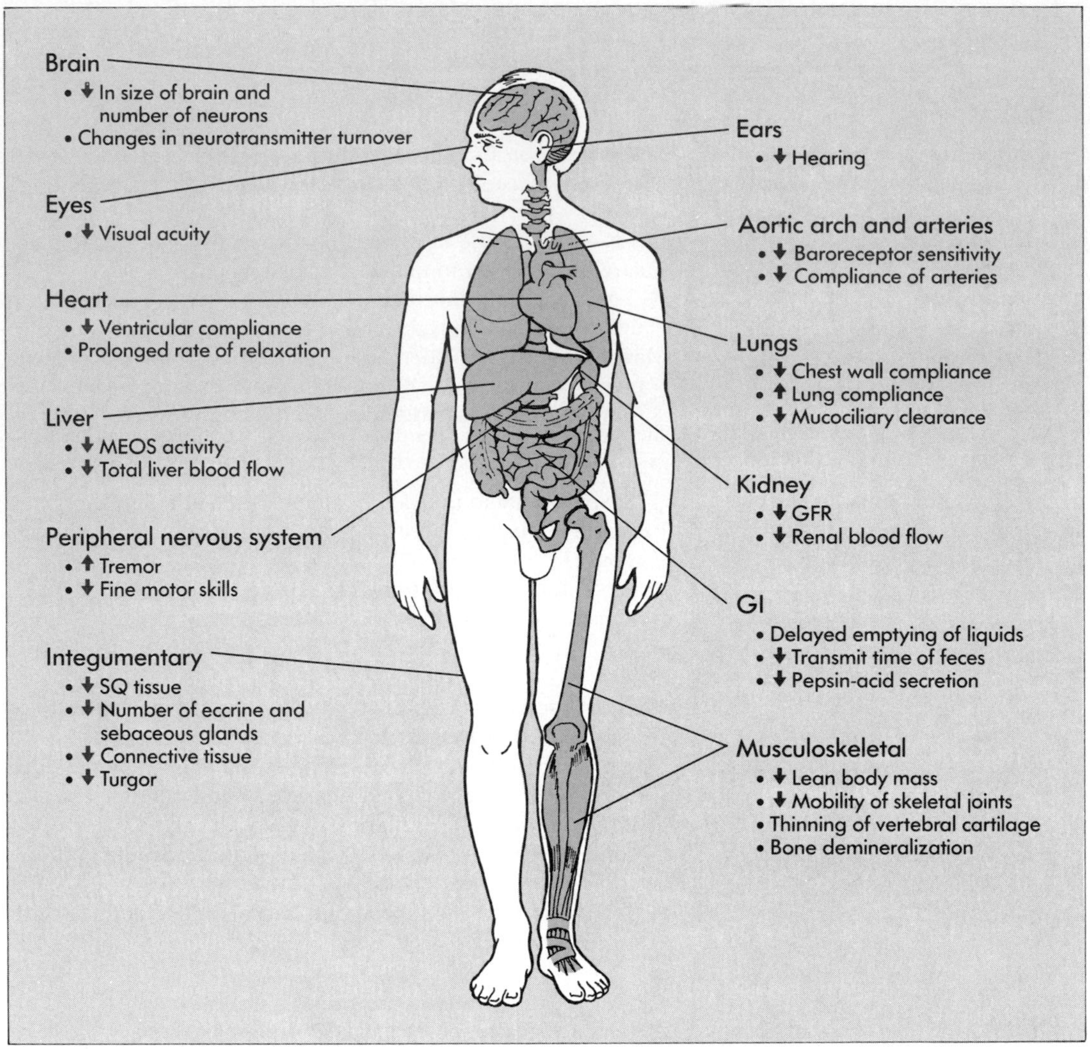

Fig. 51-3 Summary of the physiologic changes that occur in all systems and that the critical care nurse should consider in caring for the elderly patient in the critical care unit. NOTE: *MEOS,* microsomal enzyme oxidative system; *GFR,* glomerular filtration rate; *GI,* gastrointestinal.

REFERENCES

1. Munoz E and others: Diagnosis-related groups, costs, and outcome for patients in the intensive care unit, *Heart Lung* 18(6):627, 1989.
2. Henning RJ and others: Clinical characteristics and resource utilization of ICU patients: implications for organization of intensive care, *Crit Care Med* 15(3):264, 1987.
3. Brock DB, Guralnik JM, Brody JA: Demography and epidemiology of aging in the United States. In Schneider EL, Rowe JW, editors: *Handbook of the biology of aging,* New York, 1990, Academic Press.
4. National Center for Health Statistics Health, United States, Hyattsville, MD, 1991, Public Health Service.
5. Rudman D, Cohan ME: Nutritional causes of renal impairment in old age, *Am J Kidney Dis* 16(4):289, 1990.
6. Abrass IB: Biology of aging. In Wilson JD and others, editors: *Harrison's principles of internal medicine,* New York, 1991, McGraw-Hill.
7. Abrams WB: Cardiovascular drugs in the elderly, *Chest* 98:980, 1990.
8. NIH Extramural Programs, U.S. Department of Health and Human Services National Institutes of Health, Bethesda, MD, 1988, Public Health Service.
9. Weisfeldt ML, Lakatta EG, Gerstenblith G: Aging and the heart. In Braunwald E, editor: *Heart disease,* Philadelphia, 1992, WB Saunders.
10. Eghbali M and others: Collagen accumulation in heart ventricles as a function of growth and aging, *Cardiovasc Res* 23:723, 1989.
11. Wegelius O, von Knorring J: The hydroxyproline and hexosamine content in human myocardium at different ages, *Acta Med Scand Suppl* 412:233, 1964.
12. Katz AM: Heart failure. In Fozzard HA and others, editors: *The heart and cardiovascular system,* New York, 1991, Raven Press.
13. Muller RT and others: Painless myocardial infarction in the elderly, *Am Heart J* 119:202, 1990.
14. Mukerji V, Holman AJ, Alpert MA: The clinical description of angina pectoris in the elderly, *Am Heart J* 117:705, 1989.
15. Gerstenblith G and others: Echocardiographic assessment of normal adult aging population, *Circulation* 56:273, 1977.
16. Walsh RA: Cardiovascular effects of the aging process, *Am J Med* 82:34, 1987.

17. Capasso JM and others: Effects of age on mechanical and electrical performance of rat myocardium, *Am J Physiol* 245:H72, 1983.
18. Wei JY, Spurgeon HA, Lakatta EG: Excitation-contraction in rat myocardium; alterations with adult aging, *Am J Physiol* 246:H784, 1984.
19. Opie LH: *The physiology of the heart and metabolism,* New York, 1991, Raven Press.
20. Lakatta EG and others: Prolonged contraction duration in the aged myocardium, *J Clin Invest* 55:61, 1975.
21. Spurgeon HA, Steinbach MF, Lakatta EG: Prolonged contraction duration in senescent myocardium is prevented by exercise, *Am J Physiol* 244:H513, 1983.
22. Froehlich JP and others: Studies of sarcoplasmic reticulum function and contraction in young and aged rat myocardium, *J Mol Cell Cardiol* 10:427, 1978.
23. Maciel LM and others: Age-induced decreases in the messenger RNA coding for the sarcoplasmic reticulum Ca^{2+}-ATPase of the rat heart, *Circ Res* 67(1):230, 1990.
24. Bonow RO and others: Effects of aging on asynchronous left ventricular regional function and global ventricular filling in normal human subjects, *J Am Coll Cardiol* 11:50, 1988.
25. Miller TR and others: Left ventricular diastolic filling and its association with age, *Am J Cardiol* 58:531, 1986.
26. Bachman S, Sparrow D, Smith LK: Effect of aging on the electrocardiogram, *Am J Cardiol* 48:513, 1981.
27. Alberts B and others: *Molecular biology of the cell,* New York, 1989, Garland Publishing.
28. Capasso JM and others: Myocardial biochemical, contractile and electrical performance following imposition of hypertension in young and old rats, *Circ Res* 57:445, 1986.
29. Effron MB and others: Changes in myosin isoenzymes, ATPase activity, and contraction duration in rat cardiac muscle with aging can be modulated by thyroxine, *Circ Res* 60:238, 1987.
30. Cinelli P and others: Effects of age on mean heart rate variability, *Age* 10:146, 1987.
31. Ribera JM and others: Cardiac rate and hyperkinetic rhythm disorders in healthy elderly subjects: evaluation by ambulatory electrocardiographic monitoring, *Gerontology* 35:158, 1989.
32. Jose AD: Effect of combined sympathetic and parasympathetic blockage on heart rate and cardiac function in man, *Am J Cardiol* 18:476, 1966.
33. Lakatta EG: Heart and circulation. In Schneider EL, Rowe JW, editors: *Handbook of the biology of aging,* San Diego, 1990, Academic Press.
34. Frolkis VV and others: Contractile function and Ca^{2+} transport system of myocardium in ageing, *Gerontology* 34:64, 1988.
35. Rodeheffer RJ and others: Exercise cardiac output is maintained with advancing age in human subjects: cardiac dilation and increased stroke volume compensate for a diminished heart rate, *Circulation* 69:203, 1984.
36. Kennedy RD, Caird FI: Physiology of heart. In Noble RJ, Rothbaum RA, editors: *Geriatric cardiology,* Philadelphia, 1981, FA Davis.
37. Horwitz LN, Lynch RA: Managing geriatric arrhythmias. I. General considerations, *Geriatrics* 46:31, 1991.
38. Camm AJ and others: The rhythm of the heart in active elderly subjects, *Am Heart J* 99:598, 1980.
39. Fleg JL, Kennedy HL: Cardiac arrhythmias in a healthy elderly population detection by a 24-hour ambulatory electrocardiography, *Chest* 81:302, 1982.
40. Docherty JR: Cardiovascular responses in ageing: a review, *Pharmacol Rev* 42:103, 1990.
41. Yin FCP and others: Age-associated decrease in ventricular response to haemodynamic stress during beta-adrenergic blockade, *Br Heart J* 40:1349, 1978.
42. Elliott HL and others: Effects of age in the responsiveness of vascular alpha-adrenoreceptors in man, *J Cardiovasc Pharmacol* 4:388, 1982.
43. Strogatz DS and others: Correlates of postural hypotension in a community sample of elderly blacks and whites, *J Am Geriatr Soc* 39:562, 1991.
44. Applegate WB and others: Prevalence of postural hypotension at baseline in the systolic hypertension in the elderly program (SHEP) cohort, *J Am Geriatr Soc* 39:1057, 1991.
45. Smith JJ and others: The effect of age on hemodynamic response to graded postural stress in normal men, *J Gerontol* 42:406, 1987.
46. Dambrink JHA, Wieling W: Circulatory response to postural change in healthy male subjects in relation to age, *Clin Sci* 72:335, 1987.
47. Lakatta EG and others: Diminished inotropic response of aged myocardium to catecholamines, *Circ Res* 36:262, 1975.
48. Guarnieri T and others: Contractile and biochemical correlates of beta adrenergic stimulation of the aged heart, *Am J Physiol* 239:H501, 1980.
49. Scarpace PJ: Decreased beta-adrenergic responsiveness during senescence, *Fed Proc* 45:51, 1986.
50. Martinez JL and others: Age-related changes in the catecholamine content of peripheral organs in male and female F344 rats, *J Gerontol* 36:280, 1981.
51. Daly RN, Goldberg PB, Roberts J: Effects of age on neurotransmission at the cardiac sympathetic neuroeffector junction, *J Pharmacol Exp Ther* 245:798, 1988.
52. Gerstenblith G and others: Diminished inotropic responsiveness to ouabain in aged rat myocardium, *Circ Res* 44:517, 1979.
53. Bierman EL: Arteriosclerosis and aging. In Finch CE, Schneider EL, editors: *Handbook of the biology of aging,* New York, 1985, Van Nostrand Reinhold.
54. Schoenberger JA: Epidemiology of systolic and diastolic systemic blood pressure elevation in the elderly, *Am J Cardiol* 57:45c, 1986.
55. Lawn RM: Lipoprotein(a) in heart disease, *Sci Am* 266:54, 1992.
56. Rowe JW: Clinical consequences of age-related impairments in vascular compliance, *Am J Cardiol* 60:68G, 1987.
57. Kreisberg RA, Kasim S: Cholesterol metabolism and aging, *Am J Med* 82:54, 1987.
58. Davis CE and others: Lipoprotein-cholesterol distributions in selected North American populations: the Lipid Research Clinics Program Prevalence Study, *Circulation* 2:302, 1980.
59. Rose BD: *Clinical physiology of acid-base and electrolyte disorders,* New York, 1989, McGraw-Hill.
60. Hall JE, Coleman TG, Guyton AC: The renin-angiotensin system: normal physiology and changes in older hypertensives, *J Am Geriatr Soc* 37:801, 1989.
61. Crane MG, Harris JJ: Effect of aging on renin activity and aldosterone excretion, *J Lab Clin Med* 87:947, 1976.
62. Sica DA, Harford A: Sodium and water disorders in the elderly. In Zawada ET, Sica DA, editors: *Geriatric nephrology and urology,* Littleton, Mass, 1985, PSG Publishing.
63. Webster JR, Kadah H: Unique aspects of respiratory disease in the aged, *Geriatrics* 46:31, 1991.
64. Thurlbeck WM: Growth, ageing and adaptation. In Murray JF, Nadel JA, editors: *Textbook of respiratory medicine,* Philadelphia, 1988, WB Saunders.
65. Levitzky MG: Effects of aging on the respiratory system, *Physiologist* 27:102, 1984.
66. Mittman C and others: Relationship between chest wall and pulmonary compliance and age, *J Appl Physiol* 20:1211, 1965.
67. West JB: *Respiratory physiology,* Baltimore, 1990, Williams & Wilkins.
68. Rizzato G, Marazzine L: Thoracoabdominal mechanisms in elderly men, *J Appl Physiol* 28:457, 1970.
69. Gutmann E, Hanzlikova V: Fast and slow motor units in ageing, *Gerontology* 22:280, 1976.

70. Pontoppidan HH, Beecher HK: Progressive loss of protective reflexes in the airway with advance of age, *JAMA* 1974:2209, 1960.
71. Belman MJ, Gaesser GA: Ventilatory muscle training in the elderly, *J Appl Physiol* 64:899, 1988.
72. Knudson RJ and others: Changes in the normal maximal expiratory flow-volume curve with growth and aging, *Am Rev Respir Dis* 127:725, 1983.
73. Turner JM, Mead J, Wohl ME: Elasticity of human lungs in relation to age, *J Appl Physiol* 25:664, 1968.
74. Pierce JA, Hocott JB: Studies on the collagen and elastin content of the human lung, *J Clin Invest* 39:8, 1960.
75. Pierce JA, Ebert RV: Fibrous network of the lung and its change with age, *Thorax* 20:469, 1965.
76. Semmens M: The pulmonary artery in the normal aged lung, *Br J Dis Chest* 64:65, 1970.
77. Sorbini CA and others: Arterial oxygen tension in relation to age in healthy subjects, *Respiration* 25:3, 1968.
78. LeBlanc P, Ruff F, Milic-Emili J: Effects of age and body position on "airway closure" in man, *J Appl Physiol* 28:448, 1970.
79. Holland J and others: Regional distribution of pulmonary ventilation and perfusion in elderly subjects, *J Clin Invest* 47:81, 1968.
80. Knudson RJ and others: Effect of aging alone on mechanical properties of the normal adult human lung, *J Appl Physiol* 43:1054, 1977.
81. Knudson RJ and others: The maximal expiratory flow-volume curve: normal standards, variability, and effects of age, *Am Rev Respir Dis* 113:587, 1976.
82. Wahba WH: Influence of aging on lung function–clinical significance of changes from age twenty, *Anesth Analg* 62:764, 1983.
83. Weder AB: The renally compromised older hypertensive: therapeutic considerations, *Geriatrics* 46:36, 1991.
84. Gilbert BR, Vaughan ED: Pathophysiology of the aging kidney, *Clinics Geriatr Med* 6(1):12, 1990.
85. Kasiske BL: Relationship between vascular disease and age-associated changes in the human kidney, *Kidney Int* 31:1153, 1987.
86. Anderson S, Brenner BM: Effects of aging on the renal glomerulus, *Am J Med* 80:435, 1986.
87. Watters JM, McClaran JC: The elderly surgical patient. In Wilmore DW and others, editors: *In care of the surgical patient,* vol VII, Special problems, New York, 1990, Scientific American.
88. Brandt LJ: Gastrointestinal disorders in the elderly. In Rossman I, editor: *Clinical geriatrics,* ed 3, Philadelphia, 1986, JB Lippincott.
89. Williams SA, Fogel RP: Common gastrointestinal problems in the elderly, *JAMA* 87:29, 1989.
90. Altman DF: Changes in gastrointestinal, pancreatic, biliary and hepatic function in aging, *Gastroenterol Clin North Am* 19(2):227, 1990.
91. Thomson AB, Keelan M: The aging gut, *Can J Physiol Pharmacol* 64:30, 1986.
92. Bansal SK and others: Upper gastrointestinal haemorrhage in the elderly: a record of 92 patients in a joint geriatric/surgical unit, *Age Ageing* 16:279, 1987.
93. Moore JG and others: Effect of age on gastric emptying of liquid-solid meals in man, *Dig Dis Sci* 28(4):340, 1983.
94. Schuster MM: Disorders of the aging GI system, *Hosp Prac* 11:95, 1976.
95. Curran J: Overview of geriatric nutrition, *Dysphagia* 5:72, 1990.
96. Ausman LM, Russel RM: Nutrition and aging. In Schneider EL, Rowe JW, editors: *Handbook of the biology of aging,* San Diego, 1990, Academic Press.
97. Sato TG, Miwa T, Tauchi H: Age changes in the human liver of the different races, *Gerontologia* 16:368, 1970.
98. Bach B and others: Disposition of antipyrine and phenytoin correlated with age and liver volume in man, *Clin Pharmacokinet* 6:389, 1981.
99. Kampmann JP, Sinding J, Moller-Jorgensen I: Effect of age on liver function, *Geriatrics* 30:91, 1975.
100. Schmucker DL, Wang RK: Age-related changes in liver drug metabolism: structure versus function, *Proc Soc Exp Biol Med* 165:178, 1980.
101. Vestal RE, Cusack BJ: Pharmacology and aging. In Schneider EL, Rowe JW, editors: *Handbook of the biology of aging,* San Diego, 1990, Academic Press.
102. Yuen GJ: Altered pharmacokinetics in the elderly, *Clin Geriatr Med* 6:257, 1990.
103. Schwertz DW, Buschmann MT: Pharmacogeriatics, *Crit Care Q* 12:26, 1989.
104. Gilman AG and others, editors: *Goodman and Gilman's the pharmacological basis of therapeutics,* London, 1990, Pergamon Press.
105. Mooradian AD: An update of the clinical pharmacokinetics, therapeutic monitoring techniques and treatment recommendations, *Clin Pharmacokinet* 18:165, 1988.
106. Creasy WA and others: Pharmacokinetics of captopril in elderly healthy male volunteers, *J Clin Pharmacol* 26:264, 1986.
107. Hockings N, Ajayi AA, Reid JL: Age and the pharmacodynamics of angiotensin converting enzyme inhibitors, enalapril and enalaprilat, *Br J Pharmacol* 21:341, 1986.
108. Pederson KE: Digoxin interactions. The influence of quindine and verapamil on the pharmacokinetics and receptor binding of digitalis glycosides, *Acta Med Scand* 697(suppl 1):1, 1985.

109. Lynch RA, Horowitz LN: Managing geriatric arrhythmias. II. Drug selection and use, *Geriatrics* 46:41, 1991.
110. Vidt GD, Borazanian RA: Calcium channel blockers in geriatric hypertension, *Geriatrics* 46:28, 1991.
111. Wall RT: Use of analgesics in the elderly, *Clin Geriatr Med* 6:345, 1990.
112. Bertel O and others: Decreased beta-adrenoreceptor responsiveness as related to age, blood pressure and plasma catecholmines in patients with essential hypertension, *Hypertension* 2:130, 1980.
113. Kendall MJ and others: Responsiveness to beta-adrenergic receptor stimulation: the effects of age are cardioselective, *Br J Clin Pharmacol* 14:821, 1982.
114. Selkoe DJ: Aging brain, aging mind, *Sci Amer* 267:134, 1992.
115. Morris JC, McManus DQ: The neurology of aging: normal versus pathologic change, *Geriatrics* 46:47, 1991.
116. Coleman PD, Flood DG: Neuron numbers and dendritic extent in normal aging and Alzheimer's disease, *Neurobiol Aging* 8:521, 1987.
117. Lytle LD, Altar A: Diet, central nervous system, and aging, *Fed Proc* 38:2017, 1979.
118. Cotman CW: Synaptic plasticity, neurotropic factors and transplantation in the aged brain. In Schneider EL, Rowe JW, editors: *Handbook of the biology of aging,* San Diego, 1990, Academic Press.
119. Cooper JR, Bloom FE, Roth RH: *The biochemical basis of neuropharmacology,* New York, 1991, Oxford University Press.
120. Morgan DG, May PC: Age-related changes in synaptic neurochemistry. In Schneider EL, Rowe JW, editors: *Handbook of the biology of aging,* San Diego, 1990, Academic Press.
121. Gottstein U, Held K: Effects of aging on cerebral circulation and metabolism in man, *Acta Neurol Scand Suppl* 72:54, 1979.
122. Fields SD: History-taking in the elderly: obtaining useful information, *Geriatrics* 46(8):26, 1991.
123. Geokas MC: The aging process, *Ann Int Med* 113:455, 1990.
124. Marmour MF: Management of elderly patients with impaired vision. In Ebaugh FG, editor: *Management of common problems in geriatric medicine,* Menlo Park, Calif, 1981, Addison-Wesley.
125. Bartoshuk LM: Taste, robust across the age span? *Ann NY Acad Sci* 561:65, 1989.
126. Cowart BJ: Relationships between taste and smell across the adult life span, *Ann NY Acad Sci* 561:39, 1989.
127. Ferris AM, Duffy VB: Effect of olfactory deficits on nutritional status, *Ann NY Acad Sci* 561:113, 1989.
128. Goode RL: The effect of aging on the ear. In Ebaugh FG, editor: *Management of common problems in geriatric medicine,* Menlo Park, Calif, 1981, Addison-Wesley.
129. Lapiere CM: The ageing dermis: the main cause for the appearance of "old skin," *Br J Dermatol* 122(suppl 35):5, 1990.
130. Jones PL, Millman A: Wound healing and the aged patient, *Nurs Clin North Am* 25(1):263, 1990.
131. Kelly L, Mobily PR: Iatrogenesis in the elderly, *J Gerontol Nurs* 17(9):24, 1991.
132. Shenefelt PD, Fenske NA: Aging and the skin: recognizing and managing common disorders, *Geriatrics* 45(10):57, 1990.
133. Exton-Smith AN: Mineral metabolism. In Finch CE, Schneider EL, editors: *Handbook of the biology of aging,* New York, 1985, Van Nostrand Reinhold.
134. Ganong WF: *Review of medical physiology,* Norwalk, Conn, 1991, Appleton & Lange.
135. Duthie EH, Abbasi AA: Laboratory testing: current recommendations for older adults, *Geriatrics* 46:10, 1991.
136. Foreman MD, Gillies DA, Wagner D: Impaired cognition in the critically ill elderly patient: clinical implications, *Crit Care Q* 12:61, 1989.
137. Boss BJ: Normal aging in the nervous system: implications for SCI nurses, *SCI* 8(2):42, 1991.
138. Piano MR: The physiologic changes that occur with aging, *Crit Care Q* 12:1, 1989.
139. Catchen H: Repeaters: inpatient accidents among the hospitalized elderly, *Nurs Res* 37:273, 1983.
140. Evans LK, Strumpf NE: Tying down the elderly. A review of the literature on physical restraint, J Am Geriatr Soc 1:65, 1989.
141. Kapp MB: Nursing home restraints and legal liability, J Leg Med 13:1, 1992.
142. Redford JB: Preventing falls in the elderly, *Hosp Med* 35:57, 1991.
143. Warshaw GA and others: Functional disability in the hospitalized elderly, *JAMA* 248:847, 1982.
144. Patrick ML: Care of the confused elderly, *Am J Nurs* 67:2536, 1967.
145. Gutheil T, Tardiff K: Indication and contraindication for seclusion and restraint. In Tardiff K, editor: *The psychiatric uses of seclusion and restraint,* Washington, DC, 1984, APA Press.
146. Robbins LJ and others: Binding the elderly: a prospective study of the use of mechanical restraints in an acute care setting, *J Am Geriatr Soc* 35:290, 1987.
147. Gerdes L: The confused or delirious patient, *Am J Nurs* 68:1228, 1968.
148. Miller M: Iatrogenic and nursigenic effect of prolonged immobilization of the ill aged, *J Am Geriatr Soc* 23:360, 1975.

A

North American Nursing Diagnosis Association's (NANDA) Taxonomy I Revised*

INTRODUCTION TO CLASSIFICATION OF NURSING DIAGNOSES

In 1973 a group of nurses met in St. Louis and organized the First National Conference for the Classification of Nursing Diagnoses. They began the formal effort to identify, develop, and classify nursing diagnoses. Nine conferences have been held since that time with the last, the tenth, being held in 1992.

Following the first conference Gebbie (1974) identified four steps necessary for the development of a classification system; they are useful today.

The first step in developing a classification is to identify all those things which nurses locate or diagnose in patients.

The second step is to reach some agreement about consistent nomenclature which can be used to describe the domain of nursing as identified in step one.

The third step in the classification process is the grouping of identified diagnoses (the labels) into classes and subclasses so that patterns and relationships among them can emerge.

The final step in the process is the substitution of numbers or equivalent abbreviations for terminology so that data related to the various diagnoses can be manipulated more readily by hand or computer.

The first conferences were invitational. Participants were placed into working groups and asked to generate diagnoses related to a specific functional system. They relied upon their recall of patient situations to generate the signs and symptoms. Diagnoses were accepted by a majority vote of the conference participants. In 1982 the conferences were opened to the nursing community at large. The process for generating and accepting diagnoses moved through several stages incorporating submission and review by clinical experts. Acceptance, which was initially by conference participants, now requires positive vote of the membership of NANDA. No formal action was taken upon new diagnoses at the 1982 and 1984 conferences while the diagnostic review process was being evaluated. However, since that time, the Guidelines for Submission and review of new diagnoses have been developed.

After much dialogue, the participants at the first conference could not agree upon a scheme to classify the newly developed diagnoses, and so the decision was made to list the diagnoses alphabetically. Though the list was expanded over years, the alphabetic system was not changed until 1986 when the NANDA Taxonomy I was endorsed for development and testing.

The structural basis for the taxonomy was derived from the work of a group of nurse theorists during the third, fourth, and fifth conferences, chaired by Sr. Callista Roy. The nurse theorist group was asked to develop a conceptual framework for the classification of nursing diagnoses. Using an inductive methodology, they studied the alphabetic list of nursing diagnoses and generated several broad patterns that grouped the individual diagnoses. Their final work proposed the nine patterns of unitary man as the conceptual framework for the diagnostic classification system (Fifth Proceedings, Roy, p. 31, 1984). During this process, different theoretical levels of abstraction were identified among the diagnoses. Depending upon the specificity of the diagnoses, some were very abstract and general while others were specific and concrete.

At the fifth conference, a taxonomy special interest group chaired by Phyllis Kritek was charged with the task of generating an initial taxonomy for the nursing diagnoses labels. The group focused upon the existing list of diagnoses and the theorists' patterns of unitary man. The labels were separated into four levels of abstraction, Level I subsuming Levels II, III, and IV; Level II subsuming Levels III, and IV, etc.; with Level I being the most abstract and Level IV being the least abstract. During this time, members observed that Level IV diagnoses were the most useful for the practicing nurse. In the final analysis the Level I categories were identified as alterations in human responses and were categorized under the nine patterns of unitary man. This was the stage of taxonomy development at the end of the fifth conference.

*From North American Nursing Diagnosis Association: *NANDA nursing diagnoses: definitions and classifications, 1992*, Philadelphia, 1992, The Association.

Upon acceptance of the NANDA Bylaws and election of officers, the Taxonomy Committee began its work of formalizing and modifying the work that had gone before. The term "Human Response Patterns" was introduced to replace the less familiar term of "Patterns of Unitary Man." This change was introduced based on the advice of a group of reviewers who critiqued the proposed Taxonomy between the sixth and seventh conferences. The nine patterns constitute Level I concepts, the most abstract level, and provide the organizing framework for the Taxonomy. Conference participants accepted this change without debate. The purposes of a taxonomy are to provide a vocabulary for classifying phenomena in a discipline, provide new ways of looking at the discipline, and play a part in concept derivation. The Taxonomy provides a beginning classification scheme which can be used to categorize and classify nursing diagnostic labels. It is not meant for use as a theoretical framework or as an assessment framework in the strict sense of those constructs. After much discussion and work, the Taxonomy was presented to the membership at the seventh conference which endorsed Taxonomy I for development and testing.

The following are rules of classification and guidelines used by the Taxonomy Committee:

1. There is no inherent order, i.e. one pattern is not considered better than another, in the numbering of the nine patterns. The first pattern developed in the taxonomy was numbered one. It so happened that it was Exchanging, but it could have been any of the other patterns. This system of numbering was retained for the inclusion of each new diagnosis.
2. The level of abstraction (general to specific, abstract to concrete) determines the level of placement within the taxonomy. Supporting literature from the submitter, expert opinion, and nursing literature assist in making the determination of placement.
3. The diagnosis is classified by considering the definition of the pattern and the definition of the diagnosis. They must be consistent.
4. The placement of the diagnosis is conceptually consistent with current theoretical views within nursing.
5. Categories in brackets were developed by the committee to clarify why certain diagnoses were placed at a specific level or in a specific pattern and from a collaborative effort with the American Nurses' Association. It is hoped that these categories will be researched and submitted as diagnoses or that new diagnoses will be submitted to replace them. This practice was only instituted to clarify the thinking of the committee so that nurses utilizing the taxonomy could understand the placement of diagnoses.
6. The numbering system was developed to facilitate computerization of the taxonomy. At this point in the development of nursing diagnoses, one digit at each level was determined to be sufficient. In the future this may need to be changed.

This has been a brief history of the development of Taxonomy I and its subsequent revisions. NANDA is working to further develop the taxonomy and the coding of nursing diagnoses for the possible inclusion in the World Health Organization International Classification of Diseases. The draft version of Taxonomy II was presented at the 1990 NANDA Conference. No further work has been completed at this time.

DEFINITIONS FOR CLASSIFICATION OF NURSING DIAGNOSES*

Classification: Systematic arrangement in groups or categories according to established criteria; an arrangement of phenomena into groups based on their relationships.

Level of abstraction: Describes the concreteness/abstractness of a concept.

a) Very abstract concepts are theoretical, may not be directly measurable, defined by concrete concepts, inclusive of concrete concepts, disassociated from any specific instance, independent of time and space, has more general descriptors, may not be clinically useful for planning treatment.
b) Concrete concepts are observable and measurable, limited by time and space, constitute a specific category, more exclusive, names a real thing or class of things, restricted by nature, may be clinically useful for planning treatment.

Nomenclature: A system or set of terms or symbols; act or process of naming; a system of terms used in a particular science or discipline; compilation of accepted terms for describing phenomena.

Nursing Diagnosis: (Approved at the Ninth Conference): Nursing Diagnosis is a clinical judgment about individual, family, or community responses to actual and potential health problems/life processes. Nursing diagnoses provide the basis for selection of nursing interventions to achieve outcomes for which the nurse is accountable.

Related factors: Factors which appear to show some type of patterned relationship with the nursing diagnosis. Such factors may be described as antecedent to, associated with, related to, contributing to, or abetting.

Taxonomy: Type of classification; the theoretical study of systematic classifications including their bases, principles, procedures, and rules. The science of how to classify and identify.

NANDA Approved Nursing Diagnoses

This list represents the NANDA approved nursing diagnoses for clinical use and testing (1992).

*These definitions are working definitions used in the development of Taxonomy I Revised—1992 and are subject to change as work progresses.

PATTERN 1: EXCHANGING

1.1.2.1	Altered Nutrition: More than body requirements
1.1.2.2	Altered Nutrition: Less than body requirements
1.1.2.3	Altered Nutrition: Potential for more than body requirements
1.2.1.1	High Risk for Infection
1.2.2.1	High Risk for Altered Body Temperature
1.2.2.2	Hypothermia
1.2.2.3	Hyperthermia
1.2.2.4	Ineffective Thermoregulation
1.2.3.1	Dysreflexia
*1.3.1.1	Constipation
1.3.1.1.1	Perceived Constipation
1.3.1.1.2	Colonic Constipation
*1.3.1.2	Diarrhea
*1.3.1.3	Bowel Incontinence
1.3.2	Altered Urinary Elimination
1.3.2.1.1	Stress Incontinence
1.3.2.1.2	Reflex Incontinence
1.3.2.1.3	Urge Incontinence
1.3.2.1.4	Functional Incontinence
1.3.2.1.5	Total Incontinence
1.3.2.2	Urinary Retention
*1.4.1.1	Altered (Specify Type) Tissue Perfusion (Renal, cerebral, cardiopulmonary, gastrointestinal, peripheral)
1.4.1.2.1	Fluid Volume Excess
1.4.1.2.2.1	Fluid Volume Deficit
1.4.1.2.2.2	High Risk for Fluid Volume Deficit
*1.4.2.1	Decreased Cardiac Output
1.5.1.1	Impaired Gas Exchange
1.5.1.2	Ineffective Airway Clearance
1.5.1.3	Ineffective Breathing Pattern
#1.5.1.3.1	Inability to Sustain Spontaneous Ventilation
#1.5.1.3.2	Dysfunctional Ventilatory Weaning Response (DVWR)
1.6.1	High Risk for Injury
1.6.1.1	High Risk for Suffocation
1.6.1.2	High Risk for Poisoning
1.6.1.3	High Risk for Trauma
1.6.1.4	High Risk for Aspiration
1.6.1.5	High Risk for Disuse Syndrome
1.6.2	Altered Protection
1.6.2.1	Impaired Tissue Integrity
*1.6.2.1.1	Altered Oral Mucous Membrane
1.6.2.1.2.1	Impaired Skin Integrity
1.6.2.1.2.2	High Risk for Impaired Skin Integrity

PATTERN 2: COMMUNICATING

2.1.1.1	Impaired Verbal Communication

PATTERN 3: RELATING

3.1.1	Impaired Social Interaction
3.1.2	Social Isolation
*3.2.1	Altered Role Performance
3.2.1.1.1	Altered Parenting
3.2.1.1.2	High Risk for Altered Parenting
3.2.1.2.1	Sexual Dysfunction
3.2.2	Altered Family Processes
#3.2.2.1	Caregiver Role Strain
#3.2.2.2	High Risk for Caregiver Role Strain
3.2.3.1	Parental Role Conflict
3.3	Altered Sexuality Patterns

PATTERN 4: VALUING

4.1.1	Spiritual Distress (distress of the human spirit)

PATTERN 5: CHOOSING

5.1.1.1	Ineffective Individual Coping
5.1.1.1.1	Impaired Adjustment
5.1.1.1.2	Defensive Coping
5.1.1.1.3	Ineffective Denial
5.1.2.1.1	Ineffective Family Coping: Disabling
5.1.2.1.2	Ineffective Family Coping: Compromised
5.1.2.2	Family Coping: Potential for Growth
#5.2.1	Ineffective Management of Therapeutic Regimen (Individuals)
5.2.1.1	Noncompliance (Specify)
5.3.1.1	Decisional Conflict (Specify)
5.4	Health Seeking Behaviors (Specify)

PATTERN 6: MOVING

6.1.1.1	Impaired Physical Mobility
#6.1.1.1.1	High Risk for Peripheral Neurovascular Dysfunction
6.1.1.2	Activity Intolerance
6.1.1.2.1	Fatigue
6.1.1.3	High Risk for Activity Intolerance
6.2.1	Sleep Pattern Disturbance
6.3.1.1	Diversional Activity Deficit
6.4.1.1	Impaired Home Maintenance Management
6.4.2	Altered Health Maintenance
*6.5.1	Feeding Self Care Deficit
6.5.1.1	Impaired Swallowing
6.5.1.2	Ineffective Breastfeeding
#6.5.1.2.1	Interrupted Breastfeeding
6.5.1.3	Effective Breastfeeding
#6.5.1.4	Ineffective Infant Feeding Pattern
*6.5.2	Bathing/Hygiene Self Care Deficit
*6.5.3	Dressing/Grooming Self Care Deficit
*6.5.4	Toileting Self Care Deficit
6.6	Altered Growth and Development
#6.7	Relocation Stress Syndrome

#New diagnostic categories approved 1992.
*Categories with modified label terminology.

PATTERN 7: PERCEIVING

*7.1.1	Body Image Disturbance
*7.1.2	Self Esteem Disturbance
7.1.2.1	Chronic Low Self Esteem
7.1.2.2	Situational Low Self Esteem
*7.1.3	Personal Identity Disturbance
7.2	Sensory/Perceptual Alterations (Specify) (Visual, auditory, kinesthetic, gustatory, tactile, olfactory)
7.2.1.1	Unilateral Neglect
7.3.1	Hopelessness
7.3.2	Powerlessness

PATTERN 8: KNOWING

8.1.1	Knowledge Deficit (Specify)
8.3	Altered Thought Processes

PATTERN 9: FEELING

*9.1.1	Pain
9.1.1.1	Chronic Pain
9.2.1.1	Dysfunctional Grieving
9.2.1.2	Anticipatory Grieving
9.2.2	High Risk for Violence: Self-directed or directed at others
#9.2.2.1	High Risk for Self-Mutilation
9.2.3	Post-Trauma Response
9.2.3.1	Rape-Trauma Syndrome
9.2.3.1.1	Rape-Trauma Syndrome: Compound Reaction
9.2.3.1.2	Rape-Trauma Syndrome: Silent Reaction
9.3.1	Anxiety
9.3.2	Fear

REFERENCES

Gebbie, K. & Lavin, M.A. (1974). Classifying nursing diagnoses. AJN, 250-253.

Gebbie, K. (1975). *Classification of Nursing Diagnoses: Proceedings of the Second National Conference*. St. Louis: Clearinghouse for Nursing Diagnosis-NANDA. (out of print. Can obtain a copy through interlibrary loan from the Library of Congress).

Gebbie, K. & Lavin, M.A (Eds.) (1975). *Classification of Nursing Diagnoses: Proceedings of the First National Conference*. St. Louis: C.V. Mosby.

Hurley, M. (Ed.) (1986). *Classification of Nursing Diagnoses: Proceedings of the Sixth National Conference*. St Louis: C. V. Mosby.

Kim, M.J., McFarland, G.K. & McLane, A.M. (Eds.) (1984). *Classification of Nursing Diagnoses: Proceedings of the Fifth National Conference*. St. Louis: C. V. Mosby.

Kim, M.J. & Moritz, D.A. (Eds.) (1982). *Classification of Nursing Diagnoses: Proceedings of the Third and Fourth National Conferences*. New York: McGraw Hill.

McLane, A.M. (Ed.) (1987). *Classification of Nursing Diagnoses: Proceedings of the Seventh National Conference*. St. Louis: C. V. Mosby.

Roy, C. (1984). *Classification of Nursing Diagnoses: Proceedings of the Fifth National Conference*, p. 31, St. Louis: C. V. Mosby.

BIBLIOGRAPHY

Carroll-Johnson, R.M. (Ed.) (1989). *Classification of Nursing Diagnoses: Proceedings of the Eighth National Conference*. Philadelphia: J.B. Lippincott Company.

Carroll-Johnson, R.M. (Ed.) (1991). *Classification of Nursing Diagnoses: Proceedings of the Ninth National Conference*. Philadelphia: J.B. Lippincott Company.

Carroll-Johnson, R.M. (Ed.) (1993). *Classification of Nursing Diagnoses: Proceedings of the Tenth National Conference*. Philadelphia: J.B. Lippincott Company.

B

Advanced Cardiac Life Support (ACLS) Guidelines

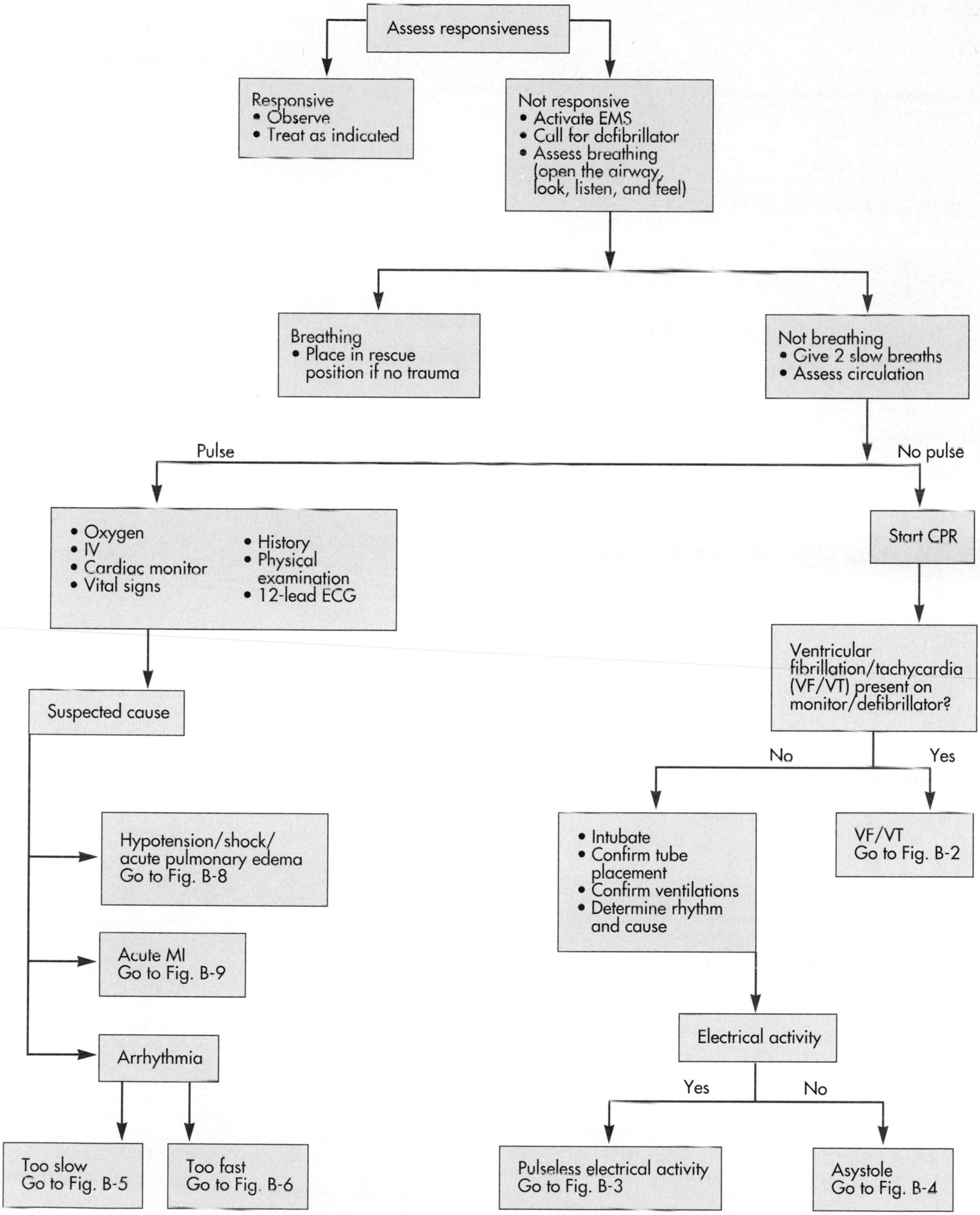

Fig. B-1 Universal algorithm for adult emergency cardiac care (ECC). (From Emergency Cardiac Care Committees and Subcommittees, American Heart Association: Guidelines for cardiopulmonary resuscitation and emergency care III: Adult advanced cardiac life support, *JAMA* 268(16):2216, 1992.)

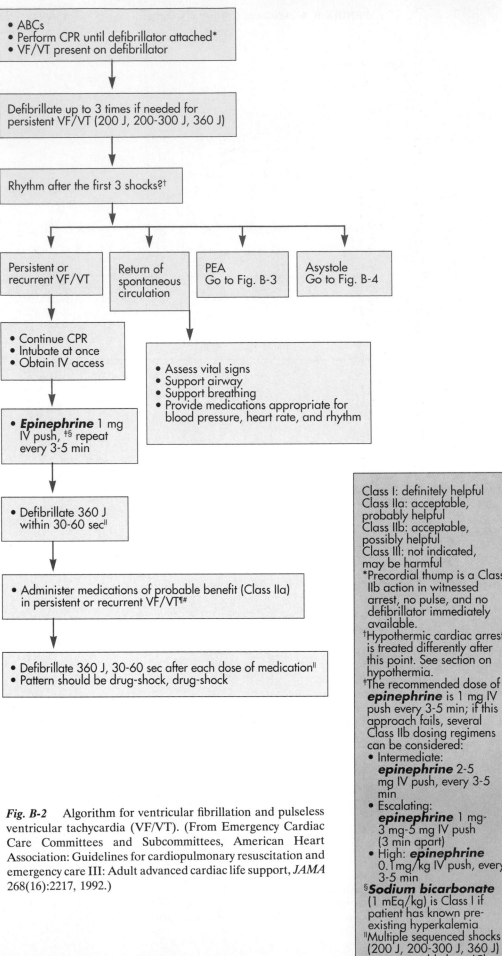

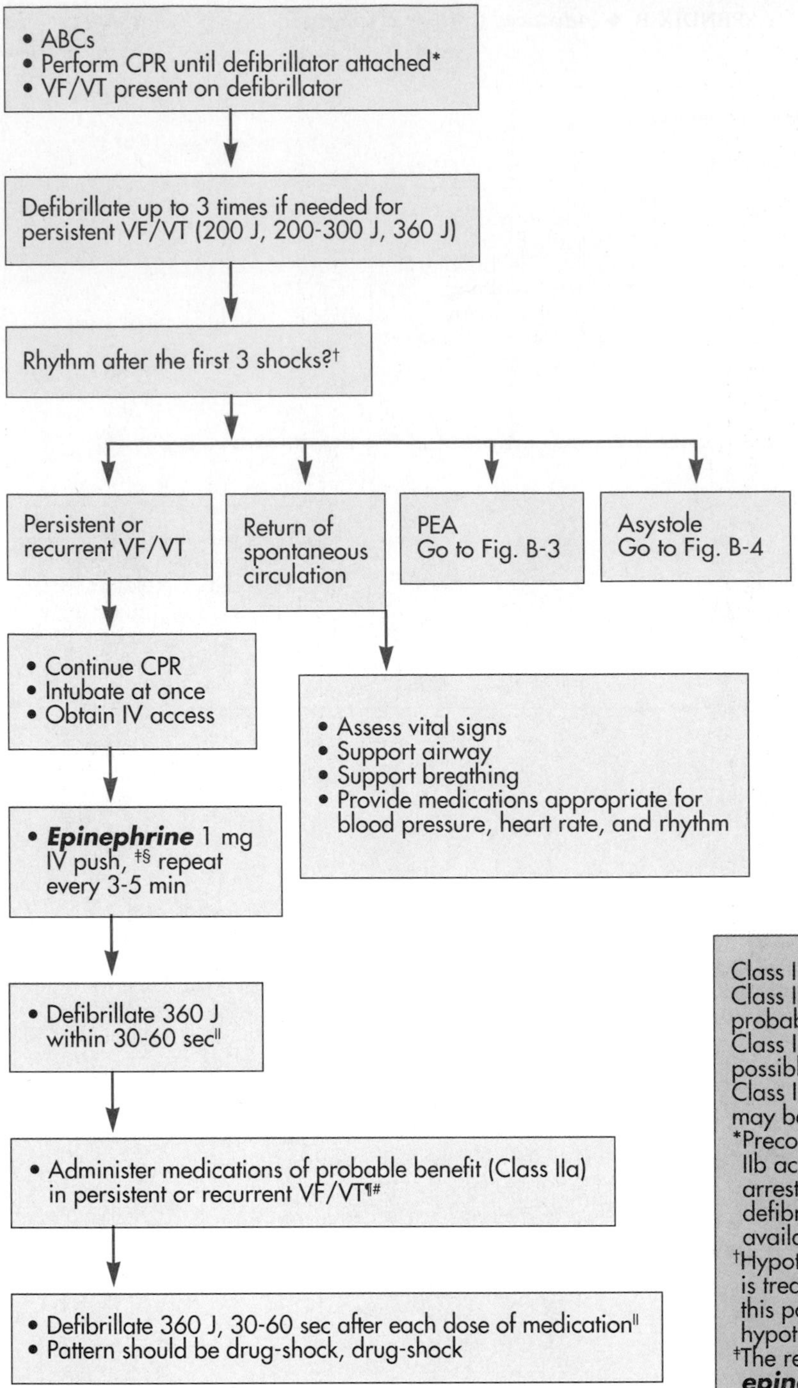
• ABCs
• Perform CPR until defibrillator attached*
• VF/VT present on defibrillator
Defibrillate up to 3 times if needed for persistent VF/VT (200 J, 200-300 J, 360 J)
Rhythm after the first 3 shocks?†
Persistent or recurrent VF/VT
Return of spontaneous circulation
PEA Go to Fig. B-3
Asystole Go to Fig. B-4
• Continue CPR
• Intubate at once
• Obtain IV access
• Assess vital signs
• Support airway
• Support breathing
• Provide medications appropriate for blood pressure, heart rate, and rhythm
• Epinephrine 1 mg IV push, ‡§ repeat every 3-5 min
• Defibrillate 360 J within 30-60 sec||
• Administer medications of probable benefit (Class IIa) in persistent or recurrent VF/VT¶#
• Defibrillate 360 J, 30-60 sec after each dose of medication||
• Pattern should be drug-shock, drug-shock

Fig. B-2 Algorithm for ventricular fibrillation and pulseless ventricular tachycardia (VF/VT). (From Emergency Cardiac Care Committees and Subcommittees, American Heart Association: Guidelines for cardiopulmonary resuscitation and emergency care III: Adult advanced cardiac life support, *JAMA* 268(16):2217, 1992.)

Class I: definitely helpful
Class IIa: acceptable, probably helpful
Class IIb: acceptable, possibly helpful
Class III: not indicated, may be harmful

*Precordial thump is a Class IIb action in witnessed arrest, no pulse, and no defibrillator immediately available.

†Hypothermic cardiac arrest is treated differently after this point. See section on hypothermia.

‡The recommended dose of **epinephrine** is 1 mg IV push every 3-5 min; if this approach fails, several Class IIb dosing regimens can be considered:

- Intermediate: **epinephrine** 2-5 mg IV push, every 3-5 min
- Escalating: **epinephrine** 1 mg-3 mg-5 mg IV push (3 min apart)
- High: **epinephrine** 0.1 mg/kg IV push, every 3-5 min

§**Sodium bicarbonate** (1 mEq/kg) is Class I if patient has known preexisting hyperkalemia

||Multiple sequenced shocks (200 J, 200-300 J, 360 J) are acceptable here (Class I), especially when medications are delayed

¶
- ***Lidocaine*** 1.5 mg/kg IV push. Repeat in 3-5 min to total loading dose of 3 mg/kg; then use
- ***Bretylium*** 5 mg/kg IV push. Repeat in 5 min at 10 mg/kg
- ***Magnesium sulfate*** 1-2 g IV in torsades de pointes or suspected hypomagnesemic state or severe refractory VF
- ***Procainamide*** 30 mg/min in refractory VF (maximum total 17 mg/kg)

#
- **Sodium bicarbonate** (1 mEq/kg IV):

Class IIa
- if known preexisting bicarbonate-responsive acidosis
- if overdose with tricyclic antidepressants
- to alkalinize the urine in drug overdoses

Class IIb
- if intubated and continued long arrest interval
- upon return of spontaneous circulation after long arrest interval

Class III
- hypoxic lactic acidosis

PEA includes
- Electromechanical dissociation (EMD)
- Pseudo-EMD
- Idioventricular rhythms
- Ventricular escape rhythms
- Bradyasystolic rhythms
- Postdefibrillation idioventricular rhythms

- Continue CPR
- Intubate at once
- Obtain IV access
- Assess blood flow using Doppler ultrasound

↓

Consider possible causes
(Parentheses = possible therapies and treatments)
- Hypovolemia (volume infusion)
- Hypoxia (ventilation)
- Cardiac tamponade (pericardiocentesis)
- Tension pneumothorax (needle decompression)
- Hypothermia (see hypothermia algorithm, Fig. B-11)
- Massive pulmonary embolism (surgery, *thrombolytics)*
- Drug overdoses such as tricyclics, digitalis, ß-blockers, calcium channel blockers
- Hyperkalemia*
- Acidosis†
- Massive acute myocardial infarction (go to Fig. B-9)

↓

- ***Epinephrine*** 1 mg IV push, *†repeat every 3-5 min

↓

- If absolute bradycardia (<60 beats/min) or relative bradycardia, give ***atropine*** 1 mg IV
- Repeat every 3-5 min up to a total of 0.4 mg/kg§

Class I: definitely helpful
Class IIa: acceptable, probably helpful
Class IIb: acceptable, possibly helpful
Class III: not indicated, may be harmful

****Sodium bicarbonate*** 1 mEq/kg is Class I if patient has known preexisting hyperkalemia.

†***Sodium bicarbonate*** 1 mEq/kg:

Class IIa
- if known preexisting bicarbonate-responsive acidosis
- if overdose with tricyclic antidepressants
- to alkalinize the urine in drug overdoses

Class IIb
- if intubated and long arrest interval
- upon return of spontaneous circulation after long arrest interval

Class III
- hypoxic lactic acidosis

‡The recommended dose of ***epinephrine*** is 1 mg IV push every 3-5 min. If this approach fails, several Class IIb dosing regimens can be considered.
- Intermediate: ***epinephrine*** 2-5 mg IV push every 3-5 min
- Escalating: ***epinephrine*** 1 mg-3 mg-5 mg IV push (3 min apart)
- High: ***epinephrine*** 0.1 mg/kg IV push every 3-5 min

§Shorter ***atropine*** dosing intervals are possibly helpful in cardiac arrest (Class IIb).

Fig. B-3 Algorithm for pulseless electrical activity (PEA) (electromechanical dissociation [EMD]). (From Emergency Cardiac Care Committees and Subcommittees, American Heart Association: Guidelines for cardiopulmonary resuscitation and emergency care III: Adult advanced cardiac life support, *JAMA* 268(16):2219, 1992.)

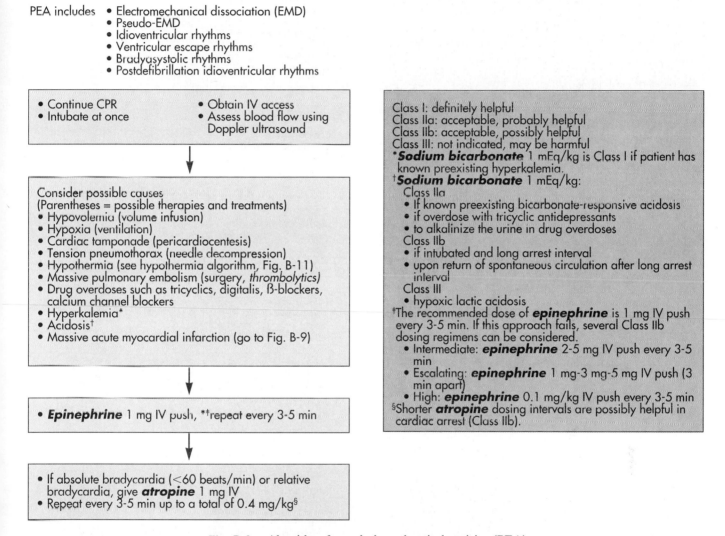

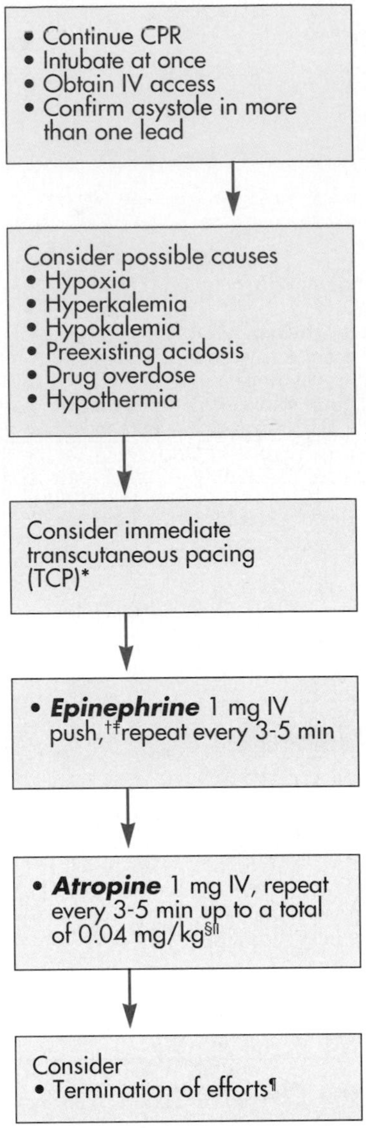

Fig. B-4 Asystole treatment algorithm. (From Emergency Cardiac Care Committees and Subcommittees, American Heart Association: Guidelines for cardiopulmonary resuscitation and emergency care III: Adult advanced cardiac life support, *JAMA* 268(16):2220, 1992.)

Class I: definitely helpful
Class IIa: acceptable, probably helpful
Class IIb: acceptable, possibly helpful
Class III: not indicated, may be harmful

*TCP is a Class IIb intervention. Lack of success may be due to delays in pacing. To be effective TCP must be performed early, simultaneously with drugs. Evidence does not support routine use of TCP for asystole.

†The recommended dose of ***epinephrine*** is 1 mg IV push every 3-5 min. If this approach fails, several Class IIb dosing regimens can be considered:
- Intermediate: ***epinephrine*** 2-5 mg IV push every 3-5 min
- Escalating: ***epinephrine*** 1 mg-3 mg-5 mg IV push, (3 min apart)
- High: ***epinephrine*** 0.1 mg/kg IV push every 3-5 min

‡***Sodium bicarbonate*** 1 mEq/kg is Class I if patient has known preexisting hyperkalemia.

§Shorter ***atropine*** dosing intervals are Class IIb in asystolic arrest.

||***Sodium bicarbonate*** 1 mEq/kg:
Class IIa
- if known preexisting bicarbonate-responsive acidosis
- if overdose with tricyclic antidepressants
- to alkalinize the urine in drug overdoses

Class IIb
- if intubated and continued long arrest interval
- upon return of spontaneous circulation after long arrest interval

Class III
- hypoxic lactic acidosis

¶If patient remains in asystole or other agonal rhythms after successful intubation and initial medications and no reversible causes are identified, consider termination of resuscitative efforts by a physician. Consider interval since arrest.

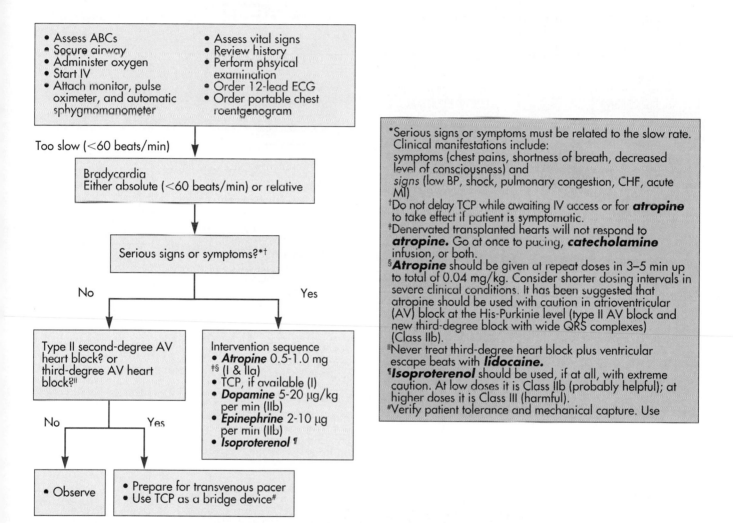

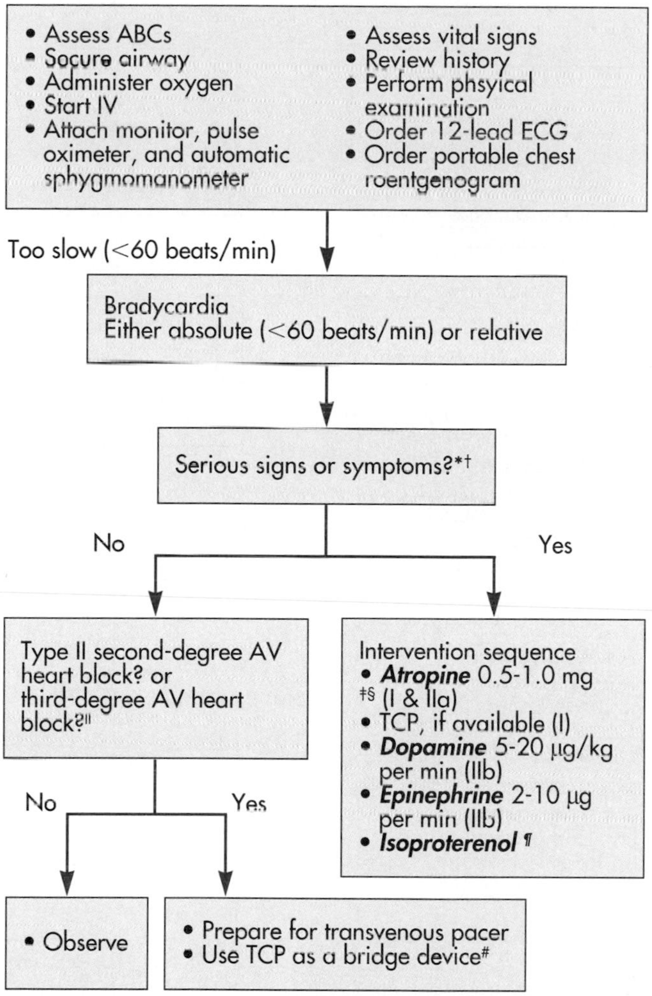
• Assess ABCs
• Secure airway
• Administer oxygen
• Start IV
• Attach monitor, pulse oximeter, and automatic sphygmomanometer
• Assess vital signs
• Review history
• Perform phsyical examination
• Order 12-lead ECG
• Order portable chest roentgenogram
Too slow (<60 beats/min)
Bradycardia
Either absolute (<60 beats/min) or relative
Serious signs or symptoms?*†
No
Yes
Type II second-degree AV heart block? or third-degree AV heart block?||
Intervention sequence
• Atropine 0.5-1.0 mg ‡§ (I & IIa)
• TCP, if available (I)
• Dopamine 5-20 μg/kg per min (IIb)
• Epinephrine 2-10 μg per min (IIb)
• Isoproterenol ¶
No
Yes
• Observe
• Prepare for transvenous pacer
• Use TCP as a bridge device#

*Serious signs or symptoms must be related to the slow rate. Clinical manifestations include:
symptoms (chest pains, shortness of breath, decreased level of consciousness) and
signs (low BP, shock, pulmonary congestion, CHF, acute MI)

†Do not delay TCP while awaiting IV access or for ***atropine*** to take effect if patient is symptomatic.

‡Denervated transplanted hearts will not respond to ***atropine.*** Go at once to pacing, ***catecholamine*** infusion, or both.

§***Atropine*** should be given at repeat doses in 3–5 min up to total of 0.04 mg/kg. Consider shorter dosing intervals in severe clinical conditions. It has been suggested that atropine should be used with caution in atrioventricular (AV) block at the His-Purkinie level (type II AV block and new third-degree block with wide QRS complexes) (Class IIb).

||Never treat third-degree heart block plus ventricular escape beats with ***lidocaine.***

¶***Isoproterenol*** should be used, if at all, with extreme caution. At low doses it is Class IIb (probably helpful); at higher doses it is Class III (harmful).

#Verify patient tolerance and mechanical capture. Use

Fig. B-5 Bradycardia algorithm (with the patient not in cardiac arrest). (From Emergency Cardiac Care Committees and Subcommittees, American Heart Association: Guidelines for cardiopulmonary resuscitation and emergency care III: Adult advanced cardiac life support, *JAMA* 268(16):2221, 1992.)

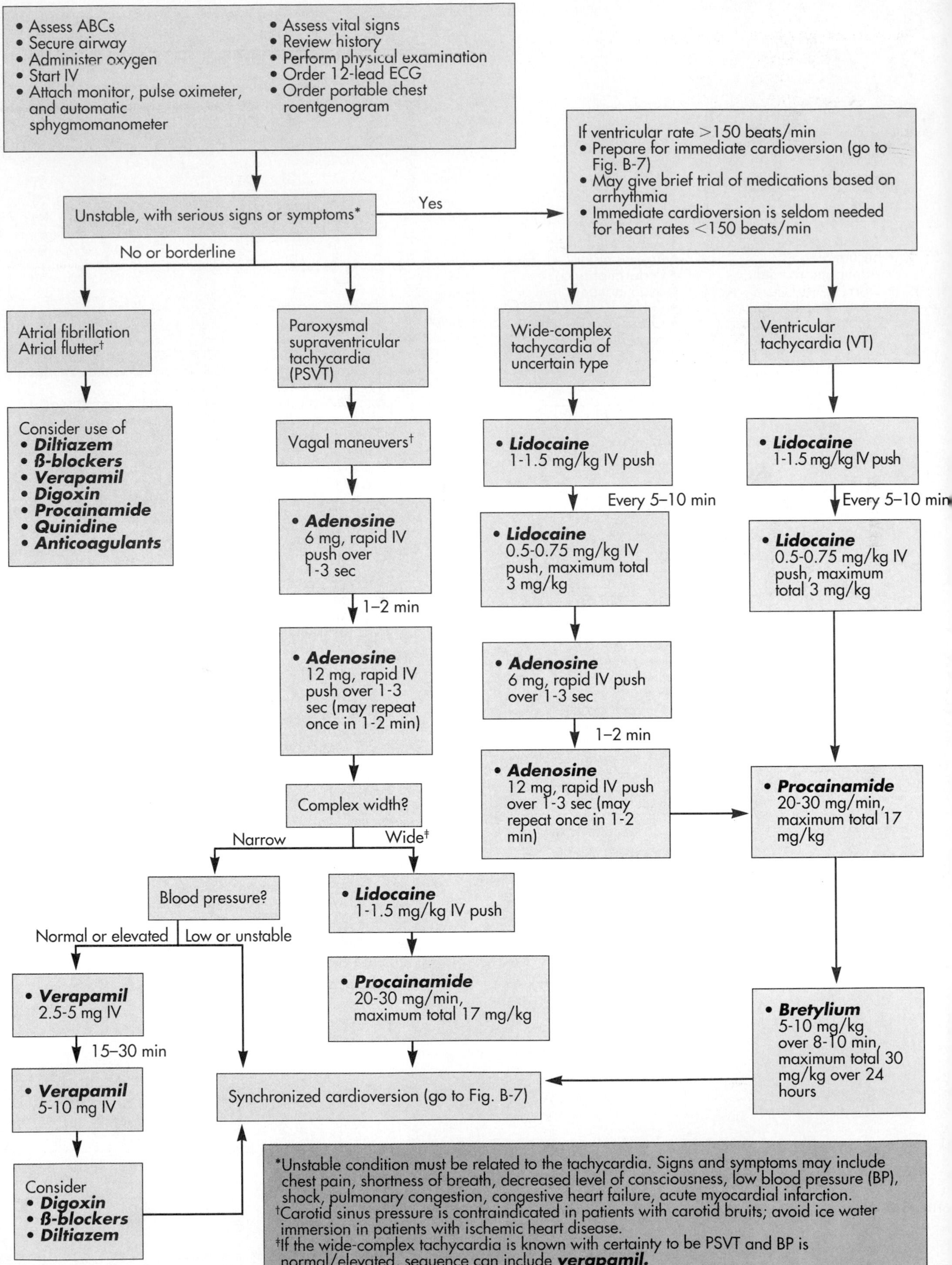

*Unstable condition must be related to the tachycardia. Signs and symptoms may include chest pain, shortness of breath, decreased level of consciousness, low blood pressure (BP), shock, pulmonary congestion, congestive heart failure, acute myocardial infarction.
†Carotid sinus pressure is contraindicated in patients with carotid bruits; avoid ice water immersion in patients with ischemic heart disease.
‡If the wide-complex tachycardia is known with certainty to be PSVT and BP is normal/elevated, sequence can include ***verapamil.***

Fig. B-6 Tachycardia algorithm. (From Emergency Cardiac Care Committees and Subcommittees, American Heart Association: Guidelines for cardiopulmonary resuscitation and emergency care III: Adult advanced cardiac life support, *JAMA* 268(16):2223, 1992.)

Tachycardia with serious signs and symptoms related to the tachycardia

↓

If ventricular rate is > 150 beats/min, prepare for immediate cardioversion.
May give brief trial of medications based on specific arrhythmias.
Immediate cardioversion is generally not needed for rates < 150 beats min.

↓

Check
- Oxygen saturation
- Suction device
- IV line
- Intubation equipment

↓

Premedicate whenever possible*

↓

Synchronized cardioversion†‡
VT§
PSVT‖
Atrial fibrillation
Atrial flutter
— 100 J, 200 J, 300 J, 360 J‡

*Effective regimens have included a sedative (e.g., ***diazepam, midazolam, barbiturates, stomidate, ketamine, methohexital***) with or without an analgesic agent (e.g., ***fentanyl, morphine, meperidine***). Many experts recommend anesthesia if service is readily available.
†Note possible need to resynchronize after each cardioversion.
‡If delays in synchronization occur and clinical conditions are critical, go to immediate unsynchronized shocks.
§Treat polymorphic VT (irregular form and rate) like VF: 200 J, 200-300 J, 360 J.
‖PSVT and atrial flutter often respond to lower energy levels (start with 50 J).

Fig. B-7 Electrical cardioversion algorithm (with the patient not in cardiac arrest). (From Emergency Cardiac Care Committees and Subcommittees, American Heart Association: Guidelines for cardiopulmonary resuscitation and emergency care III: Adult advanced cardiac life support, *JAMA* 268(16):2224, 1992.)

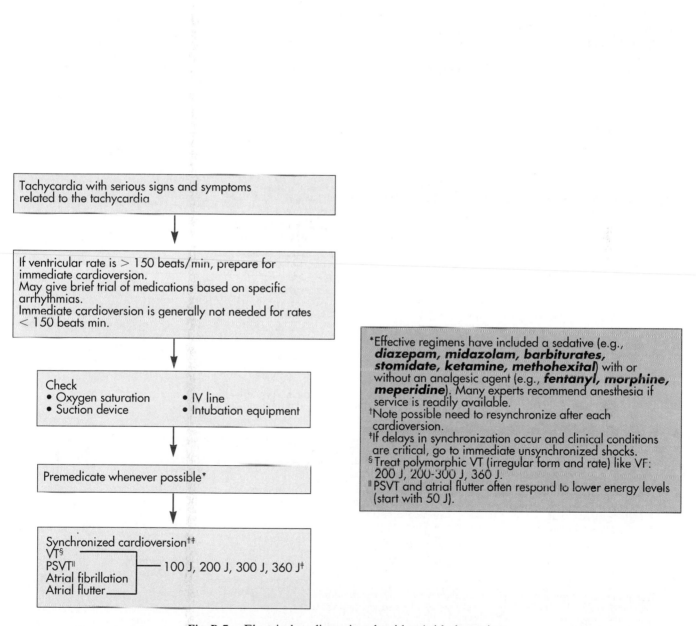

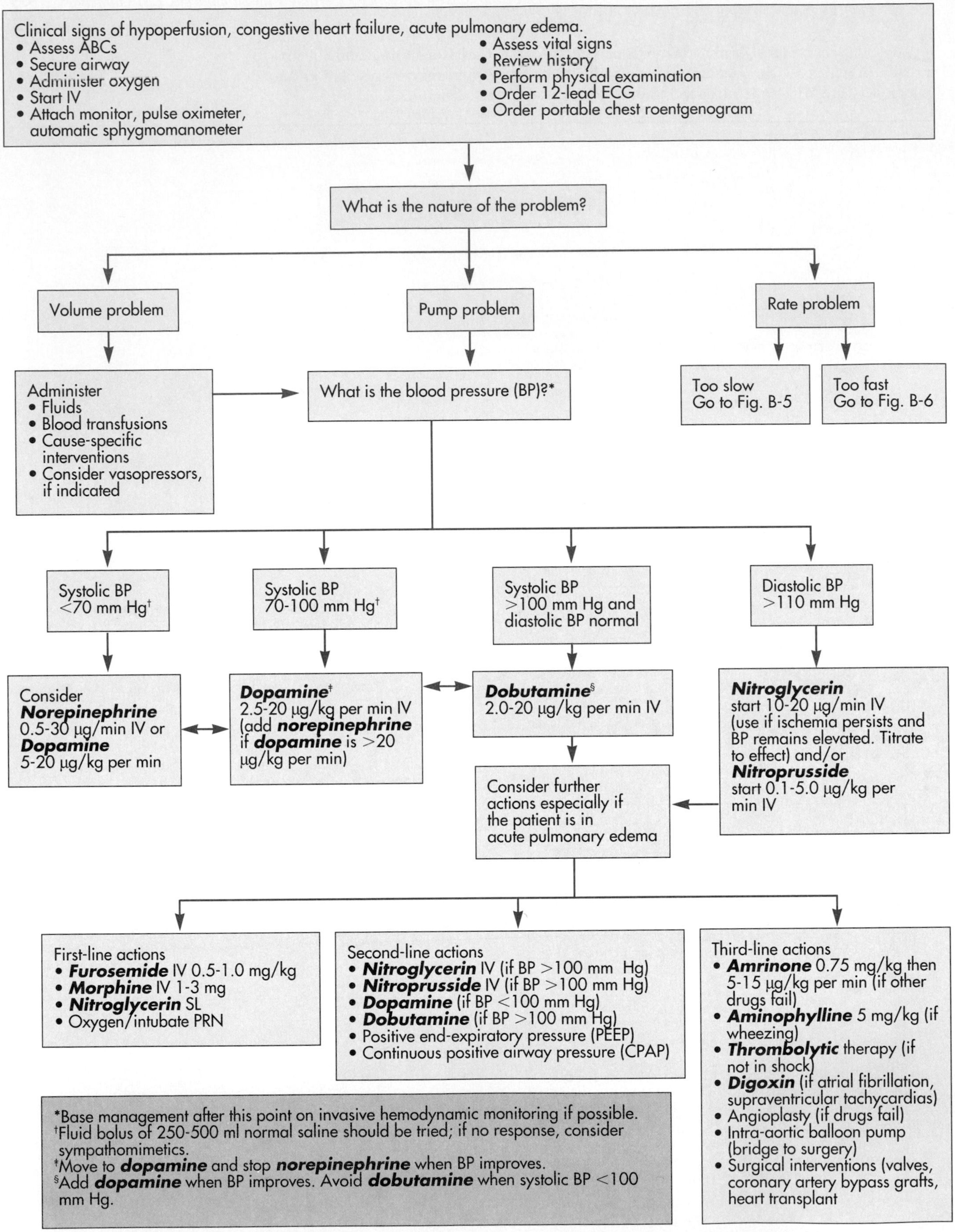

Fig. B-8 Algorithm for hypotension, shock, and acute pulmonary edema. (From Emergency Cardiac Care Committees and Subcommittees, American Heart Association: Guidelines for cardiopulmonary resuscitation and emergency care III: Adult advanced cardiac life support, *JAMA* 268(16):2227, 1992.)

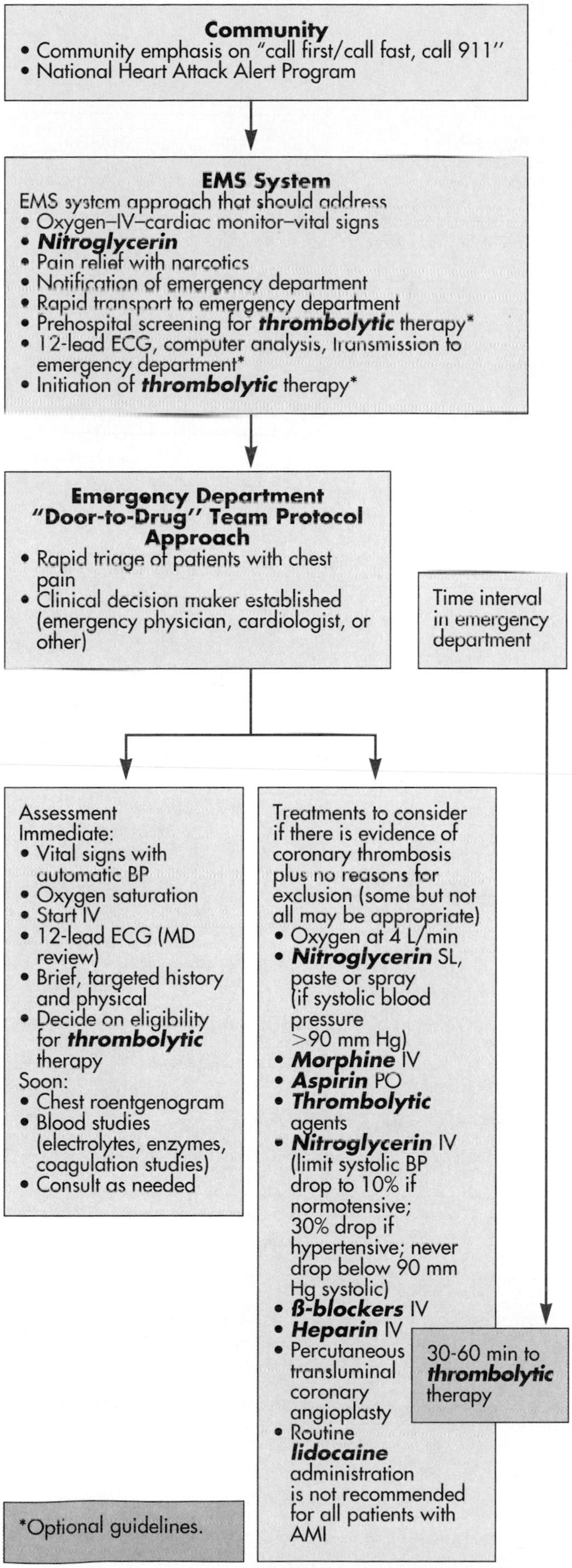
Community
• Community emphasis on "call first/call fast, call 911"
• National Heart Attack Alert Program
EMS System
EMS system approach that should address
• Oxygen–IV–cardiac monitor–vital signs
• Nitroglycerin
• Pain relief with narcotics
• Notification of emergency department
• Rapid transport to emergency department
• Prehospital screening for thrombolytic therapy*
• 12-lead ECG, computer analysis, transmission to emergency department*
• Initiation of thrombolytic therapy*
Emergency Department "Door-to-Drug" Team Protocol Approach
• Rapid triage of patients with chest pain
• Clinical decision maker established (emergency physician, cardiologist, or other)
Time interval in emergency department
Assessment
Immediate:
• Vital signs with automatic BP
• Oxygen saturation
• Start IV
• 12-lead ECG (MD review)
• Brief, targeted history and physical
• Decide on eligibility for thrombolytic therapy
Soon:
• Chest roentgenogram
• Blood studies (electrolytes, enzymes, coagulation studies)
• Consult as needed
Treatments to consider if there is evidence of coronary thrombosis plus no reasons for exclusion (some but not all may be appropriate)
• Oxygen at 4 L/min
• Nitroglycerin SL, paste or spray (if systolic blood pressure >90 mm Hg)
• Morphine IV
• Aspirin PO
• Thrombolytic agents
• Nitroglycerin IV (limit systolic BP drop to 10% if normotensive; 30% drop if hypertensive; never drop below 90 mm Hg systolic)
• ß-blockers IV
• Heparin IV
• Percutaneous transluminal coronary angioplasty
• Routine lidocaine administration is not recommended for all patients with AMI
30-60 min to thrombolytic therapy
*Optional guidelines.

Fig. B-9 Acute myocardial infarction (AMI) algorithm. Recommendations for early treatment of patients with chest pain and possible AMI. (From Emergency Cardiac Care Committees and Subcommittees, American Heart Association: Guidelines for cardiopulmonary resuscitation and emergency care III: Adult advanced cardiac life support, *JAMA* 268(16):2230, 1992.)

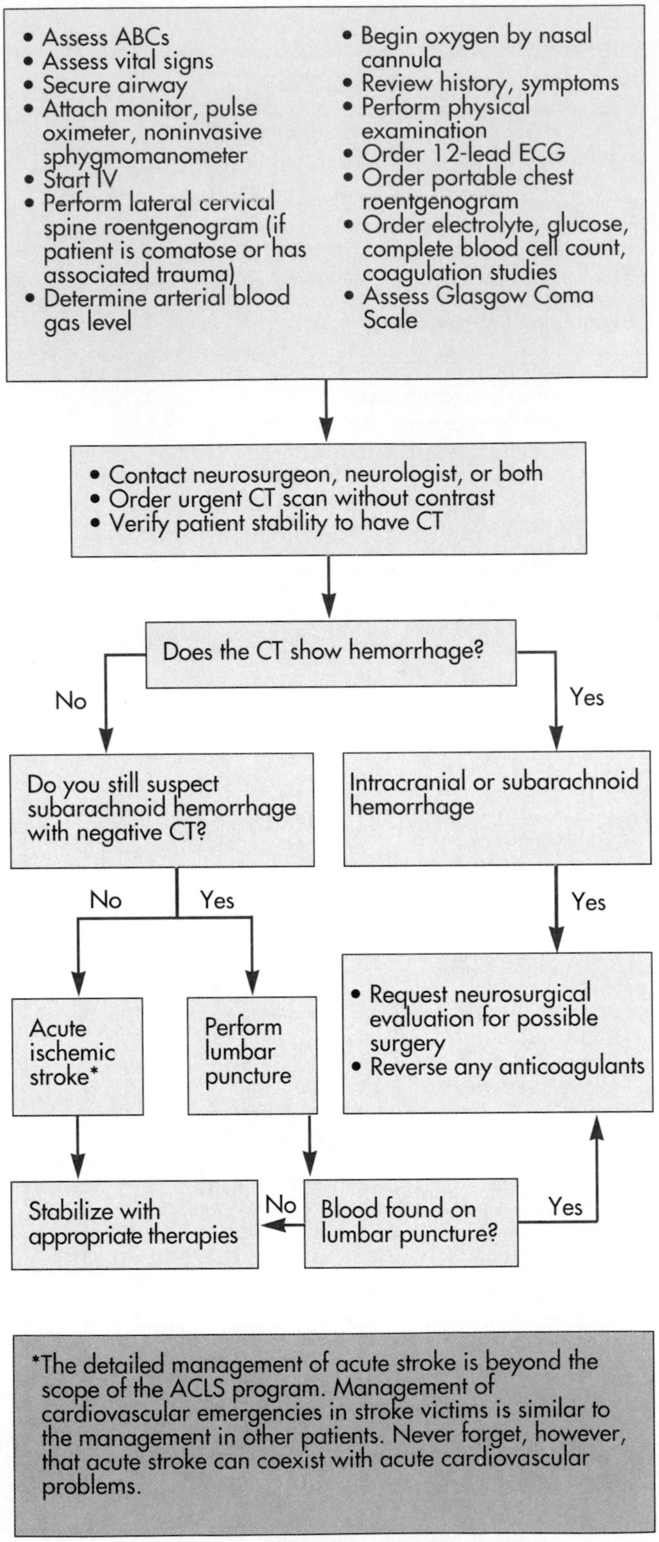

Fig. B-10 Algorithm for initial evaluation of suspected stroke. (From Emergency Cardiac Care Committees and Subcommittees, American Heart Association: Guidelines for cardiopulmonary resuscitation and emergency care IV: Special resuscitation situations, *JAMA* 268(16):2243, 1992.)

helan B-11

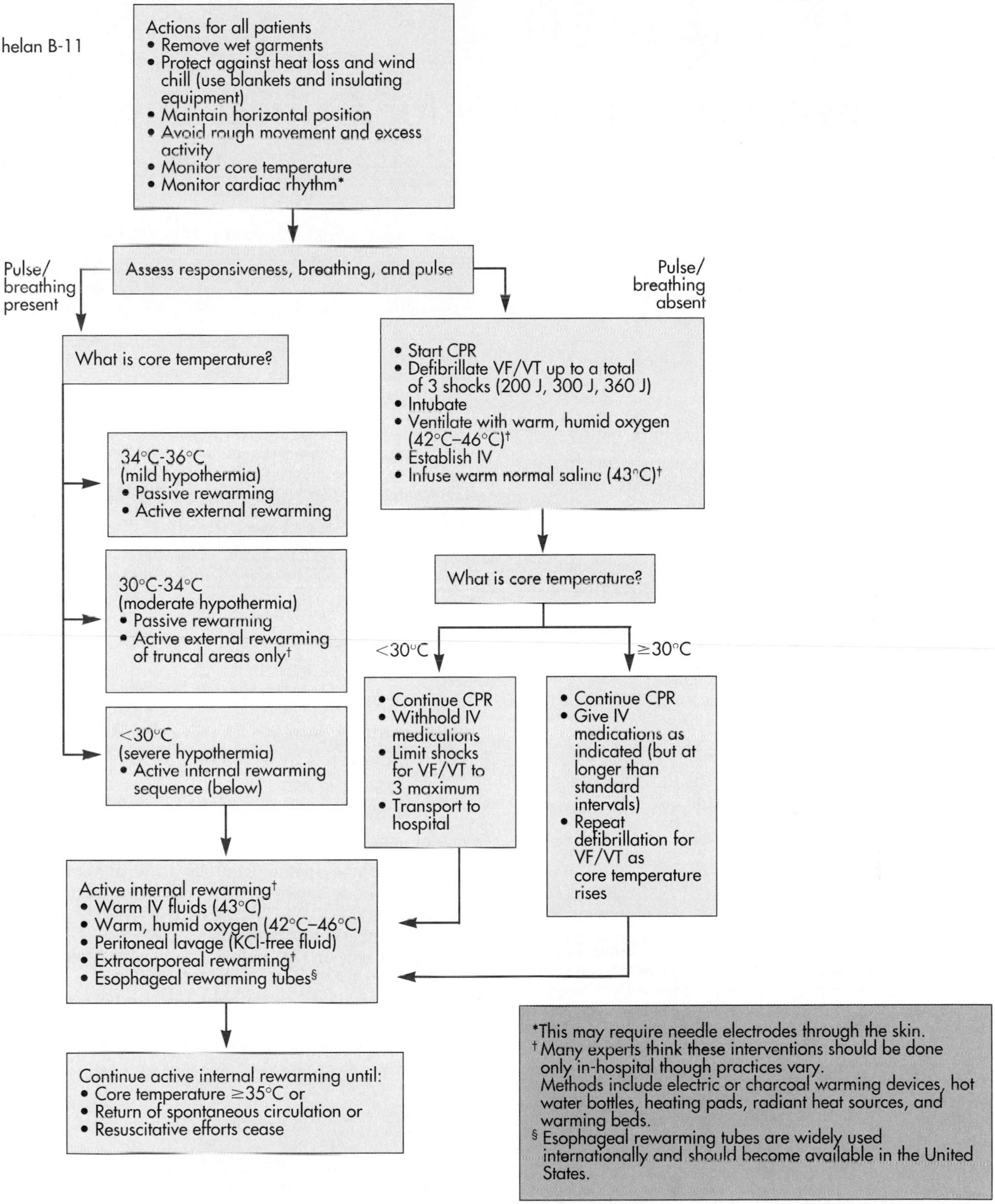

Fig. B-11 Algorithm for treatment of hypothermia. (From Emergency Cardiac Care Committees and Subcommittees, American Heart Association: Guidelines for cardiopulmonary resuscitation and emergency care IV: Special resuscitation situations, *JAMA* 268(16):2245, 1992.)

C

Physiologic Formulas for Critical Care

HEMODYNAMIC FORMULAS

Mean (Systemic) Arterial Pressure (MAP)

$$\frac{(\text{Systemic Diastolic} \times 2) + (\text{Systemic Systolic} \times 1)}{3}$$

Systemic Vascular Resistance (SVR)

$$\frac{\text{MAP} - \text{RAP}}{\text{CO}} = \text{SVR in units (Normal range 10-18 units)}$$

$$\frac{\text{MAP} - \text{RAP}}{\text{CO}} \times 80 = \text{SVR in dynes/sec/cm}^{-5} \text{ (Normal range 800-1400 dynes/sec/cm}^{-5}\text{)}$$

Systemic Vascular Resistance Index (SVRI)

$$\frac{\text{MAP} - \text{RAP}}{\text{CI}} \times 80 = \text{SVRI in dynes/sec/cm}^{-5}\text{/m}^2 \text{ (Normal range 2000-2400 dynes/sec/cm}^{-5}\text{/m}^2\text{)}$$

Pulmonary Vascular Resistance (PVR)

$$\frac{\text{PAP mean} - \text{PAWP}}{\text{CO}} = \text{PVR in units (Normal range 1.2-3.0 units)}$$

$$\frac{\text{PAP mean} - \text{PAWP}}{\text{CO}} \times 80 = \text{PVR in dynes/sec/cm}^{-5} \text{ (Normal range 100-250 dynes/sec/cm}^{-5}\text{)}$$

RAP, Right atrial pressure; *CO*, cardiac output; *CI*, cardiac index; *SV*, stroke volume; *HR*, heart rate; *PAP* mean, pulmonary artery mean pressure; *PAWP*, pulmonary artery wedge pressure; *PB*, barometric pressure; Hgb, hemoglobin; Hbo_2, oxyhemoglobin; *Qs*, shunt flow; *Qt*, total blood flow; MAP, mean arterial pressure; ICP, intracranial pressure.

*pK = 6.1 is the dissociation constant of carbonic acid.

†$Paco_2 \times .03$ converts $Paco_2$ from mm Hg to mEq/L.

‡1.25 is a constant used to take into account the normal respiratory quotient.

§47 is a constant used to correct for the normal water vapor pressure of humidified gas.

‖.003 is a constant used because 0.003 ml of oxygen will dissolve in each 100 ml of blood.

¶1.34 is a constant used because each gram of hemoglobin will carry 1.34 ml oxygen. Actually, if the hemoglobin is chemically pure (rare), each gram is capable of carrying 1.39 ml of oxygen. Because most hemoglobin has impurities, 1.34 is the accepted constant.

Pulmonary Vascular Resistance Index (PVRI)

$$\frac{\text{PAP mean} - \text{PAWP}}{\text{CI}} \times 80 = \text{PVRI in dynes/sec/cm}^{-5}\text{/m}^2 \text{ (Normal range 225-315 dynes/sec/cm}^{-5}\text{/m}^2\text{)}$$

Left Cardiac Work Index (LCWI)

Step 1. $\text{MAP} \times \text{CO} \times 0.0136 = \text{LCW}$

Step 2. $\frac{\text{LCW}}{\text{BSA}} = \text{LCWI (Normal range 3.4-4.2 kg-m/m}^2\text{)}$

Left Ventricular Stroke Work Index (LVSWI)

Step 1. $\text{MAP} \times \text{SV} \times 0.0136 = \text{LVSW}$

Step 2. $\frac{\text{LVSW}}{\text{BSA}} = \text{LVSWI (Normal range 50-62 g-m/m}^2\text{)}$

Right Cardiac Work Index (RCWI)

Step 1. $\text{PAP mean} \times \text{CO} \times 0.0136 = \text{RCW}$

Step 2. $\frac{\text{RCW}}{\text{BSA}} = \text{RCWI (Normal range 0.54-0.66 kg-m/m}^2\text{)}$

Right Ventricular Stroke Work Index (RVSWI)

Step 1. $\text{PAP mean} \times \text{SV} \times 0.0136 = \text{RVSW}$

Step 2. $\frac{\text{RVSW}}{\text{BSA}} = \text{RVSWI (Normal range 7.9-9.7 g-m/m}^2\text{)}$

Body Surface Area

Many hemodynamic formulas can be *indexed* or adjusted to body size by use of a body surface area (BSA) nomogram (Fig. C-1). To calculate BSA:

1. Obtain height and weight.
2. Mark height on the left scale and weight on the right scale.
3. Draw a straight line between the two points marked on the nomogram.

The number where the line crosses the middle scale is the BSA value.

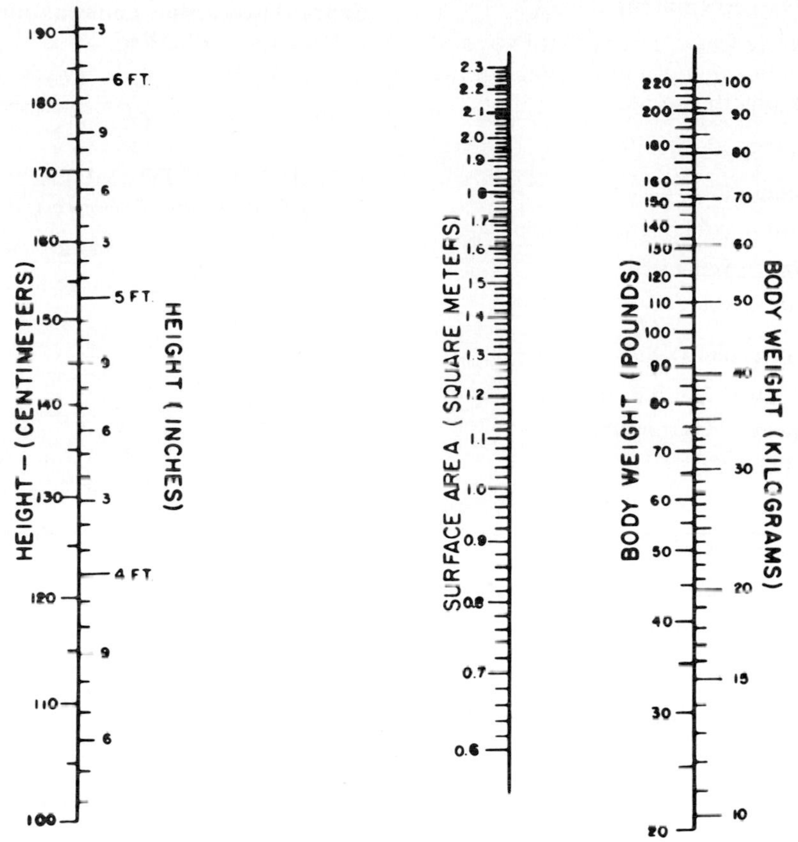

Fig. C-1 Body surface area (BSA) nomogram.

PULMONARY FORMULAS

Henderson-Hasselbach Equation (Blood pH)

$$pH = pK^{*} + \text{Log}\,\frac{HCO_3^- \text{ mEq/L (Base)}}{Paco_2 \text{ mm Hg} \times .03\dagger \text{ (Acid)}}$$

$$pH = 6.1 = \text{Log}\,\frac{HCO_3^- \text{ mEq/L (Base)}}{Paco_2 \text{ mEq/L (Acid)}}$$

Partial Pressure of Oxygen in the Alveolus (P_{AO_2}, expressed in mm Hg)

$$P_{AO_2} - PIo_2 - (Paco_2 \times 1.25)\ddagger$$

Partial Pressure of Inspired Oxygen (PIo_2, expressed in mm Hg)

$$PIo_2 = FIo_2 \times (PB - 47)\S$$

Arterial Oxygen Saturation (Sao_2)

$$\frac{Hgbo_2}{(Hgb + Hgbo_2)} \times 100$$

Normal range >92%

A-a Gradient (also known as A-a Do_2)

A-a gradient = $PAo_2 - Pao_2$ (expressed in mm Hg; normal <10 mm Hg but normal increases with age and FIo_2)

Calculation of the Arterial Oxygen Content (Cao_2)

Oxygen content is a measure of the total amount of oxygen carried in the blood—both the oxygen dissolved in plasma (Pao_2) and the oxygen bound to hemoglobin (Sao_2). Oxygen content is reported in ml/100 ml blood or as volume percent.

There are three steps in the Cao_2 calculation.

Step 1. Calculate the amount of oxygen dissolved in 100 ml of plasma:

$$Pao_2 \times .003\| = \text{ml } O_2\text{/100 ml plasma}$$

Step 2. Calculate the amount of oxygen bound to hemoglobin:

$$Hgb \times 1.34\P \times Sao_2 = \text{ml of } O_2 \text{ bound to Hgb}$$

Step 3. Add the results of Steps 1 and 2 for the Cao_2.

Example: Patient A	
Pao_2	100 mm Hg
Sao_2	.97
Hgb	15 g%

Step 1. 100 × .003 = *.3 ml* O_2 in 100 ml plasma.
Step 2. 15 g% × 1.34 × .97 = *19.5* ml O_2 bound to Hgb.
Step 3. 0.3 + 19.5 = *19.8 vol% Cao_2*.

Calculation of Venous Oxygen Content (Cvo_2)

Same steps as to calculate Cao_2, except that Pvo_2 and Svo_2 are substituted into the equation in the place of the arterial values. Hgb remains the same.

Normal range 12-15 vol%

Tissue Oxygen Consumption (Vo_2)

$(CO \times Cao_2 \times 10) - (CO \times Cvo_2 \times 10)$

Arterial − venous

Normal range 250 ml/min

Mixed Venous Oxygen Saturation (Svo_2)

$(CO \times Cao_2 \times 10) - Vo_2$

O_2 delivery − O_2 consumption

Normal range 60%-80%

Shunt (intracardiac abnormalities or decreased pulmonary ventilation)

$$\frac{Qs}{Qt} = \frac{Cco_2 - CaO_2}{Cco_2 - CvO^2}$$

NEUROLOGIC FORMULA

Cerebral Perfusion Pressure (CPP)

MAP − ICP

Normal range 80-100 mm Hg

FORMULAS

ESTIMATING CALORIC NEEDS

1. Calculate basal energy expenditure (BEE). This is the energy needed for basic life processes such as respiratory function and maintenance of body temperature.
   Women: $BEE = 655 + (9.6 \times W) + (1.7 \times H) - (4.7 \times A)$
   Men: $BEE = 66 + (13.7 \times W) + (5 \times H) - (6.8 \times A)$
   W = Current weight in kg; H = Height in cm; A = Age in yr
2. Multiply BEE by an appropriate activity factor.

Level of activity	Multiply BEE by
Bed rest	1.2
Light (e.g., sedentary office work)	1.3
Moderate (e.g., nursing)	1.4
Strenuous (e.g., manual labor)	1.5 or more

3. Multiply by an appropriate stress factor to meet the needs of the ill or injured patient.

Type of stress	Multiply the value obtained in Step 2 by
Fever	1 + 0.13/° C elevation above normal (or 0.07/° F)
Pneumonia	1.2
Major injury	1.3
Severe sepsis	1.5-1.6
Major burns	1.8-2.0

ESTIMATING PROTEIN NEEDS

Protein needs vary with degree of malnutrition and stress.

Condition	Multiply desirable body weight (kg) by
Healthy individual or well-nourished elective surgery patient	0.8-1 g protein
Malnourished or catabolic state (e.g., sepsis, major injury, burns)	1.2-2+ g protein

Example of calculation of needs

A 38-year-old male patient with pelvic, rib, and long-bone fractures; pneumothorax; and a ruptured spleen after a vehicle accident. Height 180 cm (5′11″), current weight 81.8 kg (180 lb), desirable weight 72.7 kg (160 lb).

Energy needs

1. $BEE = 66 + (13.7 \times 81.8) + (5 \times 180) - (6.8 \times 38) = 1829$ calories/day
2. Energy needs for bed rest = 1829 calories × 1.2 = 2195 calories/day
3. Energy needs for injury = 2195 calories × 1.3 = 2853 calories/day

Protein needs = 72.7 kg × 1.5 g = 109 g/day

Index

D

J

K

N

T

U